Torres and Ehrlich

Modern Dental Assisting

Torres and Ehrlich

Modern Dental Assisting

Eighth Edition

Doni L. Bird, CDA, RDH, MA
Director of Allied Dental Education
Santa Rosa Junior College
Santa Rosa, CA

Debbie S. Robinson, CDA, MS
Dental Assisting Educational Consultant
Hillsborough, NC

MOSBY
ELSEVIER

ELSEVIER
SAUNDERS

11830 Westline Industrial Drive
St. Louis, Missouri 63146

TORRES AND EHRLICH MODERN DENTAL ASSISTING, EIGHTH EDITION

Notice

Neither the Publisher nor the Authors assume any responsibility for any loss or injury and/or damage to persons or property arising out of or related to any use of the material contained in this book. It is the responsibility of the treating practitioner, relying on independent expertise and knowledge of the patient, to determine the best treatment and method of application for the patient.

The Publisher

Previous editions copyrighted 2002, 1999, 1995, 1990, 1985, 1980, 1976

ISBN-13: 978–0–7216–3907–9
ISBN-10: 0–7216–3907–0

Executive Editor: Penny Rudolph
Managing Editor: Jaime Pendill
Publishing Services Manager: Pat Joiner
Project Manager: Gena Magouirk
Designer: Julia Dummitt

Printed in China

Last digit is the print number: 9 8 7 6 5 4 3 2

Reviewers for the Eighth Edition

Roberta Albano, CDA, RDH, MEd
Springfield Technical Community College
Springfield, Massachusetts

Julie Bera, RDA, CDA, COA, MA
Grand Rapids Community College
Grand Rapids, Michigan

Ann Brunick, RDH, MS
University of South Dakota
Vermillion, South Dakota

Amelia Capers, CDA, RDH
Aiken Technical College
North Augusta, South Carolina

Patricia Capps, CDA, RDH, MS
Indiana University School of Dentistry
Indianapolis, Indiana

Jamie Carpenter, CODA
Eastland-Fairfield Career and Technical Schools
Groveport, Ohio

Carol Ann Chapman, RDH
Edison Community College
Fort Myers, Florida

Tammie Chapman, RDA
Career Centers of Texas, Forth Worth
Fort Worth, Texas

Sandra Christiansen, RDA
Dental Assistant Training School
Castro Valley, California

Deborah Clinger, CDA, EFDA
Career School of Dental Assisting
Golden Hill, Oregon

Alison Collins, CDA, MS
Northwestern Michigan College
Traverse City, Michigan

Sallie Donovan, CDA, RDA, MS
Northwestern Michigan College
Traverse City, Michigan

Donna Eastbrooks, CDA, RDH, MEd
Manor College
Jenkintown, Pennsylvania

Tammy Erickson, CDA, RDA
Herzing College–Lakeland Academy
Crystal, Minnesota

Margaret Fehrenbach, RDH, MS
Private Practice, Marquette University
Seattle, Washington

Betty Finkbeiner, CDA, RDA, MS
Washtenaw Community College
Ann Arbor, Michigan

Janet Fisher, CDA, MS
Salina Area Technical School
Salina, Kansas

Carol Giaquinto, CDA, RDH, MEd
Springfield Technical Community College
Springfield, Massachusetts

Heidi Gottfried, BA
Gateway Technical College
Kenosha, Wisconsin

Daniel Hassler, DDS
Concorde Career Institute
Lauderdale Lakes, Florida

Brandy Hoffman, CDA, CDPMA, RDA, EFDA
Career Centers of Texas–Corpus Christi Branch
Corpus Christi, Texas

Darcy Abel Hunter, RDH
Erwin Technical Center
Tampa, Florida

Janet Jaccarino, CDA, RDH
The University of Medicine and Dentistry of New Jersey
School of Health Related Professions
Newark, New Jersey

Kathy Malone, RDH, EFDA, BS
Manor College
Jenkintown, Pennsylvania

Tracy Marsh, CDA, RDA, RDH
The University of Medicine and Dentistry of New Jersey
School of Health Related Professions
Newark, New Jersey

Jill Massey, RDA
Concorde Career College
Valley Village, California

Linda McGillicuddy, CDA, BS
Truckee Meadows Community College
Reno, Nevada

Glenda Miller, CDA, EDA, BS
Florida Community College at Jacksonville
Jacksonville, Florida

Julie Muhle, CDA
Truckee Meadows Community College
Reno, Nevada

Christine Nathe, RDH, MS
University of New Mexico
Albuquerque, New Mexico

Natalie Nazworth, RDA, RDH
Texas Careers–Lubbock Campus
Lubbock, Texas

Beatrice Pena, CDA
San Antonio College of Medical and Dental Assistants
San Antonio, Texas

Sheri Sauer, CODA
Eastland-Fairfield Career and Technical Schools
Groveport, Ohio

Sandra Sims
Southern Medical and Dental Careers Institute
Cartersville, Georgia

Pam Smalley, CDA, MSW
Missouri College
St. Louis, Missouri

Diane Turner, RDA, MS
Waukesha County Technical College
Pewaukee, Wisconsin

L. Joleen Vanbibber, CDPMA
Davis Applied Technology College
Kaysville, Utah

Pamela S. Whitehouse, RDA
Western Career College/US Education Corp
Pleasant Hill, California

About the Authors

Doni L. Bird is the director of the Dental Education Programs at Santa Rosa Junior College. She has taught dental assisting at City College of San Francisco and the University of New Mexico. Before becoming a dental assisting educator, she practiced as a dental assistant in private practice and at Mount Zion Hospital and Medical Center. Doni holds Bachelor of Education and Masters in Education degrees from San Francisco State University and a degree in dental hygiene from the University of New Mexico. She is a member of the Education Committee of the Office Safety and Asepsis Research Foundation (OSAP) and also serves as a member of the Foundation Board of the California Dental Association. As a Certified Dental Assistant, she has been a member of local, state, and national dental assistants associations for the past 25 years. She served as president of the Northern California Dental Assistants Association and Chairman of the Dental Assisting National Board. She is a current member of the California Association of Dental Assisting Teachers (CADAT) and serves as a consultant in dental assisting education to the Commission on Dental Accreditation of the American Dental Association.

Debbie S. Robinson holds an Associate Degree in Dental Assisting from Broward Community College, a Bachelors Degree in Health Administration from Florida Atlantic University, and a Masters Degree in Dental Auxiliary Dental Education from University of North Carolina at Chapel Hill. She has held certifications from DANB in the General Chairside, Orthodontic Assisting, and Infection Control areas. Debbie practiced as a clinical dental assistant in the settings of a pediatric office, dental research center, and special patient care clinic. With more than 20 years of teaching in the community college and university settings. Debbie served as a Clinical Assistant Professor and Coordinator of the Dental Assisting Program and Dental Assisting Specialty Program at the University of North Carolina School of Dentistry. During her career, she has presented over 500 hours of continuing education for practicing dental assistants at local, state, and international meetings. She served as a member of the DANB test construction committee for two terms, authored and co-authored journal articles for *The Dental Assistant*, and has designed online courses for Procter and Gamble. She is currently involved in doing consulting work with community colleges and proprietary schools in the development of new dental assisting programs across the country.

Preface

In recent years, the relationship of oral health and systemic health has been clearly documented. The public is becoming more aware of the relationship between oral health and general health throughout life. The educated and clinically competent dental assistant joins the dentist and dental hygienist to assist patients in achieving maximum oral and general health.

The spectrum of knowledge and skills required of a dental assistant today requires an increasing need for knowledge of current research, of self-evaluation, and of clinical competence. The dental assistant of today must have critical thinking abilities when problem-solving or making legal and ethical decisions.

A career as a dental assistant is challenging and rewarding. To become that well-educated and clinically competent dental assistant, it requires dedication, determination, and desire. This may sound like quite a challenge, but you can do it!

The Learning Package

The eighth edition of *Modern Dental Assisting* is designed as a comprehensive learning package.

The student package includes:

- The textbook
- The Interactive Dental Office CD-ROM
- Dental Assisting Video Procedures CD-ROM
- Student Workbook
- Evolve website

The faculty package includes:

- The textbook
- The Interactive Dental Office CD-ROM
- Dental Assisting Video Procedures CD-ROM
- Instructor's Electronic Resource CD-ROM
- Transparency acetates
- Student Workbook
- Evolve website
- Instructor's Resource Manual
- Curriculum Guide

The entire package has been designed with the student and educator in mind. The ease of reading each comprehensive chapter and the additional materials provides students with the maximum opportunity to learn. The driving force in the development of this package was to create a competent dental assistant. With that goal in mind, this package meets and exceeds accreditation standards and certification requirements.

Textbook Design

Specific updated guidelines and recommendations that have been integrated in this edition are;

- CDC standards, which include the most recent scientific and clinical evidence to support these recommendations. The new recommendations are included in this textbook in a clear and easy-to-read format. Students will better understand "why" and "what" they must do to promote the highest infection-control standards for patients and dental professionals.
- Digital radiography is changing the way that dental radiography is practiced. In this edition, students will learn about the various types of digital imaging, including the advantages, disadvantages and various types of digital radiography equipment. The video CD included in this text includes footage of the way to set up a digital system and the technique used to take digital exposures.
- Stress-related ailments are common in the workplace. In dentistry, neck and shoulder pain, headaches, and hand and wrist pain can be caused by poor work habits. The student will learn how to prevent these potentially career-ending injuries by incorporating ergonomic principles into daily activities.
- Patient confidentiality is of the utmost importance and legally mandated in realms of the healthcare systems. HIPAA standards are integrated throughout the textbook to inform the student of their importance and of ways to include them into practice.
- New Current Dental Terminology (CDT) codes have been updated and published to include the most up-to-date procedures and categories of service offered in the dental practice setting.

The design for this edition also includes:

- The book is divided into 11 **parts** from historical and scientific information to the general and specialization of dentistry. Each part opener provides an introduction and lists the related chapters that are found within that section.

  Part 1: The Dental Assisting Profession
  Part 2: Sciences in Dentistry
  Part 3: Oral Health and Prevention of Dental Disease
  Part 4: Infection Control in Dentistry
  Part 5: Occupational Health and Safety
  Part 6: Patient Information and Assessment
  Part 7: Foundation of Clinical Dentistry
  Part 8: Dental Radiography
  Part 9: Dental Materials

Part 10: Comprehensive Dental Care
Part 11: Dental Administration and Communication Skills

- **Chapter Outlines** at the beginning of each chapter introduce you to the material and the order of its presentation.
- **Key Terms** are introduced throughout the chapter in bold lettering. All Key Terms are also included in a comprehensive Glossary in the back of the book. The pronunciation and definition reinforce these new terms.
- **Learning and Performance Outcomes** are introduced at the beginning of the chapter so that the learners know what is expected of them at the theoretical and performance level.
- **Procedures** present a step-by-step sequence using the correct equipment and supplies required to perform the basic to the most detailed procedure. Procedural icons are included to remind you of the preparation and precautions needed.
- **Recall Questions** are scattered throughout each chapter for students to test their immediate knowledge. Answers are available to instructors in the Instructor's Resource Manual, on the Instructor's Electronic Resource CD-ROM, and on the Evolve website for instructors.
- **Patient Education** sections offer tips and strategies to help you interact and share information with patients.
- **Legal and Ethical Implications** sections help you focus on the ethical and legal behaviors you need to know to protect yourself, your patients, and the practice for which you work.
- **Eye to the Future** sections introduce you to the cutting-edge research, future trends, and topics relating to the subject matter of the chapter.
- **Critical Thinking** questions and scenarios at the end of each chapter reinforce your ability to solve problems and make appropriate decisions.

The Interactive Dental Office CD-ROM

The interactive portion of this learning package offers exercises for the immediate application of knowledge to help the student develop and retain critical thinking and problem-solving skills. Exercises have been developed to help in the reinforcement of content within the chapters. This CD-ROM offers the student a variety of exercises and resources such as patient case studies, charting exercises, radiographic mounting exercises, numbering systems, a dental dictionary, and a quiz show game to help in the preparation of tests and national exams

Dental Assisting Video Procedures CD-ROM

Visual presentation is vital when learning clinical skills. The video CD-ROM now provides 60 short video clips of specific skills the dental assistant performs in the clinical setting. Emphasis of these videos is on the expanded functions delegated to the credentialed dental assistant. It should be noted that there may be more than one way to perform any technique correctly. Some dental assistants may perform a procedure one way while others choose to perform the same procedure using a slightly different technique. We have chosen to feature the techniques that are used by the majority of dental assisting programs.

Student Workbook

The student workbook is a supplement to the learning process. The content of the workbook matches the book chapter by chapter to help you master and apply key concepts and procedures to a clinical situation. Clinical competency forms are located within appropriate chapters of the Workbook. They allow you to evaluate your strengths and weaknesses in performing procedures. As a bonus, flash cards are located in the back of the workbook as a study tool to help in the studying process of terms, instruments, and procedures.

Instructor's Electronic Resource CD-ROM

This CD-ROM set aids the instructor by providing PowerPoint presentations for each chapter, an ExamView test bank for each chapter, the Workbook exercise answers and Recall questions and answers, transparency acetates, and the complete Instructor's Resource Manual. A second CD-ROM includes the procedural videos that are also enclosed with the textbook.

Instructor's Resource Manual

Available in print format and electronically on Evolve, the Instructor's Resource Manual is designed to save the instructor time and take the guesswork out of classroom planning and preparation. It includes the Chapter Focus, Teaching Tips, answers to the Workbook exercises, and Recall questions and answers. Also included is a Reference Guide for patient case studies from the Interactive Dental Office CD-ROM showing how the case studies on the CD-ROM correspond with the content in the textbook.

Evolve Website

Elsevier has created a website dedicated solely to support this learning package. The web site includes a *Student site* and *Instructor site.*

Student site resources include:

- Practice quizzes for every chapter
- Key Term exercises for every chapter
- Labeling exercises

- Two chapters from *Spanish Terminology for the Dental Team*
  - General Emergency Protocol
  - Taking a Patient History
- Content updates
- WebLinks

Faculty site resources include:

- Access to all the student resources
- ExamView test bank
- Downloadable versions of the Curriculum Guide and Instructor's Resource Manual
- PowerPoint lecture slides
- Dental assisting video procedures
- A complete image collection
- Answers to Workbook exercises and Recall questions and answers
- Competency skill sheets for all procedures in the book
- Internet-based course management tools hosted through Evolve

Our hope is that you are excited about the profession that you are entering. And our desire is that the learning package that we have put together fully prepares you for the challenges that your education and profession will offer.

Doni L. Bird
Debbie S. Robinson

Acknowledgments

We sincerely appreciate and thank the many reviewers who have carefully read and provided suggestions and recommendations for every facet of this learning package. Each suggestion was carefully considered and included whenever possible. We will always continue to welcome comments and requests from dental assisting educators.

We wish to thank the Health Sciences Department at Santa Rosa Junior College for allowing us the use their beautiful facility and a special thanks to the dental assisting and dental hygiene students who participated in the video and photo sessions. We extend our appreciation to the following SRJC Dental Program faculty for their participation with the videos: Kay Murphy, Marlene Wilgis, Kelly O'Shea, and Pam Rosell.

Thank you to Dr. John Featherstone at the University of California School of Dentistry for the use of his slides and research on dental caries. Many of the photographs in this edition have been the work of the talented Dr. Mark Dellinges at the University of California School of Dentistry. Many thanks also to Pamela Landry, RDA, and Dr. William Bird for their expertise and continual support.

We believe that the eighth edition of *Modern Dental Assisting* is the best and most comprehensive learning package on the market today. This is due largely to the fantastic team of professionals at Elsevier. Their total commitment and dedication to this project has been unparallel. Our sincere appreciation to Penny Rudolph, Executive Editor; Jaime Pendill, Managing Editor; Lynn Hoops, Senior Marketing Manager; Pat Joiner, Publishing Services Manager; Gena Magouirk, Project Manager; Julia Dummitt, Designer; Bruce Robison, Multimedia Producer; and Cindy Ahlheim, Multimedia Producer. The resources available for *MDA* truly make it a stand above the rest.

We especially thank our husbands, families, and dear friends who have understood the work schedule and demands for our time that this project required. Without your love and support, it would not have been possible.

DLB and *DSR*

Dedication

We dedicate this eighth edition of *Modern Dental Assisting*
to the dental assisting educators throughout the country and across the world
who have adopted *MDA* over the last 30-plus years.

In developing this edition, we have worked diligently
to present you with an educational package that you can rely on
to provide you and your students the most recent information
and the best teaching support system available today.

We admire and applaud the dedicated dental assisting
educator who strives to improve the quality of dental assisting education
and who encourages and challenges students to be the best that they can be.

Doni L. Bird
Debbie S. Robinson

Detailed Contents

PART 2: SCIENCES IN DENTISTRY

PART 4: INFECTION CONTROL IN DENTISTRY

PART 10: ASSISTING IN COMPREHENSIVE DENTAL CARE

Procedures

How to Use This Learning Package

Modern Dental Assisting is the ultimate learning package for preparing students to become dental assistants in the dental office. It provides a solid foundation for the basic and advanced clinical skills students must master in order to achieve competence, and its student-friendly style clarifies even the most complex concepts and procedures to help prepare for DANB certification.

Textbook Features

A detailed chapter Outline introduces you to the chapter material as a whole, allowing you to see at a glance how the subject material is organized. It also helps you focus on one topic at a time by showing you the relationship to other chapters in the section.

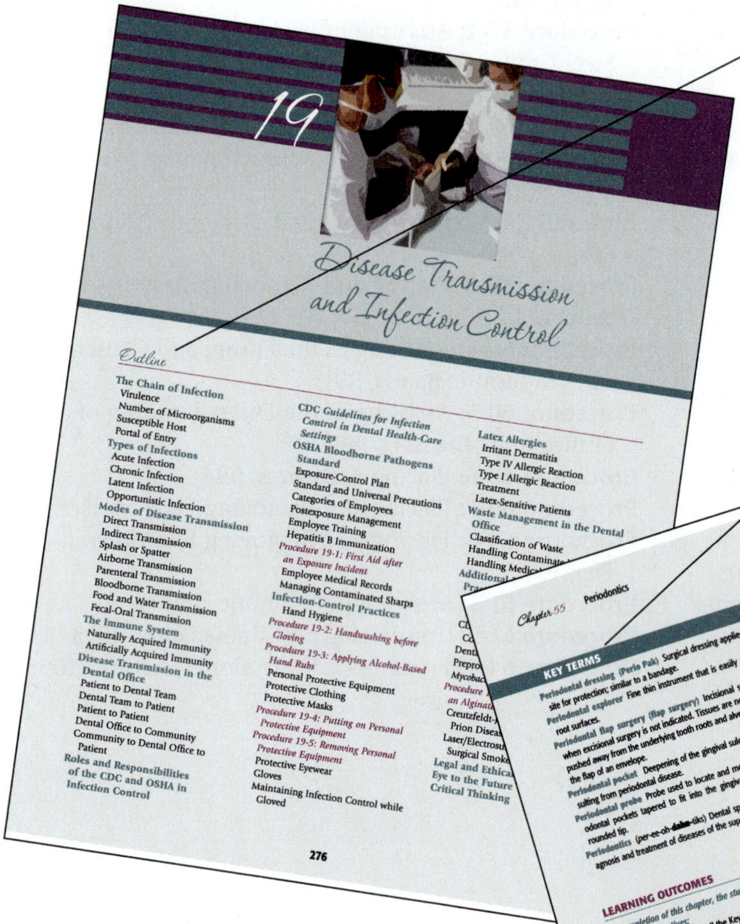

Key Terms and a complete Glossary with definitions and pronunciations reinforce new terminology. In the pronunciations, the main accented syllable is bolded. If there is a secondary accented syllable, it is italicized.

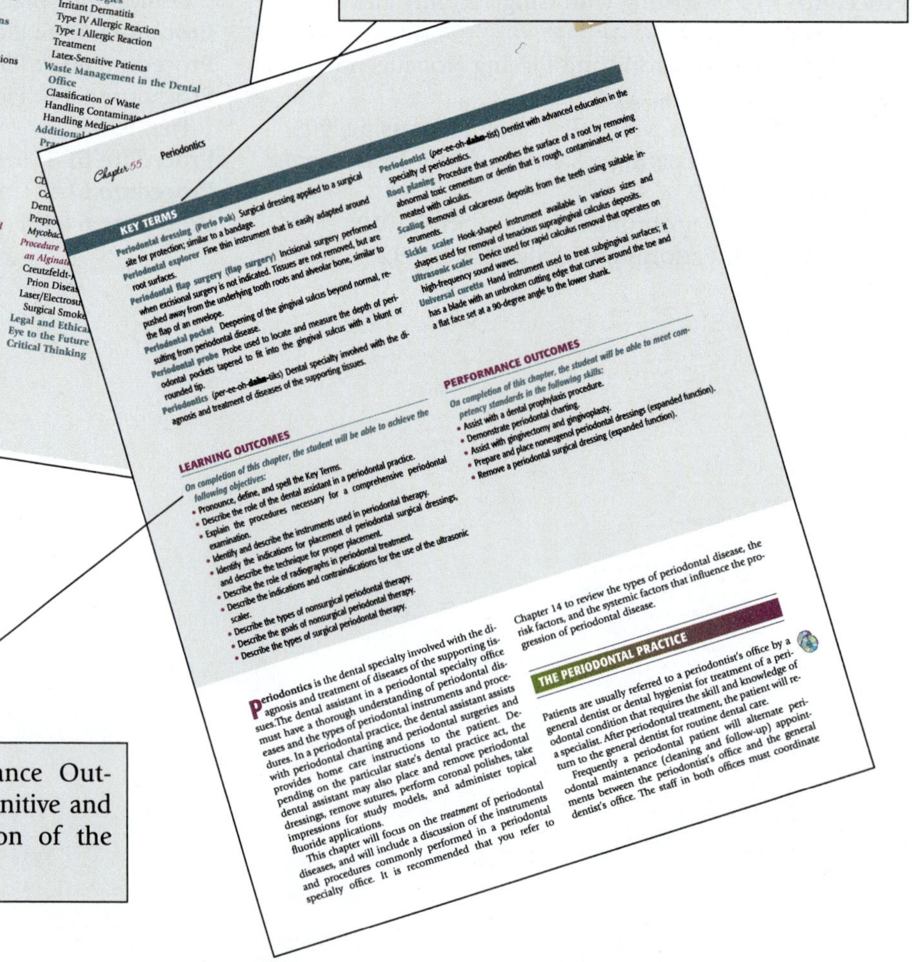

Learning Outcomes and Performance Outcomes assist you in meeting the cognitive and procedural objectives on completion of the chapter.

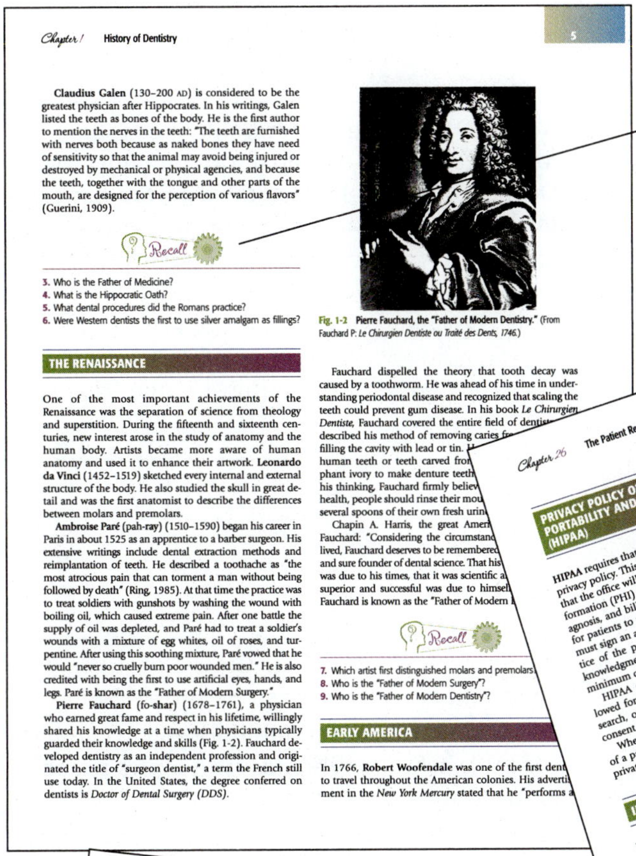

Recall Questions are interspersed throughout each chapter to help you retain the previous information before going on to the next topic. The answers to the Recall questions are available to instructors on the Evolve website and in the Instructor's Resource Manual.

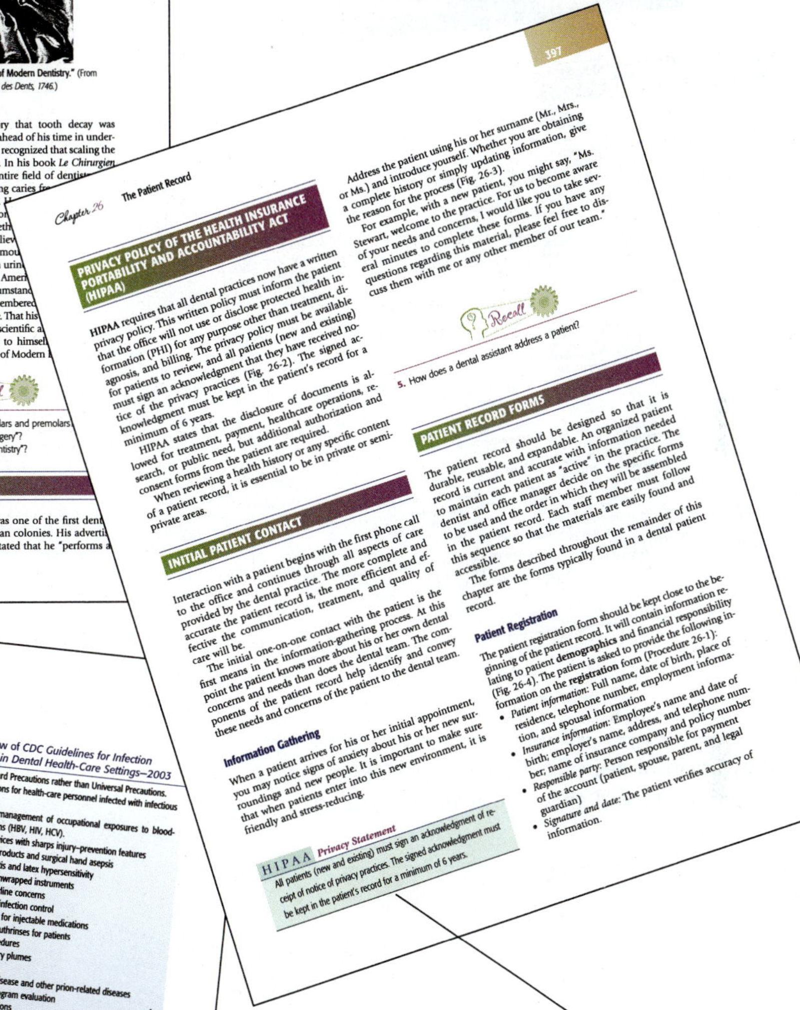

HIPAA boxes feature important information on HIPAA regulations and how they affect dental practice.

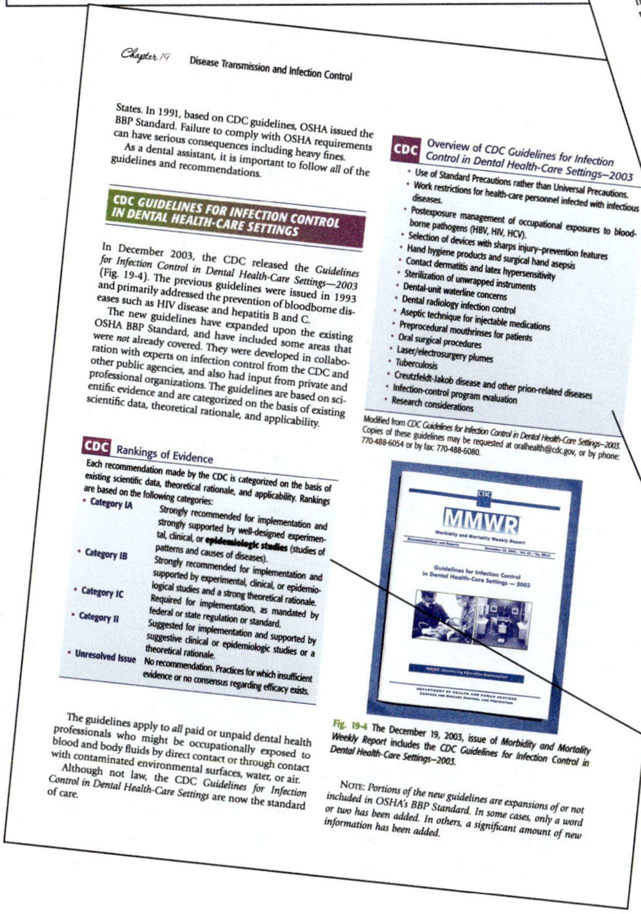

CDC boxes highlight the latest guidelines for safe dental practice.

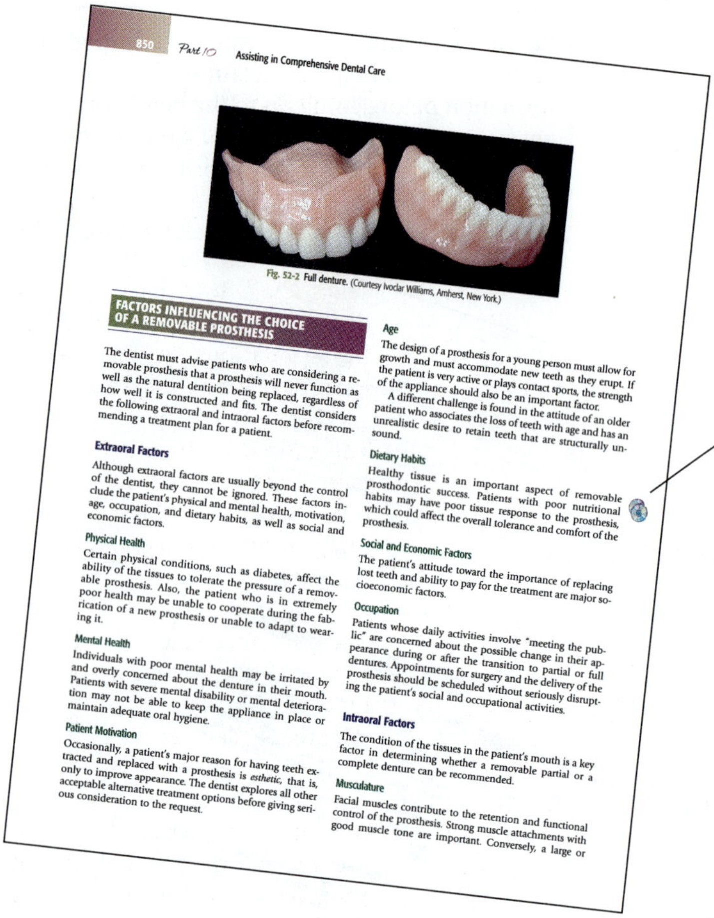

850 Part 10 Assisting in Comprehensive Dental Care

Fig. 52-2 Full denture. (Courtesy Ivoclar Williams, Amherst, New York.)

FACTORS INFLUENCING THE CHOICE OF A REMOVABLE PROSTHESIS

The dentist must advise patients who are considering a removable prosthesis that a prosthesis will never function as well as the natural dentition being replaced, regardless of how well it is constructed and fits. The dentist considers the following extraoral and intraoral factors before recommending a treatment plan for a patient.

Extraoral Factors

Although extraoral factors are usually beyond the control of the dentist, they cannot be ignored. These factors include the patient's physical and mental health, motivation, age, occupation, and dietary habits, as well as social and economic factors.

Physical Health

Certain physical conditions, such as diabetes, affect the ability of the tissues to tolerate the pressure of a removable prosthesis. Also, the patient who is in extremely poor health may be unable to cooperate during the fabrication of a new prosthesis or unable to adapt to wearing it.

Mental Health

Individuals with poor mental health may be irritated by and overly concerned about the denture in their mouth. Patients with severe mental disability or mental deterioration may not be able to keep the appliance in place or maintain adequate oral hygiene.

Patient Motivation

Occasionally, a patient's major reason for having teeth extracted and replaced with a prosthesis is *esthetic*, that is, only to improve appearance. The dentist explores all other acceptable alternative treatment options before giving serious consideration to the request.

Age

The design of a prosthesis for a young person must allow for growth and must accommodate new teeth as they erupt. If the patient is very active or plays contact sports, the strength of the appliance should also be an important factor.

A different challenge is found in the attitude of an older patient who associates the loss of teeth with age and has an unrealistic desire to retain teeth that are structurally unsound.

Dietary Habits

Healthy tissue is an important aspect of removable prosthodontic success. Patients with poor nutritional habits may have poor tissue response to the prosthesis, which could affect the overall tolerance and comfort of the prosthesis.

Social and Economic Factors

The patient's attitude toward the importance of replacing lost teeth and ability to pay for the treatment are major socioeconomic factors.

Occupation

Patients whose daily activities involve "meeting the public" are concerned about the possible change in their appearance during or after the transition to partial or full dentures. Appointments for surgery and the delivery of the prosthesis should be scheduled without seriously disrupting the patient's social and occupational activities.

Intraoral Factors

The condition of the tissues in the patient's mouth is a key factor in determining whether a removable partial or a complete denture can be recommended.

Musculature

Facial muscles contribute to the retention and functional control of the prosthesis. Strong muscle attachments with good muscle tone are important. Conversely, a large or

A CD-ROM icon in the textbook directs students to corresponding material on the Interactive Dental Office CD-ROM located in the back of the book.

Eye to the Future boxes introduce you to cutting-edge research, future trends, and topics relating to the chapter content.

Patient Education boxes offer tips and strategies to help you interact and share information with patients.

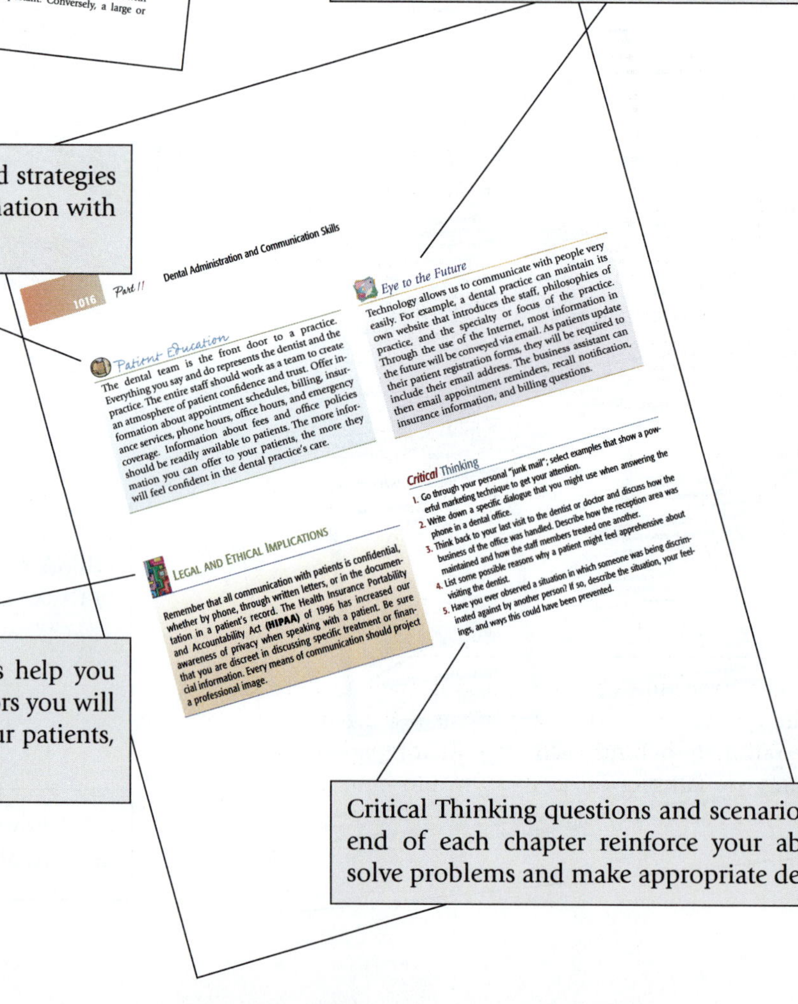

1016 Part 11 Dental Administration and Communication Skills

Patient Education

The dental team is the front door to a practice. Everything you say and do represents the dentist and the practice. The entire staff should work as a team to create an atmosphere of patient confidence and trust. Offer information about appointment schedules, billing, insurance services, phone hours, office hours, and emergency coverage. Information about fees and office policies should be readily available to patients. The more information you can offer to your patients, the more they will feel confident in the dental practice's care.

Eye to the Future

Technology allows us to communicate with people very easily. For example, a dental practice can maintain its own website that introduces the staff, philosophies of practice, and the specialty or focus of the practice. Through the use of the Internet, most information in the future will be conveyed via email. As patients update their patient registration forms, they will be required to include their email address. The business assistant can then email appointment reminders, recall notification, insurance information, and billing questions.

Legal and Ethical Implications

Remember that all communication with patients is confidential, whether by phone, through written letters, or in the documentation in a patient's record. The Health Insurance Portability and Accountability Act **(HIPAA)** of 1996 has increased our awareness of privacy when speaking with a patient. Be sure that you are discreet in discussing specific treatment or financial information. Every means of communication should project a professional image.

Critical Thinking

1. Go through your personal "junk mail"; select examples that show a powerful marketing technique to get your attention.
2. Write down a specific dialogue that you might use when answering the phone in a dental office.
3. Think back to your last visit to the dentist or doctor and discuss how the business of the office was handled. Describe how the reception area was maintained and how the staff members treated one another.
4. List some possible reasons why a patient might feel apprehensive about visiting the dentist.
5. Have you ever observed a situation in which someone was being discriminated against by another person? If so, describe the situation, your feelings, and ways this could have been prevented.

Legal and Ethical Implications boxes help you focus on the legal and ethical behaviors you will need to know to protect yourself, your patients, and the practice for which you work.

Critical Thinking questions and scenarios at the end of each chapter reinforce your ability to solve problems and make appropriate decisions.

Dental Assisting Procedures

It should be noted that there may be more than one way to perform any technique correctly. Some dental assistants may perform a procedure one way while others choose to perform the same procedure using a slightly different technique. We have chosen to feature the techniques that are used by the majority of dental assisting programs.

Procedural icons are located with each procedure to remind you at a glance of those important precautions that are required when performing the procedure.

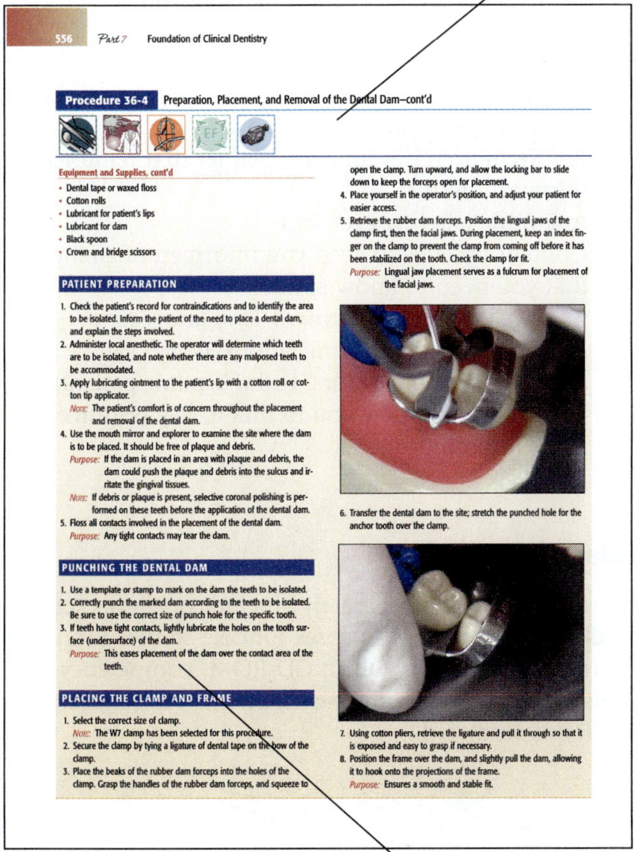

556 *Part 7* Foundation of Clinical Dentistry

Procedure 36-4 Preparation, Placement, and Removal of the Dental Dam—cont'd

Equipment and Supplies, cont'd

- Dental tape or waxed floss
- Cotton rolls
- Lubricant for patient's lips
- Lubricant for dam
- Black spoon
- Crown and bridge scissors

PATIENT PREPARATION

1. Check the patient's record for contraindications and to identify the area to be isolated. Inform the patient of the need to place a dental dam, and explain the steps involved.
2. Administer local anesthetic. The operator will determine which teeth are to be isolated, and note whether there are any malposed teeth to be accommodated.
3. Apply lubricating ointment to the patient's lip with a cotton roll or cotton tip applicator.
   Note: The patient's comfort is of concern throughout the placement and removal of the dental dam.
4. Use the mouth mirror and explorer to examine the site where the dam is to be placed. It should be free of plaque and debris.
   Purpose: If the dam is placed in an area with plaque and debris, the dam could push the plaque and debris into the sulcus and irritate the gingival tissues.
   Note: If debris or plaque is present, selective coronal polishing is performed on these teeth before the application of the dental dam.
5. Floss all contacts involved in the placement of the dental dam.
   Purpose: Any tight contacts may tear the dam.

PUNCHING THE DENTAL DAM

1. Use a template or stamp to mark on the dam the teeth to be isolated.
2. Correctly punch the marked dam according to the teeth to be isolated. Be sure to use the correct size of punch hole for the specific tooth.
3. If teeth have tight contacts, lightly lubricate the holes on the tooth surface (undersurface) of the dam.
   Purpose: This eases placement of the dam over the contact area of the teeth.

PLACING THE CLAMP AND FRAME

1. Select the correct size of clamp.
   Note: The W7 clamp has been selected for this procedure.
2. Secure the clamp by tying a ligature of dental tape on the bow of the clamp.
3. Place the beaks of the rubber dam forceps into the holes of the clamp. Grasp the handles of the rubber dam forceps, and squeeze to open the clamp. Turn upward, and allow the locking bar to slide down to keep the forceps open for placement.
4. Place yourself in the operator's position, and adjust your patient for easier access.
5. Retrieve the rubber dam forceps. Position the lingual jaws of the clamp first, then the facial jaws. During placement, keep an index finger on the clamp to prevent the clamp from coming off before it has been stabilized on the tooth. Check the clamp for fit.
   Purpose: Lingual jaw placement serves as a fulcrum for placement of the facial jaws.
6. Transfer the dental dam to the site; stretch the punched hole for the anchor tooth over the clamp.
7. Using cotton pliers, retrieve the ligature and pull it through so that it is exposed and easy to grasp if necessary.
8. Position the frame over the dam, and slightly pull the dam, allowing it to hook onto the projections of the frame.
   Purpose: Ensures a smooth and stable fit.

Step-by-step procedures in the textbook include illustrations, the equipment and supplies you will need, icons, and the rationale behind each step. At the end of many procedures are samples of how you would enter the procedure in the patient's chart.

Icon Key

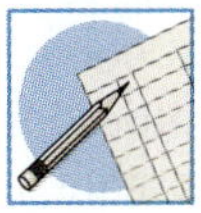

The procedure should be documented in the patient record.

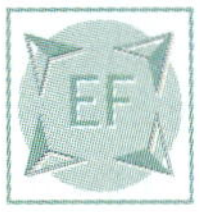

The procedure is considered an expanded function, and in some states it will be delegated to the dental assistant. Always check the regulations in the Dental Practice Acts of your state.

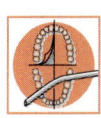

The procedure involves contact with materials that are considered hazardous. Special handling or disposal techniques are required.

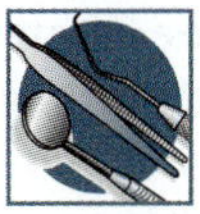

The student should be able to identify the instruments required for the procedure and document their use.

The procedure is sensitive to moisture contamination. Special precautions such as cotton roll placement, oral evacuation, and use of a dental dam must be included to avoid moisture in the oral cavity.

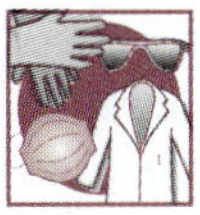

The procedure involves exposure to potentially infectious materials and requires the use of appropriate personal protective equipment, such as a mask, eyewear, and gloves.

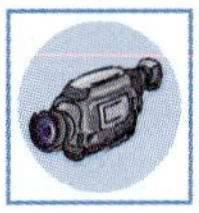

The procedure is supplemented on the Dental Assisting Video Procedures CD-ROM.

Dental Assisting Procedures CD-ROM

Sixty video clips that supplement key procedures in the text are available on the Dental Assisting Video Procedures CD-ROM located in the back of the book. Competency skill sheets that correspond to every procedure in the textbook are located in the student workbook and on the Evolve website. A video reference guide and CD tutorial can be found on the pages that follow. It should be noted that there may be more than one way to perform any technique correctly. Some dental assistants may perform a procedure one way while others choose to perform the same procedure using a slightly different technique. We have chosen to feature the techniques that are used by the majority of dental assisting programs.

Interactive Dental Office CD-ROM

The Interactive Dental Office is an exciting teaching tool for classroom and individual student use. The program features 25 patients ranging in age from 2½ to 86 years. Each patient has an examination to be charted as the doctor dictates it, plus radiographs to be mounted and evaluated. The patient cases represent a wide variety of dental conditions and procedures typically found in a general dentistry practice. Students will also be challenged with medical and dental emergencies that simulate true life emergencies. Twenty questions for each case are included, and students are given immediate and meaningful feedback with every answer. After the second incorrect answer, the student is given the correct answer and moves on to the next question. A patient case reference guide and CD tutorial can be found on the pages that follow.

This CD-ROM also includes an electronic dictionary, and review questions in a game show format that cover the topics of anatomy and physiology, business office activities, instrumentation, pathology, radiation health and safety, and workplace safety. Questions used in the games are not the same as those used in the patient cases.

Evolve Website

The Evolve website includes free learning resources available to instructors and students using *Torres and Ehrlich Modern Dental Assisting*. At the front of this textbook is a page introducing the Evolve site. All you need to get started is a computer with an Internet connection. To register as a Student or Instructor, enter the following URL: http://evolve.elsevier.com/Bird/modern. Follow the directions for either "Instructors" or "Students" to create an Evolve account. You will have to do this only one time.

Instructor Resources include:

- An all-new test bank in ExamView that allows you to randomize exams
- Power Point lecture slides that make class presentations easier
- An all inclusive image collection that allows you to create your own presentations
- Competency Sheets that correspond to every procedure in the textbook
- Answers to Recall questions in the textbook
- Answers to student Workbook questions

Student Resources include:

- Practice quizzes for each chapter that prepare you for classroom exams
- Key Term exercises for each chapter that reinforce important terms
- Anatomic labeling exercises
- Content updates to keep you informed of changes that you need to know about
- Bonus chapters from *Spanish Terminology for the Dental Team* with pronunciations, which can be used as a reference for working with Hispanic patients
- WebLinks that allow you to link to key resources for more information

Student Workbook

The workbook (sold separately) includes review exercises for all chapters, review exercises for case studies found on The Interactive Dental Office CD-ROM, competency skill sheets for all procedures in the textbook, plus 42 flashcards as a bonus study aid.

How to Use the Interactive Dental Office CD-ROM

Hello and welcome to the Interactive Dental Office brought to you by Elsevier. In the simulated dental practice of Drs. Bowman and Roberts, you can go right to work as you meet the patients, mount radiographs, chart examinations, schedule appointments, and help with patient care. But, be alert! For when you least expect it, you'll encounter real-life medical and dental emergencies. It isn't all work. You also have the opportunity to be a winner with games that test your knowledge in pathology, radiation safety, business office activities, workplace safety, oral anatomy, and dental instruments. Our goal is to provide you with the opportunities to improve the skills you'll need in your role as a member of a real dental health practice. For assistance with this program, see the Help section on the left side of the Main Menu near the Exit.

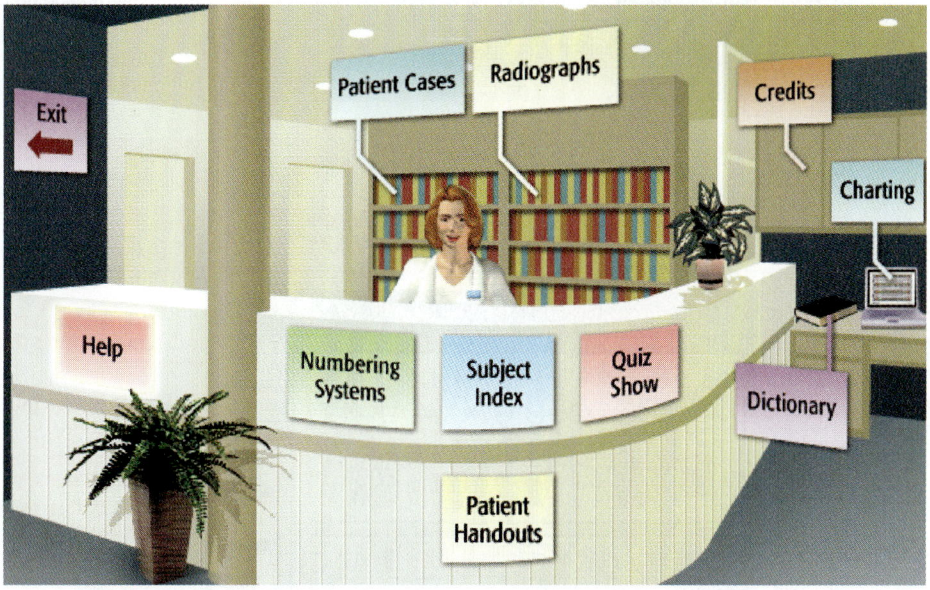

Help Section

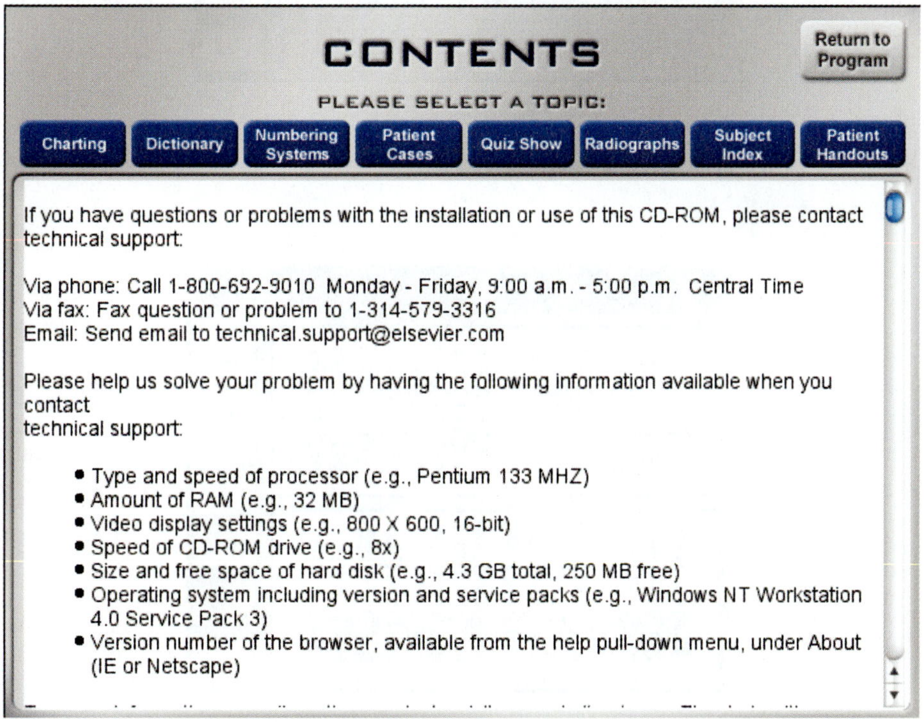

Charting

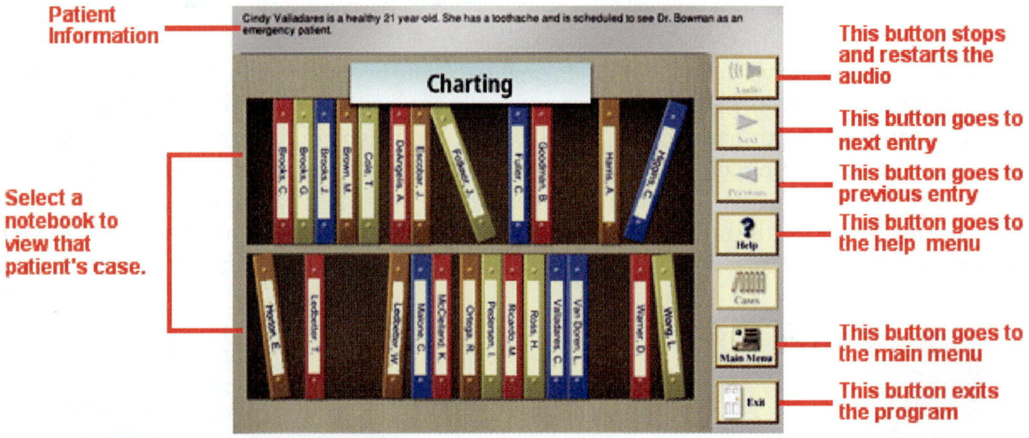
Patient Information
Cindy Valladares is a healthy 21 year-old. She has a toothache and is scheduled to see Dr. Bowman as an emergency patient.
Charting
Select a notebook to view that patient's case.
This button stops and restarts the audio
This button goes to next entry
This button goes to previous entry
This button goes to the help menu
This button goes to the main menu
This button exits the program

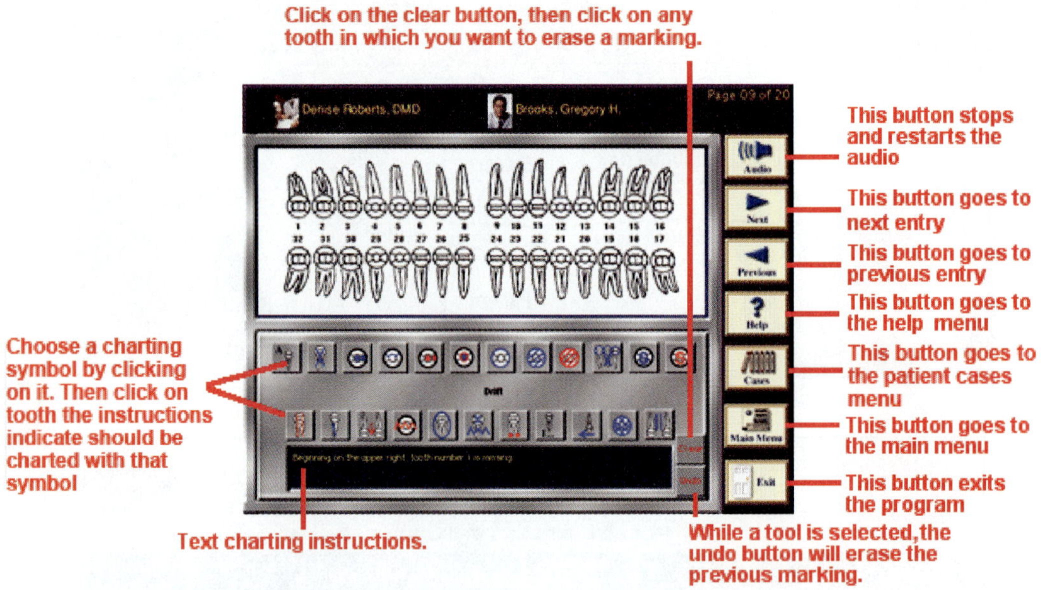
Click on the clear button, then click on any tooth in which you want to erase a marking.
Choose a charting symbol by clicking on it. Then click on tooth the instructions indicate should be charted with that symbol
Text charting instructions.
While a tool is selected, the undo button will erase the previous marking.
This button stops and restarts the audio
This button goes to next entry
This button goes to previous entry
This button goes to the help menu
This button goes to the patient cases menu
This button goes to the main menu
This button exits the program

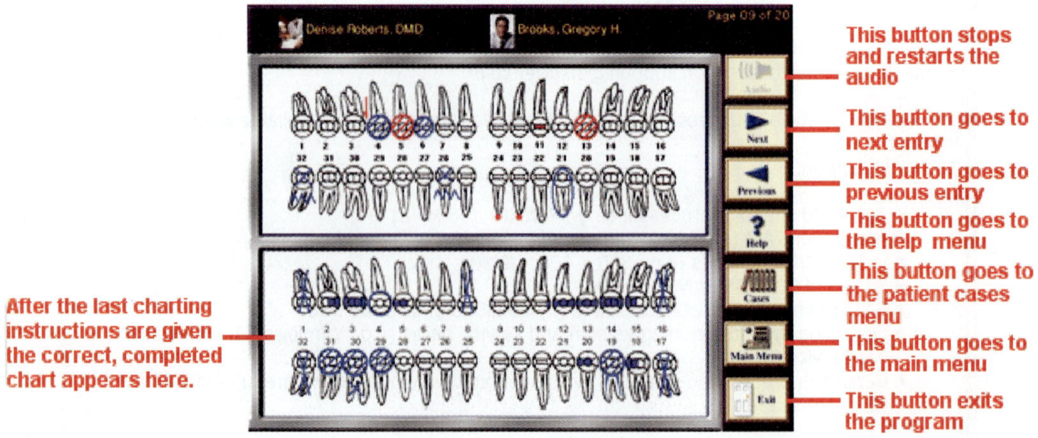
After the last charting instructions are given the correct, completed chart appears here.
This button stops and restarts the audio
This button goes to next entry
This button goes to previous entry
This button goes to the help menu
This button goes to the patient cases menu
This button goes to the main menu
This button exits the program

Dictionary

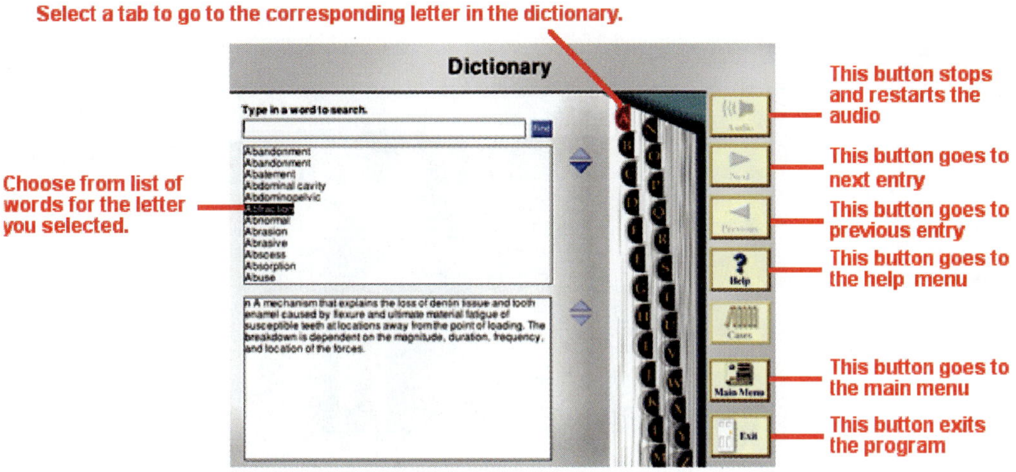
Select a tab to go to the corresponding letter in the dictionary.
Dictionary
Type in a word to search.
Choose from list of words for the letter you selected.
This button stops and restarts the audio
This button goes to next entry
This button goes to previous entry
This button goes to the help menu
This button goes to the main menu
This button exits the program

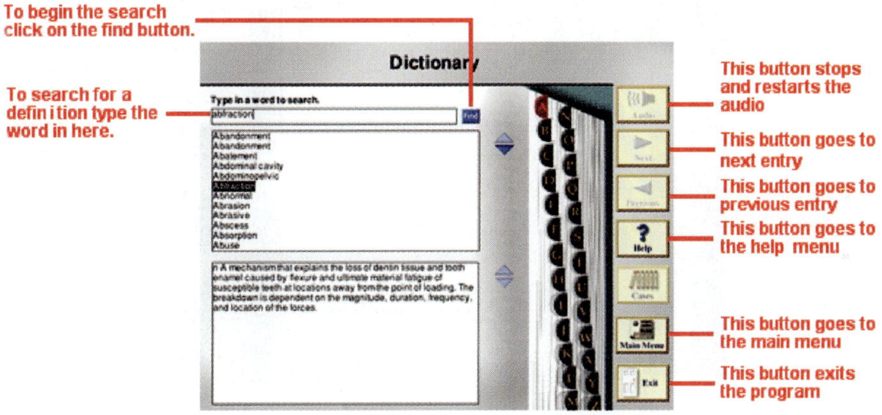
To begin the search click on the find button.
Dictionary
To search for a definition type the word in here.
This button stops and restarts the audio
This button goes to next entry
This button goes to previous entry
This button goes to the help menu
This button goes to the main menu
This button exits the program

Numbering Systems

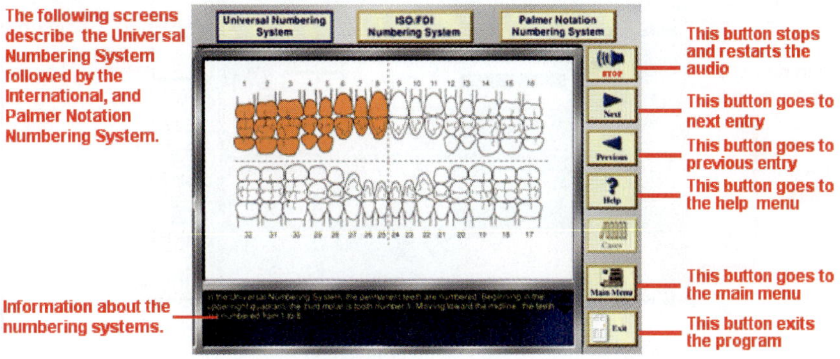
The following screens describe the Universal Numbering System followed by the International, and Palmer Notation Numbering System.
Universal Numbering System
ISO/FDI Numbering System
Palmer Notation Numbering System
Information about the numbering systems.
This button stops and restarts the audio
This button goes to next entry
This button goes to previous entry
This button goes to the help menu
This button goes to the main menu
This button exits the program

Patient Cases

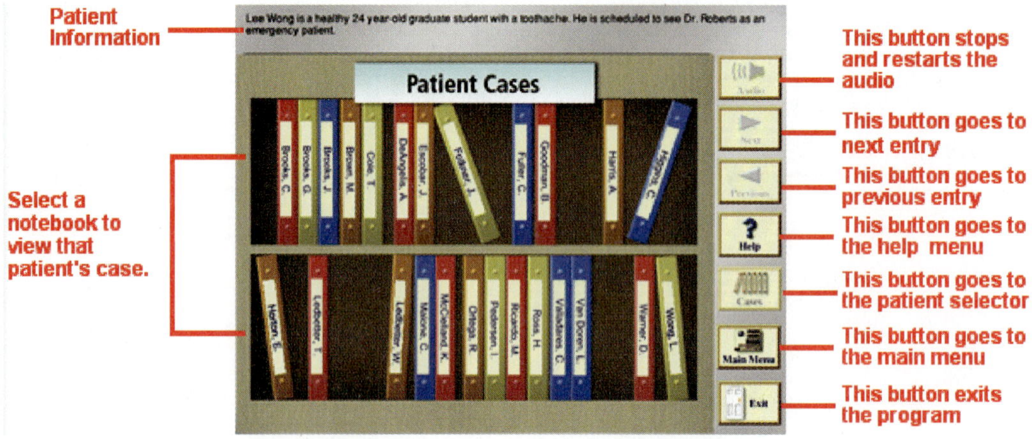
Patient Information
Select a notebook to view that patient's case.
Patient Cases
This button stops and restarts the audio
This button goes to next entry
This button goes to previous entry
This button goes to the help menu
This button goes to the patient selector
This button goes to the main menu
This button exits the program

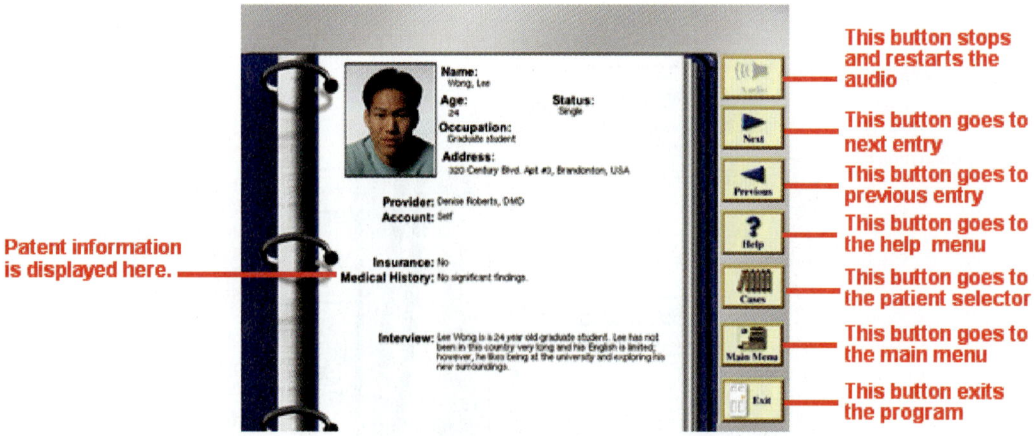
Patent information is displayed here.
Name:
Age:
Status:
Occupation:
Address:
Provider:
Account:
Insurance:
Medical History:
Interview:
This button stops and restarts the audio
This button goes to next entry
This button goes to previous entry
This button goes to the help menu
This button goes to the patient selector
This button goes to the main menu
This button exits the program

Quiz Show

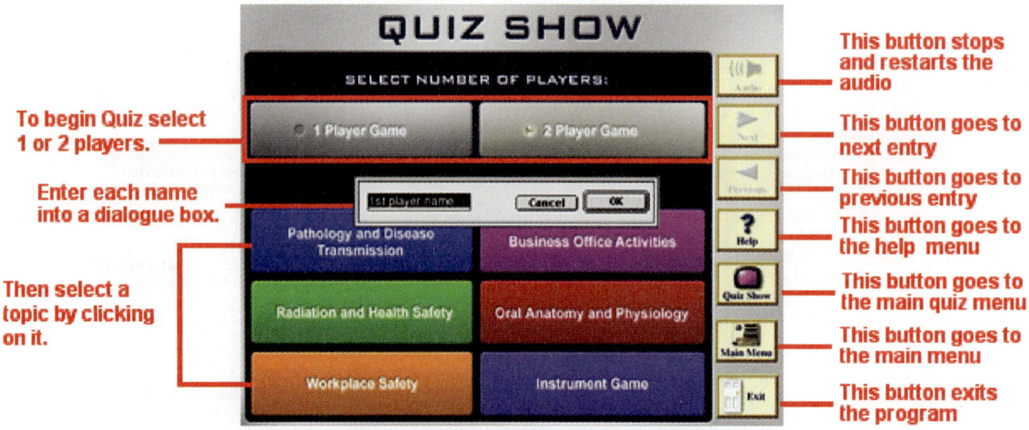
QUIZ SHOW
SELECT NUMBER OF PLAYERS:
1 Player Game
2 Player Game
Cancel
OK
Pathology and Disease Transmission
Business Office Activities
Radiation and Health Safety
Oral Anatomy and Physiology
Workplace Safety
Instrument Game
To begin Quiz select 1 or 2 players.
Enter each name into a dialogue box.
Then select a topic by clicking on it.
This button stops and restarts the audio
This button goes to next entry
This button goes to previous entry
This button goes to the help menu
This button goes to the main quiz menu
This button goes to the main menu
This button exits the program

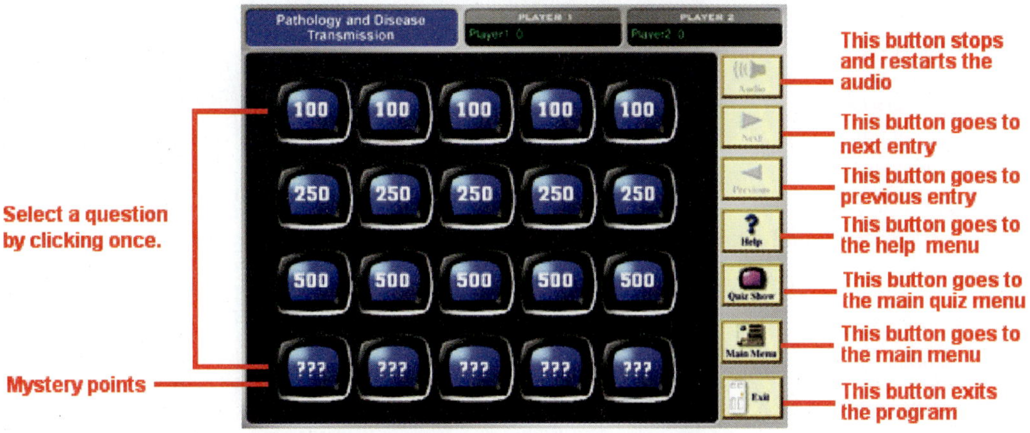
Pathology and Disease Transmission
PLAYER 1
PLAYER 2
Select a question by clicking once.
Mystery points
This button stops and restarts the audio
This button goes to next entry
This button goes to previous entry
This button goes to the help menu
This button goes to the main quiz menu
This button goes to the main menu
This button exits the program

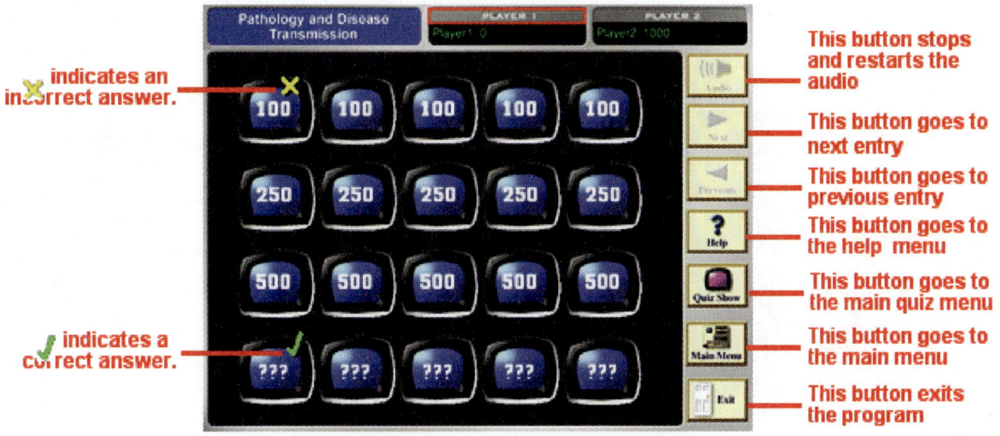
Pathology and Disease Transmission
PLAYER 1
PLAYER 2
indicates an incorrect answer.
indicates a correct answer.
This button stops and restarts the audio
This button goes to next entry
This button goes to previous entry
This button goes to the help menu
This button goes to the main quiz menu
This button goes to the main menu
This button exits the program

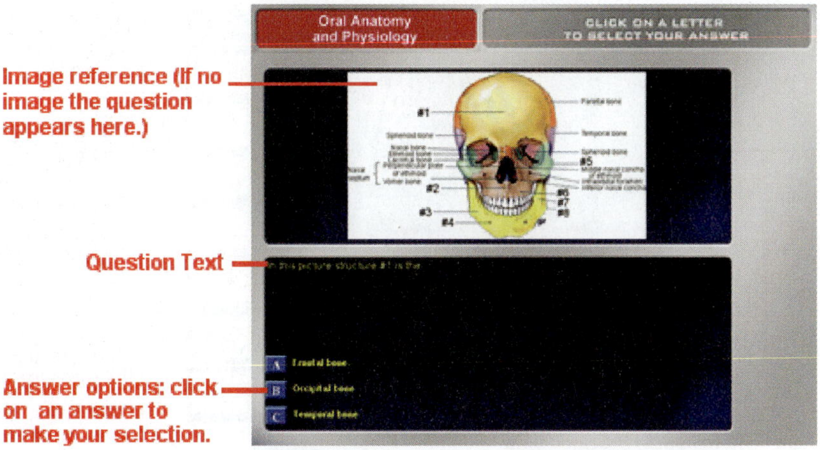
Oral Anatomy and Physiology
CLICK ON A LETTER TO SELECT YOUR ANSWER
Image reference (If no image the question appears here.)
Question Text
Answer options: click on an answer to make your selection.
Frontal bone
Occipital bone
Temporal bone

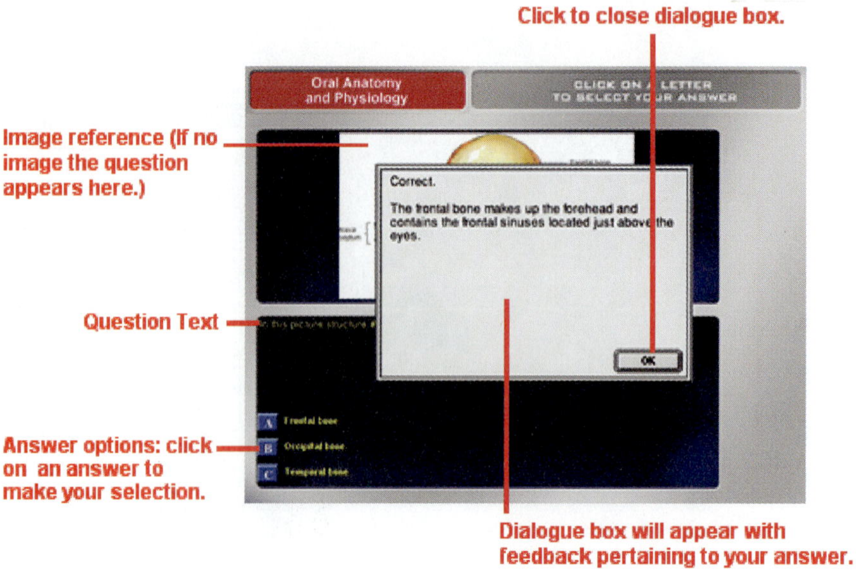
Click to close dialogue box.
Oral Anatomy and Physiology
Image reference (If no image the question appears here.)
Correct.
The frontal bone makes up the forehead and contains the frontal sinuses located just above the eyes.
OK
Question Text
Answer options: click on an answer to make your selection.
Dialogue box will appear with feedback pertaining to your answer.

Radiographs

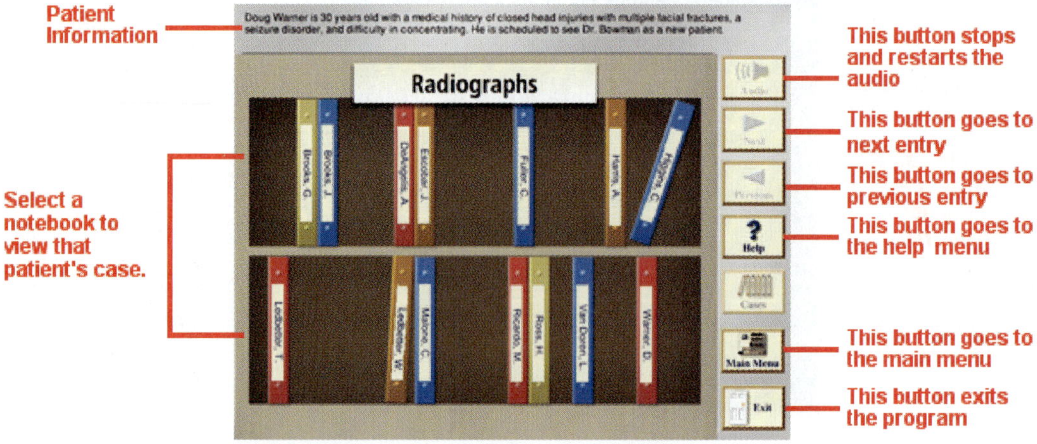
Patient Information
Doug Warner is 30 years old with a medical history of closed head injuries with multiple facial fractures, a seizure disorder, and difficulty in concentrating. He is scheduled to see Dr. Bowman as a new patient.
Radiographs
Select a notebook to view that patient's case.
This button stops and restarts the audio
This button goes to next entry
This button goes to previous entry
This button goes to the help menu
This button goes to the main menu
This button exits the program

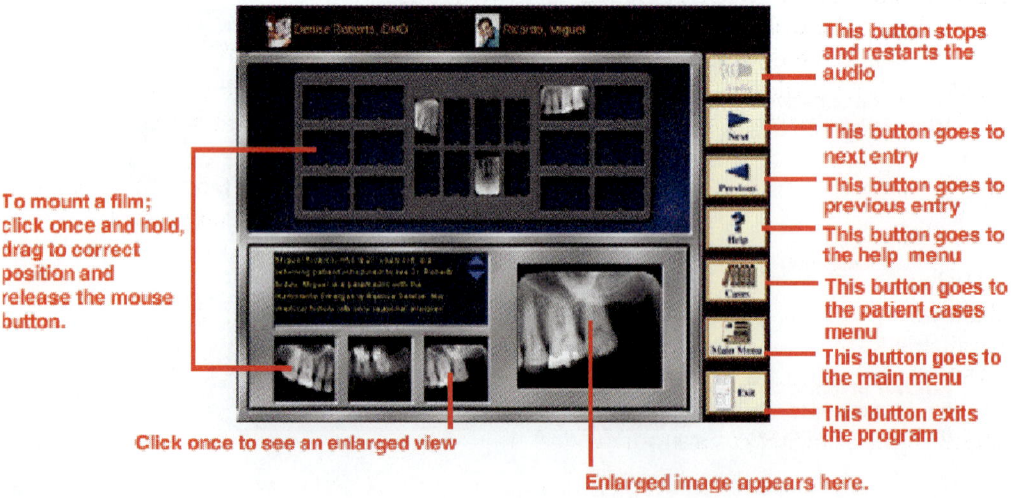
To mount a film; click once and hold, drag to correct position and release the mouse button.
This button stops and restarts the audio
This button goes to next entry
This button goes to previous entry
This button goes to the help menu
This button goes to the patient cases menu
This button goes to the main menu
This button exits the program
Click once to see an enlarged view
Enlarged image appears here.

Subject Index

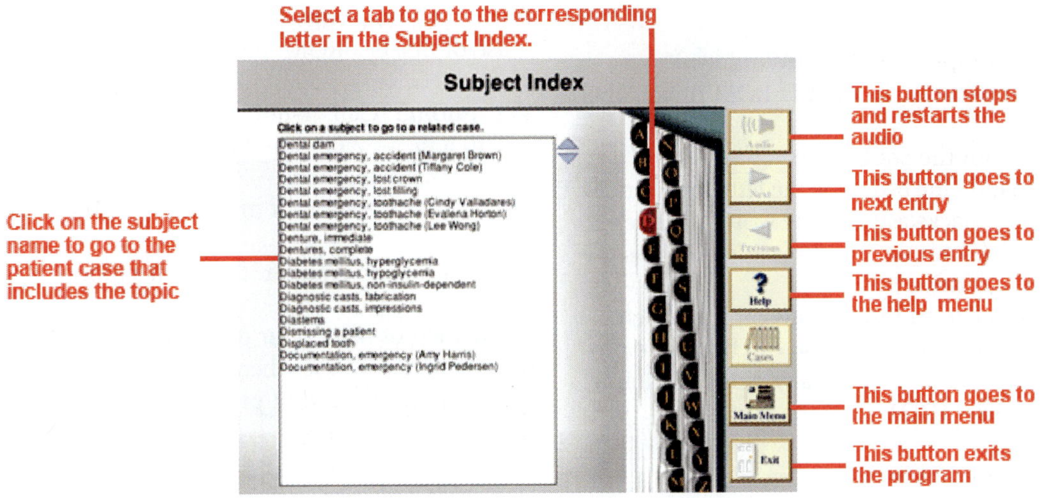

Patient Handouts

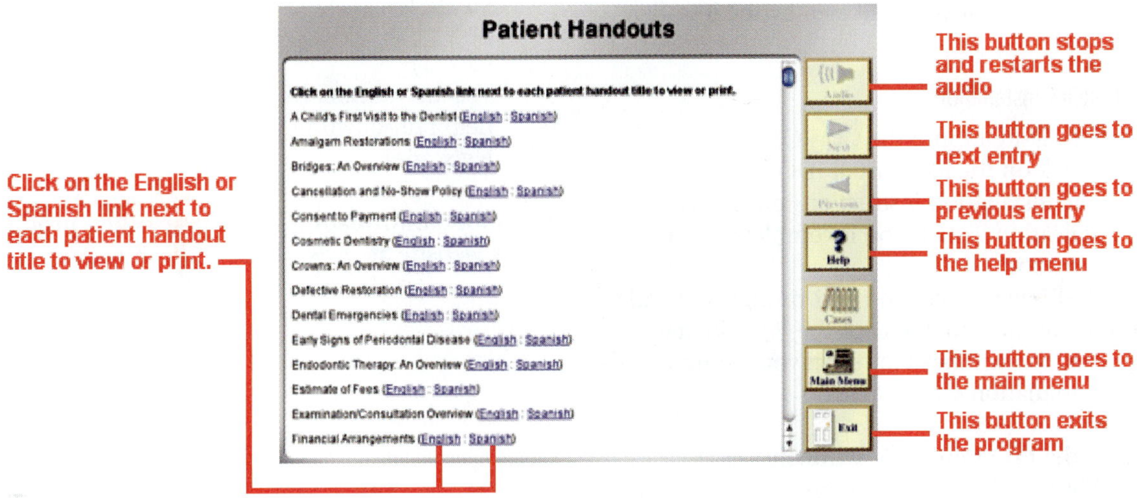

NOTE: Customizable versions of the Patient Handouts in Microsoft Word are available on this disk in both English and Spanish. To access the customizable documents, go to the Patient Handouts folder by double-clicking **My Computer,** right-clicking the **CD Drive,** and selecting **Explore.**

Minimum System Requirements

Macintosh:

G3 PowerPC or Higher
OSX 10.1.2 and above
64MB or more available RAM
Hard disk with 150 MB free space
CD-ROM drive
800 × 600 or larger 16-bit or higher color monitor
Optional: Printer

Windows:

Pentium III or higher
Windows 98, 2000, XP
64 MB or more available RAM
Hard disk with 150 MB free space
CD-ROM drive
800 × 600 or larger 16-bit or higher color monitor
Windows-compatible sound card
Optional: Printer

Installation Instructions

PC CD-ROM Installation

1. Turn on your computer and start Windows.™
2. Insert the compact disc in the CD-ROM drive, label side up.
3. Choose Run from the Start menu.
4. In the Command Line box, type the letter of your CD drive, a colon, a backslash and the word "setup.exe"; then click O.K. (Example:d:\setup.exe, where d is the letter of your CD drive.)
5. Follow the installation instructions on the screen.
6. Once installation is complete you can begin the program from the Start menu at any time. (Example: Start – Programs – IDO)

UN-installing the Program for PC

1. Select the uninstall program from the Start menu. (Example: Start – Programs – IDO)
2. For Windows 95-98 users, double-click on the "Uninstall Interactive Dental Office" icon located in the IDO folder, which was created by the installer.

Macintosh CD-ROM Installation

1. Insert the CD-ROM into the CD-ROM drive.
2. Double click on the file "Install IDO _ƒ"
3. Follow the installation instructions on the screen
4. After application installation is complete quit the install application.
5. If DO NOT have QuickTime 4.02 or higher installed in your computer, double-click the "QuickTime 4.02 Mac" icon. You will need to restart your computer after this installation.

UN-installing the Program for Macintosh

1. Drag " IDO _ƒ" folder to trash can
2. Empty Trash.

Getting Help

If you have questions or problems with the installation or use of this CD-ROM, please contact technical support:

Via phone: Call 1-800-692-9010 Monday — Friday, 5:30 a.m. — 7:00 p.m. Central Time

Via fax: Fax question or problem to 1-314-579-3316

Via email: Send email to technical.support@elsevier.com

Please help us solve your problem by having the following information available when you contact technical support:

- Type and speed of processor (e.g., Pentium 133 MHz)
- Amount of RAM (e.g., 64 MB)
- Video display settings (e.g., 800 × 600, 16-bit)
- Speed of CD-ROM drive (e.g., 8×)
- Size and free space of hard disk (e.g., 4.3 GB total, 250 MB free)
- Operating system including version and service packs (e.g., Windows NT Workstation 4.0 Service Pack 3)
- Version number of the browser, available from the help pull-down menu, under About (IE or Netscape)

For more information regarding other products, visit our website at www.us.elsevierhealth.com.

The Interactive Dental Office CD-ROM

Patient Case Study Reference Guide

The Interactive Dental Office CD-ROM features 25 patient case studies. The patient cases represent a wide variety of dental conditions and procedures typically found in a general dentistry practice. Content from many chapters is integrated throughout the case studies; however, we are listing a reference to the chapter in which the topic covered in most detail within the case study can be found.

Patient	Related Chapter(s)
Christopher Brooks **Age:** 7 **Marital Status:** Single **Occupation:** Student **Address:** 3871 South Dockside Drive Harborville, USA **Provider:** Denise Roberts, DMD **Account:** Gregory Brooks **Insurance:** Yes **Medical History:** No significant findings **Interview:** Chris Brooks, the son of Gregory and Jessica Brooks, is a healthy 7 year old. Dr. Roberts has been his dentist for as long as he can remember, and he enjoys coming to see her. Chris is a Cub Scout who likes playing sports and going to ball games with his dad.	Chapter 59: Dental Sealants
Gregory H. Brooks **Age:** 35 **Marital Status:** Married **Occupation:** Sales Representative **Address:** 3871 South Dockside Drive Harborville, USA **Provider:** Denise Roberts, DMD **Account:** Self **Insurance:** Yes **Medical History:** No significant findings **Interview:** Greg Brooks is a 35-year-old sales representative who really enjoys his work and his family. In fact, he likes just about everything except going to the dentist! His wife has finally convinced him to see Dr. Roberts.	Chapter 53: Dental Implants

Patient	Related Chapter(s)
Jessica Brooks **Age:** 29 **Marital Status:** Married **Occupation:** Not presently employed **Address:** 3871 South Dockside Drive Harborville, USA **Provider:** Denise Roberts, DMD **Account:** Gregory Brooks (husband) **Insurance:** Yes **Medical History:** Jessica is $6\frac{1}{2}$ months pregnant at the time of her recall visit. **Interview:** Jessica Brooks is the wife of Greg Brooks and the mother of Chris. She had been teaching school; however, now she is pregnant and plans to stay home for a while after the baby is born. Like her son, Chris, Jessica is a longtime patient of Dr. Roberts.	Chapter 48: General Dentistry
Margaret Brown **Age:** $2\frac{1}{2}$ **Marital Status:** Single **Occupation:** **Address:** 2300 Harborview Terrace, Apt 302 Harborville, USA **Provider:** David Bowman, DDS **Account:** Roger Brown (father) **Insurance:** No **Medical History:** No significant findings **Interview:** Maggie is a very active $2\frac{1}{2}$-year-old who wants to do things her way! She has never been to the dentist; however, this changes very quickly when she falls in the bathtub and bumps her mouth.	Chapter 57: Pediatric Dentistry
Tiffany Cole **Age:** 8 **Marital Status:** Single **Occupation:** Student **Address:** 3321 Homestead Circle Brandonton, USA **Provider:** Denise Roberts, DMD **Account:** Clifford Cole (father), 823 Sandy Dune Street Harborville, USA **Insurance:** No **Medical History:** No significant findings **Interview:** Tiffany Cole is a healthy 8-year-old who enjoys school, loves to read, and likes playing soccer. Tiffany's parents are divorced, and she lives with her mother; however, her dad is actively involved in her life, including bringing her to see Dr. Roberts.	Chapter 42: Extraoral and Digital Radiography

Patient	Related Chapter(s)
Antonio DeAngelis **Age:** 72 **Marital Status:** Married **Occupation:** Retired **Address:**1818 Sandy Drive Harborville, USA **Provider:** Denise Roberts, DMD **Account:** Self **Insurance:** No **Medical History:** Takes medication for hypertension and high cholesterol. **Interview:** Antonio DeAngelis, who is 72 years old, is married and a long time resident of the community. He is seeing Dr. Roberts as a new patient because his previous dentist retired. Mr. DeAngelis, who is also retired, considers himself to be in good health and particularly enjoys fishing with his grandchildren.	Chapter 54: Endodontics
Jose Escobar Age: 78 **Marital Status:** Widower **Occupation:** Retired **Address:** 1700 Carlton Terrace, #105 Brandonton, USA **Provider:** David Bowman, DDS **Account:** Patient is responsible for account; however, finances are being managed by his daughter, Mrs. Warren Thompson. **Insurance:** **Medical History:** A year ago patient had a stroke, resulting in hemiparesis (slight paralysis) on the left side of his body. **Interview:** Jose Escobar, a 78-year-old widower, lives in a nursing home. His daughter, Emily Thompson, manages her father's finances and takes him wherever he needs to go, including to see Dr. Bowman.	Chapter 52: Removable Prosthodontics
Janet Folkner **Age:** 78 **Marital Status:** Married **Occupation:** Housewife **Address:** 3300 Meadowview Gardens, #518 Harborville, USA **Provider:** David Bowman, DDS **Account:** Peter Folkman (husband) **Insurance:** No **Medical History:** Heart pacemaker, arthritis. No known allergies. **Interview:** Janet Folkner, age 78, and her husband, Peter Folkner, recently moved into a nearby retirement community. Mrs. Folkner, who has retained most of her teeth, has not been to the dentist for several years because of concerns about finances. Now she is scheduled to see Dr. Bowman as a new patient.	Chapter 55: Periodontics

Patient	Related Chapter(s)
Charles Fuller **Age:** 54 **Marital Status:** Divorced **Occupation:** Unemployed, on disability **Address:** 6712 Hightower Arms, Apt 814 Brandonton, USA **Provider:** David Bowman, DDS **Account:** Self **Insurance:** No **Medical History:** Heart murmur, damaged heart valve, cardiac catheterization, history of chest pain, mature onset diabetes, and severe hypertension. **Interview:** Charles Fuller is a 54-year-old US army veteran with problems! He is divorced, in poor health, and unable to work. He has no children or immediate family. In addition to all of this, he also has severe dental problems.	Chapter 56: Oral and Maxillofacial Surgery
Bret Goodman **Age:** 4 **Marital Status:** Single **Occupation:** **Address:** 1520 Valley Road Brandonton, USA **Provider:** Denise Roberts, DMD **Account:** Helena Goodman (mother) **Insurance:** No **Medical History:** No significant findings **Interview:** Bret Goodman is an active 4-year-old who loves to run, climb, and explore! His mother is a single parent and takes good care of Bret; however, Bret has baby bottle mouth (BBM) and has already received extensive dental care. Because of poor cooperation with his previous dentist, Ms. Goodman decided to bring Bret to Dr. Roberts for dental care.	Chapter 57: Pediatric Dentistry
Amy Harris **Age:** 35 **Marital Status:** Single **Occupation:** Investment Broker **Address:** 1100 Shoreside Condominiums, Unit 10 Harborville, USA **Provider:** David Bowman, DDS **Account:** Self **Insurance:** Yes **Medical History:** No significant findings **Interview:** Amy Harris is 35 years old, single, and a highly successful investment broker. Dr. Bowman has been her dentist since Ms. Harris moved here 10 years ago.	Chapter 45: Dental Cements

Patient	Related Chapter(s)
Chester Higgins **Age:** 74 **Marital Status:** Married **Occupation:** Retired postal worker **Address:** 330 Pikeville Road Brandonton, USA **Provider:** David Bowman, DDS **Account:** Self **Insurance:** No **Medical History:** Allergic to penicillin and sulfa drugs. Angina pectoris. **Interview:** Chester Higgins, who is 74, is a retired postal worker. Generally in good health, Mr. Higgins and his wife travel as much as possible. Dr. Bowman has been Chester Higgins' dentist for many years and they share a common interest in stamp collecting.	Chapter 50: Fixed Prosthodontics
Evalena Horton **Age:** 32 **Marital Status:** Single **Occupation:** The Hightower Supermarket, part-time clerk **Address:** 1799 Hamilton Circle Brandonton, USA **Provider:** David Bowman, DDS **Account:** Self **Insurance:** No **Medical History:** Rheumatic fever with heart valve damage. **Interview:** Evalena Horton, who is 32 years old, works part-time as a clerk at the Hightower Supermarket. Although shy and somewhat timid, she enjoys this work because it allows her to keep up with what is going on in town! One thing Evalena definitely does not like is going to the dentist.	Chapter 47: Laboratory Materials and Procedures
Todd Ledbetter **Age:** 11 **Marital Status:** Single **Occupation:** Student **Address:** 629 Channel Way Harborville, USA **Provider:** Denise Roberts, DMD **Account:** Arthur K. Ledbetter (father) **Insurance:** Yes, dual coverage **Medical History:** No significant findings **Interview:** Todd Ledbetter, who is 11 years old, recently moved here with his family. He is already involved in several sports; however, his greatest enthusiasm is "surfing the net." It has been 12 months since Todd's last dental visit, and he is scheduled to see Dr. Roberts.	Chapter 28: Oral Diagnosis and Treatment Planning

Patient	Related Chapter(s)
Wendy Ledbetter **Age:** 18 **Marital Status:** Single **Occupation:** Student **Address:** 629 Channel Way Harborville, USA **Provider:** Denise Roberts, DMD **Account:** Arthur K. Ledbetter (father) **Insurance:** Yes, dual coverage **Medical History:** Juvenile onset diabetes. Uses insulin by injection. **Interview:** Wendy Ledbetter, who is 18 years old, completed high school and her orthodontic treatment just before the family moved here. Although Wendy likes the community, she is really excited about going away to college in the fall.	Chapter 31: Assisting in a Medical Emergency
Crystal Malone **Age:** 25 **Marital Status:** Single **Occupation:** Unemployed **Address:** 1855 Rogers Street Brandonton, USA **Provider:** Denise Roberts, DMD **Account:** Warren Malone (father) **Insurance:** Father has insurance. **Medical History:** No significant findings **Interview:** Crystal Malone, is 25 years old, single, and a recent college graduate with a drama degree. She is concerned about the appearance of her teeth because she plans to be an actress. Her father, Warren Malone, is still paying her expenses while Crystal is getting her career started.	Chapter 48: General Dentistry
Kevin McClelland **Age:** 11 **Marital Status:** Single **Occupation:** Student **Address:** 970 Broadview Circle, Apt 250 Middleburg, USA **Provider:** David Bowman, DDS **Account:** Douglas McClelland (father) **Insurance:** No **Medical History:** History of epilepsy. Updated history notes difficulty with medication. **Interview:** Kevin McClelland is 11 years old and is a long time patient of Dr. Bowman's. Currently Kevin is also undergoing orthodontic treatment. Although he doesn't much care for sports, Kevin does share Todd Ledbetter's enthusiasm for computers!	Chapter 60: Orthodontics

<table>
<tr><th>Patient</th><th>Related Chapter(s)</th></tr>
<tr><td>Raul Ortega Jr.
Age: 5
Marital Status: Single
Occupation:
Address:
717 Terrace Garden Court
Middleburg, USA
Provider: David Bowman, DDS
Account: Raul Ortega Sr.
Insurance: No
Medical History: No significant findings
Interview:
Raul Ortega Jr. is a bright, active 5 year old. He likes to watch TV (when his parents let him) and to shoot baskets with his older brother (when he'll let him). Raul has baby bottle mouth (BBM), and Dr. Bowman is his dentist.</td><td>Chapter 57: Pediatric Dentistry</td></tr>
<tr><td>Ingrid Pedersen
Age: 18
Marital Status: Single
Occupation: Student
Address:
2020 Northshore Drive
Harborville, USA
Provider: Denise Roberts, DMD
Account: Father, Lars Pedersen
Insurance: Yes
Medical History: History of asthma, carries an inhaler. Pollen allergies. No antibiotic allergies.
Interview:
Ingrid Pedersen is 18 years old, has recently graduated from high school, and is getting ready to leave for college. Although her father is still responsible for her account, Ingrid works part-time at the Biggie Burger Shop to earn extra money.</td><td>Chapter 56: Oral and Maxillofacial Surgery</td></tr>
<tr><td>Miguel Ricardo
Age: 27
Marital Status: Married
Occupation: Paramedic
Address:
Box 522 Farmdale Rd.
Brandonton, USA
Provider: Denise Roberts, DMD
Account: Self
Insurance: Yes, dual coverage
Medical History: Seasonal allergies
Interview:
Miguel Ricardo is 27 years old, married, and a paramedic with the Emergency Rescue Service. In his spare time, Miguel coaches the local Little League Team, and they had a championship team last year!</td><td>Chapter 48: General Dentistry</td></tr>
</table>

Patient	Related Chapter(s)
Harriet Ross **Age:** 84 **Marital Status:** Widow **Occupation:** **Address:** 1600 Harborview Oaks, Apt 33 Harborville, USA **Provider:** Denise Roberts, DMD **Account:** Self; however, funds are managed by her niece Miss Catherine Dowdell. **Insurance:** No **Medical History:** Heart condition, edema in lower legs and ankles, arthritis, a profound hearing loss, and increasing forgetfulness. **Interview:** Harriet Ross is an 84-year-old widow. Mrs. Ross has not seen Dr. Roberts recently because she wasn't feeling well. Now she wants an upper denture to improve her appearance. Catherine Dowdell lives with her aunt and helps her by fixing meals, running errands, providing transportation, and managing all financial matters.	Chapter 56: Oral and Maxillofacial Surgery
Cindy Valladares **Age:** 21 **Marital Status:** Single **Occupation:** College student (part-time waitress) **Address:** Straton Hall, Room 512 University Heights, USA **Provider:** David Bowman, DDS **Account:** Self **Insurance:** No **Medical History:** No significant findings **Interview:** Cindy Valladares is 21 years old, a full-time college student, and a part-time waitress at the El Rancho Steak House. After completing her undergraduate education, Cindy plans to go on medical school.	Chapter 54: Endodontics
Louisa Van Doren **Age:** 68 **Marital Status:** Married **Occupation:** Retired **Address:** 789 Curtis Street Brandonton, USA **Provider:** David Bowman, DDS **Account:** James David Van Doren (husband) **Insurance:** No **Medical History:** Hypertension, maturity onset diabetes, osteoporosis **Interview:** Louisa Van Doren, who is 68 years old, and her husband James David Van Doren recently retired to the area. Mrs. Van Doren has received extensive dental care in the past and is anxious to find a new dentist. Although her health is not too good, Mrs. Van Doren is already extremely active in her church.	Chapter 55: Periodontics

Patient	Related Chapter(s)
Douglas Warner Jr. **Age:** 30 **Marital Status:** Single **Occupation:** Unemployed **Address:** PO Box 501 Brandonton, USA **Provider:** David Bowman, DDS **Account:** Mrs. Douglas Howard Warner, Sr. (mother) **Insurance:** No **Medical History:** Injured 6 months ago in a motorcycle accident. He sustained closed head injuries with multiple facial fractures requiring surgical fixation. He now takes medication for a seizure disorder and has difficulty concentrating. **Interview:** Doug Warner, who is 30 years old and single, was injured 6 months ago in a motorcycle accident in which he was not wearing a helmet. Doug was recently released from a rehabilitation facility, is unemployed, and is living at home with his mother.	Chapter 48: General Dentistry
Lee Wong **Age:** 24 **Marital Status:** Single **Occupation:** Graduate student **Address:** 320 Century Blvd. Apt #3 Brandonton, USA **Provider:** Denise Roberts, DMD **Account:** Self **Insurance:** No **Medical History:** No significant findings **Interview:** Lee Wong is a 24 year old graduate student. Lee has not been in this country very long, and his English is limited; however, he likes being at the university and exploring his new surroundings.	Chapter 56: Oral and Maxillofacial Surgery

How to Use the Dental Assisting Video Procedures CD-ROM

This CD-ROM includes dental assisting procedures vital for the education of the dental assisting student. Simply go to the main menu and use the cursor to click the section you wish to view.

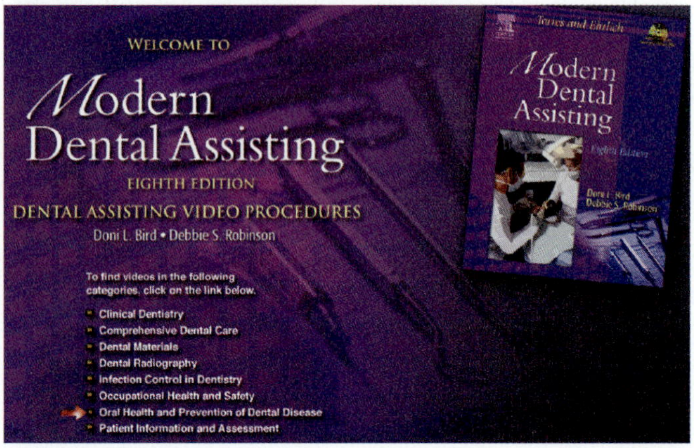
WELCOME TO
Modern
Dental Assisting
EIGHTH EDITION
DENTAL ASSISTING VIDEO PROCEDURES
Doni L. Bird • Debbie S. Robinson
To find videos in the following categories, click on the link below.
Clinical Dentistry
Comprehensive Dental Care
Dental Materials
Dental Radiography
Infection Control in Dentistry
Occupational Health and Safety
Oral Health and Prevention of Dental Disease
Patient Information and Assessment
Modern
Dental
Assisting

Another page will appear with a menu of video procedures. The selected video procedure will begin playing in the video screen on the right.

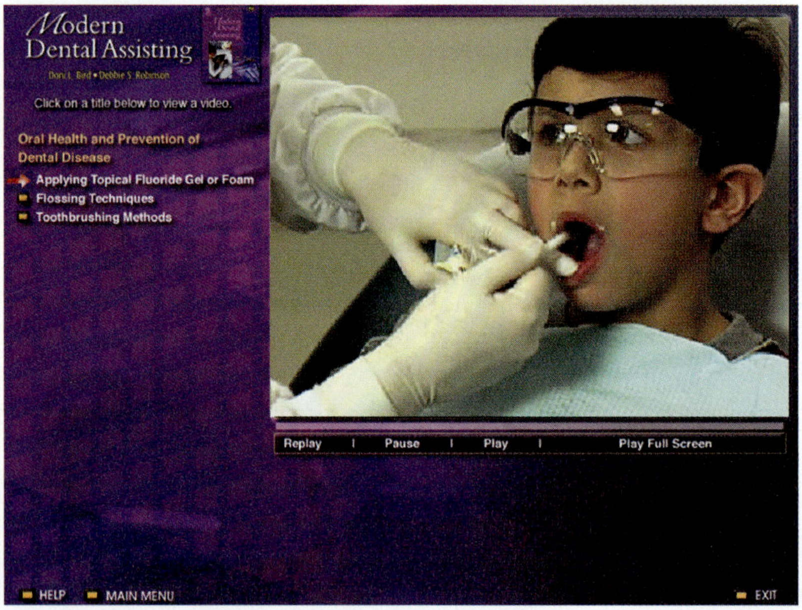

To navigate the video clip, click on the Play or Re-play button to view the clip and Pause to stop the clip. To view the video full screen, select the Play Full Screen button (the Spacebar will return screen to normal view).

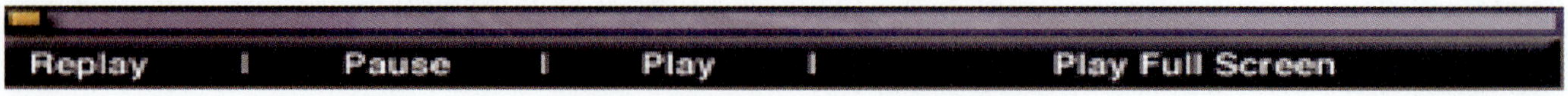

Once a video segment is finished, you may choose another selection from the Main Menu or Exit the program. For more information regarding the CD-ROM click the Help button.

Minimum System Requirements

PC CD-ROM

PC Based Pentium PIII 700 or Celeron 1 GHz or higher
Windows ME, XP Home and Pro
128 MB RAM
16X CD-ROM Drive
Video Card with 16-bit or higher color (24 or 32 bit is best)
Display Resolution of 800 × 600 or greater
Sound Card and Speakers
* May work with Windows 98SE but is not officially supported by Microsoft.

Macintosh CD-ROM

Power PC G4 500MHZ, I-MAC, I-Book
Macintosh OS 10.X and higher
128 MB RAM
16X CD-ROM Drive
Video Card with 16 bit or higher color (24 or 32 bit is best)
Display Resolution of 800 × 600 or greater
Sound Card and Speakers

Operation Instructions

PC CD-ROM Operation

This is a self-executing Microsoft Windows CD-ROM; simply insert disk, and it will play automatically.

If the auto insert feature on your CD drive is disabled or the CD fails to start automatically, you can start manually by:

You may start the presentation by clicking on the "Start" button on the taskbar>
Select "Run">
Click "Browse">
Look for the disk named "Dental" and highlight the "Dental.exe" program in the CD root directory>
Click "Open">
Click "OK"

Macintosh CD-ROM Operation

Find the disk named "Dental" and click to view contents. Apple OS X users can select the "EULA.app."

If you do not have QuickTime™ installed then you will be prompted to do so from the program.

Apple Quicktime™ is the video player utilized for the Macintosh platform. A free version is included on this CD. The CD will automatically check your system to determine whether the player is present. If the player is not installed, it will install it for you. Please follow all prompts as you may be required to restart your computer upon installation completion. If your system does not have QuickTime™ player and the installer does not run automatically, you may install it manually by running the QuickTime™ Installer located within the QuickTime™ directory on this CD.

Getting Help

If you have questions or problems with the installation or use of this CD-ROM, please contact technical support:

Via phone: Call 1-800-692-9010 Monday — Friday, 5:30 a.m. — 7:00 p.m. Central Time

Via fax: Fax question or problem to 1-314-579-3316

Email: Send email to technical.support.elsevier.com

Please help us solve your problem by having the following information available when you contact technical support:

- Type and speed of processor (e.g., Pentium 133 MHz)
- Amount of RAM (e.g., 64 MB)
- Video display settings (e.g., 800 × 600, 16-bit)
- Speed of CD-ROM drive (e.g., 8×)
- Size and free space of hard disk (e.g., 4.3 GB total, 250 MB free)
- Operating system including version and service packs (e.g., Windows NT Workstation 4.0 Service Pack 3)
- Version number of the browser, available from the help pull-down menu, under About (IE or Netscape)

For more information regarding other products, visit our website at www.us.elsevierhealth.com.

If You Have Difficulty Viewing Video

For Windows PC Users Only

This CD ROM uses Direct X, a free standard component included with the Windows operating systems listed above. It does not have to be installed or altered if already present. You do not need to install any additional software to view this disk.

If your operating system was not listed above, you may not have Direct X installed. You may obtain a free copy of the latest version of Direct X by visiting the link below. Please be sure to install the correct version for your operating system. Full instructions and installation notes are available on the Microsoft website.

All information regarding Direct X, as well as links to free downloads can be found at:

http://www.microsoft.com/directx

Video Topics and Corresponding Textbook Chapters

CATEGORIES/VIDEO TITLES	CORRESPONDING TEXTBOOK CHAPTER
Clinical Dentistry	
Applying a Topical Anesthetic	Chapter 37
Assisting with Local Anesthesia	Chapter 37
Dental Dam Placement and Removal	Chapter 36
Identifying and Attaching Handpieces	Chapter 35
Positioning the High-Volume Evacuator	Chapter 36
Transferring Instruments (Single-Handed)	Chapter 33
Comprehensive Dental Care	
Applying Dental Sealants	Chapter 59
Assembling and Placing a Matrix Band and Universal Retainer	Chapter 49
Coronal Polishing	Chapter 58
Fabricating a Custom Acrylic Provisional Crown	Chapter 51
Noneugenol Periodontal Dressing	Chapter 55
Placing an Intermediate Restoration	Chapter 48
Placing and Removing Retraction Cord	Chapter 50
Removing a Periodontal Dressing	Chapter 55
Suture Removal	Chapter 56
Dental Materials	
Constructing a Vacuum-Formed Tray	Chapter 47
Mixing Alginate and Taking Preliminary Impressions	Chapter 46
Mixing and Transferring Amalgam	Chapter 43
Mixing Zinc Phosphate for Permanent Cementation	Chapter 45
Pouring Dental Models Using Inverted-Pour Method	Chapter 47
Removing Cement	Chapter 45
Dental Radiography	
Assembling the XCP Instruments	Chapter 41
Automatic Processing of Dental Radiographs	Chapter 39
Bisecting Technique	Chapter 41
Maxillary Canine Exposure	
Maxillary Incisor Exposure	
Mandibular Canine Exposure	
Mandibular Incisor Exposure	
Maxillary Premolar Exposure	
Maxillary Molar Exposure	
Mandibular Premolar Exposure	
Mandibular Molar Exposure	

CATEGORIES/VIDEO TITLES	CORRESPONDING TEXTBOOK CHAPTER
Bite-Wing Technique	Chapter 41
Molar Exposure	
Premolar Exposure	
Digital Radiography	Chapter 41
Setting Up the Digital System	
Maxillary Canine Exposure	
Maxillary Molar Exposure	
Bite-Wing Exposure	
Duplicating Radiographs	Chapter 39
Manual Processing of Dental Radiographs	Chapter 39
Mounting Dental Radiographs	Chapter 41
Occlusal Technique (Maxillary/Mandibular)	Chapter 41
Paralleling Technique	Chapter 41
Maxillary Canine Exposure	
Maxillary Central/Lateral Incisor Exposure	
Mandibular Canine Exposure	
Mandibular Incisor Exposure	
Maxillary Premolar Exposure	
Maxillary Molar Exposure	
Mandibular Premolar Exposure	
Mandibular Molar Exposure	
Positioning Patient for Panoramic Radiography	Chapter 42
Positioning the Patient to Take Radiographs	Chapter 41
Preparing Panoramic Equipment	Chapter 42
Preparing the Operatory/Equipment to Take Radiographs	Chapter 41

Infection Control in Dentistry

Autoclaving Instruments	Chapter 21
Handwashing Techniques	Chapter 19
Operating the Ultrasonic Cleaner	Chapter 21
Placing and Removing Surface Barriers	Chapter 20
Treatment Room Cleaning and Disinfection	Chapter 20

Occupational Health and Safety

Body-Strengthening Exercises	Chapter 25

Oral Health and Prevention of Dental Disease

Applying Topical Fluoride Gel or Foam	Chapter 15
Flossing Techniques	Chapter 15
Toothbrushing Methods	Chapter 15

Patient Information and Assessment

Taking a Patient's Blood Pressure	Chapter 27

Part 1

The Dental Assisting Profession

Dental assistants are important members of the dental healthcare team. A career as a dental assistant is exciting, challenging, and very rewarding. The educated dental assistant can look forward to job satisfaction, variety, and financial reward. It is a career that offers opportunities for recent high school graduates as well as individuals who may be older and wish to return to school and change careers.

Professionalism is difficult to define. It is an attitude that is apparent in everything said and done by a person, at and away from the office. Professionalism distinguishes people who "have a job" from those who "pursue a career." By always behaving in a professional manner, the dental assistant earns respect and acknowledgment as a dental healthcare professional.

This section is designed to provide an overview of the dental profession. It begins with a look at dentistry through the ages, introduces the other members of the dental healthcare team, and discusses the legal and ethical standards expected of a dental professional.

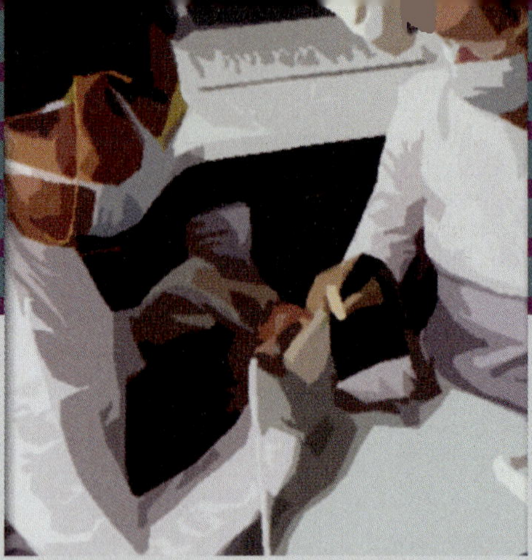

1 History of Dentistry

Outline

KEY TERMS

Commission on Dental Accreditation of the American Dental Association Commission that accredits dental, dental assisting, dental hygiene, and dental laboratory educational programs.

Dental treatise (**tree**-tiz) Formal article or book based on dental evidence and facts.

Forensic dentistry (fo-**ren**-zik) Area of dentistry that establishes the identity of an individual based on dental evidence such as dental records, impressions, bite marks, etc.

Periodontal disease (*pair*-e-o-**don**-tul) Infections and other conditions of the structures that support the teeth (gums and bone).

Preceptorship (pre-**sep**-tor-ship) Study under the guidance of a dentist or other professional.

Silver amalgam paste (a-**mal**-gum) A mixture of mercury, silver, and tin.

LEARNING OUTCOMES

On completion of this chapter, the student will be able to achieve the following objectives:

- Pronounce, define, and spell the Key Terms.
- Describe the role of Hippocrates in history.
- State the basic premise of the Hippocratic Oath.
- Name the first woman to graduate from a college of dentistry.
- Name the first woman to practice dentistry in the United States.
- Name the first African-American woman to receive a dental degree in the United States.
- Discuss the contributions of Horace H. Hayden and Chapin A. Harris.
- Describe two major contributions of G.V. Black.
- Name the first dentist to employ a dental assistant.
- Name the first female dental assistant.
- Name the scientist who discovered radiographs.
- Name the physician who first used nitrous oxide for tooth extractions.
- Discuss the purpose and activities of the National Museum of Dentistry.

Dentistry has a long and fascinating history. From the earliest times, humans have suffered from dental pain and have sought a variety of means to alleviate it. As they developed tools, humans also cleaned and cared for their teeth and oral cavity. The early toothbrushes ranged from wooden sticks with frayed ends for scraping the tongue to ivory-handled brushes with animal-hair bristles for cleaning the teeth.

It is easy to believe that the ideas and techniques used in dentistry today have been recently discovered or invented. Actually, many of the remarkable techniques in modern dentistry can be traced to the earliest times in every culture. People may think of "cosmetic dentistry" as a relatively new field, but skulls of ninth-century Mayans have numerous inlays of decorative jade and turquoise on the front teeth. Skulls of the Incas discovered in Ecuador have gold pounded into prepared holes in the teeth, similar to modern gold inlay restorations. As early as the sixth century BC, the Etruscans were able to make false teeth using gold and cattle teeth (Fig. 1-1). More than 2200 years ago, a cleft palate was repaired on a child in China. Muhammad introduced basic oral hygiene into the ritual of Islam in the seventh century AD. He recognized the value of **Siwak,** a tree twig containing natural minerals, as an oral hygiene device.

As B.W. Weinberger noted in *Dentistry: An Illustrated History* (Ring, 1995), a profession that is ignorant of its past experiences has lost a valuable asset because "it has missed its best guide to the future." Table 1-1 lists major highlights in the history of dentistry.

Table 1-1 ***Highlights in the History of Dentistry***

Date	Group/Individual	Event
3000–2151 BC	Egyptians	Hesi-Re is earliest dentist known by name.
2700 BC	Chinese	Chinese Canon of Medicine refers to dentistry.
900–300 BC	Mayans	Teeth receive attention for religious reasons or self-adornment.
460–322 BC	Greeks	Hippocrates and Aristotle write about tooth decay.
166–201 AD	Romans	Restore decayed teeth with gold crowns.
570–950	Muslims	Use Siwak as a primitive toothbrush.
1510–1590	Ambroise Paré	Writes extensively about dentistry, including extractions.
1678–1761	Pierre Fauchard	Becomes "Father of Modern Dentistry."
1728–1793	John Hunter	Performs first scientific study of teeth.
1826	M. Taveau	Introduces amalgam as "silver paste."
1844	Horace Wells	Uses nitrous oxide for relief of dental pain.
1859		American Dental Association is founded.
1885	C. Edmund Kells	Employs first dental assistant.
1895	G.V. Black	Becomes "Grand Old Man of Dentistry"and perfects amalgam.
1895	W.C. Roentgen	Discovers x-rays.
1908	Frederick McKay	Discovers that fluoride is connected with prevention of dental caries.
1913	Alfred C. Fones	Establishes first dental hygiene school in Bridgeport, Connecticut.
1923		American Dental Hygiene Association is founded.
1924		American Dental Assistants Association is founded.
1947		Dental Assisting National Board is founded.
1970	Congress	Creates Occupational Safety and Health Administration.
1978	*Journal of the American Dental Association*	Publishes a report on infection control for dental offices.
1982		First hepatitis B vaccine becomes commercially available.
2000		*Oral Health in America: A Report of the Surgeon General* is released.
2003	Centers for Disease Control and Prevention	Releases *Guidelines for Infection Control in Dental Health-Care Settings–2003.*

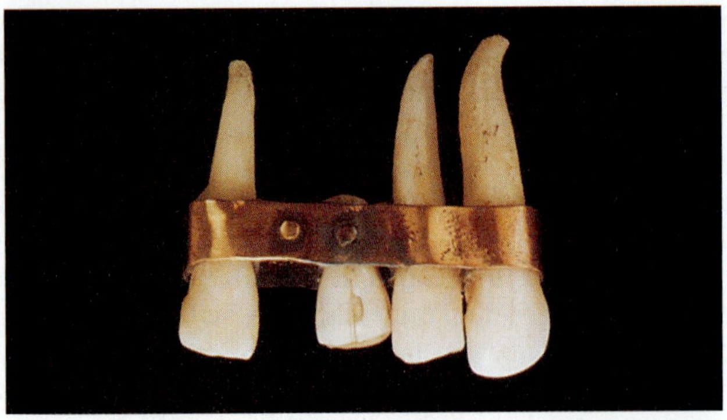

Fig. 1-1 Ancient Etruscan gold-banded bridge with built-in calf's tooth. (From Ring M: *Dentistry: an illustrated history,* New York, 1985, Mosby/Abrams.)

EARLY TIMES

The Egyptians

As long as 4600 years ago in Egypt, physicians began to specialize in healing certain parts of the body. A physician named **Hesi-Re** was the earliest dentist whose name is known. He practiced about 3000 BC and was called "Chief of the Toothers and the Physicians." Three teeth fastened together with gold wire, apparently an early fixed bridge, were found with the remains of an Egyptian who lived about 3100 BC.

A radiograph of the skull of Thuya, mother-in-law of Pharaoh Amenhotep III, showed bone loss in her jaws, an indication of **periodontal disease.** Some dental problems have been attributed to the Egyptian diet, which was primarily vegetarian. Grain was ground with stone pestles, which mixed sand and grit into the food, resulting in severe wear of the *occlusal* (biting) tooth surfaces and exposure of the pulp.

Recall

1. Who was Hesi-Re?
2. How long has dental disease existed?

The Greeks

During the fifth century BC in Greece, the practice of medicine and dentistry was based on the worship practices of the priesthood. Priests would give patients a sleeping potion and perform healing rituals. During this period, **Hippocrates** (460–377 BC) began to outline a rational approach to treating patients. He suggested that four main fluids in the body—blood, black bile, yellow bile, and phlegm—along with heat, cold, dry air, and wet air, must remain in balance or disease would occur. His approach to treatment of patients earned him the title **Father of Medicine.**

Hippocrates stressed the importance of keeping the teeth in good condition. His writings described the teeth, their formation, and their eruption, as well as diseases of the teeth and methods of treatment. He also developed a dentifrice and mouthwash. The famous **Hippocratic Oath,** a solemn obligation to refrain from wrongdoing and to treat patients with confidentiality and to the best of one's ability, still serves as the basis of the code of ethics for medical and dental professions.

Aristotle (384–322 BC), the great philosopher, referred to teeth in many of his writings. However, he mistakenly stated that the gingiva was responsible for tooth formation and that men had 32 teeth and women had only 30. Many of his erroneous ideas were not corrected until the Renaissance.

Diocles of Carystus, an Athenian physician of Aristotle's time, recommended rubbing the gums and teeth with bare fingers and "finely pulverized mint" to remove adherent food particles. Other materials used to clean the teeth included pumice, talc, emery, ground alabaster, coral powder, and iron rust.

The Chinese

By 2000 BC, the Chinese were practicing dentistry. They used arsenic to treat decayed teeth. This probably relieved the toothache. About the second century AD, the Chinese developed a **silver amalgam paste** for fillings, more than a thousand years before dentists in the West. In the eleventh century, **T'ing To-t'ung** and **Yu Shu** described the entire process of chewing and swallowing. Their description of the process was accurate, but they were incorrect about what happened to the food when it reached the stomach. They believed digestion was a result of vapors arising from the spleen.

The Romans

When the medical profession in Rome was just beginning, dentistry was already being practiced. Several Roman physicians wrote extensively about dental treatment, although many people still believed that a "toothworm" was responsible for toothaches. In addition to extracting teeth, the Romans were skilled in restoring decayed teeth with gold crowns and replacing missing teeth by means of fixed bridgework.

The Romans had a high regard for oral hygiene and developed tooth-cleaning powders made of eggshells, bones, and oyster shells mixed with honey. Dinner guests of upper-class Romans picked their teeth between each course with elaborately decorated toothpicks of metal, often gold, and were invited to take their gold toothpicks home as gifts.

Cornelius Celsus (25 BC–50 AD) wrote *De Medicina,* a digest of medical and surgical science from the earliest times to the period of Augustus Caesar. This book contains the earliest record of orthodontic treatment.

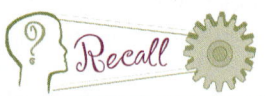

Claudius Galen (130–200 AD) is considered to be the greatest physician after Hippocrates. In his writings, Galen listed the teeth as bones of the body. He is the first author to mention the nerves in the teeth: "The teeth are furnished with nerves both because as naked bones they have need of sensitivity so that the animal may avoid being injured or destroyed by mechanical or physical agencies, and because the teeth, together with the tongue and other parts of the mouth, are designed for the perception of various flavors" (Guerini, 1909).

Recall

3. Who is the Father of Medicine?
4. What is the Hippocratic Oath?
5. What dental procedures did the Romans practice?
6. Were Western dentists the first to use silver amalgam as fillings?

THE RENAISSANCE

One of the most important achievements of the Renaissance was the separation of science from theology and superstition. During the fifteenth and sixteenth centuries, new interest arose in the study of anatomy and the human body. Artists became more aware of human anatomy and used it to enhance their artwork. **Leonardo da Vinci** (1452–1519) sketched every internal and external structure of the body. He also studied the skull in great detail and was the first anatomist to describe the differences between molars and premolars.

Ambroise Paré (pah-**ray**) (1510–1590) began his career in Paris in about 1525 as an apprentice to a barber surgeon. His extensive writings include dental extraction methods and reimplantation of teeth. He described a toothache as "the most atrocious pain that can torment a man without being followed by death" (Ring, 1985). At that time the practice was to treat soldiers with gunshots by washing the wound with boiling oil, which caused extreme pain. After one battle the supply of oil was depleted, and Paré had to treat a soldier's wounds with a mixture of egg whites, oil of roses, and turpentine. After using this soothing mixture, Paré vowed that he would "never so cruelly burn poor wounded men." He is also credited with being the first to use artificial eyes, hands, and legs. Paré is known as the "Father of Modern Surgery."

Pierre Fauchard (fo-**shar**) (1678–1761), a physician who earned great fame and respect in his lifetime, willingly shared his knowledge at a time when physicians typically guarded their knowledge and skills (Fig. 1-2). Fauchard developed dentistry as an independent profession and originated the title of "surgeon dentist," a term the French still use today. In the United States, the degree conferred on dentists is *Doctor of Dental Surgery (DDS).*

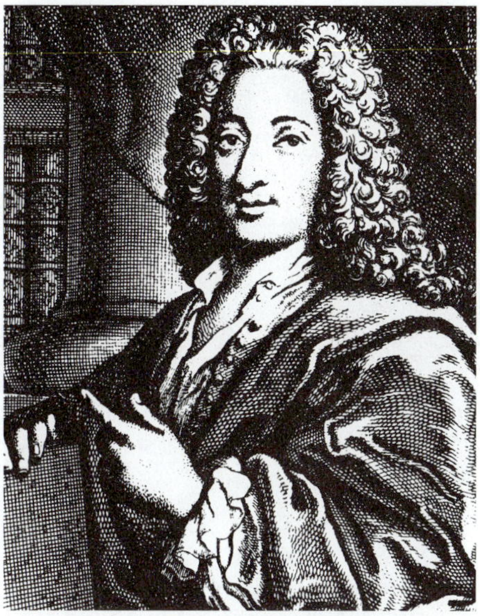

Fig. 1-2 **Pierre Fauchard, the "Father of Modern Dentistry."** (From Fauchard P: *Le Chirurgien Dentiste ou Traité des Dents, 1746.*)

Fauchard dispelled the theory that tooth decay was caused by a toothworm. He was ahead of his time in understanding periodontal disease and recognized that scaling the teeth could prevent gum disease. In his book *Le Chirurgien Dentiste,* Fauchard covered the entire field of dentistry and described his method of removing caries from a tooth and filling the cavity with lead or tin. He suggested using either human teeth or teeth carved from hippopotamus or elephant ivory to make denture teeth. Although advanced in his thinking, Fauchard firmly believed that to ensure good health, people should rinse their mouth every morning with several spoons of their own fresh urine.

Chapin A. Harris, the great American dentist, said of Fauchard: "Considering the circumstances under which he lived, Fauchard deserves to be remembered as a noble pioneer and sure founder of dental science. That his practice was crude was due to his times, that it was scientific and comparatively superior and successful was due to himself" (Ring, 1985). Fauchard is known as the "Father of Modern Dentistry."

Recall

7. Which artist first distinguished molars and premolars?
8. Who is the "Father of Modern Surgery"?
9. Who is the "Father of Modern Dentistry"?

EARLY AMERICA

In 1766, **Robert Woofendale** was one of the first dentists to travel throughout the American colonies. His advertisement in the *New York Mercury* stated that he "performs all

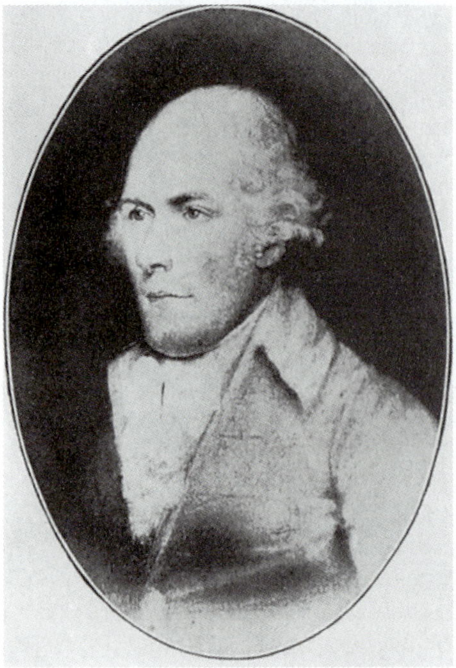

Fig. 1-3 **John Greenwood, dentist to George Washington.** (From Kock CRD: *History of dental surgery*, vol 3, Fort Wayne, Indiana, 1910, National Art Publishing.)

operations upon the teeth, sockets, gums and palate, likewise fixes artificial teeth, so as to escape discernment" (Ring, 1985). A short time later, **John Baker** arrived from Cork County, Ireland, where he studied dentistry. Although he was a physician, Baker practiced dentistry in Boston, New York, Philadelphia, and many other colonial cities. George Washington was one of his patients.

Paul Revere (1735–1818), the famous colonial patriot, was a silversmith by trade, but he studied dentistry as an apprentice under Dr. Baker in Boston. When Baker moved to New York in 1768, Revere took over his practice. However, Revere was primarily interested in using his skills as a silversmith to make artificial teeth and surgical instruments. After six years of part-time practice, he gave up dental practice.

Paul Revere is credited with beginning the science of **forensic dentistry,** performing the first identification of a corpse based on dental history. Dr. Joseph Warren was killed at the Battle of Bunker Hill in 1775 and was buried by the British in a mass grave. A year later the bodies were exhumed but were unrecognizable. Revere studied the skulls and identified Warren's body on the basis of a two-unit bridge he had made.

Isaac Greenwood (1730–1803) is regarded as the first native-born American dentist. Like Paul Revere, Greenwood had many trades and studied dentistry under Dr. John Baker. Greenwood's second son, **John Greenwood** (1760–1819), served in the colonial army at age 14 and in 1785 began to practice dentistry in New York City. He was one of George Washington's dentists (Fig. 1-3).

Recall

10. Who was John Baker's famous patient?
11. Which famous colonial patriot first used forensic evidence?
12. Who was Robert Woofendale?

EDUCATIONAL AND PROFESSIONAL DEVELOPMENT IN THE UNITED STATES

In the early days, there were no colleges for dentistry in the United States. Dentists learned their profession through a **preceptorship**, studying and learning under the direction of a skilled professional. During 1839 and 1840, Horace Hayden and Chapin A. Harris set the foundation for the profession of dentistry.

Horace H. Hayden (1769–1844) was inspired by his own dentist, John Greenwood, and became a reputable dentist. He lectured to medical students on the topic of dentistry and wrote for professional journals. **Chapin A. Harris** (1806–1860), a preceptorial student of Hayden, was instrumental in establishing the first nationwide association of dentists in the United States. His book, *The Dental Art: A Practical Treatise on Dental Surgery,* was reissued during 74 years in 13 editions; no other **dental treatise** can match this record. Together in 1840, Hayden and Harris established the first dental college in the world, the **Baltimore College of Dental Surgery,** now the University of Maryland, School of Dentistry.

Dr. Green Vardiman Black (1836–1915), known worldwide as **G.V. Black,** earned the title of the "Grand Old Man of Dentistry" through his unmatched contributions to the profession (Figs. 1-4 and 1-5). Dr. Black believed that dentistry should stand as a profession independent from and equal to that of medicine. He invented numerous machines for testing metal alloys and dental instruments. He taught in dental schools, became a dean, and wrote more than 500 articles and several books. Two of his major contributions to dentistry were (1) the principle of *extension for prevention,* in which the margins of a filling were extended to within reach of a toothbrush for cleaning the tooth, and (2) standardized rules of cavity preparation and filling.

A man of vision, Black told his dental students at Northwestern University, "The day is surely coming, and perhaps within the lifetime of you young men before me, when we will be engaged in practicing preventive, rather than reparative, dentistry" (Ring, 1985).

Wilhelm Conrad Roentgen (**rent**-ken) (1845–1923) was a Bavarian physicist who discovered x-rays, or radiographs, in 1895 (Fig. 1-6). His discovery revolutionized di-

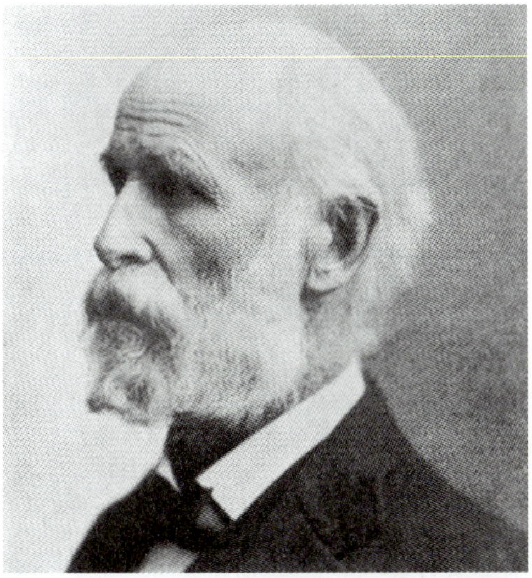

Fig. 1-4 **G.V. Black, the "Grand Old Man of Dentistry."** (From Kock CRD: *History of dental surgery,* vol 1, Chicago, 1909, National Art Publishing.)

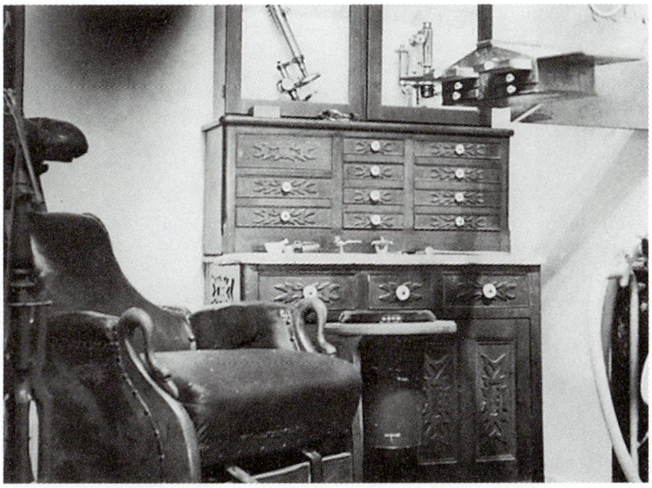

Fig. 1-5 **Black's dental treatment room, as reconstructed in a Smithsonian exhibit.**

agnostic capabilities and forever changed the practice of medicine and dentistry (see Chapter 38).

Horace Wells (1815–1848) is the dentist credited with the discovery of inhalation anesthesia in 1844, one of the most important medical discoveries of all time. Before this innovation, the only remedies for pain were brute force, alcohol (brandy, rum, whiskey), and opium. The oral drugs could not be properly dosed, and patients were generally undermedicated or overmedicated. If an operation lasted more than 20 minutes, it was possible for the patient to die of exhaustion or shock. Realizing the potential for pain-free dental surgery using nitrous oxide, Wells said, "Let it be as free as the air we breathe" (Ring, 1985) (see Chapter 37).

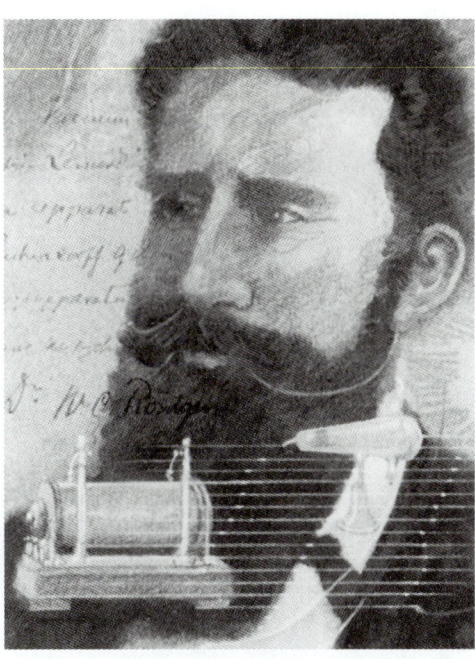

Fig. 1-6 **Roentgen discovered the early potential of a radiograph beam in 1895.** (Courtesy Eastman-Kodak, Rochester, New York.)

Recall

13. Who founded the first dental school in America?
14. Who earned the title of "Grand Old Man of Dentistry"?
15. Who was the first dentist to use nitrous oxide?

Women in Dentistry

In the eighteenth and early nineteenth centuries, dental schools throughout the world did not accept women. Yet, many women broke those barriers and led the way for other women to follow as dental professionals (Figs. 1-7 and 1-8). Today, women represent almost 50 percent of students in some dental schools. It is projected that by the year 2020, 20 percent of all dental practitioners in the United States will be women. Today, women are active in dental associations, specialty organizations, public health, and the military (Table 1-2).

Ida Gray (1867–1953) was the first black woman in the county to earn a formal DDS degree, and the first black woman to practice dentistry in Chicago. She graduated from the University of Michigan, School of Dentistry and practiced dentistry in Chicago until she retired in 1928. In 1929 she married William Rollins and used the name of Dr. **Ida Gray-Rollins** for the rest of her life.

History of Dental Assisting

C. Edmund Kells (1856–1928), a New Orleans dentist, is usually credited with employing the first dental assistant

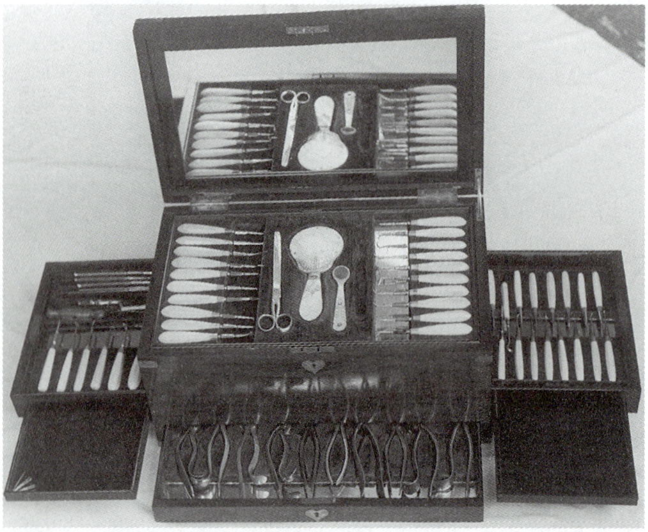

Fig. 1-7 **Dental instrument kit belonging to Nellie E. Pooler Chapman. She practiced dentistry in Nevada City, California. She died in 1906.** (Courtesy University of California San Francisco, School of Dentistry.)

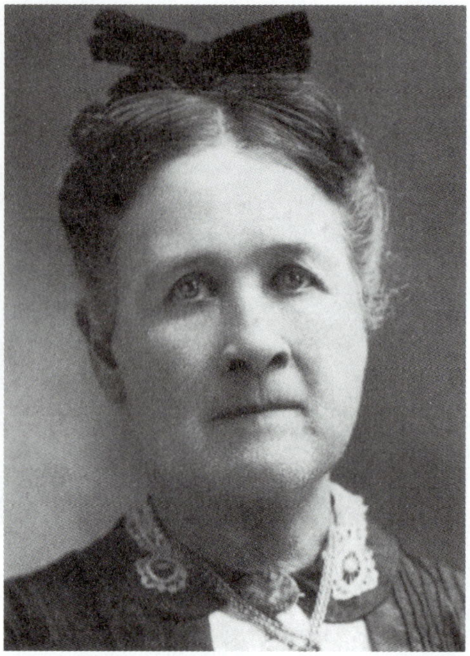

Fig. 1-8 **Lucy B. Hobbs-Taylor, the first female graduate of dental school.** (Courtesy Kansas State Historical Society.)

Table 1-2 ***Highlights of Women in Dentistry***

Date	Group/Individual	Event
1859	Emeline Robert Jones	First woman to establish a regular dental practice in the U.S.
1866	Lucy B. Hobbs-Taylor	First woman to graduate from a recognized dental college; received credit for time as a preceptor in her husband's practice.
1869	Henriette Hirschfeld	First woman to complete the full dental curriculum.
1870	Nellie E. Pooler Chapman	First woman to practice dentistry in California.
1873	Emilie Foeking	First female graduate of the Baltimore College of Dental Surgery. Wrote a thesis titled *"Is Woman adapted to the dental profession?"*
1876	Jennie D. Spurrier	First female dentist in Illinois. Her first patient needed an extraction, for which she was paid 50 cents. She had it engraved with the date and *"My first."*
1885	Malvina Cueria	First female dental assistant.
1890	Ida Gray-Rollins	First African-American female dental graduate from a U.S. dental college.
1892	Mary Stillwell-Kuedsel	Founded the Women's Dental Association of the U.S. with 12 charter members.
1906	Irene Newman	First dental hygienist.
1927	M. Evangeline Jordan	Author of the first textbook on pediatric dentistry.
1951	Helen E. Myers	U.S. Army's first female dentist.
1975	Jeanne C. Sinkford	First female dean of a dental school.
1991	Geraldine T. Morrow	First female president of the American Dental Association.

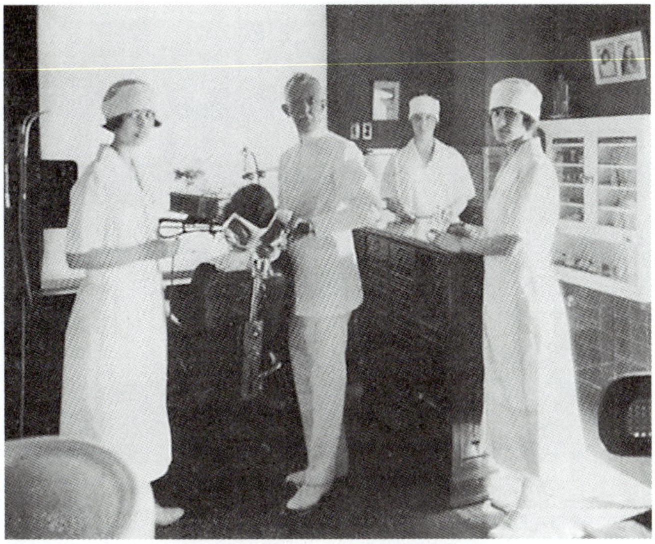

Fig. 1-9 **C. Edmund Kells and his "working unit," about 1900. Assistant on the left is keeping cold air on the cavity, while assistant on the right mixes materials and "secretary" records details.** (From Kells CE: *The dentist's own book,* St Louis, 1925, Mosby.)

(Fig. 1-9). In 1885 the first "lady assistant" was really a "lady in attendance" who made it respectable for a woman patient to visit a dental office unaccompanied. The assistant helped with office duties, and by 1900, Kells was working with both a chairside dental assistant and a secretarial assistant. Soon other dentists saw the value of dental assistants and began to train dental assistants in their own offices.

In 1930 a curriculum committee was formed to draft courses of training to be used as educational guides. In 1948 the Certifying Board of the American Dental Assistants Association was established (now the Dental Assisting National Board, DANB). By 1950, there were one- and two-year programs for dental-assisting education.

History of Dental Hygiene

The first person to become a dental hygienist was **Irene Newman,** a dental assistant in Bridgeport, Connecticut, in the early 1900s. At that time a dentist, **Alfred C. Fones,** believed that women could be trained to provide preventive services and thus give the dentist time to provide more complex procedures. Dr. Fones trained Irene Newman in dental hygiene and then developed a school for dental hygienists in 1913 (Fig. 1-10). The school exists today as the University of Bridgeport, Fones School of Dental Hygiene.

Dental Accreditation

By 1900 the profession of dentistry had become well established, and dental schools were being developed across the country (Fig. 1-11). The educational requirements for dentists, dental hygienists, and dental assistants have increased dramatically over the years.

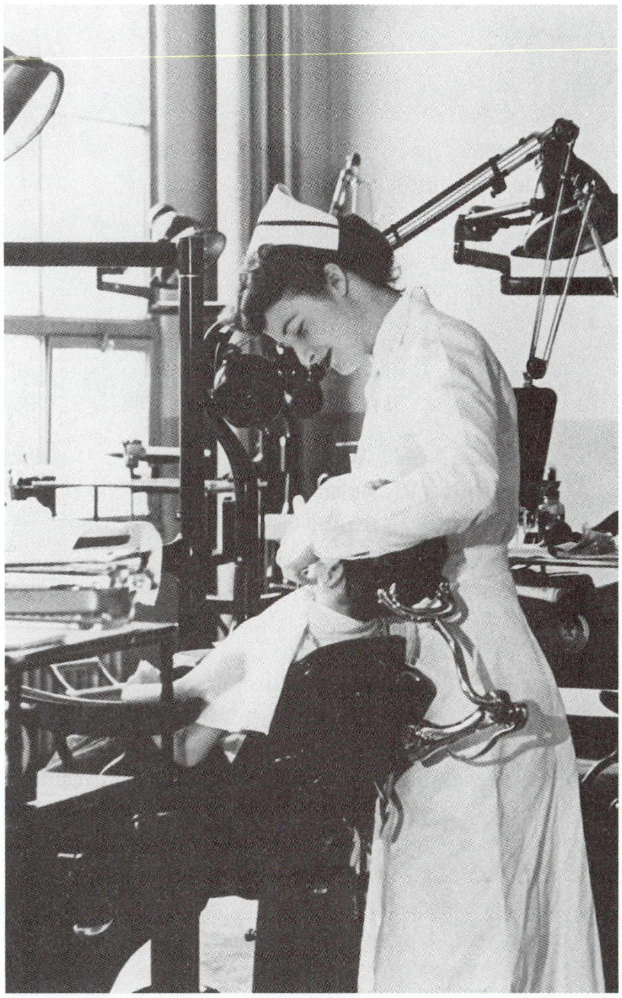

Fig. 1-10 **Dental hygienist during the 1960s working in a standing position.** (From Daniel SJ, Harfst SA: *Mosby's dental hygiene: concepts, cases, and competencies*–2004 update. St. Louis, 2004, Mosby; Courtesy Fr. Edward J. Dowling, S.J. Marine Historical Collection, University of Detroit, Mercy, Detroit.)

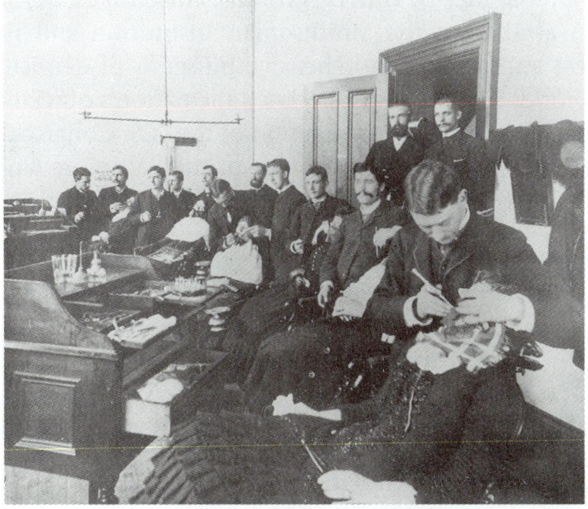

Fig. 1-11 **Dental students at University of California San Francisco, School of Dentistry treat patients in the dental clinic in the early 1900s.** (Courtesy University of California San Francisco, School of Dentistry.)

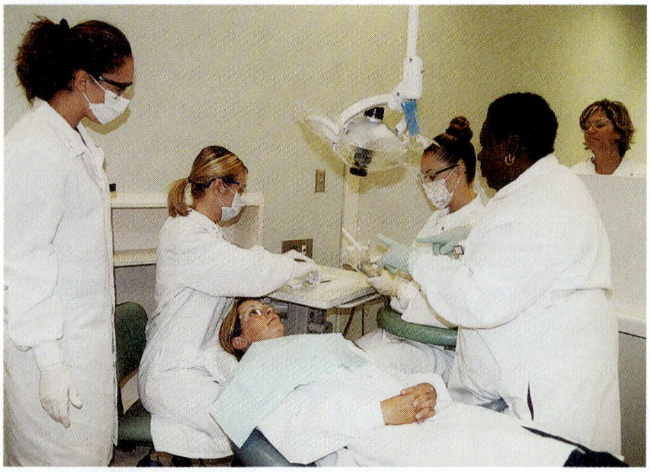

Fig. 1-12 Modern dental-assisting students practicing chairside skills with their instructor in an accredited dental-assisting program.

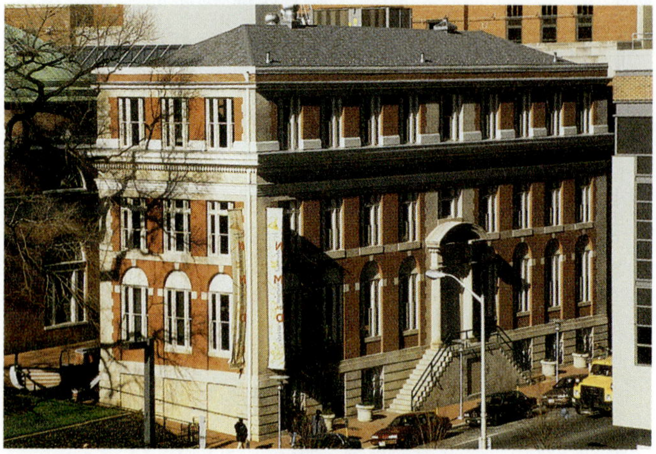

Fig. 1-13 Dr. Samuel D. Harris National Museum of Dentistry. (Courtesy National Museum of Dentistry, Baltimore, Maryland.)

Today, the **Commission on Dental Accreditation of the American Dental Association** is responsible for the evaluation and accreditation of dental educational programs in the United States. These include graduate dental programs, postgraduate specialty programs, and residency programs for dentists. The Commission also sets standards for educational programs in dental assisting, dental hygiene, and dental laboratory technology.

To maintain accreditation status, schools are reviewed every seven years through a comprehensive self-study and a visit by members of an accreditation team. The accreditation process provides assurance to the students and the public that the program continues to meet the high standards set forth by the dental profession (Fig. 1-12).

National Museum of Dentistry

The **Dr. Samuel D. Harris National Museum of Dentistry** is an affiliate of the Smithsonian Institution and is the largest and most comprehensive museum of dentistry in the world. In 2003 it was declared the nation's official dental museum by a joint resolution of the U.S. Congress. The museum is built on the grounds of the Baltimore College of Dental Surgery in Baltimore, Maryland, the world's first dental college. The museum's name honors Dr. Samuel D. Harris, a retired pediatric dentist who in 1992 was instrumental in founding the museum (Fig. 1-13).

The museum provides many interactive exhibits, historic artifacts, and engaging educational programs. The visitors learn about the heritage and future of dentistry, achievements of dental professionals, and the importance of oral health in a healthy life. To obtain more information, visit the web site: http://www.dentalmuseum.umaryland.edu/.

Recall

16. Who was the first dentist to use a dental assistant?
17. Who founded dental hygiene education in America?
18. Who was the first woman in the world to graduate from dental school?
19. Who was the first African-American female dentist in the United States?
20. Where is the Dr. Samuel D. Harris National Museum of Dentistry located?

LEGAL AND ETHICAL IMPLICATIONS

The public views the profession of dentistry with respect and trust. As important members of the oral healthcare profession, dental assistants should remember the trials and errors, the struggles, and the contributions made over the years to advance the dental profession.

Remember, to learn we must stand on the shoulders of those before us.

Eye to the Future

History shows that humans have always tried to improve the appearance of their teeth, and to end dental pain and tooth loss. Artificial teeth that were once made from wood or ivory are now created from highly esthetic porcelain. Once-painful dental treatments are now accomplished virtually pain free. Advances in equipment design, dental materials, anesthesia, and diagnostic techniques have made modern dentistry a more exact science.

These are especially interesting, challenging, and exciting times to be entering the dental healthcare profession.

Critical Thinking

1. What would you say to a 50-year-old patient who was reluctant to come to the dentist because of his negative experiences in the dental office as a child?
2. What would you tell the mother of a child who thinks dental decay began when soft drinks and candy were discovered?
3. Historically, who can be role models for young women today who face discrimination in their career choices?
4. What would you say to someone who does not understand why you are studying the history of dentistry?
5. Why is the Hippocratic Oath important today?

2

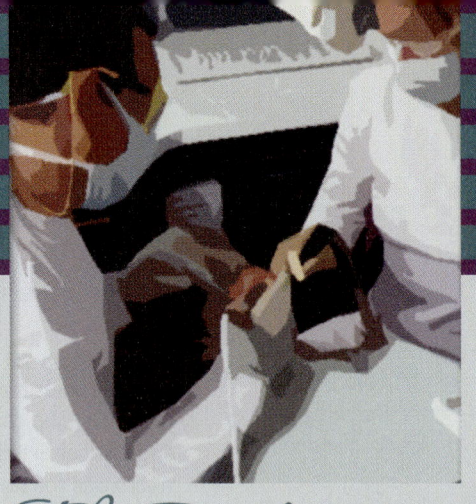

The Professional Dental Assistant

Outline

KEY TERMS

American Dental Assistants Association (ADAA) Professional organization that represents the profession of dental assisting.

Certified dental assistant (CDA) The nationally recognized credential of the dental assistant who has passed the DANB certification examination and keeps up current practice through continuing education.

Dental Assisting National Board (DANB) National agency responsible for administering the certification examination and issuing the credential of certified dental assistant.

HIPAA The Health Insurance Portability and Accountability Act of 1996 specifies federal regulations ensuring privacy regarding a patient's health-care information.

Professional Person who meets the standards of a profession.

LEARNING OUTCOMES

On completion of this chapter, the student will be able to achieve the following objectives:

- Pronounce, define, and spell the Key Terms.
- Discuss the concept of professionalism.
- Demonstrate the characteristics of a professional dental assistant.
- Demonstrate the personal qualities of a professional dental assistant.
- Describe the role and purpose of the American Dental Assistants Association (ADAA).
- Describe the benefits of membership in the ADAA.
- Describe the role of the Dental Assisting National Board (DANB).
- Explain where to obtain information about the DANB.
- Identify the purpose of the Health Insurance Portability and Accountability Act of 1996 (HIPAA).

A highly skilled dental assistant is a vital member of the dental healthcare team. Reducing patient anxiety, making decisions, simplifying treatment procedures, and improving the quality of patient care are all part of a dental assistant's day (Fig. 2-1).

You chose an exciting and challenging career when you decided to become a professional dental assistant. A career in dental assisting offers variety, job satisfaction, opportunity for service, and financial reward. It is a career that requires dedication, personal responsibility, integrity, and a commitment to continuing education.

CHARACTERISTICS OF A PROFESSIONAL DENTAL ASSISTANT

Becoming a dental assistant is more than acquiring the knowledge and developing the skills necessary to perform a variety of duties. Becoming a dental assistant is about becoming a **professional.**

Professionalism is an attitude that is apparent in everything you do and say, in and out of the dental office. Professionalism is what distinguishes people who "have a job" from those who "pursue a career." The public's expectations of healthcare workers are higher than expectations of individuals in other occupations. The dental assistant must demonstrate patience and compassion when communicating with patients and other team members. When you demonstrate your professionalism, you receive respect and acknowledgment from your colleagues and patients as a valued member of the dental healthcare team.

Professional Appearance

When the dental assistant has a professional appearance, it promotes the patient's confidence in the entire office and improves his or her dental experience. The essential aspects of a professional appearance are (1) good health, (2) good grooming, and (3) appropriate dress.

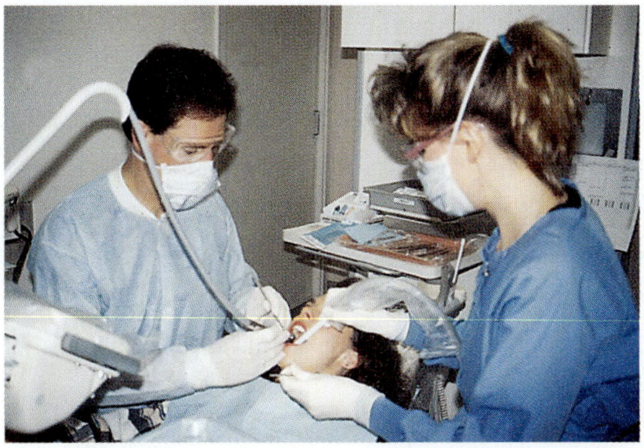

Fig. 2-1 The dental assistant is an important member of the dental healthcare team.

Guidelines for a Professional Appearance

- Uniform or scrubs should be clean, pressed, and in good repair.*
- Shoes and laces should be clean and in good condition.*
- Hair should be styled so that it stays out of your face.*
- Jewelry should be avoided.*
- Fingernails should be clean and short.*
- Artificial fingernails should not be worn; they can harbor bacteria.*
- Perfumes and body scents should not be worn.
- Tobacco products should not be used.
- Makeup should be subtle and natural.
- Avoid tattoos, body piercings, bright fingernail polish, and extreme hairdos.
- Bathe each day and use deodorant.
- Maintain good oral hygiene.

*Special implications for infection control and prevention of disease transmission.

To stay in *good health,* you must get an adequate amount of rest, eat well-balanced meals, and exercise enough to keep fit. Dental assisting is a physically demanding profession.

Good grooming requires paying attention to the details of your personal appearance. Personal cleanliness involves taking a daily bath or shower, using a deodorant, and practicing good oral hygiene. Do not use perfume or cologne. You are working in very close personal proximity to coworkers and patients who may be allergic to or irritated by some scents. Avoid the use of tobacco products because the odor lingers on your hair and clothing, and is offensive in a professional setting.

Appropriate dress involves wearing clothing appropriate for the type of position in which the dental assistant is working (see Chapter 3). Regardless of the type of professional wear, it must be clean, wrinkle-free, and worn over appropriate undergarments (Fig. 2-2). In any dental position, excessive makeup and jewelry are not considered appropriate for a professional appearance. Infection-control requirements must also be considered when selecting clinical wear (see Chapter 19).

Recall

1. Name the three essential aspects of a professional appearance.

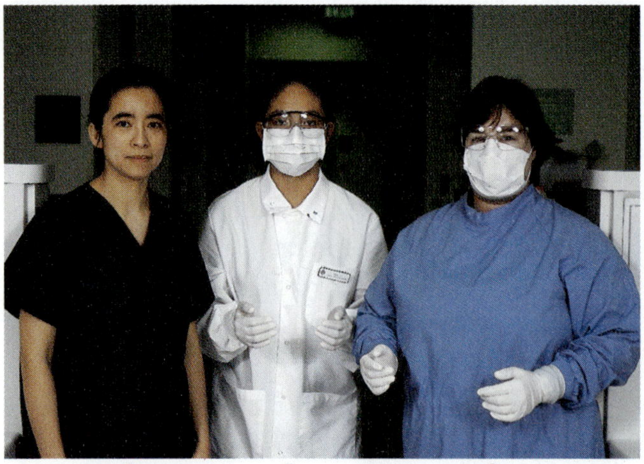

Fig. 2-2 The professional dental assistant's attire may vary depending on the duties performed. **A,** Scrubs are acceptable at times. **B,** Full personal protective wear is indicated for chairside procedures. **C,** Surgical gowns may be indicated for surgery or hospital dentistry.

Knowledge and Skills

Depending on the type of dental practice, the duties of a dental assistant will vary. Ideally, dental assistants should have both front-desk and chairside (clinical) skills. This is very convenient when a team member is absent from the office. Generally, dental assistants will choose to stay in the position they prefer. Regardless of the type of dental practice, the day of a dental assistant is never boring or "routine."

Teamwork

Teamwork is extremely important in a dental office. The letters in the word *team* mean that "Together, Everyone Accomplishes More." Dental assistants should offer to do an absent colleague's work and should be willing to help coworkers when other tasks are completed. When there are several assistants in an office, each should be able and willing to substitute for the others in an emergency.

Many Roles of Dental Assistants

Chairside dental assistant

Works directly with the dentist in the treatment area. Primary responsibilities in this role include, but are not limited to, the following:

- Seating and preparing for patients
- Charting
- Instituting infection-control procedures
- Mixing and passing dental materials
- Assisting the dentist during procedures
- Ensuring patient comfort
- Exposing and processing radiographs
- Pouring and trimming models, as well as performing other laboratory procedures
- Providing patient education
- Providing postoperative instructions to patients
- Overseeing inventory control, and ordering dental supplies
- Ensuring compliance with OSHA regulations

Expanded-functions dental assistant

Delegation of the following functions varies among states, depending on the individual state's dental practice act:

- Placing dental sealants
- Taking impressions
- Fabricating temporary crowns and bridges
- Placing retraction cord

Expanded-functions dental assistant–cont'd

- Applying fluoride
- Applying topical anesthetic
- Placing and removing dental dams
- Placing and removing matrices and wedges
- Applying liners, varnishes, and bases
- Placing, carving, and finishing amalgam or composite restorations
- Removing sutures
- Placing and removing periodontal dressings
- Performing additional functions as specified in the dental practice act of the state in which the dental assistant is employed. It is important to be aware of the laws of the state in which you practice.

Administrative assistant

Also known as the *secretarial assistant, business assistant,* or *receptionist.* The administrative assistant is responsible for the efficient operation of the business office, including the following duties:

- Greeting patients and answering the phone
- Scheduling patient visits
- Managing patient records
- Managing accounts receivable and accounts payable
- Managing the recall system
- Maintaining privacy of patient information
- Overseeing and monitoring practice marketing activities

Attitude

Patients, coworkers, and employers appreciate the dental assistant who has a good attitude. It is important to show a willingness to get along by avoiding criticism of others, showing appreciation for what others have done, and being willing to pitch in and help. The dental office can be a stressful place for patients and staff, so it is important to maintain a positive attitude.

Dedication

Professional dental assistants are dedicated to their dental practice, their patients, and the profession of dental assisting. Dedication is possible only if the assistant truly cares for people, is empathetic to their needs, and maintains a positive attitude.

Responsibility and Initiative

The dental assistant can demonstrate work responsibility by (1) arriving on time, (2) staying for the full shift, (3) being a cooperative team member, and (4) not asking to leave early. Assistants should understand what is expected in their regular job and, if time permits, should volunteer to help others who may be overworked.

You can show a willingness to learn additional skills by asking questions and observing others. Show initiative by finding tasks to perform without being asked. Show responsibility by calling the office when you are ill or unavoidably late. *Do not* discuss your personal problems in the dental office with either your patients or other staff members.

Recall

2. How can you show that you are a responsible person?

Confidentiality

Everything that is said or done in the dental office must remain confidential. Dental assistants have access to a vast amount of personal and financial information about their patients. Such information must be held in strict confidence and must not be discussed with others. Breaches of confidentiality can result in lawsuits against all parties involved.

You cannot reveal the identity of a patient or any information from his or her records without the patient's written consent. *Never* discuss patients with anyone outside the dental office.

Check Your Personal Qualities as a Dental Assistant

How do I interact with patients?

- Am I friendly? Do I have a pleasant attitude?
- Do I listen more than I talk?
- Am I courteous?
- Am I considerate, respectful, and kind?
- Do I control my temper?
- Do I try to see the other person's point of view?

Am I responsible?

- Am I dependable?
- Am I attentive to details?
- Am I calm in an emergency?
- Am I responsible for my own actions?
- Do I tend to blame others or find fault with others?
- Do I offer to help others without being asked?
- Do I avoid office gossip?

There is a new set of federal privacy laws called **HIPAA** (Health Insurance Portability and Accountability Act of 1996). These new laws affect all types of healthcare providers regarding methods that must be taken to ensure that patient privacy is protected while health information is shared among healthcare providers. You will learn the details of these new laws in Chapter 63.

Personal Qualities

Most people do not enjoy a visit to the dentist, and many are stressed or intimidated. The dental assistant must (1) demonstrate sensitivity to the patient's needs, (2) show empathy, (3) say "the right thing at the right time," and (4) *be sincere.*

Again, avoid discussing aspects of your personal life with your patients. By learning to be a good listener, you will develop sensitivity for the opinions and concerns of others. It is nearly impossible to build *rapport* (good relations) with the patients in your office if they do not trust you.

PROFESSIONAL ORGANIZATIONS

American Dental Assistants Association

The **American Dental Assistants Association (ADAA)** is the organization that represents the profession of dental assisting. The ADAA was formed in 1924 by **Juliette A. Southard** (Fig. 2-3). Her vision was of "an educated, efficient dental assistant with her own place in the profession of dentistry."

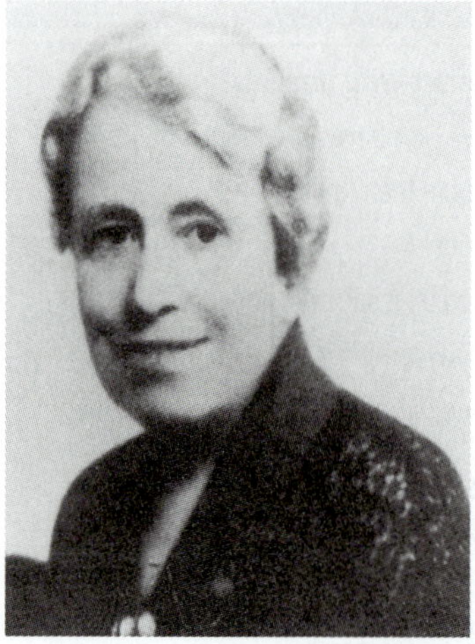

Fig. 2-3 Juliette A. Southard, founder of the ADAA. (Courtesy ADAA.)

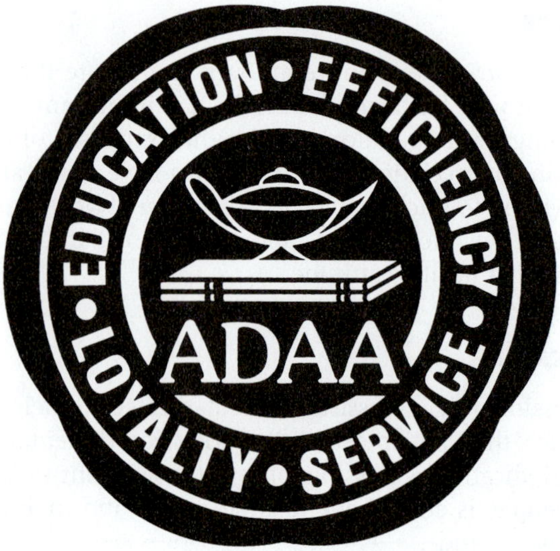

Fig. 2-4 The ADAA seal. (Courtesy ADAA.)

ADAA Mission Statement

To advance the careers of dental assistants and to promote the dental-assisting profession in matters of education, legislation, credentialing, and professional activities that enhance the delivery of quality dental healthcare to the public.

The ADAA is a national nonprofit corporation based in Chicago. Membership is *tripartite,* which means when you join the ADAA, you become a member of (1) the state component, (2) the local component, and (3) the national organization (Fig. 2-4).

By becoming a member of the ADAA, dental assistants can be proactive and take leadership positions within organized dentistry and the healthcare profession.

Benefits of Membership

By joining the ADAA, you can grow personally and professionally and keep abreast of legislative issues and current information. ADAA members have the opportunity to attend local, state, and national meetings, where they can participate in workshops, earn continuing education credit, hear prominent speakers, and establish lifelong friendships with other dental assistants.

Other benefits of membership include a subscription to *The Dental Assistant,* the journal of the ADAA; professional liability, accidental death and dismemberment, and medical insurance options; awards and scholarships; membership loan program; credit card options; and other discounts. Student membership is available for those enrolled in formal training programs.

Where to Obtain More Information: ADAA

American Dental Assistants Association
35 East Wacker Drive, Suite 1730
Chicago, IL 60601-2211
Phone: 312-541-1550
Fax: 312-541-1496
www.dentalassistant.org

Participating in ADAA activities develops your "people skills" and teaches leadership. You can influence the future of your profession and show that you are serious about your career.

Recall

3. What is the purpose of the ADAA?

Dental Assisting National Board

The **Dental Assisting National Board (DANB)** is the national agency responsible for testing dental assistants and issuing the credential of **certified dental assistant (CDA).** The DANB operates independently from the American Dental Association and the ADAA. Certification is a voluntary credential and is not mandatory in all states, although some states require a dental assistant to be a CDA to legally perform specific "expanded functions" within the state.

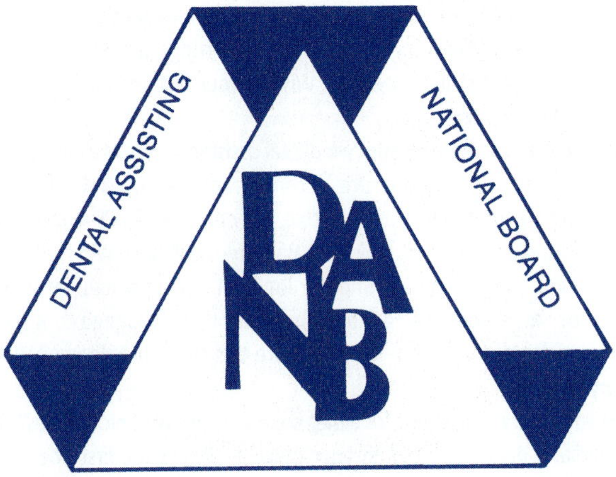

Fig. 2-5 Official logo of the DANB. (Courtesy DANB.)

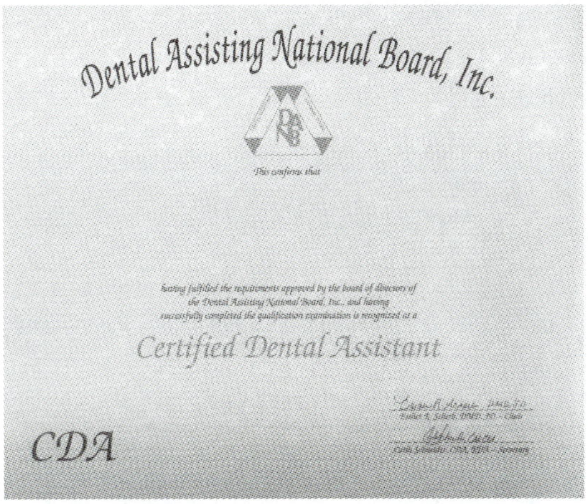

Fig. 2-6 Official certificate of CDA. (Courtesy DANB.)

By becoming DANB-certified, dental assistants demonstrate their commitment to excellence. In addition, a CDA in the dental office promotes the image of professionalism.

In order for dental assistants to teach in an ADA-accredited dental-assisting program, they must be currently certified by the DANB.

Certified Dental Assistant

To become a certified dental assistant (CDA), an assistant must take and pass a national written examination administered by the DANB. Successful completion of the DANB examination entitles the assistant to use the CDA credential, wear the official certification pin (Fig. 2-5), and display the CDA certificate (Fig. 2-6). The DANB examination consists of three major categories: radiology, infection control, and general chairside. The applicant must pass all three categories in order to become a CDA.

To remain currently certified, the CDA must complete a specified number of continuing education hours and pay a renewal fee each year.

Specialty Certification

For those dental assistants who are not in a general dentistry practice, the DANB also offers specialized certification, including *certified dental practice management administrator* (CDPMA) and *certified orthodontic assistant* (COA) (Box 2-1).

Recall

4. What credential is issued by the DANB?

5. Where can you obtain additional information about the DANB?

Box 2-1 Summary of Dental Assisting National Board Eligibility Pathways

Pathway I

Graduation from a dental-assisting or dental hygiene program accredited by the ADA Commission on Dental Accreditation *and*

Cardiopulmonary resuscitation (CPR) certification earned within 2 years prior to the examination date on which application is being made.

Pathway II

High school graduation or equivalent *and*

Minimum of two (2) years full-time work experience (at least 3500 hours accumulated over a 24-month period) as a dental assistant verified by dentist-employer *or*

At least 3500 hours of a combination of full- and part-time or only part-time work experience earned over a minimum of 24 months and a maximum of 48 months as a dental assistant verified by dentist-employer *and*

Cardiopulmonary resuscitation (CPR) certification earned within 2 years prior to the examination date on which application is being made.

Pathway III

Status as a current or previous DANB CDA or graduation from a DDS or DMD program accredited by the ADA or foreign dental degree program *and*

Cardiopulmonary resuscitation (CPR) certification earned within 2 years prior to the examination date for which application is being made.

From *DANB 2004 Candidate Guide,* Dental Assisting National Board, Inc., 2004.

Where to Obtain More Information: DANB

Dental Assisting National Board
676 North St. Clair Street, Suite 1880
Chicago, IL 60611
Phone: 800-FOR-DANB or 312-642-3368
Fax: 312-642-1475
www.danb.org

Eye to the Future

In the past, dentists were able to handle their practices with only one dental assistant. As times have changed, so has the practice of dentistry. The increased demand for dental care and the shortage of dental professionals have created more opportunities for qualified dental assistants. The current demand for educationally qualified dental assistants is at an all-time high. Employment opportunities are abundant and extremely varied. The future is promising and challenging for the educationally qualified dental assistant.

Critical Thinking

1. Imagine yourself as a nervous dental patient entering the dental office to have your wisdom teeth extracted. The dental assistant who greets you has long red artificial fingernails, dangling earrings, a tattoo on her arm, and long hair over her shoulders. What is your first impression of the office and the dentist?
2. Dr. Barrientos is interviewing two dental assistants for a chairside position in his new office. Both are recent graduates of a local dental-assisting program. Both seem capable, but only one is a CDA and a member of ADAA. Who do you think Dr. Barrientos will hire? Why?
3. While you and a friend are having lunch at a local restaurant, you remember an embarrassing but funny event that happened to a patient in your dental office. You want to share this story, but do you? Why or why not?
4. Do you have a preference for either administrative or clinical duties? Why?
5. Claudia, a dental assistant in your office, is always the first one out the door at 5 PM. You always stay and finish up, but you are tired of Claudia's irresponsible behavior. How do you handle this situation?

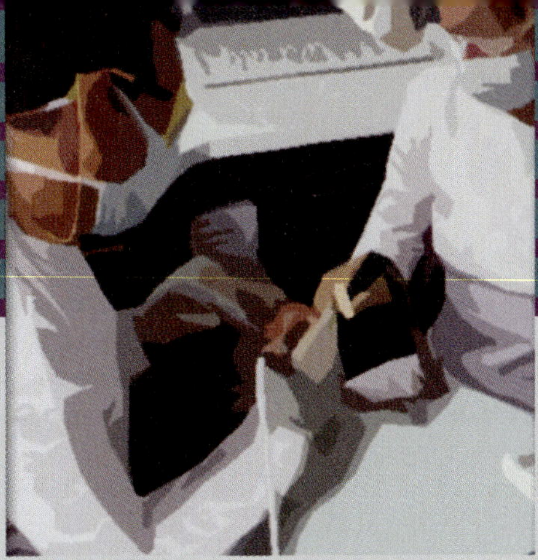

3 The Dental Healthcare Team

Outline

Dentist
Dental Specialists
Registered Dental Hygienist
Dental Assistant
- Clinical Dental Assistant
- Sterilization Assistant
- Expanded-Functions Dental Assistant
- Business Assistant

Dental Laboratory Technician
Supporting Services
Legal and Ethical Implications
Eye to the Future
Critical Thinking

KEY TERMS

Certified dental technician A dental laboratory technician who has passed a written national examination and who performs dental laboratory services such as fabricating crowns, bridges, and dentures, as specified by the dentist's written prescription.

Dental assistant Oral healthcare professional trained to provide supportive procedures to the dentist and patients.

Dental equipment technician Specialist who installs and maintains dental equipment.

Dental hygienist (hy-**jen**-ist) Licensed oral healthcare professional who provides preventive, therapeutic, and educational services.

Dental laboratory technician Professional who performs dental laboratory services such as fabricating crowns, bridges, and dentures, as specified by the dentist's written prescription. Most frequently trained on the job as apprentices.

Dental public health Specialty that promotes oral health through organized community efforts.

Dental spa A new trend in dentistry that treats patients to a variety of amenities, including massages and herbal masks, in a spalike atmosphere.

Dental supply person Representative of a dental supply company who provides dental supplies, product information, services, and repairs.

Dentist Oral healthcare provider licensed to practice dentistry.

Detail person Representative of a specific company who provides information concerning the company's product.

Endodontics (*en*-do-**don**-tiks) Dental specialty that diagnoses and treats diseases of the pulp.

Oral and maxillofacial radiology (*ray*-dee-**ol**-o-gee) Dental specialty that deals with the diagnosis of disease through various forms of imaging, including x-ray films (radiographs).

Oral and maxillofacial surgery (mak-*sil*-o-**fay**-shul) Dental surgical specialty that diagnoses and treats conditions of the mouth, face, upper jaw (maxilla), and associated areas.

Oral pathology (pa-**thol**-o-gee) Dental specialty that diagnoses and treats diseases of the oral structures.

Orthodontics (orth-o-**don**-tiks) Specialty within dentistry that focuses on preventing, intercepting, and correcting skeletal and dental problems.

Pediatric dentistry (pee-dee-**a**-trik) Dental specialty concerned with neonatal through adolescent patients as well as patients with special needs in these age groups.

Periodontics (*per*-ee-oh-**dahn**-tiks) Dental specialty involved with the diagnosis and treatment of diseases of the supporting tissues.

Prosthodontics (*pros*-tho-**don**-tiks) Dental specialty that provides restoration and replacement of natural teeth.

LEARNING OUTCOMES

On completion of this chapter, the student will be able to achieve the following objectives:

- Pronounce, define, and spell the Key Terms.
- Name the members of the dental healthcare team and describe their roles.
- Identify the minimal educational requirements for each member of the dental healthcare team.
- Describe the supportive services provided by other members of the dental healthcare team.
- Describe the various roles and responsibilities of a dental assistant.
- Name and describe each of the recognized dental specialties.

The purpose of the dental healthcare team is to provide quality oral healthcare for the patients in the practice. The **dentist** is the individual who is legally responsible for the care of the patients and the supervision of all other members of the team. The dentist is often referred to as the leader of the team.

The dental healthcare team consists of the following:

- Dentist (general dentist or specialist)
- Dental assistant (clinical, expanded functions, business)
- Dental hygienist
- Dental laboratory technician

Roles and Responsibilities of Dental Healthcare Team Members

Dentist or dental specialist

- Is legally responsible for the care of the patient.
- Assesses the patient's oral health needs as related to physical and emotional well-being.
- Uses up-to-date diagnostic skills.
- Uses current techniques and skills in all aspects of patient care.
- Provides legally required supervision for dental auxiliaries.

Clinical dental assistant (chairside assistant, circulating assistant)

- Seats and prepares patients.
- Maintains and prepares treatment rooms and instruments.
- Assists dentist at chairside during patient treatment.
- Prepares and delivers dental materials.
- Provides postoperative patient instructions.
- Oversees infection-control program.
- Performs radiographic procedures.
- Performs basic laboratory procedures (e.g., pouring impressions to create diagnostic casts).
- Provides assurance and support for the patient.

Expanded-functions dental assistant

- Performs only those intraoral (inside mouth) procedures that are legal in the state in which the EFDA practices.
- Check with your state board of dentistry for a current listing of dental assistant duties.

Dental hygienist

- Assesses the periodontal status of patients, including measurement of the depth of periodontal pockets and conditions of the oral tissues.
- Performs dental prophylaxis (e.g., removal of plaque from crowns and root surfaces).
- Performs scaling and root-planing procedures.
- Exposes, processes, and evaluates the quality of radiographs.
- Performs additional procedures, such as administration of local anesthetic and administration of nitrous oxide if allowed by the state.

Business assistant (administrative assistant, secretarial assistant, receptionist)

- Greets patients and answers the phone.
- Makes and confirms appointments.
- Manages patient records, payroll, insurance billing, and financial arrangements.
- Ensures that patient privacy measures are in place and followed.
- Oversees patient relations.

Dental laboratory technician

- Performs laboratory work only under licensed dentist's prescription.
- Constructs and repairs prosthetic devices (e.g., full and partial dentures).
- Constructs restorations (e.g., crowns, bridges, inlays, veneers).

DENTIST

The dentist trained in the United States must graduate from a dental university approved by the Commission on Dental Accreditation of the American Dental Association. Most dentists also have an undergraduate degree before being admitted to a dental university. Dental education programs usually last 4 academic years.

The training in the dental university includes dental sciences and intensive clinical practice on patients in the university's clinic. When dentists graduate from a dental university, they are awarded either the *Doctor of Dental Surgery* (DDS) or the *Doctor of Medical Dentistry* (DMD), depending on which dental school they attended. Before going into practice, all dentists must pass a *written* national board examination. Dentists are then required to take a *clinical* board examination in the state in which they choose to practice.

Dentists have a variety of practice options available to them. Some will choose to practice alone, some may choose to have a practice partner, and others may enter a large group practice. Other options for dentists include the military, public health, community clinics, research, teaching, or returning to school for specialty training.

Although a general dentist is trained and legally permitted to perform all dental functions, many dentists prefer to refer more difficult cases to specialists who have advanced training in certain areas. Most dentists are members of their professional organization, the *American Dental Association (ADA)*.

DENTAL SPECIALISTS

The ADA recognizes nine specialties. Depending on the type of specialty, the additional education to become a specialist varies from two to six years. Most dentists who are specialists will also belong to a professional organization for their specialty in addition to membership in the ADA.

Recall

1. Name the members of the dental healthcare team.
2. Name the nine dental specialties.

Dental Specialties Recognized by the American Dental Association

1. **Dental public health** involves developing policies at county, state, and national levels for programs to control and prevent disease. Examples include dental public health professionals involved with fluoridation issues, community oral health education, and Head Start programs. Dental public health also includes dental screenings within a community to assess the needs of the community. In dental public health, the community is the patient rather than the individual.
2. **Endodontics** involves the cause, diagnosis, prevention, and treatment of diseases and injuries of the pulp and associated structures. The common term for much of the treatment is *root canal.* The specialist is an *endodontist.* (See Chapter 54.)
3. **Oral and maxillofacial radiology** became the first new dental specialty in 36 years when it was granted recognition by the ADA in 1999. The *dental radiologist* uses new and sophisticated imaging techniques to locate tumors and infectious diseases of the jaws, head, and neck, and assists in the diagnosis of patients with trauma and temporomandibular disorders. (See Chapter 42.)
4. **Oral and maxillofacial surgery** involves the diagnosis and surgical treatment of diseases, injuries, and defects of the oral and maxillofacial regions. It involves much more than tooth extractions. The specialist is an *oral and maxillofacial surgeon.* (See Chapter 56.)
5. **Oral pathology** involves the nature of diseases affecting the oral cavity and adjacent structures. A major function is to perform biopsies and work closely with oral surgeons to provide a diagnosis. The specialist is an *oral pathologist.* (See Chapter 17.)
6. **Orthodontics** involves the diagnosis, treatment, and prevention of malocclusions of the teeth and associated structures. This specialty entails much more than fitting of braces. The specialist is an *orthodontist.* (See Chapter 60.)
7. **Pediatric dentistry** involves the oral healthcare of children from birth to adolescence. The *pediatric dentist* often treats children with emotional and behavioral problems. (See Chapter 57.)
8. **Periodontics** involves the diagnosis and treatment of diseases of the oral tissues supporting and surrounding the teeth. The specialist is a *periodontist.* (See Chapter 55.)
9. **Prosthodontics** involves the restoration and replacement of natural teeth with artificial constructs such as crowns, bridges, and dentures. The specialist is a *prosthodontist.* (See Chapters 50, 52, and 53.)

REGISTERED DENTAL HYGIENIST

Generally, a *registered dental hygienist (RDH)* removes deposits on the teeth, exposes radiographs, places topical fluoride and dental sealants, and provides patients with home care instructions (Fig. 3-1). The duties delegated to the dental hygienist vary from state to state. In many states, dental hygienists are allowed to administer local anesthesia. It is important for dental hygienists to have a thorough understanding of the laws of the state in which they practice. There are employment opportunities for dental hygienists in private and specialty dental offices, health clinics, school systems, research facilities, public health departments, educational programs, and marketing and sales of dental products.

The minimal education required for a dental hygienist is two academic years of college study and an associate degree in an ADA-accredited dental hygiene program. Dental hygiene is also offered in bachelor's and master's degree programs.

The RDH must pass both written national or regional board examinations and clinical state board examinations to be licensed by the state in which he or she plans to practice. In most states, the RDH is required to work under the supervision of a licensed dentist.

Dental hygienists may be members of their professional organization, the *American Dental Hygienists Association (ADHA)*. For additional information on dental hygiene, visit the website at http://www.adha.org.

Recall

3. What is the minimal length of education for dental hygiene licensure?

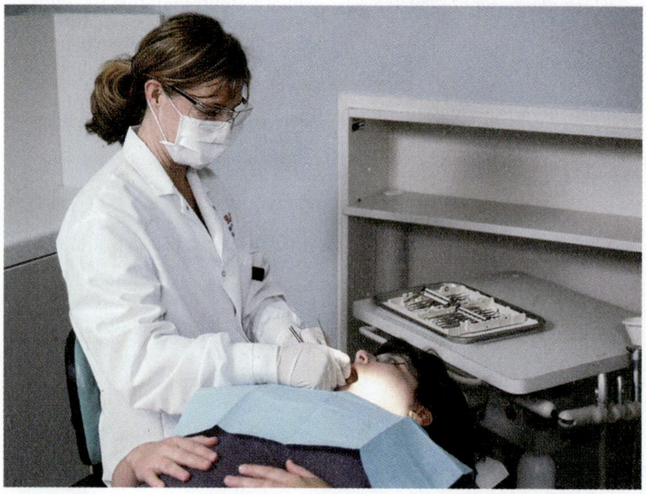

Fig. 3-1 Dental hygienist performing an oral prophylaxis.

DENTAL ASSISTANT

As an educationally qualified **dental assistant,** you will be able to assume many activities that do not require the professional skill and judgment of the dentist. However, the responsibilities assigned to you as a dental assistant are limited by the regulations of the dental practice act of the state in which you practice (see Chapter 5).

Although not all states require formal education for dental assistants, minimal standards for schools accredited by the Commission on Dental Accreditation require a program of approximately one academic year in length, conducted in a post–high-school educational institution. The curriculum must include didactic, laboratory, and clinical content. Dental assistants may also receive training at vocational schools or proprietary schools accredited through the state's Board of Dentistry.

As modern dentistry changes and procedures and techniques become more complex, the role of the dental assistant will continue to evolve. Many important and varied roles are available within dentistry for dental assistants. Each dental practice is unique and has specific needs, and the educationally qualified dental assistant is quick to adapt to new situations as the need arises.

Clinical Dental Assistant

The clinical dental assistant is directly involved in patient care. The role of the clinical dental assistant is usually defined as *chairside* or *circulating assistant.*

Chairside Assistant

The chairside assistant works primarily with the dentist who uses four-handed dentistry techniques. The term *four-handed dentistry* describes the seated dentist and chairside

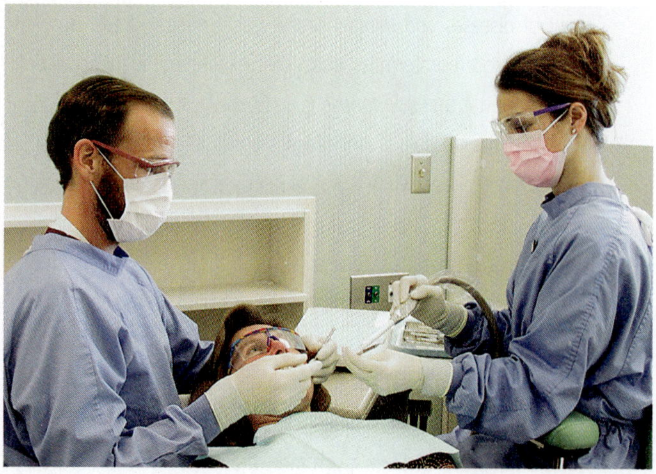

Fig. 3-2 Dentist and chairside dental assistant working together.

assistant working as an efficient team (Fig. 3-2). The chairside assistant mixes dental materials, exchanges instruments, and provides oral evacuation during dental procedures. An equally important role of the chairside dental assistant is to make the patient comfortable and relaxed.

Circulating Assistant

The circulating assistant serves as an extra pair of hands where needed throughout the clinical areas of the practice. This is referred to as *six-handed dentistry* (Fig. 3-3).

In many practices, the circulating assistant is responsible for seating and dismissing patients as well as preparing and caring for instruments and treatment rooms.

Sterilization Assistant

In many offices, the responsibility for sterilization procedures is delegated to a specific individual. In other offices, all dental assistants share this important responsibility. The sterilization assistant efficiently and safely processes all instruments and manages biohazard waste. Other responsibilities include weekly monitoring of sterilizers and maintenance of sterilization monitoring reports (Fig. 3-4). The sterilization assistant is also responsible for the selection of infection-control products and performing quality-assurance procedures (see Chapters 20 and 21).

Expanded-Functions Dental Assistant

An expanded-functions dental assistant (EFDA) has received additional training and is legally permitted to provide certain intraoral patient care procedures beyond the duties traditionally performed by a dental assistant (Fig. 3-5). Duties delegated to the EFDA vary according to the dental practice act in each state. It is important that a dental assistant only performs functions allowed by state law (see Chapter 5).

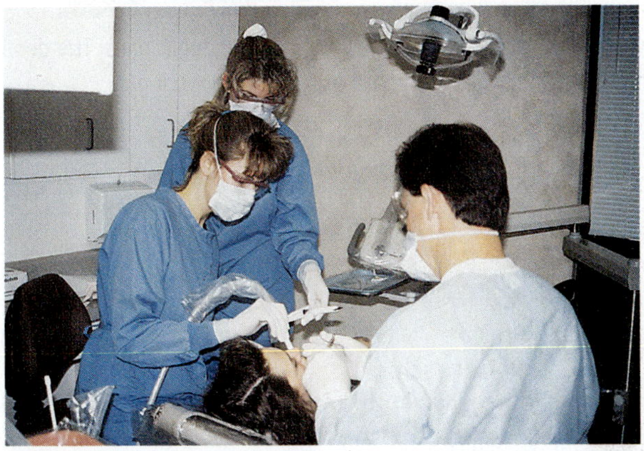

Fig. 3-3 Chairside dental assistant supported by a circulating dental assistant.

Business Assistant

Business assistants, also known as *administrative assistants, secretarial assistants,* and *receptionists,* are primarily responsible for the smooth and efficient operation of the business office (Fig. 3-6). Two or more assistants may work in the business area of a dental office. The duties of a business assistant include controlling appointments, communicating on the phone, coordinating financial arrangements with patients, and handling dental insurance claims. It is not uncommon for a chairside dental assistant to move into a business office position. It is very helpful when the individual at the desk has an excellent understanding of how the clinical practice functions.

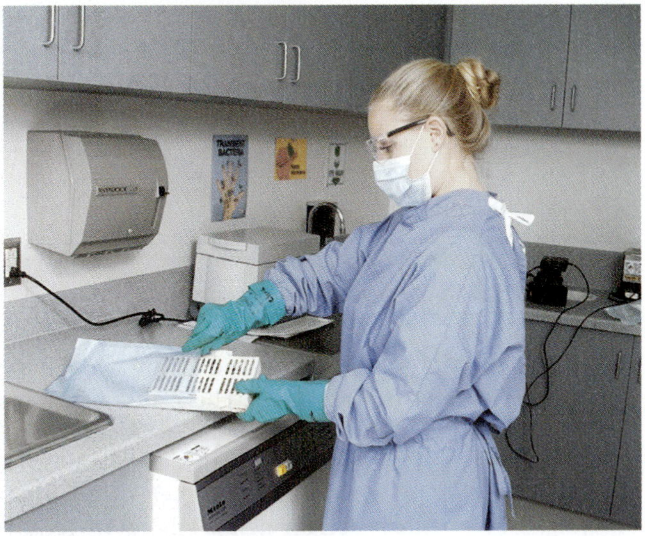

Fig. 3-4 A sterilization assistant is an important member of the team.

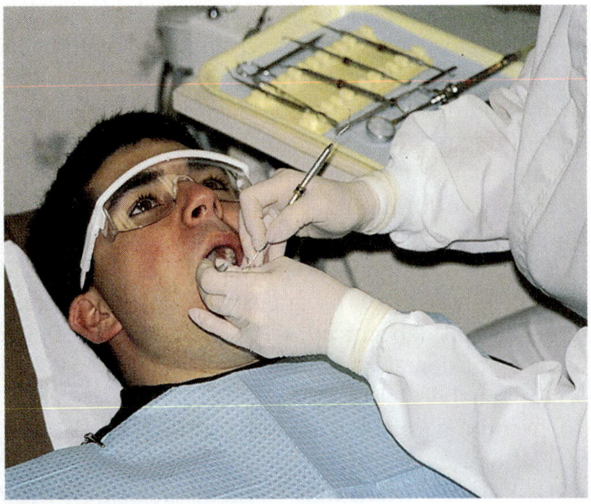

Fig. 3-5 EFDA removing excess cement. (Courtesy Pamela Landry, RDA.)

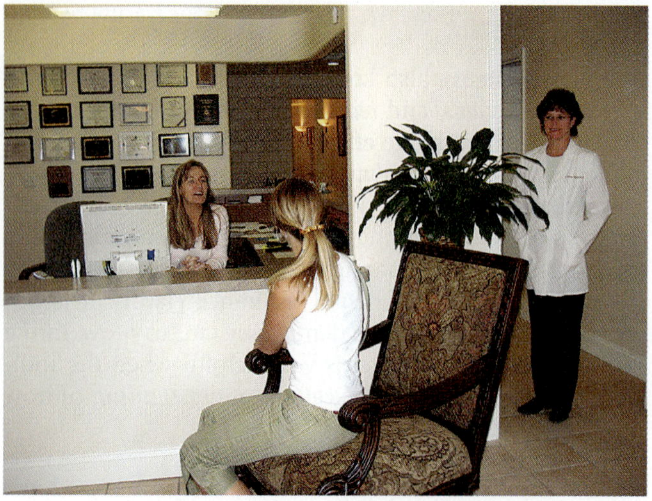

Fig. 3-6 A patient is greeted by the business assistant before meeting the dental hygienist. (Courtesy Dr. Peter Pang, Sonoma, California.)

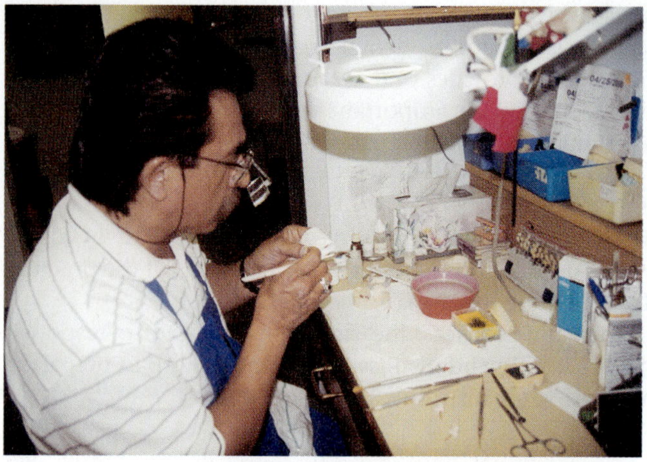

Fig. 3-7 Dental laboratory technician fabricating a crown.

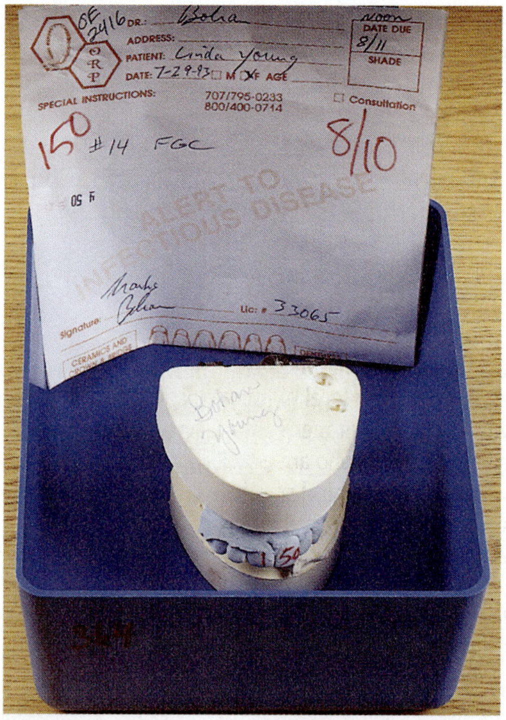

Fig. 3-8 Laboratory dental cases are stored in work pans. The dentist's written laboratory prescription is posted on the work pan.

DENTAL LABORATORY TECHNICIAN

The *dental laboratory technician* usually does not work in the dental office with the other team members, although some dental offices have "in-house" laboratories. Many dental technicians choose to be employed in private laboratories, and others choose to own and operate their own laboratory (Fig. 3-7). In either case, the dental laboratory technician may legally perform only those tasks specified by the *written prescription* of the dentist (Fig. 3-8). Dental technicians make crowns, bridges, and dentures from impressions taken by the dentist and sent to the dental laboratory. The dental assistant often communicates with the dental laboratory technician regarding the length of time needed to return a case, or to relay special instructions from the dentist about a case. It is important to have a good working relationship with the dental laboratory.

In most states, dental laboratory technicians are not required to have formal education. They can receive their training through apprenticeship, commercial schools, or ADA-accredited programs. Many have received their training in ADA-accredited programs that are two years in length. Dental laboratory technicians have extensive knowledge of dental anatomy and materials and also excellent manual dexterity.

To become a **certified dental technician (CDT),** the dental laboratory technician must pass a written examination. Dental technicians may be members of their professional organization, the *American Dental Laboratory Technician Association (ADLTA).*

Recall

4. What is the minimal length of education for an ADA-accredited dental-assisting program?
5. What is the minimal length of education for an ADA-accredited dental laboratory technician program?
6. What is required before a dental laboratory technician can perform a task?

SUPPORTING SERVICES

Often, people in these positions are former dental assistants, dental hygienists, or dental laboratory technicians. Although not official members of the dental healthcare team, the following individuals are important and provide necessary services and support to the dental office. The **dental supply person** is a representative from a dental supply company who routinely calls on dental offices. This person provides services such as taking orders for supplies, providing new product information, and helping to arrange for service and repairs. The dental supply person visits the dental office frequently.

The **detail person** is a representative of a *specific company,* often a drug or dental product manufacturer, who visits the dental office to provide the dentist with information concerning the specific company's product.

The **dental equipment technician** is a specialist who installs and maintains dental equipment. This service may be provided under a maintenance contract or on an as-needed basis. Sometimes, the dental supply person and the equipment technician work for the same company, and one phone call is all that is necessary.

Legal and Ethical Implications

There may be occasions when you will be asked to perform tasks that are beyond your level of training, or are illegal in your state. Always remember that there are many opportunities in the field of dentistry for those who are educationally qualified without having to sacrifice your ethical standards.

All truly successful dental health professionals have a passion for their profession and pride in the quality of care they deliver. You can demonstrate pride in your profession by becoming a member of your professional organization, the ADAA. A frequently quoted saying in dentistry is *"patients don't care how much you know, until they know how much you care."*

Eye to the Future

Because many people fear going to the dentist, a new trend in dentistry called **dental spas** is spreading across the country. Dental spas are most prevalent in cosmetic dental practices. To ease the patient's anxiety and avoid the sterile feel and smell of traditional dental offices, dental spas offer a soothing and peaceful atmosphere. Scented aromatherapy candles are often located throughout the office. A wide variety of amenities are offered in dental spas, including warm paraffin baths for the hands, massaging back pads, soft fleece blankets, assorted teas, and warm aromatherapy neck pillows. Each room often has its own cable television and a large selection of videos. At the end of the dental procedure, patients are offered a warm lemon-scented towel and a cool, refreshing bottle of water. Spa dentistry puts patients at ease during dental treatment. Whether spa dentistry is a fad or an emerging trend in dentistry remains to be seen.

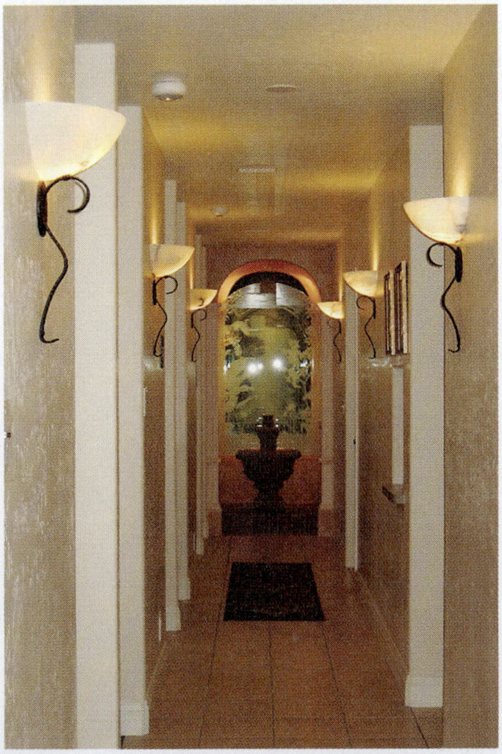

A

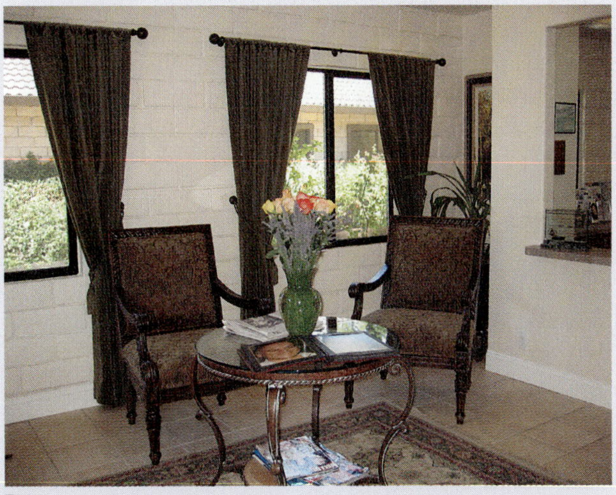

B

A, The entrance to the treatment areas of a modern dental spa-type office. **B,** The reception area of a modern dental spa-type office. (Courtesy Dr. Peter Pang, Sonoma, California.)

Critical Thinking

1. Dentistry is an excellent profession with many opportunities for the person who is willing to accept responsibilities and high standards. The professional dental assistant must be willing to accept responsibilities. How do you think you will fit into the dental profession?
2. Do you have a preference for a business office position or chairside position? Why?
3. Do you think you might want to work for a specialist? If so, which one and why?
4. Did you learn anything in this chapter that surprised you? If so, what?
5. Where would you like to see yourself in 10 years?
6. Are any dental spas located in your area?

4

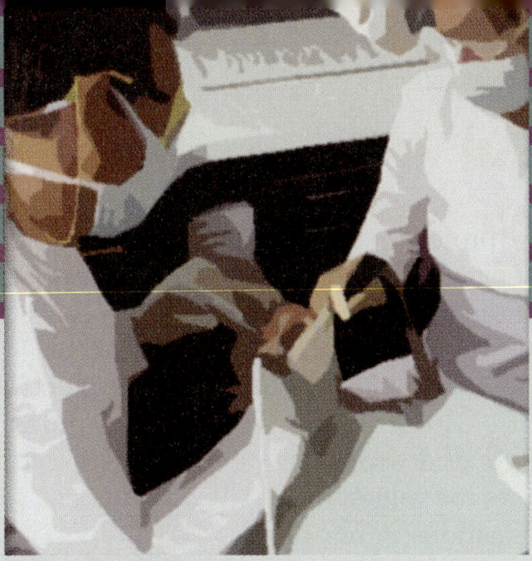

Dental Ethics

Outline

Sources for Ethics
Basic Principles of Ethics
- Regard for Self-Determination (Autonomy)
- To "Do No Harm" (Nonmaleficence)
- Promotion of Well-Being (Beneficence)
- Regard for Justice

Confidentiality
Professional Code of Ethics
Applying Ethical Principles
Ethical Dilemmas
- Case Study

Steps for Solving Ethical Dilemmas
Legal and Ethical Implications
Eye to the Future
Critical Thinking

KEY TERMS

Code of ethics Voluntary standards of behavior established by a profession.

Ethics Moral standards of conduct; rules or principles that govern proper conduct.

HIPAA The Health Insurance Portability and Accountability Act of 1996 specifies federal regulations ensuring privacy regarding a patient's health-care information.

Laws Minimum standards of behavior established by statutes for a population or profession.

LEARNING OUTCOMES

On completion of this chapter, the student will be able to achieve the following objectives:

- Pronounce, define, and spell the Key Terms.
- Explain and give examples of the basic principles of ethics.
- Discuss the American Dental Assistants Association Code of Ethics.
- Explain the difference between being "legal" and being "ethical."
- Describe the steps in ethical decision making.
- Give examples of ethical dilemmas for each principle of ethics.
- Give examples of personal ethics and unethical behaviors.
- Develop case studies involving ethical dilemmas.

Dental assistants are oral healthcare professionals. As members of a profession, they must practice according to both ethical and legal standards that the public expects from healthcare providers. The connection between law and ethics is very close. Chapter 5 will discuss the legal aspects of dental practice.

Ethics deals with moral conduct (right and wrong behavior, "good" and "evil"). Ethics includes the values, high standards of conduct, and personal obligations in our interactions with other professionals and patients. There are very few absolutes and many gray areas regarding ethics. Ethical issues are subject to individual interpretation as to the right or wrong of particular situations. Ethical behavior is important to dental healthcare professionals as they provide dental care to their patients (Fig. 4-1).

As a general rule, *ethical standards* are always of a higher order than the minimum legal standards established by the law. A behavior can be unethical and still be legal, but it cannot be illegal and still be ethical. The study of ethics seeks to answer two basic questions:

1. *What* should I do?
2. *Why* should I do it?

Ethics refers to what you *should* do, not what you must do. The law deals with what you *must* do (see Chapter 5).

Recall

1. What is the difference between ethics and law?

SOURCES FOR ETHICS

Ethical decisions have been present in every part of our lives. Ethics are involved in the way we treat other humans, animals, and the environment. You have been learning personal ethics throughout your life in a variety of ways from the sources listed in the next column.

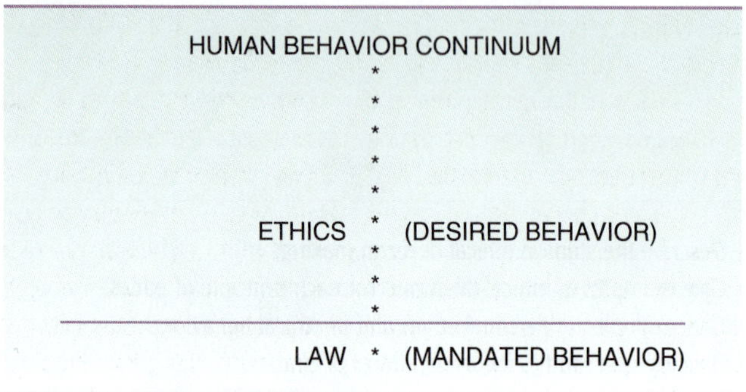

Fig. 4-1 Human behavior continuum. (Courtesy Dr. Harold Werner. From Hall JK: *Nursing ethics and law,* Philadelphia, 1996, Saunders.)

1. Basic instinct (tells you "right" from "wrong")
2. Parents ("How would you feel if someone did that to you?")
3. Teachers ("Study hard; don't cheat")
4. Religion ("Do unto others as you would have them do unto you")
5. Other people's behavior

BASIC PRINCIPLES OF ETHICS

Actions and decisions of healthcare providers are guided by ethical principles.

The following four basic principles of ethics have been developed over time. These principles guide healthcare providers by helping to identify, clarify, and justify moral (ethical) choices (Box 4-1).

Regard for Self-Determination (Autonomy)

Self-determination includes the right to privacy, freedom of choice, and the acceptance of responsibility for one's actions. Autonomy encourages a person's freedom to think, judge, and act independently without undue influence. People are free to do what they like, as long as they do not break the law or cause harm to others. For example, patients have the right to participate in decisions relating to dental care, or they have the right to refuse recommended treatments.

To "Do No Harm" (Nonmaleficence)

This principle comes from Hippocrates' dictate to "do no harm." It is the most basic element in morality. It relates to all levels of interpersonal and professional behavior. For example, if an action causes harm (physical or mental) to another, it cannot be considered moral. An example of this principle in practice might be when a patient wants the dentist to provide a treatment that the dentist believes is not in the best interest of the patient. The dentist is bound by the ethical principle to "do no harm."

Box 4-1 Basic Ethical Principles

Principle	Description
Autonomy	Self-determination, right to freedom of choice, self-responsibility
Nonmaleficence	To do no harm
Beneficence	To do good or provide a benefit
Justice	Fairness

Promotion of Well-Being (Beneficence)

This principle is based on the idea that actions are ethical as long as they will benefit a person or community. Sometimes, not *causing* harm is not enough, and one wants to help others. Volunteering in dental health education programs is an example of this type of behavior.

Regard for Justice

This principle involves treating people fairly and giving people what they deserve and are entitled to receive. This concept is demonstrated in the philosophy that all patients should receive the same quality of dental care regardless of their socioeconomic status, ethnicity, education, or ability to pay.

CONFIDENTIALITY

Confidentiality is a very important issue in the health profession. Patients have a right to privacy concerning their healthcare and treatment choices (Fig. 4-2). Healthcare professionals have an obligation to respect a patient's privacy. However, there are conflicts that will arise surrounding the principle of confidentiality. There are legal requirements to report cases of suspected child abuse or elder abuse to protect the individuals from harm. There can be issues when dealing with adolescents, who may or may not be adults according to the legal system. Often, the patient's right to confidentiality has to be balanced against the rights of other individuals. In any situation, the healthcare provider must explain to the patient that there are professional and legal responsibilities that exist for disclosure, and try to help the patient as much as possible.

In addition to moral and ethical principles for patient confidentiality, the **HIPAA** (Health Insurance Portability and Accountability Act of 1996) has very definite legal requirements for confidentiality of patients' health information (see Chapter 63).

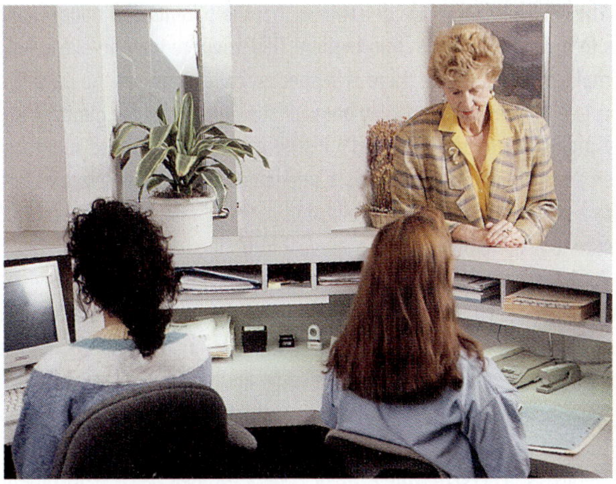

Fig. 4-2 Patients have the right to expect confidentiality of their conversations in the dental office.

HIPAA *Summary of the Health Insurance Portability and Accountability Act of 1996*

The Health Insurance Portability and Accountability Act (HIPAA) of 1996 was signed into law by President Bill Clinton on August 21, 1996. Conclusive regulations were issued on August 17, 2000, to take effect by October 16, 2002. HIPAA requires that the transactions of all patient health care information be formatted in a standardized electronic style. In addition to protecting the privacy and security of patient information, HIPAA includes legislation on the formation of medical savings accounts, the authorization of a fraud- and abuse-control program, the easy transport of health insurance coverage, and the simplification of administrative terms and conditions.

HIPAA encompasses privacy requirements that can be broken down into three types–privacy standards, patients' rights, and administrative requirements.

1. **Privacy Standards.** A central concern of HIPAA is the careful use and disclosure of protected health information (PHI), which generally is electronically controlled health information that is able to be distinguished individually. PHI also refers to verbal communication, although the HIPAA Privacy Rule is not intended to hinder necessary verbal communication. The U.S. Department of Health and Human Services (USDHHS) does not require restructuring, such as soundproofing, architectural changes, and so forth, but some caution is necessary when exchanging health information by conversation.

An Acknowledgment of Receipt of Notice of Privacy Practices, which allows patient information to be used or divulged for treatment, payment, or health care operations (TPO), should be procured from each patient. A detailed and time-sensitive authorization can also be issued, which allows the dentist to release information in special circumstances other than TPOs. A *written consent* is also an option. Dentists can disclose PHI *without* acknowledgment, consent, or authorization in very special situations, for example, perceived child abuse, public health supervision, fraud investigation, or law enforcement with valid permission (e.g., a warrant). When divulging PHI, a dentist must try to disclose only the *minimum necessary* information, to help safeguard the patient's information as much as possible.

It is important that dental professionals adhere to HIPAA standards because healthcare providers (as well as healthcare clearinghouses and healthcare plans) who convey *electronically* formatted health information via an outside billing service or merchant are considered *covered entities.* Covered entities may be dealt serious civil and criminal penalties for violation of HIPAA legislation. Failure to comply with HIPAA privacy requirements may result in civil penalties of up to $100 per offense with an annual maximum of $25,000 for repeated failure to comply with the same requirement. Criminal penalties resulting from the illegal mishandling of private health information can range from $50,000 and/or 1 year in prison to $250,000 and/or 10 years in prison.

Continued

HIPAA Summary of the Health Insurance Portability and Accountability Act of 1996—cont'd

2. **Patients' Rights.** HIPAA allows patients, authorized representatives, and parents of minors, as well as minors, to become more aware of the health information privacy to which they are entitled. These rights include, but are not limited to, the right to view and copy their health information, the right to dispute alleged breaches of policies and regulations, and the right to request alternative forms of communicating with their dentist. If any health information is released for any reason other than TPO, the patient is entitled to an account of the transaction. Therefore, it is important for dentists to keep accurate records of such information and to provide them when necessary.

The HIPAA Privacy Rule determines that the parents of a minor have access to their child's health information. This privilege may be overruled, for example, in cases where there is suspected child abuse or the parent consents to a term of confidentiality between the dentist and the minor. The parents' rights to access their child's PHI also may be restricted in situations when a legal entity, such as a court, intervenes and when a law does not require a parent's consent. For a full list of patients' rights provided by HIPAA, be sure to acquire a copy of the law and to understand it well.

3. **Administrative Requirements.** Complying with HIPAA legislation may seem like a chore, but it does not need to be so. It is recommended that you become appropriately familiar with the law, organize the requirements into simpler tasks, begin compliance early, and document your progress in compliance. An important first step is to evaluate the current information and practices of your office.

Dentists will need to write a *privacy policy* for their office, a document for their patients detailing the office's practices concerning PHI. The ADA's *HIPAA Privacy Kit* includes forms that you (the dentist) can use to customize your privacy policy. It is useful to try to understand the role of healthcare information for your patients and the ways in which they deal with the information while they are visiting your office. Train your staff; make sure they are familiar with the terms of HIPAA and your office's privacy policy and related forms. HIPAA requires that you designate a *privacy officer,* a person in your office who will be responsible for applying the new policies in your office, fielding complaints, and making choices involving the minimum necessary requirements. Another person with the role of *contact person* will process complaints.

A *Notice of Privacy Practices*—a document detailing the patient's rights and the dental office's obligations concerning PHI—also must be drawn up. Further, any role of a third party with access to PHI must be clearly documented. This third party is known as a *business associate* (BA) and is defined as any entity who, on behalf of the dentist, takes part in any activity that involves exposure of PHI. The *HIPAA Privacy Kit* provides a copy of the USDHHS "Business Associate Contract Terms," which provides a concrete format for detailing BA interactions.

The main HIPAA privacy compliance date, including all staff training, was April 14, 2003, although many covered entities who submitted a request and a compliance plan by October 15, 2002, were granted one-year extensions. Contact your local branch of the ADA for details. It is recommended that dentists prepare their offices ahead of time for all deadlines, which includes preparing privacy polices and forms, business associate contracts, and employee training sessions.

For a comprehensive discussion of all of these terms and requirements, a complete list of HIPAA policies and procedures, and a full collection of HIPAA privacy forms, contact the American Dental Association for a *HIPAA Privacy Kit.* The relevant ADA website is www.ada.org/goto/hipaa. Other websites that may contain useful information about HIPAA are:

USDHHS Office of Civil Rights: www.hhs.gov/ocr/hipaa

Work Group on Electronic Data Interchange: www.wedi.org/SNIP

Phoenix Health: www.hipaadvisory.com

USDHHS Office of the Assistant Secretary for Planning and Evaluation: http://aspe.os.dhhs.gov/admnsimp/

Data from: *HIPAA Privacy Kit;* and http://www.ada.org.

Recall

2. What are the four basic principles of ethics?

PROFESSIONAL CODE OF ETHICS

All professions (e.g., dental, medical, legal), including the ADAA, have a written code of ethics. These are *voluntary* standards that are set by members of the profession. They are not laws. The Code of Ethics serves as a method of self-regulation within the profession. Remember that the code states the "ideal behavior." Most professional codes of ethics are revised periodically to keep them consistent with the times, but there is no change in the moral intent or overall idealism.

Professional organizations establish a Code of Ethics for the following reasons:

1. To demonstrate the standard of care the public can expect from its members.
2. To increase the ethical consciousness and ethical responsibility of its members.
3. To guide its members in making informed ethical decisions.
4. To establish a standard for professional judgment and conduct.

Recall

3. What establishes a guide to professional behavior?

ADAA: Principles of Ethics and Code of Professional Conduct

- Abide by the bylaws of the Association.
- Maintain loyalty to the Association.
- Pursue the objectives of the Association.
- Hold in confidence the information entrusted to you by the Association.
- Maintain respect for the members and employees of the Association.
- Serve all members of the Association in an impartial manner.
- Recognize and follow all laws and regulations relating to activities of the Association.
- Exercise and insist on sound business principles in the conduct of affairs of the Association.
- Use legal and ethical means to influence legislation or regulation affecting members of the Association.
- Issue no false or misleading statements to fellow members or the public.
- Refrain from disseminating malicious information concerning the Association or any member or employee of the Association.
- Maintain high standards of personal conduct and integrity.
- Do not imply Association endorsement of personal opinions or positions.
- Cooperate in a reasonable and proper manner with staff and members.
- Accept no personal compensation from fellow members, except as approved by the Association.
- Promote and maintain the highest standards of performance in service to the Association.
- Assure public confidence in the integrity and service of the Association.

APPLYING ETHICAL PRINCIPLES

We face ethical issues every day in our personal and professional lives. Listed below are examples of applying ethical principles.

- A woman chooses not to have dental radiographs because she is afraid of radiation exposure. She has the right to accept or refuse radiographs. She also has the right to be fully informed about her oral healthcare, and her dentist would likely explain the risks of undetected conditions by not having dental radiographs. The dentist is facing an ethical dilemma that involves the principle of autonomy.
- Several dental assistants in your office enjoy gossiping about the receptionist. By refusing to participate in office gossip, you are applying the principle of doing no harm.
- A student in your dental-assisting class is struggling with her studies. You could ignore the student because you have too much to do, or you could apply the principle of well-being by offering to help her study.
- You find a wallet containing a large amount of cash and identification of the owner. By returning the wallet and the cash, you are applying the principle of justice.

ETHICAL DILEMMAS

There is a difference between an everyday problem that can be solved by applying an ethical principle, and an *ethical dilemma.* An ethical dilemma occurs when one or more ethical principles are in conflict. For example, an ethical dilemma occurs when the principle of avoiding harm is in conflict with the principle of autonomy in a specific situation.

Case Study

A patient who has had a recent heart attack wishes to have some veneers placed on her front teeth immediately because she is going on a cruise in three weeks. The dentist wants to wait awhile for her medical condition to stabilize before beginning the cosmetic procedure. The patient is very insistent about her wishes. The dentist now has an ethical dilemma to solve.

In the case study above, the conflict is between the patient's ethical right to *self-determination (autonomy),* and the dentist's ethical obligation to "do no harm."

Ethical dilemmas are different from a situation in which a dentist knowingly charges an insurance company for a procedure that was not performed. That clearly involves unethical and illegal behavior.

Another example of principles in conflict is when the dentist believes a treatment is in the best interest of the patient, and the patient chooses another option (autonomy versus "do no harm"). The dentist may choose to perform the procedure that the patient prefers *only* if that procedure is within the standards of patient care. It would be unethical under the principle of "do no harm" for the dentist to perform a procedure that is below the standard of care just because the patient wants it. For example, a patient may want to have all of his healthy teeth extracted so he does not have to brush and floss (autonomy). In this case, it would be unethical for a dentist to comply with the patient's wishes.

STEPS FOR SOLVING ETHICAL DILEMMAS

Many ethical dilemmas do not have quick or easy solutions. When an ethical dilemma is particularly complex, it can help to use the following steps as a "roadmap." It sometimes helps to write down the alternatives to evaluate all the options.

1. ***Identify the alternatives.*** Answer these questions: What alternatives do I have? What are the likely outcomes of each alternative?
2. ***Determine the professional implications.*** With each alternative, determine what "should" and "should not" be done professionally. You must carefully consider all specific professional obligations relevant to the situation.
3. ***Rank the alternatives.*** Then select the best alternative. If you think two alternatives are equal, you must choose one or the other. This step allows you to know that you have done your best given the circumstances.
4. ***Choose a course of action.*** When you follow these steps and make a judgment and a decision about what should and should not be done ethically and professionally, you will be more comfortable with your decision.

Legal and Ethical Implications

You may be faced with a situation in which your dentist/employer's conduct violates ethical standards. Before you make any judgments, be absolutely certain of all information and circumstances. If there are violations of ethical conduct, you must answer the following questions:

1. Do you want to remain at your job under these circumstances?
2. Should you discuss the situation with your employer?
3. Should you seek other employment?
4. If you remain, will it affect you in the future with other employers?

These decisions are difficult, especially if you like your employer and enjoy your job. A dental assistant is not *legally* obligated to report questionable actions of the dentist or to attempt to alter the circumstances. However, as an *ethical* dental assistant, you have to live with the decisions you make. You will not want to participate in substandard care or unlawful practices that may be harmful to patients.

Eye to the Future

You may be faced with ethical dilemmas daily when you are working in a dental practice. Many professional ethical judgments are straightforward. When you are faced with more complex issues, however, remember the steps for solving ethical dilemmas. Remember also that choosing the correct alternative is not the always the easiest choice, but it is always the best choice.

Critical Thinking

1. Susan, the office manager in your dental office, enjoys sharing personal information about the dentist and his wife with members of the staff. You are uncomfortable with her behavior, but you know she is responsible for your evaluation so you are reluctant to speak to her. What can you do?
2. You have just begun working for Dr. Wong as a dental assistant. You know that confidential papers, case histories, and the appointment book should be kept from curious eyes to protect patients as well as the dentist and office staff. The receptionist does not always follow these practices, however, and insists there are no ethical issues with any of the patients. Is there anything you can do to protect your patients' privacy?
3. The president of the local dental assistants society asks you to volunteer for the upcoming dental screenings at an urban school on Saturday. You had planned to spend some time with friends you have not seen in awhile. You know volunteers are hard to find and this is a worthwhile project, but it has been weeks since you and your friends got together. What will you do? Why?

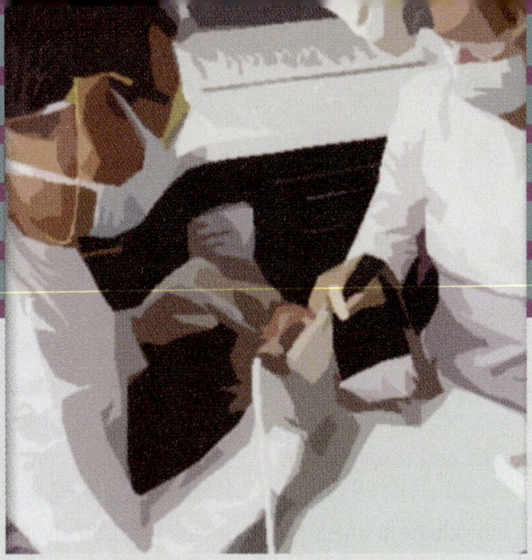

5 Dentistry and the Law

Outline

Statutory Law
- Contract Law
- Tort Law

State Dental Practice Act
- Board of Dentistry
- Expanded Functions and Supervision
- Unlicensed Practice of Dentistry

Dentist-Patient Relationship
- Duty of Care/Standard of Care
- Abandonment
- Patient Responsibilities
- Due Care

Malpractice
- Acts of Omission and Commission
- Doctrine of *res ipsa loquitur*

Risk Management
- Avoiding Malpractice Lawsuits
- "Silence Is Golden"
- Guidelines for Informed Consent
- Patient Referral
- Guarantees
- Contributory Negligence

Patient Records

Procedure 5-1: Correcting a Chart Entry

- Ownership of Dental Records and Radiographs

Reporting Child Abuse and Neglect
- Immunity

Legal and Ethical Implications

Eye to the Future

Critical Thinking

KEY TERMS

Abandonment Termination by the dentist of the dentist-patient relationship without reasonable notice to the patient.

Administrative law Category of law that involves regulations established by government agencies.

Board of dentistry State agency that adopts rules and regulations and implements the specific state's dental practice act.

Civil law Category of law that deals with the relations of individuals, corporations, or other organizations.

Contract law Category of law that involves an agreement for services in exchange for a payment (contract).

Criminal law Category of law that involves violations against the state or government.

Dental auxiliary (awg-**zil**-yah-ree) Dental assistants, dental hygienists, and dental laboratory technicians.

Direct supervision Level of supervision in which the dentist is physically present when the dental auxiliary performs delegated functions.

Due care Just, proper, and sufficient care; or the absence of negligence.

Expanded functions Specific intraoral functions delegated to an auxiliary that require increased skill and training.

Expressed contract A contract that is established through verbal or written words.

Felony A major crime, such as fraud or drug abuse. Conviction can result in imprisonment of one year or more.

General supervision Level of supervision in which the dental auxiliary performs delegated functions according to the instructions of the dentist, who is not necessarily physically present.

Implied consent Consent in which the patient's action indicates consent for treatment.

Implied contract Contract that is established by actions, not words.

Informed consent Permission granted by a patient after being informed about the details of a procedure.

Infraction Minor offense that usually results in only a fine.

Licensure License to practice in a specific state.

Malpractice Professional negligence.

Continued

KEY TERMS—cont'd

Mandated reporters Designated professionals who are required by law to report known or suspected child abuse.

Misdemeanor Offense that may result in imprisonment of six months to one year.

Patient of record Individual who has been examined and diagnosed by the dentist and has had treatment planned.

Reciprocity (re-si-**prah**-si-tee) System that allows individuals in one state to obtain a license in another state without retesting.

Res gestae Statements made by a person present at the time of an alleged negligent act that are admissible as evidence in a court of law.

Res ipsa loquitur (Latin phrase for "the thing speaks for itself")

Respondeat superior (Latin for "Let the master answer") Legal doctrine that holds an employer liable for acts of the employee.

Standard of care The level of knowledge, skill, and care comparable to that of other dentists treating similar patients under similar conditions.

State dental practice act Document of law that specifies the legal requirements to practice dentistry in a particular state.

Statutory law Law enacted by legislation through U.S. Congress, state legislature, or local legislative bodies.

Tort law Law involving an act that brings harm to a person or damages to property.

Written consent Consent that involves a written explanation of the diagnostic findings, prescribed treatment, and reasonable expectations about treatment results.

LEARNING OUTCOMES

On completion of this chapter, the student will be able to achieve the following objectives:

- Pronounce, define, and spell the Key Terms.
- Explain the purpose of the state dental practice act.
- Explain the purpose for licensing dental health professionals.
- Describe the types of dental auxiliary supervision.
- Explain the circumstances required for patient abandonment.
- Explain the principle of contributory negligence.
- Describe the differences between civil and criminal law.
- Describe ways to prevent malpractice suits.
- Describe the difference between written and implied consent.
- Describe the procedure for obtaining consent for minor patients.
- Describe the procedure for documenting informed consent.
- Explain when it is necessary to obtain an informed refusal.
- Describe the exceptions for disclosure.
- Demonstrate how to make corrections on a patient's record.
- Give an example of *respondeat superior.*
- Give an example of *res gestae.*
- Discuss the indications of child abuse and neglect.

Every state government has the responsibility to protect the health, welfare, and safety of its citizens. To do this, regulations are written and legislation is passed. When the U.S. Congress, a state legislature, or a local legislative body passes legislation, it becomes **statutory law.** As a dental assistant, you must understand the law in order to protect yourself, the dentist, and the patient.

STATUTORY LAW

There are two types of statutory law, criminal law and civil law. **Criminal law** involves crimes against society. In criminal law, a governmental agency such as law enforcement or the board of dentistry initiates legal action. **Civil law** involves crimes against an individual with another individual initiating legal action (i.e., lawsuit).

Criminal law seeks to punish the offender, while civil law seeks to compensate the victim. For example, a dental assistant who performs a procedure that is not legal is in violation of criminal law. Insurance fraud is another criminal act that may be committed in a dental office.

Criminal offenses are classified as follows:

- **Felony:** Major crime, such as insurance fraud or drug abuse in the dental setting. Conviction may result in imprisonment for one year or more.
- **Misdemeanor:** A lesser offense that may result in a variety of penalties, including fines, loss or suspension of the license to practice dentistry, mandatory continuing education, counseling, or community service. An example of a misdemeanor is a dentist who violates a regulation of the dental practice act such as failing to follow infection-control regulations.
- **Infraction:** Minor offense (e.g., traffic violation) that usually results in only a fine. For example, if a dentist does not pay his or her license renewal fee on time, a penalty fee would be added to the original renewal fee.

Civil law is concerned with the relations of individuals, corporations, or other organizations. Classifications of civil law that affect the practice of dentistry are as follows:

- **Contract law** involves a binding agreement between two or more people. This could involve employment contracts or contracts for patient treatment.
- **Tort law** involves acts (intentional or unintentional) that bring harm to a person or damages to property. An exam-

ple would be a malpractice suit in which a patient alleges that a dentist caused harm or damage to him or her.

- **Administrative law** involves regulations established by government agencies, for example, violations of the Occupational Safety and Health Administration (OSHA). The regulations of the dental practice act are examples of administrative law.

Contract Law

For a contract or agreement to be *binding,* it must be between two competent people. This eliminates mentally incompetent persons, those under the influence of alcohol or drugs, and minors. The agreement must also include an exchange of a service for payment. When the dentist accepts the patient and the patient arrives for care, the dentist has the legal obligation under contract law to provide dental care. A contract can be either *expressed* or *implied,* as follows:

- **Expressed contracts** are established through the written word or verbal agreement. Expressed contracts are commonly used when the required treatment is extensive or will take a long period of time to complete (e.g., orthodontics or full-mouth reconstruction).
- **Implied contracts** are established by *actions,* not words. Most dental contracts are implied contracts. For example, if a patient comes to the dentist with a toothache and allows the dentist to examine him or her, it is implied that the patient wants treatment.

Tort Law

A **tort** is a civil wrong. A tort can be *intentional* or *unintentional.* For example, a breach of confidentiality is an intentional tort. However, if a dental assistant mounts radiographic films on the wrong side and the dentist notices and corrects the error, no harm is done to the patient and no tort would occur. However, a tort would occur if the dentist extracts a tooth on the wrong side of the mouth as a result of not noticing the error.

In addition, a tort can be an act of *omission* (i.e., not doing something that should have been done) or an act of *commission* (i.e., doing something that should not have been done). For example, failing to recognize periodontal disease, or not taking radiographs would be an act of *omission.* Taking out the wrong tooth or causing nerve injury during an extraction would be an act of *commission.*

Recall

1. What are the two types of statutory law?
2. What is the difference between an act of omission and an act of commission?
3. What is the difference between an expressed contract and an implied contract?

STATE DENTAL PRACTICE ACT

To protect the public from incompetent dental healthcare providers, each state has established a **state dental practice act.** The dental practice act specifies the legal requirements for the practice of dentistry within each state. It may be a single law or a compilation of laws that regulate the practice of dentistry. Regulations regarding dental assistants vary greatly from state to state. It is important to have a clear understanding of the law in *your* state as it relates to dental assisting and the practice of dentistry. Each state's dental practice act is now accessible on the Internet. You will find links to each state's dental practice act at http://www.ada.org.

Board of Dentistry

An administrative board, usually called the **board of dentistry,** interprets and implements state regulations.

The governor of the state usually appoints the members of the state board of dentistry, also referred to as the *dental board* in some states. In addition to having licensed dentists as board members, some states have dental hygienists, dental assistants, and consumers as members of the board.

The board adopts rules and regulations that define, interpret, and implement the intent of the dental practice act. The board is also responsible for enforcement of regulations for practice of dentistry within the state.

Licensure (having a license to practice in a specific state) is one method of supervising individuals who practice in the state. The purpose of licensure is to protect the public from unqualified or incompetent practitioners. The requirements for licensure vary from state to state, but dentists and dental hygienists *must* be licensed by the state in which they practice.

An increasing number of states are requiring either licensing or registration for dental assistants in their states. It is essential to understand the requirements for practice

A Typical Dental Practice Act Includes:

1. Requirements for licensure
2. Requirements for license renewal
3. Grounds for suspension or revocation of a license
4. Requirements for continuing dental education
5. Duties to be delegated to dental assistants and dental hygienists
6. Infection-control regulations
7. Requirements for the use of radiation and qualifications for health professionals who expose dental radiographs

in your state. In every state, any person who practices dentistry without a license is guilty of an illegal act.

Some states have a reciprocity agreement with another state. **Reciprocity** is an agreement between two or more states to allow a dentist or dental hygienist who is licensed in one state to receive, usually without further examination, a license to practice in any of the other states in the reciprocity agreement. Reciprocity agreements are usually between states with adjoining borders and similar testing requirements. States without reciprocity agreements require dentists and dental hygienists licensed in another state to take their state board examination.

The state board of dentistry has the authority not only to *issue* licenses but also to *revoke, suspend,* or *deny renewal* of a license. Most states will take action if the licensed person has a felony conviction or a misdemeanor involving drug addiction, moral corruptness, incompetence, or mental/physical disability that may cause harm to patients.

Recall

4. What is the purpose of licensure?
5. What authority does a state board of dentistry have?
6. What is meant by reciprocity?

Expanded Functions Delegated to Qualified Dental Assistants*

- Inspecting oral cavity with mouth mirror
- Applying topical anesthetics
- Polishing coronal surfaces of teeth
- Assisting with administration of nitrous oxide
- Applying topical anticarcinogenic agents
- Fitting trial endodontic file points
- Determining root length and endodontic file length
- Making impressions for intraoral appliances
- Making impressions for study casts
- Removing sutures
- Performing preliminary oral examinations
- Placing and removing matrices and wedges
- Placing and removing temporary or sedative restorations
- Placing and removing temporary crowns and bridges
- Preparing teeth for etching
- Placing and removing rubber dams
- Placing and removing periodontal dressings
- Placing, condensing, and carving amalgam restorations
- Placing and finishing composite resin restorations
- Applying cavity liners and bases
- Applying pit-and-fissure sealants
- Placing and removing orthodontic arch wires, brackets, and bands

* Check with your state's board of dentistry for information pertaining to your state. Locate your state's dental practice act on the Internet at http://www.ada.org.

Expanded Functions and Supervision

Expanded functions are specific intraoral tasks delegated to qualified dental auxiliaries who have increased skill and training. When these functions are included in the dental practice act, the dentist may delegate them to the dental assistant. Some states require additional education, certification, or registration to perform these functions.

As with all functions performed by the dental assistant, expanded functions are included in the doctrine of ***respondeat superior*** ("Let the master answer"). This means that the employer is responsible for any harm caused by the actions of the employee while the employee is carrying out the business of the employer. In a dental practice, this means that the patient may sue the dentist for an error committed by the dental assistant.

However, the employee is also responsible for his or her own actions, and the injured patient may also file suit against the dental assistant. The dentist's liability insurance cannot be counted on to provide complete coverage for the dental assistant. Many dental assistants who provide direct patient care choose to carry their own liability insurance.

In states that allow the dentist to delegate expanded functions to a **dental auxiliary** (dental assistant or dental hygienist), the rules in the state dental practice act are usually specific regarding the types of auxiliary supervision that the dentist must provide. The following terms are used often in dental practice acts:

- A **patient of record** is an individual who has been examined and diagnosed by a licensed dentist and has had his or her treatment planned by the dentist.
- **Direct supervision** generally means that the dentist has delegated a specific procedure to be performed for a patient of record by a legally qualified dental auxiliary (who meets the requirements of the state board of dentistry). The dentist must examine the patient before delegating the procedure and again when the procedure is complete. *The dentist must be physically present in the office at the time the procedures are performed.*
- **General supervision** (indirect supervision) generally means that the dentist has authorized and delegated specific procedures that may be performed by a legally qualified dental auxiliary for a patient of record.

Exposing radiographs and recementing a temporary crown that has become dislodged are examples of functions that are often delegated under general supervision.

Recall

7. What does *respondeat superior* mean?
8. What is the difference between direct supervision and general supervision?

Unlicensed Practice of Dentistry

As a dental assistant, you may legally perform *only* those functions that have been delegated to you under the dental practice act of the state in which you practice. Performing procedures that are not legal is the same as practicing dentistry without a license, which is a *criminal act.* Ignorance of the dental practice act is no excuse for illegally practicing dentistry. *If the dentist asks you to perform an expanded function that is not legal in your state and you choose to do so, you are committing a criminal act.*

Dentist's Duty of Care to the Patient

1. Be properly licensed.
2. Use reasonable skill, care, and judgment.
3. Use standard drugs, materials, and techniques.
4. Use "standard precautions" in treatment of all patients.
5. Maintain confidentiality of all information.
6. Obtain and update patients' medical-dental health history.
7. Make appropriate referrals, and request consultation when indicated.
8. Maintain a level of knowledge and competence in keeping with advances in the dental profession.
9. Do not exceed the scope of practice or allow assistants under general supervision to perform unlawful acts.
10. Complete patients' care in a timely manner.
11. Do not use experimental procedures.
12. Obtain informed consent from the patient or guardian before beginning an examination or treatment.
13. Arrange for patients' care during a temporary absence.
14. Give adequate instructions to patients.
15. Achieve reasonable treatment results.

DENTIST-PATIENT RELATIONSHIP

Duty of Care/Standard of Care

The concept of *duty of care* (also known as the **standard of care**) is commonly misunderstood among dental professionals. Many assume it is a law or regulation and it provides specific steps that a dentist must follow. It is, in fact, not a black-and-white rule at all. Instead, it is a legal *concept* that provides general boundaries within which a dentist must perform in a given situation.

The standard of care that a dentist must meet is simply the customary practice of reputable dentists who have similar training and experience, who practice in similar disciplines, and/or who practice in the same area or a similar locality (e.g., urban or remote rural). When a dentist fails to meet the standard of care and the patient is injured, the dentist may be held liable for malpractice.

The duty of care owed by a dentist to a patient includes (1) being licensed; (2) using reasonable skill, care, and judgment; and (3) using standard drugs, materials, and techniques. The dentist may refuse to treat a patient; however, this action must *not* be based on the patient's race, color, or creed.

In addition, the Americans with Disabilities Act protects patients with infectious diseases such as human immunodeficiency virus (HIV) infection. For example, a patient with HIV cannot be refused treatment simply because of the disease. The only exception would be the HIV patient who has a special condition (e.g., severe periodontal disease) that requires the care of a specialist, and the dentist would refer any patient with the same condition to a specialist, regardless of HIV status. In other words, a patient cannot be refused treatment based *only* on HIV status (see Chapter 19).

Abandonment

Abandonment refers to discontinuation of care after treatment has begun, but before it has been completed. The dentist may be liable for abandonment if the dentist ends the dentist-patient relationship without giving the patient reasonable notice. Even if a patient refuses to follow instructions and fails to keep appointments, the dentist may not legally refuse to give the patient another appointment. The dentist may not dismiss or refuse to treat a patient of record without giving the patient written notification of termination. After notification, care must continue for a reasonable length of time, usually 30 days, to allow the patient time to find another dentist. It could even be considered abandonment if a dentist left the area for a weekend without making arrangements with another dentist to be available for emergencies, or without leaving a number for the patient to call for care.

Patient Responsibilities

The patient also has legal duties to the dentist. The patient is legally required to pay a reasonable and agreed-on fee for services. The patient also is expected to cooperate and follow instructions regarding treatment and home care.

Due Care

Due care is a legal term meaning proper and sufficient care or the absence of negligence. The dentist has a legal obligation to use due care in treating patients. This obligation applies to all treatment procedures.

When administering and prescribing drugs, due care implies that the dentist is familiar with the drug and its properties. The dentist must also have adequate information regarding the patient's health to know whether the drug is suitable for the patient or whether the patient's health record contraindicates its use. Therefore a complete, up-to-date health history is essential.

Recall

9. What is meant by abandonment?

10. Can a dentist refuse to treat a patient because he or she has HIV infection?

MALPRACTICE

Although patients may bring a lawsuit against the dentist, it does not mean that they will win. The following four conditions, sometimes called the "four Ds," must *all* be present for a malpractice lawsuit to be successful:

1. Duty. A dentist-patient relationship must exist to establish the duty.
2. Derelict (lacking a sense of duty, negligent). Negligence occurred as a result of not meeting the standard of care.
3. Direct cause. The negligent act was the direct cause of the injury.
4. Damages. Pain and suffering, loss of income, and medical bills are included in damages.

If a dentist injects local anesthetic on the wrong side of a patient's mouth, for example, probably no grounds exist for a malpractice suit because no "damages" occurred to the patient. Although there might have been negligence ("derelict"), all four conditions were not present.

Acts of Omission and Commission

Malpractice is *professional negligence,* or the failure to use due care or the lack of due care. In dentistry, the two types of malpractice are acts of omission and acts of commission.

An act of omission is failure to perform an act that a "reasonable and prudent professional" *would* perform. An example would be a dentist who fails to diagnose periodontal disease because the dentist did not take radiographs or perform a periodontal probing.

An act of commission is performance of an act that a "reasonable and prudent professional" *would not* perform. An example would be a dentist who administers 15 cartridges of a local anesthetic to a small child, resulting in life-threatening overdose.

Doctrine of *res ipsa loquitur*

Sometimes an expert witness is not necessary in a malpractice suit. Under the doctrine of ***res ipsa loquitur*** ("the act speaks for itself") the evidence is clear. For example, the dentist extracted the wrong tooth, or broke an instrument during a root canal and left the instrument in the tooth.

Recall

11. What are the "four Ds" necessary for a successful malpractice suit?

12. What does *res ipsa loquitur* mean?

RISK MANAGEMENT

In this age of increasing *litigiousness* (proneness to engage in lawsuits), the dental team must constantly be aware of the need to avoid unnecessary malpractice risks in the dental practice. The major areas of risk management (prevention of lawsuits) involve (1) maintaining accurate and complete records, (2) gaining informed consent, and (3) doing everything possible to maintain the highest standards of clinical excellence.

Legal authorities note that the primary factor in avoiding legal problems with patients is maintaining a climate of *good rapport* and *open communication* with all patients. When patients become angry or frustrated and believe they are not being heard, they are more likely to file a lawsuit.

Avoiding Malpractice Lawsuits

Prevention and good communication with the patient are the best defenses against malpractice. Patients are less

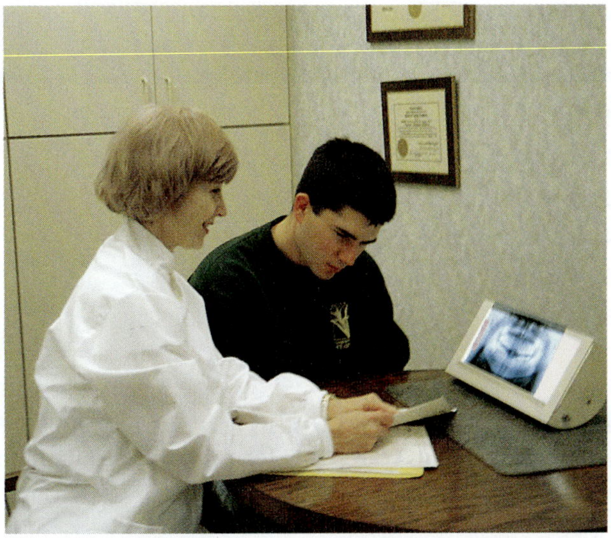

Fig. 5-1 An important role of the dental assistant is to help maintain good communication with the patient. (Courtesy Pamela Landry, RDA.)

likely to initiate a lawsuit when they have a clear understanding of the following:

1. The planned treatment
2. Reasonable treatment results
3. Potential treatment complications
4. Their financial obligations

The dental assistant plays an important role in the prevention of malpractice litigation by being aware of signs of patient dissatisfaction and alerting the dentist (Fig. 5-1).

Recall

13. What are the best defenses against a malpractice suit?

"Silence Is Golden"

The dental assistant must never make critical remarks about dental treatment rendered by an employer or another dentist. The dental assistant should never discuss other patients and should also avoid discussing the dentist's professional liability insurance.

Under the concept of ***res gestae*** ("part of the action"), statements made spontaneously by anyone (including the dental assistant) at the time of an alleged negligent act are admissible as evidence and may be damaging to the dentist and dental assistant in a court of law. Comments such as "whoops" or "uh-oh" may unnecessarily frighten the patient and should be avoided.

Recall

14. What is meant by *res gestae?*

Guidelines for Informed Consent

The patient should be informed about the following:

- Nature of the proposed treatment, including the cost and expected time for healing.
- Benefits of the proposed treatment, as well as the consequences of *not* having the treatment.
- Common, severe risks associated with the proposed treatment.
- Reasonable alternatives to the proposed treatment, including risks and benefits of each alternative.

Guidelines for Informed Consent

The concept of **informed consent** is based on the idea that it is the patient who must pay the bill and endure the pain and suffering that may result from treatment. Therefore the patient has the right to know all important facts about the proposed treatment.

Informed Patient Consent

Informed consent to dental treatment is based on the information provided by the dentist. Two things must occur for the patient to give informed consent: *being informed* and *giving consent.* This means that the dentist must give the patient enough information about his or her condition and all available treatment options. The patient and dentist then discuss these options and the patient chooses the most suitable treatment alternative.

When a patient enters a dentist's office, the patient gives **implied consent,** at least for the dental examination. Provided the patient is capable, implied consent is given when the patient agrees to treatment or at least does not object to treatment. In a court of law, implied consent is a less reliable form of consent in a malpractice suit. **Written consent** is the preferred means of obtaining and documenting the patient's consent and understanding of the procedure.

Informed Refusal

If a patient refuses the proposed treatment, the dentist must inform the patient about the likely consequences and obtain the patient's informed refusal.

However, obtaining the patient's informed refusal does not release the dentist from the responsibility of providing the standard of care. A patient may not consent to substandard care, and the dentist may not legally or ethically agree to provide such care. For example, if a patient refuses radiographs, the dentist may refer the patient to another provider because the dentist believes radiographs are a necessary standard of care. Another dentist, however, may be willing to treat the patient without radiograph films and may request that the patient sign a written and dated informed refusal for radiographs. This statement is then filed with the patient's record.

Exceptions to Disclosure

The dentist does not have a duty to disclose information about the proposed treatment in the following situations:

1. The patient asks not to be advised.
2. The procedure is simple and straightforward, and life-threatening risks are remote (e.g., death from a filling).
3. The treatment risk is minor and rarely results in serious side effects (e.g., discomfort while biting down as radiograph films are taken).
4. The information would be so upsetting that the patient would be unable to weigh risks and benefits rationally; this is known as the *therapeutic exception.*

Informed Consent for Minors

The parent, custodial parent, or legal guardian must give consent for minor children. When parents live separately, the child's personal information form should indicate which parent is the custodial parent. When separated parents share custody, the child's record should contain letters from each parent providing consent and authorization to treat. Asking in advance for a parent's or custodial parent's "blanket" consent for emergency treatment avoids confusions and delays should the child require emergency care when a parent or guardian is not present.

Documenting Informed Consent

Most states do not require a specific means for documenting discussions on informed consent. At the minimum, the patient's record should indicate that the patient received information about the risks, benefits, and alternatives and consented to or refused the proposed treatment.

When the treatment is extensive, invasive, or risky, a written informed consent document is recommended. The patient, the dentist, and a witness should sign the written consent form. The patient should receive a copy of the form, and the original should be kept in the patient's chart.

Content of Informed Consent Forms

Informed consent is a *process,* not only a form. It involves face-to-face discussion between the dentist and the patient. There should be enough time available to answer all of the patient's questions and concerns.

There are many types of commercial informed consent forms available from professional organizations and insurance companies. Many dentists choose to develop their own forms. In any case, the form should contain the following:

- The nature of the proposed treatment
- Benefits and alternatives
- Risks and potential consequences of not performing treatment
- Other information as necessary for the particular case

The form should be signed by the patient, the dentist, and a witness. The patient should receive a copy of the form, and the original should be kept in the patient's chart.

The informed consent form and discussion do not absolutely protect the dentist against the patient who alleges that he or she was not fully informed about a procedure. However, thorough documentation greatly increases the dentist's chance of defense against such allegations.

Clinical Situations That Require Written Informed Consent

1. New drugs are used.
2. Experimentation or clinical testing is involved.
3. Patient's identifiable photograph is used.
4. General anesthetic is administered.
5. Minors are treated in a public program.
6. Treatment takes more than one year to complete.

Recall

15. What is the difference between implied consent and written consent?

Patient Referral

Dentists usually refer a patient who has an unusual case or a condition beyond their scope of expertise. The dentist must inform the patient that the needed treatment cannot be properly performed in the office and requires the services of a specialist. The dentist should assist the patient in finding an appropriate specialist.

Failure to Refer

Many malpractice claims involve the failure of the general dentist to refer the patient to a specialist when the patient's oral condition requires special attention.

Failure to recognize periodontal disease and refer patients to a periodontist is a very common cause for this type of malpractice suit. Periodontal disease is a silent disease and patients rarely experience pain, and are often not even aware that a problem exists. Therefore, it is important that the general dentist establishes a patient's baseline oral condition and uses it to compare any changes in periodontal health over time.

When a patient is referred to a specialist, thoroughly document the referral in the patient's chart. Include a description of the problem, reasons for referral, the name and specialty of the referral dentist, and whether or not the patient has agreed to be referred.

Guarantees

Outcomes of dental care cannot be completely predicted. Neither the dentist nor the staff should make a promise or claim about the outcome of care, because this could be interpreted as a "guarantee." It is unethical to make guarantees, and in some states it is illegal.

Contributory Negligence

The patient's record should include notation of any broken appointments or last-minute cancellations. These actions may be interpreted as "contributory negligence" on the part of the patient. Contributory negligence occurs when the patient's action (or lack of action) negatively affects the treatment outcome. Documentation of broken and cancelled appointments helps protect the practice from legal recourse should a patient claim negligence against the dentist.

For example, a dentist and dental hygienist explain the need for improved home care to a patient and document the instructions on the patient's chart. At each visit, however, the patient's home care remains unimproved despite continued warnings. The patient's periodontal condition continues to decline. The patient's lack of home care is contributory negligence, leading to the development of periodontal disease.

Recall

16. Why should broken appointments be noted on the patient's chart?

PATIENT RECORDS

Records regarding patient care are referred to as the *dental chart* or *patient record.* These records are important legal documents that must be protected and handled with care (see Chapter 26). All examination records, diagnoses, radiographs, consent forms, updated medical histories, copies of medical and laboratory prescriptions, and correspondence to or about a patient are filed together in the patient's folder. Financial information is *not* included in the patient chart.

Patient records are acceptable in court and clearly show the date and the details of services rendered for each patient. Nothing should be left to memory. Incomplete or unclear records are damaging evidence in a malpractice

Guidelines for Charting Entries in Clinical Records

1. Keep a separate chart for each patient. Do not use a "group" chart for an entire family.
2. Business and financial information is not part of the clinical record. Do not include these records in the chart.
3. It is better to chart too much information than too little.
4. Make the chart entry during the examination or patient visit. The longer the time between the procedure and the charting entry, the greater the chance for errors.
5. Write legibly, and record the entry accurately in ink. Date and initial the entry.
6. The chart entry should be sufficiently complete to indicate that nothing was neglected; this includes the reason for the visit, details of the treatment provided, and a record of all instructions to the patient, prescriptions, and referrals.
7. Never change the chart after a problem arises. If a charting error occurs, correct it properly (see Fig. 5-2).

Procedure 5-1 Correcting a Chart Entry

Goal

To gain competency in correcting an error on a patient's record.

PROCEDURAL STEPS

1. Using an ink pen, draw a single line through the previous entry. Initial and date the change.
   Purpose: To ensure the original entry is still readable, and the change is permanent.
2. Write the corrected entry in ink on the next available line.
3. Initial and date the new entry.
   Purpose: To identify the individual responsible for the chart entry.

DATE	TOOTH	SERVICE RENDERED
~~2/10/xx~~		~~exam, adult prophy 2/15/xx DDA~~
2/10/xx	3	X-ray, remove amal restoration. Place
		sedative treatment. If pain persists,
		refer to endodontist. 2/15/xx DDA

Fig. 5-2 The original entry is readable with only a line through it when a charting error is corrected.

Indicators of Child Abuse and Neglect

Behavioral indicators

1. Child is wary of adult contacts.
2. Child is apprehensive when other children cry.
3. Child is afraid to go home.
4. Child is frightened of parents.
5. Child exhibits overly compliant, passive, and undemanding behaviors to avoid confrontation with abuser.
6. Child lags in development of motor skills, toilet training, socialization, or language. (Developmental lags may also result from physical abuse, medical neglect, or nutritional deficiency.)

Dental neglect or abuse

1 Untreated rampant caries that are easily detectable by a layperson
2. Untreated pain, infection, bleeding, or trauma affecting orofacial region
3. Injuries or tears to labial frenum, indicating forced feedings
4. Cigarette burns or bitemarks
5. Cuts, bleeding, or finger marks on ears or "cauliflower ear"
6. Bald or sparse spots on scalp, indicating malnutrition or hair pulling

Other indicators

1. Child is dirty, is unkempt, or has poor oral hygiene.
2. Child is dressed inappropriately for weather to conceal bruises or injuries (for example, long sleeves on a hot day).
3. Child shows evidence of poor supervision, such as repeated falls down stairs, repeated ingestion of harmful substances, or being left alone in a car or on the street.
4. Mentally or physically disabled children are especially vulnerable and are often targets for abuse because of the difficulties caregivers face associated with meeting the needs of these patients.

case. Every entry in a chart should be made as if the chart will be seen in a court of law (Procedure 5-1).

Patient records must never be altered. If an error is made on the patient's chart, it must be corrected properly (Fig. 5-2). The dental assistant should never use white correction fluid or attempt to cover up the original entry.

Ownership of Dental Records and Radiographs

The dentist technically "owns" all patient records and radiographs. According to some state laws, however, patients have the right to *access* (review) and *retrieve* (remove) their records and radiographs.

Original records and radiographs are not allowed to leave the practice without the dentist's permission. In most situations, duplicate radiographs and a photocopy of the record will satisfy the patient's needs. If a disagreement arises with the patient on this subject, the dental assistant should not attempt to make a decision, but should refer the matter to the dentist immediately.

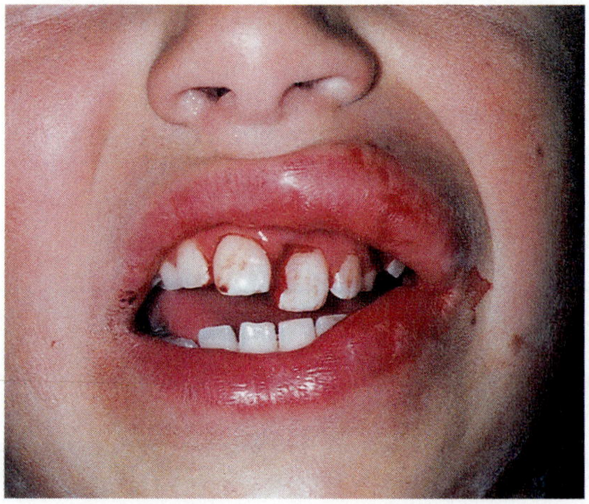

Fig. 5-3 This boy was a victim of child abuse.

REPORTING CHILD ABUSE AND NEGLECT

Cases of child abuse and neglect are increasingly reported throughout the United States. Approximately 65% of child abuse injuries involve the head, neck, or mouth areas (Fig. 5-3). Therefore, dental personnel are appropriate healthcare providers to identify signs of abuse in their pediatric patients. In many states, dental professionals are required by law to report known or suspected cases of child abuse.

The primary intent of reporting abuse is *to protect the child.* It is equally important to provide help for the parents. Parents may be unable to ask for help directly, and child abuse may be a means of revealing family problems. The report of abuse may lead to changes in the home and lower the risk of abuse.

Child abuse is legally defined as any act of omission or commission that endangers or impairs a child's physical or emotional health and development. These acts include (1) physical abuse and corporal punishment resulting in injury, (2) emotional abuse, (3) emotional deprivation, (4) physical neglect or inadequate supervision, and (5) sexual abuse or exploitation.

In states that identify dental professionals as **mandated reporters,** dental assistants must report suspected child abuse if they observe signs of abuse or if they have reasonable suspicion of abuse. The report may be made to a child protection agency, such as a county welfare or probation department, or to a police or sheriff's department.

Immunity

In states that legally mandate the reporting of child abuse, immunity is granted from criminal or civil liability for reporting as required. This means that the dental assistant cannot be sued for reporting suspicions in an attempt to protect the child.

Recall

17. What is the primary purpose of reporting suspected cases of child abuse?

18. What are mandated reporters?

LEGAL AND ETHICAL IMPLICATIONS

The practice of dentistry is subject to a variety of laws and regulations that are meant to protect the public. Dental assisting is a highly skilled profession that requires education and competence in a variety of procedures.

As a dental assistant, you should have a general understanding of how laws affect the practice of dentistry and how you can minimize the risk of malpractice liability. Legally and ethically, you must be aware of the laws that govern the practice of dentistry in your state and always practice within the law.

Eye to the Future

The number of lawsuits in dentistry increases each year. Remember that you may still be involved in a malpractice suit or may be called to testify even if you are no longer employed in the practice.

Critical Thinking

Mrs. Jensen has been a patient in your office for more than 10 years. At best, she has been difficult and demanding. She has failed to keep some appointments and often arrives late for other appointments. When Mrs. Jensen phoned the office to make an appointment, the receptionist told her that Dr. Klein would no longer be able to treat her. Mrs. Jensen became very angry and threatened to call her attorney.

1. Does Mrs. Jensen have a basis for legal action? If so, under what grounds?
2. Even though the receptionist told Mrs. Jensen that she could not be seen again in the dental office, is Dr. Klein still liable? Why or why not?
3. What would have been a better way to dismiss Mrs. Jensen from the practice?

Part 2

Sciences in Dentistry

The sciences form the foundation for your career as a dental assistant. The human body is wonderful, complex, and fascinating. As you study the information in this section, think about your own body. It will make this information even more relevant to you.

The chapters in this section provide an overview of basic human anatomy and physiology. You will be able to identify the structures of the oral cavity, and understand how the teeth begin to develop before birth. You will use your knowledge of the dentition every day in your career as a dental assistant.

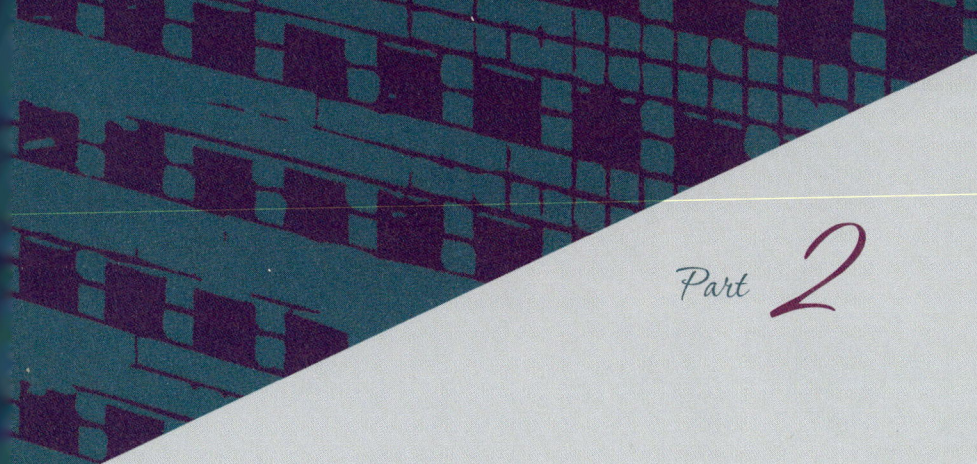

6

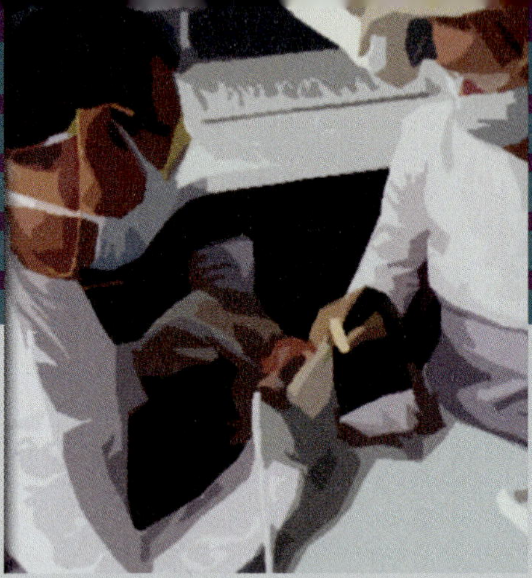

General Anatomy

Outline

Planes and Body Directions
Structural Units
- Cells
- Tissues
- Organs
- Body Systems

Body Cavities
Body Regions
Legal and Ethical Implications
Eye to the Future
Critical Thinking

KEY TERMS

Abdominal cavity Space in the body that contains the stomach, liver, gallbladder, spleen, and most of the intestines.

Abdominopelvic Pertaining to part of the ventral cavity that contains the abdominal and pelvic cavities.

Anatomical (anatomic) position (*an*-eh-**tom**-i-kul, *an*-eh-**tom**-ik) The body standing erect with face forward, feet together, arms hanging at the sides, and palms forward.

Anatomy (ah-**nat**-eh-mee) Study of the shape and structure of the human body.

Anterior Toward the front.

Appendicular (*ap*-pen-**dik**-u-ler) Pertaining to the body region that consists of the arms and legs.

Axial (**ak**-see-al) Pertaining to the body region that comprises the head, neck, and trunk.

Connective tissue The major support material of the body.

Cranial cavity (**kray**-nee-ul) Space in the body that houses the brain.

Cytoplasm (**si**-toe-*plaz*-em) Gel-like fluid inside the cell.

Differentiation Term for the specialization function of cells.

Distal Farther away from the trunk of the body; opposite of proximal.

Dorsal cavity Space in the back of the body that contains the cranial and spinal cavities.

Epithelial tissue (*ep*-i-**thee**-lee-ul) Type of tissue that forms the covering of all body surfaces.

Frontal plane Vertical plane that divides the body into anterior (front) and posterior (back) portions. Also known as the **coronal plane.**

Horizontal plane Plane that divides the body into superior (upper) and inferior (lower) portions.

Medial Toward or near the midline of the body.

Midsagittal plane Imaginary line that divides the patient's body into right and left sides.

Muscle tissue Tissue with the ability to lengthen or shorten to provide movement to body parts.

Nerve tissue Responsible for coordinating and controlling body activities.

Nucleus (**noo**-klee-us) "Control center" of the cell.

Organelle (*or*-guh-**nel**) Specialized part of a cell that performs a specific function.

Parietal (pah-**rye**-ih-tul) Pertaining to the walls of a body cavity.

Pelvic cavity Space in the body that contains portions of the large and small intestines, the rectum, urinary bladder, and reproductive organs.

Physiology (*fiz*-ee-**ahl**-eh-jee) Study of the functions of the human body.

Planes Three imaginary lines used to divide the body into sections.

Posterior Toward the back.

Proximal Closer to the trunk of the body. Opposite of distal.

Spinal cavity Space in the body that contains the spinal cord.

KEY TERMS—cont'd

Superior Above another portion, or closer to the head.
Thoracic cavity Space in the body that contains the heart, lungs, esophagus, and trachea.
Ventral cavity Space in the front of the body that contains the thoracic cavity and the abdominopelvic cavity.
Visceral (**vis**-er-ul) Pertaining to internal organs or the covering of organs.

LEARNING OUTCOMES

On completion of this chapter, the student will be able to achieve the following objectives:

- Pronounce, define, and spell the Key Terms.
- Explain the difference between anatomy and physiology.
- Identify the planes and associated body directions used to divide the body into sections.
- Identify the four levels of organization in the human body.
- Describe the components of a cell.
- Identify and describe the four types of tissues in the human body.
- Name and locate the two major body cavities and their components.
- Name and locate the two reference regions of the body.

It is important for the dental assistant to understand the basic structure and anatomy of the human body. **Anatomy** is the scientific study of the *shape* and *structure* of the human body. **Physiology** is the scientific study of how the body *functions* (see Chapter 7). The studies of anatomy and physiology are closely related because one continuously influences the other. Remember that *function affects structure,* and *structure affects function.*

To communicate effectively as a health professional, you must first begin by learning certain basic terms that relate to the anatomy of the body. This chapter deals with terms used to describe directions and regions of the body. You are learning a new vocabulary that will continue to grow as you progress through the book. The basic anatomic reference systems are (1) planes and body directions, (2) structural units, and (3) body cavities.

PLANES AND BODY DIRECTIONS

The terms used to describe *directions* in relation to the whole body are easier to understand if you think of them as *pairs of opposite directions,* such as up and down, left and right, or front and back (Table 6-1).

When describing the human body, it is assumed that the body is in "anatomical position." **Anatomical** (or **anatomic**) **position** is the body standing erect with face forward, feet together, arms hanging at the sides, and palms forward (Fig. 6-1).

To help visualize the relationships of internal body parts, three imaginary lines called **planes** are used to divide the body into sections.

1. The **midsagittal plane,** also known as the *median plane* or *midline plane,* is the vertical plane that divides the body into equal left and right halves.
2. The **horizontal plane,** also known as the *transverse plane,* divides the body into **superior** (upper) and *inferior* (lower) portions.

Table 6-1 ***Directional Terms for the Human Body***

Term	Definition	Example
Superior	Above another part, or closer to head	Nose is superior to mouth
Inferior	Below another part, or closer to feet	Heart is inferior to neck
Proximal	Closer to a point of attachment, or closer to trunk of body	Elbow is proximal to wrist
Distal	Farther from a point of attachment, or farther from trunk of body	Fingers are distal to wrist
Lateral	The side, or away from the midline	Ears are lateral to eyes
Medial	Toward or nearer the midline	Nose is medial to ears
Dorsal	On the back	Spine is on dorsal side of body
Ventral	On the front	Face is on ventral side of body
Anterior	Toward the front	Heart is anterior to spine
Posterior	Toward the back	Ear is posterior to nose

3. The **frontal plane,** also known as the *coronal plane,* is any vertical plane at right angles to the midsagittal plane that divides the body into **anterior** (front) and **posterior** (back) portions.

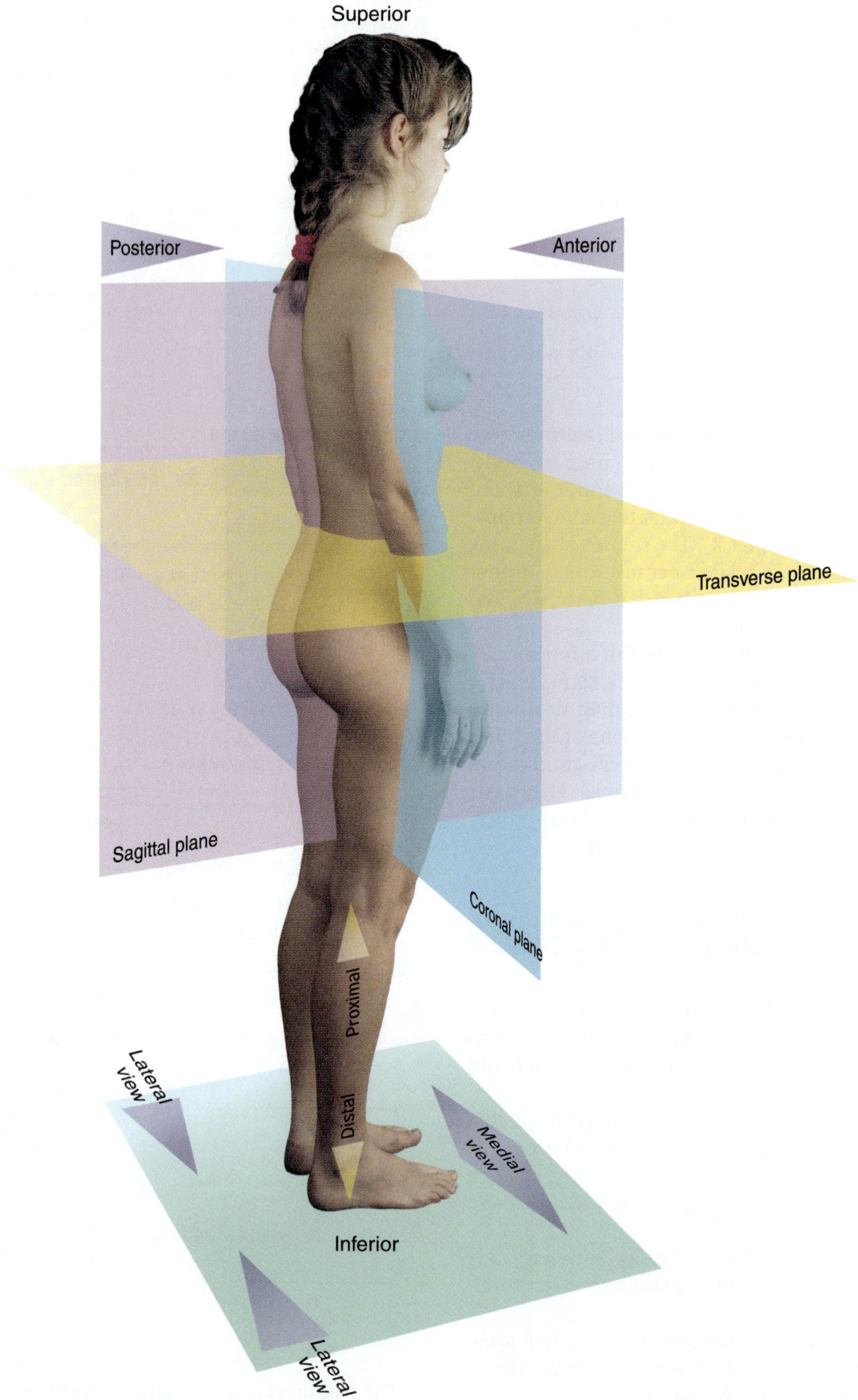

Fig. 6-1 Body in anatomical (anatomic) position. (From Abrahams PH, Marks SC Jr, and Hutchins RT: *McMinn's color atlas of human anatomy,* St Louis, 2003, Mosby.)

Recall

1. What is the difference between anatomy and physiology?
2. What three imaginary lines are used to divide the body into sections?

STRUCTURAL UNITS

The human body is incredibly complex. However, the study of anatomy is not difficult when it is broken down into small units.

The study of the human body begins with the smallest units and builds systematically to larger and larger units, finally resulting in the complete body. The human body has four organizational levels. Beginning with the simplest to the most complex, they are (1) cells, (2) tissues, (3) organs, and (4) body systems (Fig. 6-2).

Cells

Cells are the basic units of structure of the human body. Every human life begins as a single cell, a fertilized egg. This single cell divides into 2 cells, then 4, 8, 16, and so on, until the adult human body is complete and has an estimated 75 trillion cells. Each tiny cell has the following unique capabilities: (1) to react to stimuli and transform nutrients into energy, (2) to grow, and (3) to reproduce (Fig. 6-3).

Cells have different shapes. Some cells are shaped like columns, and others are shaped like cubes or spheres. For example, red blood cells resemble shallow saucers; nerve cells look like threads; and cheek cells resemble flat paving stones. The life span of cells varies depending on the type. For example, cells in the lining of the intestines die after one and a half days; red blood cells die after 120 days; and nerve cells can live for 100 years.

Different types of cells have different functions; brain cells, for example, have a different function than blood cells. The term for this specialized function of cells is **differentiation.** The human body contains many types of cells, each with a specific purpose.

Cell Membrane

Each cell has a thin membrane that surrounds it. This membrane serves two purposes:

1. The cell membrane helps the cell maintain its form and separates the cell contents from the surrounding environment. Imagine the cell membrane as being similar to the thin white membrane that lines the inside of an eggshell and holds the rest of the egg in place.
2. The cell membrane has special physical and chemical properties that allow it to recognize and interact with other cells. Basically it "decides" what may enter or leave the cell. For example, nutrients are allowed to pass though, and waste products are allowed to leave. This maintains a healthy balance for the cell to survive.

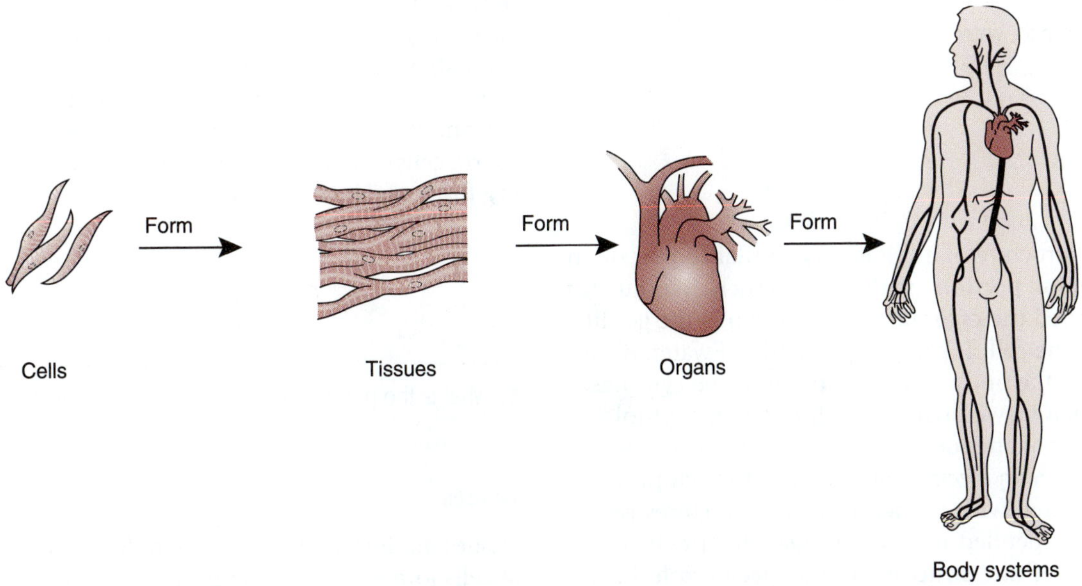

Fig. 6-2 Organizational levels of the body. The human body develops from the simplest to the most complex forms.

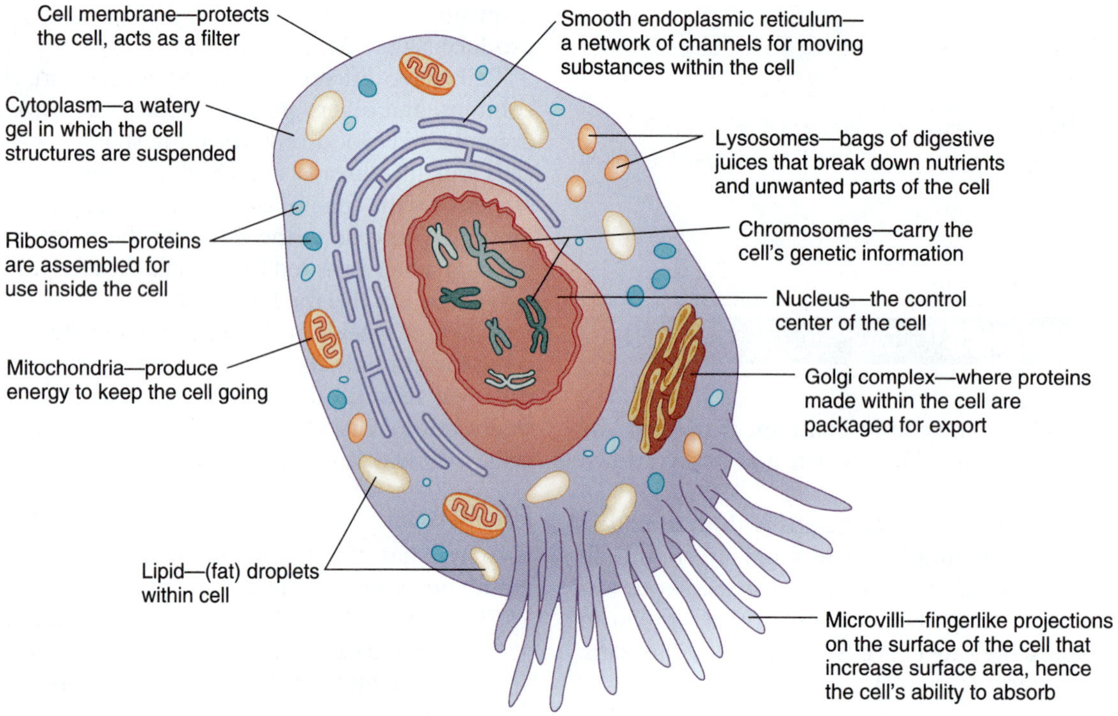
Cell membrane—protects the cell, acts as a filter
Cytoplasm—a watery gel in which the cell structures are suspended
Ribosomes—proteins are assembled for use inside the cell
Mitochondria—produce energy to keep the cell going
Lipid—(fat) droplets within cell
Smooth endoplasmic reticulum—a network of channels for moving substances within the cell
Lysosomes—bags of digestive juices that break down nutrients and unwanted parts of the cell
Chromosomes—carry the cell's genetic information
Nucleus—the control center of the cell
Golgi complex—where proteins made within the cell are packaged for export
Microvilli—fingerlike projections on the surface of the cell that increase surface area, hence the cell's ability to absorb

Fig. 6-3 Basic human cell.

Visualizing the Semipermeable Function of the Cell

Visualize a teabag in a cup of water. The teabag paper acts as a semipermeable membrane that holds the tea leaves in the bag. It does, however, permit the water to enter the bag. The smallest particles mix with the water, which carries them back through the porous teabag into the cup of water. We know that this occurs by the color and flavor change in the water.

Cytoplasm

The overall structure of a cell is very similar to that of an egg; the major portion of the cell (much like an egg white) is called the **cytoplasm.** Cytoplasm is the gel-like fluid inside the cell. It consists primarily of water. About two thirds of the body's water is found in the cytoplasm of cells. When viewed with an ordinary light, cytoplasm appears homogeneous and empty. However, when viewed through an electron microscope, the cytoplasm is highly organized with numerous small structures called **organelles** suspended in it. Each organelle, or "little organ," has a definite structure and a specific role in the function of a cell. Organelles manufacture, modify, store, and transport proteins and also dispose of cellular wastes.

Nucleus

The "control center" of the cell is called the **nucleus,** which can be compared to an egg yolk. The nucleus directs the metabolic activities of the cell. All cells have at least one nucleus at some time during their existence. Some cells (e.g., red blood cells) lose their nucleus as they mature. Other cells (e.g., skeletal muscle cells) have more than one nucleus.

The nucleus of every cell contains a complete set of the body's chromosomes, which contain *DNA* (deoxyribonucleic acid) and *RNA* (ribonucleic acid), two chemicals that carry all genetic information.

Human life begins as the result of cell division. For this reason, all the cells in your body (except for the egg or sperm cells) contain the same information as the fertilized egg from which you began.

Recall

3. What is the portion of the cell that carries genetic information?

Tissues

Tissues are formed when many millions of the same type of cells join together to perform a specific function for the body. There are four main tissue types in the human body: (1) epithelial, (2) connective, (3) muscle, and (4) nerve tissue (Box 6-1).

Epithelial tissue forms a covering for the external and internal body surfaces (e.g., the skin on the outside of the body, and the lining of the oral cavity and intestines). The purposes of epithelial cells are to (1) provide protection, (2) produce secretions, and (3) regulate the passage of materials across them. Some epithelial cells are *specialized,* meaning they have special functions associated with skin color, hair, nails, mucus production, and sweat regulation.

Connective tissue is the major support material of the body. It provides support for the body and connects its

Box 6-1 Types of Tissues and Functions in the Human Body

Epithelial tissue

Covering and lining

Skin protects the body from exposure to disease-causing organisms.

Epithelium lines internal organs and body cavities (e.g., nose, mouth, stomach).

Glandular or secretory

Epithelial tissues secrete substances such as digestive juices, hormones, milk, perspiration, and mucus.

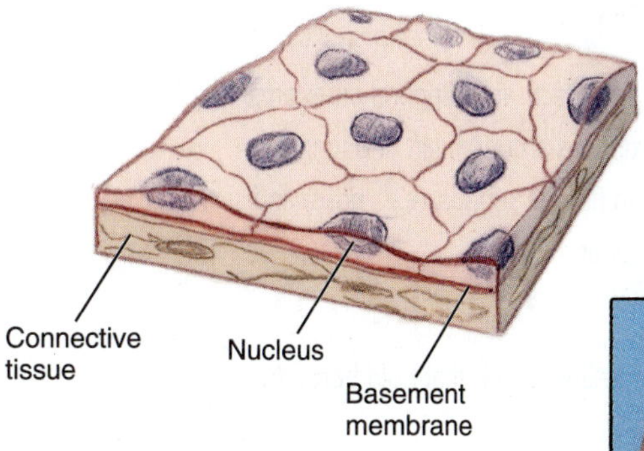

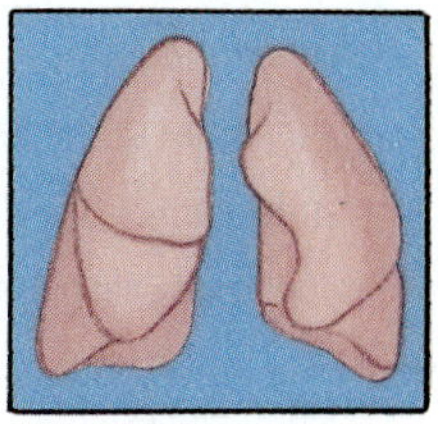

Simple squamous ("scaly") epithelium.

Muscle tissue

Striated

Also called **skeletal** and *voluntary,* these muscles are attached to bones, tendons, or other muscles.

Striated (striped) muscles are responsible for voluntary movement.

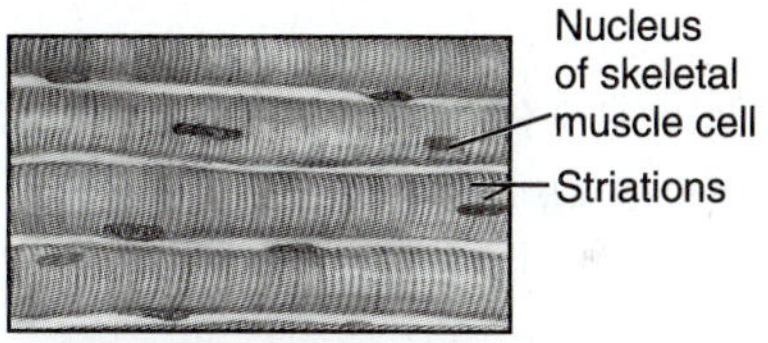

Smooth

Also known as **visceral,** *nonstriated,* and *involuntary,* these muscles provide involuntary movements (e.g., digestion).

Smooth muscles are in visceral (internal) organs as well as in hollow body cavities.

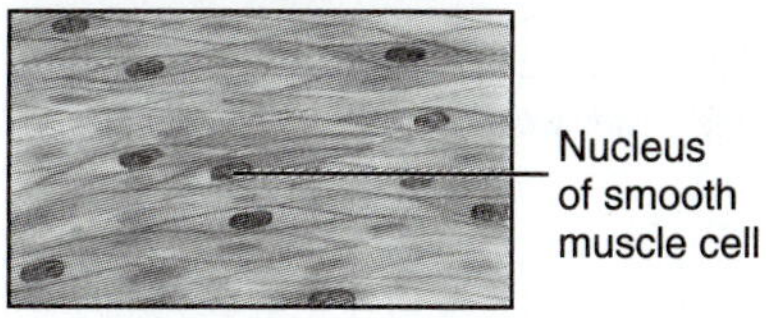

Cardiac

Tissue makes up the walls of the heart.

Muscles help pump blood out of the heart.

Even though muscle has striations, movement is involuntary.

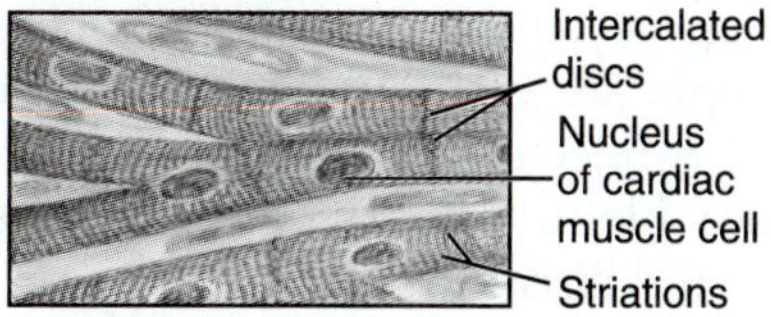

Nerve tissue

Neuronal

Tissue reacts to environmental stimuli.

Nerves carry messages (impulses) to and from the brain.

Tissues are found in the brain, spinal cord, and sense organs.

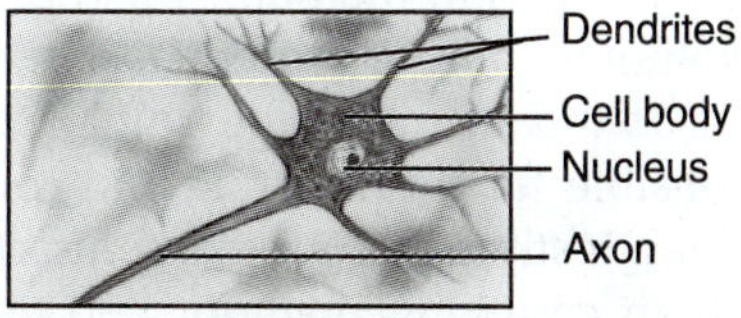

Art from Applegate EJ: *The anatomy and physiology learning system,* ed 2, Philadelphia, 2000, Saunders.

Continued

Box 6-1 Types of Tissues and Functions in the Human Body—cont'd

Connnective tissue

Adipose (fat)

Tissues store fat.

Tissues provide energy source when needed.

Fat cushions, supports, and insulates the body.

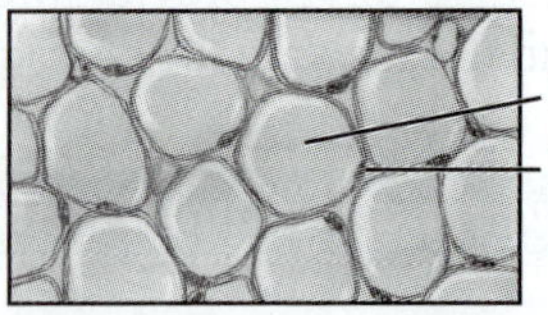

Supportive

Osseous tissue (bone) protects and supports other organs (e.g., spinal column, ribs around heart and lungs).

Cartilage provides firm flexible support (e.g., nose) and serves as a shock absorber at the joints.

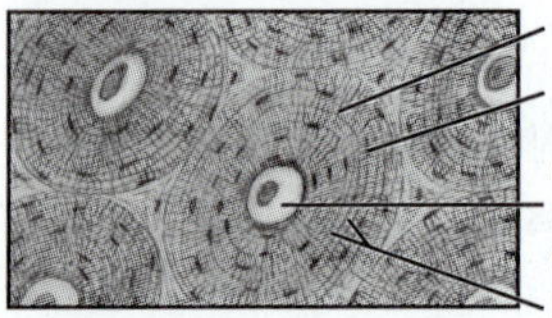

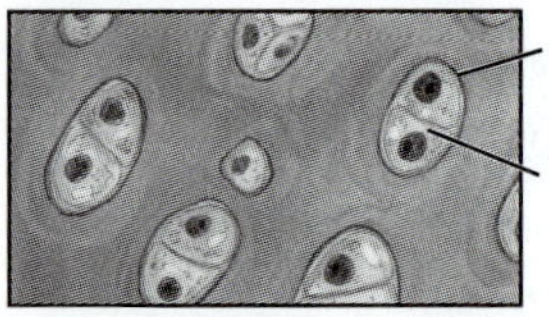

Dense fibrous

Ligaments are strong flexible bands that hold bones together at the joints.

Tendons are white glossy bands that attach skeletal muscles to the bones.

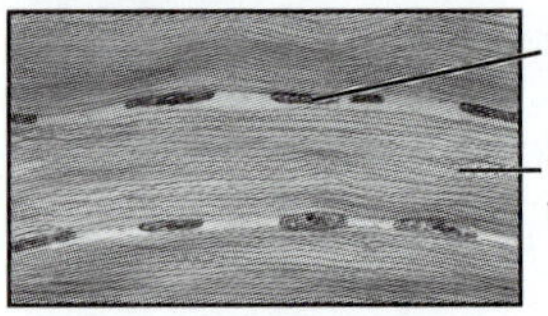

Vascular

Blood transports nutrients and oxygen to body cells and carries away waste products.

Lymph transports tissue fluid, proteins, fat, and other materials from the tissues to the capillaries.

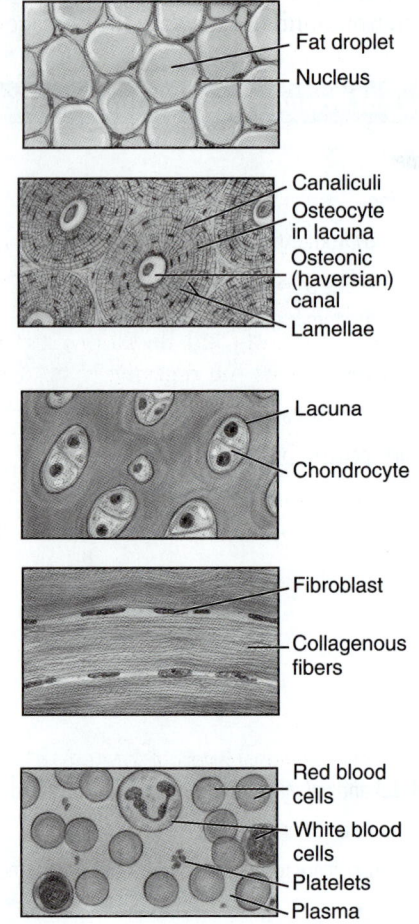

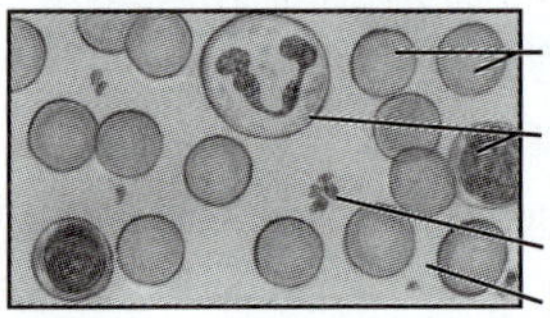

Art from Applegate EJ: *The anatomy and physiology learning system,* ed 2, Philadelphia, 2000, Saunders.

organs and tissues. Fat, tendons, ligaments, bone, cartilage, blood, and lymph are all types of connective tissue. Specific types of connective tissue can store fat, destroy bacteria, produce blood cells, and develop antibodies against infection and disease.

Muscle tissue has the ability to lengthen and shorten and thus move body parts. The skeletal muscles are either *voluntary* or *involuntary.* For example, when you decide when to move your arms or legs, the muscle movement is voluntary. However, the beating of your heart, churning of your stomach, and changes in the pupils of your eyes are controlled by involuntary muscle movements.

Nerve tissue is found in the brain, spinal cord, and nerves. It is responsible for coordinating and controlling many body activities. It stimulates muscle contraction and plays a major role in emotions, memory, and reasoning. Nerve tissue also has the unique ability to react to environmental changes, such as heat, cold, light, or pressure. Nerve tissue also carries messages from all areas of the body to the brain and from the brain to all areas of the body. To perform these functions, cells in nerve tissue need to communicate with each other by way of electrical nerve impulses.

Recall

4. What are the four types of tissues in the human body?

Organs

Organs are formed when several types of tissues group together to perform a single function. For example, the stomach is an organ that contains each of the four tissue types (nerve, connective, muscle, epithelial) and performs the digestive function in the body. The heart and lungs are also organs that contain all four major tissue types.

Body Systems

A body system is composed of a group of organs working together to perform a major function to keep the body healthy and functional. For example, the digestive system is responsible for ingestion of food, digestion, and absorption of nutrition. Organs of the digestive system include the esophagus, stomach, and small and large intestines. Each organ has its specific job to do, and when each of the digestive organs performs its function as required, the proper digestion, absorption, and elimination of food occur. There are 10 major body systems (see Chapter 7).

Recall

5. What are the four organizational levels of the human body, from simplest to most complex?

BODY CAVITIES

The organs of the body are located in areas called *body cavities.* There are two main body cavities (Fig. 6-4).

The cavity located in the back of the body is known as the **dorsal cavity.** The cavity located in the front of the body is called the **ventral cavity.** Each of the two major body cavities is further divided into smaller cavities. **Parietal** refers to the walls of a body cavity.

The dorsal cavity is divided into the **cranial cavity,** which contains the brain, and the **spinal cavity,** which contains the spinal cord. The cranial and spinal cavities join with each other to form a continuous space.

The ventral cavity is much larger than the dorsal cavity and is subdivided into the **thoracic cavity** and the **abdominopelvic** (abdominal and pelvic) cavity. The thoracic cavity contains the heart, lungs, esophagus, and trachea. The **abdominal cavity** houses the stomach, liver, gallbladder, spleen, and most of the intestines. The **pelvic cavity** contains portions of the small and large intestines, the rectum, urinary bladder, and internal reproductive organs.

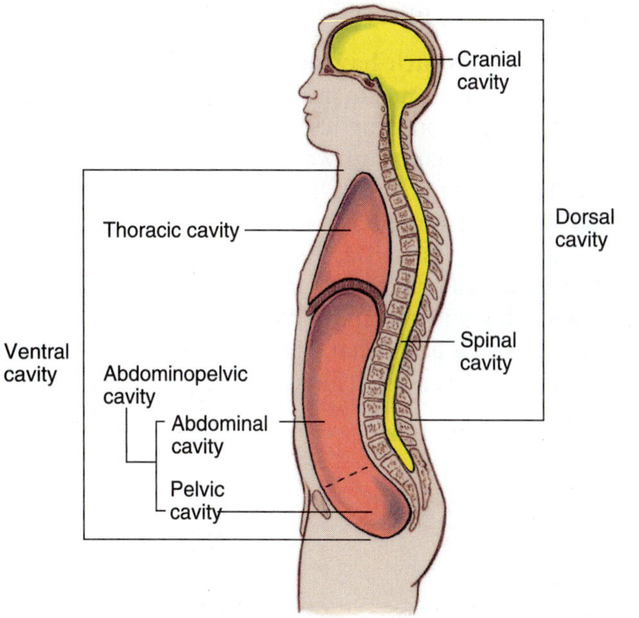

Fig. 6-4 **Spaces within the body that house specific organs are referred to as *body cavities.*** (From Applegate EJ: *The anatomy and physiology learning system,* ed 2, Philadelphia, 2000, Saunders.)

BODY REGIONS

For reference, the body is divided into two major regions. The **axial** division consists of the head, neck, and trunk, and the **appendicular** region comprises the arms and legs.

Recall

6. What are the two major body cavities?
7. Which components make up the axial and appendicular regions of the human body?

LEGAL AND ETHICAL IMPLICATIONS

A wise person once said, "Patients don't care how much you know, until they know how much you care." Never forget that your patients are more than cells, organs, and body systems. They are the most important people in the dental office. Treat patients as you would want to be treated in the healthcare environment.

Eye to the Future

Oral health research has identified the precise genetic errors that lead to many craniofacial syndromes. Because of this ongoing research, we can now provide essential information to women who are pregnant or want to become pregnant, and educate them about the risks of drugs, certain medications, alcohol, and cigarette smoking, as well as the importance of nutrients like folic acid. Research is mastering the arts of diagnostic screening and detection. We are well on the way to replacement of genes that will lead to the ability to repair or correct genetic defects even before birth.

Critical Thinking

1. Why is the study of general anatomy included in a dental-assisting textbook?
2. What types of tissues make up the skin?
3. Do you think cellular research is important? Why or why not?

7

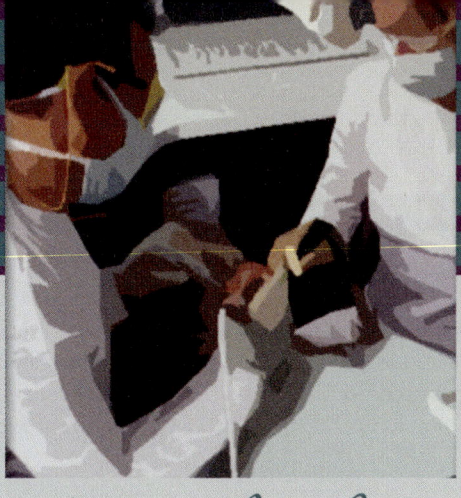

General Physiology

Outline

KEY TERMS

Apocrine sweat glands Large sweat glands that are found under the arms, around the nipples, and in the genital region.

Appendicular skeleton (*ap*-pen-**dik**-u-ler) Portion of the skeleton that consists of the upper extremities and shoulder girdle plus the lower extremities and pelvic girdle.

Arteries Large blood vessels that carry blood away from the heart.

Articulation (*ahr*-tik-u-**lay**-shun) Another term for *joint.*

Axial skeleton (**ak**-see-ul) Portion of the skeleton that consists of the skull, spinal column, ribs, and sternum.

Bone marrow Gelatinous material that produces white blood cells, red blood cells, or platelets.

Cancellous bone (kan-**sel**-us) Lightweight, spongy bone found in the interior of bones.

Capillaries A system of microscopic vessels that connects the arterial and venous systems.

Cartilage Tough, connective, nonvascular, elastic tissue.

Central nervous system (CNS) The brain and spinal cord.

Compact bone Hard, dense, strong bone that forms the outer layer of the bones, where it is needed for strength; also known as *cortical bone.*

Integumentary system (in-teg-yu-**men**-ta-ree) The skin system.

Involuntary muscles Muscles that function automatically without conscious control.

Joints Structural areas where two or more bones come together.

Muscle insertion Location where the muscle ends; the portion away from the body's midline.

Muscle origin Location where the muscle begins; the portion toward the body's midline.

Neurons Direct nerve impulses.

Osteoblasts (**os**-te-o-*blasts*) Cells that form bone.

Pericardium (*per*-i-**kahr**-dee-um) Double-walled sac that encloses the heart.

Periosteum (*per*-e-**ahs**-tee-um) Specialized connective tissue covering all bones of the body.

Peripheral nervous system (PNS) Cranial nerves and spinal nerves.

Peristalsis (*per*-i-**stahl**-sis) Rhythmic action that moves food through the digestive tract.

Continued

KEY TERMS—cont'd

Plasma A straw-colored fluid that transports nutrients, hormones, and waste products.

Red blood cells Cells that contain the blood protein *hemoglobin,* which plays an essential role in oxygen transport; also known as *erythrocytes.*

Sebaceous glands Oil glands that keep the hair and skin soft and are associated with sex hormones.

Sharpey's fibers Tissues that anchor the periosteum to the bone.

Sudoriferous glands (soo-do-**rif**-er-us) Sweat glands that are widely distributed over the body and provide heat regulation.

Veins Blood vessels that carry blood to the heart.

White blood cells Cells that have the primary function of fighting disease in the body; also known as *leukocytes.*

LEARNING OUTCOMES

On completion of this chapter, the student will be able to achieve the following objectives:

- Pronounce, define, and spell the Key Terms.
- Name and locate each of the 10 body systems.
- Explain the purpose of each body system.
- Describe the components of each body system.
- Explain how each body system functions.
- Describe the signs and symptoms of common disorders related to each body system.
- Give examples of conditions that require interaction of the body systems.

The human body is the most incredible creation, with its senses and strengths, an ingenious defense system, and mental capabilities. The human body is a masterpiece more amazing than science fiction.

The study of the human body is as old as human history, because people have always had a fascination about how the body is put together, how it works, why it becomes diseased, and why it wears out.

Physiology is the study of how living organisms *function.* It continues beyond the study of anatomy into how the body works, what it can do, and why (see Chapter 6).

The human body has 10 systems: (1) skeletal (2) muscular, (3) cardiovascular (including lymphatic and immune systems), (4) nervous, (5) respiratory, (6) digestive, (7) endocrine, (8) urinary, (9) integumentary (skin), and (10) reproductive. Each system has specific organs within it, and each body system performs specific functions. When all 10 systems are functioning well, the person is healthy (Table 7-1). This chapter summarizes each of these body systems, their components and functions, and the disorders that affect them.

Table 7-1 ***Major Body Systems***

Body System	Components	Major Functions
Skeletal system	206 bones	Protection, support, and shape; hematopoietic; storage of certain minerals
Muscular system	Striated, smooth, and cardiac muscle	Holding body erect, locomotion, movement of body fluids, production of body heat, communication
Cardiovascular system	Heart, arteries, veins, blood	Respiratory, nutritive, excretory
Lymphatic and immune systems	White blood cells; lymph fluid, vessels, and nodes; spleen and tonsils	Defense against disease, conservation of plasma proteins and fluid, lipid absorption
Nervous system	Central and peripheral nervous systems, special sense organs	Reception of stimuli, transmission of messages, coordinating mechanism
Respiratory system	Nose, paranasal sinuses, pharynx, epiglottis, larynx, trachea, bronchi, and lungs	Transport of oxygen to cells, excretion of carbon dioxide and some water wastes
Digestive system	Mouth, pharynx, esophagus, stomach, intestines, and accessory organs	Digestion of food, absorption of nutrients, elimination of solid wastes
Urinary system	Kidneys, ureters, bladder, and urethra	Formation and elimination of urine, maintenance of homeostasis

SKELETAL SYSTEM

The skull, spine, and rib cage form the **axial skeleton** and account for 80 of the 206 bones in the human body. The shoulders, arms, hands, hips, legs and feet form the **appendicular skeleton.** The skull has 28 bones and is discussed in detail in Chapter 9 (Fig. 7-1).

The axial skeleton (80 bones) consists of the skull, spinal column, ribs, and sternum. Its function is to protect

Table 7-1 ***Major Body Systems—cont'd***

Body System	Components	Major Functions
Integumentary system	Skin, hair, nails, and sweat and sebaceous glands	Protection of body, regulation of body temperature
Endocrine system	Adrenals, gonads, pancreas, parathyroids, pineal, pituitary, thymus, and thyroid	Integration of body functions, control of growth, maintenance of homeostasis
Reproductive system	*Male:* testes, penis *Female:* ovaries, fallopian tubes, uterus, vagina	Production of new life

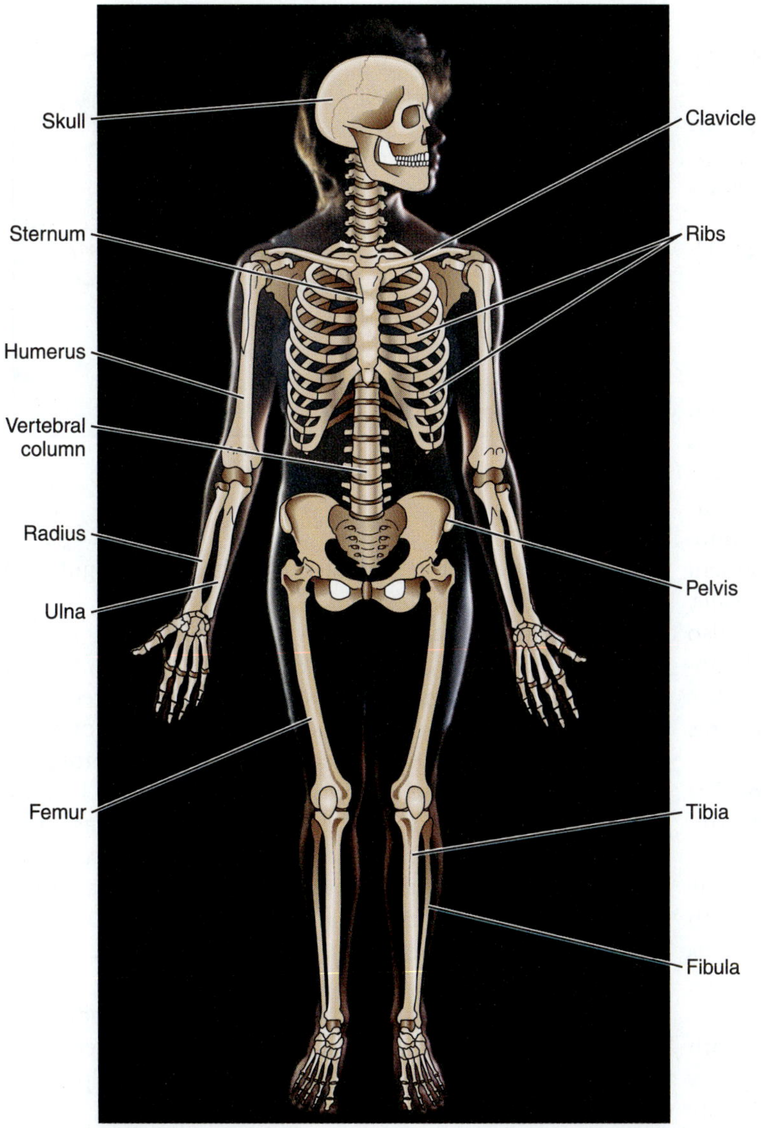

Fig. 7-1 **The skeletal system.** (From Chester G: *Modern medical assisting,* Philadelphia, 1998, Saunders.)

Box 7-1 Disorders of the Skeletal System

Examples of disorders	Signs and symptoms
Arthritis: inflammation of a joint. More than 100 forms are known, all having different causes.	Swelling and pain, usually with structural changes involved. Mobility impairment and difficulty in performing daily tasks.
Gout: inflammatory joint reaction caused by accumulation of uric acid crystals. The area usually affected is the big toe.	The joint usually becomes red, warm, shiny, swollen, and very sensitive to the touch.
Osteomyelitis: infection of the bone, caused by bacteria, fungi, or contaminated foreign material such as an artificial joint.	Sudden onset of fever, limited movement, and severe pain in the body part involved.
Osteoporosis: age-related disease in which the bones demineralize, resulting in loss of bone density and fractures.	Frequent fractures, especially of vertebrae, wrist, or hip. Back pain and decrease in height.
Sprain: injury to a joint. The joint is usually stretched beyond its normal range of movement.	Pain, swelling, bruising, abnormal movement, and joint weakness (depending on severity).
Fracture: broken bones caused by stress on the bone. Fractures can occur in any bone in the body and are classified by the type of fracture.	Severe pain, swelling, and disfigurement, depending on the type of fracture.

the major organs of the nervous, respiratory, and circulatory systems.

The appendicular skeleton (126 bones) consists of the upper extremities and shoulder area plus the lower extremities and pelvic area. It protects the organs of digestion and reproduction.

Many disorders can affect the skeletal system (Box 7-1).

Bone

The bones of the human body only weigh approximately 20 pounds. The bones of the body allow us to stand and walk, and they protect internal organs. The skull protects the brain, and the rib cage shields the heart and lungs. Bone is a living connective tissue that is capable of repairing itself when injured. It consists of an organic component (the cells and matrix) and an inorganic component (minerals). The minerals, primarily *calcium* and *phosphate,* give rigidity to bone. These minerals stored in bones also act as reservoirs to maintain essential blood mineral concentrations when the body's supply is inadequate. The three layers of bone are (1) periosteum, (2) compact bone, and (3) cancellous bone and marrow (Fig. 7-2).

The **periosteum** (Latin for "surrounding the bone") is the first layer of the bone. It is a thin layer of whitish connective tissue and contains nerves and blood vessels. It supplies the cells from which the hard bone below the periosteum is built up. It is necessary for bone growth and repair, for nutrition, and for carrying away waste. It is the periosteum that is responsible for the life of the bone and is capable of repair. The inner layer is loose connective tissue containing **osteoblasts,** or cells associated with bone formation. The periosteum is anchored to bone by **Sharpey's fibers,** which penetrate the underlying bone

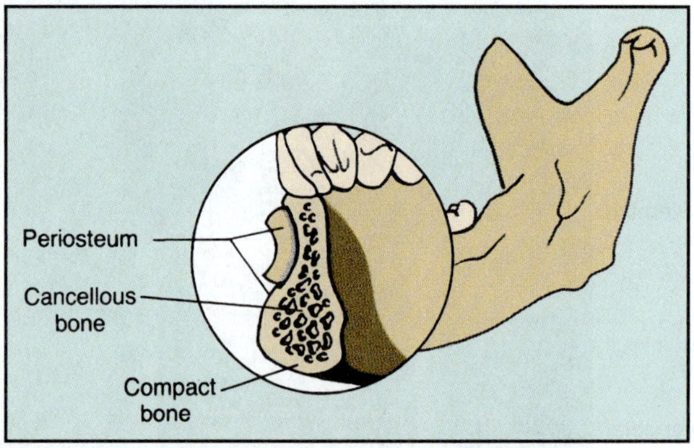

Fig. 7-2 The structure of bone.

matrix. Beneath the periosteum is the dense, rigid compact bone.

Compact bone, also known as *cortical bone,* is hard, dense, and very strong (Fig. 7-3; see also Fig. 7-2). It forms the outer layer of the bones, where it is needed for strength. This layer of bone is so dense that surgeons must use a saw or bone bur instead of a knife to cut through it.

Cancellous bone, also known as *spongy bone,* is found inside the bone. It is lighter in weight and not as strong as compact bone. The *trabeculae* (plural of *trabecula*) are bony spicules in cancellous bone that form a honeycomb pattern of spaces that are filled with *bone marrow.* The trabeculae appear as a weblike structure in a radiograph (see Fig. 7-3).

Bone marrow is a gelatinous material that produces either white blood cells (which fight infection), red blood cells (which carry oxygen), or platelets (which help to stop bleeding).

A

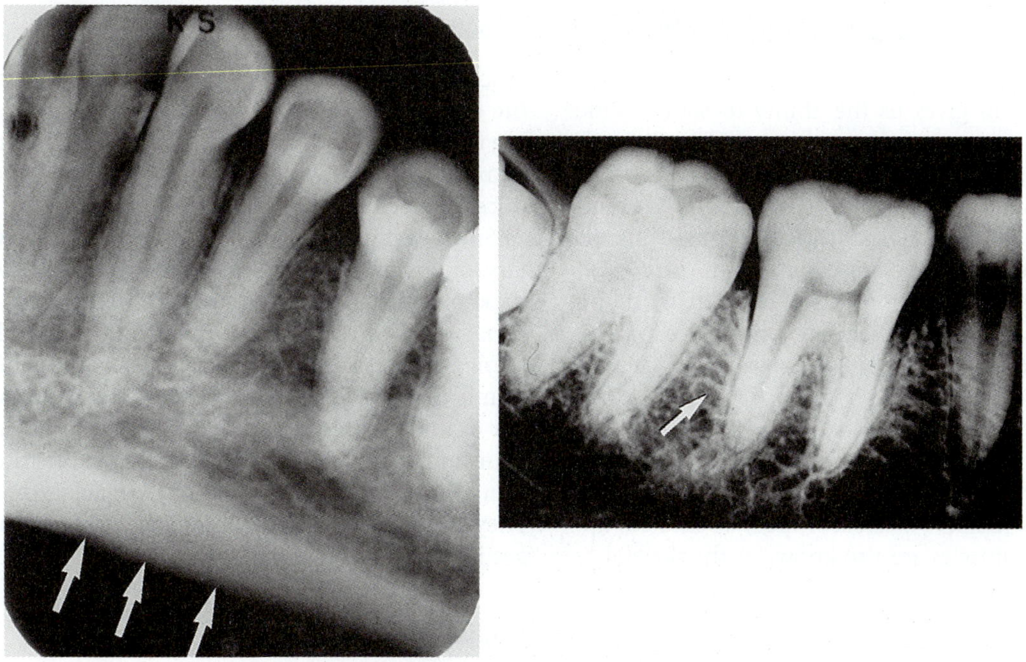

B

Fig. 7-3 **A, Cortical bone appears hard and dense. B, Cancellous bone forms trabeculae.** (From Haring JI, Lind LJ: *Radiographic interpretation for the dental hygienist,* Philadelphia, 1993, Saunders.)

Cartilage

Cartilage is also strong but more elastic than bone. It is found where bones join together. Cartilage is a tough, nonvascular (not associated with blood), connective tissue. In addition to the ends of bone, cartilage forms the nose and ears.

Recall

1. What are the two divisions of the skeleton?
2. What is the connective tissue that covers all bones?
3. What are the two types of bone and their features?
4. Where is cartilage found?

Joints

Joints, or **articulations,** are areas where two bones come together. The three basic types of joints are as follows:

1. *Fibrous joints,* such as the sutures of the skull, do not move. A *suture* is the jagged line where the bones articulate and form a joint that does not move.
2. *Cartilaginous joints* are made of connective tissue and cartilage. They only move very slightly. An example is the joints between the bones of the vertebrae.
3. *Synovial joints* are the movable joints and make up most of the joints in the body. Some synovial joints are lined with a fibrous sac called a *bursa.* The bursa is filled with *synovial fluid* and acts as a cushion to ease movement (Fig. 7-4). Examples of synovial joints include the knee and elbow (hinge type) and the hips and shoulders (ball-and-socket type).

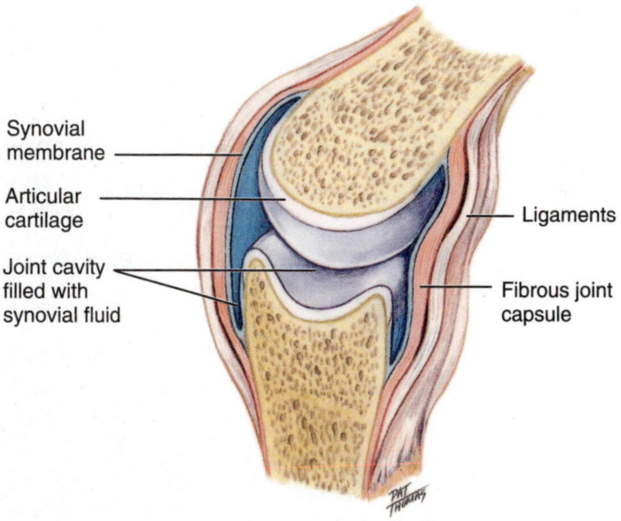

Fig. 7-4 **Generalized structure of a synovial joint.** (From Applegate EJ: *The anatomy and physiology learning system,* Philadelphia, 2000, Saunders.)

Recall

5. *Articulation* is another term for what structure?

MUSCULAR SYSTEM

The muscular system gives us the ability to stand, walk, run, jump, move our eyes, smile, and frown (Figs. 7-5 and 7-6). In order for muscles to make the body move, they must work together. Each muscle consists of muscle tissue, connective tissue, nerve tissue, and vascular (blood) tissue. Many disorders can affect the muscular system (Box 7-2).

The muscular system is composed of more than 600 individual muscles. However, there are only three *types of muscles.* These muscle types are *striated, smooth,* and *cardiac.*

Striated Muscle

Striated muscles are so named because dark and light bands in the muscle fibers create a striped, or striated, appearance. Striated muscles are also known as the skeletal or voluntary muscles. These muscles attach to the bones of the skeleton and make voluntary bodily motion possible. *Voluntary muscles* are so named because we have conscious (voluntary) control over these muscles. For example, you decide when to move your arms or legs.

Smooth Muscle

Smooth muscle fibers move the internal organs, such as the digestive tract, blood vessels, and secretory ducts leading from glands. In contrast to the marked contraction and relaxation of the striated muscles, smooth muscles produce relatively slow contraction.

Smooth muscles are also known as unstriated, involuntary, or visceral muscles. *Unstriated muscles* do not have the dark and light bands that produce the striped appearance seen in striated muscles. **Involuntary muscles** are so named because they are under the control of the autonomic nervous system and are not controlled voluntarily. For example, you do not decide when to begin digesting your lunch. *Visceral muscles* are so named because they are found in all the visceral (internal) organs except the heart. They are also found in hollow structures, such as the digestive and urinary tracts.

Cardiac Muscle

Cardiac muscle is striated in appearance but resembles smooth muscle in its action. Cardiac muscle forms most of

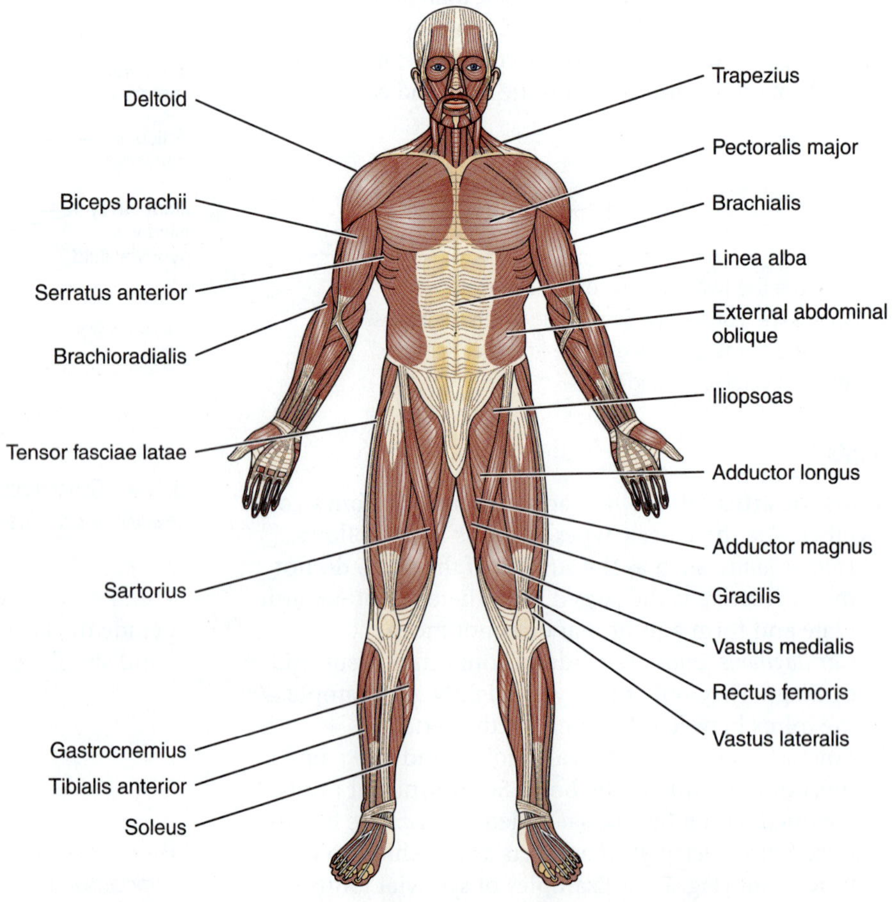

Fig. 7-5 **Muscles of the body, anterior view.** (From Chester G: *Modern medical assisting,* Philadelphia, 1998, Saunders.)

the walls of the heart, and contraction of this muscle results in the heartbeat. Over a lifetime, the heart will have beaten 4 billion times and have pumped 600,000 tons of blood. Physiologists think the reason that the cardiac muscle is so durable is that the cardiac muscle combines the power of the striated voluntary muscles with the steady reliability of the smooth, involuntary ones. Moreover, the cardiac fibers connect with each other and create a mutually supportive network of communications.

Recall

6. What are the three types of muscle tissue?
7. What distinguishes the appearance of each muscle type?

Muscle Function

Muscles are the only body tissues that have the ability to contract and relax. *Contraction* is the tightening of a muscle, during which it becomes shorter and thicker. *Relaxation*

Box 7-2 Disorders of the Muscular System

Examples of disorders	Signs and symptoms
Contusions: soft tissue trauma.	Swelling, tenderness, and localized hemorrhage and bruising can cause restriction in range of motion but no loss of joint stability.
Strain: injury of a muscle that has been stretched beyond its capacity.	Small blood vessels around the area rupture, causing swelling of the area. The area becomes tender with possible painful muscle spasms.
Progressive muscular dystrophy: includes nine types, all with unknown causes.	Progressive muscle atrophy with organ involvement and weakness.
Sprain: injury to a joint that has been stretched beyond its normal range of motion, resulting in a tear.	Depending on the severity of the damage, it may include pain of the affected area, swelling, bruising, abnormal motion, and joint weakness.

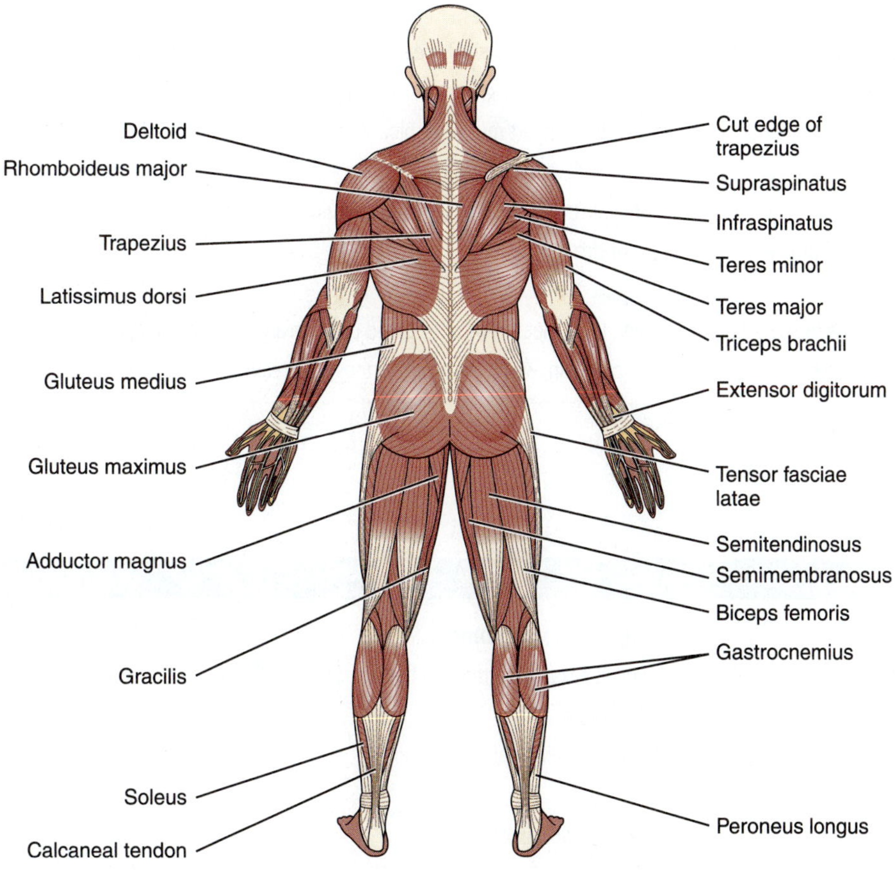

Fig. 7-6 Muscles of the body, posterior view. (From Chester G: *Modern medical assisting*, Philadelphia, 1998, Saunders.)

occurs when a muscle returns to its original form or shape. The muscles of the body are arranged in opposing pairs so that when one muscle contracts, the other muscle relaxes. These opposing actions make motion possible.

Muscle origin is the place where the muscle begins (originates). This position is the more fixed attachment or the portion of the muscle that is toward the midline of the body.

Muscle insertion is the place where the muscle ends (inserts). This position is the more movable attachment or the portion of the muscle that is away from the midline of the body.

Recall

8. What are four disorders of the muscular system?

CARDIOVASCULAR SYSTEM

The cardiovascular system consists of the (1) circulatory system, (2) heart, and (3) lymphatic system. These systems provide life-sustaining functions for the survival of body cells and tissues. Disorders of the heart and lymphatic system have specific signs and symptoms (Boxes 7-3 and 7-4).

Circulatory System

The two primary functions of the circulatory system are as follows:

1. Transport (a) oxygen and nutrients *to* the body cells, (b) carbon dioxide and waste products *from* the body cells, and (c) hormones and antibodies throughout the body.
2. Regulate body temperature and maintain chemical stability.

Box 7-3 Disorders of the Heart

Examples of disorders	Signs and symptoms
Cardiomyopathy: heart muscle disease. Cause is unknown; usually leads to heart failure.	Fatigue, weakness, heart failure, chest pain, and shortness of breath.
Coronary artery disease: caused by a build-up of cholesterol plaques in coronary arteries, reducing blood flow to the heart.	Chest pain, shortness of breath. Pain may radiate to neck, jaw, arm, or back. Ashen or gray color and anxiety are also common.
Endocarditis: inflammation of the endocardial layer of the heart; can be caused by bacteria, virus, tuberculosis, or cancer.	High fever, heart murmurs, blood clots, joint pain, fatigue, shortness of breath, and chest pain.
Heart failure: the heart can no longer pump an adequate supply of blood. Can be caused by disease, congenital problems, hypertension, lung disease, or valve problems.	Breathlessness, weakness, fatigue, dizziness, confusion, hypotension, or death.
Pericarditis: inflammation of the pericardial layer of the heart. Can be caused by bacteria, virus, tuberculosis, or cancer.	High fever, heart murmurs, blood clots, enlarged spleen, fatigue, joint pain, weight loss, or shortness of breath.

Box 7-4 Disorders of the Lymphatic System

Examples of disorders	Signs and symptoms
Lymphangitis: inflammation of peripheral lymphatic vessels, usually caused by an infection.	Red streaks that extend up the arm or leg, with enlarged, tender lymph nodes.
Lymphadenopathy: swelling or enlargement of one or more lymph nodes; can result from infection, inflammation, or neoplasm.	Painful swelling of lymph nodes.
Lymphedema: swelling of soft tissues due to increased amount of lymph.	Painful swelling of limbs.

Heart

Each day the heart pumps 4000 gallons of blood at a speed of 40 miles per hour through 70,000 miles of vessels (Fig. 7-7). The heart is a hollow muscle with four chambers. Heart size varies from individual to individual but is about the size of a closed fist. The heart is protected by the thoracic cavity and located between the lungs and above the diaphragm. The heart is enclosed in a double-walled membranous sac known as the **pericardium.** Pericardial fluid between the layers prevents friction when the heart beats.

Heart Chambers

The heart functions as a double pump; the right side pumps blood to the lungs, and the left side sends blood to the rest of the body. The coronary vessels supply blood for the heart muscle (Fig. 7-8). Each side is subdivided into an upper and a lower chamber, for a total of four chambers. The upper chambers, the *atria,* receive blood. The lower chambers, the *ventricles,* pump blood.

Heart Valves

One-way valves prevent the backflow of blood and separate the chambers of the heart by opening and closing with each heartbeat (Fig. 7-9). The *tricuspid valve* (with three "cusps," or triangular segments) is between the right atrium and ventricle. The *mitral valve* has two cusps and lies between the left atrium and ventricle. Two *semilunar valves* have three crescent-shaped flaps. The *pulmonary semilunar valve* allows blood to flow from the right ventricle into the pulmonary artery. Blood flows from the left ventricle into the aorta through the *aortic semilunar valve.*

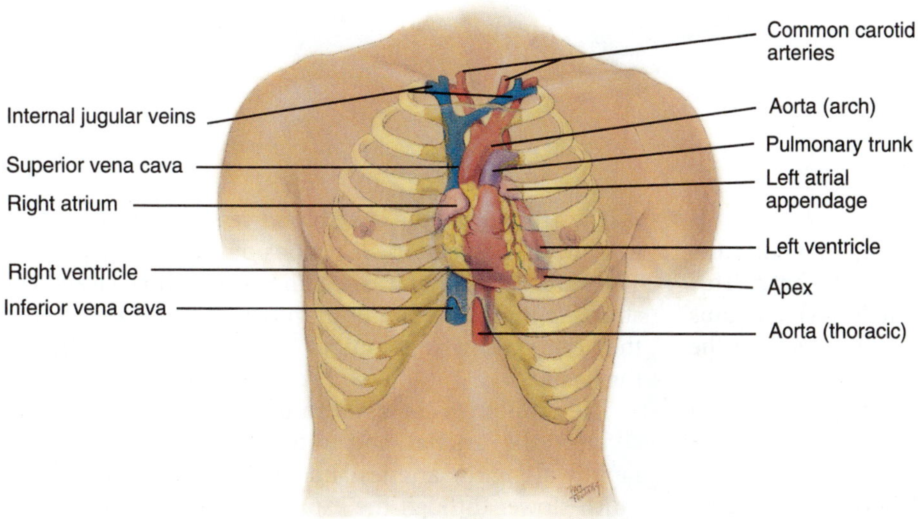

Fig. 7-7 **The heart and great vessels.**

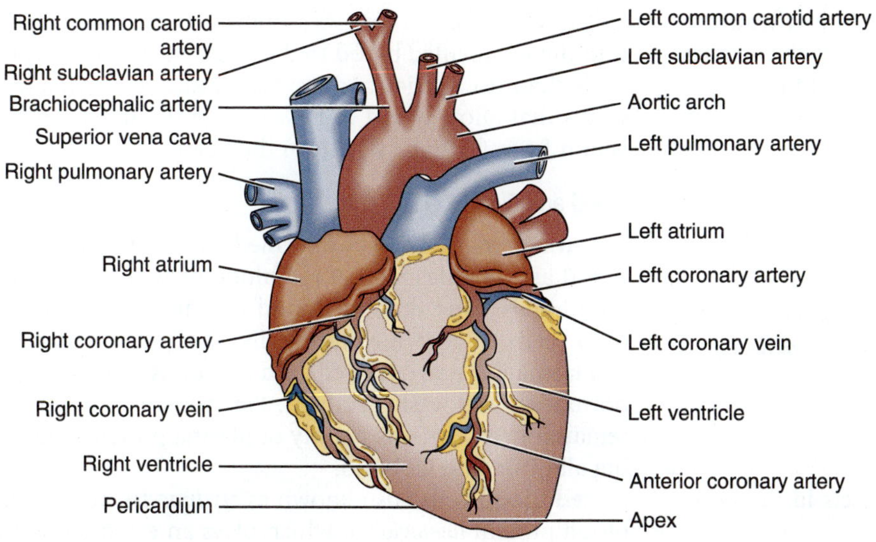

Fig. 7-8 **Coronary vessels.** (From Chester G: *Modern medical assisting,* Philadelphia, 1998, Saunders.)

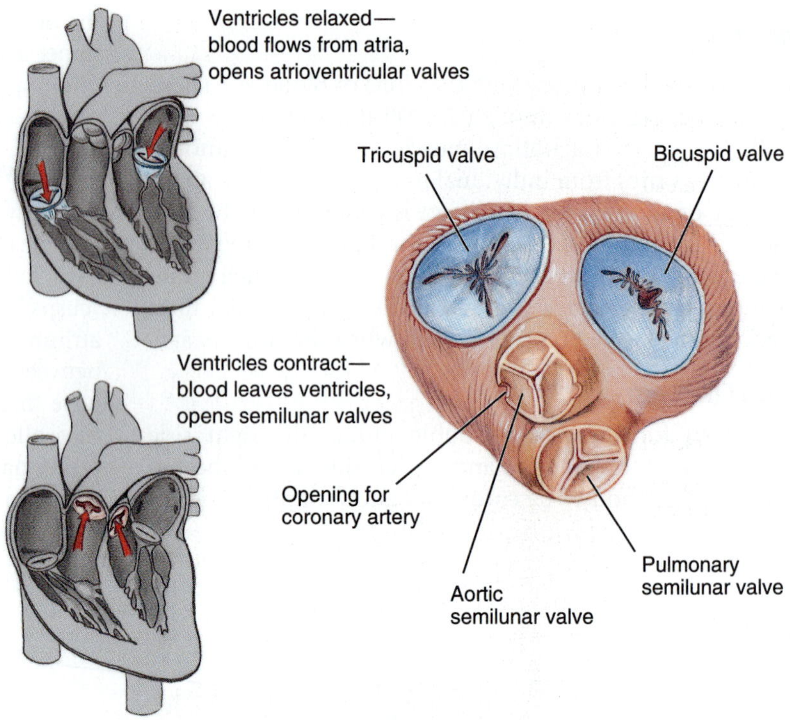

Fig. 7-9 Heart valves, superior view. (From Applegate EJ: *The anatomy and physiology learning system,* ed 2, Philadelphia, 2000, Saunders.)

Blood Flow Through the Heart

The *right atrium* receives blood from the superior and inferior venae cavae, the largest veins that enter the heart. This blood comes from all tissues (except the lungs), contains waste materials, and is oxygen-poor. Blood flows from the right atrium into the right ventricle.

The *right ventricle* receives blood from the right atrium and pumps it into the pulmonary artery, which carries it to the lungs.

The *left atrium* receives oxygenated blood from the lungs through the four pulmonary veins. (These are the only veins in the body that contain oxygen-rich blood.) Blood flows from here into the left ventricle.

The *left ventricle* receives blood from the left atrium. Blood then goes into the aorta, the largest of the arteries, and is pumped to all parts of the body, except the lungs.

Recall

9. What are the two primary functions of the circulatory system?
10. What are the upper and lower chambers of the heart?

Blood Vessels

There are three major types of blood vessels in the body: the arteries, veins, and capillaries.

The **arteries** are the large blood vessels that carry blood away from the heart to all regions of the body (Fig. 7-10). The walls of the arteries are composed of three layers. This structure makes arteries both muscular and elastic so that they can expand and contract with the pumping beat of the heart.

The **capillaries** are a system of microscopic vessels that connect the arterial and venous system. Blood flows rapidly along the arteries and veins; however, this flow is much slower through the expanded area provided by the capillaries. This slower flow allows time for the exchange of oxygen, nutrients, and waste materials between the tissue fluids and the surrounding cells.

The **veins** form a low-pressure collecting system to return the waste-filled blood to the heart. Veins have thinner walls than do arteries and are less elastic. The veins have valves that allow blood to flow toward the heart but prevent it from flowing away from the heart.

Blood and Blood Cells

The three main types of formed elements present in blood are: (1) plasma, (2) red blood cells, and (3) white blood cells. One drop of blood contains 5 million red blood cells, 7500 white blood cells, and 300,000 platelets.

Plasma is a straw-colored fluid that transports nutrients, hormones, and waste products. Plasma is 91% water. The remaining 9% consists mainly of plasma proteins, including albumin and globulin.

Red blood cells, also known as *erythrocytes,* contain the blood protein *hemoglobin,* which plays an essential role in

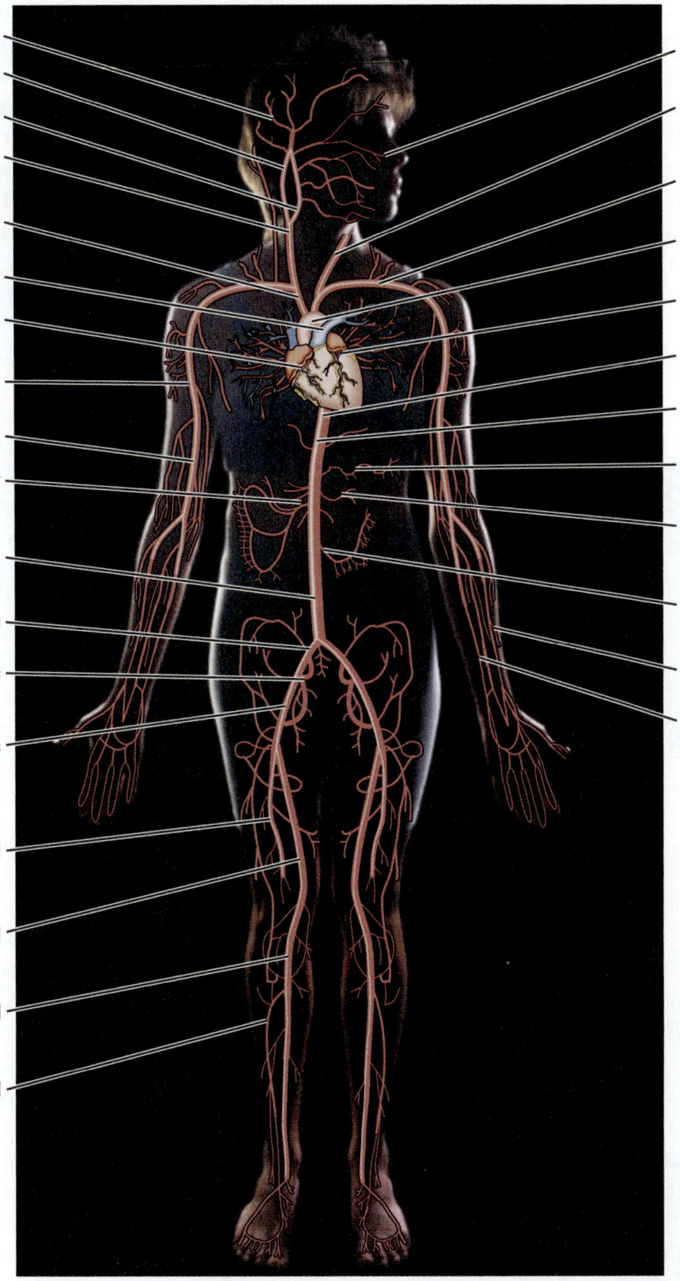

Fig. 7-10 Arteries carry blood from the heart to the body. (From Chester G: *Modern medical assisting,* Philadelphia, 1998, Saunders.)

oxygen transport. Erythrocytes are produced by the red bone marrow. When erythrocytes are no longer useful, they are destroyed by macrophages in the spleen, liver, and bone marrow.

White blood cells, also known as *leukocytes,* have the primary function of fighting disease in the body. The five major groups of leukocytes are as follows:

1. *Basophils* have imprecisely understood functions.
2. *Eosinophils* increase in number in allergic conditions.
3. *Lymphocytes* are important in the immune process to protect the body.
4. *Monocytes* act as *macrophages* and dispose of dead and dying cells and other debris.
5. *Neutrophils* fight disease by engulfing germs.
6. *Thrombocytes,* also known as *platelets,* are the smallest formed elements of the blood. They are manufactured in the bone marrow and play an important role in the clotting of blood.

Recall

11. What are the names and functions of the three main types of blood vessels?

Blood Typing and Rh Factor

The safe administration of blood from donor to recipient requires typing and cross-matching. *Blood typing* is based on the antigens and antibodies found in the blood. The most important classifications are A, AB, B, and O. Patients who receive blood incompatible with their own may experience a serious and possibly fatal reaction.

The *Rh factor,* named for its discovery through research with rhesus monkeys, is an additional antigen present on the surface of the red blood cells of some individuals. In addition to matching these blood types, the Rh factor must also be matched according to whether it is positive or negative. A person whose blood contains the factor is *Rh positive.* A person whose blood does *not* contain the factor is *Rh negative.* Anti-Rh antibodies are not naturally found in plasma as in blood types but do develop if exposed to the Rh factor. For example, an Rh-negative mother who gives birth to an Rh-positive baby will not have a blood reaction with the first pregnancy, but after the mixing of blood during delivery, the mother will develop anti-Rh antibodies in

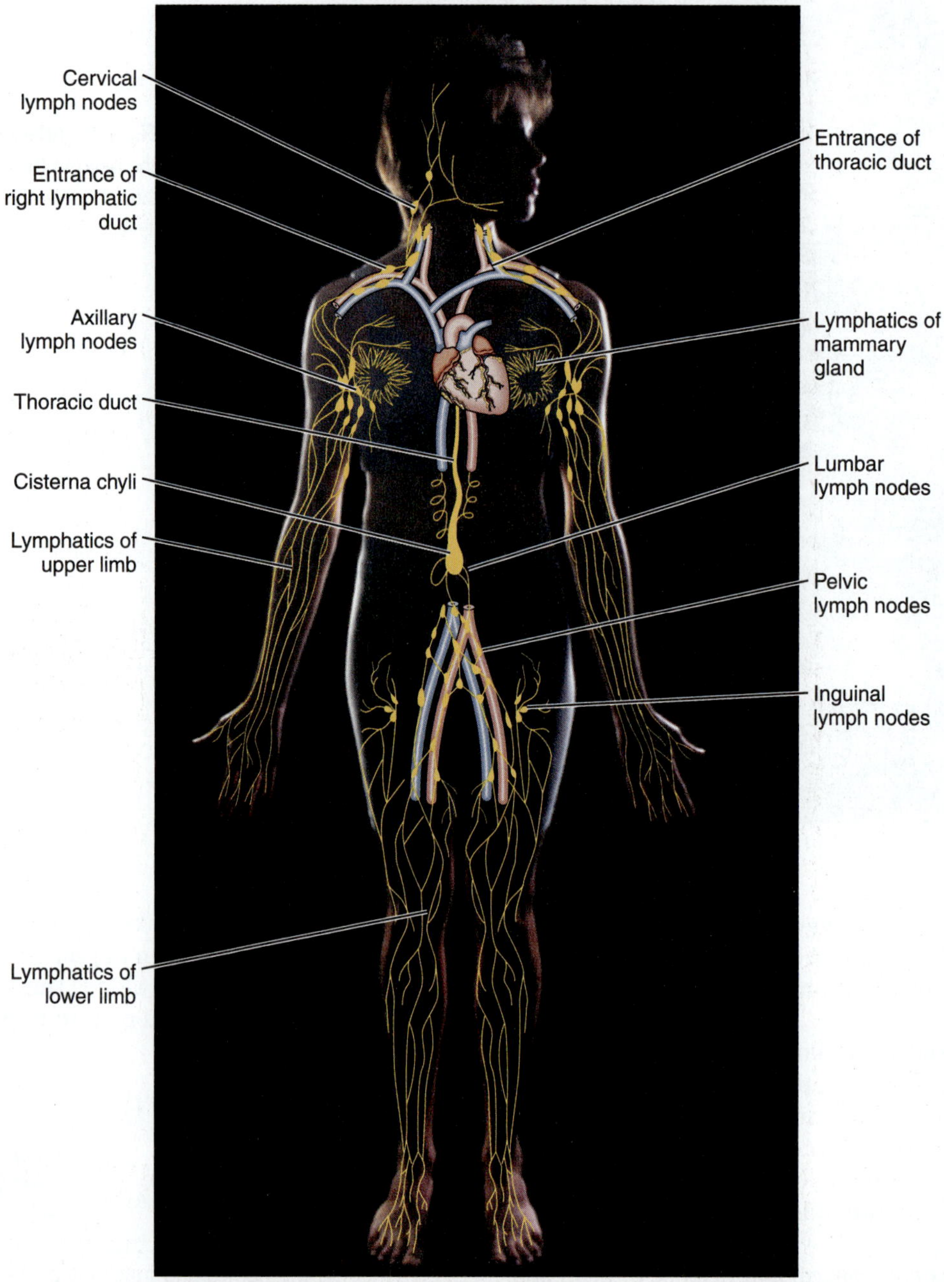

Fig. 7-11 Lymphatic system. (From Chester G: *Modern medical assisting,* Philadelphia, 1998, Saunders.)

her serum. A subsequent Rh-positive fetus may develop erythroblastosis fetalis if maternal anti-Rh antibodies react with fetal Rh antigen. This condition can cause the death of the fetus. Immediately after the delivery of Rh-positive babies, Rh-negative mothers are given an injection of anti-Rh gamma globulin to prevent the development of anti-Rh antibodies.

Lymphatic System

The structures of the lymphatic system include the lymph vessels, lymph nodes, lymph fluid, and lymphoid organs (Fig. 7-11). The drainage vessels absorb excess protein from tissues and return it to the bloodstream. The lymphoid organs contribute to the immune system to assist with destruction of harmful microorganisms. (See also Chapter 19 for a discussion of immunity and how it relates to disease transmission.) Fluid leaves circulatory capillaries to bathe tissues and cells to keep them moist. This same clear, light-yellow fluid, called *lymph,* is reabsorbed by the lymphatic system and returned to the blood through the veins. This one-way flowing system moves fluid toward the heart.

Lymph Vessels

Lymph capillaries are thin-walled tubes that carry lymph from the tissue spaces to the larger *lymphatic vessels.* Like veins, lymphatic vessels have valves to prevent the backflow of fluid. Lymph fluid always flows toward the thoracic cavity, where it empties into veins in the upper thoracic region. Specialized lymph vessels, called lacteals, are located in the small intestine. The *lacteals* aid in the absorption of fats from the small intestine into the bloodstream.

Lymph Nodes

Lymph nodes are small round or oval structures located in lymph vessels. They fight disease by producing antibodies, which are part of the immune reaction. In acute infections the lymph nodes become swollen and tender as a result of the collection of lymphocytes gathered to destroy the invading substances (see Box 7-4).

The major lymph node sites of the body include *cervical nodes* (in the neck), *axillary nodes* (under the arms), and *inguinal nodes* (in the lower abdomen).

Lymph Fluid

Lymph, also known as *tissue fluid,* is a clear and colorless fluid. Lymph flows in the spaces between the cells and tissues so that it can carry the substances from these tissues back into the bloodstream.

Lymphoid Organs

Tonsils

The tonsils are masses of lymphatic tissue located in the upper portions of the nose and throat, where they form a protective ring of lymphatic tissue (Fig. 7-12).

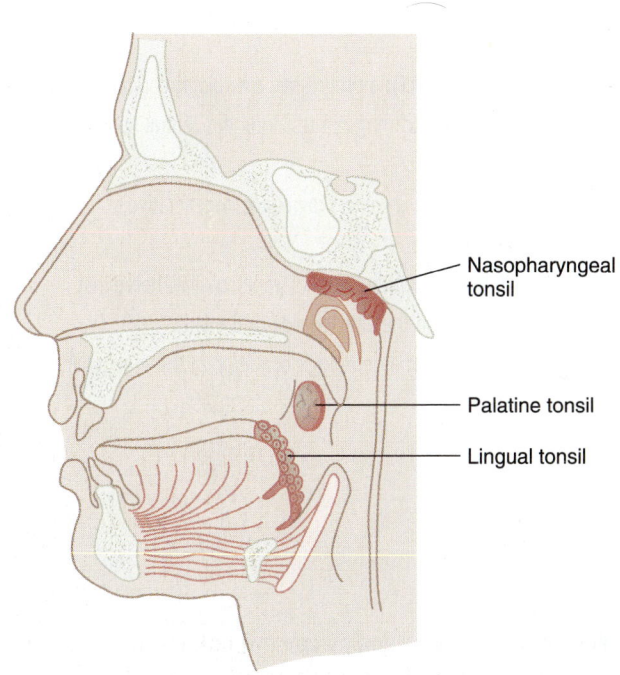

The *nasopharyngeal tonsils,* also known as *adenoids,* are found in the nasopharynx. The *palatine tonsils* are located in the oropharynx between the anterior and posterior pillars of fauces (throat) and are visible through the mouth. The *lingual tonsils* are located on the back of the tongue.

All these tonsils are removed during a tonsillectomy. Tonsils place lymphocytes into lymph to destroy invading microorganisms and may become infected in the process.

Spleen

The spleen is the largest of the lymphoid organs. It is about the size of a clenched fist and is located in the upper-left quadrant of the abdomen, just below the diaphragm and behind the stomach. The spleen produces lymphocytes and monocytes, which are important components of the immune system. It also filters microorganisms and other debris not destroyed by the lymphatic system.

Other splenic functions include storing red blood cells, maintaining the appropriate balance between cells and plasma in the blood, and removing and destroying nonviable (worn-out) red blood cells.

Recall

12. What is the primary function of the lymphatic system?
13. What tissues make up the lymphatic system?

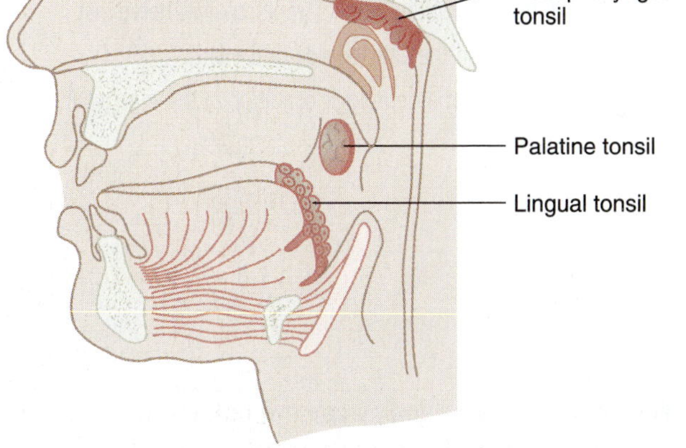

Fig. 7-12 The tonsils.

NERVOUS SYSTEM

The nervous system is the communication system of the body. Instructions and directions are sent out by this system to the various organs in the body. The nervous system can be compared to computer communications, with the brain and spinal cord as the main computer and the nerves as the cables that carry messages to and from this center. Many disorders can affect the nervous system (Box 7-5).

The nervous system is composed of the central and the peripheral nervous systems. The **central nervous system (CNS)** consists of the brain and spinal cord (Fig. 7-13). The **peripheral nervous system (PNS)** consists of the cranial nerves and the spinal nerves. The PNS also includes the autonomic nervous system, which is divided into the *sympathetic* and *parasympathetic* nervous systems.

Recall

14. What two systems make up the nervous system?
15. What are the two divisions of the autonomic nervous system?

Neurons

The basic function of the **neurons** is to direct communication or nerve impulses. Neurons have the properties of *excitability,* the ability to respond to a stimulus, and *conductivity,* transmission of an impulse.

The three types of neurons may be described according to their functions, as follows:

1. *Sensory neurons* emerge from the skin or sense organs and carry impulses toward the brain and spinal cord.

Box 7-5 Disorders of the Nervous System

Examples of disorders	Signs and symptoms
Head injury: can be caused by a blunt trauma to the head or a break in the skull.	Symptoms vary, depending on the area of the brain involved in the injury, but can include bleeding, swelling, or increased intracranial pressure.
Brain tumors: can be benign (noncancerous) or malignant (cancerous).	Depends on the location of the tumor, which exerts pressure on surrounding tissues.
Migraine headache: vasodilation and increased blood flow to the head.	Throbbing sensation, severe head pain, nausea, vomiting, and blurred vision.
Cerebrovascular accident: interruption of blood flow to the brain; can be caused by a hemorrhage or a blood clot and is commonly called a *stroke.*	Numbness, altered mental status, vertigo, loss of muscle coordination, and others.
Epilepsy: seizures.	Grand mal: rigid and jerking motions. Petit mal: stare, amnesia for event.
Multiple sclerosis (MS): a progressive neurologic condition with demyelination and scarring of sites along the central nervous system.	Visual problems and sensory, motor, and emotional problems can occur.
Alzheimer's disease: chronic, progressive degenerative disease with no cure.	Loss of recent memory for events, persons, and places. Over time, confusion and disorientation increase, leading to physical deterioration and death.
Bell's palsy: paralysis of the facial (seventh cranial) nerve that causes distortion on the affected side of the face.	The person may not be able to open an eye or close the mouth. The condition may be unilateral or bilateral.
Trigeminal neuralgia: a neurologic condition of the trigeminal facial nerve.	Also known as *tic douloureux.* Severe pain caused by inflammation of the trigeminal (fifth cranial) nerve. This pain, which has been described as excruciating, stabbing, and searing, may last for a few seconds; however, the initial incident is usually followed by other episodes, often of increasing severity. Depending on which of the three nerve branches is affected, the pain could occur around the eyes and over the forehead; in the upper lip, nose, and cheek; or in the tongue and lower lip.
Parkinson's disease: a slowly progressive, degenerative, neurologic disorder.	Resting tremors of hands, rigidity of movement, shuffling gait, masklike face, and stooped appearance.

2. *Motor neurons* carry impulses away from the brain and spinal cord and toward the muscles and glands.
3. *Associative neurons* carry impulses from one neuron to another.

A *synapse* is the space between two neurons or between a neuron and a receptor organ. A *neurotransmitter* is a chemical substance that allows the impulse to jump across the synapse from one neuron to another.

Some nerves have a white protective covering called the *myelin sheath.* The nerves covered with myelin are referred to as the *white matter.* Nerves that do not have the protective myelin sheath are gray and make up the *gray matter* of the brain and spinal cord.

Recall

16. What are the three types of neurons, according to their function?

Central Nervous System

The brain is enclosed in the cranium for protection, whereas the vertebrae protect the spinal cord.

Brain

The brain is the primary center for regulating and coordinating body activities, and each part of the brain controls different aspects of body functions. The largest part of the brain is the *cerebrum,* which is divided into the right and left cerebral hemispheres. The brain is organized so that the left side of the brain controls the right side of the body and the right side of the brain controls the left side of the body.

Spinal Cord

The spinal cord carries all the nerves that affect the limbs and lower part of the body. The spine is the pathway for impulses going to and from the brain. *Cerebrospinal fluid* flows throughout the brain and around the spinal cord.

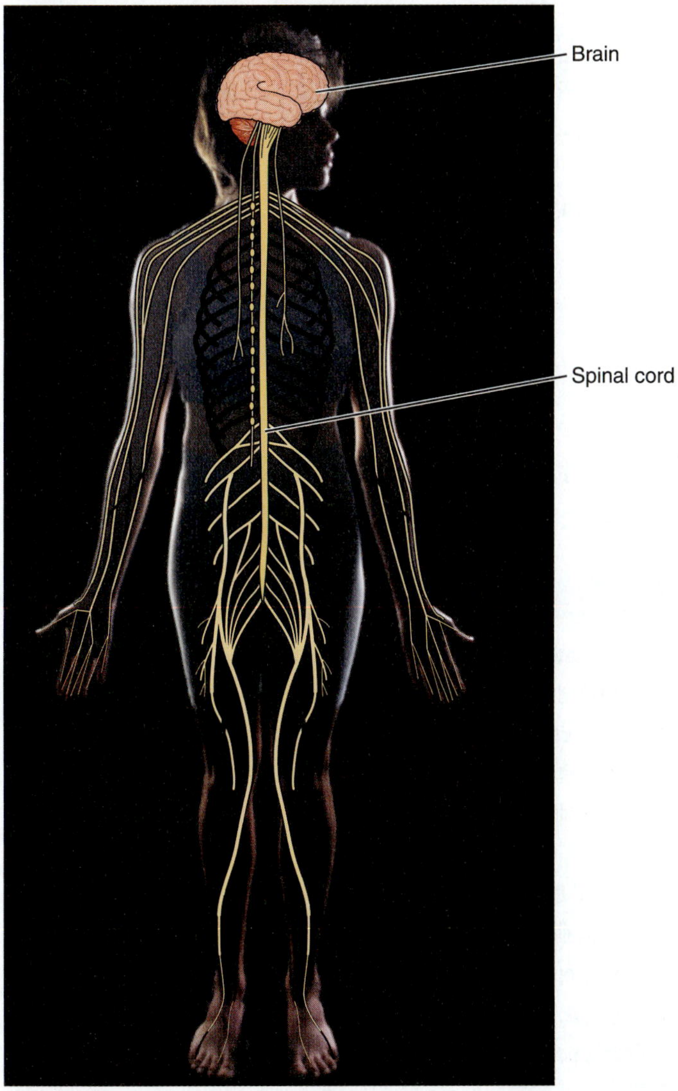

Fig. 7-13 The central nervous system (CNS). (From Chester G: *Modern medical assisting,* Philadelphia, 1998, Saunders.)

Its primary function is to cushion these organs from shock and injury.

Peripheral Nervous System

The PNS consists of the nerves that branch out from the brain and spinal cord. The PNS has two divisions. The *autonomic nervous system* (ANS) controls unconscious activities, such as breathing, heart rate, body temperature, blood pressure, and pupil size. The *somatic nervous system* (SNS) controls conscious activities.

RESPIRATORY SYSTEM

The term *respiration* means "breathing" or "to breathe." The respiratory system delivers *oxygen* to the millions of cells in the body and transports the waste product *carbon dioxide* out of the body. The respiratory system comprises the nose, paranasal sinuses, pharynx, epiglottis, larynx, trachea, alveoli, and lungs. Disorders of the respiratory system have specific signs and symptoms (Box 7-6).

Structures

Nose

Air enters the body through the nostrils (*nares*) of the nose and passes through the *nasal cavity* (Fig. 7-14). The nose is divided by a wall of cartilage called the *nasal septum.*

The nose and respiratory system are lined with mucous membrane, which is a specialized form of epithelial tissue. The incoming air is filtered by the *cilia,* which are thin hairs attached to the mucous membrane just inside the nostrils.

Mucus secreted by the mucous membranes helps to moisten and warm the air as it enters the nose. (Notice the difference in spelling between *mucous,* the name of the membrane, and *mucus,* the secretion of the membrane.)

Pharynx

After passing through the nasal cavity, the air reaches the pharynx, which is commonly known as the *throat.* The three divisions of the pharynx are the nasopharynx, oropharynx, and laryngopharynx.

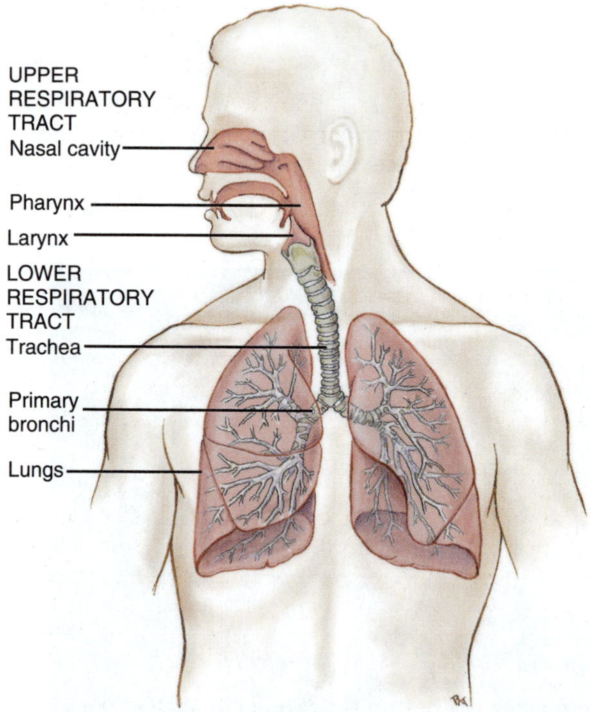

Fig. 7-14 Conducting passages of the respiratory system.

Box 7-6 Disorders of the Respiratory System

Examples of disorders	Signs and symptoms
Tonsillitis: inflammation of the tonsils. Adenoids may also be involved.	Severely dry, scratchy, and sore throat. May include fever, chills, headache, muscle aches, and general body aching.
Sinusitis: acute inflammation of a sinus.	Fever, chills, nasal obstruction, pain, and tenderness over the affected sinus.
Pneumonia: acute inflammation of the lungs. It can be viral, bacterial, or nonbacterial.	Fever, chills, productive cough, and general malaise.
Pharyngitis (sore throat): inflammation of the throat caused by virus, bacteria, or irritants.	Sore red throat, chills, high temperature, headache, and difficulty in swallowing.
Tuberculosis: infectious disease caused by infected droplets containing the tubercle bacteria.	Early symptoms include low-grade fever, chills, night sweats, weakness, and fatigue. Later, coughing of sputum containing blood and chest pain.
Lung cancer: strong relationship between smoking and air pollutants.	Cough, pain, shortness of breath, weight loss, and general malaise.

The *nasopharynx* is located behind the nose and above the soft palate. The *eustachian tube,* the narrow tube leading from the middle ear, opens into the nasopharynx.

The *oropharynx* extends from the soft palate above to the level of the epiglottis below. This is the part of the throat that is visible when one is looking into the mouth. This opening leads both to the stomach and to the lungs. If a patient aspirates an object during treatment, such as a sharp tooth fragment, it could go to the lung or the digestive system. (As used here, *aspirate* means to inhale or swallow accidentally.)

The *laryngopharynx* extends from the level of the epiglottis above to the larynx below. The nasopharynx contains the adenoids; the oropharynx contains the palatine tonsils.

Epiglottis

The oropharynx and laryngopharynx serve as a common passageway for both food from the mouth and air from the nose. During swallowing, the epiglottis acts as a lid and covers the larynx so that food does *not* enter the lungs.

Larynx

The larynx, also known as the *voice box,* contains the vocal bands, which make speech possible. The larynx is protected and held open by a series of cartilaginous structures. The largest cartilage forms the prominent projection in front of the neck commonly known as the "Adam's apple."

Trachea

Air passes from the larynx to the trachea. The trachea extends from the neck into the chest, directly in front of the esophagus. It is protected and held open by a series of C-shaped cartilaginous rings.

Lungs

The trachea divides into two branches called *bronchi.* Each bronchus leads to a lung, where it divides and subdivides into increasingly smaller branches; *bronchioles* are the smallest of these branches. *Alveoli* are the tiny grapelike clusters found at the end of each bronchiole. The walls of the alveoli are very thin and are surrounded by a network of capillaries. During respiration, the exchange of gases between the lungs and the blood takes place in the alveoli. The oxygen from the air passes through the thin walls of the alveoli into the bloodstream, and carbon dioxide passes from the blood into the alveoli to be expelled into the air.

Recall

17. What is the function of the respiratory system?

DIGESTIVE SYSTEM

The digestive system works like an assembly line in reverse. It takes in whole foods and breaks them down into their chemical components. Food that has been eaten is broken down by digestive juices into small absorbable nutrients that generate energy and provide the body with the nutrients, water, and electrolytes necessary for life. The digestive system functions under involuntary control. We decide what and when we eat, but once we swallow our food, our digestive system takes over without our conscious thought. Disorders of the digestive system range from common (e.g., gastroesophageal reflux) to life-threatening (e.g., peritonitis) (Box 7-7).

Digestive Process

The digestive system provides nutrition for the body through the following five basic actions:

1. *Ingestion.* Food is taken into the mouth.

Box 7-7 Disorders of the Digestive System

Examples of disorders	Signs and symptoms
Gastroesophageal reflux: backward flow of gastric juices into esophagus.	Heartburn and difficulty swallowing.
Peptic ulcer: erosion of the gastric mucosa that exposes it to gastric juice and pepsin.	Feeling of pressure, burning, heaviness, or hunger; change in appetite and weight loss.
Ulcerative colitis and Crohn's disease: chronic inflammatory process of bowel resulting in poor absorption of nutrients.	Abdominal pain, cramping, or diarrhea with weight loss; may have anemia, fatigue; possibly bloody stools, pain, and cramping.
Hemorrhoids: varicose or dilated veins in the anal canal.	Itching and pain and burning with defecation.
Peritonitis: inflammation of the lining of the abdominal cavity; a life-threatening condition.	Fever, acute pain, cramping, signs of shock, tenderness, and rigid or distended abdomen.

2. *Digestion.* The digestive process begins in the mouth with *mastication* (chewing), mixing the food with saliva, and swallowing it. A digestive enzyme called *salivary amylase* begins the process of breaking down carbohydrates into simpler forms that the body can use. After the food is swallowed, the churning action of the stomach mixes it with gastric juice. The digestion of carbohydrates continues in the stomach, and the digestion of protein begins.
3. *Movement.* After swallowing, **peristalsis** occurs, the rhythmic wavelike contractions that move the food through the digestive tract.
4. *Absorption.* The nutritional elements in the gastrointestinal tract pass through its lining and into the bloodstream. Most absorption of nutrients occurs in the small intestines.
5. *Elimination.* In the large intestine, excess water is absorbed, and the solid by-products of digestion are eliminated from the body in feces.

Structures

The major structures of the digestive system are the mouth, pharynx, esophagus, stomach, small intestine, large intestine, liver, gallbladder, and pancreas (Fig. 7-15).

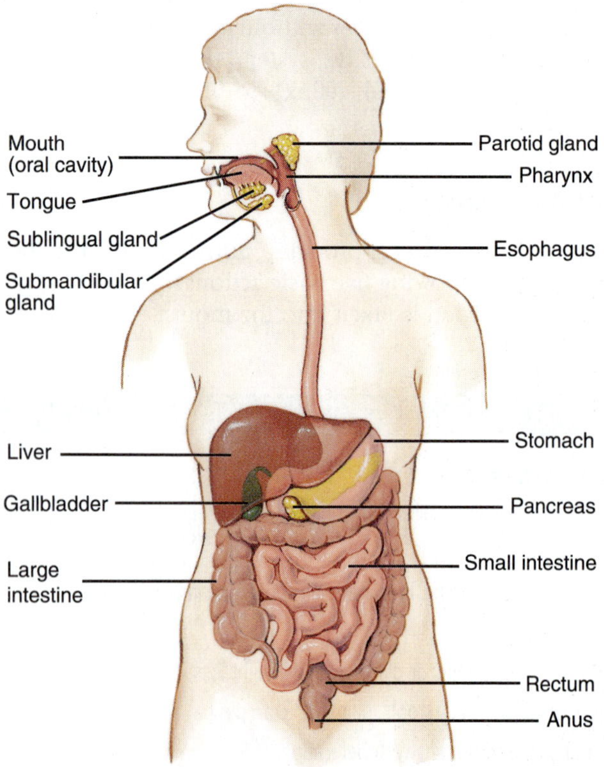

Fig. 7-15 Major structures of the digestive system. (From Applegate EJ: *The anatomy and physiology learning system,* ed 2, Philadelphia, 2000, Saunders.)

Mouth

The *mouth,* known as the oral region of the head, has many structures associated with it. Each of these structures is discussed in detail in Chapter 10.

Pharynx

The *pharynx* is a fibromuscular tube that connects the nasal and oral cavities to the larynx and esophagus. It serves as a passageway for food and air.

Esophagus

The *esophagus* is a tubelike structure approximately 10 inches in length that transports food from the pharynx to the stomach.

Stomach

The *stomach* is a saclike organ that lies in the abdominal cavity just under the diaphragm. Glands within the stomach produce the gastric juices that aid in digestion and the mucus that forms the protective coating of the stomach lining.

Small Intestine

The *small intestine* extends from the stomach to the first part of the large intestine. It consists of three parts: the duodenum, jejunum, and ileum.

Large Intestine

The *large intestine* extends from the end of the small intestine to the anus. It is divided into four parts: the cecum, colon, sigmoid colon, and rectum and anus.

Liver, Gallbladder, and Pancreas

The *liver* is located in the right upper quadrant of the abdomen. It removes excess *glucose* (sugar) from the bloodstream and stores it as *glycogen* (starch). When the blood sugar level is low, the liver converts the glycogen back into glucose and releases it for use by the body.

The liver destroys old erythrocytes, removes poisons from the blood, and manufactures some blood proteins. It also manufactures *bile,* a digestive juice.

The *gallbladder* is a pear-shaped sac located under the liver. It stores and concentrates the bile for later use. When needed, bile is emptied into the duodenum of the small intestine.

The *pancreas* produces pancreatic juices, which contain digestive enzymes. These juices are emptied into the duodenum of the small intestine.

Recall

18. What is the role of the digestive system?
19. What are the five actions of the digestive system?

ENDOCRINE SYSTEM

The endocrine system uses chemical messengers called *hormones* that move through the bloodstream and can reach every cell in the body.

Hormones help maintain a constant environment inside the body, adjusting the amount of salt and water in the tissues, sugar in the blood, and salt in sweat to suit the particular conditions that exist. Hormones produce both long-term changes, such as a child's growth and sexual maturation, and rhythmic ones, such as the menstrual cycle. They trigger swift, dramatic responses in the body whenever illness or injury strikes or whenever the brain perceives danger. Hormones have a lot to do with emotions such as fear, anger, joy, and despair.

The hormones are secreted directly into the bloodstream (not through a duct). The endocrine glands include the *thyroid* and *parathyroid, ovaries, testes, pituitary, pancreas,* and *adrenal medulla.* The major endocrine glands are scattered throughout the body but are considered to be one system (Fig. 7-16).

The system itself is interrelated, and the secretion from one gland can affect glands elsewhere. Many disorders can affect the endocrine system (Box 7-8).

Recall

20. What are the primary functions of the endocrine system?

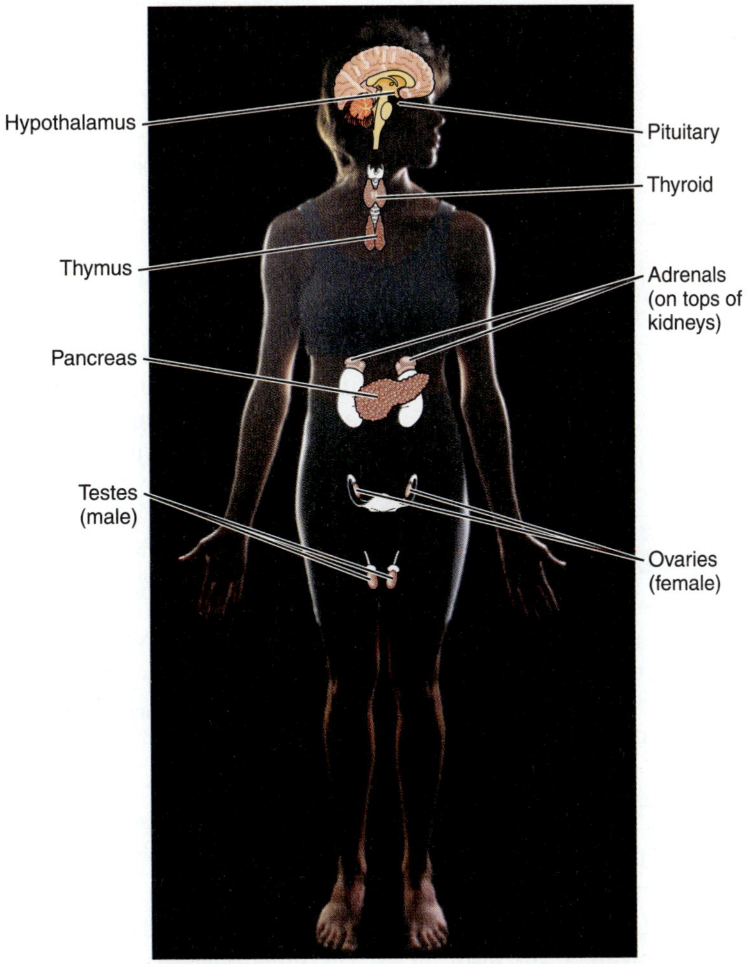

Fig. 7-16 Endocrine glands. (From Chester G: *Modern medical assisting,* Philadelphia, 1998, Saunders.)

Box 7-8 Disorders of the Endocrine System

Examples of disorders	Signs and symptoms
Hypothyroidism: decreased level of activity of the thyroid gland.	Decreased level of metabolism, sensitivity to cold, weight gain, or thick hair.
Hyperthyroidism: excessive level of activity of the thyroid gland.	Nervousness, agitation, irritability, inability to concentrate, heat intolerance, or weight loss with increased appetite.
Diabetes mellitus: impaired glucose uptake by the cells.	Type I diabetes: insulin dependence, weight loss, fatigue, and frequent urination. Type II diabetes: no insulin dependence; symptoms less severe than Type I and may include blurred vision.

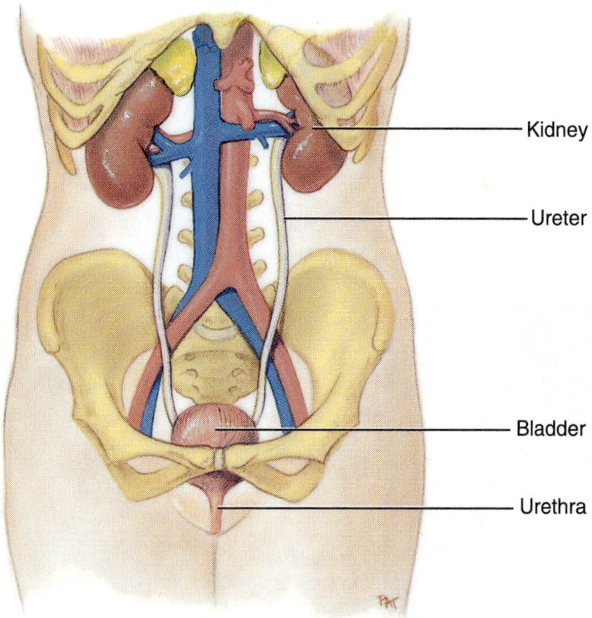

Fig. 7-17 The urinary system. (From Chester G: *Modern medical assisting,* Philadelphia, 1998, Saunders.)

URINARY SYSTEM

The urinary system is also known as the *excretory system* (Fig. 7-17). Its principal function is to maintain fluid volume and composition of the body fluids. To accomplish this, gallons of fluid are filtered out of the bloodstream and through tubules of the kidneys. Waste products leave the body in the form of urine, and the needed substances are returned to the blood. Disorders of the urinary system range from incontinence to renal failure (Box 7-9).

The urinary system consists of (1) the *kidneys,* where urine is formed to carry away waste materials from the blood; (2) the *ureters,* which transport the urine from the kidneys; (3) the *bladder,* where the urine is stored until it can be eliminated; and (4) the *urethra,* through which the bladder is emptied to the outside through the process of urination. The kidneys require a large blood supply and are connected close to the body's main artery, the aorta. More than two pints of blood pass through the kidneys every minute.

Box 7-9 Disorders of the Urinary System

Examples of disorders	Signs and symptoms
Renal failure: loss of kidney function.	Rapid retention of fluid and metabolic wastes.
Urinary incontinence: inability to control urination; bladder pressure increases.	Incontinence during coughing, sneezing, or laughing. Can be a symptom of urinary tract infection and other diseases, including Parkinson's disease and multiple sclerosis.
Cystitis: inflammation of the bladder.	Painful urination, urgency, low back pain, and fever.

Recall

21. What is the primary function of the urinary system?

INTEGUMENTARY SYSTEM

The skin is the body's first line of defense against disease. The **integumentary system,** or *skin system,* has many important functions, as follows:

1. Helps to regulate body temperature

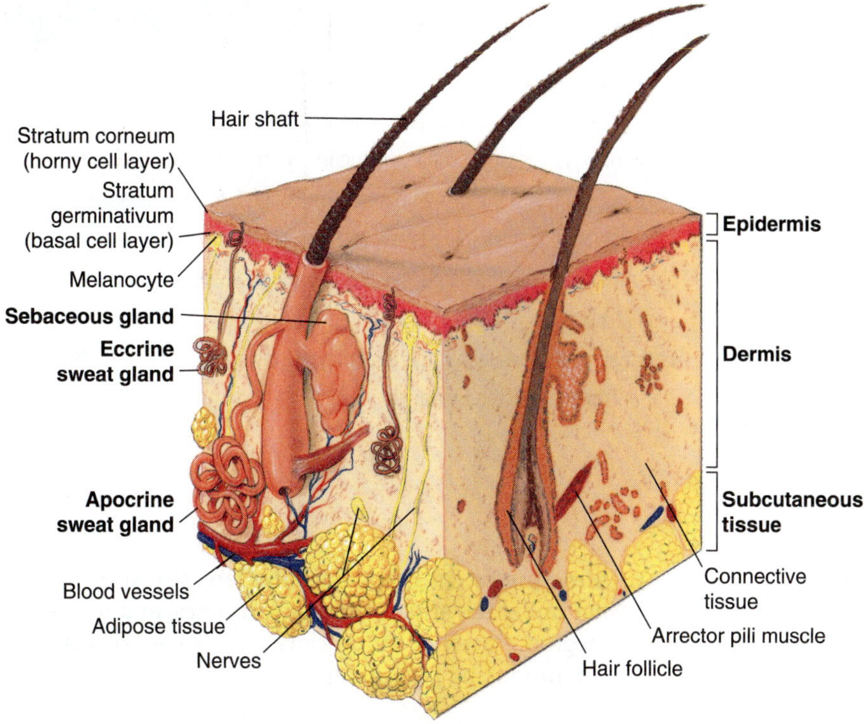

Fig. 7-18 **Structure and layers of the skin.** (From Jarvis C: *Physical examination and health assessment,* ed 3, Philadelphia, 2000, Saunders.)

Box 7-10 Disorders of the Integumentary System

Examples of disorders	Signs and symptoms
Abscess: usually the result of a wound allowing bacteria to invade the dermis.	Red, tender nodule that enlarges and becomes more painful as it grows.
Acne: one of the most common skin diseases. Inflammation of the sebaceous glands causing pimples and/or blackheads.	The face and upper body are the most common sites. The inflamed lesions are papules, pustules, and cysts.
Eczema: nonspecific dermatitis; may be acute or chronic.	Severe itching, and symptoms may include weeping vesicles and crusted patches.
Basal cell carcinoma: most common of all human cancers. Primary cause is exposure to sun radiation.	A pearly, nodular border. The tumor enlarges, developing a central crater that continually repeats the cycle of eroding, crusting, bleeding, and healing.

2. Provides a barrier that prevents bacteria from entering the body
3. Excretes liquids and salts
4. Provides sensitivity to touch
5. Uses ultraviolet rays from the sun to convert chemicals into the vitamin D necessary for absorption of calcium

Disorders of the integumentary system range from abscess to carcinoma (Box 7-10).

Skin Structures

The skin is composed of different layers, including the epidermis, dermis, and subcutaneous fat (Fig. 7-18).

Epidermis

The *epidermis* is the outer layer of the skin. It has no blood supply of its own. The cells receive their nutrients from vessels in the underlying tissue. As new cells are pushed to the surface, the older cells die and are *sloughed* (cast) off.

Dermis

The *dermis* is a thick connective tissue layer that gives bulk to the skin. The dermal layer contains many free nerve endings and receptors, which allow for detection of touch, temperature, and pain. With age the connective tissue becomes less elasticized, and wrinkles develop.

Box 7-11 Disorders of the Female Reproductive System

Examples of disorders	Signs and symptoms
Vaginitis: inflammation of the vagina.	Vaginal discharge, itching, and pain, especially on urination.
Ovarian tumors: enlargements of normal ovarian structures.	Feeling of pelvic pressure, urinary frequency, constipation, and backache.
Toxic shock syndrome: infection related to menstruation and tampon use.	Flulike symptoms for the first 24 hours. Onset of high fever, headache, sore throat, vomiting, generalized rash, and hypotension.
Pelvic inflammatory disease (PID): inflammation of several reproductive organs.	Foul-smelling vaginal discharge and abdominal pain. General symptoms of an infection.
Breast cancer: uncontrolled growth of cancer cells within the breast. These cells spread to other areas of the body.	Abnormal mass of tissue in the breast; may see dimpling, nipple retraction, or enlargement of the breast.

Subcutaneous Fat

Subcutaneous fat is a layer of loose connective tissue that anchors the skin to underlying organs. It insulates the body against heat loss and cushions underlying organs. The distribution of subcutaneous fat is responsible for the differences in body contours between men and women.

Skin Appendages

The skin has a number of appendages, including hair, nails, and glands.

Hair

Hair is found on almost all skin surfaces. It is enclosed in a follicle and consists of a root and a shaft. The bulk of the shaft is made of dead material and protein. Hair and skin color are determined by the melanin produced in the epidermis.

Nails

As with hair, *nails* primarily consist of nonliving matter. Nails contain a root and a body. The body is the visible portion, and the root is covered by skin called the *cuticle.* The extensive blood supply in the underlying dermis gives nails their pink color.

Glands

The three types of glands in the skin are sebaceous, sudoriferous, and apocrine sweat glands.

Sebaceous glands are found in all areas of the body except for the palms of the hands and the soles of the feet. They are oil glands that keep the hair and skin soft. They are also associated with sex hormones and become active during puberty. Sebaceous activity decreases with age, which is why hair and skin become dry as aging occurs.

Sudoriferous glands are distributed all over the body and provide heat regulation by secreting sweat. Sweat is also produced in response to stress.

Apocrine sweat glands are the largest glands and are found under the arms, around the nipples, and in the genital region. Bacterial action causes the secretions to break down, producing body odor.

Recall

22. What are four functions of the skin?
23. What are the appendages to the skin?

Reproductive System

Female

The female reproductive system consists of the external and internal genitalia. The external genitalia consist of the *mons pubis, labia majora* and *labia minora, vulva,* and *clitoris.* The internal genitalia consist of the *ovaries, fallopian tubes, uterus,* and *vagina.* Fertility, the normal functioning of the reproductive system, begins at puberty (the onset of menstruation) and ceases at menopause. Many disorders can affect the female reproductive system (Box 7-11).

Male

The male reproductive system produces and transports sperm. This system consists of the *testes, excretory ducts,* and accessory organs. The accessory organs include the *prostate* and *seminal vesicles.* In the male, several organs serve as parts of both the urinary tract and the reproductive system. A disorder may interfere with the function of either system or both systems (Box 7-12).

Box 7-12 Disorders of the Male Reproductive System

Examples of disorders	Signs and symptoms
Testicular cancer: rare; usually occurs in men younger than 40. Most common type of cancer in men between 20 and 35 years of age.	Begins as a painless lump in the testicle; may spread through lymphatic system to lymph nodes in abdomen, chest, neck, or lungs.
Orchitis: infection or inflammation of one or both testes.	Pain in the involved testes. High temperature with red, swollen, and tender testes.
Epididymitis: inflammation or infection of the epididymis.	Pain and tenderness in the groin area and scrotum. High fever and symptoms of urinary tract infection may be present.
Prostate cancer: cause is unknown; third leading cause of cancer death in men; more common in men more than 40 years old.	Urinary frequency, difficulty in urinating, and urinary retention.

THE INTERACTION OF THE TEN BODY SYSTEMS

Body systems do not operate independently; they exert important effects on each other. For example, when you exercise hard, your muscular system needs extra oxygen, so your respiratory system works harder than usual to supply it. The ovaries and testes clearly belong to the reproductive system. However, since one of their functions is to produce hormones, they are also components of the endocrine system. The muscular system quite clearly depends on the skeletal system. A healthy respiratory system is of no value if the circulatory system fails. When something happens in one system, the event usually affects other systems. For example, if your nervous system reacts to upsetting information while you are eating, your digestive system may not function as well as usual.

Legal and Ethical Implications

Oral health is a necessary component for overall general health. New research is pointing to associations between chronic oral infections and heart and lung diseases, stroke, low birthweight, and premature births. There is a recognized association between periodontal disease and diabetes. You cannot be healthy without oral health. Oral health and general health are not separate entities. The risk factors that affect general health, such as tobacco use and poor nutrition, also affect oral health.

In this country today there are inequities and disparities that prevent people from achieving optimal oral health. The barriers to oral health include lack of access to care, whether because of limited income or lack of insurance, transportation, or the flexibility to take time off from work to see a dentist. Individuals with disabilities and those with complex health problems may face additional barriers to care.

There are many challenges remaining to meet the social, political, and economic barriers to oral health and general well-being.

Eye to the Future

As a dental assistant, you need a strong foundation in anatomy and physiology. This information can help you both personally and professionally. For example, it is important for you to understand how the muscular system works so you can protect the muscles in your neck and back from fatigue and strain while assisting during long procedures. You also will see patients with muscular problems who will need your understanding and assistance.

You will be better prepared to assist during a medical emergency in the dental office when you understand the circulatory and respiratory systems. Prescription medications may adversely affect a patient's dental treatment. You should be alert for signs and symptoms of various systemic disorders in yourself and your family as well as in your patients.

Critical Thinking

1. The respiratory system is exposed to the atmosphere and is susceptible to airborne infections, contaminants, and irritants. What can you do to protect your respiratory system?
2. If a patient with severe arthritis in her hands came into your dental office, what dental-related difficulties might she experience?
3. When 80-year-old Mrs. McBride comes into the office, the receptionist comments on how nice her hair looks. Mrs. McBride thanks the receptionist and then mentions that her hair used to be much softer and had more shine when she was younger. Do you think Mrs. McBride's hair has actually changed? Why or why not?
4. Mr. Cardono has been a patient in your office for several years. While you update his health history, Mr. Cardono states that his immunity must be down because he recently has had several severe sore throats and colds. Which body system is responsible for the decline in his immunity?

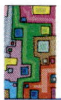

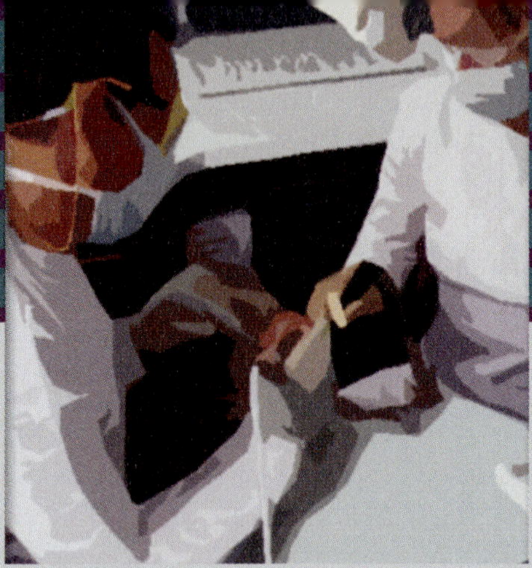

8 Oral Embryology and Histology

Outline

Oral Embryology
- Prenatal Development
- Embryonic Development of the Face and Oral Cavity
- Developmental Disturbances
- Facial Development after Birth
- Life Cycle of a Tooth

Oral Histology
- Crown
- Root
- Enamel
- Dentin
- Cementum
- Pulp
- Periodontium

Legal and Ethical Implications

Eye to the Future

Critical Thinking

KEY TERMS

Alveolar crest Highest point of the alveolar ridge.

Alveolar socket Cavity within the alveolar process that surrounds the root of a tooth.

Ameloblasts (a-**mel**-o-*blasts*) Cells that form enamel.

Anatomic crown Portion of the tooth that is covered with enamel.

Apex Tapered end of each root tip.

Apical foramen Natural opening in the root.

Cementoblasts (se-**men**-toe-*blasts*) Cells that form cementum.

Cementoclasts (se-**men**-toe-*klasts*) Cells that resorb cementum.

Cementum Specialized, calcified connective tissue that covers the anatomic root of a tooth.

Clinical crown That portion of the tooth that is visible in the oral cavity.

Conception Union of the male sperm and female ovum.

Coronal pulp Soft tissue that lies within the crown portion of the tooth.

Cortical plate Dense outer covering of spongy bone that makes up the central part of the alveolar process.

Dental lamina Thickened band of oral epithelium that follows the curve of each developing arch.

Dental papilla Small nipple-shaped elevation.

Dental sac Connective tissue that envelops the developing tooth.

Dentin Hard portion of the root that surrounds the pulp and is covered by enamel on the crown and by cementum on the root.

Dentinal fiber Fibers found in dentinal tubules.

Dentinal tubules Microscopic canals found in dentin.

Deposition The process by which the body adds new bone.

Embryo An organism in the earliest stages of development.

Embryology (*em*-bre-**ahl**-eh-jee) The study of prenatal development.

Embryonic period (*em*-bre-**on**-ik) Stage of human development that occurs from the beginning of the second week to the end of the eighth week.

Enamel lamellae Thin, leaflike structures that extend from the enamel surface toward the detinoenamel junction and consist of organic material with little mineral content.

Enamel organ Part of a developing tooth destined to produce enamel.

Enamel spindles The ends of odontoblasts (dentin-forming cells) that extend across the detinoenamel junction a short distance into the enamel.

Enamel tufts The hypocalcified or uncalcified ends of groups of enamel prisms that start at the detinoenamel junction and may extend to the inner third of the enamel.

Exfoliation (eks--*fo*-le-**a**-shun) The normal process of shedding the primary teeth.

Fetal period Stage of human development that starts at the beginning of the ninth week and ends at birth.

Fibroblasts Type of cell in connective tissue responsible for the formation of the intercellular substance of pulp.

KEY TERMS—cont'd

Gestation (jes-**ta**-shun) Stage of human development that starts at fertilization and ends at birth.

Histology (his-**tahl**-eh-jee) The study of the structure and function of body tissues on a microscopic level.

Hunter-Schreger bands Alternating light and dark bands in the enamel that are produced when enamel prisms intertwine or change direction.

Hydroxyapatite Mineral compound that is the principal inorganic component of bone and teeth.

Hyoid arch The second branchial arch, which forms the styloid process, stapes of the ear, stylohyoid ligament, and part of the hyoid bone.

Lamina dura Thin, compact bone that lines the alveolar socket; also known as the *cribriform plate.*

Lining mucosa Mucous membrane that covers the inside of the cheeks, vestibule, lips, soft palate, and underside of the tongue and acts as a cushion for underlying structures.

Mandibular arch (man-**dib**-u-ler) The lower jaw.

Masticatory mucosa (**mas**-ti-kah-*tor*-ee) Mucous membrane that covers the hard palate, dorsum of the tongue, and gingiva.

Meiosis (mi-**oh**-sis) Reproductive cell production that ensures the correct number of chromosomes.

Modeling Bone changes that involve deposition and resorption of bone and occur along articulations as they increase in size and shape to keep up with the growth of the surrounding tissues; also known as *displacement.*

Odontoblasts (o-**don**-to-blasts) Cells that form dentin.

Odontogenesis (o-*don*-to-**jen**-eh-sis) Formation of new teeth.

Osteoblasts (**os**-te-o-*blasts*) Cells that form bone.

Osteoclasts (**os**-te-o-*klasts*) Cells that resorb bone.

Periodontium (*per*-e-oh-**don**-she-um) Structures that surround, support, and are attached to the teeth.

Preimplantation period Stage of development during the first week after fertilization.

Prenatal development (pre-**nay**-tul) Stage of human development that starts at pregnancy and ends at birth.

Primary cementum Cementum that covers the root of the tooth and is formed outward from the cementodentinal junction for the full length of the root.

Primary dentin Dentin that forms before eruption and makes up the bulk of the tooth.

Primary palate The shelf separating the oral and nasal cavities.

Prisms A calcified column or rod.

Pulp chamber The space occupied by the pulp.

Radicular pulp The other portion of pulp known as root pulp.

Remodeling Growth and change in shape of existing bone that involves deposition and resorption of bone.

Resorption (re-**sorp**-shun) The body's processes of eliminating existing bone or hard tissue structure.

Secondary cementum Cementum that is formed on the apical half of the root; also known as *cellular cementum*.

Secondary dentin Dentin that forms after eruption and continues at a very slow rate throughout the life of the tooth.

Secondary palate The final palate formed during embryonic development.

Specialized mucosa Mucous membrane on the tongue in the form of lingual papillae, which are structures associated with sensations of taste.

Stomodeum The primitive mouth.

Stratified squamous epithelium (**skwa**-mus) Layers of flat, formed epithelium.

Striae of Retzius Incremental rings that represent variations in deposition of the enamel matrix during tooth formation.

Succedaneous (*suk*-se-**day**-ne-us) Permanent teeth that replace primary teeth.

Tertiary dentin Dentin that forms in response to irritation and appears as a localized deposit on the wall of the pulp chamber; also known as *reparative dentin.*

Tooth buds Enlargements produced by the formation of dental lamina.

Zygote Fertilized egg.

LEARNING OUTCOMES

On completion of this chapter, the student will be able to achieve the following objectives:

- Pronounce, define, and spell the Key Terms.
- Define embryology and histology.
- Describe the three periods of prenatal development.
- Discuss prenatal influences on dental development.
- Describe the function of osteoclasts and osteoblasts.
- Describe the steps in the formation of the palate.
- Describe the stages in development of a tooth.
- Discuss genetic and environmental factors that can affect dental development.
- Discuss the life cycle of a tooth.
- Explain the difference between the clinical and anatomic crowns.
- Name and describe the tissues of the teeth.
- Name and describe the three types of dentin.
- Describe the structure and location of the dental pulp.
- Name and describe the components of the periodontium.
- Describe the functions of periodontal ligaments.
- Describe the types of oral mucosa and give an example of each.

Embryology is the study of **prenatal development** throughout the stages before birth. The first part of this chapter discusses development with emphasis on the formation of the teeth and structures of the oral cavity. Learning about the development of the oral structures is the foundation for later understanding of developmental problems that may occur in these structures.

Histology is the study of the structure and function of the tissues on a *microscopic level.* The second part of this chapter covers the histology of the teeth, their supporting structures, and the oral mucosa, which surrounds the teeth and lines the mouth. By understanding the histology of the oral tissues, the dental assistant can better understand the disease processes that occur in the oral cavity.

ORAL EMBRYOLOGY

Pregnancy begins with **conception,** which is also known as *fertilization.* **Gestation,** the period from fertilization to birth, has an average duration of 9 months from conception to birth, or 40 weeks from the last menstrual period (LMP). The due date is usually figured by a convenient rule of thumb; count back three months from the day the LMP began, then add a year and a week. The date you come up with is just a guide; the baby may arrive anywhere from two weeks earlier to two weeks later. The sex of the baby is established at conception, and will be apparent in a few weeks. This little 1-inch being weighs only about .04 ounce (1 gram), and could fit comfortably on a tablespoon.

A physician usually describes prenatal development in weeks on the basis of the date of the LMP. In embryology, *developmental age* is based on the date of conception, which is assumed to have occurred two weeks after the LMP. The developmental ages noted in this chapter are based on the date of conception.

Prenatal Development

Prenatal development consists of three distinct periods: preimplantation, embryonic, and fetal (Fig. 8-1).

The **preimplantation period** takes place during the first week. At the beginning of the week, an ovum (egg) is penetrated by and united with a sperm during fertilization (Fig. 8-2). The penetration of the egg by a sperm cell has an immediate effect on the surface of the egg: the outer coating of the egg changes, so that no other sperm cell can enter. The union of the egg and sperm subsequently forms a fertilized egg, or **zygote.** In the zygote, the 23 chromosomes in the sperm unite with the 23 chromosomes in the egg, providing a new life with a full complement of 46 chromosomes. These chromosomes will determine its inherited characteristics and direct its growth and development. The process of joining each parent's chromosomes is called **meiosis.** Meiosis ensures that the future embryo will have the correct number of chromosomes.

The **embryonic period** extends from the beginning of the second week to the end of the eighth week, and the new individual is known as an **embryo.** This period is the *most critical time* because during these weeks, development begins on all major structures of the body. The cells begin to *proliferate* (increase in number), *differentiate* (change

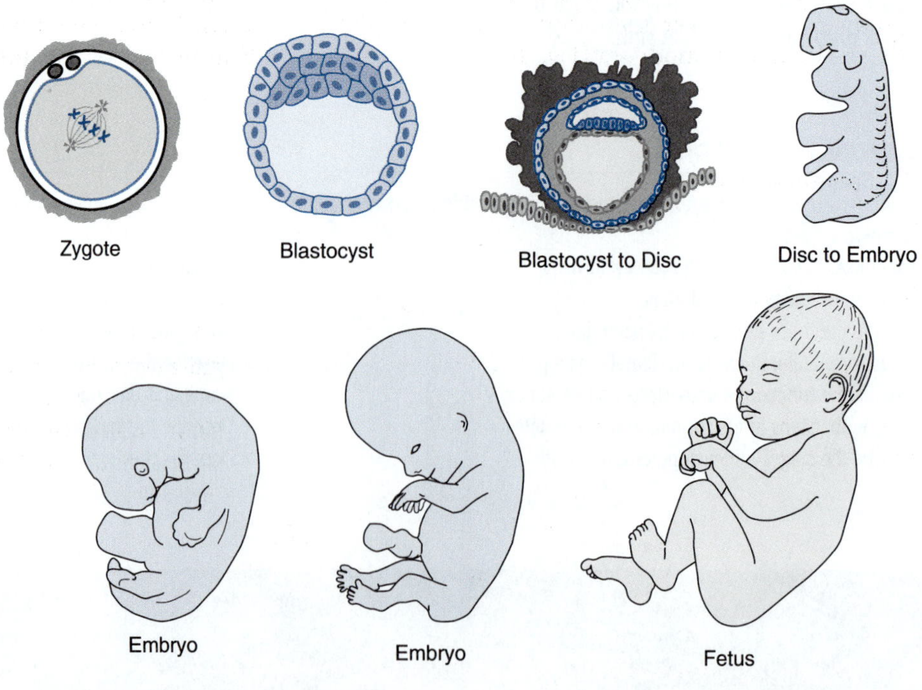

Fig. 8-1 Periods and structures in prenatal development. Note that the size of the structures is neither accurate nor comparative. (Modified from Bath-Balogh MB, Fehrenbach MJ: *Illustrated dental embryology, histology, and anatomy,* ed 2, St Louis, 2005, Saunders.)

into tissues and organs), and *integrate* (form systems). Many of these key developments occur before the mother even knows she is pregnant. At about the end of the eighth week of pregnancy, a baby graduates from embryo to fetus. This name change signifies a change in the baby's level of development. While an embryo, the baby looks very much like a tadpole, but as a fetus, it has a distinctly human appearance.

The **fetal period** continues from the ninth week and lasts until birth. During the fetal phase, the body systems continue to develop and mature. It has distinguishable ears, arms, hands, legs, and feet, as well as the fingerprints and footprints that will set it apart from other human beings. Because all the organ systems are formed during the embryonic period, the fetus is less vulnerable than the embryo to malformations caused by radiation, viruses, and drugs (Box 8-1). The fetal stage is a period of growth and maturation (Fig. 8-3).

Recall

1. What are the three periods of prenatal development?
2. Which period of prenatal development is the most critical, and why?

Embryonic Development of the Face and Oral Cavity

The face and its related tissues begin to form during the fourth week of prenatal development within the embryonic period. During this time, the rapidly growing brain of the embryo bulges over the oropharyngeal membrane, beating heart, and **stomodeum** (Fig. 8-4).

Primary Embryonic Layers

During the third week of development, the cells of the embryo form the three primary embryonic layers: the *ectoderm, mesoderm,* and *endoderm.* The cells within each layer multiply and differentiate into the specialized cells needed to form the organs and tissues of the body.

Recall

3. What are the three primary embryonic layers?

Early Development of the Mouth

In the fourth week, the stomodeum (primitive mouth) and the primitive pharynx merge, and the stomodeum develops into part of the mouth. By the beginning of the fifth week, the embryo is approximately 5 mm. The heart is prominent and bulging (Fig. 8-5).

The site of the face is indicated from above by the region just in front of the bulging forebrain (future forehead) and from below by the first pair of branchial arches (future jaws).

Branchial Arches

By the end of the fourth week, six pairs of branchial arches have formed. The first two of these arches give rise to the structures of the head and neck (see Chapter 9).

The *first branchial arch,* also known as the **mandibular arch,** forms the bones, muscles, and nerves of the face. The first arch also forms the lower lip, the muscles of

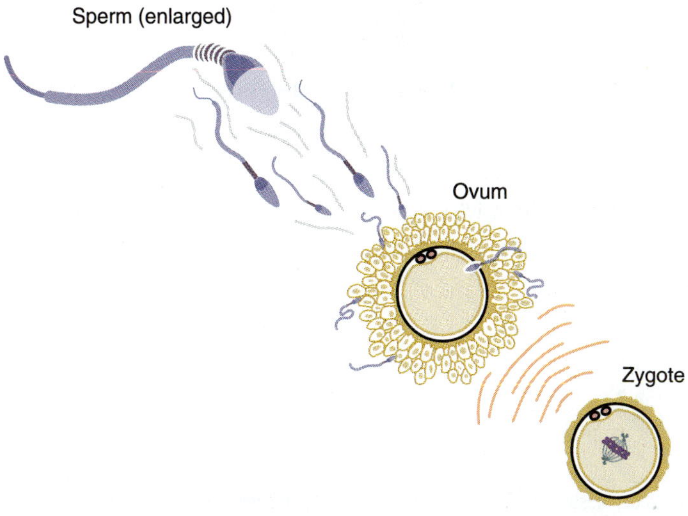

Fig. 8-2 **Sperm fertilizes the ovum and unites with it to form the zygote after the process of meiosis and during the first week of prenatal development. Chromosomes from the ovum and sperm join to form a zygote—a new individual.** (From Bath-Balogh MB, Fehrenbach MJ: *Illustrated dental embryology, histology, and anatomy,* ed 2, St Louis, 2005, Saunders.)

Box 8-1 Developmental Disturbances

Developmental period

Examples of disturbances

Preimplantation period

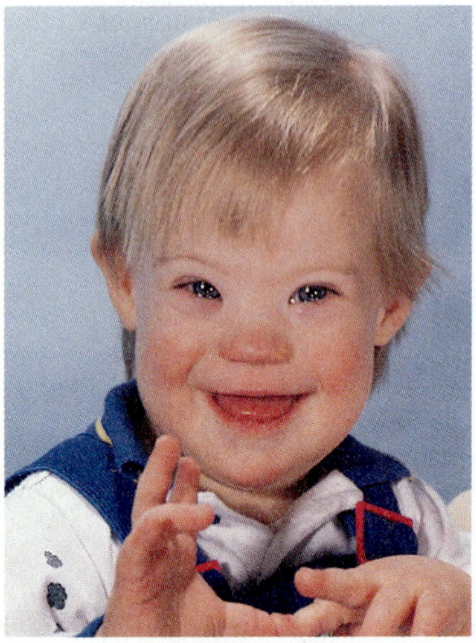

Child with Down syndrome.

- If any disturbances occur in meiosis during fertilization, major congenital malformations result. *Down syndrome* is caused by an extra chromosome. A child with this syndrome has a flat, broad face with wide-set eyes, a flat-bridged nose, oblique eyelid fissures, and other defects. An affected child can have various levels of mental retardation. Children with Down syndrome have increased levels of periodontal (gum) disease and abnormally shaped teeth.
- Implantation may occur outside the uterus; this is called *ectopic pregnancy* (ek-**top**-ik). Most such pregnancies occur in the fallopian tube. Tubal pregnancies usually rupture, causing loss of the embryo and threatening the life of the pregnant woman.

Embryonic period

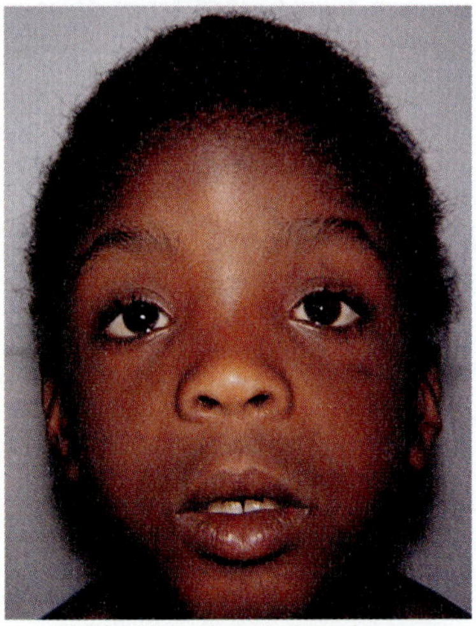

Child with fetal alcohol syndrome.

Developmental disturbances during this period may cause major congenital malformations.

- Caused by the *rubella virus* (roo-**bell**-ah), German measles in the mother can result in cardiac defects and deafness in the child.
- Exposure to high levels of radiation may result in cell death and retardation of mental development and physical growth.
- Fetal alcohol syndrome can occur when pregnant women ingest alcohol.

Fetal period

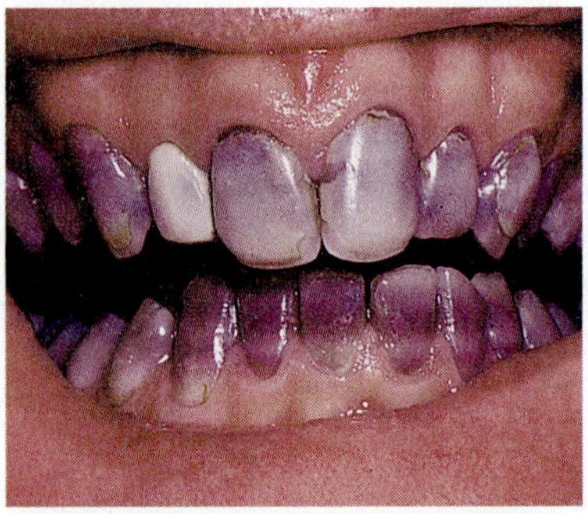

Endogenous developmental stain: tetracycline.

- In *amniocentesis* (**am**-nee-o-sen-**tee**-sis), a common prenatal diagnostic procedure, amniotic fluid is sampled during the 14th to 16th weeks to determine if a birth defect is present in the fetus.
- When pregnant women take the systemic antibiotic *tetracycline* (**tet**-rah-**si**-kleen) during the fetal period, permanent staining of the child's primary teeth may result.

Figures from Zitelli BJ and Davis HW: *Atlas of pediatric physical diagnosis,* ed 4, St Louis, 2002, Mosby; and Daniel SJ and Harfst SA: *Mosby's dental hygiene: concepts, cases, and competencies,* 2004 update, St Louis, 2004, Mosby. (Courtesy Dr. George Taybos, Jackson, MS.)

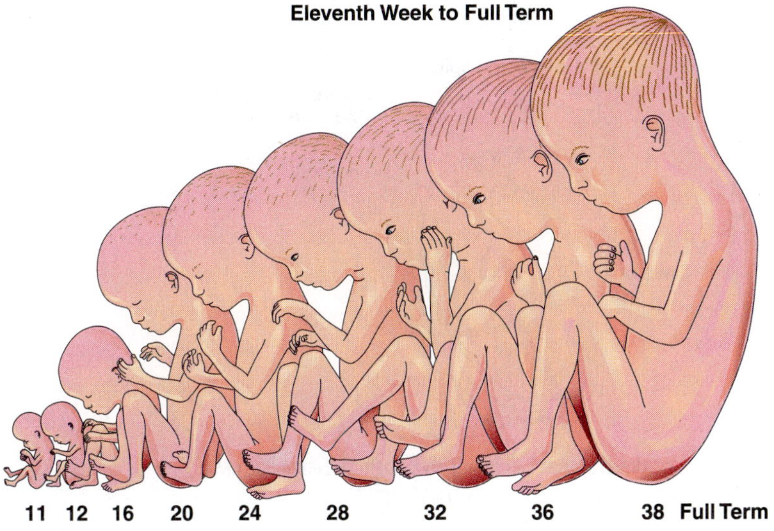

Fig. 8-3 A fetus at various weeks of development.

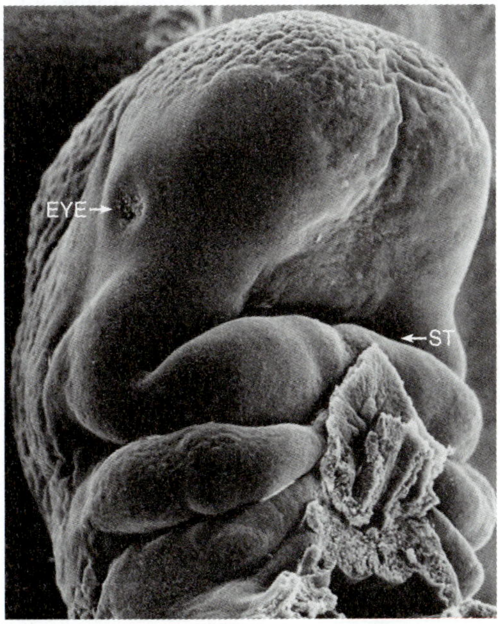

Fig. 8-4 Scanning electron micrograph of the head and neck of an embryo at four weeks showing development of the brain, face, and heart. Note the stomodeum (ST), or "primitive mouth," and the developing eye.

Structures Formed by Specialized Cells of Primary Embryonic Layers

Ectoderm (outer layer)	Mesoderm (middle layer)	Endoderm (inner layer)
Skin, brain, spinal cord	Bones, muscles	Lining of digestive system
Hair, nails	Circulatory system	Lining of lungs
Enamel of teeth	Kidneys, ducts	Parts of urogenital system
Lining of oral cavity	Reproductive system	
	Lining of abdominal cavity	
	Dentin, pulp, and cementum of teeth	

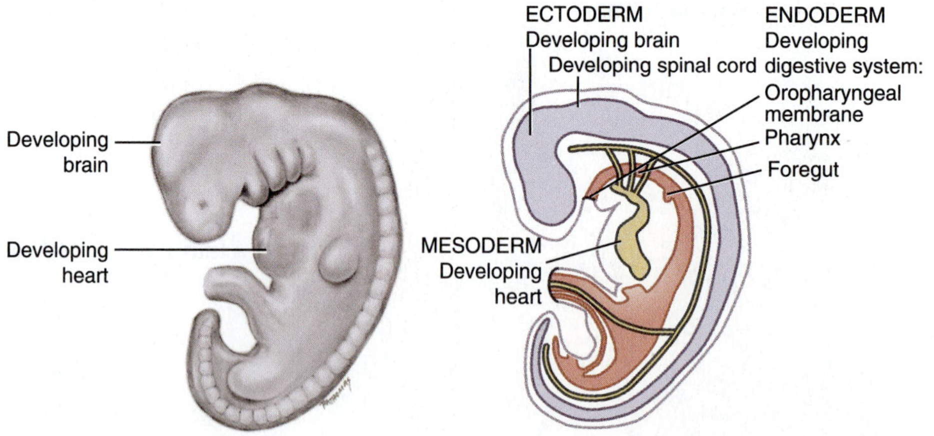

Fig. 8-5 A human embryo during the fifth week of development. (From Bath-Balogh M, Fehrenbach MJ: *Illustrated dental embryology, histology, and anatomy,* ed 2, St Louis, 2005, Saunders.)

mastication, and the anterior portion of the alveolar process of the mandible.

The *second branchial arch,* also known as the **hyoid arch,** forms the styloid process, stapes of the ear, stylohyoid ligament, and part of the hyoid bone. The second arch also forms the side and front of the neck, and some muscles of facial expression.

The *third branchial arch* forms the body of the hyoid and the posterior tongue. The *fourth, fifth,* and *sixth branchial arches* form the structures of the lower throat, including the thyroid cartilage, and the muscles and nerves of the pharynx and larynx.

Recall

4. Which branchial arch forms the bones, muscles, nerves of the face, and lower lip?
5. Which branchial arch forms the side and front of the neck?

Hard and Soft Palates

The formation of the palate takes several weeks to occur. It is formed from two separate embryonic structures, the **primary palate** and the **secondary palate.** This process begins in the fifth week of prenatal development. The hard and soft palates are formed by the union of the primary and secondary palates. This fusion makes a Y-shaped pattern in the roof of the mouth. This pattern is visible in the bony hard palate of an infant; however, the bones continue to fuse, and these lines are no longer visible on the adult hard palate.

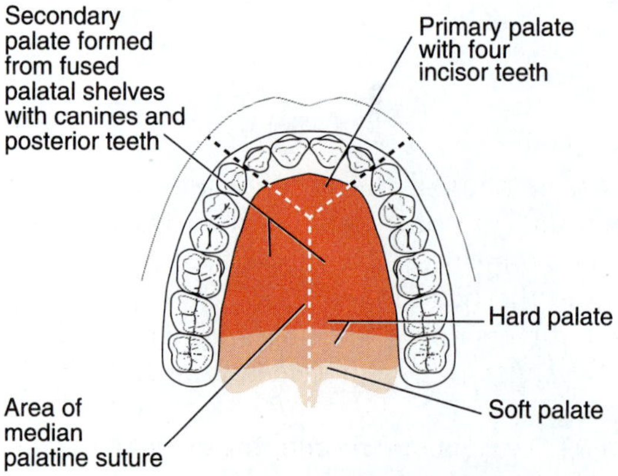

Fig. 8-6 Adult palate and developmental divisions. (From Bath-Balogh M, Fehrenbach MJ: *Illustrated dental embryology, histology, and anatomy,* ed 2, St Louis, 2005, Saunders..)

Fusion usually begins from the anterior during the ninth week. The palate is then completed during the twelfth week within the fetal period. Thus the palate is developed in three consecutive stages: (1) formation of the primary palate, (2) formation of the secondary palate, and (3) fusion of the palate (Fig. 8-6). Any disruption in the process may result in a cleft lip or cleft palate (Fig. 8-7) (see Chapter 10).

Recall

6. What are the three stages of palate formation?

A 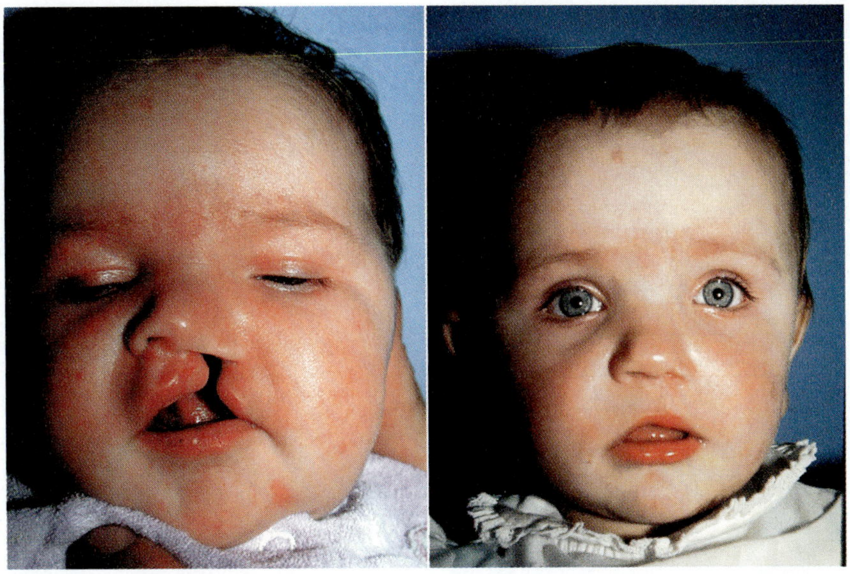 B

Fig. 8-7 **A,** An infant with a left unilateral complete cleft lip and palate. **B,** The infant after corrective surgeries are performed. (From Kaban L, Trolis M: *Pediatric oral and maxillofacial surgery,* Philadelphia, 2004, Saunders.)

Facial Development

The development of the human face occurs primarily between the fifth and eighth weeks. The face develops from the frontonasal process, which covers the forebrain, and the first branchial arch. The forward growth of the structures of the mouth produces striking age-related changes in the silhouette of the developing head, as follows:

- In the embryo at one month, the overhanging forehead is the dominant feature.
- During the second month, there is rapid growth of the nose and upper jaw, while the lower jaw appears to lag behind.
- In the third month, the fetus definitely resembles a human, although the head is still disproportionately large.
- At four months, the face looks human, the hard and soft palates are differentiated, and formation has begun on all the primary dentition (arrangement and number of teeth).
- During the last trimester, fat is laid down in the cheeks; these "sucking pads" give a healthy full-term fetus the characteristic round contour of the face.

Recall

7. When does the development of the human face occur?

Tooth Development

When the embryo is five to six weeks old, the first signs of tooth development are found in the anterior mandibular region (Table 8-1). Shortly after the mandibular anteriors develop, the anterior maxillary teeth begin to develop, and the process of tooth development progresses toward the posterior in both jaws.

By the seventeenth week, all primary teeth are developed and the development of the permanent teeth has begun.

At birth, there are normally 44 teeth in various stages of development. Enamel formation is well underway on all primary dentition and may be just beginning on the permanent first molars.

Recall

8. At birth, how many teeth are in various stages of development?

Developmental Disturbances

Disturbances in any stage of dental development may cause a wide variety of *anomalies* (abnormalities). Developmental disturbances can be caused by both genetic and environmental factors (see Box 8-1 and Chapter 17).

Table 8-1 ***Stages of Tooth Development***

Stage/Time Span*	Microscopic Appearance	Main Processes Involved	Description
Initiation stage/sixth to seventh weeks	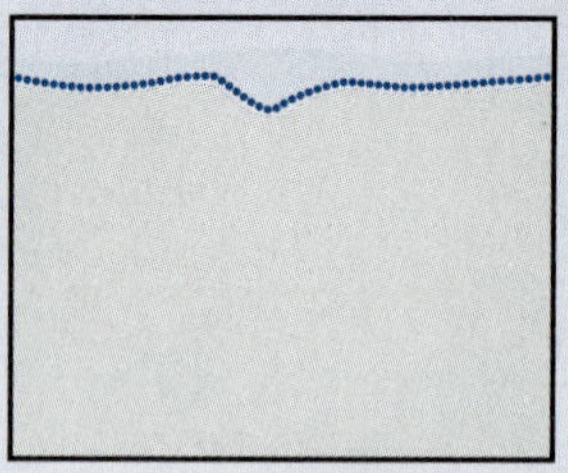	Induction	Ectoderm lining stomodeum gives rise to oral epithelium and then to dental lamina, adjacent to deeper mesenchyme and neural crest cells and separated by a basement membrane.
Bud stage/eighth week	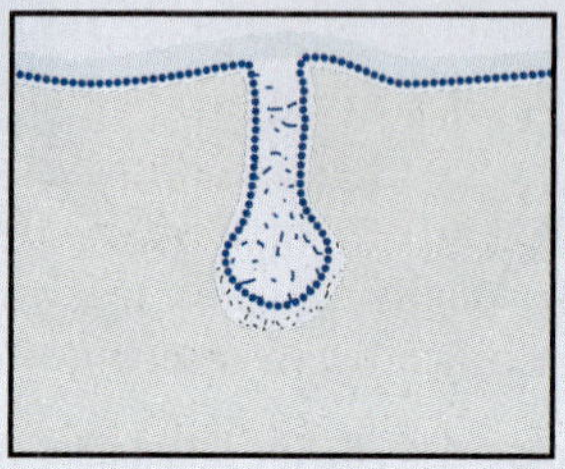	Proliferation	Growth of dental lamina into bud that penetrates growing mesenchyme
Cap stage/ninth to tenth weeks	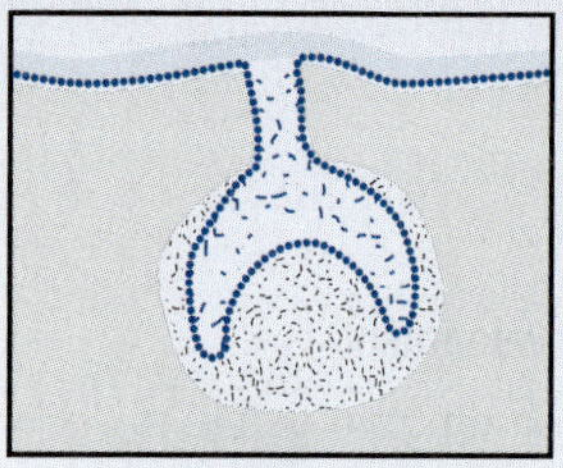	Proliferation, differentiation, morphogenesis	Enamel organ forms into cap, surrounding mass of dental papilla from the mesenchyme and surrounded by mass of **dental sac** also from the mesenchyme; formation of the tooth germ.
Bell stage/eleventh to twelfth weeks	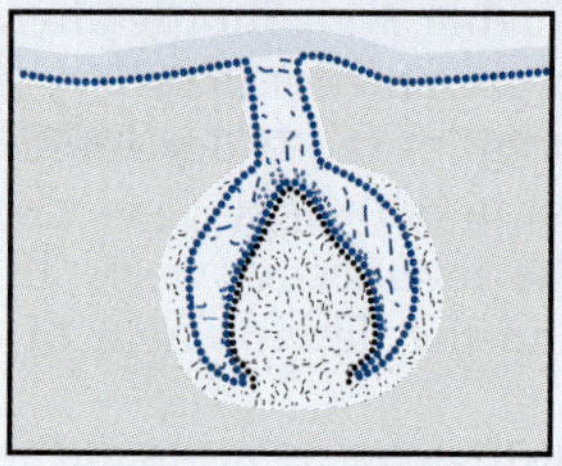	Proliferation, differentiation, morphogenesis	Differentiation of enamel organ into bell with four cell types and dental papilla into two cell types.
Apposition stage/varies per tooth	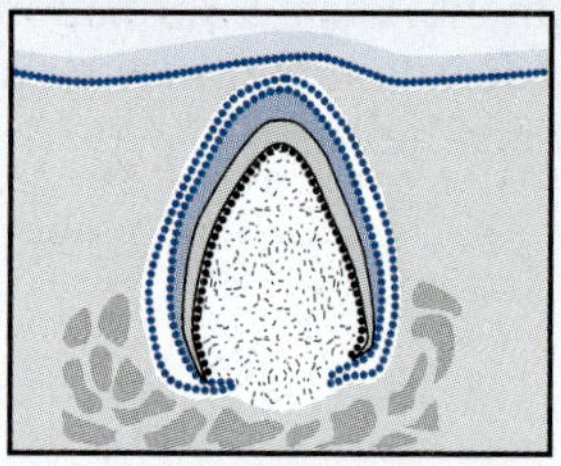	Induction, proliferation	Dental tissues secreted as matrix in successive layers.
Maturation stage/varies per tooth	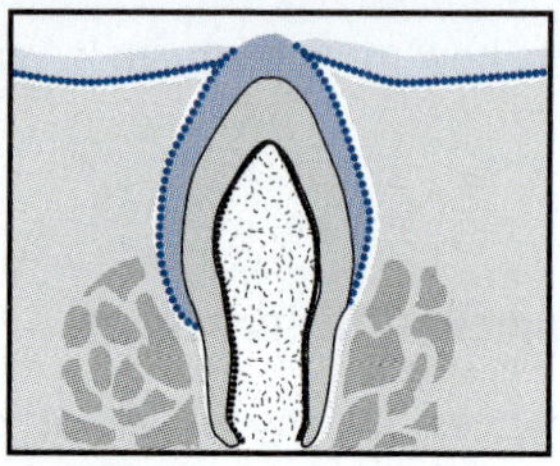	Maturation	Dental tissues fully mineralize to their mature levels.

From Bath-Balogh MB, Fehrenbach MJ: Illustrated dental embryology, histology, and anatomy, *ed 2, St Louis, 2005, Saunders.*
**Note that these are approximate prenatal time spans for the development of the primary dentition.*

Genetic Factors

In prenatal tooth development, the genetic factor that is most often a concern is tooth and jaw size. A child may inherit large teeth from one parent and a small jaw from the other, or small teeth and a large jaw. A large discrepancy in the size relationship of teeth and jaws may cause malocclusion (poor tooth position or contact) as the child develops.

Less common genetic factors appear in the dentition as anomalies.

Environmental Factors

Adverse environmental influences are called *teratogens* and include infections, drugs, and exposure to radiation. Drugs taken during pregnancy may cause birth defects. Such drugs include prescribed medication, over-the-counter remedies such as aspirin and cold tablets, and abused drugs including alcohol. Antibiotics, particularly tetracycline, taken during pregnancy may result in a yellow-gray-brown stain on the primary teeth. Women of childbearing age should avoid teratogens from the time of their first menstrual period.

The mother's dental health is also of concern. Toxins from a dental infection may be dangerous to both mother and child (e.g., toxins from periodontal disease in the mother are linked to low birth weight in the infant). Fever in the mother during pregnancy will leave marks in the developing teeth of the fetus.

Good nutrition *before* pregnancy helps to carry mother and child through the first weeks, which are critical for the developing child. This is also the time when morning sickness affects many expectant mothers, and some women find it difficult to eat.

Recall

9. What are the two major categories of factors that can adversely influence dental development?

Facial Development After Birth

The shape of the face changes considerably from newborn to adult (Fig. 8-8). After the immediate postnatal period, most facial growth takes place in predictable *growth spurts,* which occur during youth and early adolescence. Facial bones grow and are reshaped to achieve normal growth and development. This process involves the **deposition** of new bone in some areas and **resorption** of existing bone from other areas.

Deposition is the process of "laying down" or adding new bone. **Osteoblasts** are the cells responsible for new bone formation. Examples of new bone formation include healing of a fractured bone and creation of new bone to fill the socket left after tooth extraction.

Resorption occurs when the body removes bone. **Osteoclasts** are the cells responsible for this process, in which bone cells are resorbed (taken away) by the body. The roots of primary teeth resorb before the tooth is lost. Resorption also occurs with loss of bone from the alveolar ridge during periodontal disease.

Known Teratogens Involved in Congenital Malformations

Drugs: Ethanol, tetracycline, phenytoin (Dilantin), lithium, methotrexate, aminopterin, diethylstilbestrol, warfarin, thalidomide, isotretinoin (retinoic acid), androgens, progesterone

Chemicals: Methylmercury, polychlorinated biphenyls

Infections: Rubella, herpes simplex, human immunodeficiency virus (HIV), syphilis

Radiation: High levels of ionizing type*

Modified from Bath-Balogh MB, Fehrenbach MJ: *Illustrated dental embryology, histology, and anatomy,* ed 2, St Louis, 2005, Saunders.
*Diagnostic levels of radiation should be avoided but have not been directly linked to congenital malformations.

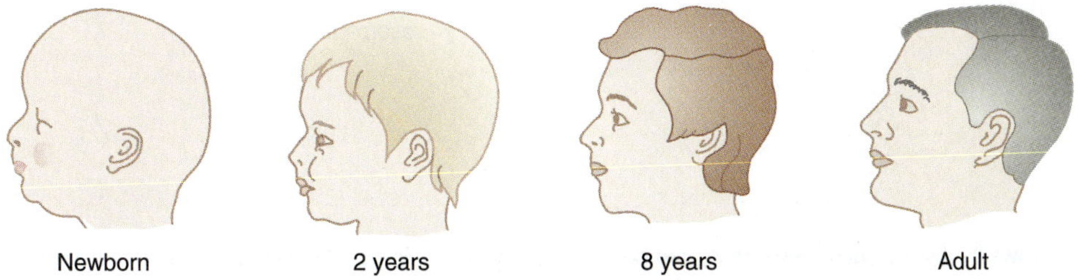

Fig. 8-8 Changes in facial contours from birth to adulthood.

Modeling, also known as *displacement,* describes the bone changes that occur along the articulations (joints) of the bones as they increase in size and shape to keep up with the growth of surrounding tissues.

Remodeling describes the growth and changes in shape of existing bone. Modeling and remodeling involve both the deposition and resorption of bone (Fig. 8-9).

Tooth Movement

Remodeling occurs in response to forces placed on the tooth within its socket. To understand this concept, imagine yourself standing in a swimming pool. As you step forward, the water moves from in front of you and fills in the space in back of you. Similarly, when force is applied to a tooth and the tooth moves, the bone in front will be *resorbed* and will be *deposited* in back of the tooth to fill in the space (Fig. 8-10).

Recall

10. What is the process of adding bone?
11. What is the process of bone loss or removal?

Life Cycle of a Tooth

The process of tooth formation is called **odontogenesis,** and it is divided into three primary periods: growth, calcification, and eruption (see Table 8-1).

Growth Periods

The growth periods are divided into three stages: bud, cap, and bell.

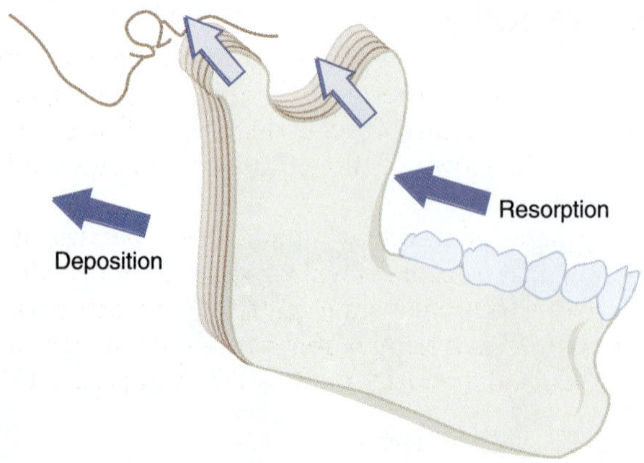

Fig. 8-9 The mandible grows by displacement, resorption, and deposition. Notice how space is created to accommodate the third molar.

Bud stage

The bud stage, also known as *initiation,* is the beginning of development for each tooth. This stage follows a definite pattern, and it takes place at a different time for each type of tooth.

Initiation starts with the formation of the **dental lamina,** which is a thickened band of oral epithelium that follows the curve of each developing dental arch. Almost as soon as the dental lamina is formed, it produces 10 enlargements in each arch. These are the **tooth buds** for the *primary teeth.*

The *permanent teeth* develop similarly. The dental lamina continues to grow in a posterior direction to produce tooth buds for the three permanent molars, which will develop distal to the primary teeth on each quadrant. The tooth bud for the first permanent molar forms at about the seventeenth week of fetal life; the tooth buds for the second molars form about six months after birth; and buds for the third molars form at about five years.

The **succedaneous teeth** are the *permanent* teeth that replace the primary teeth. These teeth develop from tooth buds in the deep portion of the dental lamina on the lingual side of the primary teeth. These begin to form as early as 24 weeks.

Cap stage

During the cap stage, also known as *proliferation,* the cells of the tooth grow and increase in number. This growth causes regular changes in size and proportion of the developing tooth, and the solid-looking tooth bud changes into a hollow, caplike shape.

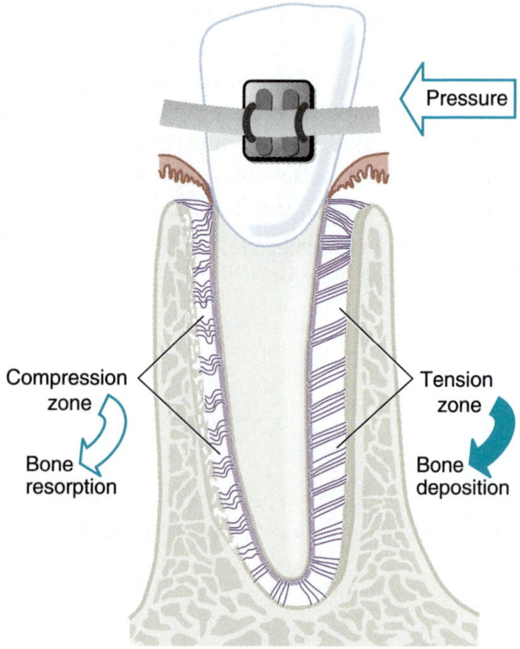

Fig. 8-10 **Process of orthodontic tooth movement.** (From Bath-Balogh MB, Fehrenbach MJ: *Illustrated dental embryology, histology, and anatomy,* ed 2, St Louis, 2005, Saunders.)

The primary embryonic ectoderm layer, which has differentiated into *oral epithelium*, becomes the **enamel organ**, which will eventually form the enamel of the developing tooth. The primary embryonic mesoderm layer, now differentiated into connective tissue known as *mesenchyme*, becomes the **dental papilla**, which will form the pulp and **dentin** of the tooth. As the enamel organ and dental papilla of the tooth develop, the mesenchyme surrounding them condenses to form a capsulelike structure called the **dental sac.** This sac will give rise to the cementum and periodontal ligament.

Bell stage

During the bell stage, the cells differentiate and become specialized in a process called *histodifferentiation*, as follows:

- The epithelial cells become **ameloblasts,** which are the enamel-forming cells.
- The peripheral cells of the dental papilla become **odontoblasts,** which are the dentin-forming cells.
- The inner cells of the dental sac differentiate into **cementoblasts,** which are cementum-forming cells.

As the tooth continues to develop, the dental organ continues to change. It assumes a shape described as resembling a bell. As these developments take place, the dental lamina, which thus far has connected the dental organ to the oral epithelium, breaks apart.

The basic shape and relative size of each tooth are established during the process of *morphodifferentiation*. The *dentinoenamel junction* (DEJ) and the *cementodentinal junction* are formed and act as a blueprint for the developing tooth.

In accordance with this pattern, the ameloblasts deposit enamel and the odontoblasts deposit dentin to give the completed tooth its characteristic shape and size. This process starts at the top of the tooth and moves downward toward the future root. The development of the root, or roots, begins after the enamel and dentin formation has reached the future *cementoenamel junction* (CEJ).

As part of this process, the inner cells of the dental sac differentiate into cementoblasts, which produce the cementum to cover the developing root.

Recall

12. What are the three primary periods in tooth formation?
13. What are the three stages in the growth period?

Calcification

Calcification is the process by which the structural outline formed during the growth stage is hardened by the deposit of calcium and other mineral salts.

The enamel is built layer by layer by the ameloblasts working outward from the DEJ, starting at the top of the crown of each tooth and spreading downward over its sides.

Pits and fissures

If the tooth has several cusps, a cap of enamel forms over each cusp. As growth continues, the cusps eventually *coalesce* (fuse together) to form a solid enamel covering for the occlusal surface of the tooth.

Pits and fissures may be formed during this process. A *fissure* is a fault along a developmental groove on the occlusal surface that is caused by incomplete or imperfect joining of the lobes during the formation of the tooth. A *pit* results when two developmental grooves cross each other, forming a deep area that is too small for the bristle of a toothbrush to clean. The enamel may be particularly thin, and these areas are often inaccessible for cleaning and are thus sites where decay frequently begins (see Chapter 59).

Eruption of Primary Teeth

Once it has passed through the previous stages, a tooth must be able to achieve its normal position. *Eruption* is the movement of the tooth into its functional position in the oral cavity.

Eruption of the primary dentition takes place in chronologic order, as does the permanent dentition later (Fig. 8-11). This process involves active eruption, which is the actual vertical movement of the tooth. We know *how* tooth eruption occurs, but *why* it occurs is still uncertain. No one can specify the exact forces that "push" teeth through the soft tissues.

Active eruption of a primary tooth has many stages in the movement of the tooth (Fig. 8-12). The period of tissue disintegration causes an inflammatory response known as "teething," which may be accompanied by tenderness and swelling of the local tissues.

Shedding of Primary Teeth

Shedding, or **exfoliation,** is the normal process by which the primary teeth are lost as the succedaneous (permanent) teeth develop.

When it is time for a primary tooth to be lost, osteoclasts cause the resorption of the root, beginning at the **apex** and continuing in the direction of the crown. Eventually the crown of the tooth is lost because of lack of support.

The process of shedding is intermittent because at the same time that osteoblasts replace resorbed bone, odontoblasts and cementoblasts are replacing resorbed portions of the root. Thus a primary tooth may tighten after being loose. Finally, the primary tooth will be lost (Fig. 8-13).

Eruption of Permanent Teeth

The process of eruption for a succedaneous tooth is the same as for the primary tooth. The permanent tooth erupts into the oral cavity in a position lingual to the roots of the

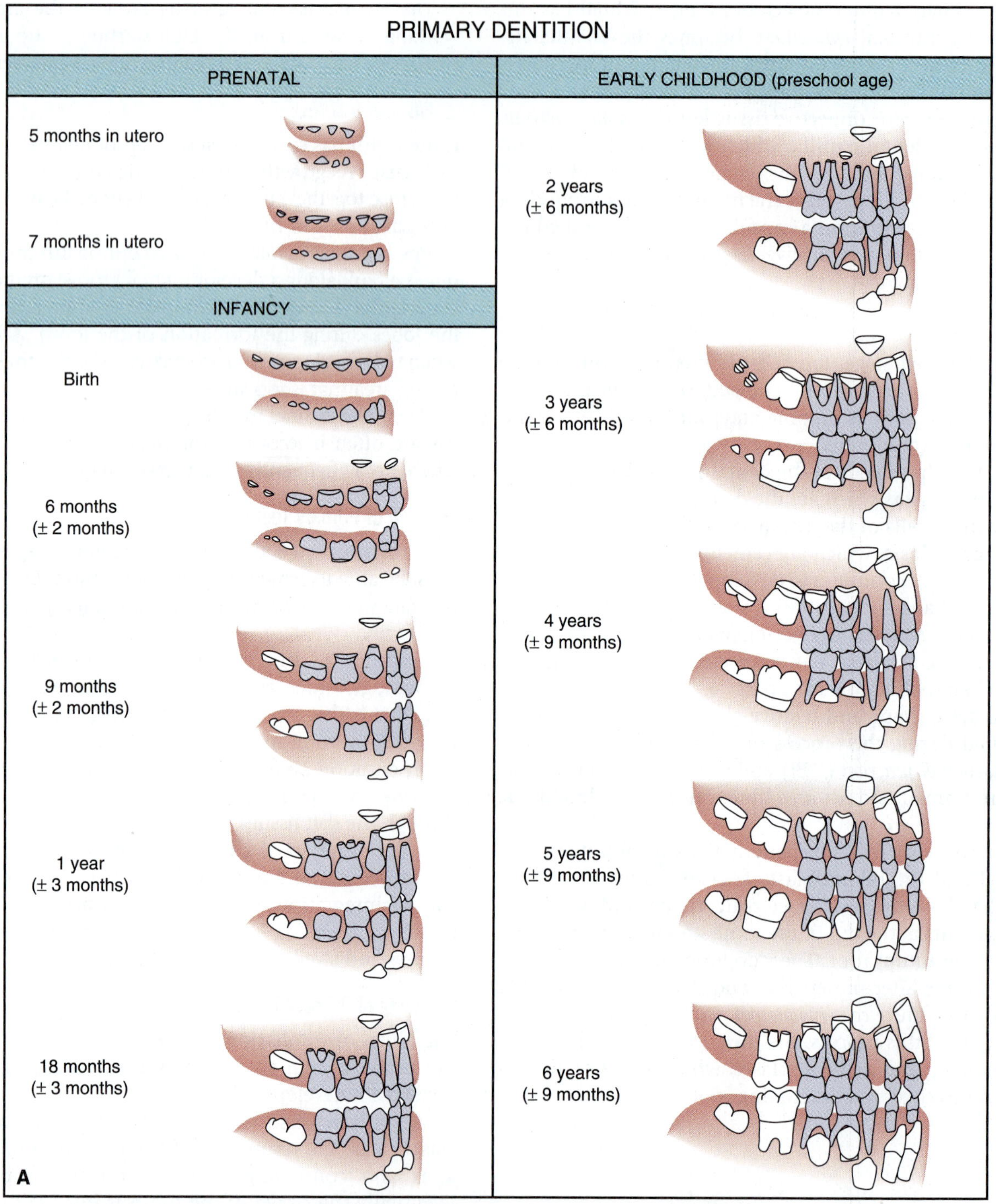

Fig. 8-11 A, Chronologic order of eruption of the primary dentition. (From Bath-Balogh MB, Fehrenbach MJ: *Illustrated dental embryology, histology, and anatomy,* ed 2, St Louis, 2005, Saunders.)

shedding (or shed) primary anterior tooth or between the roots of the shedding primary posterior tooth (Fig. 8-14).

When a permanent tooth starts to erupt before the primary tooth is fully shed, problems in spacing can arise. Thus it is important for children with retained primary teeth to seek dental consultation early.

Recall

14. When a tooth has several cusps, what structures are formed when the cusps join together?

15. What is the name of the process by which teeth move into the oral cavity?

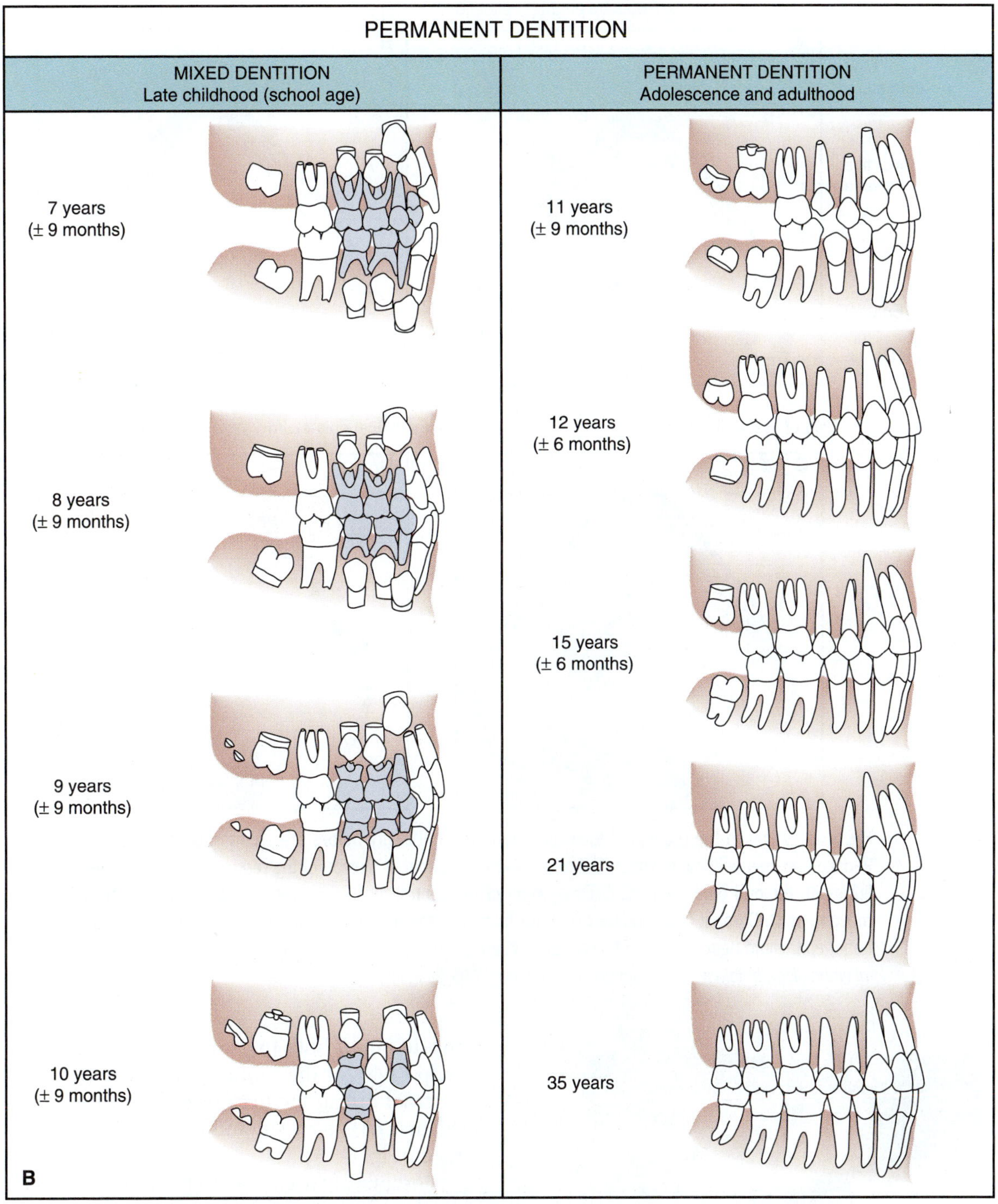

Fig. 8-11, cont'd B, Permanent dentition. (From Bath-Balogh MB, Fehrenbach MJ: *Illustrated dental embryology, histology, and anatomy,* ed 2, St Louis, 2005, Saunders.)

ORAL HISTOLOGY

Oral histology is the study of the *structure and function* of the teeth and oral tissues. This section discusses anatomic parts and histology of the teeth, the supporting structures, and the oral mucosa, which surrounds the teeth and lines the mouth.

Each tooth consists of a crown and one or more roots. The size and shape of the crown and the size and number of roots vary according to the type of tooth (see Chapter 11).

Crown

The crown has dentin covered by enamel, and each root has dentin covered by cementum. The inner portion of

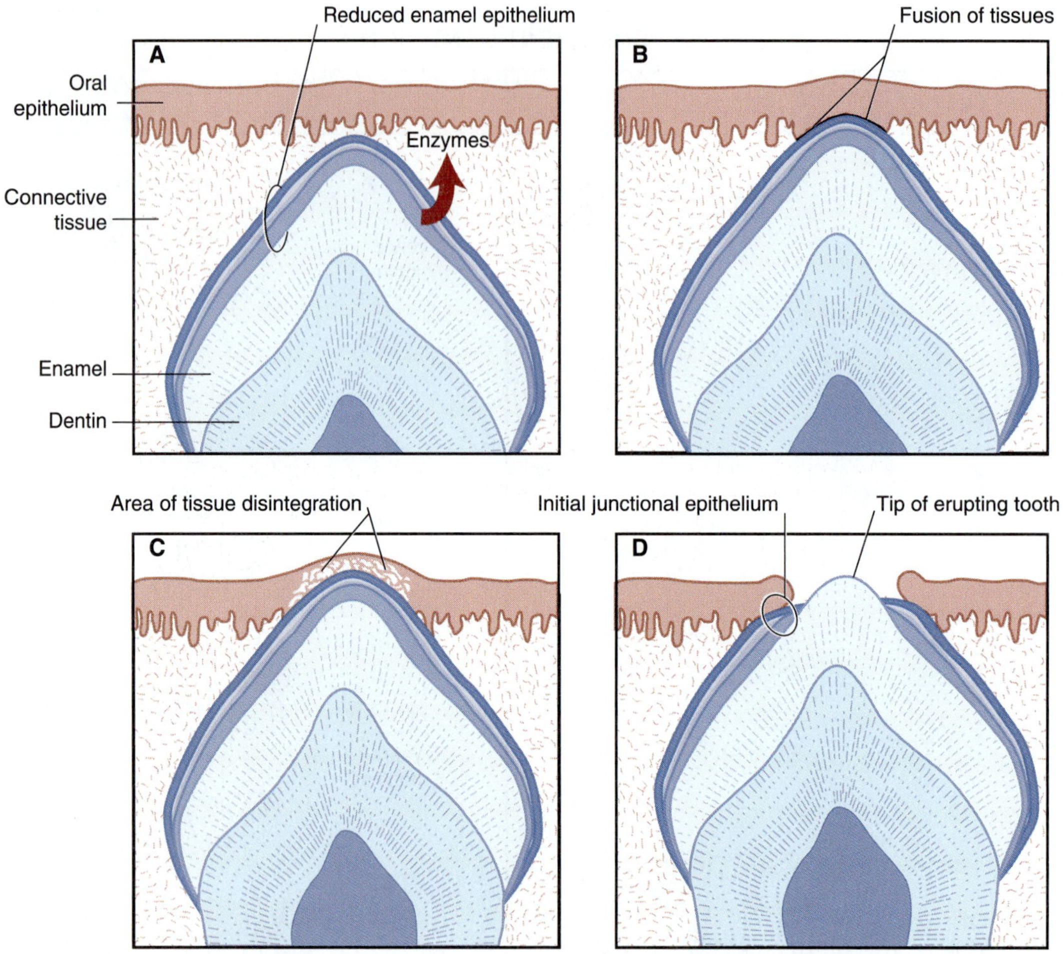

Fig. 8-12 Stages in the process of tooth eruption. **A,** Oral cavity before the eruption process begins. Reduced enamel epithelium covers the newly formed enamel. **B,** Fusion of the reduced enamel epithelium with the oral epithelium. **C,** Disintegration of the central fused tissue, leaving a tunnel for tooth movement. **D,** Coronal fused tissues peel back from the crown during eruption, leaving the initial junctional epithelium near the cementoenamel junction. (From Bath-Balogh MB, Fehrenbach MJ: *Illustrated dental embryology, histology, and anatomy,* ed 2, St Louis, 2005, Saunders.)

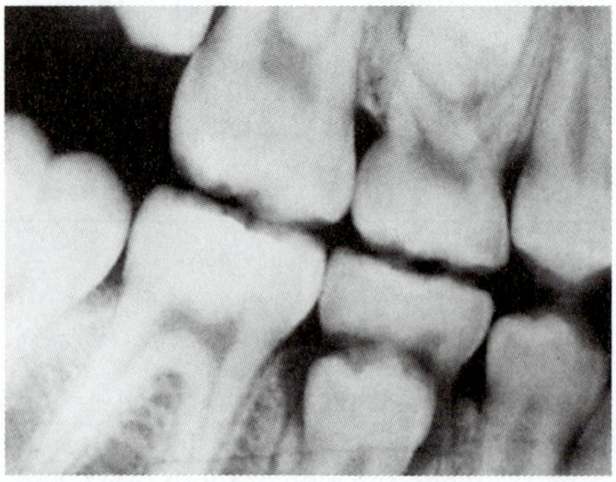

Fig. 8-13 Radiograph showing normal resorption of the roots of a mandibular primary molar before being shed.

the dentin of both the crown and the root also covers the pulp cavity of the tooth close to the CEJ. The CEJ is the external line at the neck or cervix of the tooth where the enamel of the crown and cementum of the root usually meet (Fig. 8-15).

Portions of the crown are usually defined in more specific ways. The **anatomic crown** is the portion of the tooth *covered with enamel* (Fig. 8-16). The size of the anatomic crown remains constant throughout the life of the tooth, regardless of the position of the gingiva. The **clinical crown** is the portion of the tooth that is *visible in the mouth.* The clinical crown varies in length during the life cycle of the tooth depending on the level of the gingiva. The clinical crown is shorter as the tooth erupts into position and is longer as the surrounding tissues recede. The phrase "long in the tooth," referring to old age, comes from the process of the clinical crown becoming longer as the gingiva recedes around the tooth.

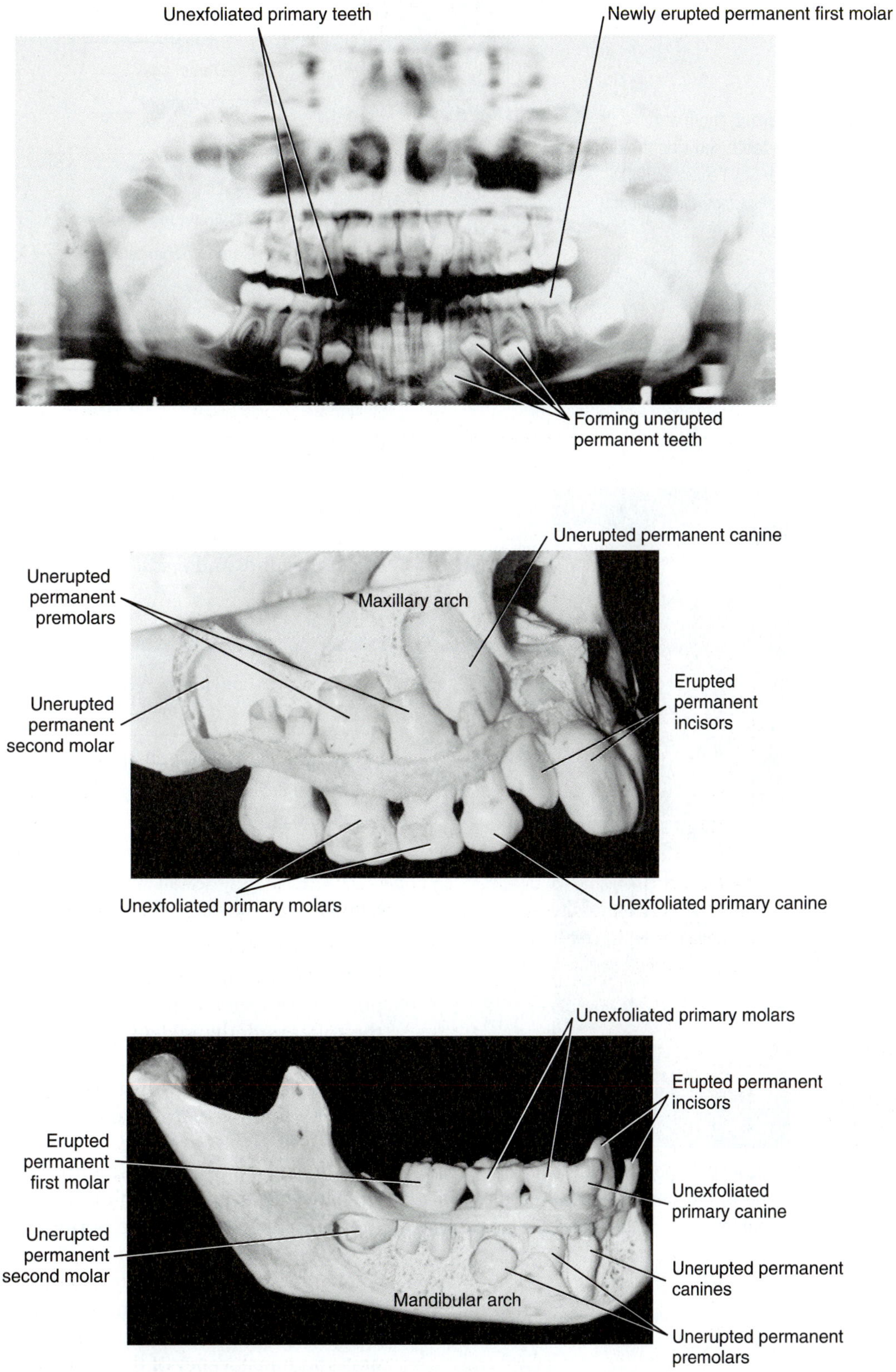

Fig. 8-14 Examples of mixed dentition with the primary and permanent teeth erupting. (From Bath-Balogh MB, Fehrenbach MJ: *Illustrated dental embryology, histology, and anatomy,* ed 2, St Louis, 2005, Saunders.)

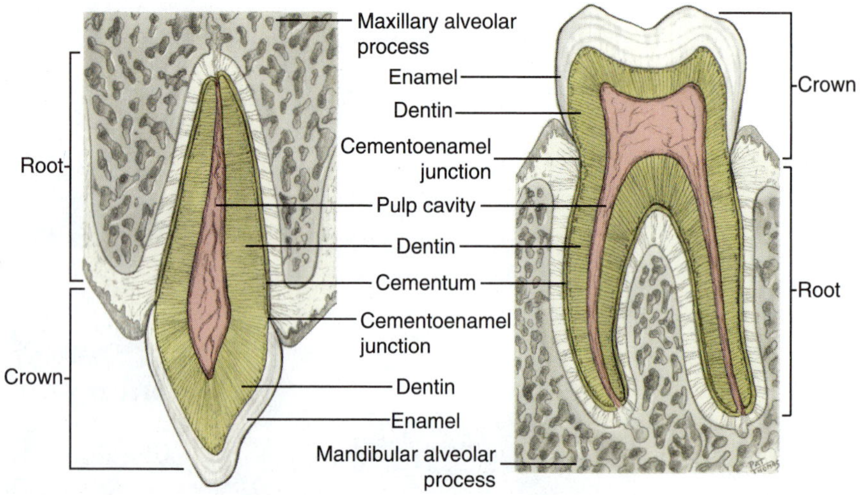

Fig. 8-15 Anterior (top or front) tooth and posterior (bottom or back) tooth showing the dental tissues. (From Bath-Balogh MB, Fehrenbach MJ: *Illustrated dental embryology, histology, and anatomy,* ed 2, St Louis, 2005, Saunders.)

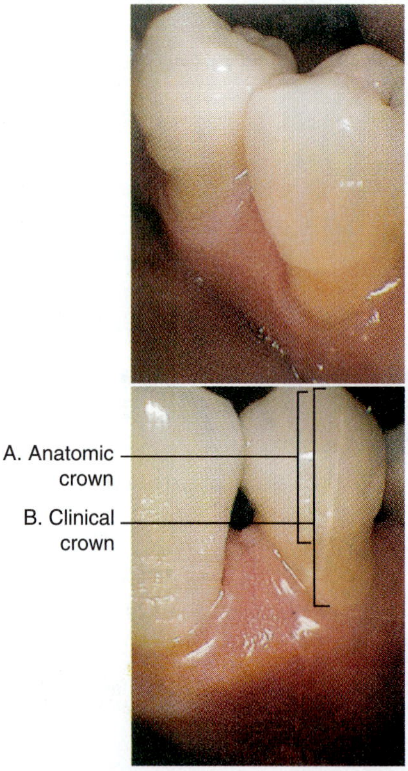

Fig. 8-16 A, The anatomic crown is the portion of the tooth covered with enamel and remains the same. B, The clinical crown is the portion of the tooth visible in the mouth and may vary due to changes in the position of the gingiva.

Root

The root of the tooth is that portion normally embedded in the alveolar process and is covered with **cementum.** Depending on the type of tooth, the root may have one, two, or three branches. *Bifurcation* means division into two roots. *Trifurcation* means division into three roots.

The tapered end of each root tip is known as the apex. Any structure or object that is situated at the apex is said to be *apical.* Anything surrounding the apex is *periapical* (*peri-* means around, and *apical* refers to the apex).

Recall

16. What is the difference between the anatomic crown and the clinical crown?

17. Where is the CEJ?

Enamel

Enamel, which makes up the anatomic crown of the tooth, is the hardest material in the body. This hardness is important because enamel forms the protective covering for the softer underlying dentin. It also provides a strong surface for crushing, grinding, and chewing food.

Enamel is able to withstand crushing stresses to about 100,000 pounds per square inch. Although enamel is strong, it is also very brittle, and this brittleness may cause the enamel to fracture or chip. Along with enamel's strength, however, the cushioning effect of the dentin and the springlike action of the **periodontium** enable enamel to withstand most of the pressures brought against it.

Enamel is *translucent* (allows some light to pass through it) and ranges in color from yellow to grayish white. These variations in shade are caused by differences in the thickness and translucency of the enamel and in the color of the dentin beneath it.

Enamel, which is formed by ameloblasts, consists of 96 to 99 percent inorganic matter and only 1 to 4 percent organic matrix. **Hydroxyapatite,** which consists primarily of calcium, is the most abundant mineral component.

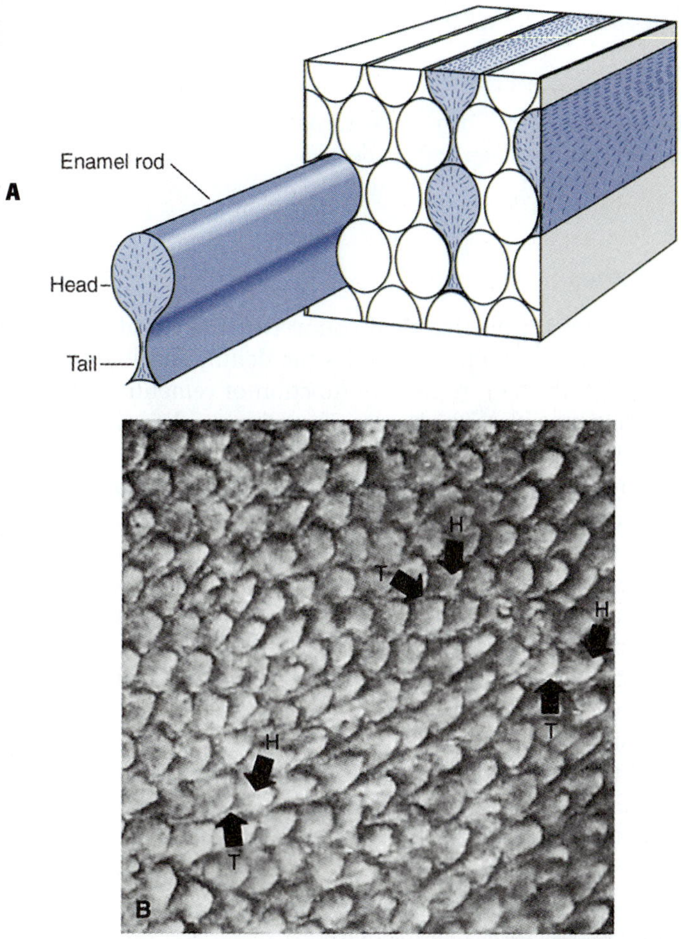

Fig. 8-17 **Enamel rod, the basic unit of enamel. A, Relationship of the rod to enamel. B, Scanning electron micrograph of enamel showing head (H) and tail (T).** (From Bath-Balogh MB, Fehrenbach MJ: *Illustrated dental embryology, histology, and anatomy,* ed 2, St Louis, 2005, Saunders.)

Hydroxyapatite is the material that is lost in the process of dental decay (see Chapter 13).

Enamel is similar to bone in its hardness and mineral content. Unlike bone, however, mature enamel does not contain cells that are capable of remodeling and repair. Nevertheless, some remineralization is possible (see Chapter 15).

Enamel is composed of millions of calcified enamel **prisms,** which are also known as *enamel rods.* These extend from the surface of the tooth to the DEJ. The enamel prisms tend to be grouped into rows organized around the circumference of the long axis of the tooth. The prisms within each row follow a course that is generally perpendicular to the surface of the tooth. This organization into rows is clinically important, because enamel tends to fracture along the interfacial planes of adjacent groups of prisms.

The diameter of a prism is approximately 5 to 8 microns, depending on its location (1 micron is one millionth of a meter). In cross-section, the prisms appear to be keyhole-shaped structures consisting of a head and a tail (Fig. 8-17). If you were to hold a handful of straws together and look at the ends, they would resemble the structure of enamel rods.

Each prism appears to be encased in a *prism sheath,* and an *interprismatic substance,* also known as an *interrod substance,* holds the sheathed prisms together. Of all these hard structures, the prisms are hardest and the interprismatic substance is weakest. These differences make it possible to "acid-etch" the teeth for the direct bonding of restorative materials (see Chapter 43).

Hunter-Schreger bands, which microscopically appear as alternating light and dark bands in the enamel, are caused by enamel prisms intertwining or changing direction.

The **striae of Retzius,** also known as the *strips of Retzius,* are incremental rings, like growth rings of a tree, representing variations in the deposition of the enamel matrix during formation of the tooth. Enamel produced prenatally contains only a few of these incremental lines; however, the shock of birth is registered as a ring known as the *neonatal* line.

Enamel tufts start at the DEJ and may extend to the inner third of the enamel. Microscopically they have the appearance of tufts of grass. Enamel tufts are the hypocalcified or uncalcified ends of groups of enamel prisms.

Enamel lamellae are thin, leaflike structures that extend from the enamel surface toward the DEJ. These lamellae consist of organic material with little mineral content. (The singular form is *lamella.*)

Enamel spindles are the ends of odontoblasts (dentin-forming cells) that extend across the DEJ a short distance into the enamel.

Recall

18. What is the hardest substance in the human body?
19. What is the most abundant mineral component in enamel?

Dentin

Dentin makes up the main portion of the tooth structure and extends almost the entire length of the tooth. It is covered by enamel on the crown and by cementum on the root.

In the primary teeth, dentin is very light yellow. In the permanent teeth, it is light yellow and somewhat transparent. The color may darken with age.

Dentin is a mineralized tissue that is harder than bone and cementum but not as hard as enamel. Although hard, dentin has elastic properties that are important in the support of enamel, which is brittle.

Dentin is composed of 70 percent inorganic material and 30 percent organic matter and water. The rapid penetration and spreading of the caries in dentin are caused in part by its high content of organic substances.

Dentin is formed by the odontoblasts, beginning at growth centers along the DEJ and proceeding inward toward what will become the pulp chamber of the tooth. The internal surface of the dentin forms the walls of the pulp cavity. The odontoblasts line these walls, and from there they continue to form and repair the dentin.

Dentin is penetrated through its entire thickness by microscopic canals called **dentinal tubules** (Fig. 8-18). Each dentinal tubule contains a **dentinal fiber.** These fibers, which terminate in a branching network at the junction with the enamel or cementum, transmit pain stimuli and make dentin an excellent thermal conductor.

Because of the dentinal fibers within the dentin, it is considered to be a living tissue. During operative procedures, dentin must be protected from dehydration and thermal shock. When 1 mm of dentin is exposed, about 30,000 dentinal fibers are exposed, and thus 30,000 living cells may be damaged.

Because it is capable of continued growth and repair, dentin consists of the following three major types:

- **Primary dentin,** which is formed before eruption, forms the bulk of the tooth.
- **Secondary dentin** begins formation after eruption and continues at a very slow rate throughout the life of the tooth. This results in the gradual narrowing of the pulp chamber with age.
- **Tertiary dentin,** also known as *reparative dentin,* is formed in response to irritation and appears as a localized deposit on the wall of the pulp chamber. This may occur in response to *attrition* (wearing away of tooth through normal use), erosion, dental caries, dental treatment, or other irritants.

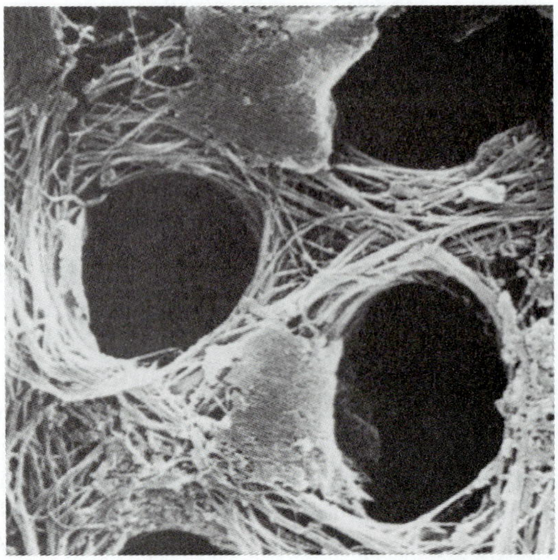

Fig. 8-18 Scanning electron micrograph of dentinal tubules.

Recall

20. How does dentin transmit sensations of pain?
21. What are the three types of dentin?

Cementum

Cementum is bonelike rigid connective tissue that covers the root of the tooth. It overlies the dentin and joins the enamel at the CEJ. A primary function of cementum is to anchor the tooth to the bony socket with attachment fibers within the periodontium.

Cementum is light yellow and is easily distinguishable from enamel by its lack of luster and its darker hue. It is somewhat lighter in color than dentin.

Cementum, which is formed by cementoblasts, is not quite as hard as dentin or bone. Unlike bone, cementum does not resorb and form again. This difference is important because it makes orthodontic treatment possible. However, cementum is capable of some repair by the deposition of new layers.

As the root develops, **primary cementum,** also known as *acellular cementum,* is formed outward from the cementodentinal junction for the full length of the root. After the tooth has reached functional occlusion, **secondary cementum,** also known as *cellular cementum,* continues to form on the apical half of the root.

As a result, the cervical half of the root is covered with a thin layer of primary cementum, and the apical half of the root has a thickened cementum covering. This continued growth in the apical area assists in maintaining the total length of the tooth by compensating for the enamel lost by attrition.

Recall

22. What are the two types of cementum?

Pulp

The inner aspect of the dentin forms the boundaries of the **pulp chamber** (Fig. 8-19). As with the dentin surrounding it, the contours of the pulp chamber follow the contours of the exterior surface of the tooth.

At the time of eruption, the pulp chamber is large; however, because of the continuous deposition of dentin, it becomes smaller with age.

The part of the pulp that lies within the crown portion of the tooth is called the **coronal pulp.** This structure includes the *pulp horns,* which are extensions of the pulp that project toward the cusp tips and incisal edges.

The other portion of the pulp is more apically located and is referred to as the **radicular pulp,** or the *root pulp.* During the development of the root, the continued deposition of dentin causes this area to become longer and narrower.

The radicular portion of the pulp in each root is continuous with the tissues of the periapical area via an **apical foramen.** In young teeth, the apical foramen is not yet fully formed, and this opening is wide. With increasing age and exposure of the tooth to functional stress, however, secondary dentin decreases the diameter of the pulp chamber and the apical foramen.

The pulp is made up of blood vessels and nerves that enter the pulp chamber through the apical foramen. The blood supply is derived from branches of the dental arteries and from the periodontal ligament.

The pulp also contains connective tissue, which consists of cells, intercellular substance, and tissue fluid. **Fibroblasts,** one type of cell in connective tissue, are responsible for the formation of the intercellular substance of the pulp.

The tissue fluid interchange between the pulp and dentin serves the important functions of keeping tissue supplied with moisture and nutrients. The rich blood supply also has an important defense function in responding to a bacterial invasion of the tooth.

The nerve supply of the pulp receives and transmits pain stimuli. When the stimulus is weak, the response by the pulpal system is weak, and the interaction goes unnoticed. When the stimulus is great, the reaction is stronger, and pain quickly calls attention to the threatened condition of the tooth.

Recall

23. What type of tissue makes up the pulp?
24. What cells form the intercellular substance of the pulp?

Periodontium

The **periodontium** supports the teeth in the alveolar bone. The periodontium consists of *cementum, alveolar bone,* and the *periodontal ligaments.* These tissues also protect and nourish the teeth. The periodontium is divided into two major units: the attachment apparatus and the gingival unit.

Attachment Apparatus

The attachment apparatus consists of the cementum (see earlier discussion), the alveolar process, and periodontal ligaments (Fig. 8-20). These tissues work together to support, maintain, and retain the tooth in its functional position within the jaw.

Alveolar process

The alveolar processes are the extensions of the bone from the body of the mandible and the maxilla that support the teeth in their functional positions in the jaws (Fig. 8-21). Osteoblasts are responsible for the formation of this bone, and osteoclasts are responsible for resorption and remodeling of the bone.

The alveolar process develops in response to the growth of the developing teeth. After teeth have been lost, bone from the alveolar process is resorbed, and the ridge decreases in size and changes in shape.

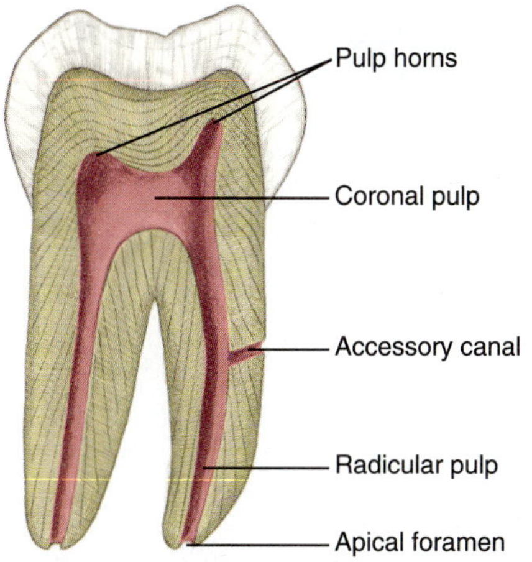

Fig. 8-19 The dental pulp. (From Bath-Balogh MB, Fehrenbach MJ: *Illustrated dental embryology, histology, and anatomy,* ed 2, St Louis, 2005, Saunders.)

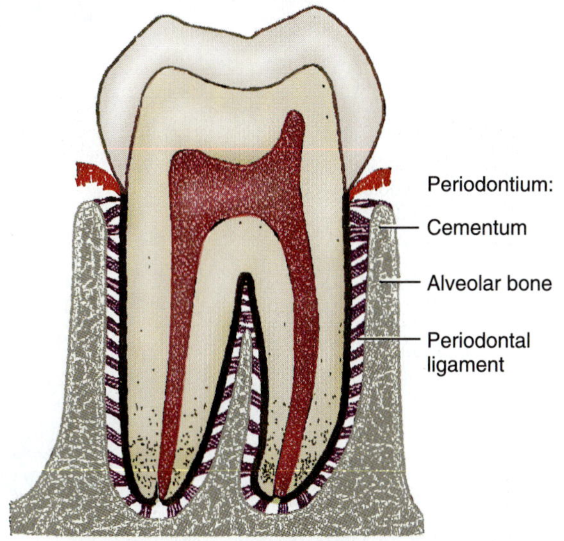

Fig. 8-20 Periodontium of the tooth with its components identified. (From Bath-Balogh MB, Fehrenbach MJ: *Illustrated dental embryology, histology, and anatomy,* ed 2, St Louis, 2005, Saunders.)

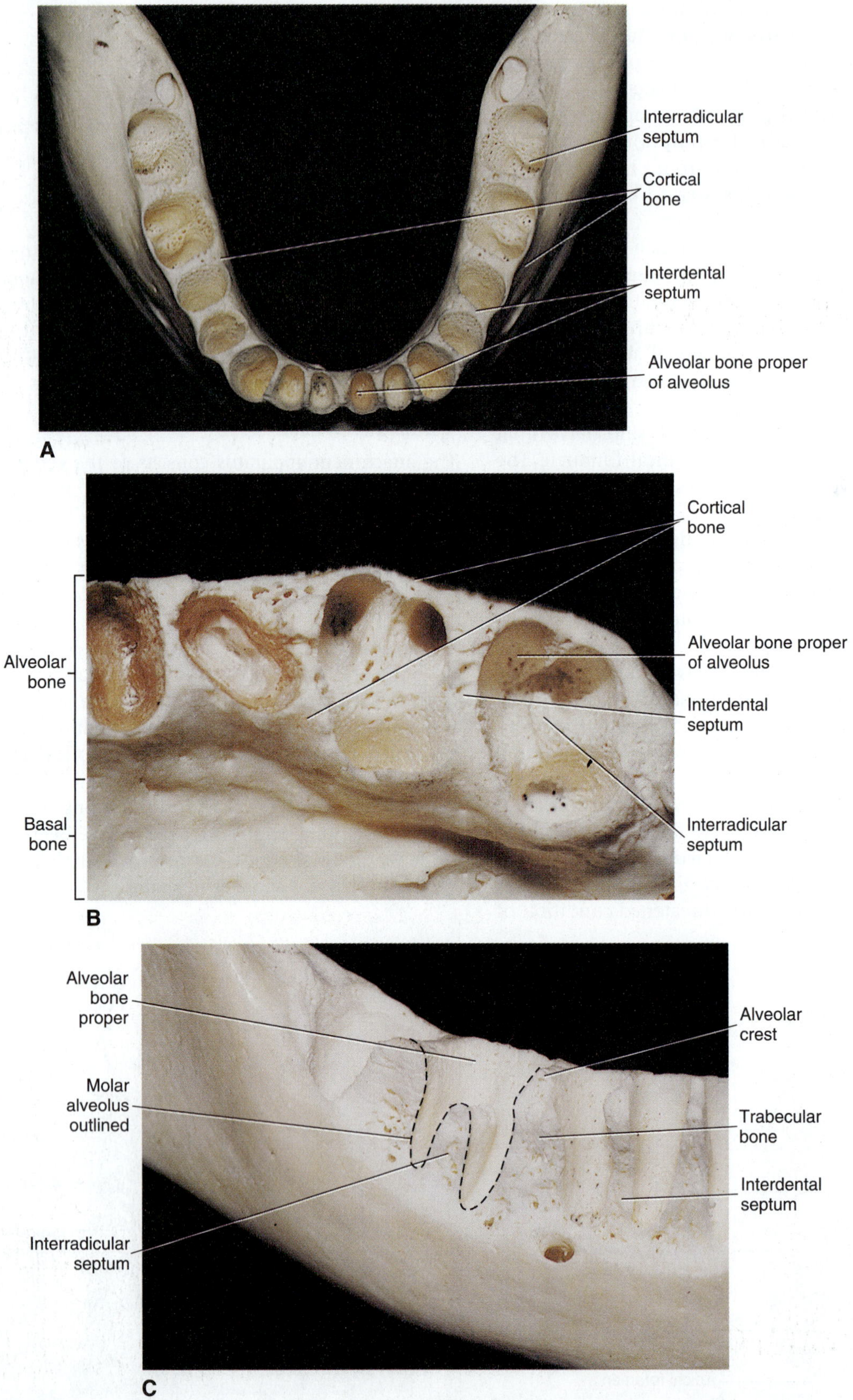

Fig. 8-21 Anatomy of the alveolar bone. **A,** Mandibular arch with the teeth removed. **B,** Portion of the maxilla of a skull with the teeth removed. **C,** Cross-section of the mandible with the teeth removed. (From Bath-Balogh MB, Fehrenbach MJ: *Illustrated dental embryology, histology, and anatomy,* ed 2, St Louis, 2005, Saunders.)

The **cortical plate** is the dense outer covering of the spongy bone that makes up the central part of the alveolar process. The cortical plate provides strength and protection and is where the skeletal muscles attach. The cortical plate of the mandible is denser than that of the maxilla and has fewer openings for the passage of nerves and vessels. This structural difference affects the technique of injection for local anesthetic and extractions.

The **alveolar crest** is the highest point of the alveolar ridge. At this location, alveolar bone fuses with the cortical plates on the facial and lingual sides of the crest of the alveolar process. In a healthy mouth, the distance between the CEJ and the alveolar crest is fairly constant (Fig. 8-22). Early periodontal disease results in a flattening of the alveolar crest.

The **alveolar socket** is the cavity within the alveolar process that surrounds the root of a tooth. The tooth does not actually contact the bone at this point. Instead, it is suspended in place within the socket by the periodontal ligaments. The bony projection separating one socket from another is called the *interdental septum.* The bone separating the roots of a multirooted tooth is called the *interradicular septum.*

The **lamina dura,** also known as the *cribriform plate,* is thin, compact bone that lines the alveolar socket. The lamina dura is pierced by many small openings, which allow the blood vessels and nerve fibers in the bone to communicate freely with those in the periodontal ligament. On a dental radiograph, the lamina dura appears as a thin white line around the root of the tooth (see Chapter 41).

Recall

25. What are the functions of osteoblasts and osteoclasts?

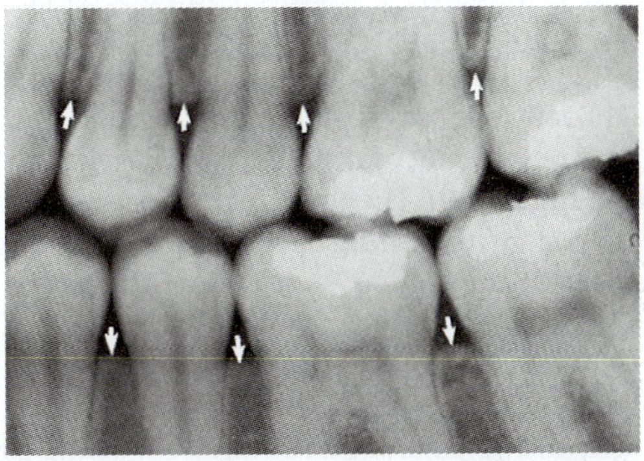

Fig. 8-22 The alveolar crest as it appears in a radiograph. (From Haring JI, Lind LJ: *Radiographic interpretation for the dental hygienist,* Philadelphia, 1993, Saunders.)

Periodontal ligament

The periodontal ligament is dense connective tissue organized into fiber groups that connects the cementum covering the root of the tooth with the alveolar bone of the socket wall.

At one end the fibers are embedded in cementum; at the other end they are embedded in bone. These embedded portions become mineralized and are known as *Sharpey's fibers.*

The periodontal ligament ranges in width from 0.1 to 0.38 mm, with the thinnest portion around the middle third of the root. With age, the width of these ligaments tends to narrow.

Supportive and Protective Functions. The fiber groups are designed to support the tooth in its socket and hold it firmly in normal relationship to the surrounding soft and hard tissues. This arrangement allows the tooth to withstand the pressures and forces of mastication.

Sensory Function. The nerve supply for the ligament comes from the nerves just before they enter the apical foramen. Also, nerve fibers in the surrounding alveolar bone provide the tooth with the protective "sense of touch." Notice how it feels when you bite into food.

The nerve fibers also act as the sensory receptors necessary for the proper positioning of the jaws during normal function.

Nutritive Function. The ligaments receive their nutrition from the blood vessels that also supply the tooth and its alveolar bone. The blood vessels enter the dental pulp through the apical foramen and from the vessels that supply the surrounding alveolar bone.

Formative and Resorptive Functions. The fibroblasts of the periodontal ligament permit the continuous and rapid remodeling that is required for these fiber groups. The cementoblasts and **cementoclasts** (cementum-resorbing cells) are also involved in these remodeling functions, as are the osteoblasts and osteoclasts.

Periodontal ligament fiber groups

The periodontal ligament has three different types of fiber groups (Fig. 8-23). The *periodontal* fiber groups support the tooth in its socket; the *transseptal* fiber groups support the tooth in relation to the adjacent teeth; and the *gingival* fiber groups support the gingiva surrounding the tooth.

Periodontal Fiber Groups. *Alveolar crest fibers* run from the crest of the alveolar bone to the cementum in the region of the CEJ. Their primary function is to retain the tooth in the socket and to oppose lateral forces.

Horizontal fibers course at right angles to the long axis of the tooth, from the cementum to the bone. Their primary function is to restrain lateral tooth movement.

Oblique fibers run in an upward direction, from cementum to the bone. These fiber bundles are the most numerous fibers and constitute the main attachment of the tooth. Their primary function is to resist forces placed on the long axis of the tooth.

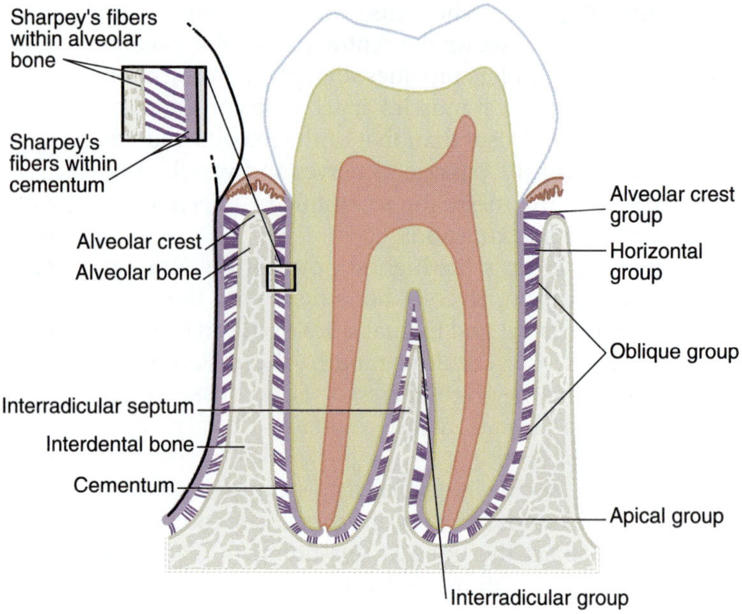

Fig. 8-23 Periodontal fiber groups. (From Bath-Balogh MB, Fehrenbach MJ: *Illustrated dental embryology, histology, and anatomy,* ed 2, St Louis, 2005, Saunders.)

Apical fibers radiate outward from the apical cementum and insert into the surrounding bone. Their primary functions are to (1) prevent the tooth from tipping, (2) resist luxation (twisting), and (3) protect the blood, lymph, and nerve supplies.

Interradicular fibers are found only in multirooted teeth. They course from the cementum of the root and insert into the interradicular septum. Their primary function is to help resist tipping and twisting.

Transseptal Fiber Groups. The *transseptal fibers,* also known as *interdental fibers,* are located interproximally above the crest of the alveolar bone between the teeth. These fibers originate in the cervical cementum of one tooth and insert into the cervical cementum of the adjacent tooth. Their primary function is to support the interproximal gingiva and to aid in securing the position of the adjacent tooth.

Gingival Fiber Groups. The *gingival fibers* are considered to be part of the periodontal ligaments even though they *do not* support the tooth in relation to the jaws. They function to support the marginal gingival tissues to maintain their relation to the tooth (Fig. 8-24). This function is similar to a sphincterlike "pulling of purse strings."

The gingival fibers are located in the *lamina propria* (connective tissues of the gingiva) and *do not* insert into the alveolar bone. The gingival fibers are divided into the following four groups:

- *Dentogingival fibers* extend from the cervical cementum outward and upward into the lamina propria.
- *Alveologingival fibers* extend upward from the alveolar crest into the lamina propria.
- *Circular fibers* form a band around the neck of the tooth and are interlaced by other groups of fibers in the unattached gingiva.
- *Dentoperiosteal fibers* extend facially and lingually from the cementum, pass over the crest of the alveolar bone, and insert into the periosteum of the alveolar process. Their primary function is to support the tooth and gingiva.

Recall

26. What is the primary function of the periodontal ligaments?
27. To which structures are the periodontal ligaments attached?

Gingival Unit

Oral mucosa almost continuously lines the oral cavity. Oral mucosa is composed of **stratified squamous epithelium** overlying connective tissue. The oral mucosa has ducts of salivary glands in various regions of the oral cavity. Although oral mucosa is present throughout the mouth, different types of mucosal tissues are present in different regions of the mouth. The three main types of oral mucosa in the oral cavity are **lining, masticatory,** and **specialized mucosa** (Fig. 8-25).

Lining mucosa

Lining mucosa is noted for its softer texture, moist surface, and ability to stretch and be compressed, acting as a cushion for the underlying structures. Lining mucosa covers the inside of the cheeks, vestibule, lips, soft palate, and ventral surface (underside) of the tongue. Run your tongue over

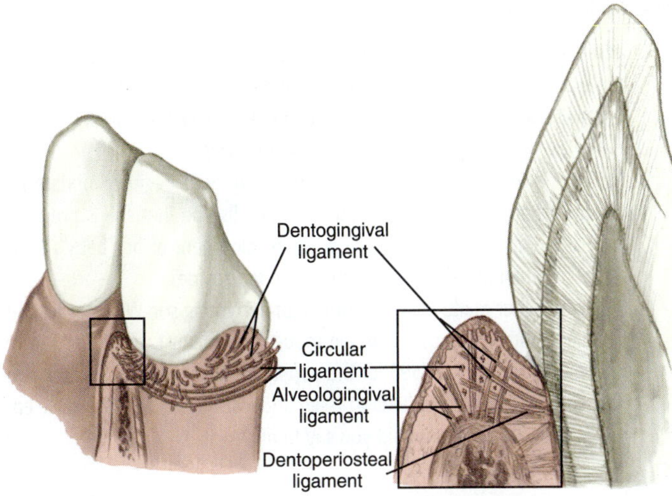

Fig. 8-24 Some of the fiber subgroups of the gingival fiber group: circular, dentogingival, alveologingival, and dentoperiosteal ligaments. (From Bath-Balogh MB, Fehrenbach MJ: *Illustrated dental embryology, histology, and anatomy,* ed 2, St Louis, 2005, Saunders.)

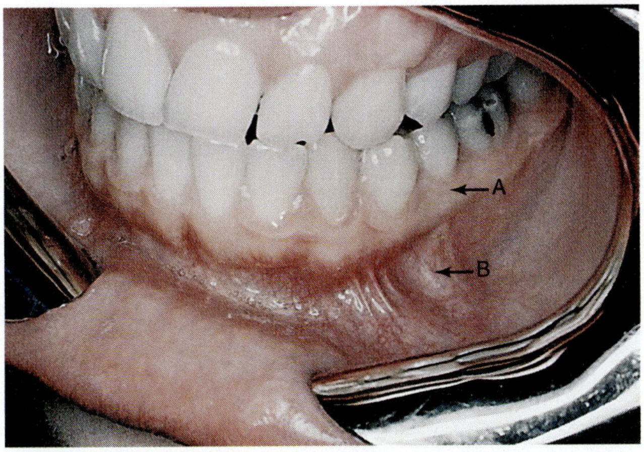

Fig. 8-25 A, **A dense masticatory type of mucosa makes up the gingiva. B, The delicate lining type of mucosa covers the vestibule.**

these areas and notice how soft and smooth these tissues are. Beneath the lining mucosa is the *submucosa,* which contains blood vessels and nerves.

Because lining mucosa is not attached to bone, it moves freely. The abundant blood supply and the thinness of the tissue give lining mucosa a brighter red color than masticatory mucosa.

Masticatory mucosa

Masticatory mucosa is noted for its rubbery surface texture and resiliency. Masticatory mucosa includes the attached gingiva, hard palate, and dorsum (upper surface) of the tongue (see Chapter 10).

Masticatory mucosa is light pink and is *keratinized,* which means that it has a tough, protective outer layer. Lining mucosa lacks this protective layer.

There is no submucosa beneath the masticatory mucosa. The masticatory mucosa is firmly affixed to the bone and does not move. Run your tongue across the roof of your mouth and compare the texture of the mucosa on your palate with that on the inside of your cheeks. This tissue is a dense covering designed to withstand the vigorous activity of chewing and swallowing food.

Specialized mucosa

The top surface, or *dorsal* surface, of the tongue has both a masticatory and *specialized mucosa* present in the form of lingual papillae. The *papillae* are associated with sensations of taste (see Chapter 10).

Recall

28. List the three types of oral mucosa, and provide an example of each.

LEGAL AND ETHICAL IMPLICATIONS

The most critical time of development is during the embryonic period because this is when the major organs are forming. Frequently a woman is not yet aware that she is pregnant. Therefore a woman should always be concerned about good nutrition and a healthy lifestyle in case she might be pregnant.

As a healthcare professional, do you think that you have any ethical responsibilities for providing pregnant patients with information about dental development?

Eye to the Future

Medical technology has made it possible to detect fetal abnormalities at an early stage of a child's development. This has opened a new frontier of medicine: treating sick babies before they are born. Infants with various disorders have been saved from severe illness, retardation, and even death. Until recently, the only access to the fetus has been through the placenta. A new technique can correct some deficiencies with an injection into the amniotic fluid that allows the fetus to swallow the medication. Guided by computers and ultrasound images and using sensitive instruments, physicians can now give blood transfusions to babies while they are still in the uterus. In other cases, physicians can drain excess fluid from the baby's brain, and can successfully perform fetal surgery.

Critical Thinking

1. A nine-year-old child arrives in your office for an emergency appointment. He was in a bicycle accident and chipped his two front teeth. The child's mother asks you if you think the chip in the teeth will eventually repair itself. How would you explain the situation to her?
2. Leanne Morris is a patient in your office. As you begin to update her health history, Leanne is very excited and tells you that she is pregnant. She asks you questions regarding the development of her baby's teeth. What information would the dentist want to provide?
3. Karen Kelleher made an appointment for her young son Willy because his primary tooth was loose, and she thought the dentist might need to remove it. When they arrived for the appointment, the tooth was no longer loose. Mrs. Kelleher was embarrassed and insisted it had been loose earlier in the week. What would you say to her?

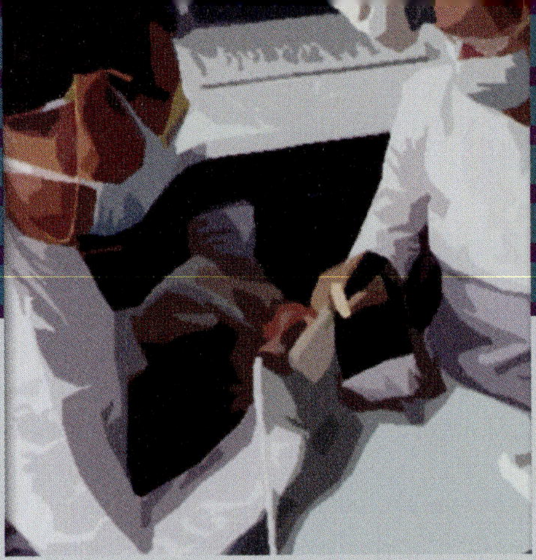

9 Head and Neck Anatomy

Outline

KEY TERMS

Alveolar process Part of the maxillary bones that form the support for teeth of the maxillary arch.

Articular disc (ar-**tik**-u-ler) Cushion of dense, specialized connective tissue that divides the articular space into upper and lower compartments; also known as the *meniscus.*

Articular eminence Raised portion of the temporal bone just anterior to the glenoid fossa.

Articular space Space between the capsular ligament and between the surfaces of the glenoid fossa and the condyle.

Buccal (**buke**-ul, **buh**-kul) Region of the head that refers to structures closest to the inner cheek.

Circumvallate lingual papillae (sur-kum-**va**-let **lin**-gwul pah-**pi**-lay) Large tissue projections on the tongue.

Condyloid process The posterior process of each ramus; articulates with a fossa in the temporal bones to form the temporomandibular joint; also known as the *mandibular condyle.*

Coronal suture Line of articulation between the frontal bone and parietal bones.

Cranium (**kray**-nee-um) Eight bones that cover and protect the brain.

External auditory meatus Bony passage of the outer ear.

Foramen A small round opening in a bone through which blood vessels, nerves, and ligaments pass; plural *foramina.*

Foramen magnum Large opening in the occipital bone that connects the vertical canal and cranial cavity.

Fossa (**fos**-ah, **faw**-seh) Wide, shallow depression on the lingual surfaces of anterior teeth.

Continued

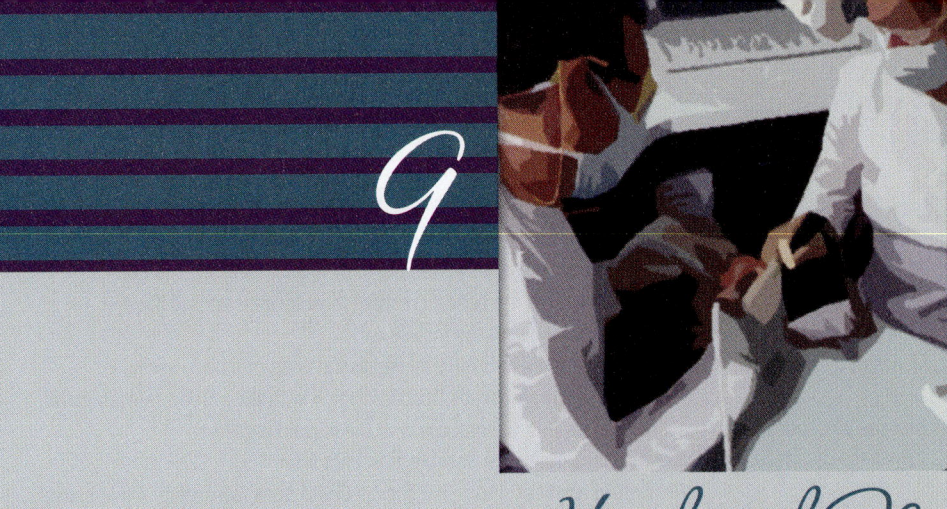

KEY TERMS—cont'd

Frontal Region of the head pertaining to the forehead.

Frontal process Process of the zygomatic bone that extends upward to articulate with the frontal bone at the outer edge of the orbit.

Glenoid fossa Area of the temporal bone where condyles of the mandible articulate with the skull.

Greater palatine nerve (**pa**-lah-tine) Nerve that serves the posterior hard palate and posterior lingual gingiva.

Hamulus A hook-shaped process.

Infraorbital (*in*-frah-**or**-bi-tul) Region of the head below the orbital region.

Lacrimal bones (**lak**-ri-mul) Paired facial bones that help form the medial wall of the orbit.

Lambdoid suture Line of junction between the occipital and parietal bones.

Lateral pterygoid plate Point of origin for internal and external pterygoid muscles.

Lymphadenopathy (*lim*-fad-**nop**-athy) Disease or swelling of the lymph nodes.

Masseter (ma-**se**-tur) The strongest and most obvious muscle of mastication.

Mastoid process Projection on the temporal bone located behind the ear.

Maxillary tuberosity Large rounded area on the outer surface of the maxillary bones in the area of the posterior teeth.

Meatus The external opening of a canal.

Medial pterygoid plate Plate that ends in the hook-shaped hamulus.

Mental Region of the head pertaining to or located near the chin.

Mental protuberance Part of the mandible that forms the chin.

Nasal Region of the head pertaining to or located near the nose.

Nasal conchae Projecting structures found in each lateral wall of the nasal cavity and extending inward from the maxilla; singular *concha.*

Occipital (ok-**sip**-i-tul) Region of the head overlying the occipital bone and covered by the scalp.

Oral Region of the head pertaining to or located near the mouth.

Orbital Region of the head pertaining to or located around the eye.

Ossicles The bones of the middle ear.

Parietal (pah-**rye**-ih-tul) Pertaining to the walls of a body cavity.

Parotid duct (pah-**rot**-id) Duct associated with the parotid salivary gland, which opens into the oral cavity at the parotid papilla.

Process A prominence or projection on a bone.

Pterygoid process Process of the sphenoid bone, consisting of two plates.

Sagittal suture Suture that is located at the midline of the skull where the two parietal bones are joined.

Sphenoid sinuses Sinuses that are located in the sphenoid bone.

Sternocleidomastoid (*stir*-no-*kli*-doe-**mass**-toid) Major cervical muscle.

Styloid process Process that extends from the undersurface of the temporal bone.

Symphysis menti (**sim**-fa-sis **men**-tee) The separation of the mandible at the chin that occurs at birth.

Temporal Region of the head superior to the zygomatic arch.

Temporal process Process that articulates with the zygomatic process of the temporal bone to form the zygomatic arch, which creates the prominence of the cheek.

Temporomandibular joint (TMJ) (*tem*-pa-ro-man-**dib**-u-ler) Joint on each side of head that allows for movement of the mandible.

Trapezius (trah-**pee**-zee-us) Major cervical muscle.

Trigeminal nerve The nerve that is the primary source of innervation for the oral cavity.

Zygomatic Region of the head pertaining to or located near the zygomatic bone (cheek bone).

Zygomatic arch The arch formed when the temporal process of the zygomatic bone articulates with the zygomatic process of the temporal bone.

Zygomatic process The process of the maxillary bones that extends upward to articulate with the zygomatic bone.

LEARNING OUTCOMES

On completion of this chapter, the student will be able to achieve the following objectives:

- Pronounce, define, and spell the Key Terms.
- Identify the regions of the head.
- Locate and identify the bones of the cranium and face.
- Locate and identify the muscles of the head and neck.
- Identify and trace the routes of the blood vessels of the head and neck.
- Identify the components of the temporomandibular joint.
- Describe the action of the temporomandibular joint.
- Identify the location of major and minor salivary glands and associated ducts.
- Describe and locate the divisions of the trigeminal nerve.
- Identify the location of major lymph node sites of the body.
- Identify and locate the paranasal sinuses of the skull.
- Integrate the knowledge about head and neck anatomy into clinical practice.

In this chapter, you will learn the anatomic basis for the clinical practice of dental assisting. You will learn names and locations of bones of the skull and face, facial nerves, lymph nodes, and salivary glands. You will be able to identify muscles of the head and neck, including the facial muscles, which create facial expressions and help to open and close the mouth and swallow food.

Afterward, you will find that your knowledge of anatomic landmarks is a necessity as you begin to mount radiographs.

REGIONS OF THE HEAD

The head can be divided into 11 regions: **frontal, parietal, occipital, temporal, orbital, nasal, infraorbital, zygomatic, buccal, oral,** and **mental.** As you continue this chapter, you will find references to these regions of the head (Fig. 9-1).

Recall

1. What are the 11 regions of the head?

BONES OF THE SKULL

The human skull is divided into two sections, the cranium and the face. The **cranium** is composed of eight bones that cover and protect the brain; the face consists of 14 bones (Box 9-1). Specific anatomic terms are used to describe landmarks on these bones (Box 9-2).

Box 9-1 Bones of the Skull

Bone	Number	Location
8 bones of the cranium		
Frontal	1	Forms the forehead, most of the orbital roof, and the anterior cranial floor
Parietal	2	Form most of the roof and upper sides of the cranium
Occipital	1	Forms the back and base of the cranium
Temporal	2	Form the sides and base of the cranium
Sphenoid	1	Forms part of the anterior base of the skull and part of the walls of the orbit
Ethmoid	1	Forms part of the orbit and the floor of the cranium
14 bones of the face		
Zygomatic	2	Form the prominence of the cheeks and part of the orbit
Maxillary	2	Form the upper jaw
Palatine	2	Form the posterior part of the hard palate and the floor of the nose
Nasal	2	Form the bridge of the nose
Lacrimal	2	Form part of the orbit at the inner angle of the eye
Vomer	1	Forms the base for the nasal septum
Inferior conchae	2	Form part of the interior of the nose
Mandible	1	Forms the lower jaw
6 auditory ossicles		
Malleus, incus, stapes	6	Bones of the middle ear

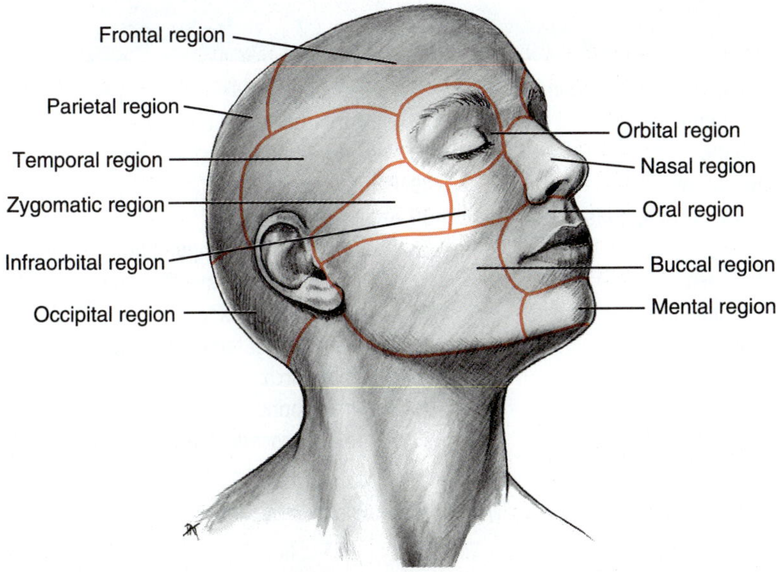

Fig. 9-1 **Regions of the head: frontal, parietal, occipital, temporal, orbital, nasal, infraorbital, zygomatic, buccal, oral, and mental.** (From Fehrenbach MJ, Herring SW: *Illustrated anatomy of the head and neck,* ed 2, Philadelphia, 2002, Saunders.)

Box 9-2 Terminology of Anatomic Landmarks of Bones

Term	Definition
Foramen	A natural opening in a bone through which blood vessels, nerves, and ligaments pass
Fossa	A hollow, grooved, or depressed area in a bone
Meatus	The external opening of a canal
Process	A prominence or projection on a bone
Suture	The jagged line where bones articulate and form a joint that does not move
Symphysis	The site where bones come together to form a cartilaginous joint
Tubercle	A small, rough projection on a bone
Tuberosity	A large, rounded process on a bone

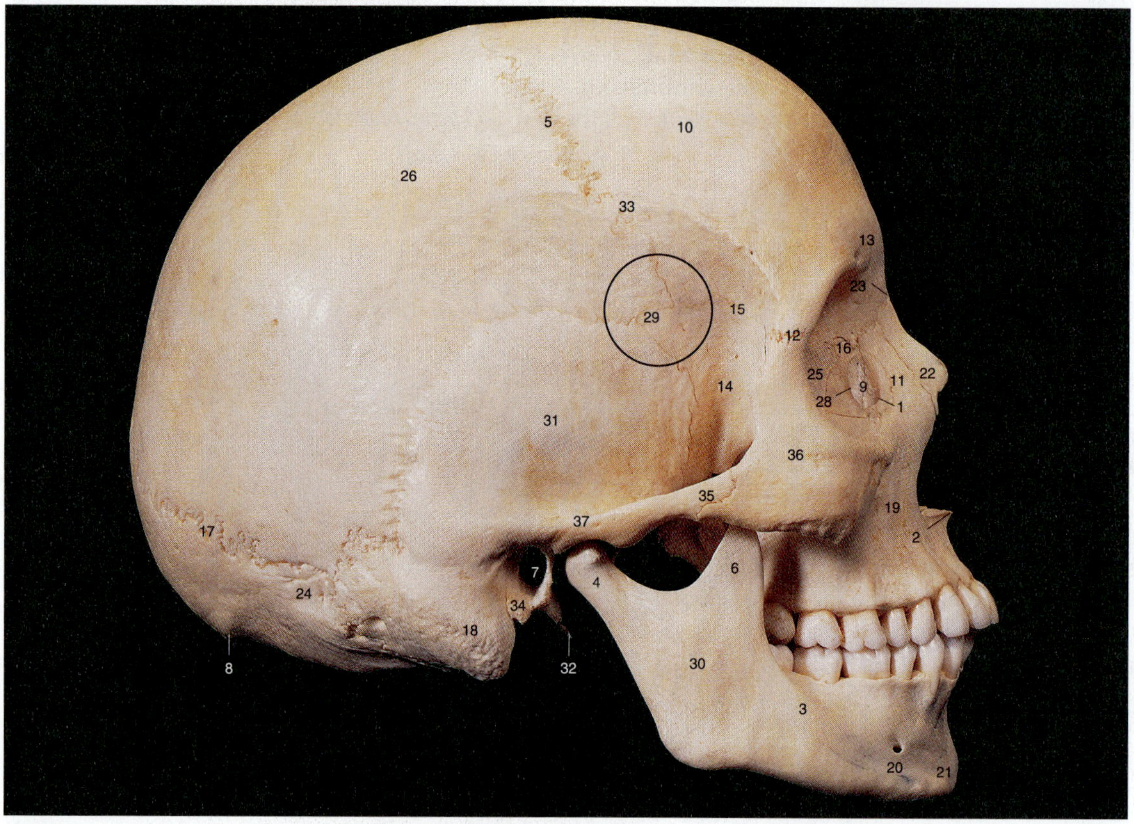

1 Anterior lacrimal crest
2 Anterior nasal spine
3 Body of mandible
4 Condyle of mandible
5 Coronal suture
6 Coronoid process of mandible
7 External acoustic meatus of temporal bone
8 External occipital protuberance (inion)
9 Fossa for lacrimal sac
10 Frontal bone
11 Frontal process of maxilla
12 Frontozygomatic suture
13 Glabella
14 Greater wing of sphenoid bone
15 Inferior temporal line
16 Lacrimal bone
17 Lambdoid suture
18 Mastoid process of temporal bone
19 Maxilla
20 Mental foramen
21 Mental protuberance
22 Nasal bone
23 Nasion
24 Occipital bone
25 Orbital part of ethmoid bone
26 Parietal bone
27 Pituitary fossa (sella turcica)
28 Posterior lacrimal crest
29 Pterion (encircled)
30 Ramus of mandible
31 Squamous part of temporal bone
32 Styloid process of temporal bone
33 Superior temporal line
34 Tympanic part of temporal bone
35 Zygomatic arch
36 Zygomatic bone
37 Zygomatic process of temporal bone

Fig. 9-2 **Lateral view of the skull.** (From Abrahams PH, Marks SC Jr, Hutchings RT: *McMinn's color atlas of human anatomy,* ed 5, St Louis, 2003, Mosby.)

Bones of the Cranium

The cranial bones are the *single frontal, occipital, sphenoid,* and *ethmoid bones* and the *paired parietal* and *temporal bones*.

Parietal Bones

The two parietal bones form most of the roof and upper sides of the cranium. The two parietal bones are joined at the **sagittal suture** at the midline of the skull. The line of articulation between the frontal bone and the parietal bones is called the **coronal suture** (Fig. 9-2). In a newborn, the anterior *fontanelle* is the soft spot where the sutures between the frontal and parietal bones have not yet closed. This spot disappears as the child grows and the sutures close.

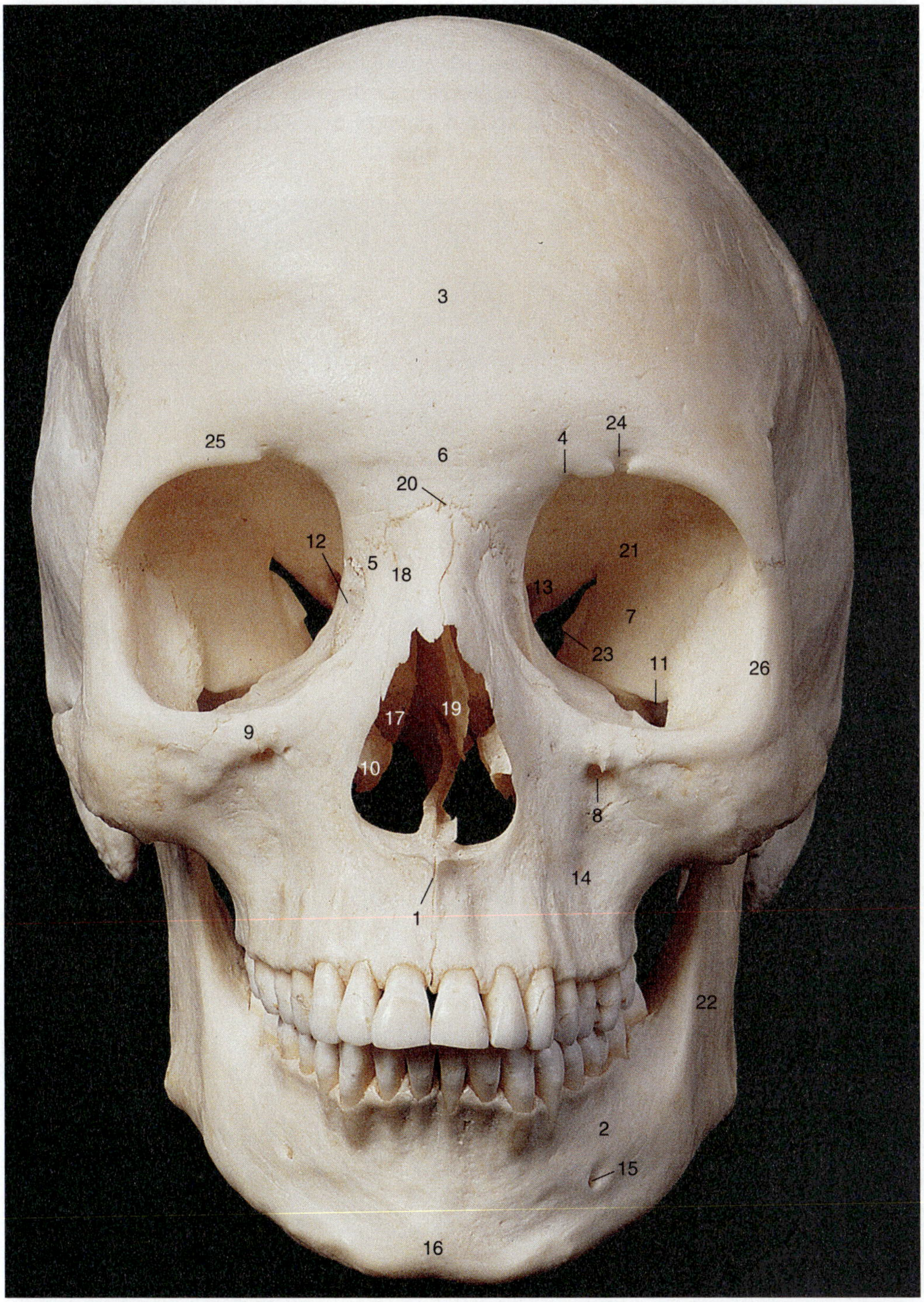

1 Anterior nasal spine
2 Body of mandible
3 Frontal bone
4 Frontal notch
5 Frontal process of maxilla
6 Glabella
7 Greater wing of sphenoid bone
8 Infraorbital foramen
9 Infraorbital margin
10 Inferior nasal concha
11 Inferior orbital fissure
12 Lacrimal bone
13 Lesser wing of sphenoid bone
14 Maxilla
15 Mental foramen
16 Mental protuberance
17 Middle nasal concha
18 Nasal bone
19 Nasal septum
20 Nasion
21 Orbit (orbital cavity)
22 Ramus of mandible
23 Superior orbital fissure
24 Supraorbital foramen
25 Supraorbital margin
26 Zygomatic bone

Fig. 9-3 Frontal view of the skull. (From Abrahams PH, Marks SC Jr, Hutchings RT: *McMinn's color atlas of human anatomy,* ed 5, St Louis, 2003, Mosby.)

Frontal Bone

The frontal bone forms the forehead, part of the floor of the cranium, and most of the roof of the orbits. (The *orbit* is the bony cavity protecting the eye.) The frontal bone contains the two *frontal sinuses,* with one located above each eye (Fig. 9-3).

Occipital Bone

The occipital bone forms the back and base of the cranium (Fig. 9-4). It joins the parietal bones at the **lambdoid suture.** The spinal cord passes through the **foramen magnum** of the occipital bone. (A **foramen** is a natural, small, round opening in a bone through which blood vessels, nerves, and ligaments pass; plural *foramina.*)

Temporal Bones

The paired temporal bones form the sides and base of the cranium (see Fig. 9-2). Each temporal bone encloses an ear and contains the **external auditory meatus,** which is the bony passage of the outer ear. (A **meatus** is the external opening of a canal.)

The **mastoid process** is a projection on the temporal bone located just behind the ear. (A **process** is a prominence or projection on a bone.) The mastoid process is composed of air spaces that communicate with the middle ear cavity.

The lower portion of each temporal bone bears the **glenoid fossa** for articulation with the mandible. (A **fossa** is a hollow, grooved, or depressed area in a bone.)

The **styloid process** extends from the undersurface of the temporal bone.

1 External occipital protuberance (inion)
2 Highest nuchal line
3 Inferior nuchal line
4 Lambda
5 Lambdoid suture
6 Occipital bone
7 Parietal bone
8 Parietal foramen
9 Sagittal suture
10 Superior nuchal line

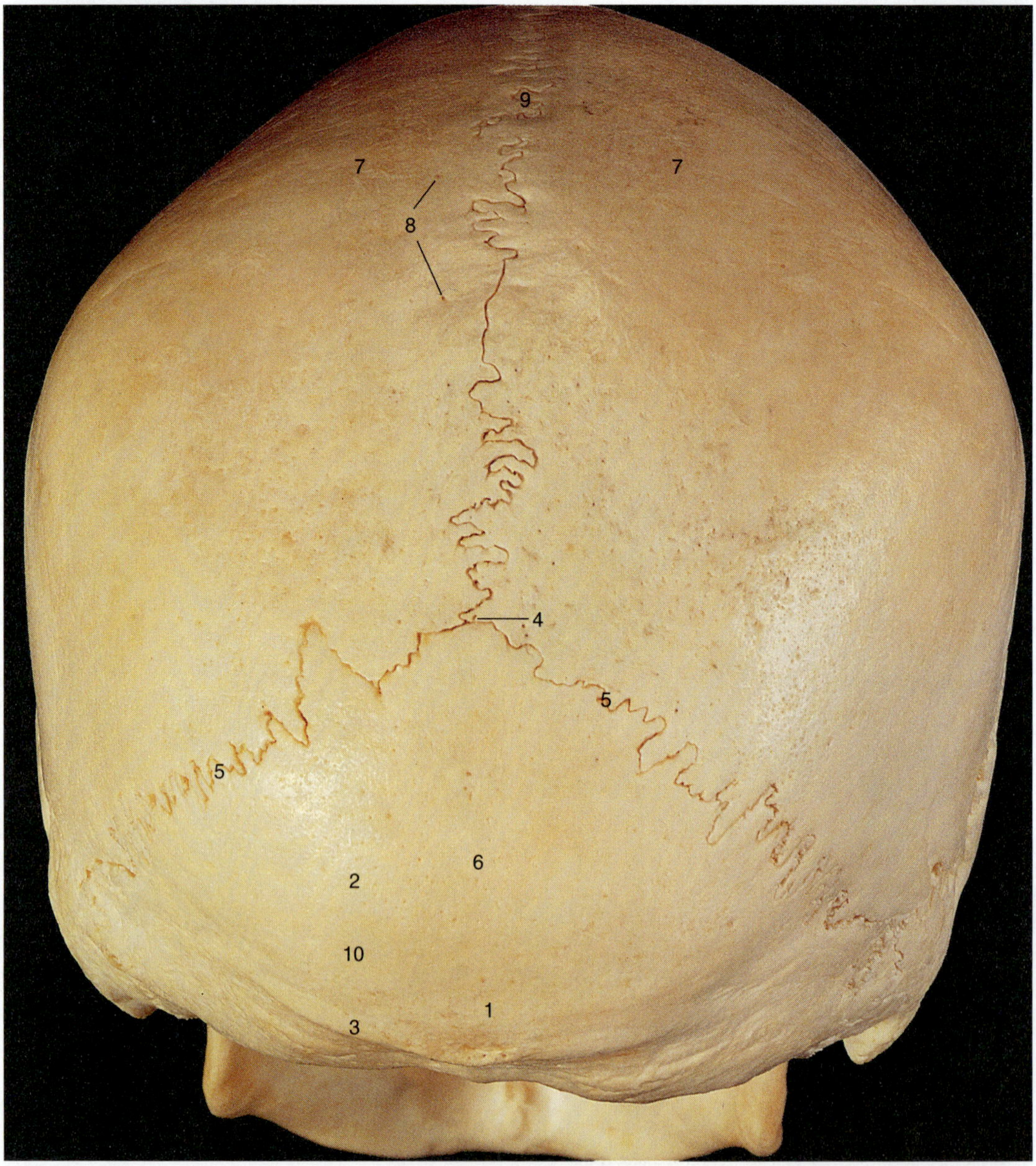

Fig. 9-4 Posterior view of the skull. (From Abrahams PH, Marks SC Jr, Hutchings RT: *McMinn's color atlas of human anatomy,* ed 5, St Louis, 2003, Mosby.)

Sphenoid Bone

The sphenoid bone is made up of a body and paired greater and lesser wings. It forms the anterior part of the base of the skull (see Fig. 9-2).

Each *greater wing* articulates with the temporal bone on either side and anteriorly with the frontal and zygomatic bones to form part of the orbit. Each *lesser wing* articulates with the ethmoid and frontal bones and also forms part of the orbit.

The **sphenoid sinuses** are located in the sphenoid bone just posterior to the eye. The **pterygoid process,** which extends downward from the sphenoid bone, consists of two plates (Fig. 9-5). The **lateral pterygoid plate** is the point of origin for the internal and external pterygoid muscles. The **medial pterygoid plate** ends in the hook-shaped **hamulus,** which is visible on some dental radiographs.

Ethmoid Bone

The ethmoid bone forms part of the floor of the cranium, the orbit, and the nasal cavity. This complex bone contains honeycomb-like spaces and the *ethmoid sinuses.* The *medial concha* and *superior concha,* which are scroll-like structures, extend from the ethmoid bone.

Auditory Ossicles

The six auditory **ossicles** are the bones of the middle ear. Each ear contains one *malleus, incus,* and *stapes.*

Recall

2. What bone forms the forehead?
3. What bone forms the back and base of the cranium?

Bones of the Face

When looking at an anterior view of the skull, the bones you see are the **lacrimal bone,** *nasal bone, vomer, nasal conchae, zygomatic bone, maxilla,* and *mandible* (Fig. 9-6).

Zygomatic Bones

The two zygomatic bones, also known as the *malar bones,* form the prominence of the cheek and the lateral wall and floor of the orbit. The **frontal process** of the zygomatic bone extends upward to articulate with the frontal bone at the outer edge of the orbit (see Fig. 9-3).

The zygomatic bones rest on the maxillary bones, and each articulates with the right or left zygomatic process. The **temporal process** of the zygomatic bone articulates with the zygomatic process of the temporal bone to form the **zygomatic arch,** which creates the prominence of the cheek. The zygomatic bones are useful in identifying maxillary radiographs.

Maxillary Bones

The two maxillary bones, also known as the *maxillae* (singular *maxilla*), form the upper jaw and part of the hard palate. The maxillary bones are joined together at the midline by the *maxillary suture.* The **zygomatic process** of the maxillary bones extends upward to articulate with the zygomatic bone.

The maxillary bones contain the *maxillary sinuses.* The **alveolar process** of the maxillary bones forms the support for the teeth of the maxillary arch. The **maxillary tuberosity** is a larger, rounded area on the outer surface of the maxillary bones in the area of the posterior teeth. The maxillary tuberosity is also a useful landmark when mounting maxillary radiographs.

Palatine Bones

The two palatine bones are not strictly considered facial bones but are considered here for ease of learning. Each palatine bone consists of two plates, the horizontal and vertical plates (Fig. 9-7).

The *horizontal plates* of the palatine bones form the posterior part of the hard palate of the mouth and the floor of the nose. The *vertical plates* form part of the lateral walls of the nasal cavity. Anteriorly, they articulate (join) with the maxillary bone.

Nasal Bones

The two nasal bones form the bridge of the nose. Superiorly, they articulate with the frontal bone and make up a small portion of the nasal septum (see Fig. 9-3).

Lacrimal Bones

The two **lacrimal bones** make up part of the orbit at the inner angle of the eye. These small, thin bones lie directly behind the frontal processes of the maxillary bones (see Fig. 9-3).

Vomer

The vomer is a single, flat bone that forms the base for the nasal septum (see Fig. 9-6).

Nasal Conchae

Each lateral wall of the nasal cavity has three projecting structures that extend inward from the maxilla, called the nasal conchae (singular *concha*). Each concha extends scroll-like into the nasal cavity. The superior, middle, and inferior **nasal conchae** are formed from the ethmoid bone (see Fig. 9-6).

Recall

4. What bones form the cheek?
5. What bones form the upper jaw and hard palate?

1 Apex of petrous part of temporal bone
2 Articular tubercle
3 Carotid canal
4 Condylar canal (posterior)
5 Edge of tegmen tympani
6 External acoustic meatus
7 External occipital crest
8 External occipital protuberance
9 Foramen lacerum
10 Foramen magnum
11 Foramen ovale
12 Foramen spinosum
13 Greater palatine foramen
14 Horizontal plate of palatine bone
15 Hypoglossal (anterior condylar) canal
16 Incisive fossa
17 Inferior nuchal line
18 Inferior orbital fissure
19 Infratemporal crest of greater wing of sphenoid bone
20 Jugular foramen
21 Lateral pterygoid plate
22 Lesser palatine foramina
23 Mandibular fossa
24 Mastoid foramen
25 Mastoid notch
26 Mastoid process
27 Medial pterygoid plate
28 Median palatine (intermaxillary) suture
29 Occipital condyle
30 Occipital groove
31 Palatine grooves and spines
32 Palatine process of maxilla
33 Palatinovaginal canal
34 Petrosquamous fissure
35 Petrotympanic fissure
36 Pharyngeal tubercle
37 Posterior border of vomer
38 Posterior nasal aperture (choana)
39 Posterior nasal spine
40 Pterygoid hamulus
41 Pyramidal process of palatine bone
42 Scaphoid fossa
43 Spine of sphenoid bone
44 Squamotympanic fissure
45 Squamous part of temporal bone
46 Styloid process
47 Stylomastoid foramen
48 Superior nuchal line
49 Transverse palatine (palatomaxillary) suture
50 Tuberosity of maxilla
51 Tympanic part of temporal bone
52 Vomerovaginal canal
53 Zygomatic arch

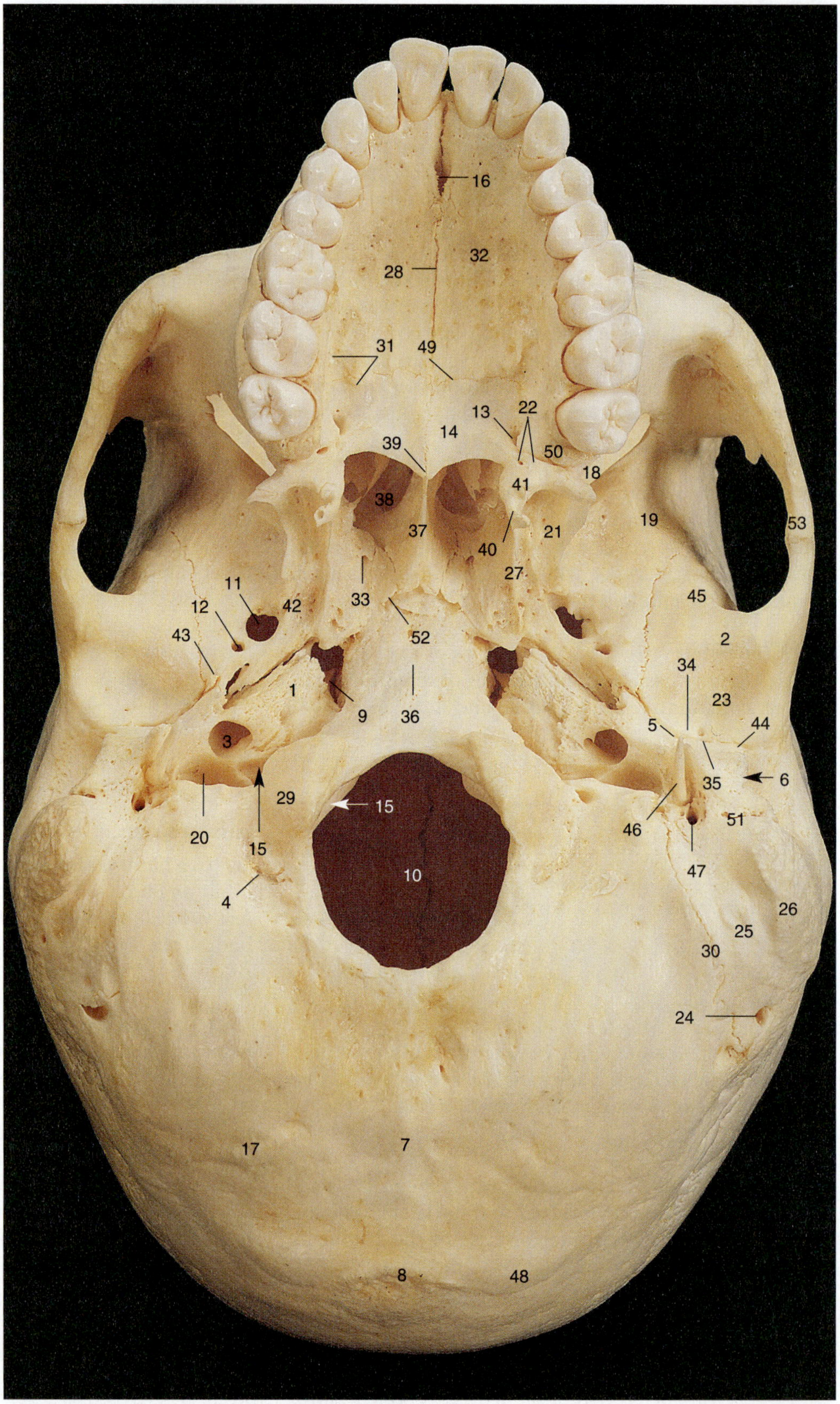

Fig. 9-5 View of external base of the skull. (From Abrahams PH, Marks SC Jr, Hutchings RT: *McMinn's color atlas of human anatomy,* ed 5, St Louis, 2003, Mosby.)

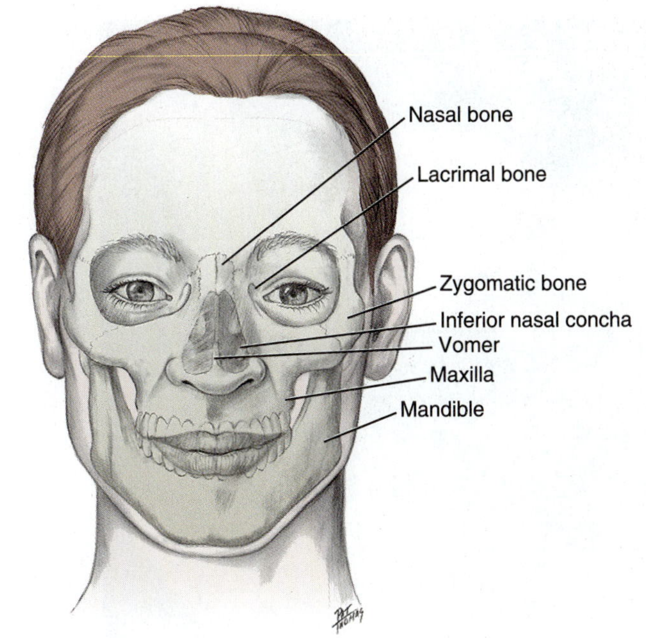

Fig. 9-6 **Anterior view of the facial bones and overlying facial tissue.** (From Fehrenbach MJ, Herring SW: *Illustrated anatomy of the head and neck,* ed 2, Philadelphia, 2002, Saunders.)

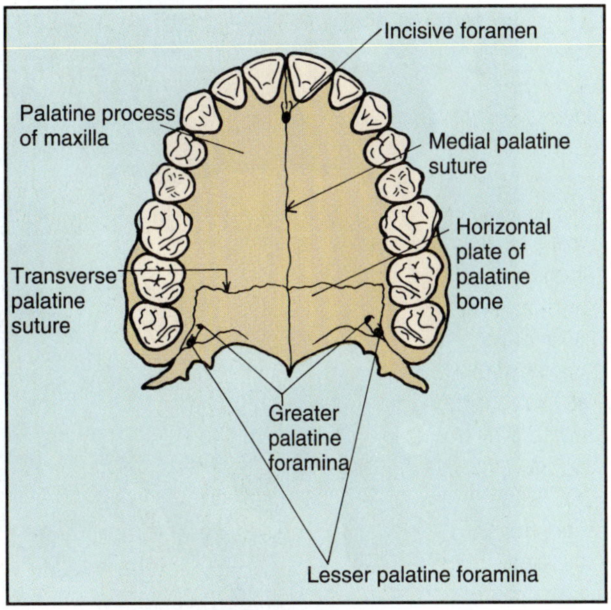

Fig. 9-7 **Bones and landmarks of the hard palate.**

Mandible

The mandible forms the lower jaw and is the movable bone of the skull. The **alveolar process** of the mandible supports the teeth of the mandibular arch (Fig. 9-8).

The U-shaped mandible, which is the strongest and longest bone of the face, develops prenatally as two parts; in early childhood, however, it ossifies (hardens) into a single bone. This symphysis is located at the midline and forms the **mental protuberance,** commonly known as the *chin.*

A mental **foramen** is located on the facial surface on the left and right between the apices of the first and second mandibular premolars. Other structures include the following:

1. *Genial tubercles,* small rounded and raised areas on the inner (medial) surface of the mandible near the symphysis
2. *Mylohyoid ridge,* on the lingual surface of the body of the mandible
3. *Angle of the mandible,* the area where the mandible meets the ramus
4. *Mandibular notch,* on the border of the mandible just anterior to the angle of the mandible
5. *Ramus,* the upright portion at each end of the mandible
6. *Coronoid process,* the anterior portion of each ramus
7. *Condyloid process,* the posterior process of each ramus; articulates with a fossa in the temporal bones to form the temporomandibular joint; also known as the *mandibular condyle*
8. *Sigmoid notch,* the structure separating the coronoid and condyloid processes
9. *Mandibular foramen,* on the lingual surface of each ramus
10. *Oblique ridge,* on the facial surface of the mandible near the base of the ramus
11. *Retromolar area,* the portion of the mandible directly posterior to the last molar on each side

Hyoid Bone

The hyoid bone is unique because it does not articulate with any other bone. Instead, the hyoid is suspended between the mandible and the larynx, where it functions as a primary support for the tongue and other muscles.

The hyoid bone is shaped like a horseshoe and consists of a central body with two lateral projections. Externally, its position is noted in the neck between the mandible and the larynx. The hyoid is suspended from the styloid process of the temporal bone by two *stylohyoid ligaments.*

Recall

6. What is the only movable bone in the skull?
7. Where is the mental foramen located?

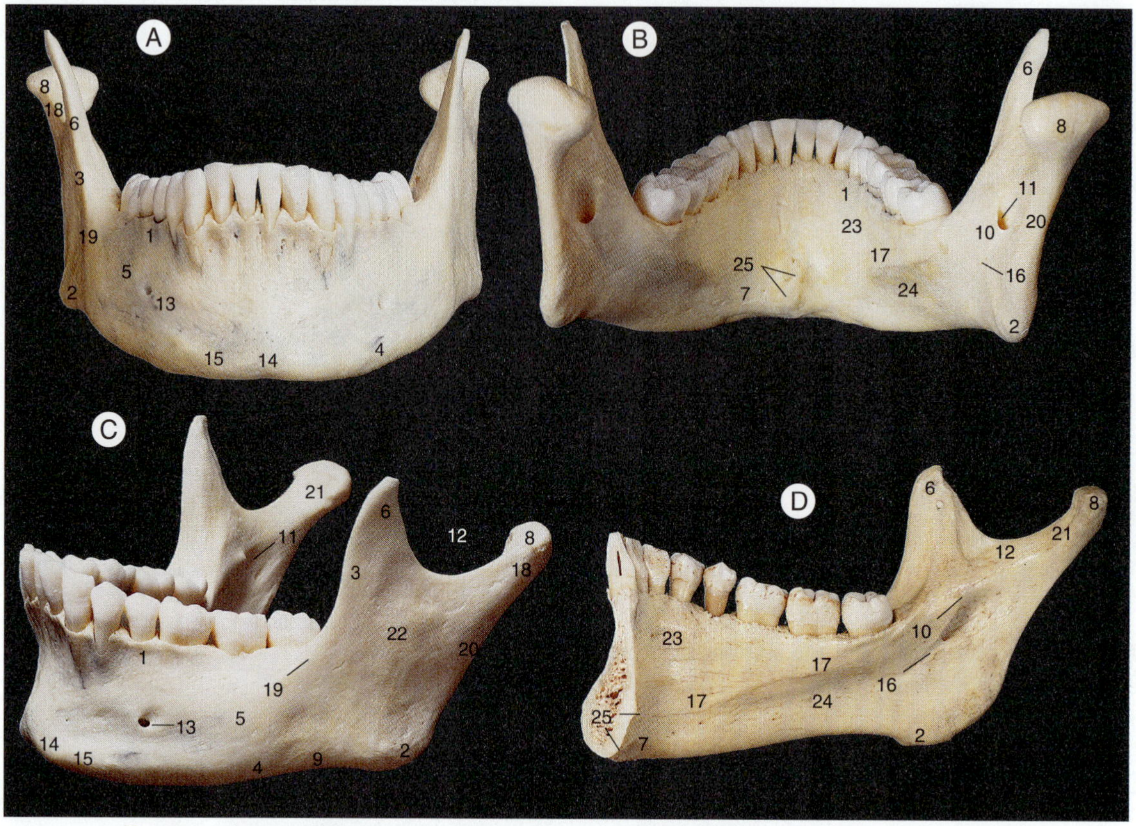

Fig. 9-8 The mandible. **A,** From the front. **B,** From behind and above. **C,** From the left and front. **D,** Internal view from the left. (From Malamed S: *Handbook of local anesthesia,* ed 5, St. Louis, 2004, Mosby. Data from Abrahams PH, Marks SC Jr, Hutchings RT: *McMinn's color atlas of human anatomy,* ed 5, St Louis, 2003, Mosby.)

1. Alveolar part
2. Angle
3. Anterior border of ramus
4. Base
5. Body
6. Coronoid process
7. Digastric fossa
8. Head
9. Inferior border of ramus
10. Lingula
11. Mandibular foramen
12. Mandibular notch
13. Mental foramen
14. Mental protuberance
15. Mental tubercle
16. Mylohyoid groove
17. Mylohyoid line
18. Neck
19. Oblique line
20. Posterior border of ramus
21. Pterygoid fovea
22. Ramus
23. Sublingual fossa
24. Submandibular fossa
25. Superior and inferior mental spines (genial tubercles)

Postnatal Development

At birth, the cranial vault is large, and the cranial base and face are small. The face lacks vertical dimension because the teeth have not yet erupted (Figs. 9-9 and 9-10).

Fusion of Bones

Several bones of the skull have not fused as single bones at the time of birth. For example, the frontal bone is separated by an interfrontal suture, and various components of the temporal, occipital, sphenoid, and ethmoid will fuse during infancy and early childhood.

Development of the Facial Bones

Mandible

At birth, the mandible is in two halves separated by the **symphysis menti.** During the first year of life, the symphysis menti fuses; later the condylar process lengthens. The chin (mental protuberance) reaches full development after puberty. Males have a more pronounced development of the chin than females.

Maxilla

At birth, the maxilla is entirely filled with the developing tooth buds (see Chapter 11). The vertical growth of the upper face is caused largely by the dentoalveolar development and the formation of the maxillary sinuses.

Differences Between Male and Female Skulls

Generally speaking, female skulls tend to be smaller and lighter with thinner walls. The female forehead usually retains a rounded anterior contour, and the teeth are smaller, with rounded incisal edges. Male skulls are

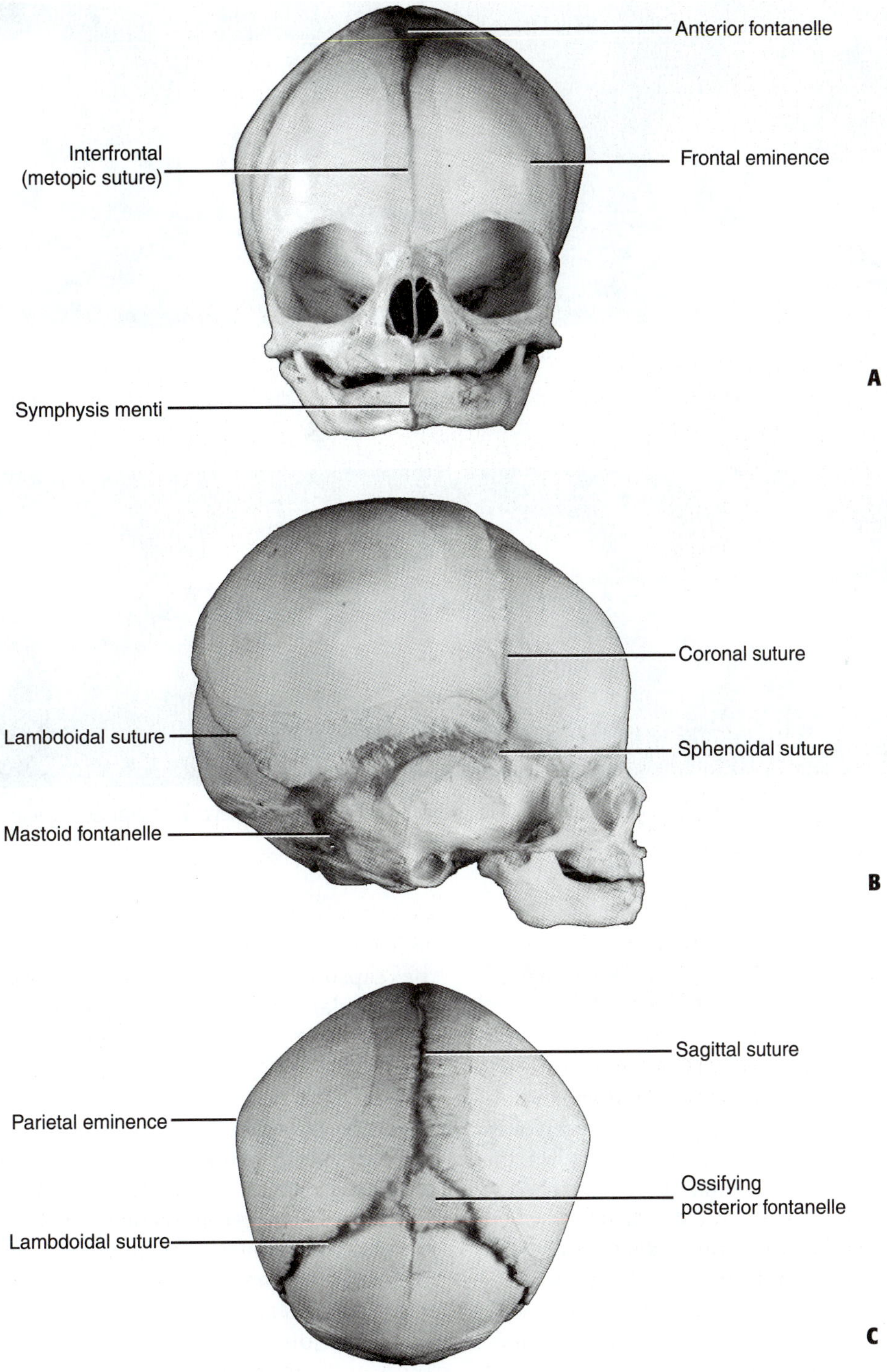

Fig. 9-9 The fetal skull. A, Anterior view. B, Lateral view. C, Posterior view. (From Liebgott B: *The anatomical basis of dentistry,* ed 2, St. Louis, 2001, Mosby.)

larger and heavier and have more rugged muscle markings and prominences. The male teeth are larger and squared incisally, and the forehead is flatter as a result of the developing frontal sinuses, which are larger in men.

Recall

8. What is the difference between the teeth of males and females?

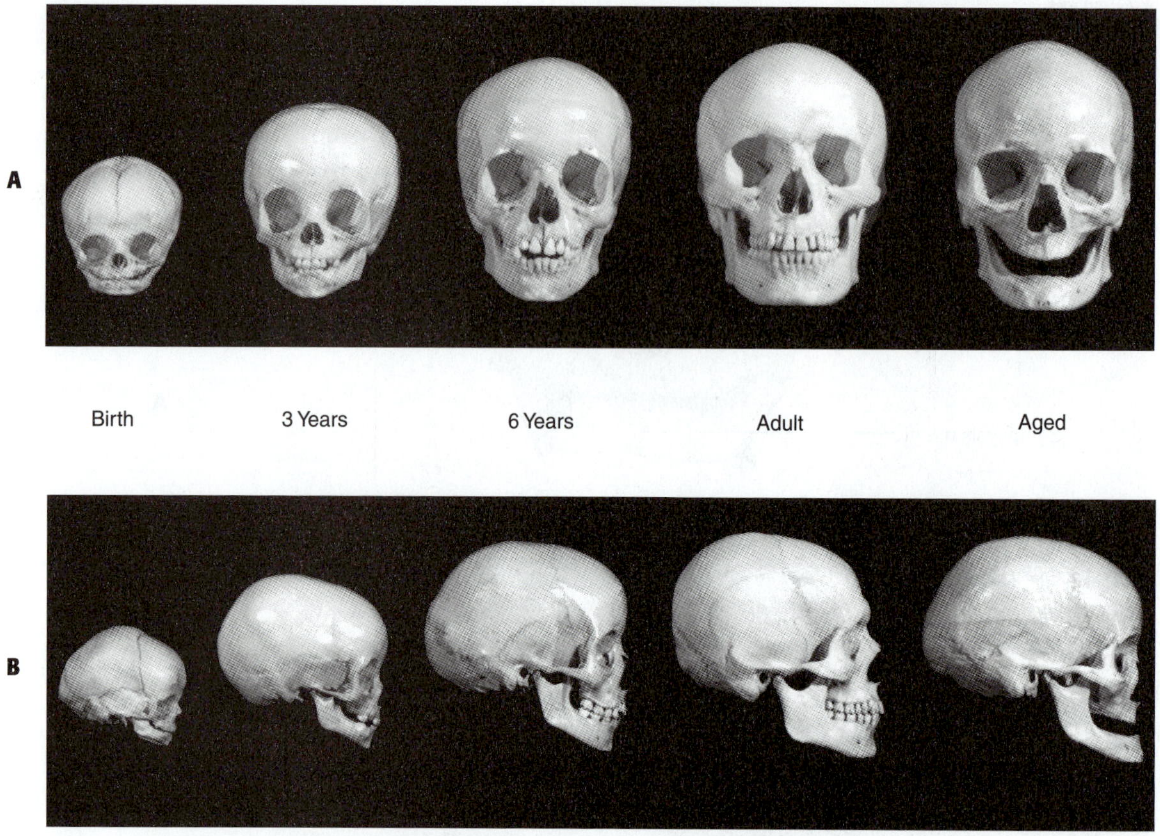

Fig. 9-10 Stages of postnatal development of the human skull. **A,** Anterior view. **B,** Lateral view. (From Liebgott B: *The anatomical basis of dentistry,* ed 2, St. Louis, 2001, Mosby.)

TEMPOROMANDIBULAR JOINTS

The **temporomandibular joint (TMJ)** is a joint on each side of the head that allows for movement of the mandible for speech and *mastication* (chewing). The TMJ receives its name from the two bones that enter into its formation, the *temporal bone* and the *mandible.* The mandible is attached to the cranium by the ligaments of the TMJ. The mandible is held in position by the muscles of mastication (Fig. 9-11). The TMJ is made up of the following three bony parts:

1. The glenoid fossa, which is lined with fibrous connective tissue, is an oval depression in the temporal bone just anterior to the external auditory meatus.
2. The **articular eminence** is a raised portion of the temporal bone just anterior to the glenoid fossa.
3. The **condyloid process** of the mandible lies in the glenoid fossa.

Capsular Ligament

A fibrous joint capsule completely encloses the TMJ. The capsule wraps around the margin of the temporal bone's articular eminence and articular fossa superiorly. Inferiorly the capsule wraps around the circumference of the mandibular condyle, including the condylar neck.

Articular Space

The **articular space** is the area between the capsular ligament and between the surfaces of the glenoid fossa and the condyle.

The **articular disc,** also known as the *meniscus,* is a cushion of dense, specialized connective tissue that divides the articular space into upper and lower compartments. These compartments are filled with *synovial fluid,* which helps lubricate the joint and fills the synovial cavities.

Jaw Movements

The TMJ performs two basic types of movement, a hinge action and a gliding movement (Fig. 9-12). With these two types of movement, the jaws can open and close and shift from side to side.

Hinge Action

The hinge action is the first phase in mouth opening, and only the lower compartment of the joint is used. During

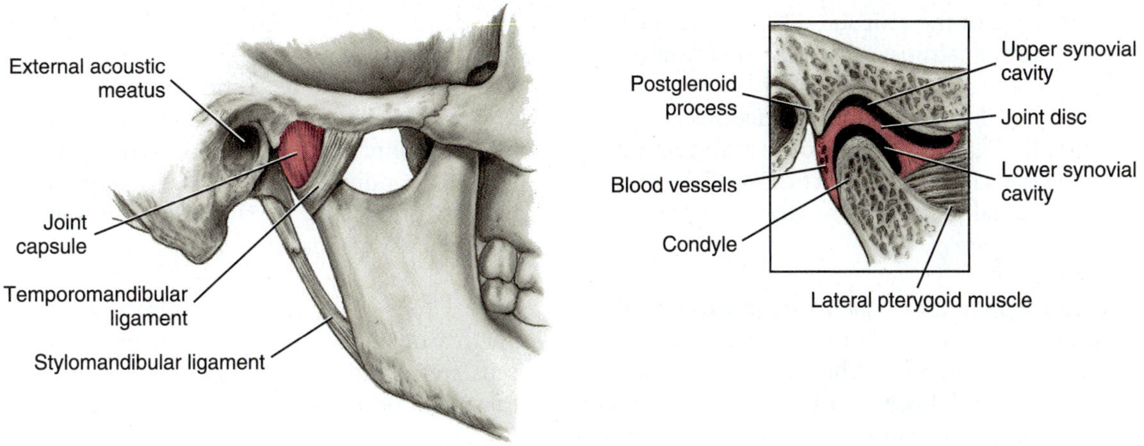

Fig. 9-11 **Lateral view of the joint capsule of the temporomandibular joint and its lateral temporomandibular ligament. Note on the insert that the capsule has been removed to show the upper and lower synovial cavities and their relationship to the articular disc.** (From Fehrenbach MJ, Herring SW: *Illustrated anatomy of the head and neck,* ed 2, Philadelphia, 2002, Saunders.)

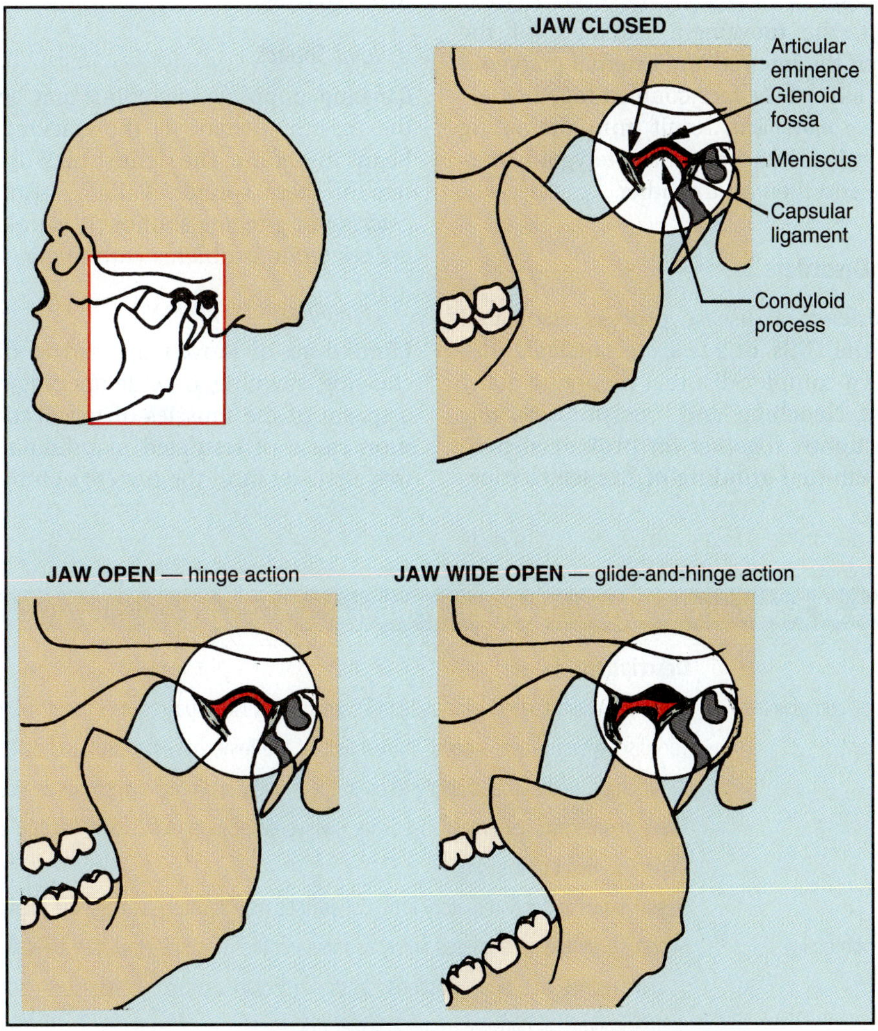

Fig. 9-12 **Hinge and gliding actions of the temporomandibular joint.**

hinge action, the condylar head rotates around a point on the undersurface of the articular disc, and the body of the mandible drops almost passively downward and backward.

The jaw is opened by the combined actions of the external pterygoid, digastric, mylohyoid, and geniohyoid muscles. The jaw is closed by the action of the temporal, masseter, and internal pterygoid muscles.

Gliding Movement

The gliding movement allows the lower jaw to move forward or backward. It involves both the lower and the upper compartments of the joint. The condyle and articular disc "glide" forward and downward along the articular eminence (projection). This movement occurs only during protrusion and lateral movements of the mandible and in combination with the hinge action during the wider opening of the mouth.

Protrusion is the forward movement of the mandible. This happens when the internal and external pterygoid muscles on both sides contract together. The reversal of this movement is the backward movement of the mandible, called *retrusion.*

Lateral movement, the movement sideways, of the mandible occurs when the internal and external pterygoid muscles on the same side of the face contract together.

Side-to-side *grinding movements* result from alternating contractions of the internal and external pterygoid muscles, first on one side and then on the other.

Temporomandibular Disorders

A patient may experience a disease process associated with one or both of the TMJs, or a *temporomandibular disorder (TMD).* TMD is a complex disorder involving many factors, such as stress, clenching, and bruxism. *Clenching* is holding the teeth tightly together for prolonged periods. *Bruxism* is the habitual grinding of the teeth, especially at night. TMD can also be caused by trauma to the jaw, systemic diseases such as osteoarthritis, or wear from aging (Box 9-3).

The diagnosis and treatment of TMD can be difficult (Fig. 9-13). Frequently, the diagnosis of TMD requires a multidisciplinary approach. For a complete analysis of the patient's condition, some cases require involvement of dentists, physicians, psychiatrists, psychologists, neurologists, neurosurgeons, and others.

Symptoms

One reason TMD is difficult to diagnose is that the symptoms are so varied. Pain, joint sounds, and limitations of movement occur most often.

Pain

Patients with TMD may report a wide range of pains, including headaches, pain in and around the ear (when no infection is present), pain on chewing, and pain in the face, head, and neck. *Spasms* ("cramps") of the muscles of mastication can become part of a cycle that results in tissue damage, increased pain, muscle tenderness, and more spasms.

Joint Sounds

Clicking, popping, or crepitus may be heard when opening the mouth. *Crepitus* is the cracking sound that may be heard in a joint. The dentist may use a stethoscope to listen for these sounds. Patients also report hearing these *cracking* or *grinding* sounds. It is unknown if joint sounds are related to problems with the jaws.

Limitations of Movement

Limitations of movement lead to difficulty and pain on chewing, yawning, or wide opening of the mouth. *Trismus,* a spasm of the muscles of mastication, is the most common cause of restricted mandibular movement. Trismus may severely limit the patient's ability to open the mouth.

Box 9-3 Categories of Temporomandibular Disorders (TMDs)

Category	Description
Acute masticatory muscle complaints	These are characterized by muscle inflammation, muscle spasms, and protective muscle splinting.
Articular disc derangement	The disc, which allows smooth movement of the joint, may be displaced or damaged. This may cause clicking sounds, limited ability to open the mouth, and other symptoms associated with TMDs.
Extrinsic trauma	These injuries from external causes may involve dislocation of the joint, fracture of the bones, and internal derangement of the joint.
Joint diseases	Degenerative and inflammatory forms of arthritis may severely damage the joint.
Chronic mandibular hypomobility	*Hypomobility* means a limited ability to move. In the mandible, this may be influenced by damage to the joint (either the bony portions or the articular capsule), contracture (shortening) of muscles of mastication, or damage to the articular disc.

Patients' descriptions of this condition include a jaw that "gets stuck," "locks," or "goes out."

Causes

TMDs are often considered to be stress-related. Frequently, oral habits such as clenching the teeth or bruxism are important contributing factors. Other causes of TMDs include (1) accidents involving injuries to the jaw, head, or neck, (2) diseases of the joint, including several varieties of arthritis, and (3) *malocclusion,* in which the teeth come together in a manner that produces abnormal strain on the joint and surrounding tissues.

Recall

9. What are the two basic types of movement by the TMJ?
10. What symptoms might a patient with a TMD have?

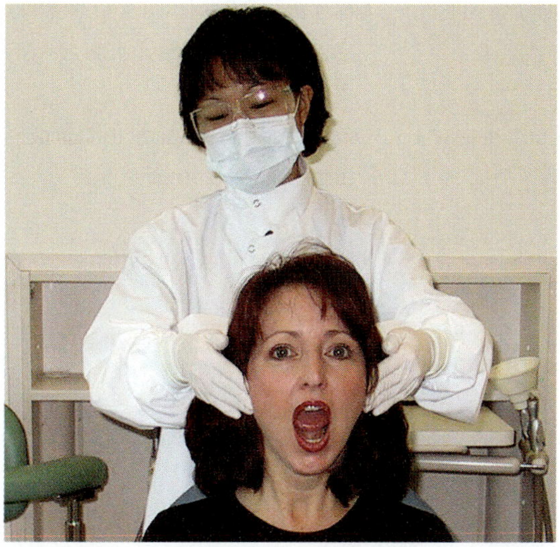

Fig. 9-13 Palpation of the patient during movements of both temporomandibular joints.

MUSCLES OF THE HEAD AND NECK

To perform a thorough patient examination, it is necessary to determine the location and action of many muscles of the head and neck. Malfunction of muscles may be involved in malocclusion, TMD, and even spread of dental infections.

Muscles must *expand* and *contract* to make movements possible. Each muscle has a point of origin that is fixed (nonmovable) and a point of insertion (movable). The muscles of the head and neck are divided into seven main groups: (1) muscles of the neck, (2) muscles of facial expression, (3) muscles of mastication, (4) muscles of the tongue, (5) muscles of the soft palate, (6) muscles of the floor of the mouth, and (7) muscles of the pharynx. There are also groups of muscles of the ears, eyes, and nose that are not included in this book.

Major Muscles of the Neck

The two muscles of the neck discussed in this text are both superficial and are easily palpated on the neck. These cervical muscles are the **sternocleidomastoid** and **trapezius.** These muscles can become quite painful when dental assistants use improper posture while assisting (Box 9-4 and Fig. 9-14).

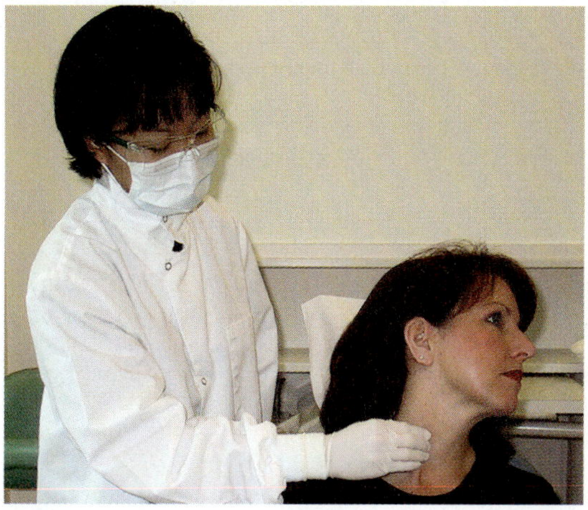

Fig. 9-14 Palpation of the sternocleidomastoid muscle by having the patient turn the head to the opposite side.

Box 9-4 Major Muscles of the Neck

Muscle	Origin	Insertion	Function
Sternocleidomastoid	Clavicle (collarbone) and lateral surfaces of sternum	Posterior and inferior to external acoustic meatus	Divides neck region into anterior and posterior cervical triangles; serves as landmark of neck during extraoral examination
Trapezius	External surface of occipital bone	Lateral third of clavicle and parts of scapula	Lifts clavicle and scapula (shoulder blade), as when shoulders are shrugged

Major Muscles of Facial Expression

The muscles of facial expression are paired muscles (left and right) and originate from the bone and insert on skin tissue. These muscles cause wrinkles at right angles to the muscle's action line. The seventh cranial (facial) nerve innervates all the muscles of facial expression (Box 9-5 and Fig. 9-15).

Major Muscles of Mastication

The muscles of mastication are four pairs of muscles attached to the mandible and include the *temporal*, **masseter**, *internal (medial) pterygoid*, and *external (lateral) pterygoid* (see Fig. 9-15).

These muscles work with the TMJ to make all movements of the mandible possible. The mandibular division of the fifth cranial (trigeminal) nerve innervates all muscles of mastication (Box 9-6).

Muscles of the Floor of the Mouth

The muscles of the floor of the mouth are the *digastric, mylohyoid, stylohyoid,* and *geniohyoid* (Fig. 9-16). These muscles are located between the mandible and the hyoid bone (Box 9-7). Different nerve branches innervate the muscles on the floor of the mouth.

Extrinsic Muscles of the Tongue

The tongue has two groups of muscles, *intrinsic* (within the tongue) and *extrinsic*. The intrinsic muscles are responsible for shaping the tongue during speech, chewing, and swallowing. The extrinsic muscles assist in the movement and functioning of the tongue and include the *genioglossus, hyoglossus, styloglossus,* and *palatoglossus* (Fig. 9-17). All the muscles of the tongue are innervated by the hypoglossal nerve except the palatoglossus. The palatoglossus muscle is

Box 9-5 Major Muscles of Facial Expression

Muscle	Origin	Insertion	Function
Orbicularis oris	From muscle fibers around mouth; no skeletal attachment	Into itself and surrounding skin	Closes and puckers lips; aids in chewing and speaking by pressing lips against teeth
Buccinator	Posterior portion of alveolar processes of maxillary bone and mandible	Fibers of orbicularis oris, at angle of mouth	Compresses cheeks against teeth and retracts angle of mouth
Mentalis	Incisive fossa of mandible	Skin of chin	Raises and wrinkles skin of chin and pushes up lower lip
Zygomatic major	Zygomatic bone	Into fibers of orbicularis oris	Draws angles of mouth upward and backward, as in laughing

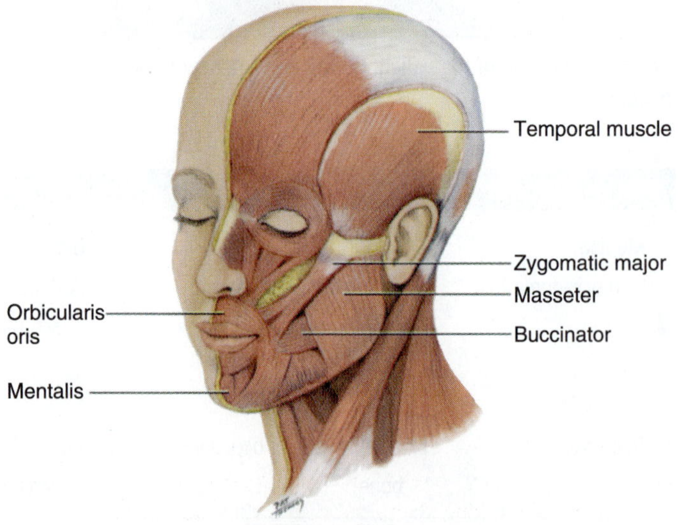

Fig. 9-15 **Major muscles of facial expression and mastication.** (From Applegate EG: *Anatomy and physiology learning system,* ed 2, Philadelphia, 2000, Saunders.)

Box 9-6 Major Muscles of Mastication

Muscle	Origin	Insertion	Function
Temporal	Temporal fossa of temporal bone	Coronoid process and anterior border of mandibular ramus	Raises mandible and closes jaws
Masseter	Superficial part: lower border of zygomatic arch Deep part: posterior and medial side of zygomatic arch	Superficial part: angle and lower lateral side of mandibular ramus Deep part: upper lateral ramus and mandibular coronoid process	Raises mandible and closes jaws
Internal (medial) pterygoid	Medial surface of lateral pterygoid plate of sphenoid bone, palatine bone, and tuberosity of maxillary bone	Into inner (medial) surface of ramus and angle of mandible	Closes jaw: acting with lateral pterygoid on same side, pulls mandible to one side; medial and lateral pterygoids on both sides act together to bring lower jaw forward*
External (lateral) pterygoid	Originates from two heads; upper head originates from greater wing of sphenoid bone	Into neck of condyle of mandible and into articular disc and capsular ligament of TMJ	Depresses mandible to open jaw*

*When both pterygoid muscles contract together, the main action is to bring the lower jaw forward, thus causing protrusion of the mandible. If only one lateral pterygoid muscle is contracted, the lower jaw shifts to the opposite side, causing lateral deviation of the mandible.

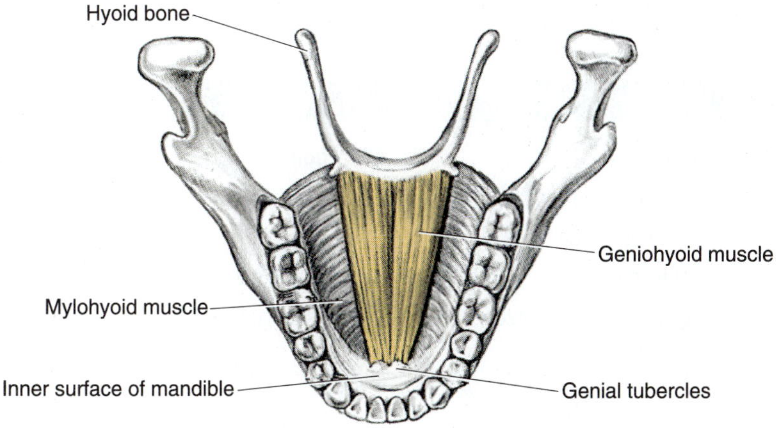

Fig. 9-16 View from above the floor of the oral cavity showing the origin and insertion of the geniohyoid muscle. (From Fehrenbach MJ, Herring SW: *Illustrated anatomy of the head and neck,* ed 2, Philadelphia, 2002, Saunders.)

discussed with the palate. Muscles of the tongue and the floor of the mouth attach to the hyoid bone (Box 9-8).

Muscles of the Soft Palate

The soft palate has two major muscles called the *palatoglossus* and *palatopharyngeus* (Box 9-9). The *pharyngeal plexus* innervates both these muscles.

Recall

11 Which cranial nerve innervates all muscles of mastication?
12. What is the name of the horseshoe-shaped bone where the muscles of the tongue and the floor of the mouth attach?

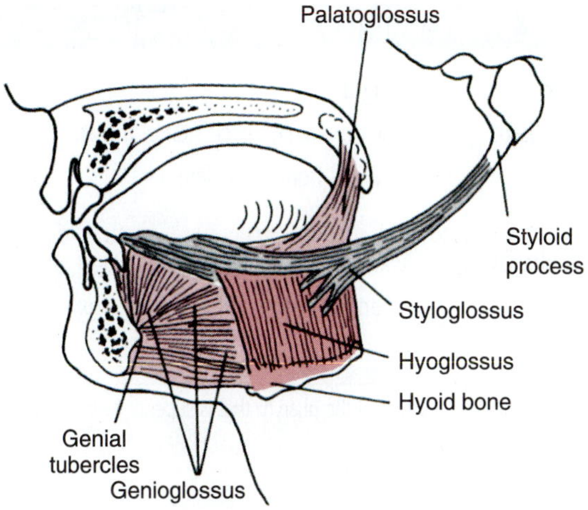

Fig. 9-17 Extrinsic muscles of the tongue.

Box 9-7 Muscles of the Floor of the Mouth

Muscle	Origin	Insertion	Function	Innervation
Mylohyoid	Left and right portions are joined at the midline. Each portion originates on mylohyoid line of mandible	Body of hyoid bone	Forms floor of mouth; elevates (raises) tongue and depresses (lowers) jaw	Posterior belly: facial nerve Anterior belly: mandibular branch of trigeminal nerve
Digastric	Anterior belly: lower border of mandible Posterior belly: mastoid process of temporal bone	Body and great horn of hyoid bone	Each digastric muscle demarcates superior portion of anterior cervical triangle, forming (with the mandible) a submandibular triangle on each side of neck	Anterior belly: facial nerve Posterior belly: facial nerve (seventh cranial nerve)
Stylohyoid	Styloid process of temporal bone	Body of hyoid bone	Assists in swallowing by raising hyoid bone	Facial nerve
Geniohyoid	Medial (inner) surface of mandible, near symphysis	Body of hyoid bone	Draws tongue and hyoid bone forward	Hypoglossal nerve

Box 9-8 Extrinsic Muscles of the Tongue

Muscle	Origin	Insertion	Function
Genioglossus	Medial (inner) surface of mandible, near symphysis	Hyoid bone and inferior (lower) surface of tongue	Depresses and protrudes tongue
Hyoglossus	Body of hyoid bone	Side of tongue	Retracts and pulls down side of tongue
Styloglossus	Styloid process of temporal bone	Side and undersurface of tongue	Retracts tongue

Box 9-9 Major Muscles of the Soft Palate

Muscle	Origin	Insertion	Function
Palatoglossus	Anterior arch on each side of throat; arises from soft palate	Along posterior side of tongue	Elevates base of tongue, arching tongue against soft palate; depresses soft palate toward tongue
Palatopharyngeal	Posterior border of thyroid cartilage and connective tissue of pharynx	Thyroid cartilage and wall of pharynx	Forms posterior pillar of fauces; serves to narrow fauces and helps to shut off nasopharynx*

*The nasopharynx is the portion of the pharynx that is superior to the level of the soft palate.

SALIVARY GLANDS

The salivary glands produce *saliva,* which lubricates and cleanses the oral cavity and aids in digestion of food by an enzymatic process. Saliva also helps maintain the integrity of tooth surfaces through a process of *remineralization.* In addition, saliva is involved in the formation of dental plaque, and it supplies the minerals for supragingival calculus formation. These processes are discussed in detail in Chapters 13 and 15.

The salivary glands produce two types of saliva. *Serous* saliva is watery, mainly protein fluid. *Mucous* saliva is very thick, mainly carbohydrate fluid. Salivary glands are classified by their size as either major or minor (Fig. 9-18).

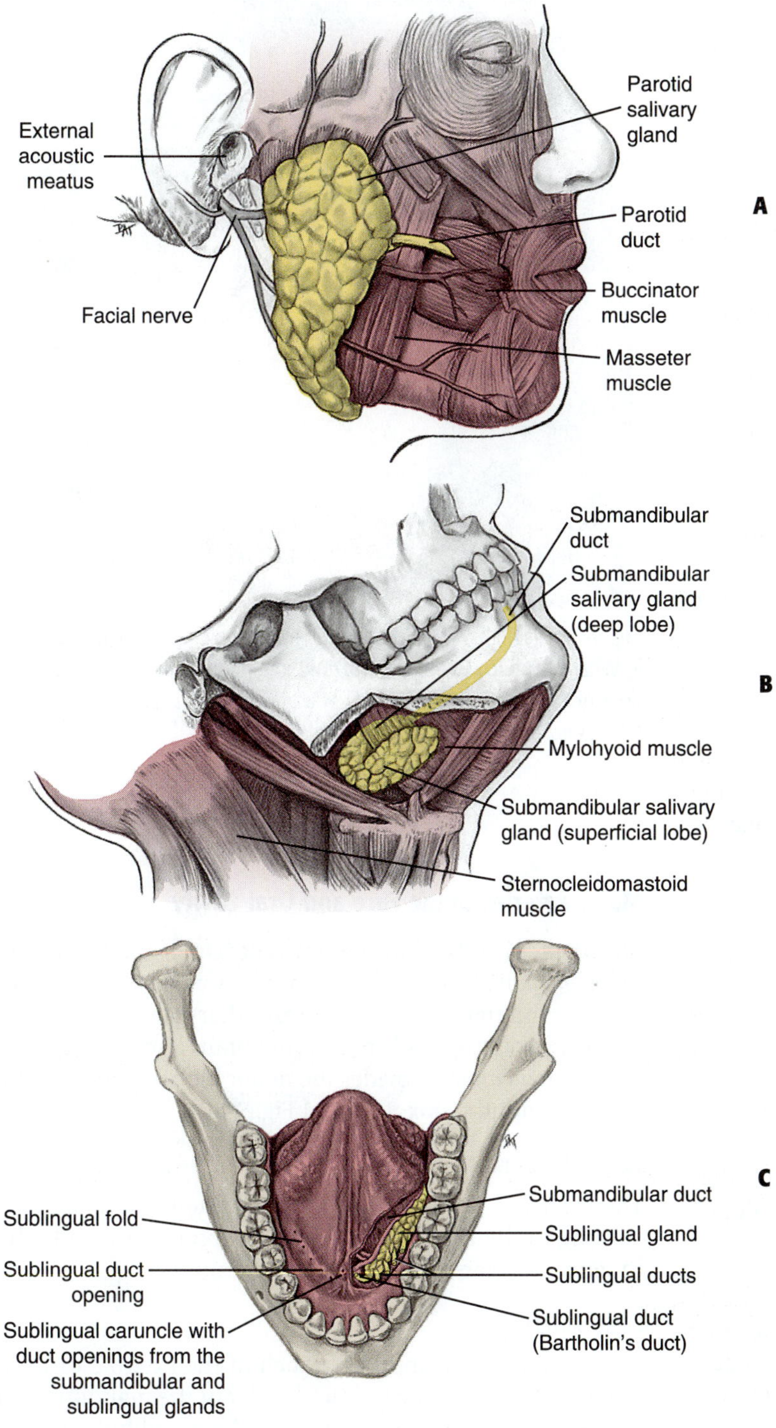

Fig. 9-18 **Major salivary glands. A, Parotid salivary glands. B, Submandibular salivary gland. C, Sublingual salivary gland. Note that the tongue is elevated and the tissues sectioned in the highlighted area.** (**A** and **B** from Fehrenbach MJ, Herring SW: *Illustrated anatomy of the head and neck,* ed 2, Philadelphia, 2002, Saunders.)

Minor Salivary Glands

The minor salivary glands are smaller and more numerous than the major salivary glands. The minor glands are scattered in the tissues of the buccal, labial, and lingual mucosa; the soft palate; the lateral portions of the hard palate; and the floor of the mouth. The *von Ebner's salivary gland* is associated with the **circumvallate lingual papillae** on the tongue.

Major Salivary Glands

The three large paired salivary glands are the *parotid,* the *submandibular,* and the *sublingual* glands.

The *parotid salivary gland* is the largest of the major salivary glands but provides only 25 percent of the total volume of saliva. It is located in an area just below and in front of the ear. Saliva passes from the parotid gland into the mouth through the **parotid duct,** also known as *Stensen's duct.*

The *submandibular salivary gland,* about the size of a walnut, is the second largest salivary gland. The gland provides 60 to 65 percent of the total volume of saliva. It lies beneath the mandible in the *submandibular fossa,* posterior to the sublingual salivary gland. The gland releases saliva into the oral cavity through the *submandibular duct,* also known as *Wharton's duct,* which ends in the sublingual caruncles. The ducts visible in the oral cavity are shown in Chapter 10.

The *sublingual salivary gland* is the smallest of the three major salivary glands. It only provides 10 percent of total salivary volume. The gland releases saliva into the oral cavity through the *sublingual duct,* also known as *Bartholin's duct.* Other smaller ducts of the sublingual gland open along the sublingual fold. A stone, or *sialolith,* may also block the salivary glands in the duct opening, preventing saliva from flowing into the mouth. Salivary stones may be removed surgically (Fig. 9-19).

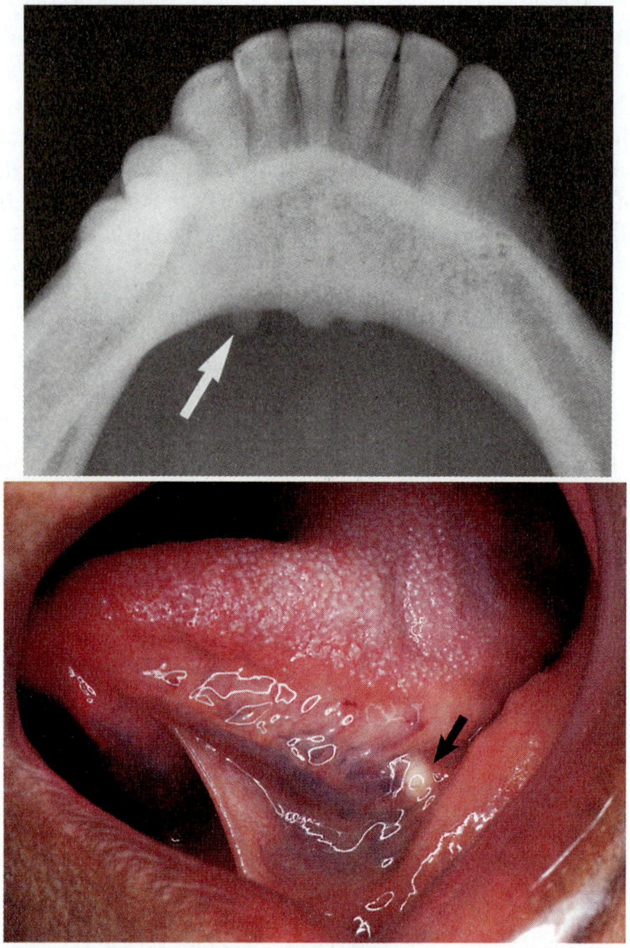

A

B

Fig. 9-19 Sialoliths. **A,** Occlusal radiograph showing a sialolith *(arrow)* in Wharton's duct. **B,** Sialolith *(arrow)* in a minor salivary gland on the floor of the mouth. (From Ibsen O, Phelan J, eds: *Oral pathology for the dental hygienist,* ed 4, St. Louis, 2004, Saunders.)

Recall

13. Which of the major salivary glands is the largest?
14. What is another name for the parotid duct?

BLOOD SUPPLY TO THE HEAD AND NECK

It is important to be able to locate the larger blood vessels of the head and neck, because these vessels may become compromised due to disease or during a dental procedure such as a local anesthetic injection. Blood vessels may also spread infection in the head and neck area.

Major Arteries of the Face and Oral Cavity

The *aorta* ascends from the left ventricle of the heart. The *common carotid artery* arises from the aorta and subdivides into the internal and external carotid arteries. The *internal carotid artery* supplies blood to the brain and eyes. The *external carotid artery* provides the major blood supply for the face and mouth (Box 9-10 and Fig. 9-20).

External Carotid Artery

The branches of the external carotid artery are named according to the areas they supply. The branches supply the tongue, face, ears, and wall of the cranium.

Facial Artery

The facial artery is another branch of the external carotid. It enters the face at the inferior border of the mandible and can be detected by gently palpating the mandibular notch.

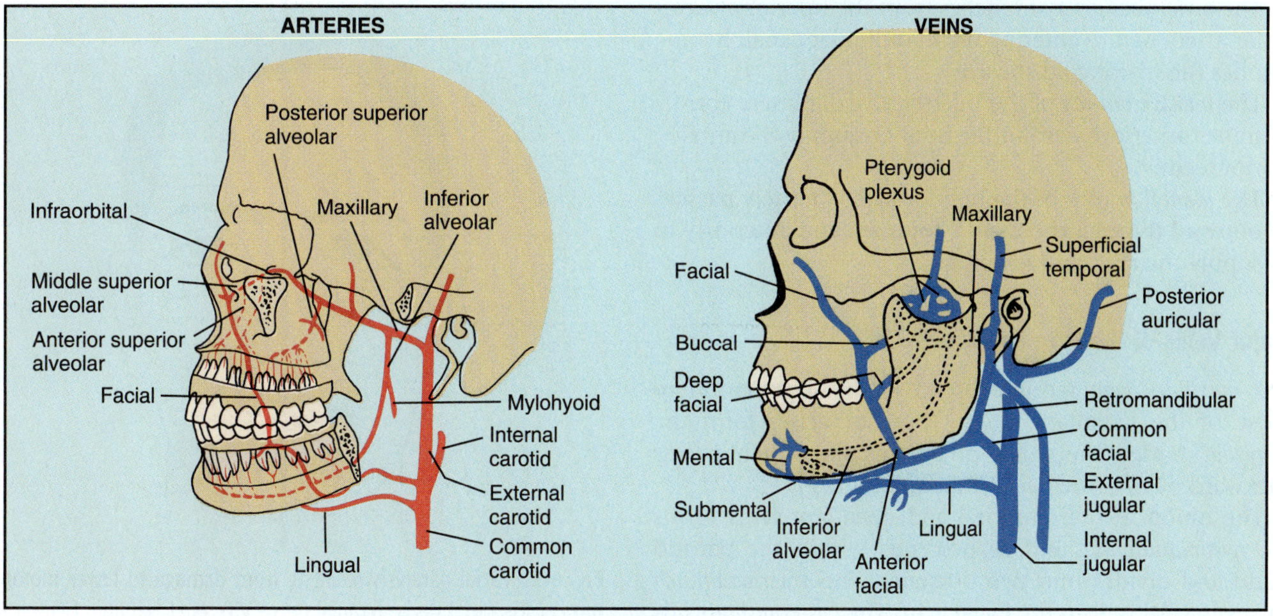

Fig. 9-20 Major arteries and veins of the face and oral cavity.

Box 9-10 Major Arteries to the Face and Mouth

Structure	Blood Supply
Muscles of facial expression	Branches and small arteries from maxillary, facial, and ophthalmic arteries
Maxillary bones	Anterior, middle, and posterior alveolar arteries
Maxillary teeth	Anterior, middle, and posterior alveolar arteries
Mandible	Inferior alveolar arteries
Mandibular teeth	Inferior alveolar arteries
Tongue	Lingual artery
Muscles of mastication	Facial arteries

The facial artery passes forward and upward across the cheek toward the angle of the mouth. Then it continues upward alongside the nose and ends at the medial *canthus* (inner corner) of the eye. The facial artery has six branches that supply the pharyngeal muscles, soft palate, tonsils, posterior tongue, submandibular gland, muscles of the face, nasal septum, nose, and eyelids.

Lingual Artery

The lingual artery is also a branch of the external carotid. It has several branches to the entire tongue, floor of the mouth, lingual gingiva, and a portion of the soft palate and tonsils.

Maxillary Artery

The maxillary artery is the larger of the two terminal branches of the external carotid. It arises behind the angle of the mandible and supplies the deep structures of the face. The maxillary artery divides into three sections: *mandibular, pterygoid,* and *pterygopalatine.*

The *pterygoid artery* supplies blood to the temporal muscle, masseter muscle, pterygoid muscles, and buccinator muscles. The pterygoid artery divides into the following five branches:

1. *Anterior* and *middle superior alveolar arteries,* with distribution to the maxillary incisors and cuspid teeth and to the maxillary sinuses
2. *Posterior superior alveolar artery,* with distribution to the maxillary molars and premolars and gingivae
3. *Infraorbital artery,* with distribution to the face
4. *Greater palatine artery,* with distribution to the hard palate and lingual gingiva
5. *Anterior superior alveolar artery,* with distribution to the anterior teeth

Mandibular Artery

The mandibular artery is behind the ramus of the mandible and branches into the following five arteries:

1. The *lingual artery* has distribution along the surface of the tongue
2. The *inferior alveolar artery* descends close to the medial surface of the mandibular ramus to the mandibular foramen, then continues along the mandibular canal. Opposite the first premolar, it divides into the incisive and mental branches.

3. The *mylohyoid artery* branches from the inferior alveolar artery before entering the mandibular canal. It supplies the mylohyoid muscle.
4. The *incisive branch* of the inferior alveolar artery continues anteriorly within the bone to supply the anterior teeth.
5. The *mental branch* of the inferior alveolar artery passes outward through the mental foramen and anteriorly to supply the chin and lower lip.

Major Veins of the Face and Mouth

The *maxillary vein* receives branches that correspond to those of the maxillary artery. These branches form the *pterygoid plexus.* The trunk of the maxillary vein passes backward behind the neck of the mandible.

The union of the temporal and maxillary veins forms the *retromandibular vein.* It descends within the parotid gland and divides into two branches. The *anterior branch* passes inward to join the facial vein. The *posterior branch* is joined by the posterior auricular vein and becomes the external jugular vein.

The *external jugular vein* empties into the *subclavian vein.* The *facial vein* begins near the side of the nose. It passes downward and crosses over the body of the mandible with the facial artery. It then passes outward and backward to unite with the anterior division of the retromandibular vein to form the *common facial vein,* which enters the internal jugular vein.

The *deep facial vein* courses from the pterygoid plexus to the facial vein. The *lingual veins* begin on the dorsum (top), sides, and undersurface of the tongue. They pass backward, following the course of the lingual artery and its branches, and terminate in the internal jugular vein.

The *internal jugular vein,* which corresponds to the common carotid artery, empties into the *superior vena cava,* which returns blood from the upper portion of the body to the right atrium of the heart.

Recall

15. What artery is behind the ramus and branches into five arteries?

16. What artery supplies the maxillary molars and premolars and gingivae?

NERVES OF THE HEAD AND NECK

A thorough understanding of the nerves of the head and neck is important in relation to the use of local anesthesia during dental treatment and as the nerves can relate to certain conditions of the face, such as facial paralysis (Fig. 9-21). Also, certain disorders of the nervous system can affect the head and neck region.

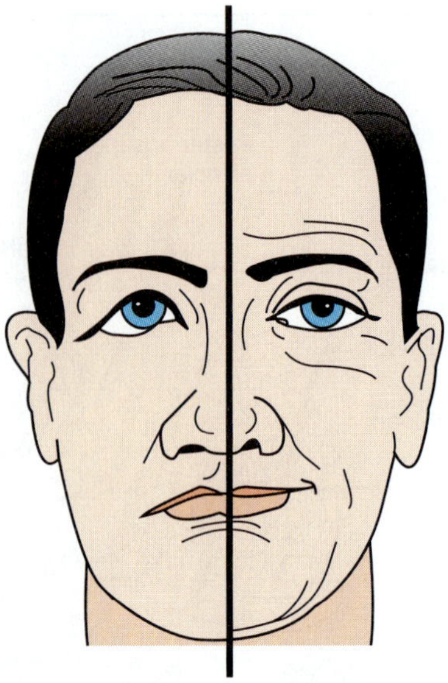

Fig. 9-21 Facial paralysis resulting from damage to lower motor neurons of the facial nerve (cranial nerve VII). (Redrawn from Liebgott B: *The anatomical basis of dentistry,* ed 2, St. Louis, 2001, Mosby; and Wilson-Pauwels L, Akesson EJ, Stewart PA: *Cranial nerves: Anatomy and clinical comments,* Toronto, 1998, BC Decker.)

Cranial Nerves

There are 12 pairs of *cranial nerves,* all of which are connected to the brain. These nerves serve both sensory and motor functions. The cranial nerves are generally named for the area or function they serve and are identified with Roman numerals I to XII (Fig. 9-22).

Innervation of the Oral Cavity

The **trigeminal nerve** is the primary source of innervation for the oral cavity (Figs. 9-23 and 9-24).

The trigeminal nerve subdivides into three main divisions: the *ophthalmic, maxillary,* and *mandibular.* The ophthalmic nerve is not discussed in this chapter.

Maxillary Division of Trigeminal Nerve

The maxillary division of the trigeminal nerve supplies the maxillary teeth, periosteum, mucous membranes, maxillary sinuses, and soft palate. The maxillary division subdivides to provide the following innervation:

1. The *nasopalatine nerve,* which passes through the incisive foramen, supplies the mucoperiosteum palatal to the maxillary anterior teeth. (*Mucoperiosteum* is periosteum having a mucous membrane surface.)

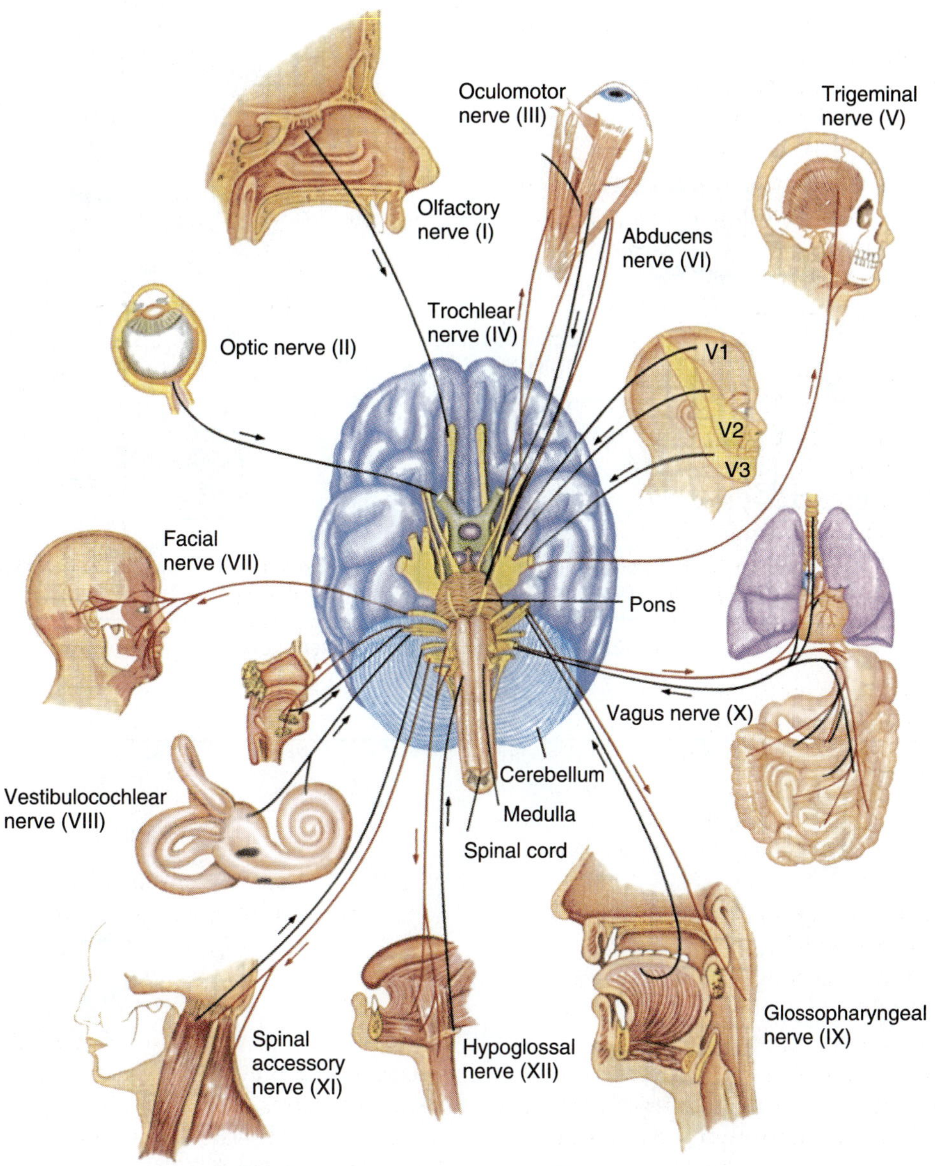

Nerve	Type	Function
I Olfactory	Sensory	Sense of smell
II Optic	Sensory	Sense of sight
III Oculomotor	Motor	Movement of eye muscles
IV Trochlear	Motor	Movement of eye muscles
V Trigeminal	Motor	Movement of muscles of mastication and other cranial muscles
	Sensory	General sensations for face, head, skin, teeth, oral cavity, and tongue
VI Abducens	Motor	Movement of eye muscles
VII Facial	Motor	Facial expression, functions of glands and muscles
	Sensory	Sense of taste on tongue
VIII Vestibulocochlear	Sensory	Senses of sound and balance
IX Glossopoharyngeal	Motor	Functioning of parotid gland
	Sensory	General sensation on skin around ear
X Vagus	Motor	Moves muscles in soft palate, pharynx, and larynx
	Sensory	General sensation on skin around ear and sense of taste
XI Accessory	Motor	Movement of muscles of the neck, soft palate, and pharynx
XII Hypoglossal	Motor	Movement of muscles of the tongue

Fig. 9-22 The 12 cranial nerves.

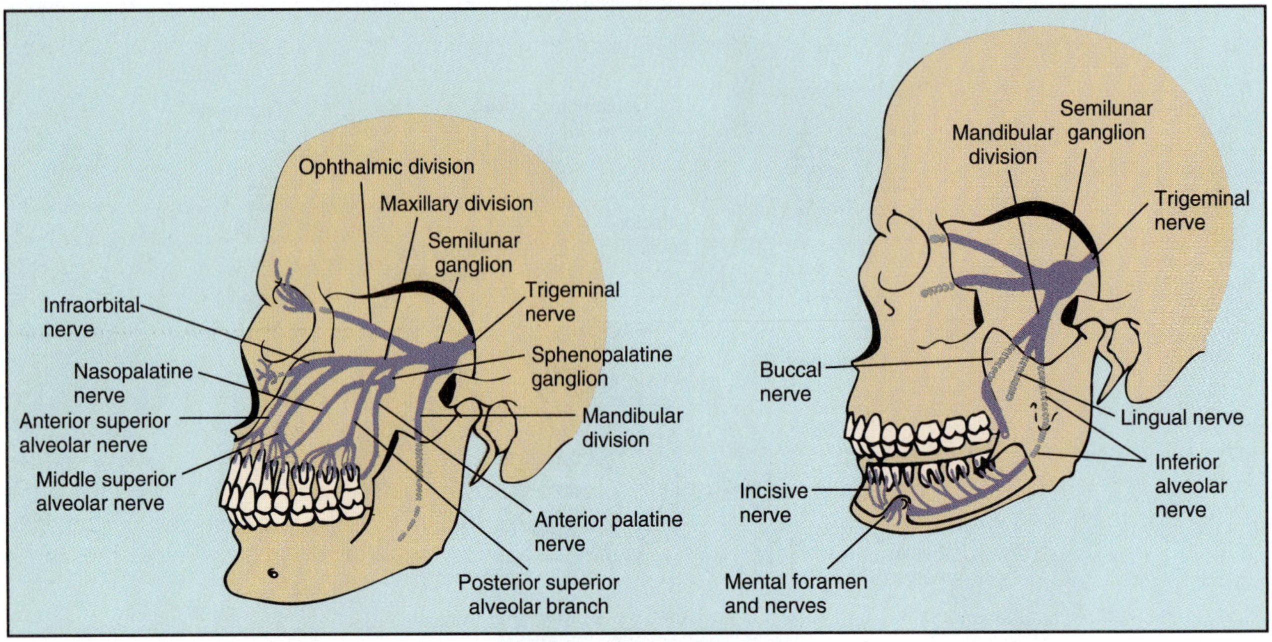

Fig. 9-23 Maxillary and mandibular innervation.

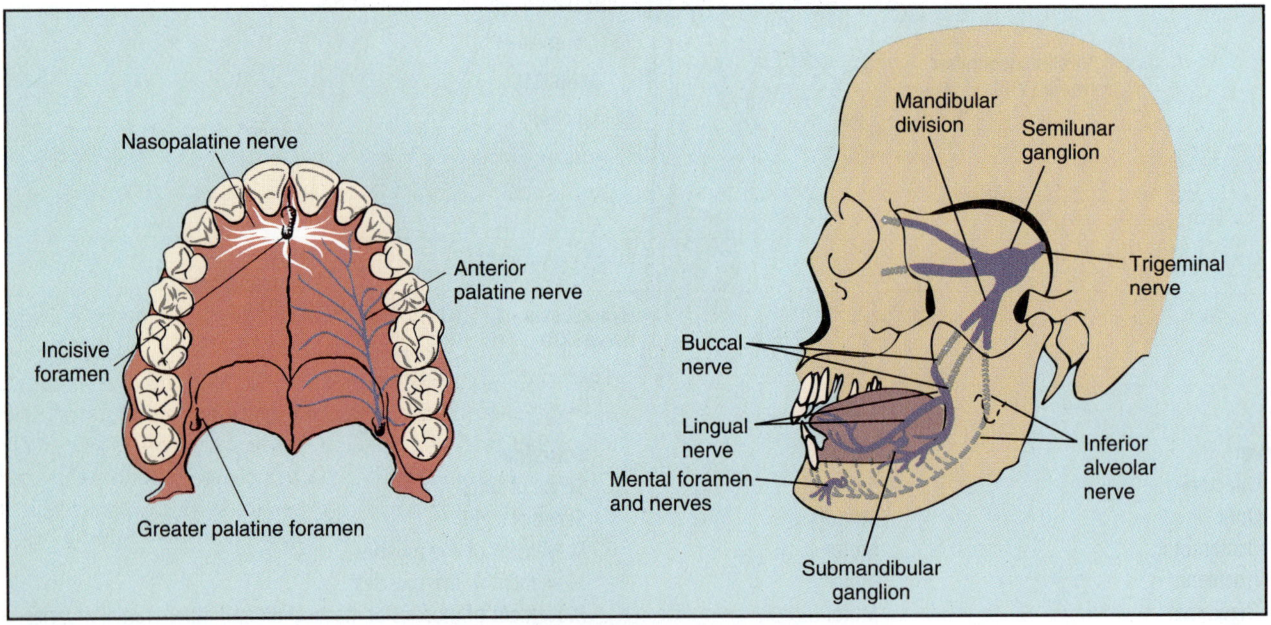

Fig. 9-24 Palatal, lingual, and buccal innervation.

2. The **greater palatine nerve,** which passes through the posterior palatine foramen and forward over the palate, supplies the mucoperiosteum, intermingling with the nasopalatine nerve.
3. The *anterior superior alveolar nerve* supplies the maxillary central, lateral, and cuspid teeth, plus their periodontal membranes and gingivae. This nerve also supplies the maxillary sinus.
4. The *middle superior alveolar nerve* supplies the maxillary first and second premolars, the mesiobuccal root of the maxillary first molar, and the maxillary sinus.
5. The *posterior superior alveolar nerve* supplies the other roots of the maxillary first molar and the maxillary second and third molars. It also branches forward to serve the lateral wall of the maxillary sinus.

Clinical Considerations: Facial Paralysis

The removal of an impacted third molar could be complicated by the relationship of the location of the nerves in the area to the tooth. For example, if the dentist damaged the nerve while attempting to remove the tooth, paralysis of the tongue or lip could result. Depending on the extent of the injury to the nerve, the paralysis could be temporary or permanent.

Mandibular Division of Trigeminal Nerve

The mandibular division of the trigeminal nerve subdivides to provide the following innervation:

1. The *buccal nerve* (long buccal) supplies branches to the buccal mucous membrane and to the mucoperiosteum of the mandibular molars.
2. The *lingual nerve* supplies the anterior two thirds of the tongue and branches to supply the lingual mucous membrane and mucoperiosteum.
3. The *inferior alveolar nerve* subdivides into the following:
   a. The *mylohyoid nerve* supplies the mylohyoid muscles and the anterior belly of the digastric muscle.
   b. *Small dental nerves* supply the molar and premolar teeth, alveolar process, and periosteum.
   c. The *mental nerve* moves outward and anteriorly through the mental foramen and supplies the chin and mucous membrane of the lower lip.
   d. The *incisive nerve* continues anteriorly within the bone and gives off small branches to supply the incisor teeth.

Recall

17. How many pairs of cranial nerves are connected to the brain?
18 Which division of the trigeminal nerve subdivides into the buccal, lingual, and inferior alveolar nerves?

LYMPH NODES OF THE HEAD AND NECK

A dental professional must examine and palpate the lymph nodes of the head and neck very carefully during an extraoral examination. Enlarged lymph nodes could indicate infection or cancer. The lymph nodes for the oral cavity drain intraoral structures such as the teeth, as well as the eyes, ears, nasal cavity, and deeper areas of the throat. Often a patient needs a referral to a physician when lymph nodes are palpable due to a disease process in these other regions.

Structure and Function

Lymph nodes are small round or oval structures located in lymph vessels. They fight disease by producing antibodies, which are part of the immune reaction. In acute infections, the lymph nodes become swollen and tender as a result of the collection of lymphocytes gathered to destroy the invading substances.

The major lymph node sites of the body include *cervical nodes* (in the neck), *axillary nodes* (under the arms), and *inguinal nodes* (in the lower abdomen). The lymph nodes of the head are classified as being *superficial* (near the surface) or *deep*. All the nodes of the head drain either the right or the left tissues in the area, depending on their location.

Superficial Lymph Nodes of the Head

There are five groups of superficial lymph nodes in the head: the occipital, retroauricular, anterior auricular, superficial parotid, and facial nodes (Fig. 9-25, *A*).

Deep Cervical Lymph Nodes

The deep cervical lymph nodes are located along the length of the internal jugular vein on each side of the neck, deep to the sternocleidomastoid muscle (Fig. 9-25, *B*).

Lymphadenopathy

When a patient has an infection or cancer in a region, the lymph nodes in that region will respond by increasing in size and becoming very firm. This change in size and consistency is termed **lymphadenopathy.** It results from an increase in both the size of individual lymphocytes (lymphocyte cells are the body's main defense) and the overall cell count in the lymphoid tissue. With an increase in the size and number of lymphocytes, the body is better able to fight the disease process.

The dentist will make an appropriate referral to a physician when any enlarged lymph nodes are found during an examination (see Fig. 9-13).

Recall

19 During what type of dental examination are lymph nodes palpated?
20. What is the term for enlarged or palpable lymph nodes?

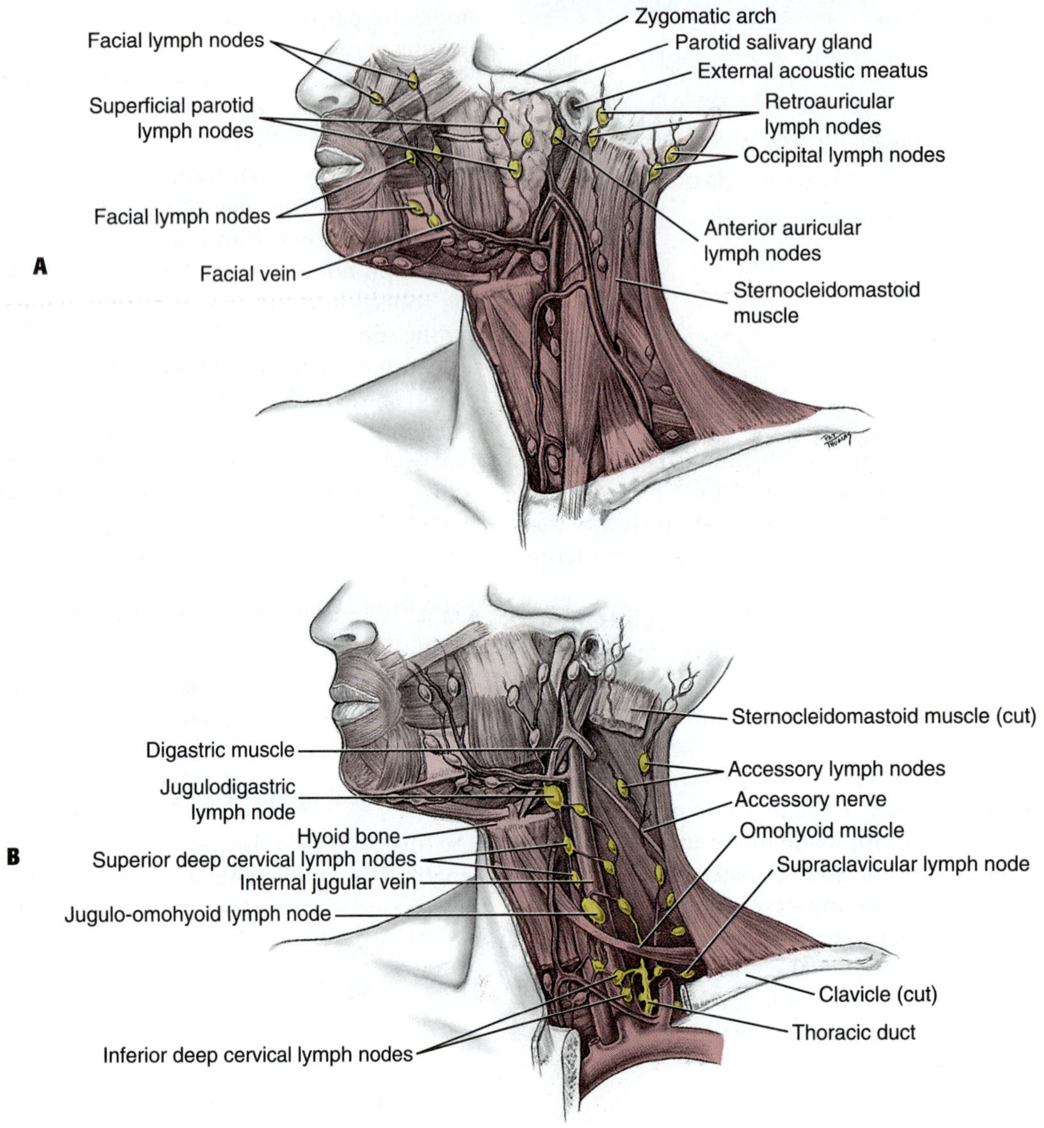

Fig. 9-25 A, Superficial lymph nodes of the head and associated structures. B, Deep cervical lymph nodes and associated structures. (From Fehrenbach MJ, Herring SW: *Illustrated anatomy of the head and neck*, ed 2, Philadelphia, 2002, Saunders.)

Clinical Considerations: Toothaches and Sinus Pain

A patient who is suffering from a toothache on the maxillary arch may actually have an infected sinus. The roots of the maxillary teeth lie in close proximity to the sinus floor. Because the teeth and the maxillary sinus share a common nerve supply, sinusitis (inflammation of the sinus) may cause a generalized aching of the maxillary teeth.

PARANASAL SINUSES

The paranasal sinuses are air-containing spaces within the skull that communicate with the nasal cavity (Fig. 9-26). (A *sinus* is an air-filled cavity within a bone.) The functions of the sinuses include (1) producing mucus, (2) making the bones of the skull lighter, and (3) providing resonance, which helps to produce sound.

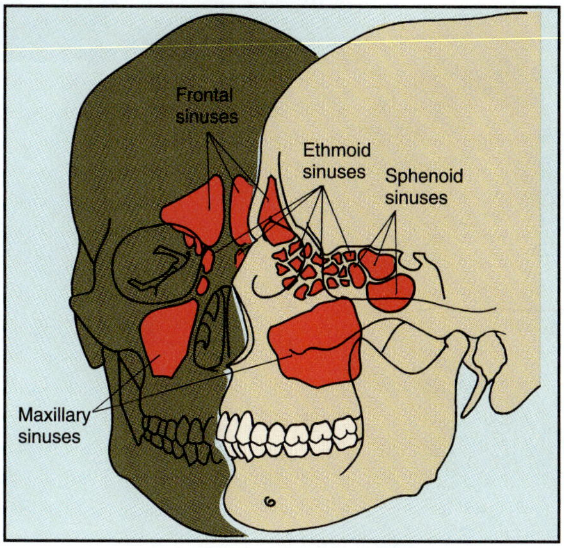

Fig. 9-26 The paranasal sinuses.

The sinuses are named for the bones in which they are located, as follows:

1. *Maxillary sinuses,* the largest of the paranasal sinuses
2. *Frontal sinuses,* located within the forehead just above the left and right eyes
3. *Ethmoid sinuses,* irregularly shaped air cells separated from the orbital cavity by a very thin layer of bone
4. *Sphenoid sinuses,* located close to the optic nerves, where an infection may damage vision

Eye to the Future

Saliva has long been recognized for its protective and lubricating properties. Today, saliva is recognized as the strongest link between oral and systemic health. Changes in salivary flow and function are extremely sensitive to subtle changes in general health.

The ancients once used salivary flow as a type of lie-detector test. A person suspected of a crime was given a mouthful of dry rice. If anxiety reduced the flow of saliva, and the suspect could not swallow the rice, the verdict was guilty as charged. The term *cotton mouth* is still used today to describe a dry mouth caused by anxiety.

Recent research has found a new role for saliva as an effective laboratory tool. Saliva is now being used for inexpensive, noninvasive, and easy-to-use diagnostic aids for oral and systemic diseases. For example, the HIV antibodies in saliva have led to the development of test kits. These test kits provide the sensitivity of a blood test, without the discomfort of a needle stick. In laboratory tests, saliva is also reliable in diagnosing viral hepatitis A, B, and C. Saliva has also been used as a diagnostic aid for Alzheimer's disease, cystic fibrosis, diabetes, and diseases of the adrenal cortex. Saliva is also proving to be an effective tool to monitor levels of hormones, medications, and illicit drugs.

Research is continuing to develop more sensitive and specific tests that someday will relate components in saliva to areas such as genetic defects, nutritional status, and age-specific changes.

Critical Thinking

1. While reading the newspaper, you notice an advertisement for an automobile with an "occipital headrest" on the passenger side. What type of headrest do you think this could be? Why?
2. If your dental-assisting program has one or more skulls that you can look at, compare the sizes of the skulls and the shapes of the teeth. See if you can determine if it is the skull of a male or female.

10

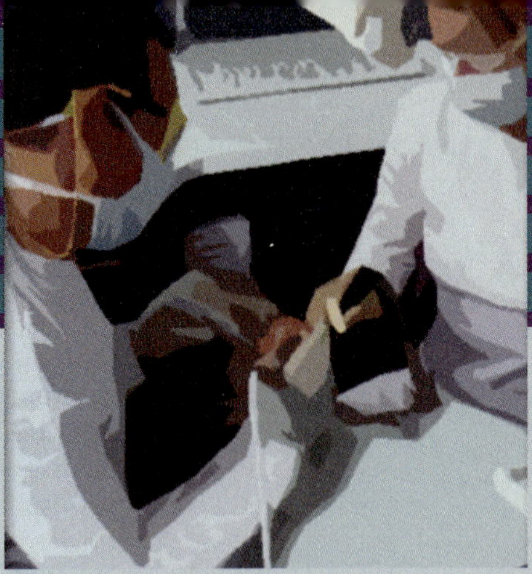

Landmarks of the Face and Oral Cavity

Outline

KEY TERMS

Ala (**ah**-la) Winglike tip of the outer side of each nostril; plural *alae.*

Angle of the mandible The lower posterior of the ramus.

Angular cheilosis Inflammation at the corners of the mouth that may be caused by a nutritional deficiency of the B complex vitamins, but most commonly is a fungal condition.

Anterior faucial pillar Anterior arch of the soft palate.

Anterior naris (**na**-ris) The nostril; plural *nares.*

Buccal vestibule Area between the cheeks and the teeth or alveolar ridge.

Canthus (**kan**-thus) Fold of tissue at the corner of the eyelids.

Filiform papillae Threadlike elevations that cover most of the tongue.

Fordyce's spots (**for**-dies-ez) Normal variations that may appear on the buccal mucosa.

Frenum (**fre**-num) Band of tissue that passes from the facial oral mucosa at the midline of the arch to the midline of the inner surface of the lip; also called *frenulum;* plural *frenula.*

Fungiform papillae Knoblike projections on the tongue.

Gingiva (**jin**-jeh-vah) Masticatory mucosa that covers the alveolar processes of the jaws and surrounds the necks of the teeth; plural *gingivae.*

Glabella (glah-**bel**-ah) Smooth surface of the frontal bone; also the anatomic part directly above the root of the nose.

Incisive papilla Pear-shaped pad of tissue that covers the incisive foramen.

Isthmus of fauces The opening between the two arches of the soft palate.

Labia The gateway to the oral cavity commonly known as "lips."

Labial commissure (**lay**-bee-ul) The angle at the corner of the mouth where the upper and lower lips join.

Labial frenum Band of tissue that passes from the facial oral mucosa at the midline of the arch to the midline of the inner surface of the lip; also called *frenulum;* plural *frenula.*

Linea alba Normal variation noted on the buccal mucosa.

Lingual frenum The thin fold of mucous membrane that extends from the floor of the mouth to the underside of the tongue.

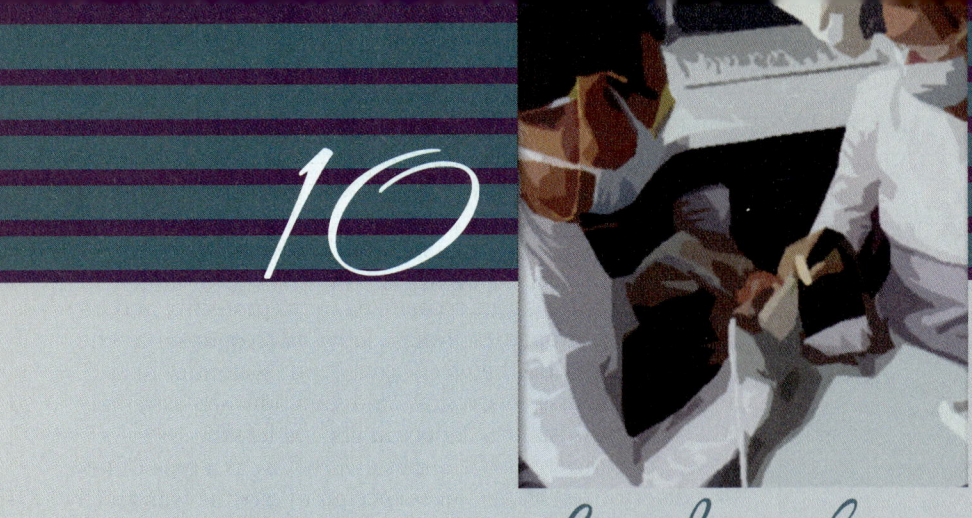

KEY TERMS—cont'd

Mental protuberance Part of the mandible that forms the chin.

Mucobuccal fold Base of the vestibule where the buccal mucosa meets the alveolar mucosa.

Mucogingival junction Distinct line of color change in the tissue where the alveolar membrane meets with attached gingivae.

Nasion (**nay**-ze-on) Midpoint between the eyes just below the eyebrows.

Nasolabial sulcus The groove extending upward between each labial commissure and nasal ala.

Oral cavity proper The space on the tongue side within the upper and lower dental arches.

Parotid papilla Small elevation of tissue located on the inner surface of the cheek.

Philtrum (**fil**-trum) Rectangular area from under the nose to the midline of the upper lip.

Posterior faucial pillar Posterior arch of the soft palate.

Root Facial landmark commonly called the "bridge" of the nose.

Septum (**sep**-tum) Tissue that divides the nasal cavity into two nasal fossae.

Tragus (**tray**-gus) Cartilaginous projection anterior to the external opening of the ear.

Uvula Pear-shaped projection at the end of the soft palate.

Vallate papillae The largest papillae on the tongue, arranged in the form of a V.

Vermilion border (ver-**mil**-yun) Darker-colored border around the lips.

Vestibule Space between the teeth and the inner mucosal lining of the lips and cheeks.

Zygomatic arch The arch formed when the temporal process of the zygomatic bone articulates with the zygomatic process of the temporal bone.

LEARNING OUTCOMES

On completion of this chapter, the student will be able to achieve the following objectives:

- Pronounce, define, and spell the Key Terms.
- Name and identify the landmarks of the face.
- Name and identify the landmarks of the oral cavity.
- Describe the structures found in the vestibular region of the oral cavity.
- Describe the area of the oral cavity proper.
- Describe the characteristics of normal gingival tissue.
- Locate and describe the functions of the taste buds.

The dental assistant must be thoroughly knowledgeable about the landmarks of the face and oral cavity. In addition to being useful reference points for dental radiography and other procedures, facial features provide essential landmarks for many deeper structures. Any deviation from normal in surface features may be clinically significant.

You may want to examine your own face and mouth or those of a partner. An operatory with a dental chair and light is an ideal setting. However, using a flashlight and tongue depressor in the laboratory setting is also adequate for intraoral inspection.

LANDMARKS OF THE FACE

The *face* is defined as the part of the head visible in a frontal view that is anterior to the ears and all that lies between the hairline and the chin.

Regions of the Face

The facial region can be subdivided into nine areas, as follows (Fig. 10-1):

1. *Forehead,* extending from the eyebrows to the hairline
2. *Temples,* or temporal area posterior to the eyes
3. *Orbital area,* containing the eye and covered by the eyelids
4. *External nose*
5. *Zygomatic (malar) area,* the prominence of the cheek
6. *Mouth* and *lips*
7. *Cheeks*
8. *Chin*
9. *External ear*

Features of the Face

The dental assistant should be able to identify the following important facial landmarks (Fig. 10-2):

1. The outer **canthus** of the eye is the fold of tissue at the outer corner of the eyelids.
2. The inner *canthus* of the eye is the fold of tissue at the inner corner of the eyelids.
3. The **ala** of the nose is the winglike tip on the outer side of each nostril.
4. The **philtrum** is the rectangular area between the two ridges running from under the nose to the midline of the upper lip.
5. The **tragus** of the ear is the cartilaginous projection anterior to the external opening of the ear.

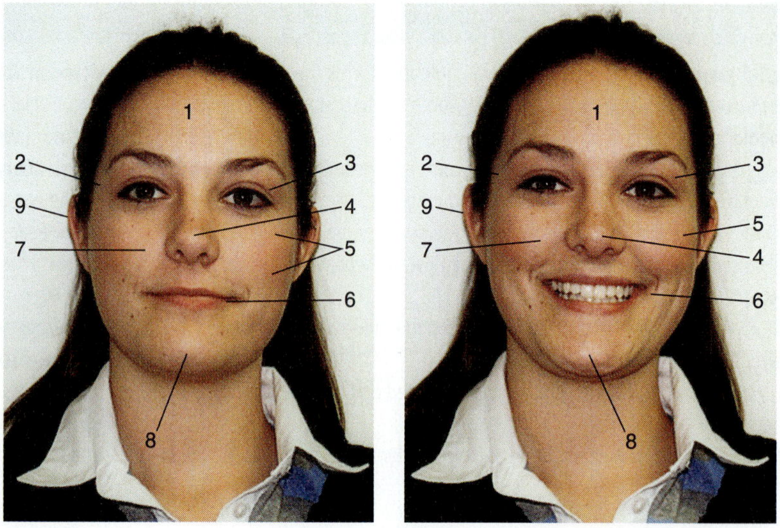

Fig. 10-1 Regions of the face. **A,** At rest. **B,** Smiling.

6. The **nasion** is midpoint between the eyes just below the eyebrows. On the skull, this is the point where the two nasal bones and the frontal bone join.
7. The **glabella** is the smooth surface of the frontal bone; also the anatomic area directly above the root of the nose.
8. The **root** is commonly called the "bridge" of the nose.
9. The **septum** is the tissue that divides the nasal cavity into two nasal fossae.
10. The **anterior naris** is the nostril.
11. The **mental protuberance** of the mandible forms the chin.
12. The **angle of the mandible** is the lower posterior of the ramus.
13. The **zygomatic arch** creates the prominence of the cheek.

Recall

1. What are the nine regions of the face?

Skin

The skin of the face is thin to medium in relative thickness. It is soft and movable over a layer of loose connective tissue. The skin around the external ear and the ala of the nose is fixed to underlying cartilage. Facial skin contains many sweat and sebaceous glands. The connective tissue below the skin contains variable amounts of fat that smooth out the contours of the face, particularly between the muscles of facial expression (see Chapter 9). Located within the connective tissue are sensory and motor nerves of facial expression.

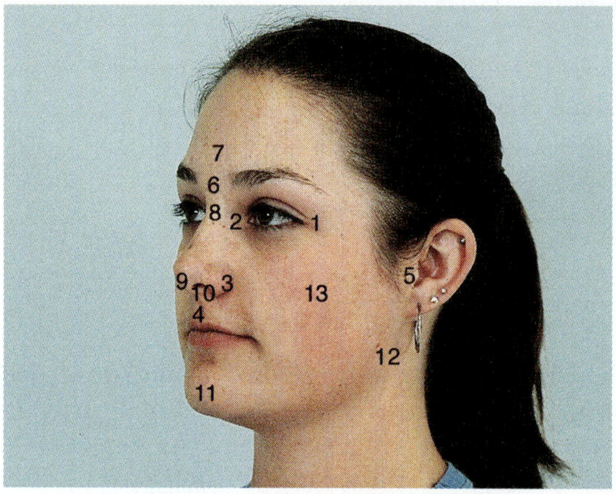

Fig. 10-2 Landmarks of the face.

Lips

The lips, also known as **labia,** provide the gateway to the oral cavity. They are formed externally by the skin and internally by mucous membrane (Fig. 10-3). The lips are outlined by the **vermilion border,** which is darker in color from the surrounding skin. Grasp your upper or lower lip between your thumb and forefinger to feel the pulsations of the labial branches of the facial artery.

The **labial commissure** is the angle at the corner of the mouth where the upper and lower lips join. The upper and lower lips are continuous at the angles of the mouth and blend with the cheeks.

The **nasolabial sulcus** is the groove extending upward between each labial commissure and nasal ala.

Recall

2. What is the area of color change around the border of the lips?

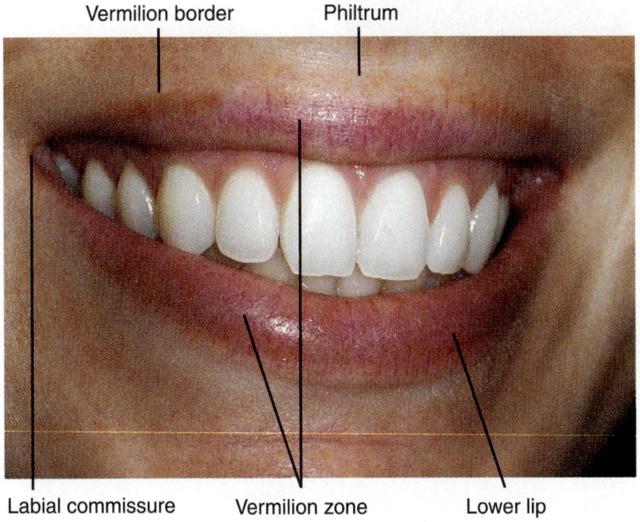

Fig. 10-3 Frontal view of the lips.

Clinical Considerations with the Lips

The dentist will examine the lips before examining the oral cavity because the lips may have a variety of lesions or diseases.

Normally, there is a distinct border between the lips and the surrounding skin of the face called the vermilion border. During a clinical examination, the dentist will look for any disappearance of the vermilion border of the lips. When this occurs, it could simply be caused by scar tissue from past injuries, or changes caused by exposure to the sun. However, changes in the vermilion border may also be associated with oral cancer. A biopsy is the only way to determine if the cells are cancerous.

An inflammation or cracking at the corners of the mouth could be a condition called **angular cheilosis,** which is associated with vitamin B deficiency. Herpes labialis, or cold sores, may be present on the lips and be very painful.

THE ORAL CAVITY

The entire oral cavity is lined with *mucous membrane* tissue. This type of tissue is moist and adapted to meet the needs of the area it covers.

The oral cavity consists of the following two areas:

1. The **vestibule** is the space between the teeth and the inner mucosal lining of the lips and cheeks.
2. The **oral cavity proper** is the space on the tongue side within the upper and lower dental arches.

Vestibules

The intraoral vestibule begins on the inside of the lips and then extends from the lips onto the alveolar process of both arches. The vestibules are lined with mucosal tissue (Fig. 10-4). The vestibular mucosa is thin, red, and loosely bound to the underlying alveolar bone. The base of each vestibule, where the buccal mucosa meets the alveolar mucosa, is termed the **mucobuccal fold** (Fig. 10-5).

There is a distinct line of color change in the tissue where the alveolar membrane meets with attached gingivae. This line is called the **mucogingival junction** (Fig. 10-6). The attached gingiva is a lighter color and has a stippled surface.

The inside surface of the cheeks forms the side walls of the oral cavity. The **buccal vestibule** is the area between the cheeks and the teeth or alveolar ridge. (*Buccal* means pertaining to the cheek.) A small elevation of tissue called the **parotid papilla** is located on the inner surface of the cheek on the buccal mucosa, just opposite the second maxillary molar. The parotid papilla protects the opening of the parotid duct (Stensen's duct) of the parotid salivary gland (see Fig. 10-5).

Fordyce's spots (or *granules*) are normal small yellowish elevations that may appear on the buccal mucosa. Another normal variation noted on the buccal mucosa is the **linea alba.** This white ridge of raised tissue extends horizontally at the level where the maxillary and mandibular teeth come together (Fig. 10-7).

Labial and Other Frenula

A *frenum*, or *frenulum* (plural *frenula*), is a narrow band of tissue that connects two structures. The *maxillary* **labial frenum** passes from the oral mucosa at the midline of the maxillary arch to the midline of the inner surface of the upper lip. The *mandibular labial frenum* passes from the oral mucosa at the midline of the mandibular arch to the midline of the inner surface of the lower lip.

In the area of the first maxillary permanent molar, the *buccal frenum* passes from the oral mucosa of the outer surface of the maxillary arch to the inner surface of the cheek. The **lingual frenum** passes from the floor of the mouth to the midline of the ventral border of the tongue (see Fig. 10-5).

Recall

3. What type of tissues cover the oral cavity?
4. What are the two regions of the oral cavity?
5. What is the name of the structure that passes from the oral mucosa to the facial midline of the mandibular arch?

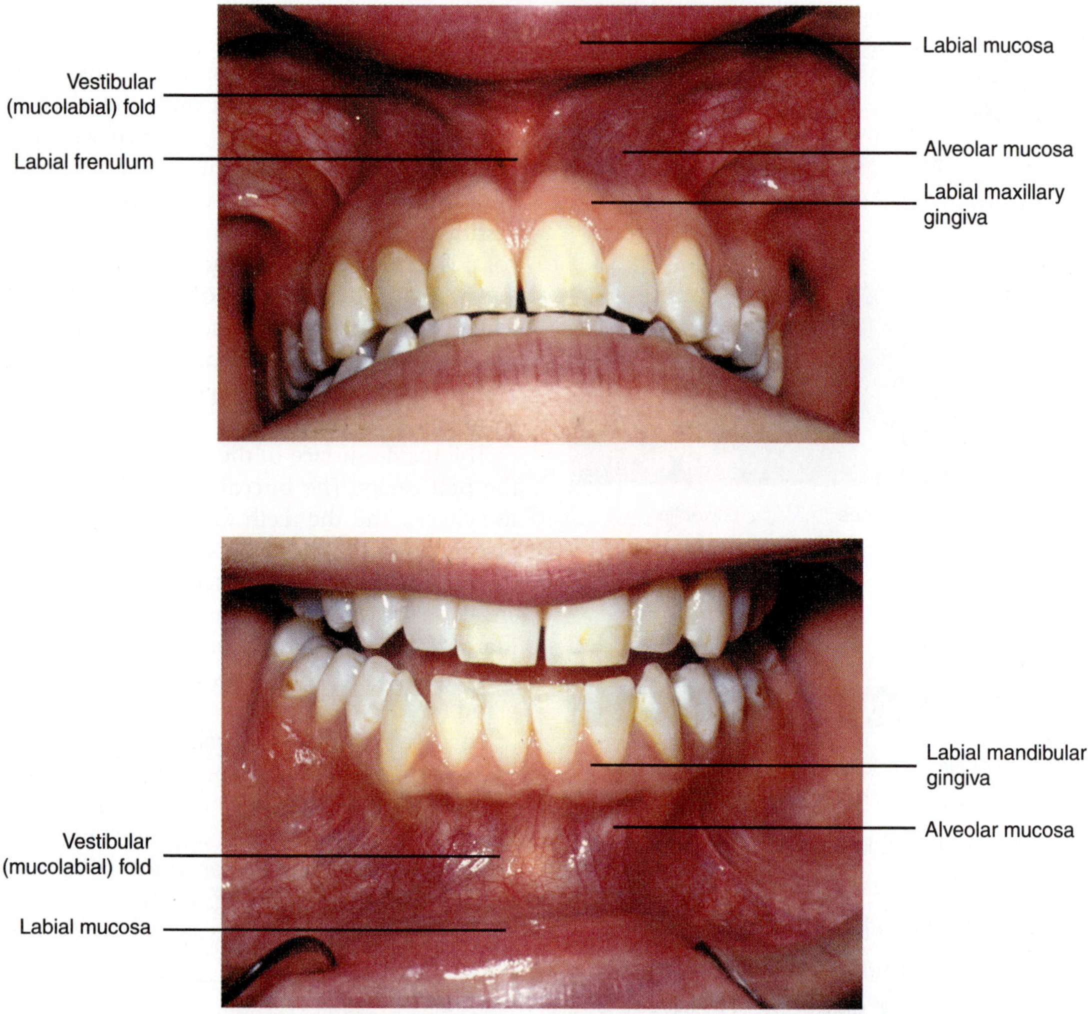

Fig. 10-4 Vestibule and vestibular tissue of the oral cavity. (From Liebgott B: *The anatomical basis of dentistry,* ed 2, St Louis, 2001, Mosby.)

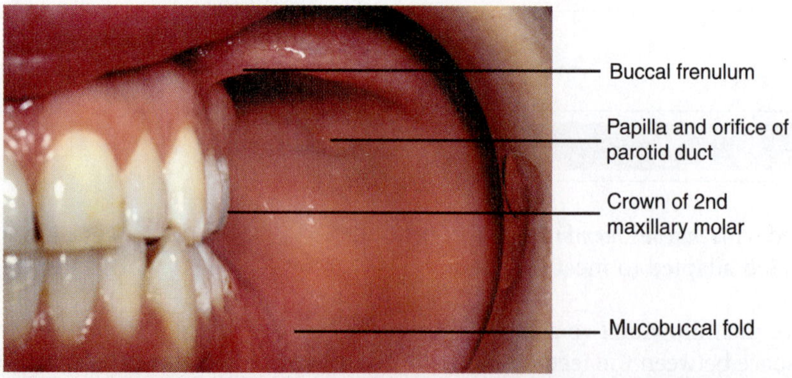

Fig. 10-5 Buccal vestibule and buccal mucosa of the cheek. The opening of the parotid duct is seen opposite the second maxillary molar. (From Liebgott B: *The anatomical basis of dentistry,* ed 2, St Louis, 2001, Mosby.)

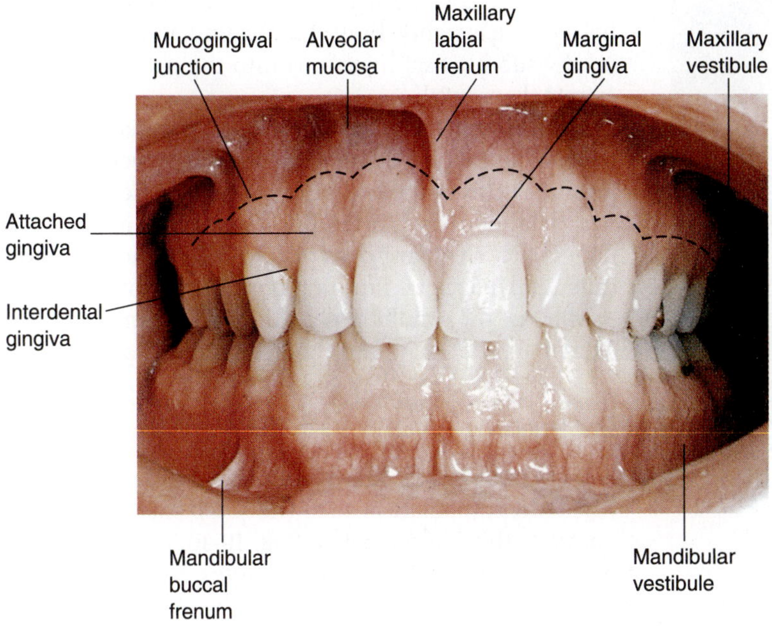

Fig. 10-6 View of gingivae and associated anatomic landmarks.

Gingiva

The **gingiva** (plural *gingivae*), commonly referred to as the "gums," is masticatory mucosa that covers the alveolar processes of the jaws and surrounds the necks of the teeth (see Fig. 10-6). Normal gingival tissue has the following characteristics:

- Gingiva surrounds the tooth like a collar and is self-cleansing.
- Gingiva is firm and resistant and tightly adapted to the tooth and bone.
- The surfaces of the attached gingiva and interdental papillae are stippled and resemble the rind of an orange.
- The color of the gingival surface varies according to the individual's pigmentation (Fig. 10-8).

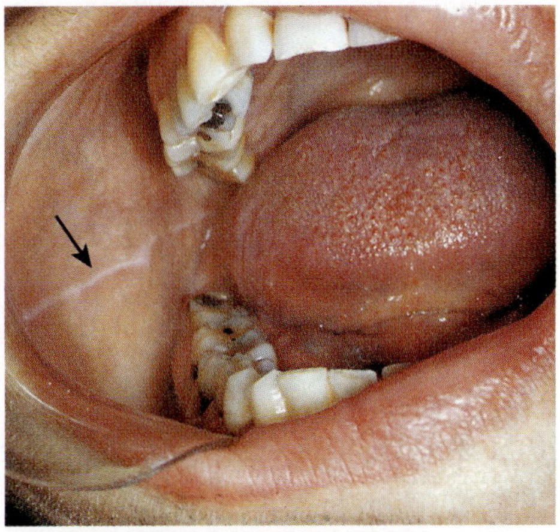

Fig. 10-7 **Linea alba.** (From Ibsen O, Phelan J: *Oral pathology for the dental hygienist,* ed 4, St Louis, 2004, Saunders.)

Unattached Gingiva

Unattached gingiva, also known as *marginal gingiva* or *free gingiva,* is the border of the gingiva surrounding the teeth in collarlike fashion (Fig. 10-9).

The unattached gingiva, which is usually light pink or coral, is not bound to the underlying tissue of the tooth. It consists of the tissues from the top of the gingival margin to the base of the gingival sulcus. The unattached gingiva is usually about 1 mm wide, and it forms the soft wall of the gingival sulcus. (The *sulcus* is the space between the tooth and the gum where popcorn husks become lodged.) The unattached gingiva is the first tissue to respond to inflammation.

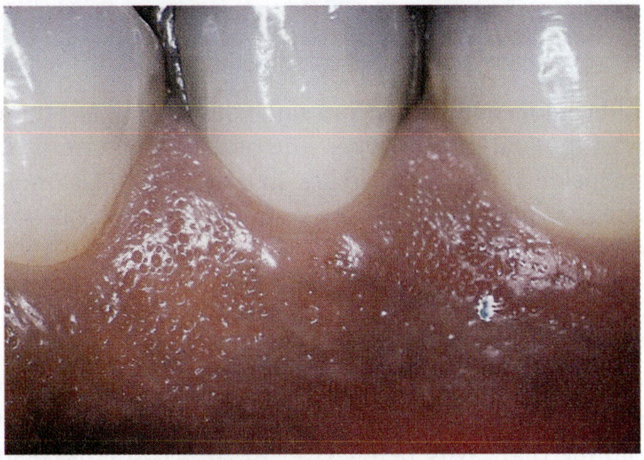

Fig. 10-8 It is normal for the color of the gingiva to vary according to the pigmentation of the individual.

Interdental Gingiva

The interdental gingiva, also known as *interdental papilla* (plural *papillae*), is the extension of the free gingiva that fills the interproximal embrasure between two adjacent teeth.

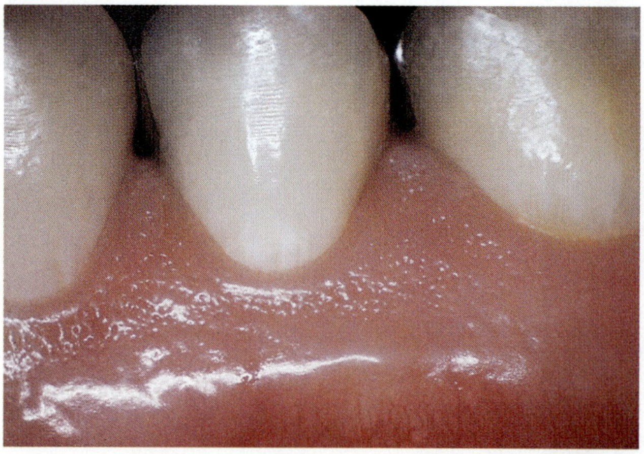

Fig. 10-9 Close-up view of gingivae and associated anatomic landmarks.

Gingival Groove

The gingival groove, also known as the *free gingival groove,* is a shallow groove that runs parallel to the margin of the unattached gingiva and marks the beginning of the attached gingiva.

Attached Gingiva

The attached gingiva extends from the base of the sulcus to the mucogingival junction. It is a stippled, dense tissue that is self-protecting, firmly bound, and resilient.

Recall

6. What is the anatomic term for the gums?
7. What is another term for unattached gingiva?
8. What is another term for interdental gingiva?

THE ORAL CAVITY PROPER

Hold your teeth together, and with your tongue, feel the areas of the oral cavity proper. The oral cavity proper is the area inside of the dental arches. In back of your last molar, there is a space that links the vestibule and the oral cavity proper.

Hard Palate

With your tongue, feel your hard palate, or roof of your mouth. The hard palate separates the nasal cavity above from the oral cavity below (Fig. 10-10, *A*). The nasal surfaces are covered with *respiratory mucosa,* and the oral surfaces are covered with *oral mucosa.* The mucosa of the hard palate is tightly bound to the underlying bone, which is why submucosal injections into the palatal area can be extremely painful.

Behind the maxillary central incisors is the **incisive papilla,** a pear-shaped pad of tissue that covers the incisive foramen. This is the site of injection for anesthesia of the nasopalatine nerve. Extending laterally from the incisive papilla are irregular ridges or folds of masticatory mucosa called palatal *rugae.* Running posteriorly from the incisive papilla is the midline palatal *raphe.* Numerous minor palatal glands open onto the palatal mucosa as small pits.

Soft Palate

Move your tongue to the back of your hard palate, and feel where the soft palate begins. The soft palate is the movable posterior third of the palate (Fig. 10-10, *B*). It has no bony support and hangs into the pharynx behind it. The soft palate ends with a pear-shaped hanging projection of tissue called the **uvula** (see Fig. 10-10, *B*).

The soft palate is supported posteriorly by two arches, the *fauces.* The *anterior arch* runs from the soft palate down to the lateral aspects of the tongue as the **anterior faucial pillar.** The *posterior arch* is the free posterior border of the soft palate and is called the **posterior faucial pillar** (Fig. 10-10, *B*). The opening between the two arches is called the **isthmus of fauces** and contains the palatine tonsil.

Recall

9. What is the pear-shaped pad of tissue behind the maxillary incisors?
10. What is the hanging projection of tissue at the border of the soft palate?

Tongue

The tongue is composed mainly of muscles. It is covered on top with a thick layer of mucous membrane and thousands of tiny projections called *papillae.* Inside the papillae are the sensory organs and nerves for both taste and touch. On a healthy tongue, the papillae are usually pinkish-white and velvety smooth.

The tongue is one of the body's most versatile organs and is responsible for a number of functions: (1) speaking, (2) positioning food while eating, (3) tasting and tactile sensations, (4) swallowing, and (5) cleansing the oral cavity. After eating, notice how your tongue moves from crevice to crevice, seeking out and removing bits of retained food in your mouth.

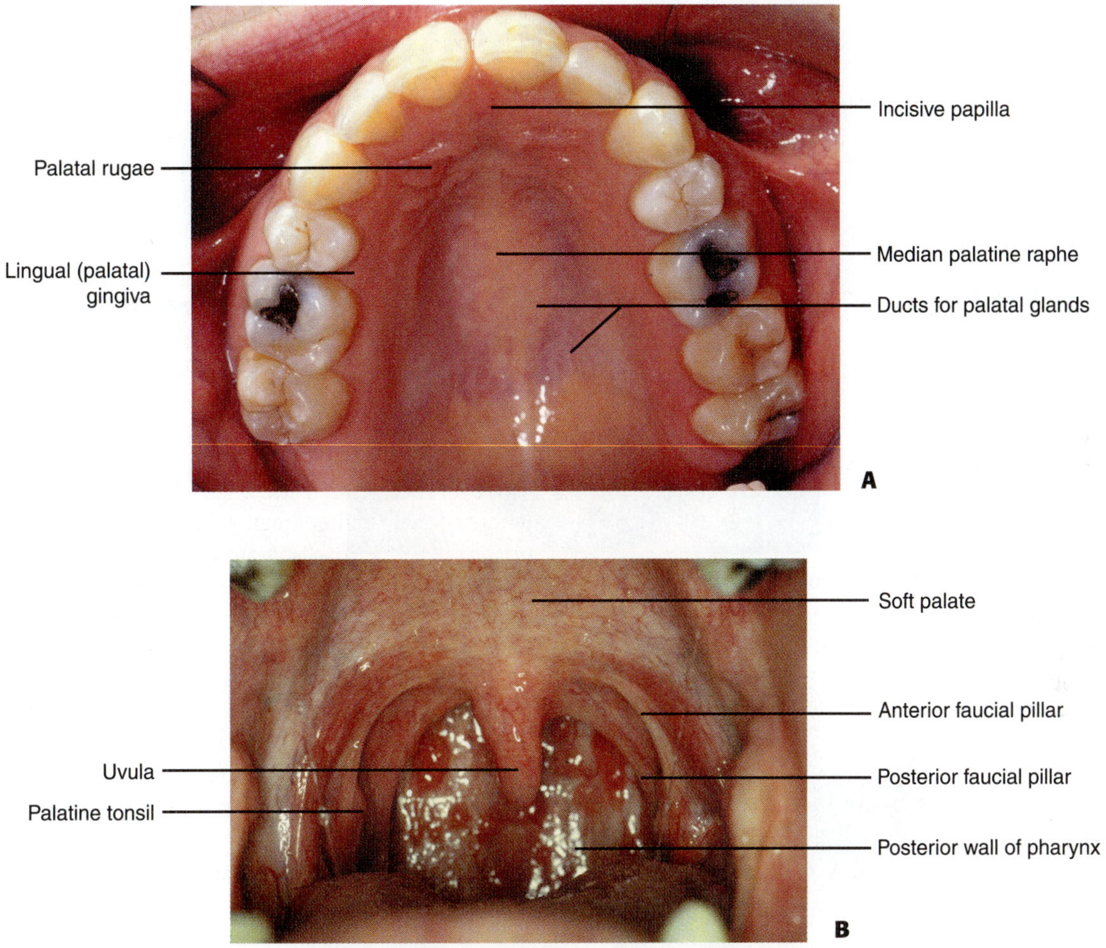

Fig. 10-10 A, Surface features of the hard palate. B, Surface features of the soft palate. (From Liebgott B: *The anatomical basis of dentistry,* ed 2, St Louis, 2001, Mosby.)

Clinical Considerations with the Gag Reflex

When working in a patient's mouth, the dental assistant must be very careful not to accidentally trigger the gag reflex. Touching the membranes of the soft palate, the fauces, and the posterior portion of the tongue can trigger the gag reflex and cause gagging or vomiting.

The anterior two thirds of the tongue, called the body, is found in the oral cavity. The *root* of the tongue is the posterior part that turns vertically downward to the pharynx. The *dorsum* is the superior (upper) and posterior roughened aspects of the tongue. It is covered with small papillae of various shapes and colors (Fig. 10-11).

The *sublingual surface* of the tongue is covered with thin, smooth, transparent mucosa through which many underlying vessels can be seen (Fig. 10-12). There are two small papillae on either side of the lingual frenulum (frenum) just behind the central incisors. Through these papillae into the mouth are the openings of the submandibular ducts. The saliva enters the oral cavity through these ducts. Salivary glands are discussed in detail in Chapter 9.

On either side of the lingual surface are two smaller *fimbriated folds.* The **lingual frenum** is the thin fold of mucous membrane that extends from the floor of the mouth to the underside of the tongue.

Recall

11. What is the term for the upper surface of the tongue?

12. What is the thin fold of mucous membrane that extends from the floor of the mouth to the underside of the tongue?

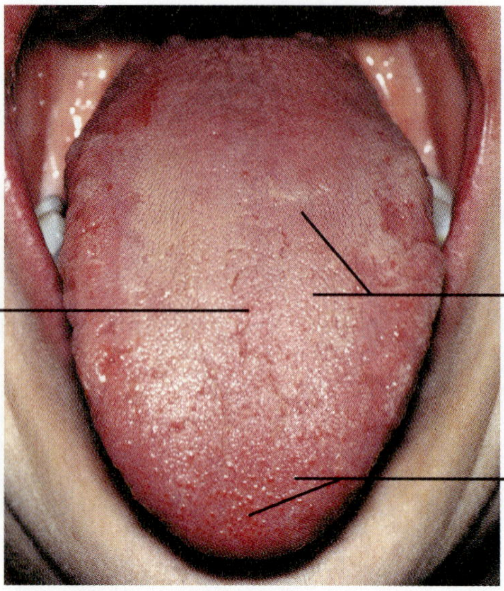

Fig. 10-11 Dorsum of the tongue. (From Liebgott B: *The anatomical basis of dentistry,* ed 2, St Louis, 2001, Mosby.)

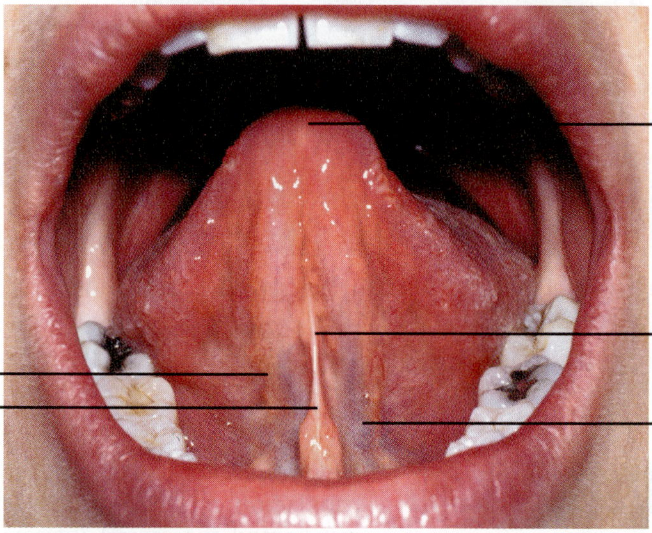

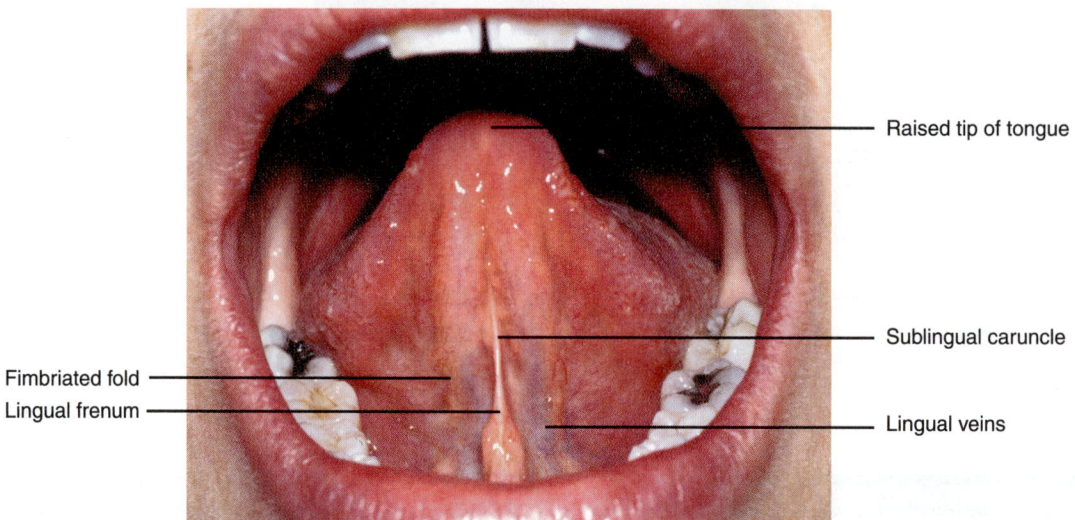

Fig. 10-12 Sublingual aspect of the tongue. (From Liebgott B: *The anatomical basis of dentistry,* ed 2, St Louis, 2001, Mosby.)

Clinical Considerations with the Lingual Frenula

The mobility of the tongue can be severely limited when the lingual frenum is unusually short. When this occurs, speech can be difficult for the patient, and performing dental procedures such as radiographs and impressions can be difficult for the operator. The condition is commonly called "tongue tied," and can be easily corrected with a surgical procedure called a lingual frenectomy in which the lingual frenulum is cut.

Taste Buds

The taste buds are the organs that allow us to enjoy the flavors of food and give us warning when foods are too hot. They are located on the dorsum (top side) of the tongue. Saliva is necessary to stimulate the taste buds to detect flavors. If your mouth were dry, you could not taste anything.

The taste buds are located on the **fungiform papillae** and in the trough of the large **vallate papillae,** which form a V on the posterior portion of the tongue. The sense of *touch* is provided by the numerous **filiform papillae** that cover the entire surface of the tongue. The filiform papillae do not contain any taste receptors.

Although there are thousands of flavors, it is believed that there are only four primary tastes that combine to create all flavors. These primary tastes are salty, sweet, sour, and bitter.

You may notice that some substances taste sweet when they enter the mouth but taste bitter by the time they reach the back. Saccharin is an example of one such substance. Of the four primary tastes, the one that is most easily distinguished is bitter. It is thought that this unmistakable taste serves as a protective mechanism. Many deadly toxins taste bitter, and a person spits them out before they can do harm.

Teeth

Humans have two sets of teeth during a lifetime. The teeth sit in bony sockets called *alveoli,* within the alveolar process of the maxilla and mandible. The portion of the tooth that is visible in the oral cavity is called the crown and is surrounded by a cuff of gingival tissue. Dental anatomy is discussed in detail in Chapters 11 and 12.

Eye to the Future

You can help prevent the early signs of aging by protecting your lips and the skin on your face from drying and chapping. Drying of the skin can be caused by soaps and detergents, dry indoor air, and exposure to sun or windy weather. Even the face masks you wear in the dental office can cause irritation to your face. You should gently pat, not vigorously rub, your skin dry after washing. Use emollient creams or lotions liberally and regularly to soften and moisturize your skin.

Critical Thinking

1. The dentist asked you to take an alginate impression of the maxillary and mandibular arches on Mr. Wong, but you are having a difficult time moving the patient's tongue out of the way to seat the impression tray. Mr. Wong tells you that he is "tongue tied." What does this mean?
2. Sixteen-year-old Letecia Williams is in your office complaining of a painful bump on her palate in back of her upper front teeth. She explained that she had eaten very hot pizza and burned the roof of her mouth. What is the normal oral landmark the pizza may have burned?
3. Thirteen-year-old Ronnie is curious about the sensation of taste. He asks you to explain how the tongue can taste sweet and sour. How would you answer?

11

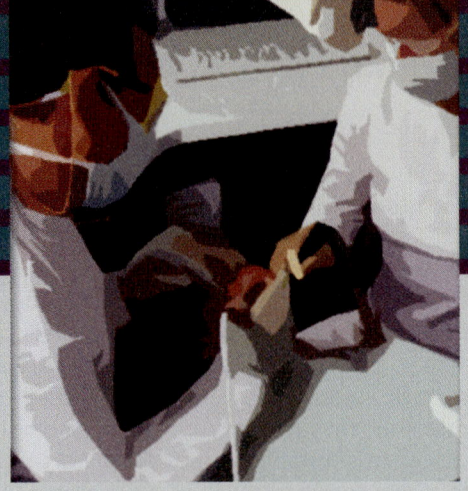

Overview of the Dentitions

Outline

Dentition Periods
- Primary Dentition
- Mixed Dentition
- Permanent Dentition

Dental Arches
- Quadrants
- Sextants
- Anterior and Posterior Teeth

Types and Functions of Teeth
- Incisors
- Canines
- Premolars
- Molars

Tooth Surfaces

Anatomic Features of Teeth
- Contours
- Contacts
- Height of Contour
- Embrasures

Angles and Divisions of Teeth
- Line and Point Angles
- Divisions into Thirds

Occlusion and Malocclusion
- Angle's Classification

Stabilization of the Arches
- Closure
- Curve of Spee
- Curve of Wilson

Tooth-Numbering Systems
- Universal/National System
- International Standards Organization System
- Palmer Notation System

Legal and Ethical Implications

Eye to the Future

Critical Thinking

KEY TERMS

Angle's classification System developed by Dr. Edward H. Angle, used to describe and classify occlusion and malocclusion.

Anterior Toward the front.

Apical third Division of the root nearest the tip of the root.

Buccal surface Tooth surface closest to the inner cheek.

Buccolingual division Lengthwise division of the crown in a labial or buccal-lingual direction, consisting of the *facial* or *buccal/labial* third, *middle* third, and *lingual* third.

Centric occlusion Maximum contact between the occluding surfaces of the maxillary and mandibular teeth.

Cervical third Division of the root nearest the neck of the tooth.

Concave Curved inward.

Contact area Area of the mesial or distal surfaces of a tooth that touches the adjacent tooth in the same arch.

Convex Curved outward.

Curve of Spee Curvature formed by the maxillary and mandibular arches in occlusion.

Curve of Wilson Cross-arch curvature of the occlusal plane.

Deciduous (di-**si**-jeh-wus) Pertaining to first dentition of 20 teeth, often called "baby teeth" or primary teeth.

Dentition (den-**ti**-shun) Natural teeth in the dental arch.

Distal surface Surface of tooth distant from the midline.

KEY TERMS—cont'd

Distoclusion A class II malocclusion in which the mesiobuccal cusp of the maxillary first molar occludes (by more than the width of a premolar) mesial to the mesiobuccal groove of the mandibular first molar.

Embrasure (im-**bray**-zhur) Triangular space in a gingival direction between the proximal surfaces of two adjoining teeth in contact.

Facial surface Tooth surface closest to the face. Facial surfaces closest to the lips are called *labial surfaces,* and facial surfaces closest to the inner cheek are called *buccal surfaces;* therefore, the term *facial* can be substituted for *labial* and *buccal,* and vice versa.

Functional occlusion Contact of the teeth during biting and chewing movements.

Incisal surface Chewing surface of anterior teeth.

Interproximal space (in-ter-**prok**-sih-mul) The area between adjacent tooth surfaces.

Labial surface Tooth surface closest to the lips.

Labioversion The inclination of the teeth to extend facially beyond the normal overlap of the incisal edge of the maxillary incisors over the mandibular incisors.

Line angle Junction of two walls in a cavity preparation.

Lingual surface Surface of mandibular and maxillary teeth closest to the tongue; also called *palatal surface.*

Linguoversion Position in which the maxillary incisors are behind the mandibular incisors.

Malocclusion (**mal**-o-*klu*-zhun) Occlusion that is deviated from a class I normal occlusion.

Mandibular arch (man-**dib**-you-ler) The lower jaw.

Masticatory surface (**mas**-ti-kah-*tor*-ee) The chewing surface of the teeth.

Maxillary arch (**max**-sah-lair-ee) The upper jaw.

Mesial surface Surface of the tooth toward the midline.

Mesioclusion (**me**-zee-o-*klu*-zhun) Term used for class III malocclusion.

Mesiodistal division Lengthwise division of the crown in a mesial-distal (front-to-back) direction, consisting of the *mesial* third, *middle* third, and *distal* third.

Middle third Division of the root in the middle.

Mixed dentition A mixture of permanent teeth and primary teeth that occurs until all primary teeth have been lost, usually between the ages of 6 and 12.

Neutroclusion An ideal mesiodistal relationship between the jaws and the dental arches.

Occlusal surface Chewing surface of posterior teeth.

Occlusion (oh-**klu**-zhun) The natural contact of the maxillary and mandibular teeth in all positions.

Occlusocervical division Crosswise division of the crown that is parallel to the occlusal or incisal surface and consists of the *occlusal* third, *middle* third, and *cervical* third.

Palatal surface Lingual surface of maxillary teeth.

Point angle Angle formed by the junction of three surfaces.

Posterior Toward the back.

Primary dentition The first set of 20 primary teeth.

Proximal surfaces The surfaces next to each other when teeth are adjacent in the arch.

Quadrant One quarter of the dentition.

Sextant One sixth of the dentition.

Succedaneous teeth (*suk*-se-**day**-ne-us) Permanent teeth that replace primary teeth.

LEARNING OUTCOMES

On completion of this chapter, the student will be able to achieve the following objectives:

- Pronounce, define, and spell the Key Terms.
- Explain how the size and shape of teeth determine the functions of different types of teeth.
- Name and identify the location of each tooth surface.
- Utilize terminology to identify landmarks of the teeth.
- Explain the differences between primary, mixed, and permanent dentitions.
- Explain the terms *occlusion, centric occlusion,* and *malocclusion.*
- Explain Angle's classification of malocclusion.
- Name and describe the three primary systems of tooth numbering.
- Identify teeth using the Universal/National system, the Palmer Notation System, and the ISO/FDI system.

In this chapter you will learn the names and location of the various types of teeth in the human dentition. You will also learn their functions and how they relate to each other in the same dental arch and to the teeth in the opposing arch. In preparation for learning dental charting, you will learn the common systems of tooth numbering, as well as the patterns of tooth eruption.

DENTITION PERIODS

During a lifetime people have two sets of teeth, the primary dentition and the permanent dentition. **Dentition** describes the natural teeth in the dental arch. Although there are only two sets of teeth, there are *three dentition periods.* These periods are *primary, mixed, and permanent.*

The first set of 20 primary teeth is called the **primary dentition,** commonly referred to as the "baby teeth." You may also hear the term **deciduous** dentition. This is an older and less frequently used dental term to describe the primary dentition.

The *permanent dentition* refers to the 32 secondary teeth, or "adult teeth." The permanent teeth that replace the primary teeth are called **succedaneous teeth,** meaning that these teeth "succeed" (come after) deciduous teeth. Because there are 20 primary teeth, there are also 20 succedaneous teeth. Molars are *not* succedaneous teeth because the premolars replace the primary molars.

The **mixed dentition** period takes place between ages of about 6 to 12 years of age. Until a child is about the age of 6, the primary dentition is in place. At about that same age, the first permanent teeth begin to emerge into the mouth and there is a mixture of permanent teeth and primary teeth until about age 12 when all the primary teeth have been lost (Table 11-1).

Primary Dentition

Only primary teeth are present in the mouth during the primary dentition period. This period occurs between approximately 6 months and 6 years of age (Table 11-2). The primary dentition period begins with the eruption of the primary mandibular central incisors and ends when the first permanent mandibular molar erupts (Fig. 11-1).

Mixed Dentition

While in the mixed dentition period, children lose their primary teeth, and the permanent teeth begin to erupt. During this period of time, children have both primary and permanent teeth in their mouth (Fig. 11-2). The mixed dentition period begins with the eruption of the first permanent tooth, and ends with the shedding of the last primary tooth.

The mixed dentition period is often a difficult time for children because color differences between the primary and permanent teeth become apparent (primary teeth are whiter than permanent teeth), and they may notice the difference in the crown size between the larger permanent teeth and the smaller primary teeth. Some children may notice crowding of the teeth as they shift positions during eruption.

Decisions regarding dental treatment are often based on the dentition period. For example, orthodontic treatment may be started or delayed because of the expected growth and expansion of the jawbones and movement of the teeth. Children experience noticeable changes in their facial contours as the jawbones begin to grow to accommodate the larger permanent teeth.

Permanent Dentition

The permanent dentition is adult dentition (Fig. 11-3). This period begins at about 12 years of age when the last primary tooth is shed (Box 11-1).

After eruption of the permanent canines and premolars, and the eruption of the second permanent molars, the permanent dentition is complete at about age 14 to 15, except for the third molars, which are not completed until about age 18 to 25. It includes eruption of all the permanent teeth, except for teeth that are congenitally (from the time of birth) missing or impacted and cannot erupt (usually the third molars). Growth of the jawbones slows and eventually stops. Minimal growth of the jaw occurs overall during the permanent dentition period because puberty has passed.

Table 11-1 ***Dentition Periods and Clinical Considerations***

Dental Period	Approximate Time Span	Teeth Marking Start of Period	Dentition Present	Growth of Jawbones
Primary dentition period	6 months to 6 years	Eruption of primary mandibular central incisor	Primary	Beginning
Mixed dentition	6 years to 12 years	Eruption of permanent mandibular first molar	Primary and permanent	Fastest and most noticeable
Permanent dentition period	After 12 years	Shedding of primary maxillary second molar	Usually permanent	Slowest and least noticeable

From Bath-Balogh M, Fehrenbach M: Illustrated dental embryology, histology, and anatomy, *Philadelphia, 1997, Saunders.*

Table 11-2 ***Primary Dentition in Order of Eruption***

Dentition	Date of Eruption	Date of Exfoliation
Maxillary Teeth		
Central incisor	6-10 months	6-7 years
Lateral incisor	9-12 months	7-8 years
First molar	12-18 months	9-11 years
Canine	16-22 months	10-12 years
Second molar	24-32 months	10-12 years
Mandibular Teeth		
Central incisor	6-10 months	6-7 years
Lateral incisor	7-10 months	7-8 years
First molar	12-18 months	9-11 years
Canine	16-22 months	9-12 years
Second molar	20-32 months	10-12 years

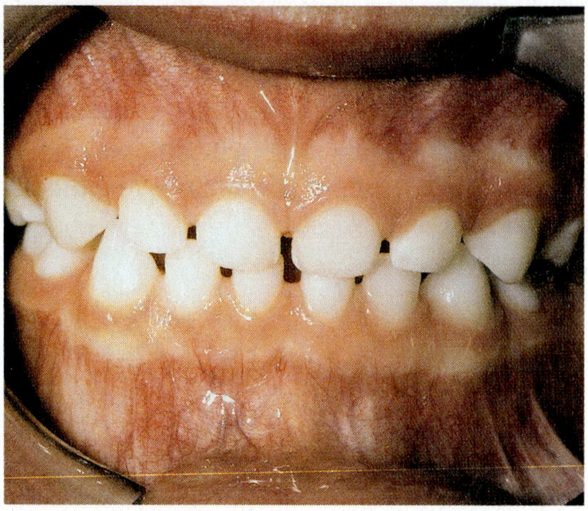

Fig. 11-1 Facial and buccal view of a primary dentition.

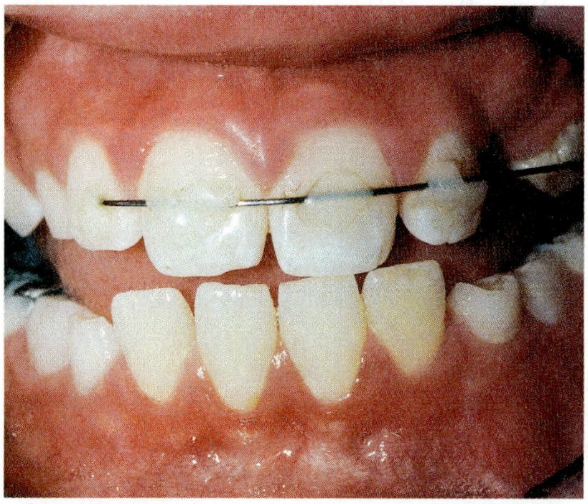

Fig. 11-2 Facial and buccal view of a mixed dentition.

Box 11-1 Permanent Dentition in Order of Eruption

Dentition	Eruption date
Maxillary teeth	
First molar	6-7 years
Central incisor	7-8 years
Lateral incisor	8-9 years
First premolar	10-11 years
Second premolar	10-12 years
Canine	11-12 years
Second molar	12-13 years
Third molar	17-21 years
Mandibular teeth	
First molar	6-7 years
Central incisor	6-7 years
Lateral incisor	7-8 years
Cuspid	9-10 years
First premolar	10-11 years
Second premolar	12-13 years
Second molar	11-13 years
Third molar	17-21 years

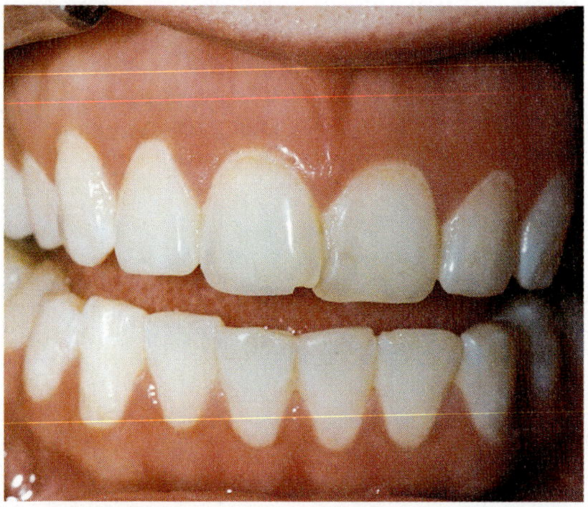

Fig. 11-3 Facial and buccal view of a permanent dentition.

DENTAL ARCHES

In the human mouth there are two dental arches, the maxillary and the mandibular. The layperson may refer to the maxillary arch as the upper jaw and the mandibular arch as the lower jaw.

- The **maxillary arch** *(upper arch)*, which is actually part of the skull, is not capable of movement. The teeth in the upper arch are set in the *maxilla*, the maxillary bone.
- The **mandibular arch** *(lower arch)* is movable through the action of the temporomandibular joint, and it applies force against the immovable maxillary arch (see Chapter 9).

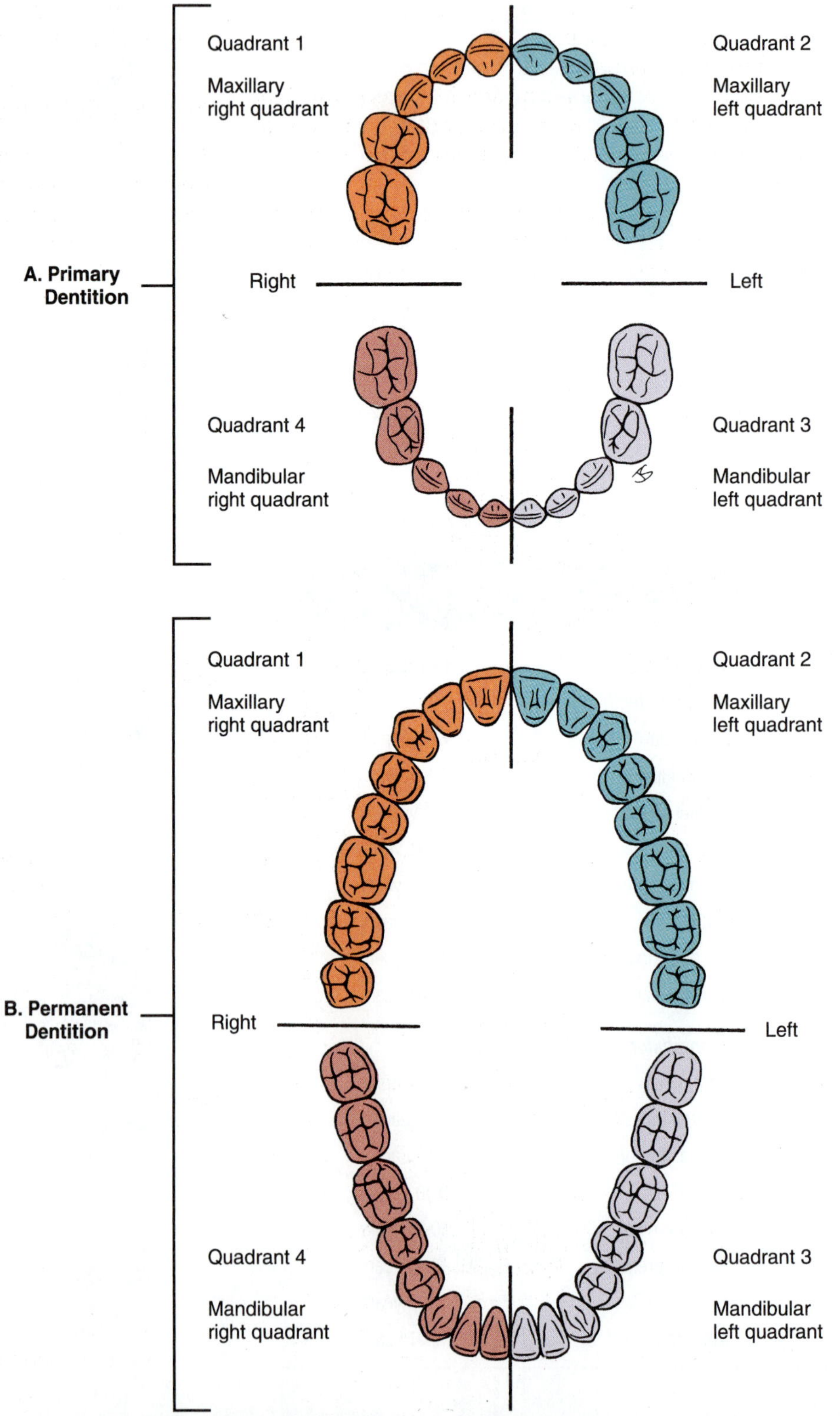

Fig. 11-4 A, Primary dentition separated into quadrants. B, Permanent dentition separated into quadrants. (From Finkbeiner B, Johnson C: *Comprehensive dental assisting,* St Louis, 1995, Mosby.)

When the teeth of both arches are in contact, the teeth are in *occlusion.*

Quadrants

When the maxillary and mandibular arches are each divided into halves, the resulting four sections are called **quadrants,** as follows:

1. Maxillary right quadrant
2. Maxillary left quadrant
3. Mandibular left quadrant
4. Mandibular right quadrant

Each quadrant of permanent dentition contains *eight* permanent teeth (4 × 8 = 32), and a quadrant of primary dentition contains *five* teeth (4 × 5 = 20) (Fig. 11-4).

As the dental assistant looks into the patient's oral cavity, the directions are reversed. This is the same concept as when two people face each other and shake hands.

Sextants

Each arch can also be divided into sextants rather than quadrants. A **sextant** is one sixth of the dentition. There are three sextants in each arch. The dental arch is divided as follows (Fig. 11-5):

1. Maxillary right posterior sextant
2. Maxillary anterior sextant
3. Maxillary left posterior sextant
4. Mandibular right posterior sextant
5. Mandibular anterior sextant
6. Mandibular left posterior sextant

Anterior and Posterior Teeth

To assist in describing their location and functions, the teeth are classified as being **anterior** (toward the front) or **posterior** (toward the back).

The anterior teeth are the incisors and canines. These are the teeth that are usually visible when people smile. The

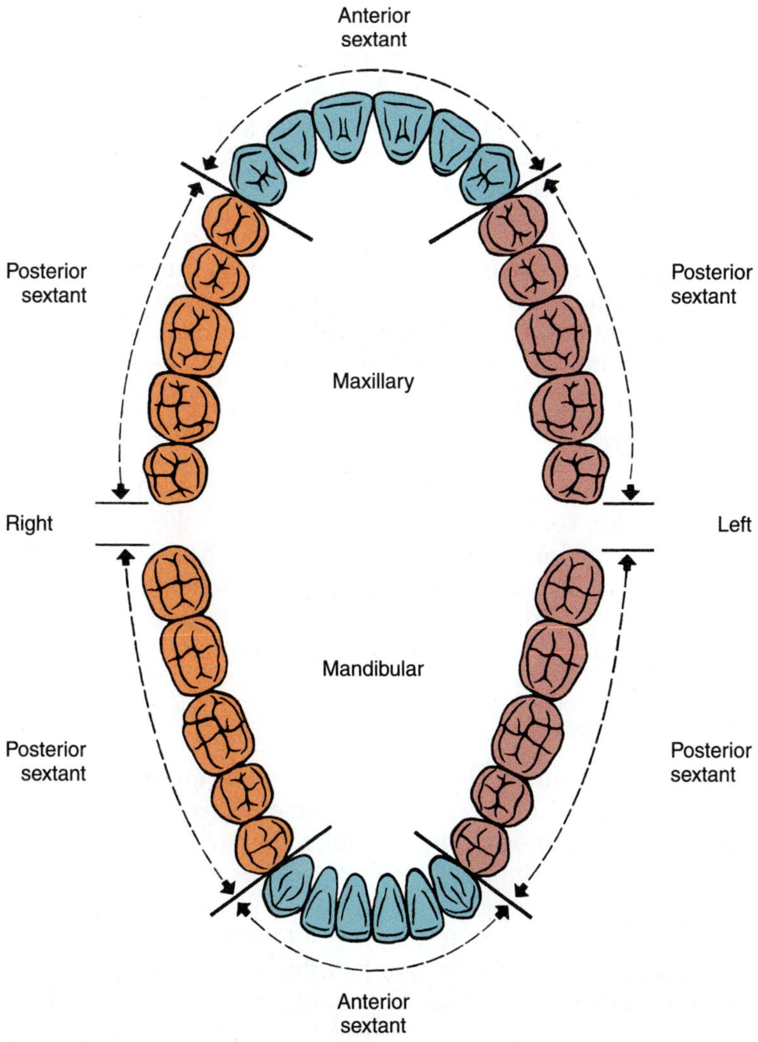

Fig. 11-5 Permanent dentition separated into sextants. (From Finkbeiner B, Johnson C: *Comprehensive dental assisting,* St Louis, 1995, Mosby.)

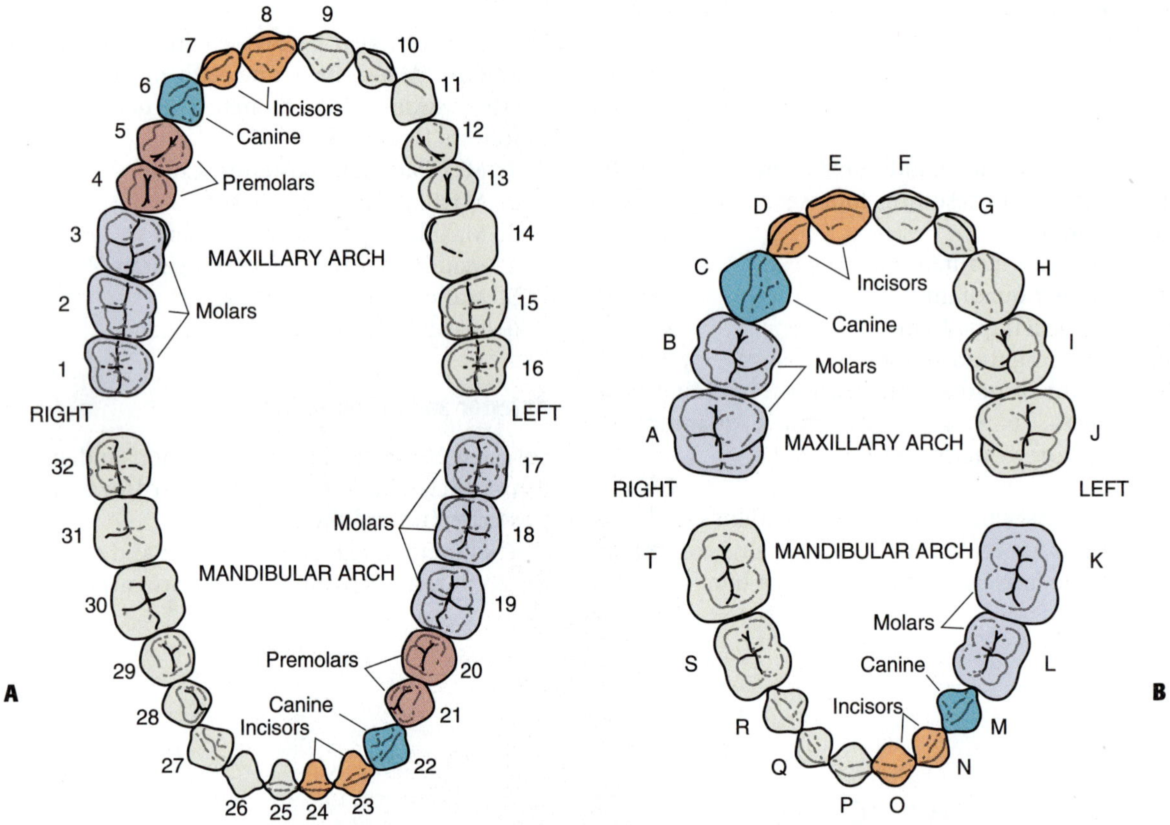

Fig. 11-6 A, Occlusal view of the permanent dentition. The types of teeth are identified using the Universal/National System. B, Occlusal view of the primary dentition. (From Bath-Balogh M, Fehrenbach MJ: *Illustrated dental embryology, histology, and anatomy,* ed 2, St Louis, 2005, Saunders.)

anterior teeth are aligned in a gentle curve. The posterior teeth are the premolars and molars. These teeth are aligned with little or no curvature and appear to be in an almost straight line. Remembering how these teeth are aligned in the dental arch will be important when you begin exposing radiographs.

Recall

1. What are the two sets of teeth that people have in their lifetime?
2. How many teeth are in each dentition?
3. What is the term for the four sections of the divided dental arches?
4. What are the terms for the front teeth and for the back teeth?

TYPES AND FUNCTIONS OF TEETH

Humans are omnivorous, which means they eat both meat and plants. To accommodate this variety in diet, human teeth are designed for cutting, tearing, and grinding different types of food.

The permanent dentition is divided into four types of teeth: *incisors, canines, premolars, and molars.* The primary dentition has incisors, canines, and molars. There are no premolars in the primary dentition (Fig. 11-6).

Incisors

Incisors are single-rooted teeth with a relatively sharp, thin edge. Located at the front of the mouth, they are designed to cut food without the application of heavy forces (an incisor is something that makes an incision, or cut). The tongue side, or lingual surface, is shaped like a shovel to aid in guiding the food into the mouth.

Canines

The canines, also known as cuspids, are located at the "corner" of the arch. They are designed for cutting and tearing foods, which require the application of force. These teeth in dogs are designed for tearing food or protecting themselves.

The canines are the longest teeth in the human dentition. They are also some of the best-anchored and most stable teeth because they have the longest root. Canines are usually the last teeth to be lost. Because of its sturdy crown, long root, and location in the arch, the canine is referred to as the "cornerstone" of the dental arch.

Premolars

There are four maxillary and four mandibular premolars. The premolars are a cross between canines and molars. You may hear the older term *bicuspids* used occasionally. This term is inaccurate because it refers to *two* ("bi") cusps, and some premolars have three cusps. Therefore the newer term *premolar* is preferred. The pointed buccal cusps hold the food while the lingual cusps grind it. Premolars are not as long as canines, and they also have a broader surface for chewing food. (There are no premolars in the primary dentition.)

Molars

Molars are much larger than premolars, usually having four or more cusps. The function of the 12 molars is to chew or grind up food. There are four or five cusps on the occlusal (biting) surface of each molar, depending on its location.

Maxillary and mandibular molars differ greatly from each other in shape, size, number of cusps, and roots. The unique characteristics of each tooth will be discussed in Chapter 12.

Recall

5. What are the four types of teeth?
6. Which tooth is referred to as the "cornerstone" of the dental arch?

TOOTH SURFACES

Imagine each tooth as being similar to a box with sides. Each tooth has five surfaces: (1) facial, (2) lingual, (3) masticatory (occlusal), (4) mesial, and (5) distal. Some surfaces of the tooth are identified by their relationship to other orofacial structures (Fig. 11-7).

The **facial surface** is the surface closest to the face. The facial surfaces closest to the lips are also termed **labial surfaces.** The facial surfaces closest to the inner cheek are also termed **buccal surfaces.** Therefore the term *facial* can be substituted for *labial* and *buccal,* and vice versa.

The **lingual surface** is the surface of mandibular and maxillary teeth that is closest to the tongue. The lingual surface of maxillary teeth may also be referred to as the **palatal surface,** because that surface is near the palate.

The **masticatory surface** is the chewing surface. On anterior teeth, it is the **incisal surface** (or *incisal edge*), and it is the **occlusal surface** for posterior teeth.

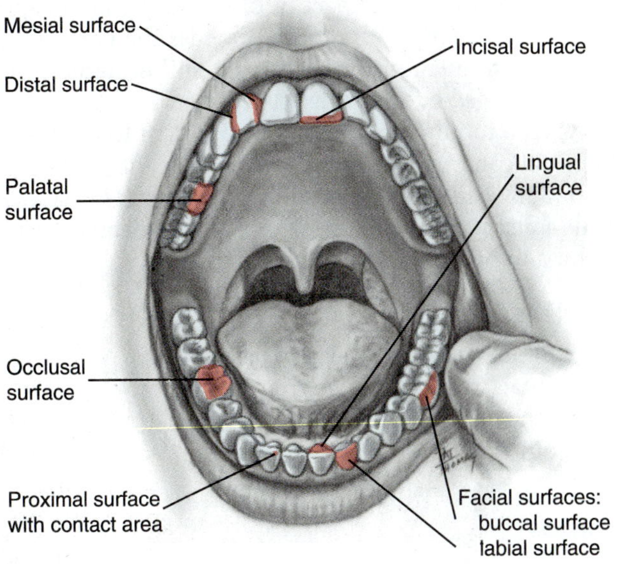

Fig. 11-7 **Surfaces of the teeth and their relationships to other oral cavity structures, to the midline, and to other teeth.** (From Bath-Balogh M, Fehrenbach MJ: *Illustrated dental embryology, histology, and anatomy,* ed 2, St Louis, 2005, Saunders.)

The **mesial surface** is the surface of the tooth *toward* the midline. The **distal surface** is the surface of the tooth *distant from* the midline.

When teeth are adjacent (next) to each other in the arch, the surfaces adjacent to each other are termed **proximal surfaces.** For example, the distal surface of the first molar and the mesial surface of the second molar are proximal surfaces. The area between adjacent tooth surfaces is called the **interproximal space.**

ANATOMIC FEATURES OF TEETH

All teeth have contours, contacts, and embrasures. These anatomic features of the teeth help to maintain their position in the arch and to protect the tissues during mastication.

Contours

All teeth have a curved surface except when the tooth is fractured or worn. Some surfaces are *convex* (curved outward); others are *concave* (curved inward). Although the general contours vary, the general principle that the *crown of the tooth narrows toward the cervical line* is true for all types of teeth.

Facial and Lingual Contours

The curvatures found on the facial and lingual surfaces provide natural passageways for food. This action protects the gingiva from the impact of foods during mastication. The normal contour of a tooth provides the gingiva with adequate stimulation for health, but still protects it from being damaged by food (Fig. 11-8, *A*).

When a tooth is restored, it is important to return it to a normal contour. With *inadequate contour,* the gingiva may be traumatized by food pushing against it (Fig. 11-8, *B*). With *overcontouring,* the gingiva will lack adequate stimulation and be difficult to clean (Fig. 11-8, *C*).

Mesial and Distal Contours

The contours of the mesial and distal surfaces provide normal contact and *embrasure* form. The contours tend to be self-cleansing and further contribute to self-preservation of the tooth.

Contacts

The **contact area** is the area of the mesial or distal surfaces of a tooth that touches the adjacent tooth in the same arch. The *contact point* is the *exact spot* at which the teeth actually touch each other. The terms *contact* and *contact area* are frequently used interchangeably to refer to the contact point.

The crown of each tooth in the dental arches should be in contact with its adjacent tooth or teeth. A proper contact relationship between adjacent teeth serves the following three purposes:

1. Prevents food from being trapped between the teeth.
2. Stabilizes the dental arches by holding the teeth in either arch in positive contact with each other.
3. Protects the interproximal gingival tissue from trauma during mastication.

Height of Contour

The height of contour is the "bulge," or widest point, on a specific surface of the crown. The contact areas on the mesial and distal surfaces are usually considered the height of contour on the proximal surfaces. The facial and lingual surfaces also have a height of contour (Fig. 11-9).

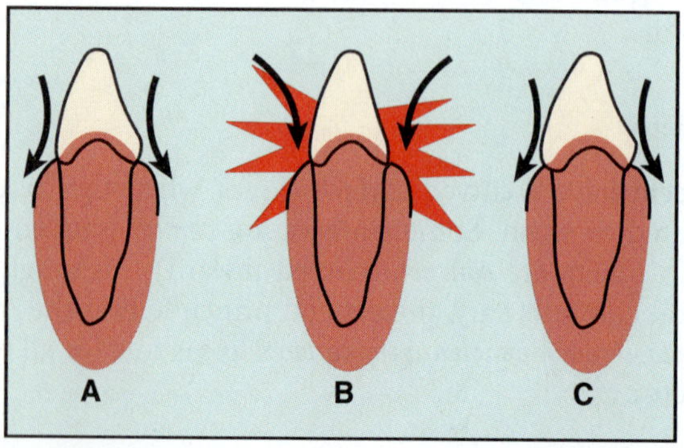

Fig. 11-8 Tooth contours. **A,** Normal contour. **B,** Inadequate contour. **C,** Overcontouring.

Embrasures

An **embrasure** is a triangular space near the gingiva between the proximal surfaces of two adjoining teeth. Embrasures are continuous with the interproximal spaces between the teeth. All tooth contours, including contact areas and embrasures, are important in the function and health of the oral tissues (Fig. 11-10).

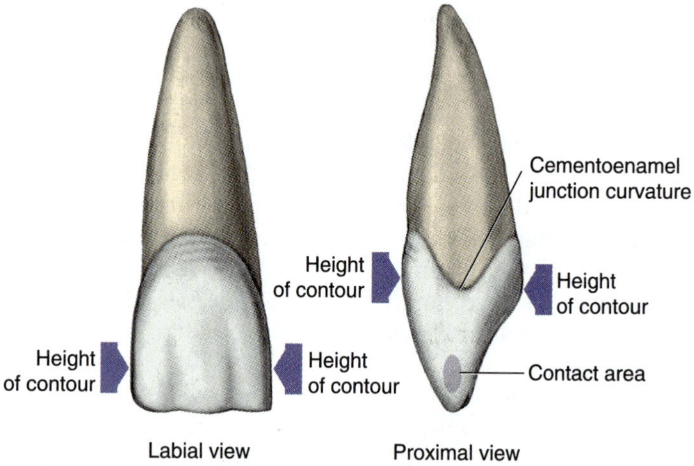

Fig. 11-9 Example of a permanent anterior tooth with the contact area and height of contour identified. (From Bath-Balogh M, Fehrenbach MJ: *Illustrated dental embryology, histology, and anatomy,* ed 2, St Louis, 2005, Saunders.)

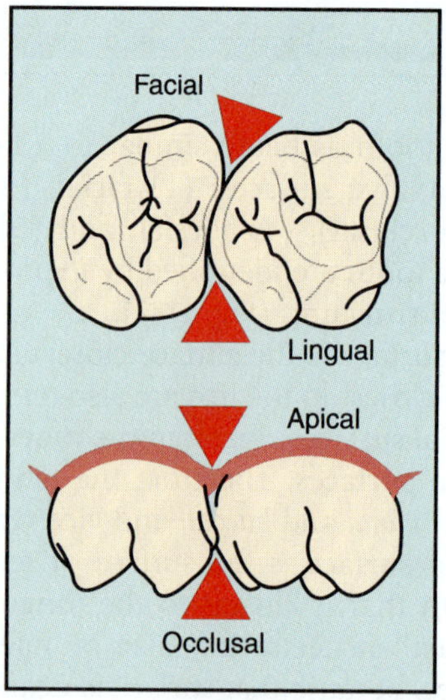

Fig. 11-10 Embrasures may diverge facially, lingually, occlusally, or apically.

Recall

7. What are the five surfaces of the teeth?
8. What is the name for the space between adjacent teeth?
9. What is the name of the area where adjacent teeth physically touch?
10. What is the name of the triangular space toward the gingiva between adjacent teeth?

ANGLES AND DIVISIONS OF TEETH

In order to better describe the teeth, the crowns and roots of the teeth have been divided into thirds, and junctions of the crown surfaces are described as **line angles** and **point angles.** Actually, there are no angles or points on the teeth. Line and point angles are used only as descriptive terms to indicate specific locations.

Line and Point Angles

A line angle is formed by the junction of two surfaces and derives its name from the combination of the two surfaces that join. For example, on an anterior tooth, the junction of the mesial and labial surfaces is called the *mesiolabial line angle* (Fig. 11-11).

A point angle is that angle formed by the junction of *three* surfaces at one point. These angles also get their name from the combination of names of the surfaces forming it. For example, the junction of the mesial, buccal, and occlusal surface of a molar is called the *mesiobuccoocclusal point angle.*

When combining these words, the last two letters of the first word are dropped and the letter *o* is substituted.

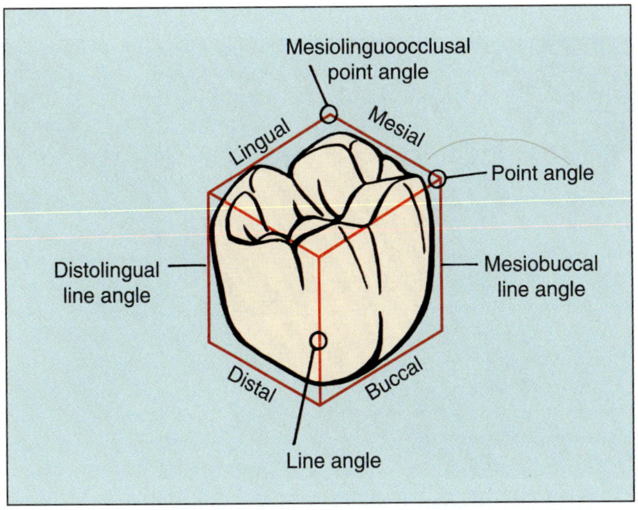

Fig. 11-11 Line and point angles.

Divisions into Thirds

To help identify a specific area of the tooth, each surface is divided into imaginary thirds (Fig. 11-12). These thirds are named according to the areas they approximate.

The *root* of the tooth is divided crosswise into thirds: the **apical third** (nearest the tip of the root), **middle third,** and **cervical third** (nearest the neck of the tooth).

The *crown* of the tooth is divided into thirds in three divisions:

1. **Occlusocervical division.** The crosswise division parallel to the occlusal or incisal surface. The occlusocervical division consists of the *occlusal* third, *middle* third, and *cervical* third.
2. **Mesiodistal division.** The lengthwise division in a mesial-distal (front-to-back) direction. The mesiodistal division consists of the *mesial* third, *middle* third, and *distal* third.
3. **Buccolingual division.** The lengthwise division in a labial or buccal-lingual direction. The buccolingual division consists of the *facial* or *buccal/labial* third, *middle* third, and *lingual* third.

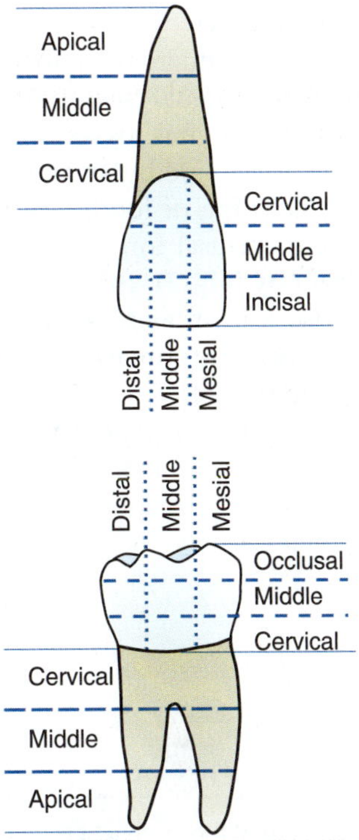

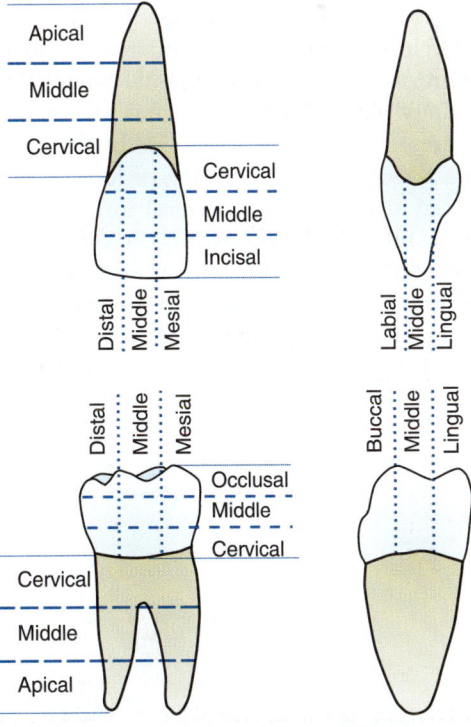

Fig. 11-12 An anterior tooth and a posterior tooth, with designations for crown and root thirds. (From Bath-Balogh M, Fehrenbach MJ, *Illustrated dental embryology, histology, and anatomy,* ed 2, St Louis, 2005, Saunders.)

Recall

11. What is the term for the junction of two tooth surfaces?
12. What is the name for the third of the tooth nearest the end of the root?

OCCLUSION AND MALOCCLUSION

Occlusion is defined as the relationship between the maxillary and mandibular teeth when the upper and lower jaws are in a fully closed position. Occlusion also refers to the relationship between the teeth in the same arch. Occlusion-related problems could affect the teeth, joints, and muscles of the head and neck and cause periodontal trauma.

Occlusion develops in a child as the primary teeth erupt. Habits such as thumb sucking or improper swallowing habits can affect the occlusion.

Proper occlusion of the erupting permanent teeth depends on the occlusion of the primary teeth as they are shed. Correction of improper occlusion is discussed in Chapter 60.

Centric occlusion occurs when the jaws are closed in a position that produces maximal stable contact between the occluding surfaces of the maxillary and mandibular teeth. In this position the condyles are in the most posterior, unstrained position in the glenoid fossa.

Centric occlusion serves as the standard for a normal occlusion. In normal occlusion, the lingual cusps of the posterior maxillary teeth fit into the central fossae of the occlusal surfaces of the posterior mandibular teeth. This positioning allows effective grinding of food. Centric occlusion widely distributes the occlusal forces and affords the greatest comfort and stability (Fig. 11-13).

Functional occlusion, also known as *physiologic occlusion,* is the term used to describe the contact of the teeth during biting and chewing movements.

Malocclusion refers to abnormal or malpositioned relationships of the maxillary teeth to mandibular teeth when they are in centric occlusion. Treatment of malocclusion is discussed in Chapter 60.

Recall

13. What is the name for the position of the teeth when they are in chewing movements?
14. What is the term for teeth that are in poor occlusion?

Angle's Classification

Angle's classification system was developed by Dr. Edward H. Angle to describe and classify occlusion and malocclusion. The basis of this system is that the *permanent maxillary first molar* is the key to occlusion. Angle's system assumes that a patient is occluding in a centric position (Table 11-3).

Class I

In class I, or **neutroclusion,** an ideal mesiodistal relationship exists between the jaws and the dental arches. The mesiobuccal cusp of the permanent maxillary first molar occludes with the mesiobuccal groove of the mandibular first molar.

Class I may include the situation in which the anterior or individual teeth are malaligned in their position in the arch. However, the relationship of the permanent first molars determines the classification.

Class II

In class II, or **distoclusion,** the mesiobuccal cusp of the maxillary first molar occludes (by more than the width of a premolar) mesial to the mesiobuccal groove of the mandibular first molar. The mandibular dental arch is in a *distal* relationship to the maxillary arch. This frequently gives the appearance of protrusion of the maxillary anterior teeth over the mandibular anterior teeth.

The major group of class II malocclusion has two subgroups, *division 1* and *division 2,* based on the position of the anterior teeth, shape of the palate, and resulting profile.

Division 1

The lips are usually flat and parted, with the lower lip tucked behind the upper incisors. The upper lip appears

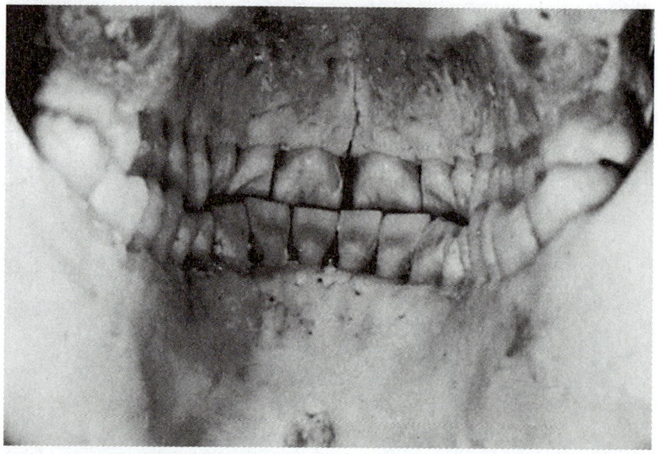

Fig. 11-13 Lingual view of the teeth in centric occlusion. (From Ash M, Nelson S: *Wheeler's dental anatomy, physiology, and occlusion,* ed 8, St Louis, 2003, Saunders.)

short and drawn up over the protruding anterior teeth of the maxillary arch.

Also in class II, division 1, the maxillary incisors are in **labioversion.** Labioversion is the inclination of the teeth to extend facially beyond the normal overlap of the incisal edge of the maxillary incisors over the mandibular incisors.

Division 2

Class II, division 2 includes class II malocclusions in which the maxillary incisors are *not* in labioversion. The maxillary central incisors are nearly normal anteroposteriorly, and they may be slightly in linguoversion. The maxillary lateral incisors may be tipped labially and mesially.

Linguoversion refers to the position of the maxillary incisors as being behind the mandibular incisors. Normally, the maxillary incisors slightly overlap the front of the mandibular incisors.

Class III

In a class III malocclusion, or **mesioclusion,** the body of the mandible must be in an abnormal *mesial* relationship to the maxilla. This frequently gives the appearance of protrusion of the mandible.

The mesiobuccal cusp of the maxillary first molar occludes in the interdental space between the distal cusp of the mandibular first permanent molar and the mesial cusp of the mandibular second permanent molar.

Recall

15. What is the technical term for class III malocclusion?
16. What classification is neutroclusion?

Table 11-3 ***Angle's Classifications of Malocclusion***

Class	Model	Arch Relationships	Descriptions
Class I	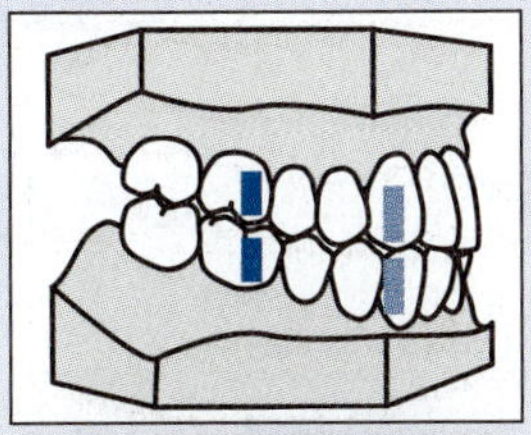	**Molar:** MB cusp of the maxillary first molar occludes with the MB groove of the mandibular first molar. **Canines:** Maxillary occludes with the distal half of the mandibular canine and the mesial half of the mandibular first premolar.	Dental malalignment(s) present (see text), such as crowding or spacing. Mesognathic profile.
Class II	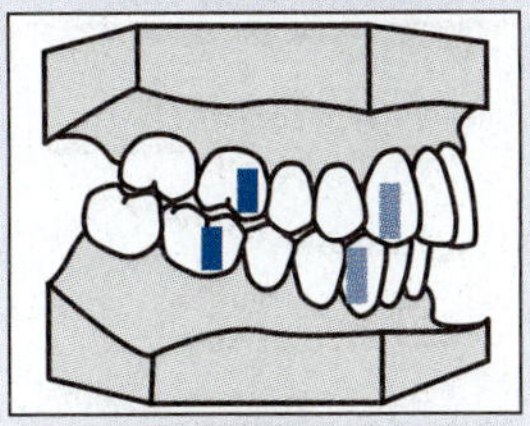 **Division 1**	**Molar:** MB cusp of the maxillary first molar occludes (by more than the width of a premolar) mesial to the MB groove of the mandibular first molar. **Canines:** Distal surface of the mandibular canine is distal to the mesial surface of the maxillary canine by at least the width of a premolar.	**Division 1:** Maxillary anteriors protrude facially from the mandibular anteriors, with deep overbite. Retrognathic profile.
	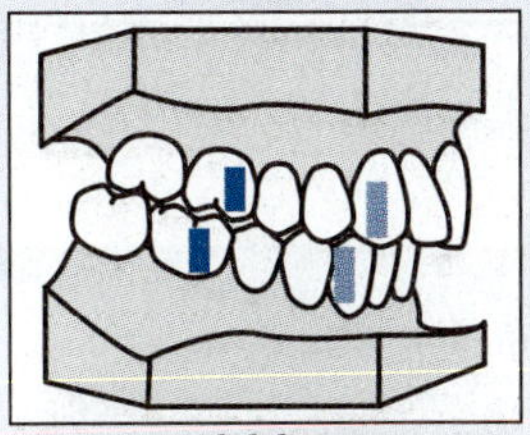 **Division 2**		**Division 2:** Maxillary central incisors are either upright or retruded, and lateral incisors are either tipped labially or overlap the central incisors with deep overbite. Mesognathic profile.
Class III	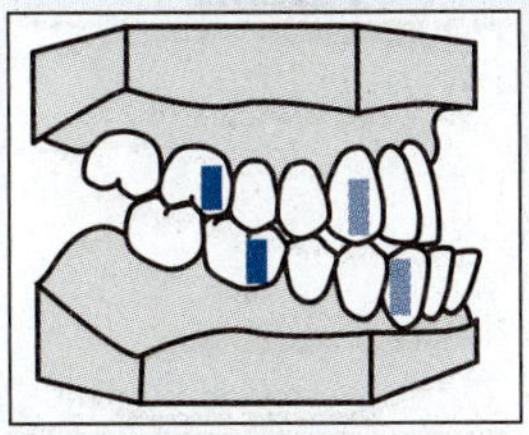	**Molar:** MB cusp of the maxillary first molar occludes (by more than the width of a premolar) distal to the MB groove of the mandibular first molar. **Canines:** Distal surface of the mandibular canine is mesial to the mesial surface of the maxillary canine by at least the width of a premolar.	Mandibular incisors in complete crossbite. Prognathic profile.

From Bath-Balogh M, Fehrenbach MJ: Illustrated dental embryology, histology, and anatomy, *ed 2, St Louis, 2005, Saunders.*
NOTE: This system deals with the classification of the permanent dentition.
MB, *mesiobuccal.*

STABILIZATION OF THE ARCHES

In a healthy mouth with properly maintained dentition, the dental arches will remain stable and efficient. However, malocclusion or the loss of one or more teeth may greatly reduce the functioning and stability of the dentition (Fig. 11-14).

Closure

The anterior teeth are not designed to support fully the occlusal forces on the entire dental arch; therefore, as the jaws close, the stronger posterior teeth come together first. After they have assumed most of the load, the more delicate anterior teeth come together.

Curve of Spee

The occlusal surfaces of the posterior teeth do not form a flat plane. Those of the mandibular arch form a slightly curved plane, which appears **concave** (curved inward, like the inside of a bowl). The maxillary arch forms a curved plane that appears **convex** (curved outward, like the outside of a bowl). The curvature formed by the maxillary and mandibular arches in occlusion is known as the **curve of Spee** (Fig. 11-15, *A*). On a radiograph, the occlusal line of the teeth appears to be smiling.

Curve of Wilson

The **curve of Wilson** is the cross-arch curvature of the posterior occlusal plane. The downward curvature of the arc is defined by a line drawn across the occlusal surface of the left mandibular first molar, extending across the arch and through the occlusal surface of the right mandibular first molar (Fig. 11-15, *B*).

Recall

17. What is the name for the curve of the occlusal plane?

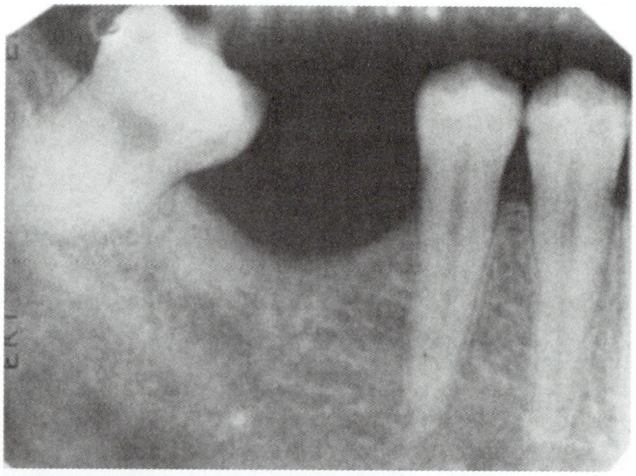

Fig. 11-14 Radiograph showing the mesial drift of the mandibular second molar after the first molar has been lost.

A

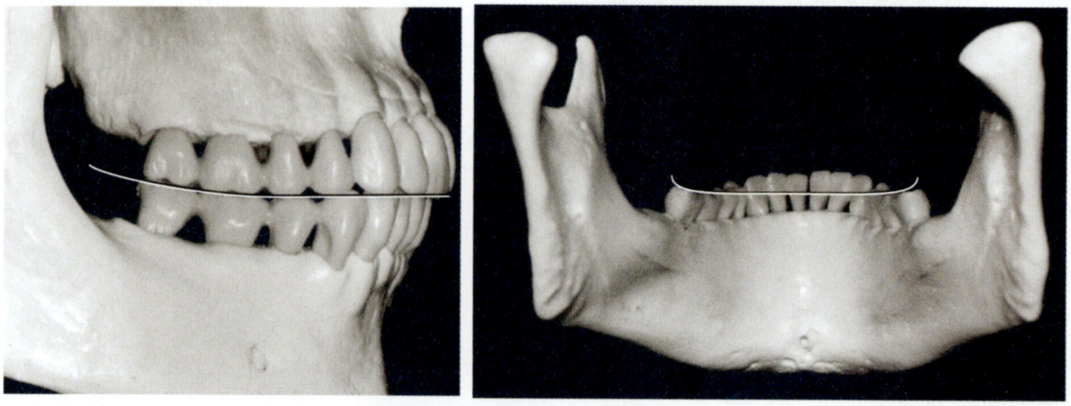

B

Fig. 11-15 Curves noted in the dental arch. **A,** Curve of Spee. **B,** Curve of Wilson. (From Bath-Balogh M, Fehrenbach MJ: *Illustrated dental embryology, histology, and anatomy,* ed 2, St Louis, 2005, Saunders.)

TOOTH-NUMBERING SYSTEMS

Numbering systems are used as a simplified means of identifying the teeth for charting and descriptive purpose. Three basic numbering systems are used, and the dental assistant must be familiar with each system (Table 11-4).

Universal/National System

The system most often used in the United States is the Universal/National System, approved by the American Dental Association (ADA) in 1968. In the Universal/National system, the permanent teeth are numbered from 1 to 32. Numbering begins with the upper-right third molar (tooth #1), works around to the upper-left third molar (tooth #16), drops to the lower-left third molar (tooth #17), and works around to the lower-right third molar (tooth #32) (see Fig. 11-6, *A*).

The primary teeth are lettered with capital letters from *A* to *T*. Lettering begins with the upper-right second primary molar (tooth A), works around to the upper-left second primary molar (tooth J), drops to the lower-left second primary molar (tooth K), and works around to the lower-right second primary molar (tooth *T*) (see Fig. 11-6, *B*).

Table 11-4 ***Tooth Designation Systems***

Tooth Name	Universal System	ISO/FDI System	Palmer Method
Permanent Dentition			
Maxillary teeth			
Maxillary right third molar	1	18	8┘
Maxillary right second molar	2	17	7┘
Maxillary right first molar	3	16	6┘
Maxillary right second premolar	4	15	5┘
Maxillary right first premolar	5	14	4┘
Maxillary right canine	6	13	3┘
Maxillary right lateral incisor	7	12	2┘
Maxillary right central incisor	8	11	1┘
Maxillary left central incisor	9	21	└1
Maxillary left lateral incisor	10	22	└2
Maxillary left canine	11	23	└3
Maxillary left first premolar	12	24	└4
Maxillary left second premolar	13	25	└5
Maxillary left first molar	14	26	└6
Maxillary left second molar	15	27	└7
Maxillary left third molar	16	28	└8
Mandibular teeth			
Mandibular left third molar	17	38	┌8
Mandibular left second molar	18	37	┌7
Mandibular left first molar	19	36	┌6
Mandibular left second premolar	20	35	┌5
Mandibular left first premolar	21	34	┌4
Mandibular left canine	22	33	┌3

Continued

Table 11-4 Tooth Designation Systems—cont'd

Tooth Name	Universal System	ISO/FDI System	Palmer Method
Permanent Dentition, cont'd			
Mandibular teeth, cont'd			
Mandibular left lateral incisor	23	32	┌2
Mandibular left central incisor	24	31	┌1
Mandibular right central incisor	25	41	1┐
Mandibular right lateral incisor	26	42	2┐
Mandibular right canine	27	43	3┐
Mandibular right first premolar	28	44	4┐
Mandibular right second premolar	29	45	5┐
Mandibular right first molar	30	46	6┐
Mandibular right second molar	31	47	7┐
Mandibular right third molar	32	48	8┐
Primary Dentition			
Maxillary teeth			
Maxillary right second molar	A	55	E┘
Maxillary right first molar	B	54	D┘
Maxillary right canine	C	53	C┘
Maxillary right lateral incisor	D	52	B┘
Maxillary right central incisor	E	51	A┘
Maxillary left central incisor	F	61	└A
Maxillary left lateral incisor	G	62	└B
Maxillary left canine	H	63	└C
Maxillary left first molar	I	64	└D
Maxillary left second molar	J	65	└E
Mandibular teeth			
Mandibular left second molar	K	75	┌E
Mandibular left first molar	L	74	┌D
Mandibular left canine	M	73	┌C
Mandibular left lateral incisor	N	72	┌B
Mandibular left central incisor	O	71	┌A
Mandibular right central incisor	P	81	A┐
Mandibular right lateral incisor	Q	82	B┐
Mandibular right canine	R	83	C┐
Mandibular right first molar	S	84	D┐
Mandibular right second molar	T	85	E┐

From Bath-Balogh M, Fehrenbach MJ: Illustrated dental embryology, histology, and anatomy, *ed 2, St Louis, 2005, Saunders.*

International Standards Organization System

To meet the needs for a numbering system that could be used internationally as well as by electronic data transfer, the World Health Organization accepted the International Standards Organization (ISO) system for teeth. In 1996 the ADA also accepted the ISO system in addition to the Universal/National system. The ISO system is based on the Fédération Dentaire Internationale (FDI) system and is used in most other countries.

The ISO/FDI system uses a two-digit tooth-recording system. The first digit indicates the quadrant, and the second digit indicates the tooth within the quadrant, with numbering from the midline toward the posterior. The permanent teeth are numbered as follows:

- The maxillary right quadrant is digit 1 and contains teeth #11 to #18.
- The maxillary left quadrant is digit 2 and contains teeth #21 to #28.
- The mandibular left quadrant is digit 3 and contains teeth #31 to #38.
- The mandibular right quadrant is digit 4 and contains teeth #41 to #48.

The primary teeth are numbered as follows:

- The maxillary right quadrant is digit 5 and contains teeth #51 to #55.
- The maxillary left quadrant is digit 6 and contains teeth #61 to #65.
- The mandibular left quadrant is digit 7 and contains teeth #71 to #75.
- The mandibular right quadrant is digit 8 and contains teeth #81 to #85.

The digits should be pronounced separately. For example, the permanent canines are teeth #1-3 ("number one-three"), #2-3 ("number two-three"), #3-3 ("number three-three"), and #4-3 ("number four-three").

To avoid miscommunication internationally, the ISO/FDI system also has designation of areas in the oral cavity (Box 11-2). A two-digit number designates these, and at least one of the two digits is zero (0). In this system, for example, 00 ("zero-zero") designates the whole oral cavity, and 01 ("zero-one") indicates the maxillary area only.

Box 11-2 ISO/FDI System for Designations of Oral Cavity

Oral cavity region	Designation
Whole oral cavity	00
Maxillary area	01
Mandibular area	02
Upper right quadrant	10
Upper left quadrant	20
Lower left quadrant	30
Lower right quadrant	40
Upper right sextant	03
Upper anterior sextant	04
Upper left sextant	05
Lower left sextant	06
Lower anterior sextant	07
Lower right sextant	08

Palmer Notation System

In the Palmer Notation System, each of the four quadrants is given its own tooth bracket made up of a vertical line and a horizontal line (Fig. 11-16). The Palmer method is a shorthand diagram of the teeth as if viewing the patient's teeth from the outside. The teeth in the right quadrant would have the vertical midline bracket to the right of the tooth numbers or letters, just as when looking at the patient. The midline is to the right of the teeth in the right quadrant.

Examples of Palmer Notation System

Maxillary right lateral incisor 2┘
Maxillary left first premolar └4
Mandibular right third molar 8┐
Mandibular left central incisor ┌1

For example, if the tooth is a maxillary tooth, the number or letter should be written above the horizontal line of the bracket, thus indicating an upper tooth. Conversely, a mandibular tooth symbol should be placed below the line, indicating a lower tooth.

The number or letter assigned to each tooth depends on its position relative to the midline. For example, central incisors, the teeth closest to the midline, have the lowest number 1 for permanent teeth and the letter A for primary teeth. All central incisors, maxillary and mandibular, are given the number 1. All lateral incisors are given the number 2, all canines are given the number 3, premolars are numbers 4 and 5, molars are 6 and 7, and the third molars are number 8.

The Palmer Notation System for Permanent Teeth

Maxillary Right	Maxillary Left
8 7 6 5 4 3 2 1	1 2 3 4 5 6 7 8
8 7 6 5 4 3 2 1	1 2 3 4 5 6 7 8
Mandibular Right	Mandibular Left

Tooth Numbers	
Central incisors	#1
Lateral incisors	#2
Canines	#3
1st premolar	#4
2nd premolar	#5
1st molar	#6
2nd molar	#7
3rd molar	#8

Examples of Charting

- 1┘ Maxillary right central incisor
- 2┐ Mandibular right lateral incisor
- └4 Maxillary left first premolar
- ┌8 Mandibular left third molar

The Palmer Notation System for Primary Teeth

Maxillary Right	Maxillary Left
E D C B A	A B C D E
E D C B A	A B C D E
Mandibular Right	Mandibular Left

Examples of Charting

- A┘ Maxillary right central incisor
- B┐ Mandibular right lateral incisor
- └C Maxillary left canine
- ┌D Mandibular left first primary molar

Tooth Letters	
Central incisors	A
Lateral incisors	B
Canines	C
1st primary molar	D
2nd primary molar	E

Fig. 11-16 Palmer Notation System.

Legal and Ethical Implications

Extreme care must be taken when entering tooth numbers on records or carrying out verbal instructions regarding a specific tooth. Errors have resulted in the extraction of the wrong tooth.

Remember that all dental records are legal documents. Learn the charting systems, and make your charting entries accurately. You may have to explain them in a court of law.

Eye to the Future

Primary teeth hold a substantial supply of stem cells in their dental pulp. Scientists at the National Institute of Dental and Craniofacial Research found that the stem cells stay alive in the tooth for a brief period after it is outside of the child's mouth. This creates the possibility of collecting these cells for research.

Stem cells may help repair damage to major organs, encourage bone regeneration, and cause specialized dentin formation. This research was published in the online version of *Proceedings of the National Academy of Sciences.*

Critical Thinking

1. While you are taking radiographs of 6-year-old Melissa's teeth, her mother expresses concern that Melissa's erupting permanent teeth look yellow compared to her nice white baby teeth. What could you say to Melissa's mother about her child's teeth?
2. You and another dental assistant are planning to speak to a group of young mothers about dental health and the importance of primary teeth. What information would you include in your presentation about primary teeth?
3. Dr. Ortega asks you to take a radiograph of tooth letters K and T. Which teeth are these?
4. Dr. Lane has just extracted the maxillary left third molar and the mandibular left third molar. What Universal tooth numbers would you enter on the insurance form?

12

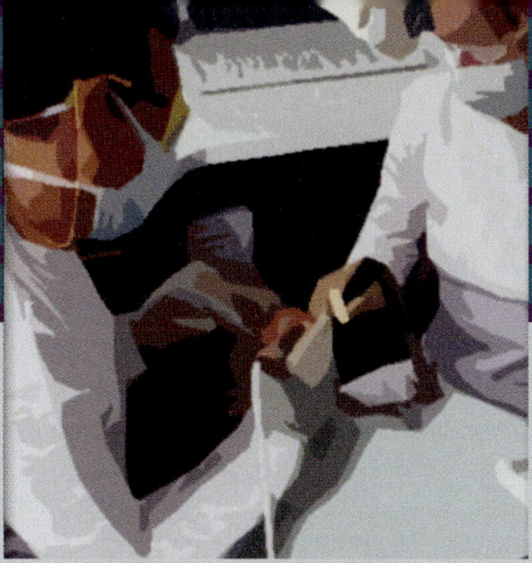

Tooth Morphology

Outline

Anterior Permanent Dentition
- Permanent Incisors
- Permanent Canines

Posterior Permanent Dentition
- Permanent Premolars
- Permanent Molars

Primary Dentition
- Primary Incisors
- Primary Canines
- Primary Molars

Eye to the Future

Critical Thinking

KEY TERMS

Bicanineate A two-cusp type of mandibular second premolar.

Bifurcated Divided into two.

Bifurcation Area in which two roots divide.

Canine eminence (**em**-ih-nen[t]s) External vertical bony ridge on the labial surface of the canines.

Central groove Most prominent developmental groove on posterior teeth.

Cingulum (**sin[g]**-gu-lum) Raised, rounded area on the cervical third of the lingual surface.

Cusp Major elevation on the masticatory surface of canines and posterior teeth.

Cusp of Carabelli The fifth supplemental cusp found lingual to the mesiolingual cusp.

Diastema (*dye*-uh-**stee**-muh) A space between two teeth.

Fossa (**fos**-ah, **faw**-seh) Wide, shallow depression on the lingual surface of anterior teeth.

Furcation (fur-**kay**-shun) Area between two or more root branches.

Imbrication lines (im-breh-**kay**-shun) Slight ridges that run mesiodistally in the cervical third of teeth.

Incisal edge Ridge on permanent incisors that appears flattened on labial, lingual, or incisal view after tooth eruption.

Inclined cuspal planes Sloping areas between the cusp ridges.

Mamelon (**mam**-ah-lon) Rounded enamel extension on the incisal ridge of incisors.

Marginal groove A developmental groove that crosses a marginal ridge and serves as a spillway, allowing food to escape during mastication.

Marginal ridge Rounded, raised border on the mesial and distal portions of the lingual surface of anterior teeth and the occlusal table of posterior teeth.

Molars Teeth located in the posterior aspect of the upper and lower jaws.

Morphology (mor-**fah**-leh-jee) Study of the form and shape, as of the teeth.

Nonsuccedaneous (non-*suk*-se-**day**-ne-us) Pertaining to a permanent tooth that does not replace a primary tooth.

Pegged laterals Incisors with a pointed or tapered shape.

Succedaneous (*suk*-se-**day**-ne-us) Permanent teeth that replace primary teeth.

Triangular groove A developmental groove that separates a marginal ridge from the triangular ridge of a cusp.

Tricanineate A three-cusp type of mandibular second premolar.

Trifurcated Divided into three.

Trifurcation Area in which three roots divide.

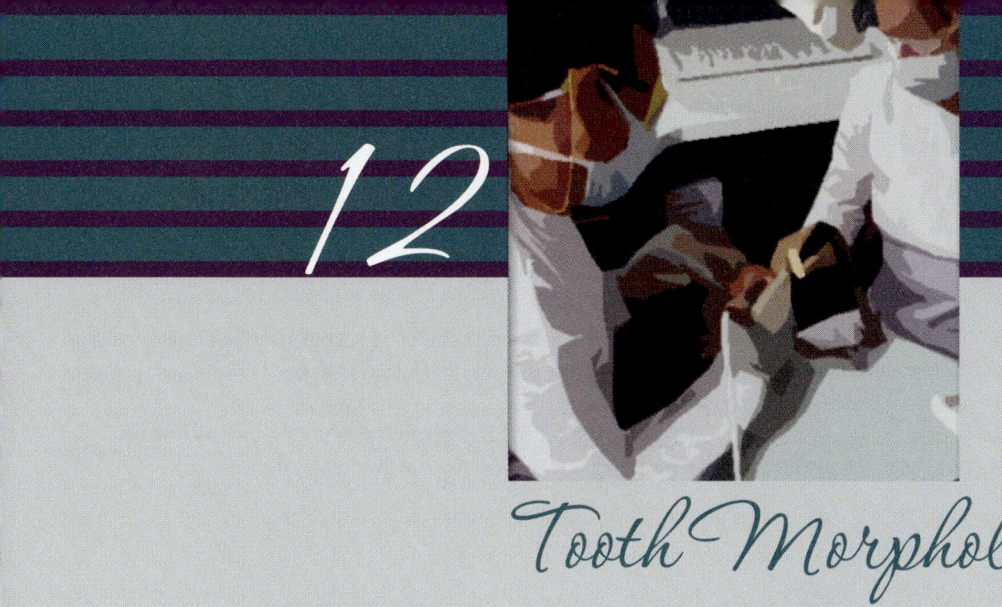

LEARNING OUTCOMES

On completion of this chapter, the student will be able to achieve the following objectives:

- Pronounce, define, and spell the Key Terms.
- Identify each tooth using the correct terms and Universal/National System code numbers.
- Identify the location of each permanent tooth.
- Use the correct terminology when discussing features of the permanent dentition.
- Describe the general and specific features of each tooth in the permanent dentition.
- Discuss clinical considerations of each tooth in the permanent dentition.
- Compare and contrast the features of the primary and permanent dentitions.
- Describe the general and specific features of the primary dentition.
- Discuss clinical considerations of the primary dentition.

A thorough understanding of tooth **morphology** (the shape of teeth) is especially useful in the following clinical situations:

- Mounting dental radiographs (see Chapter 41)
- Assisting in charting a mouth with missing teeth and teeth that have "drifted"
- Selecting temporary crowns from a box with a variety of shapes (Fig. 12-1)
- Forming matrix bands before application (see Chapter 48)
- Selection of rubber dam clamps (Chapter 36)
- Fabrication of temporary crowns and bridges (Chapter 51)

As you study tooth morphology, remember that there is always a certain amount of normal variation among individual teeth. Every tooth may not meet all the criteria for identification. When you understand the characteristics of each tooth, however, you will be able to differentiate among teeth as well as between the left teeth and the right teeth in any particular group.

ANTERIOR PERMANENT DENTITION

The permanent anterior teeth include the two *central incisors,* two *lateral incisors,* and two *canines.* The central incisors are closest to the midline, the lateral incisors are the second teeth from the midline, and the canines are the third teeth from the midline. All anterior teeth are **succedaneous,** which means they replace primary teeth of the same type.

The anterior teeth play an important role in a person's appearance (Fig. 12-2). The size, shape, color, and position of the anterior teeth directly relate to how a person looks. Many people are extremely self-conscious about the appearance of their front (anterior) teeth. The anterior teeth also play an important role in speech and are necessary for *s* and *t* sounds.

All anterior teeth have a **cingulum,** a rounded, raised area on the cervical third of the lingual surface. The lingual surface has rounded, raised borders on the mesial and distal surfaces called **marginal ridges.** Some anterior teeth

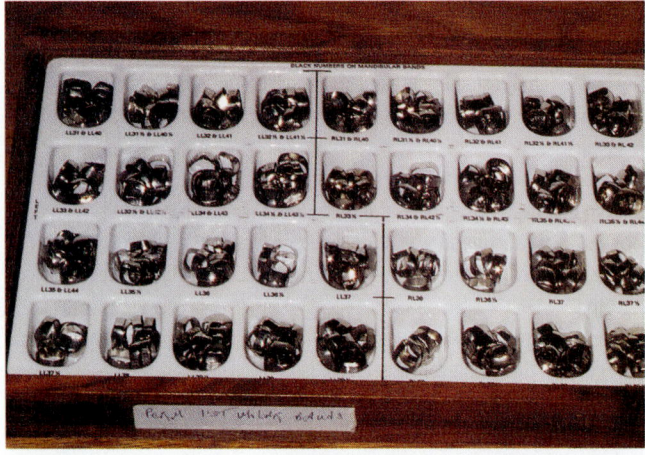

Fig. 12-1 Stainless steel crowns are available in a variety of sizes for each tooth.

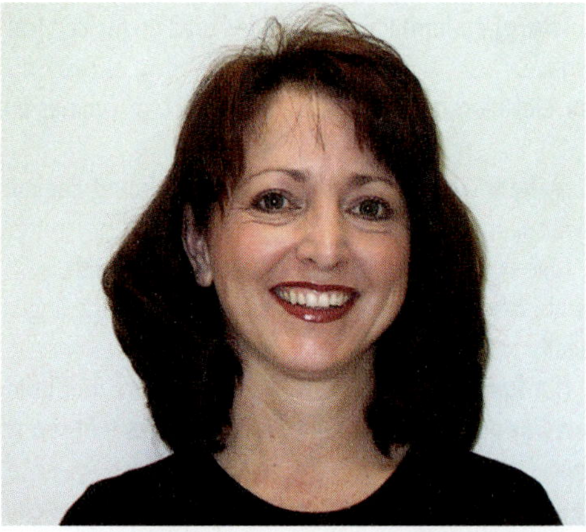

Fig. 12-2 Attractive teeth are important for a nice smile.

have a **fossa,** a wide, shallow depression on the lingual surfaces (Fig. 12-3).

Rub your tongue up and down on the lingual side of your front teeth. The bump or raised area you feel near the gingiva is the cingulum, and the deeper area is the fossa.

The tooth descriptions in this chapter are accompanied by the Universal/National System number (#) for the teeth (Box 12-1). The Universal/National System for Primary Teeth is shown in Box 12-2.

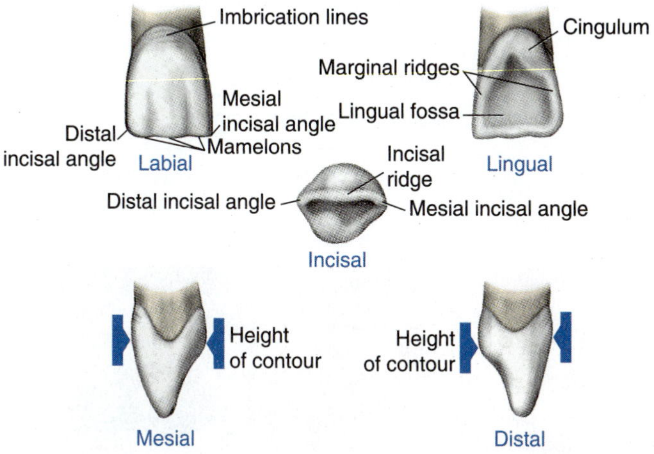

Fig. 12-3 Various views of a newly erupted permanent maxillary incisor showing its features.

Permanent Incisors

There are eight permanent incisors—four maxillary and four mandibular. The maxillary group comprises two central incisors and two lateral incisors, as does the mandibular group. These teeth complement each other in form and function. The central incisors erupt about a year or so before the lateral incisors

Maxillary Central Incisors

The *maxillary central incisors* (#8 and #9) have unique anatomic features (Fig. 12-4). They are larger than mandibular central incisors in all dimensions, especially in width (mesiodistally). The labial surfaces are more rounded from the incisal aspect. The root of the maxillary central is shorter than the roots of other permanent maxillary teeth. The marginal ridges, lingual fossa, and cingulum are more prominent on the maxillary central incisor than on the mandibular central incisor.

When an incisor is newly erupted, the incisal portion is rounded and called the *incisal ridge.* The term *edge* implies an angle formed by the merging of two flat surfaces. Therefore, an **incisal edge** does not exist on an incisor until occlusal wear has created a flattened surface on the incisal portion. The incisal edge is also known as the *incisal surface* or *incisal plane.* The incisal edges of maxillary incisors have a lingual inclination (slant). The incisal edges of the mandibular incisors have a labial inclination. The incisal planes of the mandibular and maxillary incisors are

Box 12-1 Universal Numbering System for Permanent Teeth

No.	Maxillary teeth	No.	Mandibular teeth
1	Maxillary right third molar	32	Mandibular right third molar
2	Maxillary right second molar	31	Mandibular right second molar
3	Maxillary right first molar	30	Mandibular right first molar
4	Maxillary right second premolar	29	Mandibular right second premolar
5	Maxillary right first premolar	28	Mandibular right first premolar
6	Maxillary right canine	27	Mandibular right canine
7	Maxillary right lateral incisor	26	Mandibular right lateral incisor
8	Maxillary right central incisor	25	Mandibular right central incisor
9	Maxillary left central incisor	24	Mandibular left central incisor
10	Maxillary left lateral incisor	23	Mandibular left lateral incisor
11	Maxillary left canine	22	Mandibular left canine
12	Maxillary left first premolar	21	Mandibular left first premolar
13	Maxillary left second premolar	20	Mandibular left second premolar
14	Maxillary left first molar	19	Mandibular left first molar
15	Maxillary left second molar	18	Mandibular left second molar
16	Maxillary left third molar	17	Mandibular left third molar

Box 12-2 Universal Lettering System for Primary Teeth

Letter	Maxillary teeth	Letter	Mandibular teeth
A	Maxillary right second molar	T	Mandibular right second molar
B	Maxillary right first molar	S	Mandibular right first molar
C	Maxillary right canine	R	Mandibular right canine
D	Maxillary right lateral incisor	Q	Mandibular right lateral incisor
E	Maxillary right central incisor	P	Mandibular right central incisor
F	Maxillary left central incisor	O	Mandibular left central incisor
G	Maxillary left lateral incisor	N	Mandibular left lateral incisor
H	Maxillary left canine	M	Mandibular left canine
I	Maxillary left first molar	L	Mandibular left first molar
J	Maxillary left second molar	K	Mandibular left second molar

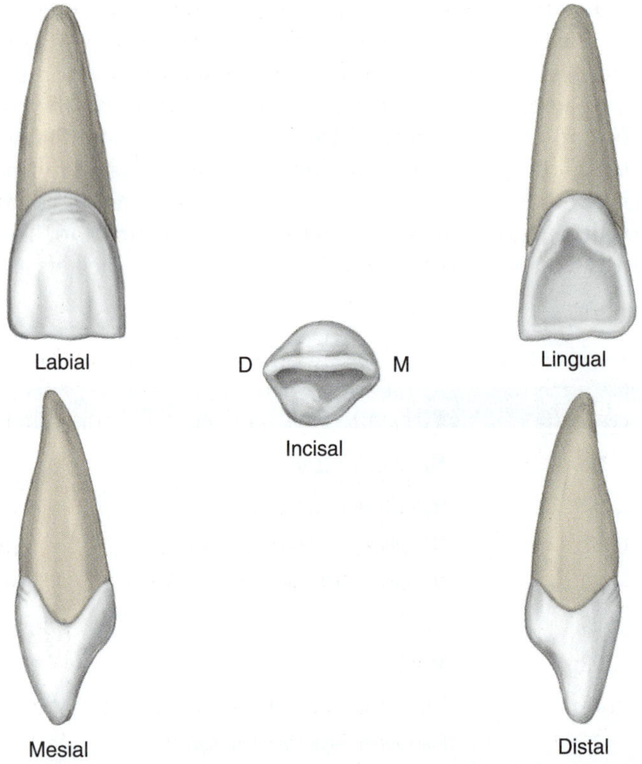

Fig. 12-4 Various views of a permanent maxillary right central incisor. (From Bath-Balogh M, Fehrenbach MJ: *Illustrated dental embryology, histology, and anatomy,* ed 2, St Louis, 2005, Saunders.)

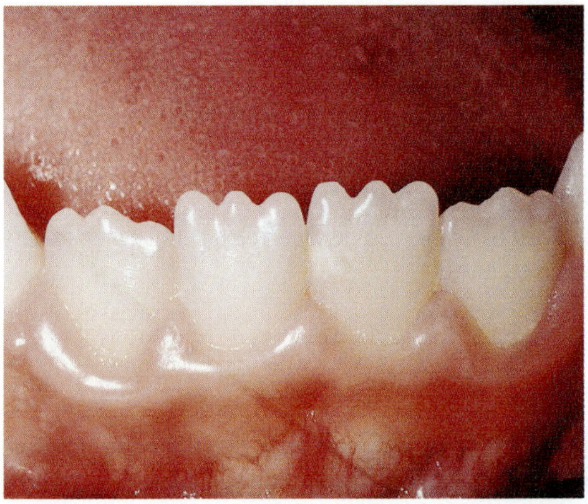

Fig. 12-5 Mamelons are the rounded portions of the incisal edge of these lower central incisors.

parallel with each other and work together to create a cutting action like the blades of a pair of scissors.

When newly erupted, the central and lateral incisors have three **mamelons,** or rounded enamel extensions on the incisal ridge, or edge (Fig. 12-5). The mamelons usually undergo attrition (wearing away of a tooth surface) shortly after eruption. Then the *incisal ridge* appears flattened and becomes the *incisal edge.*

Maxillary Lateral Incisors

The *maxillary lateral incisors* (#7 and #10) are smaller than the central incisors in all dimensions except root length (Fig. 12-6). They usually erupt after the maxillary central incisors. The crown of a maxillary lateral incisor has a single root that is relatively smooth and straight but may curve slightly to the distal. Remember this feature; it will be helpful when you are mounting radiographs.

The lateral incisors vary in form more than any other tooth except the third molars, and frequently they are congenitally missing. It is not uncommon to find maxillary lateral incisors with a pointed or tapered shape; such teeth are called **pegged laterals** (Fig. 12-7). Because of the vari-

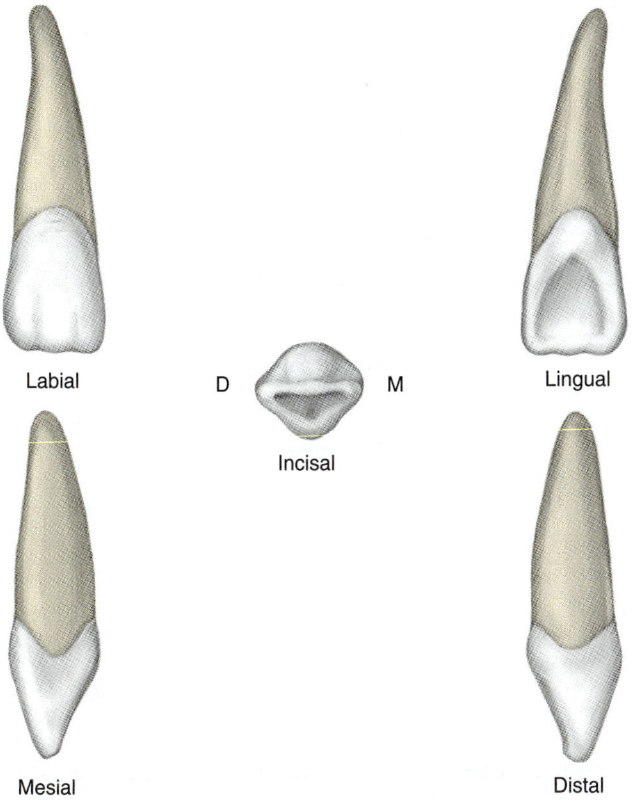

Fig. 12-6 **Various views of a permanent maxillary right lateral incisor.** (From Bath-Balogh M, Fehrenbach MJ: *Illustrated dental embryology, histology, and anatomy,* ed 2, St Louis, 2005, Saunders.)

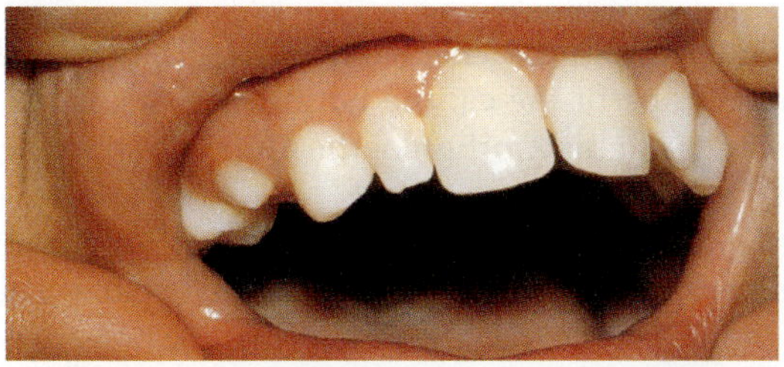

Fig. 12-7 **Pegged maxillary lateral incisor. Note the conical shape. The maxillary third molars differ considerably in size, contour, and relative position from the other teeth.** (From Ibsen OC, Phelan JA: *Oral pathology for the dental hygienist,* ed 4, St Louis, 2004, Saunders.)

ations in form, the permanent maxillary lateral incisors can present challenges during preventive, restorative, and orthodontic procedures. Often, unattractive open contacts (spaces between teeth) called **diastemas** occur in this area because of the variations in the size and shape of the lateral incisor and its position in the arch. Fortunately today there are dental materials and techniques available to correct these conditions.

Recall

1. How many anterior teeth are in the permanent dentition?
2. What is the term for the permanent teeth that replace primary teeth?
3. What is the term for the rounded, raised area on the cervical third of the lingual surface on anterior teeth?
4. What feature do newly erupted central and lateral incisors have on the incisal ridge?

Mandibular Incisors

The permanent *mandibular incisors* are the smallest teeth of the permanent dentition and the most symmetric. The central and lateral incisors of the mandibular arch closely resemble each other.

Unlike the maxillary central and lateral incisors, the mandibular lateral incisor is larger than the mandibular central incisor. The lower, mandibular incisors generally erupt before the upper, maxillary incisors. It is rare for developmental disturbances to occur with mandibular incisors.

Supragingival tooth deposits such as plaque, calculus, and stain tend to collect in the lingual concavity of the mandibular incisors. The buildup of these deposits is increased by the release of saliva, with its mineral contents, from the *sublingual* and *submandibular salivary glands* in the floor of the mouth.

Mandibular central incisors

The *mandibular central incisors* (#24 and #25) are the smallest teeth in the dental arches. They have a small centered cingulum, subtle lingual fossa, and equally subtle marginal ridges.

The crown of a mandibular central incisor is narrower on the lingual surface than on the labial surface (Fig. 12-8). Developmental horizontal lines on anterior teeth, or **imbrication lines,** and developmental depressions are usually not obvious.

Mandibular lateral incisors

The *mandibular lateral incisors* (#23 and #26) are slightly larger than the mandibular central incisors but otherwise are similar. The lateral teeth usually erupt after the mandibular central incisors. The mesial side of the crown is often longer than the distal side, causing the incisal ridge, which is straight, to slope downward in a distal direction. This helps to distinguish the right mandibular lateral incisor from the left incisor (Fig. 12-9).

Permanent Canines

The permanent canines are the four anterior teeth located at the corners of each quadrant for each dental arch (Fig. 12-10, *A*). They are commonly referred to as the "cornerstone"

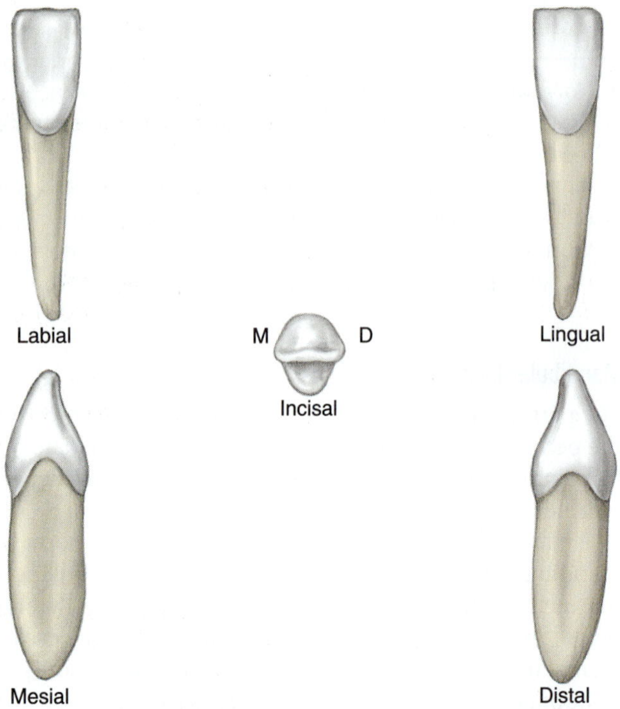

Fig. 12-8 **Various views of a permanent mandibular right central incisor.** (From Bath-Balogh M, Fehrenbach MJ: *Illustrated dental embryology, histology, and anatomy,* ed 2, St Louis, 2005, Saunders.)

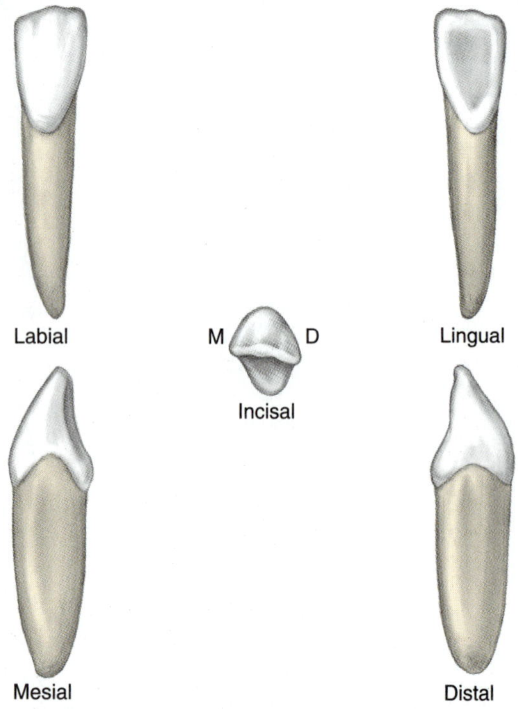

Fig. 12-9 **Various views of a permanent mandibular right lateral incisor.** (From Bath-Balogh M, Fehrenbach MJ: *Illustrated dental embryology, histology, and anatomy,* ed 2, St Louis, 2005, Saunders.)

Clinical Considerations with Incisors

The maxillary and mandibular incisors function together in a scissor-like action. The anterior teeth are the most noticeable in a person's smile.

Knowing the location of the grooves and ridges and understanding the characteristics is important to the dental assistant when constructing temporary crowns or bridges, or when finishing and polishing existing restorations.

of the dental arches. These teeth are the most stable in the mouth. Their name is derived from the Latin word for dog *(canus)* because canines resemble dogs' teeth. The permanent canines are the longest teeth in the dentition. The canine has a particularly long, thick root. The root is usually the same length as/twice the length of the crown. The crown of the canine is shaped in a manner that promotes cleanliness. Because of the self-cleansing shape and the sturdy anchorage in the jaws, the canines are usually the last teeth to be lost.

Another important characteristic of the canines is the cosmetic value of the **canine eminence**. This is the bony ridge over the labial portion of the roots of the canines that forms facial contours.

Patients commonly call the canines their "eyeteeth" and often notice the normal slightly deeper yellow color of their canines compared with their incisors.

You may hear the term *cuspid* in place of *canine.* This is an older term that was used because they were the only teeth in the permanent dentition with one cusp. A **cusp** is a major elevation on the masticatory surface of a canine or posterior tooth.

Maxillary Canines

The *maxillary canines* (#6 and #11) usually erupt after the mandibular canines, after the maxillary incisors, and possibly after the maxillary premolars. The maxillary canines have a larger and more developed cusp than the mandibular canines (see Fig. 12-10, *B*).

Similar to the other anterior teeth, each canine has an incisal edge. Different from the incisors is the cusp tip, which is in line with the long axis of the root. The cusp tip is sharper on a maxillary canine. Because of the cusp tip, the

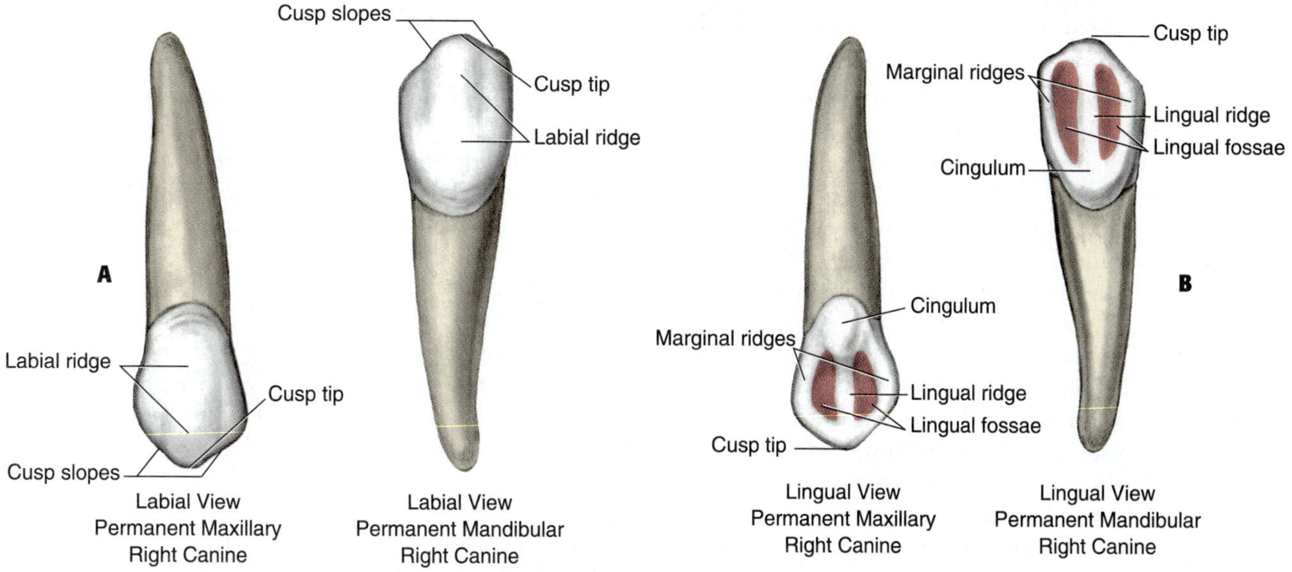

Fig. 12-10 Views of permanent mandibular and maxillary canines. A, Labial view. B, Lingual view. (From Bath-Balogh M, Fehrenbach MJ: *Illustrated dental embryology, histology, and anatomy,* ed 2, St Louis, 2005, Saunders.)

Clinical Considerations with Canines

The maxillary and mandibular canines look very similar to each other. The four canines are commonly referred to as the "cornerstone" of the dental arches. The location and shape of these teeth make them almost self-cleaning, and they frequently last throughout a person's life, or are the last teeth a person loses. The canines are also very important in establishing a natural facial contour.

incisal edge of the canine is divided into two cusp slopes, or ridges, rather than being nearly straight across as is an incisor. The mesial cusp slope is usually shorter than the distal cusp slope in both maxillary and mandibular canines when they first erupt. The length of these cusp slopes and the cusp tip can change with attrition.

Mandibular Canines

The *mandibular canines* (#22 and #27) usually erupt before the maxillary canines and after most of the incisors have erupted.

A mandibular canine closely resembles a maxillary canine. Although the entire tooth is usually as long, a mandibular canine is narrower labiolingually and mesiodistally than a maxillary canine. The crown of the tooth can be as long as or longer than that of a maxillary canine. The lingual surface of the crown of the mandibular canine is smoother than that of the maxillary canine and has a less-developed cingulum and two marginal ridges (Fig. 12-11).

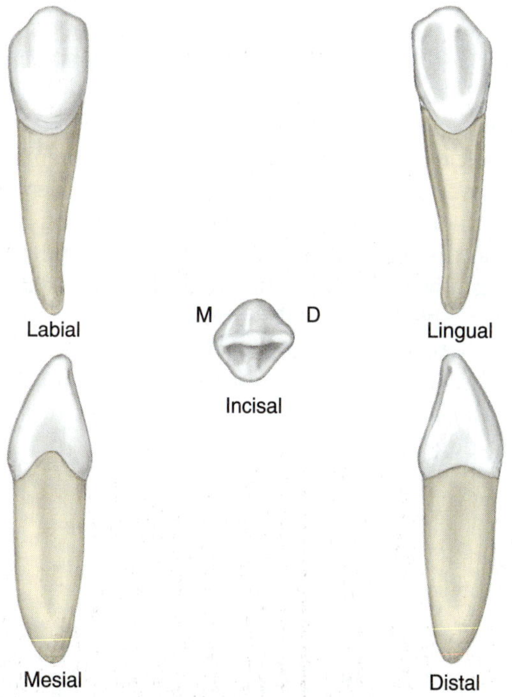

Fig. 12-11 Various views of a permanent mandibular right canine. (From Bath-Balogh M, Fehrenbach MJ: *Illustrated dental embryology, histology, and anatomy,* ed 2, St Louis, 2005, Saunders.)

Recall

5. Which teeth are the longest ones in the permanent dentition?
6. Which teeth are the smallest ones in the permanent dentition?
7. What is the name for the developmental horizontal lines on anterior teeth?

POSTERIOR PERMANENT DENTITION

The permanent posterior teeth include the *premolars* and **molars.** The crown of each posterior tooth has an occlusal surface and marginal ridges on the mesial and distal surfaces (Fig. 12-12).

The occlusal surfaces have two or more cusps. Imagine each cusp as a mountain with sloping areas, or cusp ridges, extending from the top of the mountain; between the ridges are sloping areas called **inclined cuspal planes.** Each cusp usually has four inclined cuspal planes. Some inclined planes are important in the occlusion of the teeth.

The marginal ridges border the occlusal surface and create an inner occlusal table. Each shallow, wide depression on the occlusal table is a fossa. One type of fossa on posterior teeth, the *central fossa,* is located where the cusp ridges converge in a central point, where the grooves meet. Another type of fossa is the *triangular fossa,* which has a triangular shape at the convergence of the cusp ridges and is associated with the termination of the triangular grooves.

Sometimes located in the deepest portions of the fossa are occlusal *developmental pits.* Each pit is a sharp pinpoint depression where two or more grooves meet.

Developmental grooves are also found on the occlusal table (Fig. 12-13). The developmental grooves on each different posterior tooth type are located in the same place and mark the junction among the developmental lobes. The grooves are sharp, deep, V-shaped linear depressions. The most prominent developmental groove on posterior teeth is the **central groove,** which generally travels mesiodistally and divides the occlusal table in half.

Other developmental grooves include **marginal grooves,** which cross marginal ridges and serve as a spillway, allowing food to escape during mastication. **Triangular grooves** separate a marginal ridge from the triangular ridge of a cusp.

Permanent Premolars

Each quadrant of the arch has a *first premolar* and a *second premolar.* The first premolar is distal to the canine. The second premolar is behind the first premolar. These teeth occlude with opposing teeth when the jaws are brought together. Premolars are efficient as grinding teeth, and they function similar to molars. The permanent premolars are succedaneous and replace the primary first and second molars. The crowns of the premolars are shorter than the crowns of the anterior teeth. The buccal surface of the premolars is rounded, and there is a prominent vertical buccal ridge in the center of the crown. There are two buccal depressions on each side of the buccal ridge. Premolars are *always* anterior to molars.

Maxillary First Premolars

Each maxillary first premolar has two cusps (buccal and lingual) and two roots (facial and lingual) (Fig. 12-14). A maxillary first premolar (#5 and #12) is larger than a maxillary second premolar (#4 and #13). Both maxillary premolars erupt earlier than the mandibular premolars.

The buccal cusp is long and sharp to assist the canine with tearing. The facial cusp of the maxillary first premolar

Clinical Considerations with Posterior Teeth

The permanent posterior teeth are responsible for the major portion of chewing. The pits and grooves on these teeth make them very susceptible to tooth decay. The occlusal surfaces should be carefully checked at each recall for signs of decay. Dental sealants are often placed on posterior teeth soon after they erupt. Dental sealants are discussed in Chapter 59.

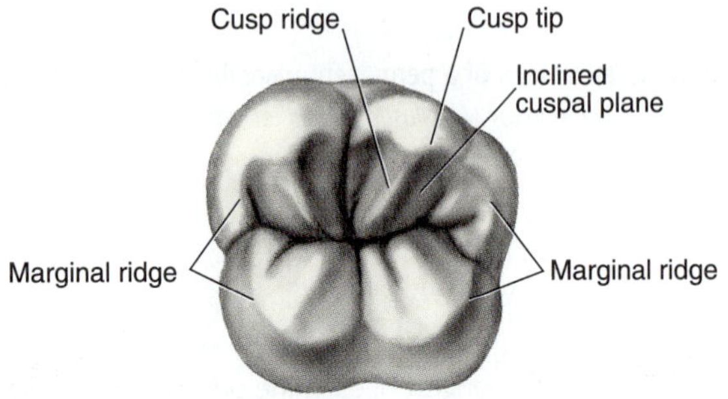

Fig. 12-12 Occlusal surface on a permanent posterior tooth and its features. (From Bath-Balogh M, Fehrenbach MJ: *Illustrated dental embryology, histology, and anatomy,* ed 2, St Louis, 2005, Saunders.)

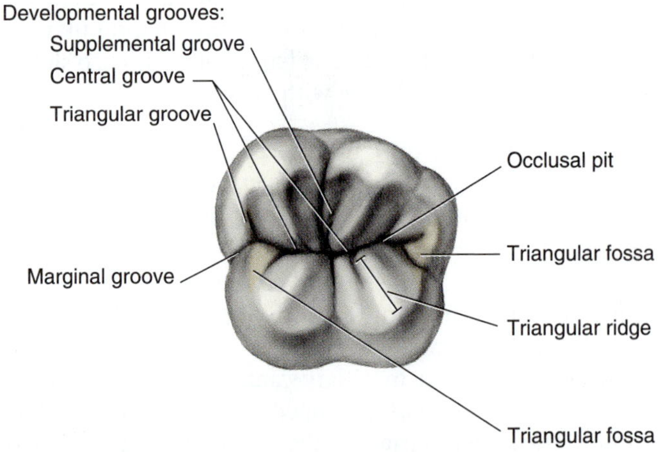

Fig. 12-13 Other features of the occlusal table on a permanent posterior tooth, including the central groove. (From Bath-Balogh M, Fehrenbach MJ: *Illustrated dental embryology, histology, and anatomy,* ed 2, St Louis, 2005, Saunders.)

is much more prominent in size than the lingual cusp. It is longer and wider across and is similar to the canine from the facial side. The central groove extends between the mesial and distal grooves. The mesial marginal ridges border the mesial groove, and the distal marginal ridge borders the distal groove.

The maxillary first premolar has a **bifurcated** root. This means that the root is divided into two roots—one buccal and one lingual. A **furcation** is an area between two or more root branches. Some first premolars have roots that are joined together, or *fused*. The roots are shorter in length and resemble the roots of the molars.

Clinical Considerations with Premolars

The maxillary and mandibular premolars work with the molars in the chewing of food. The first premolars help the canines in shearing or cutting bits of food. The premolars also support the corners of the mouth and cheeks. When people lose all of their molars, they can usually still chew if they still have their premolars. Unfortunately, it is very noticeable when a person smiles and is missing one or more maxillary premolars.

Modified from Bath-Balogh M, Fehrenbach MJ: *Illustrated dental embryology, histology, and anatomy*, ed 2, St Louis, 2005, Saunders.

Maxillary Second Premolars

Each maxillary second premolar (#4 and #13) has two cusps (buccal and lingual) and one root.

The maxillary second premolar differs from the first premolar in the following ways:

- The cusps, one buccal and one lingual, are more equal in length on the second premolar.
- The lingual cusp is larger than, almost the same height as, the buccal cusp on the maxillary second premolar.
- The mesiobuccal cusp slope is shorter than the distobuccal cusp slope on the second premolar.
- The cusps of the secondary premolar are not as sharp as those of the maxillary first premolar.
- The second premolar has only one root and therefore only one root canal.
- The second premolar has a very slight depression on the mesial root.
- The second premolar is wider buccolingually than mesiodistally.

Mandibular First Premolars

The mandibular first premolars (#21 and #28) have a long and well-formed buccal cusp and a small, nonfunctioning lingual cusp. The lingual cusp may be small.

The mandibular first premolars are smaller and shorter than the mandibular second premolars (Fig. 12-15). The

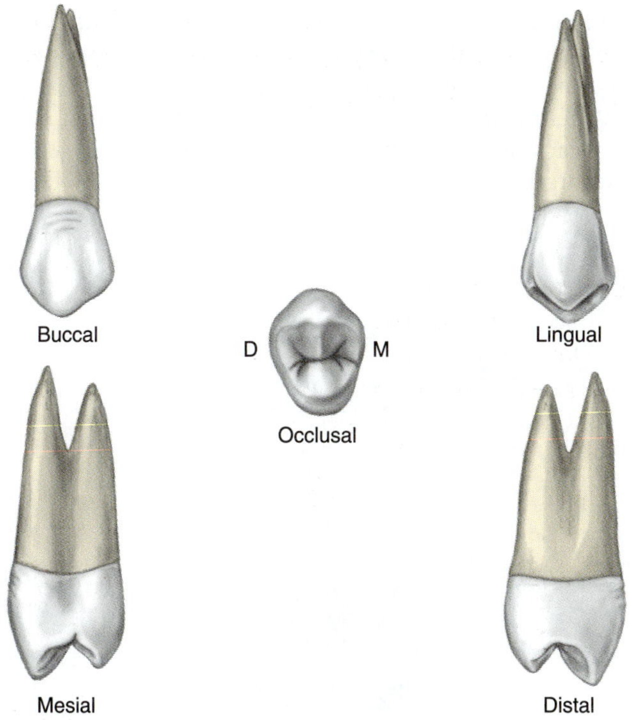

Fig. 12-14 Various views of a permanent maxillary first premolar. (From Bath-Balogh M, Fehrenbach MJ: *Illustrated dental embryology, histology, and anatomy*, ed 2, St Louis, 2005, Saunders.)

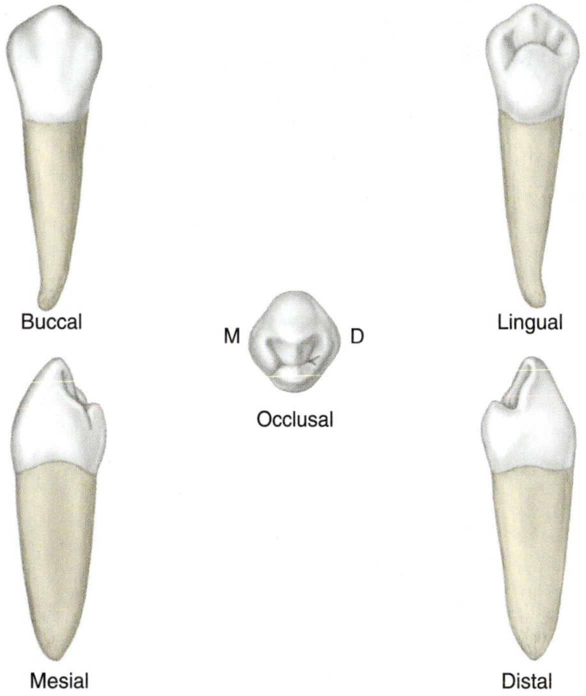

Fig. 12-15 Various views of a permanent mandibular right first premolar. (From Bath-Balogh M, Fehrenbach MJ: *Illustrated dental embryology, histology, and anatomy*, ed 2, St Louis, 2005, Saunders.)

mandibular premolars do not resemble each other as much as do the maxillary premolars. Generally, both mandibular premolars erupt into the oral cavity later than do the maxillary premolars.

The permanent premolars also have an equal buccolingual and mesiodistal width when viewed from the occlusal, making the outline almost round. In addition, both types of premolars have a similar buccal outline of both the crown and the root.

The mesial and distal contact areas of mandibular premolars are nearly the same level. The crowns incline lingually bringing the cusps into proper occlusion with the teeth on the opposing arch.

Mandibular Second Premolars

The permanent mandibular second premolars (#20 and #29) erupt distal to the mandibular first premolars. Thus they are the succedaneous replacements for the primary mandibular second molars (Fig. 12-16).

There are two forms of the mandibular second premolar: the *three-cusp type,* or **tricanineate** form, and the *two-cusp type,* or **bicanineate** form. The more common three-cusp type has one large buccal cusp and two smaller lingual cusps. Less often they have a larger buccal cusp and a single smaller lingual cusp. The three-cusp type also appears more angular from the occlusal view, and the two-cusp type appears more rounded.

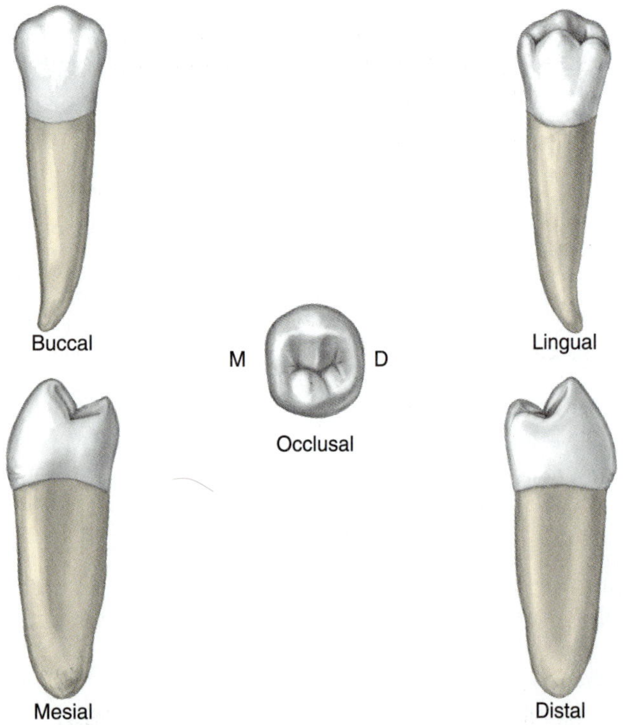

Fig. 12-16 Various views of a permanent mandibular second premolar. (From Bath-Balogh M, Fehrenbach MJ: *Illustrated dental embryology, histology, and anatomy,* ed 2, St Louis, 2005, Saunders.)

In tricanineate premolars, the groove pattern is typically Y-shaped. In the two-cusp type, the groove pattern may be either U-shaped (also called C-shaped) or H-grooved, depending on whether the central developmental groove is straight mesiodistally or curved bucally at its ends (Fig. 12-17).

Both types of mandibular second premolars have more supplemental grooves than the mandibular first premolars. The single root of the mandibular second premolar is larger and longer than that of a first mandibular premolar but shorter than that of the maxillary premolars.

Recall

8. What feature borders the occlusal table of a posterior tooth?

9. What are the pinpoint depressions where two or more grooves meet?

10. Which teeth are frequently extracted as part of orthodontic treatment?

11. What are the two forms of mandibular second premolars?

Permanent Molars

There are 12 molars in the permanent dentition, three in each quadrant. The permanent molars are the largest teeth in the dentition. The name *molar* comes from the Latin word for "grinding," one of the functions of the molar teeth. There are three types of molars: the first molar, second molar, and third molar. The first and second molars are also called the 6-year and 12-year molars, respectively, because of the approximate ages at eruption.

The molar crowns have four or five short, blunt cusps, and each molar has two or three roots that help to support the larger crown (Fig. 12-18).

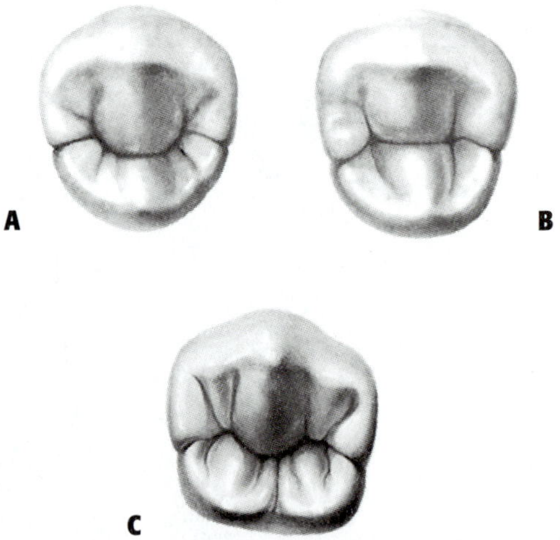

Fig. 12-17 Occlusal views of a permanent mandibular second premolar, A, U-type. B, H-type, C, Y-type. (From Zeisz RD, Nuckolls J: *Dental anatomy,* St Louis, 1949, Mosby.)

Maxillary Molars

The *maxillary molars* assist the mandibular molars in performing the major portion of the work of mastication. They are usually the first permanent teeth to erupt into the maxillary arch. Because of both their size and their "anchorage" in the jaws, the molars are the largest and strongest maxillary teeth. Each maxillary molar usually has four major cusps, with two cusps on the buccal portion of the occlusal table and two on the lingual.

Each maxillary molar has three well-separated and well-developed roots. A tooth with three roots is said to be **trifurcated,** which means divided into thirds. A **trifurcation** is the area at which the three roots divide. Because maxillary molars are trifurcated, the three divisions are usually located on the mesial, buccal, and distal surfaces. They provide the tooth with maximum anchorage against occlusal forces. All maxillary molars are wider buccolingually than mesiodistally.

Maxillary first molars

The maxillary first molars (#3 and #14) are the first permanent teeth to erupt into the maxillary arch (Fig. 12-19). They erupt distal to the primary maxillary second molars and thus are **nonsuccedaneous,** meaning they *do not* replace the primary teeth.

The maxillary first molar is the largest tooth in the maxillary arch and also has the largest crown in the permanent dentition. This molar is composed of five developmental lobes, two buccal and three lingual.

Four of the cusps are well-developed functioning cusps (mesiolingual, distolingual, mesiobuccal, and distobuccal), and the fifth supplemental cusp is of little practical use. The fifth cusp is called the **cusp of Carabelli.** When present, this cusp is found lingual to the mesiolingual cusp. However, it is often so poorly developed that it is scarcely distinguishable.

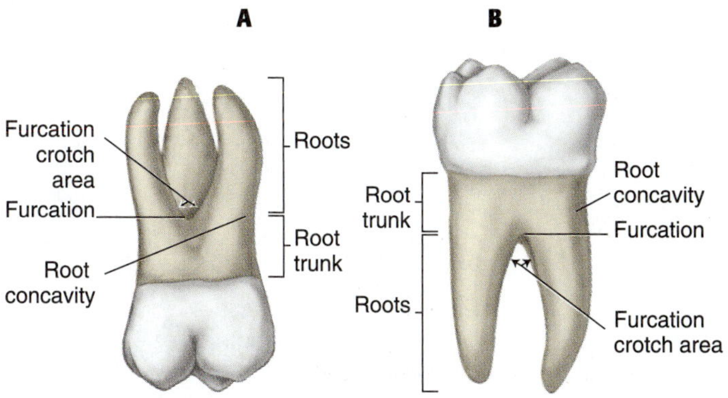

Fig. 12-18 A, Maxillary first molar. B, Mandibular first molar. (From Bath-Balogh M, Fehrenbach MJ: *Illustrated dental embryology, histology, and anatomy,* ed 2, St Louis, 2005, Saunders.)

Maxillary second molars

The maxillary second molars (#2 and #15) supplement the first molars in function (Fig. 12-20). These molars erupt distal to the permanent maxillary first molars and are nonsuccedaneous.

The crown is somewhat shorter than that of the first molar, and the maxillary second molar usually has four cusps (mesiobuccal, distobuccal, mesiolingual, and distolingual). No fifth cusp is present. There are three roots

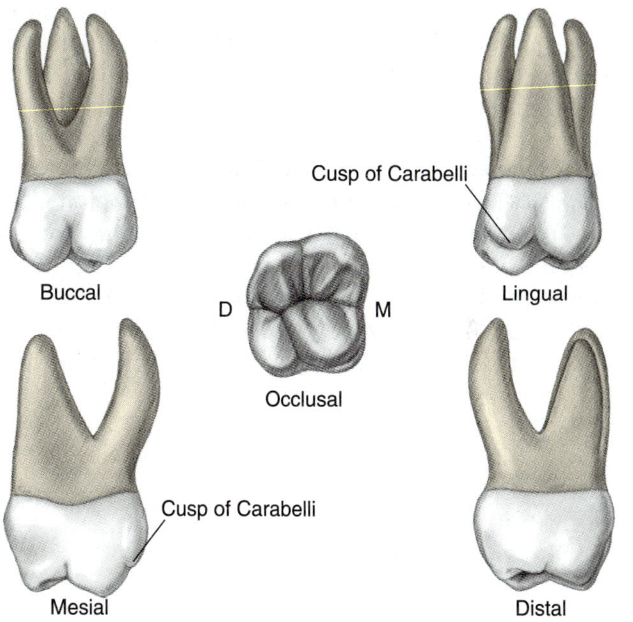

Fig. 12-19 Various views of a permanent maxillary right first molar. (From Bath-Balogh M, Fehrenbach MJ: *Illustrated dental embryology, histology, and anatomy,* ed 2, St Louis, 2005, Saunders.)

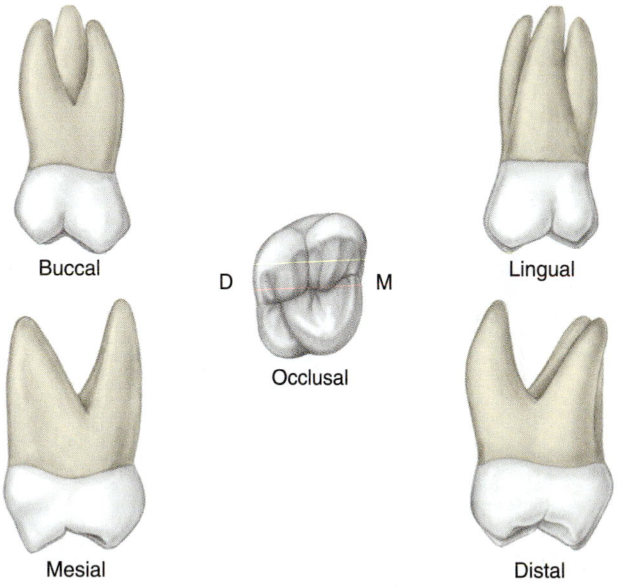

Fig. 12-20 Various views of a permanent maxillary right second molar. (From Bath-Balogh M, Fehrenbach MJ: *Illustrated dental embryology, histology, and anatomy,* ed 2, St Louis, 2005, Saunders.)

(mesiobuccal, distobuccal, and lingual). The roots of the secondary molars are smaller than the roots of the first molars. The lingual root is still the largest and longest.

The buccal groove is located farther distally on the buccal surface of the second than the first maxillary molar. The mesiobuccal cusp of the second maxillary molar is longer and has a less sharp cusp tip than the distobuccal cusp.

Maxillary third molars

The maxillary third molars (#1 and #16) often appear as a developmental anomaly. The maxillary third molar differs considerably in size, contour, and relative position from the other teeth. Maxillary third molars are more likely than other teeth in the arch to be out of position. They are seldom as well developed as the maxillary second molar, to which they bear some resemblance.

The third molar supplements the second molar in function. Its fundamental design is similar, but the crown is smaller, and the roots usually are shorter. The roots of this tooth tend to fuse, and the result is a single, tapered root (Figs. 12-21 and 12-22). People sometimes refer to this tooth as the "wisdom" tooth because it is the last to erupt.

Recall

12. What is the term for a tooth with three roots?
13. What is the term for a tooth that does not replace a primary tooth?
14. What is the name of the fifth cusp on a maxillary first molar?

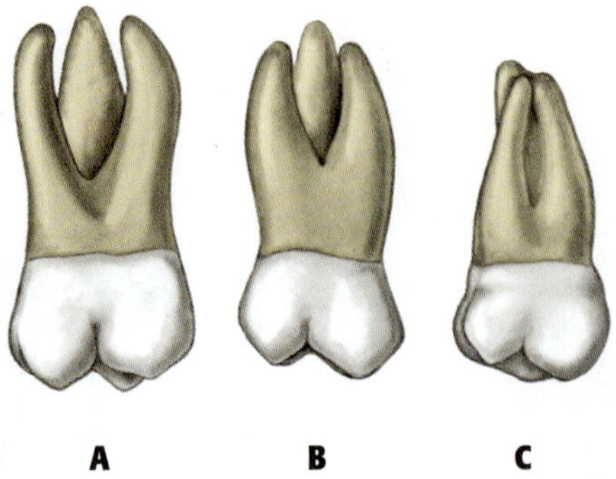

Fig. 12-21 **Buccal views of permanent maxillary right molars. A, First molar. B, Second molar. C, Third molar. Notice how the roots tend to be closer together when the molars are farther distally. Third molar roots are often fused.** (Modified from Brand RW, Isselhard DE: *Anatomy of orofacial structures,* ed 7, St Louis, 2003, Mosby.)

Mandibular Molars

The *mandibular molars* erupt six months to one year before the corresponding permanent maxillary molars. The crown of a mandibular molar has four or five major cusps, of which there are always two lingual cusps of about the same width. All mandibular molars are wider mesiodistally than buccolingually,

Each mandibular molar has *two* well-developed roots: one mesial and one distal. As mentioned earlier, a tooth with two roots is bifurcated, which means divided into two. Each root has its own root canal. A **bifurcation** is the area at which the two roots divide.

Clinical Considerations with Maxillary Molars

- The roots of the maxillary molars are in close proximity to the walls and floor of the sinus. On rare occasions, the maxillary sinus may be accidentally perforated by an instrument during surgical removal of a maxillary molar.
- Because the maxillary molar roots are close to the sinus, some patients confuse the pain caused by a sinus infection with pain related to their maxillary teeth, and vice versa. Diagnostic tests are necessary to determine the cause.
- If the maxillary first molar is lost to caries or periodontal disease, the second molar can tip and drift into the open space, causing difficulty in chewing and furthering periodontal disease.
- Third molars often present oral hygiene problems for patients because this area is difficult to reach with a toothbrush.

Modified from Bath-Balogh M, Fehrenbach MJ: *Illustrated dental embryology, histology, and anatomy,* ed 2, St Louis, 2005, Saunders.

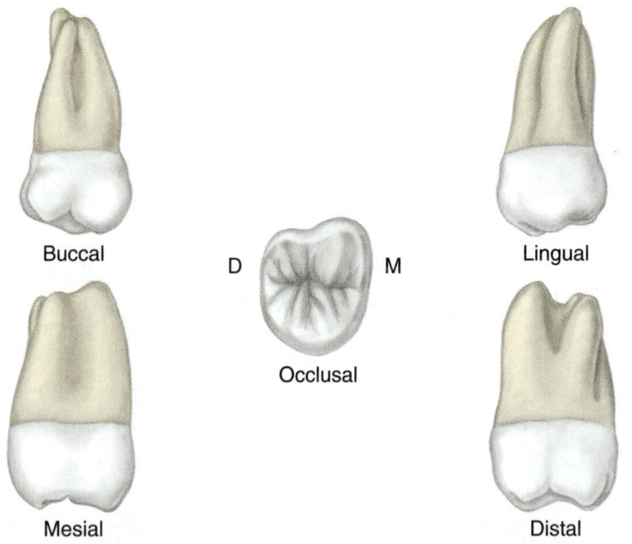

Fig. 12-22 **Various views of permanent maxillary right third molars.** (From Bath-Balogh M, Fehrenbach MJ: *Illustrated dental embryology, histology, and anatomy,* ed 2, St Louis, 2005, Saunders.)

Mandibular first molars

The permanent mandibular first molars (#19 and #30) erupt between six and seven years of age. These teeth are usually the first permanent teeth to erupt in the oral cavity (Fig. 12-23). They erupt distal to the primary mandibular second molars and thus are nonsuccedaneous.

The two roots, mesial and distal, of a mandibular first molar are larger and more divergent than those of a second molar, leaving the roots widely separated buccally. Usually both roots are the same length. However, if one is longer it is the mesial root, which is also wider and stronger than the distal root. When this molar has three roots, the mesial root has both buccal and lingual branches.

The mesiobuccal cusp is the largest, widest, and highest cusp on the buccal portion. The distobuccal cusp is slightly smaller, shorter, and sharper than the mesiobuccal cusp. The distal cusp is the lowest cusp and is slightly sharper than the other two.

Mandibular second molars

The mandibular second molars (#18 and #31) erupt between 11 and 12 years of age (Fig. 12-24). These teeth erupt distal to the permanent first molars and thus are nonsuccedaneous.

The crown of the mandibular second molar is slightly smaller than that of the first molar in all directions. The crown has four well-developed cusps (mesiolingual, distolingual, mesiobuccal, and distobuccal) and two roots (mesial and distal).

The two roots of the mandibular second molar are smaller, shorter, less divergent, and closer together than those of the first molar. These roots are not as broad buccolingually as those of the first molar and are not as widely separated.

The mesiolingual cusp and distolingual cusp have the same size and shape as the buccal cusps.

Mandibular third molars

The mandibular third molars (#17 and #32) are similar to the maxillary third molars in that they vary greatly in shape and have no standard form. There is no typical mandibular third molar. This molar is usually smaller in all dimensions than the second molar. The third molar usually consists of four developmental lobes.

The crown of a mandibular third molar tapers distally when viewed from the mesial aspect. The occlusal outline of the crown is more oval than rectangular, although the crown frequently resembles that of a second molar. The two mesial cusps are larger that the two distal cusps. The occlusal surface appears very wrinkled (Fig. 12-25).

A mandibular third molar usually has two roots that are fused, irregularly curved, and shorter than those of a mandibular second molar. Third molars are frequently impacted.

Third molars often present with anomalies in form and position. A common anomaly is that the multiple roots are fused to form a single root (Fig. 12-26).

Recall

15. How many roots do mandibular molars have?

16. Which teeth are referred to as the "wisdom" teeth?

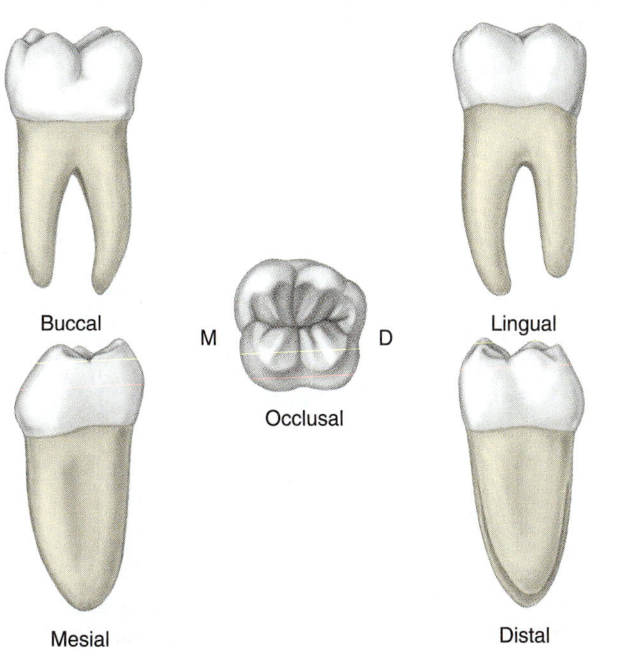

Fig. 12-23 **Various views of a permanent mandibular right first molar.** (From Bath-Balogh M, Fehrenbach MJ: *Illustrated dental embryology, histology, and anatomy,* ed 2, St Louis, 2005, Saunders.)

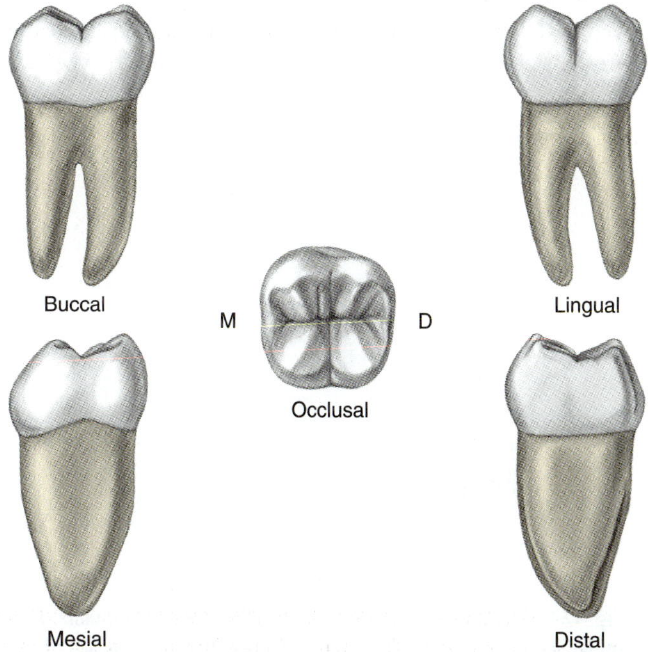

Fig. 12-24 **Various views of a permanent mandibular right second molar.** (From Bath-Balogh M, Fehrenbach MJ: *Illustrated dental embryology, histology, and anatomy,* ed 2, St Louis, 2005, Saunders.)

Clinical Considerations with Mandibular Molars

The mandibular molars can present difficulty in positioning the oral evacuator because of the lingual inclination of the crowns. In addition, patients often have problems with their oral hygiene because of the lingual inclination of the molar teeth, and they may miss cleaning the lingual gingiva with the toothbrush.

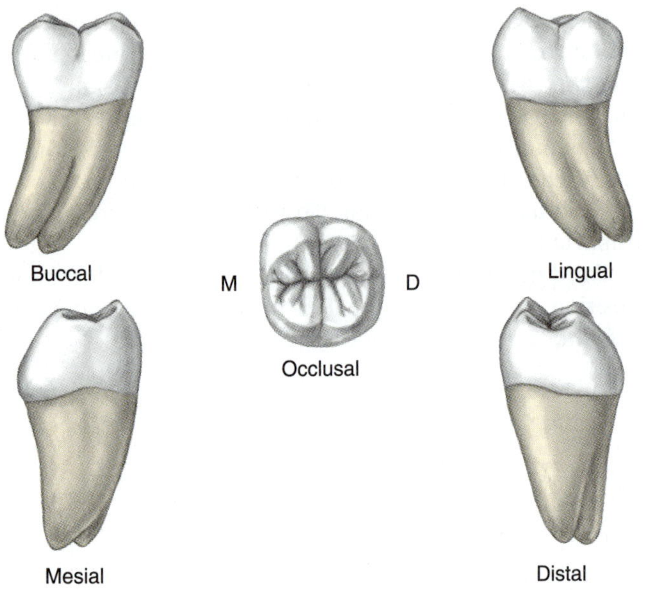

Fig. 12-25 Various views of the permanent mandibular right third molar. (From Bath-Balogh M, Fehrenbach MJ: *Illustrated dental embryology, histology, and anatomy,* ed 2, St Louis, 2005, Saunders.)

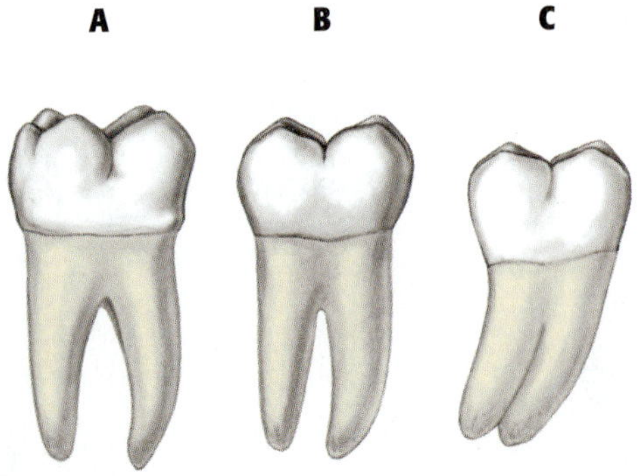

Fig. 12-26 Buccal views of permanent mandibular right molars. A, First molar. B, Second molar. C, Third molar. Note that the roots are closer together and become shorter from the first molar to the third molar. Third molar roots are often fused. (Modified from Brand RW, Isselhard DE: *Anatomy of orofacial structures,* ed 7, St Louis, 2003, Mosby.)

PRIMARY DENTITION

There are 20 primary teeth in the primary dentition, 10 in the maxillary arch and 10 in the mandibular arch. These teeth include incisors, canines, and molars. The primary teeth are numbered in the Universal/National System by using the capital letters *A* through *T.*

The primary teeth are smaller overall and have whiter enamel than the permanent teeth. This is because of the increased opacity of the enamel, which covers the underlying dentin. The crown of any primary tooth is short in relation to its total length. The crowns are narrower at the *cementoenamel junction* (CEJ). The roots of primary teeth are also narrower and longer than the crown.

The pulp chambers and pulp horns in primary teeth are relatively large in proportion to those of the permanent teeth. There is a thick layer of dentin between the pulp chambers and the enamel, especially in the primary mandibular second molar. However, the enamel layer is relatively thin (Fig. 12-27).

Primary Incisors

The deciduous incisors are smaller than their permanent successors in the size of both their crowns and roots. The roots are twice as long the crowns and taper toward the apex.

Maxillary Central Incisors

The crown of the primary maxillary central incisor (*E* and *F*) is wider mesiodistally than incisocervically, the opposite of its permanent successor. It is the only tooth of either dentition with this crown dimension.

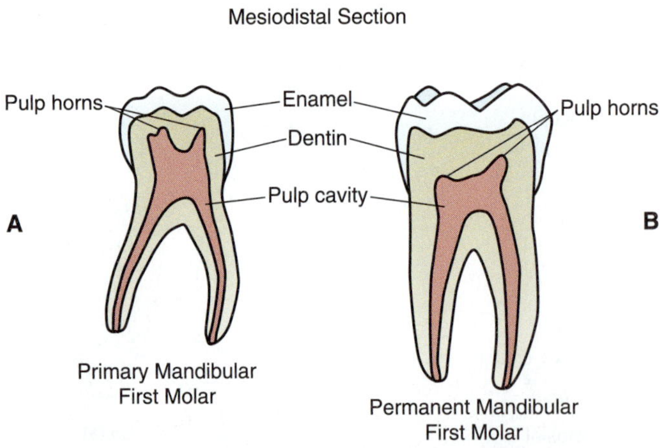

Fig. 12-27 A, Primary mandibular molar. B, Permanent mandibular molar. (From Bath-Balogh M, Fehrenbach MJ: *Illustrated dental embryology, histology, and anatomy,* ed 2, St Louis, 2005, Saunders.)

The primary maxillary incisors have no mamelons. These teeth rarely have developmental depressions or imbrication lines. The cingulum and marginal ridges are more prominent than on the permanent successor, and the lingual fossa is deeper (Fig. 12-28).

Maxillary Lateral Incisors

The crown of the primary maxillary lateral incisor (*D* and *G*) is similar to that of the central incisor but is much smaller in all dimensions (Fig. 12-29).

The incisal angles on the lateral incisor are also more rounded than on the central incisor. The lateral root is longer in proportion to its crown, and its apex is sharper.

Mandibular Central Incisors

The crown of the primary mandibular incisor (*O* and *P*) resembles the primary mandibular lateral incisor more than its permanent central successor (Fig. 12-30).

The mandibular central incisor is extremely symmetric. It is also not as constricted at the CEJ as the primary maxillary incisor. Its mesial and distal outlines from the labial aspect also show that the crown tapers evenly from the contact areas.

Clinical Considerations with Primary Teeth

- Some parents think that the "baby teeth" are only temporary and are not really important because these teeth will be replaced by permanent ones. However, when primary teeth are lost prematurely, there can be serious problems with tooth alignment, spacing, and occlusion for the child later on. The primary teeth play an important role in "saving" space for the permanent teeth.
- In addition to providing for chewing, appearance, and speech for about 5 to 11 years, primary teeth support the cheeks and lips and a normal facial appearance.
- Because the enamel and dentin are thinner in primary teeth, decay can travel quickly through the enamel to the pulp, possibly causing loss of the tooth.
- Early dental health education and dental care are essential for keeping the primary dentition healthy.
- Primary teeth are essential for the formation of clear speech.

Modified from Bath-Balogh M, Fehrenbach MJ: *Illustrated dental embryology, histology, and anatomy,* Philadelphia, 1997, Saunders.

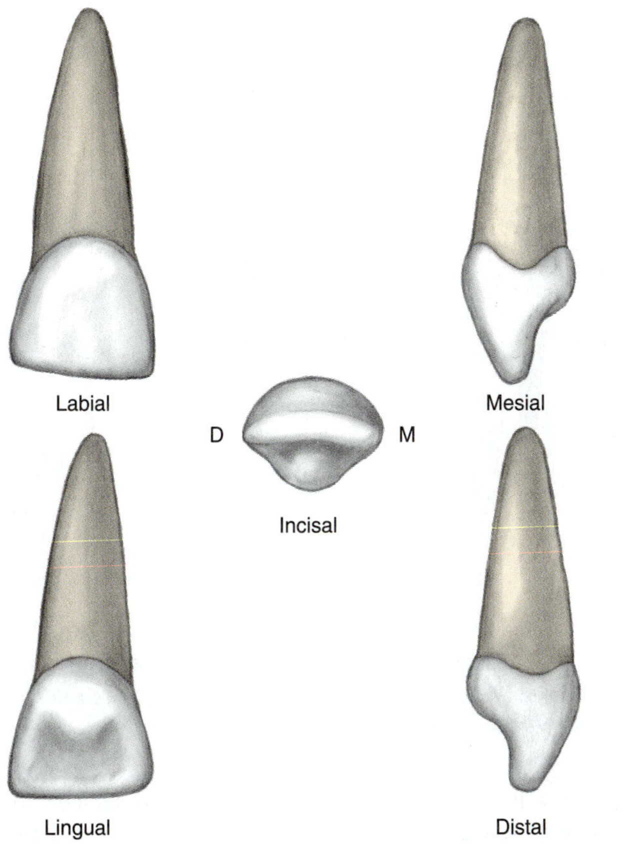

Fig. 12-28 Various views of a primary maxillary right central incisor. (From Bath-Balogh M, Fehrenbach MJ: *Illustrated dental embryology, histology, and anatomy,* ed 2, St Louis, 2005, Saunders.)

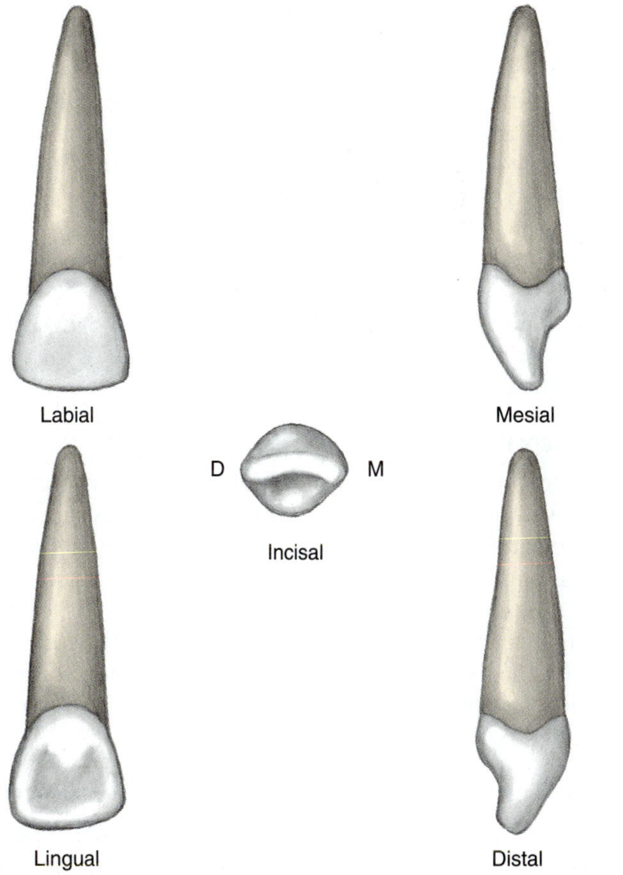

Fig. 12-29 Various views of a primary maxillary lateral incisor. (From Bath-Balogh M, Fehrenbach MJ: *Illustrated dental embryology, histology, and anatomy,* ed 2, St Louis, 2005, Saunders.)

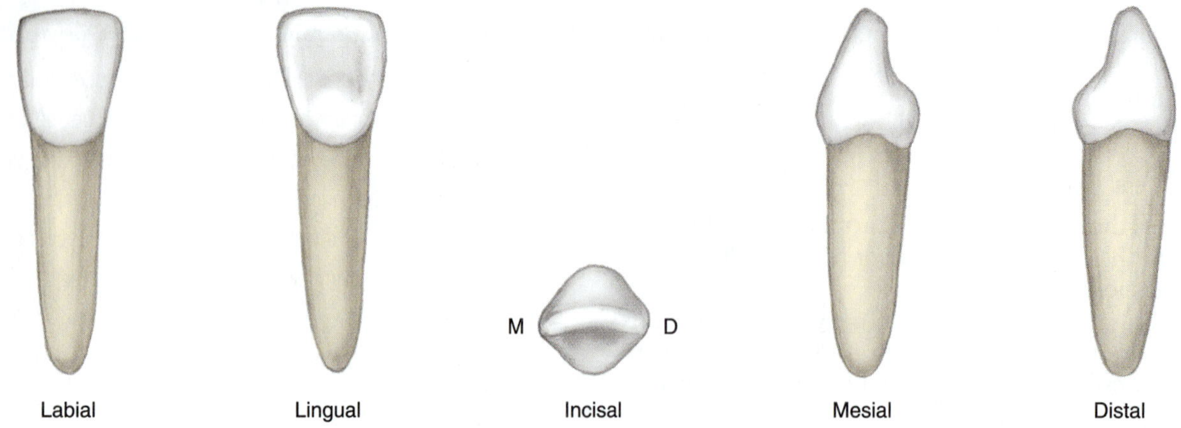

Fig. 12-30 Various views of a primary mandibular central incisor. (From Bath-Balogh M, Fehrenbach MJ: *Illustrated dental embryology, histology, and anatomy,* ed 2, St Louis, 2005, Saunders.)

The lingual surface of the mandibular central incisor appears smooth and tapers toward the prominent cingulum. The marginal ridges are less pronounced than those of the primary maxillary incisor.

Mandibular Lateral Incisors

The crown of the primary lateral incisor (*Q* and *N*) is similar in form to that of the central incisor in the same arch but is wider and longer (Fig. 12-31).

The incisal edge of the mandibular lateral incisor slopes distally, and the distoincisal angle is more rounded. The root may have a distal curvature in its apical third and usually has a distal longitudinal groove.

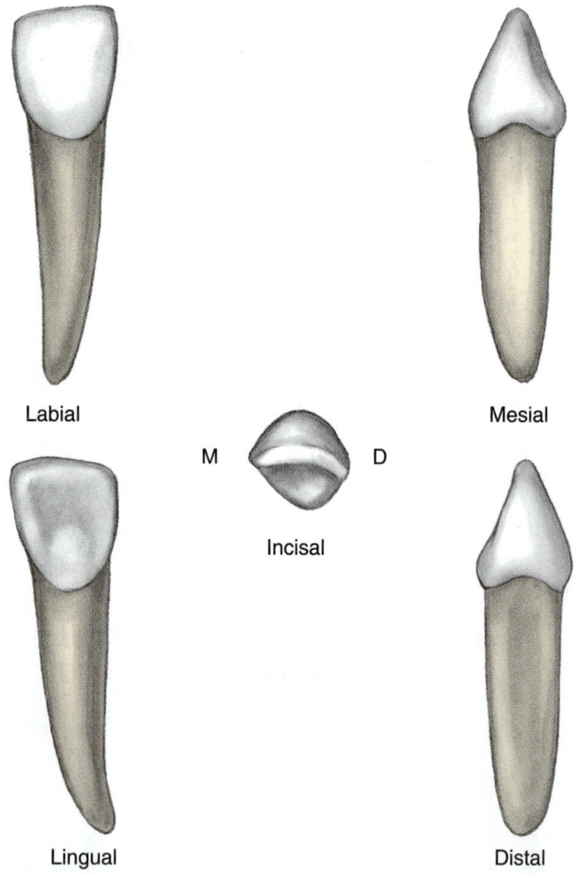

Fig. 12-31 Various views of a primary mandibular lateral incisor. (From Bath-Balogh M, Fehrenbach MJ: *Illustrated dental embryology, histology, and anatomy,* ed 2, St Louis, 2005, Saunders.)

Primary Canines

There are four primary canines, two in each dental arch. These primary canines differ from the outline of their permanent successors in the following ways.

Maxillary Canines

The crown of the primary maxillary canine (*C* and *H*) has a relatively longer and sharper cusp than that of its permanent successor when first erupted (Fig. 12-32). The mesial and distal outlines of the primary maxillary canine are rounder.

On the lingual surface the cingulum is well developed, as are the lingual ridge and marginal ridges. The mesiolingual and distolingual fossae are shallow. The root is inclined distally, is twice as long as the crown, and is more slender than the root of its successor.

Mandibular Canines

The primary mandibular canine (*M* and *R*) resembles the primary maxillary canine, although some dimensions are different. This tooth is much smaller labiolingually (Fig. 12-33).

The distal cusp slope is much longer than the mesial cusp slope. The lingual surface of the primary mandibular canine is marked by a shallow lingual fossa. The incisal edge is straight and is centered over the crown labiolingually. The root is long, narrow, and almost twice the length of the crown, although shorter and more tapered than the root of a primary maxillary canine.

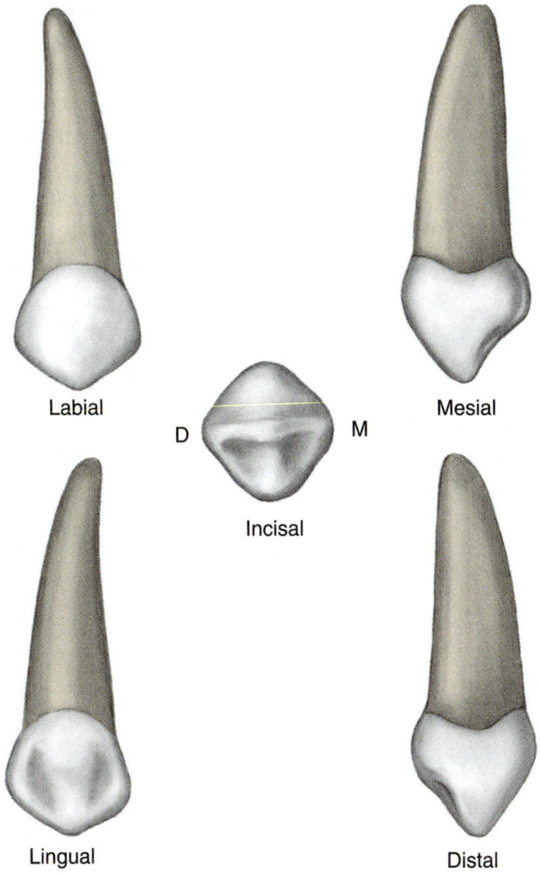

Fig. 12-32 Various views of a primary maxillary canine. (From Bath-Balogh M, Fehrenbach MJ: *Illustrated dental embryology, histology, and anatomy*, ed 2, St Louis, 2005, Saunders.)

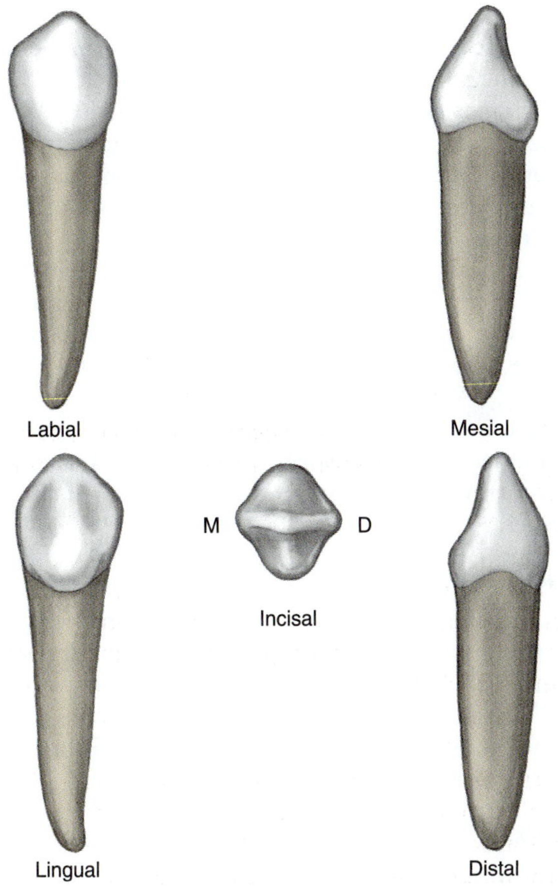

Fig. 12-33 Various views of a primary mandibular canine. (From Bath-Balogh M, Fehrenbach MJ: *Illustrated dental embryology, histology, and anatomy*, ed 2, St Louis, 2005, Saunders.)

Recall

17. How thick is the enamel covering on a primary tooth?
18. What method of identification is used in the Universal/National System for the primary dentition?

Primary Molars

The primary dentition has a total of eight primary molars. Each quadrant has a first primary molar and a second primary molar. Each molar crown is wider than it is tall. The permanent premolars replace the primary molars when they are exfoliated.

Maxillary First Molars

The crown of the primary maxillary first molar (*B* and *I*) does not resemble any other crown of either dentition (Fig. 12-34). The height of contour on the buccal surface is at

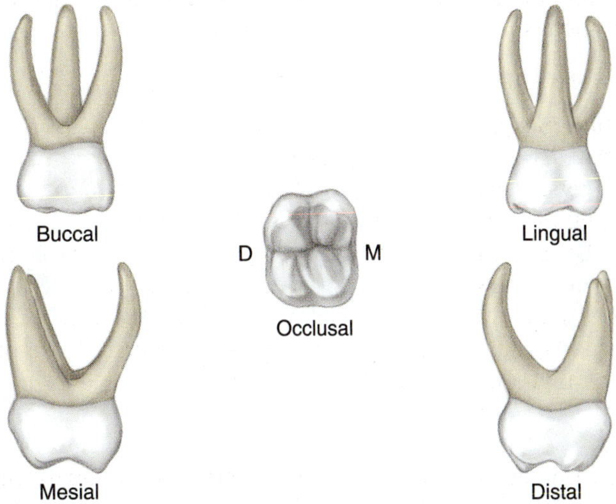

Fig. 12-34 Various views of a primary maxillary first molar. (From Bath-Balogh M, Fehrenbach MJ: *Illustrated dental embryology, histology, and anatomy*, ed 2, St Louis, 2005, Saunders.)

the cervical one third of the tooth, and on the lingual side it is at the middle one third.

The occlusal table may have four cusps (mesiobuccal, mesiolingual, distobuccal, and distolingual); the two mesial cusps are the largest cusps, and the two distal cusps are very small. The primary maxillary first molar frequently has only three cusps because the distolingual cusp may be absent. The occlusal table also has a very prominent transverse ridge.

This tooth also has an H-shaped groove pattern and three fossae: central, mesial triangular, and distal triangular. The central groove connects the central pit with the mesial pit and distal pit at each end of the occlusal table.

The primary maxillary first molar has three roots, which are thinner and have greater flare than the permanent maxillary first molar. The lingual root is the longest and most divergent.

Maxillary Second Molars

The primary maxillary second molar (*A* and *J*) is larger than the primary maxillary first molar (Fig. 12-35). This tooth most closely resembles the form of the permanent maxillary first molar but is smaller in all dimensions. The second molar usually has a cusp of Carabelli, the minor fifth cusp.

Mandibular First Molars

The crown of the primary mandibular first molar (*L* and *S*) is unlike any other tooth of either dentition (Fig. 12-36). The tooth has a prominent buccal cervical ridge, also on the mesial half of the buccal surface, similar to other primary molars. The height of contour on the buccal surface is at the cervical one third of the tooth, and on the lingual side it is at the middle one third. The mesiolingual line angle of the crown is rounder than other line angles.

The primary mandibular first molar has four cusps; the mesial cusps are larger. The mesiolingual cusp is long, pointed, and angled into the occlusal table. A transverse ridge passes between the mesiobuccal and mesiolingual cusps. The tooth has two roots, which are positioned similarly to those of other primary and permanent mandibular molars.

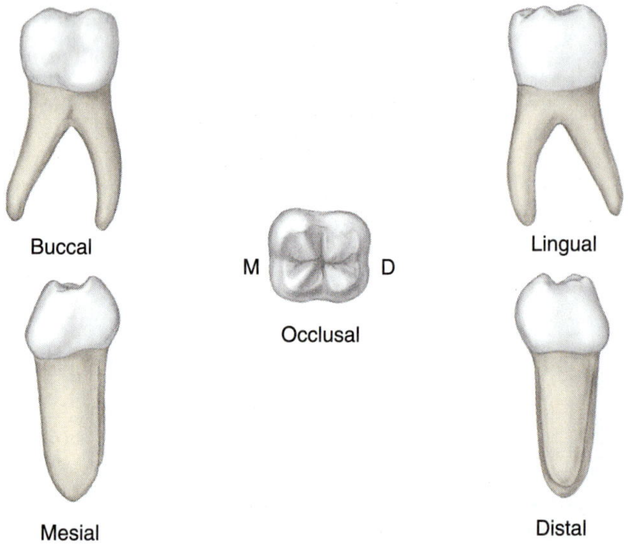

Fig. 12-36 Various views of a primary mandibular first molar. (From Bath-Balogh M, Fehrenbach MJ: *Illustrated dental embryology, histology, and anatomy,* ed 2, St Louis, 2005, Saunders.)

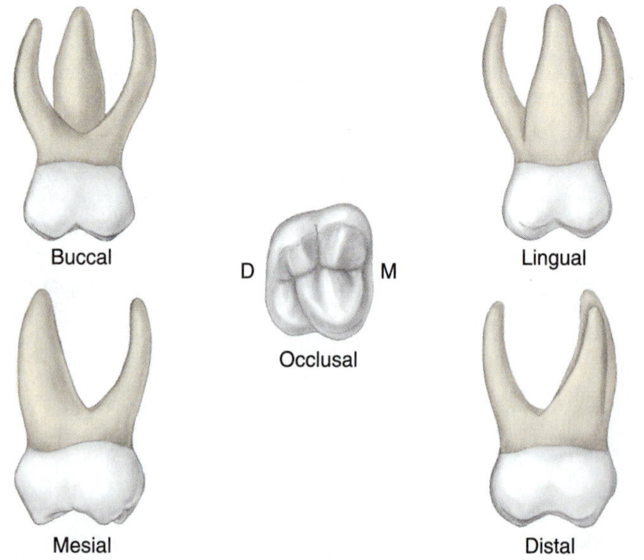

Fig. 12-35 Various views of a primary maxillary second molar. (From Bath-Balogh M, Fehrenbach MJ: *Illustrated dental embryology, histology, and anatomy,* ed 2, St Louis, 2005, Saunders.)

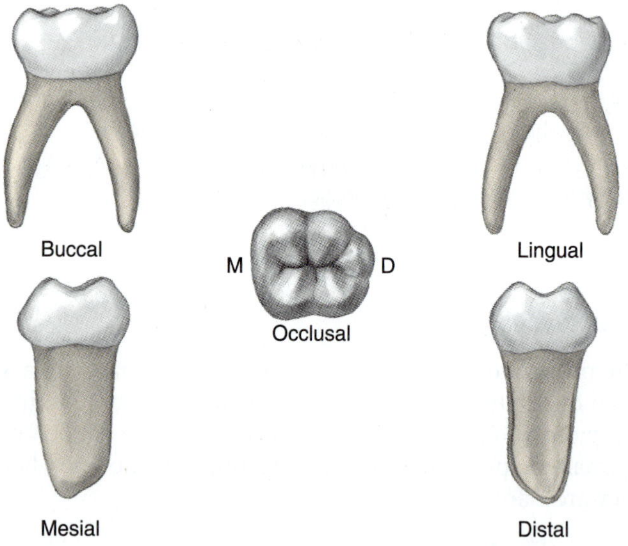

Fig. 12-37 Various views of a primary mandibular second molar. (From Bath-Balogh M, Fehrenbach MJ: *Illustrated dental embryology, histology, and anatomy,* ed 2, St Louis, 2005, Saunders.)

Mandibular Second Molars

The primary mandibular second molar (*K* and *T*) is larger than the primary mandibular first molar (Fig. 12-37). Because it has five cusps, the second molar most closely resembles the form of the permanent mandibular first molar that erupts distal to it. The three buccal cusps are nearly equal in size, however, and the primary mandibular second molar has an overall oval occlusal shape.

Recall

19. Do primary anterior teeth have mamelons?
20. Which primary molar has an H-shaped groove pattern on the occlusal surface?
21. Which primary mandibular molar is the largest?

Eye to the Future

As a practicing dental assistant, you will be surprised at how often your knowledge of tooth morphology and the other dental sciences will directly relate to patient care and your understanding of dental treatment plans.

For example, while exposing radiographs or making impressions, you may notice that the anatomy of the lingual surfaces of the patient's maxillary anterior teeth has an unusually smooth, glassy appearance. You may see few if any stains or lines on the teeth and may notice a slight loss of occlusal anatomy on the posterior teeth. These are common oral manifestations associated with bulimia. The erosion is caused by the acidic gastric fluids from chronic vomiting and movement of the tongue.

A good topic for discussion is how to approach a patient who may have an eating disorder and the steps necessary to regain the patient's oral health.

Critical Thinking

1. Eight-year-old Ricky Martinez is at your dental office for a six-month checkup. While you are waiting for Dr. Miller to come to the treatment room, Ricky asks you why the edges on your front teeth are flat and his have "ruffled edges." What would you tell Ricky?
2. Mrs. Little is in your dental office for her four-year-old daughter Rochelle's checkup. During your conversation with Mrs. Little, it becomes apparent that she does not know the importance of the primary dentition to Rochelle's oral health. What would you tell her?
3. Dr. Berger asks you to obtain a radiograph of tooth T. To which tooth is she referring?
4. A young mother brings her 4-year-old son into your dental office with a toothache. The mother is shocked and embarrassed when the dentist tells her that the decay had gone into the pulp chamber. Another dentist saw the child just over a year ago. How do you think this happened?

Part 3

Oral Health and Prevention of Dental Disease

"The mouth is the gateway to the rest of the body, a mirror of our overall well-being."

Harold C. Slavkin, DDS
Former Director, National Institute of Dental and Craniofacial Research
Dean, University of Southern California, School of Dentistry

The U.S. Surgeon General's report *Oral Health in America (www.nidcr.nih.gov/sgr/sgrohweb.home.htm)* has alerted Americans to the full meaning of oral health and its importance to general health and well-being. A major theme of this report is that **oral health means much more than healthy teeth.** It means being free of chronic oral-facial pain, oral and pharyngeal (throat) cancers, oral soft tissue lesions, birth defects such as cleft lip and palate, and scores of other diseases and disorders. **You cannot be healthy without oral health.** *Oral health* and *general health* should not be interpreted as separate entities. Oral health is a critical component of health.

Every day in the United States, millions of people, including children, working families, and the elderly, live in constant pain as a result of oral disease or injury to the mouth. The chapters in this section discuss the two most important infectious dental diseases–*dental caries* and *periodontal disease*–and describe effective measures to improve oral health and prevent oral disease. Also discussed in this section is the role of nutrition in general health and how it relates to oral health in particular.

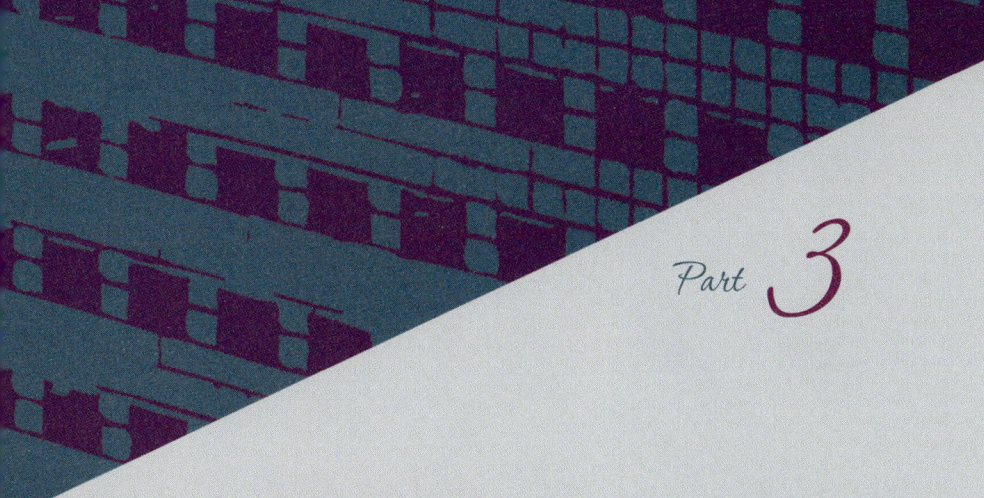

13

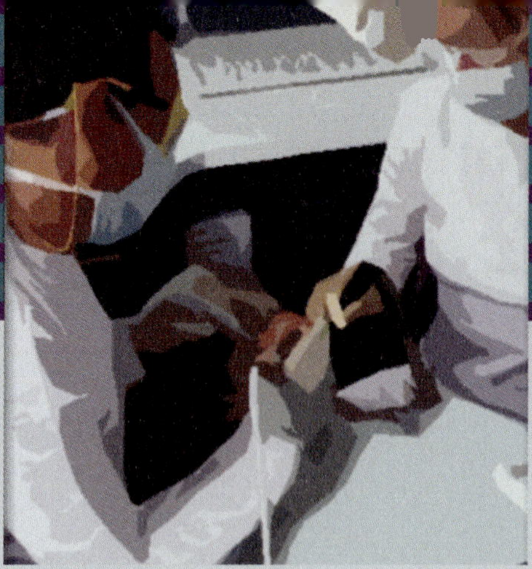

Dental Caries

Outline

KEY TERMS

Caries (**kar**-eez) Tooth decay.

Cavitation (ka-veh-**tay**-shun) Formation of a cavity or hole.

Demineralization (de-mi-neh-ra-leh-**zay**-shun) Loss of minerals from the tooth.

Fermentable carbohydrates (fur-**men**-teh-bull) Simple carbohydrates, such as sucrose, fructose, lactose, and glucose.

Incipient caries (in-**sip**-ee-ent) Tooth decay that is beginning to form or become apparent.

Lactobacilli (*lak*-toe-bah-**sil**-eye) Bacteria that produce lactic acid from carbohydrates.

Mutans streptococci (*strep*-toe-**kok**-si) Type of bacteria primarily responsible for caries.

Pellicle (**pe**-leh-kul) Thin film coating of salivary materials deposited on tooth surfaces.

Plaque (**plak**) Soft deposit on teeth that consists of bacteria and bacterial byproducts.

Rampant caries (**ram**-punt) Decay that develops rapidly and is widespread throughout the mouth.

Remineralization Replacement of minerals in the tooth.

Xerostomia (zir-oh-**sto**-me-ah) Dryness of the mouth caused by reduction of saliva.

LEARNING OUTCOMES

On completion of this chapter, the student will be able to achieve the following objectives:

- Pronounce, define, and spell the Key Terms.
- Name the most common chronic disease in children.
- Recognize dental caries as an infectious disease.
- Explain the process of dental caries.
- Identify the risk factors for dental caries.
- Explain the purpose of caries activity tests.
- Describe the modes of transmission of dental caries.
- Identify the infective agent in the caries process.
- Explain the role of saliva in oral health.
- Describe the relationship between diet and dental caries.
- Explain the remineralization process.
- Distinguish between root caries and smooth surface caries.
- Describe the advantages and disadvantages of the laser caries detection device.

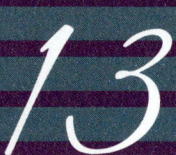

Dental **caries** (tooth decay) is now the single most common chronic disease in children. In fact, there are five times more children in the United States with untreated dental disease than with childhood asthma. This results in more than 50 million missed school hours every year.

Dental caries is an infectious bacterial disease that has plagued humankind since the beginning of recorded history. Since the late 19th century, dentists have been fighting tooth decay by drilling out the decayed tooth structure and filling the tooth with a restorative material. Today, the emphasis in fighting dental caries is shifting from the traditional approach of restoring (filling) teeth to the new strategies of reducing dental caries. Advances in science and new technologies have placed the emphasis on *prevention* and *early intervention*. This chapter discusses the process of tooth decay and the science and practice of caries prevention.

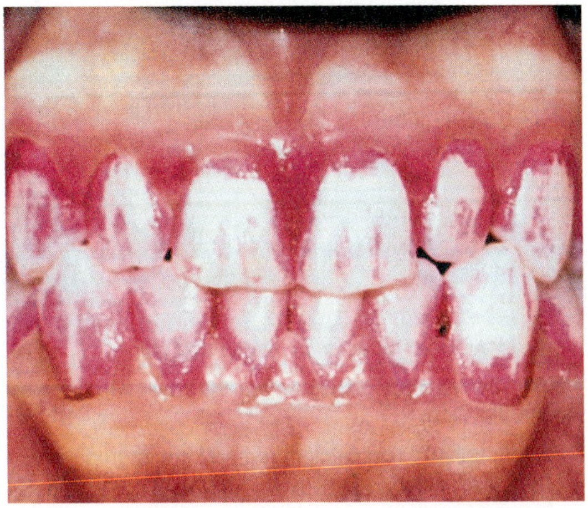

Fig. 13-1 Dental plaque made visible with disclosing agent.

BACTERIAL INFECTION

Certain bacteria in the mouth can metabolize **fermentable carbohydrates** and generate acids as waste products of their metabolism. The two specific groups of bacteria in the mouth that are responsible for dental caries are the **mutans streptococci** (MS) (*Streptococcus mutans*) and the **lactobacilli** (LB).

MS are considered to be the *major pathogenic* (disease-producing) bacteria and are found in relatively large numbers in the dental plaque. The presence of LB in a patient's mouth indicates that the patient has a high sugar intake. MS and LB, either separately or together, are the primary causative agents of dental caries.

It is important to note that the oral cavity of a newborn does not contain MS. However, the bacteria are transmitted through contact with saliva (most frequently the mother's saliva) to the infant. Mothers are the most common source of the disease-causing MS because of the close and frequent contact between mother and child during the first few years. For example, a mother may taste food on a spoon before giving it to her baby. Science has proved that when mothers have high counts of MS in their mouths, their infants also have high counts of the same bacteria in their mouths. Therefore women should be certain their own mouths are healthy.

Remember, dental caries is an infectious disease. When the number of caries-causing bacteria in the mouth increases, the risk for developing dental caries also increases.

Recall

1. What two types of bacteria primarily cause dental caries?
2. Which of the above two types of bacteria is most responsible for dental caries?

Dental Plaque

Dental **plaque** is a colorless, soft, sticky coating that adheres to the teeth (Fig. 13-1). If toothbrushing and flossing are not thorough, plaque will remain attached to the tooth. Even self-cleansing movements of the tongue, or rinsing and spraying the mouth with water or mouthwash will not dislodge the plaque.

If you were to look at plaque under a microscope, you would see colonies of bacteria embedded in an adhesive substance called the **pellicle**. Formation of plaque on a tooth concentrates millions of microorganisms on that tooth. A milligram of wet plaque may contain as many as 200 to 500 million microorganisms. A similar amount of saliva flowing in the oral cavity contains less than 1 percent of this number of organisms, so it is clear that the bacteria in the plaque attached to the tooth are a major part of the problem.

Enamel Structure

To understand the process of how bacterial infection leads to the caries process, it is important to review the structure of the enamel. Enamel is the most highly mineralized tissue in the body and is stronger than bone. Refer to Chapter 8 for an in-depth discussion of the structure of enamel.

Enamel consists of microscopic crystals of hydroxyapatite arranged in structural layers or rods, also known as *prisms*. The crystals are surrounded by water, and primary teeth have slightly more water than permanent teeth. The water in the enamel allows acids to flow into the tooth and minerals to flow out of the tooth. Carbonated apatite, a mineral in enamel, makes it easier for the tooth structure to dissolve (Fig. 13-2).

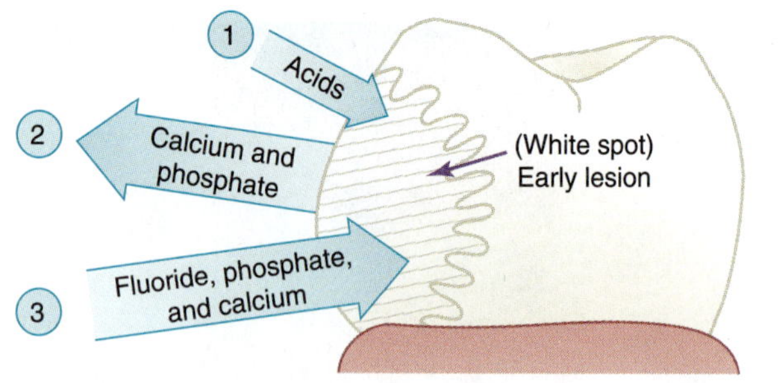

1. The tooth is attacked by acids in plaque and saliva.
2. Calcium and phosphate dissolve from the enamel in the process of demineralization.
3. Fluoride, phosphate, and calcium re-enter the enamel in a process called remineralization.

Fig. 13-2 Chemical interchange of carbonated apatite and acid.

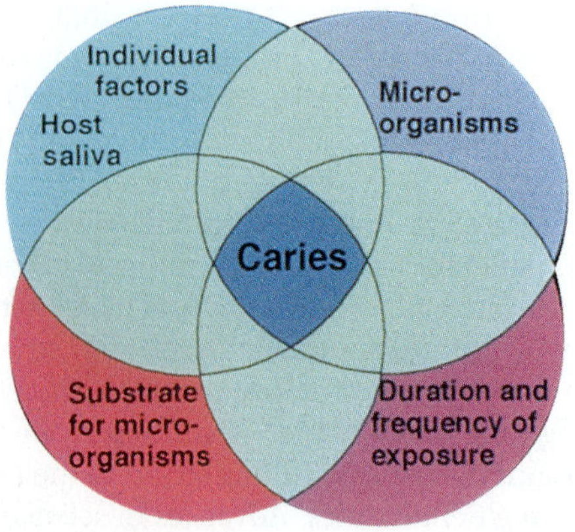

Fig. 13-3 Factors involved in the formation of carious defects. (Courtesy Ivoclar, Vivadent, Amhurst, NY.)

Recall

3. What is the soft, sticky bacterial mass that adheres to the teeth?
4. What is the mineral in the enamel that makes the crystal easier to dissolve?

THE CARIES PROCESS

Dental caries is a disease caused by multiple factors (Fig. 13-3). For caries to develop, the following three factors must occur at the same time:

1. A susceptible tooth
2. Diet rich in fermentable carbohydrates
3. Specific bacteria (regardless of the other factors, caries cannot occur without bacteria)

The bacteria in dental plaque feed on the fermentable carbohydrates found in a regular diet. Just as wastes are a byproduct of eating, the bacteria produce acids as a byproduct of their metabolism. As fermentable carbohydrates are consumed more frequently, more acid is produced and the risk for decay increases. Acid from the plaque travels into the tooth and dissolves the minerals underneath the enamel or dentin surface. If this process progresses, decay develops.

Carious lesions can occur in four general areas of the tooth, as follows:

1. *Pit* and *fissure caries* occurs primarily on the occlusal surfaces, the buccal and lingual grooves of posterior teeth, and the lingual pits of the maxillary incisors.
2. *Smooth surface caries* occurs on intact enamel other than pits and fissures.
3. *Root surface caries* occurs on any surface of the root.
4. *Secondary caries,* or *recurrent caries,* occurs on the tooth surrounding a restoration.

Recall

5. What are the three factors necessary for the formation of dental caries?

Stages of Caries Development

It can take months or even years for a carious lesion to develop. Carious lesions occur when more minerals are lost from the enamel than are deposited. However, dental caries is not simply a continual, cumulative loss of minerals in the tooth. Rather, caries is a dynamic, ongoing process characterized by *alternating periods* of demineralization and remineralization.

Demineralization is the dissolving of the calcium and phosphate from the hydroxyapatite crystals. In **remineralization,** calcium and phosphate are redeposited in previously demineralized areas. The processes of demineralization and remineralization may occur without loss of tooth structure.

Carious lesions develop in two distinct stages, as follows:

1. The first stage, the **incipient caries** or *incipient lesions,* occurs when caries begin to demineralize the enamel (Fig. 13-4, *A*).
2. The second stage, the *overt lesion,* or *frank lesion,* is characterized by **cavitation,** the development of a cavity or hole (Fig. 13-4, *B*).

At times the onset of the incipient lesion is followed rapidly by the development of cavitation, with multiple lesions throughout the mouth. This condition is known as **rampant caries** (Figs. 13-5 and 13-6; also see Fig. 13-4, *C*). Usually, rampant caries occurs after excessive and frequent intake of sucrose or after **xerostomia** (dry mouth).

A

B

C

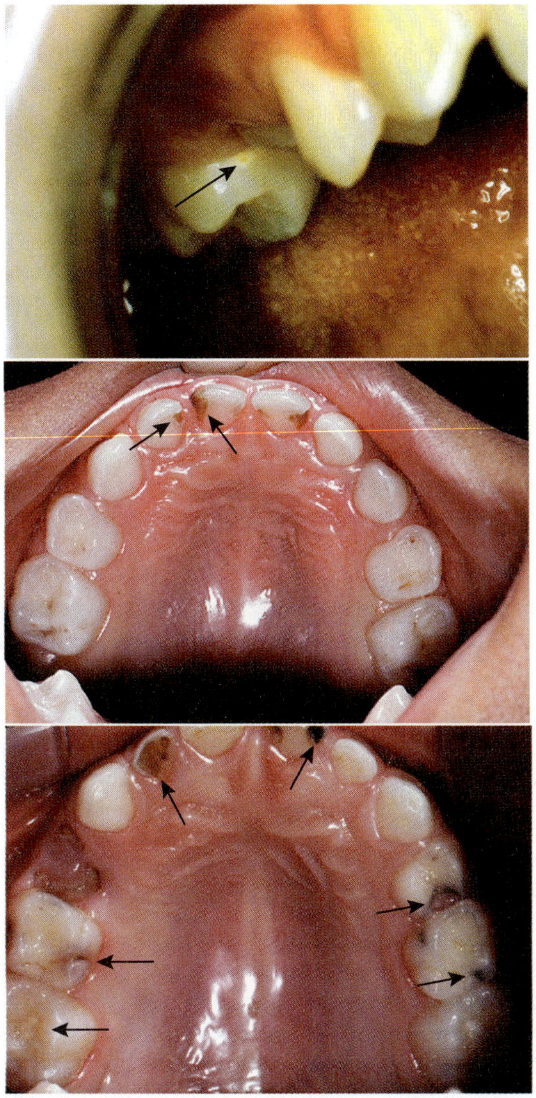

Fig. 13-4 **A,** Early carious lesion, or white spot of demineralization. **B,** Overt carious lesión. **C,** Rampant caries. (**A,** Courtesy Dr. John Featherstone, University of California, San Francisco School of Dentistry; **B** and **C,** Courtesy Dr. Frank Hodges, Santa Rosa, Calif.)

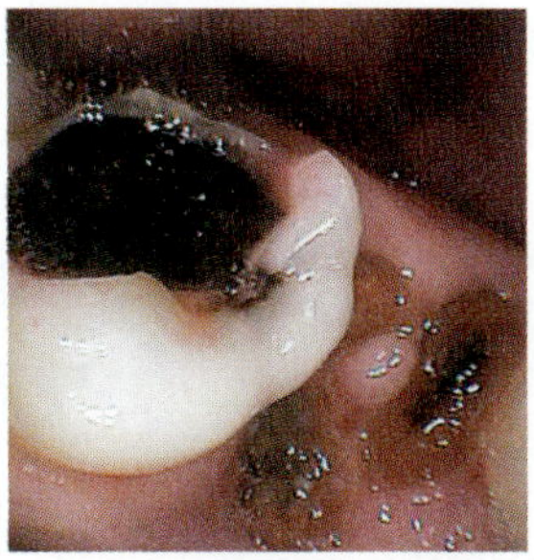

Fig. 13-5 Severely decayed molar on a child.

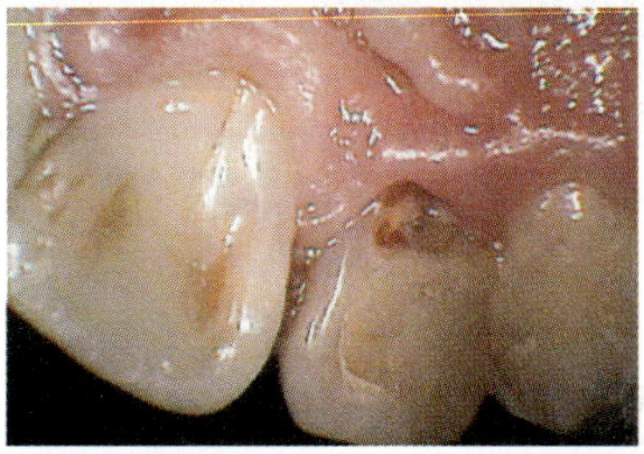

Fig. 13-6 Decay on the lingual surface of a maxillary lateral incisor.

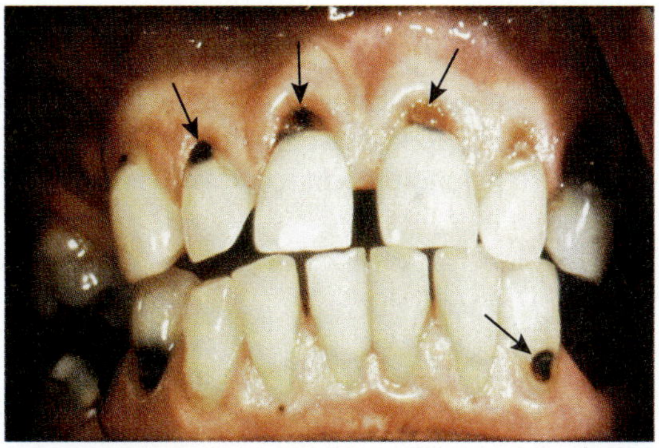

Fig. 13-7 Root surface caries. (Courtesy Dr. John Featherstone, University of California, San Francisco, School of Dentistry.)

Recall

6. What is the term for the dissolution of calcium and phosphate from the tooth?
7. What is the term for rapid and extensive formation of caries?

Root Caries

Root caries is becoming more prevalent and is a particular concern for elderly persons, who often have gingival recession exposing the root surfaces. People are living longer and keeping their teeth longer, and older people often take medications that reduce salivary flow.

Carious lesions on root surfaces form more quickly than do coronal caries because the cementum on the root surface is softer than enamel or dentin. Also, the root lesions have a different clinical appearance. As with coronal caries, root caries undergoes periods of demineralization and remineralization (Fig. 13-7).

Secondary (Recurrent) Caries

Secondary, or recurrent, caries starts to form in the tiny spaces between the tooth and the margins of a restoration. Bacteria are able to thrive in these areas. This type of caries

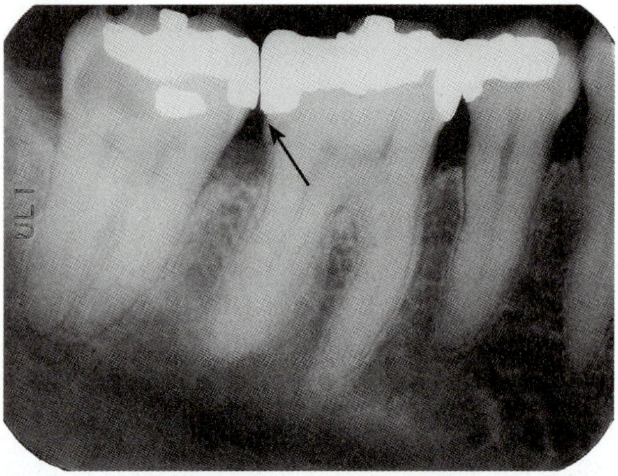

Fig. 13-8 Radiograph showing recurrent decay *(arrow)* under an amalgam restoration.

is very difficult to diagnose because it cannot easily be seen or be detected with an explorer. Radiographs are required to detect this type of caries.

When dental restorations need to be replaced, the reason is usually recurrent caries under the existing restoration. New restorative materials that bond to the tooth structure may help prevent recurrent decay from occurring by eliminating the tiny space between tooth and filling material where microleakage can occur. Restorative materials that slowly release fluoride can also help to prevent secondary caries (Fig. 13-8).

Recall

8. What is the term for caries occurring under or adjacent to existing dental restorations?

THE IMPORTANCE OF SALIVA

Saliva is a crucial substance that provides *physical, chemical,* and *antibacterial* protective measures for the teeth.

The ***physical protection*** is dependent on the water content in the saliva and the amount or flow of saliva. If enough saliva is present, it provides a cleansing effect. The fluid dilutes and removes acid components in the dental plaque. If the saliva is thick, it is less effective than a thinner or more watery saliva in clearing carbohydrates.

The ***chemical protection*** provided by the saliva is especially important because saliva contains calcium, phosphate, and fluoride. Saliva keeps calcium in the mouth, ready to be used during remineralization. Saliva also includes buffers, bicarbonate, phosphate, and small proteins that neutralize acids after ingestion of fermentable carbohydrates.

The ***antibacterial protection*** provided by saliva depends on substances within the saliva, such as immunoglobulins, that work against the bacteria. However, if the bacterial count becomes very high, these substances may not be able to provide sufficient antibacterial protection.

If salivary function is reduced because of illness, medications, or radiation therapy, the teeth are at increased risk for decay.

Recall

9. What are the three protective mechanisms produced by saliva?

DIAGNOSIS OF CARIES

Accurately diagnosing early dental caries is a challenge for the dentist. The following methods are used for detecting dental caries, and each has specific limitations. (Detection of dental caries is also discussed in Chapter 28.)

Dental Explorer

When a sharp explorer tip is pressed into an area of suspected caries, it will "stick" when being removed. New research shows that this technique is not effective in diagnosing carious lesions on teeth that have been exposed to fluoride because the enamel is harder.

Radiographs

Although useful for detection of interproximal caries, early caries on occlusal surfaces is not visible on radiographs. In addition, the extent of caries can easily be misdiagnosed because the caries is often two times deeper and more widespread than it appears on radiographs.

Visual Appearance

The appearance of dark-stained grooves in the teeth may indicate caries, although the dark grooves may also simply be stain caused by coffee or tea. A gray shadowing underneath enamel can also indicate decay.

Indicator Dyes

Special dyes are available for use during operative procedures; these products, when applied to the inside of a preparation, can indicate through a color change whether there is still decay remaining.

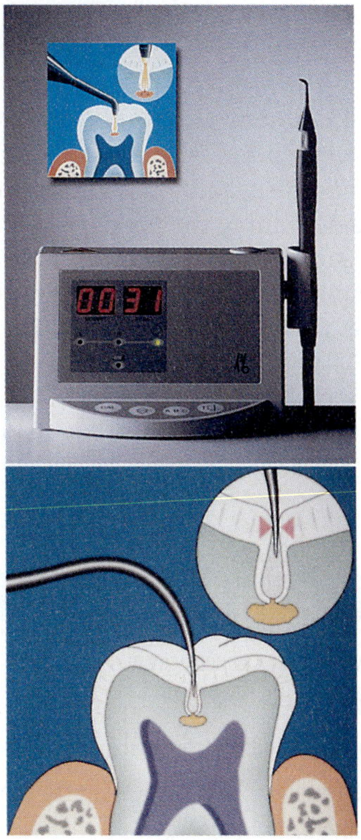

Fig. 13-9 The DIAGNOdent directs a laser beam into the occlusal surface. (Courtesy KaVo America, Lake Zurich, Ill.)

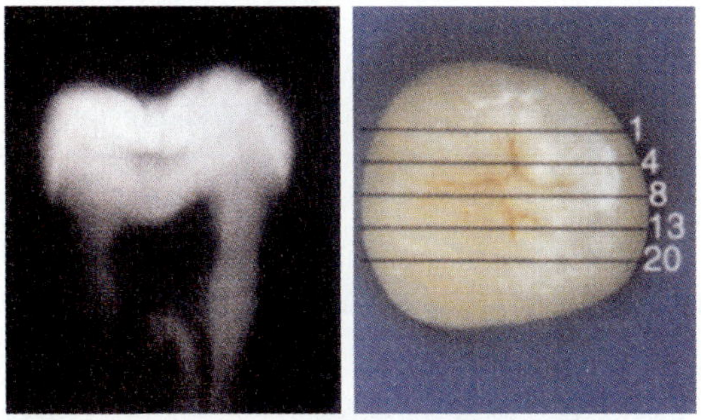

Fig. 13-10 Visual and radiographic appearance of seemingly intact molar. (Courtesy KaVo America, Lake Zurich, Ill.)

Laser Caries Detector

The laser caries detector is a newly developed device used to diagnose caries and reveal bacterial activity under the enamel surface (Fig. 13-9).

A small, battery-operated unit directs a laser beam into the tooth. When the laser beam passes through a change in the density of the tooth, it gives off a fluorescent light of different wavelengths. A clean, healthy tooth exhibits little or no fluorescence, resulting in very low readings. However, carious tooth structure shows higher degrees of fluorescence. The larger the amount of decay, the higher the readings.

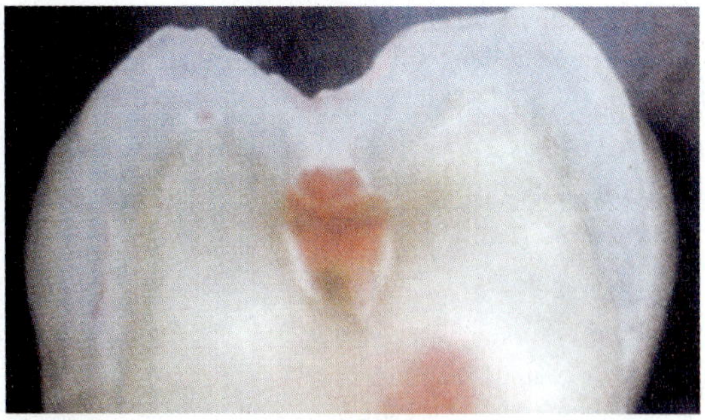

Fig. 13-11 Cross-section of molar showing decay. (Courtesy KaVo America, Lake Zurich, Ill.)

Benefits of Caries Risk Assessment

Testing is easily done.

In-office testing is cost-effective.

Dental assistants can perform tests.

Plans for prevention can be individualized.

Patients are motivated to undergo treatment.

The laser caries detector is equally effective in both primary and permanent teeth (Figs. 13-10 and 13-11). The laser wavelength is translated into a number from 0 to 99 that appears on the face of the unit.

There are limitations to the use of the laser. For example, it cannot be used to diagnose interproximal caries because of the limited access of those surfaces. It cannot detect caries under dental sealants or under an amalgam restoration, although it will detect decay around the occlusal margins of a restoration.

METHODS OF CARIES INTERVENTION

Even though the dentist restores (fills) the carious teeth, there is still the risk for further decay. This is because restoring teeth has no effect on the bacteria still living in the mouth. Dental caries occurs when there are more disease-causing agents (e.g., bacteria, fermentable carbohydrates) in the mouth than protective agents (e.g., saliva, fluoride). The caries process can be interrupted or prevented in the following ways:

- *Fluoride.* Various forms of fluoride are available to strengthen teeth against solubility and acid.
- *Antibacterial therapy.* Products such as chlorhexidine mouthrinses are effective agents against bacteria in the oral cavity.
- *Decreased fermentable carbohydrates.* Another intervention is reducing the amount and frequency of fermentable carbohydrates in the diet.

- *Increased salivary flow.* Chewing sugarless gum, including newer types with the noncariogenic sweetener *xylitol,* increases the flow of saliva (Fig. 13-12).

These methods of caries intervention are discussed in greater detail in Chapter 15.

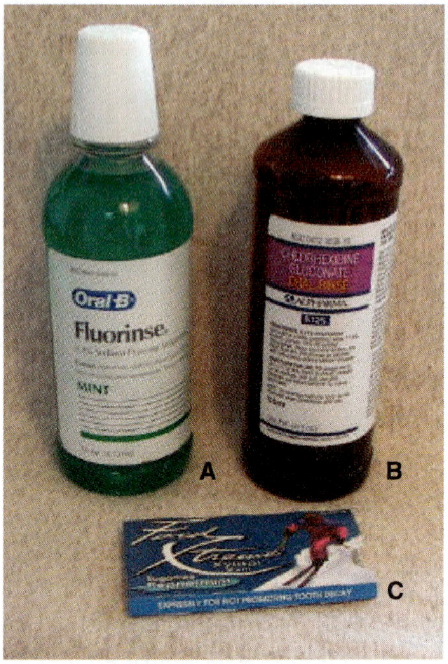

Fig. 13-12 Preventive measures against caries. **A,** Fluoride rinse. **B,** Chlorhexidine rinse. **C,** Xylitol gum.

RISK ASSESSMENT FOR CARIES

Caries risk assessment tests are used to detect the number of MS and LB present in the saliva. High bacterial counts indicate a high caries risk, and low counts indicate a low risk for caries. By determining the patient's risk for developing dental caries, and by beginning appropriate preventive treatment, dental caries can be prevented from ever forming. Procedure 13-1 reviews the steps in the caries risk assessment.

Patients with high numbers of bacteria in the mouth are very likely to develop carious lesions if preventive measures are not provided.

Candidates for Caries Risk Testing

- New patients with signs of caries activity
- Pregnant patients
- Patients experiencing sudden increase in incidence of caries
- Individuals taking medications that may affect the flow of saliva
- Patients with xerostomia
- Patients with upcoming chemotherapy
- Patients who consume fermentable carbohydrates frequently
- Patients with diseases of the immune system

Procedure 13-1 Performing Caries Risk Assessment

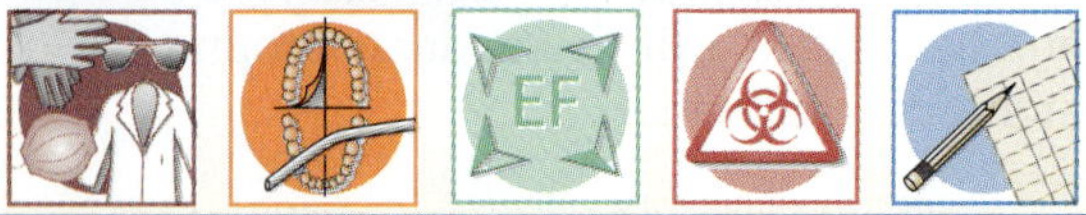

Goal

To perform a caries risk assessment using the Caries Risk Test (CRT, Ivoclar) and comparing the density of mutans streptococci (MS) and lactobacilli (LB) colonies with the corresponding evaluation pictures.

Equipment and Supplies

- CRT kit
- Paraffin pellet
- $NaHCO_3$ tablet (sodium, hydrogen, carbonate)
- Pipette
- Agar carrier
- Test vial
- Evaluation chart
- Paper cup
- Pen with waterproof ink
- Culture incubator

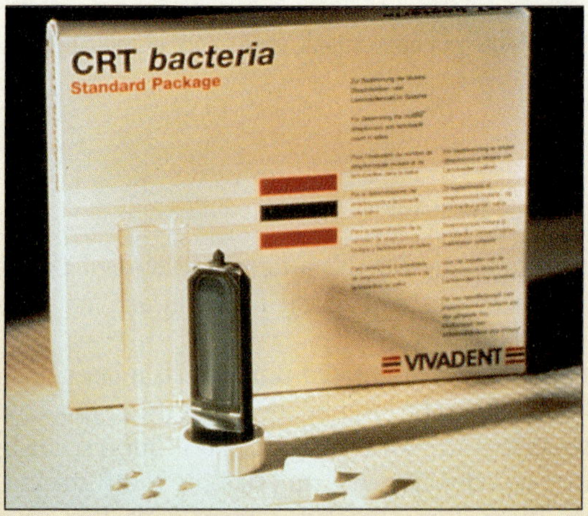

Procedure 13-1 Performing Caries Risk Assessment—cont'd

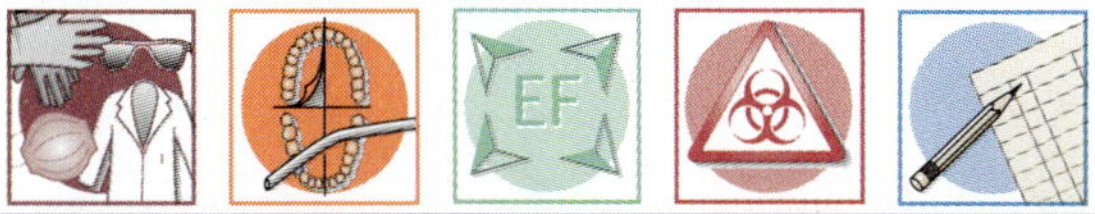

PROCEDURAL STEPS

1. Explain the procedure to the patient.
   Purpose: To educate the patient about the process of caries risk assessment.
2. Have the patient chew the paraffin wax pellet.
   Purpose: To stimulate salivation.

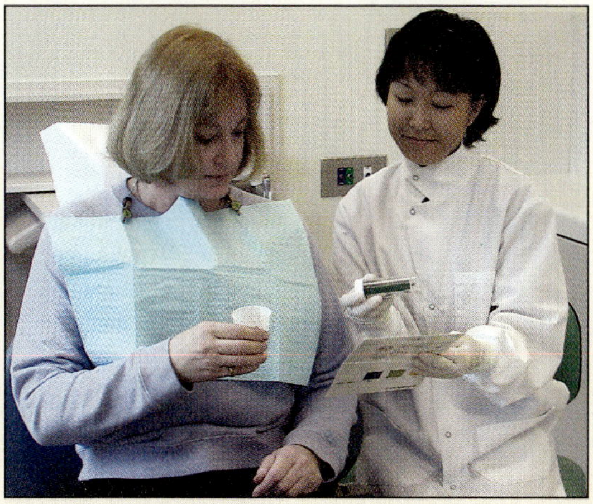

3. Have the patient expectorate into the paper cup.
   Purpose: To collect the saliva sample.

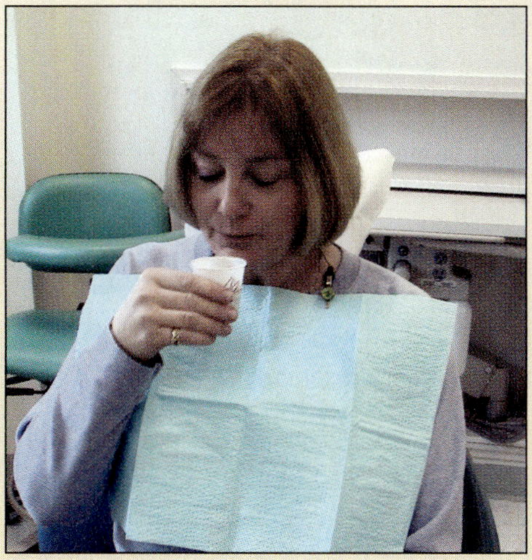

4. Remove the agar carrier from the test vial and place an $NaHCO_3$ tablet at the bottom of the vial.
   Purpose: The $NaHCO_3$ tablet will determine the buffer capacity of the saliva.

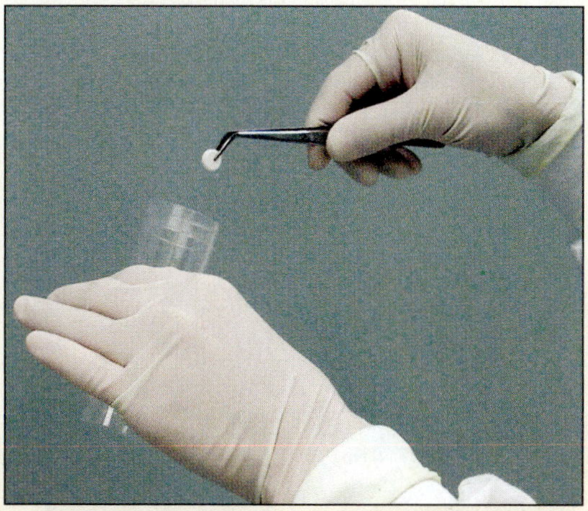

5. Carefully remove the protective foils from the two agar surfaces. Do not touch the agar.
   Purpose: To prevent contamination of the agar surfaces.

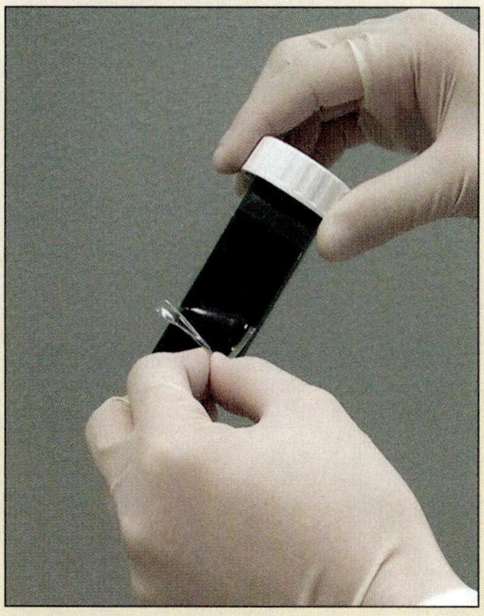

continued

Procedure 13-1 Performing Caries Risk Assessment—cont'd

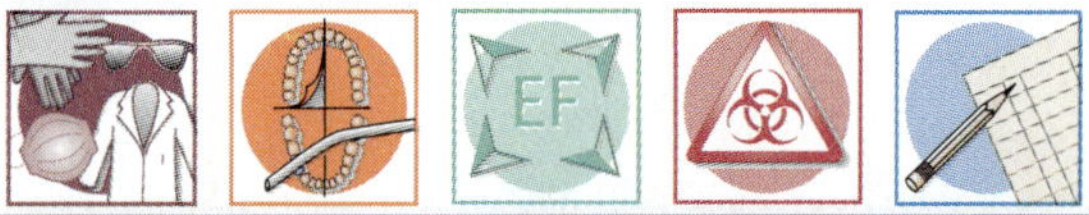

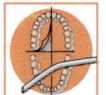

PROCEDURAL STEPS, cont'd

6. Thoroughly wet both agar surfaces using a pipette. Avoid scratching the agar surface. Hold the carrier at an angle while wetting.
   Purpose: One side is sensitive to MS, and the other side is sensitive to LB.

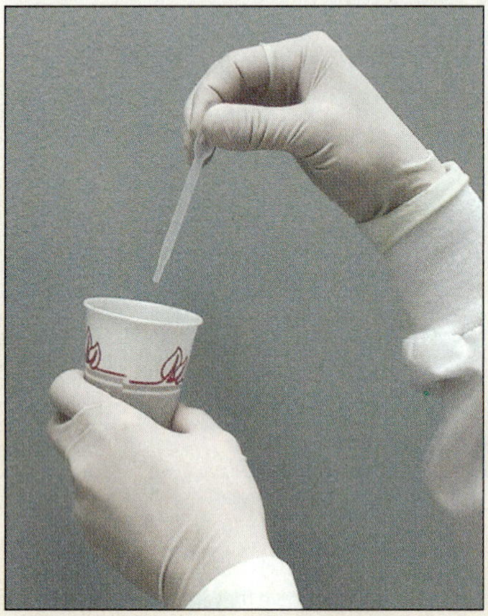

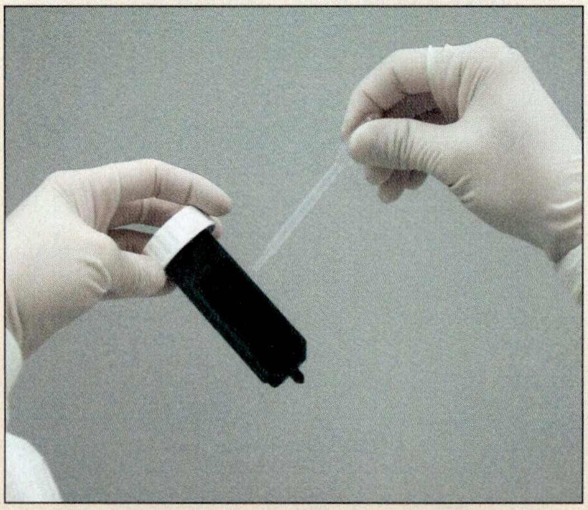

7. Slide the agar carrier back into the vial and close the vial tightly.
   Purpose: To prevent cross-contamination of the sample.

8. Use a waterproof pen to note the name of the patient and the date on the lid of the vial.

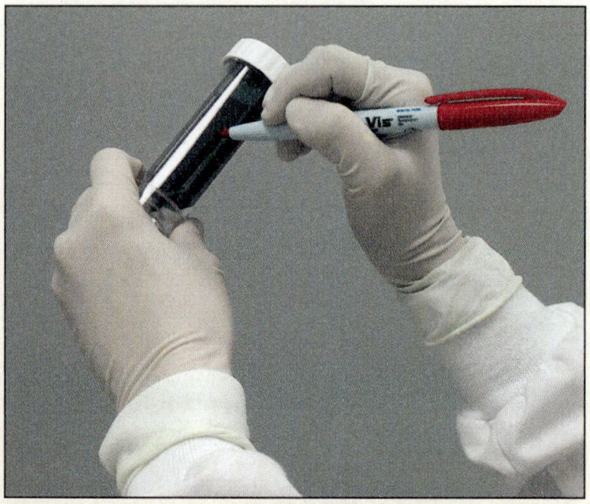

9. Place the test vial upright in the incubator. Incubate at 37° C (99° F) for 49 hours.
   Purpose: To allow the bacteria on the agar strips to grow.

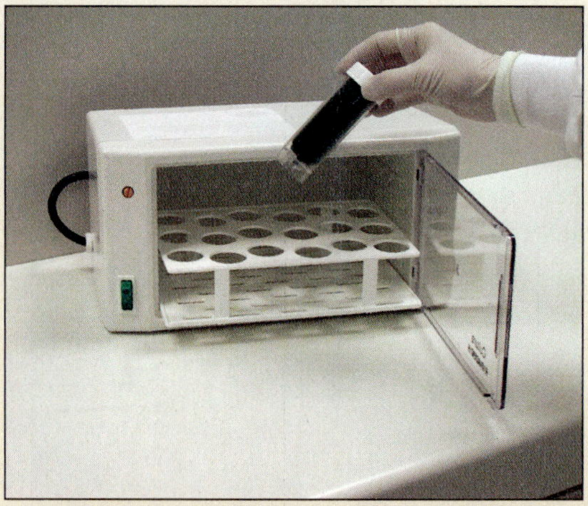

10. Remove the vial from the incubator.

Procedure 13-1 Performing Caries Risk Assessment—cont'd

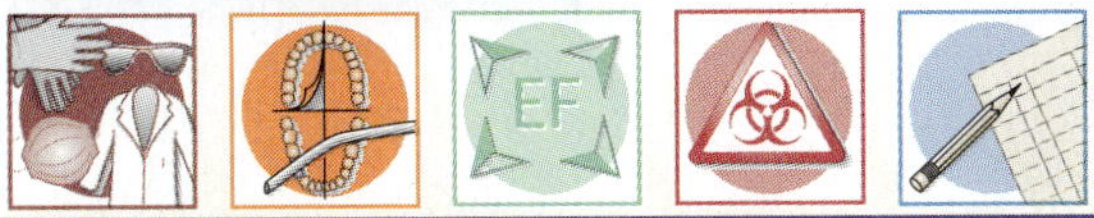

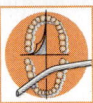

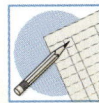

11. Compare the density of the bacterial colonies with the corresponding evaluation pictures on the chart included in the CRT kit.
    Tip: Hold the agar carrier at a slight angle under a light source to see the colonies clearly.

    A. Compare the density of the MS colonies

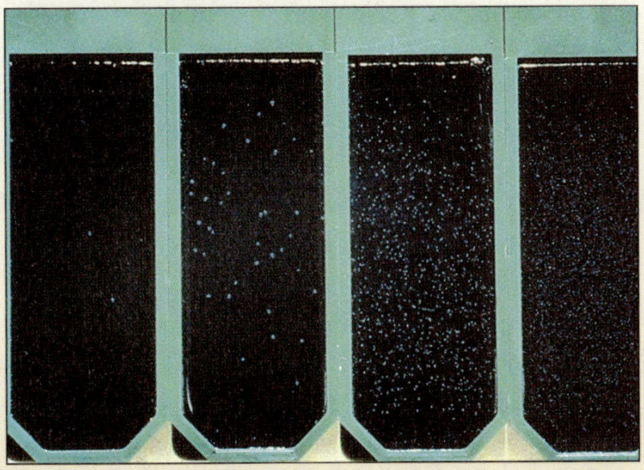

    B. Compare the density of the LB colonies

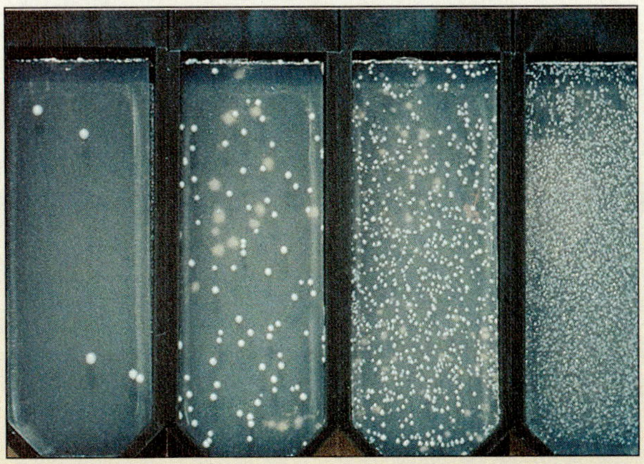

Legal and Ethical Implications

When should a carious lesion be observed, treated with some preventive measure, or actually restored? There is no single answer to this question. This is an individual decision that the dentist must make for each patient, and it is based on sound professional judgment.

The dentist must analyze the patient's diet, dental history, and oral hygiene regimen to determine which approach to tooth restoration is necessary. People with a high caries rate may need immediate restorations of lesions. On the other hand, for lesions that have been dormant for many years, the dentist may choose to watch for additional time without dental intervention.

There are varying professional opinions about whether or not to restore small initial carious lesions in teeth. The opinions range from the conservative preference for remineralizing initial lesions to a more aggressive approach of restoring all carious lesions. Each dentist must make his or her own decisions on the basis of the individual patient's history and needs.

Eye to the Future

Diagnosis of dental caries has become more challenging as knowledge of the disease has changed. More factors involved in the caries process have been identified. Risk factors are better understood, and better methods for detection are being developed. Most important, strategies for the prevention of dental caries must continue to be formulated.

In the future, it is anticipated that advances in molecular biology will provide dental professionals with a rapid method of assessing a patient's risk for dental caries before the patient leaves the dental chair. Someday there will likely be a vaccine to prevent dental caries.

Critical Thinking

1. Mr. Johnstone comes into your office complaining of pain in a lower right first molar. The tooth has a large amalgam restoration that was placed 10 years ago. As you begin to take the radiograph, you do not see any visible decay. What is a possible cause for his pain?
2. The Hatrick twins are in your dental office for a routine checkup. Mrs. Hatrick informs you that they both eat the same amount of sweets. However, Christie eats her sweets all at once, whereas Carol divides her sweets throughout the day. Which of the twins is most likely to have tooth decay? Why?
3. As a dental assistant, you have been asked to speak to a group of pregnant women regarding their dental health. Why is it important for these pregnant women to have excellent dental health before their babies are born?

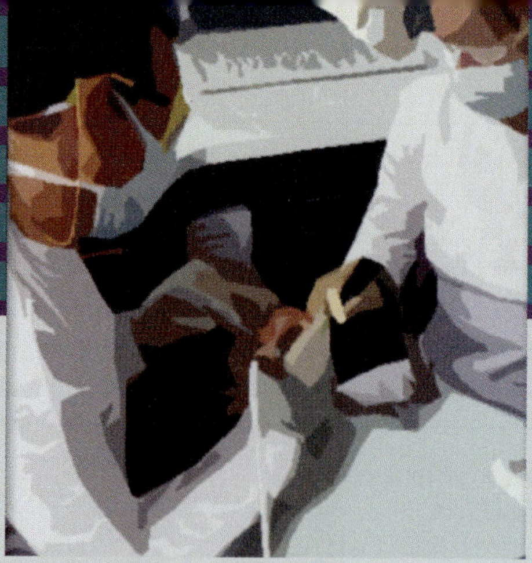

14 Periodontal Disease

Outline

KEY TERMS

Calculus (**kal**-kyou-lus) Calcium and phosphate salts in saliva that become mineralized and adhere to tooth surfaces.

Gingivitis (*jin*-jih-**vi**-tis) Inflammation of the gingival tissue.

Periodontal (per-ee-oh-**don**-tul) Referring to the periodontium.

Periodontitis (per-ee-oh-*don*-**ti**-tis) Inflammatory disease of the supporting tissues of the teeth.

Periodontium (*per*-e-oh-**don**-she-um) Structures that surround, support, and are attached to the teeth.

Perioscopy (per-ee-**os**-co-py) Procedure using a dental endoscope subgingivally.

Plaque (**plak**) Soft deposit on teeth that consists of bacteria and bacterial byproducts.

Subgingival (*sub*-**jin**-jih-vul) Referring to the area below the gingiva.

Supragingival (*soo*-pruh-**jin**-jih-vul) Referring to the area above the gingiva.

LEARNING OUTCOMES

On completion of this chapter, the student will be able to achieve the following objectives:

- Pronounce, define, and spell the Key Terms.
- Name and describe the tissues of the periodontium.
- Describe the prevalence of periodontal disease.
- Name the structures that make up the periodontium.
- Identify systemic factors influencing periodontal disease.
- Identify and describe the two main types of periodontal diseases.
- Explain the significance of plaque and calculus in periodontal disease.
- Identify the risk factors that contribute to periodontal disease.
- Describe the systemic conditions that are linked to periodontal disease.
- Describe the clinical characteristics of gingivitis.
- Describe the progression of periodontitis.

Periodontal disease is an infectious process that involves inflammation. Periodontal diseases involve the structures of the periodontium (Box 14-1).

The **periodontium** is made up of the structures that surround, support, and are attached to the teeth (Fig. 14-1).

Box 14-1 Structures of the Periodontium

Name	Description
Gingivae	Commonly referred to as *gums.* This mucosa covers the alveolar process of the jaws and surrounds the necks of the teeth.
Epithelial attachment	Tissue at the base of the sulcus where the gingiva attaches to the tooth.
Sulcus	Space between the tooth and the free gingiva.
Periodontal ligaments	Dense connective fibers that connect the cementum covering the root of the tooth with the alveolar bone of the socket wall.
Cementum	Covers the root of the tooth. The primary function of the cementum is to anchor the tooth to the bony socket with the attachments of the periodontal ligaments.
Alveolar bone	The bone that supports the tooth in its position within the jaw. The *alveolar socket* is the cavity in the bone that surrounds the tooth.

From Robinson D, Bird D: *Essentials of dental assisting,* ed 3, Philadelphia, 2001, Saunders.

Periodontal disease causes a breakdown of the periodontium, resulting in loss of tissue attachment and destruction of the alveolar bone.

This chapter discusses the various types of periodontal diseases, including the causes and common signs and symptoms. Chapter 55 discusses the dental specialty of periodontics, including periodontal charting, instrumentation, treatment procedures, and surgical techniques.

PREVALENCE

Periodontal diseases are the leading cause of tooth loss in adults. Almost 75 percent of American adults have some form of periodontal disease, and most are unaware of the condition. Almost all adults and many children have calculus on their teeth.

Fortunately, with early detection and treatment of periodontal disease, most people can keep their teeth for life.

SYSTEMIC CONDITIONS LINKED TO PERIODONTAL DISEASE

Certain systemic conditions increase the patient's susceptibility to periodontal disease, and periodontal disease, in turn, may actually increase a patient's susceptibility to certain systemic conditions.

Cardiovascular Disease

Individuals with periodontal disease have a higher incidence of coronary heart disease. This results in a greater occurrence of strokes and heart attacks. Individuals with

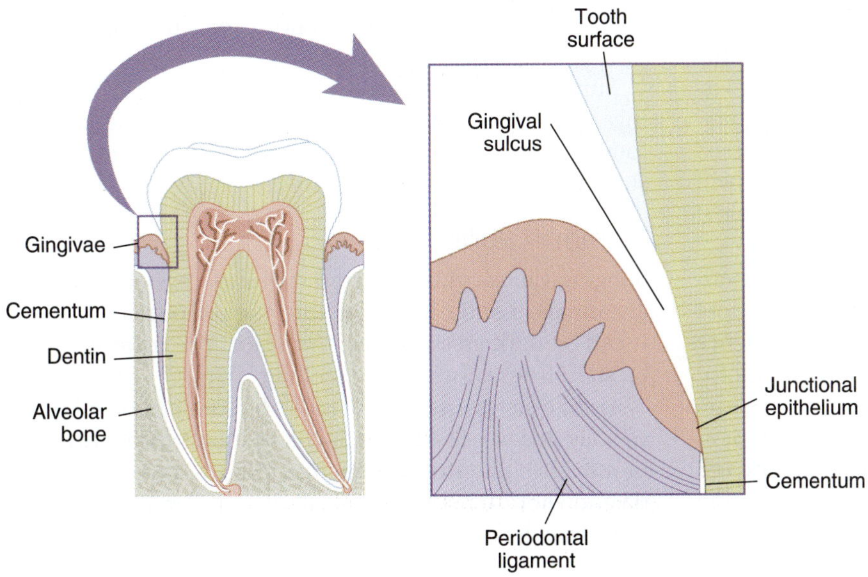

Fig. 14-1 Structures of the periodontium: junctional epithelium, gingival sulcus, periodontal ligaments, and cementum.

severe periodontal disease have 3 times the risk for stroke and 3.6 times the risk for coronary heart disease when compared with individuals without periodontal disease. Studies show that oral bacteria can easily spread into the bloodstream, attach to fatty plaques in the coronary arteries, and contribute to clot formation and heart attacks.

Preterm Low Birth Weight

Preterm birth is defined as a pregnancy of less than 37 weeks, and low birth weight is less than 5.5 pounds. Preterm birth and low birth weight are the two most significant predictors of the health and survival of an infant. Other risk factors such as smoking, alcohol use, and drug use also contribute to preterm low-birth-weight (PLBW) infants. Women with severe periodontal disease have 7 times the risk for PLBW babies as women with little or no periodontal disease. The cause of this association may be linked to certain biochemicals that are produced with periodontal disease, such as *prostaglandin* E_2, which may create hormones that cause early uterine contraction and labor.

Respiratory Disease

Individuals with periodontal disease may also be at greater risk for respiratory infections. It appears that the bacteria colonized in the mouth may alter the respiratory epithelium, leaving it more susceptible to pneumonia. In addition, patients who already have chronic bronchitis, emphysema, and chronic obstructive pulmonary disease may have their existing conditions aggravated by inhaling bacteria from the mouth into the lungs. These bacteria multiply in the respiratory tract and cause infections.

Dental Plaque

Plaque is a soft mass of bacterial deposits that covers the tooth surfaces. When the plaque layer is thin, it is not visible, but it will stain pink when a disclosing agent (erythrosine stain) is applied. (Staining plaque is discussed further in Chapter 15.) If not removed, the plaque will continue to build up and appear as a sticky white material (Fig. 14-2).

Although plaque is the primary factor in causing periodontal disease, the type of bacteria, the amount of time bacteria are left undisturbed on the teeth, and the patient's response to the bacteria are all critical factors in the risk for developing periodontal disease. Plaque cannot be removed simply by rinsing the mouth. The bacteria in dental plaque cause inflammation by producing enzymes and toxins that destroy the periodontal tissues and lower the host defenses.

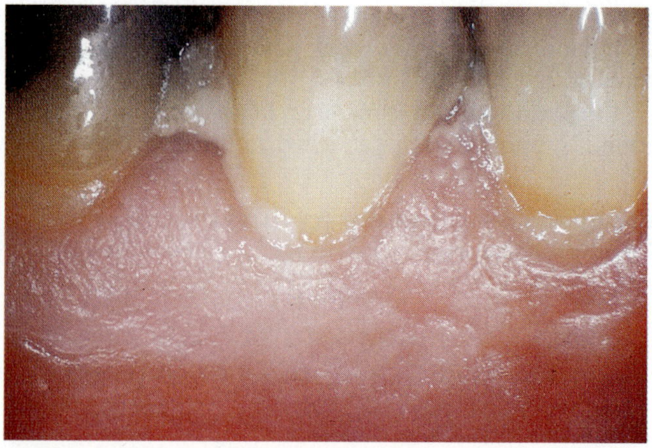

Fig. 14-2 Buildup of bacterial plaque on the teeth affects the gingival tissues.

Calculus

The calcium and phosphate salts in the saliva form **calculus,** commonly called "tartar." Calculus is a hard, stonelike material that attaches to the tooth surface. The surface of calculus is porous and rough and provides an excellent surface on which additional plaque can grow. Calculus can also penetrate into the cementum on root surfaces. It cannot be removed by the patient and must be removed by the dentist or the dental hygienist with scaling instruments. Regular, effective plaque control measures can minimize or eliminate the buildup of calculus. Plaque control measures are discussed in Chapter 15.

Calculus is usually divided into **supragingival** and **subgingival** types, even though both types often occur together.

Supragingival Calculus

Supragingival calculus is found on the clinical crowns of the teeth, above the margin of the gingiva. It is readily visible as a yellowish-white deposit that may darken over time (Fig. 14-3).

Supragingival calculus occurs frequently near the openings of Wharton's ducts (on the lingual surfaces of the lower anterior teeth) and Stensen's ducts (on the buccal surfaces of the maxillary molars).

Subgingival Calculus

Subgingival calculus forms on root surfaces below the gingival margin and can extend into the periodontal pockets. It can be dark green or black in color. The color is caused by stain from subgingival bleeding.

Unlike supragingival calculus, the location of subgingival calculus is not site-specific. It is found throughout the mouth. Subgingival calculus provides a reservoir for bacteria and endotoxins. Subgingival calculus covered by plaque can cause greater disease than plaque alone.

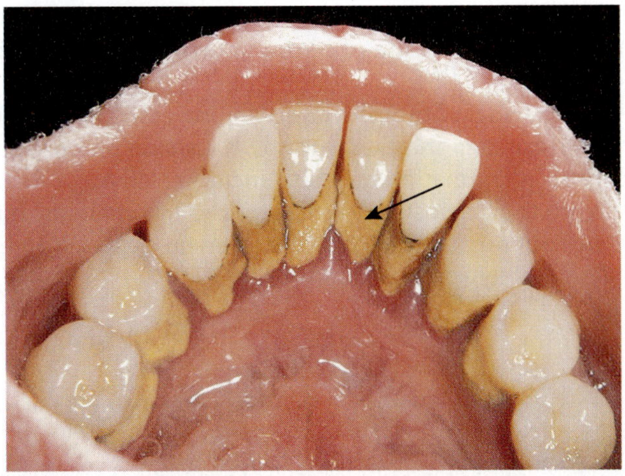

Fig. 14-3 **Heavy calculus deposits on the lingual surfaces of the lower anterior teeth.** (Courtesy Dr. Edward J. Taggart, San Francisco, Calif.)

Tooth Deposits

Acquired pellicle Thin film of protein that quickly forms on teeth. It can be removed by coronal polishing with an abrasive agent such as "prophy" paste.

Materia alba Soft mixture of bacteria and salivary proteins, also known as "white material." It is visible without the use of a disclosing agent and is common in individuals with poor oral hygiene.

Food debris Particles of food that are impacted between the teeth after eating. Food debris does not simply become plaque. If fermentable carbohydrates are present, however, the food debris may contribute to dental caries.

Other Risk Factors

The vast majority of periodontal diseases begin as an inflammation caused by an accumulation of bacterial plaque. However, periodontal diseases may also be triggered by other factors such as malocclusions, certain medications (such as for blood pressure), and serious nutritional deficiencies.

Disease-causing bacteria are necessary for periodontal disease to begin, but they are not totally responsible for the destruction of the periodontium. Other risk factors alter the body's response to the bacteria present in the mouth. The risk factors involved will determine the onset, degree, and severity of the periodontal disease. This is why there is a great deal of variability in each individual's susceptibility to periodontal disease and success in treatment of the disease.

Periodontal disease is a complex interaction of bacterial infection and risk factors; the more risk factors an individual has, the greater the susceptibility for periodontal disease (Box 14-2).

Box 14-2 Common Risk Factors for Periodontal Disease

Risk Factor	Rationale
Smoking	Smokers have greater loss of attachment, bone loss, periodontal pocket depths, calculus formation, and tooth loss. Periodontal treatments are less effective in smokers than in nonsmokers.
Diabetes mellitus	Diabetes is a strong risk factor for periodontal disease. Individuals with diabetes are three times more likely to have attachment and bone loss. Persons who have their diabetes under control have less attachment and bone loss than those with poor control.
Poor oral hygiene	Lack of good oral hygiene increases the risk of periodontal disease in all age groups. Excellent oral hygiene greatly reduces the risk of severe periodontal disease.
Osteoporosis	There is an association between alveolar bone loss and osteoporosis. Women with osteoporosis have increased alveolar bone resorption, attachment loss, and tooth loss compared with women without osteoporosis. Estrogen deficiency also has been linked to decreases in alveolar bone.
HIV/AIDS	There is increased gingival inflammation around the margins of all the teeth. Often patients with HIV/AIDS will develop necrotizing ulcerative periodontitis (NUP).
Stress	Psychological stress is associated with depression of the immune system, and studies show a link between stress and periodontal attachment loss. Research is still ongoing to determine the link between psychological stress and periodontal disease.
Medications	Some medications, such as tetracycline and nonsteroidal anti-inflammatory drugs (NSAIDs), have a beneficial effect on the periodontium, and others have a negative effect. Decreased salivary flow (xerostomia) can be caused by more than 400 medications, including diuretics, antihistamines, antipsychotics, antihypertension agents, and analgesics. Antiseizure drugs and hormones such as estrogen and progesterone can cause gingival enlargement.
Local factors	Overhanging restorations, subgingival placement of crown margins, orthodontic appliances, and removable partial dentures also may contribute to the progression of periodontal disease.

TYPES

The term *periodontal disease* includes both gingivitis and periodontitis.

Gingivitis and periodontitis are the two basic forms of periodontal disease, and each has a variety of forms. It is important to have a clear understanding of the characteristics of the healthy periodontium as a foundation on which to recognize signs of disease. You may want to review the appearance of healthy oral tissues presented in Chapter 10.

Gingivitis

Gingivitis is inflammation of the gingival tissue. It may be the most common human disease and is one of the easiest to treat and control. Areas of redness and swelling characterize gingivitis, and the gingiva tends to bleed easily. In addition, there may be changes in the gingival contour and loss of tissue adaptation to the teeth (Table 14-1).

Gingivitis is found only in the epithelium and gingival connective tissues. There is *no* tissue recession or loss of connective tissue or bone associated with gingivitis (Fig. 14-4).

Other types of gingivitis are associated with puberty, pregnancy, and the use of birth control medications (Fig. 14-5 and Box 14-3).

When female hormone levels are increased, some subgingival bacteria increase, such as *Bacteroides* species, and gingival inflammation may also increase. Although this is believed to be associated with increases in female sex hormone secretions, the success of treatment depends on excellent oral hygiene (Fig. 14-6).

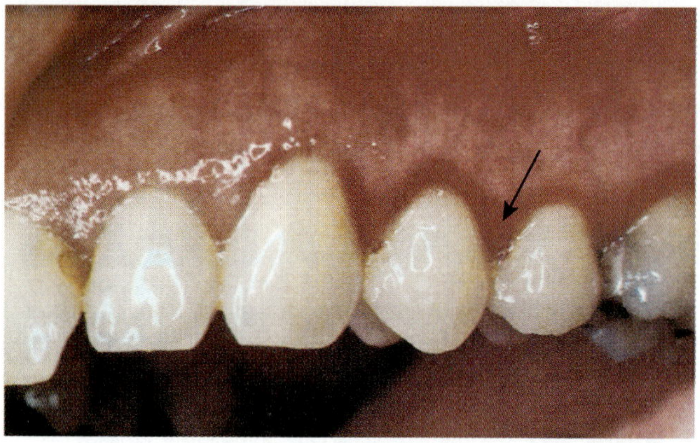

Fig. 14-4 Gingivitis type I.

Table 14-1 *Terminology Used to Describe Observations Associated with Clinical Assessment of Gingiva*

Characteristic	Terminology	Description	Example
Gingival color	Location:	Generalized or localized	Localized slight marginal redness on linguals of numbers 18, 19, 30, 31; all other areas coral pink, uniform in color
	Distribution:	Diffuse, marginal, or papillary	
	Severity:	Slight, moderate, severe	
	Quality:	Red, bright red, pink, cyanotic	
Gingival contour	Location:	Generalized or localized	Localized moderately cratered papilla on numbers 6-11, 22-27; all other areas within normal limits
	Distribution:	Diffuse, marginal, or papillary	
	Severity:	Slight, moderate, severe	
	Quality:	Bulbous, flattened, punched-out, cratered	
Consistency of gingiva	Location:	Generalized or localized	Generalized moderate marginal sponginess more severe on facial numbers 8, 9; all other areas coral pink with moderate, generalized melanin pigmentation
	Distribution:	Diffuse, marginal, or papillary	
	Severity:	Slight, moderate, severe	
	Quality:	Firm (fibrotic), spongy (edematous)	
Surface texture of gingiva	Location:	Generalized or localized	Localized smooth gingiva on facial numbers 7, 8; all other areas with generalized stippling
	Distribution:	Diffuse, marginal, or papillary	
	Quality:	Smooth, shiny, eroded, stippling	

From Darby M, Walsh M: Dental hygiene theory and practice, *ed 2, St Louis, 2003, WB Saunders.*

Recall

1. What is dental plaque?
2. What is calculus?
3. The term *periodontal disease* includes both ____________ and ____________.

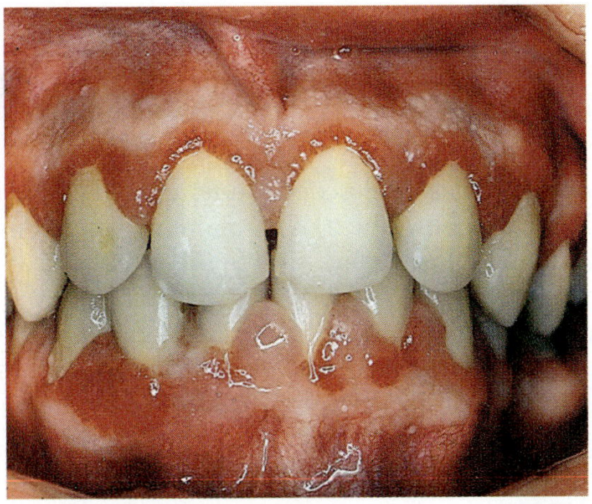

Fig. 14-5 Medication-induced gingivitis. (From Perry D, Beemsterboer P, Taggart E: *Periodontology for the dental hygienist,* Philadelphia, 2001, WB Saunders.)

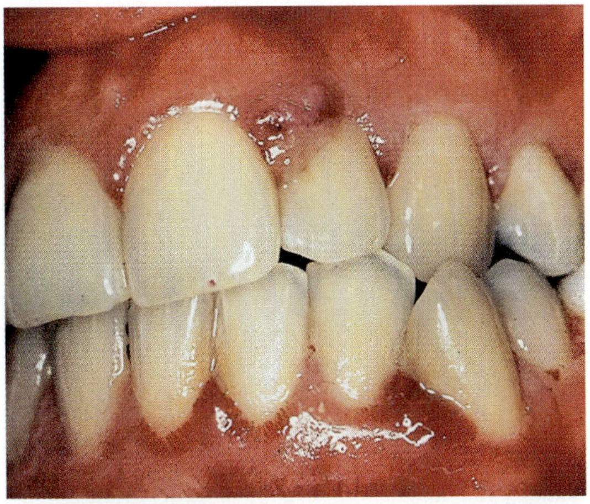

Fig. 14-6 Pregnancy gingivitis. (From Perry D, Beemsterboer P, Taggart E: *Periodontology for the dental hygienist,* Philadelphia, 2001, WB Saunders.)

Box 14-3 Characteristics of Plaque-Induced Gingival Diseases

I. Dental Plaque–Induced Gingivitis

*Dental Plaque–Induced Gingivitis**

Inflammation of the gingiva with plaque present at the gingival margin. Characterized by absence of attachment loss; clinical redness; bleeding upon provocation; changes in contour, color, and consistency. No radiographic evidence of crestal bone loss. Local contributing factors may enhance susceptibility.

II. Plaque–Induced Gingival Diseases Modified by Systemic Factors

Endogenous Sex Steroid Hormone Gingival Disease

Includes puberty-associated gingivitis, pregnancy-associated gingivitis, and menstrual cycle gingivitis; characterized by an exaggerated response to plaque, reflected by intense inflammation, redness, edema, and enlargement with absence of bone and attachment loss; in pregnancy may progress to a pyogenic granuloma (pregnancy tumor).

Diabetes Mellitus–Associated Gingivitis

Found in children with poorly controlled type 1 diabetes mellitus. Characteristics similar to plaque-induced gingivitis, but severity is related to control of blood glucose levels rather than plaque control.

Hematologic (Leukemic) Gingival Diseases

Swollen, glazed, and spongy gingival tissues that are red to deep purple in color; enlargement is first observed in the interdental papilla; plaque may exacerbate condition but is not necessary for it to occur.

Drug-Influenced Gingival Enlargement

Occurs as a result of the use of phenytoin, cyclosporine, and calcium channel blockers such as nifedipine and verapamil. Onset is usually within 3 months of drug use and is more common in younger age groups. Characterized by an exaggerated response to plaque resulting in gingival overgrowth (most commonly occurring in the anterior area and beginning in the interdental papilla); found in gingiva with or without bone loss but is not associated with loss of attachment.

Gingival Diseases Associated with Nutrition

Associated with a severe vitamin C deficiency and scurvy. Gingiva appears red, bulbous, spongy, and hemorrhagic.

* Williams R: Periodontal disease: The emergence of a new paradigm, *Compendium* 19(suppl):4, 1999.
From Darby M, Walsh M: *Dental hygiene theory and practice,* ed 2, St Louis, 2003, WB Saunders.

Gingivitis is painless and often unrecognized until a dental professional emphasizes its importance. Improved daily oral hygiene practices will reverse gingivitis.

Periodontitis

Periodontitis is inflammation of the supporting tissues of the teeth. It is the extension of the inflammatory process from the gingiva into the connective tissue and alveolar bone that support the teeth (Fig. 14-7). As the disease progresses, there is destruction of the connective tissue attachment at the base of a periodontal pocket.

At one time it was believed that periodontitis progressed slowly and at a constant rate. All individuals were thought to be equally susceptible to periodontitis. These concepts have been found to be overly simplistic and partially inaccurate. The current view of periodontitis is that there are several forms of the disease, all of which are infections caused by groups of microorganisms living in the oral cavity. All forms of periodontal disease, however, appear to be related to changes in the many types of bacteria in the oral cavity (Fig. 14-8).

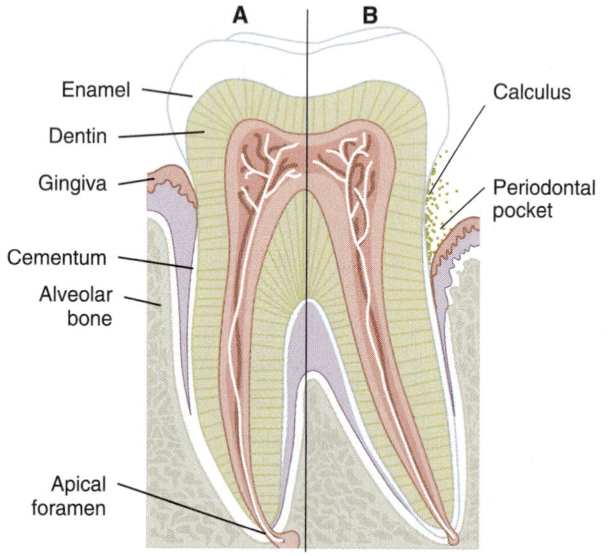

Fig. 14-7 Cross-section of a tooth and associated anatomical structures. **A,** Illustrates the depth of a normal gingival sulcus. **B,** Illustrates a periodontal pocket.

DESCRIPTION OF PERIODONTAL DISEASE

Periodontal disease is described in terms of the severity of the disease and how much of the mouth is affected:

- If less than 30 percent of sites in the mouth are affected, the disease is considered *localized.*
- If more than 30 percent of sites in the mouth are affected, the disease is considered *generalized* (Fig. 14-9).
- The severity of the disease is determined by the amount of lost attachment, as follows:
  - Slight or early
  - Moderate
  - Severe or advanced

The American Academy of Periodontology has identified seven basic case types of periodontal disease based on the severity of the disease and the amount of tissue destruction that has occurred at the time of examination (Box 14-4).

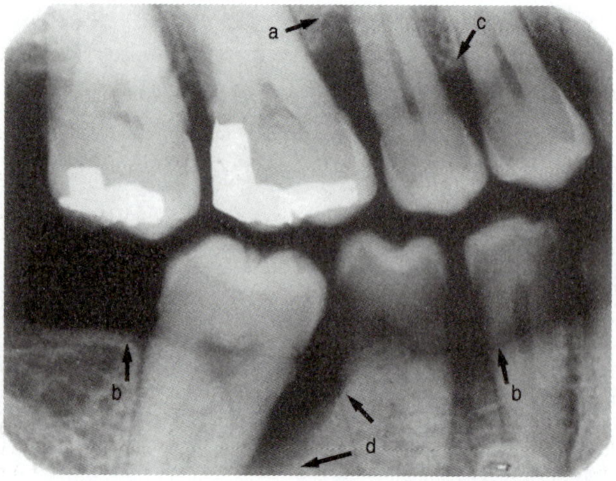

Fig. 14-8 The arrows indicate varying amounts of bone loss due to periodontal disease. (From Miles DA, et al: *Radiographic imaging for dental auxiliaries,* ed 3, Philadelphia, 1999, WB Saunders.)

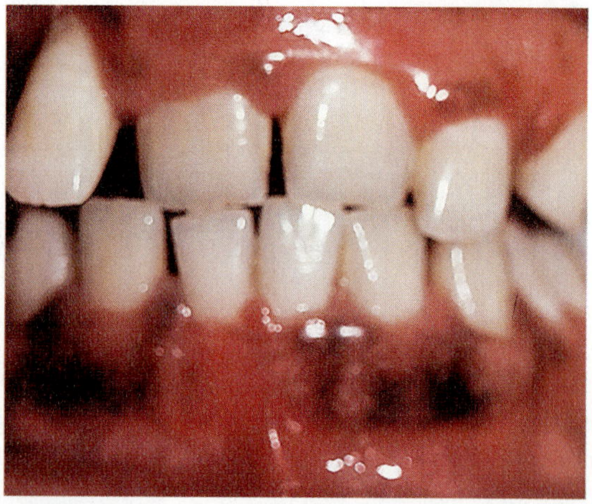

Fig. 14-9 Generalized early-onset periodontitis. (From Perry D, Beemsterboer P, Taggart E: *Periodontology for the dental hygienist,* Philadelphia, 2001, WB Saunders.)

Box 14-4 Characteristics of Periodontitis

I. Chronic Periodontitis[*]

Onset at any age but is most prevalent in adults. Characterized by inflammation of the supporting structures of the teeth, loss of clinical attachment due to destruction of the periodontal ligament, and loss of adjacent bone. Prevalence and severity increases with age. The following levels of chronic periodontal classifications have been identified:

- **Slight or Early Periodontitis:** Progression of gingival inflammation into the alveolar bone crest and early bone loss resulting in slight attachment loss of 1 to 2 mm with periodontal probing depths of 3 to 4 mm.
- **Moderate Periodontitis:** A more advanced state of the previous condition, with increased destruction of periodontal structures, clinical attachment loss up to 4 mm, moderate-to-deep pockets (5-7 mm), moderate bone loss, tooth mobility, and furcation involvement not exceeding class I in molars.
- **Severe or Advanced Periodontitis:** Further progression of periodontitis with severe destruction of the periodontal structures, clinical attachment loss over 5 mm, increased bone loss, increased pocket depth (usually 7 mm or greater), increased tooth mobility, and furcation involvement greater than class I in molars.

II. Aggressive Periodontitis[†]

Occurs prior to age 35 and is associated with rapid rate of progression of tissue destruction, host defense defects, and composition of subgingival flora. The following subclassifications have been identified:

- **Prepubertal Periodontitis:** Onset occurs between eruption of the primary teeth and puberty; occurs in localized forms usually not associated with a systemic disease and generalized forms usually accompanied by alteration of neutrophil functioning; clinically manifests as attachment loss around primary and/or permanent teeth.

II. Aggressive Periodontitis[†]—cont'd

- **Juvenile Periodontitis:** Localized and generalized forms. Generalized form (GJP) occurs late in the teenage years with a variable microbial etiology that may include *Actinobacillus actinomycetemcomitans (Aa)* and *Porphyromonas gingivalis (Pg)* and affects most teeth.

Localized form is associated with less acute clinical signs of inflammation than would be expected based on the severity of destruction. The localized form (LJP) is associated with bone and attachment loss confined mostly to permanent first molars and/or incisors. Age of onset is at or around puberty; associated with *Actinobacillus actinomycetemcomitans (Aa)* and neutrophil dysfunction.

III. Necrotizing Periodontal Diseases[‡]

- Necrotizing ulcerative gingivitis (NUG): A gingival infection of complex etiology (e.g., plaque, temporary depression of polymorphonuclear neutrophil (PMN) functioning, stress, poor diet) characterized by sudden onset of pain, necrosis of the tips of the gingival papillae (punched out appearance), and bleeding. Secondary features include fetid breath and a pseudomembrane covering. Fusiform bacteria, *Prevetella intermedia,* and spirochetes have been associated with gingival lesions.
- Necrotizing ulcerative periodontitis (NUP): Characterized by necrosis of gingival tissues, periodontal ligament, and alveolar bone. Associated with immune disorders such as HIV infection and individuals on immunosuppressive therapies; characteristics include severe and rapid periodontal destruction. Extensive necrosis of the soft tissue occurs simultaneously with alveolar bone loss, resulting in a lack of deep pocket formation.

*Slavkin HC: Building a better mousetrap: Toward an understanding of osteoporosis, *Journal of the American Dental Association* 150:1632, 1999.
†Fedi P, Vernino A, Gray J: *The periodontic syllabus,* Philadelphia, 2000, Lippincott Williams and Wilkins.
‡Armitage G: Development of a classification system for periodontal diseases and conditions, *Annals of Periodontology* 4:1, 1999.
From Darby M, Walsh M: *Dental hygiene theory and practice,* ed 2, St Louis, 2003, WB Saunders.

SIGNS AND SYMPTOMS

The following signs and symptoms are most often seen in patients with periodontal disease:

- Red, swollen, or tender gingiva
- Bleeding gingiva while brushing or flossing
- Loose or separating teeth
- Pain or pressure when chewing
- Pus around the teeth or gingival tissues

Recall

4. What is the definition of periodontitis?
5. How many basic types of periodontal disease have been identified by the American Academy of Periodontology?
6. How is the severity of periodontal disease determined?

Legal and Ethical Implications

One of the most common types of malpractice lawsuits alleges that the dentist failed to diagnose and inform a patient that he or she had periodontal disease.

A common scenario is that the dentist had discussed the need for improved oral hygiene care with the patient at every visit but did not document those conversations. Years later, when the resulting periodontal disease became a serious problem, the patient did not recall these instructions and denied being told about the causes of periodontal disease. It is important to observe and chart the patient's oral hygiene status. Be certain to document all home care instructions that have been given to the patient. In addition, it is important to document that the patient has been clearly informed about the potential for future periodontal disease if the home care does not improve.

Critical Thinking

1. Laura Sinclair is a 24-year-old patient in your dental practice. During her routine checkup, the dentist notices that Laura has some slight bleeding around the molars and slightly reddish gingival margins around other teeth. Laura insists her home care practices have not changed. What other factors might be involved in causing this mild gingivitis in Laura?
2. Roger Fernandez is a 63-year-old man who has come into your office for a new patient examination. His medical history indicates he is taking medications for his type 1 diabetes mellitus. Based on this information, do you think you might see any unusual conditions in his oral tissues? If so, what and why?
3. A pregnant patient has been scheduled to come into your office for an emergency appointment. The receptionist tells you and the dentist that this patient is very concerned about her painful and bleeding gums, which she never had before. What is your first impression as to the possible cause of this pregnant patient's problems?

Eye to the Future

Traditionally, nonsurgical examination of the sulcus has been limited to the use of explorers and radiographs. **Perioscopy** is a new procedure that uses a miniature dental endoscope with video, lighting, and magnification technology. It enables the operator to look into a deep subgingival pocket to explore the gingival sulcus and to see the precise location of root deposits, granulation tissue, caries, and root fractures. The goal of periodontal therapy is to get the root surfaces as clean as possible so that the tissues can heal, and now with the perioscope the operator can actually see any remaining calculus that might have been missed. In addition, the perioscope enables the operator and patient to look at defects (magnified up to 46 times) on enamel and cementum and identify initial decay and/or cracks that were previously camouflaged.

A miniature camera is attached to a tiny probe and then gently placed into the sulcus. The images are immediately displayed on a chairside video screen for the operator and patient to see.

To maintain sterility, a disposable sterile sheath is placed around the perioscope for each patient use. There is very little discomfort during the procedure, and often the patient does not require the use of local anesthesia. This device may one day become a new standard of care in the diagnosis and treatment of periodontal disease worldwide.

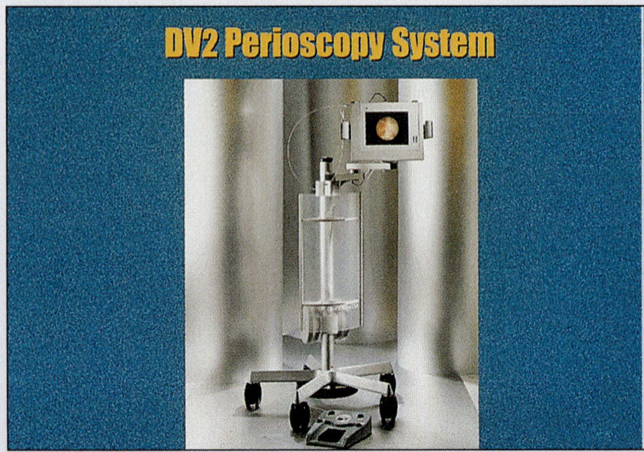

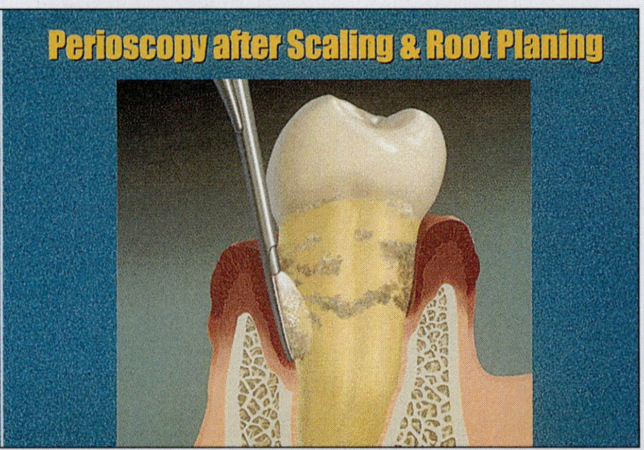

Perioscopy: state of the art technology. (Courtesy DentalView, Inc.)

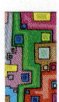

15

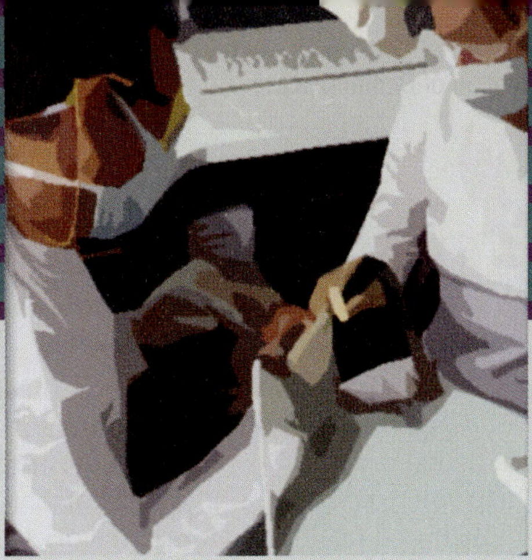

Preventive Dentistry

Outline

KEY TERMS

Dental sealant Coating that covers the occlusal pits and fissures of teeth.

Disclosing agent Coloring agent that makes plaque visible when applied to teeth.

Pontic (**pon**-tik) Artificial tooth that replaces a missing natural tooth.

Preventive dentistry Program of patient education, use of fluorides, application of dental sealants, proper nutrition, and plaque control.

Systemic fluoride Fluoride that is ingested and then circulated throughout the body.

Topical fluoride Fluoride that is applied directly to the tooth.

LEARNING OUTCOMES

On completion of this chapter, the student will be able to achieve the following objectives:

- Pronounce, define, and spell the Key Terms.
- Explain the goal of preventive dentistry.
- Describe the components of a preventive dentistry program.
- Describe the effect of water fluoridation on the teeth.
- Identify sources of systemic fluoride.
- Assist patients in understanding the benefits of preventive dentistry.
- Discuss techniques for educating patients in preventive care.
- Discuss three methods of fluoride therapy.
- Describe the effects of excessive amounts of fluoride.
- Describe the purpose of a fluoride needs assessment.
- Explain the steps in analyzing a food diary.
- Compare and contrast the methods of toothbrushing techniques.
- Describe the process for cleaning a denture.

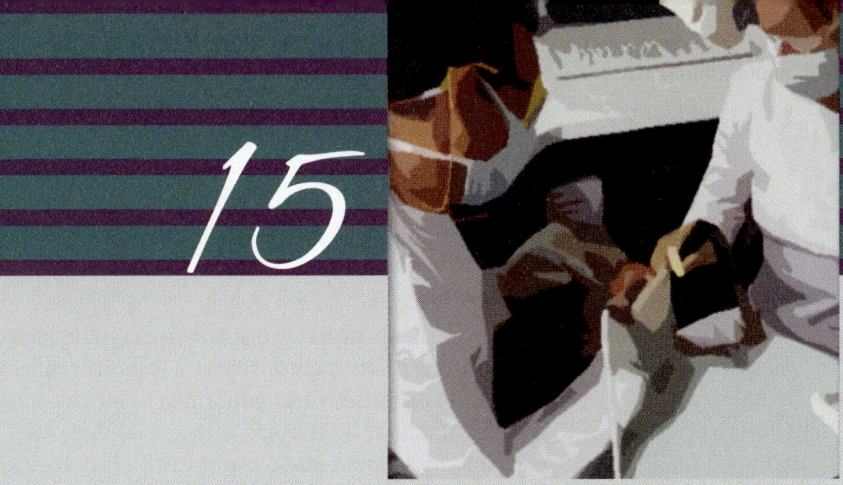

It is the goal of **preventive dentistry** to help people have maximum oral health throughout their lives. To achieve this goal, dental professionals must work together with their patients to prevent new and recurring disease. As discussed in Chapters 13 and 14, the various types of bacteria found in dental plaque are responsible for *dental caries* and *periodontal disease,* the two most common dental diseases.

The information in this chapter will help you to educate patients on how to achieve and maintain their oral health.

PARTNERS IN PREVENTION

To prevent dental disease, a *partnership* must exist between the patient and the dental healthcare team. As a dental assistant, your first step is to help patients understand what causes dental disease and how to prevent it. The next step is to motivate patients to change their behaviors and become partners in recognizing and preventing dental disease in themselves and their families. For example, mothers can be taught to simply lift their children's lips and look for any stains, white spots, or dark areas on the children's teeth (Fig. 15-1).

Optimum oral health can become a reality by partners working together in a comprehensive preventive dentistry program that includes the following (Box 15-1):

- Patient education
- Use of fluorides
- Application of dental sealants
- Proper nutrition
- Plaque control program

Recall

1. What is the goal of preventive dentistry?
2. What are the two most common dental diseases?

PATIENT EDUCATION

As a dental professional, your job is to help patients develop and maintain sound dental habits throughout their lives. To accomplish this, you must educate, encourage, and assist patients to change attitudes and modify behaviors that work against good oral health (Fig. 15-2).

The dental assistant can be a dynamic force in creating the desire for preventive dental care. Most patients have a high regard for their dentist and dental assistant. If you make the patient an active and responsible partner rather than a passive object, you can set the stage for the patient's more responsible behavior.

For a preventive program to be effective, patient education must be reinforced and repeated periodically. Very few people master a skill after just one lesson. On subsequent visits, review the patient's new oral health practices and be

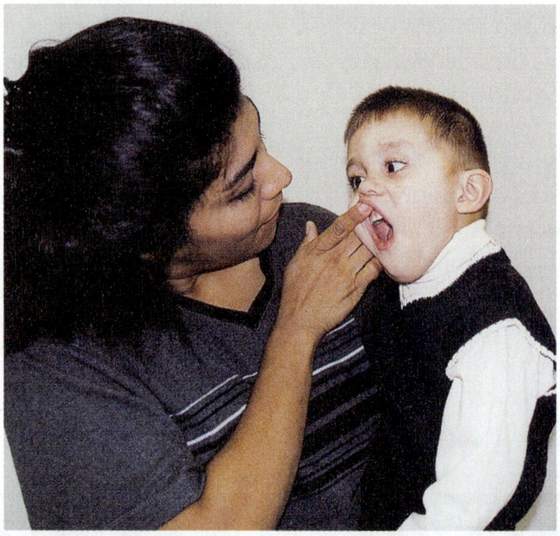

Fig. 15-1 The mother lifts the child's lip and looks for early signs of decay.

Box 15-1 Comprehensive Preventive Dentistry Program

Component	Description
Nutrition	Dietary counseling extends beyond the narrow scope of limiting sugar consumption and may include a discussion of nutrition from the standpoint of oral health as well as general health.
Patient education	Education motivates patients, provides them with information, and assists them in developing the skills necessary to practice good oral hygiene.
Plaque control	Daily removal of bacterial plaque from the teeth and adjacent oral tissues.
Fluoride therapy	Includes professionally applied fluorides, at-home fluoride therapy, and the consumption of fluoridated community water.
Sealants	Sealants are most frequently applied to the difficult-to-clean occlusal surfaces of the teeth. Decay-causing bacteria are then prevented from reaching into occlusal pits and fissures.

sure to compliment them on their successes (no matter how small). When you relate well with your patients and communicate effectively in a calm and nonthreatening manner, you can win their trust and confidence. Most important, you will influence another person to adopt healthy behaviors.

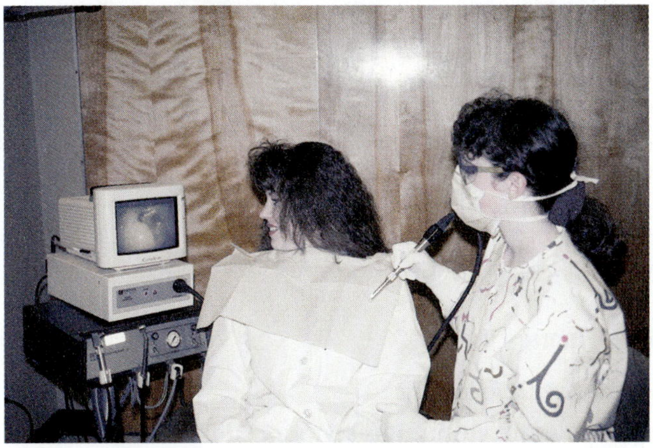

Fig. 15-2 **The dental assistant uses the intraoral camera to assist with patient education.**

Recall

3. What is the goal of a patient education program?
4. What is the initial step in a patient education program?

DENTAL SEALANTS

A **dental sealant** is a plastic-like coating that is applied over the occlusal pits and grooves of the teeth. Sealants are used to protect the difficult-to-clean occlusal surfaces of the teeth from the bacteria that cause decay (Fig. 15-3).

Dental sealants are an important component in preventive dentistry. In several states the application of dental sealants is delegated to the dental assistant as an expanded function (see Chapter 59).

Recall

5. What are dental sealants?

Patient Education Guidelines

1. *Listen carefully* to learn how patients perceive their dental health-care needs. Each patient will have different needs. Because you are so aware of the importance of good dental health, the patient's perception and your perception of the patient's dental needs may be very different.
2. *Instruct the patient on how to remove plaque.* This is the initial instruction for most patients. Because plaque is not visible on most teeth, you must use a **disclosing agent.** It is a very effective aid for a patient to actually see the plaque on the teeth. Disclosing agents are available in tablet or liquid form. This is the time to explain the relationship of plaque to dental disease (caries and periodontal disease). You must customize the message for each patient.
3. *Assess the patient's motivations and needs.* Then combine the patient's motivating factors with the patient's needs to make recommendations for oral health care. For instance, when a patient's immediate concern is staining on the front teeth, it is not effective to emphasize the plaque on the lingual surface of the molars.
4. *Select the home care aids.* With the patient's needs identified, select a toothbrush, toothbrushing method, interproximal cleaning aids (such as dental floss), and a dentifrice (toothpaste).
5. *Keep the instruction simple.* If you select a style of communication that is comfortable for the individual patient, you are more likely to have the desired impact. Help the patient make any necessary improvements in his or her technique. Comment positively on the patient's efforts.
6. *Reinforce home care* during the patient's return visits for dental treatment. People tend to regress in their home care efforts, so expect periodic set-backs. When these occur, help patients achieve their goals in a positive and helpful manner.

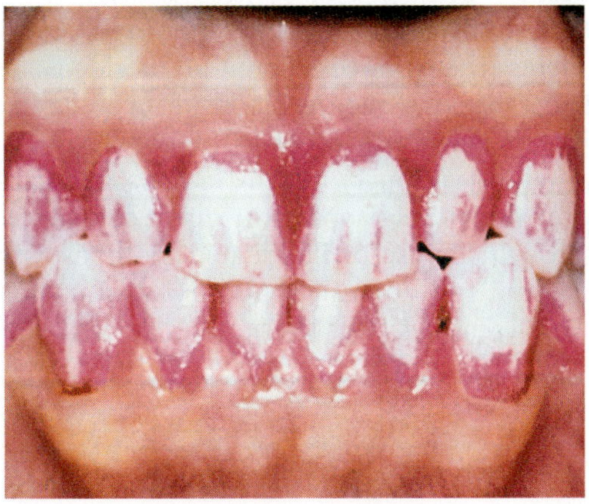

Disclosing solution shows heavy plaque formation throughout the mouth.

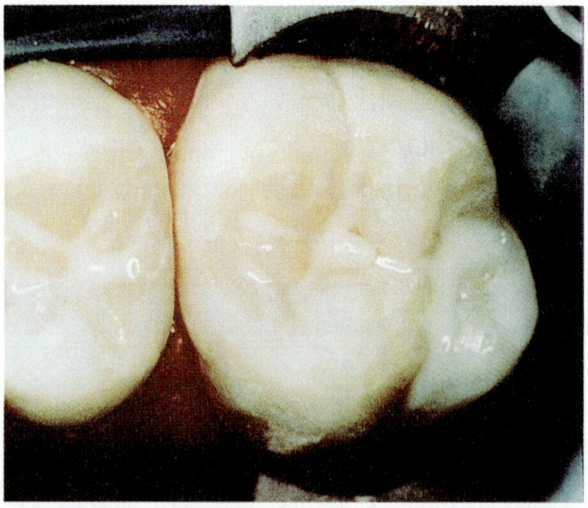

Fig. 15-3 This molar is protected from decay with a dental sealant. (Courtesy 3M Espe Co, St Paul, Minn.)

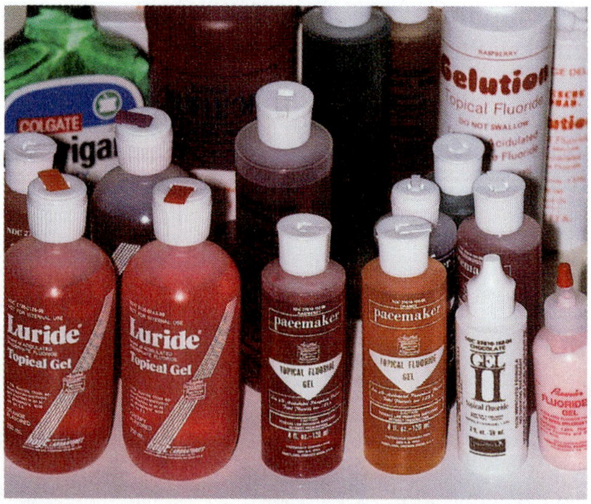

Fig. 15-4 Topical forms of fluoride.

FLUORIDE

Since the 1950s, fluoride has been the primary weapon to combat dental caries. *Slowing demineralization* and *enhancing remineralization* of tooth surfaces are now considered to be the most important ways that fluoride controls the caries process (see Chapter 13).

Fluoride, sometimes referred to as "nature's cavity fighter," is a mineral that occurs naturally in food and water. To achieve the maximum cavity prevention benefits of fluoride, an ongoing supply of both systemic and topical fluoride must be available throughout life. Based on the patient's needs, various ways are available to receive fluoride therapy, including the following:

- Prescription-strength fluorides that are applied in the dental office
- Nonprescription-strength, over-the-counter products for home use
- Consumption of fluoridated bottled water or community water

Systemic fluoride is ingested in water, food, beverages, or supplements. The required amount of fluoride is absorbed through the intestine into the bloodstream and transported to the tissues where it is needed. The body excretes excess systemic fluoride through the skin, kidneys, and feces.

Topical fluoride is applied in direct contact with the teeth through the use of fluoridated toothpaste, fluoride mouthrinses, and topical applications of rinses, gels, foams, and varnishes (Fig. 15-4).

Recall

6. What is the process by which fluoride prevents decay?
7. What are the two routes or means by which the body receives fluoride?

How Fluoride Works

Preeruptive Development

Before a tooth erupts, it is surrounded by a fluid-filled sac. The fluoride present in this fluid strengthens the enamel of the developing tooth and makes it more acid-resistant.

Before birth, the source of systemic fluoride is from the mother's diet. After birth and before the teeth erupt, the child ingests systemic fluoride.

Posteruptive Development

After eruption of teeth, fluoride continues to enter the enamel and strengthen the structure of the enamel crystals. These fluoride-enriched crystals are *less acid-soluble* than the original structure of the enamel.

After eruption, an ongoing supply of fluoride from both systemic and topical sources is important for the remineralization process.

Safe and Toxic Levels

Fluorides used in the dental office have been proved to be safe and effective *when used as recommended.* Chronic overexposure to fluoride, even at low concentrations, can result in dental *fluorosis* in children younger than 6 years with developing teeth (Fig. 15-5). Abuse of high-concentration gels or solutions of fluoride or accidental ingestion of a concentrated fluoride preparation can lead to a toxic reaction. Acute fluoride poisoning is rare.

Precautions

To protect patients from receiving too much fluoride, an evaluation of their current fluoride intake should be made. For example, a child may live in an area with community water fluoridation, attend a preschool with a fluoride rinse program, and use a fluoride toothpaste at home. The den-

A

B

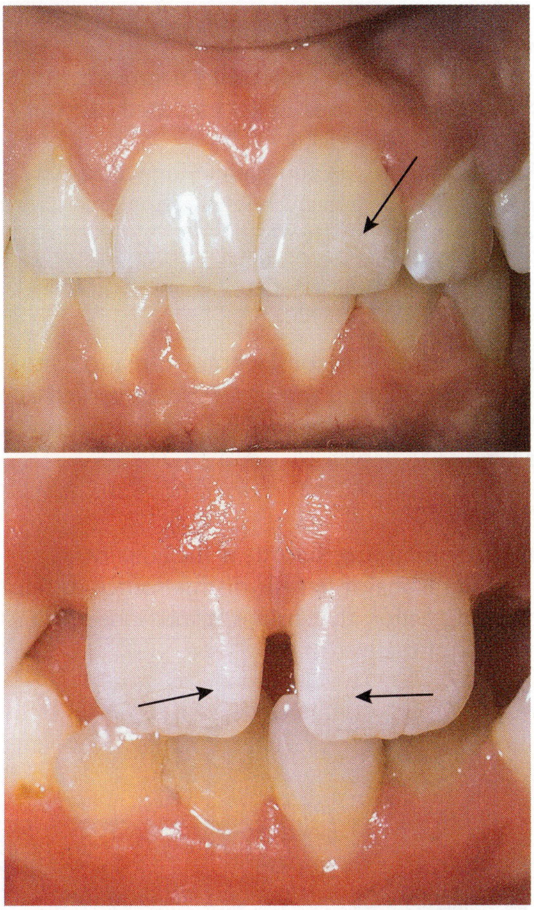

Fig. 15-5 **A,** Mild fluorosis. **B,** Moderate fluorosis.

tist will consider these multiple sources of fluoride before prescribing additional fluoride supplements or office treatments for this child.

A particular area of concern involves young children who may consume excessive fluoride by swallowing fluoridated toothpaste, which may cause fluorosis. Adult supervision of young children during toothbrushing is necessary, and the child should be instructed not to swallow the toothpaste. Fluoride in drinking water, fluoride toothpaste, fluoride rinses, and professionally applied treatments provide a cumulative effect, and the amount taken in should be monitored.

Recall

8. What is the name of the dental condition that results from too much fluoride?

9. What precautions are necessary for children using fluoridated toothpaste?

Fluoride Needs Assessment

This assessment will help us determine your individual need for a specific fluoride therapeutic program that can help you keep your teeth for life.

Please put a check mark in front of any of the following statements that apply to you.

__ No fluoride in your drinking water as a child.
__ No fluoride in your drinking water now.
__ Drink filtered or bottled water.
__ Have receding gums or history of gum disease.
__ Have multiple fillings or crowns.
__ Strong family history of dental decay.
__ Currently wear orthodontic braces.
__ Have sensitivity to hot, cold, or touch.
__ Use home care whitening products.
__ Limited hand dexterity.
__ Use of strong breath mints or sugar-containing chewing gum, lozenges, or hard candy between meals.
__ Visit dental office regularly.
__ Currently undergoing (or history of) chemotherapy.
__ Suffer from acid reflux.
__ Teeth that do not feel clean or that trap food.
__ Dental work done in the past year.
__ Snack frequently between meals.
__ Sip on beverages throughout the day (other than water).
__ Use tobacco products of any type.
__ Grind teeth frequently.
__ Brush less than twice daily.
__ Floss less than once daily.

(Modified from Oral-B Laboratories.)

Fluoride Needs Assessment

A "fluoride needs assessment" is often used to help patients become more involved in their caries prevention program. The assessment strengthens the dental partnership process by gathering relevant information from the patient and then, in turn, educating the patient on why fluoride is important and how it plays a role in the risk for future caries. Using the fluoride needs assessment has the following advantages:

- Saves time by identifying risk factors
- Opens communication between the dental professional and the patient
- Helps "individualize" patient fluoride therapies
- Allows the dentist to more accurately determine the appropriate fluoride therapy

Sources of Fluoride

Fluoridated Water

Until recently, it was believed that water fluoridation was effective in preventing tooth decay by systemic uptake and incorporation into the enamel of developing teeth. It has now been proved that the major effects of water fluoridation are *topical* and not systemic. Topical uptake means the fluoride diffuses into the surface of the enamel of an *erupted tooth* rather than being incorporated into unerupted teeth during development.

For more than 40 years, fluoride has been safely added to communal water supplies. Most major cities in the United States have fluoridated water, and there are continuing efforts to fluoridate water in communities without fluoridation. From a public health standpoint, fluoridation of public water supplies is a good way to deliver fluoride to lower socioeconomic populations that may not otherwise have access to topical fluoride products such as fluoridated toothpaste and mouthrinses.

Approximately *one part per million* (ppm) of fluoride in drinking water has been specified as the safe and recommended concentration to aid in the control of dental decay. This is approximately equivalent to one drop of fluoride in a bathtub of water. Recommended optimum concentrations vary from 0.7 to 1.2 ppm depending on the climate. Lower concentrations are usually recommended in hot areas, where people consume larger quantities of water.

The levels of fluoride in controlled water fluoridation are so low that there is *no danger* of ingesting an acutely toxic quantity of fluoride in water. Communities in some states, however, have water that naturally contains more than twice the optimum level of fluoride, and fluorosis is often seen in patients who live in these areas (see Chapter 17).

Sources of Systemic Fluoride

Foods and Beverages

Because many processed foods and beverages are prepared with fluoridated water, they must be considered a source of dietary fluoride in children who drink them regularly. In addition, many brands of bottled water contain fluoride. Persons who want the benefits of fluoride must be sure to check labels.

Prescribed Dietary Supplements

The dentist may prescribe dietary fluoride supplements in the form of tablets, drops, or lozenges for children ages 6 months to 16 years who live in areas with no source of fluoridated water (Fig. 15-6). Before prescribing supplements, the dentist considers the following factors:

- Fluoride level of the child's drinking water
- Child's exposure to multiple water sources (for example, a child whose home water source is not fluoridated but whose daycare center or school is in a fluoridated area)
- All potential sources of fluoride, because many juice products and prepared foods marketed for young children contain fluoride
- Whether the parents and patient are willing to cooperate on an ongoing basis, because supplementation is recommended until age 16

Sources of Topical Fluoride

Topical fluoride is available in home care products such as fluoridated toothpastes and mouthrinses, as well as in professional topical fluoride applications used in the dental office (Fig. 15-7; Tables 15-1 and 15-2).

Toothpastes

Toothpaste containing fluoride is the *primary source* of topical fluoride. A major benefit of this source of fluoride is the brushing action that brings it into close contact with the surfaces of the teeth.

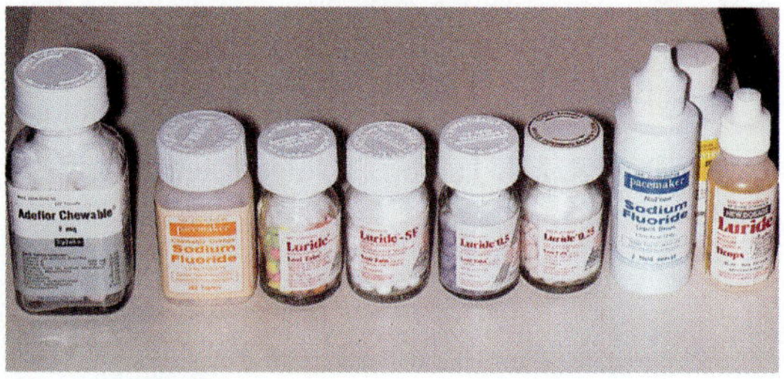

Fig. 15-6 Fluoride can be dispensed by the dentist in a tablet form.

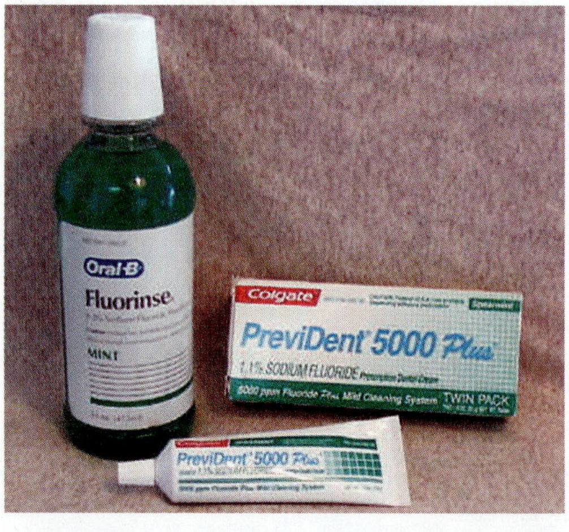

Fig. 15-7 Prescription-strength (0.2% sodium fluoride) mouthrinse and (1.1% sodium fluoride) dentifrice are effective in preventing dental decay.

Table 15-1 ***Types of Professionally Applied Fluorides***

Type	Form	Application Technique	Comments
Sodium fluoride (NaF) pH = neutral	Solution 2%	Paint-on	Use cotton rolls to absorb excess solution.
Sodium fluoride (NaF) pH = neutral	Gel 2%	Tray	Do not allow the patient to swallow the gel.
Sodium fluoride (NaF) pH = neutral	Foam 2%	Tray	Patients are less likely to swallow this because of the consistency. Use less in the tray than the gel.
Acidulated phosphate fluoride (APF) pH 3.0-3.5	Solution 1.23%	Paint-on	Avoid use on patients with ceramic and composite restorations. Use cotton rolls to absorb excess solution.
Acidulated phosphate fluoride (APF) pH 3.0-3.5	Gel 1.23%	Paint-on or tray	Avoid use on patients with ceramic and composite restorations. Take care not to overfill tray.
Acidulated phosphate fluoride (APF) pH 3.0-3.5	Foam	Tray	Avoid use on patients with ceramic and composite restorations. Smaller amounts are needed for tray.

Table 15-2 ***Fluoride Therapies for Home Use***

Patient Problem	Type of Therapy	Active Ingredient	Benefits
Adult Caries			
Patient compliance	Toothpaste	1.1% neutral sodium fluoride (NaF)	Helps prevent tooth decay
Exposed roots	Prescription therapy		Safe for restorations and ceramic crowns
Root caries			Applies fluoride while brushing
Xerostomia (dry mouth)			Alcohol free
Adult Caries			
Exposed roots	Brush-on gel	1.1% neutral NaF	Arrests 91% of early root caries
Root caries	Prescription therapy		Helps prevent tooth decay
Xerostomia (dry mouth)			Safe for restorations and ceramics
			Alcohol free
Caries			
Requires high concentration of fluoride	Dental rinse	0.2% neutral NaF	Up to 55% reduction in caries with weekly use
Difficulty brushing	Prescription therapy		Highest concentration home fluoride rinse
Patient compliance			Safe for restorations
			Once a week
Dentinal Sensitivity and Decay			
Exposed dentin	Home care gel	0.4% stannous fluoride (SnF)	Reduces hypersensitivity
Caries risk			Prevents caries
			Available without a prescription

Continued

Table 15-2 ***Fluoride Therapies for Home Use—cont'd***

Patient Problem	Type of Therapy	Active Ingredient	Benefits
Exposed Roots			
After scaling	Home care rinse	0.63% SnF (dilutes to 0.1%)	Helps prevent demineralization of exposed roots
After root planing		Rx	Helps prevent plaque accumulation
After periodontal surgery			Reduces *Mutans streptococci* count in saliva
			Reduces caries
			Alcohol free
Hypersensitivity			
Temporary sensitivity during whitening	Dentin desensitizer	1.09% NaF	Rapid temporary relief at home
Sensitivity due to loss of temporary crowns	Rx	0.4% SnF	One-minute applications
Temporary sensitivity at home		0.14% hydrogen fluoride	
Orthodontic Calcification			
Caries in children	Oral rinse	0.044% NaF and acidulated phosphate topical solution	Helps prevent demineralization
			Enhances remineralization
			Alcohol free
			Available over the counter
	Gel	1.1% NaF and acidulated phosphate	Safe, effective against white spots
	Rx		Helps reduce decalcification
			Promotes remineralization
			Safe for orthodontic appliances
Caries Prevention			
Children	Anticavity fluoride rinse	0.05% neutral NaF	Up to 71% fewer adult root caries
Adolescents			Up to 40% fewer cavities in children
Adults			Freshens breath
			Available over the counter

Daily brushing with fluoride-containing toothpaste is of benefit to patients of all age groups (Fig. 15-8). Children younger than 6 or 7 years should be carefully supervised because ingestion of the fluoride-containing toothpaste may cause dental fluorosis. There are now training toothpastes available for very young children that do not contain fluoride (Fig. 15-9).

Additional types of toothpastes are available on the market, including some that contain whitening and desensitizing agents.

Mouthrinses

Mouthrinses containing fluoride may be recommended as an additional source of topical fluoride for high-risk patients.

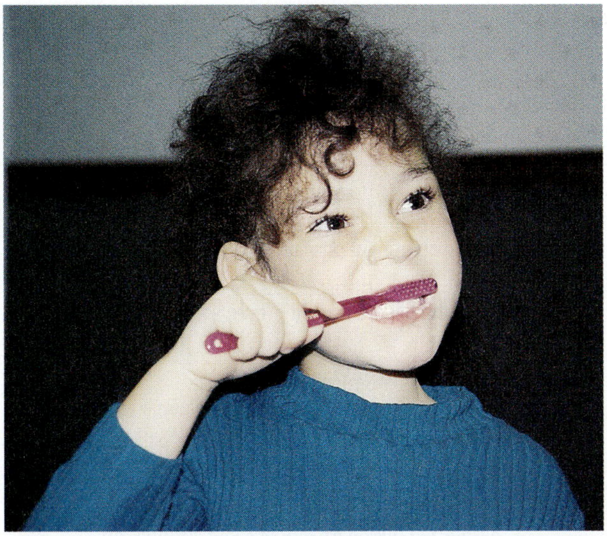

Fig. 15-8 Children must be carefully supervised while brushing to make sure they do not swallow fluoride-containing toothpaste.

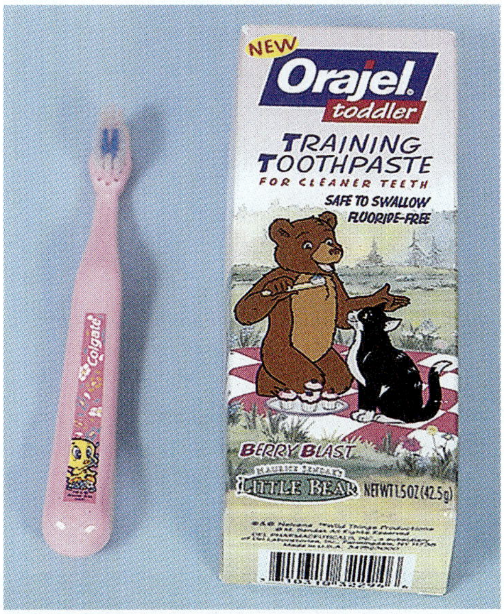

Fig. 15-9 Training toothpaste for young children.

Over-the-counter nonprescription rinses generally contain 0.05% sodium fluoride and are designed for daily use. *Prescription rinses* generally contain 0.63% stannous fluoride or 0.2% sodium fluoride. Fluoride rinses are often used for their antiplaque properties. Stannous fluoride is also effective in decreasing dental *hypersensitivity* (extreme sensitivity of the tooth, such as to hot and cold).

Fluoride mouthrinses are most effective when used after brushing and flossing. Approximately 10 ml of solution should be swished vigorously for 1 minute and then spit out. The patient should be instructed not to eat or drink for 30 minutes after using the mouthrinse. Because of the chance of ingesting excessive fluoride, the adult patient must be cautioned not to swallow the mouthrinse, and children should be closely supervised.

Also available on the market are mouthrinses containing antimicrobial properties that show promise for the prevention and control of periodontal diseases (Fig. 15-10).

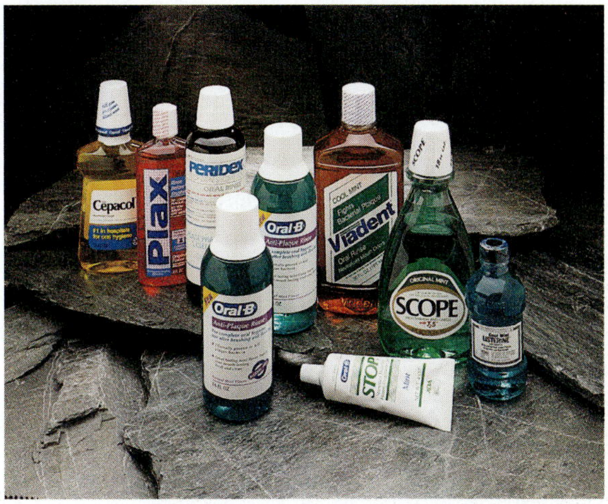

Fig. 15-10 Various chemotherapeutic products available to consumers. (Courtesy Oral-B Laboratories.)

Gels

Gels containing varying concentrations of sodium fluoride are available for home use. Gels with a higher concentration (2%) require a prescription, and those products containing a lower concentration (1.1%) may be purchased over the counter.

High-risk patients can use these at home by brushing or applying with a reusable custom tray. The patient is instructed to use the tray at bedtime. A small amount of the brush-on gel is placed in the tray, and the tray is placed over the teeth for 5 minutes.

NOTE: If water in the area is fluoridated, the patient is instructed to rinse with water after using the gel, to prevent consumption of excess fluoride. If the water is not fluoridated, the patient is told to spit out the excess but not to rinse with water after the application. Any small amounts of fluoride swallowed provide extra dietary fluoride.

Professional Applications

Professional topical fluoride applications may be recommended for some children soon after the eruption of the permanent teeth and for some high-risk patients. This treatment can be performed by the dentist, hygienist, or qualified dental assistant (Procedure 15-1).

Procedure 15-1 Applying Topical Fluoride Gel or Foam

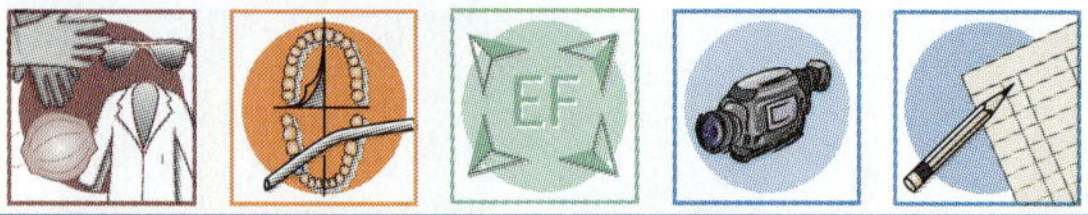

Goal

To apply a topical fluoride gel or foam competently and effectively.

Equipment and Supplies

- Fluoride gel or foam
- Disposable trays of appropriate size
- Saliva ejector
- Cotton rolls
- Air-water syringe
- Timer

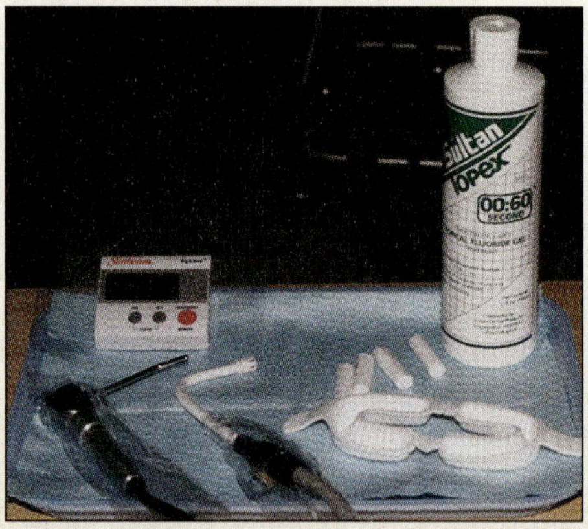

PROCEDURAL STEPS

Selecting the Tray

1. Select a disposable tray that is the appropriate size for the patient's mouth. The tray must be long and sufficiently deep to cover all erupted teeth completely without extending beyond the distal surface of the most posterior tooth.

   Purpose: Trays are available in sizes to fit primary, mixed, and adult dentition. If the patient's mouth can accommodate it, you may use a double-arch tray. This saves time by treating both arches at the same time. Remember, trays are discarded after a single use, and if you try a tray in the mouth but do not use it, that tray must be discarded.

Preparing the Teeth

1. Check to see whether calculus is present; if it is not, no preparation is required.

   Purpose: Fluoride diffuses easily through the acquired pellicle and bacterial plaque.
2. If calculus is present, request that the dentist or dental hygienist remove it.

   Purpose: Calculus prevents the fluoride from reaching the enamel of the tooth.

   Note: The presence of plaque will not affect the uptake of fluoride.

Applying the Topical Fluoride

1. Seat the patient in an upright position, and explain the procedure.

   Purpose: Having the patient upright prevents the gel from going into the throat.
2. Instruct the patient not to swallow the fluoride.
3. Select the appropriate tray and load it with a minimal amount of the fluoride, following the guidelines according to the patient's age.

   Reminder: Containers that are handled with gloved hands during the appointment should be surface-disinfected during treatment room cleanup. An alternative is to wear gloves while handling the container.

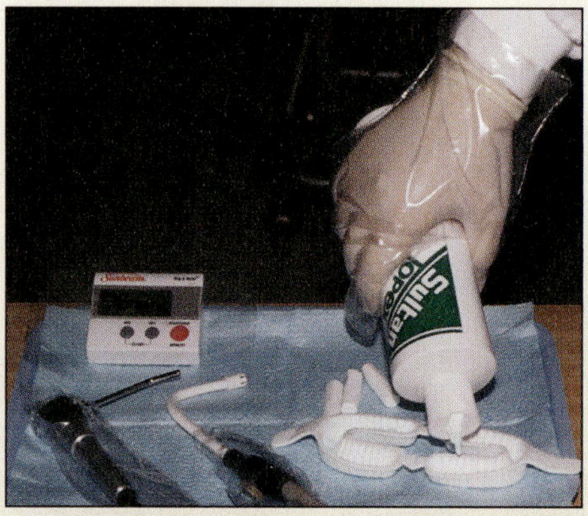

4. Dry the teeth using air from the air-water syringe.

   Purpose: For the fluoride to be maximally effective, the teeth must be dry when the fluoride is applied.

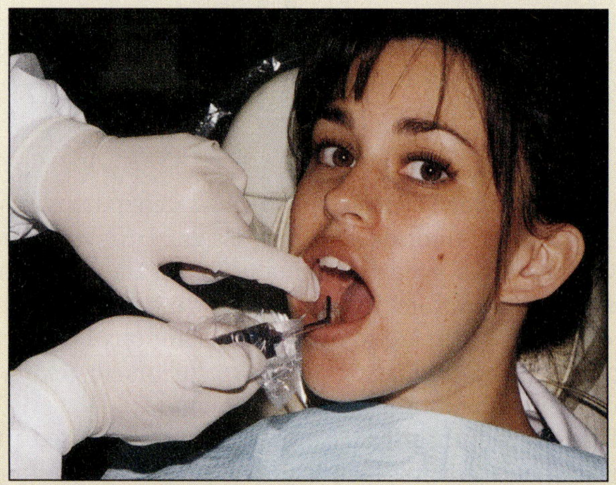

Procedure 15-1 Applying Topical Fluoride Gel or Foam—cont'd

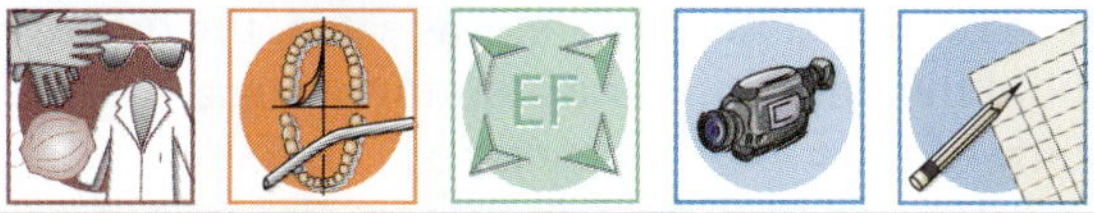

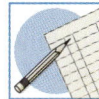

Applying the Topical Fluoride, cont'd

5. Insert the tray, and place cotton rolls between the arches. Ask the patient to bite up and down gently on the cotton rolls.
   Purpose: To squeeze the fluoride over all tooth surfaces.

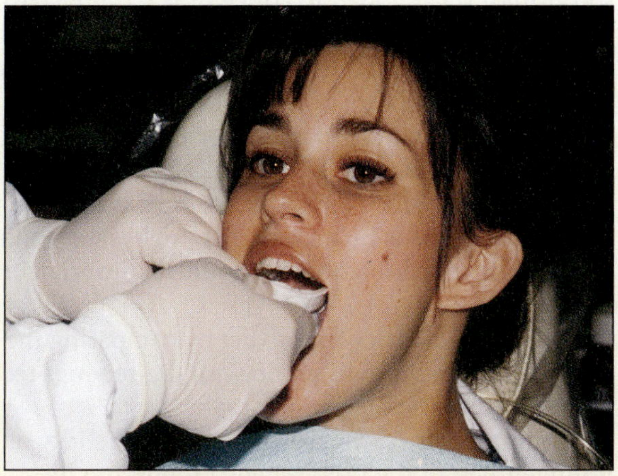

6. Promptly place the saliva ejector and tilt the patient's head forward.
   Purpose: To prevent the patient from swallowing the fluoride.

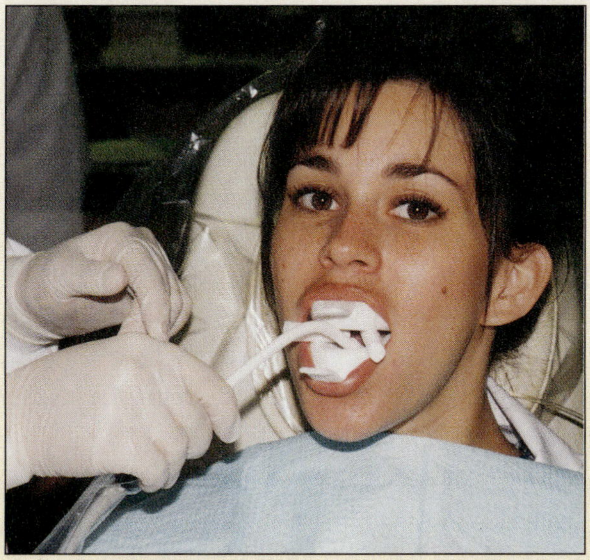

7. Set the timer for the appropriate amount of time based on the manufacturer's instructions. During this time, do *not* leave the patient unattended.
8. On completion, remove the tray, but do not allow the patient to rinse or swallow. Promptly use the saliva ejector or high-volume oral evacuator tip to remove excess saliva and solution.
   Purpose: Removing excess saliva and fluoride solution will make the patient more comfortable and less likely to rinse with water.
9. Instruct the patient not to rinse, eat, drink, or brush the teeth for at least 30 minutes.
   Purpose: These activities could disturb the action of the fluoride.

Documentation

Date	Procedure	Operator
1/25/05	Applied APF fluoride gel. Instructed patient not to eat for 30 min.	CDH/46

NUTRITION AND DENTAL CARIES

Dental caries cannot occur without dietary sugars. Sucrose is more *cariogenic* (caries-causing) than other types of sugars, although maltose, lactose, glucose, and fructose also have high caries-producing abilities. Flour and starches alone are not usually cariogenic, but when starch is mixed with sugar, as in cookies, the chance for developing dental decay increases.

Sugar Substitutes

Initially, artificial sweeteners were developed for the 10 million patients with diabetes in the United States and for people who struggle with obesity. In recent years the use of artificial sweeteners has significantly increased. The principal sugar substitutes available are *saccharine* (Sweet'N Low), *aspartame* (NutraSweet and Equal), *sorbitol*, *xylitol*, and *mannitol*.

Of these sugar substitutes, saccharine, aspartame, sorbitol, and mannitol are *noncariogenic*, which means that they do not *cause* dental caries. Xylitol is the only one of the artificial sweeteners that actually *prevents caries* (anticariogenic).

Xylitol

The exact mechanism by which xylitol prevents tooth decay is still being studied, but it is believed that bacteria cannot use xylitol to produce acid and that it may inhibit the growth of *S. mutans*. Xylitol is derived from birch trees, corn cobs, oats, bananas, and certain mushrooms. Its cost is about 10 times that of sucrose. Therefore, although products containing xylitol are significantly better, they are more expensive than products with other types of artificial sweeteners (Fig. 15-11).

Dietary Analysis

A dietary analysis is done to determine whether the patient's current food intake is affecting his or her dental health. It is a quick and easy procedure in which the patient maintains a *food diary* that includes everything eaten each day for 1 week. The listing includes all meals, supplements, gum, snacks, and fluoridated water. The patient must also record the time the food was eaten, the quantity in household measures, and the amount of sugar that was added to any of the foods or beverages.

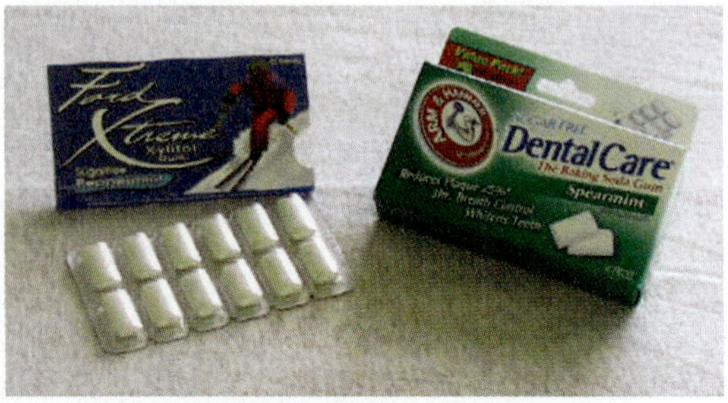

Fig. 15-11 Ford Xtreme Xylitol gum and Sugar Free Dental Care gum containing xylitol and sorbitol.

If the patient's food diary reveals any diet-related oral problems such as high sugar intake or frequent snacks, some form of dietary counseling is indicated.

Steps for Analyzing a Food Diary

1. Note the time when meals and snacks were eaten.
2. Note the foods sweetened with added sugar, including soft drinks, sugar added to coffee or tea, candy, pastry, cough drops, and fruits. Note *all* carbonated beverages, including soft drinks and beer (even those considered "diet" drinks), because of their acidity.
3. Note any dried fruit, such as berries, dates, prunes, and raisins, because they are highly concentrated sweets. However, fresh fruits such as apples or oranges are not concentrated sweets because of their high water content.
4. Arrange the remaining foods into the appropriate food groups.
5. Evaluate the adequacy of the diet by comparing the servings from each food group with the servings recommended in the dietary guide.
6. Determine the frequency and consistency (sticky or nonretentive) of the presweetened foods and determine their likelihood of contributing to the patient's oral health problems.
7. From the information in the food diary, determine the need for dietary counseling with the patient. For exam-

Hard Facts About Soft Drinks

1. Large sizes mean more calories, more sugar, and more acid in a single serving. A 64-ounce "big cup" has more than five 12-ounce cans in a single serving.
2. Soft drinks have no nutritional value. In regular sodas, all the calories come from sugar.
3. Sugar in sodas combines with bacteria in the mouth to form acid.
4. Diet or "sugar-free" sodas contain their own acid. The acid attacks the teeth. Each acid attack lasts about 20 minutes.
5. In addition to tooth decay, heavy soda consumption has been linked to diabetes, obesity, and osteoporosis.
6. Teenagers today drink three times more soda than teenagers 20 years ago, often as a substitute for milk.
7. One fifth of all 1- and 2-year-old children drink sodas.
8. Sealants protect only the chewing surfaces of teeth. Decay caused by sodas tends to occur on smooth tooth surfaces, where sealants cannot reach.

(Modified from the Minnesota Dental Association.)

ple, a patient with rampant caries and a diet high in sweets is in need of comprehensive dietary counseling. Conversely, a patient with slight caries and minimal sugar intake would likely need only minimal dietary counseling.

Recall

10. What is the key dietary factor that relates to dental caries?
11. What information must a patient include in a food diary?
12. How do sugar-free sodas relate to dental caries?

PLAQUE CONTROL PROGRAM

Patients cannot remove all the plaque on their teeth every day, but they can keep plaque under control by brushing, flossing, using interdental cleaning aids, and using antimicrobial solutions. The dental assistant can work with the patient to develop a program of oral hygiene strategies to be followed routinely at home.

The goal is to thoroughly remove plaque *at least* once daily. After plaque has been thoroughly removed, it takes about 24 hours to form again. The techniques selected must be based on the needs and abilities of the individual patient.

A wide variety of oral hygiene products are currently available. It is important for dental assistants to remain up to date on the newest products on the market so that they can advise patients, make recommendations, and answer questions.

Toothbrushes and Toothbrushing

Choosing the size and style of a toothbrush is a personal decision. The two basic types of toothbrushes are *manual* and *automatic*. When used properly, both types are effective in the removal of dental plaque.

Manual Toothbrushes

Toothbrushes come in many styles of head size, tuft shape, and angle and shape of handle (Fig. 15-12). There is not one "ideal" toothbrush for everyone.

In general, dental professionals recommend soft-bristled brushes, because these bristles are gentler to the soft tissues and any exposed cementum or dentin. Soft bristles also adapt to the contours of the tooth better than hard bristles.

The bristles may be nylon or natural. *Nylon* is preferred because the ends are rounded and polished, which makes the toothbrush safer.

The most important factor to ensure is that the toothbrush readily removes plaque without causing tissue damage. Toothbrushes should be replaced as soon as the bristles show signs of wear or begin to splay outward, usually after about 8 to 12 weeks. Some people choose to discard their toothbrush after an illness; however, there is no scientific basis for this practice.

Automatic Toothbrushes

Automatic, or powered, toothbrushes are gaining in popularity. As with manual toothbrushes, various types of automatic brushes are available.

Automatic brushes have larger handles, which contain a rechargeable battery. The larger handle also makes them useful for patients with physical disabilities. In addition, automatic toothbrushes may have some motivational value for children.

Automatic toothbrushes use one of several motions, including back and forth, up and down, or circular. Other models of automatic toothbrushes feature pulsating and ultrasonic action (Fig. 15-13). Some types have a timing device that sounds every 30 seconds to remind the user to change quadrants in the mouth (Box 15-2).

Toothbrushing Methods

Regardless of the toothbrush a patient chooses, it can only remove plaque thoroughly when it is used properly. Table 15-3 summarizes the following five toothbrushing methods that are most commonly taught to patients: Bass method, modified Bass (rolling stroke) method, modified Stillman's method, Charters' method, and Fones' method. Of these methods, the modified Bass is most frequently recommended.

When reviewing toothbrushing technique with patients, observe their toothbrushing technique before recommending a particular brushing method. When patients have healthy gingivae and few plaque deposits, you should not recommend a totally new brushing technique but merely coach them to continue their safe, effective pattern of brushing. You may be able to offer tips to patients on how to better reach a specific area of the mouth if they have plaque retention in that area. Many patients require only minor modifications to the technique they are using.

Ask patients to demonstrate their brushing technique for you. It is helpful to have a large hand mirror so that patients can observe their own technique. You can provide tips while they are brushing (Fig. 15-14). Whenever possible, give patients written materials that reinforce the concepts you presented in the oral health lesson. Patients will frequently ask, "How often should I brush?" The most commonly accepted answer among dental professionals is to brush twice a day. Patients will also ask about the proper length of time to brush. Often patients will brush for only 1 minute or less. Some dental professionals recommend at least 3 minutes, whereas others recommend five to ten strokes in each area. It is best to customize your instructions based on the patient's oral health status and history of compliance with oral health instructions.

Examples of manual toothbrushes

Product and company	Toothbrush design	Product and company	Toothbrush design
Crest Complete Procter & Gamble Co. Cincinnati, Ohio	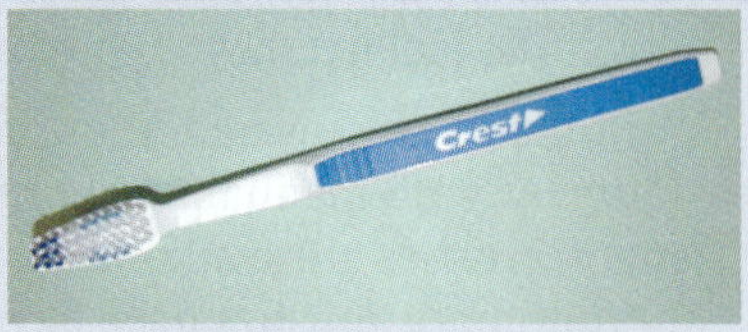	**Mentadent ProCare Flexible Handle** Chesebrough-Ponds USA, Co. Greenwich, Conn.	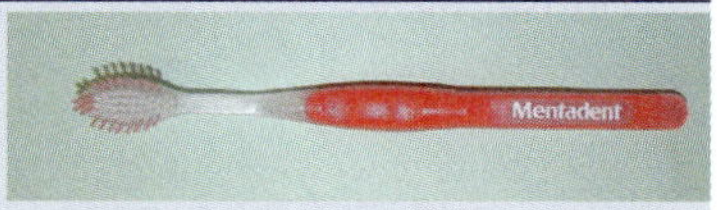
Crest Triple Effect Procter & Gamble Co. Cincinnati, Ohio	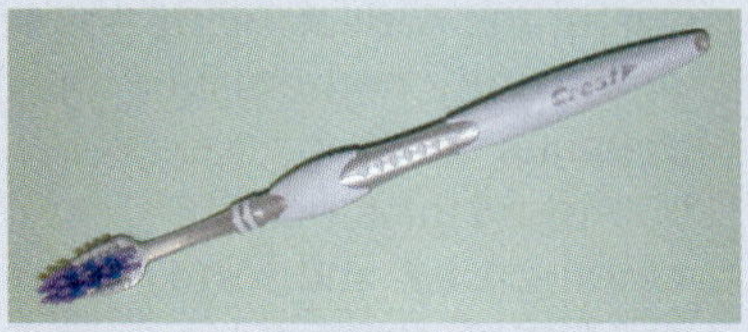	**Oral-B Cross Action** Oral-B Laboratories Belmont, Calif.	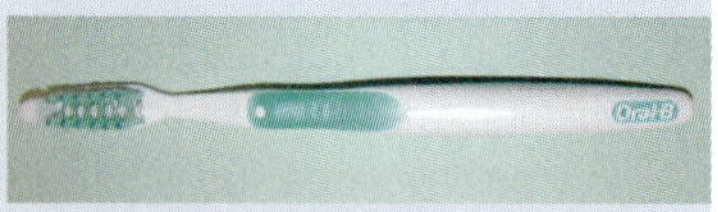
Reach Personal Products Co. Division of McNeil-PPC, Inc. Skillman, N.J.	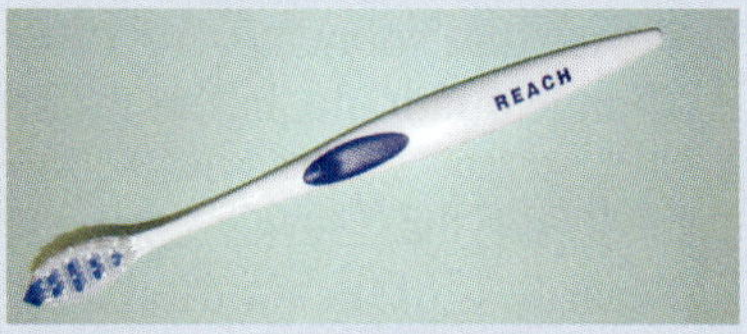	**Oral-B Advantage** Oral-B Laboratories Iowa City, Iowa	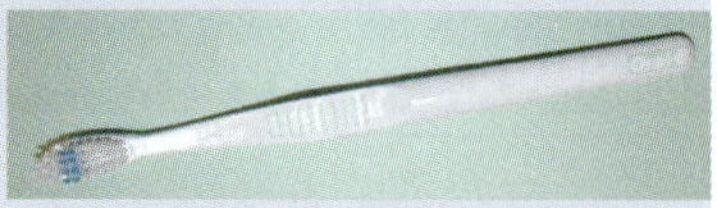
Butler GUM John O. Butler Co. A Sunstar Company Chicago, Ill.	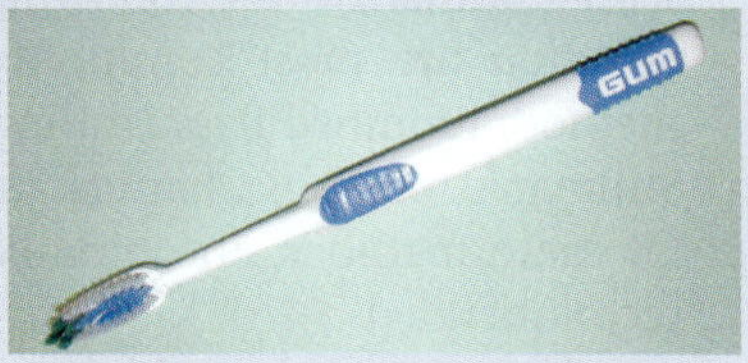	**Colgate Total** Colgate-Palmolive Co. New York, N.Y.	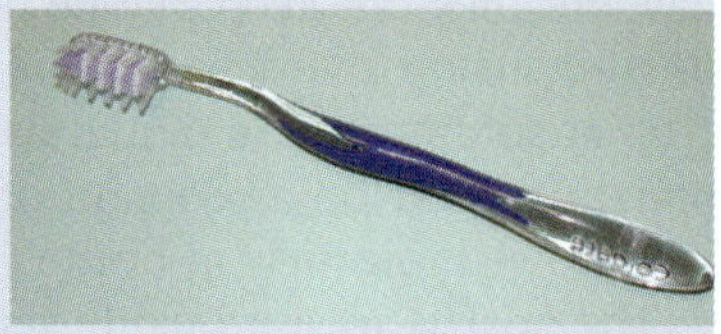
		Colgate Plus Colgate-Palmolive Co. New York, N.Y.	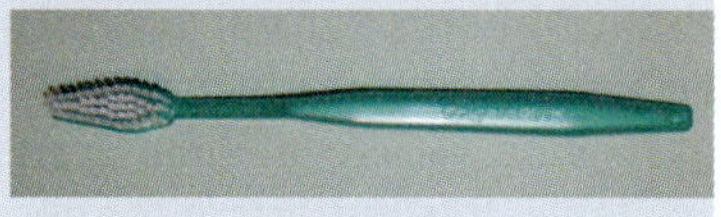

Fig. 15-12 **Examples of manual toothbrushes.** (From Daniel SJ, Harfst SA: *Mosby's dental hygiene: concepts, cases, and competencies,* St Louis, 2002, Mosby.)

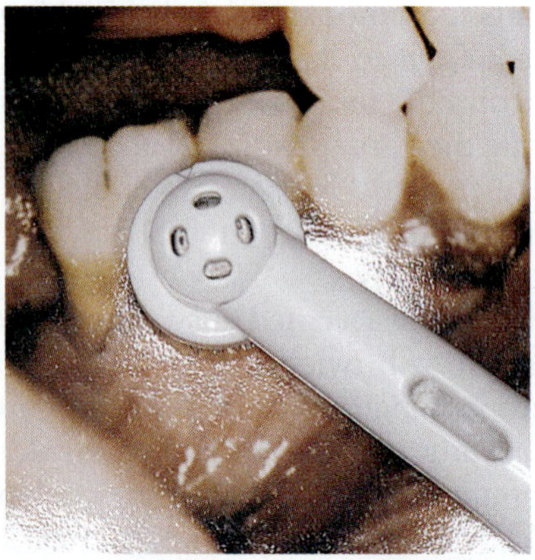

Fig. 15-13 **The proper adaptation of the brush head of a powered toothbrush.** (From Daniel SJ, Harfst SA: *Mosby's dental hygiene: concepts, cases, and competencies,* St Louis, 2002, Mosby.)

Box 15-2 Examples of Powered Toothbrushes

Product and company	Description
Oral-B Braun	
3-D Plaque Remover Oral-B Laboratories Iowa City, Iowa	Oscillating, small circulating brush head. Some units include dual oscillating and back-and-forth motion.
Butler GUM	
Pulse Plaque Remover John O. Butler Co. A Sunstar Company Chicago, Illinois	Brush tufts move up and down. Uses disposable AA batteries rather than rechargeable battery.

Box 15-2 Examples of Powered Toothbrushes—cont'd

Product and company	Description
Colgate Actibrush	
Colgate-Palmolive Co. New York, New York	Small, round, soft-bristle head with oscillating movement.
Crest Spin Brush	
Procter & Gamble Cincinnati, Ohio	The brush head is a combination of stationary bristles on the posterior two-thirds and small, round oscillating bristles on the anterior one-third of the head. Disposable AA batteries are used to operate the brush.
Interplak	
Powered Brush Bausch & Lomb Tucker, Georgia	Individual brush tufts rotate and counter-rotate. Choice of either large or small brush head.
Rotadent	
Prodentec Batesville, Arkansas	Small rotating brush. Choice of flat or pointed brush head.
SynchroSonic	
Waterpik Technologies Fort Collins, Colorado	Brush head vibrates with sound.
Sonicare	
Philips Oral Healthcare Snoqualmie, Washington	Brush head vibrates with sound.

From Daniel SJ, Harfst SA: *Mosby's dental hygiene: concepts, cases, and competencies–2004 update,* St Louis, 2004, Mosby.

Toothbrushing Precautions

Patients should be cautioned about damage that may be caused by vigorously scrubbing the teeth with any toothbrush. Over time this may cause abnormal *abrasion* (wear) of the tooth structure, gingival recession, and exposure of the root surface (Fig. 15-15).

Toothbrushing for Unusual Conditions

Even when an unusual or painful oral condition exists, the patient must be encouraged to brush wherever possible. It is inadvisable to go for prolonged periods without removing plaque. However, the following conditions may require a temporary departure from the routine oral care:

- *Acute oral inflammation* or a *traumatic lesion* may make brushing painful. Patients should be instructed to brush all areas of the mouth that are not affected and to resume regular oral hygiene practices as soon as possible. Rinsing with a warm, mild saline solution can encourage healing and remove debris.
- *After periodontal surgery,* patients receive instructions concerning brushing where sutures or dressings are placed. Direct or vigorous brushing of a periodontal dressing could dislodge it. Patients may be instructed to brush only the occlusal surfaces and to use *very light* strokes over the dressing. The other teeth and gingiva should be brushed as usual.
- *After dental extractions,* patients are often reluctant to brush their teeth. However, the teeth adjacent to the extraction site need cleaning as soon as possible to reduce bacterial collections and to promote healing. Patients are usually instructed to avoid the surgical site but to brush the other teeth as usual.
- *After dental restorations,* patients are often reluctant to brush a new crown or new fixed bridge. Specific oral hygiene instructions should be given to the patient at the time of the visit. Most often, patients will be instructed to brush all areas of their mouth normally.

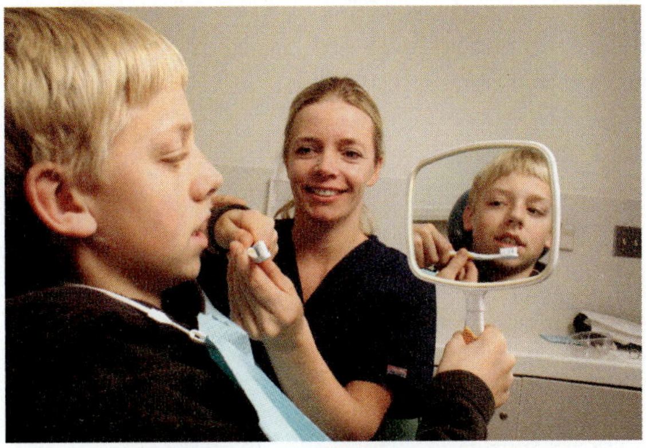

Fig. 15-14 Observing toothbrushing technique.

Table 15-3 ***Tooth-Brushing Methods***

Method	Description	Considerations	Initial Brush
Bass	• Bristles placed directly into sulcus at 45-degree angle to the tooth • Gentle short strokes in sulcus • Followed by "rolling stroke" method since Bass method cleans only sulcus	• Good plaque removal from gingival margin and sulcus • Limited cleaning on remainder of tooth surface • Easy to learn	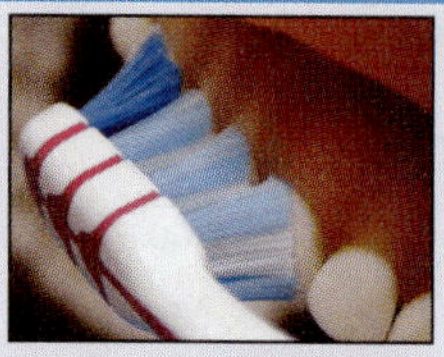
Rolling stroke	• Bristles are placed against attached gingiva at a 45-degree angle to the tooth • Brush is rolled slowly by flexing wrist to drag bristles against tooth with gentle, firm motion • Brush is rolled at least five times for each area	• Used for removing plaque at gingival margin and clinical crown • Limited plaque removal at gingival margin	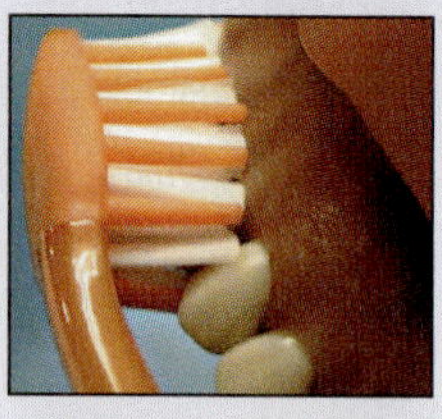
Modified Stillman's	• Bristles are placed onto the attached gingiva at a 45-degree angle to the tooth • Bristles are pressed (enough to cause slight gingival blanching) and vibrated to promote circulation • A "rolling stroke" is added to cleanse the tooth • The action is repeated sequentially throughout the mouth • In the anterior lingual area, place the heel or toe of the brush on the gingiva, rotating and sweeping toward incisal edges	• Good gingival stimulation • Good (clinical crown) coronal and interproximal cleaning • Limited sulcular cleaning • Dexterity required	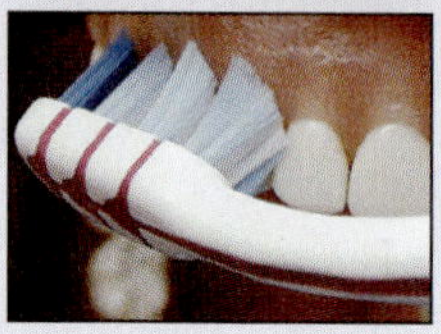
Charters'	• Side of brush is placed against tooth with bristles facing occlusally • Brush is slid to a 45-degree angle at the gingival margin • Bristles are then pressed into the margin and proximal areas and vibrated for at least 10 strokes for each area of the mouth • A "rolling stroke" is recommended before use of this technique to cleanse the coronal surface	• Good interproximal cleaning • Limited sulcular cleaning • Useful around orthodontic bands, fixed prostheses	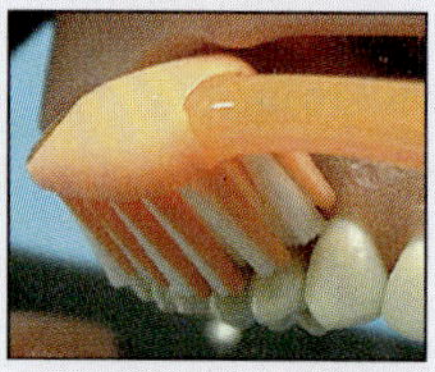
Fones'	• With teeth closed, brush is placed against the cheek with bristles directed to the posterior teeth • Circular strokes are used in a quick sweeping motion • Anterior teeth are placed end-to-end and cleansed in the same manner • In-and-out strokes are used to cleanse the palatal and lingual areas	• Easy to learn first technique for children • Possibly detrimental for vigorous adult brushers	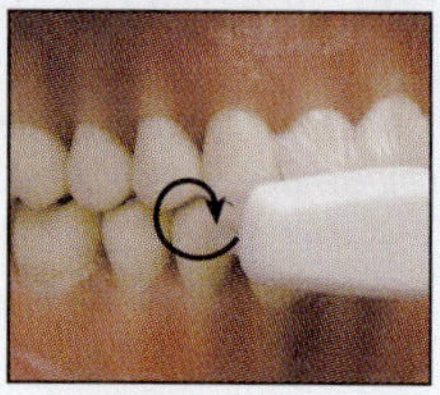
Horizonal/Scrub	• Bristles are placed at a 90-degree angle to the tooth, and brush is moved back and forth or in a large circular motion	• Removes plaque successfully from facial and lingual surfaces (unless a hard brush is used) • If a hard brush is used, there is the potential for damage to the tooth structure and to the soft tissues • Inability to access interproximal areas	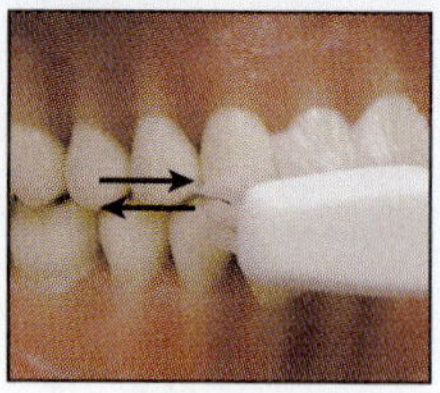

From Daniel SJ, Harfst SA: Mosby's dental hygiene: concepts, cases, and competencies, *St Louis, 2002, Mosby.*

Recall

13. What can patients do daily to remove plaque?
14. Which type of toothbrush bristles is usually recommended?
15. Which method of toothbrushing is generally recommended?

Dental Floss or Tape

When used properly, dental floss or tape removes bacterial plaque and thus reduces interproximal bleeding (Fig. 15-16 and Procedure 15-2). Dental floss is circular in shape, and dental tape is flat. Dental floss can be purchased in various colors and flavors, although these do not perform better than plain floss.

Both floss and tape are available in waxed or unwaxed varieties, and patients should be encouraged to use the type they prefer. Some patients dislike unwaxed floss because it is thinner and tends to shred or tear on older dental restorations. Research has shown that there is no difference in the effectiveness of waxed or unwaxed floss for plaque removal.

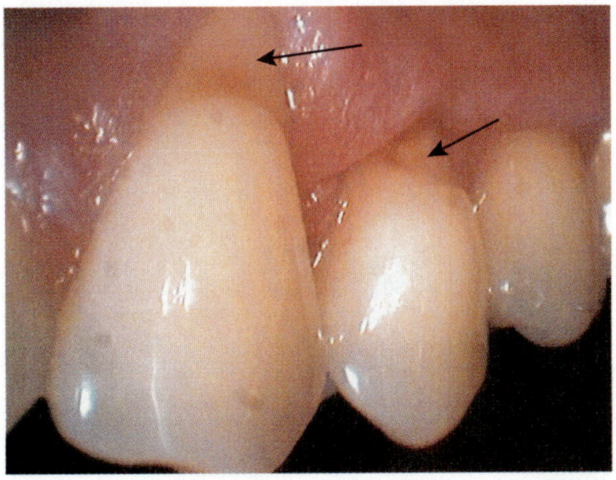

Fig. 15-15 **Improper brushing techniques can result in abrasion of the tooth surface and cause gingival recession.** (Courtesy Dr. Robert Meckstroth.)

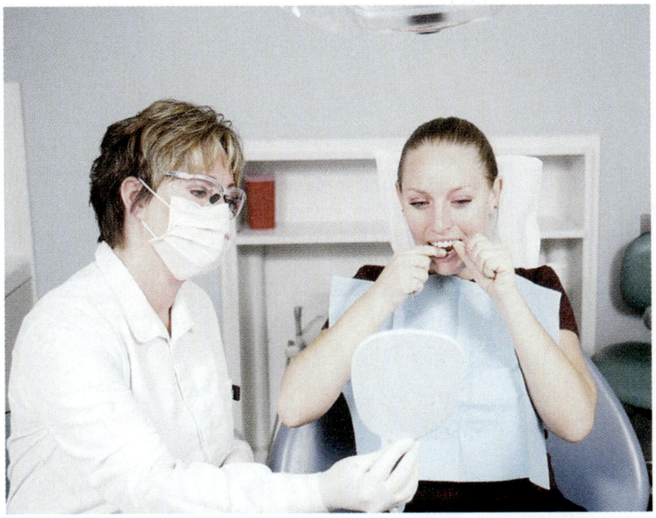

Fig. 15-16 **The dental assistant helps the patient with flossing.**

When to Floss

Dental floss should be used *before* toothbrushing for the following reasons:

- When plaque has been removed from proximal surfaces, the fluoride in the dentifrice used during brushing is able to reach the proximal surfaces for prevention of dental caries.
- When brushing is done first, the mouth may feel "clean." Thus the patient may see no need to floss or may not want to take the additional time to floss.

Recall

16. What is the difference between dental floss and dental tape?
17. Which is more effective, waxed or unwaxed dental floss?

Interdental Aids

Special devices are recommended as aids for cleaning between teeth with large or open interdental spaces and under fixed bridges (Fig. 15-17). These are aids to flossing but do not replace it in all areas of the oral cavity (Fig. 15-18, *A* and *B*).

End-Tuft Brushes

Interdental brushes are made from soft nylon filaments formed into a narrow cone shape. They are useful to clean areas that are hard to reach with a regular toothbrush, such as orthodontic appliances, fixed bridges, space maintainers, and proximal tooth surfaces next to open embrasures.

Bridge Threaders

Bridge threaders are used to pass dental floss under the **pontic** ("false" tooth) of a fixed bridge (Fig. 15-19). They are used with regular dental floss. A piece of dental floss is looped through the circular part of the bridge threader. Then the straight part of the threader is slipped under the pontic, and the floss is pulled through.

Automatic Flossers

Automatic flossers are designed for patients who have difficulty manipulating dental floss (Fig. 15-20). These battery-operated devices have one-use, replaceable, thin rubber filament tips. The tip is inserted into the interproximal space. When the button on the handle is pressed, the rubber tip vibrates against the interproximal tooth surfaces.

Procedure 15-2 Assisting the Patient with Dental Floss

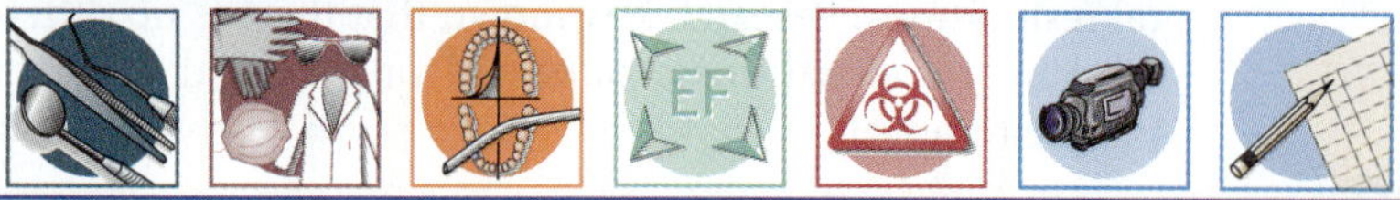

Goal

To teach a patient how to use dental floss effectively.

Equipment and Supplies

- Hand mirror for patient
- Dental floss

PROCEDURAL STEPS

Preparing the Floss

1. Cut a piece of floss about 18 inches long. Wrap the excess floss around your middle or index fingers of both hands, leaving 2 to 3 inches of working space exposed.

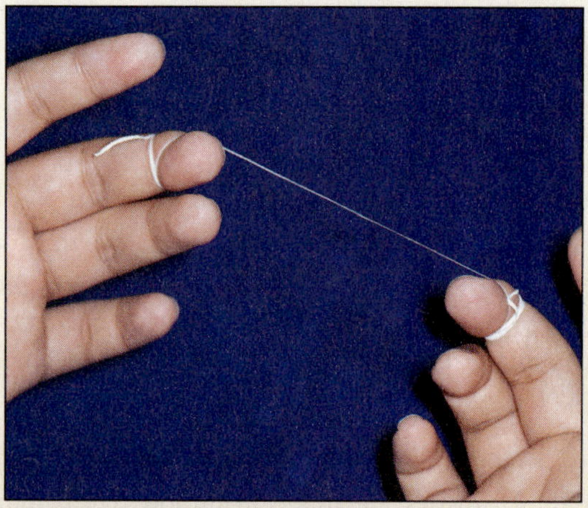

2. Stretch the floss tightly between your fingers and use your thumb and index finger to guide the floss into place.
3. Hold the floss tightly between the thumb and forefinger of each hand. These fingers control the floss, and they should be no more than ½ inch apart.

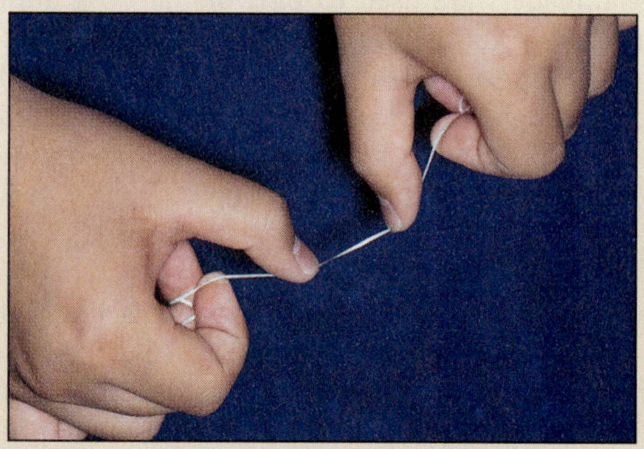

Flossing the Teeth

1. Pass the floss gently between the patient's teeth, using a sawing motion. Guide the floss to the gumline. Do not force or snap the floss past the contact area.
   Purpose: The floss may cut or injure the tissue.
2. Curve the floss into a C shape against one tooth. Slide it gently into the space between the gingiva and the tooth. Use both hands to move the floss up and down on one side of the tooth.
   Purpose: To remove plaque from the difficult-to-reach proximal areas.
3. Repeat these steps on each side of all the teeth in both arches, including the posterior surface of the last tooth in each quadrant.

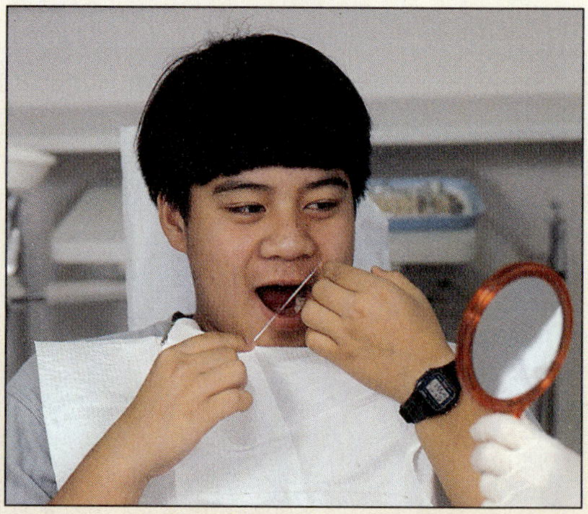

4. As the floss becomes frayed or soiled, move a fresh area into the working position.
   Note: This procedure is described as it would be performed by the patient at home.

Documentation

Date	Procedure	Operator
2/20/05	Provided flossing demonstration and instruction. Patient practiced technique and did well.	DLB/120

Modified from Policy to Practice: *OSAP's Guide to the Guidelines,* OSAP, Annapolis, Md, 2004.

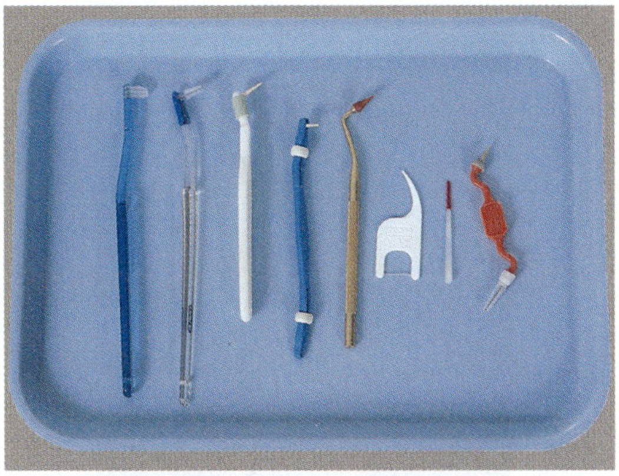

Fig. 15-17 Types of interdental aids.

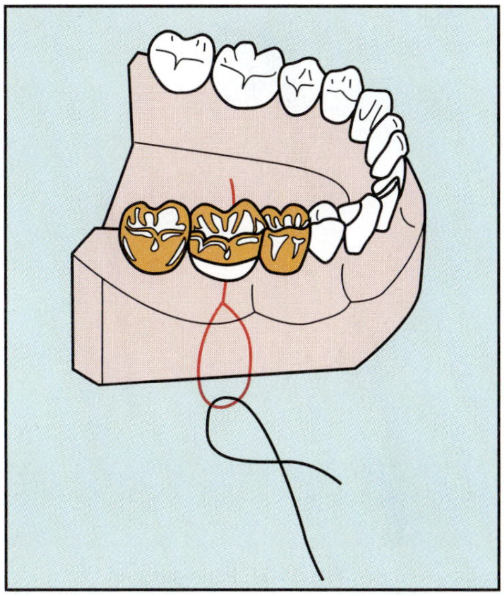

Fig. 15-19 A bridge threader is used as an aid to clean under a fixed bridge.

A

B

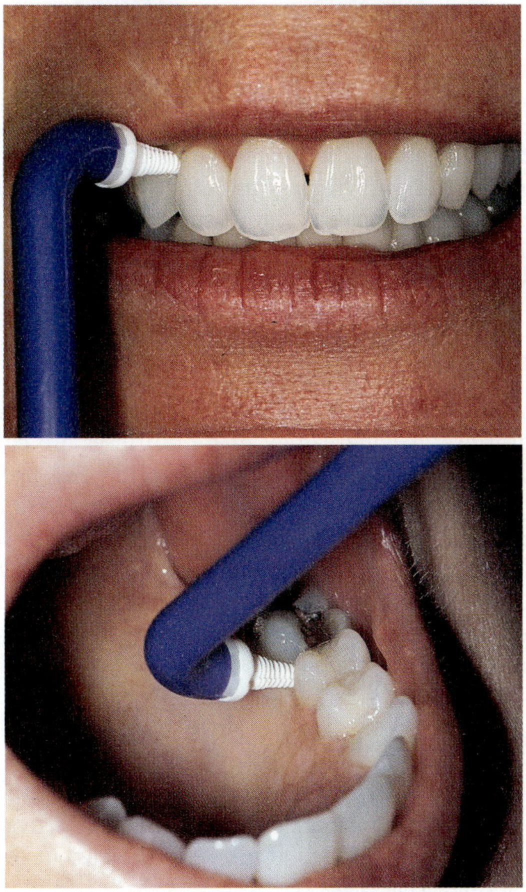

Fig. 15-18 An interdental hygienic aid. **A,** Anterior teeth. **B,** Cleaning posterior interproximal areas that are difficult to reach.

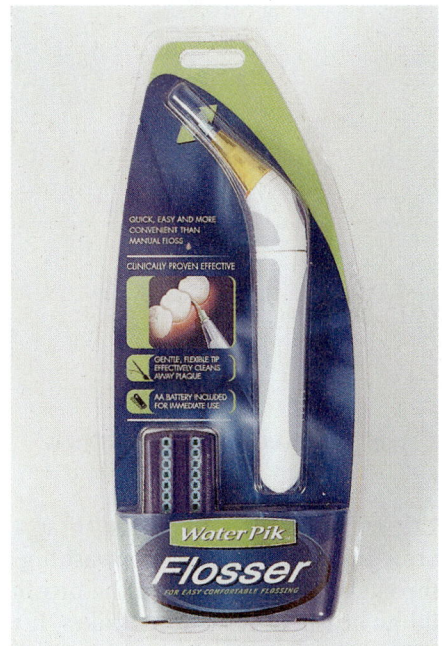

Fig. 15-20 Automatic flosser.

Perio-Aid

A perio-aid is a handle with holes in the end designed to hold toothpicks (Fig. 15-21). The patient can clean difficult-to-reach areas of the mouth with the toothpick. It is especially useful in interproximal areas of gingival recession or after periodontal surgery.

To use a perio-aid, a firm, round toothpick is inserted into an opening at either end of the handle, and the excess length is broken off. The end of the toothpick is then carried to the area to be cleaned by simply holding the device with one hand.

Dentures

Patients who have full or partial dentures will need to use a denture brush to clean all areas of the denture

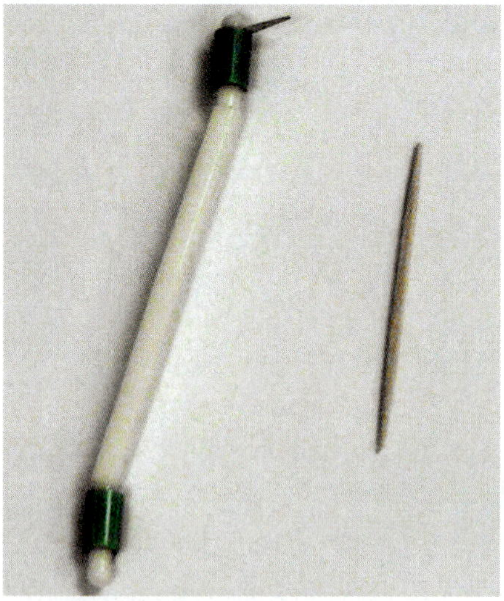

Fig. 15-21 Perio-aid.

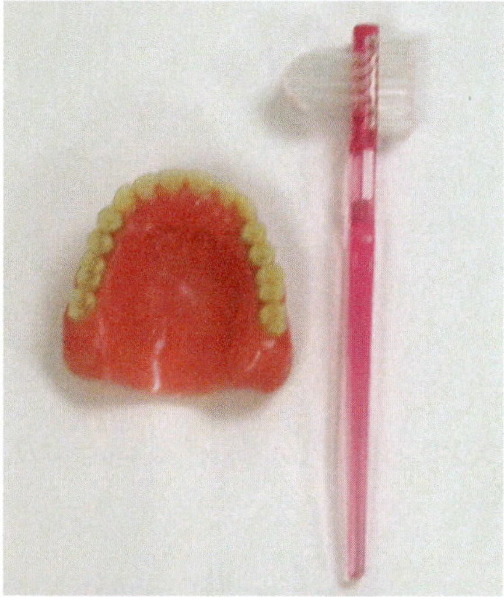

Fig. 15-22 Denture and denture brush.

(Fig. 15-22). A nonabrasive cleaner such as a commercial denture cleaner, mild soap, dishwashing liquid, or mild toothpaste should be used on the brush. The denture should be brushed with short strokes. It is always a good idea to put water or a towel in the sink so that the dentures will not break if they are dropped.

Toothpaste

Toothpaste (dentifrice) contains ingredients designed to remove food residue and has abrasives to remove stain. Highly polished tooth surfaces will stain less readily and remain clean longer. In addition, most brands of toothpaste now contain fluoride. They also contain flavoring agents to give the mouth a fresh and clean feeling (Fig. 15-23).

Some toothpastes now contain a compound that reduces calculus formation when they are used regularly af-

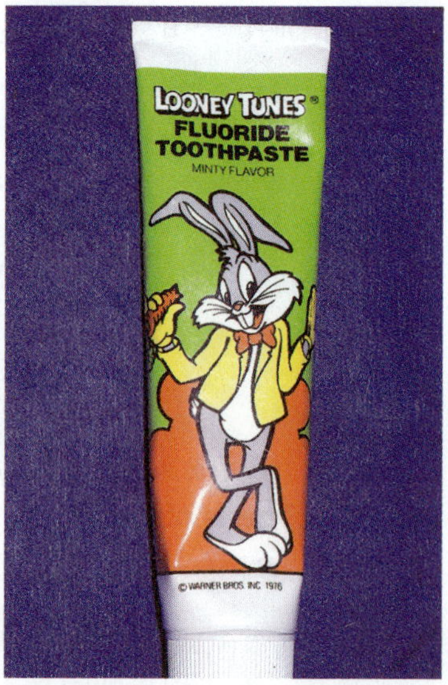

Fig. 15-23 Toothpaste for children.

ter dental prophylaxis. However, this compound will not remove existing calculus. This "tartar-control" toothpaste may be helpful for those individuals who accumulate excessive calculus between regular cleaning appointments (Table 15-4).

Mouthrinses

Many patients like the feeling of freshness provided by a mouthrinse. A wide variety of mouthrinses are currently available, and some also contain fluoride. Because many mouthrinses also contain alcohol as an ingredient, recovering alcoholics are advised to read the label and select a mouthrinse that does not contain alcohol (Fig. 15-24).

Rinsing the mouth with water is recommended after meals and snacks when toothbrushing and interdental cleaning are not possible.

Oral Irrigation Devices

Oral irrigators deliver a pulsating stream of water or chemical agent through a nozzle to the teeth and gingivae. Oral irrigation can be applied at home by the patient or in the dental office (Fig. 15-25).

Oral irrigation helps to reduce bacterial levels in subgingival areas. For selected patients, oral irrigation can supplement other oral hygiene techniques.

Recall

18. What cleaners can be used to clean dentures?
19. Will "tartar-control" toothpaste remove calculus?
20. If you cannot brush and floss after lunch, what should you do?

Table 15-4 ***Types of Toothpastes***

Type	Active Ingredient	How It Works	Comments
Fluoride/anticaries	Sodium fluoride	Assists in remineralization of the teeth	Excellent choice for caries prevention. Young children must be supervised to prevent them from swallowing the toothpaste.
Antigingivitis	Triclosan and sodium fluoride	Antimicrobial action on the bacteria in the plaque	ADA-approved as a decay-preventive dentifrice that also helps to reduce gingivitis, plaque, and calculus.
Desensitizing	Potassium nitrate	Blocks the openings to the exposed dentinal tubules	These take several weeks to work.
Whitening	Hydrogen peroxide or carbamide peroxide	Mild abrasive that removes surface stain and provides a gentle polish	Some patients notice tissue irritation. The degree of whitening varies among patients.
Baking soda	Sodium bicarbonate	Mild abrasive	May provide some antimicrobial effect.
Tartar control	Sodium hexametaphosphate or pyrophosphate	Inhibits calcification of deposits on the teeth	The major effect is on supragingival calculus.

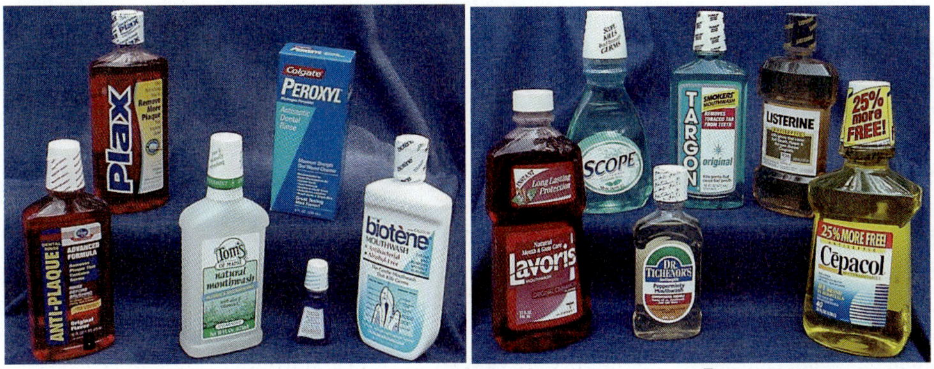

A B

Fig. 15-24 **Mouthrinses. A, Two prerinses *(left)* and several alcohol-free mouthrinses *(right)*. B, Familiar brands of mouthrinses containing alcohol in amounts ranging from 8% to 27%.** (Courtesy Dr. W.B. Stilley II, Brandon, Miss; From Daniel SJ, Harfst SA: *Mosby's dental hygiene: concepts, cases, and competencies–2004 update,* St Louis, 2004, Mosby.)

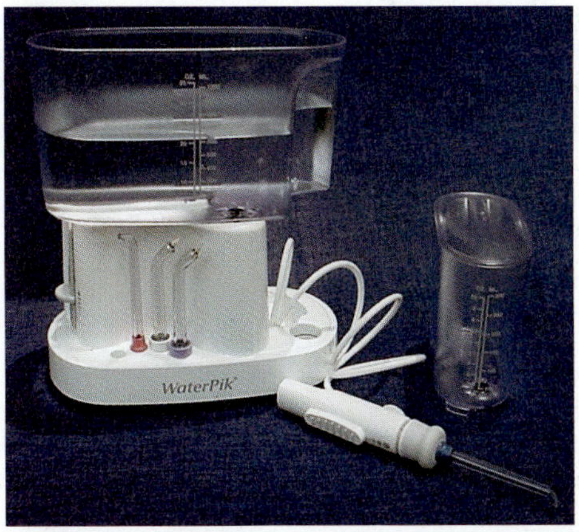

Fig. 15-25 **Irrigator. Unit is shown with supragingival and marginal irrigation tips and two reservoirs. The larger reservoir is on top of the unit and is designed for water. The smaller reservoir is designed for chemotherapeutic agents (e.g., chlorhexidine) and is tinted to reduce light degradation.** (Courtesy Waterpik Technologies, Fort Collins, Colo.)

General Guidelines for Home Care Products

The ADA Council on Dental Therapeutics conducts an independent review of the scientific evidence of the research claims and evaluation of home care products. When a products meets the appropriate standards, it is given the ADA Seal of Acceptance (Fig. 15-26). The ADA's Seal of Acceptance provides a quality assurance guarantee for consumers and professionals.

You can check the ADA's website (www.ada.org) to receive current information on toothbrushes, dentifrices, interproximal aids, and products for the prevention of gingivitis and caries.

Fig 15-26 The American Dental Association's Seal of Acceptance.

LEGAL AND ETHICAL IMPLICATIONS

Despite the powerful evidence in support of water fluoridation, it is frequently the subject of vigorous opposition. The issue of water fluoridation gives dental professionals the chance to promote oral health at the community level. The American Dental Association has a long-standing policy that dentists should work to promote fluoridation in their communities. However, not all dental professionals are comfortable in this role.

Dentists, dental assistants, and dental hygienists should at least educate their patients about what fluoridation is and who benefits from it. They can encourage patients to support the issue with a vote. Dental professionals should know the concentration of fluoride in their community's drinking water supply. This information may be obtained from the state or local health department.

Remember that fluoridation is a political issue. Success in a fluoridation campaign requires the use of the media, publicity, education, door-to-door canvassing, telephone calls, and "getting out the vote" on election day.

Critical Thinking

1. Corey Kendall is a 16-year-old patient in your office. Corey is very conscious about her health and weight. She has a moderately high rate of decay but insists she does not eat candy. When you review her food diary, you notice she consumes large amounts of diet colas and has dried fruit for snacks. What recommendations would you make for Corey? What information would you give her regarding diet colas?
2. Mr. Hahn Tran is a 62-year-old patient in your office. He has several older restorations in his mouth that need to be replaced. Mr. Tran does not floss now because the unwaxed floss he previously used shredded and got caught between his teeth. What suggestions do you have for Mr. Tran?
3. Recently, several patients have been asking about the benefits of an automatic toothbrush compared with the manual brushes they currently use. How will you respond to these inquiries?

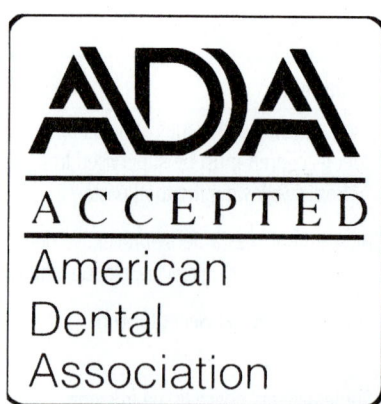

16

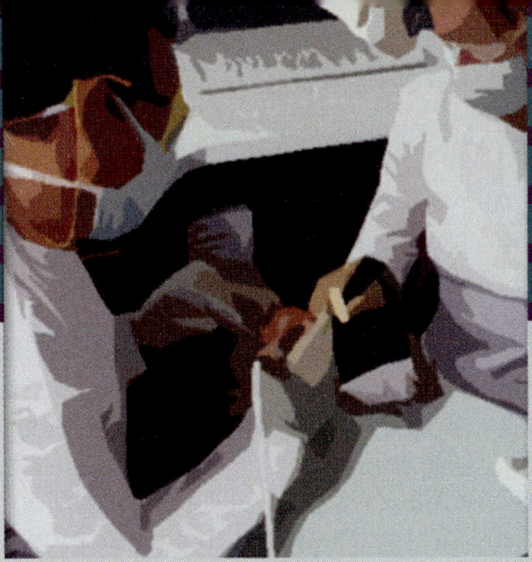

Nutrition

Outline

- **Recommended Dietary Allowances (RDAs)**
- **Food Guide Pyramid**
- **Carbohydrates**
  - Foods That Cause Tooth Decay
- **Proteins**
- **Fats (Lipids)**
  - Cholesterol
  - Antioxidants
- **Vitamins**
- **Minerals**
- **Water**
- **Diet Modification**
- **Dietary Analysis**
- **Reading Food Labels**
  - Product Label Information
  - Labeling Ingredients
  - Label Claims
  - Organic Foods
- **Eating Disorders**
  - Bulimia
  - Anorexia Nervosa
  - Female Athlete Triad
  - Management of Eating Disorders
- **Healthy Habits**
- **Patient Education**
- **Legal and Ethical Implications**
- **Eye to the Future**
- **Critical Thinking**

KEY TERMS

Amino acids (ah-**me**-no) Compounds in proteins used by the body to build and repair tissue.

Anorexia nervosa (a-neh-**rek**-see-ah ner-**voh**-sah) Eating disorder caused by an altered self-image.

Bulimia (boo-**lee**-me-ah) Eating disorder characterized by binge eating and self-induced vomiting.

Cariogenic Producing or promoting tooth decay.

Fats Lipids.

Nutrients (**new**-tree-unts) Organic and inorganic chemicals in food that supply energy.

Organic (or-**ga**-nik) Describes food products that have been grown without the use of chemical pesticides, herbicides, or fertilizers.

Triglycerides Neutral fats.

LEARNING OUTCOMES

On completion of this chapter, the student will be able to achieve the following objectives:

- Pronounce, define, and spell the Key Terms.
- Explain how diet and nutrition can affect oral conditions.
- Explain why the study of nutrition is important to the dental assistant.
- Describe the three types of proteins.
- List the six areas of the Food Guide Pyramid.
- Explain the meaning of "recommended dietary (daily) allowance."
- Describe the difference between vitamins and minerals.
- Describe the role of carbohydrates in the daily diet.
- Explain the need for minerals in the diet.
- Discuss the health and oral implications of eating disorders.
- Explain how to interpret food labels.
- Explain the criteria for a food to be considered "organic."
- Explain the relationship between frequency and amount of cariogenic foods in causing tooth decay.

You probably have heard the expression, "You are what you eat." This is true because food is used to build and repair the body. Food choices must therefore be based on sound information and knowledge.

Although good nutrition is important for everyone, it is particularly critical for pregnant women, young children, and elderly persons. Malnutrition during these crucial periods may result in physical or mental disabilities. Well-nourished persons are usually better able to heal and ward off infections than poorly nourished individuals.

As a dental assistant, you will be discussing nutrition and food choices with patients in a variety of circumstances (Fig. 16-1), including the following situations:

- Counseling patients about the prevention of tooth decay
- Counseling patients regarding their diet after oral surgery or other dental procedures
- Performing dietary analysis with patients
- Counseling patients who have orthodontic appliances regarding food choices

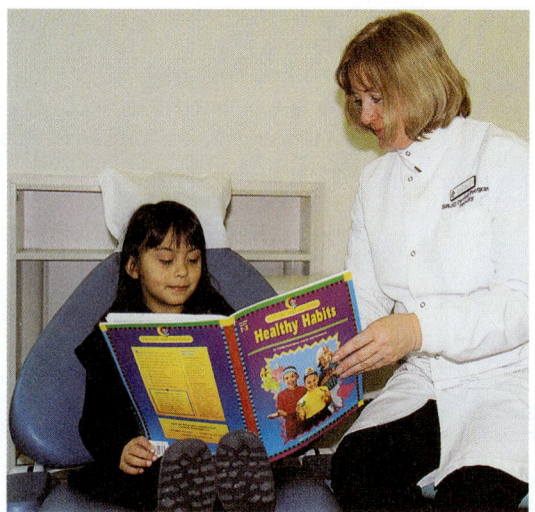

Fig. 16-1 The dental assistant discusses nutrition and dental health with her patient.

The study of *nutrition* is the science of how the body uses food for development, growth, repair, and maintenance. **Nutrients** are the components in food that are needed by the body.

This chapter discusses the six primary nutrients, new dietary guidelines, antioxidants, food labels, and "right" eating habits for your patients and yourself (Box 16-1).

RECOMMENDED DIETARY ALLOWANCES (RDAs)

The RDAs are the levels of essential nutrients that are needed by individuals on a daily basis. These recommendations are based on scientific knowledge about each nutrient, as determined by the Food and Nutrition Board of the National Academy of Sciences. The RDAs are reevaluated and reissued approximately every 4 years to keep up with emerging research.

FOOD GUIDE PYRAMID

The Food Guide Pyramid is a visual "outline" of what to eat each day. It is not a rigid prescription, but a general guide that lets you choose a healthful diet that is right for

Six Key Nutrients

Carbohydrates	Water
Proteins	Vitamins
Fats	Minerals

Box 16-1 Functions of Five Major Nutrients

Carbohydrates	Proteins	Fats/Lipids	Vitamins	Minerals
Energy Bulk Make other compounds	Provide structure Regulate body processes: Enzymes Hormones Carrier molecules Fluid and electrolyte balance Energy	Energy Essential fatty acids Transport for fat-soluble vitamins Structure components Insulation Cushions organs	Function with enzymes	Component of body structures Part of enzyme molecules Part of organic molecules (hemoglobin) Fluid and electrolyte balance

From Applegate E: *The anatomy and physiology learning system,* ed 2, Philadelphia, 2000, Saunders.

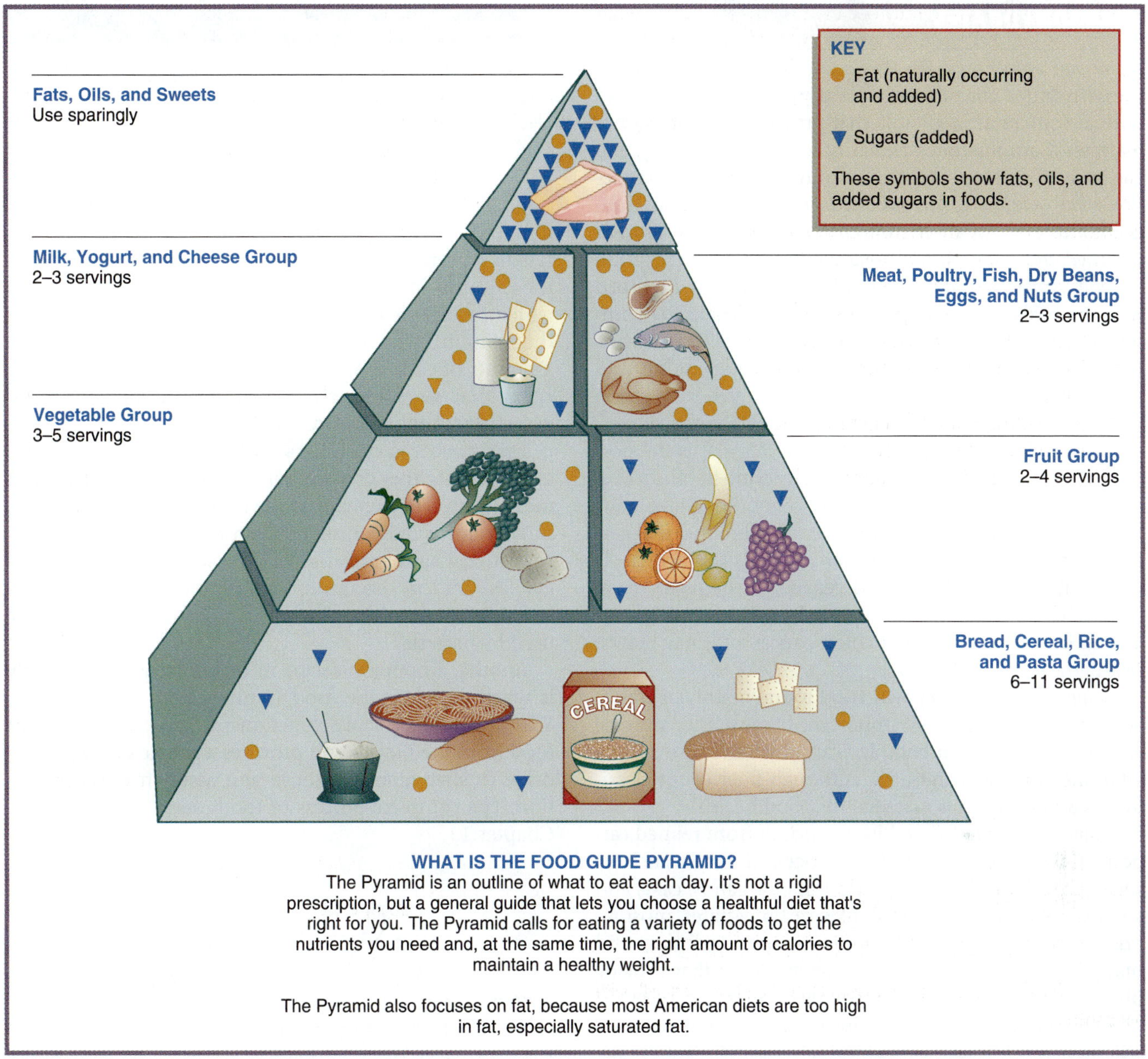

Fig. 16-2 Food Guide Pyramid. (From US Department of Agriculture and US Department of Health and Human Services, 1996.)

you. The pyramid calls for eating a variety of foods to get the nutrients you need and the right amount of calories to maintain a healthy weight (Fig. 16-2).

The largest sections of the pyramid represent foods that should be consumed in the greatest quantities. The *grain group,* the largest section, forms the base at the bottom of the pyramid. The *sweets and fats group,* the smallest section, is found at the top. The purpose of the Food Guide Pyramid is to show how the proportions of each basic food group contribute to a balanced diet.

Two symbols, a circle and a triangle, are used on the pyramid. The *circle* indicates fat that occurs naturally or is added to food. The *triangle* indicates sugar that is added. These symbols show how fat and sugar, even though they come mainly from fats, oils, and sweets, can occur in any of the five basic food groups.

Each of these food groups provides some, but *not all,* of the nutrients you need. Foods in one group can't replace those in another. No one food group is more important than another for good health—you need them all.

You can discuss the Food Guide Pyramid with patients to help them understand how to achieve healthful eating habits. Eating a healthful diet is necessary to look better, feel better, have more energy, and have a more positive outlook on life.

CARBOHYDRATES

Carbohydrates are primarily plant products in origin. No animal sources are available that provide adequate carbohydrates. Carbohydrates are easily converted to energy, and the body uses them as the chief source of energy.

Carbohydrates are divided into three groups based on the complexity of their molecules: *simple sugars, complex carbohydrates* (starch), and *dietary fiber.* With the exception of fiber, carbohydrates are easily digested and absorbed into the body. Simple sugars are absorbed first; the complex sugars must be processed before they can be absorbed in the intestinal tract. Dietary fiber is indigestible and passes through the intestinal tract unchanged. Each group has a specific function in health.

Dietary fiber is commonly called *roughage.* It is the portion of the plant that is eaten but cannot be absorbed. Fiber is classified by its water solubility. Roughage adds bulk to the intestinal tract and is beneficial for normal gastrointestinal functioning. *Water-soluble fiber,* which is found in oat bran, fruits, and vegetables, helps to lower cholesterol. *Insoluble fiber,* which is found in whole grains and beans, helps to prevent colon cancer and may reduce heart attack risk (Table 16-1).

Complex carbohydrates, which are found mainly in grains, vegetables, and fruits, are important because they provide energy. Foods high in complex carbohydrates also supply vitamins, minerals, and fiber. Although fiber is not classified as a nutrient, it is essential for good health.

Simple sugars are formed in the mouth from refined carbohydrates that are found in processed foods such as sugar, syrup, jelly, bread, crackers, cookies, candy, cake, and soft drinks. In contrast to complex carbohydrates, most refined carbohydrates supply only "empty" calories, and many are high in fat. *Empty calories* are those that provide only calories and no other nutrients or fiber.

Although it may be wise to lower dietary fat, consumers should be cautioned to read food labels carefully. In many low-fat or reduced-fat foods, fat is replaced with sugars. As a result, although the fat content of a food is less, the calorie count may be the same or higher than in the original higher fat version of the food.

Sources of Carbohydrates

Cereal grains: wheat, corn, oat, rice, barley, buckwheat

Sweets: table sugar, honey, maple and corn syrups

Vegetables: green leafy vegetables, dried beans and peas

Foods That Cause Tooth Decay

Any food that contains sugars or other carbohydrates that can be metabolized by bacteria in plaque is described as being **cariogenic** (producing or promoting dental decay). For instance, refined carbohydrates, such as candy and other sweets, are cariogenic.

A major factor in determining the cariogenicity of a carbohydrate is how long the food stays in the mouth. Sugary liquids such as soft drinks leave the mouth quickly and are not as cariogenic as sticky foods, such as raisins or caramels, which adhere to the teeth and stay in the mouth longer. Furthermore, the frequency with which cariogenic foods are eaten is more important than the amount. The child that snacks all day on small amounts of cariogenic food is far more likely to develop decay than the child that eats a larger amount of cariogenic food, but only once a day.

Foods such as crackers, although not sweet, are cariogenic because they contain refined carbohydrates that stick to the teeth. They remain in the mouth long enough to be broken down into sugars that can be used by the bacteria in plaque. Complex carbohydrates, such as fruits and vegetables, are less cariogenic because they clear the mouth before they are converted into simple sugars that can be used by bacteria.

Another important factor in determining cariogenicity is whether or not the food stimulates the flow of saliva. *Salivary flow* serves two functions: it speeds clearance of food from the mouth and provides a source of dietary fluoride to strengthen the tooth and assist in remineralization. The complete process of tooth decay is described in Chapter 13.

Recall

1. What are nutrients?
2. What are the three types of carbohydrates?
3. What is meant by cariogenicity?

PROTEINS

Proteins are the only nutrients that can build and repair body tissues, and this is their primary function. Proteins are composed of **amino acids,** which are used in the building and repair process. There are 20 amino acids, *eight* of which are essential in the adult for normal growth and maintenance of tissues. These *essential* amino acids must come from food.

Proteins are classified as being either complete, partially complete, or incomplete.

Table 16-1 ***Dietary Fiber in Some Common Foods***

Food	Amount	Weight (grams)	Calories	Dietary Fiber (grams)
Fruit				
Apple, with peel	1 medium	138	80	3.9
Apple juice	1 cup	228	116	0.7
Banana, peeled	1 medium	110	100	2.5
Orange, peeled	1 medium	145	67	3.1
Prunes, dried	3 medium	8	60	3.5
Vegetables, Cooked				
Potato with skin, baked	1 large	200	220	3.9
Carrots, sliced	1 cup	150	60	5.0
Broccoli	1 spear	180	53	6.2
Green beans	1 cup	130	40	3.3
Corn	1 cup	164	134	7.7
Peas	1 cup	160	130	7.4
Vegetables, Raw				
Celery	1 cup	120	19	2.0
Carrots	1 medium	72	31	2.0
Tomato	1 medium	120	24	2.0
Lettuce, chopped	1 cup	56	53	0.8
Cauliflower	1 cup	100	24	2.7
Legumes and Nuts				
Navy beans, cooked	1 cup	190	225	13.0
Lima beans, cooked	1 cup	170	170	9.2
Lentils, cooked	1 cup	200	215	8.7
Pecans, dried, halves	1 cup	108	720	6.5
Walnuts, English, chopped	1 cup	120	770	8.4
Peanut butter, regular	1 tablespoon	16	95	1.0
Bread and Pasta				
White bread	1 slice	28	75	0.5
Whole wheat bread	1 slice	28	70	2.4
Spaghetti, cooked	1 cup	130	190	1.0
Brown rice, cooked	1 cup	195	232	2.8
White rice, cooked	1 cup	205	223	0.6

From Applegate E: The anatomy and physiology learning system, *ed 2, Philadelphia, 2000, Saunders.*

Sources of Protein

Complete proteins: meat, fish, poultry, eggs, dairy products

Partially complete proteins: grains, vegetables

Incomplete proteins: corn, gelatin

- A *complete protein* contains a well-balanced mixture of all eight essential amino acids. If it is the sole source of protein in the diet, a complete protein will support life and normal growth.
- A *partially complete* protein supplies an unbalanced mixture of essential amino acids. If it is the sole source of protein, a partially complete protein will maintain life but will not support normal growth.
- An *incomplete protein* will not support life or normal growth. It must not be the sole source of protein because the protein is missing or extremely low in one or more of the essential amino acids.

Each gram of protein supplies 4 calories.

Recall

4. What is an amino acid?
5. How many of the amino acids are essential?
6. What is a complete protein?

FATS (LIPIDS)

Most fats in the diet are **triglycerides,** or *neutral fats,* which occur in both animal and plant food. **Fats,** also called *lipids,* have six important functions in the body, as follows:

1. Fats are important sources of energy.
2. Fats provide essential fatty acids.
3. Fats transport vitamins.
4. Fats provide heat insulation.
5. Fats are components of cell membranes and *myelin,* the covering around nerve fibers.
6. Fats form protective cushions around the body organs.

Although fats are essential components of a healthy diet, excessive amounts are not desirable. Most Americans need to reduce their intake of dietary fat. The American Heart Association recommends that no more than 30 percent of the daily calorie intake should be in the form of fats.

In general, however, 40 percent or more of the calories in the average American diet comes from fat. This overconsumption of fats is unhealthy and related to cardiovascular disease, obesity, diabetes, and some cancers.

Sources of Antioxidants

Vitamin E: soy beans, almonds, oatmeal, chick peas (garbanzo beans), hazel nuts, rye flour, wheat germ, sunflower seeds

Vitamin C: peppers, oranges, Brussels sprouts, strawberries, tangerines, broccoli, lemons, raspberries, cabbage, grapefruit, black currants, cauliflower

Beta-carotene: carrots, sweet potatoes, pumpkin, kale, winter squash, spinach, cantaloupe, apricots, mustard greens

Seasonings: nutmeg, thyme, rosemary, sesame, cloves, green tea, oregano, pepper

Cholesterol

Cholesterol is a fat typically found in saturated fats (from animal sources). It is also manufactured within the body. Confusion often exists between "good fat" and "bad fat." The *good* fats in our diet are *polyunsaturated* and *monounsaturated* fats. The *bad* dietary fats are *cholesterol* and *saturated* fats.

Body fat is also divided into two categories. The "good" fat is *high-density lipoprotein (HDL);* the "bad" fat is *low-density lipoprotein (LDL).* The levels of HDL and LDL can often be successfully changed through diet.

It is important to understand the differences between the types of fat and the meaning of numbers used to identify fat content. Many foods that are high in saturated fats are also high in cholesterol. The recommendation is that cholesterol be limited to less than 250 mg per day, which is the amount in one egg yolk. Table 16-2 compares some common sources of fats and cholesterol.

Antioxidants

Recent research indicates that cholesterol itself may not be the problem in the development of heart disease. Rather, the problem may be the way in which the cholesterol reacts with the oxygen (*oxidizes*) in blood.

In addition to lowering the dietary intake of cholesterol, increasing the intake of antioxidants may be beneficial. The antioxidant vitamins E and C and beta-carotene can prevent cholesterol from oxidizing and damaging the arteries. Many fruits and vegetables and certain seasonings contain naturally occurring antioxidants.

Recall

7. Which systemic diseases are related to excess fat in the diet?
8. Which cholesterol is "good," and which is "bad"?

Table 16-2 ***Common Sources of Fat and Cholesterol***

Food	Amount	Weight (grams)	Total Calories	Total Fat (grams)	Saturated Fat (grams)	Cholesterol (milligrams)
Milk, nonfat	1 cup	244	86	0.4 (4%)*	0.3 (3%)*	4
Milk, 2%	1 cup	244	121	4.8 (36%)	2.9 (2%)	22
Milk, whole	1 cup	244	151	8.2 (49%)	5.0 (30%)	33
Egg, hard boiled	1 whole	50	79	5.6 (64%)	1.7 (19%)	274
Cream cheese	1 ounce	28.3	100	10.0 (90%)	6.3 (57%)	31.4
Mayonnaise	1 tablespoon	13.8	99	10.9 (99%)	1.7 (15%)	8.1
Butter	1 tablespoon	14.2	102	11.5 (100%)	7.2 (63%)	31.1
Cheese, American	1 ounce	28.3	107	9.0 (76%)	5.7 (48%)	27.3
Cheese, cheddar	1 ounce	28.3	115	9.2 (72%)	5.8 (45%)	27.3
Sirloin steak	3 ounces	85	240	15.0 (66%)	6.4 (24%)	74
Ground beef	3 ounces	85	230	16.0 (63%)	6.2 (24%)	74
Chicken breast (no skin)	3 ounces	86	142	3.0 (19%)	0.9 (6%)	73
Fried chicken	3 ounces	85	187	7.8 (38%)	2.1 (10%)	79.6
Frankfurter	2 ounces	57	183	16.6 (82%)	6.1 (30%)	29
Turkey, roasted	3 ounces	85	145	4.2 (26%)	1.4 (9%)	65
Cod, broiled	3 ounces	85	97	0.9 (8%)	0.8 (7%)	51
Tuna salad	½ cup	102	188	9.5 (45%)	1.6 (8%)	40
Avocado	1 medium	201	324	30.8 (86%)	4.9 (14%)	0

**Percentage of the total calories represented by the fat. From Applegate E:* The anatomy and physiology learning system, *ed 2, Philadelphia, 2000, Saunders.*

VITAMINS

Vitamins are organic substances that occur in plant and animal tissues. They are essential in minute amounts for the human body to maintain growth and good health. Vitamins do not *supply* energy, but they are needed to *release* energy from the carbohydrates, fats, and proteins.

Many vitamins function with enzymes in the chemical reactions in the body. To date, 13 vitamins have been discovered. Of these, four are *fat-soluble,* and nine are *water-soluble.* The *fat-soluble vitamins* (A, D, E, and K) are stored in body fat and are not destroyed by cooking.

The *water-soluble vitamins* (B and C), which are naturally present in food, are easily destroyed during food preparation. These water-soluble vitamins are not stored in the body and therefore must be consumed each day. Because of their similar functions, all the water-soluble vitamins except vitamin C are often grouped together and referred to as the *B-complex vitamins* (Table 16-3).

Recall

9. Which type of vitamin is stored in the body and is not destroyed by cooking?

10. Which vitamins are referred to as the B-complex vitamins?

11. Which vitamins are fat-soluble?

Table 16-3 ***Vitamins: Best Sources, Primary Functions, Deficiency Symptoms, and Toxicity***

U.S. RDA*	Sources	Functions	Deficiency Symptoms†	Toxicity
Vitamin A (Carotene)				
5000 IU	Yellow or orange fruits and vegetables, green leafy vegetables, oatmeal, liver, dairy products	Formation and maintenance of skin, hair, and mucous membranes; sight in dim light; bone and tooth growth	Night blindness, dry scaly skin, frequent fatigue	Toxic in high doses, although beta-carotene is nontoxic
Vitamin B_1 (Thiamine)				
1.5 mg	Cereal, oatmeal, meat, rice, pasta, whole grains, liver	Release of energy from carbohydrates, growth and metabolism	Heart irregularities, fatigue, nerve disorders, mental confusion	Not toxic; high doses excreted by kidneys
Vitamin B_2 (Riboflavin)				
2 mg	Whole grains, green leafy vegetables, organ meats, milk, eggs	Release of energy from proteins, fats, and carbohydrates	Cracks in corners of mouth, rash, anemia	No toxic effects reported
Vitamin B_6 (Pyridoxine)				
2 mg	Fish, poultry, lean meats, bananas, prunes, dried beans, whole grains, avocados	Building of body tissue, metabolism of proteins	Convulsions, dermatitis, muscular weakness, skin cracks, anemia	Possible nerve damage in hands and feet with long-term megadoses
Vitamin B_{12} (Cobalamin)				
6 μg	Meats, milk products, seafood	Cell development, nervous system functioning, metabolism of proteins and fats	Anemia, nervousness, fatigue	No toxic effects reported
Biotin				
0.3 mg	Cereal/grain products, yeast, legumes, liver	Metabolism of proteins, fats, and carbohydrates	Nausea, vomiting, depression, hair loss, dry scaly skin	No toxic effects reported
Folate (Folic Acid, Folacin)				
0.4 mg	Green leafy vegetables, organ meats, dried peas, beans, and lentils	Genetic material development, red blood cell production	Gastrointestinal disorders, anemia, cracks on lips	Some evidence of toxicity in large doses
Niacin				
20 mg	Meat, poultry, fish, cereal, peanuts, potatoes, dairy products, eggs	Metabolism of proteins, fats, and carbohydrates	Skin disorders, diarrhea, indigestion, general fatigue	Physician's care for nicotinic acid form

Data from U.S. Food and Drug Administration, American Institute for Cancer Research, and U.S. Department of Agriculture/Human Nutrition Information Service.
**RDA, recommended dietary (daily) allowance for adults and children over 4 years;* IU, *international units;* mg, *milligrams;* μg, *micrograms.*
†*Many of these symptoms can also be attributed to problems other than vitamin deficiency. If you have these symptoms and they persist, see your physician.*

Table 16-3 Vitamins: Best Sources, Primary Functions, Deficiency Symptoms, and Toxicity—cont'd

U.S. RDA*	Sources	Functions	Deficiency Symptoms†	Toxicity
Pantothenic Acid				
10 mg	Lean meats, whole grains, legumes, vegetables, fruits	Release of energy from fats and carbohydrates	Fatigue, vomiting, stomach distress, infections, muscle cramps	No toxic effects reported
Vitamin C (Ascorbic Acid)				
60 mg	Citrus fruits, berries, vegetables, peppers	Structure of bone, cartilage, muscle, and blood vessels; maintenance of capillaries and gums; absorption of iron	Swollen or bleeding gums, slow wound healing, fatigue, depression, poor digestion	Nausea, cramps, and diarrhea with 1 g or more
Vitamin D				
400 IU	Fortified milk/margarine, butter, eggs, fish, sunlight	Bone and tooth formation; maintenance of cardiac and nervous system function	*Children:* rickets and other bone deformities *Adults:* calcium loss from bones	Diarrhea and weight loss possible with high intake
Vitamin E				
30 IU	Multigrain cereals, nuts, wheat germ, vegetable oils, green leafy vegetables	Protection of blood cells, body tissues, and essential fatty acids	Muscular wasting, nerve damage, anemia, reproductive failure	Relatively nontoxic
Vitamin K				
‡—	Green leafy vegetables, fruit, dairy and grain products	Blood clotting	Bleeding disorders in newborns and patients taking blood-thinning medications	Not toxic as found in food

‡*There is no RDA for vitamin K.*

MINERALS

Minerals are essential elements that are needed in small amounts to maintain health and function and must be supplied by the diet. Minerals and vitamins are found in all foods except those that are highly refined. They are found in all tissues and fluids, and they account for 4 percent of the body weight. Of the many minerals used by the body, 14 are considered to be essential.

Minerals are the components of the bones and teeth that make them rigid and strong. They also play an important part in maintaining the body's water-electrolyte balance.

Minerals are usually classified according to the amounts required by the body. The minerals that are needed in larger amounts (100 mg/day or more) are *sodium, potassium, calcium, chloride, phosphorus,* and *magnesium.* The *trace elements,* which are needed in smaller amounts (no more than a few milligrams a day), include iron, zinc, copper, selenium, chromium, manganese, iodine, and fluorine (Table 16-4).

Table 16-4 Minerals: Best Sources, Primary Functions, Deficiency Symptoms, and Toxicity

Adult RDA*	Sources	Functions	Deficiency Symptoms†	Toxicity Symptoms
Calcium (Ca^{2+}, Ca^{++})				
800-1000 μg	Milk and milk products, green leafy vegetables, soy products, sardines, salmon	Muscle and nervous system function, blood coagulation, bone and tooth formation	Poor bone growth and tooth development *Children:* dental caries, rickets *Adults:* soft and brittle bones	Kidney stones
Chloride (Cl^-)				
750 mg	Salt, fish, vegetables	Fluid and acid-base balance, activation of gastric enzymes	Growth retardation, psychomotor deficits, memory loss	Disturbances in acid-base balance
Magnesium (Mg^{2+}, Mg^{++})				
280-350 mg	Dark green vegetables, nuts, soybeans, whole grains, bananas, apricots, seafood	Bone and tooth formation, protein synthesis, lipid metabolism	Rare except in disease states Confusion, hallucinations, poor memory, muscle weakness, cramps	Drowsiness, weakness, lethargy *Severe:* skeletal paralysis, respiratory depression, coma, death
Phosphorus (PO_4)				
800 mg	Milk and milk products, eggs, meats, legumes, whole grains	Bone and tooth formation, energy metabolism, acid-base balance	*Malabsorption (rare):* anorexia, weakness, stiff joints, fragile bones	Muscle spasms
Potassium (K^+)				
2000 mg	Milk and milk products, apricots, oranges, bananas, greens, meats, legumes	Fluid and acid-base balance, transmission of nerve impulses, enzyme reactions	Impaired growth, hypertension, bone fragility, central nervous system changes	*Hyperkalemia* (excess potassium in blood), cardiac disturbances
Sodium (Na^+)				
500 mg	*Major:* salt (sodium chloride) *Minor:* milk, vegetables	Acid-base balance, cell membrane permeability, impulse transmission	Weight loss, central nervous system abnormalities	Hypertension, leading to cardiovascular and kidney diseases
Chromium (Cr^{3+})				
50-200 μg	Liver, whole grains, cheese, legumes	Enzyme activation, glucose removal	Weight loss, central nervous system abnormalities	Inhibited insulin activity
Copper (Cu^{2+}, Cu^{++})				
1.5-3 mg	Shellfish, liver, nuts, whole grains, raisins	Red blood cell production, lipid metabolism	Anemia, bone fragility, impaired immune response	Neuron and liver cell damage from copper accumulation

Data from U.S. Food and Drug Administration, American Institute for Cancer Research, and U.S. Department of Agriculture/Human Nutrition Information Service.
*RDA, *recommended dietary (daily) allowance for adults and children over 4 years;* IU, *international units;* mg, *milligrams;* μg, *micrograms.*
†*Many of these symptoms can also be attributed to problems other than mineral deficiency. If you have these symptoms and they persist, see your physician.*

Table 16-4 Minerals: Best Sources, Primary Functions, Deficiency Symptoms, and Toxicity—cont'd

U.S. RDA*	Sources	Functions	Deficiency Symptoms†	Toxicity
Fluorine (F^-)				
1.5-4 mg	Foods cooked in fluoridated water, fish, gelatin	Bone and tooth formation	Increased susceptibility to caries	Fluorosis, mottling of teeth
Iodine (I^-)				
150 μg	*Major:* iodized salt *Minor:* fish, seaweed, vegetables	Energy metabolism, normal cell functioning	Goiter, cretinism (infants of iodine-deficient mothers)	Minimal toxic effect with normal thyroid functioning
Iron (Fe^{3+})				
10-15 mg	Organ meats, cereals, green leafy vegetables, whole grains	Hemoglobin formation, growth and development	Iron deficiency anemia, behavioral changes	Cirrhosis, diabetes, pigmentation, joint pain
Manganese (Mn^{2+})				
‡—	Nuts, whole grains, vegetables and fruits, coffee, tea, cocoa, egg yolk	Normal bone structure, reproduction, normal functioning of cells and central nervous system	None observed in humans	Iron-deficiency anemia through inhibiting effect on iron absorption; pulmonary changes, anorexia, apathy, impotence, headaches, leg cramps, speech impairment; resembles Parkinson's disease in advanced stages of toxicity
Selenium (Se)				
‡—	Protein-rich foods (meat, eggs, milk), whole grains, seafood, liver and other meats, egg yolks, garlic	Part of an enzyme system; acts as an antioxidant with vitamin E to protect the cell from oxygen	Keshan disease (a human cardiomyopathy) and Kashin-Bek disease (an endemic human osteoarthropathy)	Physical defects of the fingernails and toenails, hair loss
Zinc (Zn^{2+})				
12-15 mg	Whole grains, wheat germ, crabmeat, oyster, liver and other meats, brewer's yeast	Involvement in protein synthesis; essential for normal growth and sexual development, wound healing, cell division and differentiation, smell acuity	Depressed immune function, poor growth, dwarfism, impaired skeletal growth, delayed sexual maturation, acrodermatitis	Severe anemia, nausea, vomiting, abdominal cramps, diarrhea, fever, hypocupremia (low blood serum copper), malaise, fatigue

‡*There is no RDA for manganese or selenium*

WATER

Water, often called "the forgotten nutrient," is a significant component of saliva. Saliva contains supersaturated concentrations of calcium and phosphate and can promote remineralization of the early carious lesion. Water is also important because it helps to build tissue, aids in regulating body temperature, and acts as a lubricant for joints and mucous membranes.

The body is approximately 80 percent water, and humans can live longer without food than without water. Approximately two thirds of body weight is water. The body loses water daily in urine, feces, sweat, and expiration (exhaling). Life-threatening electrolyte imbalances can result from extensive water loss caused by vomiting, diarrhea, burns, or excessive perspiration.

The recommended daily allowance of water for an adult is about 64 ounces. Foods and other fluids satisfy most of the daily requirements for water. All foods contain some water. Vegetables and fruits are more than 80 percent water and meats are 40 to 60 percent water.

Recall

12. Which minerals are present in the largest quantities?
13. What is often called "the forgotten nutrient"?

DIET MODIFICATION

Diet modification provided by members of the dental team is usually focused on dental health and not intended to replace the services of a registered dietitian. Patients with dietary issues related to underlying medical conditions need to be referred to a physician and registered dietitian.

The patient's lifestyle and background must be considered when making recommendations. Remember, if your dietary recommendations are compatible with the patient's normal diet, the patient is more likely to comply.

Diet Recommendations in Dentistry

Diet	Recommendations
Dental caries	Limit frequency of eating cariogenic foods.
	Avoid crackers, donuts, potato chips between meals.
	Eat fruits for dessert and snacks.
	Eat raw vegetables for snacks.
	Avoid sticky or retentive foods.
	Avoid slowly dissolving candies.
	Use sugar-free gum.
Periodontal disease	Avoid soft, mushy foods.
	Avoid popcorn.
	Eat plenty of fruits high in vitamin C.
	Eat fresh rather than canned, mushy vegetables.
	Eat plenty of dairy products for calcium for bone health.
	Avoid nuts.
New dentures	Encourage chewing.
	Begin by chewing on molar teeth.
	Work up to biting with incisors.
	Cut food into smaller pieces.
	Nuts may be difficult to chew.
	Eat plenty of dairy products for calcium for bone health.
	Eat casseroles, lasagna, and other soft foods to increase nutrients.
Oral surgery	Eat soft foods or process foods in a blender if needed.
	Avoid spicy foods.
	Maintain nutrient levels to promote healing.
	Eat hot cereals, rice, pasta, soft bread, soups with rice.
Orthodontics	Avoid chewy or sticky foods.
	Eat soft foods.
	Avoid hard foods like apples, raw carrots, etc.
	Eat plenty of dairy products for calcium for bone health.

DIETARY ANALYSIS

A dietary analysis is used to help patients understand the role of nutrition in their dental and general health. To do this, ask the patient to keep a diet diary for about 3 days. The patient's cooperation is essential in performing this analysis because the patient must record *every* food eaten, including the amount, how it was prepared, and when it was eaten.

The dental team then reviews the completed diary with the patient using a dietary analysis form (Fig. 16-3). Information from the diet diary is divided into groups on the analysis form and compared with the recommended number of servings per day. Empty calories and cariogenic foods are highlighted.

Always suggest modifications in a *positive* manner. The review of the dietary analysis should *never* be phrased in critical terms or stated in any way to make the patient un-

Patient's name ______________________ Date __________

Food	Veg	Fruit	Meat	Milk	Bread	Other
Orange juice		1				
Coffee						1
Toast					1	
Butter						1
Jam						1
Pizza	1			1	1	
Diet soda						1
Candy bar						1
Chicken, roasted			1			
Baked potato	1					
Butter						1
Sour cream						1
Broccoli	1					
Cheese sauce				1		
Ice cream				1		
Totals	3	1	1	3	2	7

Fig. 16-3 Sample dietary analysis form.

comfortable. A collection of nutrition labels from food boxes is helpful in making the patient aware of how much sugar and fat is consumed.

READING FOOD LABELS

In 1995 the U.S. Department of Agriculture (USDA) required that all food products contain a nutrition fact label (Fig. 16-4). These labels are an excellent source of nutrition information. Every food label must include the following nutrition facts:

- Individual serving size
- Number of servings per container
- Total calories
- Calories derived from fat content
- Percentage of daily value (% of RDA)

Product Label Information

Begin with the *serving size.* This information is given in both common household units and metric units. The serving size is uniform across product lines so that you can easily compare similar foods.

The *amount* of each nutrient in the food is expressed in two ways: as a percentage of the RDA and by weight of the serving size. By using the percentage of daily values, you can easily determine whether a food contributes a large or a small amount of a particular nutrient. Remember that if you eat more or less than the serving size on the label, you will need to adjust the amounts of the nutrients accordingly. For example, the label on ice cream indicates 150 calories per serving, but the serving size is only $^1/_2$ cup. The average dish of ice cream actually eaten may be 500 or 600 calories.

Labeling Ingredients

Almost all foods are required to have the ingredients listed on the package. The ingredients are listed in descending order of weight to indicate the proportion of any ingredient. For example, after reading a label on a fruit drink, you may find that only 5 percent of the drink is fruit juice (see Fig. 16-4).

Artificial coloring must also be named in the list of ingredients. It is no longer acceptable to simply state "Color

NUTRITION FACTS

Serving size 1 1/4 cup (30 g)
Servings per container about 16

Amount per serving	Cereal	Cereal with 1/2 cup skim milk
Calories	110	160
Calories from fat	0	0
	% Daily value**	
Total fat 0 g*	0%	0%
Saturated fat 0 g	0%	1%
Cholesterol 0 mg	0%	1%
Sodium 270 mg	11%	14%
Total carbohydrate 26 g	9%	11%
Dietary fiber less than 1 g	0%	0%
Sugars 3 g		
Other carbohydrate 22 g		
Protein 2 g		
Vitamin A	0%	6%
Vitamin C	10%	10%
Calcium	0%	15%
Iron	50%	50%
Thiamin	25%	25%
Niacin	25%	25%
Vitamin B_6	25%	25%
Folate	25%	25%
Vitamin B_{12}	25%	30%

*Amount in cereal. One half cup skim milk contributes an additional 40 calories, less than 5 mg cholesterol, 65 mg sodium, 6 g total carbohydrate (6 g sugars) and 4 g protein.
**Percent daily values are based on a 2,000 calorie diet. Your daily values may be higher or lower depending on your calorie needs:

	Calories:	2000	2500
Total fat	Less than	65 g	80 g
Saturated fat	Less than	20 g	25 g
Cholesterol	Less than	300 mg	300 mg
Sodium	Less than	2400 mg	2400 mg
Total carbohydrate		300 g	375 g
Dietary fiber		25 g	30 g

Calories per gram:
Fat 9 • Carbohydrate 4 • Protein 4

Fig. 16-4 Nutrition facts label.

added." The government has also set strict conditions under which statements such as "low-fat" and "a good source of fiber" can be used as part of the front label on the product.

Label Claims

Examples of nutrient claims include "high-fiber," "reduced calories," and "cholesterol-free." Usually, these claims make a comparison with the "regular" version of the product. For example, a *reduced-fat* claim on a jar of peanut butter means that the peanut butter has at least 25 percent less fat than the regular peanut butter. A *light* salad dressing has at least 50 percent less fat or one-third fewer calories than the regular dressing.

Other labels show that a food is high or low in a certain nutrient. For example, *low-fat* Italian salad dressing has 3 g of fat or less per 2-tablespoon (30-g) serving, and *fat-free* Italian salad dressing has less than 0.5 of fat per serving (Fig. 16-5).

Organic Foods

In 1990 the USDA proposed rules regarding the labeling of food that was "organically grown." Now, foods with the **organic** label must have been grown without the use of chemical pesticides, herbicides, or fertilizers. Also, the use of hormones in organic seed preparation is prohibited.

In addition, there are regulations regarding meat, poultry, and milk. As with plants, the use of hormones is prohibited during the organic animal's growth or the product's preparation for consumption. Organic milk must have no added vitamins or chemicals, and preparations are closely monitored.

Regulations regarding labeling of organic products protect the consumer by ensuring the products are in fact "organic."

EATING DISORDERS

On the flip side of the obesity epidemic in the United States is the serious threat caused by eating disorders. Influences of the media, the fashion industry, and perceived cultural values have led to a preoccupation with being thin. Such influences have contributed to a society of weight-conscious adolescents and adults and an increase in eating disorders. Eating disorders have serious medical, oral, and psychological implications and can be life-threatening. Eating disorders commonly occur during adolescence and adulthood and include *anorexia nervosa* and *bulimia* (the two most common), as well as other related disorders such as *binge eating, compulsive overeating, female athlete triad,* and *chronic dieting syndrome.* The majority of those who suffer from eating disorders are 14 to 25 years old, white, and affluent. The occurrence of eating disorders is much more common in females; the ratio of females to males is 10:1 (Table 16-5).

Bulimia

Bulimia is often referred to as "bingeing and purging" disorder. Often this pattern occurs when an individual is only slightly overweight and tries to lose weight by dieting but fails to achieve the desired results. This person believes that self-worth is related to being thin.

Usually the pattern begins with some form of upset or stress, after which the individual finds comfort in eating a huge amount of high-calorie food. The eating binge is followed by guilt and behaviors that may include self-induced vomiting, food abstinence, the use of laxatives and enemas, and excessive exercise.

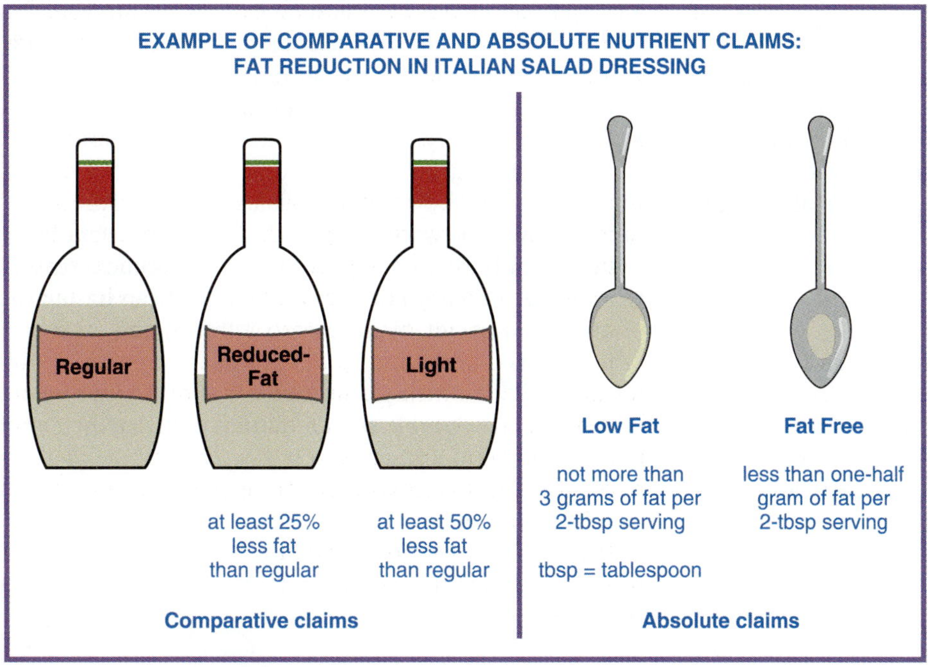

Fig. 16-5 Comparative versus absolute nutrient claims. (From Kinn ME, Woods M: *The medical assistant: administrative and clinical,* ed 8, Philadelphia, 1999, Saunders.)

Table 16-5 ***Common Diet-Related Disorders***

Disorders	Major Dietary Components	Corrective Dietary Measures
Allergies	Wide variety of foods are possible allergens: wheat, milk, eggs, chocolate most common	Eliminate or restrict food sources of allergen
Anemia	Deficiency of iron, vitamin B_{12}, or folacin	Increase amount of deficient nutrient
Anorexia nervosa	Starvation, fear of becoming fat, altered body image	High-calorie diet, psychotherapy, behavior modification
Atherosclerosis	High cholesterol, high saturated fat, excessive calories	Control calories, decrease total fat in diet to 30% to 35% of calories, change to more unsaturated fats, lower cholesterol content of diet, stress complex carbohydrates rather than simple sugars
Bulimia	Binge eating, self-induced vomiting	Regular diet, behavior modification, psychotherapy
Cancer of the colon	Low fiber	Increase dietary fiber and fluids
Cirrhosis of the liver	Excessive ingestion of alcohol or nutrients	Reduce dietary level of excessive nutrient or substance
Constipation/diverticulosis	Poor fiber intake, poor fluid intake	Increase dietary fiber and fluids
Diabetes mellitus	Obesity, excessive sugar consumption	Control calories and carbohydrates
Hypertension	Obesity, high salt intake	Control calories, decrease sodium intake
Obesity	Excessive calorie intake, inadequate physical activity	Decrease calories, increase activity, behavior modification, group therapy

From Kinn ME, Woods M: The medical assistant: administrative and clinical, *ed 8, Philadelphia, 1999, Saunders.*

Most bulimic individuals want help and will often make attempts to get into a treatment program. In the dental office, bulimic individuals are easily recognized because they will often have severe wear on the lingual surfaces of their teeth caused by the stomach acid from repeated vomiting (see Chapter 17).

Anorexia Nervosa

Anorexia nervosa is characterized by self-starvation. These individuals are usually female and in their early to middle 20s. They have an abnormal fear of becoming fat and have a severely distorted image of their body. Without medical intervention persons with anorexia nervosa will become extremely malnourished, lose excessive amounts of weight, and die.

Physical signs of possible anorexia nervosa include muscle wasting, amenorrhea (stopping menstruation), dry skin, constipation, brittle nails, and thin brittle hair. Because calcium intake is usually decreased, there is often a decrease in the strength of the teeth and health of the periodontal tissues.

Female Athlete Triad

This condition affects young female athletes and is characterized by an eating disorder that includes restrictive dieting, overexercising, weight loss, and a lack of body fat. It results in osteoporosis (bone thinning) and amenorrhea. Dental risks include enamel decalcification, increased caries, and increase periodontal and soft tissue inflammation.

Management of Eating Disorders

Anorexia nervosa and bulimia are considered psychiatric diseases with serious medical, dental, and nutritional complications. Dental professionals are often the first healthcare providers to diagnose an eating disorder. In addition to providing dental care and education, the dentist is obligated to assist the patient in obtaining psychotherapy and medical care.

Successful management of these disorders requires a team approach including psychiatrists, psychologists, physicians, nurses, dietitians, social workers, and dentists. The road to recovery is often long and expensive.

Recall

14. Which governmental agency regulates the labeling of food products?

15. What criteria are used to determine whether a product is "organic"?

16. What are the two most serious eating disorders?

HEALTHY HABITS

As a dental assistant, you can educate your patients regarding the following five healthy habits for a long life:

- *Eat right.* Consume five servings of fruits and vegetables daily, plus generous portions of grain, beans, and dairy products.
- *Keep bones strong.* Include sufficient calcium in your diet. If you do not receive enough direct sunlight, take a daily supplement for vitamin D, which helps your body absorb calcium more effectively.
- *Protect immune system.* Be sure to eat whole grains, green leafy vegetables, seafood, lean meats, and moderate amounts of vegetable oils to receive vitamins E and B_6 and the trace mineral zinc. These substances help your body to fight infection and chronic disease.
- *Maintain a healthy body weight.* Excess fat can hasten the onset of diabetes, heart disease, arthritis, and other problems.
- *Exercise.* Combine aerobic exercises such as walking or running with simple stretch training to strengthen your muscles.

Patient Education

As a dental assistant, you can help your patients prevent dental disease. You can teach them how to adjust their diet and make healthier food choices. For teaching to be effective, it is important to have a thorough understanding of the material you are going to discuss and the rationale behind it. The following tips are helpful when providing nutrition information to patients:

- Use pictures and charts to illustrate your points.
- Remember that ethnic and cultural foods are important to patients.
- Encourage patients to play an active role in the learning process.
- Invite patients to call the office whenever questions or concerns arise.

LEGAL AND ETHICAL IMPLICATIONS

- Information you provide to the patient during dietary counseling should be documented in the patient's record.
- Dental assistants should not counsel patients beyond the scope of dentistry (i.e., weight control, eating disorders). If you see signs of nutrition-related diseases or deficiencies, notify the dentist so that the patient may be referred to a physician for a diagnosis.

Eye to the Future

Research today is focusing on nutrition as a tool to help prevent chronic disease and prolong life. Already, advances in genetic engineering have resulted in lower-fat meats, tomatoes with good flavor year round, and virus-resistant vegetables. Fortification is being used to boost the amount of nutrients in foods and to add nutrients to foods that do not usually contain them. For example, orange juice is now being fortified with calcium and vitamin D. The science of nutrition will continue to evolve.

Critical Thinking

1. Using the Food Guide Pyramid, analyze your own dietary habits. Are there any areas in which you need to improve?
2. Linda Hines is a 17-year-old patient in your dental office. While sitting in the reception area, Linda notices a poster of the Food Guide Pyramid on the wall and asks you what it means. How would you explain the concept of the pyramid?
3. Leanne is an energetic cheerleader in a local high school. She is very conscious about her appearance, especially her weight. She does not appear malnourished and does not exhibit any oral manifestations of bulimia. She tells you that she tries to "watch her diet." Would you have any suggestions or recommendations for Leanne?
4. The label on a bag of "light" potato chips indicates there are only 100 calories per serving. What is the other important piece of information you should know before eating that bag of potato chips?

17

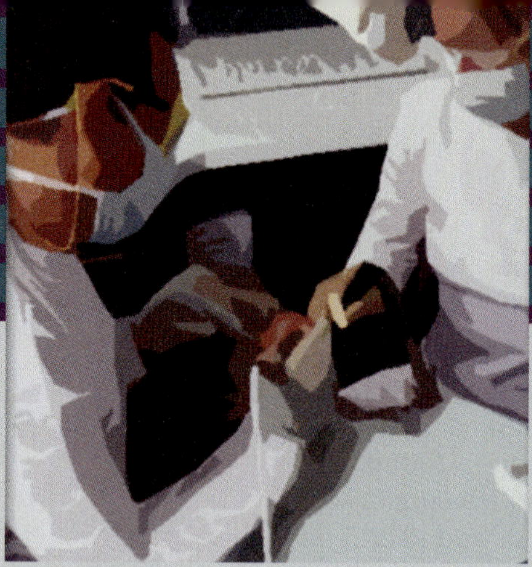

Oral Pathology

Outline

Making a Diagnosis
- Historical Diagnosis
- Clinical Diagnosis
- Radiographic Diagnosis
- Microscopic Diagnosis
- Laboratory Diagnosis
- Therapeutic Diagnosis
- Surgical Diagnosis
- Differential Diagnosis
- Acute/Chronic Inflammation

Oral Lesions
- Lesions Extending Below Mucosal Surface
- Lesions Extending Above Mucosal Surface
- Lesions Even with Mucosal Surface
- Raised or Flat Lesions

Diseases of the Oral Soft Tissues
- Leukoplakia
- Lichen Planus
- Candidiasis
- Aphthous Ulcers
- Cellulitis

Conditions of the Tongue

Oral Cancer
- Leukemia
- Smokeless Tobacco
- Therapy for Oral Cancer
- Dental Implications of Radiation Therapy
- Dental Implications of Chemotherapy

Human Immunodeficiency Virus (HIV) and Acquired Immunodeficiency Syndrome (AIDS)
- Oral Manifestations
- Hairy Leukoplakia
- Kaposi's Sarcoma
- Herpes Simplex
- Herpes Zoster
- Human Papillomavirus

Developmental Disorders
- Genetic Factors
- Environmental Factors
- Disturbances in Jaw Development
- Disturbances in Lip, Palate, and Tongue Development
- Disturbances in Tooth Development and Eruption
- Disturbances in Enamel Formation
- Disturbances in Dentin Formation
- Abnormal Eruption of the Teeth

Miscellaneous Disorders
- Abrasion
- Attrition
- Bruxism
- Bulimia
- Orofacial Piercings

Patient Education

Legal and Ethical Implications

Eye to the Future

Critical Thinking

KEY TERMS

Abscess (**ab**-*ses*) Localized area of pus originating from an infection.

Acute inflammation Minimal and short-lasting injury to tissue.

Biopsy (**bye**-ahp-see) Removal of tissue from living patients for diagnostic examination.

Candidiasis (kan-duh-**die**-ah-sis) Superficial infection caused by a yeastlike fungus.

Carcinoma (kar-sih-**no**-muh) Malignant tumor in epithelial tissue.

Cellulitis (sel-yuh-**lie**-tis) Inflammation of cellular or connective tissue.

Chronic inflammation Continuous injury or irritation to tissue.

Congenital disorders (kun-**jeh**-nih-tul) Disorders that are present at birth.

Cyst (**sist**) Closed cell or pouch with a definite wall.

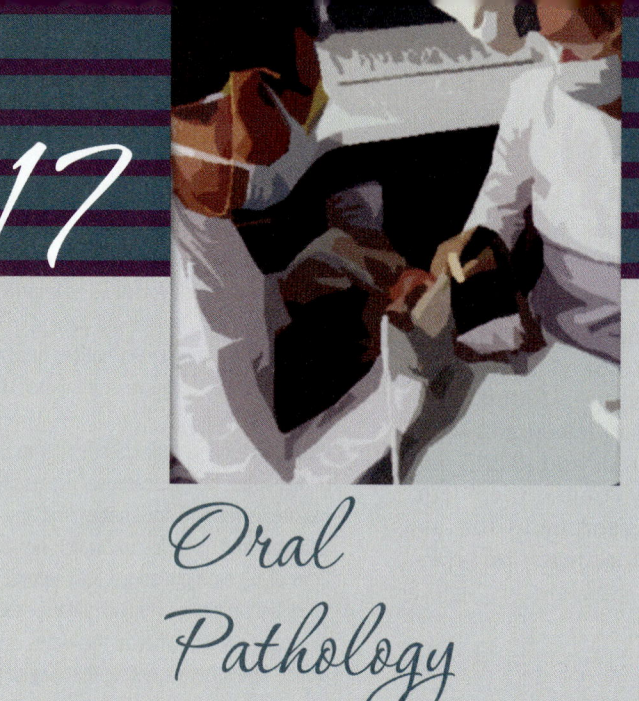

KEY TERMS—cont'd

Ecchymosis (e-ki-**mo**-sis) Technical term for bruising.
Erosion Wearing away of tissue.
Inflammation Protective response of the tissues to irritation or injury.
Glossitis (glaw-**sigh**-tus) Inflammation of the tongue.
Granuloma (gran-yuh-**lo**-muh) A granular tumor or growth.
Hematoma (he-muh-**toe**-muh) Swelling or mass of blood collected in one area or organ.
Lesion (**lee**-zhun) An area of pathology.
Leukemia (lu-**kee**-me-ah) A progressive disease in which the bone marrow produces an increased number of immature or abnormal white cells.
Leukoplakia (lew-ko-**play**-kee-ah) Formation of white spots or patches on the oral mucosa.
Lichen planus (**li**-kun, **li**-chun) Benign, chronic disease affecting the skin and oral mucosa.
Lymphadenopathy (lim-*fad*-e-**nop**-athy) Disease or swelling of the lymph nodes.
Lymphoma (lim-**fo**-ma) Malignant disorder of the lymphoid tissue.
Metastasize (muh-**tas**-tah-size) To spread (disease) from one part of the body to another.
Pathology (pa-**tha**-lah-jee) The study of disease.
Petechia (pe-**teak**-e-a) Small, pinpoint red spot on the skin or mucous membrane.
Sarcoma (sar-**ko**-ma) Malignant tumor in connective tissue such as muscle or bone.
Xerostomia (*zir*-oh-**sto**-me-ah) Dryness of the mouth caused by reduction of saliva.

LEARNING OUTCOMES

On completion of this chapter, the student will be able to achieve the following objectives:

- Pronounce, define, and spell the Key Terms.
- Explain why oral pathology is important for the dental assistant.
- Explain why categories of diagnostic information are necessary.
- Describe the warning symptoms of oral cancer.
- Describe the types of oral lesions.
- Name five lesions that are associated with HIV/AIDS.
- Describe the appearance of lesions associated with the use of smokeless tobacco.
- Describe three conditions associated with the tongue.
- Identify two oral conditions related to nutritional factors.
- Recognize developmental disorders of the dentition.
- List and define three anomalies that affect the number of teeth.
- List and define five anomalies related to the shape of the teeth.
- Define, describe, and identify the developmental anomalies discussed in this chapter.
- Describe the oral conditions of a patient with bulimia.
- Describe the classic signs of inflammation.
- Differentiate between chronic and acute inflammation.

Oral **pathology** is the study of diseases in the oral cavity. Only a dentist or physician may diagnose pathologic *(disease)* conditions, but it is important for the dental assistant to be able to recognize the differences between normal and abnormal conditions that appear in the mouth. For example, while taking radiographs or impressions, the dental assistant might notice a lesion in the patient's mouth that appears abnormal. Then the dentist would be informed so that a diagnosis could be made.

Many *systemic diseases* as well as *infectious diseases* have oral manifestations (signs and symptoms). The dental assistant should also understand how oral abnormalities affect the patient's general health and planned dental treatment.

Before you can recognize the abnormal conditions, you must have a solid understanding of the appearance of the normal oral conditions. You might want to review the appearance of normal oral tissues in Chapter 10.

The dental assistant should understand the terms used to describe pathologic conditions and record preliminary identification and descriptions of lesions. You should use these terms in the clinical setting so that they become part of your everyday professional vocabulary. You then can communicate effectively with other professionals.

In addition to pathologic conditions, this chapter includes conditions that are variations of normal but not considered pathologic.

MAKING A DIAGNOSIS

Making an accurate diagnosis is much like putting a puzzle together—many pieces are necessary. To make an accurate diagnosis, the dentist must rely on a variety of types of information. Remember, one piece of information alone usually is not enough to make a diagnosis. There are eight sources of information that can be used to make a final diagnosis. These are *historical, clinical, radiographic, laboratory, microscopic, surgical, therapeutic,* and *differential findings.* Imagine each of these findings as pieces of a puzzle leading to a diagnosis.

Historical Diagnosis

Personal history, family history, medical and dental histories, and history of the lesion are often useful in making a diagnosis. Family histories are important because of genetic disorders such as dentinogenesis imperfecta (Fig. 17-1). Melanin pigmentation of the gingiva is common in dark-skinned individuals (Fig. 17-2). Medical histories can give information about medication the patient may be taking that could have an effect on the oral tissues.

Clinical Diagnosis

A clinical diagnosis is based on the clinical appearance of the lesion, including the color, size, shape, and location. Examples of conditions diagnosed on the basis of clinical appearance are fissured tongue (Fig. 17-3), maxillary and mandibular tori and torus palatinus (Fig. 17-4), and median rhomboid glossitis (Fig. 17-5).

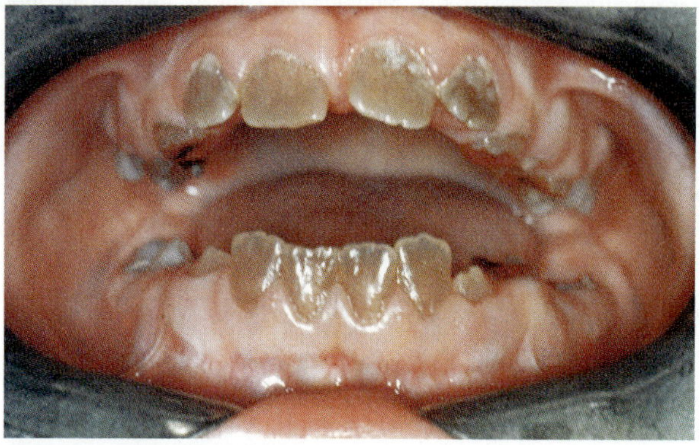

Fig. 17-1 Dentinogenesis imperfecta. (From Ibsen O, Phelan J: *Oral pathology for the dental hygienist,* ed 4, St Louis, 2004, WB Saunders.)

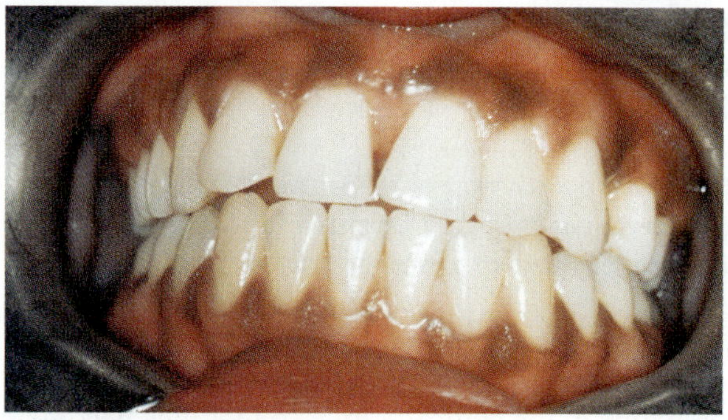

Fig. 17-2 Melanin pigmentation. (From Ibsen O, Phelan J: *Oral pathology for the dental hygienist,* ed 4, St Louis, 2004, WB Saunders.)

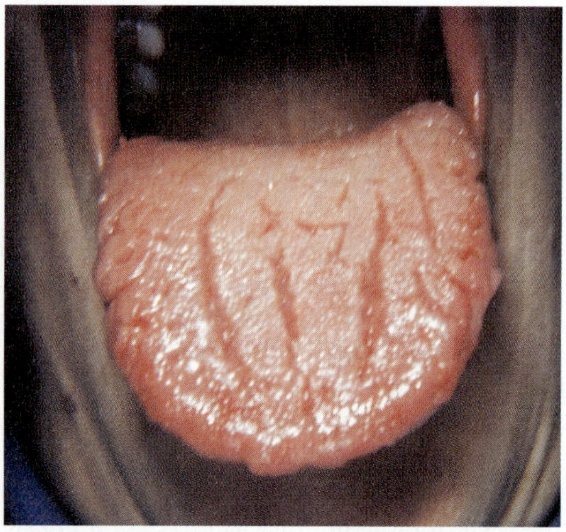

Fig. 17-3 Fissured tongue. (From Ibsen O, Phelan J: *Oral pathology for the dental hygienist,* ed 4, St Louis, 2004, WB Saunders.)

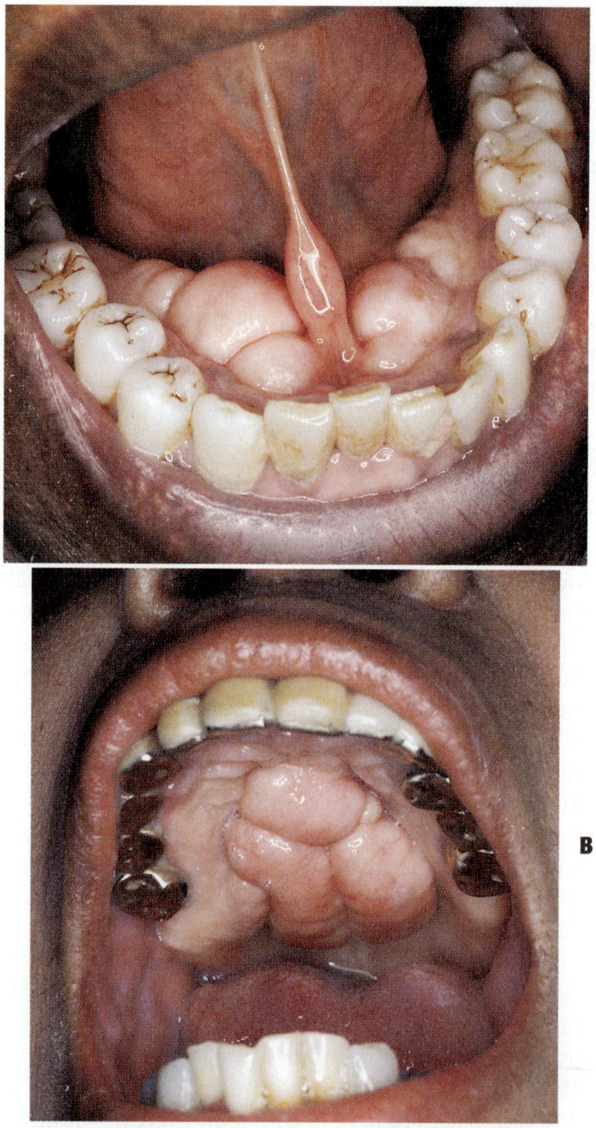

A

B

Fig. 17-4 A, Clinical appearance of bilateral mandibular tori. B, Clinical appearance of lobulated torus palatinus. (From Ibsen O, Phelan J: *Oral pathology for the dental hygienist,* ed 4, St Louis, 2004, WB Saunders.)

Radiographic Diagnosis

Radiographs are excellent in providing information about periapical pathology (Fig. 17-6), internal resorption (Fig. 17-7), and impacted teeth (Fig. 17-8).

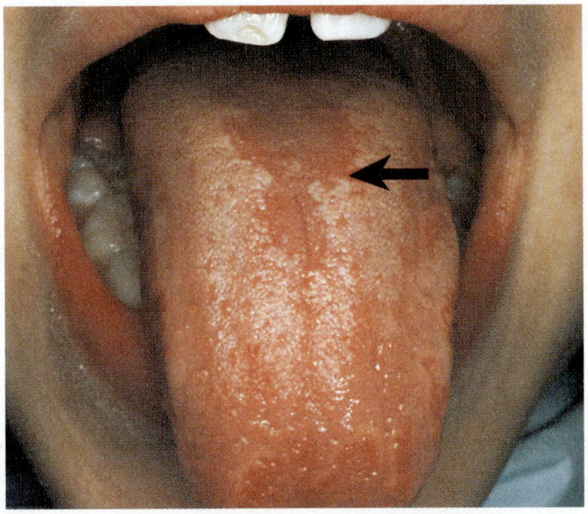

Fig. 17-5 **Median rhomboid glossitis *(arrow).*** (From Ibsen O, Phelan J: *Oral pathology for the dental hygienist,* ed 4, St Louis, 2004, WB Saunders.)

A

B

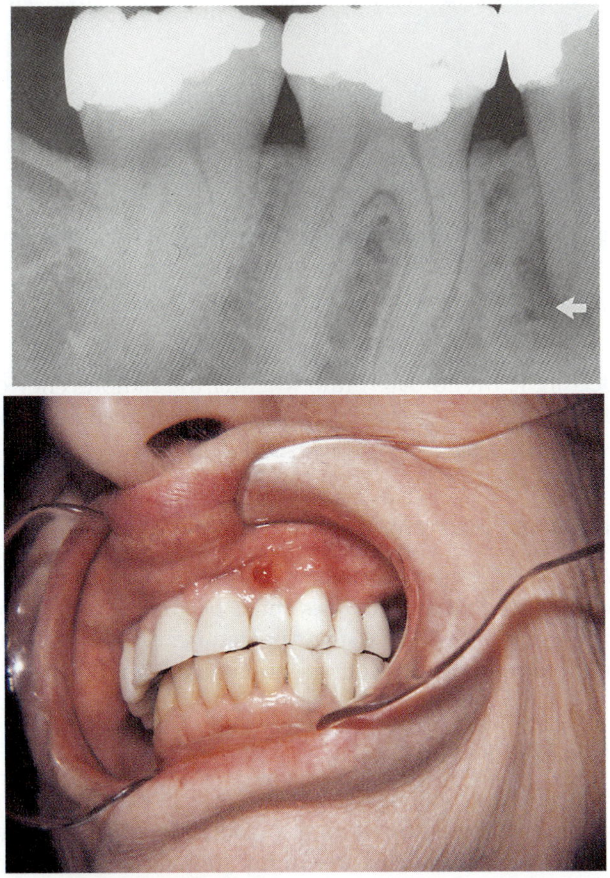

Fig. 17-6 **Periapical pathology.** (From Ibsen O, Phelan J: *Oral pathology for the dental hygienist,* ed 4, St Louis, 2004, WB Saunders.)

Microscopic Diagnosis

When a suspicious lesion is present, tissue is removed from the lesion and sent to a pathology laboratory, where it is evaluated microscopically (called **biopsy**). This procedure is very often used to make the definitive (final) diagnosis. For example, a white lesion cannot be diagnosed on the basis of the clinical appearance alone. A biopsy must be taken to determine whether or not the lesion is malignant (Fig. 17-9).

Laboratory Diagnosis

Blood chemistries and other laboratory tests including urinalysis can provide information that leads to a diagnosis. Cultures done in the laboratory can be used to diagnose types of oral infections.

Therapeutic Diagnosis

Therapeutic diagnosis is made by providing a treatment (therapy) and seeing how the condition responds. For example, angular cheilitis (Fig. 17-10) could be caused by a

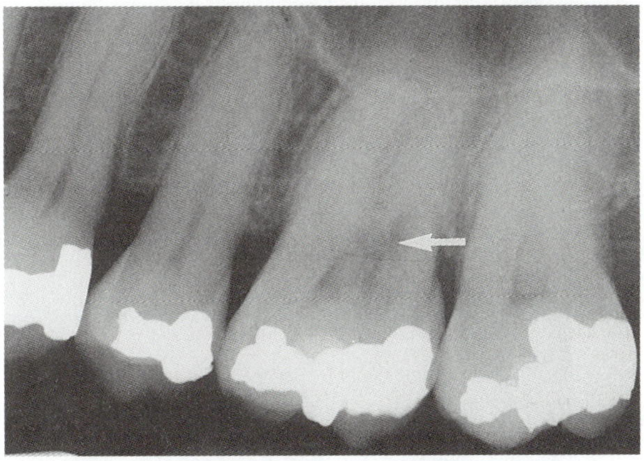

Fig. 17-7 **Internal resorption *(arrow).*** (From Ibsen O, Phelan J: *Oral pathology for the dental hygienist,* ed 4, St Louis, 2004, WB Saunders.)

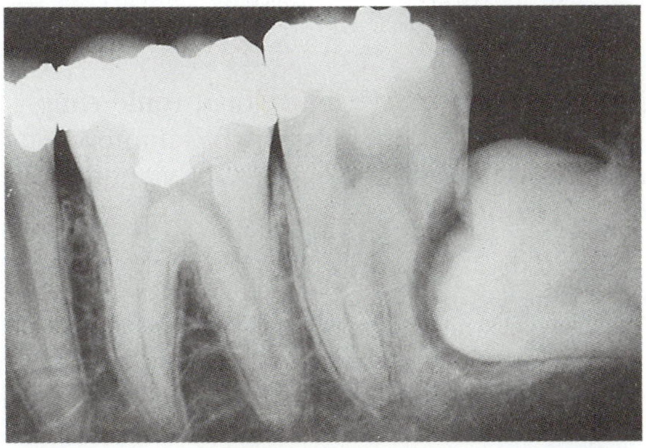

Fig. 17-8 **Horizontal impaction of the third molar.** (From Ibsen O, Phelan J: *Oral pathology for the dental hygienist,* ed 4, St Louis, 2004, WB Saunders.)

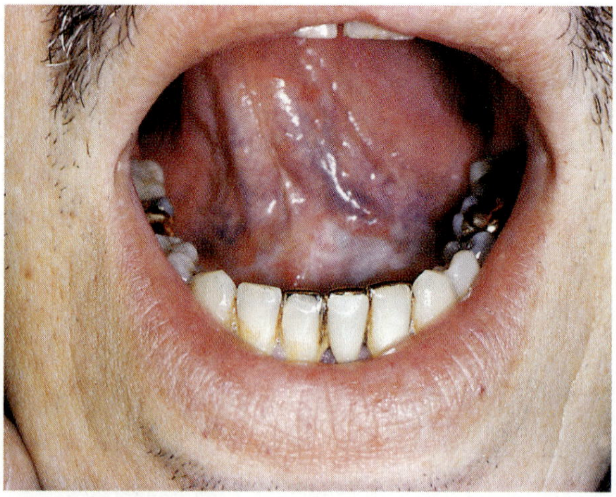

Fig. 17-9 A white lesion is seen on the anterior floor and ventral surface of the tongue. (From Ibsen O, Phelan J: *Oral pathology for the dental hygienist,* ed 4, St Louis, 2004, WB Saunders.)

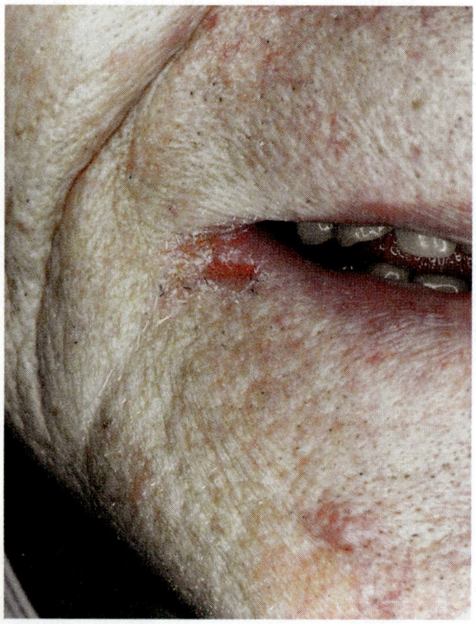

Fig. 17-10 Angular cheilitis. (From Ibsen O, Phelan J: *Oral pathology for the dental hygienist,* ed 4, St Louis, 2004, WB Saunders.)

lack of the B complex vitamins, or it could simply be a fungal infection. If the angular cheilitis improves after the patient is given an antifungal cream, the vitamin deficiency theory can be ruled out.

Surgical Diagnosis

A diagnosis is made based on the findings from a surgical procedure. For example, on a radiograph a traumatic bone cyst (Fig. 17-11) also looks like a static bone cyst (Fig. 17-12). However, one condition would require treatment, whereas the other would not. Surgically opening the area and in-

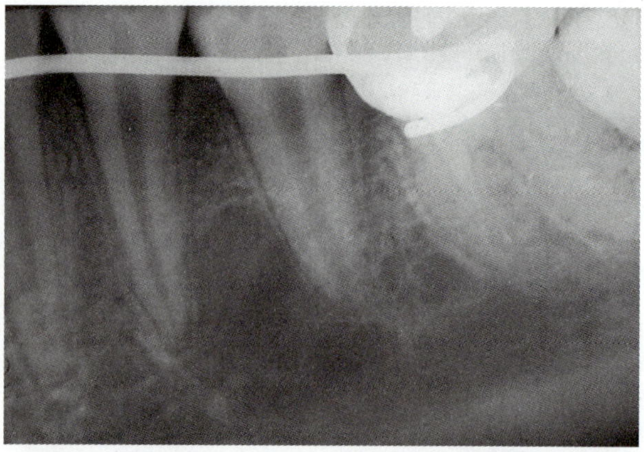

Fig. 17-11 Traumatic bone cyst. (Courtesy Dr. Edward V. Zegarelli. From Ibsen O, Phelan J: *Oral pathology for the dental hygienist,* ed 4, St Louis, 2004, WB Saunders.)

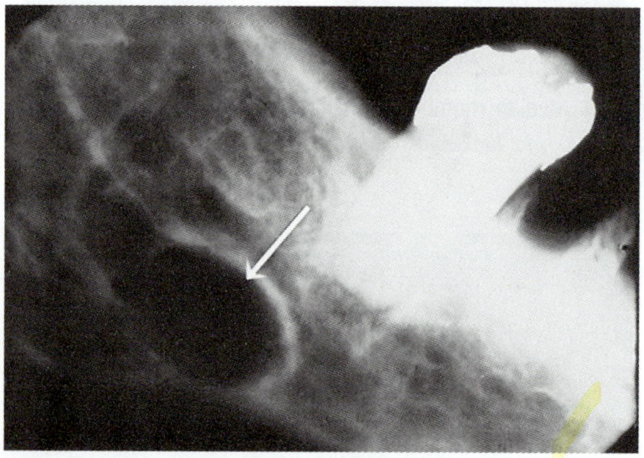

Fig. 17-12 Arrow points to static bone cyst. (Courtesy Dr. Edward V. Zegarelli. From Ibsen O, Phelan J: *Oral pathology for the dental hygienist,* ed 4, St Louis, 2004, WB Saunders.)

specting it would determine whether the radiolucency on the radiograph was indeed a condition that needed further treatment or not.

Differential Diagnosis

When there are two or more possible causes for a condition, a differential diagnosis must be made. The dentist will determine which tests or procedures should be done to rule out the incorrect cause and make a final diagnosis.

Acute/Chronic Inflammation

Inflammation is the body's protective response to irritation or injury. The inflammatory response is determined by the extent and duration of the injury. Inflammation can be acute or chronic. For example, **acute inflammation** occurs if the injury to the tissue is minimal and short-lasting and

Classic Signs of Inflammation

Redness	Heat
Swelling	Pain

the tissue begins to repair quickly. **Chronic inflammation** occurs when the injury or irritation to the tissue continues. Inflammation of a specific tissue is described by the suffix *-itis* added to the name of the tissue (e.g., gingivitis, periodontitis, pulpitis). Refer to Chapter 14 for a discussion of gingival and periodontal inflammatory diseases.

ORAL LESIONS

Lesion is a broad term for abnormal tissues in the oral cavity. A lesion can be a wound, sore, or any other tissue damage caused by injury or disease. It is important to identify the type of lesion in order to make a diagnosis. Lesions of the oral mucosa are classified as to whether they extend below or extend above the mucosal surface and whether or not they lie flat or even with the mucosal surface.

Lesions Extending Below Mucosal Surface

An *ulcer* is a break of the mucosa that looks like a punched-out area, similar to a crater. An ulcer may be as small as 2 mm or as large as several centimeters.

An **erosion** of the soft tissue is a shallow injury in the mucosa caused by mechanical trauma, such as chewing. (*Trauma* means wound or injury.) The margins may be ragged and red and quite painful.

An **abscess** is a collection of pus in a specific area. Abscesses are commonly found at the apex of a tooth (periapical abscess). An abscess may be caused by bacteria in a badly decayed tooth or by bacteria resulting from a severe periodontal infection (see Chapter 14).

A **cyst** is a fluid or semisolid, fluid-filled sac. The material within the cyst is not always infectious. In dentistry, a cyst may form around the crown of an unerupted tooth (Fig. 17-13).

Lesions Extending Above Mucosal Surface

Blisters, also known as *vesicles,* are filled with a watery fluid. (They look like the blisters that appear on feet as a result of poorly fitting shoes.) They are rarely seen in the oral cavity because they tend to rupture, leaving ulcers with ragged edges.

A *pustule* looks like a blister, but it contains pus. A **hematoma** is also similar to a blister, but it contains blood.

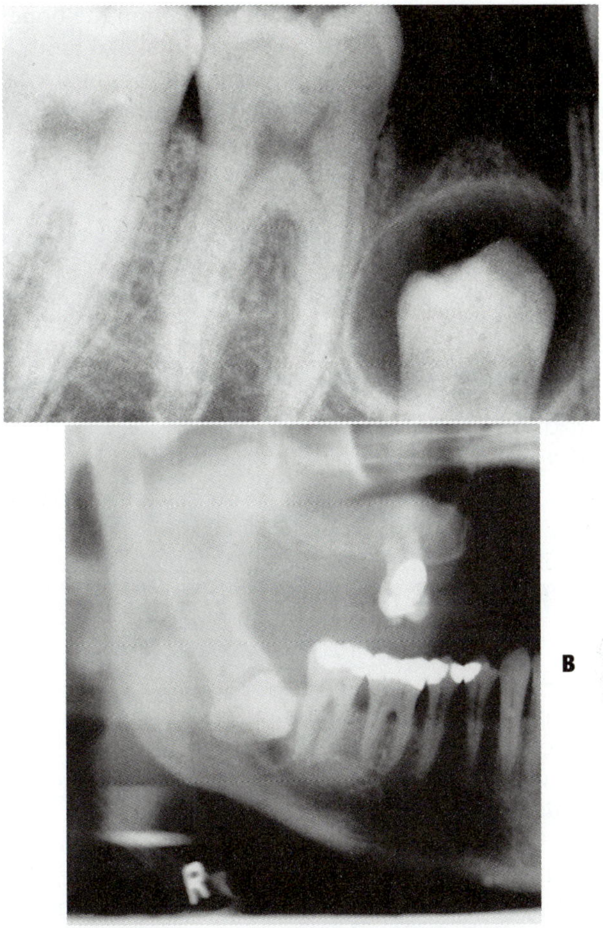
A
B

Fig. 17-13 Radiographs of dentigerous cysts around the crown of an unerupted bicuspid *(A)* and an impacted third molar *(B).* (From Ibsen O, Phelan J: *Oral pathology for the dental hygienist,* ed 4, St Louis, 2004, WB Saunders.)

A *plaque* is any patch or flat area that is slightly raised from the surface. (*Note:* This is *not* the same as dental plaque, which is discussed in Chapter 13.)

Lesions Even with Mucosal Surface

These lesions lie flat or even with the surface of the oral mucosa and are well-defined areas of discoloration. An **ecchymosis,** which is the medical term for *bruising,* is an example of this type of lesion.

Raised or Flat Lesions

Nodules, which could be either below the surface or slightly elevated, are small, round, solid lesions. When palpated, a nodule feels like a pea beneath the surface.

Granuloma is a term with many meanings. In dentistry, it is often used to describe a type of nodule that contains granulation tissue. (The suffix *-oma* means tumor or neoplasm.) A granuloma may appear on the gingival surface as a swollen mass. It may also be located within the bone as a periapical granuloma at the apex of a nonvital tooth.

Tumors are also known as *neoplasms.* A tumor is any mass of tissue that grows beyond the normal size and serves no useful purpose. A tumor may be *benign* (not life-threatening) or *malignant* (life-threatening).

Recall

1. Which lesions are below the mucosal surface?
2. Which lesions extend above the mucosal surface?
3. What lesion is even with the mucosal surface?

DISEASES OF THE ORAL SOFT TISSUES

Leukoplakia

Leukoplakia is a general term meaning "white patch." It may occur anywhere in the mouth. Very little pain is associated with leukoplakia unless there is also ulceration and secondary infection.

The lesions vary in appearance and texture from a fine, white transparency to a heavy, thick, warty plaque. To be classified as leukoplakia, the lesion should be firmly attached to the underlying tissue, and rubbing or scraping with an instrument should not remove it.

The cause of leukoplakia is unknown, but the presence of the disease is often linked to chronic irritation or trauma. Such injury may result from the use of smokeless tobacco, poorly fitting dentures, or cheek biting (Fig. 17-14).

Leukoplakia often appears before the development of a malignant lesion, so early diagnosis and treatment are important.

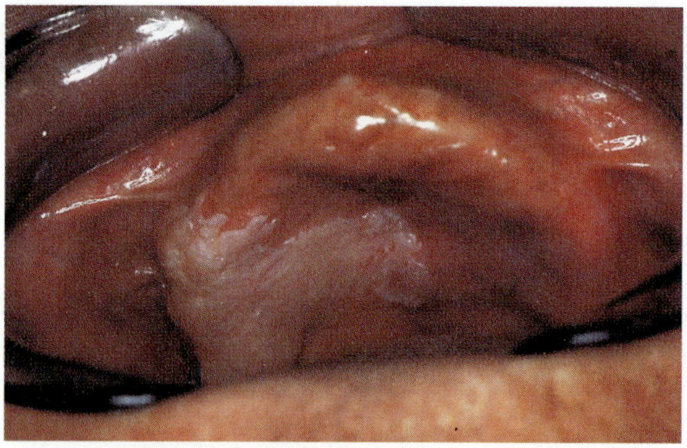

Fig. 17-14 Leukoplakia. (From Ibsen O, Phelan J: *Oral pathology for the dental hygienist,* ed 4, St Louis, 2004, WB Saunders.)

Lichen Planus

Lichen planus is a benign, chronic disease that affects the skin and oral mucosa. Many factors have been implicated in lichen planus, but the cause remains unknown.

On the oral mucosa the patchy white lesions have a characteristic pattern of circles and interconnecting lines called *Wickham's striae* (Fig. 17-15). A second type of lichen planus can cause erosive lesions on the gingiva. This type of lesion tends to worsen with emotional stress.

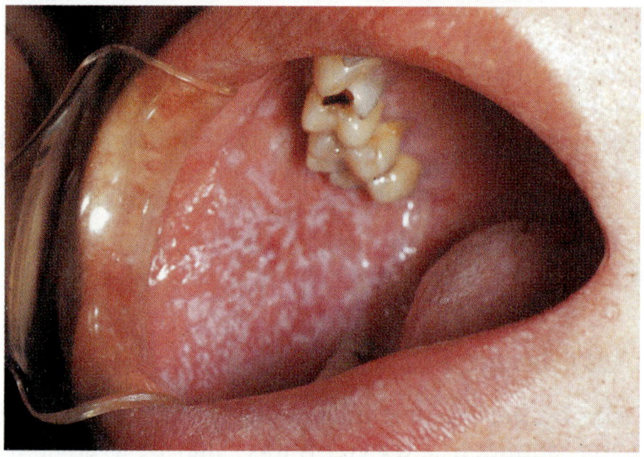

Fig. 17-15 Lichen planus on the buccal mucosa. (Courtesy Dr. Edward V. Zegarelli. From Ibsen O, Phelan J: *Oral pathology for the dental hygienist,* ed 4, St Louis, 2004, WB Saunders.)

Candidiasis

Candidiasis is a superficial infection caused by the yeast-like fungus *Candida albicans.* It is the most common oral fungal infection, but it does not usually occur in the healthy general population.

Candidiasis can result from antibiotic therapy, diabetes, xerostomia (dry mouth), and weakened immunologic reactions. It can also be the initial clinical manifestation for patients with acquired immunodeficiency syndrome (AIDS; see later discussion in this chapter).

Candidiasis is accompanied by discomfort or pain, *halitosis* (unpleasant breath odor), and *dysgeusia* (distorted sense of taste). Diaper rash, vaginitis, and thrush are also common types of candidiasis.

Pseudomembranous Candidiasis

In pseudomembranous candidiasis, also known as *thrush,* creamy white plaques (resembling cottage cheese or curdled milk) form in the mouth (Fig. 17-16). The patient frequently complains of a burning sensation, an unpleasant taste, or the feeling of "blisters forming in the mouth." These "blisters" generally prove to be the pseudomembranous plaques. (*Pseudomembranous* is a term describing a false membrane or tissue.)

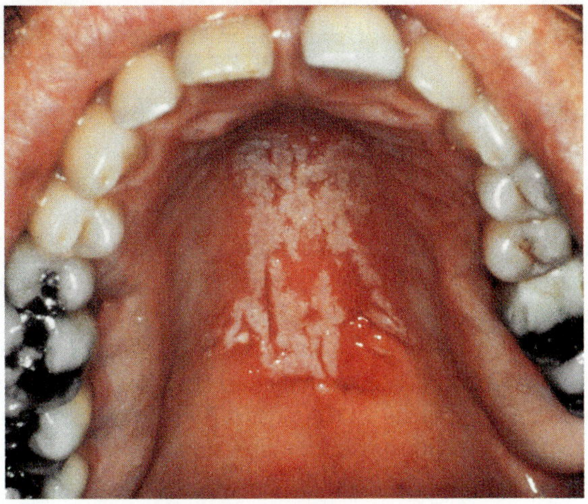

Fig. 17-16 Pseudomembranous candidiasis. (From Ibsen O, Phelan J: *Oral pathology for the dental hygienist,* ed 4, St Louis, 2004, WB Saunders.)

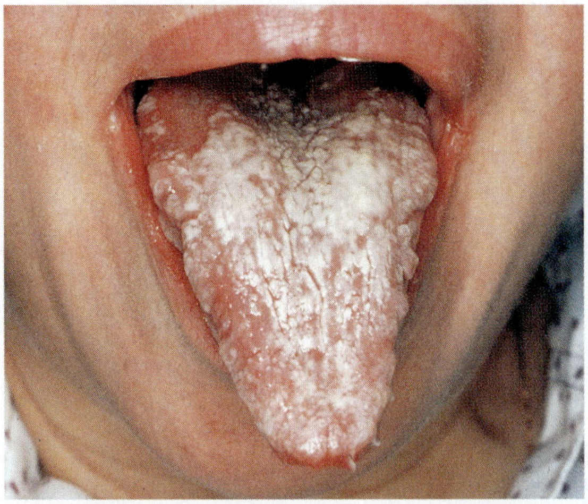

Fig. 17-17 Chronic hyperplastic candidiasis. The white appearance of the tongue did not wipe off, and it disappeared with antifungal treatment. (From Ibsen O, Phelan J: *Oral pathology for the dental hygienist,* ed 4, St Louis, 2004, WB Saunders.)

The plaques can be scraped off; they rarely bleed when they are removed. When bleeding is present, the patient likely has an additional mucosal problem. When this condition is seen in babies, it is called *infantile candidiasis.*

Hyperplastic Candidiasis

Hyperplastic candidiasis appears as a white plaque that cannot be removed by scraping. This form is most often found on the buccal mucosa in patients infected with human immunodeficiency virus (HIV) (Fig. 17-17).

In most patients, antifungal therapy begins to resolve the infection within 2 to 3 days, with complete clearing after 10 to 14 days. If the lesions are still present after this time or if they recur quickly, further investigation is necessary to rule out endocrine disturbances or immunologic deficiencies.

Atrophic Candidiasis

In atrophic candidiasis, also known as *erythematous candidiasis,* smooth red patches may appear on the dorsal areas of the tongue and palate. Atrophic candidiasis usually appears after the patient has been taking a broad-spectrum antibiotic. The patient may complain that the mouth feels scalded or burned, "like swallowing something too hot."

In most patients, antifungal therapy begins to resolve the infection within 2 to 3 days, with complete clearing after 10 to 14 days. If the lesions are still present after this time or if they recur quickly, further investigation is necessary to rule out endocrine disturbances or immunologic deficiencies.

Aphthous Ulcers

Aphthous ulcers, also known as "canker sores," are a common form of oral mucosal ulceration.

Recurrent aphthous ulcer (RAU) is a disease that causes recurring outbreaks of blister-like sores inside the mouth and on the lips. These sores appear on the lining mucosa of the cheeks, edge of the tongue, floor of the mouth, palates, and soft, red portion of the lip.

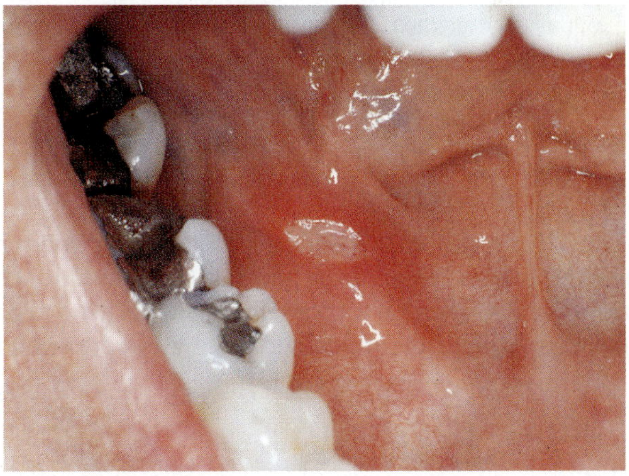

Fig. 17-18 Minor aphthous ulcer. (From Ibsen O, Phelan J: *Oral pathology for the dental hygienist,* ed 4, St Louis, 2004, WB Saunders.)

In the early stages of an outbreak, the patient experiences a burning sensation, followed by the formation of small blisters. When the blister breaks, the typical ulcer forms. It is small and oval, and the center is yellow to gray and surrounded by a red margin.

Minor RAU is the mildest form of involvement and represents 90 percent of all cases. Patients usually experience recurring episodes fewer than six times a year, and the lesions typically heal within 7 to 10 days (Fig. 17-18).

Major RAU, which occurs in only about 10 percent of cases, is characterized by more frequent outbreaks of larger, deeper ulcers that take longer to heal. This is found most often in patients with a compromised immune system.

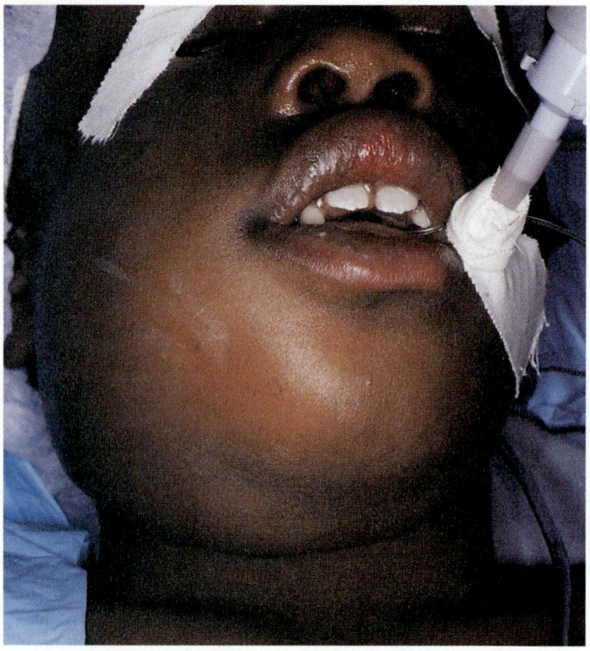

Fig. 17-19 Cellulitis. Swelling is caused by increased local edema associated with a dental infection. The patient was hospitalized for treatment of the swelling. (From Ibsen O, Phelan J: *Oral pathology for the dental hygienist,* ed 4, St Louis, 2004, WB Saunders.)

The patient with RAU is often debilitated (weakened) because these sores make eating and drinking quite difficult. Various agents, such as topical anesthetic agents for pain control and drugs to promote healing, may be prescribed.

Cellulitis

Cellulitis is a condition in which an inflammation is *uncontrolled* within a localized area. It spreads throughout the soft tissue or organ (Fig. 17-19).

Cellulitis is associated with oral infections, such as abscessed teeth. Swelling usually develops rapidly. The patient has a high fever, the skin usually becomes very red, and the area is characterized by severe throbbing pain as the inflammation localizes.

Cellulitis can be dangerous because it can travel quickly to sensitive tissues such as the eye or brain.

Recall

4. What type of condition appears as a white patch or area?
5. What condition is caused by yeast-like fungal infection?
6. What is another term for "canker sore"?
7. What is the condition in which inflammation causes severe pain and high fever?

CONDITIONS OF THE TONGUE

Glossitis is the general term used to describe inflammation and changes to the tongue. A condition called *black hairy tongue* may be caused by an oral flora imbalance after the administration of antibiotics. In this condition, the filiform papillae become elongated so that they resemble hairs. These elongated papillae become stained by food and tobacco, producing the name "black hairy" tongue (Fig. 17-20).

In *geographic tongue* the surface of the tongue loses areas of the filiform papillae in irregularly shaped patterns. The smooth areas resemble a map, thus the name "geographic" tongue. Over days or weeks the smooth areas and the whitish margins seem to change locations across the surface of the tongue by healing on one border and extending on another (Fig. 17-21).

Geographic tongue affects 1 to 3 percent of the population. The condition occurs at all ages, and women are affected almost twice as often as men.

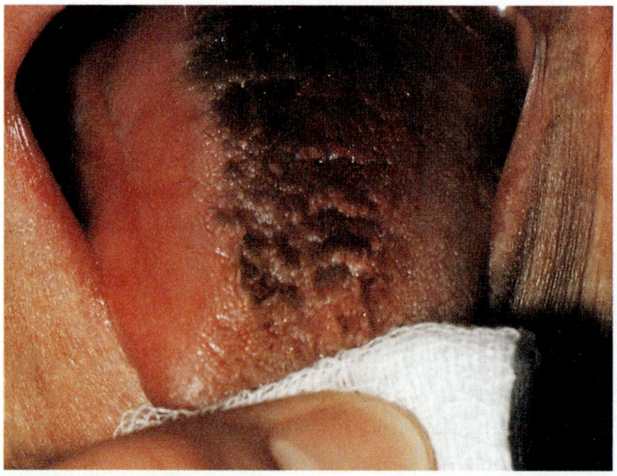

Fig. 17-20 Black hairy tongue. (From Ibsen O, Phelan J: *Oral pathology for the dental hygienist,* ed 4, St Louis, 2004, WB Saunders.)

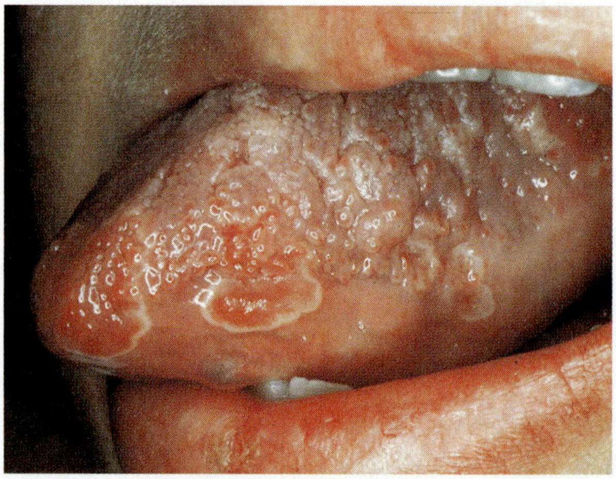

Fig. 17-21 Geographic tongue. (From Ibsen O, Phelan J: *Oral pathology for the dental hygienist,* ed 4, St Louis, 2004, WB Saunders.)

Fissured tongue is considered a variation of normal, and its cause is unknown (Fig. 17-22). Theories include a vitamin deficiency or chronic trauma over a long period. The top of the tongue appears to have deep fissures or grooves that become irritated if food debris collects in them. The patient with a fissured tongue is advised to brush the tongue gently with a soft toothbrush to keep the fissures clean of debris and irritants. No treatment is indicated for this condition.

Pernicious anemia is a condition in which the body does not absorb vitamin B_{12}. People who have this condition show signs of anemia, weakness, pallor, and fatigue on exertion. Other signs can include nausea, diarrhea, abdominal pain, and loss of appetite.

The oral manifestations of pernicious anemia include *angular cheilitis* (ulceration and redness at the corners of the lips), mucosal ulceration, loss of papillae on the tongue, and a burning and painful tongue (Fig. 17-23).

Recall

8. What is the term for an inflammation of the tongue?
9. What is the condition in which a pattern on the tongue changes?
10. What is the condition in which the body does not absorb vitamin B_{12}?

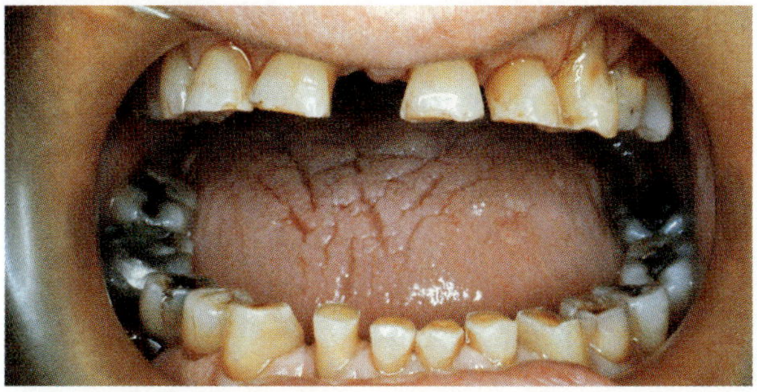

Fig. 17-22 Fissured tongue and attrition. (From Ibsen O, Phelan J: *Oral pathology for the dental hygienist,* ed 4, St Louis, 2004, WB Saunders.)

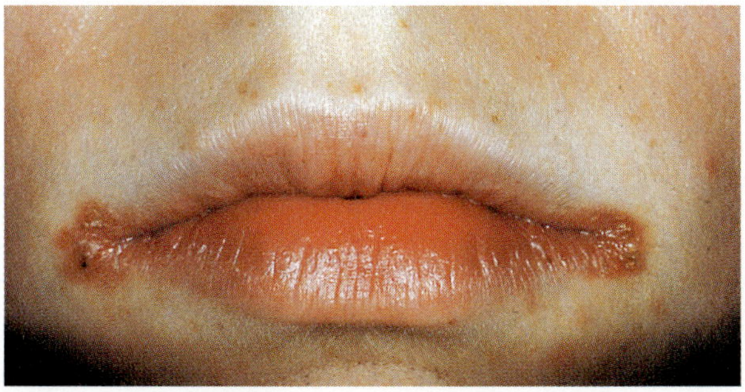

Fig. 17-23 Angular cheilitis. (From Ibsen O, Phelan J: *Oral pathology for the dental hygienist,* ed 4, St Louis, 2004, WB Saunders.)

ORAL CANCER

Oral cancer is one of the 10 most frequently occurring cancers in the world. In the United States, the site most often affected is the vermilion border of the lip (Fig. 17-24).

In the early stages most oral cancers are not painful, and therefore they frequently go undetected. Oral cancers are frequently fatal if not detected early enough or if left untreated (Box 17-1).

Box 17-1 Appearance of Early Cancer

Type of lesion	Clinical appearance
White areas	These lesions may vary from a filmy, barely visible change in the mucosa to a heavy, thick area of white tissue. Fissures or ulcers in a white area are most indicative of a malignancy. *Leukoplakia,* a white patch that cannot be wiped off, may be associated with chemical agents or tobacco.
Red areas	These lesions may have a velvety texture, sometimes with small ulcers. The term *erythroplakia* is used to designate lesions that appear as bright red patches.
Ulcers	These lesions may have flat or raised margins. Palpation may reveal *induration* (hardening).
Masses	Papillary masses, sometimes with ulcerated areas, occur as elevations above the surrounding tissues. Other masses may occur below the normal mucosa and may only be found by palpation.
Pigmentation	Black or brown pigmented areas may be located on mucosa where pigmentation does not normally occur.

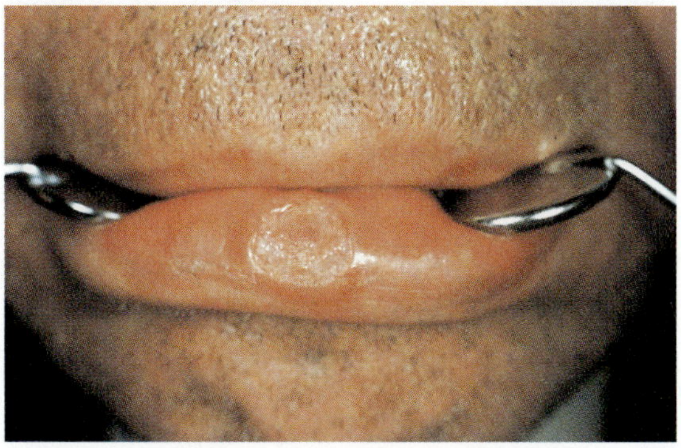

Fig. 17-24 Clinical appearance of squamous cell carcinoma of the lower lip. (From Ibsen O, Phelan J: *Oral pathology for the dental hygienist,* ed 4, St Louis, 2004, WB Saunders.)

A **carcinoma** is a malignant neoplasm (growth) of the epithelium (tissue lining the mouth) that tends to invade surrounding bone and connective tissue. Cancers quickly **metastasize** (spread) to other regions of the body, usually the neck and cervical lymph nodes.

Carcinomas occur on the lips, tongue, cheeks, and floor of the mouth. The lesions usually appear first as a white or ulcerated area, although some types may also appear as a velvety smooth red lesion.

An *adenocarcinoma* is a malignant tumor that comes from the glands underlying the oral mucosa (the prefix *adeno-* meaning "gland"). This tumor first appears clinically as a lump or bulge beneath overlying normal mucosa.

A **sarcoma** is a malignant neoplasm that comes from supportive and connective tissue such as bone. An *osteosarcoma* is a malignant tumor involving the bone. In the mouth the affected bones are those of the jaws. Although the cancer may start in the bone, it often spreads and involves the surrounding soft tissues (Fig. 17-25).

Oral Cancer Warning Signs

- Any sore in the mouth that does not heal
- Any lumps or swelling on the neck, lips, or oral cavity
- White or rough-textured lesions on the lips or oral cavity
- Numbness in or around the oral cavity
- Dryness in the mouth for no apparent reason
- Burning sensation or soreness in the oral cavity for no apparent reason
- Repeated bleeding in a specific area of the oral cavity for no apparent reason
- Difficulty speaking, chewing, or swallowing

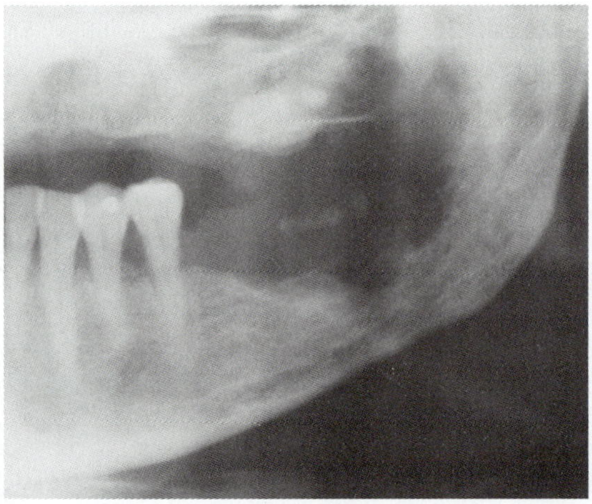

Fig. 17-25 Left side of a panoramic radiograph showing destruction of the mandible by squamous cell carcinoma. (From Ibsen O, Phelan J: *Oral pathology for the dental hygienist,* ed 4, St Louis, 2004, WB Saunders.)

Leukemia

Leukemia is a cancer of the blood-forming organs. It is characterized by rapid growth of immature *leukocytes* (white blood cells). Oral symptoms may be among the first indications of leukemia. These symptoms include hemorrhage, ulceration, enlargement, spongy texture, and magenta coloration of the gingiva (Fig. 17-26). Enlargement of lymph nodes, symptoms of anemia, and general bleeding tendencies also are typical.

Smokeless Tobacco

Smokeless tobacco, in the form of chewing tobacco or snuff, presents a serious health hazard. It is a major concern because of the high rates of precancerous leukoplakia and oral cancer occurring among users of smokeless tobacco. In addition, cancers of the pharynx, larynx, and esophagus occur 400 to 500 times more frequently among users than among nonusers.

Smokeless tobacco is also linked to serious irritation of the oral mucosa and an increased incidence of tooth loss from periodontal disease (Fig. 17-27).

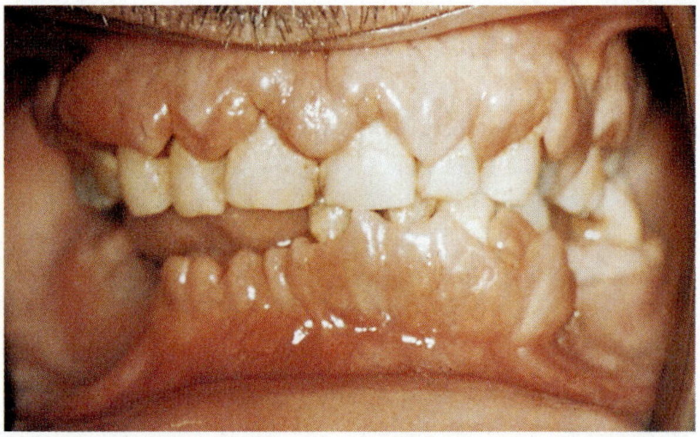

Fig. 17-26 Leukemia. (From Ibsen O, Phelan J: *Oral pathology for the dental hygienist,* ed 4, St Louis, 2004, WB Saunders.)

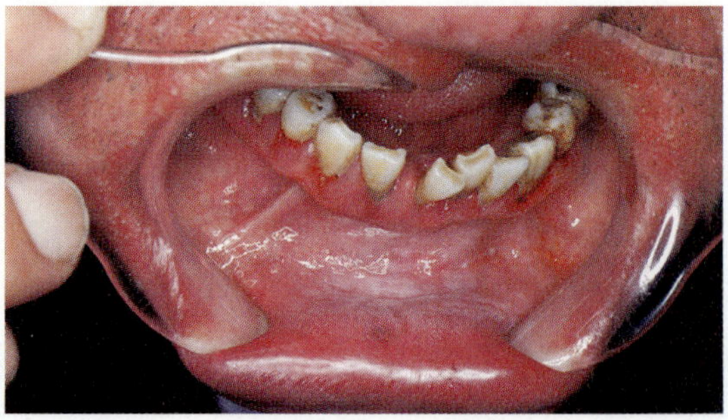

Fig. 17-27 Tobacco chewer's white lesion. Note the rough texture of the surface. (From Ibsen O, Phelan J: *Oral pathology for the dental hygienist,* ed 4, St Louis, 2004, WB Saunders.)

Recall

11. What type of cancer affects the blood-forming organs?
12. What is a common precancerous lesion among users of smokeless tobacco?
13. What is the term for a malignant lesion in the epithelial tissue of the oral cavity?

Recall

14. What causes radiation caries?
15. What is the term for a lack of saliva?

Therapy for Oral Cancer

Oral cancers are treated by surgery, radiation therapy, or chemotherapy. Often a combination of these three is used.

Dental Implications of Radiation Therapy

Because radiation for treatment of head and neck cancer affects the salivary glands, blood vessels, and bones of the jaws, patients receiving this treatment can be expected to develop specific dental problems, such as radiation mucositis and postradiation **xerostomia** (Fig. 17-28).

Xerostomia

If the radiation affects the major salivary glands, there can be irreversible destruction of these glands. When this occurs, saliva can no longer be produced and the patient will suffer from severe xerostomia (dry mouth). The lack of adequate saliva and the reduced blood supply to the tissues also can precipitate oral infection, delay healing, and make it difficult to wear dentures. Saliva substitutes can be used by the patient for some relief.

Radiation Caries

Caused by the lack of saliva, caries usually appears first in the cervical areas of the teeth. The teeth also may become extremely sensitive to hot and cold stimuli.

Osteoradionecrosis

Radiation also causes a decreased blood supply to the bones of the jaw. This can result in osteonecrosis (death of the bone). Patients should not have teeth extracted after they have been treated with head or neck radiation, because the jaw could be fractured and the wound may fail to heal as a result of osteoradionecrosis. To avoid osteoradionecrosis, it may be necessary to extract the patient's teeth before the radiation treatment.

Dental Implications of Chemotherapy

Chemotherapeutic agents are powerful drugs that destroy or deactivate rapidly dividing cancer cells. The significant side effects of these drugs frequently involve the oral tissues (Box 17-2).

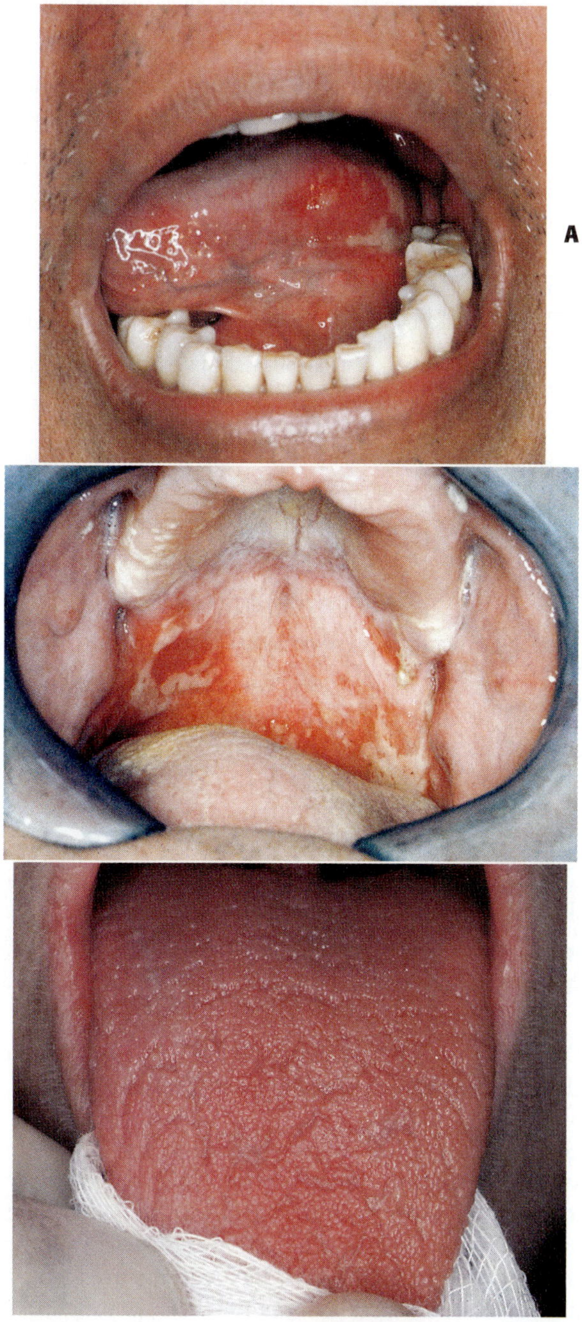

A

B

C

Fig. 17-28 **A** and **B,** Radiation mucositis. **C,** Postradiation xerostomia. (From Ibsen O, Phelan J: *Oral pathology for the dental hygienist,* ed 4, St Louis, 2004, WB Saunders.)

Box 17-2 Dental Implications of Chemotherapy

Side effect	Appearance
Mucositis	Inflammatory change in the oral mucosa in which the mucosa takes on a whitish appearance
Aphthous ulcers	Common side effect of most chemotherapeutic agents
Transient reactions	**Cheilitis** (inflammation of corners of the lips), **glossitis** (inflammation of the tongue), and **paresthesia** (abnormal burning or tingling sensation or loss of sensation) are less common and transient reactions. (*Transient* means the condition will disappear without additional treatment.)
Xerostomia	Dryness of the mouth is caused by the lack of normal salivary secretions and is another transient phenomenon in chemotherapy. Recovery usually occurs within 10 days.
Delayed healing	Because chemotherapeutic drugs act on all dividing cells, interference with healing may be anticipated when the drug is administered during the healing period.
Dentinal malformation	Chemotherapy in children during dentinal development can be expected to produce dental defects.

Oral Lesions Associated with HIV Infection

- Candidiasis
- Herpes simplex infection
- Herpes zoster
- Hairy leukoplakia
- Human papillomavirus (HPV) lesions
- Atypical gingivitis and periodontitis
- Other opportunistic infections reported:
  - *Mycobacterium avium, Mycobacterium intracellulare*
  - Cytomegalovirus
  - *Cryptococcus neoformans*
  - *Klebsiella pneumoniae*
  - *Enterobacter cloacae*
  - *Histoplasma capsulatum*
- Kaposi's sarcoma
- Non-Hodgkin's lymphoma
- Aphthous ulcers
- Mucosal pigmentation
- Bilateral salivary gland enlargement and xerostomia
- Spontaneous gingival bleeding resulting from thrombocytopenia

From Ibsen O, Phelan J: *Oral pathology for the dental hygienist,* ed 4, St Louis, 2004, WB Saunders.

HUMAN IMMUNODEFICIENCY VIRUS (HIV) AND ACQUIRED IMMUNODEFICIENCY SYNDROME (AIDS)

AIDS is the end-stage disease for an individual infected with HIV. Oral lesions are prominent features of AIDS and HIV infection.

Some of these lesions are known to be indicators of developing immunodeficiency and predictors of the development of AIDS in individuals who are HIV-positive. Lesions develop because the immune system is compromised when the T-helper cells become depleted as a result of the disease. Causes of oral lesions include opportunistic infections, tumors, and autoimmune-like diseases.

Oral Manifestations

Because the patient's immune system is severely damaged, death is usually caused by an opportunistic infection. An **opportunistic infection** is one that normally would be controlled by the immune system but that cannot be controlled because the immune system is not functioning properly due to HIV/AIDS or other causes.

It is important to remember that some of the lesions that look like those common with HIV and AIDS infection may also be caused by other disorders.

HIV Gingivitis

A bright red line along the border of the free gingival margin characterizes HIV gingivitis, also known as *atypical gingivitis.* Some patients may have progression of the bright red line from the free gingival margin over the attached gingival and alveolar mucosa. Other patients have petechia-like patches over the gingiva. (**Petechiae** are small, pinpoint bruises.)

HIV Periodontitis

The periodontal lesions of HIV periodontitis, also known as *AIDS virus–associated periodontitis,* resemble those ob-

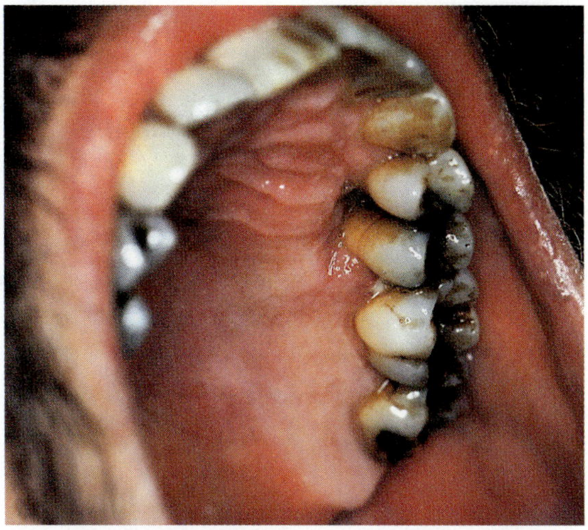

Fig. 17-29 Atypical periodontal disease in a patient with HIV infection. (From Ibsen O, Phelan J: *Oral pathology for the dental hygienist,* ed 4, St Louis, 2004, WB Saunders.)

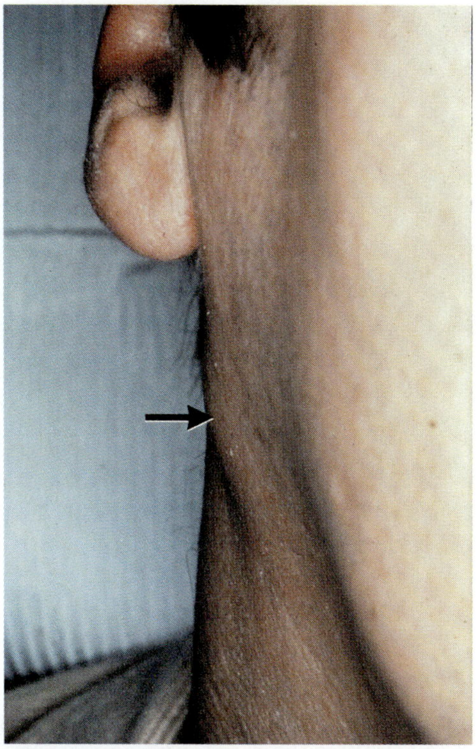

Fig. 17-30 Lymphadenopathy. (From Ibsen O, Phelan J: *Oral pathology for the dental hygienist,* ed 4, St Louis, 2004, WB Saunders.)

served in acute necrotizing gingivitis superimposed on rapidly progressive periodontitis (Fig. 17-29). Other symptoms include interproximal necrosis and cratering, marked swelling and intense erythema over the free and attached gingiva, intense pain, and spontaneous bleeding and bad breath.

Cervical Lymphadenopathy

Cervical **lymphadenopathy** is the enlargement of the cervical (neck) nodes (Fig. 17-30). Lymphadenopathy, meaning disease or swelling of the lymph nodes, is indicative of a systemic problem and is frequently seen in association with AIDS.

Candidiasis

Candidiasis, as discussed earlier, is often the initial oral sign of the progression from HIV-positive status to AIDS. In a patient with a compromised immune system, candidiasis can be a very debilitating and serious disorder (Fig. 17-31).

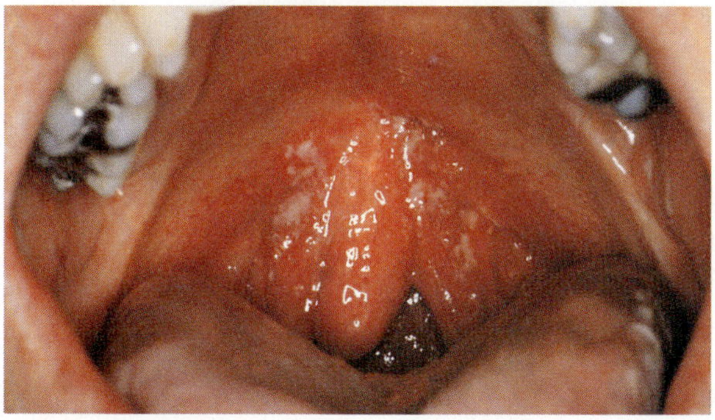

Fig. 17-31 Candidiasis in a patient with HIV infection. Removable plaques are present on the mucosa of the soft palate. (From Ibsen O, Phelan J: *Oral pathology for the dental hygienist,* ed 4, St Louis, 2004, WB Saunders.)

Lymphoma

Lymphoma is the general term used to describe malignant disorders of the lymphoid tissue. In the immunocompromised individual, lymphoma may occur as a solitary lump or nodule, a swelling, or a nonhealing ulcer that occurs anywhere in the oral cavity. The swelling may be ulcerated or may be covered with intact, normal-appearing mucosa.

Usually painful, the lesion grows rapidly in size and may be the first evidence of lymphoma. Diagnosis must be made from a biopsy because this condition closely resembles other oral diseases (Fig. 17-32).

Hairy Leukoplakia

Most individuals with hairy leukoplakia are positive for HIV, and it can be an important *early* sign of the change to AIDS status. Hairy leukoplakia is a white plaque usually found on one side or sometimes on both sides on the lateral borders (sides) of the tongue (Fig. 17-33).

Hairy leukoplakia may spread to cover the entire dorsal surface of the tongue. It can also develop on the buccal mucosa, where it generally has a flat appearance.

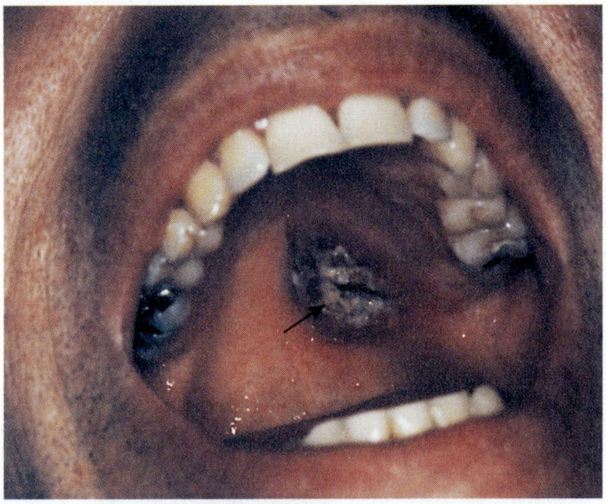

Fig. 17-32 **Intraoral lymphoma in a patient with AIDS.** (From Ibsen O, Phelan J: *Oral pathology for the dental hygienist,* ed 4, St Louis, 2004, WB Saunders.)

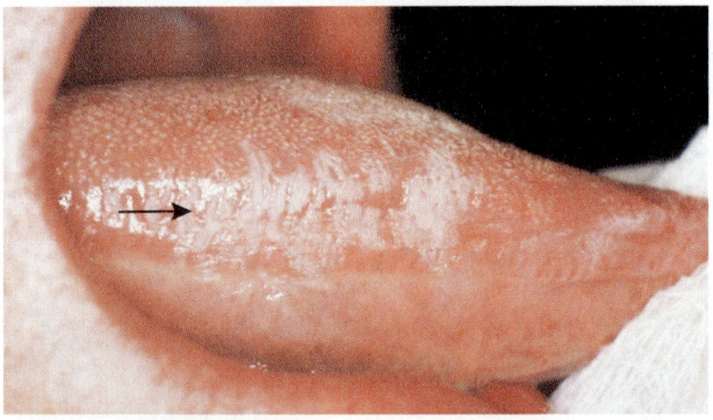

Fig. 17-33 **Hairy leukoplakia on the lateral borders of the tongue.** (From Ibsen O, Phelan J: *Oral pathology for the dental hygienist,* ed 4, St Louis, 2004, WB Saunders.)

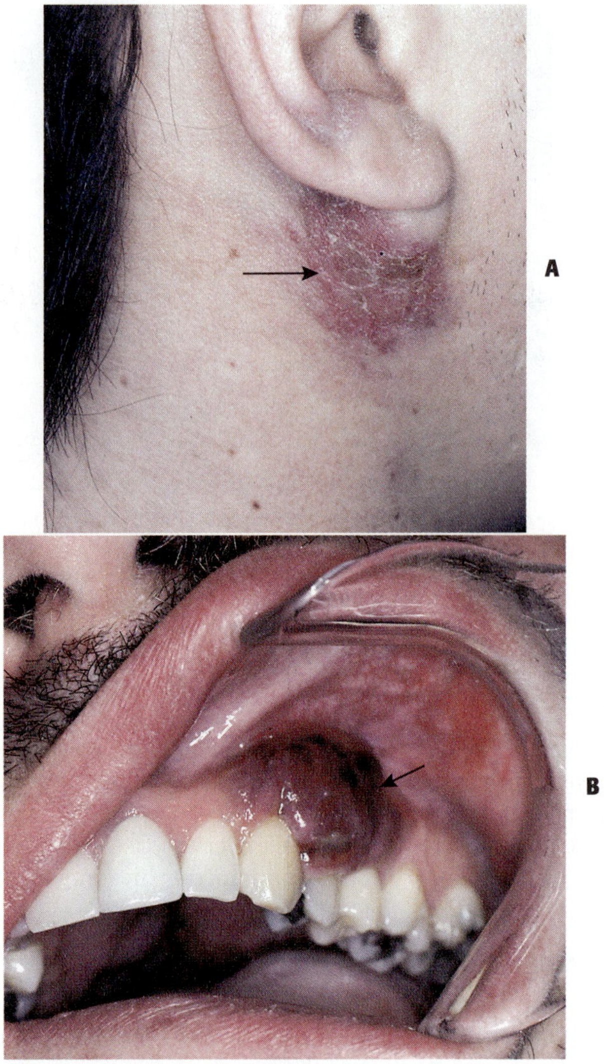

Fig. 17-34 **Kaposi's sarcoma in a patient with AIDS. A, Skin. B, Gingivae.** (From Ibsen O, Phelan J: *Oral pathology for the dental hygienist,* ed 4, St Louis, 2004, WB Saunders.)

Kaposi's Sarcoma

Kaposi's sarcoma is one of the opportunistic infections that occur in patients with HIV infection. Oral lesions of Kaposi's sarcoma may appear as multiple bluish, blackish, or reddish blotches that are usually flat in the early stages.

At present, no effective treatment exists for Kaposi's sarcoma. Surgical excision to decrease the size of the lesion is sometimes attempted, as well as radiation treatment and chemotherapy.

Kaposi's sarcoma is one of the intraoral lesions used to diagnose AIDS (Fig. 17-34).

Herpes Simplex

Herpes simplex lesions usually occur on the lip. In immunocompromised patients, however, the lesions may occur throughout the mouth (Fig. 17-35).

The herpes virus causes an ulcer-like lesion. A lesion that persists for longer than 1 month is particularly significant as an indicator of AIDS. Patients who do *not* have HIV or AIDS also may have herpes.

Herpes Zoster

In the immunocompromised patient the latent herpes zoster virus, also known as *shingles,* may cause intraoral manifestations in the form of blisters. The blisters break and form ulcers.

These lesions are generally present on both sides of the mouth and are very painful. A complaint of pain coming from the teeth, without apparent dental cause, is an early symptom of herpes zoster.

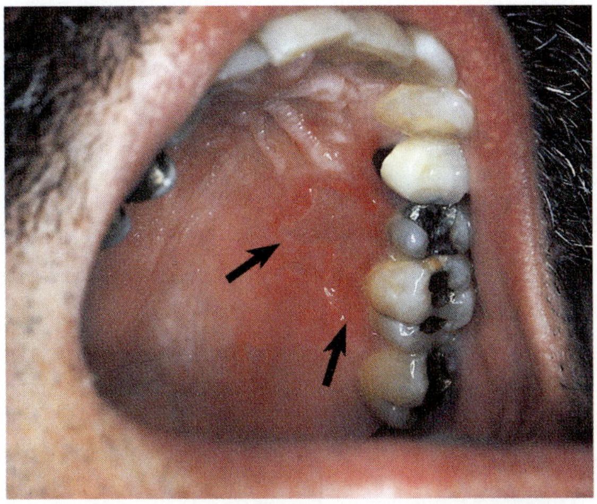

Fig. 17-35 Herpes simplex ulceration of the hard palate in a patient with HIV infection. Arrows point the to periphery of the ulcer. (From Ibsen O, Phelan J: *Oral pathology for the dental hygienist,* ed 4, St Louis, 2004, WB Saunders.)

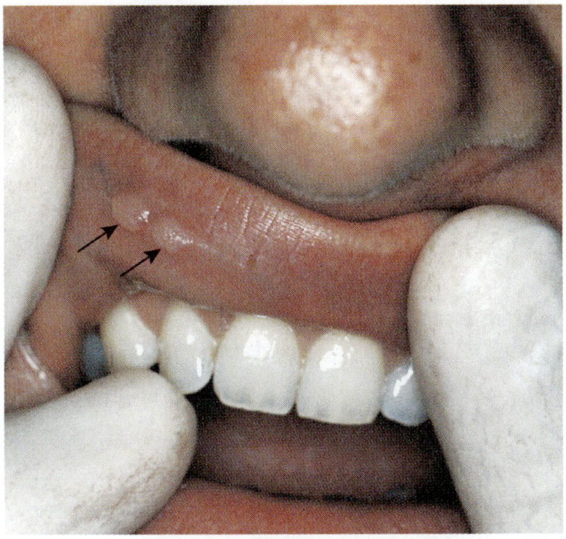

Fig. 17-36 Papillary lesion of the upper lip caused by human papillomavirus in a patient with HIV infection. (From Ibsen O, Phelan J: *Oral pathology for the dental hygienist,* ed 4, St Louis, 2004, WB Saunders.)

Human Papillomavirus

Human papillomaviruses are responsible for warts such as oral papillomas. These appear most often in immunocompromised individuals. The warts are a common finding in patients with early HIV infection.

Diagnosis is made based on history, clinical appearance, and biopsy. These warts appear spiky, and some have a raised, cauliflower-like appearance. Other lesions are well defined, have a flat surface, and essentially disappear when the mucosa is stretched.

Although surgery or carbon dioxide laser excision can remove these warts, they frequently recur after removal (Fig. 17-36).

Recall

16. What is the condition frequently seen on the lateral border of the tongue of patients with HIV/AIDS?
17. Which opportunistic infection is seen as purplish lesions on the skin or oral mucosa of patients with HIV/AIDS?
18. What is the malignant condition that involves the lymph nodes of HIV/AIDS patients?

DEVELOPMENTAL DISORDERS

The development of the human body is an extremely complex process. When cells in the body divide, there is the chance for developmental disorders to occur. The result is usually a deformity of part of the body.

Inherited disorders are different from developmental disorders because they are caused by an *abnormal gene* in an individual and are transmitted from parent to child through the egg or sperm.

Congenital disorders are present at birth. They can be either inherited or developmental, but the exact cause of most congenital abnormalities is unknown.

Developmental disturbances are influenced by both *genetic* and *environmental* factors (Table 17-1).

Genetic Factors

Malformations are often caused by genetic factors, such as abnormalities in the chromosomes. The size of the teeth and jaw are common genetic factors. A child can inherit large teeth from one parent and a small jaw from the other, or a child may inherit small teeth and a large jaw.

Environmental Factors

Environmental factors that have a negative effect on development are called *teratogens.* Examples of teratogens are infections, drugs, and exposure to radiation. Women of childbearing age should avoid teratogens from the time of their first missed menstrual period if they could be pregnant.

During the pregnancy, fever and disease in the mother will affect the developing teeth of the fetus. Some drugs taken during pregnancy may cause birth defects. Such drugs include certain prescribed medications, over-the-counter remedies such as aspirin and cold tablets, and drugs of abuse, including alcohol.

Table 17-1 ***Dental Developmental Disturbances***

Disturbance	Stage	Description	Etiologic Factors	Clinical Ramifications
Anodontia	Initiation stage	Absence of single or multiple teeth	Hereditary, endocrine dysfunction, systemic disease, excess radiation exposure	May cause disruption of occlusion and aesthetic problems. May need partial or full dentures, bridges, and/or implants to replace teeth.
Supernumerary teeth	Initiation stage	Development of one or more extra teeth	Hereditary	Occurs commonly between the maxillary centrals, distal to third molars, and premolar region. May cause crowding, failure of normal eruption, and disruption of occlusion.
Macrodontia/ microdontia	Bud stage	Abnormally large or small teeth	Developmental or hereditary	Commonly involves permanent maxillary lateral incisor and third molars.
Dens in dente	Cap stage	Enamel organ invaginates into the dental papilla	Hereditary	Commonly affects the permanent maxillary lateral incisor. Tooth may have deep lingual pit and need endodontic therapy.
Gemination	Cap stage	Tooth germ tries to divide	Hereditary	Large single-rooted tooth with one pulp cavity and exhibits "twinning" in crown area. Normal number of teeth in dentition. May cause problems in appearance and spacing.
Fusion	Cap stage	Union of two adjacent tooth germs	Pressure on area	Large tooth with two pulp cavities. Extra tooth in dentition. May cause problems in appearance and spacing.
Tubercle	Cap stage	Extra cusp due to effects on enamel organ	Trauma, pressure, or metabolic disease	Common or permanent molars or cingulum of anterior teeth.
Enamel pearl	Apposition and maturation stages	Sphere of enamel on root	Displacement of ameloblasts to root surface	May be confused with calculus deposit on root.
Enamel dysplasia	Apposition and maturation stages	Faulty development of enamel from interference involving ameloblasts	Local or systemic or hereditary	Pitting and intrinsic color changes in enamel.
Dentinal dysplasia	Apposition and maturation stages	Faulty development of dentin from interference with odontoblasts	Local or systemic or hereditary	Intrinsic color changes and changes in thickness of dentin possible. Problems in function or aesthetics.
Concrescence	Apposition and maturation stages	Union of root structure of two or more teeth by cementum	Traumatic injury or crowding of teeth	Common with permanent maxillary molars.

Known Teratogens Involved in Congenital Malformations

Drugs

Ethanol, tetracycline, phenytoin (Dilantin), lithium, methotrexate, aminopterin, diethylstilbestrol, warfarin, thalidomide, isotretinoin (retinoic acid), androgens, progesterone

Chemicals

Methylmercury, polychlorinated biphenyls

Infections

Rubella virus, herpes simplex virus, human immunodeficiency virus, syphilis microbe

Radiation

High levels of ionizing type*

*Note that diagnostic levels of radiation should be avoided but have not been directly linked to congenital malformations.
From Bath-Balogh MB, Fehrenbach M: *Illustrated dental embryology, histology, and anatomy,* ed 2, St Louis, 2005, WB Saunders.

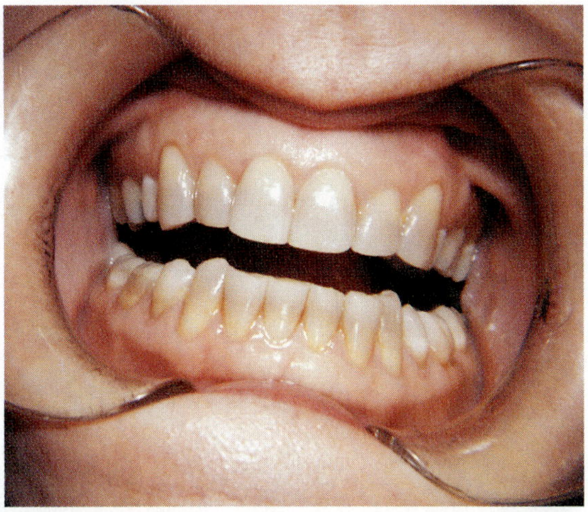

Fig. 17-37 Discoloration of teeth caused by tetracycline ingestion. (From Ibsen O, Phelan J: *Oral pathology for the dental hygienist,* ed 4, St Louis, 2004, WB Saunders.)

Antibiotics, particularly tetracycline, taken during pregnancy may result in a yellow-gray-brown stain on the primary teeth (Fig. 17-37) (see Chapter 58).

Recall

19. What is the difference between developmental disorders and inherited disorders?
20. What is a congenital disorder?

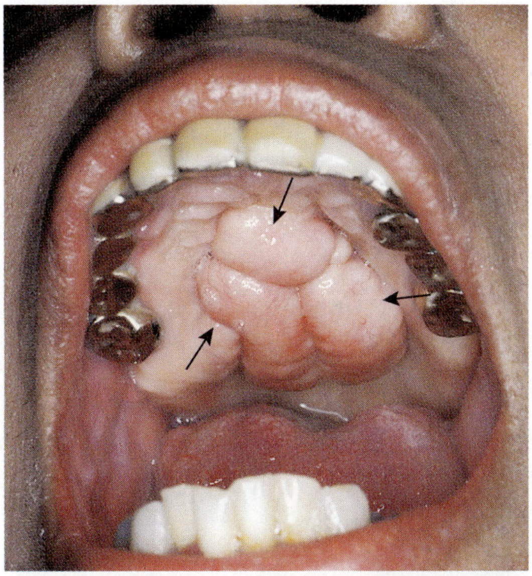

Fig. 17-38 Torus palatinus. (From Ibsen O, Phelan J: *Oral pathology for the dental hygienist,* ed 4, St Louis, 2004, WB Saunders.)

Disturbances in Jaw Development

Macrognathia is a condition characterized by abnormally large jaws. This occurs most often in the mandible, and the result is a class III malocclusion (see Chapter 60).

Micrognathia is a condition characterized by abnormally small jaws. This occurs most often in the mandible, and the result is a class II malocclusion.

An *exostosis* is a benign bony growth projecting outward from the surface of a bone (plural *exostoses*). An exostosis also may be referred to as a torus, defined as a bulging projection (plural *tori*).

A *torus palatinus* is a bony overgrowth in the midline of the hard palate (Fig. 17-38). A *torus mandibularis* is a bony overgrowth on the lingual surface of the mandible near the premolar and molar area. These growths are not harmful; however, it may be necessary to remove them so that a full or partial denture may be placed and worn comfortably (Fig. 17-39).

Disturbances in Lip, Palate, and Tongue Development

A *cleft lip* results when the maxillary and medial nasal processes fail to fuse (Fig. 17-40).

A *cleft palate* results when the palatal shelves fail to fuse with the primary palate. This disturbance may be hereditary or environmental. A *cleft uvula* is the mildest form of

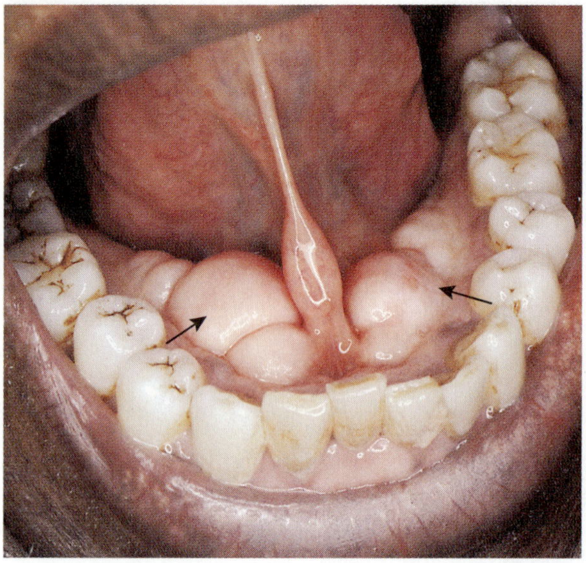

Fig. 17-39 Bilateral mandibular tori. (From Ibsen O, Phelan J: *Oral pathology for the dental hygienist,* ed 4, St Louis, 2004, WB Saunders.)

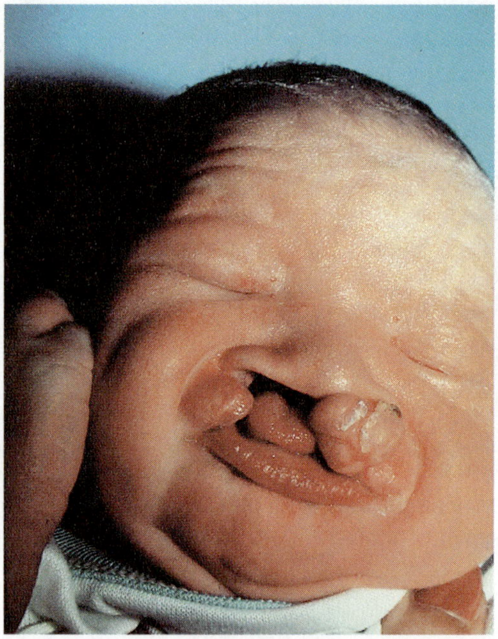

Fig. 17-40 A newborn with bilateral complete cleft lip and palate. Note severe angulation of the premaxillary segment. (From Ibsen O, Phelan J: *Oral pathology for the dental hygienist,* ed 4, St Louis, 2004, WB Saunders.)

cleft palate. Cleft palate, with or without cleft lip, occurs in 1 per 2500 live births.

Ankyloglossia, also known as *tongue-tie,* results in a short lingual frenum that extends to the apex of the tongue. This limits the movement of the tongue (Fig. 17-41).

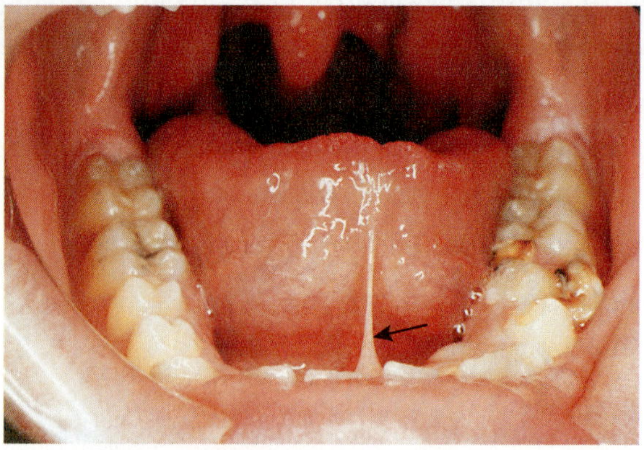

Fig. 17-41 Ankyloglossia. The short frenum is attached near the tip of the tongue. (From Ibsen O, Phelan J: *Oral pathology for the dental hygienist,* ed 4, St Louis, 2004, WB Saunders.)

Recall

21. What is the term for abnormally large jaws?
22. What is the term for bony growths in the palate?
23. What is a more common term for ankyloglossia?

Disturbances in Tooth Development and Eruption

An *ameloblastoma* is a tumor composed of remnants of the dental lamina that failed to disintegrate after the tooth buds were formed.

Anodontia is the congenital absence of teeth. It may be partial or total and may affect the primary or permanent dentition or both. The teeth most often involved are third molars, followed by maxillary lateral incisors and second premolars (Fig. 17-42).

Supernumerary teeth are any teeth in excess of the 32 normal permanent teeth. These teeth may be normal in size and shape, but they are most frequently small and poorly developed (Fig. 17-43).

Macrodontia is the term used to describe abnormally large teeth. It may affect the entire dentition or may appear in only two teeth, such as the maxillary central incisors.

Microdontia is the term used to describe abnormally small teeth. When microdontia affects an entire dentition, it is frequently associated with other defects, such as congenital heart disease or Down syndrome.

Dens in dente, or "a tooth within a tooth," is a developmental anomaly that results in the formation of a small, toothlike mass of enamel and dentin within the pulp. On a radiograph, this resembles a tooth within another tooth (Fig. 17-44).

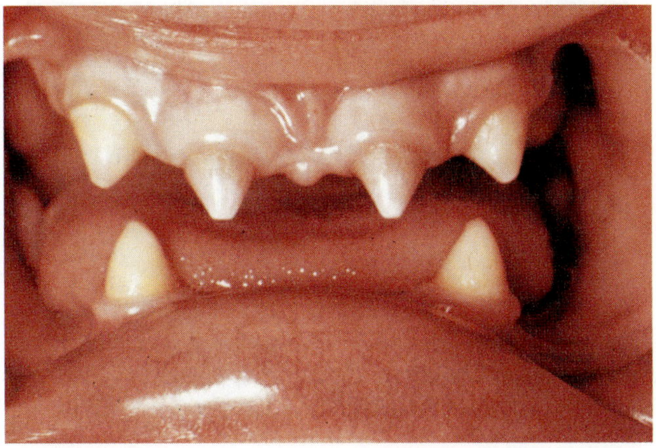

Fig. 17-42 Partial anodontia. (From Ibsen O, Phelan J: *Oral pathology for the dental hygienist,* ed 4, St Louis, 2004, WB Saunders.)

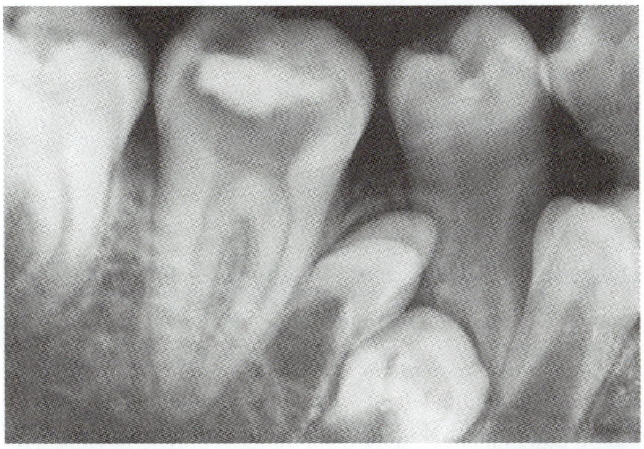

Fig. 17-43 Radiograph showing unerupted supernumerary teeth. (From Ibsen O, Phelan J: *Oral pathology for the dental hygienist,* ed 4, St Louis, 2004, WB Saunders.)

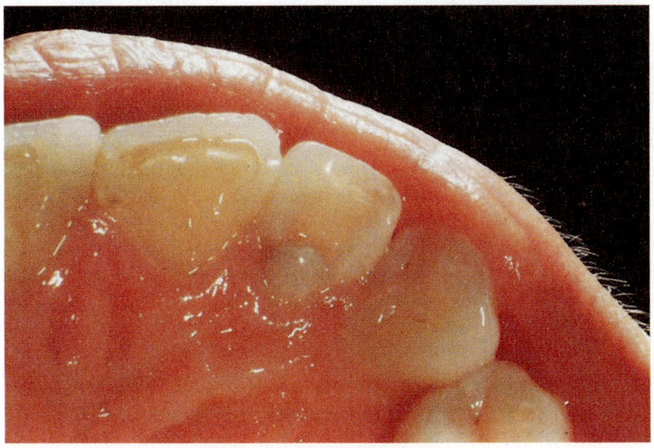

Fig. 17-44 Dens in dente.

Variation in form may include extra, missing, or fused cusps or anomalies of roots. The most common variations, however, are in the form of peg-shaped teeth. *Hutchinson's incisors,* a variety of peg-shaped teeth, are usually associated with maternal syphilis (Fig. 17-45).

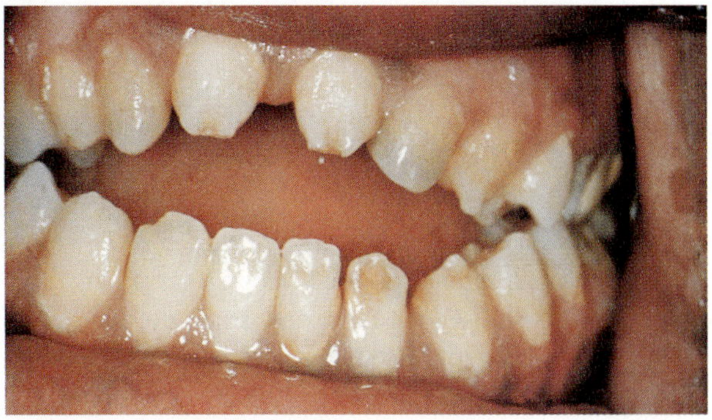

Fig. 17-45 Hutchinson's incisors. (From Ibsen O, Phelan J: *Oral pathology for the dental hygienist,* ed 4, St Louis, 2004, Saunders.)

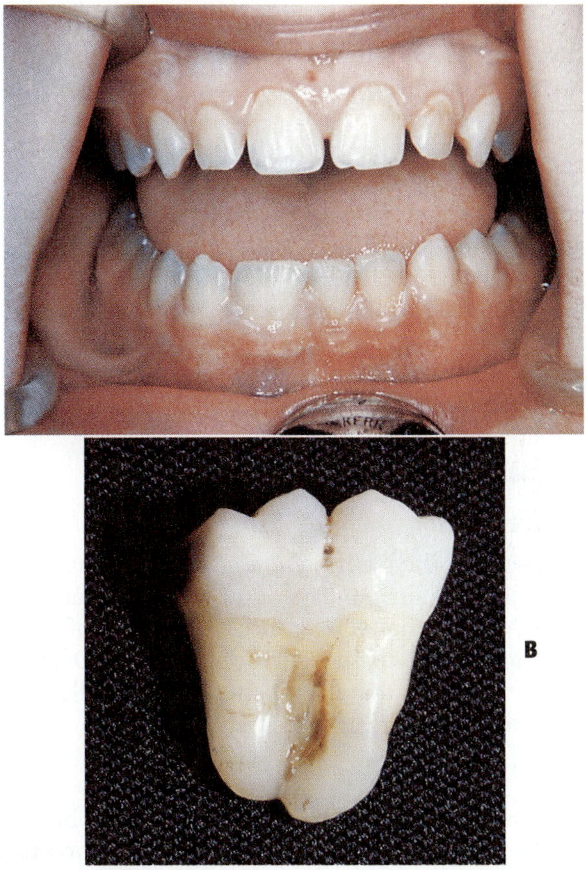

A

B

Fig. 17-46 A, Clinical picture of fusion involving a permanent lateral incisor. B, Fusion of mandibular molars. (From Ibsen O, Phelan J: *Oral pathology for the dental hygienist,* ed 4, St Louis, 2004, WB Saunders.)

Fusion is the joining together of the dentin and enamel of two or more separate developing teeth. Fusion of teeth leads to a reduced number of teeth in the dental arch (Fig. 17-46).

Gemination is an attempt by the tooth bud to divide. When this attempt is not successful, an incisal notch indicates it.

Twinning means that the tooth bud division is complete, and the result is the formation of an extra tooth. This tooth is usually a mirror image of its adjacent partner in the dental arch.

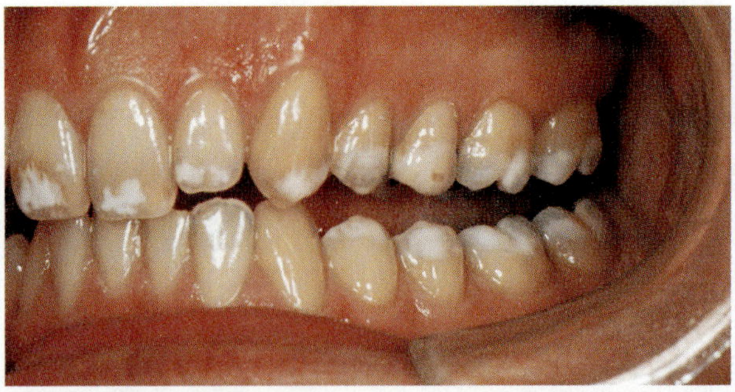

Fig. 17-47 **Note loss of enamel in these teeth in a patient with hypocalcified amelogenesis imperfecta.** (From Ibsen O, Phelan J: *Oral pathology for the dental hygienist,* ed 4, St Louis, 2004, WB Saunders.)

Recall

24. What is the dental term for "tooth within a tooth"?
25. What is the term used for abnormally small teeth?
26. What term is used to describe two teeth joining together?

Disturbances in Enamel Formation

Amelogenesis imperfecta is a hereditary abnormality in which there are defects in the enamel formation (Fig. 17-47).

Hypocalcification is the incomplete calcification or hardening of the enamel of a tooth.

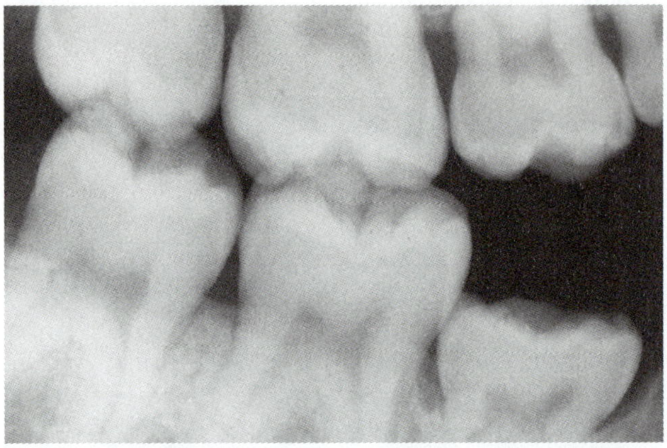

Fig. 17-48 **A radiograph of ankylosis of a deciduous molar.** (From Ibsen O, Phelan J: *Oral pathology for the dental hygienist,* ed 4, St Louis, 2004, WB Saunders.)

Disturbances in Dentin Formation

Dentinogenesis imperfecta is a hereditary condition that affects the formation of dentin. It is found in both the primary and the permanent dentition. Teeth having dentinogenesis imperfecta are opalescent and have an almost amber color. Soon, however, the enamel tends to chip away from the dentin, and the weakened teeth become worn down (see Fig. 17-1).

Abnormal Eruption of the Teeth

Premature Eruption

Natal teeth are the teeth present at birth. Neonatal teeth erupt within the first 30 days of life. The teeth most often involved are the mandibular incisors. Because of the lack of root formation, these teeth are soon shed. Often they will be removed so that the infant does not swallow them if they are shed.

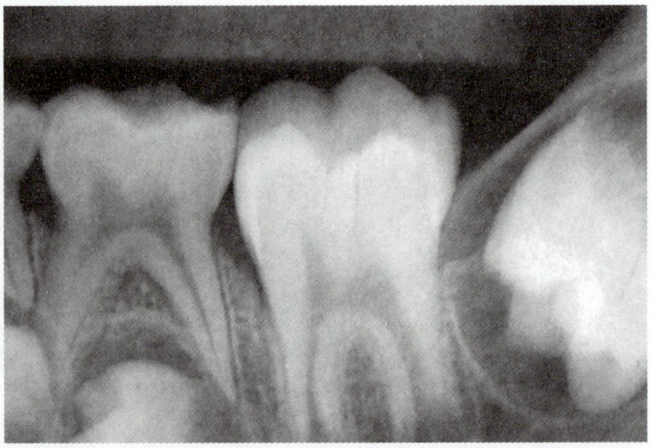

Fig. 17-49 **Impactions in mixed dentition visible on a dental radiograph.**

Ankylosis

Ankylosed teeth are deciduous teeth in which bone has fused to cementum and dentin. This prevents the exfoliation of the deciduous tooth and the eruption of the underlying permanent tooth. Deciduous molars are the most often affected by ankylosis (Fig. 17-48).

Impaction

Impaction is the term used to describe any tooth that remains unerupted in the jaws beyond the time at which it should normally erupt (Fig. 17-49). The following three processes may cause impaction:

1. Premature loss of primary teeth
2. Shifting of the developing tooth into a horizontal or other abnormal position
3. Shifting of the developing tooth into a position from which it cannot erupt because of the presence of other teeth, a lack of jaw space, or abnormally large tooth crowns

Impactions and their treatment are discussed further in Chapter 56.

Recall

27. Which teeth are most often affected by ankylosis?
28. What is the hereditary condition that affects the dentin?

MISCELLANEOUS DISORDERS

Abrasion

Abrasion is the abnormal wearing away of tooth structure. Abrasion is caused by a repetitive habit, such as improper tooth brushing, most often a back-and-forth scrubbing motion using excessive pressure. The use of an abrasive dentifrice or a hard-bristled toothbrush may also cause abrasion (Fig. 17-50).

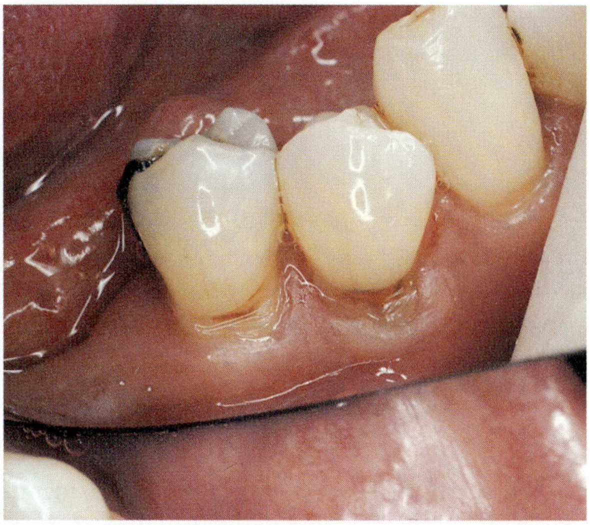

Fig. 17-50 Abrasion at the cervical area of mandibular premolars caused by toothbrushing. (From Ibsen O, Phelan J: *Oral pathology for the dental hygienist,* ed 4, St Louis, 2004, WB Saunders.)

Attrition

Attrition is the normal wearing away of tooth structure during chewing (Fig. 17-51). Attrition is normal and occurs with age on the incisal, occlusal, and proximal surfaces of the teeth. It occurs in both deciduous and permanent dentitions.

A diet of more fibrous food causes a greater rate of attrition. Attrition is made worse by bruxism, as well as by the use of chewing tobacco. The rate of attrition appears to be greater in men than in women.

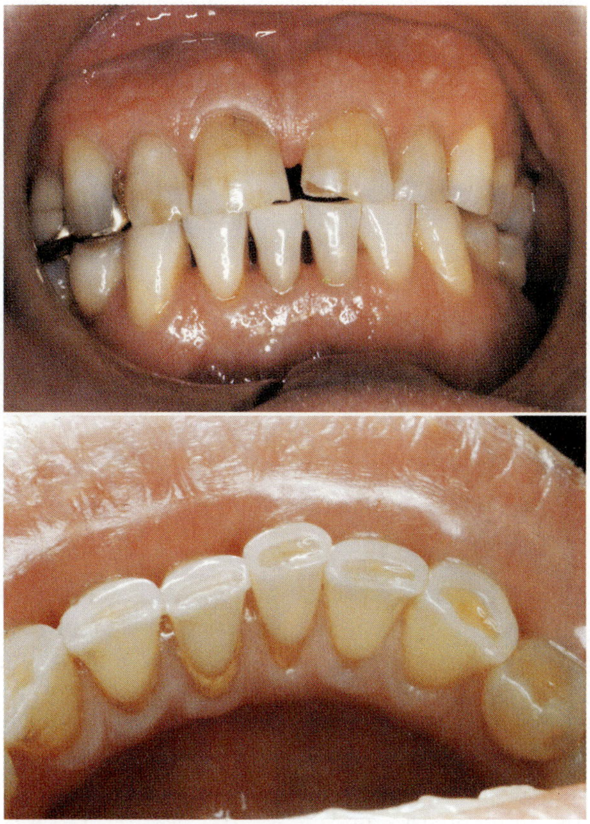

A

B

Fig. 17-51 A, Attrition of adult dentition. B, Attrition of adult dentition (incisal view). (From Ibsen O, Phelan J: *Oral pathology for the dental hygienist,* ed 4, St Louis, 2004, WB Saunders.)

Bruxism

Bruxism is an oral habit characterized by involuntary gnashing, grinding, and clenching of the teeth. It is usually performed during sleep and is often associated with stress or tension. Bruxism causes abnormal wear of the teeth (Fig. 17-52).

Bruxism also damages the periodontal ligament and associated supporting structures and is a major factor contributing to temporomandibular joint disorders.

In addition to stress reduction techniques, a night guard or removable splint is frequently used as a temporary aid in the treatment of bruxism. The purpose of this splint is to reduce the damage caused by the grinding while the patient is asleep.

Bulimia

Bulimia is an eating disorder characterized by food bingeing followed by self-induced vomiting. The dental profes-

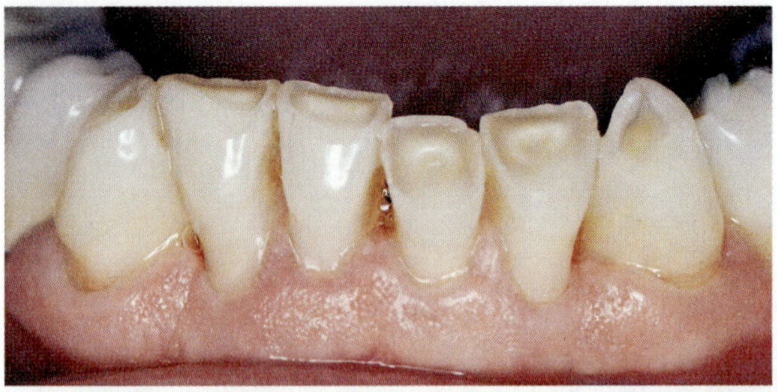

Fig. 17-52 **Attrition of the mandibular anterior teeth resulting from bruxism.** (From Ibsen O, Phelan J: *Oral pathology for the dental hygienist,* ed 4, St Louis, 2004, WB Saunders.)

sional is often the first healthcare professional to identify a patient with bulimia, because of the pattern of erosion on the lingual surfaces of the teeth (Fig. 17-53).

Generally, the person with bulimia maintains a normal body weight but is secretive about eating habits. Vomiting after eating is a component of bulimia but not of anorexia nervosa, another eating disorder. Generalized erosion of the lingual surfaces of the teeth is common and results from the acid produced by frequent vomiting (see Chapter 16).

Dental management of the patient with bulimia requires minimizing the effects of the stomach acids on tooth enamel by encouraging the daily use of a fluoride rinse and fluoridated toothpaste. Rinsing the mouth with water and thoroughly cleaning the teeth immediately after vomiting also lessen the effect of the acid. However, the patient should be encouraged to seek professional treatment to end the eating disorder.

Orofacial Piercings

Piercing parts of the face and oral cavity followed by the insertion of various objects has recently become popular among some segments of the population. The dental complications of this practice can include chipped teeth, broken teeth, and serious infections at the site of the piercings. Infection can spread throughout the head and neck area with serious results.

Recall

29. What is the difference between attrition and abrasion?
30. What is an oral indication of bulimia?
31. What are three potential complications of orofacial piercing?

A

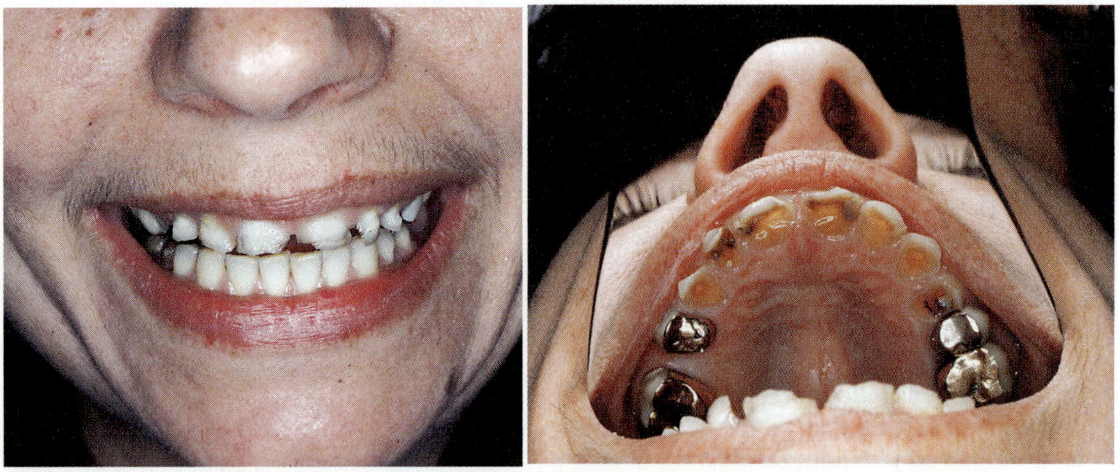

B

Fig. 17-53 **Erosion caused by bulimia. A, Decreased tooth size. B, Erosion of maxillary lingual surfaces.** (From Ibsen O, Phelan J: *Oral pathology for the dental hygienist,* ed 4, St Louis, 2004, WB Saunders.)

Patient Education

You will probably see patients with piercings of the tongue, lips, or other oral areas. As a dental assistant, you may have the opportunity to educate your patients about how piercing can be dangerous.

The mouth contains millions of bacteria, and infection is a common complication of oral piercing. Pain and swelling are other side effects of piercing. The tongue, the most popular piercing site in the mouth, could swell large enough to close off the airway. Piercing can also cause uncontrollable bleeding or nerve damage.

Even if the piercing injury itself does not cause problems, other hazards are created by the jewelry inserted. People can choke on any studs, barbells, or hoops that come loose in the mouth. Chipped or cracked teeth can result from contact with the jewelry.

Educate patients that this fashion statement involves more than just deciding on the style or placement of jewelry. The decision to pierce oral structures could have major consequences for oral health as well.

Legal and Ethical Implications

Always carefully check the medical histories of all your patients before each appointment. Many patients take medications that can cause changes in the oral tissues. For example, antianxiety medications, antipsychotic medications, and antihistamines can cause xerostomia. Drugs such as prednisone can increase the risk for candidiasis and other oral infections. Other medications can cause gingival hyperplasia. By being alert, you can play an important role in the patient's care.

Eye to the Future

Today surgery, radiation therapy, and chemotherapy are used to treat oral cancer. Unfortunately, radiation therapy and chemotherapy can cause several serious oral conditions. In the future, perhaps more effective and less damaging therapies will be developed. Better yet, perhaps there will be a significant reduction in the number of oral cancers as a result of less smoking and alcohol use, along with improved treatment technologies. An oral cancer examination should be part of every routine dental examination. The key to long-term survival is early recognition and diagnosis.

Critical Thinking

1. Rex Ryan is a 32-year-old man in your practice. His medical history indicates that he is HIV-positive. While exposing radiographs, you notice several purplish areas on his neck and also on his palate. What do you think these purplish areas could be?
2. Blanche Jones is an 82-year-old woman who lives alone. She is very thin and sometimes appears quite weak. She is in your office complaining about her burning tongue. While the dentist is doing the examination, you notice that her tongue is smooth and very red. What could be the problem?
3. Jason is a 16-year-old patient who is in your office for his annual dental checkup. He is a pitcher on his high school baseball team. He admits to using smokeless tobacco. What type of lesions do you expect to see in his mouth?

Part 4

Infection Control in Dentistry

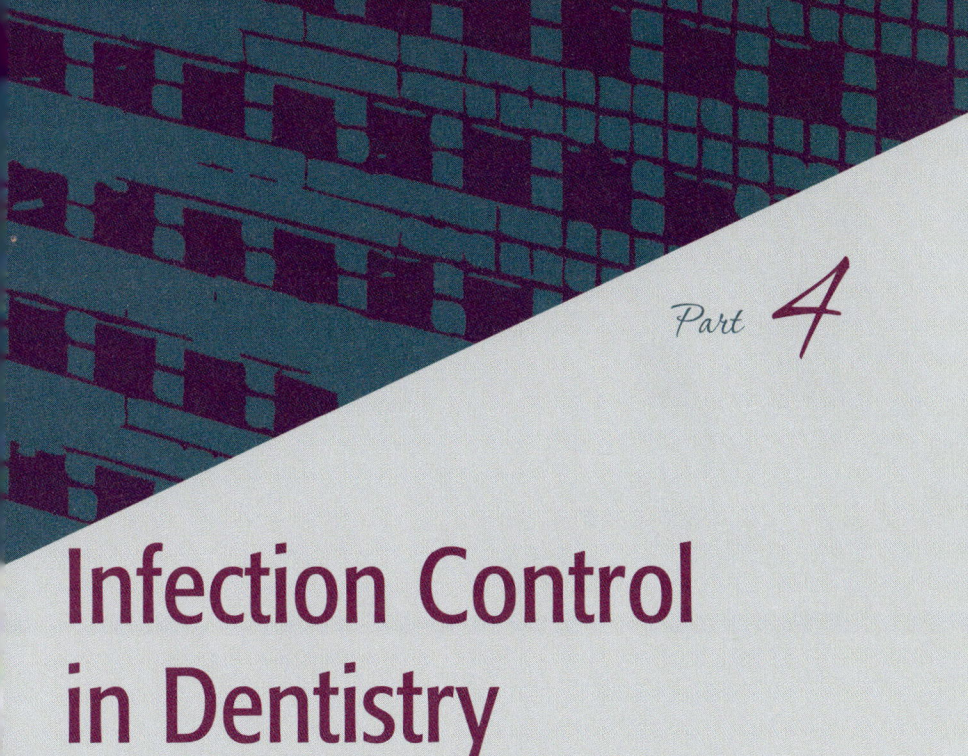

The Centers for Disease Control and Prevention (CDC) has recently released the new *Guidelines for Infection Control in Dental Health-Care Settings.* These guidelines are now the standard for infection control in dentistry. This section will provide a comprehensive overview of these new guidelines.

Dental staff and patients may be exposed to a wide variety of disease-causing microorganisms that may be transmitted in the dental office. Diseases such as hepatitis, human immunodeficiency virus (HIV) infection, herpes, and tuberculosis have been joined by new diseases such as West Nile virus and severe acute respiratory syndrome (SARS). The microbiology chapter in this section will provide you with the necessary foundation to understand the organisms that cause disease and introduce you to some of the diseases of concern for dentistry.

As new diseases evolve, dental healthcare professionals must adopt the newest and most effective infection-control techniques to prevent transmission in the dental setting.

The step-by-step procedures in the following chapters will guide you through instrument processing, surface and equipment disinfection, and personal protective wear. The Occupational Safety and Health Administration (OSHA) Bloodborne Pathogens Standard (BBP), the most important infection-control law in dentistry, is discussed in detail.

18

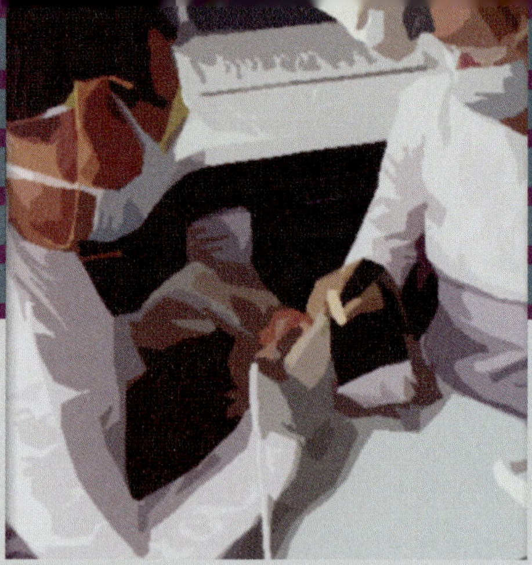

Microbiology

Outline

KEY TERMS

Aerobes (**air**-ohbz) Bacteria that require oxygen to grow.

Anaerobes (**an**-air-ohbz) Bacteria that grow in the absence of oxygen and are destroyed by oxygen.

Bacilli (singular *bacillus*) Rod-shaped bacteria that cause tuberculosis and other diseases.

Candida A common yeast found in the oral cavity, gastrointestinal tract, female genital tract, and sometimes the skin.

Chancre A painless ulcerating sore.

Cocci Spherical bacterial cells that reproduce by dividing into two; singular *coccus.*

Coronavirus (co-**ro**-na-*vi*-rus) Type of virus that causes respiratory infections.

Creutzfeldt-Jakob disease (**kroits**-fuhlt–**yah**-kop) Rare chronic brain disease with onset in middle to late life (40 to 60 years).

Endospore A resistant, dormant structure formed inside of some bacteria that can withstand adverse conditions.

Facultative anaerobes Organisms that can grow with or without oxygen.

Fungi Plants, such as mushrooms, yeasts, and molds, that lack chlorophyll; singular *fungus.*

Gram-negative Classification of bacteria that do not hold a dye stain under a microscope.

Gram-positive Classification of bacteria that hold a dye stain and appear dark purple under a microscope.

Gram's stain Four-step staining process developed by Hans Christian Gram used for separating bacteria into groups.

Gram-variable Classification of bacteria that are not consistently stained.

Herpesvirus A virus that causes infections in humans, such as herpes, cytomegalovirus, chickenpox, shingles, mononucleosis, measles, and Kaposi 's sarcoma.

Latent Dormant or suppressed.

Microbiology The study of microorganisms.

Nonpathogenic (*non*-pa-thuh-**jeh**-nik) Pertaining to microorganisms that do *not* produce disease.

Oral candidiasis (kan-dah-**die**-uh-sis) A *Candida* yeast infection of the oral mucosa.

Pathogens (**pa**-thuh-jehns) Disease-producing microorganisms.

Percutaneous (per-ku-**tan**-e-us) Through the skin, such as a needlestick, cut, or human bite.

Petri plate A small flat dish made of thin glass or plastic containing sterile solid medium for the culture of microorganisms; also called *petri dish.*

Prions (**pry**-ons) Infectious particles of proteins that lack nucleic acids.

Protozoa (pro-tuh-**zo**-uh) Single-celled microscopic animals without a rigid cell wall.

Provirus Virus that is hidden during the latency period.

Spirochetes Spiral-shaped bacteria.

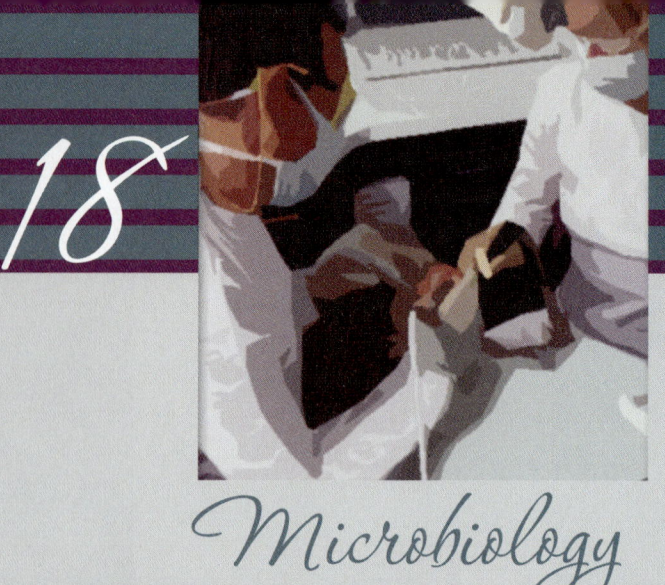

KEY TERMS—cont'd

Staphylococci Cocci that form irregular groups or clusters.
Streptococci Cocci that form chains as they divide.
Tyndallization (*tin*-duhl-i-**zay**-shun) Intermittent, or fractional, sterilization.
Virulent (**veer**-uh-luhnt) Capable of causing serious disease.
Viruses Ultramicroscopic infectious agents that contain either DNA or RNA.

LEARNING OUTCOMES

On completion of this chapter, the student will be able to achieve the following objectives:

- Pronounce, define, and spell the Key Terms.
- Discuss the contributions of early pioneers in microbiology.
- Explain why the study of microbiology is important for the dental assistant.
- Identify the types of bacteria according to their shape.
- List the major groups of microorganisms.
- Describe the differences among aerobes, anaerobes, and facultative anaerobes.
- Identify diseases caused by chlamydiae.
- Identify the most resistant form of life known, and explain how it survives.
- Compare viruses with bacteria, and name diseases caused by each.
- Explain why specificity in viruses is important.
- Describe how prions differ from viruses and bacteria.
- Name the bloodborne pathogens of concern in dentistry.
- Name two diseases caused by prions.
- Describe the symptoms of SARS.
- Explain how SARS is spread.
- Describe the symptoms of West Nile virus.
- Explain how West Nile virus is spread.
- Explain how each type of hepatitis is transmitted.
- Describe the effect of HIV on the immune system.
- Identify methods of HIV transmission.

The dental assistant needs a foundation in microbiology in order to understand the nature of **pathogens** (disease-producing microorganisms) and how to prevent the transmission of disease in the dental office. This knowledge helps the assistant to make important decisions regarding infection-control products and procedures (see Chapter 19). It is important to note that the two most common oral diseases, *dental caries* (decay) and *periodontal disease*, are caused by bacterial infections.

Microbiology is the study of microorganisms (*micro-* means microscopically small, and *bio-* means living organisms). Because of their microscopic size, the existence of microorganisms is usually unnoticed unless they cause illness. Most people experience common colds in the winter months, and many others experience life-threatening illnesses caused by microorganisms.

Fortunately, most microorganisms are **nonpathogenic** (do not produce human illness). In fact, microorganisms are valuable allies in many ways. Microorganisms used in the production of flavorful cheeses and yogurt, for example, are very beneficial. Other microorganisms are used in disposal of waste products, fertilization of soil, and production of lifesaving drugs.

PIONEERS IN MICROBIOLOGY

Aristotle (384–322 BC) introduced the earliest belief that life was "spontaneously generated" from nonliving matter. This theory remained unchallenged for more than 2000 years. According to his theory, living things arose from muck, decaying food, warm rain, or even dirty shirts.

Antony van Leeuwenhoek (**lay**-vuhn-hoak) (1632–1723) was a Dutch merchant and amateur scientist. He used a primitive microscope to observe stagnant water and scrapings from the teeth. His microscope was simple; it consisted of a small lens mounted between two thin plates of metal. Through the lens of about magnification 300, van Leeuwenhoek could see small life-forms he called "animalcules." After 20 years of careful observation, he reported his findings to the Royal Society of London.

John Tyndall (**tin**-duhl) (1820–1893) was an English physicist who explained the need for prolonged heating to destroy microbial life in broth. He discovered that bacteria existed in heat-stable and heat-sensitive forms. Prolonged or intermittent heating was needed to destroy the heat-stable form. Intermittent heating, now called **tyndallization,** killed both forms. Almost simultaneously, German botanist Ferdinand Cohn (1828–1898) described the heat-stable forms as **endospores,** which are formed during the life cycle of certain bacteria (see Chapter 21).

Joseph Lister (1827–1912) was an English surgeon who recognized the role of airborne microorganisms in postsurgical infections. By applying carbolic acid to dressings and using an aerosol of carbolic acid during surgery, he lowered the risk of infection after surgery.

Robert Koch (1843–1910) was a German physician who provided the techniques and discipline necessary to guide future microbiologists. He developed the use of a two-part dish for growing bacteria and a technique for isolating pure colonies of bacteria (Fig. 18-1). The two-part dishes

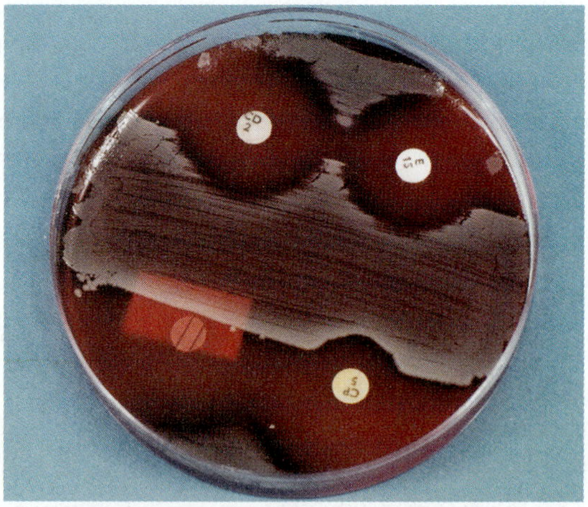

Fig. 18-1 Colonies of bacteria are growing in the culture medium in this Petri plate. (From Samaranayake LP: *Essential microbiology in dentistry,* ed 2, New York, 2002, Churchill Livingstone.)

Koch's Postulates

1. The microbial agent must be found in every case of the disease.
2. The microorganism must be isolated and grown in pure culture.
3. The microorganism must cause the same disease when inoculated into a susceptible animal.
4. The same microbial agent must be recovered from the inoculated animal.

were named **Petri plates** after Julius Petri (1852–1921), a German bacteriologist. Petri plates are still used in microbiology labs today.

To prove that a specific microorganism caused a particular disease, Koch applied guidelines that are still in use today.

Louis Pasteur (1822–1895) was a famous French chemist. He disproved the theory of spontaneous generation of life and associated living microorganisms with disease. Pasteur designed flasks shaped like swan necks (*S*-shaped) for heating broths. The curved pathway caused by the bends in the glass prevented dust particles, which contained microorganisms from the air, from entering the heated broth. Instead, the dust particles settled in the bends of the long-necked flasks, even over an extended period. When the top of a flask was removed, microorganisms once again appeared in the liquid. Pasteur's experiments put an end to the theory of spontaneous generation of life.

Pasteur's ongoing contributions to the emerging germ theory of disease earned him the title "Father of Microbiology." At the request of Napoleon III in 1863, Pasteur saved the French wine industry by showing that vats of spoiled wine contained acid-producing bacteria.

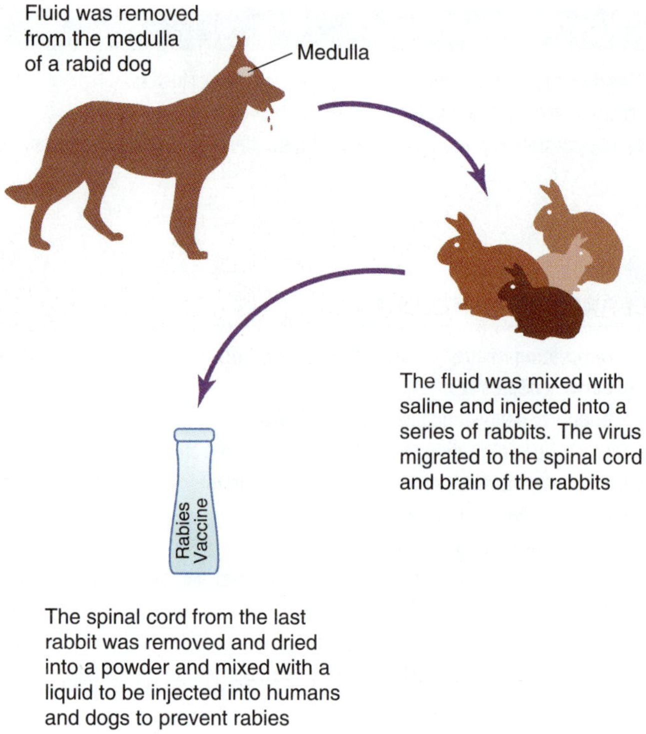

Fig. 18-2 Discovery of rabies vaccine by Louis Pasteur, 1885.

The contaminants could be destroyed at temperatures of 50° to 60° F in a short time. The process of heating grape juice to reduce microorganisms became known as *pasteurization.* Today, pathogens in milk are destroyed through pasteurization.

Pasteur prepared the first vaccine for the fatal animal disease *rabies.* Although he never isolated the actual rabies virus, he infected rabbits by inoculating them with a preparation from the medulla (a portion of the brainstem and spinal cord) of rabid dogs. The viruses migrated to the spinal cord and brain of the rabbits. Pasteur maintained the organism by successive inoculations in rabbits (Fig. 18-2). He inoculated dogs with dried, powdered rabbit medulla, suspended in broth, to prevent rabies.

The French government built the Pasteur Institute in 1888 to honor Pasteur, whose last words reportedly were, "There is still a great deal to do" (Fig. 18-3).

Recall

1. Why is microbiology important to the dental assistant?
2. Who is referred to as the "Father of Microbiology?"
3. Who recognized that airborne microorganisms were responsible for postsurgical infections?
4. Who was responsible for discovering the rabies vaccine?

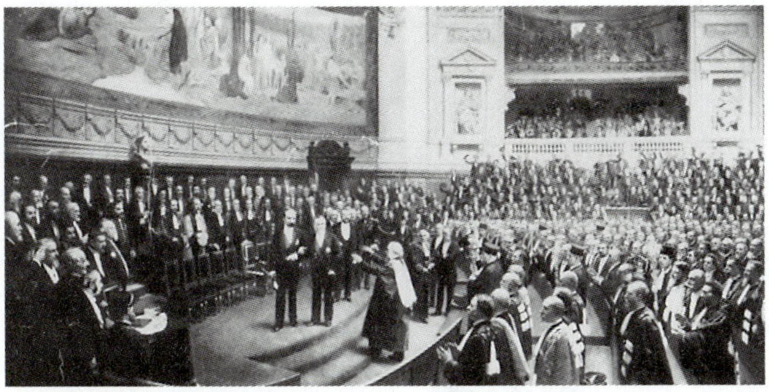

Fig. 18-3 Louis Pasteur is honored at the Sorbonne. (Courtesy National Library of Medicine.)

MAJOR GROUPS OF MICROORGANISMS

The five major groups of microorganisms are (1) *bacteria,* (2) *algae,* (3) *protozoa,* (4) *fungi,* and (5) *viruses.* Members of the first four groups are easily recognized with the aid of a light microscope used in most laboratories. Viruses, however, are so tiny they can be seen only with a powerful electron microscope.

Viruses have often been described as "perfect parasites" because they live inside cells of the host and use the resources of the cells to produce up to 10,000 offspring in as quickly as 7 hours. Viruses are responsible for most of the emerging microbial diseases today. The cells in which invading viruses live and replicate are called *host cells.*

Although not a member of the major groups, a recently discovered infectious particle is known as a *prion.* **Prions** are unique agents in that they contain abnormal protein with *no* DNA or RNA (deoxyribonucleic or ribonucleic acid). Prions are responsible for a group of chronic diseases with long incubation periods (see later discussion in the section about prions).

Bacteria

Bacteria (singular *bacterium*) are a large group of one-celled microorganisms that vary in size, shape, and arrangement of cells. Most bacteria are capable of living independently under favorable environmental conditions. Pathogenic bacteria usually grow best at 98.6° F (37° C) in a moist dark environment.

A bacterial infection can be spread by many means of transmission (see Chapter 19). Humans host a variety of bacteria at all times. The skin, respiratory tract, and gastrointestinal tract are inhabited by a great variety of harmless bacteria, called *normal flora.* They are beneficial and protect the human host by aiding in metabolism and preventing entrance of harmful bacteria.

An infection occurs when bacteria occurring naturally in one part of the body invade another part of the body and become harmful. When this occurs, normal flora are considered *opportunistic,* or causing infection. For example, the urinary tract infection, *cystitis,* is caused by contamination with *Escherichia coli,* a bacterium that is normal flora in the intestine.

Shape

Most bacteria can be classified according to their shape. When viewed under a microscope, bacteria have three shapes: (1) *spherical* (cocci), (2) *rod* (bacilli), and *spiral* (spirochetes) (Fig. 18-4).

Cocci reproduce by dividing into two. The cocci that form chains as they divide are called **streptococci.** Examples of infections caused by streptococci include pharyngitis (a severe sore throat commonly known as "strep throat"), tonsillitis, pneumonia, and endocarditis (Fig. 18-5). The cocci that form irregular groups or clusters are called **staphylococci.** Examples of infections caused by staphylococci include boils and other skin infections, endocarditis, and pneumonia (Fig. 18-6).

Bacilli (singular *bacillus*) are rod-shaped bacteria. Tuberculosis is one disease caused by a bacillus.

Spirochetes are spiral-shaped bacteria. These bacteria have flexible cell walls and are capable of movement. Lyme disease, which is transmitted to humans through the bite of an infected deer tick, is caused by a spirochete. Syphilis is also caused by a spirochete (see later discussion in the section about syphilis under Bacterial Diseases).

Gram-Positive and Gram-Negative Bacteria

Hans Christian Gram, a Danish bacteriologist, developed a four-step staining process for separating bacteria into two groups in 1884. **Gram's stain** requires the sequential use of a crystal violet dye, iodine solution, alcohol solution, and safranin dye. A physician may make a diagnosis on the basis of a Gram's stain and begin appropriate antimicrobial therapy. The classification follows:

- The bacteria that are stained by the dye are classified as **gram-positive.** They appear dark purple under the microscope (Fig. 18-7).
- The bacteria that do not hold the stain are classified as **gram-negative.** They are almost colorless and nearly invisible under the microscope (Fig. 18-8).
- The bacteria that are not consistently stained are classified as **gram-variable.** An example is the organism called *Mycobacterium tuberculosis.*

Need for Oxygen

- **Aerobes** are a variety of bacteria that require oxygen to grow.
- **Anaerobes** are bacteria that grow in the absence of oxygen and are destroyed by oxygen.
- **Facultative anaerobes** are organisms that can grow in either the presence or the absence of oxygen.

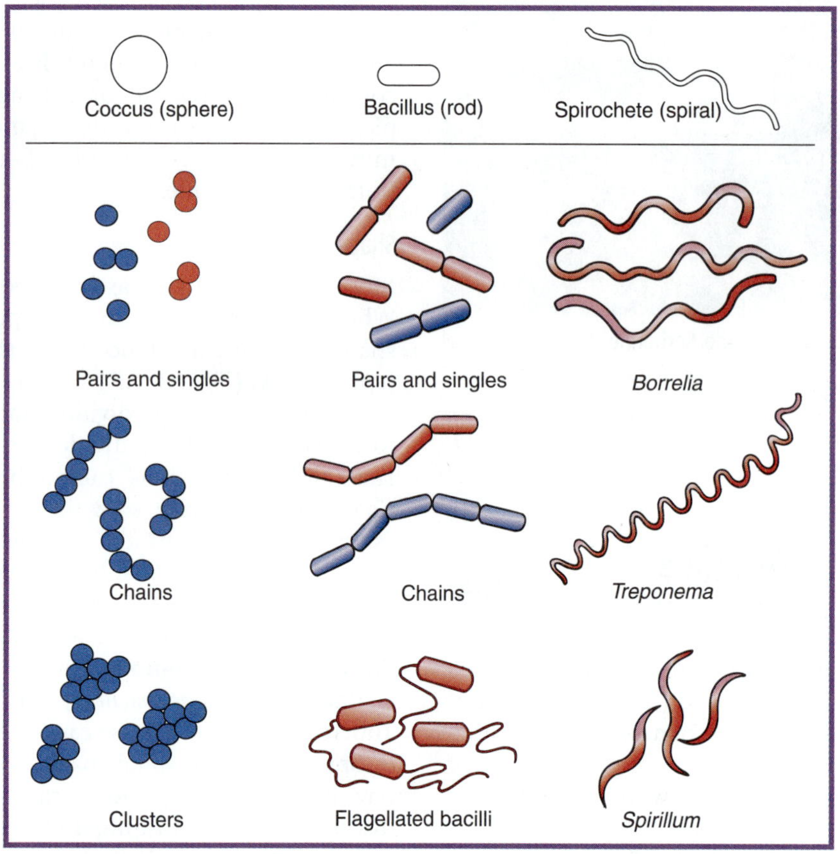

Fig. 18-4 Three basic shapes of bacteria. (From Stepp CA, Woods M: *Laboratory procedures for medical office personnel,* Philadelphia, 1998, Saunders.)

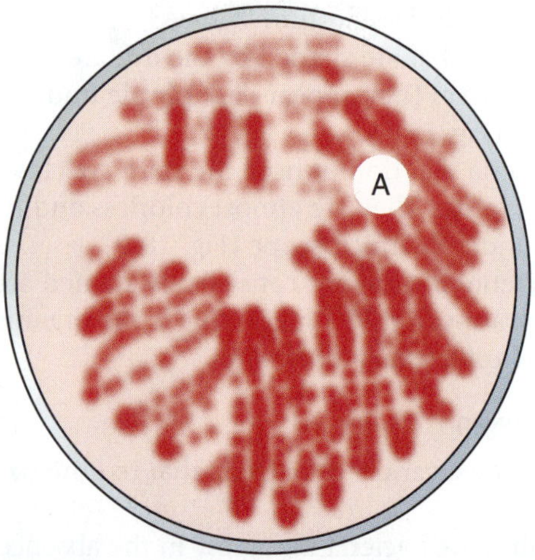

Fig. 18-5 Colonies of streptococci growing on agar medium are diagnostic for strep throat. (From Stepp CA, Woods M: *Laboratory procedures for medical office personnel,* Philadelphia, 1998, Saunders.)

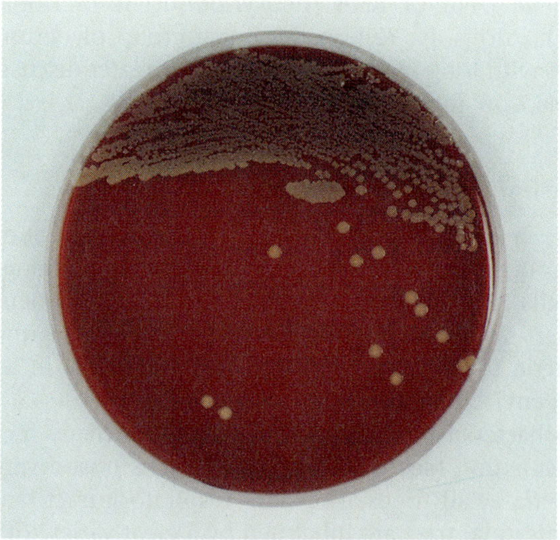

Fig. 18-6 Golden-yellow colonies of staphylococci. (From Samaranayake LP: *Essential microbiology in dentistry,* ed 2, New York, 2002, Churchill Livingstone.)

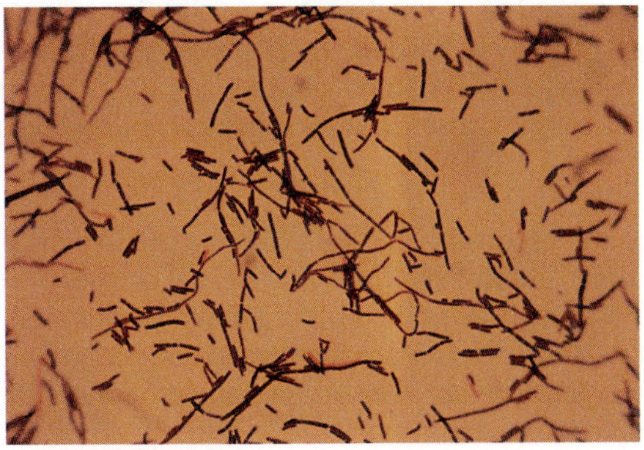

Fig. 18-7 Gram-positive stain. (From De la Maza LM, Pezzlo MT, Baron EJ: *Color atlas of microbiology,* St Louis, 1997, Mosby.)

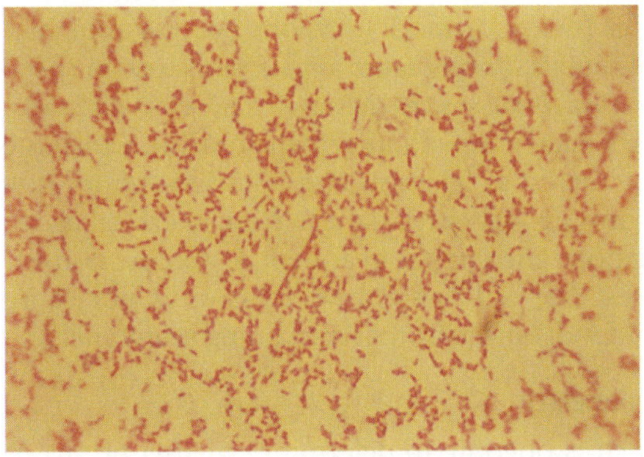

Fig. 18-8 Gram-negative stain. (From De la Maza LM, Pezzlo MT, Baron EJ: *Color atlas of microbiology,* St Louis, 1997, Mosby.)

Capsules

Some types of bacteria form a capsule that forms a protective layer covering the cell wall. *Streptococcus mutans,* which is a causative factor in dental caries, forms such a capsule.

Bacteria with this protective coating are generally **virulent** (capable of causing serious disease) because the capsule increases their ability to resist the body's defense mechanisms. The capsule may also prevent antibiotic agents from affecting the bacteria.

Spores

Under unfavorable conditions, some bacteria change into a highly resistant form called spores. Tetanus is an example of a disease caused by a spore-forming bacillus.

Bacteria remain alive in the spore form but are inactive. As spores, they cannot reproduce or cause disease. When conditions are again favorable, the bacteria become active and capable of causing disease.

Spores represent the *most resistant form* of life known. They can survive extremes of heat and dryness and even the presence of disinfectants and radiation. Because of this incredible resistance, harmless spores are used to test the effectiveness of techniques used to sterilize dental instruments (see Chapter 21).

Recall

5. What are the three primary shapes of bacteria?
6. What is the staining process for separating bacteria?
7. What is the term for bacteria that require oxygen to grow?
8. What is the most resistant form of bacterial life?

Rickettsiae

Rickettsiae are short, nonmotile (nonmovable) rods that normally live in the intestinal tract of insects such as lice, fleas, ticks, and mosquitoes. These organisms are very small and require host cells to reproduce.

The diseases caused by rickettsiae include typhus and Rocky Mountain spotted fever. These diseases are transmitted to humans through the bite of an infected insect.

Algae

Algae range from microscopic single-cell organisms to larger multiple-cell organisms such as seaweed and kelp. All algae contain chlorophyll as well as pigments that cause them to appear yellow-green, brown, or red. Algae are found in abundance in both freshwater and marine habitats. Most algae do not produce human disease.

Protozoa

Protozoa (singular *protozoon* or *protozoan*) consist of a large group of one-cell organisms that do not have a rigid cell wall. Protozoa are found in freshwater and marine habitats and in moist soil. Their diet includes bacteria, small algae, and other protozoa.

Some protozoa can remain viable as cysts for long periods outside their hosts. The thick walls of the cyst make them resistant to drying. The majority of protozoa do not cause disease, but some live in hosts and do cause damage. A small number of protozoa are responsible for intestinal infections of humans; others invade the blood, lungs, liver, or brain.

Fungi

Fungi (singular *fungus*) are plants such as mushrooms, yeasts, and molds that lack *chlorophyll,* the substance that makes plants green. Fungi are not green.

Candida is a common yeast found in the oral cavity of about half the patient population. It also is found in the gastrointestinal tract, female genital tract, and sometimes the skin. Cross-infection may occur from mother to baby and among infant siblings.

Oral candidiasis is caused by the yeast *Candida albicans.* All forms of candidiasis are considered to be opportunistic infections, especially affecting very young, very old, and very ill patients. Infants and terminally ill patients are also at risk. Candidiasis infections are common under dentures in patients with human immunodeficiency virus (HIV) infection.

Oral candidiasis is characterized by white membranes on the surface of the oral mucosa, tongue, and elsewhere in the oral cavity. The lesions may resemble thin cottage cheese; wiping reveals a raw, red, and sometimes bleeding base (Fig. 18-9). Candidiasis is treated with topical antifungal preparations such as nystatin in the form of lozenges.

Prions

Prions were discovered by Dr. Stanley Prusiner while he was doing research into **Creutzfeldt-Jakob disease** (a rare central nervous system disease causing dementia) and other degenerative disorders. Prions are defined as "small *pro*teinaceous *in*fectious particles," thus their name. Prions are composed entirely of proteins that lack nucleic acids (DNA or RNA).

The recent discovery that proteins alone can transmit an infectious disease came as a great surprise to the scientific community. Until the discovery of prions, it was believed that any agent capable of transmitting disease had to be made up of genetic material composed of nucleic acids.

A

B

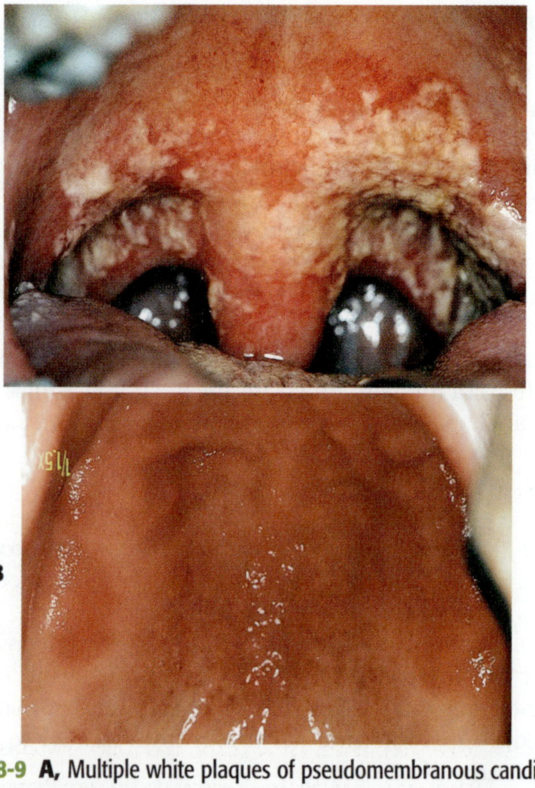

Fig. 18-9 A, Multiple white plaques of pseudomembranous candidiasis (thrush) in an HIV-infected individual. **B,** *Candida*-associated denture stomatitis showing the edentulous maxillary arch. (From Regezi JA, Sciubba JJ, Pogrel MA: *Atlas of oral and maxillofacial pathology,* St Louis, 2000, Saunders.)

Prions convert normal protein molecules into dangerous ones simply by causing the normal ones *to change their shape.* Therefore prions are a new and separate class, unlike bacteria, fungi, viruses, and all other known pathogens.

Prion Diseases

Prions are responsible for mad cow disease and are linked to human diseases such as Creutzfeldt-Jakob disease and possibly Alzheimer's disease. The known prion diseases are all fatal. These diseases are sometimes referred to as *spongiform encephalopathies.* They are so named because they frequently cause holes in the brain.

Prion diseases in humans are rare; all affect the brain and can be dormant for years. Disease has been transmitted by corneal transplant, contaminated surgical instruments, and injections of growth hormone derived from human pituitaries (before artificial hormone became available).

In animals, prions cause *scrapie* (a disease in sheep) and *bovine spongiform encephalopathy* (mad cow disease). Prion diseases may be hereditary *or* transmissible, which is of particular interest to scientists and infection-control experts.

Prions are highly resistant to heat, chemical agents, and irradiation. There is no treatment or vaccine against prion diseases. The only preventive measure is not eating suspected food, especially that containing *neural* (nerve) tissue.

Future Research

Research is ongoing to determine whether prions consisting of other proteins play a part in more common neurodegenerative conditions, including Alzheimer's disease, Parkinson's disease, and amyotrophic lateral sclerosis (Lou Gehrig's disease). All these disorders have marked similarities. As with all the prion diseases, these neuropathologic diseases occur sporadically but sometimes run in families. Also, all are usually diseases of middle to later life and share similar pathologies.

Recall

9. How are prions different from other microorganisms?

Viruses

Viruses are much smaller than bacteria. Despite their tiny size, many viruses cause fatal diseases. New and increasingly destructive viruses are being discovered and have caused the creation of a special area within microbiology called *virology* (the study of viruses and their effects).

Viruses can live and multiply only *inside* an appropriate host cell. The host cells may be human, animal, plant, or bacteria.

A virus invades a host cell, *replicates* (produces copies of itself), and then destroys the host cell so the viruses are released into the body. The various forms of viral hepatitis and HIV are discussed in more detail later in this chapter.

Specificity

Viruses can have *specificity* (preference) for particular cell types in order to replicate. Some viruses have a high degree of specificity. For example, HIV infects cells known as CD4 cells, and hepatitis virus infects only liver cells. Other viruses are able to cause disease in more than one organ. For example, the mumps virus can infect the thyroid, pancreas, testicles, and ovaries.

Unfortunately, some viruses can cross the placenta and infect the fetus. One fourth of HIV-infected mothers pass the infection on to the infant. Cytomegalovirus (CMV) infection during pregnancy is a major cause of mental retardation, blindness, and impaired hearing in children.

Latency

Some viruses establish a **latent** (dormant) state in host cells. The virus becomes integrated into the nucleic acid of the host cell and is known as a **provirus.** A latent virus can be reactivated in the future and produce more infective viral particles, followed by signs and symptoms of the disease.

Stress, infection with another virus, and exposure to ultraviolet light can reactivate the virus. Some HIV patients have experienced prolonged periods of latency and remained in good health for many years. For example, hepatitis C is known to have a latency period of 15 to 25 years.

Treatment of Viral Diseases

Viruses cause many clinically significant diseases in humans. Unfortunately, most viral diseases can be treated only *symptomatically,* that is, treating the *symptom,* not the infective cause.

Viruses cannot be grown on artificial culture media and *cannot* be destroyed by antibiotic drugs. General antibiotics are ineffective in preventing or curtailing viral infections. Even the few drugs that are effective against specific viruses have limitations because viruses often produce different types of infection, have different host cells, or can cause serious side effects.

Viruses are also capable of *mutation* (changing). Viruses can change so they are better suited to survive current conditions and resist efforts to kill them. It is very difficult to develop vaccines against viruses because of their ability to change their genetic code.

Transmission of Viral Diseases

Viral diseases are transmitted by (1) direct contact, (2) insects, (3) blood transfusions, (4) contaminated food or water, and (5) inhalation of droplets expelled by coughing or sneezing.

Viruses in the Environment

Viruses can be destroyed easily in the external environment. Widely used chemicals such as chlorine (bleach), iodine, phenol, and formaldehyde effectively destroy viruses on surfaces and objects coming into contact with the infected patient. These agents, however, are too toxic to be used internally (see Chapter 21).

VIRAL DISEASES

Viral Hepatitis

There are at least five types of viral hepatitis, each of which is caused by a different virus: hepatitis A virus (HAV), hepatitis B virus (HBV), hepatitis C virus (HCV), hepatitis D virus (HDV), and hepatitis E virus (HEV) (Table 18-1).

Frequently Asked Questions about Viral Hepatitis

Q. What is viral hepatitis?

A. Hepatitis is inflammation of the liver caused by a virus. There are five identified types of hepatitis, and each one is caused by a different virus. In the United States, hepatitis A, hepatitis B, and hepatitis C are the most common types.

Q. What are the symptoms of viral hepatitis?

A. The symptoms of newly acquired hepatitis A, B, and C are the same. If symptoms occur, they might include:

- tiredness
- loss of appetite
- nausea
- abdominal discomfort
- dark urine
- clay-colored bowel movements
- yellowing of the skin and eyes (jaundice)

Q. How long can HAV, HBV, and HCV survive outside the body?

A. HAV can live outside the body for months, depending on the environmental conditions.

HBV can survive outside the body for at least seven days and still be capable of transmitting infection.

HCV can survive outside the body and still transmit infection for 16 hours, but not longer than 4 days.

Q. How long is the HBV vaccine effective?

A. The HBV vaccine protects against chronic HBV infection for at least 15 years, even though antibodies may drop below detectable levels.

Q. Are booster doses of the HBV vaccine needed?

A. No, booster doses of the vaccine are not recommended routinely.

For more information on hepatitis and other bloodborne diseases, go to http://www.cdc.gov/ncidod/diseases/hepatitis

Modified from Centers for Disease Control and Prevention, National Center for Infectious Diseases.

Table 18-1 ***Primary Types of Hepatitis***

	A	B	C	D	E
Source of virus	fecal/oral	blood and body fluids	blood and body fluids	blood and body fluids	fecal/oral
Route of transmission	fecal/oral	percutaneous and mucosal tissues	percutaneous and mucosal tissues	percutaneous and mucosal tissues	fecal/oral
Chronic infection	no	yes	yes	yes	no
Prevention	vaccine	immunization	blood donor screening; modify risky behavior	HBV vaccine	ensure safe drinking water

Modified from Centers for Disease Control and Prevention, National Center for Infectious Diseases.

Hepatitis A

Hepatitis A virus (HAV) can affect anyone. It is spread from person to person by putting something in the mouth that has been contaminated with the stool of a person with hepatitis A. This type of transmission is called "fecal-oral." Good personal hygiene and proper sanitation can also help prevent hepatitis A. Always wash your hands after changing a diaper or using the bathroom. Hepatitis A is the least serious form of viral hepatitis. There is a vaccine available that provides long-term prevention in persons over two years of age.

Hepatitis B

Hepatitis B virus (HBV) causes a very serious disease that may result in prolonged illness, liver cancer, cirrhosis of the liver, liver failure, and even death. It is a bloodborne disease that may also be transmitted by other body fluids, including saliva.

Anyone who has ever had the disease, and some persons who have been exposed but have not actually been ill, may be carriers of HBV. This means that patients who appear to be healthy and have no history of the disease may actually be spreading the infection to others. HBV is responsible for 34 percent of all types of acute viral hepatitis. This presents a high risk for dental personnel because dental treatment brings them into contact with saliva and blood.

In addition, dental personnel may unknowingly be carriers of the disease. In this situation, there is always the risk of transmitting the infection to the patient during treatment.

Hepatitis B immunization

A highly effective vaccine is available to prevent hepatitis B. All dental personnel with a chance of occupational exposure should be vaccinated against hepatitis B. The Occupational Safety and Health Administration (OSHA) Bloodborne Pathogens Standard (BBP) (see Chapter 19) requires that an employer offer the hepatitis B vaccination, at no cost to the employee, within 10 days of initial assignment to a position in which there is chance of occupational exposure to blood and/or other body fluids. The employee has the right to refuse the offer of vaccination; however, that employee must sign a release form indicating that the employer offered the vaccine, and that the employee understands the potential risks of contracting hepatitis B.

Postvaccination testing is recommended one to six months after the third injection to be sure that the individual has developed the antibodies necessary for immunity. Should antibodies not be present, the three-dose series should be repeated.

The hepatitis B vaccine is considered safe for pregnant women.

Who Should Get the HBV Vaccine?

- All babies at birth
- All children 0-18 years of age who have not been vaccinated
- Persons of any age whose behavior puts them at risk for HBV infection
- Persons whose jobs expose them to human blood and/or body fluids

Hepatitis C

Hepatitis C virus (HCV) is most efficiently transmitted through blood transfusion or percutaneous exposure to blood. **Percutaneous** means performed through the skin. This can occur from an accidental needlestick to an employee in a dental office, or from sharing contaminated needles among injection drug users, or from contaminated tattoo needles. The carrier rate associated with HCV is higher than that associated with HBV. Unfortunately there is no vaccine against hepatitis C, nor is there a cure for the disease. However, there are effective treatments to control the effects of the disease. The primary concern of occupational exposure to HCV is through needlesticks or other percutaneous injuries.

Hepatitis D

Hepatitis D virus (HDV) is a defective virus that cannot replicate itself without the presence of HBV. Therefore, infection with HDV may occur simultaneously as a co-infection with HBV or may occur in an HBV carrier. Persons with a co-infection of HBV and HDV often have more severe acute disease and a higher risk of death compared with those infected with HBV alone. Vaccination against HBV will also prevent infection with HDV.

Hepatitis E

Hepatitis E virus (HEV) is not transmitted through bloodborne contact. It is most frequently transmitted via the fecal-oral routes through contaminated food or water. The disease is most frequently seen in the form of an epidemic in developing countries, and transmission is not a major concern in a standard dental setting.

Recall

10. Which types of hepatitis are spread by exposure to blood?

Human Immunodeficiency Virus

Human immunodeficiency virus (HIV) infection is a bloodborne viral disease. It is a disease in which the body's immune system breaks down. Acquired immunodeficiency syndrome (AIDS) is caused by HIV. When HIV enters the body, it infects special *T cells* and slowly kills them. T cells have special receptors on their surface and are primarily responsible for immunity. As more and more T cells die, the body's ability to fight the infection weakens.

A person with HIV infection may remain healthy for many years. HIV-positive people develop AIDS when they become sick with serious illnesses and infections that can occur with HIV. See Chapter 17 for the oral conditions that are frequently associated with HIV infection.

HIV is spread by sexual contact with an infected person, and by needle sharing among drug users. Before blood-donor screening for HIV, the virus was also transmitted by blood transfusion. Now that blood is screened for HIV antibodies, the blood supply is safe in this country. Babies born to HIV-infected mothers may become infected before or during birth, or through breastfeeding after birth.

In (nondental) healthcare settings, workers have been infected with HIV after being stuck with needles containing HIV-infected blood, or less frequently, after infected blood gets into the worker's bloodstream through an open cut or splashes into a mucous membrane (e.g., eyes or inside of the nose).

Types of Human Herpesviruses

Herpes simplex virus (HSV)	
Type 1 Herpes simplex virus	Causes primarily oral lesions
Type 2 Herpes simplex virus	Causes primarily genital lesions
Herpes zoster virus (HZV)	Causes herpes zoster, shingles, and chickenpox
Cytomegalovirus (CMV)	Normally latent (does not cause disease) but may become active when immune system is damaged. Once active, it is highly contagious and is transmitted in most body fluids.
Epstein-Barr virus (EBV)	Causes infectious mononucleosis and Burkitt's lymphoma, which is a malignancy of the lymph tissues

Herpesviruses

A **herpesvirus** is a double-stranded DNA virus that causes infections in humans such as herpes, CMV, chickenpox, shingles, mononucleosis, measles, and Kaposi's sarcoma. The virus may be dormant for years and then become activated and cause disease.

There are four major herpesviruses that affect humans:

1. *Herpes simplex virus* (HSV) is divided into two types: *herpes simplex virus type 1* (HSV 1), which causes primarily oral lesions, and *herpes simplex virus type 2* (HSV 2), which causes primarily genital lesions.
2. *Herpes zoster* or *varicella-zoster virus* (HZV) causes herpes zoster, shingles, and chickenpox.
3. The *cytomegalovirus* (CMV) is normally latent (does not produce disease) but may become active when the immune system is damaged (once active, it is highly contagious and is transmitted by most body fluids).
4. The *Epstein-Barr virus* (EBV) causes infectious mononucleosis and Burkitt's lymphoma, which is a malignant neoplasm involving lymphatic tissues.

Herpes Simplex Virus Type 1

Herpes simplex virus type 1 is a viral infection that causes recurrent sores on lips. Because these sores frequently develop when the patient has a cold or fever of other origin, the disease has become commonly known as *fever blisters* or *cold sores* (see Chapter 17).

Primary herpes

This disease, which is highly contagious, makes its first appearance in very young children (one to three years of age) and is known as *primary herpes.*

The child may have a slight fever, pain in the mouth, increased salivation, bad breath, and a general feeling of illness. The inside of the mouth becomes swollen, and the gingivae are inflamed.

Healing begins naturally within 3 days, and the illness is usually over in 7 to 14 days. During this time, supportive measures can be taken to make the child more comfortable, relieve the pain, and prevent secondary infection.

Recurrent herpes labialis

After this initial childhood infection, the virus of herpes simplex lies dormant and reappears later in life as the familiar recurring fever blister or cold sore (Fig. 18-10).

Recurrences tend to take place when the patient's general resistance is lowered as a result of stress, fever, illness, injury, and exposure to the sun. The use of sunscreen with a sun protection factor of 15 helps to prevent sun-induced recurrences of herpes.

Attacks may recur as infrequently as once a year or as often as weekly or even daily. As in the case of primary herpes, recurrent herpes labialis sores heal by themselves in 7 to 10 days, leaving no scar.

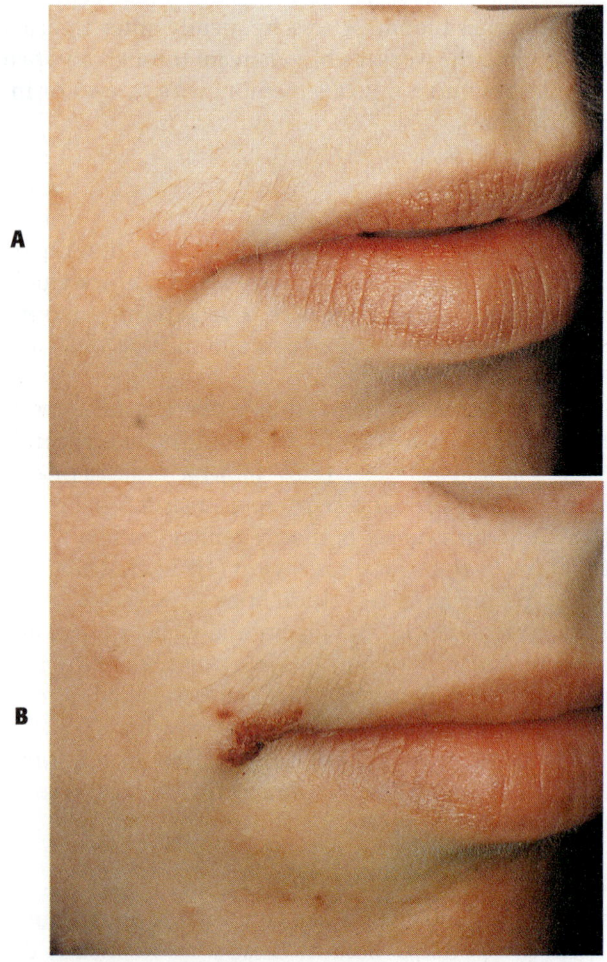

Fig. 18-10 **Herpes labialis. A, 12 hours after onset. B, 48 hours after onset.** (From Ibsen OA, Phelan JA: *Oral pathology for the dental hygienist,* ed 4, Philadelphia, 2004, Saunders.)

Herpes Simplex Virus Type 2

Herpes simplex virus type 2, also known as *genital herpes,* is one of the most common sexually transmitted diseases (STDs) in the United States. Initial symptoms, which generally appear 2 to 10 days after infection, include tingling, itching, and a burning sensation during urination.

Once a person is infected with the virus, outbreaks will recur. The disease can be transmitted only during these recurrences.

A mother with active vaginal or cervical herpetic lesions at the time of delivery can pass the virus to her newborn. About 50 percent of such newborns will be infected as they pass through the birth canal. Of the infants infected, at least 85 percent will be severely damaged or killed by the virus.

Herpes Zoster Virus

HZV (human herpesvirus type 3) causes both varicella (chickenpox) and herpes zoster (shingles). These are two different diseases but are caused by the identical organism. Chickenpox is the primary infection, and zoster is the reactivation of illness. It is a highly contagious infection in individuals who have not been previously exposed to the virus. Transmission occurs by direct contact with skin lesions or droplet infection from infectious saliva.

Cytomegalovirus

CMV (human herpesvirus type 5) rarely causes disease unless there are other factors present such as a compromised immune system. However it can infect the fetus during pregnancy. In some cases infants will be born deaf or suffer mental retardation later in life. The route of transmission of CMV is unclear.

Epstein-Barr Virus

EBV (human herpesvirus type 4) is responsible for a number of infections including infectious mononucleosis, nasopharyngeal cancer, lymphoma, and oral hairy leukoplakia (see Chapter 17). Infectious mononucleosis is an acute infectious disease that primarily affects people between the ages of 15 and 20 years. EBV is present in the saliva and is transmitted by kissing, hence it is often called the "kissing disease."

Herpes Transmission

The major transmission route for the herpesvirus is through direct contact with lesions or with infectious saliva. When oral lesions are present, the patient may be asked to reschedule his appointment for a time after the lesions have healed. Even when there are no active lesions, there is still a possibility of viral transmission through saliva or the aerosol spray from the dental handpiece.

Because there is no preventive vaccine to protect against herpes, it is essential that precautions be taken to prevent exposure.

Protective eyewear is particularly important because a herpes infection in the eye may cause blindness. Gloves protect against infection through lesions or abrasions on the hands.

West Nile Virus

The West Nile virus is commonly found in Africa, West Asia, and in the Middle East. It is believed to have been in the United States since the early summer of 1999. The virus is carried by mosquitoes and can infect humans, birds, horses, and some other mammals. It affects a person's nervous system, causing inflammation of the brain and spinal cord. Symptoms include fever, headache, tiredness, aches, and sometimes rash. Cases occur primarily in late summer or early fall. In southern climates where temperatures are milder, West Nile virus can be transmitted year-round.

Severe Acute Respiratory Syndrome

Severe acute respiratory syndrome (SARS) is a viral respiratory illness caused by a **coronavirus.** This is the same type of virus responsible for colds. SARS was first reported in Asia in 2003 where 774 people died from the disease. In the United States, only eight people had laboratory evidence of SARS infection, and these people had traveled to other parts of the world.

SARS is spread by close person-to-person contact. It is thought that the virus is transmitted by respiratory droplets spread when a person coughs or sneezes. The droplets are propelled up to three feet and land on the mucous membranes of the mouth, nose, or eyes of persons nearby. Symptoms of SARS include headache, overall discomfort, respiratory distress, and diarrhea. After two to seven days, SARS patients may develop a dry cough, and most patients develop pneumonia.

The Centers for Disease Control and Prevention (CDC) is working with state and local health departments and healthcare organizations to be prepared to respond quickly when, or if, SARS appears in the United States. The CDC has also issued alert notices to travelers who may have been exposed to cases of SARS.

Recall

11. How is HIV spread?
12. What tissues are affected by the West Nile virus?
13. How is SARS spread?

BACTERIAL DISEASES

Tuberculosis

Tuberculosis, which is caused by the bacterium *M. tuberculosis,* is the leading cause of death worldwide from infectious diseases.

Because HIV-infected patients have a weakened immune system, they are highly susceptible to tuberculosis; therefore, HIV and tuberculosis are often present together. Of the two, tuberculosis is a greater health risk for healthcare workers. One reason for this is that the rod-shaped tubercle bacillus is able to withstand disinfectants that kill many other bacteria. Tuberculosis kill time is the benchmark for the effectiveness of a surface disinfectant (see Chapter 20).

Legionnaires' Disease

The *Legionella pneumophila* bacterium (named after an epidemic of this disease during an American Legion convention in Philadelphia) is responsible for two acute bacterial diseases: *Pontiac fever* and *Legionnaires' disease.* The bacteria are transmitted through aerosolization and aspiration of contaminated water. (Chapter 24 discusses dental unit waterlines.)

There is no person-to-person transmission. The *L. pneumophila* bacteria have been found to thrive in lakes, creeks, hot tubs, spas, air-conditioning systems, shower heads, water distillation systems, and the biofilm found in dental unit waterlines (Fig. 18-11). Dental personnel have higher antibodies against *L. pneumophila* than the general public, indicating occupational exposure and resistance to this organism.

The least serious form of infection is called Pontiac fever and causes acute flulike symptoms with headache, high fever, dry cough, chills, diarrhea, chest pain, and abdominal pain.

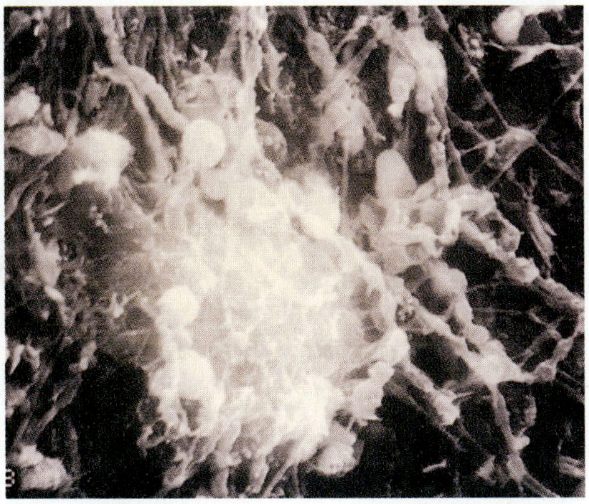

Fig. 18-11 Bacteria in biofilm taken from dental unit waterlines. (Courtesy Dr. Shannon Mills, USAF.)

The more serious form of infection is called Legionnaires' disease and causes a very severe pneumonia. In immunocompromised or elderly individuals, the disease can be fatal.

Tetanus

Tetanus, which is also known as *lockjaw,* is an extremely dangerous and often fatal disease that is caused by a spore-forming bacillus found in soil, dust, or animal or human feces.

This microbe is usually introduced into the body through a wound or break in the skin (as in a puncture wound from a soiled instrument).

The organism causing tetanus produces the severe muscle spasms and rigidity that give the disease its popular name of lockjaw. The disease can be prevented by the administration of a vaccine; however, immunity must be kept current through booster doses. (It is important that dental personnel keep all immunizations current.)

Syphilis

Syphilis, an STD, is caused by *Treponema pallidum* spirochetes. Although these bacteria are quite fragile outside of the body, there is danger of direct cross-infection in the dental operatory through contact with oral lesions.

The first stage of syphilis is the presence of a painless ulcerating sore, known as a **chancre,** which is infectious *on contact.* When it occurs on the lip, it may resemble herpes, but the crusting is darker (Fig. 18-12).

The second stage is also infectious, and immediate infection may occur through contact with an open sore. Signs of special interest to dental personnel are:

- Split papules at the corners of the mouth
- Grayish-white, moist, "mucous patches" on the tongue, roof of the mouth, tonsils, or inner surfaces of the lips (these are *highly infectious*)
- Generalized measles-type rash, poxlike pustules, oozing sores, and hair falling out of the scalp

The third stage, known as *latent syphilis,* is usually fatal, and it may occur after the disease has been dormant for 20 years.

Recall

14. What microorganism is used as the benchmark for the effectiveness of a surface disinfectant?

15. What disease is also known as lockjaw?

16. What is a sign of the first stage of syphilis?

A

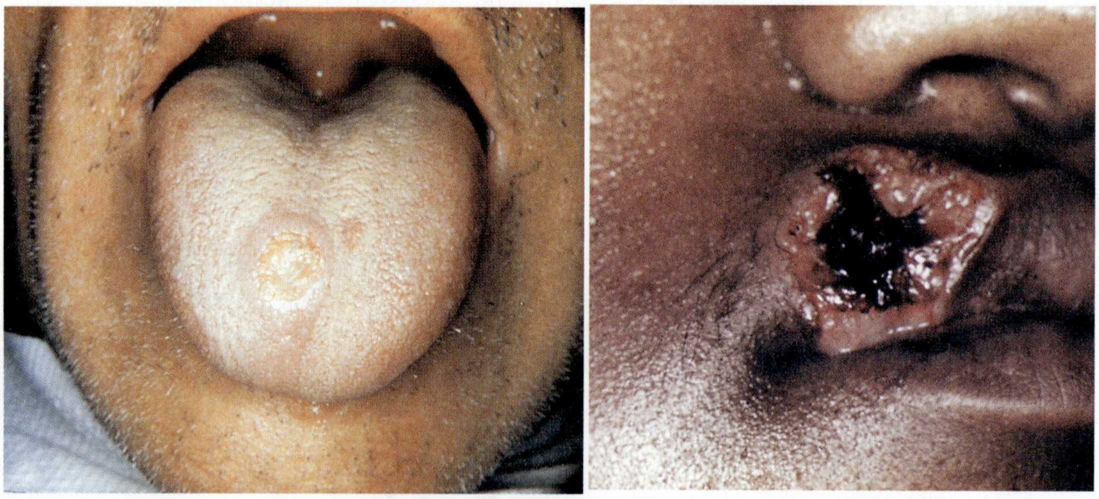

B

Fig. 18-12 **A,** Chancre on tongue seen in primary syphilis. **B,** Chancre on lip. (From Ibsen OA, Phelan JA: *Oral pathology for the dental hygienist,* ed 4, Philadelphia, 2004, Saunders. **A,** Courtesy Dr. Norman Trieger; **B,** Courtesy Dr. Edward V. Zegarelli.)

Legal and Ethical Implications

As people travel across the country and around the world, the microorganisms they carry travel with them. The patients you see in the office bring with them a variety of microorganisms.

Dental assistants must be especially aware of their daily encounters with microorganisms and the possible consequences. Understanding the microbial world is part of the dental assistant's personal and professional responsibility.

Today many patients are concerned about possible disease transmission in the dental office. To assure patients, the dental assistant should be prepared to discuss all aspects of the office's infection-control procedures. To do this requires an understanding of microbiology and the characteristics of microorganisms.

Eye to the Future

Progress in developing drugs to treat viral diseases such as HIV infection and hepatitis has been slow and difficult. This is because it is difficult to find drugs capable of killing the viruses without hurting the host cell. Antiviral agents must reach target organs without disturbing the cell functions of the host. Progress is being made in the development of drugs for the management of HIV and HCV.

Research continues to find antiviral agents that will target only the enzymes responsible for the replication of the virus in infected cells. Often, drugs used in combinations can delay or prevent the disease. The hope for a cure or prevention of all forms of hepatitis and HIV infection through vaccines lies with drugs as yet undeveloped.

Critical Thinking

1. On your next trip to the supermarket, look for the foods that have been through the process of pasteurization.
2. How would you answer a friend who asked, "Why are you studying microbiology?"
3. Do you think the world would be a better place if there were no bacteria? Why or why not?
4. Should physicians prescribe antibiotics for viral infections? Why or why not?

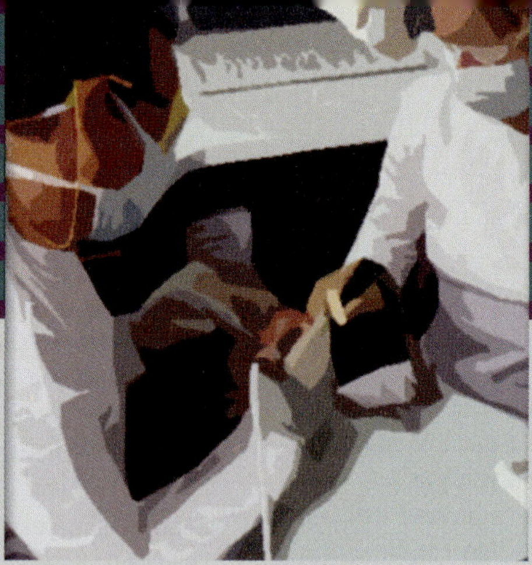

19 Disease Transmission and Infection Control

Outline

KEY TERMS

Acquired immunity Immunity that is developed during a person's lifetime.

Acute infection An infection of short duration that is often severe.

Anaphylaxis (a-neh-fah-**lak**-sis) Extreme hypersensitivity to a substance that can lead to shock and life-threatening respiratory collapse.

Artificially acquired immunity Immunity that results from a vaccination.

Bloodborne disease Disease such as HBV, HCV, or HIV infection that is caused by microorganisms such as viruses or bacteria that are carried in blood.

Bloodborne pathogens Disease-causing organisms transferred through contact with blood or other bodily fluids.

Chronic infection An infection of long duration.

Communicable disease Condition caused by an infection that can be spread from person to person or from contact with body fluids.

Contaminated waste Items such as gloves and patient napkins that may contain the potentially infectious body fluids of patients.

Direct contact Touching or contact with a patient's blood or saliva.

Droplet infection Infection that occurs through mucosal surfaces of the eyes, nose, or mouth.

Epidemiologic studies (ep-i-de-mi-o-**log**-ic) Study of the patterns and causes of diseases.

Hazardous waste Waste posing a danger to humans or the environment.

Immunity (i-**mu**-neh-tee) Ability of the body to resist disease.

Indirect contact Touching or contact with a contaminated surface or instrument.

Infectious disease Disease that is communicable.

Infectious waste Waste that is capable of transmitting an infectious disease.

Inherited immunity Immunity that is present at birth.

Latent infection (**lay**-tunt) Persistent infection with recurrent symptoms that "come and go."

Naturally acquired immunity Immunity that occurs when a person has contracted and is recovering from a disease.

Occupational exposure Any reasonably anticipated skin, eye, or mucous membrane contact or percutaneous injury with blood or any other potentially infectious materials.

OSHA Bloodborne Pathogens Standard Guidelines designed to protect employees against occupational exposure to bloodborne pathogens.

Pathogen (**pa**-thah-jen) Disease-causing organism.

Percutaneous (per-kew-**tay**-nee-us) Through the skin, such as a needlestick, cut, or human bite.

Permucosal (per-mu-**ko**-sul) Contact with mucous membranes, such as the eyes or mouth.

Personal protective equipment (PPE) Items such as protective clothing, masks, gloves, and eyewear used to protect employees.

Sharps Pointed or cutting instruments, including needles, scalpel blades, orthodontic wires, and endodontic instruments.

Standard Precautions Standard of care designed to protect healthcare providers from pathogens that can be spread by blood or any other body fluid, excretion, or secretion; expands upon the concept of Universal Precautions.

Universal Precautions Guidelines based on treating all human blood and body fluids (including saliva) as potentially infectious.

Virulence (**vir**-eh-lents) Strength of a pathogen's ability to cause disease; also known as *pathogenicity.*

LEARNING OUTCOMES

On completion of this chapter, the student will be able to achieve the following objectives:

- Pronounce, define, and spell the Key Terms.
- Describe the roles of the CDC and OSHA in infection control.
- Explain the difference between Universal Precautions and Standard Precautions.
- Describe the differences between a chronic infection and an acute infection.
- Describe the types of immunity, and give examples of each.
- Give an example of a latent infection.
- Identify links in the chain of infection.
- Describe the methods of disease transmission in a dental office.
- Describe the components of an OSHA Exposure Control Plan.
- Explain the rationale for standard precautions.
- Identify the OSHA categories of risk for occupational exposure.
- Describe the first aid necessary after an exposure incident.
- Discuss the rationale for hepatitis B vaccination for dental assistants.
- Explain the importance of hand care for dental assistants.
- Explain proper hand hygiene for dental assistants.
- Explain the advantages of alcohol-based hand rubs.
- Discuss the types of PPE needed for dental assistants.
- Demonstrate the proper sequence for donning and removing personal protective equipment.
- Identify the various types of gloves used in a dental office.
- Explain the types and symptoms of latex reactions.
- Describe the proper handling and disposal methods for each type of waste generated in dentistry.
- Explain the CDC recommendations regarding the use of a saliva ejector.
- Describe the rationale of CDC recommendations regarding Creutzfeldt-Jakob disease and other prion-related diseases.
- Describe the rationale of CDC recommendations regarding laser plumes.
- Explain the precautions necessary when treating an active tuberculosis patient.

The dental assistant is at risk of exposure to disease agents through contact with blood or other potentially infectious body fluids. In this chapter you will learn how to break the chain of infection, recognize the methods of disease transmission, and understand how the immune system provides the body with resistance to infections.

This chapter discusses the new *CDC Infection Control Guidelines* and the requirements of the **OSHA Bloodborne Pathogens (BBP) Standard.** By carefully following the infection-control and safety information in this chapter, you can minimize the risks of disease transmission to yourself, your patients, and other members of the dental team.

CDC Overview of the CDC Infection-Control Recommendations for Dentistry

- Personnel Health Elements of an Infection-Control Program
- Prevention of Transmission of Bloodborne Pathogens
- Prevention of Exposure to Blood and other Potentially Infectious Materials
- Hand Hygiene
- Personal Protective Equipment
- Contact Dermatitis and Latex Sensitivity
- Environmental Infection Control
- Dental Unit Waterlines, Biofilms, and Water Quality
- Boil-Water Notices
- Dental Handpieces and Other Devices Attached to Air and Water Lines
- Dental Radiology
- Aseptic Technique for Parenteral Medications
- Single-Use Disposable Devices
- Oral Surgical Procedures
- Handling of Extracted Teeth
- Dental Laboratory
- *Mycobacterium tuberculosis* Program Evaluation

NOTE: These recommendations are summarized in Chapters 18, 19, 20, and 21, and are available in total from the CDC at oralhealth@cdc.gov, or by phone: 770-488-6054, or by fax: 770-488-6080.

NOTE: *Throughout the text in this chapter, CDC recommendations are indicated and the category of scientific evidence is noted at the end of each recommendation.*

THE CHAIN OF INFECTION

The life and growth of **pathogens** (disease-causing organisms) is a *cycle,* or a chain. Break any link in the chain, and you break the infectious process. The chain of infection consists of four parts: (1) virulence, (2) number of microorganisms, (3) susceptible host, and (4) portal of entry (Fig. 19-1).

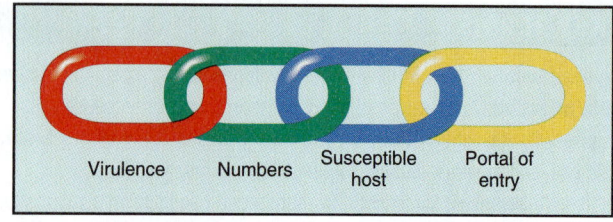

Fig. 19-1 At least one part must be removed to break the chain of infection.

Virulence

The **virulence** of an organism refers to the degree of *pathogenicity* or strength of that organism in its ability to produce disease. Because the body cannot change the virulence of microorganisms, persons must rely on their body defenses and specific immunizations, such as for hepatitis B virus (HBV). Another defense is to avoid coming in contact with microorganisms by always following the infection-control techniques described in this chapter.

Number of Microorganisms

To cause disease, there must be a high enough number of pathogenic microorganisms present to overwhelm the body's defenses. The number of pathogens may be directly related to the amount of bioburden present. *Bioburden* refers to organic materials such as blood and saliva. The use of the dental dam and high-volume evacuation helps to minimize bioburden on surfaces and thereby reduces the number of microorganisms in the aerosol.

Susceptible Host

A susceptible host is a person who is unable to resist infection by the pathogen. An individual who is in poor health, is chronically fatigued and under extreme stress, or has a weakened immune system is more likely to become infected. Therefore, staying healthy, washing the hands frequently, and keeping immunizations up-to-date will help members of the dental team to resist infection and stay healthy.

Portal of Entry

To cause infection, the pathogens must have a portal of entry, or means of entering the body. The portals of entry for *airborne pathogens* are through the mouth and nose. **Bloodborne pathogens** must have access to the blood supply as a means of entry into the body. This can occur through a break in the skin caused by a needlestick, a cut, or even a human bite. It can also occur through the mucous membranes of the nose and oral cavity.

TYPES OF INFECTIONS

Acute Infection

In an **acute infection,** symptoms are often severe and usually appear soon after the initial infection occurs. Acute infections are of *short duration.* For example, with a viral infection such as the common cold, the body's defense mechanisms usually eliminate the virus within two to three weeks.

Chronic Infection

Chronic infections are those in which the microorganism is present for a *long duration;* some may persist for life. The person may be *asymptomatic* (not showing symptoms of the disease) but may still be a carrier of the disease, as with hepatitis C virus (HCV) or human immunodeficiency virus (HIV) infection.

Latent Infection

A **latent infection** is a persistent infection in which the symptoms "come and go." Cold sores (oral herpes simplex) and genital herpes are latent viral infections.

The virus first enters the body and causes the original lesion. It then lies dormant, away from the surface, in a nerve cell, until certain conditions (such as illness with fever, sunburn, and stress) cause the virus to leave the nerve cell and seek the surface again. Once the virus reaches the surface, it becomes detectable for a short time and causes another outbreak at that site.

Another herpesvirus, *herpes zoster,* causes chickenpox. This virus may lie dormant and later erupt as the painful disease shingles.

Opportunistic Infection

Opportunistic infections are caused by normally nonpathogenic organisms and occur in individuals whose resistance is decreased or compromised. For example, an individual recovering from influenza may develop pneumonia or an ear infection. Opportunistic infections are common in patients with autoimmune disease or diabetes and in elderly persons.

MODES OF DISEASE TRANSMISSION

Before you can prevent disease transmission in the dental office, you must first understand how infectious diseases are spread.

An **infectious disease** is one that is *communicable* or *contagious.* These terms mean that the disease can be transmitted (spread) in some way from one host to another (Fig. 19-2).

Primary Modes of Disease Transmission in Dentistry

Direct contact: Touching or contact with the patient's blood or other body fluids.

Indirect contact: Touching or contact with a contaminated surface or instrument.

Droplet infection: An infection that occurs through mucosal surfaces of the eyes, nose, or mouth.

Parenteral transmission: Needlestick injuries, human bites, cuts, abrasions, or any break in the skin.

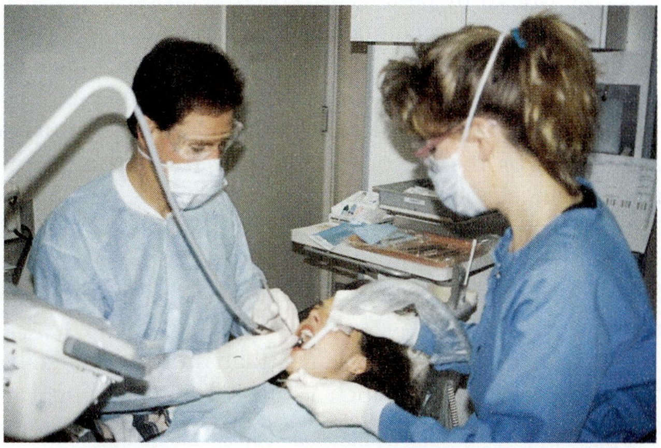

Fig. 19-2 Pathogens can be transferred from staff to patient, patient to staff, and patient to patient from contaminated equipment.

Direct Transmission

Pathogens can be transferred by coming into direct contact with the infectious lesion or infected body fluids, including blood, saliva, semen, and vaginal secretions. Many viruses and pathogenic bacteria are transmitted directly and cause hepatitis, herpes infection, HIV infection, and tuberculosis.

Exposure to blood and saliva is of particular concern for dental workers during dental treatment. Although blood may not be visible in the saliva, it often is present.

Indirect Transmission

The indirect transfer of organisms to a susceptible person can occur by handling contaminated instruments or touching contaminated surfaces and then touching the face, eyes, or mouth. It is important to wash your hands frequently to avoid indirect transmission of microorganisms.

Splash or Spatter

Blood, saliva, or nasopharyngeal (nasal) secretions can be sprayed or spattered during dental procedures. Diseases can be transmitted during a dental procedure by splashing the mucosa (mouth or eyes) or nonintact skin with blood or blood-contaminated saliva.

Intact skin, which is not broken in any way, acts as a natural protective barrier. *Nonintact skin,* in which there is a cut, scrape, or needlestick injury, provides an entrance for pathogens into the body.

Airborne Transmission

Airborne transmission, also known as *droplet infection,* is the spread of disease through droplets of moisture containing bacteria or viruses. Most of the contagious respiratory diseases are caused by pathogens carried in droplets of moisture. Some of these pathogens are carried long distances through the air and ventilation systems. Airborne transmission can also occur when someone coughs or sneezes.

Aerosols containing saliva, blood, and microorganisms are created by the use of the high-speed handpiece, air-water syringe, and ultrasonic scaler during dental procedures. Inhaling the bacteria and debris in the aerosol (without the protection of a facemask) is comparable to having someone sneeze in your face twice a minute at a distance of 1 foot.

Mists are droplet particles larger than those generated by the aerosol spray. Mists, such as those from coughing, can transmit respiratory infections. However, mists do not appear to transmit hepatitis B virus or HIV despite being inhaled.

Spatter consists of large droplet particles contaminated with blood, saliva, and other debris. Spatter is created during all restorative and hygiene procedures involving rotary and ultrasonic dental instruments. Use of the air-water syringe may also produce spatter.

Spatter droplets travel farther than the aerosol mist and tend to land on the upper surfaces of the wrist and forearms, upper arms, and chest. Droplets may also reach the necktie/collar area of the dentist, assistant, or hygienist.

Parenteral Transmission

Parenteral means through the skin, as with cuts or punctures. Parenteral transmission of bloodborne pathogens (disease-causing organisms transferred through contact with blood or other bodily fluids) can occur through needlestick injuries, human bites, cuts, abrasions, or any break in the skin.

Bloodborne Transmission

Certain pathogens, referred to as *bloodborne,* are carried in the blood and body fluids of infected individuals and can be transmitted to others. Bloodborne transmission occurs through direct or indirect contact with blood and other body fluids. Saliva is of particular concern during dental treatment because it frequently is contaminated with blood. Remember, although blood is not visible in the saliva, it may be present.

Improperly sterilized instruments and equipment can transfer all bloodborne diseases. Individuals sharing needles while using illegal drugs easily transmit these diseases to each other. Unprotected sex is another common method of transmission of bloodborne disease.

Common bloodborne microorganisms of concern in dentistry include HCV, HBV, and HIV. Because dental treatment often involves contact with blood and always with saliva, bloodborne diseases are of major concern in the dental office.

Food and Water Transmission

Many diseases are transmitted by contaminated food that has not been cooked or refrigerated properly and water that has been contaminated with human or animal fecal material. For example, tuberculosis, botulism, and staphylococcal and streptococcal infections are spread by contaminated food or water.

Fecal-Oral Transmission

Many pathogens are present in fecal matter. If proper sanitation procedures, such as handwashing after use of the toilet, are not followed, these pathogens may be transmitted directly by touching another person or transmitted indirectly by contact with contaminated surfaces or food.

Fecal-oral transmission occurs most often among healthcare and day care workers (who frequently change diapers) and by careless food handlers.

THE IMMUNE SYSTEM

The immune system is responsible for providing resistance to communicable diseases. A **communicable disease** is a condition caused by an infection that can be spread from person to person or from contact with body fluids.

Immunity allows the body to resist disease and prevent foreign bodies from causing infection. When immunity is present at birth, it is called **inherited immunity.** Immunity that is developed during a person's lifetime is called **acquired immunity.** Acquired immunity can occur either naturally or artificially (Fig. 19-3).

Naturally Acquired Immunity

Naturally acquired immunity occurs when a person previously contracted a disease and recovered. When the

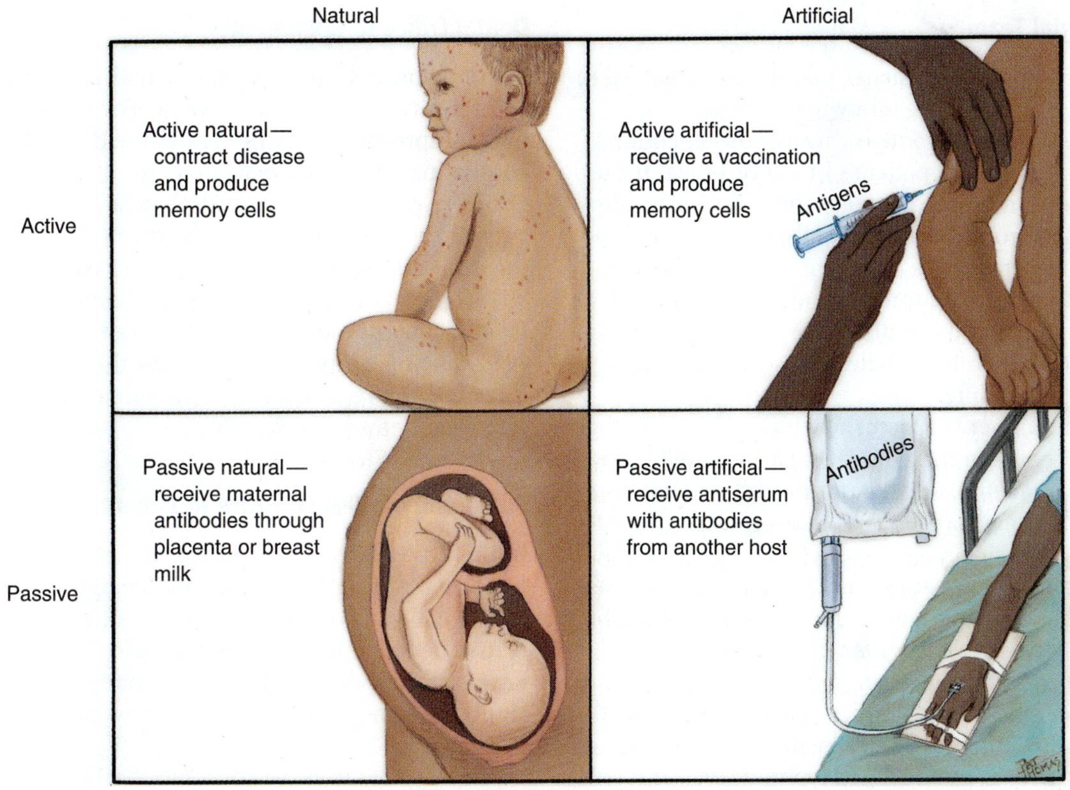

Fig. 19-3 Acquired immunity. (From Applegate EJ: *The anatomy and physiology learning system,* ed 2, Philadelphia, 2000, Saunders.)

Immunizations Strongly Recommended for Healthcare Personnel

Hepatitis B
Influenza
Measles
Mumps
Rubella
Varicella-zoster

Modified from *CDC Guidelines for Infection Control in Dental Health-Care Settings–2003.*

body was fighting the invading pathogen, it formed antibodies that provide future resistance against that particular pathogen. This form of immunity is called *active immunity,* because the body of the host is actively involved in the process.

Another type, *passive immunity,* occurs during pregnancy when the fetus receives antibodies from the mother's placenta. Passive immunity also occurs when the mother breastfeeds the infant. It is called "passive" immunity because the antibodies are acquired from an outside source.

Artificially Acquired Immunity

When the human body has not been exposed to a disease, it has not developed antibodies and is completely defenseless against the disease. However, antibodies can be introduced into the body artificially by *immunization* or *vaccination.*

A vaccine containing weakened disease-causing organisms or genetically engineered organisms is injected into the body. The harmful characteristics of the disease-producing organisms are eliminated from the vaccine to make them less likely to cause disease. The body then forms antibodies in response to the vaccine, resulting in **artificially acquired immunity.**

DISEASE TRANSMISSION IN THE DENTAL OFFICE

Disease transmission in the dental office can occur in a variety of ways as described below:

- Patient to dental team
- Dental team to patient
- Patient to patient
- Dental office to community (includes dental team's family)
- Community to dental office to patient

Patient to Dental Team

Microorganisms from the patient's mouth can be passed to the dental team through the following routes:

1. The most common route is through **direct contact** (touching) with the patient's blood or saliva. If the dental team member has cuts, abrasions, or breaks in the skin around the fingernails, microorganisms may gain entrance.
2. **Droplet infection** is through mucosal surfaces of the eyes, nose, and mouth. It can occur when the dental team member inhales aerosol generated by the dental handpiece or air-water syringe.
3. **Indirect contact** can occur when the team member touches a contaminated surface or instrument. Cuts or punctures with contaminated needles, burs, instruments, or files may also result in disease transmission.

Infection-control measures that help prevent disease transmission from the patient to the dental team member include *(1) gloves, (2) handwashing, (3) masks, (4) rubber dams,* and *(5) patient mouthrinses.*

Always remember, a patient may be a carrier of a disease. Carrier-transmitted diseases include certain types of viral hepatitis, herpes, tuberculosis, typhoid fever, and HIV, among others.

Dental Team to Patient

Fortunately, the spread of disease from a member of the dental team to a patient is very unlikely to happen. If proper procedures are not followed, however, disease transmission could occur.

Team-to-patient transmission can result if the dental team member has lesions on the hands, or if the hands are cut while in the patient's mouth, transferring microorganisms. Droplet infection of the patient can occur if the dental team member has a cold, but this can also occur outside the dental office.

Infection-control measures that help prevent team-to-patient transmission include: (1) masks, (2) gloves, (3) handwashing, and (4) immunization.

Patient to Patient

Patient-to-patient disease transmission has occurred in the medical field, but no cases of this type of transmission have yet been documented in dentistry. Although this transmission can occur, contamination from instruments used on one patient would need to be transferred to another patient.

Infection-control measures that can prevent patient-to-patient transmission include: (1) instrument sterilization, (2) surface barriers, (3) handwashing, (4) gloves, and (5) use of sterile instruments.

Dental Office to Community

Microorganisms can leave the dental office and enter the community in a variety of ways. For example, contaminated impressions may be sent to the dental laboratory, or contaminated equipment may be sent out for repair. Office-to-community transmission can also occur if members of the dental team transport microorganisms out of the office on their clothing or in their hair.

Infection-control measures that help prevent organisms from leaving the dental office include: (1) handwashing, (2) changing clothes before leaving the office, and (3) disinfecting impressions and contaminated equipment before such items leave the office.

Community to Dental Office to Patient

In this type of disease transmission, microorganisms enter the dental office through the municipal water that supplies the dental unit. Waterborne organisms colonize the inside of the dental unit waterlines and form *biofilm.* As water flows through the handpiece, air-water syringe, and ultrasonic scaler, a patient could swallow contaminated water (see Chapter 24).

Recall

1. What is the most common route of contamination?
2. What is the term for acquiring an infection through mucosal tissues?
3. What infection-control measures help prevent disease transmission from the dental team to the patient?

ROLES AND RESPONSIBILITIES OF THE CDC AND OSHA IN INFECTION CONTROL

The Centers for Disease Control and Prevention (CDC) and the Occupational Safety and Health Administration (OSHA) are federal agencies that play very important roles in infection control for dentistry (see Chapter 22).

The CDC is *not* a regulatory agency. Its role is to issue specific *recommendations* based on sound scientific evidence on health-related matters. In 1986, the CDC issued the first recommendations for the dental profession to prevent the transmission of bloodborne diseases. Although the CDC's recommendations are not law, they establish a standard of care for the dental profession.

OSHA *is* a regulatory agency. Its role is to issue specific *standards* to protect the health of employees in the United

States. In 1991, based on CDC guidelines, OSHA issued the BBP Standard. Failure to comply with OSHA requirements can have serious consequences including heavy fines.

As a dental assistant, it is important to follow *all* of the guidelines and recommendations.

CDC GUIDELINES FOR INFECTION CONTROL IN DENTAL HEALTH-CARE SETTINGS

In December 2003, the CDC released the *Guidelines for Infection Control in Dental Health-Care Settings—2003* (Fig. 19-4). The previous guidelines were issued in 1993 and primarily addressed the prevention of bloodborne diseases such as HIV disease and hepatitis B and C.

The new guidelines have expanded upon the existing OSHA BBP Standard, and have included some areas that were *not* already covered. They were developed in collaboration with experts on infection control from the CDC and other public agencies, and also had input from private and professional organizations. The guidelines are based on scientific evidence and are categorized on the basis of existing scientific data, theoretical rationale, and applicability.

CDC Rankings of Evidence

Each recommendation made by the CDC is categorized on the basis of existing scientific data, theoretical rationale, and applicability. Rankings are based on the following categories:

- **Category IA** Strongly recommended for implementation and strongly supported by well-designed experimental, clinical, or **epidemiologic studies** (studies of patterns and causes of diseases).
- **Category IB** Strongly recommended for implementation and supported by experimental, clinical, or epidemiological studies and a strong theoretical rationale.
- **Category IC** Required for implementation, as mandated by federal or state regulation or standard.
- **Category II** Suggested for implementation and supported by suggestive clinical or epidemiologic studies or a theoretical rationale.
- **Unresolved Issue** No recommendation. Practices for which insufficient evidence or no consensus regarding efficacy exists.

The guidelines apply to *all* paid or unpaid dental health professionals who might be occupationally exposed to blood and body fluids by direct contact or through contact with contaminated environmental surfaces, water, or air.

Although not law, the CDC *Guidelines for Infection Control in Dental Health-Care Settings* are now the standard of care.

CDC Overview of *CDC Guidelines for Infection Control in Dental Health-Care Settings–2003*

- Use of Standard Precautions rather than Universal Precautions.
- Work restrictions for health-care personnel infected with infectious diseases.
- Postexposure management of occupational exposures to bloodborne pathogens (HBV, HIV, HCV).
- Selection of devices with sharps injury–prevention features
- Hand hygiene products and surgical hand asepsis
- Contact dermatitis and latex hypersensitivity
- Sterilization of unwrapped instruments
- Dental-unit waterline concerns
- Dental radiology infection control
- Aseptic technique for injectable medications
- Preprocedural mouthrinses for patients
- Oral surgical procedures
- Laser/electrosurgery plumes
- Tuberculosis
- Creutzfeldt-Jakob disease and other prion-related diseases
- Infection-control program evaluation
- Research considerations

Modified from *CDC Guidelines for Infection Control in Dental Health-Care Settings–2003.* Copies of these guidelines may be requested at oralhealth@cdc.gov, or by phone: 770-488-6054 or by fax: 770-488-6080.

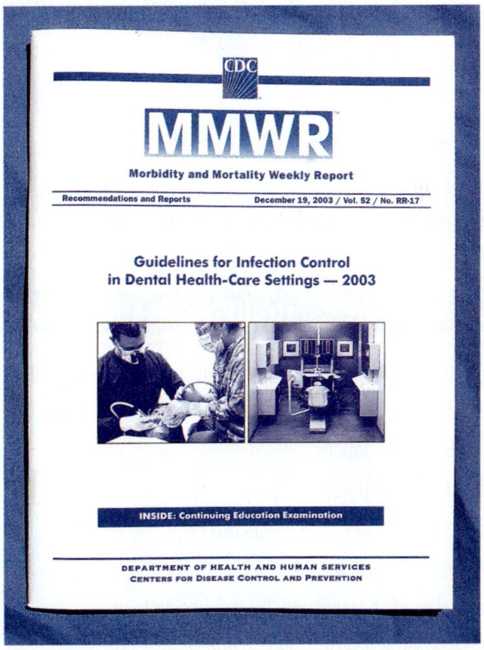

Fig. 19-4 The December 19, 2003, issue of *Morbidity and Mortality Weekly Report* includes the *CDC Guidelines for Infection Control in Dental Health-Care Settings–2003.*

NOTE: *Portions of the new guidelines are expansions of or not included in OSHA's BBP Standard. In some cases, only a word or two has been added. In others, a significant amount of new information has been added.*

OSHA BLOODBORNE PATHOGENS STANDARD

OSHA's BBP Standard is the most important infection-control law in dentistry. It is designed to protect employees against occupational exposure to bloodborne, disease-causing organisms, such as HBV, HCV, and HIV.

The BBP requires employers to protect their employees from exposure to blood and *other potentially infectious material* (OPIM) in the workplace and to provide proper care to the employee if an exposure should occur. The standard applies to any type of facility in which employees might be exposed to blood and other body fluids, including dental and medical offices, hospitals, funeral homes, emergency medical services, and nursing homes.

OSHA requires that a copy of the BBP Standard be present in every dental office and clinic. A copy of the OSHA BBP Standard may be obtained by visiting http://www.osha.gov/SLTC/bloodbornepathogens/index/html.

Exposure-Control Plan

Each dental office must have a written exposure-control plan that clearly describes how that office complies with the BBP Standard. The exposure-control plan must be reviewed and updated at least annually. A copy must be accessible to all employees.

Standard and Universal Precautions

The term *Universal Precautions* is still referred to in the OSHA BBP Standard. **Universal Precautions** is based on the concept that all human blood and body fluids (including saliva) are to be treated as if known to be infected with the **bloodborne diseases** hepatitis B, hepatitis C, or HIV infection. The rationale for this concept is that it is not possible to identify those individuals who are infectious, so Universal Precautions were to be used for all healthcare personnel and their patients.

The CDC expanded the concept and changed the term to *Standard Precautions.* **Standard Precautions** integrate and expand the elements of Universal Precautions into a standard of care designed to protect healthcare providers from pathogens that can be spread by *blood or any other body fluid, excretion, or secretion.* Saliva has always been considered a potentially infectious material in dental infection control; therefore there is no difference in clinical dental practices between Universal Precautions and Standard Precautions. Standard Precautions apply to contact with:

- Blood
- All body fluids, secretions, and excretions except sweat, regardless of whether or not they contain blood
- Nonintact skin
- Mucous membranes

Written Exposure-Control Plan Required by OSHA

General policy of implementing Centers for Disease Control and Prevention guidelines and American Dental Association infection-control recommendations

- Use of universal precautions
- Required use of personal protective equipment
- Standardized housekeeping
- Laundering of contaminated protective clothing
- Standardized policy on cleaning and disinfection
- Policy on general waste disposal
- Labeling procedure (secondary labeling)
- Policy on sterilization (including monitoring) and disinfection
- Use of sharps containers and disposal system
- Standardized handwashing protocol
- HBV vaccination
- Postexposure evaluation and medical follow-up

CDC Standard Precautions

- Wash hands before and after every patient. (IA and IC)
- Wear gloves when touching blood, body fluids, secretions, and contaminated items.
- Use care when handling sharps. (IA and IC)
- Wear a mask and eye protection, or a face shield during procedures likely to generate splashes or sprays. (IA and IC)
- Carefully handle contaminated patient-care items to prevent the transfer of microorganisms to people or equipment. (IA and IC)
- Use a mouthpiece or other ventilation device as an alternative to mouth-to-mouth resuscitation when practical. (IA and IC)
- Standard Precautions must be used in the treatment of all patients. (IA and IC)

Categories of Employees

The OSHA BBP Standard requires employers to categorize tasks and procedures during which an employee might have an occupational exposure (Table 19-1).

The BBP defines an **occupational exposure** as "any reasonably anticipated skin, eye, mucous membrane contact, or percutaneous injury with blood or any other potentially infectious materials." **Percutaneous** (through the skin, such as needlesticks, cuts, and human bites) and **permucosal** (contact with mucous membranes, such as the eyes or mouth) exposures to blood, saliva, and other body fluids pose the greatest risk for transmission of HIV, HBV, and HCV.

Postexposure Management

Despite efforts to prevent occupational exposure incidents, accidents happen. Therefore, before an accident occurs, the BBP Standard requires the employer to have a written plan. This plan explains exactly what steps the employee must follow after the exposure incident occurs and the type of medical follow-up that will be provided to the employee at no charge.

The employer must provide training to employees on the proper response to an exposure incident. Procedure 19-1 reviews first-aid steps after exposure.

Employee Training

The BBP Standard requires the dentist/employer to provide training in infection-control and safety issues to all personnel who may come in contact with blood, saliva, or contaminated instruments or surfaces. The employer must keep records of all training sessions. The record of each training session must include the date of the session, the name of the presenter, the topic, and the names of all employees who attended.

Hepatitis B Immunization

The BBP Standard requires the dentist/employer to offer the HBV vaccination series to all employees whose jobs include categories I and II tasks. The vaccine must be offered

Follow-up Measures for Exposed Worker*

Confidential medical counseling

HIV test series immediately and at 6 weeks, 12 weeks, and 6 months

HBV immune globulin (if no prior HBV vaccination)

Tetanus booster

Documentation of incident on appropriate OSHA form

*Services must be offered without charge.
From Robinson D, Bird D: *Essentials of dental assisting,* ed 3, Philadelphia, 2000, Saunders.

Table 19-1 ***Occupational Exposure Determination***

Category	Definition	Example
I	Routinely exposed to blood, saliva, or both	Dentist, dental hygienist, dental assistant, sterilization assistant, dental laboratory technician
II	May on occasion be exposed to blood, saliva, or both	Receptionist or office manager who may occasionally clean a treatment room or handle instruments or impressions
III	Never exposed to blood, saliva, or both	Financial manager, insurance clerk, or computer operator

Procedure 19-1 First Aid after an Exposure Incident

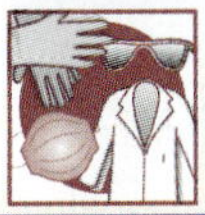
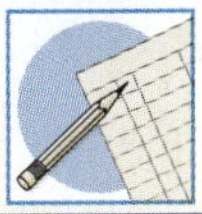

Goal

To perform appropriate first aid after an exposure incident.

Equipment and Supplies

- Soap and water
- Paper towels
- Antiseptic cream or ointment
- Adhesive bandage
- Exposure incident report form

PROCEDURAL STEPS

1. Stop operations immediately.
2. Remove your gloves.
3. If the area of broken skin is bleeding, gently squeeze the site to express a small amount of visible blood.
4. Wash your hands thoroughly, using antimicrobial soap and warm water.
5. Dry your hands.
6. Apply a small amount of antiseptic to the affected area.
   Note: Do not apply caustic agents such as bleach or disinfectant solutions to the wound.

1. Apply an adhesive bandage to the area.
2. Complete applicable postexposure follow-up steps.
   Note: The employer should be notified of the injury immediately after initial first aid is provided.

within 10 days of assignment to a category I or II job. To document compliance, the dentist/employer must obtain proof from the physician who administered the vaccination to the employee.

The employee has the right to refuse the HBV vaccine for any reason. The employee is then required to sign an *informed refusal* form that is kept on file in the dental office. Even if the employee originally signed the refusal form, the employee always has the right to reverse the decision and receive the vaccine at a later date at no charge.

CDC Postvaccine Testing

Between one and two months after the series has been completed, a blood test should be performed to ensure that the individual has developed immunity. Individuals who have not developed immunity should be evaluated by their physician to determine the need for an additional dose of HBV vaccine. Individuals who do not respond to the second three-dose series of the vaccine should be counseled regarding their susceptibility to HBV infection and precautions to take. (IA and IC)

Need for a Booster

The CDC does *not* recommend routine booster doses of the HBV vaccine, nor does it recommend routine blood testing to monitor the HBV antibody level in individuals who have already had the vaccine. This is assuming that the individual was tested after receiving the vaccine and was known to have initially developed antibodies. An exception is the immunized individual who has a documented exposure incident and for whom the attending physician orders a booster dose.

Management of an Exposure Incident*

1. Document the route(s) of exposure and the circumstances in which the incident occurred (for example, cut, needlestick, or blood splash).
2. Identify and document the *source individual* (patient whose blood or body fluid is involved in the exposure incident), unless the employer can establish that identification is not possible or is prohibited by state or local law.
3. Request that the source individual have his or her blood tested for HIV and HBV (the source individual can refuse this request).
4. Advise the employee to have his or her blood tested for HIV and HBV. (The employee has the right to refuse to be tested.) By law, the employee's blood test results are held confidential from the employer.
5. Provide medically indicated prophylaxis treatment, such as necessary injections of gamma globulin, HBV vaccine booster, tetanus booster, or a combination.
6. Provide appropriate counseling.
7. Evaluate reported illnesses after the incident.

*Employer actions as required by the OSHA BBP Standard.

Employee Medical Records

The dentist/employer must keep a confidential medical record for each employee. The employer must store these records in a locked file for the duration of employment plus 30 years.

OSHA Bloodborne Pathogens Standard Training Requirements

- Epidemiology, modes of transmission, and prevention of HBV and HIV
- Risks to the fetus from HBV and HIV
- Location and proper use of all protective equipment
- Proper work practices using Universal Precautions
- Meaning of color codes, biohazard symbol, and precautions to follow in handling infectious waste
- Procedures to follow if needlestick or other injury occurs

From Robinson D, Bird D: *Essentials of dental assisting,* ed 3, Philadelphia, 2000, Saunders.

Standard HBV Informed Refusal

OSHA Bloodborne Pathogens Standard (29CFR 1910.1030)
Hepatitis B Vaccine Declination

I understand that due to my occupational exposure to blood and other potentially infectious materials I may be at risk of acquiring hepatitis B virus (HBV) infection. I have been given the opportunity to be vaccinated with the hepatitis B vaccine, at no charge to myself. However, I decline hepatitis B vaccination at this time. I understand that by declining this vaccine, I continue to be at risk of acquiring hepatitis B, a serious disease. If in the future I continue to have occupational exposure to blood or other potentially infectious materials and I want to be vaccinated with hepatitis B vaccine, I can receive the vaccination series at no charge to me.

____________________ __________
Employee signature Date

____________________ __________
Witness signature Date

Managing Contaminated Sharps

Contaminated needles and other disposable **sharps,** such as scalpel blades, orthodontic wires, and broken glass, must be placed into a sharps container. The *sharps container* must be puncture-resistant, closable, leakproof, and color-coded or labeled with the biohazard symbol (Fig. 19-5).

Sharps containers must be located as close as possible to the place of immediate disposal. Do not cut, bend, or break the needles before disposal. Never attempt to remove a needle from a *disposable type device.*

Preventing Needlesticks

There are needles on the market that have safety guards to prevent accidental needlesticks (Fig. 19-6). Do not bend or break needles before disposal. Always use the single-handed scoop technique or some type of safety device (Fig. 19-7).

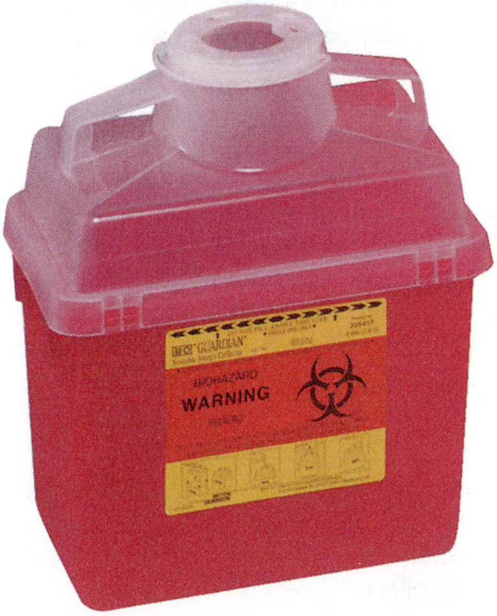

Fig. 19-5 A puncture-resistant sharps-disposal container should be located as close as possible to the area where the disposal of sharps takes place.

Recall

4. What is the purpose of the BBP Standard?
5. How often should an exposure-control plan be reviewed and updated?
6. What does the term *Standard Precautions* include?
7. What information must be included in the employee training record?
8. What must the employee do if he or she does not want the hepatitis B vaccine?

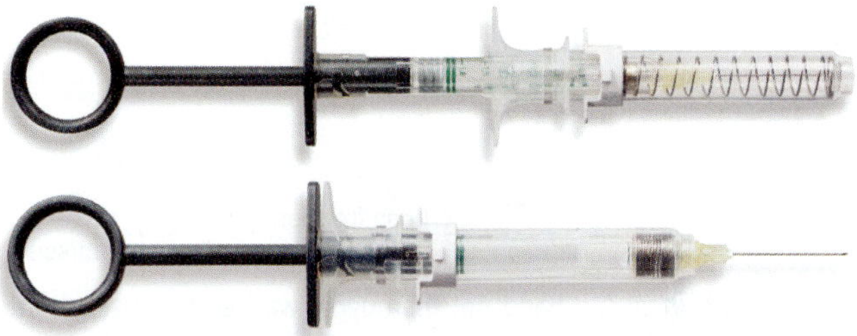
Fig. 19-6 OneShot safety syringe. A sterile, single-use barrel assembly. The plunger comes off the syringe and is autoclavable. (Courtesy Sultan Chemists Inc., Englewood, NJ.)

CDC Guidelines for Needles

Never recap used needles by using both hands or any other technique that involves directing the point of a needle toward any part of the body. (IA and IC)

Requirements for Employee Medical Records

- Employee's name and social security number
- Proof of employee's HBV vaccination or signed refusal
- Circumstances of any exposure incident (such as a needlestick) involving the employee and the name of the source individual (e.g., a patient whose blood or bodily fluid was involved in the incident)
- A copy of the postexposure follow-up procedures for any injuries sustained by that employee

These records must be retained by the employer for the duration of employment plus 30 years.
From Robinson D, Bird D: *Essentials of dental assisting,* ed 3, Philadelphia, 2000, Saunders.

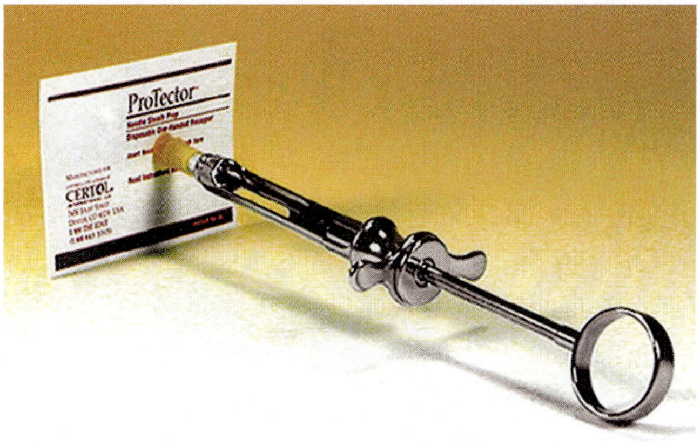

Fig. 19-7 ProTector disposable needle guard. (Courtesy Certol.)

INFECTION-CONTROL PRACTICES

Hand Hygiene

Handwashing Guidelines

You must wash your hands before you put on gloves (Procedure 19-2) and immediately after you remove gloves. Handwashing is also required if you inadvertently touch contaminated objects or surfaces while barehanded (Fig. 19-8). You should always use *liquid* soap during handwashing. Bar soap should never be used because it may transmit contamination.

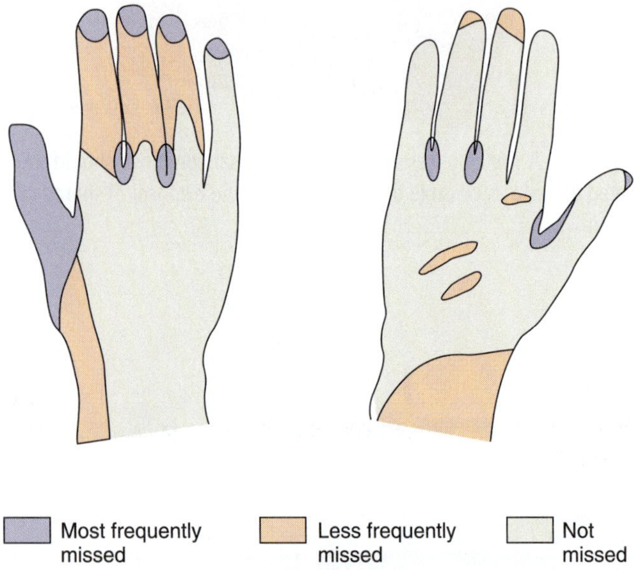

Fig. 19-8 Areas of the hand not thoroughly washed because of poor handwashing technique. (From Samaranayake LP: *Essential microbiology for dentistry,* ed 2, New York, 2002, Churchill Livingstone.)

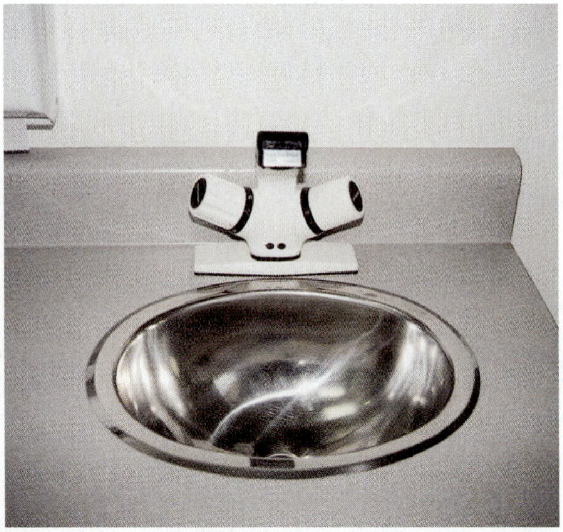

Fig. 19-9 Sensing device automatically turns the water on and off with hands-free operation.

To minimize cross-contamination, it is preferable that treatment room sinks be equipped with "hands-free" faucets that are activated electronically or with foot pedals (Fig. 19-9).

CDC Hand Hygiene in Dental Health-Care Settings

For most routine dental procedures, such as examinations and nonsurgical procedures, wash your hands with antimicrobial or nonantimicrobial soap and water. If your hands are not visibly soiled, you may use an alcohol-based, waterless hand rub. For surgical procedures, you should perform a surgical scrub using antimicrobial or nonantimicrobial soap and water, dry your hands, and apply an alcohol-based surgical hand rub with persistent activity. (IA)

OVERVIEW OF 2002 CDC HAND HYGIENE GUIDELINES

In 2002, the Centers for Disease Control and Prevention released new recommendations for hand hygiene in health-care settings. *Hand hygiene* is a term that applies to either handwashing, use of an antiseptic hand rub, or surgical hand antisepsis. Evidence suggests that hand antisepsis, the cleansing of hands with an antiseptic hand rub, is more effective in reducing nosocomial infections than plain handwashing.

Follow these guidelines in the care of all patients

- Continue to wash hands with antimicrobial or nonantimicrobial soap and water whenever the hands are visibly soiled.
- Use an alcohol-based hand rub to routinely decontaminate the hands in the following clinical situations: *(Note: If alcohol-based hand rubs are not available, the alternative is handwashing)*
  - Before and after client contact.
  - Before donning sterile gloves when inserting central intravascular catheters.
  - Before performing nonsurgical invasive procedures (e.g., urinary catheter insertion, nasotracheal suctioning).
  - After contact with body fluids or excretions, mucous membranes, nonintact skin, and wound dressings.
  - When moving from a contaminated body site (rectal area or mouth) to a clean body site (surgical wound, urinary meatus) during client care.
  - After contact with inanimate objects (including medical equipment) in the immediate vicinity of the client.
  - After removing gloves.
- Before eating and after using a restroom, wash hands with a nonantimicrobial or antimicrobial soap and water.
- Antimicrobial-impregnated wipes (i.e., towelettes) are not a substitute for using an alcohol-based hand rub or antimicrobial soap.
- If exposure to *Bacillus anthracis* is suspected or proven, wash hands with nonantimicrobial or antimicrobial soap and water. The physical action of washing and rinsing hands is recommended because alcohols, chlorhexidine, iodophors, and other antiseptic agents have poor activity against spores.

Method for decontaminating hands

When using an alcohol-based hand rub, apply product to palm of one hand and rub hands together, covering all surfaces of hands and fingers, until hands are dry. Follow the manufacturer's recommendations regarding the volume of product to use.

Follow these guidelines for surgical hand antisepsis

- Surgical hand antisepsis reduces the resident microbial count on the hands to a minimum.
- The CDC recommends using an antimicrobial soap, and scrubbing hands and forearms for the length of time recommended by the manufacturer, usually 2 to 6 minutes. The Association of Operating Room Nurses recommends 5 to 10 minutes. Refer to agency policy for time required.
- When using an alcohol-based surgical hand-rub product with persistent activity, follow the manufacturer's instructions. Before applying the alcohol solution, prewash hands and forearms with a nonantimicrobial soap and dry hands and forearms completely. After application of the alcohol-based product as recommended, allow hands and forearms to dry thoroughly before donning sterile gloves.

General recommendations for hand hygiene

- Use hand lotions or creams to minimize the occurrence of irritant contact dermatitis associated with hand antisepsis or handwashing.
- Do not wear artificial fingernails or extenders when having direct contact with clients at high risk (e.g., those in intensive-care units or operating rooms).
- Keep natural nail tips less than ¼-inch long.
- Wear gloves when contact with blood or other potentially infectious materials, mucous membranes, and nonintact skin could occur.
- Remove gloves after caring for a client. Do not wear the same pair of gloves for the care of more than one client, and do not wash gloves between uses with different clients.
- Change gloves during client care if moving from a contaminated body site to a clean body site.

From *Morbidity and Mortality Weekly Report* 51 (RR16): 1-44. October 25, 2002. Centers for Disease Control and Prevention. Available at www.cdc.gov/handhygiene.

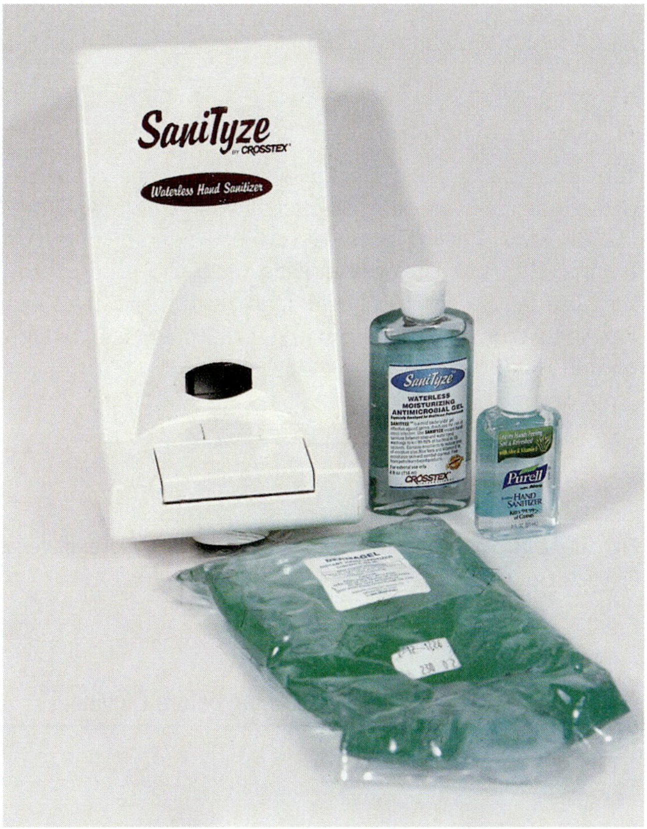

Fig. 19-10 Alcohol-based hand rub agents are available for refillable wall-mounted containers, in counter size, and in purse size. (Courtesy Crosstex.)

Alcohol-Based Hand Rubs

There is now a new category of antiseptic products on the market for hand hygiene. Waterless antiseptic agents are alcohol-based products that are available in gels, foams, or rinses (Fig.19-10). They do not require the use of water. The product is simply applied to the hands, which are then rubbed together to cover all surfaces.

These products are more effective at reducing microbial flora than plain soap, or even an antimicrobial hand wash. Concentrations of 60 to 95 percent are the most effective. Higher concentrations are actually *less effective.* In addition, these products are actually good for your skin. They contain emollients that reduce the incidence of chapping, irritation, and drying of the skin. These products are very "dose-sensitive." This means you must use the amount that is recommended. Using a smaller amount seriously decreases the effectiveness of the product.

Alcohol-based hand rubs *are not* indicated if your hands are visibly soiled or contaminated with organic matter, such as blood or saliva. In this case, you would need to wash your hands first with soap and water, and then follow with the alcohol-based product (Procedure 19-3).

Hand Care Recommendations

Healthy skin is better able to withstand the damaging effects of repeated washing and of wearing gloves. It is important to dry your hands well before donning gloves.

Dental personnel with open sores or weeping dermatitis must avoid activities involving direct patient contact and handling contaminated instruments or equipment until the condition on the hands is healed.

CDC Special Considerations for Hand Hygiene

Because rings and long fingernails can harbor pathogens, nails should be kept short and well-manicured. Rings, long nails, and artificial nails are likely to puncture examination gloves and may poke a patient during an examination. In addition, microorganisms thrive around rough cuticles and can enter the body through any break in the skin. The CDC Guidelines recommend that rings, fingernail polish, and artificial nails should not be worn at work. (II)

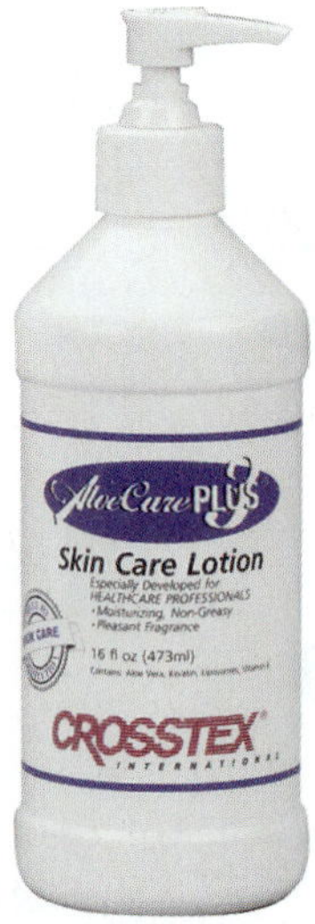

Fig. 19-11 Hand lotions must be compatible with glove material. (Courtesy Crosstex.)

Recall

9. What is the most effective hand product on the market for use on clean hands?

10. Why should long or artificial nails and rings be avoided when working in a dental office?

CDC Hand Care Products

Use hand lotions to prevent skin dryness associated with handwashing. (IA) Check the compatibility of the lotion with your gloves (Fig. 19-11). The petroleum or other oil emollients can have a harmful effect on the integrity of the gloves (see Fig. 19-22).

Store liquid hand care products in disposable closed containers or closed containers that can be washed and dried before refilling. Do not add soap or lotion to a partially empty dispenser. (IA) Refilling partially empty containers can lead to bacterial contamination.

Procedure 19-2 Handwashing before Gloving

Goal

To wash hands properly before gloving.

Equipment and Supplies

- Sink with running water
- Liquid soap in a dispenser
- Nailbrush or orange stick
- Paper towels in a dispenser

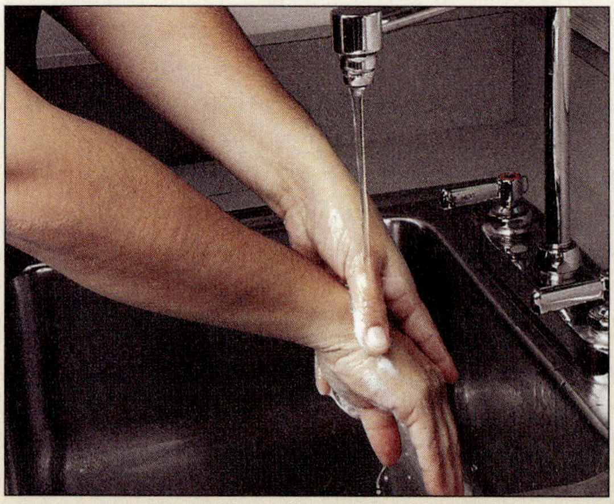

PROCEDURAL STEPS

1. Remove all jewelry, including watch and rings.
   Purpose: Jewelry is difficult to clean, can harbor microbes, and can puncture the gloves.
2. Use the foot or electronic control to regulate water flow. If this is not available, use a paper towel to grasp the faucets to turn them on and off. Discard the towel after use. Allow your hands to become wet.
   Purpose: Faucets may have been contaminated by being touched with soiled or contaminated hands.

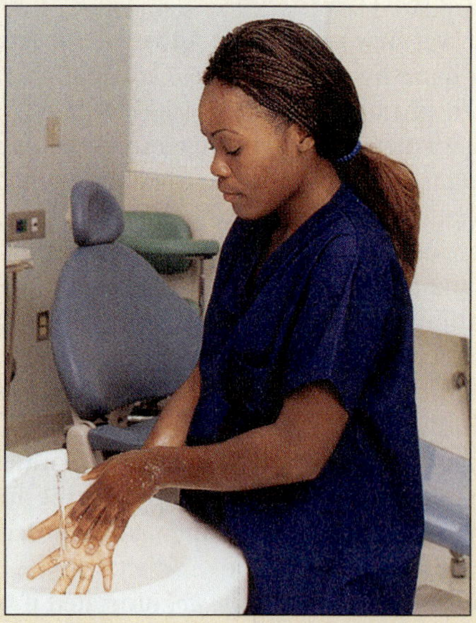

Procedure 19-2 Handwashing before Gloving–cont'd

3. Apply soap, and lather using a circular motion with friction while holding your fingertips downward. Rub well between your fingers. If this is the first handwashing of the day, use a nailbrush or an orange stick. Inspect and clean under every fingernail during this step.
   Purpose: Friction removes soil and contaminants from your hands and wrists.

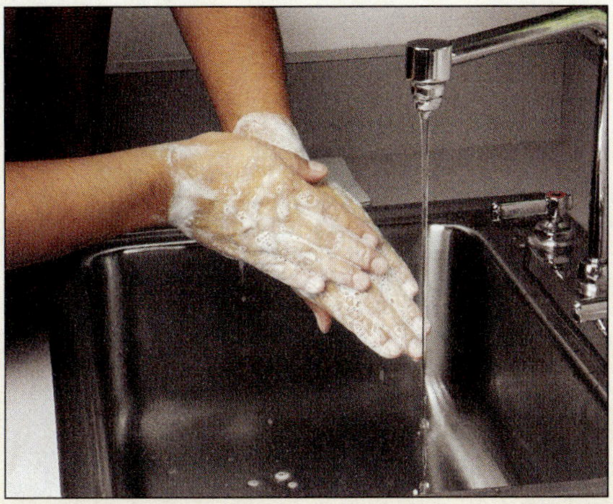

4. Vigorously rub together the lathered hands under a stream of water to remove surface debris.
   Purpose: Scrubbing the first time removes gross debris.
5. Apply more soap, and vigorously rub together lathered hands for a minimum of 10 seconds under a stream of water.
   Purpose: Secondary scrubbing removes residual debris and tenacious microorganisms, which thrive under the free edges of the fingernails.
6. Rinse the hands with cool water.
   Purpose: Cool water closes the pores.

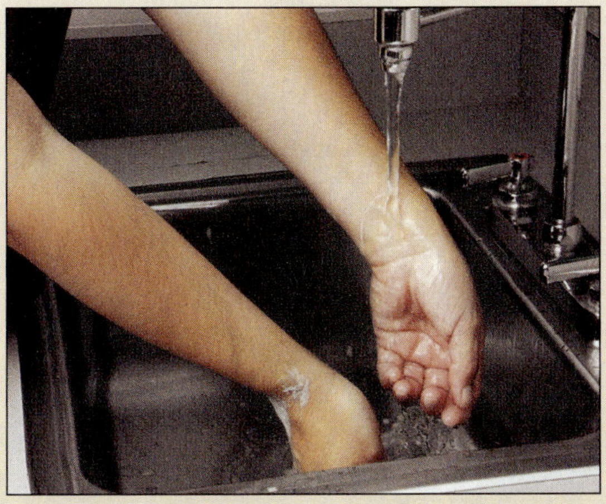

7. Use a paper towel to dry the hands thoroughly, and then dry the forearms.
   Purpose: Reusable cloth towels remain moist, contribute to microbial growth, and spread contamination.

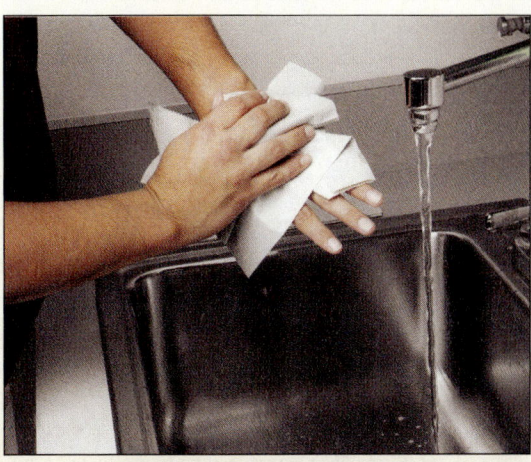

8. If water faucets are not foot-operated, turn off the faucet with a clean paper towel.
   Purpose: The faucet is dirty and will contaminate your clean hands.

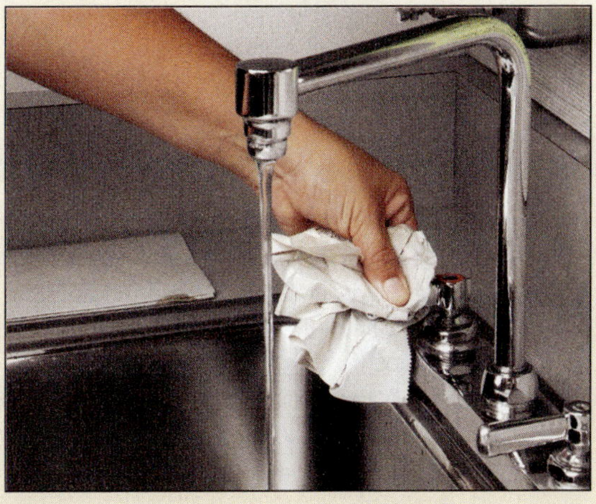

Illustrations from Young AP, Kennedy DB: *Kinn's the medical assistant: an applied learning approach,* ed 9, Philadelphia, 2003, Saunders.

Procedure 19-3 Applying Alcohol-Based Hand Rubs

Goal

To apply an alcohol-based hand rub.

Equipment and Supplies

- Alcohol-based hand rub (60 to 95 percent concentration)

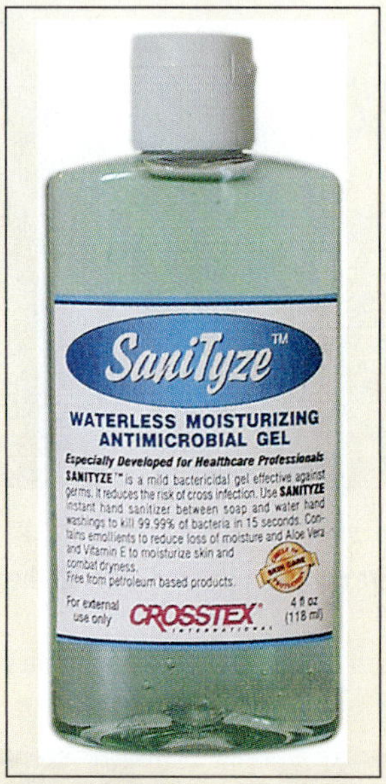

PROCEDURAL STEPS

1. Check your hands to be sure they are not visibly soiled or contaminated with organic matter, such as blood or saliva. If necessary, wash your hands with soap and water and dry them thoroughly.
   Purpose: Alcohol-based hand rubs are not effective in the presence of organic matter.
2. Read directions carefully to determine the proper amount to dispense.
   Purpose: These products are very dose-sensitive. If you use a smaller amount than is recommended, the effectiveness will be seriously decreased.
3. Dispense the proper amount of the product into the palm of one hand.

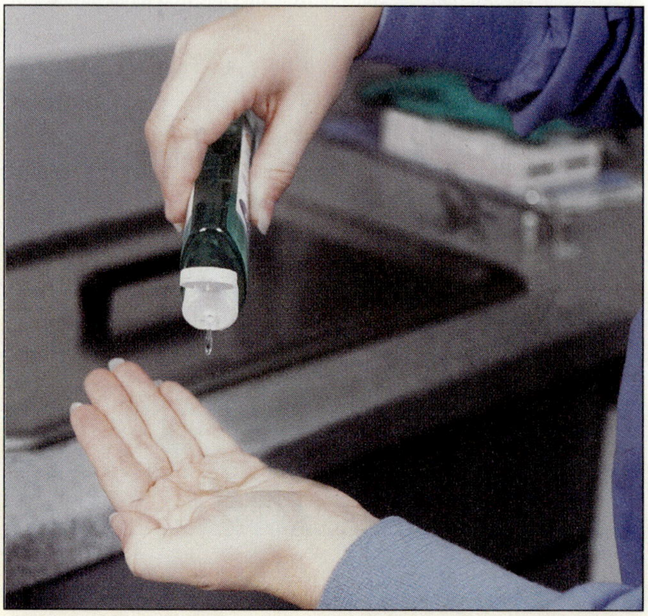

4. Rub the palms of your hands together.

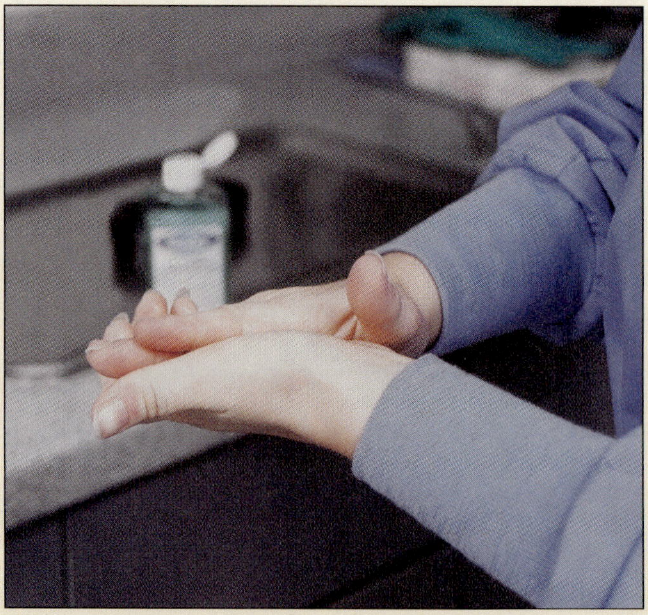

Procedure 19-3 Applying Alcohol-Based Hand Rubs—cont'd

5. Rub the product between your fingers.

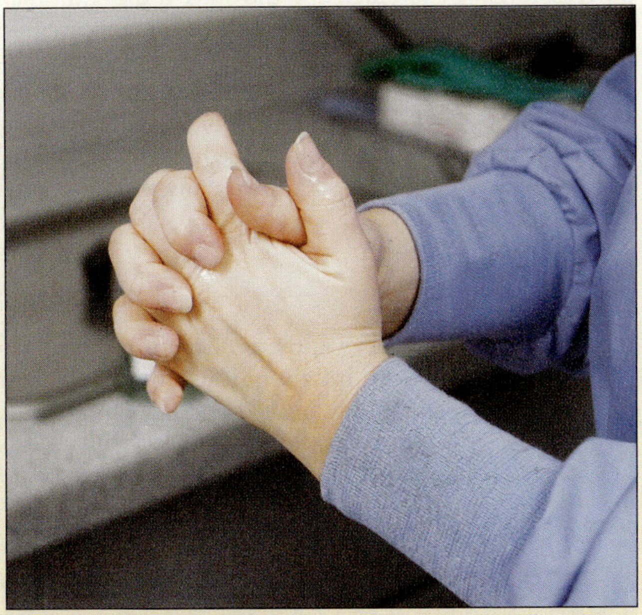

6. Rub the product over the back of your hands.
Purpose: It is important to thoroughly cover both of your hands.

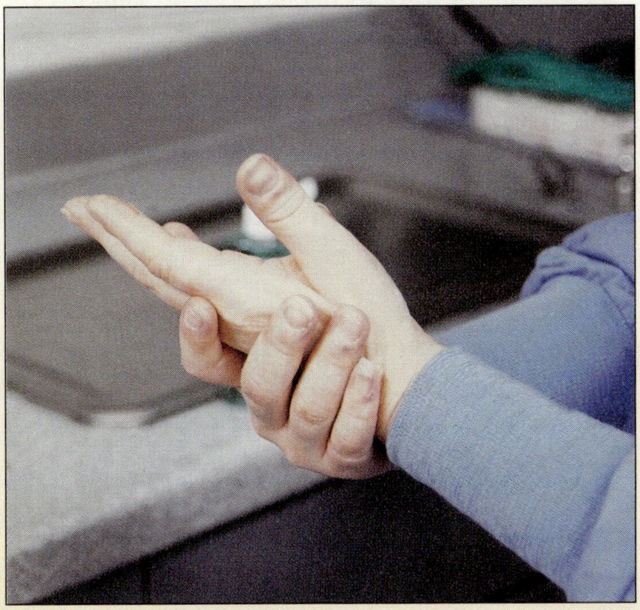

Personal Protective Equipment

OSHA's BBP Standard requires the employer to provide employees with appropriate **personal protective equipment (PPE)** without charge to the employee. Examples of PPE include protective clothing, surgical masks, face shields, protective eyewear, disposable patient-treatment gloves, and heavy-duty utility gloves.

Because dental assistants are likely to come in contact with blood and saliva, you must wear PPE whenever you are performing tasks that could produce splash, spatter, aerosol, or other contact with body fluids (Fig. 19-12).

The term *spatter* describes larger droplets in an aerosol spray. *Splatter* describes larger droplets formed when a fluid splashes. These terms are often used interchangeably to describe droplets of potentially infectious materials.

You must also wear appropriate PPE when you perform other clinical activities that require handling items contaminated with patient secretions. Examples include processing dental radiographs and handling laboratory cases, dentures and other prosthetic appliances, or contaminated equipment and surfaces.

You put on your PPE in the reverse order of what you change most frequently during the day. Gloves are changed the most often, face protection less often, and protective clothing the least often (Procedure 19-4). You remove your PPE in a manner to prevent contaminating hands, clothing, skin, and mucous membranes (Procedure 19-5).

Protective Clothing

The purpose of protective clothing is to protect the skin and underclothing from exposure to saliva, blood, aerosol, and other contaminated materials. Types of protective clothing can include smocks, pants, skirts, laboratory coats, surgical scrubs (hospital operating room clothing), scrub (surgical) hats, and shoe covers. Technically, clinic shoes and hosiery also are part of PPE.

The decision as to the type of protective clothing you should wear is based on the degree of anticipated exposure to infectious materials. For example, assisting with the high-speed handpiece during a cavity preparation carries a high risk of exposure to contaminated aerosol. Charting during an oral examination, on the other hand, carries a lower risk of exposure because it does not involve use of the handpiece or air-water syringe, which creates contaminated aerosol (Fig. 19-13).

The BBP Standard prohibits an employee from taking protective clothing home to be laundered. Laundering contaminated protective clothing is the responsibility of the employer, and many offices have a laundry service that will pick up contaminated laundry from the dental office.

Protective Clothing Requirements

1. Protective clothing should be made of fluid-resistant material. Cotton, cotton/polyester, or disposable jackets or gowns usually are satisfactory for routine dental procedures.
2. To minimize the amount of uncovered skin, clothing should have long sleeves and a high neckline.
3. The design of the sleeve should allow the cuff to be tucked inside the band of the glove.
4. During high-risk procedures, protective clothing must cover dental personnel at least to the knees when seated.
5. Buttons, trim, zippers, and other ornamentation (which may harbor pathogens) should be kept to a minimum.

NOTE: *The type and characteristics of protective clothing depend on the anticipated degree of exposure.*

Handling Contaminated Laundry

As mentioned earlier, the BBP Standard states that protective clothing may not be taken home and washed by employees. It may be laundered in the office if the equipment is available and Universal Precautions are followed for handling and laundering the contaminated clothing.

Contaminated linens that are removed from the office for laundering should be in a leakproof bag with a biohazard label or appropriately color-coded label (Fig. 19-14). Disposable gowns must be discarded daily and more often if visibly soiled (Fig. 19-15).

Protective Masks

A surgical mask is worn over the nose and mouth to protect the person from inhaling infectious organisms spread by the aerosol spray of the handpiece or air-water syringe and by accidental splashes. A mask with at least 95 percent filtration efficiency for particles 3 to 5 mi-

Guidelines for the Use of Protective Clothing

Because protective clothing can spread contamination, it is *not* worn out of the office for any reason, including travel to and from the office.

Protective clothing should be changed at least daily and more often if visibly soiled.

If a protective garment becomes visibly soiled or saturated with chemicals or body fluids, it should be changed immediately.

Protective clothing must *not* be worn in staff lounge areas or when workers are eating or consuming beverages.

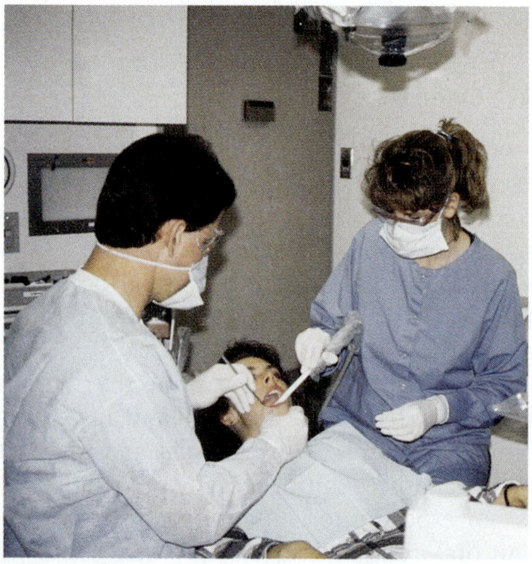

Fig. 19-12 Appropriate clinical attire consists of long-sleeved gowns, gloves, and eyewear.

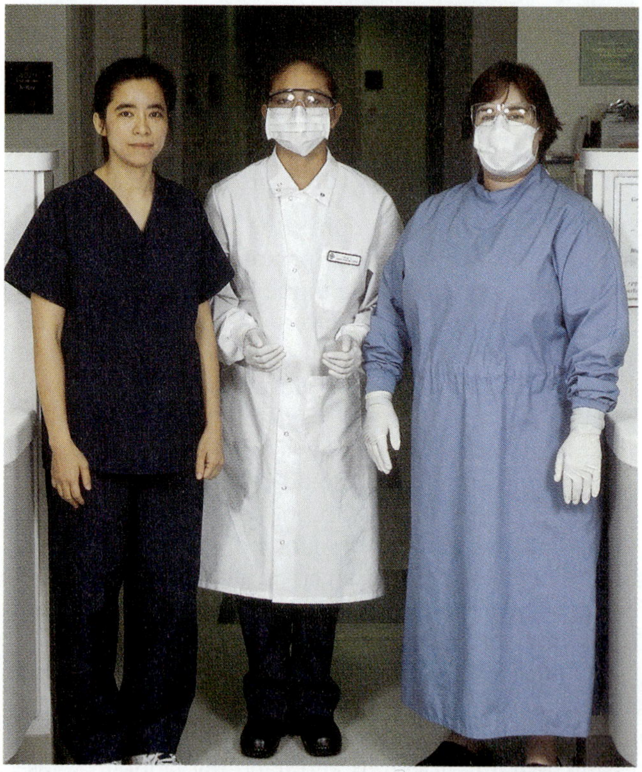

A B C

Fig. 19-13 Depending on the task, the dental assistant's attire might be scrubs, lab coats, or surgical gowns. **A,** Dental assistant in scrubs. **B,** Dental assistant in lab coat. **C,** Dental assistant in surgical gown.

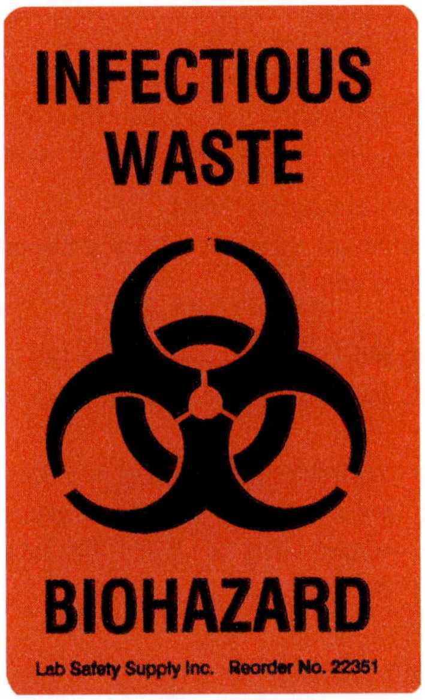

Fig. 19-14 Containers of contaminated laundry must be labeled with the universal biohazard symbol.

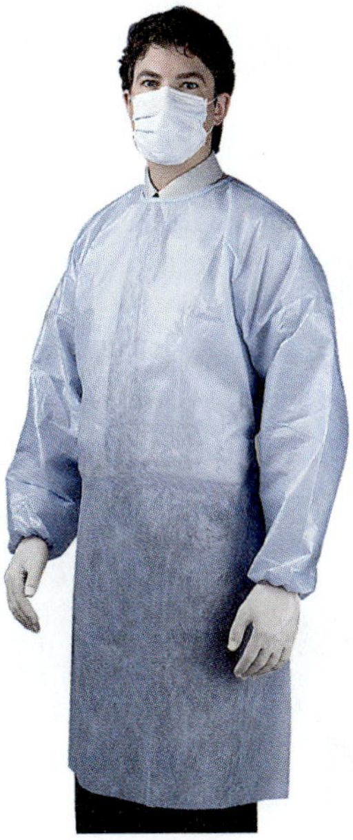

Fig. 19-15 Fluid-impervious gown. (Courtesy Crosstex.)

Procedure 19-4 Putting on Personal Protective Equipment

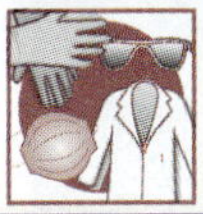

Goal

To put on PPE prior to patient care.

Equipment and Supplies

- Protective clothing
- Surgical mask
- Protective eyewear
- Gloves

PROCEDURAL STEPS

1. Put on your protective clothing over your uniform, street clothes, or scrubs.

   Note: Protective clothing could be long-sleeved lab coats, clinic jackets, or gowns.

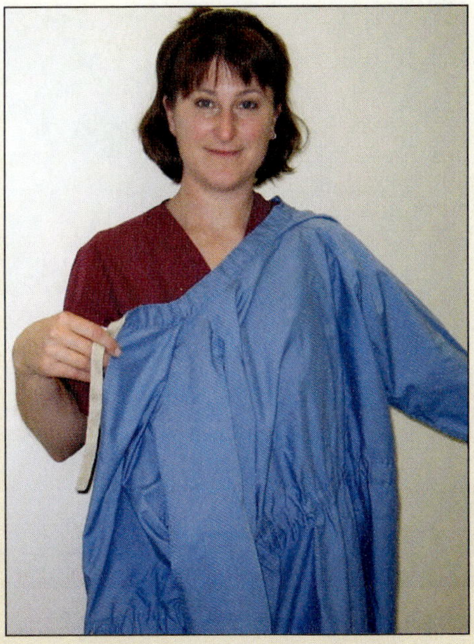

continued

Procedure 19-4 Putting on Personal Protective Equipment—cont'd

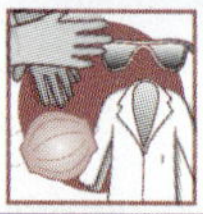

PROCEDURAL STEPS, cont'd

2. Put on your surgical mask, and adjust the fit.

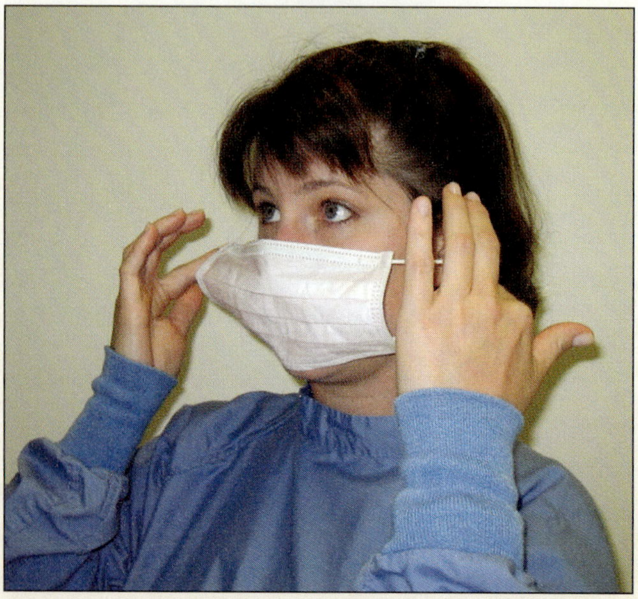

3. Put on your protective eyewear.
   Note: Eyewear should be impact-resistant and have side protection. Goggles or face shields are also acceptable.

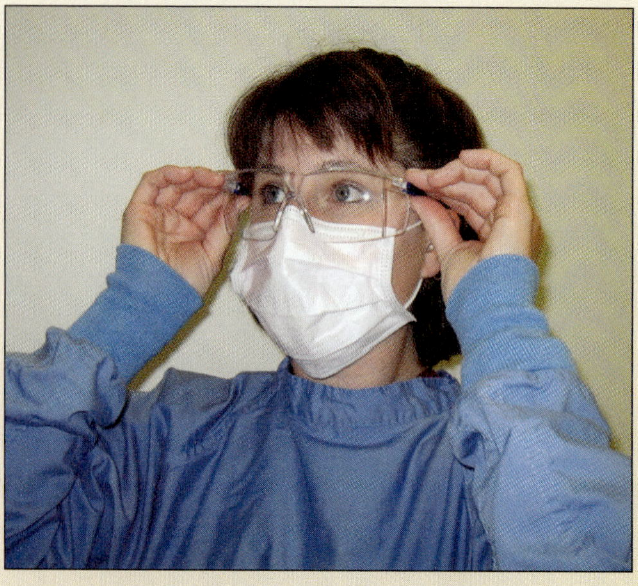

4. Thoroughly wash and dry your hands.
   Note: If your hands are not visibly soiled, you may use an alcohol-based hand rub.

5. Hold one glove at the cuff, place your opposite hand inside the glove, and pull it onto your hand. Repeat with a new glove for your other hand.
   Important Note: Regarding the sequence of putting on PPE, the *most important* step is to put on the gloves last to avoid contaminating them before they are placed in the patient's mouth.

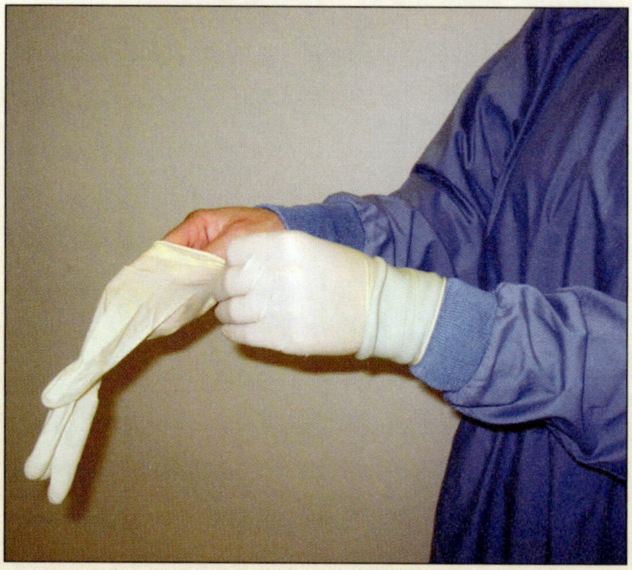

Modified from *Policy to practice: OSAP's guide to the guidelines,* Annapolis, Maryland, 2004, OSAP.

Procedure 19-5 Removing Personal Protective Equipment

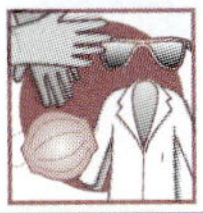

Goal

To remove personal protective wear.

Equipment and Supplies

- Protective clothing
- Surgical mask
- Protective eyewear
- Gloves

PROCEDURAL STEPS

1. Use your gloved hand to grasp the other glove at the outside cuff. Pull downward, turning the glove inside out as it pulls away from your hand.

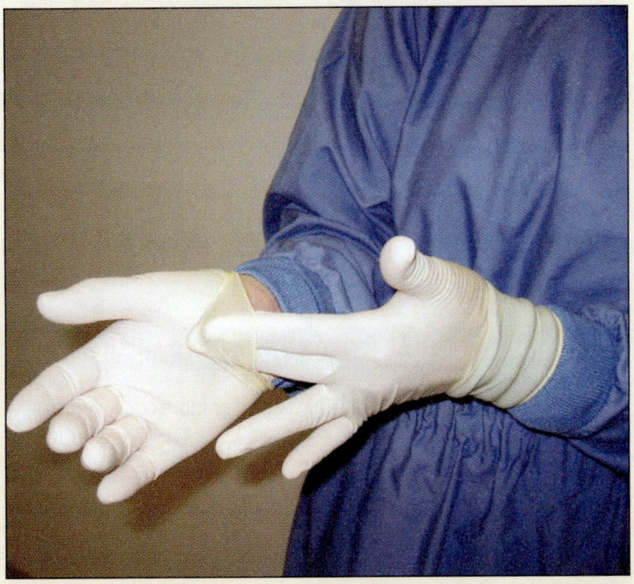

2. For the other hand, use your ungloved fingers to grasp the inside (uncontaminated area) of the cuff of the remaining glove. Pull downward to remove the glove, turning it inside out. Discard the gloves into the waste receptacle.
3. Wash and thoroughly dry hands.

   Note: If no visible contamination exists and gloves have not been torn or punctured during the procedure, you may use an alcohol-based hand rub in place of handwashing. However, if your hands are damp from perspiration or have glove powder, you may prefer to wash them with antimicrobial soap and water.

Eyewear

1. Remove eyewear by touching it only on the ear rests (which are not contaminated).

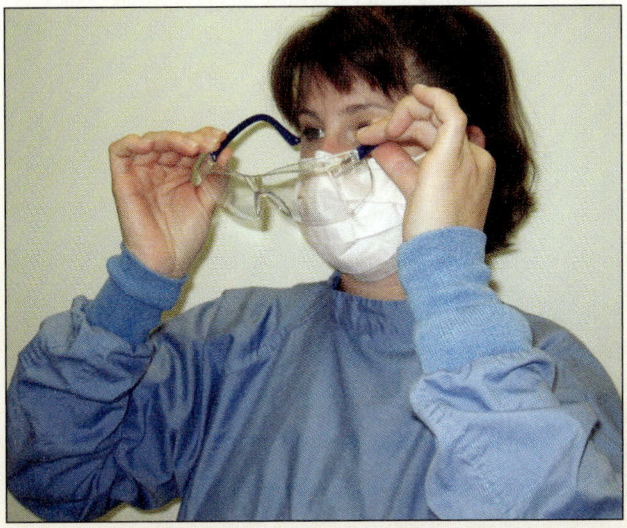

2. Place the eyewear on a disposable towel until it can be properly cleaned and disinfected.

Masks

1. Slide the fingers of each hand under the elastic strap in front of your ears and remove the mask. Discard the mask into the waste receptacle.

   Note: Be sure your fingers contact only the mask's ties or elastic strap.

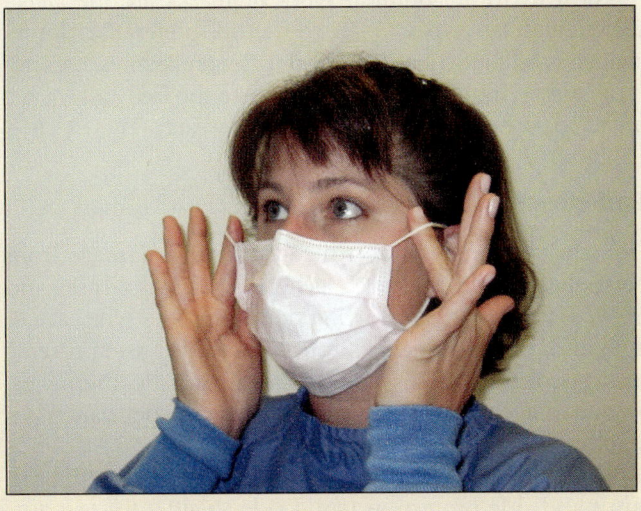

Modified from *Policy to practice: OSAP's guide to the guidelines,* Annapolis, Maryland, 2004, OSAP.

continued

Procedure 19-5 Removing Personal Protective Equipment—cont'd

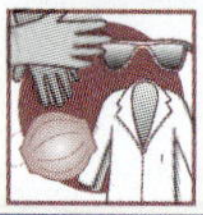

PROCEDURAL STEPS, cont'd

Protective Clothing

1. Pull the gown off, turning it inside out as it comes off.
   Note: Be careful not to allow the gown to touch underlying clothes or skin.

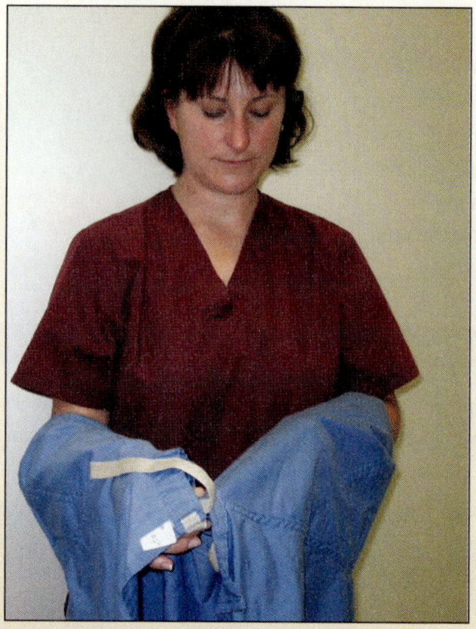

Modified from *Policy to practice: OSAP's guide to the guidelines,* Annapolis, Maryland, 2004, OSAP.

crometers (μm) in diameter should be worn whenever splash or spatter is likely. Surgical masks do not provide a perfect seal around the edges, therefore unfiltered air can pass through the edges. For that reason, it is important to select a mask that fits your face well. Masks should be changed between patients, or during patient treatment if the mask becomes wet.

The two most common types of masks are the *dome-shaped* and *flat* types. Some operators prefer the dome-shaped type, particularly during lengthy procedures, because it *conforms* ("molds") more effectively to the face and creates an air space between the mask and the wearer (Fig. 19-16).

Guidelines for the Use of Protective Masks

Masks should be changed for every patient or more often, particularly if heavy spatter is generated during the treatment or if the mask becomes damp.

Masks should be handled by touching only the side edges to avoid contact with the more heavily contaminated body of the mask.

Masks should conform to the shape of the face.

Masks should not contact the mouth when being worn because the moisture generated will decrease the mask filtration efficiency. A damp or wet mask is *not* an effective mask.

Protective Eyewear

Eyewear is worn to protect the eyes against damage from aerosolized pathogens such as herpes simplex viruses and *Staphylococcus* and from flying debris such as scrap amalgam and tooth fragments. Protective eyewear also prevents injury from splattered solutions and caustic chemicals. Such damage may be irreparable and lead to permanent visual impairment or blindness.

The BBP Standard requires the use of eyewear with both front and side protection (solid side shields) for use during exposure-prone procedures. If you wear prescription glasses, you must add protective side and bottom shields. Protective eyewear that can be worn over prescription glasses is also available. If you wear contact lenses, you must also wear protective eyewear with side shields or a face shield (Fig. 19-17).

The CDC *Guidelines* recommend that you clean your eyewear with soap and water, or if visibly soiled you can clean and disinfect reusable facial protective wear between patients.

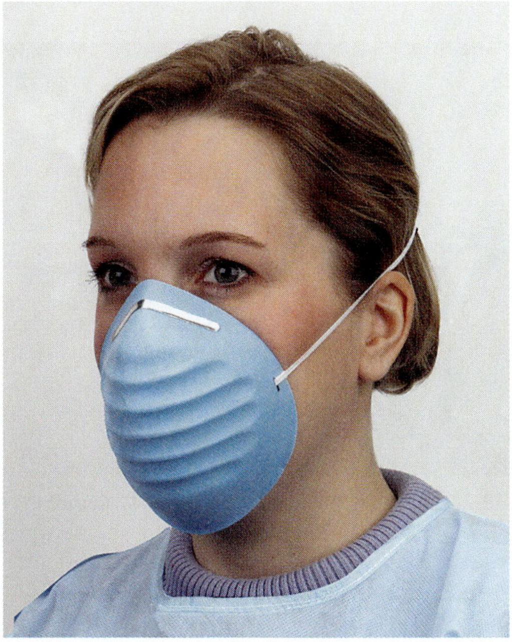

Fig. 19-16 Dome-style facemask. (Courtesy Crosstex.)

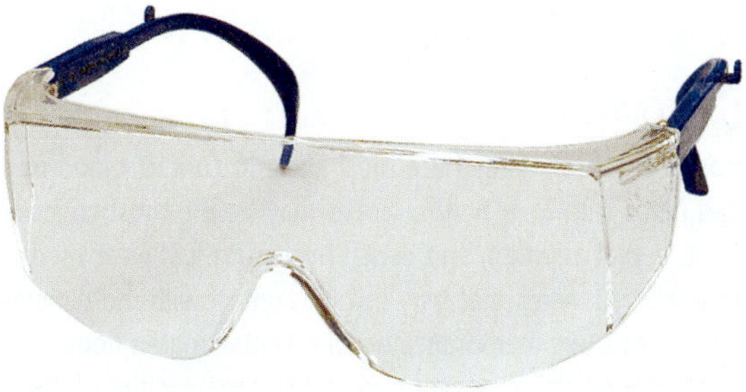

Fig. 19-17 Safety goggles with protective side shields. (Courtesy Crosstex.)

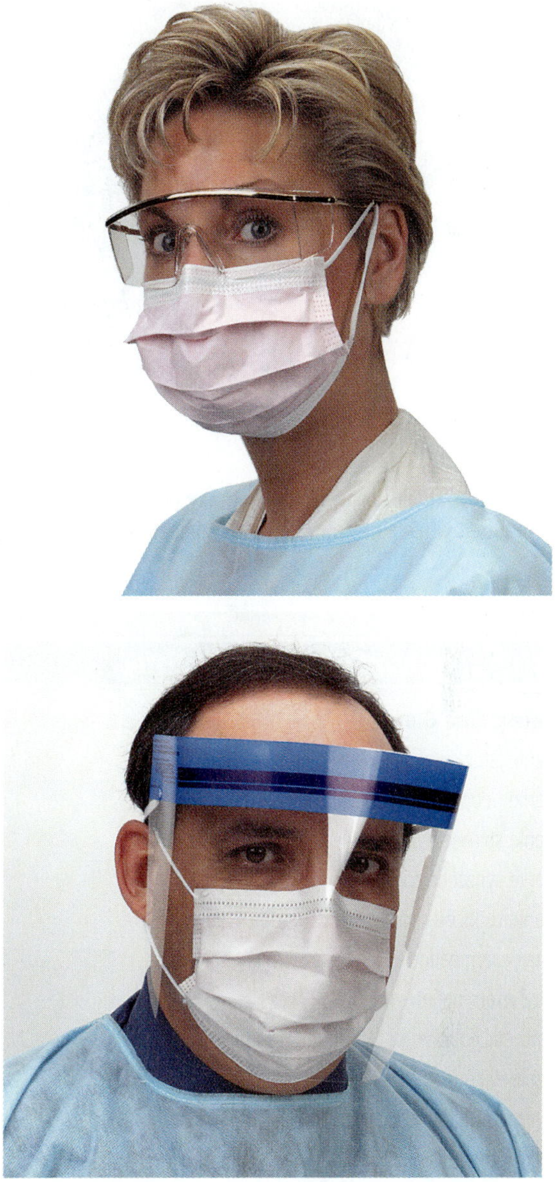

A

B

Fig. 19-18 A, Facemask and safety glasses. B, Facemask and disposable face shield. (Courtesy Crosstex.)

The two types of protective eyewear used during patient care are (1) glasses with protective side shields and (2) clear face shields (Fig. 19-18).

Face Shields

A chin-length plastic face shield may be worn as an alternative to protective eyewear. However, a shield cannot replace a facemask because the shield does not protect against inhalation of contaminated aerosols (Fig. 19-19).

When splashing or spattering of blood or other body fluids is likely during a procedure such as surgery, a face shield is often worn *in addition to* a protective mask.

Patient Eyewear

Patients should be provided with protective eyewear because they also may be subject to eye damage from (1) handpiece spatter, (2) spilled or splashed dental materials including caustic chemical agents, and (3) airborne bits of acrylic or tooth fragments (Fig. 19-20).

When certain laser treatments are performed, patients must be supplied with special filtered-lens glasses.

Recall

11. What are four examples of PPE?
12. What determines the type of PPE to be worn?
13. What are the two types of protective eyewear?

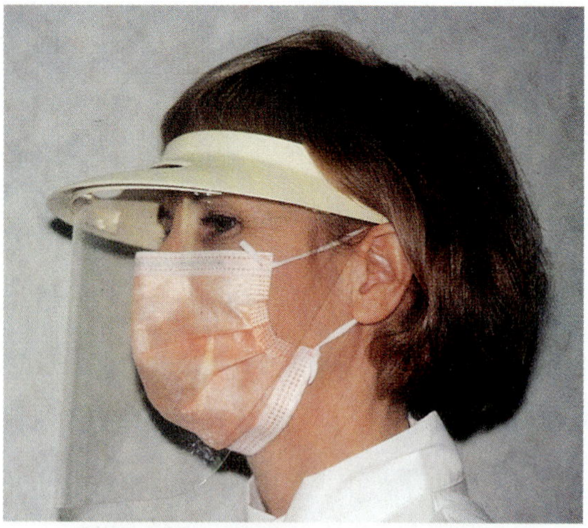

Fig. 19-19 Face shields provide adequate eye protection, but a facemask is still required when assisting with aerosol-generating procedures.

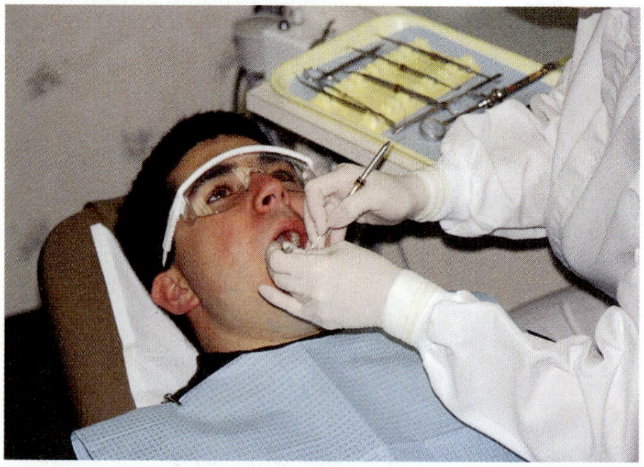

Fig. 19-20 Patients should be provided with protective eyewear.

Box 19-1 Types of Gloves in Dentistry

Patient Care Gloves

Sterile latex surgical gloves
Sterile neoprene surgical gloves*
Sterile styrene surgical gloves*
Sterile synthetic copolymer gloves*
Sterile reduced-protein latex surgeon's gloves
Latex examination gloves
Vinyl examination gloves*
Synthetic copolymer examination gloves*
Nitrile examination gloves*
Styrene-butadiene examination gloves*
Polyurethane gloves*
Powderless gloves
Flavored gloves
Low-protein gloves

Utility Gloves

Heavy latex gloves
Heavy nitrile gloves
Thin copolymer gloves
Thin plastic ("food handler") gloves

Other Gloves

Heat-resistant gloves
Dermal (cotton) gloves

*Nonlatex gloves; one should review the labeling or check with the manufacturer to confirm.
From Miller CH and Palenik CJ: *Infection control and management of hazardous materials for the dental team,* ed 3, St Louis, 2005, Mosby.

Gloves

The types of gloves used in a dental practice should be determined by the various procedures that are performed in the practice (Box 19-1).

CDC Gloves

Because dental personnel are most likely to contact blood or contaminated items with their hands, gloves may be the most critical PPE. The dentist, dental assistant, and dental hygienist must wear medical gloves during all treatments that may involve contact with the patient's blood, saliva, or mucous membranes or with contaminated items or surfaces. Wear a new pair of gloves for each patient, remove them promptly after use, and wash your hands immediately to avoid transfer of microorganisms to other patients or the environment. (IB)

Consult with the glove manufacturer regarding the chemical compatibility of the glove material and dental materials you use. (II)

Examination Gloves

Medical examination gloves usually are latex or vinyl and often are referred to as "exam gloves" or "procedure gloves." These are the gloves most frequently worn by dental personnel during patient care (Fig. 19-21).

Examination gloves are inexpensive, are available in a range of sizes from extra small to extra large, and fit either hand. These gloves are *nonsterile* and serve strictly as a protective barrier for the wearer.

Gloves Damaged During Treatment

Gloves are effective only when they are *intact* (not damaged, torn, ripped, or punctured). If gloves are damaged during treatment, change them immediately and wash

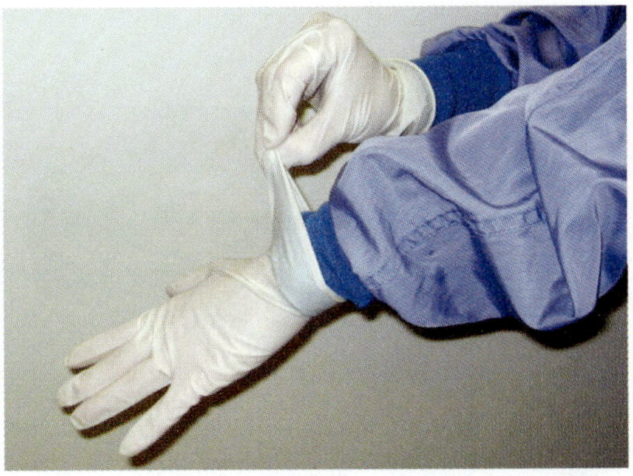

Fig. 19-21 **Nonsterile exam gloves.** (Courtesy Crosstex.)

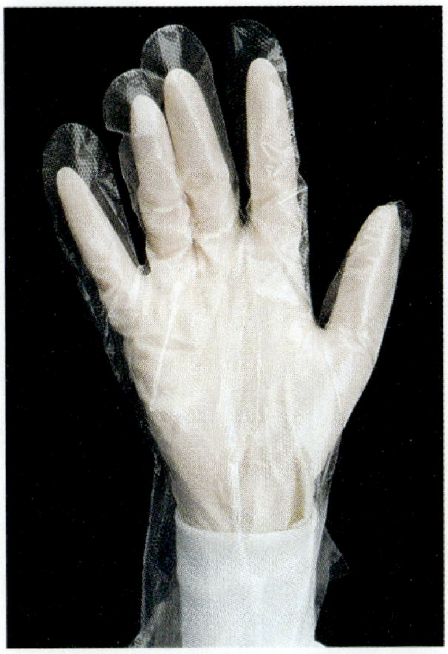

Fig. 19-22 **Overglove worn over a latex exam glove.**

Guidelines for the Use of Gloves

All gloves used in patient care must be discarded after a single use. These gloves may not be washed, disinfected, or sterilized, although they may be rinsed with water to remove excess powder.

Latex, vinyl, or other disposable medical-quality gloves may be used for patient examinations and dental procedures.

Replace torn or damaged gloves immediately.

Do not wear jewelry under gloves. (Rings harbor pathogens and may tear the glove.)

Change gloves frequently. (If the procedure is long, change gloves about once each hour.)

Remove contaminated gloves before leaving the chairside during patient care, and replace them with new gloves before returning to patient care (see "Guidelines for the Use of Overgloves").

Wash hands after glove removal and before regloving

your hands before regloving. The procedure for regloving in this situation is as follows:

1. Excuse yourself and leave the chairside.
2. Remove and discard the damaged gloves.
3. Wash hands thoroughly.
4. Reglove before returning to the chairside to resume the dental procedure.

If you leave the chairside for any reason during the treatment of a patient, overgloves should be used. You must remove your contaminated examination gloves and wash your hands *before* you leave the chairside. When you return, you should wash and dry your hands and use fresh examination gloves.

Overgloves

Overgloves, also known as "food handler gloves," are made of lightweight, inexpensive, clear plastic. These may be worn over contaminated treatment gloves *(overgloving)*

Guidelines for the Use of Overgloves

Overgloves are *not* acceptable alone as a hand barrier or for intraoral procedures.

Overgloves must be worn carefully to avoid contamination during handling with contaminated procedure gloves.

Overgloves are placed before the secondary procedure is performed and are removed *before* patient treatment is resumed.

Overgloves are discarded after a single use.

to prevent the contamination of clean objects handled during treatment (Fig. 19-22).

Infection-control procedures for use in the mixing and passing of dental materials are discussed in more detail in Chapter 47.

Sterile Surgical Gloves

Sterile gloves, which are the type used in hospital operating rooms, should be worn for invasive procedures involving the cutting of bone or significant amounts of blood or saliva, such as oral surgery or periodontal treatment.

Sterile gloves are supplied in prepackaged units to maintain sterility before use. They are provided in specific sizes and are fitted to the left or right hand. Hand preparation and the use of surgical gloves are discussed in Chapter 56.

CDC Sterile Surgeon's Gloves

The CDC *Guidelines* offer no recommendations regarding the effectiveness of wearing two pairs of gloves to prevent disease transmission during oral surgical procedures. (Unresolved issue)

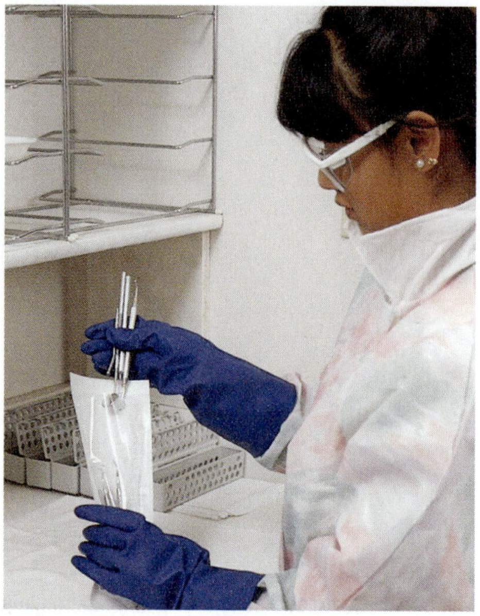

Fig. 19-23 Utility gloves are used when preparing instruments for sterilization.

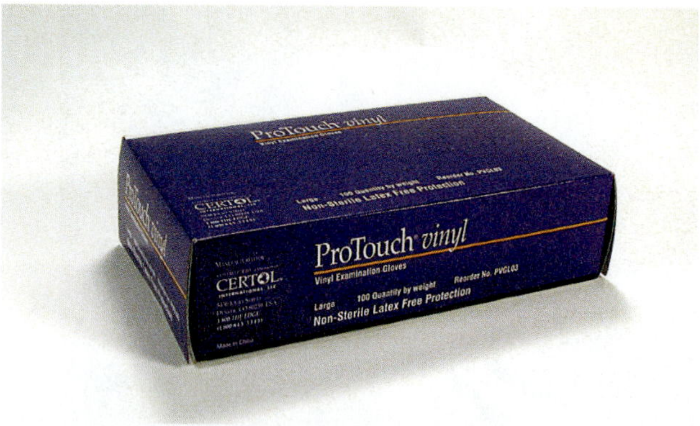

Fig. 19-24 Latex-free nitrile gloves. (Courtesy Certol.)

Utility Gloves

Utility gloves are *not* used for direct patient care. Utility gloves are worn (1) when the treatment room is cleaned and disinfected between patients, (2) while contaminated instruments are being cleaned or handled, and (3) for surface cleaning and disinfecting (Fig. 19-23). Utility gloves may be washed, disinfected, or sterilized and reused. Utility gloves must be discarded, however, when they become worn and no longer have the ability to provide barrier protection. After use, utility gloves must be considered contaminated and handled appropriately until they have been properly disinfected or sterilized. Each staff member responsible for cleanup procedures must have his or her own designated pair of utility gloves.

Non–Latex-Containing Gloves

Occasionally, healthcare providers or patients may experience serious allergic reactions to latex (see Latex Allergies section). The person who is sensitive to latex can substitute with gloves made from vinyl, nitrile, and other non–latex-containing materials (Fig. 19-24).

Maintaining Infection Control while Gloved

During a dental procedure, it may be necessary to touch surfaces or objects such as drawer handles or material containers. If you touch these with a gloved hand, both the surface and the glove become contaminated. To minimize the possibility of cross-contamination, you can use an overglove when it is necessary to touch a surface.

Opening Drawers and Cabinets

If you anticipate what materials you will need and have those items for each procedure ready and easily accessible, you will save time and minimize cross-contamination. Each surface you touch with contaminated gloves also becomes contaminated. By eliminating the need to open drawers and cabinets, you limit operatory contamination.

Set up instruments, medications, and impression materials ahead of time, and use disposable and unit-dose items whenever possible. Keep a pair of salad tongs or forceps within reach in the operatory. These simple tools can be used to open cabinets, pull out drawers, and obtain any unanticipated yet necessary items without contaminating additional items and surfaces. Appropriately disinfect the tongs or forceps between patients.

Opening Containers

During the procedure it may become necessary to open containers of materials or supplies. When opening a container, use overgloves, a paper towel, or a sterile gauze sponge to remove the lid or cap. In doing this, take care not to touch any surface of the container.

Use sterile cotton pliers to remove an item from the container. If the container or bottle is touched, it becomes contaminated and must be disinfected at the end of the procedure.

Recall

14. What may be the most critical PPE?
15. When should sterile gloves be worn?
16. When should utility gloves be worn?
17. What type of glove should be worn to open drawers during a dental procedure?

LATEX ALLERGIES

The use of natural rubber latex gloves has proved to be one of the most effective means of protecting the dental worker and the patient from the transmission of disease. However, the increased use of latex gloves and other products that contain latex in the dental office and other healthcare settings has created other problems. The number of healthcare workers and patients who have become hypersensitive to latex has increased dramatically.

CDC Guidelines for Contact Dermatitis and Latex Hypersensitivity

1. Educate dental healthcare workers regarding the signs, symptoms, and diagnoses of skin reactions associated with frequent hand hygiene and glove use. (IB)
2. Screen all patients for latex allergy (e.g., take health history and refer patient for medical consultation when latex allergy is suspected). (IB)
3. Ensure a latex-safe environment for patients and dental healthcare personnel. (IB)
4. Have emergency treatment kits with latex-free products available at all times. (II)

There are three common types of allergic reactions to latex. Irritant dermatitis involves only a surface irritation. Type I and type IV allergies involve an immune reaction.

Irritant Dermatitis

Irritant dermatitis is a *non*immunologic process (does *not* involve the body's immune system). It is caused by contact with a substance that produces a chemical irritation to the skin. The skin becomes reddened, dry, irritated, and in severe cases, cracked (Fig. 19-25).

Identifying and correcting the causes, which include the following, can reverse irritant dermatitis:

- Frequent handwashing with soaps or antimicrobial agents
- Failure to rinse the soaps or microbial agents completely from the hands
- Irritation caused by the cornstarch powder in the gloves
- Excessive perspiration on the hands while wearing gloves
- Failure to dry hands thoroughly after rinsing

Type IV Allergic Reaction

Type IV allergic reaction, the most common type of latex allergy, is a delayed contact reaction and involves the immune system. It may take 48 to 72 hours for the red, itchy rash to appear. The reactions are limited to the areas of contact and do not involve the entire body. The chemicals used to process the latex in the gloves cause an immune response; the proteins in the latex do not cause it.

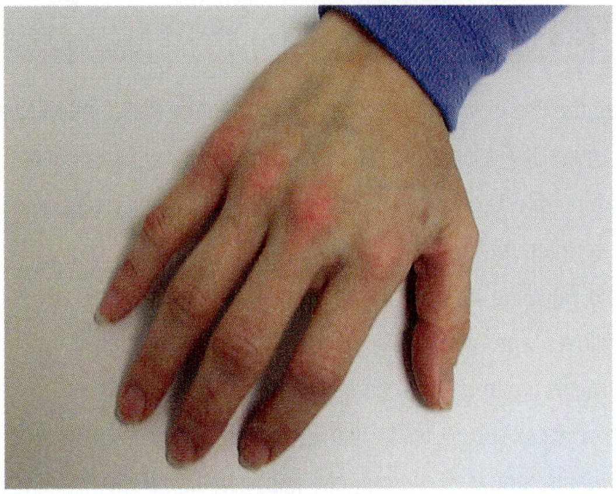

Fig. 19-25 Irritant dermatitis.

NOTE: *Chemicals such as glutaraldehyde and acrylates readily permeate (pass through) latex gloves and can irritate the skin. The irritation may be mistaken for an allergic reaction to the chemicals in the latex glove. Thus, latex gloves should never be worn when handling chemicals.*

Type I Allergic Reaction

Type I allergic reaction is the most serious type of latex allergy and can result in death. The reaction is in response to the latex *proteins* in the glove, unlike the reaction to chemical additives in type IV. A severe immunologic response occurs, usually two to three minutes after the latex allergens contact the skin or mucous membranes.

The proteins from the latex adhere to the cornstarch powder particles inside the gloves. Frequent handling of powdered latex gloves, such as during donning, and frequent removal of powdered gloves from boxes during the day cause the proteins, which are bound to the powder, to remain suspended in the air for prolonged periods. Sensitized persons can experience coughing, wheezing, runny eyes and nose, shortness of breath, and respiratory distress.

The primary cause of death associated with latex allergies is anaphylaxis. **Anaphylaxis** is the most severe form of immediate allergic reaction. Death results from closure of the airway by swelling (see Chapter 31).

Treatment

There is no specific cure for latex allergy. The only options are prevention, avoidance of latex-containing products, and treatment of the symptoms. Persons who suspect that they are allergic to latex should see a qualified healthcare

Care of Patients with Latex Allergies

Keep the use of latex-containing products in the dental office to a minimum. There is no practical way to create a "latex-free" dental office.

Allow no direct contact by the patient with latex (latex gloves or latex rubber dam material).

Avoid handling instruments with latex gloves, including wearing latex gloves when packaging instruments for sterilization if those instruments are to be used on a latex-allergic patient.

Use nonlatex substitutes for patient care: prophy cups, latex-free instruments, nonlatex tourniquets, and nonlatex stoppers in medicine droppers used for dental materials.

Use non–latex-containing blood pressure cuffs.

The latex-allergic patient should be scheduled as the first patient of the day. (Latex falls out of the air at night.)

There should be no latex in the treatment room.

The treatment room that is to be used for latex-allergic patients should be located near an outside entrance (to prevent the patient from traveling through a large dental suite where there may be latex from other activities).

Ensure that no one who has worn latex that day enters the treatment room when a latex-allergic patient is being treated (latex particles can remain on clothing, hair, shoes, etc.).

Modified from Ownby D: Presentation at 1996 OSAP Annual Symposium.

provider for a test to confirm the allergy. Once diagnosed as having a latex allergy, patients should avoid latex in all aspects of their personal and professional lives.

NOTE: *When one employee in the dental office has been diagnosed as having a latex allergy, all staff members should use practices to minimize the use of latex-containing products. These measures include use of powderless gloves by all dental staff members to minimize the risk of airborne latex particles.*

Latex-Sensitive Patients

In the healthcare setting, patients with latex allergies should be treated using alternatives to latex. Vinyl gloves and a nonlatex rubber dam should be available in all dental offices.

Recall

18. What type of response is irritant dermatitis?
19. What is the most common type of latex allergy?
20. What is the most serious type of latex allergy?
21. What type of gloves should be used for a latex-sensitive patient?

WASTE MANAGEMENT IN THE DENTAL OFFICE

Dental practices are subject to a wide variety of federal, state, and local regulations concerning waste management issues. Waste management can be confusing because agencies do not always use a consistent glossary of terms and definitions (Box 19-2).

For example, the Environmental Protection Agency (EPA) and the majority of state and local regulations do not categorize saliva or saliva-soaked items as infectious waste. However, because of the high probability that blood may be carried in saliva during dental procedures, CDC *Guidelines* and OSHA BBP Standard regulations consider saliva in dentistry to be a potentially infectious body fluid. As such, saliva-coated items should be treated as *potentially infectious waste* and disposed of as contaminated waste.

The OSHA BBP Standard requires that all waste be disposed of according to applicable federal, state, and local regulations.

CDC Guidelines for Regulated Medical Waste

1. Develop a medical-waste–management program. Disposal of regulated medical waste must follow federal, state, and local regulations. (IC)
2. Ensure that dental healthcare personnel who handle and dispose of regulated medical waste are trained in appropriate handling and disposal methods and are informed of the possible health and safety hazards. (IC)
3. Pour blood, suctioned fluids, or other liquid waste carefully into a drain connected to a sanitary sewer system, if local sewage discharge requirements are met and the state has declared this an appropriate method of disposal. Wear appropriate PPE while performing this task. (IC)

Box 19-2 Classification of Waste

Type	Examples	Handling Requirements
General waste	Paper towels, paper mixing pads, empty food containers	Discard in covered containers made of durable materials such as plastic or metal.
Hazardous waste	Waste presenting a danger to humans or the environment (toxic chemicals)	Follow your specific state and local regulations.
Contaminated waste	Waste that has been in contact with blood or other body fluids (used barriers, patient napkins)	In most states, dispose of with the general waste.
Infectious or regulated waste (biohazard)	Waste that is capable of transmitting an infectious disease	Follow your specific state and local regulations.
1. Blood and blood-soaked materials	Blood or saliva that can be squeezed out or dried blood that may flake off of an item	Containers for all three types of infectious waste must be labeled with the biohazard label.
2. Pathologic waste	Soft tissue and extracted teeth	
3. Sharps	Contaminated needles, scalpel blades, orthodontic wires, endodontic instruments (reamers and files)	Closable, leakproof, puncture-resistant containers. Containers should be color-coded red and marked with the biohazard symbol. Sharps containers should be located as close as possible to the work area.

Classification of Waste

The handling, storage, labeling, and disposal of waste depend entirely on the type of waste. For example, when reprocessing a dental treatment room, the waste should be separated into general waste containers and hazardous waste containers. The dental assistant must understand the types of waste to know what items are discarded in which container.

General Waste

General waste is all nonhazardous, nonregulated waste and should be discarded in covered containers made of durable material such as plastic or metal. For ease in handling, general waste receptacles should be lined with plastic bags. General waste includes disposable paper towels, paper mixing pads, and empty food containers.

Contaminated Waste

Waste that has been in contact with blood or other body fluids is considered **contaminated waste,** which includes used barriers and patient napkins. In most states, contaminated waste is disposed of as general waste (regular household-type waste). In a few states, however, it may be considered and defined as regulated, or infectious, waste.

Appropriate PPE should be worn when handling or disposing of contaminated waste.

Hazardous Waste

Hazardous waste poses a risk to humans and the environment. Toxic chemicals and materials are hazardous waste. Examples include scrap amalgam, spent fixer solution, and lead foil from x-ray film packets. Some items, such as extracted teeth with amalgam restorations, may be both hazardous waste (because of the amalgam) and infectious waste (because of the blood).

Handling of Extracted Teeth

Dispose of extracted teeth as regulated medical waste unless returned to the patient. When teeth are returned to the patient, the provisions of the standard no longer apply. Do not dispose of extracted teeth containing amalgam with regulated medical waste that will be incinerated. Because of the mercury in amalgam fillings, you should check your state and local regulations regarding disposal of teeth containing amalgam.

Infectious or Regulated Waste (Biohazard)

Infectious waste, also called *regulated waste* or *biohazardous waste,* is contaminated waste that is capable of transmitting an infectious disease. For waste to be infectious, pathogens must be strong enough and in sufficient numbers to infect a susceptible individual.

Infectious waste is never disposed of as general waste. It requires special handling and disposal. Most dental offices are exposed to the following three types of infectious waste:

1. *Blood and blood-soaked materials.* Blood or saliva can be squeezed out, or dried blood may flake off from the item. Gauze dripping with blood is such an item.
2. *Pathologic waste.* Soft tissue and extracted teeth are examples.
3. *Sharps.* Examples include all contaminated sharp objects used for patient care.

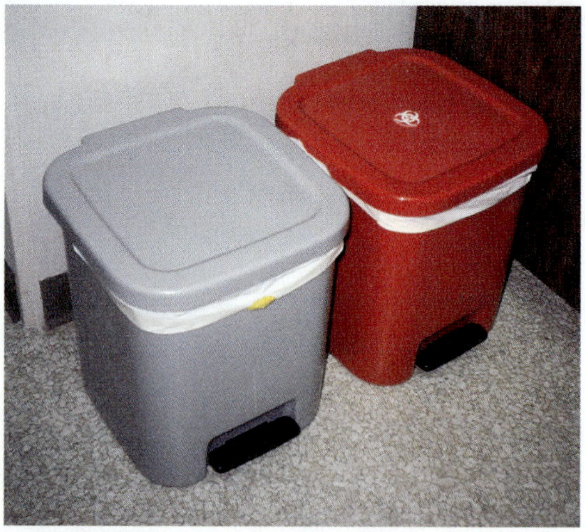

Fig. 19-26 Waste is separated into clearly marked containers. *Left,* Unregulated waste; *right,* Regulated waste.

CDC CDC Guidelines for Handling Extracted Teeth

1. Dispose of extracted teeth as regulated waste unless returned to the patient. (II)
2. Do not dispose of extracted teeth containing amalgam in regulated medical waste intended for incineration. (II)
3. Heat-sterilize teeth that do not contain amalgam before they are used for educational purposes. (IB)

Handling Contaminated Waste

Contaminated items that may contain the body fluids of patients, such as gloves and patient napkins, should be placed in a lined trash receptacle. Receptacles for contaminated waste should be covered with a properly fitted lid that can be opened with a foot pedal. Keeping the lid closed prevents air movement and the spreading of contaminants. This receptacle should not be overfilled, and it should be emptied at least once daily.

Red bags or containers should *not* be used for unregulated waste. Check the specific requirements of your local state or county health department (Fig. 19-26).

Handling Medical Waste

Medical waste is any solid waste that is generated in the diagnosis, treatment, or immunization of humans or animals in research. Infectious waste is a subset of medical waste. Only a small percentage of medical waste is infectious and needs to be regulated.

Infectious Waste

Containers of infectious waste (regulated waste), as defined earlier, must be labeled with the universal biohazard symbol, identified in compliance with local regulations, or both. Local regulations may vary regarding the return of extracted teeth to patients, especially for young children who give their tooth to the "tooth fairy."

NOTE: *Containers used for holding contaminated items also must be labeled. Examples of such containers are contaminated sharps containers, pans or trays used for holding contaminated instruments, bags of contaminated laundry, specimen containers, and storage containers.*

Disposal of Medical Waste

Once contaminated waste leaves the office, it is then regulated by the EPA and by state and local laws. Under most regulations, the manner of disposal is determined by the amount (weight) of infectious materials for disposal.

The average dental practice is categorized as a "small producer" of infectious waste, and disposal is regulated accordingly. The law requires the dentist to maintain records of the final disposal of this medical waste, including documentation of how, when, and where it was disposed.

Recall

22. What are three examples of contaminated waste?
23. What are three examples of general waste?
24. What is another term for infectious waste?
25. Which type of waste must be identified with the biohazard label?

ADDITIONAL INFECTION-CONTROL PRACTICES

OSHA BBP

- Never eat, drink, smoke, apply cosmetics or lip balm, or handle contact lenses in any area of the dental office where there is possible contamination, such as the dental treatment rooms, dental laboratory, sterilization area, or x-ray processing area.

- Never store food or drink in refrigerators that contain potentially contaminated items.

CDC Guidelines–Special Considerations

Saliva Ejectors

Backflow from low-volume saliva ejectors occurs when the pressure in the patient's mouth is less than that in the evacuator. This backflow can be a potential source of cross-contamination between patients. Although no adverse health effects associated with the saliva ejector have been reported, you should be aware that in certain situations, backflow could occur when using a saliva ejector.

CDC Saliva Ejector

Do not advise patients to close their lips tightly around the tip of the saliva ejector to evacuate oral fluids. (II)

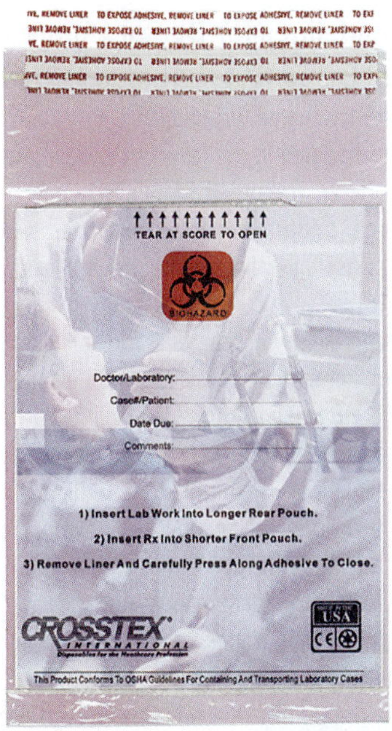

Fig. 19-27 Pouch for lab cases with the biohazard label. (Courtesy Crosstex.)

Dental Laboratory

Items that are commonly used in a dental laboratory (e.g., dentures, partials, impressions, and bite registrations) are potential sources for cross-contamination. Dental prostheses or impressions can be contaminated with bacteria, viruses, and fungi. These items should be handled in a manner to prevent exposure to dental team members, patients, and the office environment.

When cases are sent to a commercial dental laboratory, there must be effective communication between the laboratory and dental office. Written information should be provided to the laboratory regarding the type of cleaning and disinfecting solutions that were used on the impressions, models, etc. Follow the manufacturer's recommendations to ensure that the materials are not damaged or distorted because of disinfectant exposure (Fig. 19-27).

Dental prostheses or impressions should be thoroughly cleaned and disinfected before being handled in an in-office laboratory (Procedure 19-6). The best time to clean and disinfect impressions, prostheses, or appliances is as soon as possible after removal from the patient's mouth before the blood or saliva can dry (Fig. 19-28). Always check the manufacturer's recommendations regarding the stability of specific materials during disinfection. The majority of items can be disinfected with an EPA-registered hospital disinfectant.

Environmental surfaces in the laboratory should be barrier-protected or cleaned and disinfected the same as you do for the dental operatory.

Laboratory items (e.g., burs, polishing points, rag wheels, or laboratory knives) that have been used on contaminated appliances or prostheses, should be heat-sterilized, disinfected between patients, or discarded (disposable products) (Fig. 19-29).

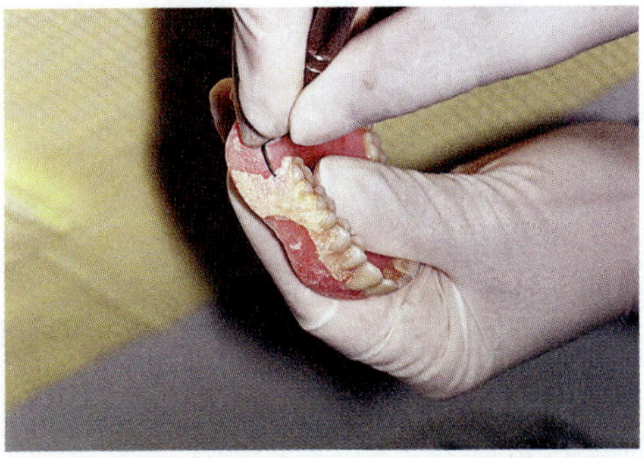

Fig. 19-28 This denture has large amounts of calculus adhering to it. (From Darby ML, Walsh MM: *Dental hygiene: theory and practice,* ed 2, St Louis, 2003, Saunders; courtesy Bertha Chan, RHD, BS.)

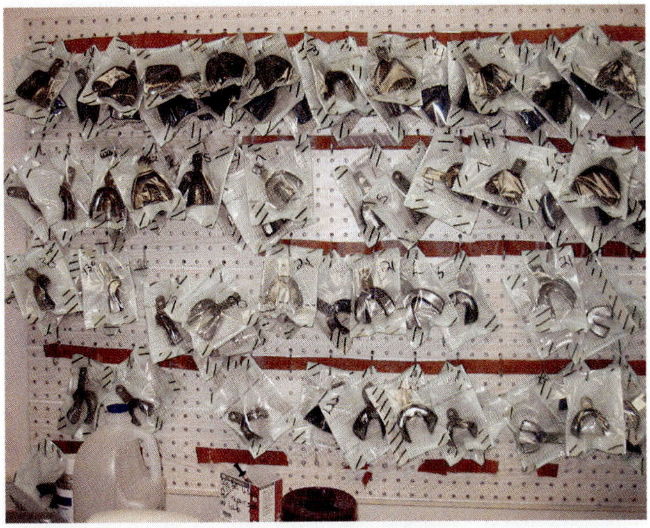

Fig. 19-29 Impression trays are heat-sterilized in individual bags.

CDC CDC Guidelines for Dental Laboratories

1. Use PPE when handling items received in the laboratory until they have been decontaminated. (IA and IC)
2. Before they are handled in the laboratory, clean, disinfect, and rinse all dental prostheses and prosthodontic materials (e.g., impressions, bite registrations, occlusal rims, and extracted teeth) by using an EPA-registered hospital disinfectant having at least an intermediate-level activity. (IB)
3. Consult with manufacturers regarding the stability of specific materials (e.g., impression materials) relative to disinfection procedures. (II)
4. Include specific information regarding disinfection techniques when laboratory cases are sent off-site and on their return. (II)
5. Clean and heat-sterilize heat-tolerant items used in the mouth (e.g., metal impression trays and face-bow forks). (IB)

   Follow manufacturers' instructions for cleaning, sterilizing, or disinfecting items that become contaminated but do not normally contact the patient (e.g., burs, polishing points, rag wheels, articulators, case pans, and lathes. If manufacturers' instructions are unavailable, clean and sterilize heat-stable items and disinfect with an EPA-registered hospital disinfectant with low- to intermediate-level activity. (II)

Modified from *Policy to practice: OSAP's guide to the guidelines,* Annapolis, Maryland, 2004, OSAP.

Preprocedural Mouthrinses

Some dental practitioners have their patients rinse with an antimicrobial mouthrinse before dental procedures. This procedure is intended to reduce the number of microorganisms released in the form of aerosol or spatter. In addition, preprocedural mouthrinsing can decrease the number of microorganisms introduced into the patient's bloodstream during invasive dental procedures. The scientific evidence is inconclusive that preprocedural mouthrinsing prevents clinical infections among dental health professionals or patients. Therefore, the CDC identifies the use of a preprocedural mouthrinse as an unresolved issue.

Mycobacterium tuberculosis

Patients infected with *M. tuberculosis* (the microorganism that causes tuberculosis [TB]) may seek dental treatment in private offices. It is important for the dental assistant to understand how to manage these patients. *M. tuberculosis* is a bacterium that is spread by airborne infective particles when the patient sneezes, coughs, or even speaks. The small particles can remain airborne for hours. Infection occurs when a susceptible person inhales the bacteria, which then travel to the lungs. TB bacteria can remain alive in the lungs for years, a condition called *latent TB infection.* Persons with latent TB usually have a reactive tuberculin

Procedure 19-6 Disinfecting an Alginate Impression

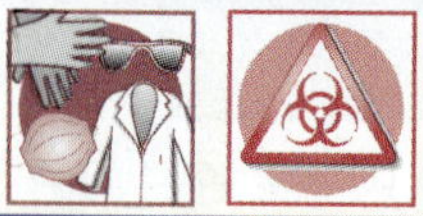

Goal

To disinfect an alginate impression.

Equipment and Supplies

- Protective clothing
- Surgical mask
- Protective eyewear
- Chemical-resistant utility gloves
- Disinfectant solution

PROCEDURAL STEPS

1. Rinse the impression under running tap water to clean it. If necessary, use a soft, camel-hair brush to remove debris.

   Purpose: To remove any blood and/or saliva.
2. Disinfect the impression using an intermediate-level hospital disinfectant for the contact time recommended on the germicide's label.

   Note: Either immersion or spraying is recommended for disinfection of impressions. Spraying uses less solution, and often you can use the same disinfectant that you use for the operatory. However, sprayed disinfectants may pool, which may prevent some surfaces from being adequately exposed to the germicide. Some organizations encourage immersion disinfection of all dental impressions.
3. If spraying is used, spray the impression thoroughly and wrap it with well-moistened paper towels. Unwrap the impression after the manufacturer's recommended contact time has elapsed.
4. If immersion is used, remove the impression after the manufacturer's recommended contact time has elapsed.
5. Rinse the disinfected impression under tap water to remove any residual germicide.
6. After a thorough rinse, gently shake the impression within the sink basin to remove the remaining water with minimal spatter.

   Note: Always check the recommendations of the impression manufacturer as to the stability of the impression material during disinfection.

skin test (TST), but they have no symptoms of active disease and are not infectious. However, they can develop disease later in life if they do not receive treatment for their latent infection. For patients with known or suspected active TB, the CDC recommends that elective dental treatment be delayed until the patient is noninfectious. For patients requiring urgent dental care, the CDC recommends referring the patient to a facility with TB engineering controls and a respiratory protection program.

CDC CDC Guidelines for *M. tuberculosis*

- All dental healthcare professionals (DHCP) should be educated regarding the signs, symptoms, and transmission of TB. (IB)
- All DHCP who could have contact with persons with suspected or confirmed cases of TB should have a baseline TST. (IB)
- Assess each patient for a history of TB, and document it on the medical history. (IB)
- Follow CDC recommendations for developing, maintaining, and implementing a TB infection-control plan. (IB)

The following applies to patients known or suspected to have active TB:

- The patient should be evaluated away from other patients and personnel. (IB)
- Elective dental treatment should be deferred until the patient is noninfectious. (IB)
- Patients who require urgent dental treatment should be referred to a facility with TB engineering controls and a respiratory protection program. (IB)

Creutzfeldt-Jakob Disease and Other Prion Diseases

Creutzfeldt-Jakob disease (CJD) belongs to a group of rapidly progressive, invariably fatal, degenerative neurological disorders. The disease can affect both humans and animals. It is thought that the disease is caused by a prion infection (see Chapter 18). Prion diseases have an incubation period (time between infection and signs of disease) of years and are usually fatal within one year of diagnosis. The CDC offers no recommendation regarding the use of special precautions in addition to Standard Precautions when treating known CJD patients. This remains an unresolved issue.

CDC Creutzfeldt-Jakob Disease

Potential infectivity of oral tissues in patients with Creutzfeldt-Jakob disease is an unresolved issue. Scientific data indicate that the risk, if any, of sporadic transmission of the disease during dental and oral surgical procedures is low to nil. No recommendation is offered regarding use of special precautions in addition to Standard Precautions when treating patients known to have Creutzfeldt-Jakob disease. (Unresolved issue)

Laser/Electrosurgery Plumes or Surgical Smoke

During surgical procedures that use a laser or an electrosurgical unit, a smoke by-product is created by the thermal destruction of the tissue. Laser plumes or surgical smoke create another potential risk for dental healthcare professionals. One concern is that the aerosolized infectious material in the laser plume may reach the nasal mucosa of the operator or other members of the dental team. However, the presence of an infectious agent in a laser plume might not be enough to cause disease from airborne exposure, especially if the agent's normal mode of transmission is not airborne. Because the effect of exposure on dental personnel from the use of dental lasers has not yet been adequately evaluated, the CDC offers no recommendations, and this remains an unresolved issue.

CDC Laser/Electrosurgery Plumes/Surgical Smoke

The effect of exposure (e.g., disease transmission or adverse respiratory effects) on DHCP from the use of lasers in dentistry has not been adequately evaluated. (Unresolved issue)

It has been suggested that the use of high-filtration surgical masks and possible full face shields, central room suction units, and mechanical smoke exhaust systems with a high-efficiency filter may reduce dental healthcare professionals' exposure to laser plumes and surgical smoke.

Recall

26. What is the BBP Standard rule regarding refrigerators in dental offices?
27. What is the CDC guideline for using saliva ejectors?
28. How does tuberculosis infection occur?
29. What is the CDC recommendation on the use of preprocedural mouthrinses?
30. Did the CDC make a recommendation on the effects of exposure to laser plumes on dental healthcare professionals? Why or why not?

Legal and Ethical Implications

The CDC *Guidelines for Infection Control in Dental Health-Care Settings–2003* apply to approximately 168,000 dentists, 218,000 dental assistants, 112,000 dental hygienists, and 53,000 dental laboratory technicians. They also apply to students, trainees, and other persons not directly involved in patient care but potentially exposed to infectious agents (e.g., administrative, clerical, housekeeping, maintenance, and volunteers). Remember that these guidelines have established the standard of care for infection control in dentistry.

Infection control is also an ethical issue for the dental assistant. Often the dental assistant is alone when performing infection-control procedures; if cross-contamination occurs, no one else may know. Always following proper infection-control procedures is a matter of personal commitment and integrity.

Patients should have absolute confidence that the infection-control procedures in the office are never compromised. This confidence is as important for the protection of the dental team members as it is for the patient.

Eye to the Future

The area of infection control in dentistry is continually evolving, and as new diseases are identified, there will be new practices and techniques to prevent their spread. While some concepts of dental infection control may seem confusing, the basic principles will remain the cornerstone for preventing disease transmission in the dental setting.

Dental professionals must remain vigilant and keep current on the latest information to ensure the health of patients, their families, and themselves.

Critical Thinking

1. How would you handle a situation in which you knew that a co-worker was not routinely following infection-control policies?
2. Mrs. James becomes offended when you put on gloves before taking her radiographs. She insists that she does not have a disease and that her previous dental assistant never wore gloves. What would you explain to her?
3. What precautions would you take if a new patient in your office said that he was allergic to latex?
4. How would you explain the CDC Guidelines and the OSHA Bloodborne Pathogens Standard to a new employee who has no formal dental-assisting education?

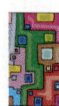

20

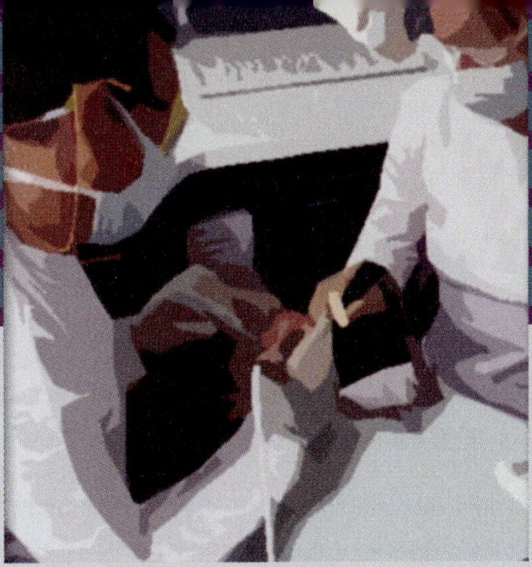

Principles and Techniques of Disinfection

Outline

KEY TERMS

Antiseptic Substance for killing microorganisms on the skin.

Bioburden Blood, saliva, and other body fluids.

Broad-spectrum activity Capable of killing a wide range of microbes.

Chlorine dioxide Effective, rapid-acting environmental surface disinfectant or chemical sterilant.

Clinical contact surface Surface touched by contaminated hands, instruments, or spatter during dental treatment.

Disinfectant Chemical used to reduce or lower the number of microorganisms on living objects.

Environmental surface Surface within a healthcare facility that is not directly involved in patient care, but may be contaminated during the course of treatment (e.g., countertops, floors, walls, instrument control panels, etc.).

Fungicidal (fun-ja-**si**-dal) A product that is capable of killing fungi.

Glutaraldehyde (glut-er-**al**-da-hide) EPA-registered high-level disinfectant.

High-level disinfectant Hospital disinfectant with tuberculocidal activity.

Hospital disinfectant Disinfectant with the ability to kill *Staphylococcus aureus, Salmonella choleraesuis,* and *Pseudomonas aeruginosa.*

Housekeeping surface Surface that is not contaminated during dental treatment (e.g., floors, walls).

Immersion disinfectant Disinfectant used for immersion (soaking) of heat-sensitive instruments.

Intermediate-level disinfectant Liquid disinfectant with EPA registration as a hospital disinfectant with tuberculocidal activity. It is used for disinfecting operatory surfaces.

Iodophor (i-**oh**-duh-for) EPA-registered, intermediate-level hospital disinfectant.

Low-level disinfectant Disinfectant that destroys certain viruses and fungi; used for general housecleaning (e.g., walls, floors).

Precleaning Removal of bioburden before disinfection.

Residual activity Action that continues long after initial application, as with disinfectants.

continued

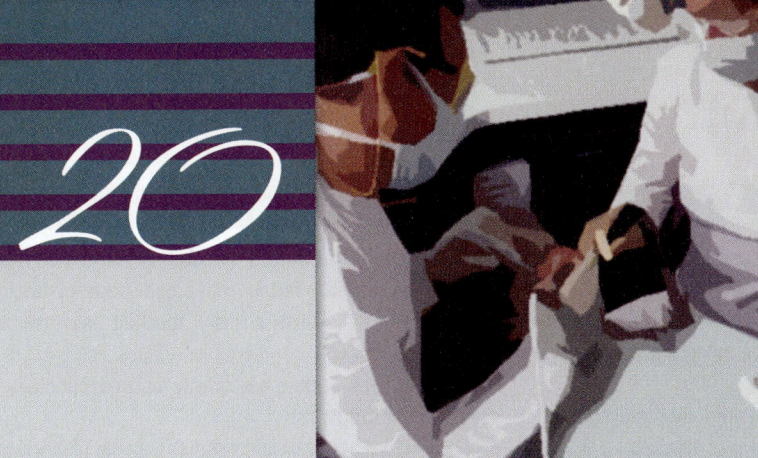

KEY TERMS—cont'd

Reuse life Time period that a disinfectant should remain effective during use and reuse.

Shelf life How long a product may be stored prior to use.

Sodium hypochlorite (hi-po-**klor**-ite) Surface disinfectant commonly known as *household bleach.*

Splash, spatter, and droplet surface Surface that does not contact members of the dental team or contaminated instruments or supplies.

Sporicidal Capable of killing bacterial spores.

Sterilant Agent that kills all microorganisms.

Sterilization (*ster*-ih-luh-**zay**-shun) Process that kills all microorganisms.

Surface barrier Fluid-resistant material used to cover surfaces likely to become contaminated.

Synthetic phenol compound (sin-**theh**-tik **fee**-nol) EPA-registered intermediate-level hospital disinfectant with broad-spectrum disinfecting action.

Touch surface Surface directly touched and contaminated during procedures.

Transfer surface Surface not directly touched, but often contacted by contaminated instruments.

Tuberculocidal (too-*bur*-ku-lo-**si**-dul) Capable of inactivating tuberculosis-causing microorganisms.

Virucidal Capable of killing some viruses.

LEARNING OUTCOMES

On completion of this chapter, the student will be able to achieve the following objectives:

- Pronounce, define, and spell the Key Terms.
- Explain why dental treatment-room surfaces need barriers or disinfection.
- List the types of surfaces in the dental office typically covered with barriers.
- Describe the two methods to deal with surface contamination.
- Explain the difference between disinfection and sterilization.
- Explain the difference between a disinfectant and an antiseptic.
- Name the government agency that is responsible for registering disinfectants.
- Identify chemical products used for intermediate-level and low-level surface disinfection, and explain the advantages and disadvantages of each.
- Demonstrate the process of cleaning and disinfecting a treatment room.
- Demonstrate the process of precleaning contaminated dental instruments.
- Explain the precautions when using chemical sterilants/disinfectants.
- Describe the CDC guidelines for disinfecting clinical contact surfaces.
- Describe the CDC guidelines for disinfecting housekeeping surfaces.

During patient treatment, dental equipment and treatment room surfaces are likely to become contaminated with saliva or aerosol containing blood and saliva. Surfaces that are touched frequently (e.g., light handles, unit controls, drawer handles) can act as reservoirs of microorganisms. When these surfaces are touched, microbial agents can be transferred to instruments, to charts, or to the nose, mouth, or eyes of dental team members or of other patients. A primary source of cross-contamination can be found when a member of the dental team touches surfaces with contaminated gloved hands.

Laboratory studies have determined that microorganisms may survive on **environmental surfaces** for different lengths of time. For example, *Mycobacterium tuberculosis* may survive for weeks, whereas the herpes simplex virus dies in a matter of minutes. It is impossible to predict accurately the life span of microorganisms on the surfaces of dental equipment. Therefore the safest approach is to assume that if the surface has had contact with saliva, blood, or other potentially infectious material, the surface contains live microorganisms.

NOTE: Throughout this chapter, the Centers for Disease Control and Prevention (CDC) recommendations are indicated and the category of scientific evidence is noted at the end of each recommendation.

CDC Rankings of Evidence

Each recommendation made by the CDC is categorized on the basis of existing scientific data, theoretical rationale, and applicability. Rankings are based on the following categories:

- **Category IA** Strongly recommended for implementation and strongly supported by well-designed experimental, clinical, or epidemiologic studies (studies of patterns and causes of diseases).
- **Category IB** Strongly recommended for implementation and supported by experimental, clinical, or epidemiologic studies and a strong theoretical rationale.
- **Category IC** Required for implementation, as mandated by federal or state regulation or standard.
- **Category II** Suggested for implementation and supported by suggestive clinical or epidemiologic studies or a theoretical rationale.
- **Unresolved Issue** No recommendation. Practices for which insufficient evidence or no consensus regarding efficacy exists.

ENVIRONMENTAL INFECTION CONTROL

The CDC *Guidelines for Infection Control in Dental Health-Care Settings—2003* divide environmental surfaces into **clinical contact surfaces** and **housekeeping surfaces.** Housekeeping surfaces include floors, walls, and sinks. Because these have much lower risk for disease transmission, cleaning and decontamination are not as rigorous as those used for clinical areas and for patient-treatment items.

CDC Recommendations for Environmental Infection Control

General Recommendations

1. Follow the manufacturers' instructions for correct use of cleaning and EPA-registered hospital disinfecting products. (IB, IC)
2. Do not use liquid chemical sterilants/high-level disinfectants for disinfection of environmental surfaces (clinical contact or housekeeping). (IB, IC)
3. Use PPE, as appropriate, when cleaning and disinfecting environmental surfaces. (IC)

Clinical Contact Surfaces

1. Use surface barriers to protect clinical contact surfaces, particularly those that are difficult to clean, and change barriers between patients. (II)
2. Clean and disinfect clinical contact surfaces that are not barrier protected, by using an EPA-registered hospital disinfectant with a low- (i.e., HIV and HBV label claims) to intermediate-level (i.e., tuberculocidal claim) activity after each patient. Use an **intermediate-level disinfectant** if visibly soiled with blood. (IB)

Housekeeping Surfaces

1. Clean housekeeping surfaces (e.g., floors, walls, and sinks) with a detergent and water or an EPA-registered hospital disinfectant/detergent on a routine basis, depending on the nature of the surface and type and degree of contamination, and as appropriate, based on the location in the facility, and when visibly soiled. (IB)
2. Clean mops and cloths after use and allow to dry before reuse, or use single-use disposable mop heads or cloths. (II)
3. Prepare fresh cleaning or EPA-registered disinfecting solutions daily and as instructed by the manufacturer. (II)
4. Clean walls, blinds, and window curtains in patient-care areas when they are visibly dusty or soiled. (II)

Things to consider when planning for cleaning and disinfection of patient-treatment areas include:

- Amount of direct patient contact
- Type and frequency of hand contact
- Potential amount of contamination by aerosol and/or spray
- Other sources of microorganisms (e.g., dust, soil, or water)

Clinical Contact Surfaces

Clinical contact surfaces can be directly contaminated either by direct spray or spatter generated during dental procedures, or by contact with the dental professional's gloved hands.

Current infection-control guidelines of the Organization for Safety and Asepsis Procedures (OSAP) recommend that clinical surfaces be classified and maintained under three categories: (1) touch, (2) transfer, and (3) splash, spatter, and droplet (Fig. 20-1).

Touch surfaces are directly touched and contaminated during treatment procedures. Touch surfaces include dental light handles, dental unit controls, chair switches, chairside computers, pens, telephones, containers of dental materials, and drawer handles.

Transfer surfaces are not directly touched but often are touched by contaminated instruments. Transfer surfaces include instrument trays and handpiece holders.

Splash, spatter, and droplet surfaces do not actually contact members of the dental team or the contaminated instruments or supplies. Countertops are a major example.

Touch and transfer surfaces should be either barrier-protected or cleaned and disinfected between patients. Splash, spatter, and droplet surfaces should be cleaned at least once daily (Box 20-1).

Surface Contamination

Two methods that deal with surface contamination are (1) to prevent the surface from becoming contaminated by the use of a **surface barrier** and (2) to preclean and disinfect the surface between patients. Each has advantages and disadvantages, and most dental offices use a combination of surface disinfection and surface barriers.

Smooth, hard surfaces such as countertops, handles, supply containers, and bottles can be quickly and easily cleaned (Fig. 20-2). Surfaces with crevices, knobs, or other difficult-to-clean features, such light handles, air-water syringe handles, and electrical switches (which can short-circuit), are better protected with surface barriers.

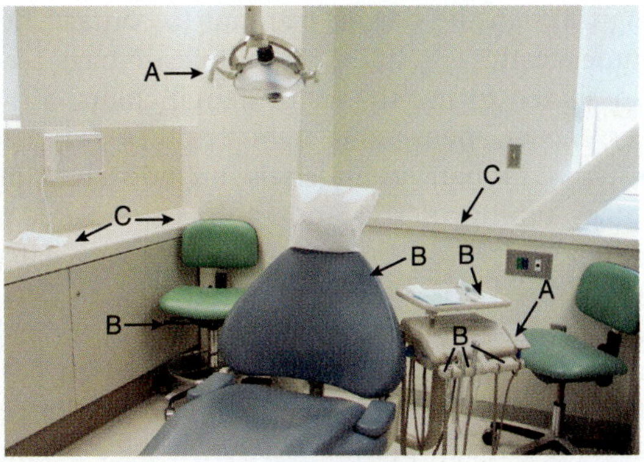

Fig. 20-1 **A,** Touch surfaces. **B,** Transfer surfaces. **C,** Splash, spatter, and droplet surfaces.

Box 20-1 Comparison of Surface Barriers and Precleaning/Disinfection

	Advantages	Disadvantages
Surface barrier	• Protects surfaces that are not easily cleaned and disinfected • Prevents contamination when properly placed • Less time-consuming • Reduces handling and storage of chemicals • Provides patient with visual assurance of cleanliness • Does not damage equipment or surfaces	• Adds plastics to the environment after disposal • May be more expensive than precleaning and disinfecting • Requires a variety of sizes and shapes • May become dislodged during treatment
Precleaning and disinfecting	• May be less expensive than surface barriers • Does not add plastic to the environment • Some dentists do not like the appearance of plastic barriers	• Requires more time and therefore may not be done properly • Not all surfaces can be adequately precleaned • Over time, some chemicals are destructive to dental equipment surfaces • No method to determine if the microbes have been removed or killed • Some disinfectants must be prepared fresh daily • Chemicals are added to the environment upon disposal

It is the responsibility of the dental assistant to make certain that equipment and treatment room surfaces are properly managed to prevent patient-to-patient disease transmission.

Surface Barriers

Placing barriers on surfaces and equipment can prevent contamination of clinical contact areas, but they are especially useful for those areas that are difficult to clean.

All surface barriers currently on the market should be resistant to fluids. Fluid-resistant barriers prevent microorganisms in saliva, blood, and other liquids from soaking through the barrier material to contact the surface underneath (Fig. 20-3). Some plastic bags are specially designed to the shapes of dental chairs, air-water syringes, hoses, pens, and light handles (Fig. 20-4). Other types of barrier materials include clear plastic wrap, bags, tubing, plastic tape, and plastic-backed paper (Figs. 20-5 and 20-6). Sticky tape as a plastic barrier is frequently used to protect smooth surfaces, such as touch pads on equipment or electrical switches on chairs and x-ray equipment. Aluminum foil can also be used because it is easily formed around any shape. Procedure 20-1 reviews steps in placing and removing barriers.

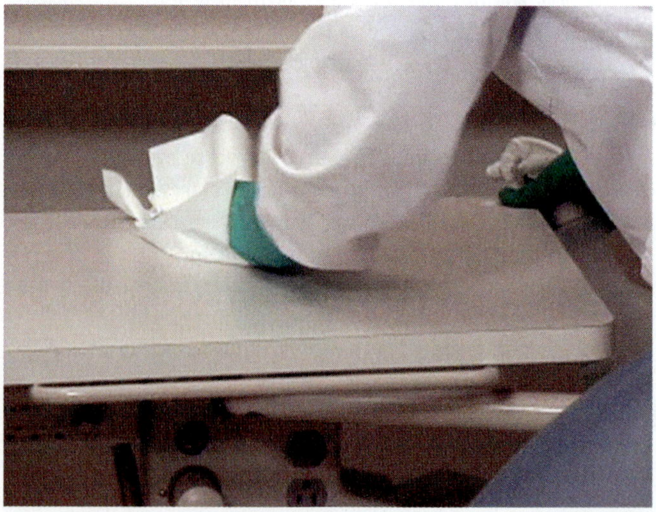

Fig. 20-2 Smooth surfaces are easily sprayed and wiped.

Between patients, while you are still gloved, you should remove and discard contaminated barriers. If you are careful when removing contaminated barriers not to touch the surface below, you do not have to clean and disinfect the surface. However, if you inadvertently do touch a surface, you will have to clean and disinfect that surface.

Even though surfaces have been covered with barriers, the surfaces should still be cleaned and disinfected at the beginning and the end of each workday.

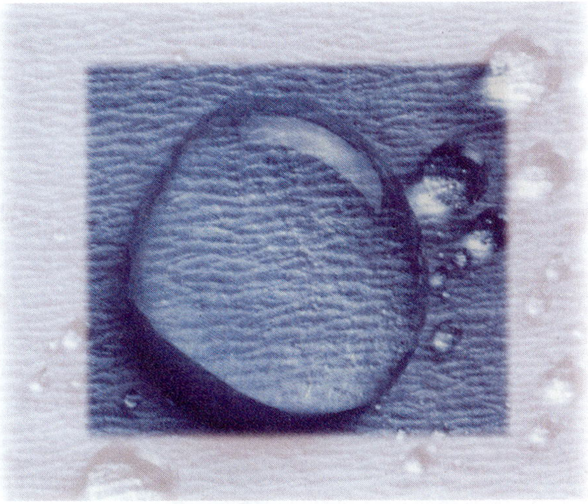

Fig. 20-3 An example of water on a fluid-resistant material. (Courtesy Crosstex.)

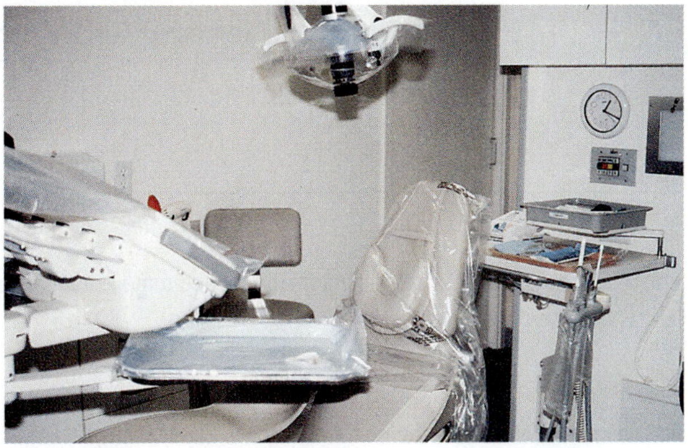

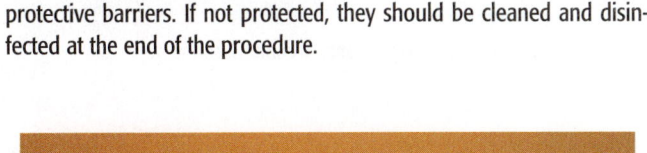

Fig. 20-4 Surfaces touched during patient care should be covered with protective barriers. If not protected, they should be cleaned and disinfected at the end of the procedure.

Surfaces Typically Protected with Barriers*

Headrest on dental chair
Control buttons on dental chair
Light handles
Light switches
Evacuator hoses and controls
X-ray control switches
Air-water syringe handles
Dental-unit control touch pads
Patient mirror handles
Handle on light-curing device
Switch on amalgamators or other automatic mixing devices
Drawer handles
Adjustment handles on operator and assistant stools
Bracket table

* If a surface cannot be easily and thoroughly cleaned and disinfected, it should have barrier protection.

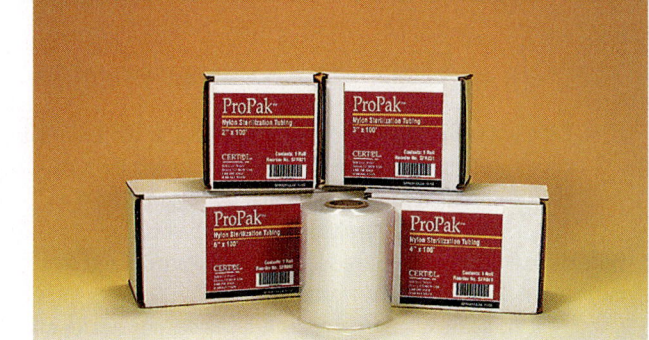

Fig. 20-5 Rolls of plastic tubing that can be cut to the desired length. (Courtesy Certol.)

Recall

1. Why must surfaces in dental treatment rooms be disinfected or protected with barriers?
2. What are the two methods that deal with surface contamination?
3. What is the purpose of surface barriers?
4. What should you do if the barrier becomes torn?

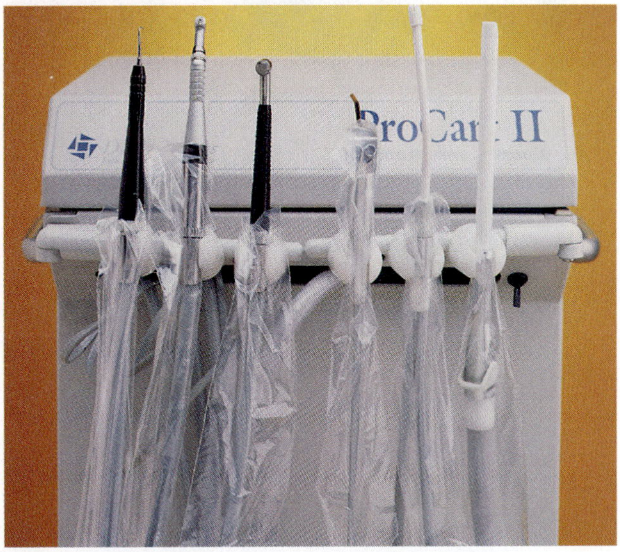

Fig. 20-6 Tube socks provide barrier protection for difficult-to-clean areas. (Courtesy Certol.)

Procedure 20-1 Placing and Removing Surface Barriers

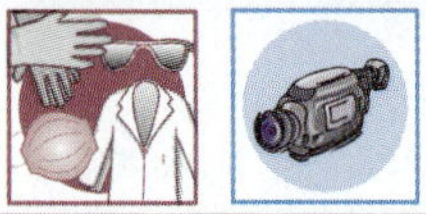

Goal

To place surface barriers before patient treatment and remove the barriers at the end of the procedure.

Equipment and Supplies

- Liquid antimicrobial hand soap
- Utility gloves
- Plastic surface barriers
- Noncontaminated surfaces in dental treatment room

PROCEDURAL STEPS

1. Wash and dry hands.
2. Select the appropriate surface barrier to be placed over the clean surface.
   Note: If the surfaces to be covered have been previously contaminated, put on your utility gloves and preclean and disinfect the surface. Then wash, disinfect, and remove your utility gloves. Wash and dry your hands before applying the surface barriers.
3. Place each barrier over the entire surface to be protected. Check that the barrier is secure and will not come off.
   Purpose: If the barrier slips out of position, the underlying surface will become contaminated and will require precleaning and disinfection, negating the barrier's purpose.

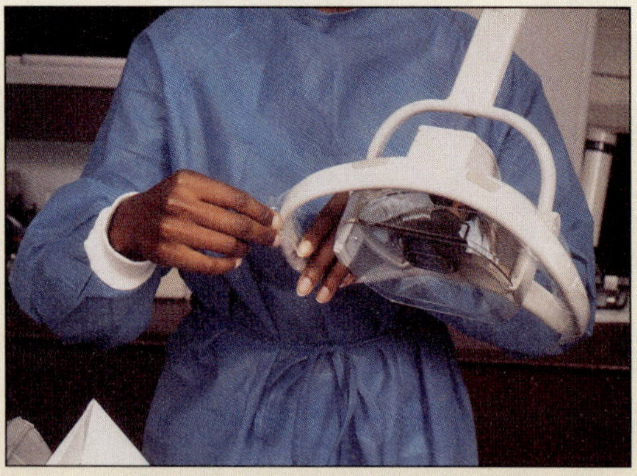

4. Wear your utility gloves to remove contaminated surface barriers after dental treatment.
   Purpose: Utility gloves protect the skin from contamination.

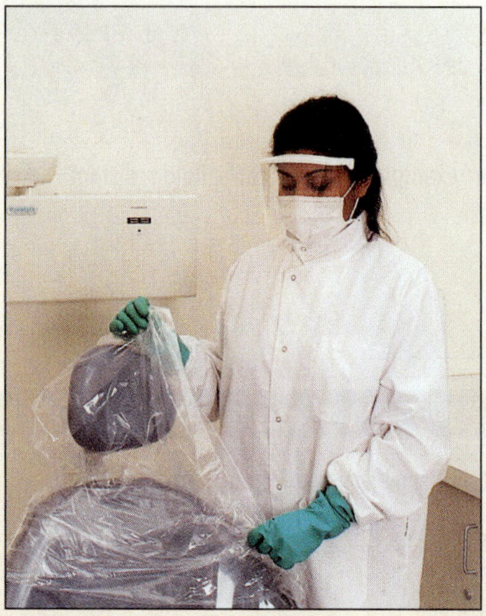

5. Very carefully remove each cover without touching the underlying surface with either the utility glove or the contaminated outside surface of the barrier.
   Purpose: If a surface is accidentally touched during the removal of the cover, the surface must be precleaned and disinfected.
6. Discard the used covers in the regular waste trash. (Check disposal laws in your state.)
   Purpose: Most states do not consider barriers to be regulated waste (requiring special disposal) unless an item is soaked or caked with blood or saliva that would be released if the item was compressed.
7. Wash, disinfect, and remove your utility gloves. Wash and dry your hands, then apply fresh surface covers for the next patient.
   Purpose: Your utility gloves are contaminated from handling the used barriers. By washing, drying, and disinfecting your utility gloves, you will know they are ready for the next use.

Precleaning and Disinfection

Although no cases of cross-infection have been linked to dental treatment room surfaces, cleaning and disinfection of these surfaces are important components in an effective infection-control program. In addition, the OSHA Bloodborne Pathogens Standard requires that contaminated work surfaces be disinfected between patient visits (see Chapter 19).

> **CDC Clinical Contact Surfaces**
>
> If barriers are not used, surfaces should be cleaned and disinfected between patients by using an EPA-registered hospital disinfectant with an HIV, HBV claim.
>
> NOTE: Under the new CDC *Guidelines,* only commercially available EPA-registered agents should be used on clinical contact surfaces in dental healthcare facilities.

Precleaning

Precleaning means to clean before disinfecting. All contaminated surfaces must be precleaned before they can be disinfected. Even if no blood is visible on the surface, it must be precleaned because even a thin layer of saliva on the surface can decrease the effectiveness of the disinfectant. Precleaning reduces the number of microbes and removes blood, saliva, and other body fluids, called **bioburden.** *Remember: If a surface is not clean, it cannot be disinfected.*

Precleaning techniques are most effective when used on contaminated surfaces that are *smooth* and *easily accessible* for cleaning. Irregular or textured surfaces are difficult or impossible to clean and therefore interfere with disinfection.

> **CDC Personal Protective Equipment (PPE)**
>
> Use PPE, as appropriate, when cleaning and disinfecting environmental surfaces. Such equipment might include gloves (e.g., puncture and chemical-resistant utility), protective clothing, protective eyewear/face shield, and mask. (IC)
>
> Because of the risks associated with exposure to chemical disinfectants and contaminated surfaces, always wear PPE to prevent occupational exposure to infectious agents and hazardous chemicals.

Regular soap and water may be used for precleaning. If you select a disinfectant that cleans as well as disinfects, however, you can save time and limit the number of products you need.

Disinfection

Disinfection is intended to kill disease-causing microorganisms that remain on the surface *after* precleaning. Spores are not killed during disinfecting procedures.

The term **disinfectant** is used for chemicals that are applied to inanimate surfaces, such as countertops and dental equipment. The term **antiseptic** is used for *antimicrobial* (organism-killing) agents that are applied to living tissue. Disinfectants and antiseptics should never be used interchangeably because tissue toxicity and damage to equipment can result.

Do not confuse disinfection with sterilization. Sterilization is the process in which all forms of life are destroyed (see Chapter 21).

Recall

5. Which regulation requires the use of surface disinfection?
6. Why must surfaces be precleaned?
7. Which type of surfaces must have barriers placed?
8. How are antiseptics different from disinfectants?

Disinfectants

Disinfectants are chemicals that destroy or inactivate most species of *pathogenic* (disease-causing) microorganisms. The Environmental Protection Agency (EPA) registers and regulates disinfectants and chemical **sterilants** according to chemical classification (Table 20-1). A sterilant kills all microorganisms.

In dentistry, *only* those products that are registered with the EPA as **hospital disinfectants** with **tuberculocidal** claims (kills the organism *M. tuberculosis*) should be used to disinfect dental treatment areas. *M. tuberculosis* is highly resistant to disinfectants (Fig. 20-7). If a disinfectant inactivates *M. tuberculosis,* it will certainly inactivate less-resistant microbial families (such as bacteria, viruses, and most fungi) on treated surfaces (Fig. 20-8). A product that is capable of killing spores would be labeled as **sporicidal.** A product that is capable of killing some viruses would be la-

> **Disinfectant Precautions**
>
> Follow the manufacturers' recommendations for:
>
> - Mixing and diluting
> - Application technique
> - Shelf life
> - Activated use life
> - All safety warnings

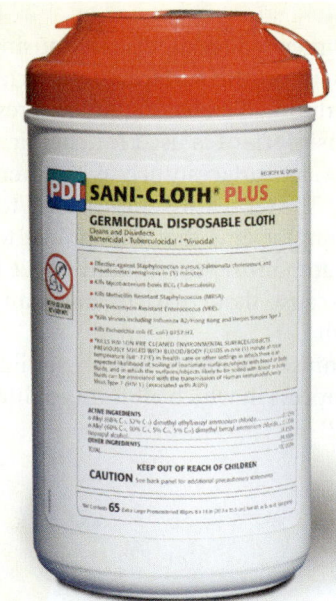

Fig. 20-7 **Disposable premoistened wipes with tuberculocidal activity.** (Courtesy Crosstex.)

Table 20-1 ***Chemical Classification of Disinfectants***

Level of Disinfection	EPA Classification	Use
High level	High level disinfectant with a relatively short contact time and a sterilant when used with a prolonged contact time	Semicritical items that cannot tolerate heat sterilization
Intermediate level	Hospital disinfectant with tuberculocidal activity	Noncritical items or surfaces that have been contaminated with blood or saliva
Low level	Nontuberculocidal	Surfaces not contaminated with blood

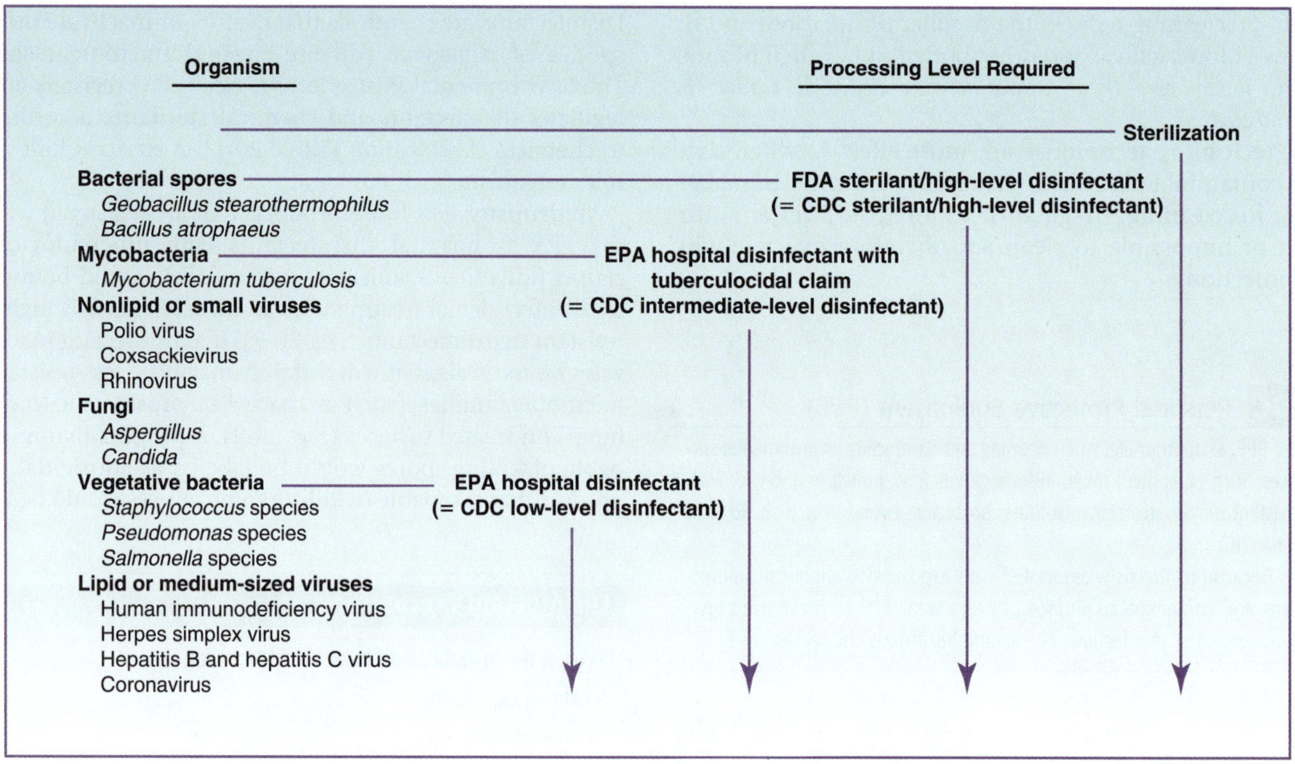

Fig. 20-8 **Decreasing order of resistance of microorganisms to germicidal chemicals.** (Modified from Bond WW, et al: Effective use of liquid germicides on medical devices: instrument design problems. In Black SS, ed: *Disinfection, sterilization and preservation,* ed 4, Philadelphia, 1991, Lea & Febiger, page 1100. From *CDC Guidelines for Infection Control in Dental Health-Care Settings–2003,* page 64.)

beled as **virucidal.** A product that is capable of killing fungi would be labeled as **fungicidal.**

A variety of chemical agents are currently marketed as surface disinfectants and instrument-immersion disinfectants. It is important to carefully read the label of every disinfectant product before you use it. These labels commonly include information about the product such as **shelf life, reuse life,** directions for use, precautionary statements on handling the product, and storage and disposal information.

Ideal surface disinfectant

The ideal surface disinfectant would rapidly kill a broad spectrum (range) of bacteria, would have residual activity and minimal toxicity, and would not damage surfaces to be treated. If a disinfectant has **residual activity,** its action continues long after the initial application. The ideal disinfectant would also be odorless and inexpensive, would work on surfaces with remaining bioburden, and would be simple to use. Unfortunately there is no ideal surface disinfectant. No current disinfectant product meets all of these criteria. Therefore, when selecting a surface disinfectant, you must carefully consider the advantages and disadvantages of various products. Often the manufacturers of dental equipment will recommend the type of surface disinfectant that is most appropriate for their dental chairs and units (Table 20-2).

Recall

9. Which agency regulates disinfectants?
10. What is the ideal disinfectant?

Table 20-2 ***EPA-Registered Surface Disinfectants for Dentistry***

Category/Active Ingredient	Contact*	Pros	Cons
Chlorines (sodium hypochlorite diluted in-office, chlorine dioxide, commercial preparations of sodium hypochlorite with added surfactants)	2-10 min 20° C or 25° C[†]	Economical; rapid, broad-spectrum activity; tuberculocidal; effective in dilute solution	Diluted solutions must be prepared daily; cannot be reused; are corrosive to some metals; may destroy fabrics; may irritate skin and other tissues; chlorine dioxide is a poor cleaner
Complex phenols ("synthetic phenols" containing multiple phenolic agents)	10 min 20° C or 25° C[†]	Broad-spectrum activity; residual activity; effective cleaner and disinfectant; tuberculocidal; compatible with metal, glass, rubber, and plastic	Extended exposure may degrade some plastics or leave etchings on glass; many preparations are limited to one day of use; may leave a residual film on treated surfaces
Dual/synergized quaternary ammonium compounds (alcohol and multiple quaternary ammonium compounds)	6 or 10 min 20° C[†]	Broad-spectrum activity; tuberculocidal; hydrophilic virus claims; low toxicity; contains detergent for cleaning	Readily inactivated by anionic detergents and organic matter; can damage some materials
Iodophors (iodine, combined with a surfactant)	10 min 20° C	Broad-spectrum activity; tuberculocidal; relatively nontoxic; effective cleaner and disinfectant; residual biocidal action	Unstable at higher temperatures; may discolor some surfaces; inactivated by alcohol and hard water; must be prepared daily; dilution and contact times are critical
Phenol-alcohol combinations (phenolic agent in an alcohol base)	10 min 20° C or 25° C[†]	Tuberculocidal; fast-acting; residual activity; some inhibit the growth of mold, mildew, and other fungi	May cause porous surfaces to dry and crack; poor cleaning capabilities
Other halogens (sodium bromide and chlorine)	5 min 20° C	Fast-acting; tuberculocidal; supplied in tablet form for simple dilution; requires minimal storage space	For use on hard surfaces only; chlorine smell

**Contact time/temperatures for tuberculocidal activity.*
[†]Varies by active ingredient or disinfectant brand.
From Infection Control in Practice, *Vol 1, No. 3, Annapolis, MD, August 2002, OSAP.*
NOTE: Glutaraldehydes and simple quaternary ammonium compounds should not be used for surface disinfection in dentistry. High-concentrations alcohols (ethyl alcohol or isopropyl alcohol of at least 70%) should be used on precleaned surfaces.

Iodophors

Iodophors are EPA-registered intermediate-level hospital disinfectants with tuberculocidal action. Iodophors are recommended for disinfecting surfaces that have been soiled with potentially infectious patient material. When used according to the manufacturer's instructions, iodophors are usually effective within 5 to 10 minutes. They may also be used as an immersion disinfectant for nonhydrocolloid impressions (Fig. 20-9).

Because iodophors are inactivated by hard water, they must be mixed with soft or distilled water. Because they contain iodine, iodophors may corrode or discolor certain metals or temporarily cause red or yellow stains on clothing and other surfaces.

Synthetic phenol compounds

Synthetic phenol compounds are EPA-registered intermediate-level hospital disinfectants with **broad-spectrum activity,** meaning they can kill a wide range of microbes. When diluted properly, phenols are used for surface disinfection, provided the surface has been thoroughly cleaned first (Fig. 20-10).

Phenols can be used on metal, glass, rubber, or plastic. They also can be used as a holding solution for instruments; however, phenols leave a residual film on treated surfaces. Synthetic phenol compound is prepared daily. Phenols may also be used to disinfect impressions; however, always check with the manufacturer of the impression material.

Sodium hypochlorite

Sodium hypochlorite is classified as an intermediate-level disinfectant and is the main ingredient in household bleach (Fig. 20-11). Sodium hypochlorite is a fast-acting, economical, and broad-spectrum disinfectant. Under the 1993 CDC *Guidelines,* it was a recommended disinfectant. However, under the new CDC *Guidelines,* because it is *not* an EPA-registered disinfectant, household bleach alone is *no longer* a recommended product for use in dental settings as a disinfectant.

There are EPA-approved disinfectant products on the market that contain sodium hypochlorite or other chlorine compounds. Always check the product label for the EPA registration number.

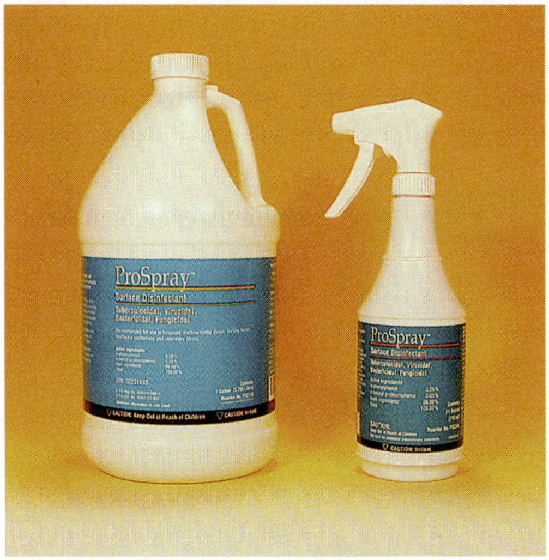

Fig. 20-10 **Synthetic phenol disinfectant.** (Courtesy Certol.)

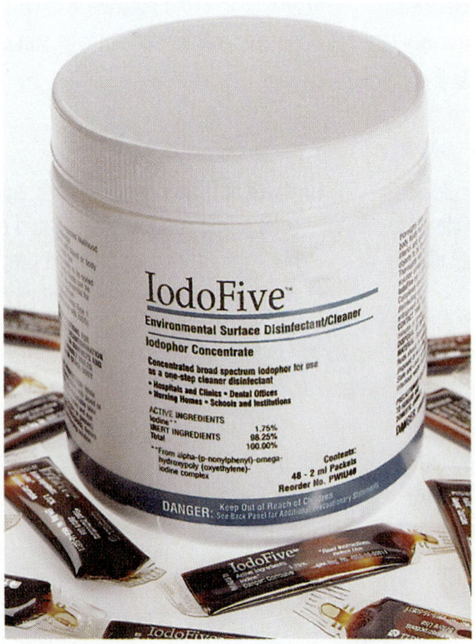

Fig. 20-9 **Iodophor surface disinfectant.** (Courtesy Certol.)

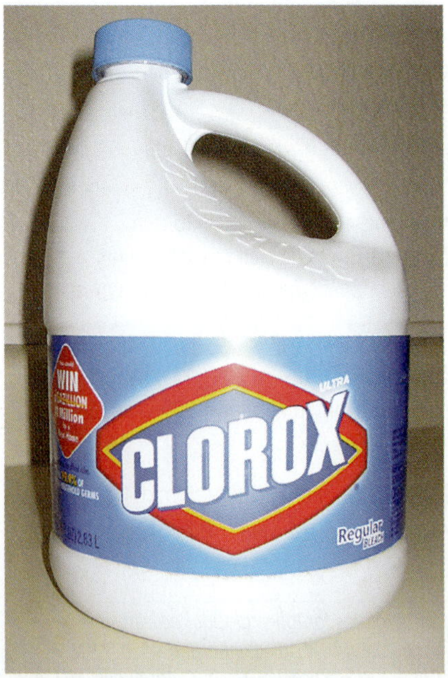

Fig. 20-11 **Sodium hypochlorite (household bleach) is a disinfectant, but because it is not EPA-registered, it should not be used in dentistry as a surface disinfectant.**

The disadvantages of sodium hypochlorite are:

- It is unstable and needs daily preparation.
- It has a strong odor and is corrosive to some metals.
- It is destructive to fabrics and may eventually cause plastic chair covers to crack.
- It is irritating to the eyes and skin.

Alcohol

Ethyl alcohol and isopropyl alcohol have been used over the years as skin antiseptics and surface disinfectants. However, alcohols are *not* effective in the presence of bioburden such as blood and saliva, and the rapid rate of evaporation limits the antimicrobial activity of the alcohol. In addition, alcohols are damaging to certain materials, such as plastics and vinyl, which are prevalent.

The American Dental Association (ADA), CDC, and OSAP do *not* recommend alcohol as an environmental surface disinfectant.

Procedure 20-2 illustrates the cleaning and disinfection of the treatment room.

Procedure 20-2 Performing Treatment Room Cleaning and Disinfection

Goal

To clean and disinfect dental treatment rooms effectively.

Equipment and Supplies

- Personal protective equipment (PPE), including utility gloves, goggles, and a mask
- Intermediate-level surface cleaner/disinfectant
- Paper towels

PROCEDURAL STEPS

1. Put on utility gloves, protective eyewear, and protective clothing.
   Purpose: To prevent contact with contaminated surfaces and chemicals.
   Note: The latex examination gloves used in patient care should *not* be used for precleaning and disinfecting procedures. The chemicals will degrade the latex glove and allow chemicals and contaminants to penetrate to the skin.
2. Make sure that the precleaning/disinfecting product has been prepared correctly and is fresh. Be certain to read and follow the manufacturer's instructions.
   Purpose: Some products are concentrated and must be diluted for use. In addition, some products must be prepared daily.

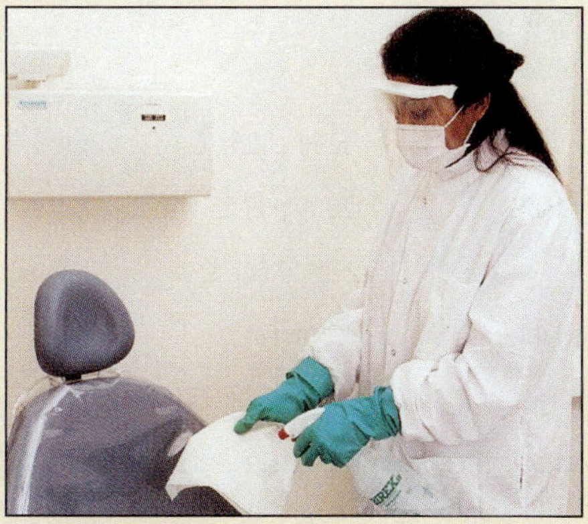

3. To preclean, spray the paper towel or gauze pad with the product and vigorously wipe the surface. You may use a small brush for surfaces that do not become visibly clean from wiping. If you are cleaning a large area, use several towels or gauze pads.
   Purpose: Overspray is reduced by spraying the product onto the towel or gauze pad. Large areas require more towels or pads to avoid spreading bioburden instead of removing it.

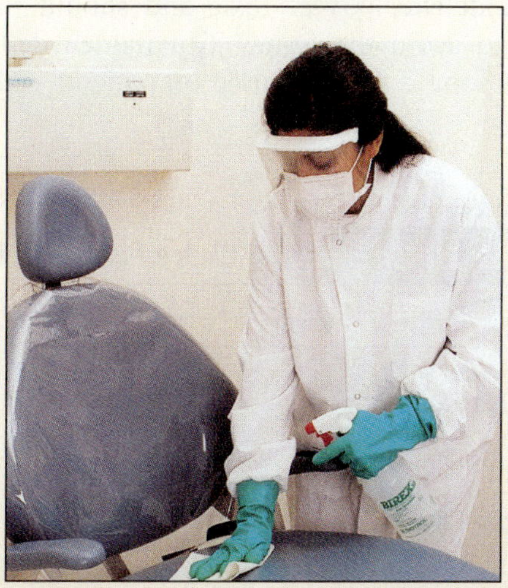

4. To disinfect, spray a fresh paper towel or gauze pad with the product. Let the surface remain moist for the manufacturer's recommended time for tuberculocidal action (usually 10 minutes).
5. If the surface is still moist after the kill time and you are ready to seat another patient, you may wipe the surface dry. Use water to rinse any residual disinfectant from surfaces that will come in contact with the patient's skin or mouth.
   Purpose: The chemicals used for precleaning and disinfecting may irritate the patient's skin or damage the patient's clothing.

Immersion disinfectants

Immersion disinfectants are chemicals on the market that can be used for sterilization or high-level disinfection. When used as a sterilant they destroy all microbial life, including bacterial endospores. Depending on the type, the time for sterilization can range from 6 hours to 30 hours. At weaker dilutions or at shorter contact time, these chemicals provide high-level disinfection, which inactivates all microorganisms *except* endospores (Table 20-3).

Most of these chemicals are toxic and can irritate the eyes, skin, and lungs. PPE must always be worn when using these chemicals. They are to be used for immersion (soaking) of heat-sensitive instruments, and should never be used as surface disinfectants.

Always keep the container lid closed to minimize fumes (Fig. 20-12).

Glutaraldehyde

Glutaraldehyde is classified as a high-level disinfectant/sterilant. It can also be used as a liquid sterilant when the immersion time is greatly increased (see Chapter 21). Times for disinfection range from 10 to 90 minutes; always read the manufacturer's recommendations. Glutaraldehyde products are useful for plastics or other items that cannot withstand heat sterilization. Some glutaraldehyde products are only effective for 28 days after activation.

Glutaraldehyde is very toxic and should be handled carefully to avoid the fumes. Glutaraldehyde-treated instruments should never be used on patients without thoroughly rinsing them with water. Prolonged contact of certain types of instruments with glutaraldehyde solutions can lead to discoloration and corrosion of the instrument surfaces and cutting edges.

Chlorine dioxide

Chlorine dioxide is classified as a high-level disinfectant/sterilant. Products containing chlorine dioxide can be used as an effective, rapid-acting, environmental surface disinfectant (3 minutes) or as a chemical sterilant (6 hours). However, chlorine dioxide products do not readily penetrate organic debris and must be used with a separate cleaner.

Other disadvantages of chlorine dioxide are (1) it must be prepared fresh daily, (2) it must be used with good ventilation, and (3) it is corrosive to aluminum containers.

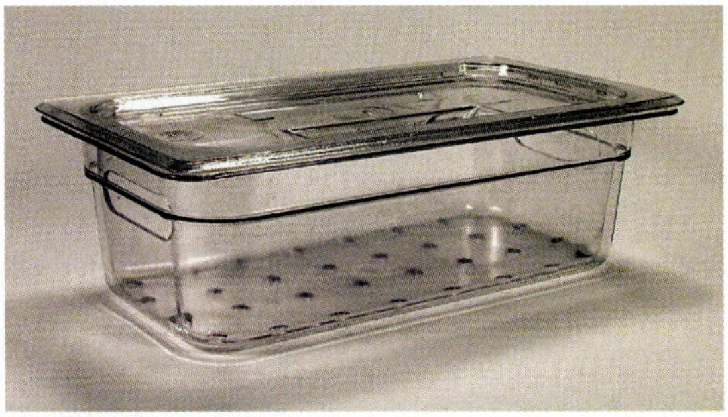

Fig. 20-12 Covered instrument tray for use with immersion disinfectants. (Courtesy Certol.)

Table 20-3 ***FDA-Cleared Instrument-Immersion Disinfectants for Dentistry***

Category/Active Ingredient	Classification	Contact Time(s)
Glutaraldehyde		
2.4%-3.4% alkaline and acidic formulations*	Sterilant	6-10 hr at 20° C, 22° C, or 25° C*
	High-level disinfectant	20-90 min at 20° C, 22° C, or 25° C*
Hydrogen peroxide, 7.3%	Sterilant	6 hr at 20° C
	High-level disinfectant	30 min at 20° C
Ortho-phthalaldehyde, 0.55%	High-level disinfectant	12 min at 20° C
Synergistic solutions		
1.12% glutaraldehyde and 1.93% phenol/phenate	Sterilant	12 hr at 25° C
	High-level disinfectant	20 min at 25° C
7.35% hydrogen peroxide and 0.23% peracetic acid	Sterilant	3 hr at 20° C
	High-level disinfectant	15 min at 20° C

**Varies by active ingredient or disinfectant brand.*

From Infection Control in Practice, *Vol 1, No. 3, Annapolis, MD, August 2002, OSAP.*

NOTE *Gluteraldehydes and simple quaternary ammonium compounds should not be used for surface disinfection in dentistry. High-concentration alcohols (ethyl alcohol or isopropyl alcohol of at least 70%) should be used on precleaned surfaces.*

Ortho-Phthalaldehyde

Ortho-Phthalaldehyde (OPA) is a chemical used in **high-level disinfectant**. It is effective in achieving high-level disinfection within 12 minutes at room temperature. It is more expensive than glutaraldehydes, but it may be a good alternative for healthcare workers with a sensitivity to glutaraldehyde. It has very little odor and does not require activation or mixing.

Disadvantages include (1) the cost, (2) that it can be used only half as long as most glutaraldehydes in dentistry, (3) that it may stain skin and fabrics, (4) that plastics turn a blue-green color where proteins have not been removed, and (5) that it does not have a sterilization claim.

Recall

11. What disinfectant can leave a reddish or yellow stain?
12. What is a disadvantage of synthetic phenols?
13. What is a more common term for sodium hypochlorite?
14. Are alcohol disinfectants effective when blood or saliva is present?
15. What are two uses of chlorine dioxide?

Housekeeping Surfaces

No scientific evidence shows that housekeeping surfaces (e.g., floors, walls, and sinks) pose a risk for disease transmission in dental healthcare settings. The majority of housekeeping surfaces need to be cleaned only with a detergent or **low-level disinfectant** (disinfectant that destroys certain viruses and fungi) and water or an EPA-registered hospital disinfectant/detergent (Fig. 20-13).

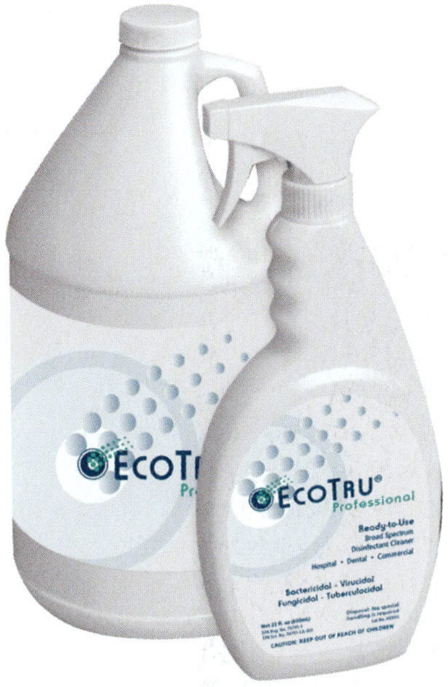

Fig. 20-13 **Fast-acting, high-level disinfectant.** (Courtesy Crosstex International.)

However, in the cleaning process, used solutions of detergents or disinfectants can be a reservoir for microorganisms, especially if prepared in dirty containers, stored for long periods of time, or prepared incorrectly. Make fresh cleaning solution each day, discard any remaining solution, and let the container dry. This will minimize bacterial contamination. When cleaning, avoid producing mists and aerosols or dispersing dust in patient-care areas.

Carpeting and Cloth Furnishings

Carpeting is more difficult to clean than nonporous hard-surface flooring, and it cannot be reliably disinfected, especially after contamination with blood and body substances. Studies have documented the presence of bacteria and fungi in carpeting. Cloth furnishings pose similar contamination risks in areas where there is direct patient care and where contaminated materials are handled, such as an operatory or instrument-processing area.

CDC Carpeting

Avoid using carpeting and cloth-upholstered furnishings in dental operatories, laboratories, and instrument-processing areas. (II)

Spills of Blood and Body Substances

The majority of blood contamination in dentistry results from spatter during dental procedures and from using rotary or ultrasonic instruments. No scientific evidence shows that human immunodeficiency virus (HIV), hepatitis B virus (HBV), or hepatitis C virus (HCV) has been transmitted from a housekeeping surface.

However, good infection-control practices and OSHA require that blood spills and other body fluids be removed and the surfaces disinfected. Always wear gloves and other PPE when decontaminating areas of spills.

CDC Managing Spills

Clean spills of blood or other potentially infectious materials and decontaminate surface with an EPA-registered hospital disinfectant with low- (i.e., HBV and HIV label claims) to intermediate-level (i.e., tuberculocidal claims) activity, depending on the size of the spill and surface porosity. (IB, IC)

Recall

16. How can you be sure that your general cleaning solutions are not contaminated?

17. What are the CDC's recommendations regarding carpeting and cloth furnishings in dental operatories, laboratories, and instrument-processing areas?

18. With what should the majority of housekeeping surfaces be cleaned?

Eye to the Future

Every day new surface disinfectants appear on the market. Yet there is still no single perfect choice for all dental practices.

Although no products on the market today meet your every need, make a list of what is important to you, and what you expect in a disinfectant. Then compare your list with the advantages and disadvantages of each product. With the rapidly changing array of products on the market, it is important that you stay up-to-date with new information as it becomes available. By becoming a member of OSAP, you will receive monthly updates of important infection-control information (http://www.osap.org).

Legal and Ethical Implications

Today, more than any time in history, patients are concerned about the risk of disease transmission in the dental office. Malpractice lawsuits have resulted from improper infection-control techniques.

All healthcare team members in the dental office must understand the importance of good infection control. Most importantly, they must follow all infection-control procedures. The best approach is to use a combination of barriers and between-patient disinfection to maintain the highest level of safety for both patients and the dental team.

Critical Thinking

1. How can you protect the electrical switches on an x-ray unit and still keep the switches free from contamination and electrical short-circuits?
2. The label on a new disinfectant states in large print that the product "will kill HIV in 30 seconds," and in smaller print it states that the tuberculocidal time is "10 minutes." How long should you leave this product on the surface to be disinfected?
3. What precautions must you take when using immersion-type disinfectants?
4. As you are removing plastic barriers from the light handle, you notice that one of the barriers has a tear in it. There is no visible blood on the handle. What would you do, and why?
5. You begin a new job in Dr. Landry's office and discover that the dental assistant is using a 1:100 solution of household bleach for surface disinfection. What would you suggest to the assistant?

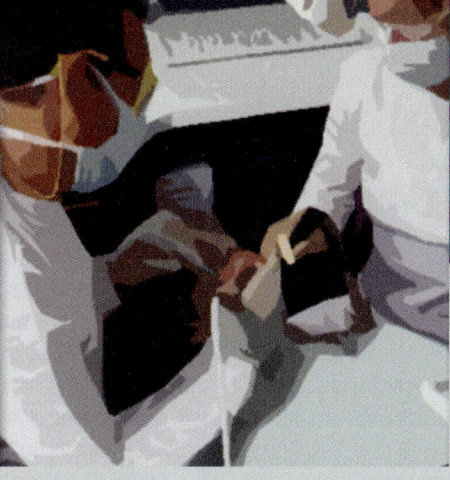

21 Principles and Techniques of Instrument Processing and Sterilization

Outline

KEY TERMS

Autoclave (**aw**-toe-klave) Instrument for sterilization by means of moist heat under pressure.

Biologic indicators Vials or strips, also known as *spore tests,* that contain harmless bacterial spores; used to determine if sterilization has occurred.

Biologic monitoring Verifies sterilization by confirming that all spore-forming microorganisms have been destroyed.

Chemical vapor sterilization (**ster**-uh-luh-**zay**-shun) Sterilization by means of hot formaldehyde vapors under pressure.

continued

KEY TERMS—cont'd

Clean area Place where sterilized instruments, fresh disposable supplies, and prepared trays are stored.

Contaminated area Place where contaminated items are brought for precleaning.

Critical instrument Item used to penetrate soft tissue or bone.

Dry-heat sterilizer Instrument for sterilization by means of heated air.

Endospore A resistant, dormant structure, formed inside of some bacteria, that can withstand adverse conditions.

Event-related packaging Instruments in packages should remain sterile indefinitely unless an event causes them to become contaminated (e.g., torn or wet packaging).

Multiparameter indicator Strips placed in packages that change colors when exposed to a combination of heat, temperature, and time. Also known as *process integrator.*

Noncritical instrument Item that comes in contact with intact skin only.

Process indicator Tapes, strips, or tabs with heat-sensitive chemicals that change color when exposed to a certain temperature.

Process integrator Strips placed in packages that change colors when exposed to a combination of heat, temperature, and time.

Semicritical instrument Item that comes in contact with oral tissues but does not penetrate soft tissue or bone.

Single-parameter indicator Tapes, strips, or tabs with heat-sensitive chemicals that change color when exposed to a certain temperature. Also known as *process indicator.*

Sterilant (**ster**-uh-lunt) Agent capable of killing all microorganisms.

Sterilization (ster-uh-luh-**zay**-shun) Process that kills all microorganisms.

Ultrasonic cleaner Instrument that loosens and removes debris by sound waves traveling through a liquid.

Use-life Period of time during which a germicidal solution is effective after having been prepared for use.

LEARNING OUTCOMES

On completion of this chapter, the student will be able to achieve the following objectives:

- Pronounce, define, and spell the Key Terms.
- Discuss the seven steps in processing dental instruments.
- Describe the three most common methods of heat sterilization and the advantages and disadvantages of each.
- Describe the precautions necessary when packaging materials for sterilization.
- Describe the steps in cleaning and sterilization of the high-speed dental handpiece.
- Explain the differences between process indicators and process integrators.
- Describe when and how biologic monitoring is done.
- Explain the primary disadvantage of flash sterilization.
- Describe the three forms of sterilization monitoring.
- Explain how sterilization failures can occur.
- Explain the limitation of chemical liquid sterilants.
- Describe the classification of instruments use to determine the type of processing.
- Explain the purpose of a holding solution.
- Understand the safety precautions necessary when operating an ultrasonic cleaner.
- Describe the Centers for Disease Control and Prevention (CDC) guidelines for sterilization and disinfection of patient-care items.
- Describe the CDC guidelines for cleaning and decontamination of instruments.
- Describe the CDC guidelines for preparation and packaging instruments for sterilization.

One of the most important responsibilities of the dental assistant is to process contaminated instruments and other patient-care items for reuse.

Instrument processing involves much more than **sterilization.** Proper processing of contaminated dental instruments is actually a seven-step process (Box 21-1). Although the seven steps are not difficult to learn, it is very important for you to have a clear understanding of *how* and *why* each step is performed.

Terms Used in Instrument Processing

Precleaning Reducing the number of microorganisms present by physically removing debris.

Sterilization Process that inactivates all microbial life, including bacterial spores, viruses, bacteria, and fungi.

Disinfection Process that kills disease-causing microorganisms, but not necessarily all microbial life.

High-level disinfection Process that kills some but not all bacterial endospores and inactivates *Mycobacterium tuberculosis.*

Intermediate-level disinfection Inactivates *M. tuberculosis* and destroys less-resistant organisms such as hepatitis B virus and human immunodeficiency virus.

Low-level disinfection Ineffective against *M. tuberculosis* and should only be used in the dental office for housekeeping purposes.

Box 21-1 Seven Steps for Instrument Processing

Step	Technique
1. Transport	Transport contaminated instruments to the processing area in a manner that minimizes the risk of exposure to persons and the environment. Use appropriate PPE and a rigid, leakproof container.
2. Cleaning	Clean instruments with a hands-free, mechanical process such as an ultrasonic cleaner or instrument washer. If instruments cannot be cleaned immediately, use a holding solution.
3. Packaging	In the clean area, wrap/package instruments in appropriate materials. Place a chemical indicator inside the package next to the instruments. If an indicator is not visible on the outside of the package, place an external process indicator on the package.
4. Sterilization	Load the sterilizer according to the manufacturer's instructions. Label packages. Do not overload the sterilizer. Place packages on their edges in single layers or on racks to increase circulation of the sterilizing agent around the instruments. Operate the sterilizer according to the manufacturer's instructions. Allow packages to cool before removing them from the sterilizer. Allow packages to cool before handling.
5. Storage	Store instruments in a clean, dry environment in a manner that maintains the integrity of the package. Rotate packages so that those with the oldest sterilization dates will be used first.
6. Delivery	Deliver packages to point of use in a manner that maintains sterility of the instruments until they are used. Inspect each package for damage. Open package aseptically.
7. Quality assurance program	An effective quality assurance program should incorporate training, record-keeping, maintenance, and use of biologic indicators.

PPE, personal protective equipment.

NOTE: *Throughout this chapter, CDC recommendations are indicated and the category of scientific evidence is noted at the end of each recommendation.*

CDC Rankings of Evidence

Each recommendation made by the CDC is categorized on the basis of existing scientific data, theoretical rationale, and applicability. Rankings are based on the following categories:

- **Category IA** Strongly recommended for implementation and strongly supported by well-designed experimental, clinical, or epidemiologic studies (studies of patterns and causes of diseases).
- **Category IB** Strongly recommended for implementation and supported by experimental, clinical, or epidemiologic studies and a strong theoretical rationale.
- **Category IC** Required for implementation, as mandated by federal or state regulation or standard.
- **Category II** Suggested for implementation and supported by suggestive clinical or epidemiologic studies or a theoretical rationale.
- **Unresolved Issue** No recommendation. Practices for which insufficient evidence or no consensus regarding efficacy exists.

CLASSIFICATION OF PATIENT-CARE ITEMS

Patient-care items are categorized into three classifications: *critical, semicritical,* and *noncritical.* The categories are based on the potential risk for infection associated with their intended use. The classifications are used to determine the *minimal* type of posttreatment processing (Box 21-2).

Critical Instruments

Critical instruments are items used to penetrate soft tissue or bone. They have the greatest risk of transmitting infection and should be sterilized by heat. Examples of critical instruments include forceps, scalpels, bone chisels, scalers, and burs.

Semicritical Instruments

Semicritical instruments touch mucous membranes or nonintact skin and have a lower risk of transmission. The majority of semicritical items in dentistry are heat-tolerant

Box 21-2 CDC Classification of Instruments and Procedures

Category	Functions and examples	Intraoral use	Risk of disease transmission	Procedure
Critical	*Function:* Touch bone or penetrate soft tissue *Examples:* Surgical and other instruments used to penetrate soft tissue or bone, including forceps, scalpels, bone chisels, scalers, and burs	Yes	Very high	Sterilization
Semicritical	*Function:* Touch mucous membranes but will not touch bone or penetrate soft tissue *Examples:* Mouth mirrors and amalgam condensers	Yes	Moderate	Sterilization or high-level disinfection
Noncritical	*Function:* Contact only with intact skin *Examples:* External dental x-ray head	No	Very low or none	Intermediate- to low-level disinfection or basic cleaning

and they should also be sterilized. If the item will be damaged by heat, it should receive, at a minimum, high-level disinfection (see Chapter 20).

Examples of semicritical items include plastic-handled brushes, high-volume evacuator (HVE) tips, rubber dam forceps, x-ray film holders, and amalgam carriers.

In dental offices today, most items used intraorally are capable of withstanding the heat of sterilization. A fundamental rule of infection control states, *"If an item can be heat-sterilized, it should be heat-sterilized."*

Noncritical Instruments

Noncritical instruments pose the least risk of transmission of infection because they contact only intact skin, which is an effective barrier to microorganisms. These items should be cleaned and processed with an Environmental Protection Agency (EPA)-registered intermediate-level or low-level disinfectant after each patient use.

Noncritical clinical devices include the position indicator device (PID) of the x-ray unit tube head, the lead apron, or the curing light that comes into contact only with intact skin.

CDC CDC Guidelines for Sterilization and Disinfection of Patient-Care Items

General Recommendations

1. Use only Food and Drug Administration (FDA)-cleared medical devices for sterilization and follow the manufacturer's instructions for correct use. (IB)
2. Clean and heat-sterilize critical dental instruments before each use. (IA)
3. Clean and heat-sterilize semicritical items before each use. (IB)
4. Allow packages to dry in the sterilizer before they are handled to avoid contamination. (IB)
5. Reprocess heat-sensitive critical and semicritical instruments by using FDA-cleared sterilant/high-level disinfectants or an FDA-cleared low-temperature sterilization method (e.g., ethylene oxide). Follow manufacturer's instructions for use of chemical sterilants/high-level disinfectants. (IB)
6. Single-use disposable instruments are acceptable alternatives if they are used only once and disposed of correctly. (IB, IC)
7. Do not use liquid chemical sterilants/high-level disinfectants for environmental surface disinfection or as holding solutions. (IB, IC)
8. Ensure that noncritical patient-care items are barrier-protected or cleaned, or if visibly soiled, cleaned and disinfected after each use with an EPA-registered hospital disinfectant. If visibly contaminated with blood, use an EPA-registered hospital disinfectant with a tuberculocidal claim (i.e., intermediate level). (IB)
9. Inform dental health-care personnel of all Occupational Safety and Health Administration (OSHA) guidelines for exposure to chemical agents used for disinfection and sterilization.

Personal Protective Equipment

To prevent disease agents from a previous patient being transferred to you, another dental team member, or the next patient, instrument processing must be performed in a consistent and disciplined manner. You must *always* use personal protective equipment (PPE), including utility gloves, mask, eyewear, and protective clothing, when processing instruments (Fig. 21-1).

Recall

1. What are the three instrument classifications used to determine the method of sterilization?
2. What PPE is necessary when processing instruments?

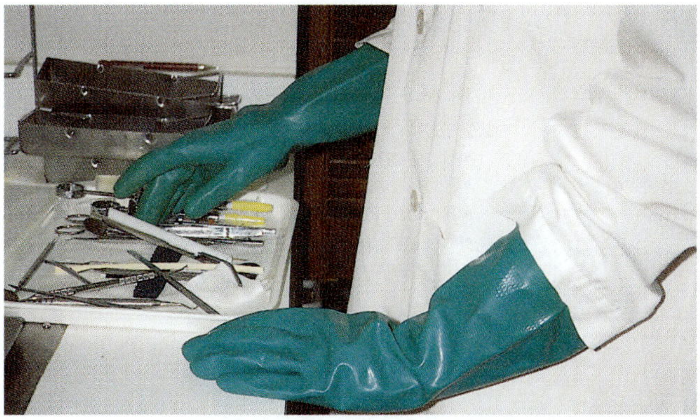

Fig. 21-1 PPE must be worn while preparing instruments for sterilization.

TRANSPORTING AND PROCESSING CONTAMINATED PATIENT-CARE ITEMS

The dental assistant can be exposed to microorganisms through contact with contaminated instruments or other patient-care items. Exposure can occur through percutaneous injury (i.e., needlesticks or cuts) or contact with the mucous membranes of the eyes, nose, or mouth.

CDC CDC Guidelines for Receiving, Cleaning, and Decontamination Procedures

1. Minimize handling of loose contaminated instruments during transport to the instrument-processing area. Use work-practice controls (e.g., carry instruments in a covered container) to minimize exposure potential. (II) Clean all visible blood and other contamination from dental instruments and devices before sterilization or disinfection procedures. (IA)
2. Use automated cleaning equipment (e.g., ultrasonic cleaner or washer-disinfector) to remove debris to improve cleaning effectiveness and decrease worker exposure to blood. (IB)
3. Use work-practice controls that minimize contact with sharp instruments if manual cleaning is necessary (e.g., long-handled brush). (IC)
4. Wear puncture- and chemical-resistant/heavy-duty utility gloves for instrument cleaning and decontamination procedures. (IB)
5. Wear appropriate PPE (e.g., mask, protective eyewear, and gown) when splashing or spraying is anticipated during cleaning. (IC)
6. Do not store critical instruments unwrapped. (IB)

INSTRUMENT-PROCESSING AREA

The instrument-processing area, or *sterilization area,* should be centrally located in the office to allow for easy access from all patient care areas. This minimizes the need to carry contaminated items through **clean areas** of the office, where sterilized instruments, fresh disposable supplies, and prepared trays are stored.

The "ideal" instrument-processing area (1) should be dedicated only to instrument processing, (2) should be physically separated from the operatories and dental laboratory, and (3) should *not* be a part of a common walkway. The area should *not* have a door or windows that open to the outside, because dust can enter the area.

The processing area should have good air circulation to control the heat generated by the sterilizers. The size of the area should accommodate all the equipment and supplies necessary for instrument processing, with multiple outlets and proper lighting, water, and an air line and vacuum line for flushing high-speed handpieces.

A deep sink should have hands-free controls for instrument rinsing and (if space permits) a foot-operated or other hands-free trash receptacle. The flooring should be an uncarpeted, seamless, hard surface. The size, shape, and accessories of the instrument-processing area vary among dental offices.

CDC CDC Guidelines for Instrument-Processing Area

1. Designate a central processing area. Divide the instrument-processing area, physically or, at a minimum, spatially, into distinct areas for 1) receiving, cleaning, and decontamination; 2) preparation and packaging; 3) sterilization; and 4) storage. Do not store instruments in an area where contaminated instruments are held or cleaned. (II)
2. Train DHCP to employ work practices that prevent contamination of clean areas. (II)

Workflow Pattern

Regardless of the size or shape of the instrument-processing area, four basic areas govern the pattern of workflow. Processing instruments should proceed in a single loop, from dirty, to clean, to sterile, to storage, without ever "doubling back" (Fig. 21-2).

If the instrument-processing area is small, you can use signs that read, "Contaminated items only," "Precleaning area," "Cleaned items only," "Sterile items only," or "Sterilization area," to separate the contaminated and clean areas. This method works well to prevent mixing of contaminated and sterile items in a small sterilization area.

Contaminated Area

All soiled instruments are brought into the **contaminated area,** the *initial receiving area,* where they are held for processing. Any disposable items not already discarded in the treatment room are removed from the instrument tray and disposed of as contaminated waste.

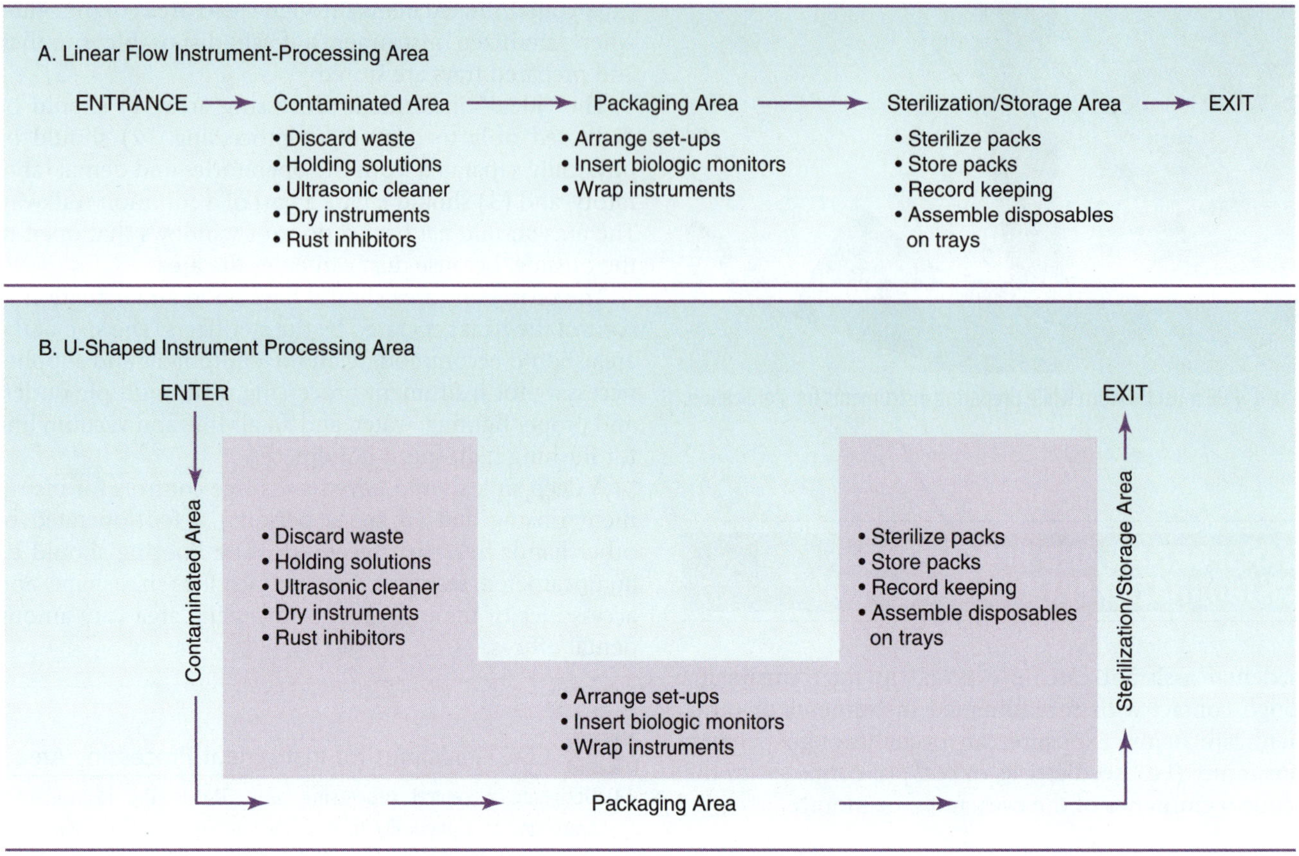

Fig. 21-2 Instrument-processing areas. **A,** Linear. **B,** U-shaped.

Thorough cleaning should be done before all disinfection and sterilization processes. It should involve removal of all debris and organic materials (e.g., blood and saliva). Methods of cleaning are described later in this chapter.

The contaminated area contains clean protective eyewear and utility gloves, counter space, a sink, a waste disposal container, holding solution, an ultrasonic cleaner, an eyewash station, and supplies for wrapping instruments before sterilization (Fig. 21-3).

NOTE: *Soiled and clean instruments are never stored in the same cabinet.*

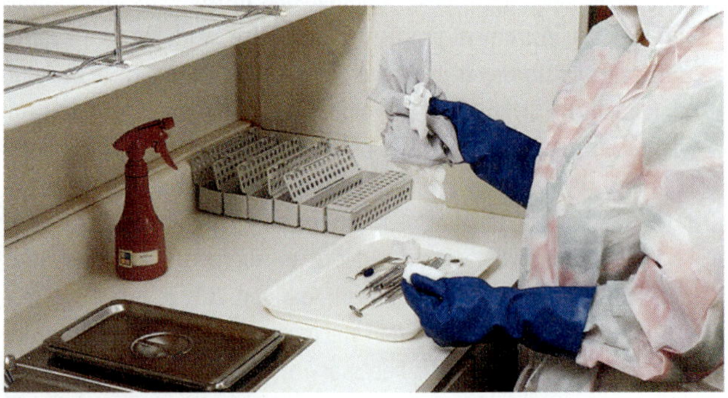

Fig. 21-3 Waste items are properly discarded.

Preparation and Packaging Area

In the preparation and packaging area, cleaned instruments and other dental supplies should be inspected, assembled into sets or trays, and wrapped or placed in packages for sterilization (Fig. 21-4).

The preparation and packaging area should have counter space and storage space for sterilized instruments, fresh disposable supplies, and prepared trays or instrument cassettes.

Clean instruments are not sterile and could still harbor pathogens. Instruments must be packaged and sterilized before being used on a patient.

Holding Solution

If the instruments cannot be cleaned immediately after the procedure, they should be placed in a holding solution to prevent the drying of blood and debris on the instruments.

The holding solution may be any noncorrosive liquid. A commercial enzymatic solution that partially dissolves organic debris may be used (Fig. 21-5). Dishwasher detergent also makes a good holding solution because it is low-cost, low-foaming, and readily available. It is neither cost-effective nor desirable to use a disinfectant alone as a holding solution.

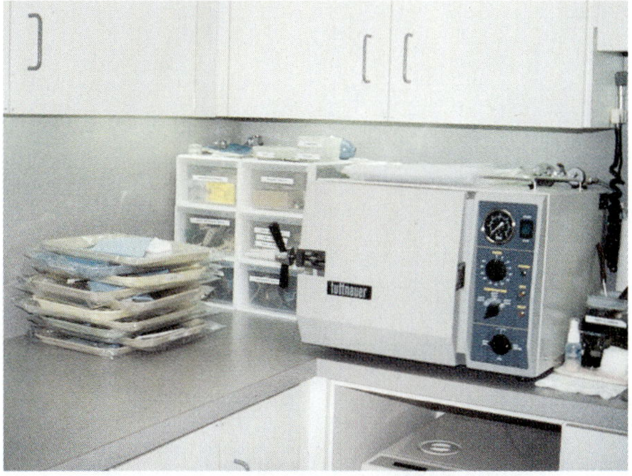

Fig. 21-4 The clean area includes the sterilizer and space to store prepared trays.

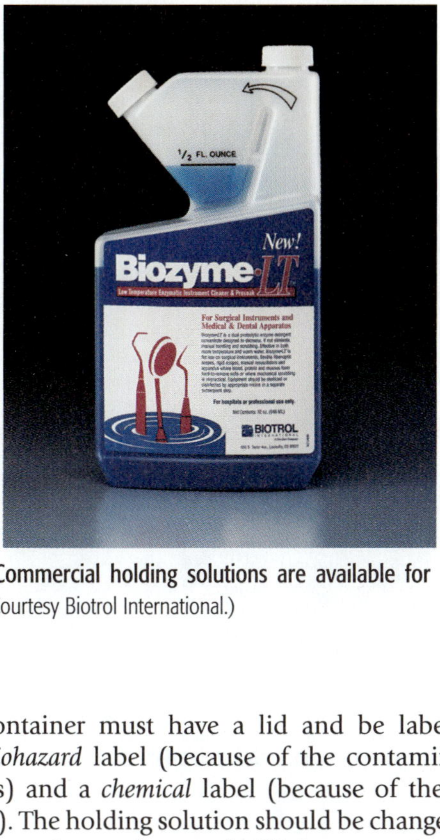

Fig. 21-5 Commercial holding solutions are available for use in precleaning. (Courtesy Biotrol International.)

The container must have a lid and be labeled with both a *biohazard* label (because of the contaminated instruments) and a *chemical* label (because of the cleaner/detergent). The holding solution should be changed at least twice daily and more frequently if it becomes clouded.

Remember, a holding solution is necessary *only* when contaminated instruments cannot be processed immediately.

PRECLEANING AND PACKAGING INSTRUMENTS

Instruments may be precleaned in one of three ways: *hand scrubbing, ultrasonic cleaning,* and *instrument washing machines.*

Hand Scrubbing

Hand scrubbing is the *least* desirable method of cleaning instruments because it requires direct hand contact with the contaminated instrument. If you absolutely must hand-scrub instruments, follow the following precautions:

- Wear goggle-type eyewear and puncture-resistant gloves, as well as your protective clothing.
- Clean only one or two instruments at a time.
- Use only a long-handled brush, preferably one with a hand guard or wide surface.
- Keep items above the waterline; fully immersing them in a basin of soapy water interferes with the ability to see the sharp ends.
- Allow instruments to air-dry, or carefully pat them with thick toweling. *Never* rub or roll the instruments in the towel, because of the risk of accidental injury.

NOTE: *Some states have specific infection-control guidelines or state OSHA plans that prohibit hand scrubbing of instruments. In these states, you must use an ultrasonic cleaner or machine cleaning.*

Ultrasonic Cleaning

Ultrasonic cleaners are used to loosen and remove debris from instruments. These cleaners also reduce the risk of hand injuries from cuts and punctures during the cleaning process (Fig. 21-6 and Procedure 21-1).

Puncture-resistant utility gloves, a mask, protective eyewear, and a protective gown should always be worn when using the ultrasonic cleaner. To further limit contact with contaminated instruments, keep a set of tongs near the ultrasonic unit for removing instruments after the cleaning cycle (Fig. 21-7).

The ultrasonic cleaner works by producing sound waves beyond the range of human hearing. These sound waves, which can travel through metal and glass containers, cause *cavitation* (formation of bubbles in liquid). The bubbles, which are too small to be seen, burst by *implosion* (bursting inward, the opposite of an explosion). The mechanical cleaning action of the bursting bubbles combined with the chemical action of the ultrasonic solution removes the debris from the instruments.

Instruments should be processed in the ultrasonic cleaner until they are visibly clean. The time may vary from 5 to 15 minutes, depending on the amount and type of material on the instruments, and the efficiency of the ultrasonic unit. Instruments in plastic or resin cassettes require slightly longer cleaning time because the cassette material absorbs some of the ultrasonic energy.

Ultrasonic Cleaning Solutions

You should use ultrasonic solutions that are specially formulated for use in the ultrasonic cleaner only (Fig. 21-8). Some ultrasonic cleaning products have enzyme activity (Fig. 21-9). Other ultrasonic cleaning products have an-

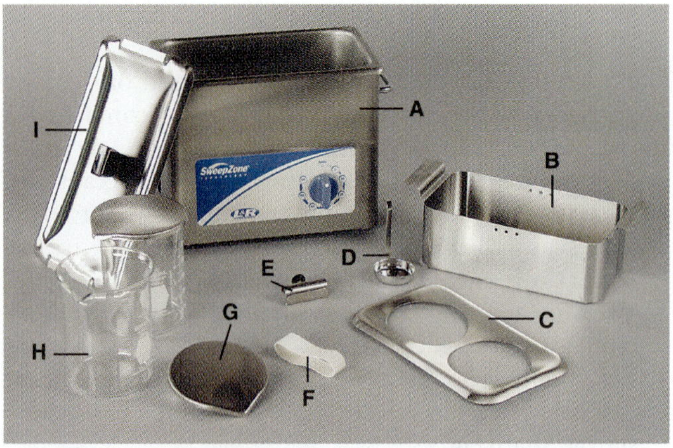

Fig. 21-6 Ultrasonic cleaning system. **A,** Ultrasonic cleaner. **B,** Instrument basket. **C,** Beaker holder. **D,** Bur tray. **E,** Suspension bracket. **F,** Beaker band. **G,** Beaker cover. **H,** Glass beaker. **I,** Cover. (Courtesy L & R Manufacturing Company, Kearny, New Jersey.)

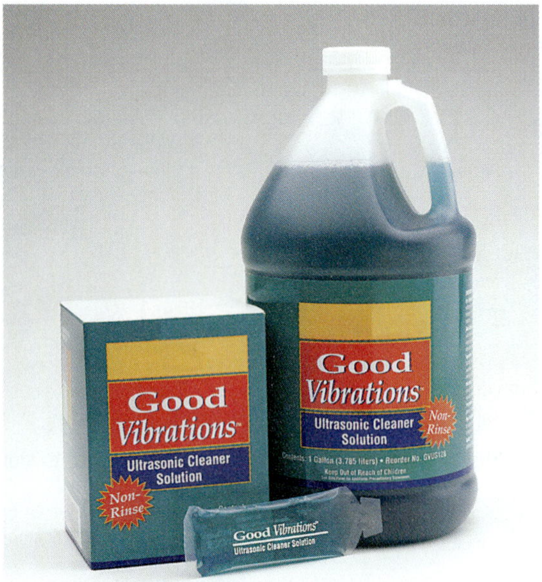

Fig. 21-8 A commercial all-purpose ultrasonic cleaner. (Courtesy Certol.)

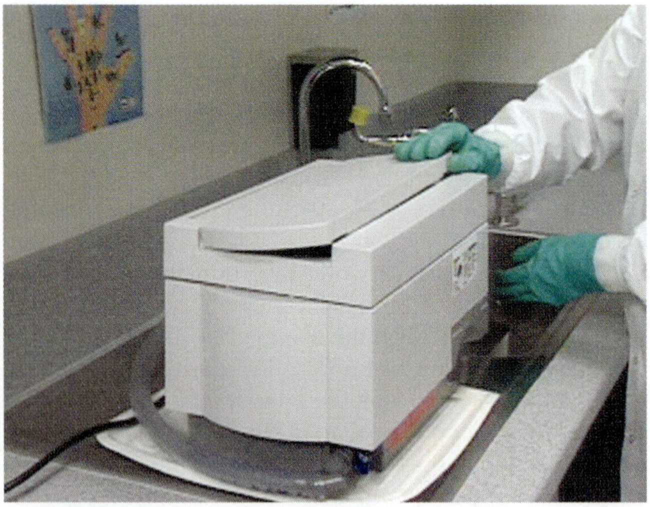

Fig. 21-7 It is important to keep the ultrasonic cleaner covered while in use to reduce spatter and contaminated aerosols.

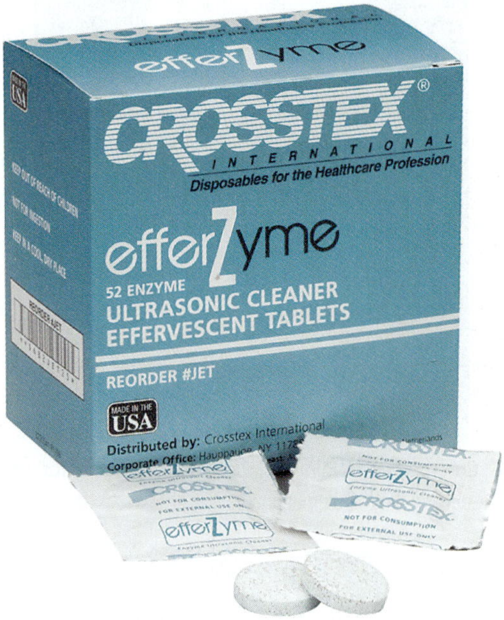

Fig. 21-9 An enzyme ultrasonic cleaner in tablet form. (Courtesy Crosstex.)

timicrobial activity, which reduces the buildup of microbes in the solutions with repeated use. The antimicrobial activity *does not disinfect* the instruments; it merely prevents the microorganisms from increasing in number.

Do *not* use other chemicals such as plain disinfectants in the ultrasonic cleaner. Some disinfectants can "fix" the blood and debris onto the instruments, making subsequent cleaning more difficult. Specific ultrasonic solutions are available that remove difficult materials, such as cements, tartar, stains, plaster, and alginate (Fig. 21-10). Refer to the ultrasonic unit manufacturer's instructions regarding the specific solution to be used.

As with the holding solution, the ultrasonic cleaning unit should be labeled with *both* a chemical label and a biohazard label because it contains a chemical *and* contaminated instruments.

Procedure 21-1 Operating the Ultrasonic Cleaner

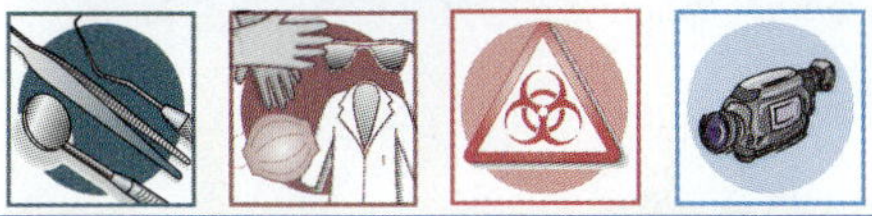

Goal

To prepare and use the ultrasonic cleaner effectively.

Equipment and Supplies

- Ultrasonic cleaning unit
- Instruments
- Ultrasonic solution
- Clean towel

PROCEDURAL STEPS

1. Put on protective clothing, mask, eyewear, and utility gloves.
   Purpose: You will be handling sharp, contaminated instruments and using a chemical ultrasonic solution that could splash in your eyes.
2. Remove the lid from the container.
   Purpose: The lid should remain on the ultrasonic device when not in use to prevent evaporation of the solution and to minimize airborne contamination.
3. Be certain the container has been filled with solution to the level recommended by the manufacturer.
   Purpose: The instruments being cleaned must be completely submerged in the solution.
4. Place loose instruments in the basket, or if using cassettes, place the cassette in the basket.
5. Replace the lid, and turn the cycle to "On." The time of the cycle may vary depending on the efficiency of the ultrasonic unit. The time ranges from 5 to 15 minutes.
   Purpose: Instruments in resin or plastic cassettes require longer cleaning times because resin and plastic absorb some of the ultrasonic energy.
6. After the cleaning cycle, remove the basket and thoroughly rinse the instruments in a sink under tap water with minimal splashing. Hold the basket at an angle to allow water to run off into the sink to minimize splashing.

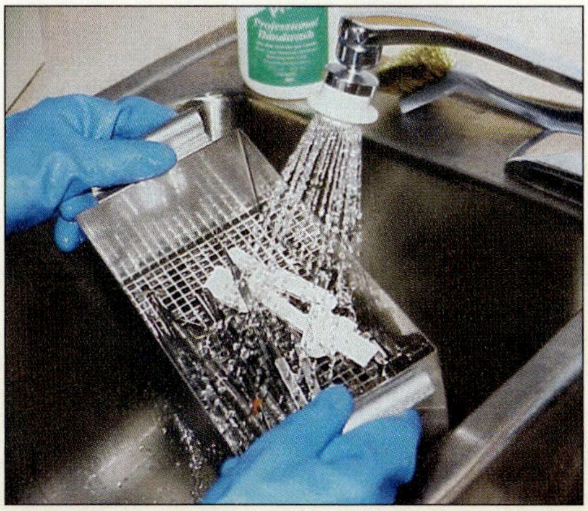

7. Gently turn the basket onto a towel, and remove the instruments or cassettes. Replace the lid on the ultrasonic cleaner.

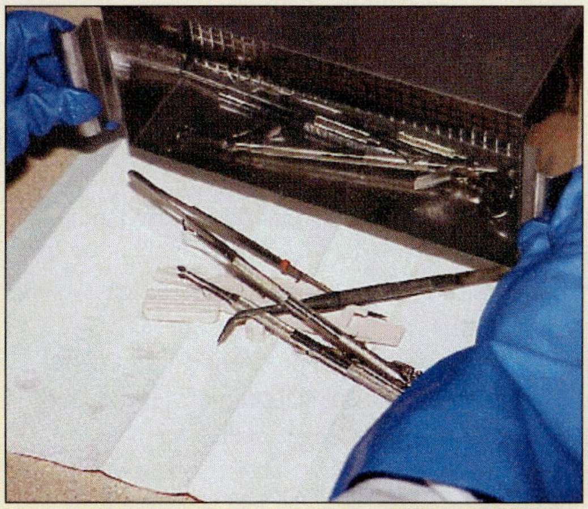

Care of the Ultrasonic Cleaner

The ultrasonic cleaner solution is *highly contaminated* and must be discarded at least once a day or sooner if it becomes visibly cloudy. When changing the solution, the inside of the pan and lid should be rinsed with water, disinfected, rinsed again, and dried. All PPE should be worn while changing solutions in the ultrasonic cleaner.

Testing the Ultrasonic Cleaner

If you notice that the instruments are not being cleaned completely after processing in the ultrasonic cleaner, the unit may not be functioning properly.

To determine whether the ultrasonic cleaner is working properly, hold a 5-by-5-inch sheet of lightweight aluminum foil vertically (like a curtain) half-submerged in

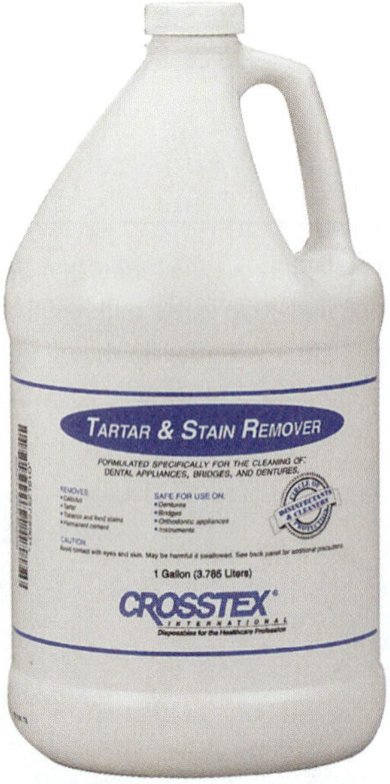

Fig. 21-10 **Special tartar and stain remover ultrasonic solution.** (Courtesy Crosstex.)

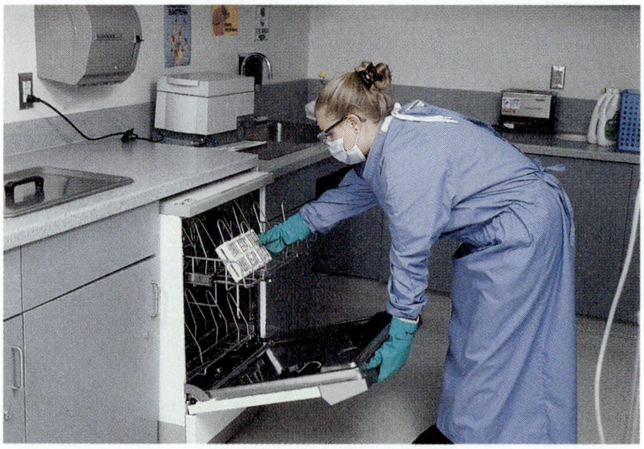

Fig. 21-11 **A Miele thermal disinfector provides safe and thorough instrument cleaning, disinfecting, and drying. Instruments must be packaged and sterilized after the cycle.**

the fresh, unused solution. Run the unit for 20 seconds, and then hold the foil up toward the light. The surfaces that were submerged into the solution should be evenly marked with a tiny pebbling effect over the entire surface. An area on the foil that is greater than ½ inch without pebbling indicates that there is a problem with the unit, and that it needs servicing by the manufacturer.

Recall

3. What is the basic rule of the workflow pattern in an instrument-processing area?
4. If instruments cannot be processed immediately, what should be done with them?
5. Name the three methods of precleaning instruments.
6. Which method of precleaning instruments is the *least* desirable?
7. How does an ultrasonic cleaner work?

Automated Washers/Disinfectors

Automated instrument washers/disinfectors look and work similar to a household dishwasher. However, the U.S. FDA must approve them for use with dental instruments (Fig. 21-11).

Automated washing/disinfecting units use a combination of very hot water recirculation and detergents to remove organic material. Then the instruments are automatically dried. These units are classified as *thermal* disinfectors because they have a disinfecting cycle that subjects the instruments to a *level of heat* that kills most vegetative microorganisms.

Instruments processed in the automatic washers/disinfectors must be wrapped and sterilized before use on a patient.

Drying, Lubrication, and Corrosion Control

Instruments and burs made of carbon steel will rust during steam sterilization. Rust inhibitors such as sodium nitrate or commercial products are available as a spray or dip solution and help to reduce rust and corrosion.

An alternative to rust inhibitors is to dry the instrument thoroughly using dry heat or unsaturated chemical vapor sterilization (see Chemical Vapor Sterilization section), which does not cause rusting.

Hinged instruments may need to be lubricated to maintain proper opening. Take care to remove all excess lubricant before heat sterilization.

Packaging Instruments

Before sterilization, the instruments should be wrapped or packaged to protect them from becoming contaminated *after* sterilization. When instruments are sterilized without being packaged, they are immediately exposed to the environment as soon as the sterilizer door is opened. They can be contaminated by aerosols in the air, dust, improper handling, or contact with nonsterile surfaces.

An additional advantage to packaging instruments is that they can be grouped into special setups, such as crown/bridge, amalgam, prophy, or composite.

CDC Guidelines for Preparation and Packaging

1. Use an internal chemical indicator in each package. If the internal indicator cannot be seen from outside the package, also use an external indicator. (II)
2. Use a container system or wrapping compatible with the type of sterilization process used and that has received FDA clearance. (IB)
3. Before sterilization of critical and semicritical instruments, inspect instruments for cleanliness, then wrap or place them in containers designed to maintain sterility during storage (e.g., cassettes and organizing trays). (IA)

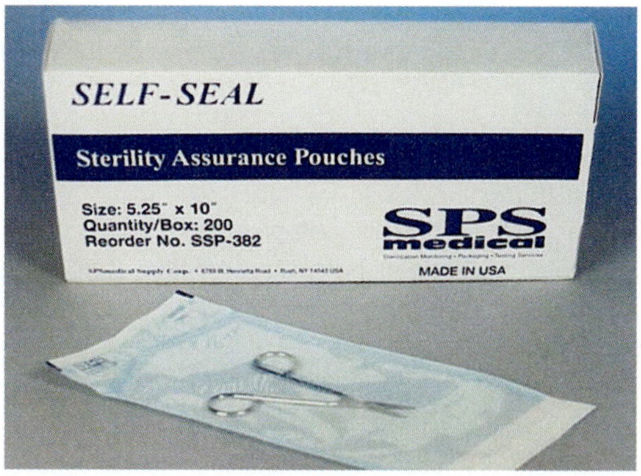

Fig. 21-12 Self-seal packages provide an excellent wrap for sterilized materials. (Courtesy SPSmedical Supply Corp.)

Box 21-3 Packaging Materials and Types of Sterilization

Packaging material	Tips
Steam sterilization	
Paper wrap	Do not use closed containers
Nylon tubing	Do not use thick cloth
Paper/plastic peel pouches	Some plastics melt
Thin cloth	
Wrapped perforated cassettes	
Dry heat sterilizers	
Paper wrap	Some paper may char
Appropriate type nylon "plastic" tube	Some plastics melt
Closed containers (use biologic indicator)	Use only materials approved for dry heat
Unsaturated chemical vapor	
Paper wrap	Do not use closed containers
Paper/plastic peel pouches	Do not use cloth (absorbs too much chemical vapor)
Wrapped perforated cassettes	Some plastics melt
	Use only materials approved for chemical vapor

Packaging Materials

Sterilization packaging materials and cassettes are medical devices and therefore must be FDA-approved. It is critical to use *only* products and materials that are labeled as "sterilization" packaging. Never substitute products such as plastic wraps, paper, or zipper-lock freezer bags that are not registered for this purpose. These products may melt or prevent the sterilizing agent from reaching the instruments inside.

Specific types of packaging material are available for each method of sterilization. You should use *only* the type of packaging material designed for the particular method of sterilization that you are using (Box 21-3).

A wide variety of sterilization packaging materials are available. Self-sealing or heat-sealed "poly" bags or tubes provide an excellent wrap (Fig. 21-12). In addition, paper wraps and cloth wraps are available. If the package is not the self-sealing type, you should only use sterilization indicator tape to seal the package.

Never use safety pins, staples, paper clips, or other sharp objects that could penetrate the packaging material.

The instruments are now ready for the sterilization process.

Sterilization of Unwrapped Instruments

An unwrapped cycle (sometimes called *flash sterilization*) is a method for sterilizing unwrapped patient-care items for immediate use. The time for unwrapped sterilization cycles depends on the type of sterilizer and the type of item (i.e., porous or nonporous) to be sterilized. Unwrapped sterilization should be used only under certain conditions.

CDC Guidelines for Sterilization of Unwrapped Instruments

1. Instruments are thoroughly cleaned and dried before sterilization.
2. Mechanical monitors are checked, and chemical indicators are used for each cycle.
3. Care is taken to avoid thermal injury to the dental professional or patients.
4. Items are aseptically transported to the point of use to maintain sterility.

Critical instruments that were sterilized unwrapped should not be stored unwrapped, and semicritical instruments should be used in a short period of time. Do not sterilize implantable devices unwrapped.

Recall

8. What prevents kitchen dishwashers from being used to preclean instruments?
9. How can instrument rusting be prevented?
10. Why should instruments be packaged before sterilization?
11. Why should you never use pins, staples, or paper clips on instrument packages?

STERILIZATION MONITORING

It is critical that dental instruments are properly sterilized. Because microorganisms cannot be seen with the naked eye, the major difficulty in sterilization is determining *when* an item is sterile.

In the early days of sterilization, a raw potato was sometimes placed in the sterilizer with the instruments and examined later to see whether it was cooked. If the potato was cooked, the load was considered sterile. As sterilization processes became more sophisticated, more scientific monitoring practices replaced the potato.

Currently, three forms of sterilization monitoring are used: *physical, chemical,* and *biologic.* All three processes are unique, have different functions, and must be used consistently to ensure sterility.

Physical Monitoring

Physical monitoring of the sterilization process involves looking at the gauges and readings on the sterilizer and recording the temperatures, pressure, and exposure time. Although correct readings do not guarantee sterilization, an incorrect reading gives you the first signal of a problem.

Remember that the temperature recorded is for the chamber, *not* the inside of the pack. Therefore, problems with overloading or improper packaging would not be detected from the reading on the gauges.

Chemical Monitoring

Chemical monitoring (external and internal) involves the use of heat-sensitive chemical that changes color when exposed to certain conditions. The two types of chemical indicators are process indicators and process integrators.

Process Indicators

Process indicators (external) are placed *outside* the instrument packages before sterilization. Examples are autoclave tape and color-change markings on packages or bags (Fig. 21-13).

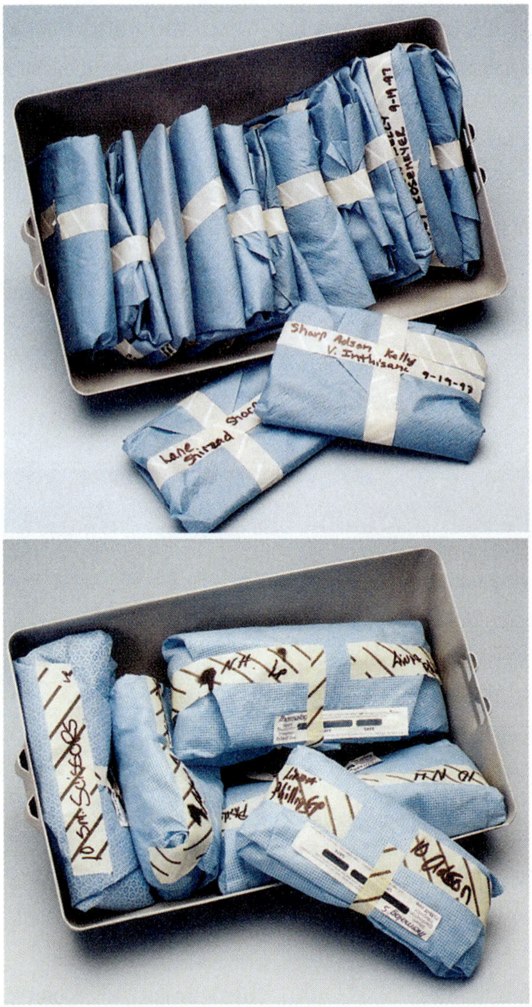

A

B

Fig. 21-13 **A,** **Unprocessed instruments.** **B,** **Wrapped instruments after processing. Note the color change in the tape.** (From Young AP, Kennedy DB: *Kinn's the medical assistant: An applied learning approach,* ed 9. Philadelphia, 2003, Saunders.)

Process indicators simply identify instrument packs that have been exposed to a certain temperature; they *do not* measure the duration or the pressure. Process indicators are also known as **single-parameter indicators.** Process indicators are useful in distinguishing between packages that were processed and those that were not processed. They can be used to prevent accidental use of unprocessed instruments.

Process Integrators

Process integrators (internal) are placed *inside* instrument packages. They respond to a combination of pressure, temperature, and time. Process integrators are also known as **multiparameter indicators.** All sterilization factors are *integrated* (Fig. 21-14).

Examples of process integrators include strips, tabs, or tubes of colored liquid. The advantage of placing integra-

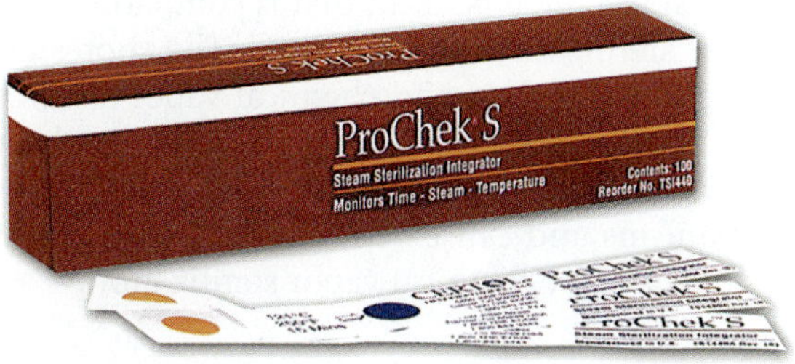

Fig. 21-14 Integrator strips used inside packs to monitor time, temperature, and pressure. (Courtesy Certol.)

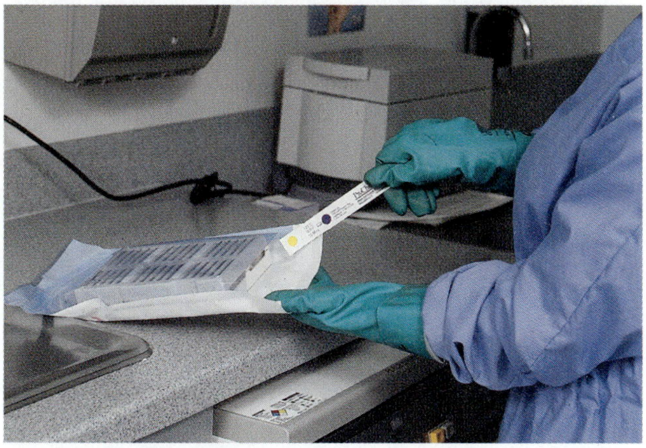

Fig. 21-15 The dental assistant inserts the integrator strip into the sterilization pouch with the instruments.

tors inside each package is assurance that the sterilizing agent penetrated the packaging (Fig. 21-15).

Limitations

Process indicators and integrators provide immediate, visual control of sterilizing conditions. They *do not indicate sterility* and are not a replacement for biologic monitoring.

Biologic Monitoring

Biologic monitoring, or *spore testing,* is the only way to determine if sterilization has occurred and all bacteria and **endospores** have been killed. The CDC, American Dental Association (ADA), and Organization for Safety and Asepsis Procedures (OSAP) recommend at least *weekly* biologic monitoring of sterilization equipment.

CDC CDC Guidelines for Sterilization Monitoring

1. Use mechanical, chemical, and biological monitors according to the manufacturer's instructions to ensure the effectiveness of the sterilization process. (IB)
2. Monitor each load with mechanical (e.g., time, temperature, and pressure) and chemical indicators. (II)
3. Place a chemical indicator on the inside of each package. If the internal indicator is not visible from the outside, also place an exterior chemical indicator on the package. (II)
4. Place items/packages correctly and loosely into the sterilizer so as not to impede penetration of the sterilant. (IB)
5. Do not use instrument packs if mechanical or chemical indicators indicate inadequate processing.
6. Monitor sterilizers at least weekly by using a biological indicator with a matching control (e.g., biologic indicator and control from the same lot number). (IB)
7. Use a biologic indicator for every sterilizer load that contains an implantable device. Verify results before using the implantable device, whenever possible. (IB)
8. Maintain sterilization records (i.e., mechanical, chemical, and biologic) in compliance with state and local regulations. (I)

Additional Reasons for Biologic Monitoring

1. Once each week, as recommended by the CDC, ADA, and OSAP
2. After the sterilizer has been serviced, to verify proper functioning
3. When you change packaging materials, to be sure the sterilizing agent is reaching the instruments
4. After an electric or power source failure, to verify proper functioning of the sterilizer
5. After training new employees, to be sure they are following proper procedures
6. For all cycles that contain any device to be implanted*

**Note:* The implant should not be placed until sterilization has been biologically monitored.

Several states also require routine biologic monitoring at weekly, monthly, or cycle-specific intervals, such as spore testing every 40 hours of use or every 30 days, whichever comes first. (Check the requirements in your state.) In addition to the recommended weekly guidelines, biologic monitoring should also be done at other times (Procedure 21-2).

Biologic indicators (BIs), also known as *spore tests,* are vials or strips of paper that contain harmless bacterial spores (spores are highly resistant to heat).

Three BIs are used in testing. Two BIs are placed inside instrument packs, and the sterilizer is operated under normal conditions. The third strip is set aside as a control.

After the load has been sterilized, all BIs are cultured. If the spores survive the sterilization cycle *(a positive culture),* a sterilization failure has occurred. If the spores are killed *(a negative culture),* the sterilization cycle was successful.

The culturing of the spore test is usually handled through the use of a mail-in monitoring service (Fig. 21-16). If in-office culturing is done, the manufacturer's instructions must be followed carefully to avoid errors (Fig. 21-17).

You must use the type of BI that is compatible with the method of sterilization you are using. The spores used to test the steam autoclave and chemical vapor sterilizer are different from the bacteria used to test the dry heat and ethylene oxide sterilizer. *Dual-species* BIs contain spores of both organisms and can be used with dry heat, ethylene oxide, autoclave, or chemical vapor sterilization.

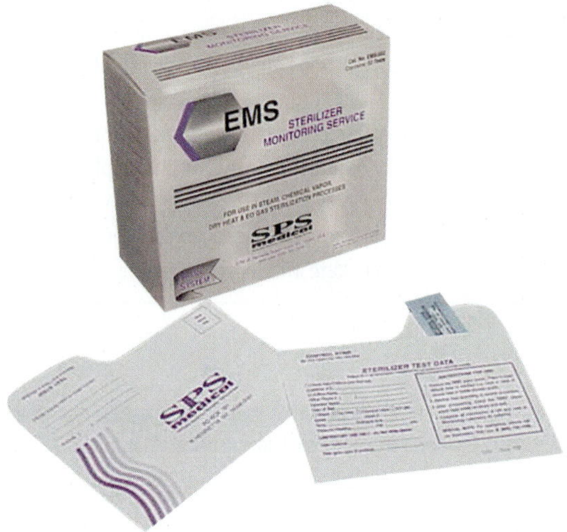

Fig. 21-16 Use of a mail-in service is a convenient method of biologic monitoring. (Courtesy SPSmedical Supply Corp.)

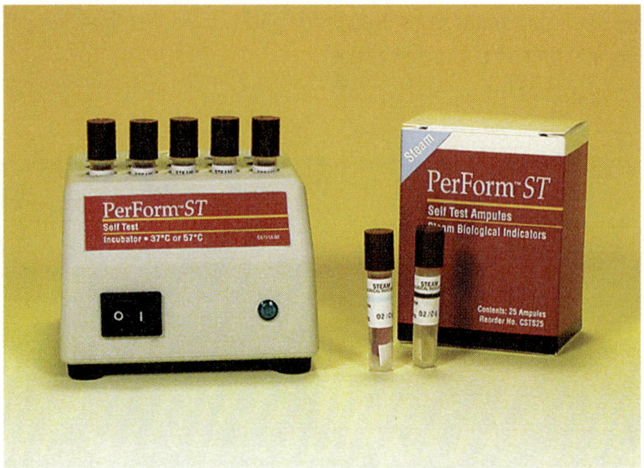

Fig. 21-17 In-office biologic monitoring system. (Courtesy Certol.)

Procedure 21-2 Performing Biologic Monitoring

Goal

To assess sterilization using BIs (spore tests).

Equipment and Supplies

- Appropriate PPE
- Instruments
- Pencil
- Dual-species BI
- Sterilization log
- Mail-in envelope

PROCEDURAL STEPS

1. While wearing all PPE, place the BI strip in the bundle of instruments and seal the package.
   Purpose: Although the instruments have been precleaned, they are still contaminated.
2. Place the pack with the BI in the center of the sterilizer load.
   Purpose: The center of the load is the most difficult for the sterilizing agent to penetrate.
3. Place the remainder of the packaged instruments into the sterilizer, and process the load through a normal sterilization cycle.
   Purpose: The monitoring evaluates what is considered the "normal" cycle.
4. Remove utility gloves, mask, and eyewear. Wash and dry hands.
   Purpose: To avoid contamination of the sterilization log.
5. In the sterilization log, record the date of the test, the type of the sterilizer, cycle, temperature, time, and the name of the person operating the sterilizer.
   Purpose: Maintaining records is part of the exposure-control program, and the specific information is necessary in the event of a sterilization failure.
6. After the load has been sterilized, remove the processed BI strip.
   Purpose: The BI has been exposed to the same sterilizing conditions as the instruments.
7. Mail the processed spore test strips and the control BI to the monitoring service.
   Purpose: It is important to obtain and maintain the results as part of the exposure-control program.

Recall

12. What are the three forms of sterilization monitoring?
13. What is a process indicator, and where is it placed?
14. What is a process integrator, and where is it placed?
15. Do process indicators and integrators ensure that an item is sterile?
16. What is the best way to determine if sterilization has occurred?

METHODS OF STERILIZATION

Sterilization destroys all microbial forms, including bacterial spores. *Sterile* is an absolute term; there is no "partially sterile" or "almost sterile."

All reusable items (critical and semicritical instruments) that come in contact with the patient's blood, saliva, or mucous membranes *must be heat-sterilized.* The three most common forms of heat sterilization in the dental office are (1) *steam sterilization,* (2) *chemical vapor sterilization,* and (3) *dry heat sterilization* (Table 21-1).

Although most reusable items can withstand heat processing, a few plastic items, such as rubber dam frames, shade guides, and x-ray film-holding devices, will be damaged by heat. For such items, a liquid **sterilant** must be used. A liquid sterilant is *not* recommended for use on any item that can withstand heat sterilization or is disposable (Table 21-2).

Steam Autoclave Sterilization

An **autoclave** is used to sterilize dental instruments and other items by means of steam under pressure. Steam sterilization involves heating water to generate steam, producing a moist heat that rapidly kills microorganisms. As the steam completely fills the sterilizing chamber, the cooler air is pushed out of an escape valve, which then closes and allows the pressure to increase. It is the *heat,* not the pressure, that actually kills the microorganisms.

In the absence of air in the autoclave, the steam creates higher temperatures than steam coming from an open pan of boiling water. The steam from a pan of boiling water cools

Table 21-1 ***Advantages and Disadvantages of Sterilization Methods***

Method of Sterilization	Advantages	Disadvantages
Steam autoclave	Short time	Damages some plastic and rubber items
	Good penetration of steam	Requires use of distilled water
	Commonly used in dental offices	May rust non–stainless steel instruments and burs
		Cannot use closed containers
Unsaturated chemical vapor	Short time	Instruments must be dry
	No corrosion	Damages some plastic and rubber items
	Instruments dry quickly following cycle	Requires special solution
		Requires good ventilation
		Cannot sterilize liquids
		Cannot use closed containers
		Cloth wrap may absorb chemicals
Dry heat oven type (static air)	No corrosion	Long sterilization time
	Can use closed containers	Instruments must be predried
	Items are dry after cycle	Damages some plastic and rubber items
		Cannot sterilize liquids
Rapid heat transfer (forced air)	Very fast	Damages some plastic and rubber items
	No corrosion	Instruments must be predried
	Items are dry after cycle	Cannot sterilize liquids

Table 21-2 ***Sterilization and Disinfection Guide for Common Dental Items***

	Steam Autoclave	Dry Heat Oven	Chemiclave	Chemical Disinfection/ Sterilization	Disposable
Angle attachments	+	+	+	+	*
Burs					
Carbon steel	–	+	+	–	++
Steel	+	+	+	–	++
Tungsten-carbide	+	++	+	+	*
Condensers	++	++	++	+	*
Dappen dishes	++	+	+	+	*
Endodontic instruments					
Broaches, files, reamers	+	++	++	—	*
Non–stainless steel metal handles	—	++	++	—	*
Stainless steel handles	++	++	++	+	*
Stainless steel with plastic handles	–	–	–	+	*
Fluoride gel trays					
Heat-resistant plastic	++	—	–	–	*
Non–heat-resistant plastic	—	—	–	–	++
Glass slabs	++	++	++	+	*
Hand instruments					
Carbon steel	–	++	++	–	*
Stainless steel	++	++	++	+	*
Handpieces					
Autoclavable	++	–	–	–	*
Contra-angles	–	–	–	+	*
Non-autoclavable	–	–	–	+	*
Prophylaxis angles	+	+	+	+	*
Impression trays					
Aluminum metal: chrome-plated	++	++	++	+	*
Custom acrylic resin	—	—	—	+	*
Plastic	—	—	—	+	++
Instruments in packs	++	+	++	*	*
Instrument tray setups					
Restorative or surgical	+	+	+	*	*
Mirrors	–	++	++	+	*
Needles	—	—	—	–	++

*+, Effective and preferred method; ++, effective and acceptable method; –, effective method, but risk of damage to materials; —, ineffective method with risk of damage to materials; *, not applicable.*

From Samaranayake LP: Essential microbiology for dentistry, *New York, 2002, Churchill Livingstone.*

Table 21-2 ***Sterilization and Disinfection Guide for Common Dental Items—cont'd***

	Steam Autoclave	Dry Heat Oven	Chemiclave	Chemical Disinfection/ Sterilization	Disposable
Orthodontic pliers					
High-quality stainless steel	++	++	++	+	*
Low-quality stainless steel	–	++	++	–	*
With plastic parts	—	—	—	+	*
Pluggers	++	++	++	+	*
Polishing wheels and discs					
Garnet and cuttle	—	–	–	—	+
Rag	++	–	+	—	*
Rubber	+	–	–	+	+
Prostheses, removable					
Rubber dam equipment	–	–	–	+	*
Carbon steel clamps	–	++	++	–	*
Metal frames	++	++	++	+	*
Plastic frames	–	–	–	+	*
Punches	–	++	++	+	*
Radiographic equipment					
Plastic film holders	–	–	–	–	++
Collimating devices	–	—	—	+	*
Rubber items					
Prophylaxis cups	+	–	–	+	++
Saliva evacuators, ejectors					
High-melting plastic	++	+	+	+	*
Low-melting plastic	–	–	–	+	++
Stainless steel clamps	++	++	++	+	*
Stones					
Diamond	+	++	++	+	*
Polishing	++	+	++	–	*
Sharpening	++	++	++	–	*
Surgical instruments					
Stainless steel	++	++	++	+	*
Ultrasonic scaling tips	+	—	—	+	*

instantly because of the surrounding room-temperature air. Manufacturers set their sterilizers (autoclaves) to reach maximum steam temperatures of approximately 250° F (121° C), with pressures of 15 or 30 pounds per square inch (psi). The steam sterilizer is used for sterilization of a variety of dental instruments and accessories, including heat-resistant plastics, dental handpieces, instruments, cotton rolls, and gauze (Fig. 21-18). Packaging material for steam sterilization must be porous enough to permit the steam to penetrate to the instruments inside. The packaging material may be fabric but most often is sealed film or paper pouches, nylon tubing, sterilizing wrap, or paper-wrapped cassettes.

Solid closed metal trays, capped glass vials, and aluminum foil *cannot* be used in an autoclave because they prevent the steam from reaching the inside of the pack.

A disadvantage of steam sterilization is that the moisture may cause corrosion on some high-carbon steel instruments. Distilled water should be used in autoclaves instead of tap water, which often contains minerals and impurities. Distilled water can minimize corrosion and pitting.

Operation Cycles

Dental office steam sterilizers usually operate through four cycles: (1) *heat-up cycle,* (2) *sterilizing cycle,* (3) *depressurization cycle,* and (4) *drying cycle.*

After the water is added, the chamber is loaded, the door is closed, the unit is turned on, and the heat-up cycle begins to generate steam. The steam pushes out the air in the chamber, and when the set temperature is reached, the sterilizing cycle begins. The temperature is maintained for the set time, usually ranging from 3 to 30 minutes (Box 21-4).

Types of Steam Sterilizers

All steam sterilizers operate in a similar manner, but different models and brands have different features. There are various sizes of chambers and mechanisms of air removal, steam generation, drying, temperature displays, and recording devices (Fig. 21-19).

Procedure 21-3 illustrates the use of an autoclave.

Flash Sterilization

Rapid or flash sterilization of dental instruments is accomplished by rapid heat transfer, steam, and unsaturated chemical vapor (Fig. 21-20).

Flash sterilization may be used *only* on instruments that are placed in the chamber *unwrapped.* This presents a com-

Box 21-4 Typical Steam Temperatures in Sterilizing Cycle

Temperature	Time
250° F (121° C)	30 minutes
250° F (121° C)	15 minutes
273° F (134° C)	10 minutes
273° F (134° C)	3 minutes

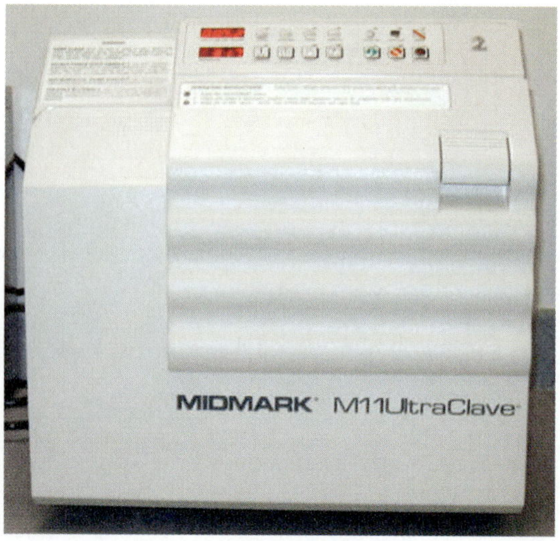

Fig. 21-18 Steam autoclave.

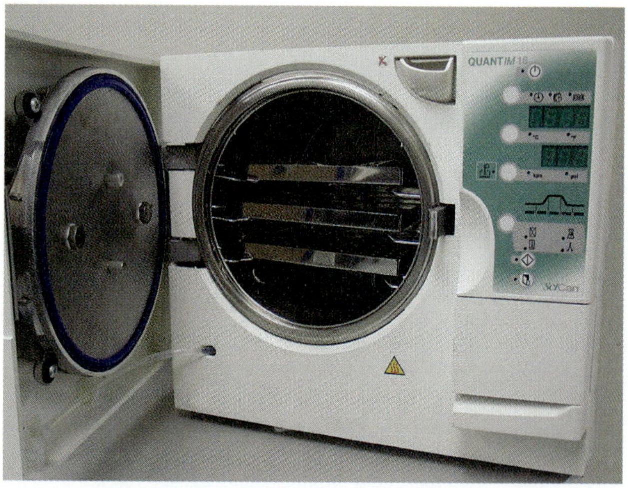

Fig. 21-19 Vacuum-type autoclave. (Courtesy SciScan.)

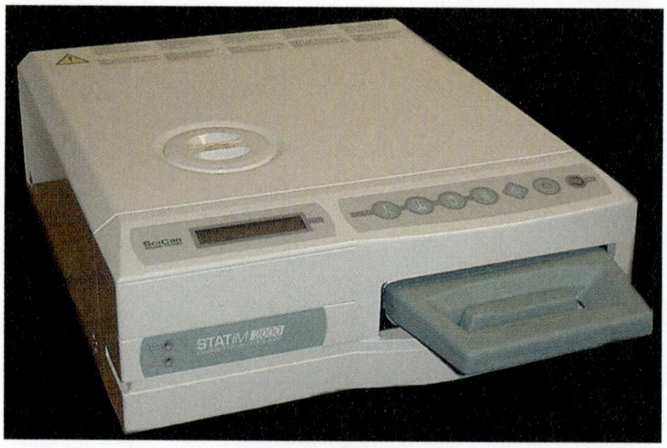

Fig. 21-20 STAT/M sterilizer. (Courtesy SciScan.)

promise because the sterility of the instruments is defeated immediately when the instruments are removed from the sterilizer.

Flash sterilization also should be used *only* for instruments that are to be *promptly* used on removal from the sterilizer. It is *always* the best policy to use a method of sterilization in which the instruments can be packaged before use and remain packaged until the time of use.

Chemical Vapor Sterilization

Chemical vapor sterilization is very similar to autoclaving, except a combination of chemicals (alcohol, formaldehyde, ketone, acetone, and water) is used instead of water to create a vapor for sterilizing (Fig. 21-21 and Procedure 21-4). OSHA requires a *material safety data sheet* (MSDS) on the chemical vapor solution because of the chemicals' toxicity.

Procedure 21-3 Autoclaving Instruments

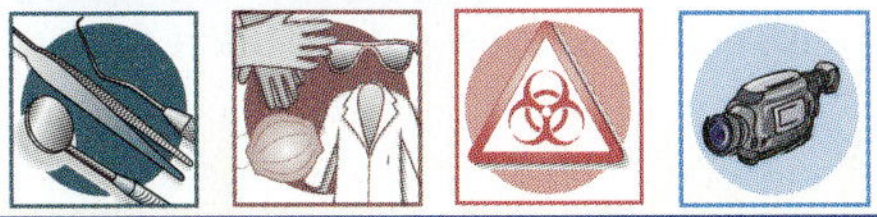

Goal

To prepare and autoclave instruments.

Equipment and Supplies

- Appropriate PPE
- Autoclaving wrapping materials
- Process integrator
- Corrosion inhibitor solution (1 percent sodium nitrate)
- Tape to seal packages
- Pen or pencil to label packages
- Oven mitt

PROCEDURAL STEPS

1. Instruments must be clean, but not necessarily dry, before wrapping for autoclaving.
   Note: The exceptions are glass slabs and dishes, rubber items, and stones. These objects must be dry before being autoclaved.
2. Non–stainless instruments and burs may be dipped in a corrosion inhibitor solution (1 percent sodium nitrate) before being wrapped.
   Note: An alternative for these instruments is sterilization by dry heat.
3. Insert the process integrator into the package.
4. Package, seal, and label the instruments.

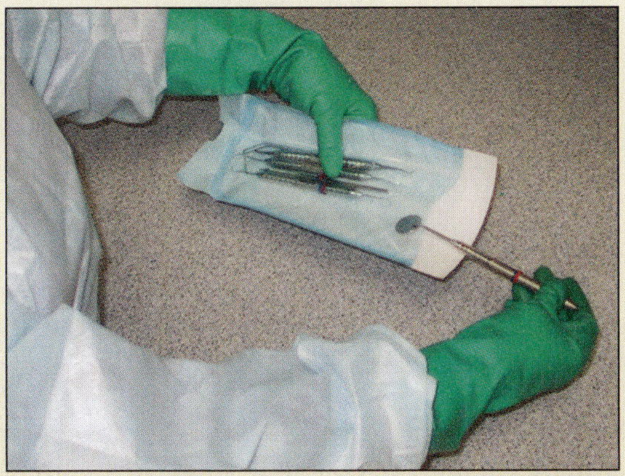

Load the Autoclave

1. Place bagged and sealed items in the autoclave.
2. Separate articles and packs from each other by a reasonable space. Tilt glass or metal canisters at an angle.
   Purpose: To permit a free flow of steam in and around all instrument packs.

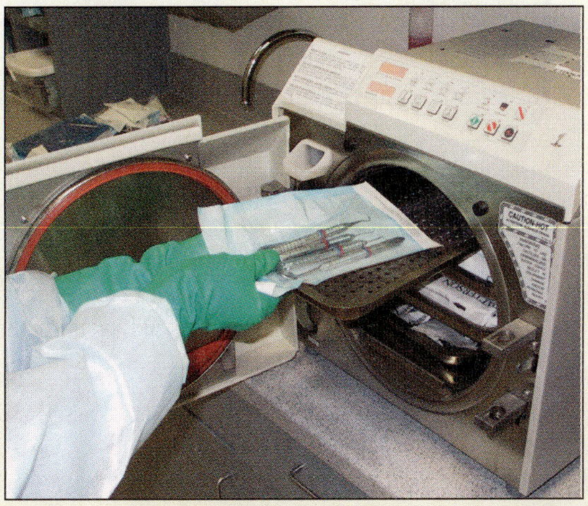

3. Place larger packs, which might block the flow of steam, at the bottom of the chamber.
   Purpose: Large loads prevent the autoclave from reaching the correct temperature and pressure and make it difficult for the steam to flow properly.
4. Never overload the autoclave.
   Purpose: Trapped air in the autoclave will inhibit the top-to-bottom flow of steam.

Operate the Autoclave

1. Read and follow the manufacturer's instructions. Most autoclaves require distilled water.
   Purpose: Tap water often contains minerals that can damage the autoclave by forming deposits on the chamber's inner surfaces and can corrode metals.

continued

Procedure 21-3 Autoclaving Instruments—cont'd

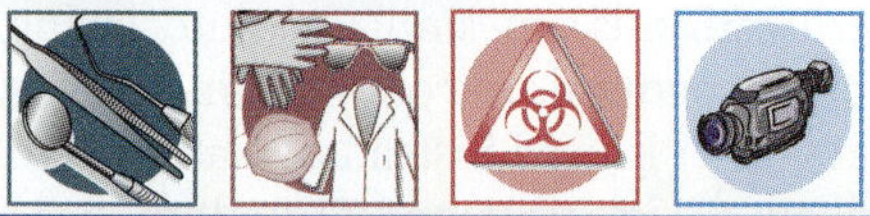

PROCEDURAL STEPS, cont'd

2. Ensure that an adequate supply of water is available. If not, add distilled water.

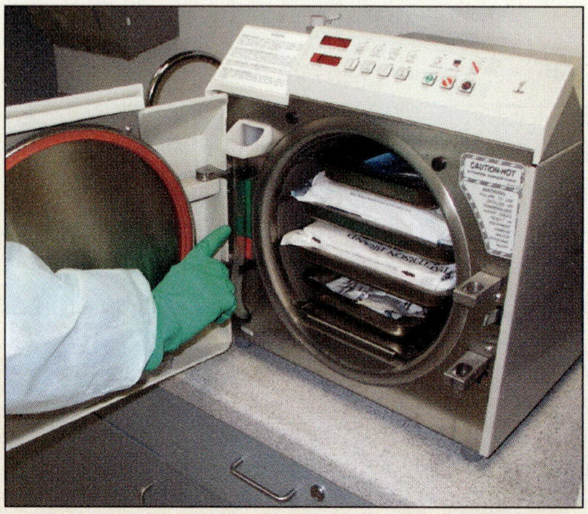

3. Set autoclave controls for the appropriate time, temperature, and pressure.

   Note: Pressure and temperature must be reached before timing begins. Duration of this warm-up time depends on the autoclave and the size of the load.

4. At the end of the sterilization cycle, vent the steam into the room. Allow the contents of the autoclave to dry and cool.

   Note: Most models vent and cool automatically. If the machine is not so equipped, open the door of the autoclave slightly after the pressure has dropped within the chamber. Do this with *extreme caution* because the contents and remaining steam are scalding. The contents should be allowed to dry and cool before they are removed.

Reassemble and Store the Trays

1. Wash your hands and put on clean examination gloves for handling sterile packs and reassembling trays.
2. Remove sealed packs from the sterilizer and place them in the clean area.

   Important Note: Work only in the clean area of the sterilization center.
3. Place the sealed packs on the tray, and add the supplies necessary to perform the procedure.
4. *Optional:* In some practices the necessary gloves and masks are added to the tray at this time. In other practices these items are stored in the treatment room.
5. Store the prepared tray in the clean area until needed in the treatment room.

Advantages

The major advantage of the chemical vapor sterilizer is that is does not rust, dull, or corrode dry metal instruments. The low water content of the vapor prevents destruction of items such as endodontic files, orthodontic pliers, wires, bands, and burs. A wide range of items can be sterilized routinely without damage.

Other advantages include the short cycle time and the availability of a dry instrument after the cycle.

Disadvantages

The primary disadvantage is that adequate ventilation is essential because residual chemical vapors containing formaldehyde and methyl alcohol can be released when

Procedure 21-4 Sterilizing Instruments with Chemical Vapor

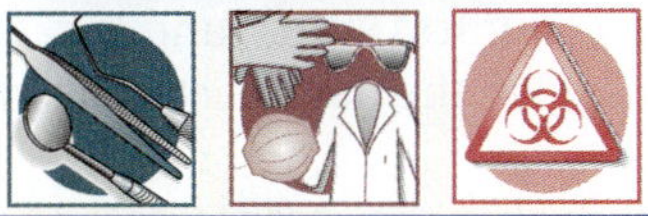

Goal

To prepare and sterilize instruments by chemical vapor sterilization.

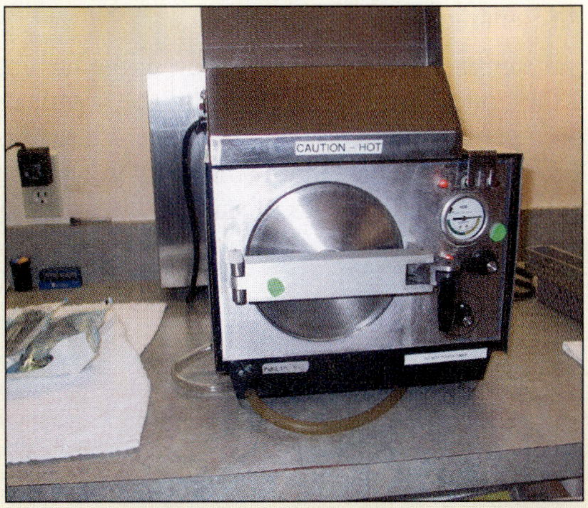

Equipment and Supplies

- Appropriate PPE
- Chemical vapor wrapping materials
- Precleaned and dried instruments
- Process integrator
- Tape to seal packages
- Pen or pencil to label packages

PROCEDURAL STEPS

Wrap the Instruments

1. Ensure that the instruments are clean and *dry* before wrapping them for chemical vapor sterilization.
   Purpose: If instruments are not absolutely dry, they will rust.
2. Insert the appropriate process integrator into the test load instrument package.
3. Take care not to create packs that are too large to be sterilized throughout.
   Purpose: Chemical vapor sterilization is not recommended for large loads or tightly wrapped instruments.

Load and Operate the Chemical Vapor Sterilizer

1. Read and follow the manufacturer's instructions.
   Important Note: Always follow the precautions in the MSDS.
2. Load the sterilizer according to the manufacturer's instructions.
   Note: This step is similar to loading an autoclave.
3. Set the controls for the appropriate time, temperature, and pressure.
   Note: Pressure and temperature must be reached before timing begins.
4. Follow the manufacturer's instructions for venting and cooling.
5. When the instruments are cool and dry, reassemble and store the preset tray.

the chamber door is opened at the end of the cycle. These vapors can temporarily leave an unpleasant odor in the area and may be irritating to the eyes.

Filtration and Monitoring of Chemical Vapors

Newer sterilizers are equipped with a special filtration device that further reduces the amount of chemical vapor remaining in the chamber at the end of the cycle. Older models can usually be retrofitted.

Formaldehyde monitoring badges also are available for employees, similar to radiation monitoring devices. The monitoring measures personal exposure to formaldehyde for a period, the badge is mailed to the monitoring service, and a laboratory analysis is sent to the employee.

Packaging

Standard packaging for chemical vapor sterilization includes film pouches or paper bags, nylon see-through tubing, sterilization wrap, and wrapped cassettes. Thick or tightly wrapped items require longer exposure because un-

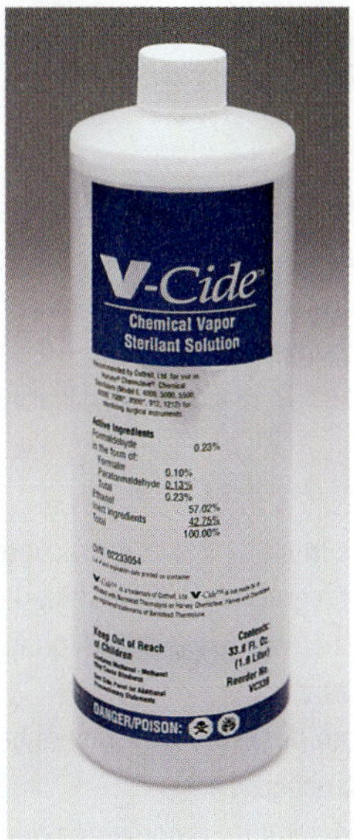

Fig. 21-21 Sterilant solution for a chemical vapor sterilizer. (Courtesy Certol.)

saturated chemical vapors are unable to penetrate as well as saturated chemical vapors under pressure.

As in autoclaving, closed containers (such as solid metal trays and capped glass vials) and aluminum foil *cannot* be used in a chemical vapor sterilizer because they prevent the sterilizing agent from reaching the instruments inside.

Pressure, Temperature, and Time

The three major factors in chemical vapor sterilization are pressure, which should measure 20 psi; temperature, which should measure 270° F (131° C); and time, which should measure 20 to 40 minutes.

Dry-Heat Sterilization

Dry-heat sterilizers operate by heating up air and transferring that heat from the air to the instruments. This form of sterilization requires higher temperatures than steam or chemical vapor sterilization. Dry-heat sterilizers operate at approximately 320° to 375° F (160° to 190° C) and vary in the time of operation depending on the manufacturer's instructions (Procedure 21-5).

The advantage of dry heat is that the instruments will not rust *if* they are thoroughly dry before they are placed in the sterilizer. Two types of dry-heat sterilizers available are *static air* and *forced air.*

Static Air Sterilizers

Static air sterilizers are similar to an oven: the heating coils are on the bottom of the chamber, and the hot air rises inside through natural convection. Heat is transferred from the *static* (nonmoving) air to the instruments in about one to two hours. The disadvantages of static dry heat are that the sterilization process is time-consuming and may not be ef-

Procedure 21-5 Sterilizing Instruments with Dry Heat

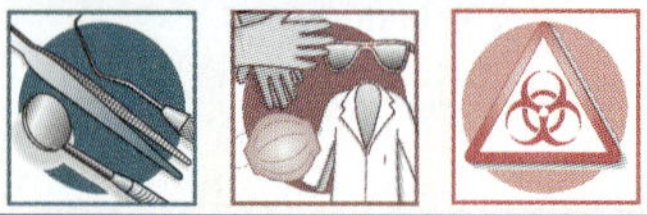

Goal

To prepare and sterilize instruments by dry-heat sterilization.

Equipment and Supplies

- Wrapping materials
- Precleaned instruments
- Process integrator for dry heat
- Tape to seal packages
- Pen or pencil to label packages

PROCEDURAL STEPS

Wrap Instruments

1. Clean and dry instruments before wrapping.
   Purpose: Wet instruments can rust during dry-heat sterilization.
2. Prepare hinged instruments, such as surgical forceps, hemostats, and scissors, with their hinges opened.
   Purpose: To allow heat to reach all areas during sterilization.

Load and Operate the Dry-Heat Sterilizer

1. Read and follow the manufacturer's instructions.
2. Insert the process integrator into the test load package.
3. Load the dry-heat chamber to permit adequate circulation of air around the packages.
   Purpose: Sterilization does not occur unless heat reaches all areas of the instruments.
4. Set the time and temperature according to the manufacturer's instructions. Allow time for the entire load to reach the desired temperature.
   Purpose: Timing does not start until the desired temperature has been reached throughout the entire load.
5. Do not place additional instruments in the load once the sterilization cycle has begun.
   Purpose: Cooler instruments will lower the temperature of the oven significantly.
6. At the end of the sterilization cycle, allow the packs to cool, then handle them very carefully.
   Purpose: Packs are very hot and could cause injury.

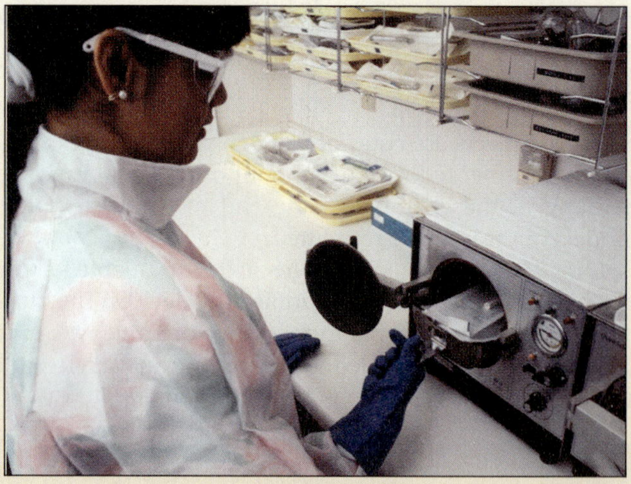

7. When the packs are cool, reassemble and store the preset tray.

fective if the operatory makes errors in calculating the correct processing time. The wrapping material must be heat-resistant. Aluminum foil, metal, and glass containers may be used. Paper and cloth packs should be avoided because they may burn or discolor from the intense heat.

Forced Air Sterilizers

Forced air sterilizers, also called *rapid heat transfer sterilizers,* circulate hot air throughout the chamber at a high velocity. This action permits a rapid transfer of heat energy from the air to the instruments, reducing the time needed for sterilization. Exposure time in forced air sterilizers, after the sterilizing temperature has been reached, ranges from 6 minutes for unpackaged items to 12 minutes for packaged items.

Sterilization Failures

A load may fail to become sterilized when direct contact for the correct time is insufficient between the sterilizing agent (chemical or steam) and all surfaces of the items being processed. Several factors can cause the sterilization process to fail, including improper instrument cleaning or packaging and sterilizer malfunction (Table 21-3).

The monitoring service will generally report a sterilization failure *(positive result)* to the dental office immediately by phone. (A positive report indicates that sterilization did *not* occur.) If the culture is negative *(negative result),* the monitoring service will mail a report to the dental office to document that the cultures were read at 24, 48, and 72 hours. (A negative report indicates that sterilization *did* occur.)

Recall

17. What causes sterilization failure?
18. What are the three most common forms of heat sterilization?
19. What is a primary disadvantage of flash sterilization?
20. What is a major advantage of chemical vapor sterilization?
21. What are the two types of dry-heat sterilization?

Chemical Liquid Sterilization

Not all items can withstand heat sterilization. Some types of plastics, such as some rubber dam frames, shade guides, and x-ray film-holding devices, are damaged by heat sterilization. Thus a liquid sterilant such as 2 percent to 3.4 percent glutaraldehyde must be used for sterilization of these items (Procedure 21-6). Sterilization in glutaralde-

Table 21-3 ***Results of Sterilization Errors***

Errors	Examples	Results
Inadequate instrument cleaning	Dried blood and/or cement remain on instruments	Organisms may be insulated from sterilizing agents
Improper packaging	Excessive wrap (too thick)	Prevents sterilizing agent from reaching instruments
	Packaging material is not compatible with type of sterilizer	Wrap may melt or sterilizing agent may not penetrate wrap
	Closed container in chemical vapor or autoclave	Sterilizing agent cannot reach inside surfaces
Improper loading of sterilizer	Overloading	Increases time to reach proper temperature and can slow the penetration to the center of the load
	No separation between packages (too close together)	May prevent sterilizing agent from reaching all items and surfaces
Improper timing	Operator error in timing	Insufficient time to sterilize
	Timing started before reaching proper temperature (in nonautomatic units)	Insufficient time to sterilize
	Dry-heat sterilizer door opened during cycle without restarting time	Insufficient time to sterilize
Improper temperature	Error in operation of sterilizer	Insufficient heat to sterilize
	Malfunction of sterilizer	Insufficient heat to sterilize

hyde requires a 10-hour contact time; anything less than 10 hours is disinfection, *not* sterilization (Fig. 21-22).

CDC Liquid Chemical Sterilants/High-Level Disinectants

When using a liquid chemical germicide for sterilization, certain poststerilization procedures are essential: 1) rinse with sterile water after removal to remove toxic or irritating residues; 2) handle using sterile gloves and dry with sterile towels; 3) deliver to the point of use in an aseptic manner.

If stored before use, the instrument should not be considered sterile and should be sterilized again just before use. In addition, the sterilization process with liquid chemical sterilant cannot be verified with biologic indicators.

In addition, these products must be used full-strength (not diluted) on precleaned instruments. Liquid sterilants may *not* be used as surface disinfectants due to the toxicity of the fumes. (IB)

Be sure that you have an MSDS for these products. All employees should be properly trained on how to handle such devices.

Ethylene Oxide Sterilization

Ethylene oxide gas is a recognized method of sterilization. This method operates at low temperatures, which is an advantage for plastic and rubber items that would melt in heat sterilizers.

However, ethylene oxide sterilization requires 4 to 12 hours for sterilization, depending on the sterilizer model. Also, at least 16 hours of poststerilization aeration is required to remove the gas molecules bound to the plastic and rubber surfaces.

Ethylene oxide is ineffective on wet items. Toxicity is a risk if the gas is not handled properly. These units are of-

Procedure 21-6 Sterilizing Instruments with Chemical Liquid

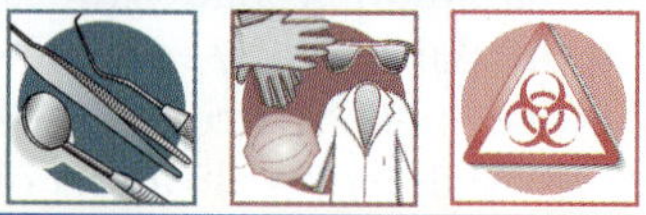

Goal

To prepare and sterilize instruments using a chemical sterilant.

Equipment and Supplies

- Appropriate PPE
- Precleaned and dried items that cannot be heat-sterilized
- Liquid chemical sterilant
- Sterile instrument tongs
- Sterile rinse water

PROCEDURAL STEPS

Prepare the Solution

1. Use utility gloves, mask, eyewear, and protective clothing when preparing, using, and discarding the solution.
   Purpose: Liquid sterilants are highly toxic and can lead to respiratory problems if not handled properly.
2. Follow the manufacturer's instructions for preparing/activating, using, and disposing of the solution.
   Purpose: In many areas, glutaraldehyde is considered a hazardous material, requires special disposal methods, and may not be dumped down the sink.
3. Prepare the solution for use as a sterilant. Label the containers with the name of the chemical, the date of preparation (to indicate the use-life), and any other information that relates to the hazards of this product. **Use-life** is the period of time during which a germicidal solution is effective after having been prepared for use.
   Purpose: Some brands remain active for 30 days; others may have a longer or shorter life.
4. Cover the container and keep it closed unless you are putting instruments in or taking them out.
   Purpose: Glutaraldehyde produces toxic fumes.

Use the Solution

1. Preclean, rinse, and dry items to be processed.
2. Place the items in a perforated tray or pan. Place the pan in the solution, and cover the container. An alternative method is to use tongs and avoid splashing.
3. Be certain that all items are fully submerged in the solution for the entire contact time.
   Purpose: The solution must be in contact with the items for the recommended contact time.
4. Rinse processed items thoroughly with water and dry. Place items in clean package.
   Note: Sterility is best maintained by rinsing with sterile water, drying with a sterile towel, and placing in a sterile container.

Maintain the Solution

1. Periodically test the glutaraldehyde concentration of the solution with a chemical test kit (available from the manufacturer).
2. Replace the solution as indicated on the instructions, or when the level of the solution is low or the solution is visibly dirty.
3. When you replace the used solution, discard all of the used solution, clean the container with a detergent, rinse with water, dry, and fill the container with a fresh solution.

Modified from Miller CH, Palenik CJ: *Infection control and management of hazardous materials for the dental team*, ed 3, St. Louis, 2005, Mosby.

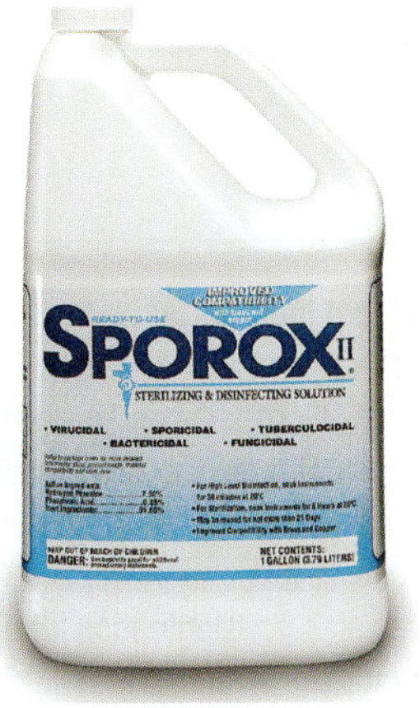

Fig. 21-22 SPOROX® II is a high-level disinfectant/sterilant used for instruments that cannot tolerate heat sterilization. (Courtesy Sultan Chemists Inc., Englewood, NJ.)

ten used in large clinics or hospital settings but rarely in private dental practices.

HANDPIECE STERILIZATION

High-speed dental handpieces rotate at speeds up to 400,000 revolutions per minute (rpm). Blood, saliva, and tooth fragments, as well as restorative materials, may lodge in the head of the handpiece, where they may be retained and transferred to another patient. Therefore, dental handpieces must be properly cleaned and heat-sterilized.

Flushing Techniques

The life expectancy of the dental handpiece depends on its frequency of use and how it is used and maintained. If debris is not removed before heat sterilization, it will bake onto the turbine and bearings. Flushing the handpiece is the best way to remove debris from the head of the handpiece.

To flush a dental handpiece, attach a pressurized handpiece cleaner to the intake tube of the handpiece (where the air passes through), and flush the head of the handpiece to remove debris. Afterward, blow out the handpiece using compressed air to remove debris before sterilization. Most handpieces should not be run without a bur in place (see Chapter 35).

Running coolant water from the dental unit through the handpiece at chairside is insufficient. Coolant water does not run through the turbine chamber, where debris can collect.

Sterilizing Techniques

Only steam sterilization and chemical vapor sterilizers are recommended, because handpiece sterilization temperatures should not exceed 275° F (135° C). Unless they will be used immediately after sterilization, handpieces should be packaged in bags, wraps, or packs to protect them from contamination before use.

Never run a handpiece "hot" out of the sterilizer, and avoid rapid cooldowns, such as running the handpiece under cold water. Handpieces use very small metal components; extreme cold changes stress the metal. If handpieces need to be cooled quickly after sterilization, use an air fan to blow room-temperature air over it (Procedure 21-7).

Procedure 21-7 Sterilizating the Dental Handpiece

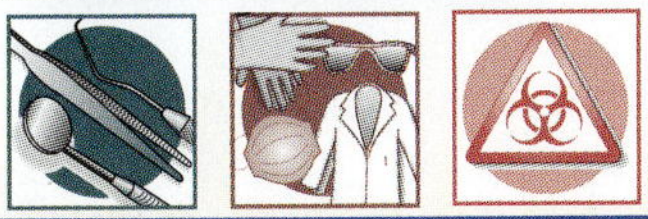

Goal

To prepare and sterilize the "sterilizable" dental handpiece.

Note: This procedure provides only an overview of general procedures for handpieces that are rated as "sterilizable" by the manufacturer. Always follow the handpiece manufacturer's instructions for maintenance and sterilization. Failure to do so can void the handpiece's warranty.

Equipment and Supplies

- Sterilizable handpiece
- Bur
- Ultrasonic cleaner (if recommended by the manufacturer)
- Lubrication (if recommended by the manufacturer)
- Cotton swab
- Isopropyl alcohol

PROCEDURAL STEPS

1. Before you remove the handpiece from the hose, with the bur still in the chuck, wipe any visible debris from the handpiece. Operate the handpiece for approximately 10 to 20 seconds to flush water and air into the lines.
   Purpose: To remove any loose debris that has become lodged in the head.
2. Remove the bur from the handpiece and then the handpiece from the hose.
   a. If the manufacturer recommends ultrasonic cleaning, follow those instructions, then thoroughly drain the handpiece, attach the hose, and briefly operate the handpiece to expel debris.
   b. If ultrasonic cleaning is not expressly recommended, scrub the handpiece thoroughly under running water with a brush and soap/detergent cleaner.

continued

Procedure 21-7 Sterilizing the Dental Handpiece—cont'd

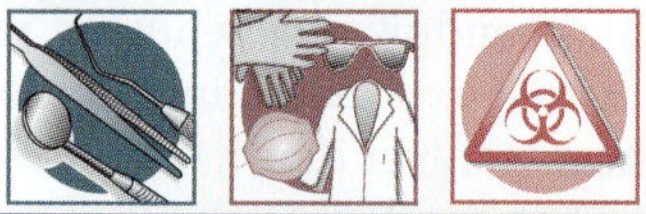

PROCEDURAL STEPS, cont'd

3. If the handpiece requires presterilization lubrication, use a handpiece cleaner recommended by the manufacturer to remove internal debris, and lubricate the handpiece.
   a. If the handpiece does not require presterilization lubrication, use a cleaner that *does not* contain a lubricant.
   b. Follow the manufacturer's instructions for each type of handpiece used.

   Purpose: To avoid overlubricating the handpiece.
4. Reattach the handpiece to an air hose, and blow out the excess lubricant from the rotating parts. Most handpieces must have a bur inserted before being operated.

   Purpose: Failure to do this can result in excess lubricant accumulating in the head and "gumming" of the excess during the heat cycle.
5. Use a cotton-tipped applicator dampened (not soaked) with isopropyl alcohol to remove all excess lubricant from fiberoptic interfaces and exposed optical surfaces. Never use strong solvents on fiberoptics.

   Purpose: Strong solvents can dissolve the epoxy binding between the fibers.
6. Be sure the handpiece is clean; then dry it and package it for sterilization. Sterilize according to the manufacturer's instructions. After the heat cycle, allow the bagged handpiece to cool and dry. Keep sterilization packaging sealed until the handpiece is to be prepared for use on a patient.

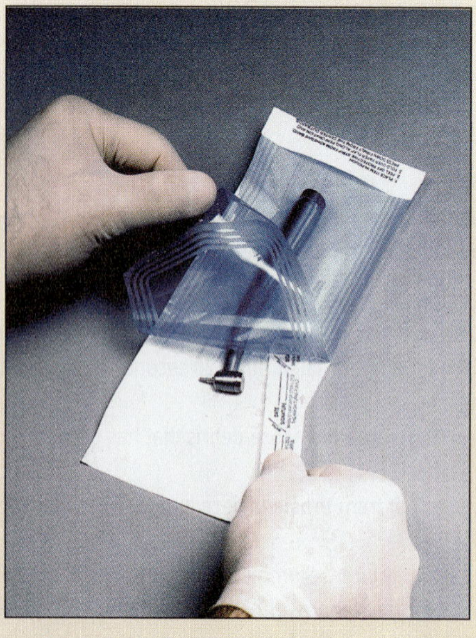

7. Flush water and air into the lines for 20 to 30 seconds before attaching the handpiece.

   Purpose: To remove any residual debris and free-floating bacteria.
8. If the handpiece does not require poststerilization measures, open the sterilized bag at chairside in front of the patient to demonstrate that a fresh handpiece is being used.
9. If the handpiece requires poststerilization lubrication, keep a separate lubricant container for use on sterilized handpieces. Lubricate the handpiece as close as possible to the actual time of use.

   Purpose: To reduce the risk of cross-contamination.
10. Open only the *end* of the sterilization packaging. Spray the lubricant into the handpiece air drive to reduce the amount of overspray and help control excess lubricant.

    Note: The dental handpiece is now ready for use.

Modified from *OSAP Focus,* no 5, 2001.

Recall

22. What is the primary disadvantage of liquid chemical sterilization?
23. How should instruments processed in a liquid chemical sterilant be rinsed?
24. How should high-speed handpieces be processed before sterilization?
25. What types of heat sterilization are appropriate for high-speed handpieces?

CDC Storage Area for Sterilized Items and Clean Dental Supplies

The storage area should contain enclosed storage for sterile items and disposable (single-use) items. Storage practices for wrapped sterilized instruments can be either date- or event-related. **Event-related packaging** means that it is assumed the contents will remain sterile indefinitely unless some event (e.g., a torn or wet package) occurs to contaminate the contents. For event-related packaging, minimally, the date of sterilization should be placed on the package, and if multiple sterilizers are used in the facility, the sterilizer used should be indicated on the outside of the packaging material. If packaging is compromised, the instruments should be recleaned, packaged in a new wrap, and sterilized again. (IB)

Clean supplies and instruments should be stored in closed or covered cabinets, if possible. Dental supplies and instruments should not be stored under sinks or in other locations where they might become wet (Fig. 21-23). (II)

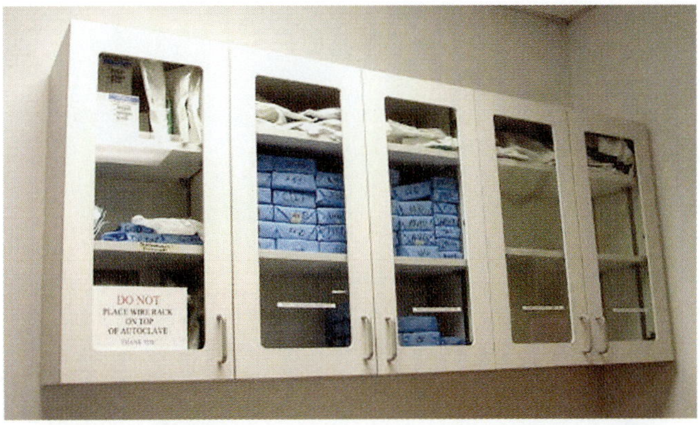

Fig. 21-23 Instruments and supplies stored in a closed cabinet.

Recall

26. What does event-related packaging mean?
27. How should clean supplies and instruments be stored?

Legal and Ethical Implications

The *CDC Guidelines for Infection Control in Dental Health-Care Settings–2003* were written to protect patients and members of the dental healthcare team from transmission of disease in the dental office. In addition, the OSHA Bloodborne Pathogens Standard requires biologic monitoring of sterilizers and maintenance of records of the results.

As a dental assistant, you are legally and ethically responsible for performing the procedures described in this chapter in a thorough and careful manner. Remember, proper instrument processing is necessary to prevent transferring microorganisms from a previous patient to the next patient or to you.

Eye to the Future

Visible light, ionizing radiation, microwave radiation, and ultraviolet (UV) rays are among the technologies being studied and applied in the area of disinfection and sterilization. Presently, *ionizing radiation* technology is being used in sterilization of heat-sensitive items and in food processing, thus reducing the number of foodborne illnesses.

UV lamps are used in surgical or inoculating hoods to reduce the number of microorganisms on surfaces. In the future, an FDA-approved light may destroy aerosols in dental operatories and sterilize all surfaces as well.

Critical Thinking

1. The dentist you work with is building a new dental office with all new equipment. She asks you to plan, design, and equip the instrument-processing area. What factors should you consider about the physical layout? What pieces of equipment should you order? What supplies will you want to have available?
2. You receive a phone call from the sterilization-monitoring company informing you that the last spore test you sent in has failed. What should you check to determine the possible cause?
3. Your friend who is not a dental assistant asks why you have to follow the *CDC Guidelines for Infection Control in Dental Health-Care Settings–2003* if the guidelines are not laws. How would you answer your friend?

Part 5

Occupational Health and Safety

The broad area of occupational health and safety is continually evolving. As new information becomes available, new rules and regulations are implemented. The dental assistant is often the person who is responsible for ensuring that the dental office is in compliance with a wide variety of federal, state, and local regulations concerning handling of hazardous chemicals, employee safety, and waste management.

In this section, you will learn the roles of the various agencies and how they interact with the dental office. You will learn how to manage chemicals in the dental office, how to identify and correctly dispose of waste materials, and why it is important to maintain the dental unit waterlines. In addition, you will learn how to prevent headaches, neck and shoulder pain, and other musculoskeletal disorders commonly associated with the practice of dental assisting.

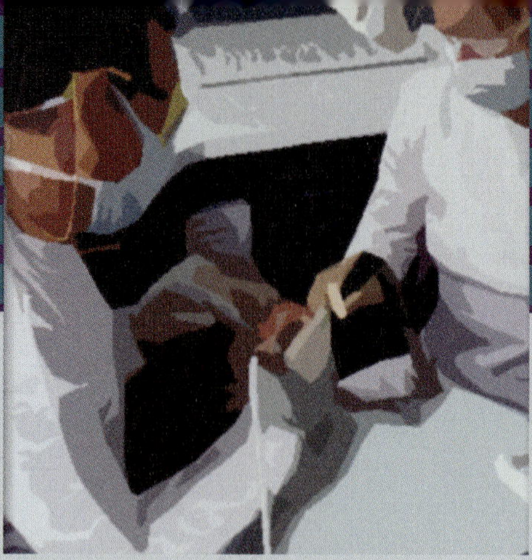

22 Regulatory and Advisory Agencies

Outline

KEY TERMS

American Dental Association (ADA) The professional organization for dentists.

Centers for Disease Control and Prevention (CDC) Federal agency that is nonregulatory and issues recommendations on health and safety.

Environmental Protection Agency (EPA) Federal regulatory agency whose responsibility it is to protect and restore the environment and public health through environmental laws.

Food and Drug Administration (FDA) Federal regulatory agency that regulates food, drugs, medical devices, animal feed and drugs, cosmetics, and radiation-emitting products (cell phones, lasers, microwaves, etc.).

National Institute for Occupational Safety and Health (NIOSH) Federal agency that is nonregulatory and provides national and worldwide leadership to prevent work-related illnesses and injuries.

National Institute of Dental and Craniofacial Research (NIDCR) Federal agency whose mission is to improve oral, dental, and craniofacial health through research, research training, and the dissemination of health information.

National Institutes of Health (NIH) One of the world's foremost research centers.

Occupational Safety and Health Administration (OSHA) Federal regulatory agency whose mission is to assure the safety and health of America's workers by setting and enforcing standards.

Organization for Safety and Asepsis Procedures (OSAP) The premier infection-control education organization in dentistry.

LEARNING OUTCOMES

On completion of this chapter, the student will be able to achieve the following objectives:

- Pronounce, define, and spell the Key Terms.
- Explain the difference between regulations and recommendations.
- Identify four professional sources for dental information.
- Name the premier infection-control educational organization in dentistry.
- Describe the role of the Centers for Disease Control and Prevention.
- Explain a primary difference between OSHA and NIOSH.
- Describe the role of the Environmental Protection Agency in relation to dentistry.
- Describe the role of the Food and Drug Administration in relation to dentistry.
- Describe the role of the National Institutes of Health.
- Describe the role of the National Institute of Dental and Craniofacial Research.

It is important for the dental assistant to recognize and understand the roles of the government agencies and professional organizations that have a direct influence on the practice of dentistry. This is especially true in the areas of infection control, chemicals, and other occupational health and safety issues. Some agencies are *regulatory* and issue rules and regulations with which dental offices must comply. Penalties for not complying with regulations may include fines, imprisonment, or suspension or revocation of licenses. Other agencies are *advisory* and have no authority for enforcement. These *nonregulatory* agencies issue recommendations that are based on strong scientific evidence and are the standard of care for dentistry today.

When you are in practice as a dental assistant, these agencies are excellent resources for information for you, and they are easily accessed on the Internet.

Government Agencies

Centers for Disease Control and Prevention (CDC)
1600 Clifton Rd.
Atlanta, GA 30333
(404) 639-3311
Division of Oral Health: 770-488-6054
Surveillance and Research: 770-488-6055
www.cdc.gov

U.S. Environmental Protection Agency (EPA)
Ariel Rios Building
1200 Pennsylvania Ave., N.W.
Washington, DC 20460
(202) 272-0167
www.epa.gov

U.S. Food and Drug Administration (FDA)
5600 Fishers Lane
Rockville, MD 20857
Center for Devices and Radiological Health: (800) 638-2041
MEDwatch: (800) FDA-1088
www.fda.gov

National Institutes of Health (NIH)
9000 Rockville Pike
Bethesda, MD 20892
(301) 496-4000
www.nih.gov

National Institute for Dental and Craniofacial Research (NIDCR)
31 Center Drive
Bethesda, MD 20892
(301) 402-2185
www. nidcr.gov

National Institute for Occupational Safety and Health (NIOSH)
Education and Information Division
4676 Columbia Parkway
Cincinnati, OH 45226
(513) 533-8377
www.cdc.gov/niosh

U.S. Occupational Safety and Health Administration (OSHA)*
200 Constitutional Ave. N.W.
Washington, DC 20210
(202) 693-1299
www.osha.gov

*Check online to see whether your state operates its own OSHA.

Professional Organizations

American Dental Association (ADA)
611 E. Chicago Ave.
Chicago, IL 60611
(312) 440-2500
www.ada.org

American Dental Assistants Association (ADAA)
203 North LaSalle St.
Chicago, IL 60601
(312) 541-1550
www.dentalassistant.org

Organization for Safety and Asepsis Procedures (OSAP)
PO Box 6297
Annapolis, MD 21401
(410) 571-0003
www.osap.org

ASSOCIATIONS AND ORGANIZATIONS

Professional organizations are a valuable resource for current infection control and other professional information.

American Dental Association

The **American Dental Association (ADA)** is the national professional organization for dentists. The ADA periodically updates its infection control recommendations as new scientific information becomes available. The ADA also publishes informational reports on emerging issues of interest to the dental community (Fig. 22-1).

Fig. 22-1 **Logo of the ADA.** (Courtesy American Dental Association.)

Organization for Safety and Asepsis Procedures

The **Organization for Safety and Asepsis Procedures (OSAP)** is dentistry's resource for infection control and safety. It is a not-for-profit organization composed of dentists, dental hygienists, dental assistants, government representatives, dental manufacturers, university professors, researchers, and dental consultants.

OSAP is a valuable resource that provides practical, scientifically sound information and recommendations on specific issues such as instrument processing, surface asepsis, dental unit waterline management, etc. OSAP's members receive a monthly newsletter on a specific issue of interest and an opportunity to receive an hour of continuing education for each newsletter reviewed.

OSAP is the premier infection-control education organization in dentistry, and all members of the dental team should consider becoming a member to keep up-to-date in the areas of infection control and dental office safety (Fig. 22-2).

State and Local Dental Societies

State and local dental societies can be helpful to you in complying with regulatory issues in your specific area. State and local dental and dental assisting societies can often answer questions and work with you or act as liaisons to the regulatory agencies.

Recall

1. What is the main difference between a recommendation and a regulation?
2. What is OSAP?

Fig. 22-2 **Logo of OSAP.** (Courtesy Organization for Safety and Asepsis Procedures.)

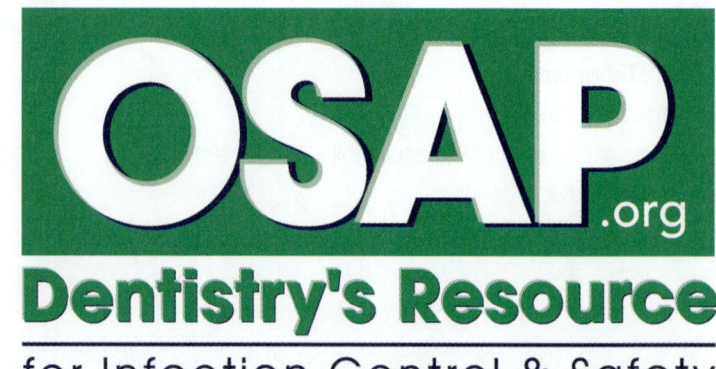

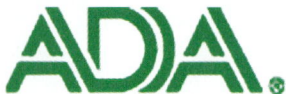

GOVERNMENT AGENCIES

Centers for Disease Control and Prevention

The **Centers for Disease Control and Prevention (CDC)** is an agency of the U.S. Department of Health and Human Services. It is recognized as the lead federal agency for protecting the health and safety of people at home and abroad. The CDC bases its public health *recommendations* on the highest quality scientific data.

The infection-control procedures practiced in dentistry today are based on the *Guidelines for Infection Control in Dental Health-Care Settings—2003* (Fig. 22-3) issued by the CDC. The CDC also has an Oral Health Services section that studies oral diseases, fluoride application, and infection control in dentistry. The CDC does *not* have the authority to make laws, but many local, state, and federal agencies use CDC recommendations to formulate laws.

The CDC has also published guidelines on preventing transmission of tuberculosis in healthcare settings, including dental offices. It publishes the *Morbidity and Mortality Weekly Report,* which provides data on health and disease trends based on reports by state health departments.

Although the CDC's national headquarters are in Atlanta, Georgia, more than 2000 CDC employees work at other locations, including 47 state health departments. About 120 employees are assigned overseas in 45 countries.

The CDC is an excellent resource of health information for the public as well as all dental professionals (Fig. 22-4).

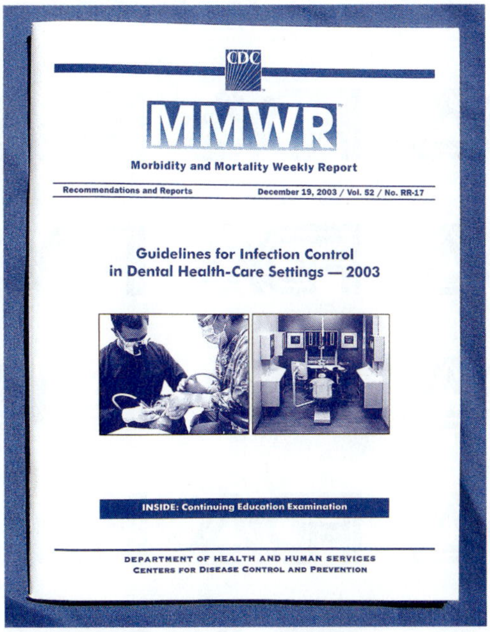
CDC

MMWR

Morbidity and Mortality Weekly Report

Recommendations and Reports December 19, 2003 / Vol. 52 / No. RR-17

Guidelines for Infection Control in Dental Health-Care Settings — 2003

INSIDE: Continuing Education Examination

DEPARTMENT OF HEALTH AND HUMAN SERVICES
CENTERS FOR DISEASE CONTROL AND PREVENTION

Fig. 22-3 ***Guidelines for Infection Control in Dental Health-Care Settings–2003.*** (Courtesy Centers for Disease Control and Prevention.)

Food and Drug Administration

The U.S. **Food and Drug Administration (FDA)** is a *regulatory* agency and is part of the U.S. Department of Health and Human Services. The FDA regulates the manufacturing and labeling of medical devices. In dentistry, the FDA must approve sterilizers, biologic and chemical indicators, ultrasonic cleaners and cleaning solutions, liquid sterilants, gloves, masks, protective eyewear, dental handpieces and instruments, dental chairs, and dental unit lights. The FDA also regulates antimicrobial handwashing products and mouthrinses (Fig. 22-5).

The FDA requires "good manufacturing practices" and reviews the safety and effectiveness of drugs and medical devices. The agency also reviews the claims on the labels of products to be certain those claims are true. All medical and dental devices to be sold in the United States must first be cleared by the FDA before being marketed (Fig. 22-6).

CDC Department of Health and Human Services
Centers for Disease Control and Prevention

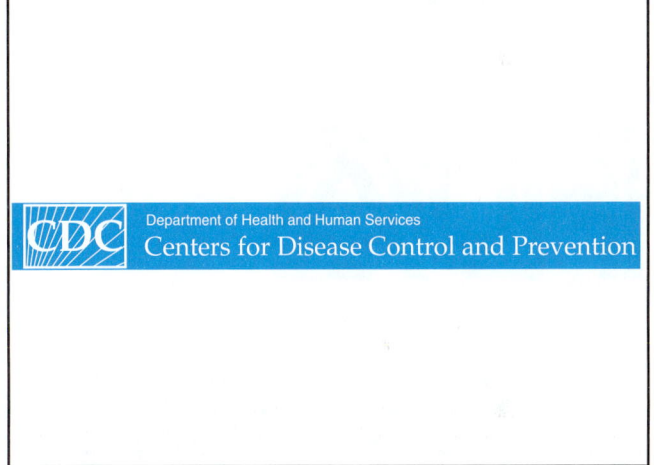

Fig. 22-4 Logo of the CDC. (Courtesy Centers for Disease Control and Prevention.)

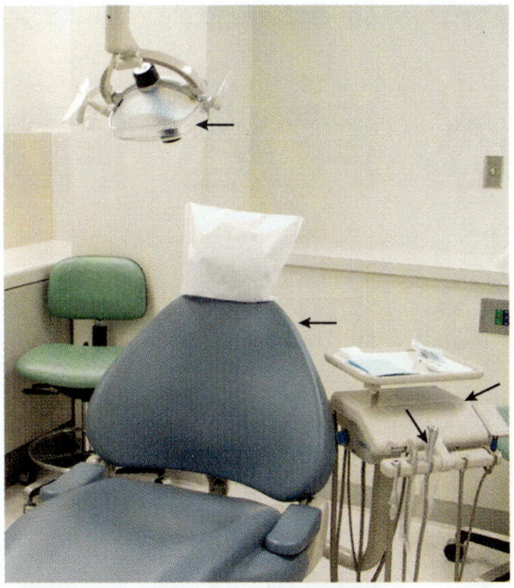

Fig. 22-5 Overview of a dental operatory showing items *(arrows)* regulated by the FDA.

U.S. Food and Drug Administration Logo Sheet 1298.01

Fig. 22-6 The FDA logo is available in a variety of sizes.

Environmental Protection Agency

The U.S. **Environmental Protection Agency (EPA)** is a *regulatory* agency. The EPA is associated with dentistry by ensuring the safety and effectiveness of disinfectants. Manufacturers of disinfectants must submit information about the safety and effectiveness of the product. The EPA reviews the manufacturer's antimicrobial claims to ensure they are supported by scientific evidence. If the manufacturer's claims meet the EPA criteria, the product receives an EPA registration number. That number must appear on the product label.

The EPA is also involved in regulating waste materials, such as chemicals and medical waste, after they leave the dental office on the way to the final disposal site (Fig. 22-7).

Occupational Safety and Health Administration

The U.S. **Occupational Safety and Health Administration (OSHA)** is a federal *regulatory* agency that is a division of the U.S. Department of Labor. OSHA's responsibility is to ensure the safety and health of America's workers. To do this, OSHA sets and enforces protective standards that employers *must* follow in order to provide a safe work place for their employees. In addition, OSHA provides training and outreach education and encourages continual improvement in workplace safety and health. In dentistry, the two most important OSHA standards are the Bloodborne Pathogens Standard (see Chapter 19), and the Hazard Communication Standard (see Chapter 23).

All states are regulated by the federal OSHA. In addition, there are 22 states that administer their own state-operated OSHA programs. In those states that administer their own OSHA programs, the state standards *must* meet or exceed federal OSHA standards.

OSHA monitors compliance with its standards through a process of investigations of the workplace. If the workplace fails to meet the requirements, a citation may be issued for each violation. Citations usually result in a fine. If a workplace fails to correct the unsafe conditions, OSHA has the legal authority to close the workplace until the problem is corrected. OSHA provides hazard information, record-keeping guidelines, and copies of standards at no cost (Fig. 22-8).

OSHA Inspections

Dental office inspections may occur:

- When an employee or patient complaint is made
- Randomly in an office with 11 or more employees
- Upon request of the dentist for a consultation visit

National Institutes of Health

The **National Institutes of Health (NIH)** is part of the U.S. Department of Health and Human Services. It is the primary federal agency for conducting and supporting medical research. NIH scientists investigate ways to prevent disease and also research the causes, treatments, and even cures for common and rare diseases. This agency provides leadership and financial support to researchers in every state and throughout the world.

The NIH supports a wide spectrum of research, from learning how the brain becomes addicted to alcohol to combating heart disease. The agency is at the forefront of new progress in medical research. Indeed, many important health and medical discoveries of the last century resulted from research supported by the NIH. The NIH translates research results into practice and communicates research findings to patients and their families, healthcare providers, and the general public (Fig. 22-9).

Fig. 22-7 Logo of the EPA. (Courtesy Environmental Protection Agency.)

Fig. 22-8 Logo of OSHA. (Courtesy Occupational Safety and Health Administration.)

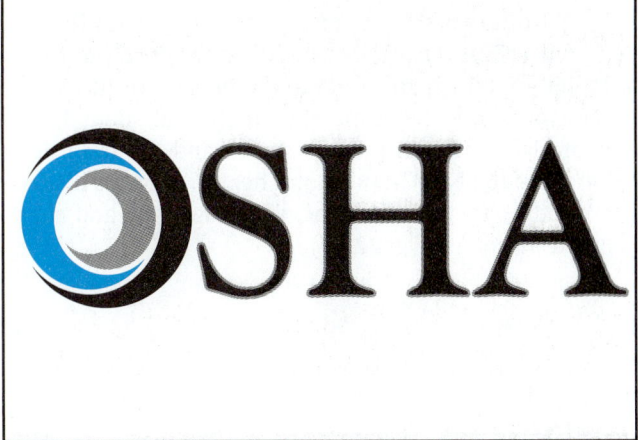

Fig. 22-9 **Logo of the NIH.** (Courtesy National Institutes of Health.)

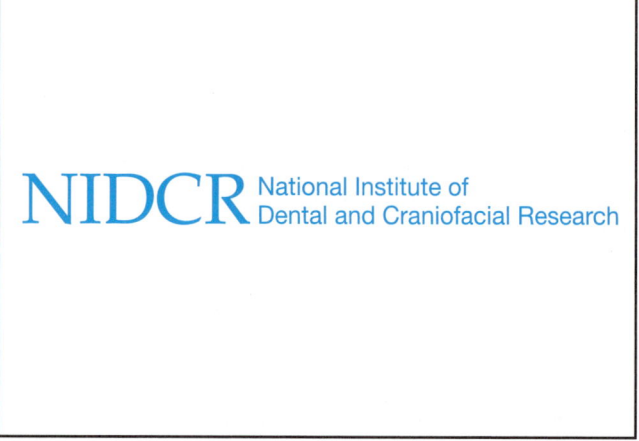

Fig. 22-10 **Logo of NIDCR.** (Courtesy National Institutes of Health.)

National Institute of Dental and Craniofacial Research

The **National Institute of Dental and Craniofacial Research (NIDCR)** is the dental research institute of the NIH. Its mission is to promote the general health of the American people by improving their oral, dental, and craniofacial health. Through research and the training of researchers, the NIDCR promotes health, prevents diseases and conditions, and develops new diagnostic and therapeutic techniques (Fig. 22-10).

Fig. 22-11 **Logo of NIOSH.** (Courtesy Centers for Disease Control and Prevention.)

National Institute for Occupational Safety and Health

Unlike OSHA, the **National Institute for Occupational Safety and Health (NIOSH)** *does not* have regulatory authority. NIOSH is the only federal institute responsible for conducting research and making *recommendations* for the prevention of work-related disease and injury. NIOSH, which is part of the CDC, conducts research on the full scope of occupational disease and injury, ranging from lung diseases in miners to preventing carpal tunnel syndrome (see Chapter 25) and allergic reactions to latex (Fig. 22-11).

In addition to conducting research, NIOSH performs the following duties:

- Investigates potentially hazardous conditions when requested by employees or employers.
- Makes recommendations and disseminates information on preventing workplace disease, injury, and disability.
- Provides training to occupational safety and health professionals.

Recall

3. What is the primary role of the CDC in dentistry?
4. What is the primary role of the FDA in dentistry?
5. What is the primary role of the EPA in dentistry?
6. What is the primary role of OSHA in dentistry?
7. What is the primary role of the NIH?
8. What is the primary role of NIDCR?

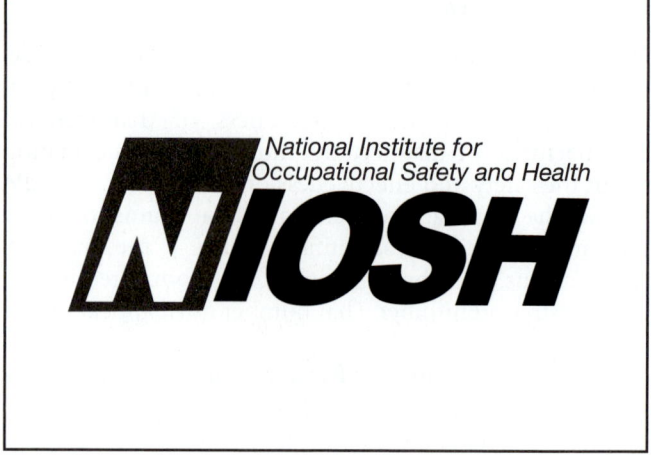

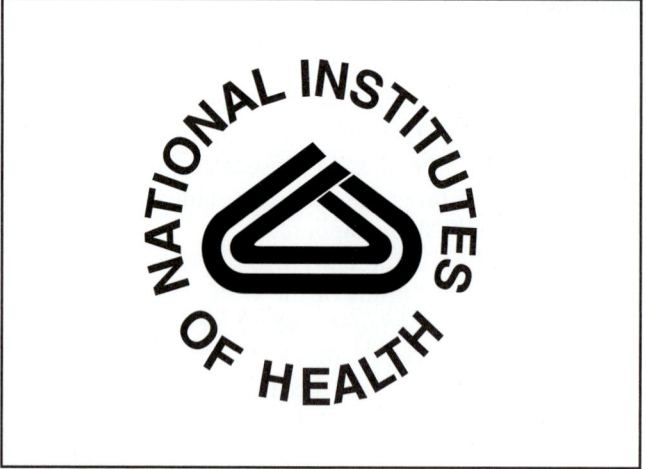

Legal and Ethical Implications

The dentist is ultimately responsible for making sure the dental office is in compliance with OSHA standards. However, it is often the responsibility of the dental assistant to maintain OSHA compliance on a day-to-day basis, and maintain the required recordkeeping. It is important that you stay current on OSHA compliance issues. The programs of most major dental meetings today offer a selection of courses on emerging diseases, occupational health, and OSHA compliance geared toward the entire dental team. In addition, you can keep up to date by reading professional journals and newsletters and by becoming a member of OSAP.

Eye to the Future

Staying current with the literature will always be important to the educated dental assistant. The Internet will continue to be an excellent resource for you to obtain information on any dental-related topic. All the professional societies and government agencies are listed on the Internet. These agencies' websites make their guidelines, recommendations, or regulations available to you with just a few keystrokes and clicks of the mouse. You can download most information directly from the websites.

PubMed is an Internet search tool that can make staying current easier and more efficient. Developed by the National Library of Medicine, PubMed provides access to more than 10 million citations, research articles, and literature reviews from journals around the world in several languages.

Critical Thinking

1. At a local dental assisting society meeting, the conversation turned to infection control. Several of the dental assistants had different opinions regarding local dental waste disposal regulations. How would you obtain accurate information regarding local regulations about dental waste removal?
2. You have been asked by a local women's group to speak about children's dental health. Where can you obtain current information on this topic to prepare for your presentation?
3. When you become a certified dental assistant or a registered dental assistant, you will need to maintain your credential with continuing education. Where will you find sources of continuing education?
4. Visit each of the federal agencies online and see the vast resources, services, and information available to you—at no cost.

23

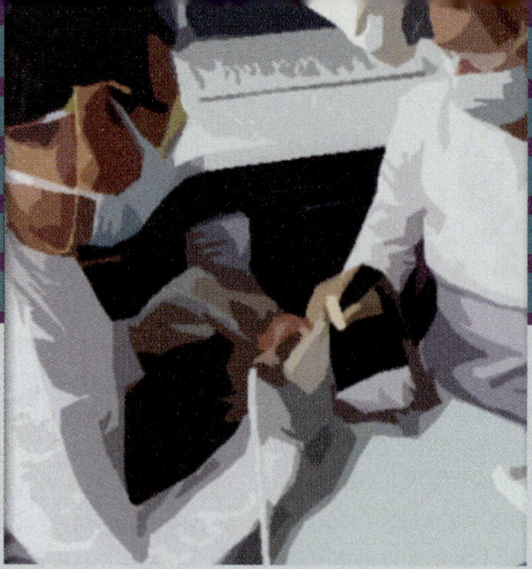

Chemical and Waste Management

Outline

KEY TERMS

Acute exposure High levels of exposure over a short period.

Chemical inventory Comprehensive list of every product used in the office that contains chemicals.

Chronic exposure Repeated exposures, generally to lower levels, over a long time.

Contaminated waste Items such as gloves and patient napkins that may contain the potentially infectious body fluids of patients.

Environmental Protection Agency (EPA) Federal regulatory agency whose responsibility it is to protect and restore the environment and public health through environmental laws.

Hazard Communication Standard Occupational Safety and Health Administration (OSHA) standard regarding employees' "right to know" about chemicals in the workplace.

Hazardous waste Waste posing a risk to humans or the environment.

Infectious waste Waste that is capable of transmitting an infectious disease.

Material safety data sheet (MSDS) Form that provides health and safety information regarding materials that contain chemicals.

Regulated waste Infectious waste that requires special handling, neutralization, and disposal.

LEARNING OUTCOMES

On completion of this chapter, the student will be able to achieve the following objectives:

- Pronounce, define, and spell the Key Terms.
- Describe potential long-term and short-term effects of exposure to chemicals.
- Explain the purpose of the OSHA Hazard Communication Standard.
- Describe three common methods of chemical exposure.
- Describe the components of a hazard communication program.
- Explain the purpose of a material safety data sheet.
- Create a label for a secondary container.
- Describe the difference between chronic and acute chemical exposure.
- Identify four methods of personal protection against chemical exposure.
- Describe in general how chemicals should be stored.
- Explain the record-keeping requirements of the Hazard Communication Standard.
- Identify types of regulated waste generated in a dental office.
- Identify types of toxic waste generated in a dental office.
- Describe how to package regulated waste for transport.

In the day-to-day practice of dentistry, the dental assistant is exposed to a wide variety of chemicals. All chemicals that are used for treatment procedures, cleaning of instruments and surfaces, disinfection and sterilization, laboratory procedures, and dental x-ray processing are capable of causing serious health consequences if they are absorbed into the body in sufficiently large amounts.

The heart, kidney, liver, and lung tissues can be seriously damaged by chemicals. Results range from short-term discomfort, such as burns or rashes, to life-threatening conditions, such as cancer or organ failure.

As a dental assistant, it is important for you to understand the proper use, storage, handling, spill cleanup, and disposal methods for all chemicals used in the dental office. In addition, you should know the first-aid procedures associated with chemicals. You must be aware of the hazardous materials that may be regulated under federal, state, or local environmental guidelines and the requirements associated with the disposal of these hazardous materials. Common examples of items that require special disposal procedures include x-ray processing solutions, lead foil backing from film packets, scrap dental amalgam, and elemental mercury.

This chapter also discusses the Occupational Safety and Health Administration (OSHA) Hazard Communication Standard and the procedures necessary to develop the safe working habits that will become part of your daily routine in the dental office.

HAZARDOUS CHEMICALS

A *hazardous chemical* is defined as any chemical that can cause either a physical or health hazard. A chemical is considered hazardous if it (1) can ignite (catch fire), (2) can react or explode when mixed with other substances, (3) is corrosive, or (4) is toxic (Fig. 23-1).

Exposure to Chemicals

The three primary methods of chemical exposure are inhalation, skin contact, and ingestion.

Inhalation of the gases, vapors, or dusts of chemicals can cause direct damage to the lungs. Some chemicals may not affect the lungs but are absorbed by them and then sent through the blood to other organs, such as the brain, liver, or kidneys, where they may cause damage.

Skin is an effective barrier against many chemicals, but some chemicals can be absorbed through the skin. In gen-

Locations of OSHA-Approved Programs

Alaska: Juneau, (907) 465-2700	Michigan: Lansing, (517) 322-1814	South Carolina: Columbia, (803) 896-4300
Arizona: Phoenix, (602) 542-5795	Minnesota: St. Paul, (651) 284-5010	Tennessee: Nashville, (615) 741-2793
California: San Francisco, (415) 703-5050	Nevada: Carson City, (775) 684-7260	Utah: Salt Lake City, (801) 530-6901
Connecticut: Wethersfield, (203) 566-5123	New Jersey: Trenton, (609) 292-2975	Vermont: Montpelier, (802) 828-5098
Hawaii: Honolulu, (808) 586-9116	New Mexico: Santa Fe, (505) 827-2850	Virgin Islands: St. Croix, (340) 773-1994
Indiana: Indianapolis, (317) 232-2678	New York: Albany, (518) 457-2741	Virginia: Richmond, (804) 786-2377
Iowa: Des Moines, (515) 281-6432	North Carolina: Raleigh, (919) 897-2900	Washington: Olympia, (360) 902-4200
Kentucky: Frankfort, (502) 564-3070	Oregon: Salem, (503) 378-3272	Wyoming: Cheyenne, (307) 777-7159
Maryland: Baltimore, (410) 767-2241	Puerto Rico: Hato Rey, (787) 754-2119	

From Miller CH, Palenik CJ: *Infection Control & Management of Hazardous Materials for the Dental Team,* ed 3, St Louis, 2005, Mosby.

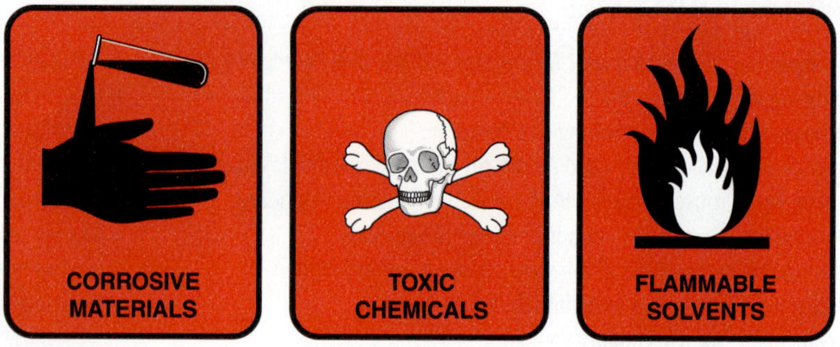

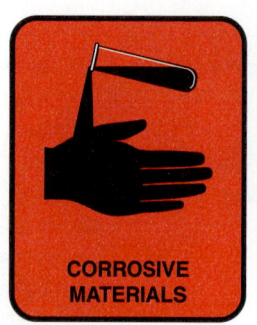

Fig. 23-1 Chemical hazard warning labels. (From Stepp CA, Woods MA: *Laboratory procedures for medical office personnel,* Philadelphia, 1998, Saunders.)

How Chemicals Enter the Body

Inhalation of chemical vapor

Absorption of chemical through the skin

Ingestion of chemical (eating or drinking)

eral, you must have *direct skin contact* with the chemical for absorption to occur. Sometimes, after repeated contact with a chemical, a skin condition called *dermatitis* may develop.

Ingestion *(swallowing)* is another way in which chemicals can enter the body. Common ways of ingesting harmful chemicals in the workplace include eating lunch in an area in which chemicals are used or eating with hands that are contaminated with chemicals. It is important to wash your hands thoroughly after contact with any chemical.

Acute and Chronic Chemical Toxicity

The potential for a chemical to cause harm and the extent of harm depend on the amount of the dose and the duration of exposure to the chemical. Chemical toxicity may be acute or chronic.

Acute chemical toxicity results from high levels of exposure over a short period. Acute toxicity is often caused by a chemical spill, in which the exposure is sudden and often involves a large amount of the chemical.

The victim of acute toxicity feels the effects immediately. Dizziness, fainting, headache, nausea, and vomiting are symptoms of acute overexposure to chemicals.

Chronic chemical toxicity results from many repeated exposures, generally to lower levels, over a much longer time (months or even years). Many effects of chronic toxicity are possible, including liver disease, brain disorders, cancer, or infertility. Always check the material safety data sheet and product label to understand the potential dangers of the chemicals in the products you use.

The difference between acute and chronic toxicity can be illustrated by considering the effects of **acute exposure** and **chronic exposure** to the same chemical. For example, a single exposure to a high concentration of benzene (acute toxicity) may cause dizziness, headache, and unconsciousness, whereas a long-term daily exposure to low levels of benzene (chronic toxicity) may eventually cause leukemia.

Recall

1. What types of health consequences could develop as a result of exposure to chemicals?
2. Why is it important for the dental assistant to understand how to handle chemicals?
3. What are three primary methods of chemical exposure?
4. What is the difference between *acute* and *chronic* chemical exposure?

Hand Protection

When using chemicals, be certain to wear utility gloves made from a *chemical-resistant* material, such as natural rubber, neoprene, or industrial-grade nitrile (Fig. 23-2).

These chemical-resistant gloves are essential because the latex gloves worn during patient care *do not* provide adequate protection when handling chemicals. When exposed to chemical disinfectants, the latex in the glove degrades and creates a *wicking* (sucking) action that will actually pull contaminants and chemicals through the glove and onto the hands.

Eye Protection

Serious damage to the eyes, even blindness, can result from chemical accidents. It is crucial to protect the eyes from fumes and splashes while pouring chemicals such as x-ray processing solutions, ultrasonic solutions, disinfectants, and sterilants.

A variety of safety eyewear is available. The ideal goggles have soft, vinyl flanges (rims) at the top and bottom and fit the face snugly (Fig. 23-3).

Protective Clothing

When caustic or staining chemicals are used, it is best to wear a rubber or neoprene apron when mixing or pouring

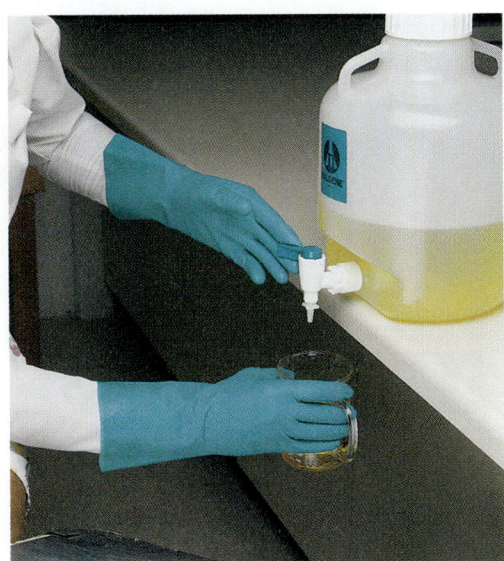

Fig. 23-2 **Clean room nitrile gloves provide protection and dexterity when handling chemicals.** (Courtesy Lab Safety Supply, Janesville, Wis.)

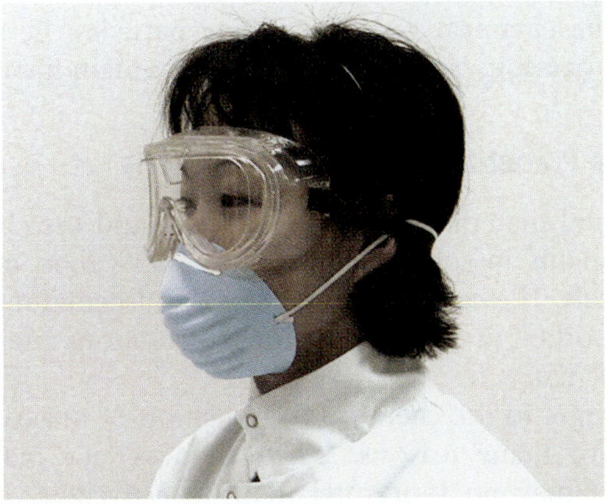

Fig. 23-3 **Dental assistant wearing chemical goggles.**

the chemical. The **material safety data sheet (MSDS)** for each product (see later discussion) provides specific information regarding the need for additional personal protective equipment (PPE).

Inhalation Protection

Depending on the quality, the masks worn during patient care may or may not provide adequate protection when working with chemicals. The proper face mask should be fluid-repellent and provide respiratory protection.

If your job requires you to pour or mix chemicals frequently, or if you are sensitive or allergic to substances, you might require a mist-respirator face mask approved by the National Institute of Occupational Safety and Health (NIOSH) (Fig. 23-4).

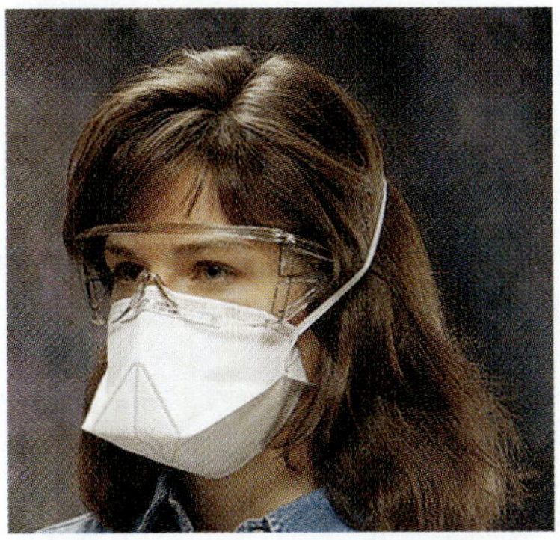

Fig. 23-4 **Disposable respirator has tapered angle to fit facial contours around nose and chin to protect against dusts and chemical mists.** (Courtesy Lab Safety Supply, Janesville, Wis.)

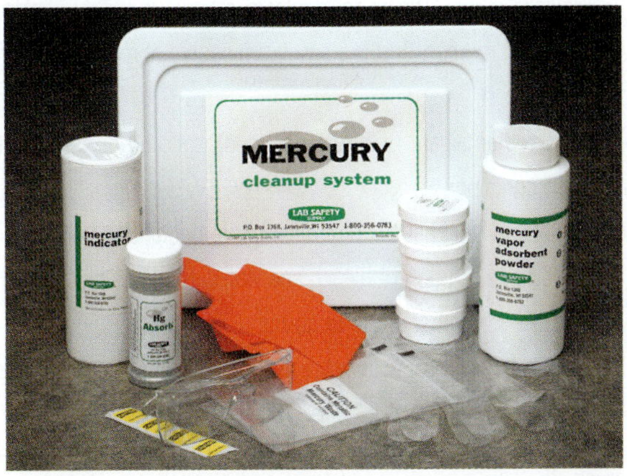

Fig. 23-5 **Mercury spill kit, with aspirator to pick up larger drops of mercury, labeled bottle for recovered mercury, base/activator product to absorb small amounts of mercury, product to absorb mercury vapors, gloves, scoop, sponge, mixing cups, spatulas, and labeled polyethylene bag for disposal.** (Courtesy Lab Safety Supply, Janesville, Wis.)

Control of Chemical Spills

Accidents and spills should not be common occurrences. Planning and practice dealing with such spills should minimize employee exposure to harmful chemicals. Refer to the MSDS for the specific product for accurate information on how to manage spills.

Mercury spill kits should be available in all dental offices in which amalgam is used. Exposure to even small amounts of mercury is very hazardous to the health of dental personnel. Mercury can be absorbed through the skin or through inhalation of mercury vapors. The spill kit for small amounts of mercury should contain mercury-absorbing powder, mercury-absorbing sponges, and a disposal bag (Fig. 23-5). A mask and utility gloves should be worn whenever cleaning up a mercury spill.

Eyewash Units

OSHA regulations require eyewash units to be installed in every workplace where chemicals are used. A variety of

Precautions When Working with Mercury

- Work in a well-ventilated space.
- Avoid direct skin contact with mercury.
- Avoid inhaling mercury vapor.
- Store mercury in unbreakable, tightly sealed containers away from heat.
- When preparing amalgam for restorations, use preloaded capsules. (This avoids exposure while measuring mercury.)
- When mixing amalgam, always close the cover before starting the amalgamator.
- Reassemble amalgam capsules immediately after dispensing the amalgam mass. (The used amalgam capsule is highly contaminated with mercury and is a significant source of mercury vapor if left open.)
- Leftover scrap amalgam (that was not used) is stored dry in a tightly closed container.
- Scrap amalgam (that has been retrieved from dental unit traps) is disinfected in a solution of bleach and water. Then it is placed in the container with other scrap amalgam.
- Clean spills using appropriate procedures and equipment. *Do not use a household vacuum cleaner or the high-volume evacuator.* (Dangerous fumes from the mercury can be released into the air.)
- Place contaminated disposable materials into polyethylene bags and seal. Dispose according to the regulations specific to your area.

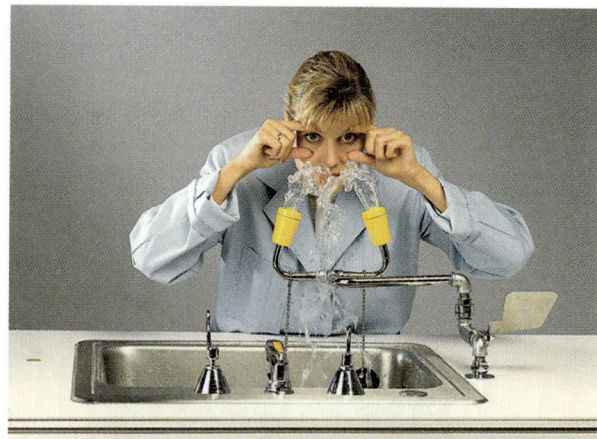

Fig. 23-6 Countertop eyewash and eye/face washes provide water to the face and eyes to gently wash away contaminants. (Courtesy Lab Safety Supply, Janesville, Wis.)

styles are available. The standard eyewash unit attaches directly to existing faucets for emergencies but still allows normal faucet use. When turned on, the eyewash unit will irrigate the eyes with a soft, wide flow of water necessary to bathe away contaminants without causing additional damage (Fig. 23-6).

Employees must be trained in the proper use of the eyewash station. The unit should be inspected frequently to ensure that it is functional. Some manufacturers of eyewash units recommend a weekly 3-minute flushing to reduce microbial content in the waterline. Always follow the manufacturer's instructions regarding proper maintenance of the eyewash unit in your office.

Ventilation

Good ventilation is necessary when dealing with any type of chemical. Many dental offices are equipped with special exhaust systems for fumes and dust in the laboratory, sterilization, and darkroom areas. For example, radiographic processing chemicals can cause contact dermatitis and irritation of the eyes, nose, throat, and respiratory system from the chemical vapors and fine particles. Be sure to keep processing tanks covered to help contain the fumes.

General Precautions for Storing Chemicals

All dental materials contain chemicals, and the chemical components in some are more hazardous than in other chemicals. The careful use and storage of dental materials are important to ensure that these preparations retain their effectiveness.

Changes in the chemical composition of materials can occur for many reasons. When changes take place, the product may no longer retain its effectiveness. A basic "safe" policy for the storage of dental medications and chemicals is to keep them in a dry, cool, dark place where they are not exposed to direct sunlight.

Follow Instructions

The manufacturer has determined the best methods of packaging and storage. The manufacturer's instructions for storage can be found on the MSDS and should be followed.

Avoid Exposure to Light

Light is the primary cause for the deterioration of sodium hypochlorite (household bleach), epinephrine, and hydrogen peroxide. This is why many chemicals are sold in dark or opaque containers. Change in color is a common sign that the chemical has deteriorated.

Check Expiration Date

The expiration date, which may be listed on the container, should be checked frequently. Products that have outlived their expiration date should be disposed of immediately.

Guidelines for Minimizing Exposure to Chemical Hazards in the Dental Office

Keep a minimum of hazardous chemicals in the office.
Read the labels and use only as directed.
Store according to the manufacturer's directions.
Keep containers tightly covered.
Avoid mixing chemicals unless consequences are known.
Wear appropriate personal protective equipment (PPE) when handling hazardous substances.
Wash hands immediately after removing gloves.
Avoid skin contact with chemicals; immediately wash skin that has come in contact with chemicals.
Maintain good ventilation.
Do not eat, drink, smoke, apply lip balm, or insert contact lenses in areas in which chemicals are used.
Keep chemicals away from open flames and heat sources.
Always have on hand an operational fire extinguisher.
Know and use proper cleanup procedures.
Keep neutralizing agents available for strong acid and alkaline solutions.
Dispose of all hazardous chemicals according to material safety data sheet (MSDS) instructions.

Rotate Inventory

Fresh supplies should always be stocked behind the current inventory to ensure that the oldest product is used first. This is the same method used to stock milk and other perishable items in a grocery store.

Recall

5. What are four methods of personal protection against chemical exposure?
6. What are the OSHA requirements regarding an eyewash unit?
7. What could be the effects of exposure to radiographic processing solutions kept in a poorly ventilated area?
8. In general, how should chemicals be stored?

Disposal of Empty Containers

Even empty containers can be hazardous because they often hold residues that can burn or explode. *Never* fill an empty container with another substance, because a dangerous chemical reaction could occur. Always follow the label instructions and the MSDS on how to dispose of empty containers.

Hazardous Waste Disposal

Substances are considered **hazardous waste** if they have certain properties or contain chemicals that could pose dangers to human health and the environment after being discarded. Regulations for proper disposal of hazardous waste vary widely among states. Even within the same state, regulations will often vary among counties or even cities. To be safe, always check the regulations specific to the area in which you work. In general, wastes are classified as "hazardous" if they have the following characteristics:

1. *Ignitable:* flammable or combustible
2. *Corrosive:* highly acidic (pH less than 2.0) or extremely basic (pH greater than 12.5). (pH is a measure of the solution's hydrogen ion concentration; water has a pH of 7.0.)
3. *Reactive:* chemically unstable or explosive, violent reaction with water, or capable of giving off toxic fumes when mixed with water
4. *Toxic:* contains arsenic, barium, chromium, mercury, lead, silver, or certain pesticides
5. *Listed by Environmental Protection Agency (EPA):* several hundred chemicals listed as hazardous

HAZARD COMMUNICATION PROGRAM

OSHA issued the **Hazard Communication Standard** to require employers to inform their employees about the *identity* and *hazards* of chemicals that they use in the workplace. The Hazard Communication Standard, also known as the "Employee Right-to-Know Law," requires employers to implement a *hazard communication program.*

The hazard communication program has the following five parts:

1. Written program
2. Inventory of hazardous chemicals
3. MSDS for every chemical
4. Proper labeling of containers
5. Employee training

Good record-keeping is also an important aspect of the program.

Written Program

The written program must identify, by name, all the employees in the office who are exposed to hazardous chemicals. It must also identify the individual who is responsible for the program. The program describes (1) staff training, (2) how chemicals are handled in the office, including all labeling and safety measures, and (3) how to respond to chemical emergencies such as spills or exposures.

Responsibilities of Dental Assistant as Coordinator of Hazard Communication Program

- Read and understand the OSHA Hazard Communication Standard.
- Implement the written hazard communication program.
- Compile a list (chemical inventory) of products in the office that contain hazardous chemicals.
- Obtain material safety data sheets (MSDSs).
- Update the MSDS file as new products are added to office inventory.
- Inform other employees of the location of MSDSs.
- Label appropriate containers.
- Provide training to other employees.

If several dentists are working in one clinic or practice, all employers must be aware of hazards and protective measures so that they can train their employees.

Chemical Inventory

The **chemical inventory** is a list of every product used in the office that contains chemicals. It includes amalgam, composites, bonding materials, etching agents, disinfectants, and impression materials, among others. Each time a new product containing a chemical is brought into the office, it must be added to the chemical list. The MSDS for that product is placed in the MSDS file. The manufacturer or distributor must provide an updated MSDS when appropriate.

The dentist will often appoint the dental assistant to be the program coordinator and to be responsible for maintaining the chemical inventory and updating the MSDS file.

Material Safety Data Sheets

MSDSs contain health and safety information about every chemical in the office (Table 23-1 and Fig. 23-7). MSDSs provide comprehensive technical information and are a resource for employees working with chemicals. They describe the physical and chemical properties of a chemical, health hazards, routes of exposure, precautions for safe handling and use, emergency and first-aid procedures, and spill control measures.

The manufacturer of a product that contains chemicals is required to supply the dental office with an MSDS for the product. However, it is the responsibility of the dental office to make sure that there is indeed an MSDS for every chemical used in the office. MSDSs often are enclosed in the package with the product. The sheets should be organized in binders so that the employees

Table 23-1 ***Sections of Material Safety Data Sheet (MSDS)***

Section	Description	Explanation
I	Product information	Identifies the name of the material, manufacturer, data on which MSDS was prepared, and who to call in case of an emergency
II	Hazardous ingredient	Identifies the hazardous ingredient; product identity must match the label; it must also include the *permissible exposure limit (PEL)* and *short-term exposure limit (STEL)* in the air
III	Physical hazard data	Identifies how the material will look and smell and some of its physical characteristics
IV	Fire and explosion data	Indicates the ignition or flash point and tells how to put out any fire that contains that material or any explosion or reactivity hazard
V	Health hazard information	Indicates symptoms of overexposure, health effects, emergency procedures, cancer-causing agents, and so on
VI	Reactivity data	Describes the stability of the product
VII	Spill or leak procedures	Describes disposal of product and how to deal with a spill or leak
VIII	Special protection information	Identifies control measures, such as ventilation, gloves, and respirator, to be taken when handling the product
IX	Special precautions	Describes special handling and storage precautions to be taken with the material and any protective measures

This is a sample format of OSHA Form 20 for MSDSs.

IDENTITY/ PRODUCT NAME: ABC LIQUID

SECTION I

MANUFACTURER'S NAME: ABC Manufacturing Company

ADDRESS: 8800-B Oakdale Office Park, Chicago, IL 60666

EMERGENCY TELEPHONE NUMBER: 1-800-224-5681

TELEPHONE NUMBER FOR INFORMATION: 1-800-341-9000

Date prepared: 1/25/20XX

SECTION II - HAZARDOUS INGREDIENTS/IDENTITY INFORMATION

HAZARDOUS COMPONENTS:	OSHA PEL	OTHER LIMITS
Eugenol	–	–
Acetic acid	10 ppm	

SECTION III - PHYSICAL/CHEMICAL CHARACTERISTICS

BOILING POINT: 491° F/255° C

SPECIFIC GRAVITY: Above 1.0

VAPOR PRESSURE: 0.1Hg@20° C

MELTING POINT: -9° C

VAPOR DENSITY: N.E.

EVAPORATION RATE: N.E.

SOLUBILITY IN WATER: Slightly soluble

APPEARANCE AND ODOR: Colorless or pale yellow liquid. Odor is oil of cloves.

SECTION IV - FIRE AND EXPLOSION HAZARD DATA

FLASH POINT (Method Used): Approx 250° F Closed cup

FLAMMABILITY (Explosive Limits): N.E. **LEL:** N.E. **UEL:** N.E.

EXTINGUISHING MEDIA: Carbon dioxide, dry chemical, or foam-type extinguishers.

SPECIAL FIRE FIGHTING PROCEDURES: Fire fighters should wear full protective clothing, including self-contained breathing apparatus. Cool containers exposed to flame with water.

UNUSUAL FIRE AND EXPLOSION HAZARDS: None

SECTION V - HEALTH HAZARD DATA

ROUTES OF ENTRY: **Inhalation?** Yes **Skin?** Yes **Ingestion?** Possible

HEALTH HAZARDS (Acute and Chronic): Liquid irritating to skin and eyes. Repeated contact may cause allergic dermatitis. Repeated daily oral dosing of large amount to rats caused liver damage. The effects in humans are unknown. Excessive exposure may result in similar effects.

CARCINOGENICITY: **OSHA REGULATED:** No

SIGNS AND SYMPTOMS OF EXPOSURE: Redness or irritation of eyes or skin.

MEDICAL CONDITIONS GENERALLY AGGRAVATED BY EXPOSURE: Known sensitization to eugenol. Open sores or wounds of the skin.

continued

Fig. 23-7 Simulated material safety data sheet (MSDS).

EMERGENCY AND FIRST AID PROCEDURES:

EYE CONTACT: Rinse with plenty of water for at least 15 minutes and seek medical attention.

SKIN CONTACT: Wash with soap and water.

INHALATION: Remove person to fresh air. Seek medical attention if irritation persists.

INGESTION: Seek medical advice.

SECTION VI - REACTIVITY DATA

STABILITY: **Unstable** ______ **Stable** __X__

CONDITIONS TO AVOID: Excessive heat, strong oxidizing agents.

INCOMPATIBILITY (Materials to Avoid): Ferric chloride, potassium permanganate.

HAZARDOUS DECOMPOSITION OR BYPRODUCTS: Forms carbon monoxide and/or carbon dioxide upon burning.

HAZARDOUS POLYMERIZATION: **May Occur** ______ **Will Not Occur** __X__

CONDITIONS TO AVOID: None

SECTION VII - PRECAUTIONS FOR SAFE HANDLING AND USE

STEPS TO BE TAKEN IN CASE MATERIAL IS RELEASED OR SPILLED: Soak material up by using sand or vermiculite, then scoop up material and place in a closed metal waste container.

WASTE DISPOSAL METHOD: Dispose of in accordance with all federal, state, and local regulations.

PRECAUTIONS TO BE TAKEN IN HANDLING AND STORING: Store in tight full containers, well sealed, protected from light. Keep away from foodstuffs and beverages. Do not expose to temperatures above 35° C.

OTHER PRECAUTIONS: Eugenol darkens and thickens upon exposure to air. Observe normal warehousing and handling precautions.

SECTION VIII - CONTROL MEASURES

RESPIRATORY PROTECTION (specify type): As with all materials, avoid casual breathing of vapors. No special respiratory protection required for the intended use of this product.

VENTILATION: Local Exhaust __X__ **Special** ______

PROTECTIVE GLOVES: Clinical Worker Gloves (Rubber)

EYE PROTECTION: Chemical Worker Goggles

OTHER PROTECTIVE CLOTHING OR EQUIPMENT: None

WORK/HYGIENIC PRACTICES: Observe normal care when working with chemicals.

Fig. 23-7, cont'd Simulated material safety data sheet (MSDS).

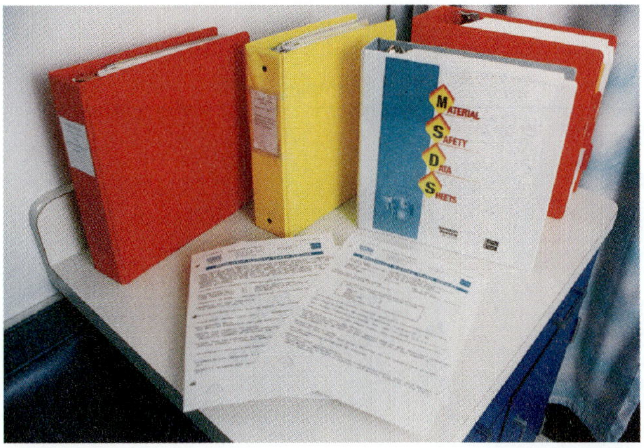

Fig. 23-8 MSDSs for quality control record-keeping. (From Kinn ME, Woods M: *The medical assistant: administrative and clinical,* ed 8, Philadelphia, 1999, Saunders.)

have ready access to them and can easily locate a particular MSDS (Fig. 23-8).

Recall

9. In general, how are chemicals determined to be hazardous?
10. What is another name for the Hazard Communication Standard?
11. What chemicals must be included in the chemical inventory?
12. What is an MSDS?

Employee Training

Employee training is essential for a successful hazard communication program. Staff training is required (1) when a new employee is hired, (2) when a new chemical product is added to the office, and (3) once a year for all continuing employees. Records of each training session must be kept on file for at least 5 years.

Although the dentist is responsible for providing the training, the dental assistant is responsible for routinely following safety precautions. The chemical training program for employees must include the following areas:

- The use of hazardous chemicals
- All safety practices, including all warnings
- Required PPE
- Safe handling and disposal methods

Outline for Hazard Communication Training Program*

1. Requirements of the Hazard Communication Standard
2. Written communication plan for the office (location, use, etc.)
3. Understanding of the hazards of the chemicals with which employees work
4. Ability to interpret warning labels and MSDS
5. Knowledge of where to obtain additional information
6. Measures to protect employees and others:
   a. Office safety procedures
   b. Available PPE
   c. Instructions for reporting accidents and emergencies
   d. Information about first aid
7. Methods and observations to detect the presence or release of a hazardous chemical
8. Question-and-answer opportunity

*On completion, employees are asked to sign a training record that will remain in the personnel file.

Labeling of Chemical Containers

Containers must be labeled to indicate what chemicals they contain and any hazards that may be present. All chemicals in the dental office must be labeled; in many cases the manufacturer's label is suitable.

When the chemical is transferred to a different container, however, the new container also must be labeled (Fig. 23-9). For example, when a concentrated chemical disinfectant is mixed fresh and placed into a spray bottle or tub *(secondary containers)*, the spray bottle or tub must be labeled. Other examples of secondary containers that hold chemicals and require labeling are automatic x-ray film processors and manual processing tanks, ultrasonic cleaning tanks, and chemical vapor sterilizers.

There is no "official" labeling system that must be used, and many approaches are available. Even a photocopy of the label from the original container attached to the new container is acceptable. The two most important considerations are that (1) the labeling system is easy to use and (2) all employees are properly trained to understand and read the label. Procedure 23-1 reviews steps in labeling a secondary container.

National Fire Protection Association Labels

The National Fire Protection Association (NFPA) has a labeling system that is frequently used to label containers of hazardous chemicals. This system consists of the use of four diamonds (blue, red, yellow, and white) that are filled with numeric ratings from 0 to 4. The categories are

Table 23-2 Types of Dental Waste

	Definition	Examples
Medical waste	Waste generated as part of treatment; can be contaminated or infectious	
Contaminated waste	Waste that has been in contact with blood or other body fluids; in most states, disposed of as general waste	Contaminated barriers Contaminated patient bibs
Infectious waste	Contaminated waste that is capable of causing an infectious disease	Blood and blood-saturated materials Pathologic waste: tissue, extracted teeth* Sharps: needles, burs
Chemical waste	Waste that poses a threat to humans or the environment	Scrap amalgam
Hazardous waste	Usually refers to toxic chemicals or materials	Lead foil
Toxic waste		Radiographic solutions†
General waste	Nonhazardous, nonregulated waste	Paper waste generated at front desk Discarded lunch bags or wraps

**If teeth contain amalgam restorations, they are* hazardous *waste as well.*
†Some states consider only fixer as toxic waste; others consider both fixer and developer as toxic.

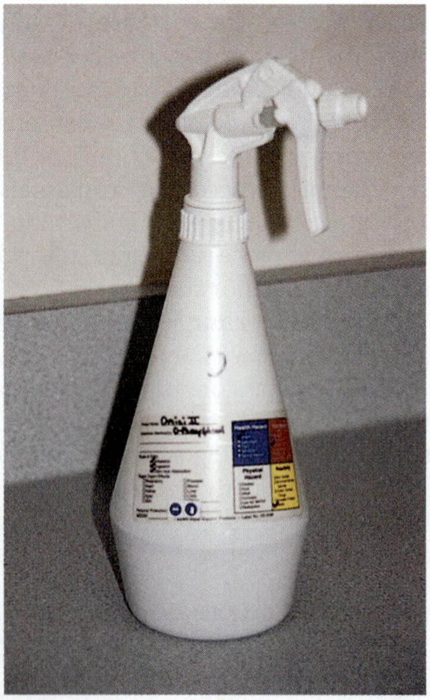

Fig. 23-9 Chemical disinfectants *not* in their original containers must be clearly labeled.

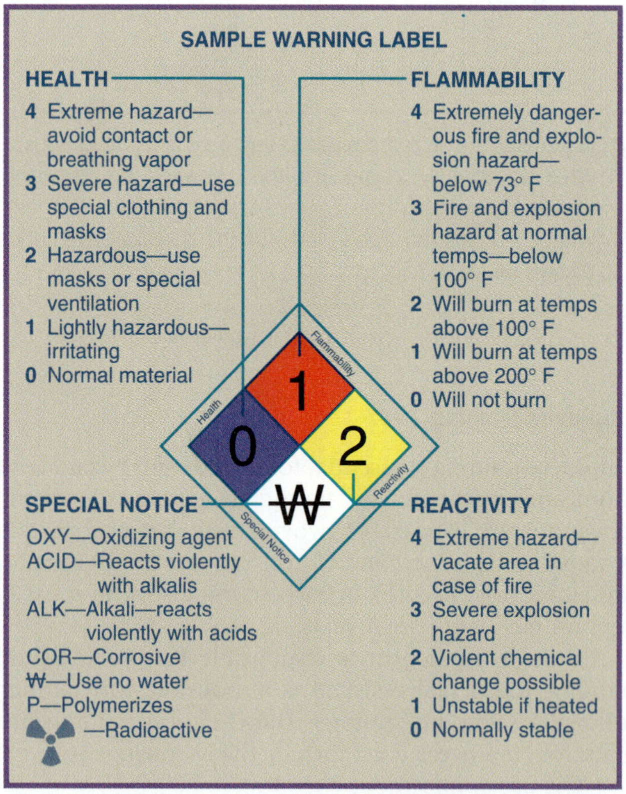

Fig. 23-10 **Numeric ratings for categories of health hazard, flammability, and reactivity and letters for special notices on chemical labels.** (From Kinn ME, Woods M: *The medical assistant: administrative and clinical,* ed 8, Philadelphia, 1999, Saunders.)

Procedure 23-1 Creating an Appropriate Label for a Secondary Container

Goal

To create a label for a secondary container according to regulations and standards for hazardous chemicals.

Equipment and Supplies

- MSDS for product to be labeled
- Pen
- NFPA chemical label

PROCEDURAL STEPS

1. Write the manufacturer's name and address on the label. (This information is found in the Product Information section of the MSDS.)
2. Write the name of the chemical(s) and the "target organ" on the label. (This information is also found in the Product Information section.)
3. Write the appropriate health hazard code in the *blue* diamond. (This information is found in the Health Hazard Data section of the MSDS.)
4. Write the appropriate flammability and explosion code in the *red* diamond. (This information is found in the Fire and Explosion section of the MSDS.)
5. Write the appropriate reactivity code in the *yellow* diamond. (This information is found in the Reactivity Data section of the MSDS.)
6. Write the appropriate specific hazard warning in the *white* diamond. (This information is found in the Precautions for Safe Handling and Use section of the MSDS.)
7. Attach the chemical label to the secondary container.

health hazard (blue), *flammability* (red), *reactivity* (yellow), and *special hazard symbols,* such as OXY for oxidizers (white) (Fig. 23-10).

Exemptions to Labeling Requirements

Certain chemicals are exempted from the standard, including tobacco and tobacco products, wood and wood products, food, drugs, cosmetics, and alcoholic beverages sold and packaged for consumer use. Drugs dispensed by a pharmacy to a healthcare provider for direct administration to a patient also are exempt from the labeling requirement, as are over-the-counter drugs and drugs intended for personal consumption by employees while in the workplace, such as aspirin and first-aid supplies.

Recall

13. What materials are exempt from labeling requirements?
14. Which employees must receive training about hazardous chemicals?
15. How long must training records be kept on file?

DENTAL OFFICE WASTE MANAGEMENT

Dental offices use certain substances that may be regulated under federal, state, or local environmental regulations. When discharged into a sewer system, these materials may impact the waste-water treatment plant or bypass through the treatment plant into a bay, ocean, river, or other waters. The environmental impact is minimized when these materials are handled, recycled, treated, or disposed of properly. Regulations vary from state to state, and many states *require* dental offices to have specific types of waste hauled away by a licensed carrier.

The dental assistant should understand the types of dental waste, how to comply with regulations, and ways to minimize the costs for disposal.

Dental Materials That May Be Regulated

- Mercury and dental amalgam
- Elemental mercury
- Amalgam capsules
- Scrap amalgam
- Amalgam traps
- Lead foil and shields
- Disinfectant solutions
- X-ray fixer solution
- X-ray developer solution

Classification of Waste

OSHA regulations apply to the handling of waste in the dental office for the protection of employees. When waste *leaves* the dental office, EPA regulations apply to the dis-

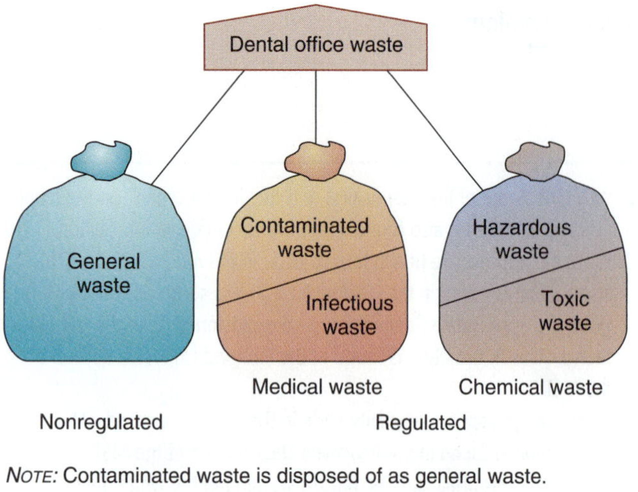

Fig. 23-11 Classification of dental waste.

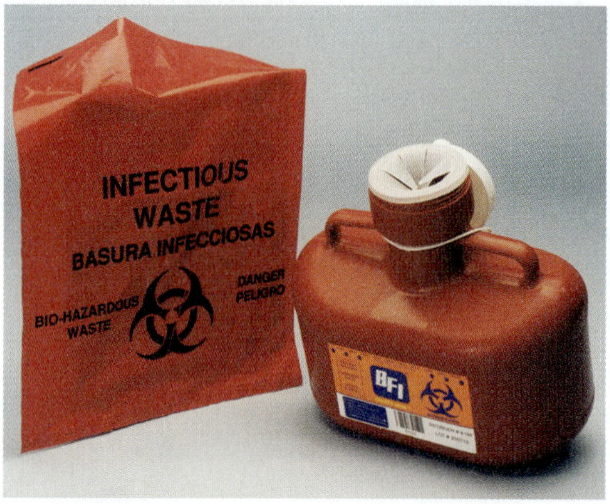

Fig. 23-12 Biohazard bag and biohazard sharps container. (From Young AP, Kennedy DB: *Kinn's the medical assistant: an applied learning approach,* ed 9, St Louis, 2003, Saunders.)

posal. All dental waste should be classified according to EPA guidelines as regulated or nonregulated (Fig. 23-11; Table 23-2).

Regulated waste includes *sharps,* such as disposable needles, scalpel blades, contaminated broken glass, disposable dental burs, and endodontic files and reamers.

Other regulated waste includes blood, blood-soaked and blood-caked items, human tissue, and pathologic waste. Regulated waste requires special disposal.

Nonregulated waste includes **contaminated waste** materials as well as saliva-soaked gauze, used patient bibs, and surface barriers.

All waste containers that hold *potentially infectious materials* (whether regulated or nonregulated) must be labeled with the *biohazard* symbol. OSHA requires this label to protect the employees, and the EPA requires this label to inform the public.

Extracted Teeth

Extracted teeth are considered to be potentially infectious materials and thus are regulated waste if they are not disinfected and returned to the patient. Many states allow the dental office to sterilize the extracted teeth. Teeth that do not contain amalgam and are going to be used for educational purposes must be heat-sterilized first.

Extracted teeth that contain amalgam restorations should *never* be heat-sterilized because the high temperatures may create toxic mercury vapors. For teeth that contain amalgam restorations, immersion in fresh, full-strength glutaraldehyde for at least 30 minutes is recommended for disinfection. After the tooth is rinsed, it can be disposed of according to local regulations.

Sharps

OSHA, the CDC, and the EPA classify sharps as **infectious waste.** According to OSHA regulations, disposable sharps must be placed in a closable, leakproof, puncture-resistant container immediately after use. The container must be labeled with the biohazard symbol and color-coded for ready identification (Fig. 23-12).

Scrap Amalgam

Scrap dental amalgam should be collected and stored in a designated, dry, airtight container.

Scrap amalgam that is *not* recycled must be managed as hazardous waste. The container of scrap amalgam that *is* recycled must be labeled with the name, address, and telephone number of the dental office and the date on which you first started collecting material in the container. Check with the mercury recycling company for any additional requirements.

In the past, scrap dental amalgam may have been kept under photographer fixer, water, or other liquid. If you encounter amalgam stored in this manner, *do not* pour the liquid down the drain under any circumstances. Contact a mercury recycler or a hazardous waste hauler for more information on how to dispose of this material properly.

Photochemical Waste

Dental offices generate two separate types of waste from x-ray processing solutions: radiographic fixer and radiographic developer (Fig. 23-13).

Radiographic Fixer

Radiographic fixer is considered a hazardous waste because of its high silver content. The two basic options for its management in the dental office are *on-site* treatment or *off-site* treatment. On-site treatment requires the installation of silver recovery systems to remove the toxic silver

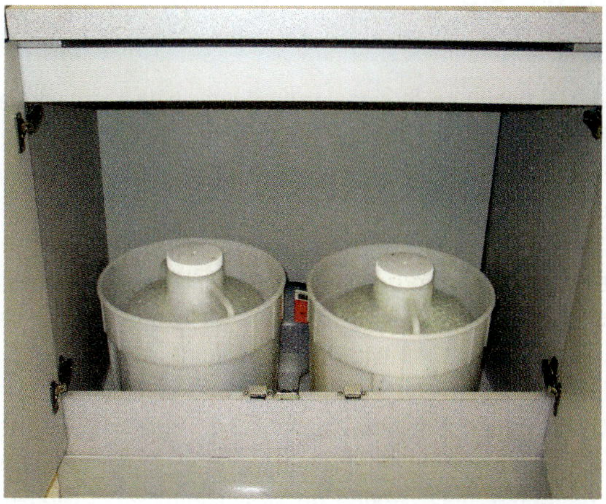

Fig. 23-13 Radiographic solutions in holding containers.

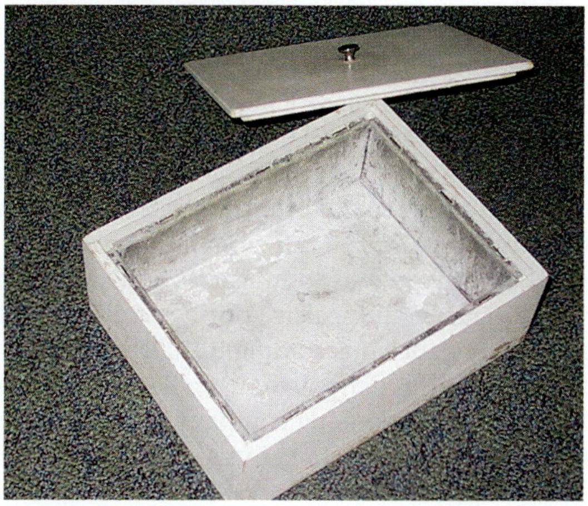

Fig. 23-14 Lead-lined wooden box is a source of lead contamination.

from the solution. Off-site treatment involves storing the used fixer and contracting with a disposal company to have it picked up. Contact your local waste-water treatment plant for specific requirements in your area.

Radiographic Developer

The developer solution may exceed the pH standard set by the local waste-water treatment plant. Products with a high or low pH are likely to be considered hazardous waste and must be managed according to local regulations.

Lead Contamination

Lead Foil

Lead foil from x-ray film packages is easily recyclable but cannot be disposed of in the garbage. Lead foil is exempt from regulation as a hazardous waste when recycled as a scrap metal, but it must be recycled through a licensed recovery facility. Eastman Kodak offers a mail-in service to recycle this material.

Lead-Lined Boxes

The U.S. Food and Drug Administration (FDA) has issued a warning to dental professionals to discontinue use of x-ray film containers lined with unpainted lead because of the potential for harmful lead exposure to patients and dental personnel (Fig. 23-14). Most of these containers are the size and shape of a shoe box, are made of wood, and are lined with lead that has not been painted or coated. Containers of this type are no longer available on the market, but the FDA believes that many may still be in use today.

Dental films stored in these boxes may be coated with a whitish film that is about 80 percent lead oxide. In many cases the level of lead on the film is highly dangerous. The lead oxide can be transferred from the film into the patient's mouth and onto the operator's hands and clothing.

The FDA cautions dental professionals *not* to use dental film that has been stored in these boxes. Wiping the film does not significantly reduce the lead levels. These boxes should be immediately discarded according to EPA regulations for disposal of scrap lead.

Always store dental film according to the manufacturer's instructions.

Disinfectants

Small quantities of spent germicidal solution containing 2 percent or less glutaraldehyde may usually be poured down the drain. Germicidal solutions with greater than 2 percent glutaraldehyde may need to be managed as a hazardous waste. Check with the local authorities on disposal methods for these chemicals.

Used or unused disinfectant with a high concentration of formaldehyde or a *flash point* less than 140° F is a hazardous waste and cannot be discharged into the sewer. Products with a red flammable label have a flash point of less than 100° F. Always check the MSDS for the flash points of other materials.

Nonhazardous Waste Management

Regular dental office waste should be recycled whenever possible. This includes aluminum, glass, newspapers, corrugated fiber, office paper, and mixed paper. The local sanitation department or garbage collection service is a source of recycling information.

Recall

16. What are three examples of regulated waste?
17. Why is x-ray (radiographic) fixer considered to be toxic?

WASTE DISPOSAL

The EPA enforces the disposal of regulated waste. If the state and local regulations are more stringent than the federal rules, the state and local regulations must be followed.

The dentist is responsible for the proper packaging, labeling, transportation, and ultimate disposal of waste generated in the dental office. All containers should be rigid, leak-resistant, impervious to moisture, and strong enough to prevent damage and leakage during handling. All containers must be labeled according to state law.

Many dental offices choose to use a licensed transporter, disposal source, or recycling company. However, the dentist is always responsible for the waste until it is either rendered nonhazardous or destroyed; therefore choosing a reputable disposal service is important.

Resources

American Dental Association (ADA)
http://www.ada.org

Environmental Protection Agency (EPA)
http://www.epa.gov/oppad001/chemregindex.htm

Food and Drug Administration (FDA)
http://www.fda.gov

National Institute for Occupational Safety and Health (NIOSH)
http://www.cdc.gov/niosh/homepage.html

Occupational Safety and Health Administration (OSHA)
http://www.osha.gov/SLTC/dentistry/index.html

Organization for Safety and Asepsis Procedures (OSAP)
http://www.osap.org

Legal and Ethical Implications

The dental health professional cannot anticipate or prevent every health and safety risk, but the risks are greatly reduced when all dental office personnel are conscious of chemical safety and infectious waste guidelines.

Use good common sense. If you are ever in doubt about the safety of a chemical product, read the MSDS, ask the dentist, or contact the manufacturer. All regulated waste must be disposed of in a manner consistent with the regulations. Always check your local and state regulations for management of dental waste if you are uncertain about disposal methods.

Your health, the health of your co-workers, and the health of the community may depend on your commitment to chemical safety.

Eye to the Future

The dental assistant who is responsible for the hazard communication program must clearly understand the basic concepts of chemical management. To do this, the coordinator must stay current with the increasing number and complexity of products in the dental office. The dental assistant/hazard communication coordinator must be vigilant in keeping the MSDS file current and complete.

Critical Thinking

1. One of your co-workers frequently eats her lunch in an area of the office in which chemicals are used. What can you say to her to convince her that this is a bad habit?
2. If you were using a chemical that had the number 4 in the red triangle on the chemical label, what would this indicate to you?
3. You have just been placed in charge of putting chemical labels on secondary containers in your dental office. What are some types of containers that should be labeled?
4. Look at the MSDSs for products usually found in the dental office. What products contain chemicals that pose hazards for (a) inhalation, (b) skin contact, and (c) flammability?
5. Go online to research regulations regarding disposal of hazardous waste in your area.

24

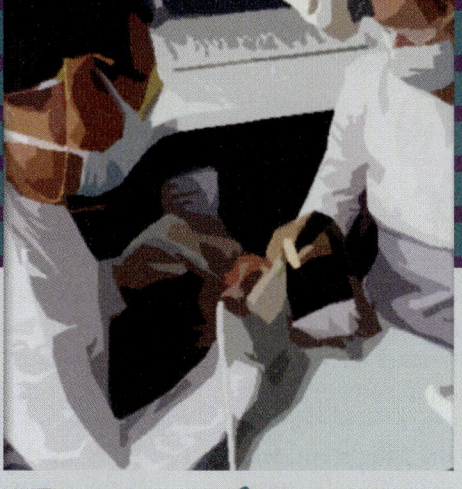

Dental Unit Waterlines

Outline

KEY TERMS

Antiretraction device A mechanism that prevents entry of fluids and microorganisms into waterlines as a result of negative water pressure; also called "suck back."

Biofilm (**buy-**oh-film) Slime-producing bacterial communities that may also harbor fungi, algae, and protozoa.

Colony-forming units (CFUs) Number of separable cells on the surface of a semisolid agar medium that create a visible colony.

Dental unit waterline (DUWL) Small-bore tubing usually made of plastic, used to deliver dental treatment water through a dental unit.

Heterotrophic bacteria (*het*-er-o-**tro**-fik) Bacteria that use organic carbon as a source of nutrients. Protozoa, fungi, and most bacteria fall into this category.

Legionella (*lee*-jeh-**nel**-a) Genus of bacteria responsible for the disease legionellosis.

Microfiltration Use of membrane filters to trap microorganisms suspended in water.

Planktonic (plank-**tah**-nik) Describes bacteria that are freely floating in water.

Self-contained water reservoir Container attached to a dental unit that is used to hold and supply water or other solutions to handpieces and air-water syringes.

LEARNING OUTCOMES

On completion of this chapter, the student will be able to achieve the following objectives:

- Pronounce, define, and spell the Key Terms.
- Explain why dental unit waterlines contain more bacteria than faucets.
- Explain the role of biofilm in dental unit waterline (DUWL) contamination.
- Discuss why there is a renewed interest in DUWL contamination.
- List the factors in bacterial contamination of dental unit water.
- Identify the primary source of microorganisms in dental unit water.
- Describe the methods to reduce bacterial contamination in dental unit waterlines.
- Describe the Centers for Disease Control and Prevention (CDC) recommendations for dental unit water quality.
- Explain the CDC recommendation for the use of saliva ejectors.

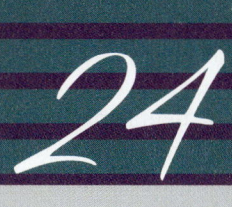

Outbreaks of waterborne disease have occurred in a broad range of facilities, including hospitals, nursing homes, schools, restaurants, community water supplies, swimming pools, and spas. Although there is no evidence of a widespread public health problem, published reports have associated illness with exposure to water from dental units. Bacteria capable of causing disease in some humans are found in dental unit waterlines, which is reason for concern (Fig. 24-1). In addition, exposing patients or dental professionals to water with extremely high bacterial counts is not in line with currently accepted infection-control principles.

In community water the number of waterborne bacteria is kept below 500 **colony-forming units (CFUs)** per milliliter (ml). The water from air-water syringes and dental handpieces frequently has levels that are hundreds or thousands of times *greater* than is permissible in drinking water. The types of bacteria found in dental unit water are frequently the same as those found in community water, but the quantity of bacteria found in the dental units are almost always higher. Research has shown that microbial counts in dental unit waterlines can reach 200,000 CFUs/ml within 5 days of installation of new lines.

This chapter provides an overview of the problem of **dental unit waterline (DUWL)** contamination, the potential health risks to patients and dental personnel, and the steps that you can take to lower the risk for DUWL contamination. You will also learn how to comply with the Centers for Disease Control and Prevention (CDC) recommendations relating to DUWLs, biofilm, and water quality.

BACKGROUND

The presence of bacteria in DUWLs was first reported more than 30 years ago. This issue is now attracting renewed attention because of the increased awareness of occupational hazards in the dental office, as well as concern about the increasing number of dental patients who have a weakened immune system.

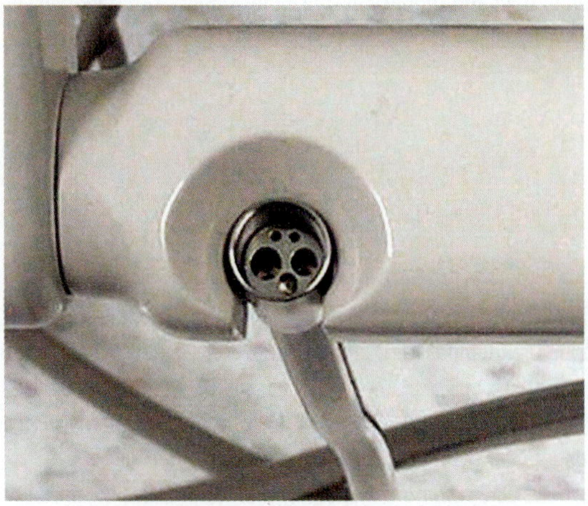

Fig. 24-1 Close-up of dental tube opening.

Studies have demonstrated that DUWLs (i.e., tubing that carries water to the high-speed handpiece, air-water syringe, and ultrasonic scaler) can become colonized with microorganisms, including bacteria, fungi, and protozoa. These microorganisms colonize and multiply on the interior surfaces of the waterline tubing and form a biofilm. (Biofilms are discussed later in this chapter.)

Several studies reveal that dental healthcare workers are exposed to *Legionella* bacteria at a much higher rate than the general public. ***Legionella*** species are harmful bacteria often found in water and moist places and are responsible for the disease *legionellosis.* Dental personnel are exposed to *Legionella* by inhaling the contaminated aerosol generated by the handpiece and the air-water syringe.

Fortunately, most dental healthcare workers are healthy and do not develop the disease. However, one dentist's death has been linked to legionellosis. Immunocompromised patients have also developed postoperative infections caused by contaminated dental water.

MICROORGANISMS IN DENTAL UNIT WATER

Waterborne and human oral microorganisms have been found in dental unit water. This indicates that *both* the incoming community water and the patient's mouth are sources of these microorganisms.

The *primary source* of microorganisms in DUWLs is the public water supply. However, saliva may be retracted back into the waterlines during treatment, a process called "backflow." The installation of **antiretraction devices** on dental units and thorough flushing of DUWLs between patients minimize this risk. The risk for backflow from saliva ejectors is discussed later in this chapter.

Dental Patients with Lowered Resistance to Disease

- Elderly patients
- Smokers
- Alcoholic patients
- Organ transplant recipients
- Blood transfusion recipients
- Patients with AIDS
- Patients with diabetes
- Patients with cancer
- Patients with autoimmune diseases
- Patients with chronic organic disorders

When the community water enters the dental office, it contains less than 500 CFUs/ml. But once that water enters DUWLs and the existing bacteria colonize and multiply within the biofilm, the CFU count greatly increases (Table 24-1).

There are two "communities" of bacteria in DUWLs. The bacterial community in the water itself is referred to as **planktonic** (free floating in the water). The other community exists in the biofilm attached to DUWL walls (Fig. 24-2).

Table 24-1 ***Sample Amounts of Bacteria in Dental Unit Water at Various U.S. Sites***

Source	CFUs/ml*
10 dental units from three offices	180,000
Tap water from three offices above	15
54 air-water syringe hoses	165,000
22 high-speed handpiece hoses	739,000
10 faucets	less than 30
4 water coolers	less than 30
11 rivers and streams	28,200
8 dental units	110,000

**Colony-forming units per milliliter.*
Modified from Miller C, Palenik C: Infection control and management of hazardous materials for the dental team, *ed 3, St Louis, 2005, Mosby.*

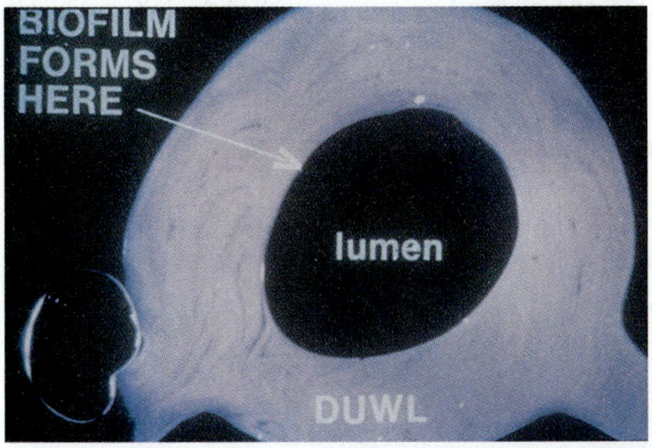

Fig. 24-2 **Cross-section of a dental unit waterline (DUWL) illustrating the formation of biofilm on the inside wall of a dental tube.** (Courtesy Dr. Shannon Mills, USAF.)

Recall

1. Are waterborne diseases limited to dentistry?
2. Is the presence of bacteria in DUWLs a recent finding?
3. Is there a widespread public health problem regarding contaminated dental water?
4. What bacteria cause the disease legionellosis?

BIOFILM

Biofilm consists of bacterial cells and other microbes that adhere to surfaces and form a protective slime layer. You may have seen or felt the biofilm slime layer that forms on the inside surface of a flower vase or a pet's water bowl.

Biofilm is found virtually in all places where moisture and a suitable surface exist. The inside of dental tubing is an especially favorable environment for biofilm to form (Fig. 24-3).

The best example of biofilm in dentistry is *dental plaque.* Biofilm is a type of "plaque" that develops inside DUWLs and causes an "infection" of the water delivery system. Biofilm can contain many types of bacteria, as well as fungi, algae, and protozoa.

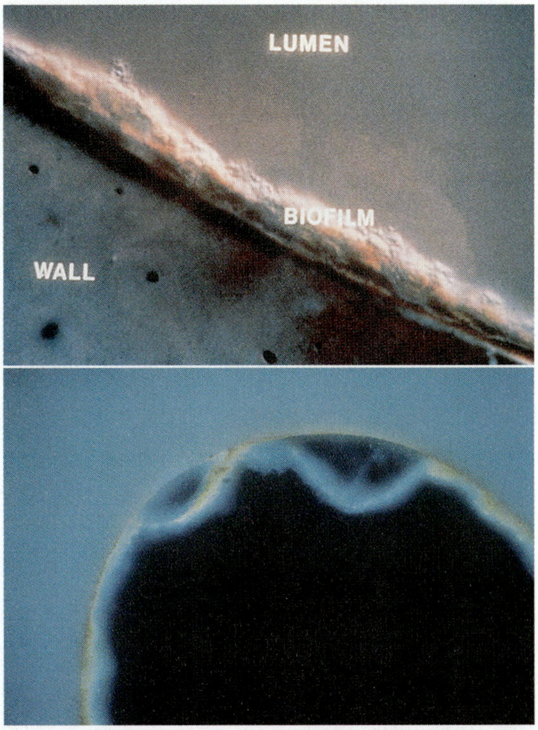

Fig. 24-3 **A, Magnification of biofilm formation on the walls of the tube. B, Magnification of cross-section of biofilm formation in DUWL.** (Courtesy Sultan Chemists, Inc, Englewood, NJ.)

NOTE: Viruses, *such as the human immunodeficiency virus (HIV)*, cannot *multiply in the DUWL.*

BIOFILM IN DENTAL WATERLINES

Water enters the dental office from municipal supplies or from wells. It is then routed to various sites within the office, including sink faucets, toilets, air conditioners, and the dental unit.

At the dental unit the water enters plastic waterlines, which pass through a multichannel control box that allows the water to be distributed to the hoses that feed various attachments, such as high-speed handpieces, air-water syringes, and ultrasonic scalers. Thus the water that enters the dental unit is the same water that supplies the entire office.

DUWLs have a narrow tube ($^{1}/_{8}$ to $^{1}/_{16}$ inch). Biofilm forms on the inside of the DUWLs as the water is flowing through the unit.

Growth-Promoting Factors

Several factors contribute to the formation of biofilm in DUWLs. The water moves at normal line pressure (slowly). Intermittent stagnation of the water inside the units typically occurs between patients, overnight, and over weekends, allowing the planktonic community of bacteria to attach to the walls of the tube. The bacteria become stabilized on a surface, and nutrients in the water feed them (Fig. 24-4).

Some dental offices have water heaters in the dental units to warm the water for the patient's comfort. The use of water heaters also may contribute to increased levels of bacterial colonization. Heating water to near body temperature for patient comfort may enhance the growth of the microorganisms. Another factor in biofilm formation in DUWLs is the maze of waterlines, where water can accumulate and become stagnant.

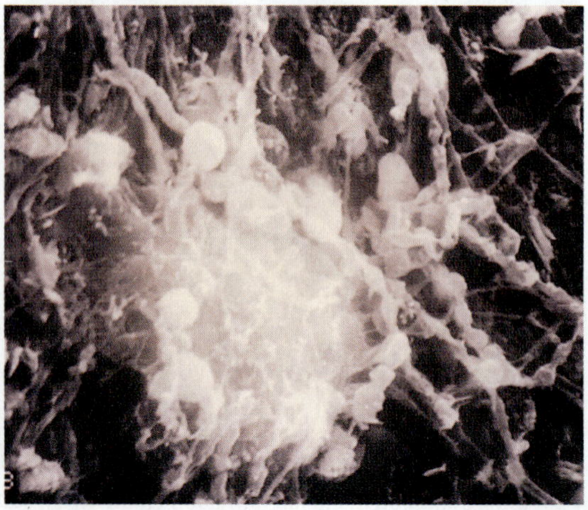

Fig. 24-4 **Bacteria in biofilm taken from dental unit waterlines.** (Courtesy Dr. Shannon Mills, USAF.)

Bacterial Characteristics

When bacteria are embedded in the protective biofilm (slime layer), they are extremely difficult to remove or kill. The bacteria in the biofilm are up to 1500 times more resistant to chemical germicides than planktonic (free-floating) bacteria.

During use of the dental handpiece or air-water syringe, some bacteria already present in the incoming public water, as well as bacteria dropping off the biofilm, are carried out (Fig. 24-5).

Recall

5. Where is biofilm found?
6. Is it appropriate to heat the water in dental units?

METHODS FOR REDUCING BACTERIAL CONTAMINATION

Complete elimination of biofilms and bacteria would be the ideal solution to the problem of DUWL contamination. Although this is not yet possible, methods for greatly reducing the level of bacterial contamination in waterlines include (1) chemical treatment regimens, (2) self-contained water reservoirs, (3) microfiltration, and (4) daily draining and drying of lines.

Self-Contained Water Reservoirs

Many manufacturers of dental units offer optional **self-contained water reservoir** systems. These systems work by supplying air pressure to the water bottle *(reservoir)*. The air pressure in the bottle forces the water from the bottle up into the DUWL and out to the handpiece and air-water

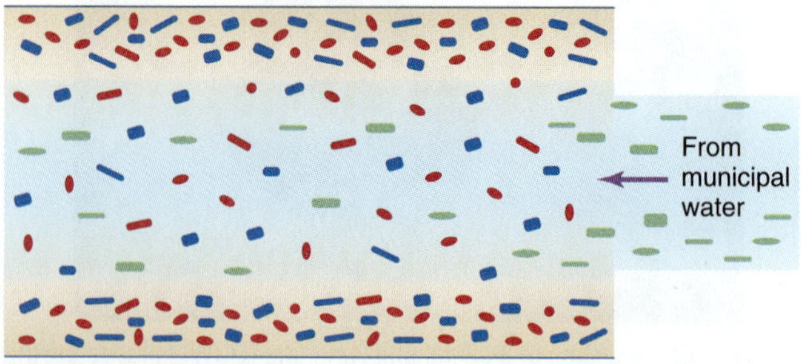

Fig. 24-5 **Bacteria in biofilm dropping into waterlines. Some bacteria are planktonic and enter directly from the municipal water supply.**

syringe (Fig. 24-6). Self-contained water systems have the following two advantages:

1. The dental personnel can select the quality of water to be used, such as distilled, tap, or sterile (Fig. 24-7).
2. Maintenance of the water system (between the reservoir bottle and the handpieces and syringes) is under the control of the dentist and staff.

Failure to follow the maintenance (cleaning and disinfection) procedures as recommended by the manufacturer may cause the water to become contaminated with even *higher than normal* counts of waterborne pathogens.

Methods to Reduce Bacterial Contamination of Dental Unit Waterlines

1. Flush waterlines for several minutes at the beginning of the day and longer after weekends.
   NOTE: Biofilms cannot be removed by flushing alone. Flushing 20 to 30 seconds between patients is recommended to eliminate material retracted from the previous patient.
2. Use a self-contained water reservoir system.
3. Use a self-contained water reservoir system combined with periodic or continuous application of chemical germicides as recommended by the equipment manufacturer.
4. Use a separate (sterile water) system for surgical procedures.
5. Purge the water from the dental lines and dry them with air at the end of each day.
6. Use microfiltration cartridges in the waterlines.
7. Stay current with new techniques and manufacturing technology for DUWLs.
8. Follow the recommendations for monitoring water quality provided by the manufacturer of the dental unit or waterline treatment product.

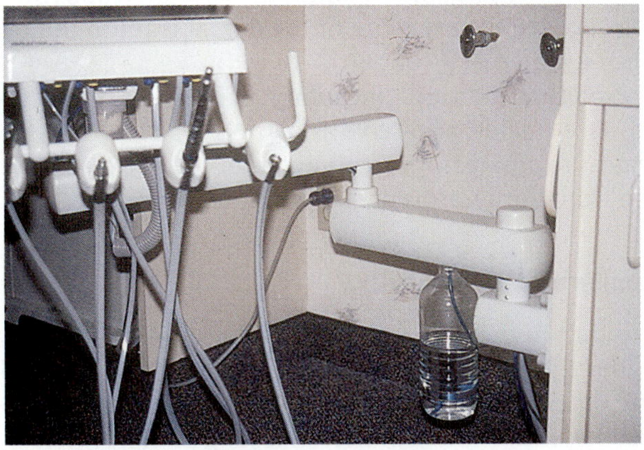

Fig. 24-6 Self-contained dental water unit. (Courtesy Dr. Ronald Johns.)

NOTE: Because the inside parts of the dental unit cannot be sterilized, the use of sterile water in the reservoir provides high-quality *water, but it will not be sterile at the point of delivery.*

Microfiltration Cartridges

A disposable in-line **microfiltration** cartridge also can dramatically reduce the bacterial contamination in the dental unit water (Fig. 24-8). This device must be inserted as close to the handpiece or air-water syringe as possible. It should be replaced at least daily on each line. The use of filtration cartridges combined with water reservoirs ensures improved water quality.

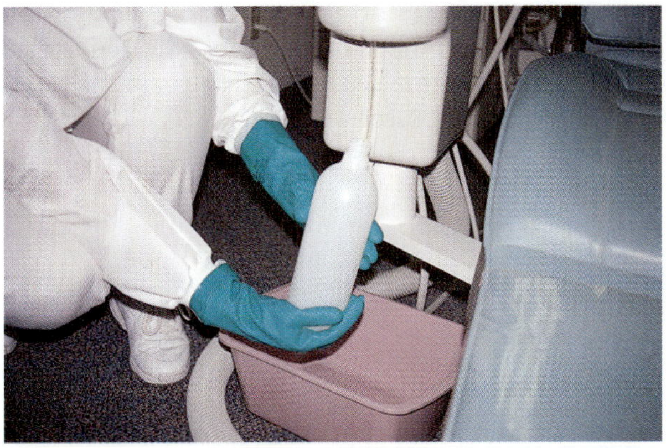

Fig. 24-7 Reservoir water bottles and lines in self-contained water systems must be cleaned and disinfected according to the manufacturer's instructions. The container under the water bottle will catch any solution drips. *NOTE: The dental assistant is careful not to touch and contaminate the neck of the bottle.* (Courtesy Pamela Landry, RDA.)

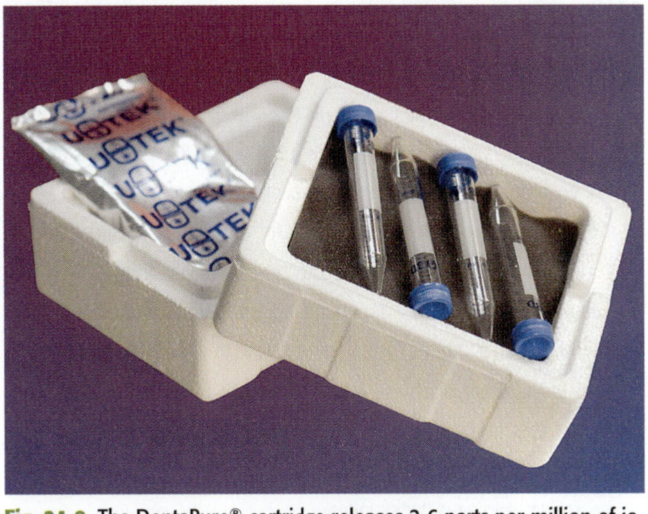

Fig. 24-8 The DentaPure® cartridge releases 2-6 parts per million of iodine as the water passes over it. The water delivered to the handpiece, 3-way water syringe, and ultrasonic scaler is treated. The cartridges are changed every 40 days. (Courtesy DentaPure, Fergus Falls, Minn.)

NOTE: Microfilters reduce the bacterial contamination of the water but do not affect *the biofilms that colonize the DUWLs.*

Chemical Agents

Chemicals can be used to help control biofilm in two ways:

1. Periodic or "shock" treatment with *biocidal* levels (levels that will kill microorganisms) of chemicals
2. Continuous application of chemicals to the system (at biocidal levels but not levels that harm humans)

Because biofilms are extremely resistant to chemical destruction, chemical treatments must be performed regularly, usually once a week. Some products now on the market provide excellent cleaning and bacterial control properties. You must take care in selecting the product to use because some chemicals can cause damage to the dental units.

Always check with the manufacturer of the dental equipment to determine the recommended chemical product and maintenance protocol.

Recall

7. Is it possible to eliminate biofilm completely?
8. If sterile water is used in the self-contained reservoir, will the water that enters the patient's mouth be sterile?
9. How often should microfilters be changed?
10. What precautions should you take when selecting a chemical for the dental unit?

CDC Recommendations for Dental Unit Waterlines, Biofilm, and Water Quality

- Use water that meets the Environmental Protection Agency (EPA) regulatory standards for drinking water (i.e., less than 500 CFU/ml of **heterotrophic bacteria**) for routine dental treatment output water.
- Consult with the dental manufacturer for appropriate methods and equipment to maintain the recommended quality of dental water.
- Follow recommendations for monitoring water quality provided by the manufacturer of the unit or waterline treatment product.
- After each patient, discharge water and air for a minimum of 20 to 30 seconds from any device connected to the dental water system that enters the patient's mouth (e.g., handpieces, ultrasonic scalers, and air-water syringes).
- Consult with the dental unit manufacturer on the need for periodic maintenance of antiretraction devices.

INFECTION CONTROL AND DENTAL UNIT WATER

Using the Proper Water

Dental unit water should *not* be used as an irrigant for surgery involving the exposure of bone. Only sterile water from special sterile water delivery systems or hand irrigation using sterile water in a sterile disposable syringe should be used in these types of surgeries.

Flushing Waterlines

All DUWLs and handpieces should be flushed every morning and from 20 to 30 seconds after each patient. Flushing temporarily reduces the microbial count in the water and helps clean the handpiece waterlines of materials that may have entered from the patient's mouth. Flushing also brings a fresh supply of chlorinated water from the main waterlines into the dental unit. *NOTE: Flushing will not remove biofilms from the lines; biofilm can form while water is moving through the lines.*

Minimizing Aerosol

Always use the high-volume evacuator when assisting with the use of the high-speed handpiece, ultrasonic scaler, and air-water syringe. This will reduce the contamination from the aerosol and spatter from the patient's saliva and from contamination with the water spray. The high-volume evacuation may also reduce exposure of the patient, as well as the dental team, to these waterborne microorganisms.

Using Protective Barriers

The rubber dam serves as a protective barrier for the patient from the dental unit water. The dam not only eliminates exposure but also greatly reduces direct contact. The dam also reduces the aerosolizing and spattering of patient microorganisms onto the dental team, but it does not reduce exposure of the dental team to the dental unit water.

Protective barriers, including masks, eye protection, and face shields, also serve as barriers for the dental team against microorganisms coming from the patient's mouth and from the aerosols and sprays of dental unit water.

Monitoring Water Quality

The only way to know whether the waterline cleaning regimen is effective is to test the water coming out of the unit. There are two options for testing dental unit water. The first is to use a commercial testing service, where you send samples of the unit water, and the results are mailed or faxed back to the dental office. A certificate is issued if the sample is below 500 CFUs. This is similar to the procedure used for monitoring the sterilizers. The second method is to use an in-office test kit (Procedure 24-1). Testing is usually done using three samples of water taken from the same dental unit. Dental handpieces should be removed before the samples are taken. With either method of monitoring, it is important that you do not contaminate the water during sampling; you should wear gloves and follow the directions of the service or the test kit very carefully (Fig. 24-9).

The CDC recommends that dental offices follow the recommendations of the manufacturer of the dental unit or the treatment product to monitor the quality of the dental unit water.

Use of Saliva Ejectors

Backflow from low-volume saliva ejectors occurs when the pressure in the patient's mouth is less than that in the evacuator. When a patient closes his or her lips around the tip of a saliva ejector, a partial vacuum is created, which can cause backflow to occur. This backflow can be a potential source of cross-contamination.

Furthermore, studies have demonstrated that gravity pulls fluid back toward the patient's mouth whenever the suction tubing holding the tip is positioned above the patient's mouth. This can also occur if you are using high-volume evacuation at the same time as the saliva ejector.

Although no adverse health effects associated with the saliva ejector have been reported, you should be aware that in certain situations, backflow could occur when using a saliva ejector.

Recall

11. What type of water must be used as an irrigant for surgery involving bone?
12. Will flushing DUWLs remove biofilm?
13. When should the high-volume evacuator be used to minimize aerosol?
14. Will the use of a rubber dam totally eliminate exposure to microorganisms?
15. What methods are available to test the quality of dental unit water?

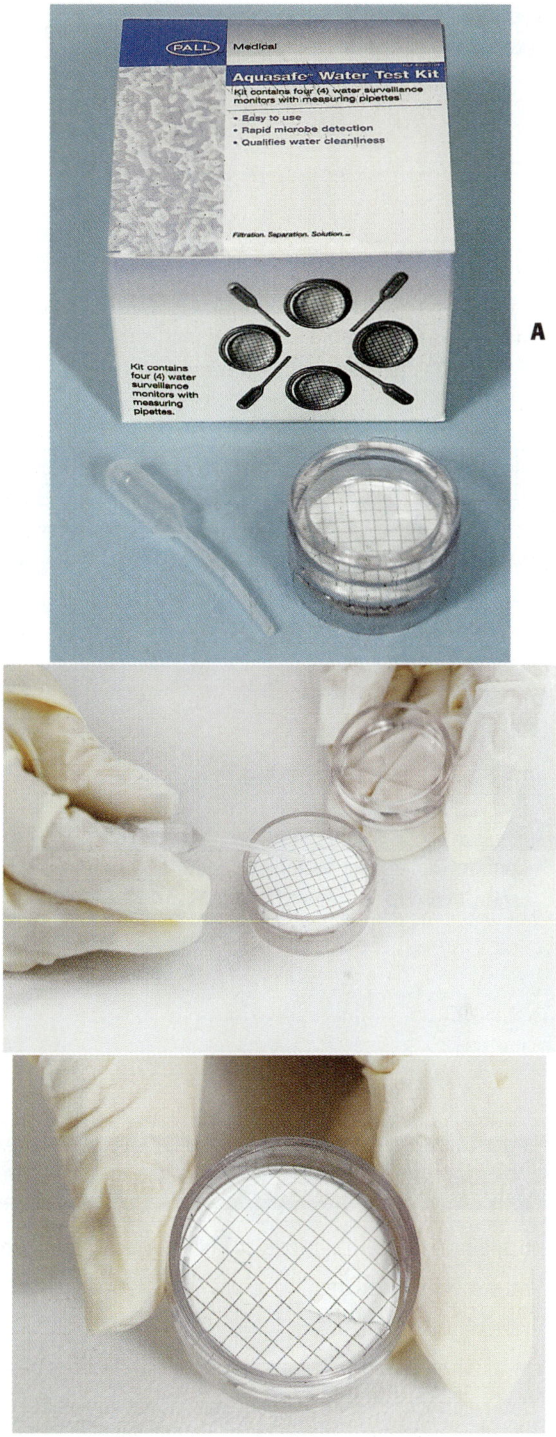

A

B

C

Fig. 24-9 **A,** Aquasafe Water Test Kit. **B,** 1 ml of dental unit water is transferred onto the surface of the test monitor. **C,** The test monitor is closed and will be checked in 48 to 72 hours. (**A** © Pall Corporation, 2004, by permission.)

Procedure 24-1 Testing Dental Unit Waterlines

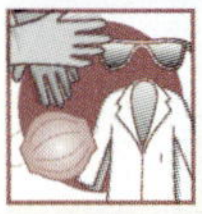 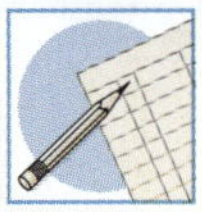

Goal

To obtain a water sample and prepare it for shipping.

Equipment and Supplies

- Testing service kit and instructions
- Clean gloves

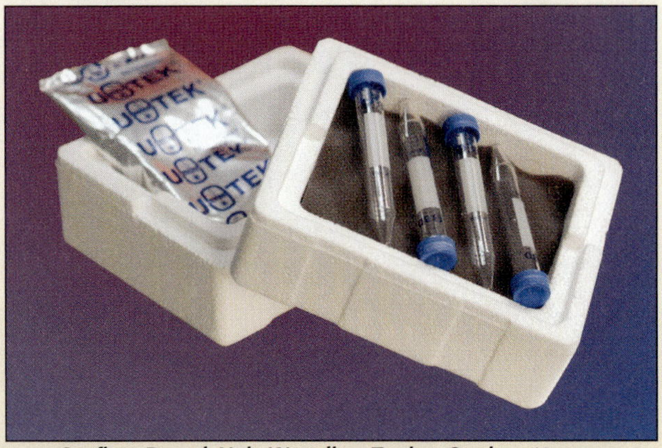

Confirm Dental Unit Waterline Testing Service. (Courtesy Confirm Monitoring Systems, Inc, Englewood, Colo.)

PROCEDURAL STEPS

1. Place refrigerant pack in the Styrofoam lid and place in freezer overnight.
2. Flush waterlines for a minimum of 2 minutes before taking samples.
   Note: Sampling should always be conducted just before any scheduled waterline maintenance or treatment.
   Purpose: To ensure that the sample is accurate.
3. Fill sterile collection vials to approximately ¾ full. *Do not touch the outlet of the waterline or the interior of the collection vial.*
   Purpose: You must not contaminate the vial.
   Note: The collection tubes contain a dehydrated chlorine neutralizer, which is visible in the bottom of the vial.
4. Use a permanent marker to label each water sample.
   Indicate the sample location and the type–e.g., Operatory 3, air-water syringe (Op3, a/w).
5. Fill out the sample submission form and enclose it with the samples.
6. Place refrigerant pack and water samples in Styrofoam shipper.
7. Place Styrofoam shipper in mailer box.
8. Complete U.S. Express Mail shipping label and affix to box.
   Note: U.S. Express Mail can be picked up by your U.S. Post Office mail carrier or taken to a post office. It must be picked up or mailed the same day the sample was taken.

CDC Recommendations for Dental Handpieces and Other Devices Attached to Air and Waterlines

Clean and heat-sterilize handpieces and other intraoral instruments that can be removed from the air and waterlines of dental units between patients.

Follow the manufacturer's instructions for cleaning, lubrication, and sterilization of handpieces and other intraoral instruments that can be removed from the air and waterlines of dental units.

Do not surface-disinfect, use liquid chemical sterilants, or use ethylene oxide on handpieces and other intraoral instruments that can be removed from the air and waterlines of dental units.

Do not advise patients to close their lips tightly around the tip of the saliva ejector to evacuate oral fluids.

Legal and Ethical Implications

As a dental assistant, you will be exposed to countless types of bacteria. However, exposure to these common microbes does *not* mean that you will develop an infection or disease.

However, when a person's immune system is compromised because of age, smoking, heavy drinking, an organ transplant, cancer, or HIV infection, that person may have more difficulty fighting off invading pathogens. It is therefore important for patients who have weakened immune systems to inform the dental personnel so that the right treatment decisions can be made. Patients should always feel free to ask questions about water quality or any other aspect of the dental practice.

To date, there has been no published scientific evidence of serious health problems for either patients or dental personnel from contact with dental unit water. Nonetheless, exposing patients or dental personnel to water of poor microbiologic quality violates universal infection-control principles.

Eye to the Future

Although the research community and dental equipment manufacturers have been working diligently on the issue of dental waterline contamination, additional research is still needed in the following areas:

- Better understanding of biofilm formation to develop new means for prevention, control, and removal
- Identification of health implications for patients, practitioners, and allied dental personnel from exposure to aerosols generated during dental procedures
- Simple, reliable, cost-effective devices for monitoring the microbial quality of water used during dental treatment

Critical Thinking

1. Mrs. Kato is coming in next week for dental treatment. She has not been to the dental office for some time because she has been receiving chemotherapy treatment for breast cancer. Are there any special considerations you should discuss with the dentist before beginning treatment of Mrs. Kato?
2. Mr. Torrence is a patient in your practice who has teeth that are extremely sensitive to cold water. On his last visit, Mr. Torrence suggested that you heat the water in the dental unit so it would be more comfortable. Do you think this is a good idea? Why or why not?
3. The staff in your dental office has decided to develop a patient information sheet to help patients understand about DUWL issues. What do you think should be included in this patient information sheet?

25

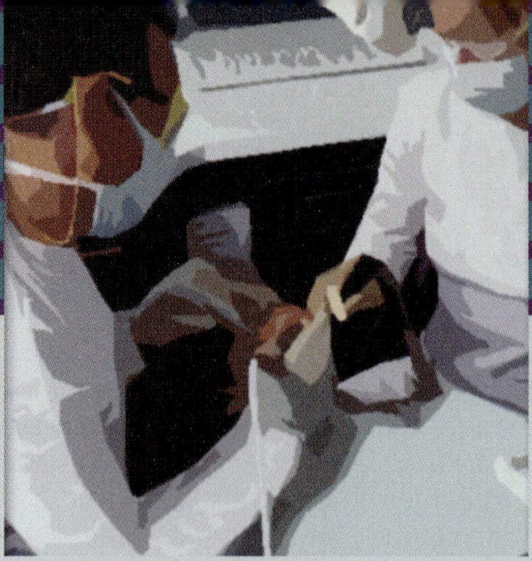

Ergonomics

Outline

KEY TERMS

Carpal tunnel syndrome (CTS) Pain associated with continued flexion and extension of the wrist.

Cumulative trauma disorders (CTDs) (**kyu**-myeh-luh-tiv) Painful conditions resulting from ongoing stresses to muscles, tendons, nerves, and joints.

Ergonomics (er-guh-**nah**-miks) Adaptation of the human body to the work environment.

Maximum horizontal reach The reach created when the upper arm is fully extended.

Maximum vertical reach The reach created by the vertical sweep of the forearm while keeping the elbow at midtorso level.

Musculoskeletal disorders (MSDs) (**mus**-kyu-loh-**skeh**-leh-tul) Painful conditions affecting both the muscles and bones, such as neck or back pain and carpal tunnel syndrome.

Neutral position The position when the body is properly aligned and the distribution of weight throughout the spine is equal.

Normal horizontal reach The reach created by the sweep of the forearm with the upper arm held at the side.

Sprains Injuries caused by a sudden twist or wrenching of a joint with stretching or tearing of ligaments.

Strains Injuries caused by extreme stretching of muscles or ligaments.

Thenar eminence (**thee**-nar **eh**-meh-nents) Fleshy mound on the palm at the base of the thumb.

LEARNING OUTCOMES

On completion of this chapter, the student will be able to achieve the following objectives:

- Pronounce, define, and spell the Key Terms.
- Describe the goal of ergonomics.
- Demonstrate the exercises that can reduce muscle fatigue and strengthen muscles.
- Demonstrate the neutral working position.
- Demonstrate the exercises to reduce eyestrain.
- Demonstrate the exercises to reduce neck strain.
- Identify common symptoms of musculoskeletal disorders.
- Identify three categories of risk factors that contribute to increased risk for injury.
- Describe the symptoms of carpal tunnel syndrome.

Many dental assistants have had to give up the career they love because of acute pain. Dental assistants often suffer with ongoing headaches, pain in the neck and shoulders, or numbness and tingling in their hands and wrists. Too often when the dental assistant finally seeks help, the pain is severe and there may be irreversible structural damage. You do not have to accept these hazards as part of your job. The key to preventing injury is to recognize and address the causes.

Ergonomics (from the Greek *ergon,* meaning "work," and *nomos,* meaning "law") deals with adaptation of the work environment to the human body. The goal of ergonomics is to help people stay healthy while performing their work more effectively. This can be done by changing workplace design, modifying instruments, strengthening muscles, taking breaks, using certain products, and providing proper training (Fig. 25-1).

This chapter discusses the common risk factors for **musculoskeletal disorders (MSDs),** the symptoms, and the techniques you can use to protect yourself from such injuries.

ERGONOMICS IN THE DENTAL OFFICE

The members of the dental team most frequently perform their work in a seated position and often use excessive motions and have unbalanced postures (Fig. 25-2). Many dental professionals experience pain associated with MSDs. Work-related symptoms range from back and joint pain to neck and shoulder pain, hand and wrist pain, and headaches.

The *early onset* of pain should alert the worker that (1) an imbalance exists and (2) if ignored, more serious damage can occur over time. When you first experience pain, you should take steps to reduce musculoskeletal inflammation and to assist healing. If you ignore the early symptoms of pain and stiffness, chronic disease may develop. It is important for the dental assistant to understand how to implement ergonomic changes and methods to prevent MSDs.

Three categories of risk factors contribute to MSDs: *posture, repetition,* and *force.*

Principle of Ergonomics

Ergonomics designs the work area and the task around the human body, rather than requiring the human to adapt to poorly designed equipment and working environments.

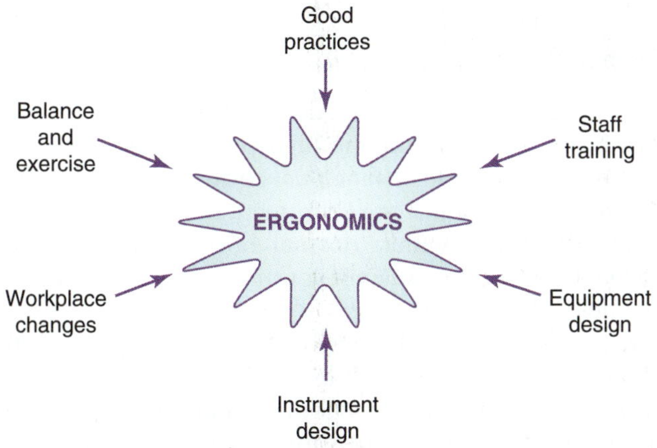

Fig. 25-1 Ergonomic factors in dentistry.

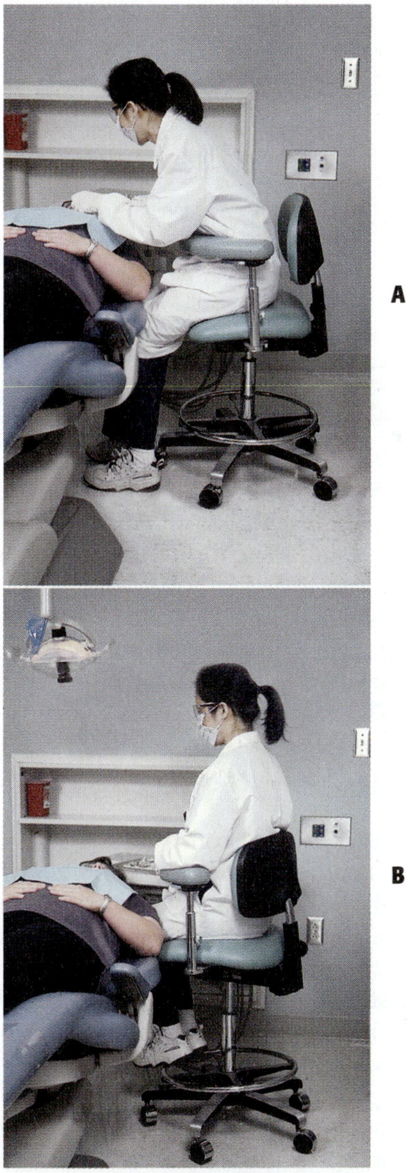

Fig. 25-2 **A,** Dental assistant in poor position. **B,** Dental assistant in proper position.

Recall

1. What is meant by "ergonomics?"
2. What is the goal of ergonomics?
3. What types of disorders are considered to be MSDs?
4. What are the three categories of risk factors that contribute to MSDs?

Ergonomic Chairside Tips

Use muscles to remain balanced for ease of movement.

Avoid prolonged, awkward positions.

Do not remain in one position for an extended time.

Do not constantly lean forward or to the side.

Remain in good physical condition.

Take breaks to stretch the neck, shoulders, and hands.

Avoid repetitive, forceful movements.

Rearrange items in the operatory for easy use.

POSTURE

Posture affects the ability of the dental assistant to reach, hold, and use equipment. Positioning also influences how long the assistant can perform a task without suffering adverse health effects.

Most dental assistants are seated while working on patients. Although sitting is generally less fatiguing than standing, any position will eventually become fatiguing over time. This may lead to low back pain.

Neutral Position

The ideal way to work is from a "neutral" position. You can establish a **neutral position** by sitting upright with your weight evenly distributed. Your legs should be separated with your feet flat on the floor when working as an operator—or flat on the footrest of the assistant's stool when assisting. Your back should be pressed against the back of the chair for lumbar support. Your hips should lean forward to rotate the pelvis backward.

The properly aligned spine resembles a gentle "S." When the spine is properly aligned, the ears, shoulders, and hips are in straight vertical alignment, providing balance, support, and equal distribution of weight throughout the spine (Fig. 25-3).

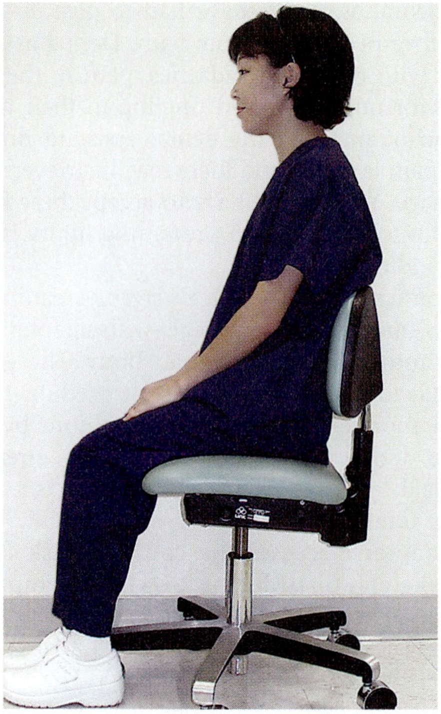

Fig. 25-3 Configuration of spine in seated dental assistant.

Deviations and Problems

Unfortunately, while assisting the dentist, the dental assistant tends to deviate from the neutral position. Such deviations include learning forward, twisting, overbending the back, and reaching. These poor postures can lead to aches, pains, numbness, and tingling. Ideally, the assistant alternates sitting and standing whenever possible.

Frequent reaching, twisting, and working with the arms in awkward positions can cause strains and sprains. **Strains** result from extreme stretching of muscles or ligaments. **Sprains** usually involve a sudden twist or wrenching of a joint with stretching or tearing of ligaments. Shoulder problems can be caused by repeatedly reaching behind the body for instruments or supplies (Fig. 25-4).

Reaching Movements

Keep frequently used items, such as the air-water syringe, handpiece, saliva ejector, and high-volume oral evacuator, within a comfortable distance, *not* above shoulder level or below the waist. Adjust the instrument tray and equipment so that items are within **normal horizontal reach,** the reach created by the sweep of your forearm with the upper arm held at your side.

Keep the operatory light within a safe **maximum vertical reach,** the reach created by the vertical sweep of your forearm while keeping your elbow at midtorso level. Other supplies used less frequently should be placed within **maximum horizontal reach,** the reach created when your upper arm is fully extended.

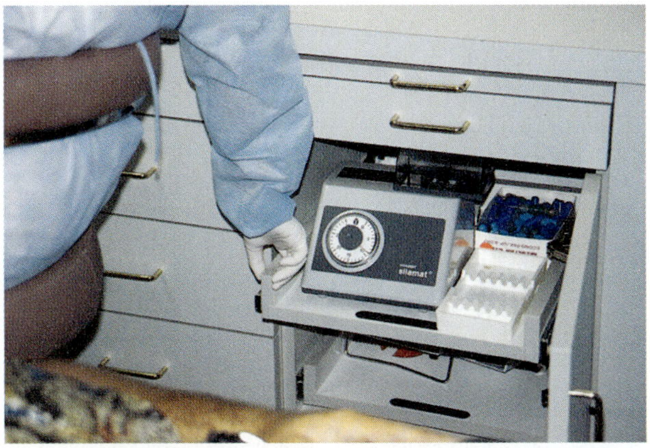

Fig. 25-4 Small pieces of equipment should be in a location that does not require twisting or bending.

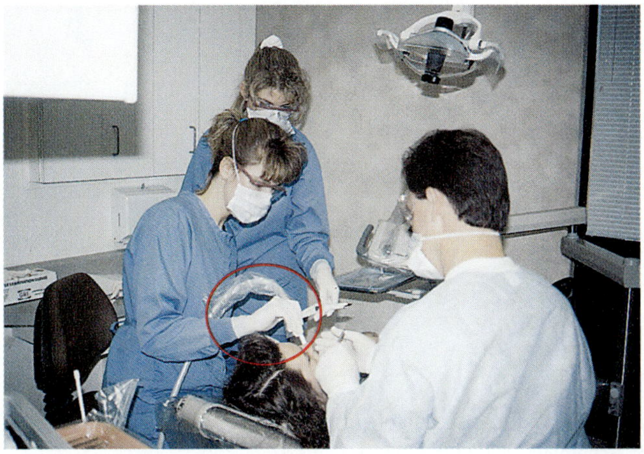

Fig. 25-5 Repetitive stress on the bend in the wrist over long periods can lead to carpal tendon injury. This dental assistant should periodically change her grasp on the oral evacuator to straighten out her wrist. She should also use the back support on her chair.

Optimal Dental Assistant Positioning

Position your head as upright as possible.

Keep your back straight and supported by a backrest.

Keep your thighs parallel to the floor.

Seat yourself at the patient's shoulder with your knees even with the edge of the headrest on the patient chair.

Keep your elbows close to your body.

Rest your feet on the chair or footrest. Avoid sitting on the edge of the chair and balancing with tiptoes on the floor; such positioning is unstable.

Remember that your eye level should be about 6 inches above the dentist's level.

Modified from *OSAP Monthly Focus* 2, 2001.

Optimal Operator Positioning

Position the head as upright as possible.

Ensure that the back is straight and supported by a backrest.

Keep elbows close to the body.

Keep thighs parallel to the floor.

Work from a 12 o'clock position (in back of the patient).

Work from a neutral position.

Reposition the patient as necessary rather than reaching, leaning, and bending for access.

Modified from *OSAP Monthly Focus* 2, 2001.

Reaches should be to the front only. Reaching behind your back and lifting can cause shoulder injury. When turning is necessary, rotate the chair rather than twisting your body.

REPETITION AND FORCE

Repetitive motion, overflexion, and overextension of the wrist can significantly increase the risk for **cumulative trauma disorders (CTDs),** particularly when the task requires force (Fig. 25-5). To help prevent common CTDs such as carpal tunnel syndrome, take periodic breaks and when scheduling patients, alternate difficult procedures with less stressful procedures.

Carpal Tunnel Syndrome

The term *carpal tunnel* refers to an anatomic area of the hand and wrist. Eight carpal bones arranged as a tunnel form this area. Inside the tunnel are nine flexor tendons and the median nerve. With improper motions the tendons swell and exert pressure on the median nerve (Fig. 25-6). Repetitive and forceful motions can lead to **carpal tunnel syndrome (CTS).**

The first symptom of CTS is often a painful tingling in one or both hands that occurs at night. A decreased ability and power to squeeze objects or make a tight fist may follow. In advanced cases the thenar muscle (located at the base of the thumb) may weaken, causing a feeling of decreased strength in the handgrip.

Other repetitive hand and wrist movements, such as knitting, gardening, or using a keyboard, can also cause CTS. Patients who are pregnant, taking oral contraceptives, have premenstrual syndrome, or suffer from rheumatoid arthritis may be more prone to develop CTS.

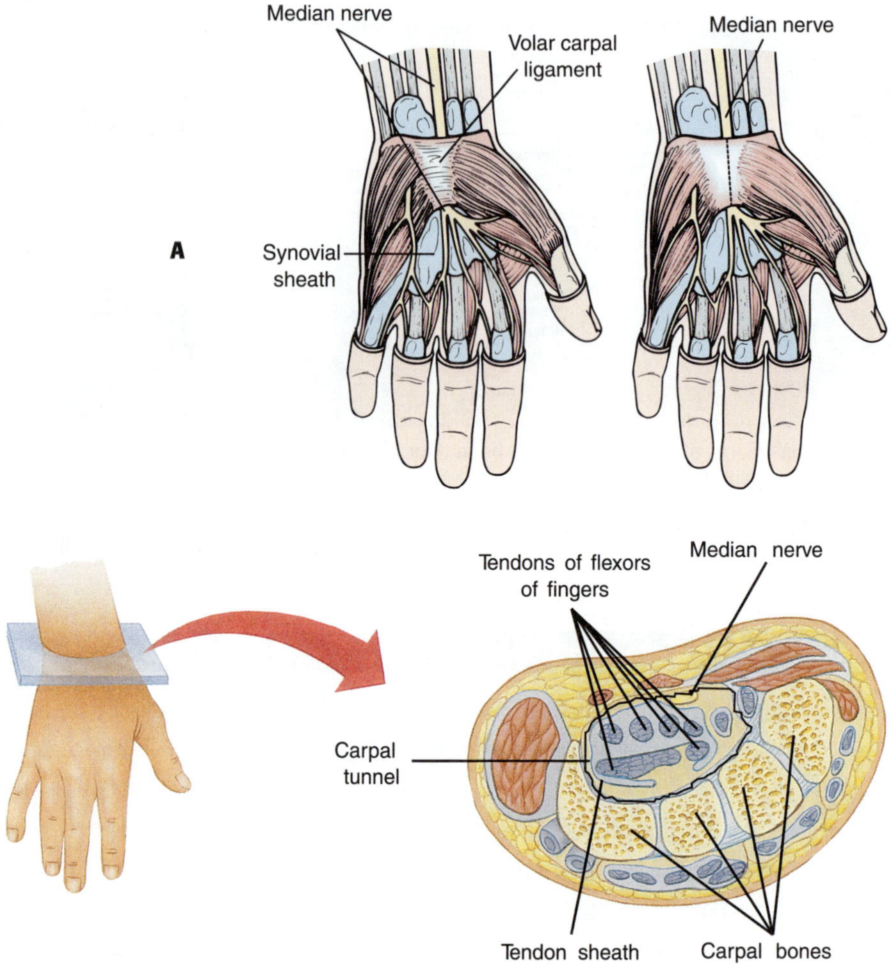

Fig. 25-6 **A,** Cross-section of wrist. **B,** Schematic view of the carpal tunnel. (From Thibodeau GA: *Anatomy and physiology,* ed 4, St Louis, 2002, Mosby.)

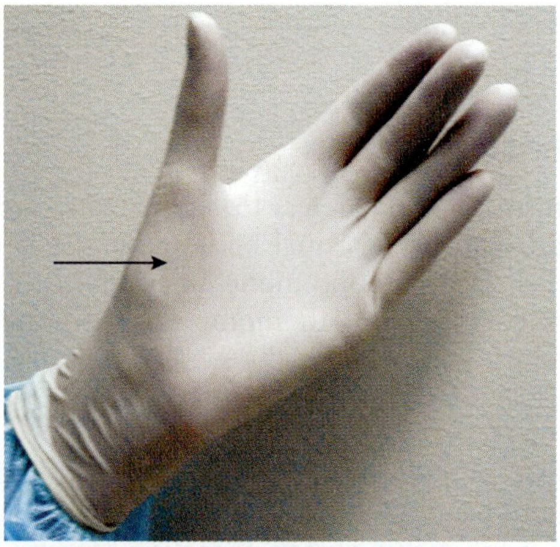

Fig. 25-7 The arrow indicates the location of the thenar eminence on a gloved hand.

Gloves

The use of *ambidextrous gloves* (gloves designed to be worn on either hand) can place excessive tension on the **thenar eminence** (the fleshy elevation on the palm at the base of the thumb) (Fig. 25-7) and hypothenar eminence by forcing the hand to work against the vertical alignment of the glove form. *Right-left gloves* that are properly sized support the hands naturally and properly position the thumb, index finger, and middle finger.

Recall

5. What is the neutral position?
6. What is meant by normal horizontal reach?
7. What type of glove is most likely to aggravate CTS?

MUSCLE-STRENGTHENING EXERCISES

Stretching and strengthening the muscles that support your back and neck and those used in the forearm, wrist, and hand will help keep these muscles strong and healthy. You should do periodic stretching throughout the workday.

Frequently resting the hands is one of the most important factors in preventing CTS. To warm the muscles and joints of your hands, slowly open and close your hands, going from a completely open position to a completely closed position, which ends with your fingers tucked into your palm (Fig. 25-8, *A* and *B*). Also press your palms together and then relax them (Fig. 25-8, *C* and *D*).

Another recommended stretching exercise is to hold one arm out in front of your body with your hand extended. With the fingers of your other hand, gently pull back on your extended fingers to increase the stretch (Fig. 25-8, *E*).

To relieve *eyestrain* caused by focusing intensely at one depth of vision for long periods, look up from the task and focus your eyes at a distance for about 20 seconds. Practice this frequently throughout the day to use your full range of vision and to lessen eyestrain.

To relieve stresses placed on the back, neck, and shoulders, perform the *full back release* (Fig. 25-9). Do head rotations for neck stiffness. *Head rotations* involve tilting the head from right to left and from forward to backward without forcing the motion beyond a range of comfort.

Shoulder shrugging can be used to stretch the shoulder muscles, which may be stressed from holding oral evacua-

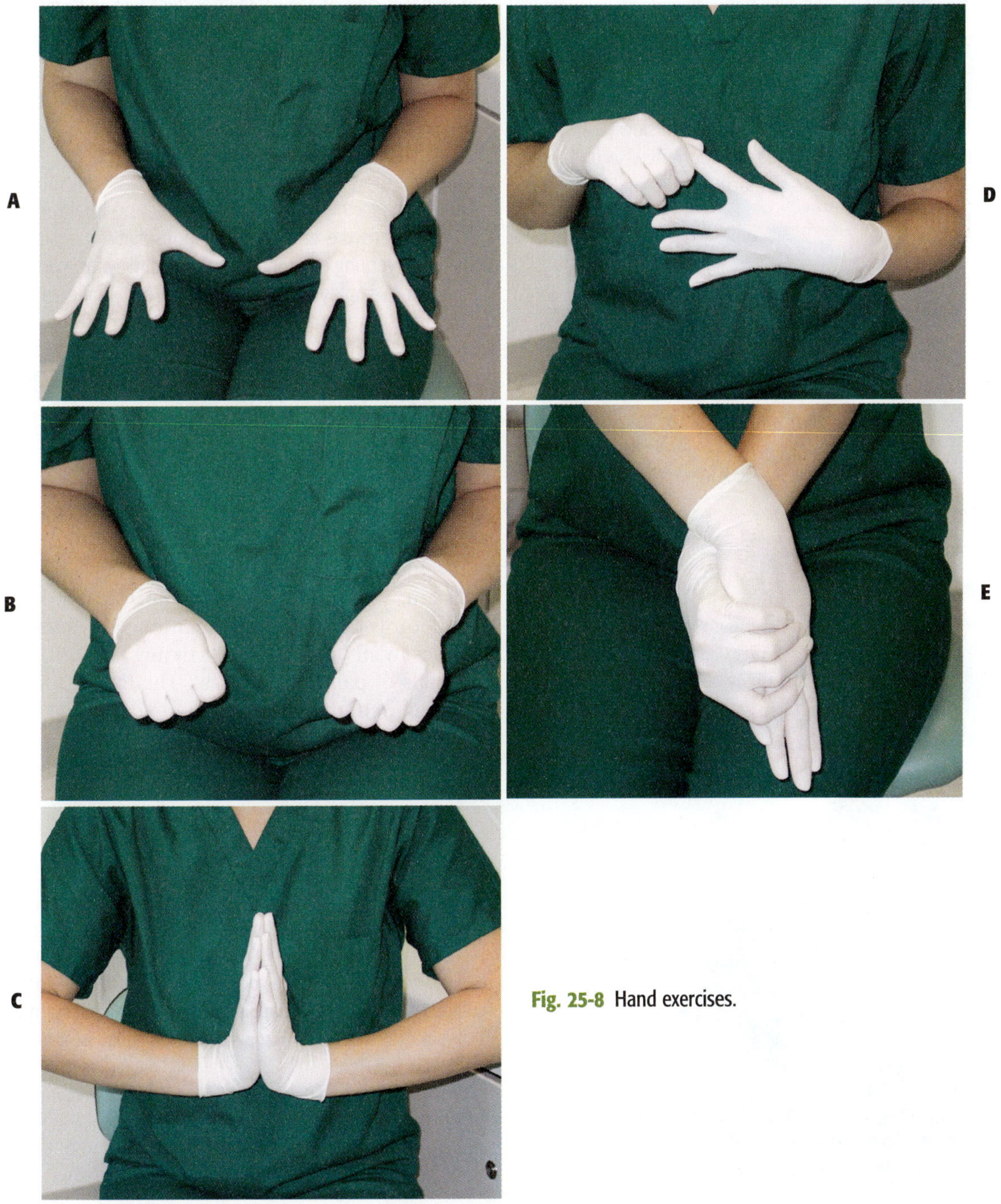

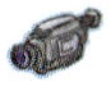

Fig. 25-8 Hand exercises.

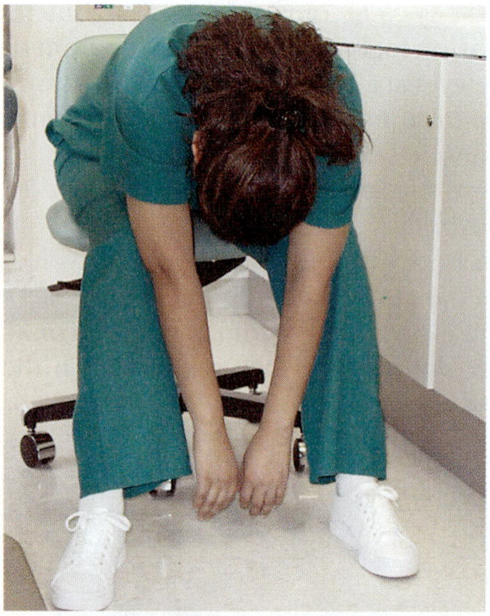

Fig. 25-9 Full back release. Let the head move down slowly, allow the arms and head to fall between the knees, hold for a few seconds, and then raise slowly by contracting the stomach muscles and rolling up. Bring the head up last.

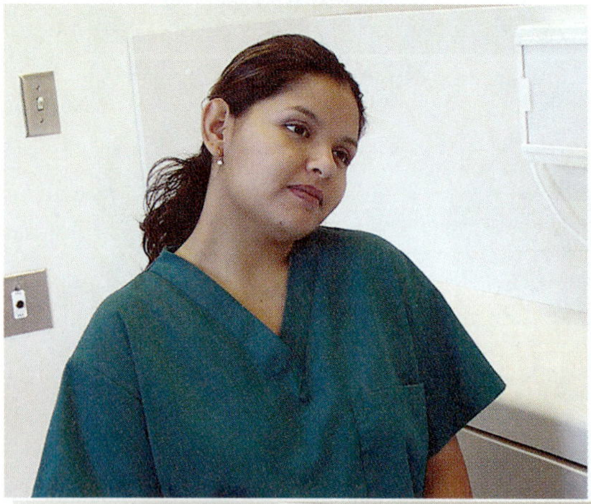

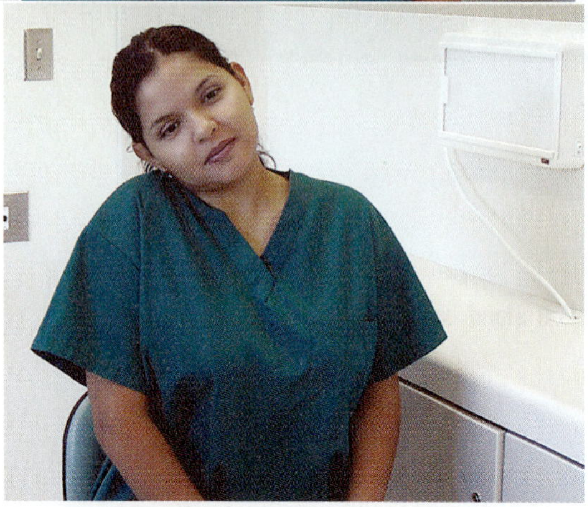

Fig. 25-10 Shoulder shrugging.

tors, instruments, and telephone handsets. Pull your shoulders up toward your ears and then roll them backward and forward in a circular motion (Fig. 25-10).

Before beginning any exercise program, you should check with your physician, particularly if you experience pain with any of the movements.

Recall

8. How can you reduce eyestrain?
9. What exercise relieves neck strain?
10. What is one of the most important factors in preventing CTS?

Legal and Ethical Implications

According to the Occupational Safety and Health Administration (OSHA), it is the employer's responsibility to ensure a safe and healthy working environment. The best way for a dental employer to protect employees from musculoskeletal injuries is to make ergonomics an important part of the practice for everyone. Some dental offices have created a separate written program to address ergonomics. Another approach is to incorporate ergonomics into the existing health and safety program.

Eye to the Future

To enjoy a healthy and pain-free career as a dental assistant, you must keep your muscles, tendons, nerves, and joints healthy. Remember to apply ergonomic principles in all of your daily activities. Do not ignore early signals of pain and stiffness. The longer the symptoms are ignored, the more severe the damage. Dentistry can be a physically stressful profession, but it is also a very rewarding profession that benefits both practitioners and patients.

Critical Thinking

1. How would you describe good posture and chairside position to a newly hired dental assistant who did not have formal training in ergonomics?
2. What exercises would you perform throughout the day to minimize the risk for MSDs?
3. What changes would you make to create a more ergonomic operatory?
4. Are there any changes you can make to your own home and/or school environment to make it more "worker friendly"?

Part 6

Patient Information and Assessment

As a student preparing to become a dental assistant, you will learn early on in your education the importance of knowing your patients. From the moment a patient walks into the dental office, the dental team takes on the shared responsibility of total care.

The chapters within this section will provide you with additional knowledge and skills necessary to your role as a dental assistant. Whether you are gathering personal information, obtaining diagnostic information such as vital signs, working with a patient who has a medically compromising condition, or assisting in a medical emergency, you are a valuable resource of the dental team.

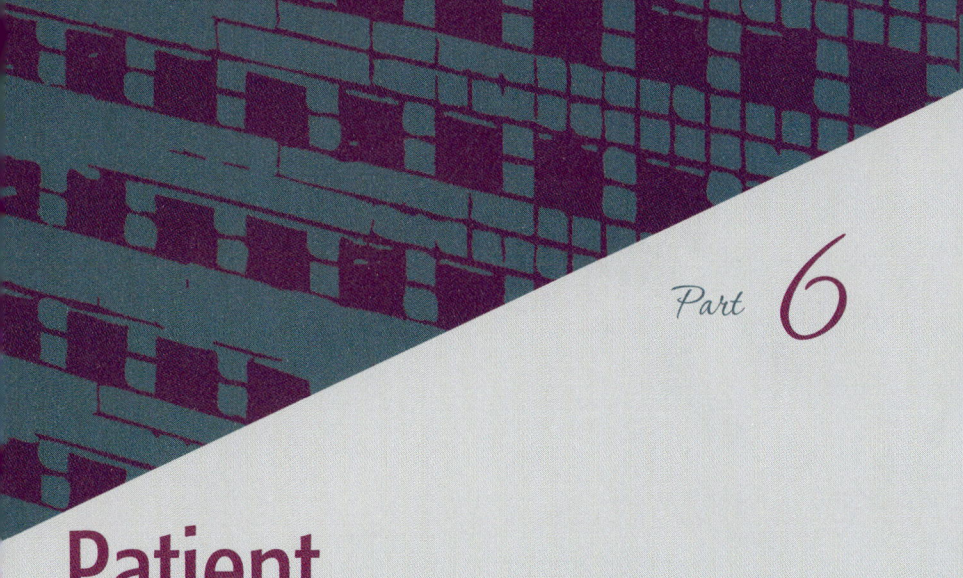

26

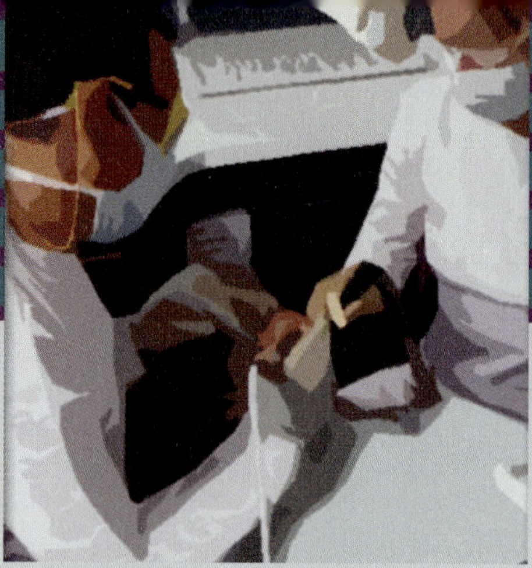

The Patient Record

Outline

KEY TERMS

Alert To bring attention to by making someone aware.

Assessment Process of making an official evaluation of someone or a situation.

Chronic Persisting over a long period of time.

Chronologic Arranged according to time of occurrence; earliest to most recent.

Demographics Personal information about patients, such as address and work; also, statistical characteristics of populations.

Diagnosis Identification or determination of the nature and cause of a disease or injury through the evaluation of a patient's history and examination.

Forensic (fo-**ren**-zik) Pertaining to the establishment of the identity of an individual based on scientific methods.

HIPAA The Health Insurance Portability and Accountability Act of 1996 specifies federal regulations ensuring privacy regarding a patient's health-care information.

Litigation (li-teh-**gay**-shun) Act of initiating legal proceedings, as in a lawsuit.

Registration The act of completing forms with personal information.

LEARNING OUTCOMES

On completion of this chapter, the student will be able to achieve the following objectives:

- Pronounce, define, and spell the Key Terms.
- Identify the purpose of a patient record.
- Describe each form in the patient record.
- Discuss the importance of the patient's medical-dental health history and its relevance to dental treatment.

PERFORMANCE OUTCOMES

On completion of this chapter, the student will be able to meet competency standards in the following skills:

- Supervise the completion of a new patient registration form.
- Obtain a completed medical-dental health history form for a new patient.
- Prepare and organize a patient record.

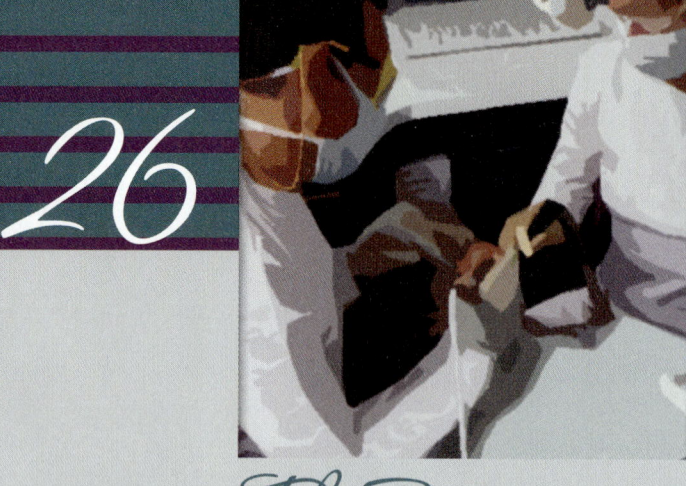

The patient record is the principal document that you will manage for each patient in a dental practice (Fig. 26-1). The information within the patient record allows the dental team to provide individualized quality care. It is important to have an organized and practical approach to the information-gathering process. The following critical information must be gathered by the dental team before providing any dental treatment or care:

- Patient registration (personal patient information)
- Medical-dental health history (patient's overall health status)
- Medical alert information (any medical concerns that exist when treating this patient)

Assessment is the process of collecting data and then evaluating or drawing conclusions from the findings. The dentist (1) assesses a patient's oral condition, (2) makes a **diagnosis,** (3) determines the type of treatment that would be best for the patient, (4) schedules appointments to provide treatment in a timely manner, and (5) follows through with the maintenance stages of the patient care process. The patient record is an important tool in monitoring patient care throughout these phases.

Recall

1. What information must the dentist have from a patient before providing dental treatment?
2. What term describes the collection of data by the dentist to make a correct diagnosis?

THE PATIENT RECORD

The dental team primarily uses the patient record to maintain information regarding a patient's dental needs and treatment. Because there is an abundance of information in a patient record, this information can take on additional meanings for the dentist.

Permanent Record

The patient record is a *permanent document* of the dentist. This permanent document, also considered a *legal document,* can be used for (1) evidence in a legal settlement or law suit, (2) as a reference tool in a **forensic** case to identify an individual by the use of the patient's radiographs or study casts, or (3) for reference to appropriate third parties, such as dental insurance companies.

Quality Assurance

The dentist uses a patient record as the primary source of information to determine the overall quality of care the patient receives. *Quality* is the key word to remember when a patient is receiving dental care.

Does the patient believe that the best and most timely treatment is being provided? This question can be extremely important if the clinical setting is a larger facility or teaching institution where many patients are seen by different clinicians. Each dental setting must promote an efficient and effective quality assurance program. The following are examples of quality assurance in the dental office:

- Routine forms completed by each patient
- Timely recall of patients for their dental needs
- Completed patient record for each "active" patient of the dental practice
- Documentation of when radiographs were taken
- Current and up-to-date emergency standards maintained by the dental team
- Current and up-to-date licenses, registrations, and training of the dental team

Risk Management

As noted earlier, the patient record provides documentation regarding a patient's condition, diagnosis, treatment, and response to treatment. For the dentist to avoid a malpractice suit in the event that **litigation** concerning the processes or outcomes of treating a patient occurs, it is imperative to have patient records organized and complete. For additional information on risk management, see Chapter 5.

Research

A complete and **chronologic** patient record can provide a source of data for research purposes. Many dental schools, public health agencies, and private practices are involved in the research of causes, distribution, and control of disease in populations. When a new research study begins, the steps taken in the patient's treatment or in the specific use of a new dental product must be accurately documented. If documentation is not complete, the data must be eliminated from the study, which would then decrease the number of examples.

Recall

3. The patient record is a permanent document of whom?
4. Why is quality assurance so important in the maintenance of a dental practice?

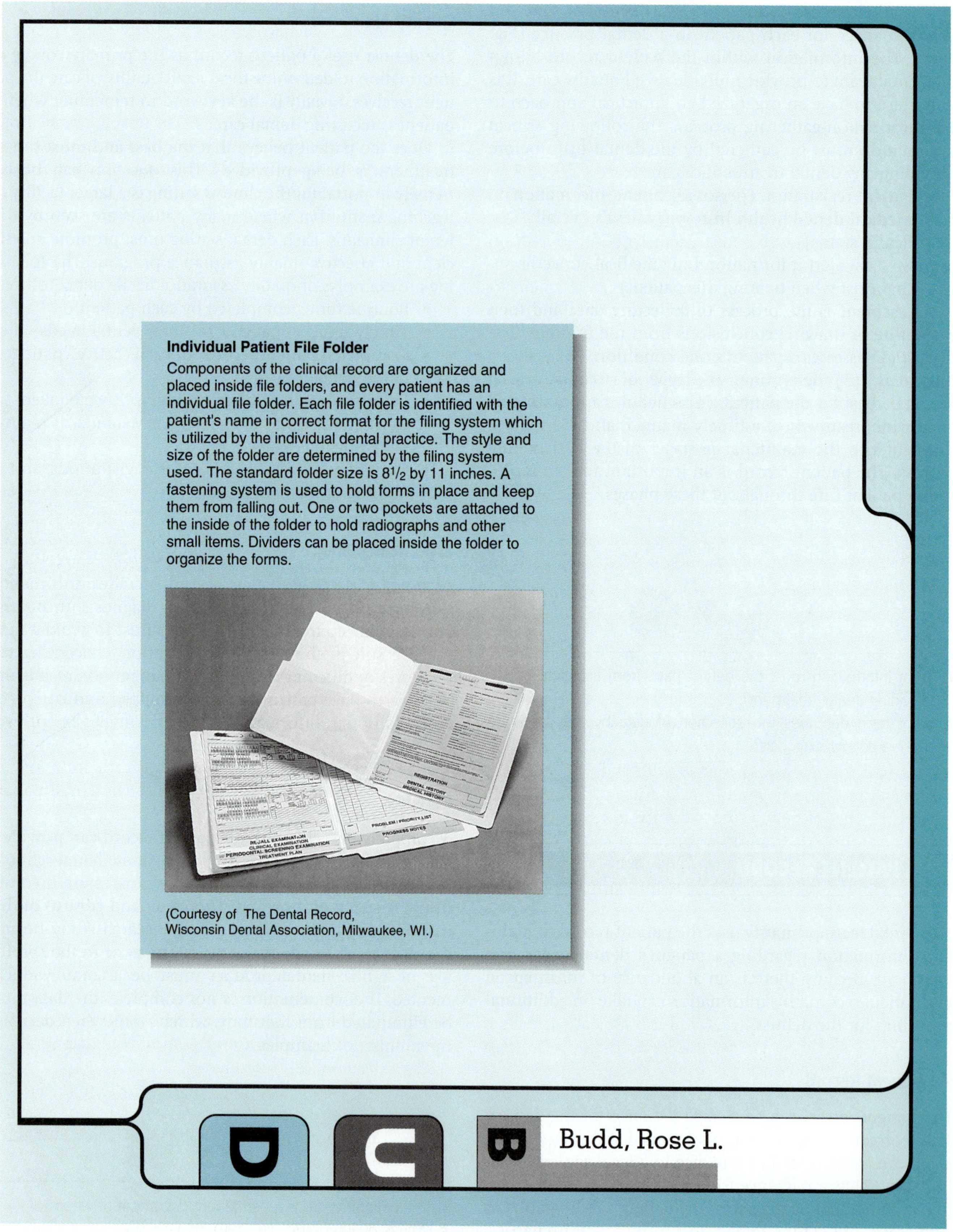
Individual Patient File Folder
Components of the clinical record are organized and placed inside file folders, and every patient has an individual file folder. Each file folder is identified with the patient's name in correct format for the filing system which is utilized by the individual dental practice. The style and size of the folder are determined by the filing system used. The standard folder size is 8½ by 11 inches. A fastening system is used to hold forms in place and keep them from falling out. One or two pockets are attached to the inside of the folder to hold radiographs and other small items. Dividers can be placed inside the folder to organize the forms.
REGISTRATION
DENTAL HISTORY
MEDICAL HISTORY
PROBLEM / PRIORITY LIST
PROGRESS NOTES
RECALL EXAMINATION
CLINICAL EXAMINATION
PERIODONTAL SCREENING EXAMINATION
TREATMENT PLAN
(Courtesy of The Dental Record, Wisconsin Dental Association, Milwaukee, WI.)
D
C
B
Budd, Rose L.

Fig. 26-1 Example of the patient record. (From Gaylor LJ: *The administrative dental assistant,* Philadelphia, 2000, Saunders.)

PRIVACY POLICY OF THE HEALTH INSURANCE PORTABILITY AND ACCOUNTABILITY ACT (HIPAA)

HIPAA requires that all dental practices now have a written privacy policy. This written policy must inform the patient that the office will not use or disclose protected health information (PHI) for any purpose other than treatment, diagnosis, and billing. The privacy policy must be available for patients to review, and all patients (new and existing) must sign an acknowledgment that they have received notice of the privacy practices (Fig. 26-2). The signed acknowledgment must be kept in the patient's record for a minimum of 6 years.

HIPAA states that the disclosure of documents is allowed for treatment, payment, healthcare operations, research, or public need, but additional authorization and consent forms from the patient are required.

When reviewing a health history or any specific content of a patient record, it is essential to be in private or semiprivate areas.

INITIAL PATIENT CONTACT

Interaction with a patient begins with the first phone call to the office and continues through all aspects of care provided by the dental practice. The more complete and accurate the patient record is, the more efficient and effective the communication, treatment, and quality of care will be.

The initial one-on-one contact with the patient is the first means in the information-gathering process. At this point the patient knows more about his or her own dental concerns and needs than does the dental team. The components of the patient record help identify and convey these needs and concerns of the patient to the dental team.

Information Gathering

When a patient arrives for his or her initial appointment, you may notice signs of anxiety about his or her new surroundings and new people. It is important to make sure that when patients enter into this new environment, it is friendly and stress-reducing.

HIPAA ***Privacy Statement***

All patients (new and existing) must sign an acknowledgment of receipt of notice of privacy practices. The signed acknowledgment must be kept in the patient's record for a minimum of 6 years.

Address the patient using his or her surname (Mr., Mrs., or Ms.) and introduce yourself. Whether you are obtaining a complete history or simply updating information, give the reason for the process (Fig. 26-3).

For example, with a new patient, you might say, "Ms. Stewart, welcome to the practice. For us to become aware of your needs and concerns, I would like you to take several minutes to complete these forms. If you have any questions regarding this material, please feel free to discuss them with me or any other member of our team."

Recall

5. How does a dental assistant address a patient?

PATIENT RECORD FORMS

The patient record should be designed so that it is durable, reusable, and expandable. An organized patient record is current and accurate with information needed to maintain each patient as "active" in the practice. The dentist and office manager decide on the specific forms to be used and the order in which they will be assembled in the patient record. Each staff member must follow this sequence so that the materials are easily found and accessible.

The forms described throughout the remainder of this chapter are the forms typically found in a dental patient record.

Patient Registration

The patient registration form should be kept close to the beginning of the patient record. It will contain information relating to patient **demographics** and financial responsibility (Fig. 26-4). The patient is asked to provide the following information on the **registration** form (Procedure 26-1):

- *Patient information:* Full name, date of birth, place of residence, telephone number, employment information, and spousal information
- *Insurance information:* Employee's name and date of birth; employer's name, address, and telephone number; name of insurance company and policy number
- *Responsible party:* Person responsible for payment of the account (patient, spouse, parent, and legal guardian)
- *Signature and date:* The patient verifies accuracy of information.

ACKNOWLEDGMENT OF RECEIPT OF NOTICE OF PRIVACY PRACTICES

****You May Refuse to Sign This Acknowledgment****

I, ________________________________, have received a copy of this office's Notice of Privacy Practices.

____
{Please Print Name}

____
{Signature}

____
{Date}

For Office Use Only

We attempted to obtain written acknowledgment of receipt of our Notice of Privacy Practices, but acknowledgment could not be obtained because:

☐ Individual refused to sign

☐ Communications barriers prohibited obtaining the acknowledgment

☐ An emergency situation prevented us from obtaining acknowledgment

☐ Other (Please Specify)

____

____

____

This Form is educational only, does not constitute legal advice, and covers only federal, not state, law (August 14, 2002).

Fig. 26-2 Example of an acknowledgment of privacy practices form. (Courtesy American Dental Association.)

Procedure 26-1 Registering a New Patient

Equipment and Supplies

- Registration form
- Black pen
- Clipboard

PROCEDURAL STEPS

1. Explain the need for the form to be completed. Give the registration form, along with a clipboard and black pen, to the patient to be completed.
2. Review the completed form for the necessary information:
   a. Full name, birth date, and name of spouse or parent
   b. Home address and telephone number
   c. Occupation, name of employer, business address, and telephone number
   d. Name and address of person responsible for payment
   e. Method of payment (cash, check, credit, assignment of benefits)
   f. Health insurance information (photocopy of both sides of insurance ID card)
   g. Name of primary insurance carrier
   h. Group policy number.

   Purpose: This information is necessary for processing financial arrangements and insurance claims.
3. Verify that the patient has provided a signature and date on the form.

Procedure 26-2 Obtaining a Medical-Dental Health History

Equipment and Supplies

- Medical-dental health history form
- Black pen
- Clipboard

PROCEDURAL STEPS

1. Explain the need for the information and the importance of fully completing the form.
2. Provide the patient with a black pen and the form on a clipboard.
3. Offer assistance to the patient in completing the form.

   Purpose: The patient may not understand the terminology or may have a language barrier.
4. Ask the patient to return the form and clipboard to you after answering all the questions.
5. Thank the patient for completing the form, and request that the patient take a seat in the reception area.
6. Review the form for errors and/or any questions that may arise before handing it to the clinical assistant.
7. Use information from the patient's medical-dental health history form to complete other documents. Remember that the information provided to you by the patient is confidential and must be maintained as such.

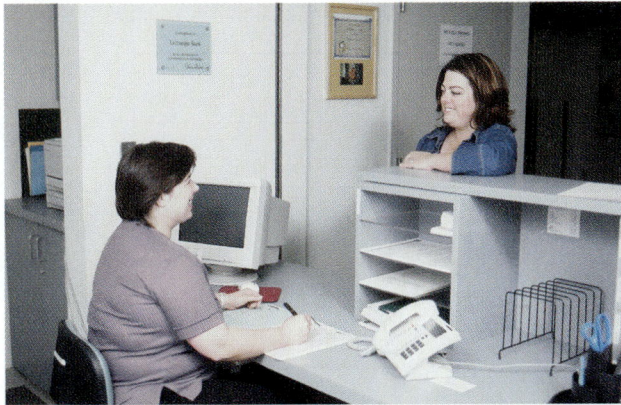

Fig. 26-3 Business assistant reviewing a patient's health history form with a new patient.

Recall

6. Where should the patient registration form be placed in a patient record?
7. To verify that the information is accurate, a patient must provide what on the form?

Medical-Dental Health History

Every patient that sees the dentist must complete a medical-dental health history form (Fig. 26-5 and Procedure 26-2). A written health history form is regarded as minimal information. The responsibility of the dental team is to review the form and initiate additional conversation and

Text continued on p. 403

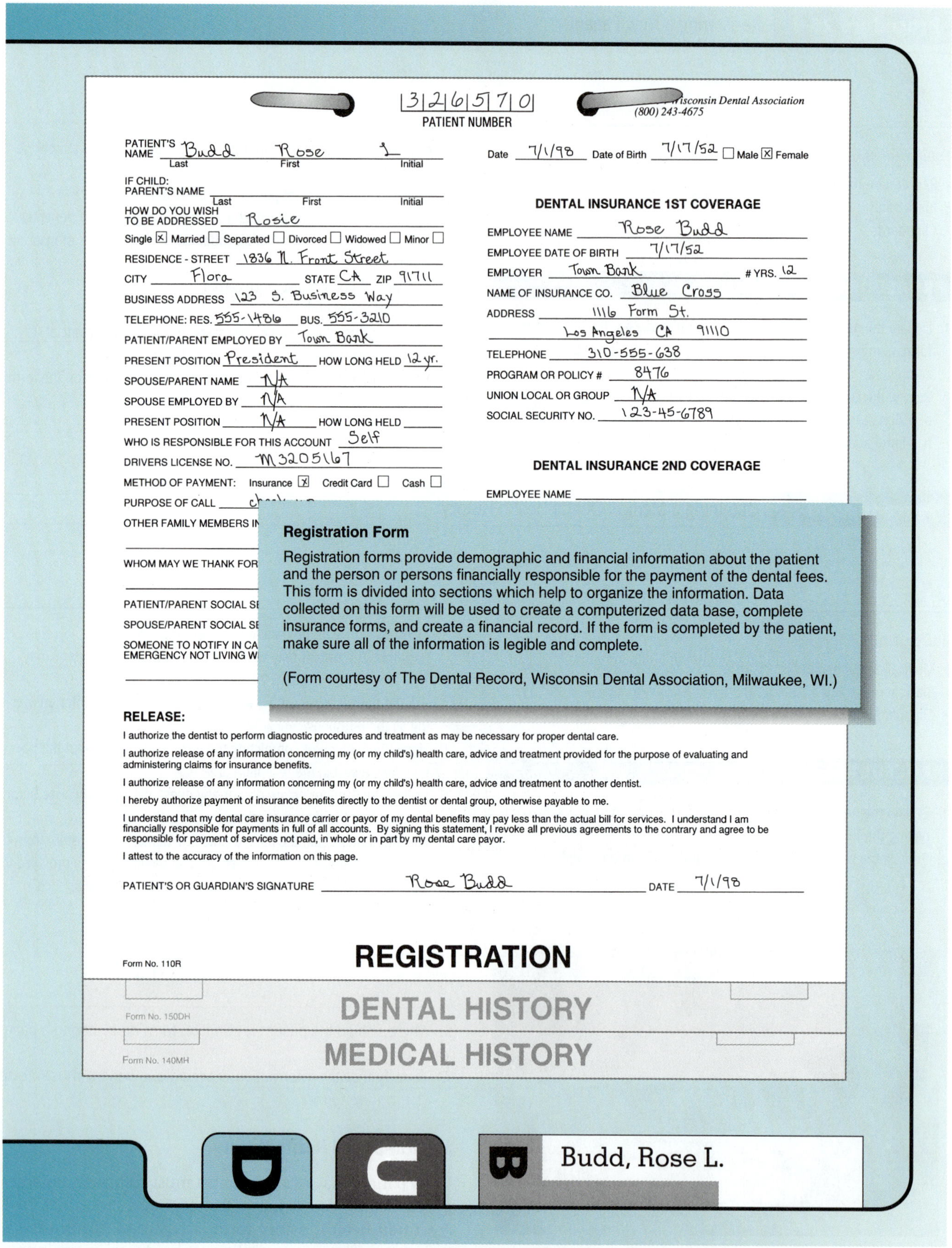

3 2 6 5 7 0
PATIENT NUMBER

Wisconsin Dental Association
(800) 243-4675

PATIENT'S NAME Budd (Last) Rose (First) L (Initial)

Date 7/1/98 Date of Birth 7/17/52 ☐ Male ☒ Female

IF CHILD: PARENT'S NAME ______ Last First Initial

HOW DO YOU WISH TO BE ADDRESSED Rosie

Single ☒ Married ☐ Separated ☐ Divorced ☐ Widowed ☐ Minor ☐

RESIDENCE - STREET 1836 N. Front Street

CITY Flora STATE CA ZIP 91711

BUSINESS ADDRESS 123 S. Business Way

TELEPHONE: RES. 555-1486 BUS. 555-3210

PATIENT/PARENT EMPLOYED BY Town Bank

PRESENT POSITION President HOW LONG HELD 12 yr.

SPOUSE/PARENT NAME N/A

SPOUSE EMPLOYED BY N/A

PRESENT POSITION N/A HOW LONG HELD ______

WHO IS RESPONSIBLE FOR THIS ACCOUNT Self

DRIVERS LICENSE NO. M3205167

METHOD OF PAYMENT: Insurance ☒ Credit Card ☐ Cash ☐

PURPOSE OF CALL checkup

OTHER FAMILY MEMBERS IN

WHOM MAY WE THANK FOR

PATIENT/PARENT SOCIAL SE

SPOUSE/PARENT SOCIAL SE

SOMEONE TO NOTIFY IN CA EMERGENCY NOT LIVING W

DENTAL INSURANCE 1ST COVERAGE

EMPLOYEE NAME Rose Budd

EMPLOYEE DATE OF BIRTH 7/17/52

EMPLOYER Town Bank # YRS. 12

NAME OF INSURANCE CO. Blue Cross

ADDRESS 1116 Form St.
Los Angeles CA 91110

TELEPHONE 310-555-638

PROGRAM OR POLICY # 8476

UNION LOCAL OR GROUP N/A

SOCIAL SECURITY NO. 123-45-6789

DENTAL INSURANCE 2ND COVERAGE

EMPLOYEE NAME ______

Registration Form

Registration forms provide demographic and financial information about the patient and the person or persons financially responsible for the payment of the dental fees. This form is divided into sections which help to organize the information. Data collected on this form will be used to create a computerized data base, complete insurance forms, and create a financial record. If the form is completed by the patient, make sure all of the information is legible and complete.

(Form courtesy of The Dental Record, Wisconsin Dental Association, Milwaukee, WI.)

RELEASE:

I authorize the dentist to perform diagnostic procedures and treatment as may be necessary for proper dental care.

I authorize release of any information concerning my (or my child's) health care, advice and treatment provided for the purpose of evaluating and administering claims for insurance benefits.

I authorize release of any information concerning my (or my child's) health care, advice and treatment to another dentist.

I hereby authorize payment of insurance benefits directly to the dentist or dental group, otherwise payable to me.

I understand that my dental care insurance carrier or payor of my dental benefits may pay less than the actual bill for services. I understand I am financially responsible for payments in full of all accounts. By signing this statement, I revoke all previous agreements to the contrary and agree to be responsible for payment of services not paid, in whole or in part by my dental care payor.

I attest to the accuracy of the information on this page.

PATIENT'S OR GUARDIAN'S SIGNATURE Rose Budd DATE 7/1/98

Form No. 110R **REGISTRATION**

Form No. 150DH **DENTAL HISTORY**

Form No. 140MH **MEDICAL HISTORY**

D C B Budd, Rose L.

Fig. 26-4 **Example of a patient registration form.** (From Gaylor LJ: *The administrative dental assistant*, Philadelphia, 2000, Saunders.)

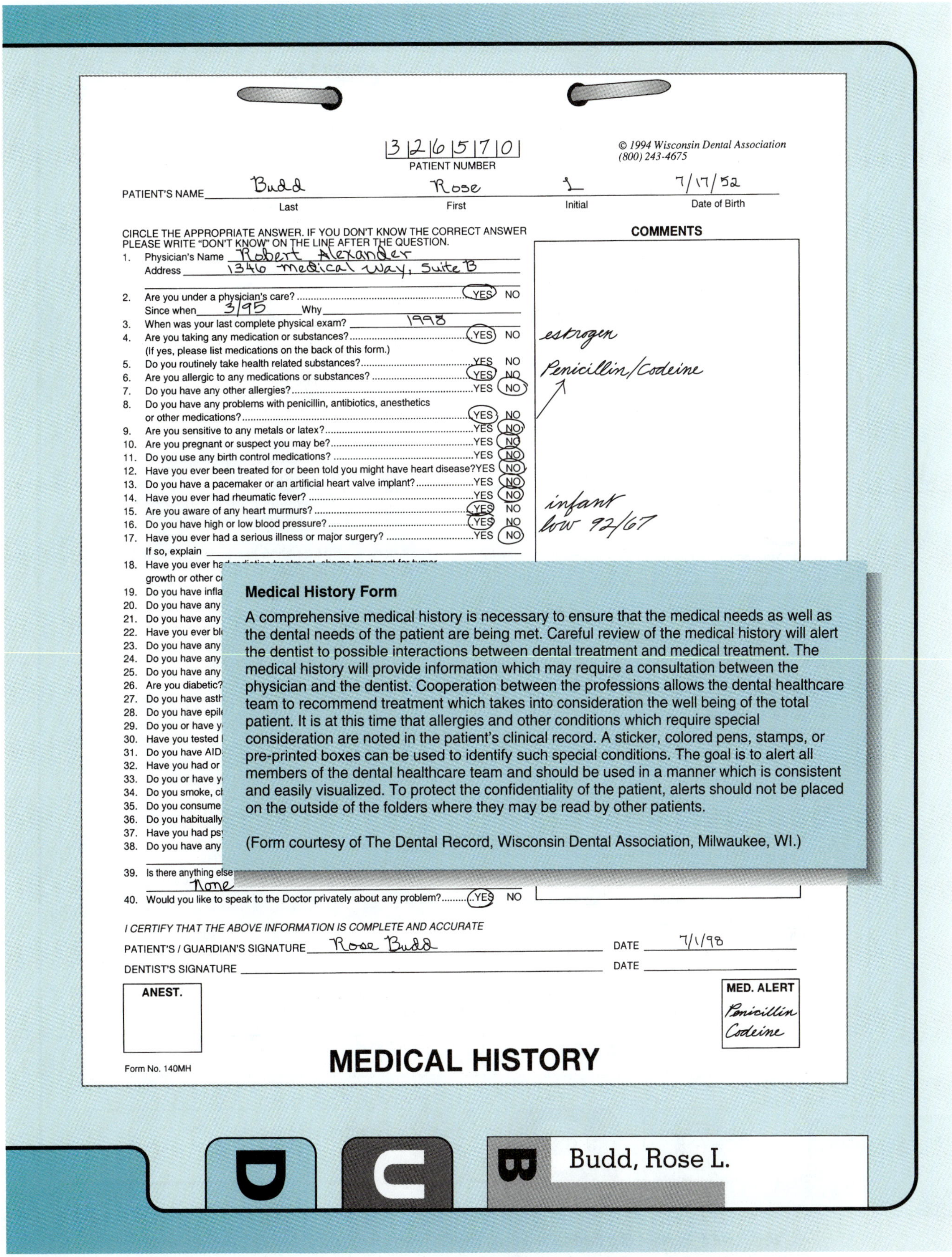

3 2 6 5 7 0
PATIENT NUMBER

© 1994 Wisconsin Dental Association
(800) 243-4675

PATIENT'S NAME Budd (Last) Rose (First) L (Initial) 7/17/52 (Date of Birth)

CIRCLE THE APPROPRIATE ANSWER. IF YOU DON'T KNOW THE CORRECT ANSWER PLEASE WRITE "DON'T KNOW" ON THE LINE AFTER THE QUESTION.

1. Physician's Name Robert Alexander
   Address 1346 Medical Way, Suite B
2. Are you under a physician's care? **YES** NO
   Since when 3/95 Why
3. When was your last complete physical exam? 1998
4. Are you taking any medication or substances? **YES** NO — estrogen
   (If yes, please list medications on the back of this form.)
5. Do you routinely take health related substances? YES NO
6. Are you allergic to any medications or substances? **YES** NO — Penicillin/Codeine
7. Do you have any other allergies? YES **NO**
8. Do you have any problems with penicillin, antibiotics, anesthetics or other medications? **YES** NO
9. Are you sensitive to any metals or latex? YES **NO**
10. Are you pregnant or suspect you may be? YES **NO**
11. Do you use any birth control medications? YES **NO**
12. Have you ever been treated for or been told you might have heart disease? YES **NO**
13. Do you have a pacemaker or an artificial heart valve implant? YES **NO**
14. Have you ever had rheumatic fever? YES **NO**
15. Are you aware of any heart murmurs? **YES** NO — infant
16. Do you have high or low blood pressure? **YES** NO — low 92/67
17. Have you ever had a serious illness or major surgery? YES **NO**
    If so, explain
18. Have you ever ha… growth or other c…
19. Do you have infla…
20. Do you have any…
21. Do you have any…
22. Have you ever bl…
23. Do you have any…
24. Do you have any…
25. Do you have any…
26. Are you diabetic?…
27. Do you have asth…
28. Do you have epil…
29. Do you or have y…
30. Have you tested…
31. Do you have AID…
32. Have you had or…
33. Do you or have y…
34. Do you smoke, c…
35. Do you consume…
36. Do you habitually…
37. Have you had ps…
38. Do you have any…
39. Is there anything else… None
40. Would you like to speak to the Doctor privately about any problem? **YES** NO

COMMENTS

I CERTIFY THAT THE ABOVE INFORMATION IS COMPLETE AND ACCURATE

PATIENT'S / GUARDIAN'S SIGNATURE Rose Budd DATE 7/1/98

DENTIST'S SIGNATURE DATE

ANEST.

MED. ALERT Penicillin Codeine

Form No. 140MH

MEDICAL HISTORY

Medical History Form

A comprehensive medical history is necessary to ensure that the medical needs as well as the dental needs of the patient are being met. Careful review of the medical history will alert the dentist to possible interactions between dental treatment and medical treatment. The medical history will provide information which may require a consultation between the physician and the dentist. Cooperation between the professions allows the dental healthcare team to recommend treatment which takes into consideration the well being of the total patient. It is at this time that allergies and other conditions which require special consideration are noted in the patient's clinical record. A sticker, colored pens, stamps, or pre-printed boxes can be used to identify such special conditions. The goal is to alert all members of the dental healthcare team and should be used in a manner which is consistent and easily visualized. To protect the confidentiality of the patient, alerts should not be placed on the outside of the folders where they may be read by other patients.

(Form courtesy of The Dental Record, Wisconsin Dental Association, Milwaukee, WI.)

D C B Budd, Rose L.

Fig. 26-5 **Example of a medical and dental health history form.** (From Gaylor LJ: *The administrative dental assistant,* Philadelphia, 2000, Saunders.)

continued

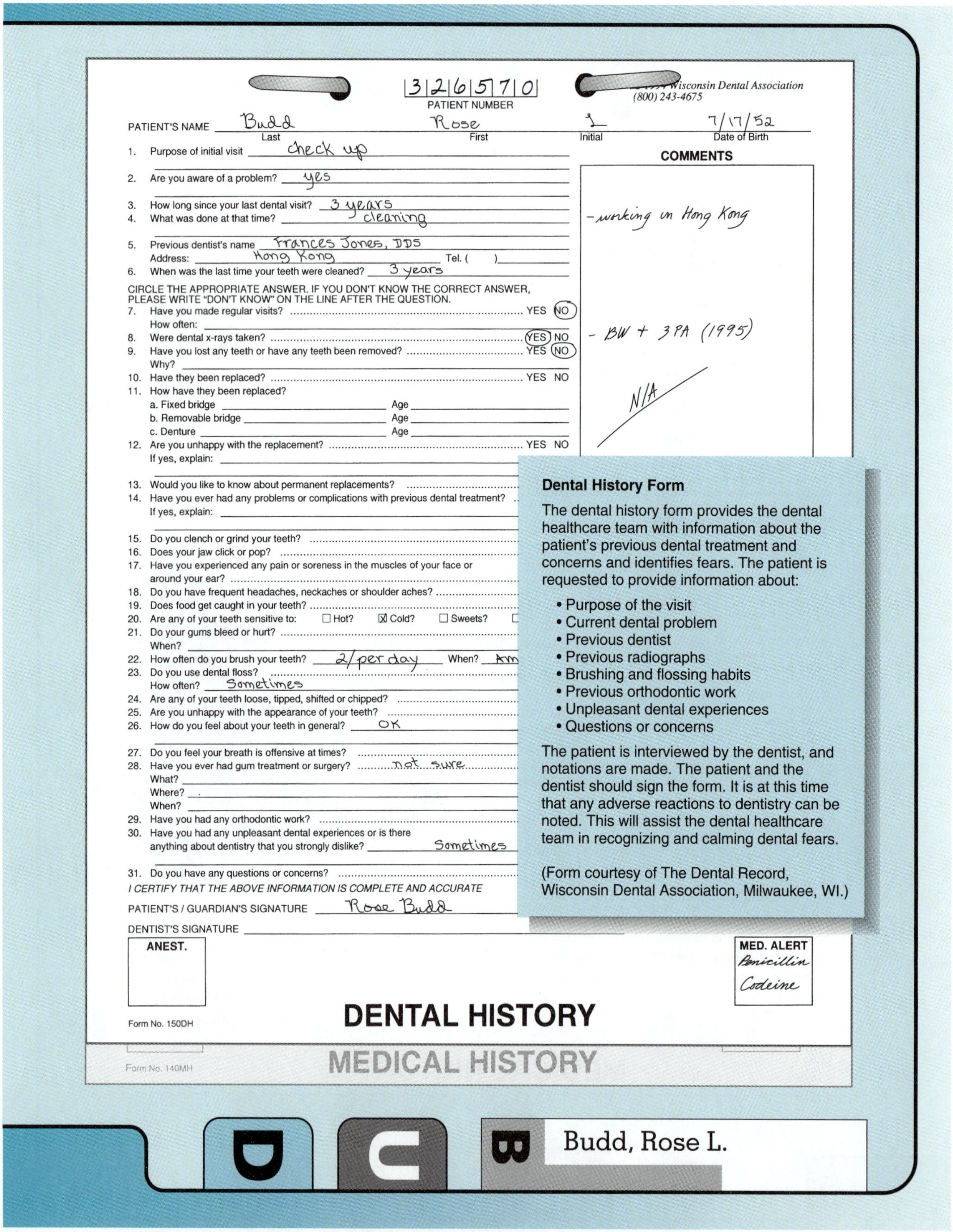

Wisconsin Dental Association
(800) 243-4675

3 2 6 5 7 0
PATIENT NUMBER

PATIENT'S NAME Budd (Last) Rose (First) L (Initial) 7/17/52 (Date of Birth)

1. Purpose of initial visit check up
2. Are you aware of a problem? yes
3. How long since your last dental visit? 3 years
4. What was done at that time? cleaning
5. Previous dentist's name Frances Jones, DDS
   Address: Hong Kong Tel. ( )
6. When was the last time your teeth were cleaned? 3 years

CIRCLE THE APPROPRIATE ANSWER. IF YOU DON'T KNOW THE CORRECT ANSWER, PLEASE WRITE "DON'T KNOW" ON THE LINE AFTER THE QUESTION.

7. Have you made regular visits? YES (NO)
   How often:
8. Were dental x-rays taken? (YES) NO
9. Have you lost any teeth or have any teeth been removed? YES (NO)
   Why?
10. Have they been replaced? YES NO
11. How have they been replaced?
   a. Fixed bridge Age
   b. Removable bridge Age
   c. Denture Age
12. Are you unhappy with the replacement? YES NO
   If yes, explain:
13. Would you like to know about permanent replacements?
14. Have you ever had any problems or complications with previous dental treatment?
   If yes, explain:
15. Do you clench or grind your teeth?
16. Does your jaw click or pop?
17. Have you experienced any pain or soreness in the muscles of your face or around your ear?
18. Do you have frequent headaches, neckaches or shoulder aches?
19. Does food get caught in your teeth?
20. Are any of your teeth sensitive to: ☐ Hot? ☒ Cold? ☐ Sweets? ☐
21. Do your gums bleed or hurt?
   When?
22. How often do you brush your teeth? 2/per day When? Am
23. Do you use dental floss?
   How often? Sometimes
24. Are any of your teeth loose, tipped, shifted or chipped?
25. Are you unhappy with the appearance of your teeth?
26. How do you feel about your teeth in general? OK
27. Do you feel your breath is offensive at times?
28. Have you ever had gum treatment or surgery? not sure
   What?
   Where?
   When?
29. Have you had any orthodontic work?
30. Have you had any unpleasant dental experiences or is there anything about dentistry that you strongly dislike? Sometimes
31. Do you have any questions or concerns?

I CERTIFY THAT THE ABOVE INFORMATION IS COMPLETE AND ACCURATE

PATIENT'S / GUARDIAN'S SIGNATURE Rose Budd

DENTIST'S SIGNATURE

COMMENTS

- working in Hong Kong

- BW + 3PA (1995)

N/A

ANEST.

MED. ALERT
Penicillin
Codeine

Form No. 150DH

DENTAL HISTORY

Form No. 140MH

MEDICAL HISTORY

D C B Budd, Rose L.

Dental History Form

The dental history form provides the dental healthcare team with information about the patient's previous dental treatment and concerns and identifies fears. The patient is requested to provide information about:

- Purpose of the visit
- Current dental problem
- Previous dentist
- Previous radiographs
- Brushing and flossing habits
- Previous orthodontic work
- Unpleasant dental experiences
- Questions or concerns

The patient is interviewed by the dentist, and notations are made. The patient and the dentist should sign the form. It is at this time that any adverse reactions to dentistry can be noted. This will assist the dental healthcare team in recognizing and calming dental fears.

(Form courtesy of The Dental Record, Wisconsin Dental Association, Milwaukee, WI.)

Fig. 26-5, cont'd Example of a medical and dental health history form. (From Gaylor LJ: *The administrative dental assistant,* Philadelphia, 2000, Saunders.)

questions to gain more insight about the patient. Once the form is completed, the patient completing the form or the patient's legal guardian must sign and date the form. The health history form is divided into medical assessment and dental assessment sections.

Medical History

The medical history section includes questions regarding the patient's past medical history, present physical condition, **chronic** conditions, allergies, and current medications. This information (1) alerts the dentist to possible medical conditions and medications that may complicate or interfere with dental treatment, and (2) aids the dentist in anticipating potential medical emergencies and identifying special treatment needs.

The dentist may also want to consult with the patient's physician regarding health concerns. The patient must sign a release-of-information form, giving consent before a consultation can take place.

Dental History

The dental history section of the form is used to obtain information about the patient's previous dental treatment and care. By asking certain questions about oral home care and previous dental experiences, the dental team can gain insight into the patient's feelings toward dentistry and information about the patient's own dental care.

Recall

8. What does the dental history section of the form provide for the dentist?

Medical Alert

When you receive a completed medical-dental health history form, one of your first priorities is to review indications of health conditions, allergic reactions, and medications that could interfere with or be life-threatening to the patient during dental treatment. An example of this would be an allergy to penicillin. The dental team would then promptly know that this patient cannot be prescribed penicillin.

On the inside cover of the patient record, medical **alerts** and other precautions that need to be followed should be noted to provide safe care to the patient (Fig. 26-6). When you receive this information, affix an "alert" sticker to the patient record on the inside cover of the patient record. By placing this inside the record, you are maintaining dentist-patient confidentiality. The alert sticker should never be placed on the outside cover.

Medical-Dental Health History Update

All patients returning for additional appointments are asked to update their medical-dental health history (Fig. 26-7). Even if a patient was seen by the dentist 3 weeks ago, the dentist would not be aware of any changes to a patient's medication regimen or medical diagnosis if it was not updated. A slight change in a medical condition could cause a reaction when receiving anesthesia or pain control methods used by the dentist. The patient's initial medical-dental health history form should be given to the patient for review. If there are any changes, a patient should record these on an additional form or a separate line in the treatment section of the patient record. The patient or parent/guardian must either indicate in writing "no change" or write in any appropriate changes in health status. The patient is then instructed to sign and date the form to indicate that the information is accurate and up to date.

Recall

9. What is an example of a medical alert?

Clinical Examination

The clinical examination form is the most detailed section in the patient record (Fig. 26-8). This form provides the dental team with past, present, and future examination data, analysis, and charting needs of the patient. This form is completed for every new patient that enters the practice, as well as at every successive appointment.

A dentist will examine the patient and dictate the findings to the dental assistant to record. Specific areas on the clinical examination form include the following (see Chapter 28 for detailed explanations of charting symbols):

- Patient's name and date of examination
- Charting system of existing restorations and present conditions
- Charting system of periodontal conditions
- Patient's chief complaint
- Occlusal evaluations
- Temporomandibular joint (TMJ) evaluations
- Comments

Specific guidelines must be followed for proper patient record management.

Treatment Plan

Once the dentist reviews the medical-dental health history form and dictates any charting or updates for the clinical

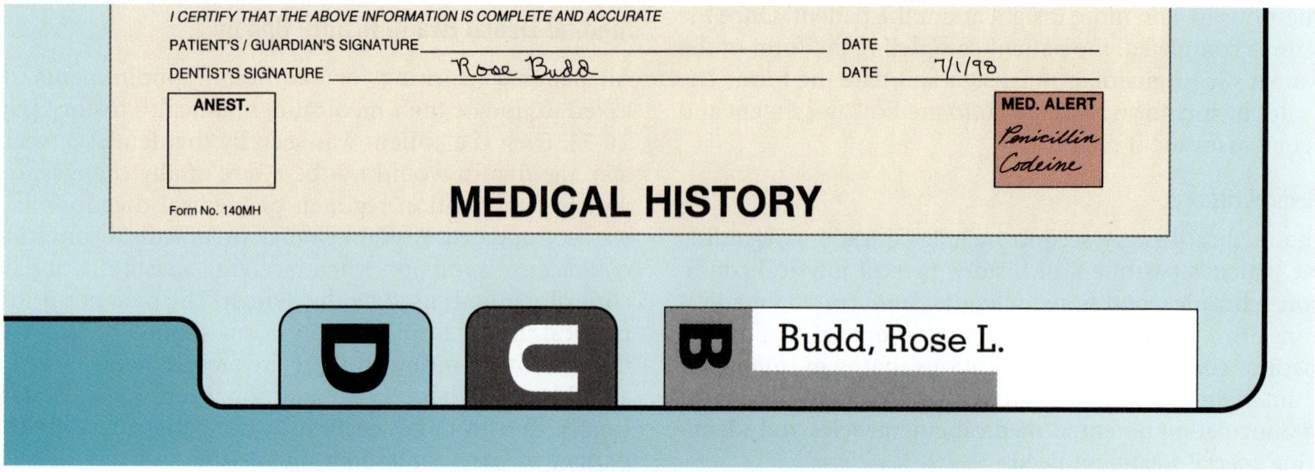

Fig. 26-6 **Always document a medical alert on the inside of the patient record *(red box).*** (From Gaylor LJ: *The administrative dental assistant,* Philadelphia, 2000, Saunders.)

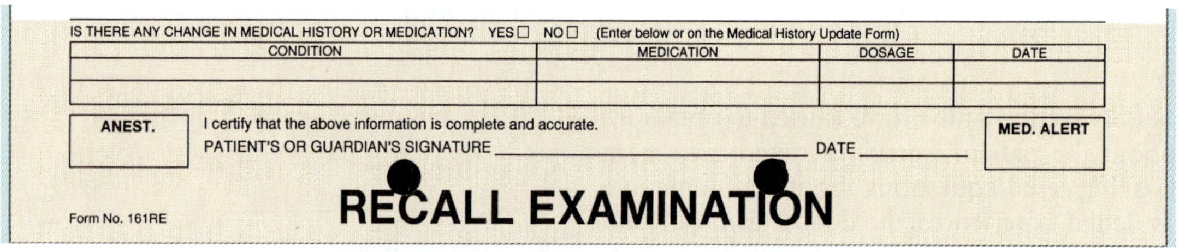

Fig. 26-7 **Example of the medical-dental health history update form *(yellow box).* Medical history update must be easily accessible.** (From Gaylor LJ: *The administrative dental assistant,* Philadelphia, 2000, Saunders.)

examination form, the dentist then records the plan of care on the treatment plan (Fig. 26-9). The treatment plan for a patient is properly sequenced to address all problems that were identified during the examination and diagnosis portion of the patient visit.

The treatment plan may need to change if financial arrangements become a factor. For example, a patient's treatment plan indicating the need for a fixed bridge might change if the patient has limited income and cannot afford the cost of a bridge. A second option of making a removable partial would then be discussed with the patient to meet the financial needs.

Progress Notes

The progress notes section of the record is where treatment is recorded (Fig. 26-10). Specific areas that should be noted on this form include the following:

- *Date:* This shows the month/day/year of treatment.
- *Tooth number:* If a specific tooth is being treated, it should be indicated by number in this section. This information provides faster reference to previous appointments.
- *Treatment:* This section of the form must be filled out completely and accurately. This written documentation is the only reference regarding treatment. All entries must be precise and legible. Following each entry, the dentist and dental assistant or the dentist and dental hygienist must sign and date the entry.

Informed Consent

The informed consent form is related to a specific treatment or procedure (Fig. 26-11). This document provides the patient with the expected outcomes of treatment and describes possible complications. These individualized forms are more commonly used when invasive or extensive treatment is required; examples of treatment may include surgical procedures, orthodontics, endodontics, periodontics, and implants.

The dentist should review the treatment plan with the patient and address any questions or concerns. Once both parties have agreed, the patient, dentist, and a witness must sign and date the forms.

Recall

10. What form in the patient record would provide knowledge to the dental team of an existing restoration?

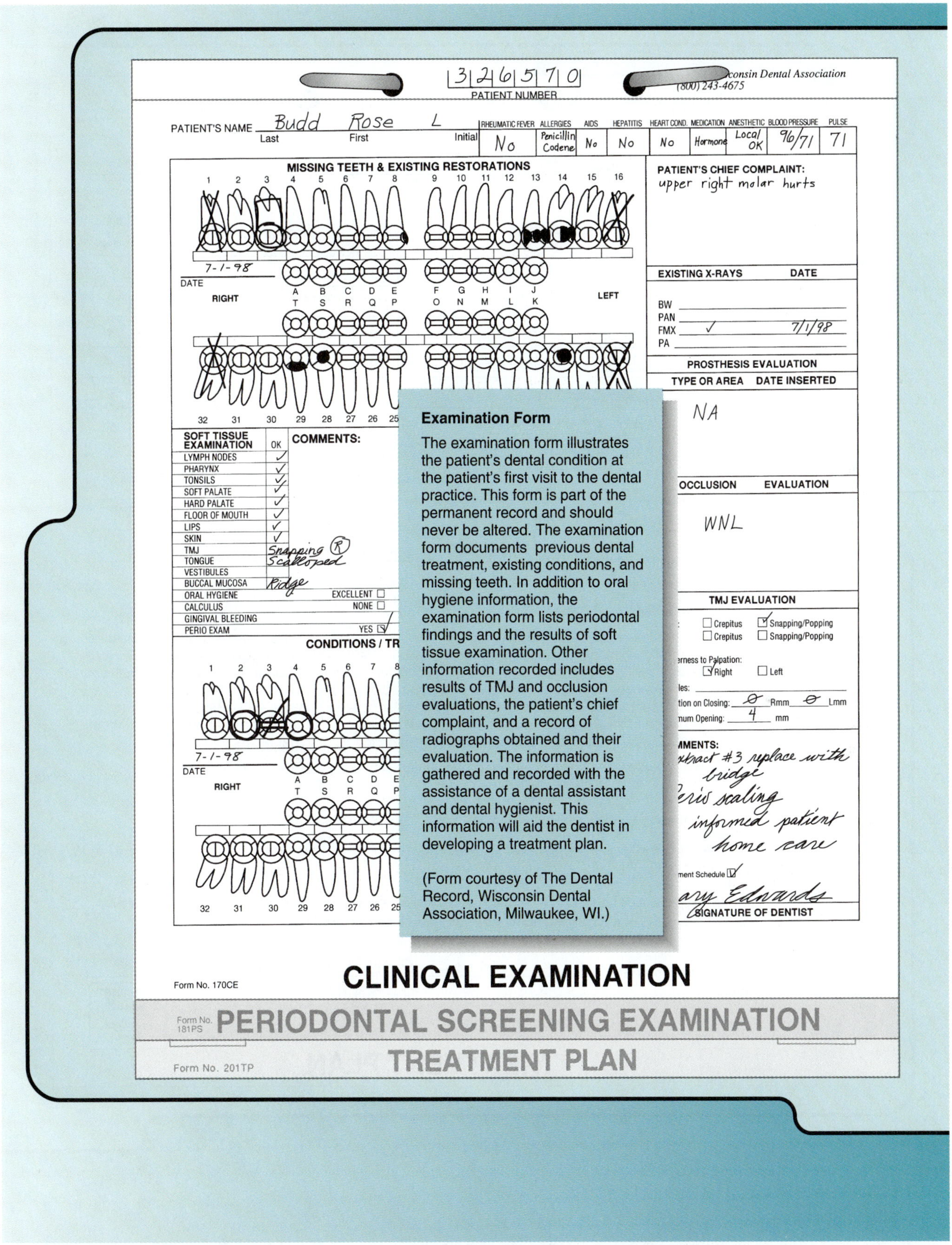

Examination Form

The examination form illustrates the patient's dental condition at the patient's first visit to the dental practice. This form is part of the permanent record and should never be altered. The examination form documents previous dental treatment, existing conditions, and missing teeth. In addition to oral hygiene information, the examination form lists periodontal findings and the results of soft tissue examination. Other information recorded includes results of TMJ and occlusion evaluations, the patient's chief complaint, and a record of radiographs obtained and their evaluation. The information is gathered and recorded with the assistance of a dental assistant and dental hygienist. This information will aid the dentist in developing a treatment plan.

(Form courtesy of The Dental Record, Wisconsin Dental Association, Milwaukee, WI.)

Fig. 26-8 **Example of a clinical examination form.** (From Gaylor LJ: *The administrative dental assistant,* Philadelphia, 2000, Saunders.)

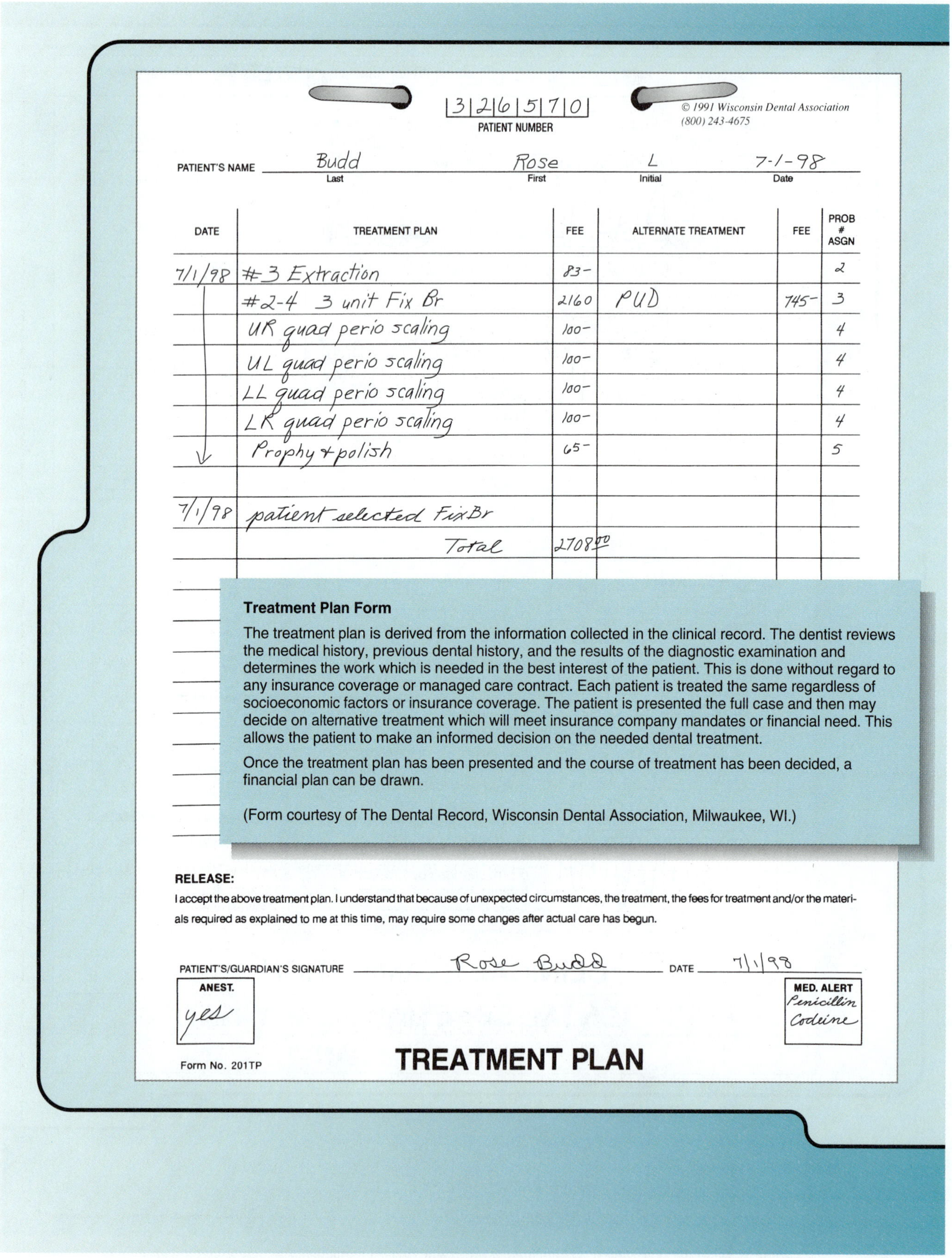

|3|2|6|5|7|0|
PATIENT NUMBER

© 1991 Wisconsin Dental Association
(800) 243-4675

PATIENT'S NAME Budd (Last) Rose (First) L (Initial) 7-1-98 (Date)

DATE	TREATMENT PLAN	FEE	ALTERNATE TREATMENT	FEE	PROB # ASGN
7/1/98	#3 Extraction	83-			2
	#2-4 3 unit Fix Br	2160	PUD	745-	3
	UR quad perio scaling	100-			4
	UL quad perio scaling	100-			4
	LL quad perio scaling	100-			4
	LR quad perio scaling	100-			4
↓	Prophy + polish	65-			5
7/1/98	patient selected FixBr				
	Total	2708.00			

Treatment Plan Form

The treatment plan is derived from the information collected in the clinical record. The dentist reviews the medical history, previous dental history, and the results of the diagnostic examination and determines the work which is needed in the best interest of the patient. This is done without regard to any insurance coverage or managed care contract. Each patient is treated the same regardless of socioeconomic factors or insurance coverage. The patient is presented the full case and then may decide on alternative treatment which will meet insurance company mandates or financial need. This allows the patient to make an informed decision on the needed dental treatment.

Once the treatment plan has been presented and the course of treatment has been decided, a financial plan can be drawn.

(Form courtesy of The Dental Record, Wisconsin Dental Association, Milwaukee, WI.)

RELEASE:

I accept the above treatment plan. I understand that because of unexpected circumstances, the treatment, the fees for treatment and/or the materials required as explained to me at this time, may require some changes after actual care has begun.

PATIENT'S/GUARDIAN'S SIGNATURE Rose Budd DATE 7/1/98

ANEST. yes

MED. ALERT Penicillin Codeine

Form No. 201TP

TREATMENT PLAN

Fig. 26-9 **Example of a treatment plan form.** (From Gaylor LJ: *The administrative dental assistant,* Philadelphia, 2000, Saunders.)

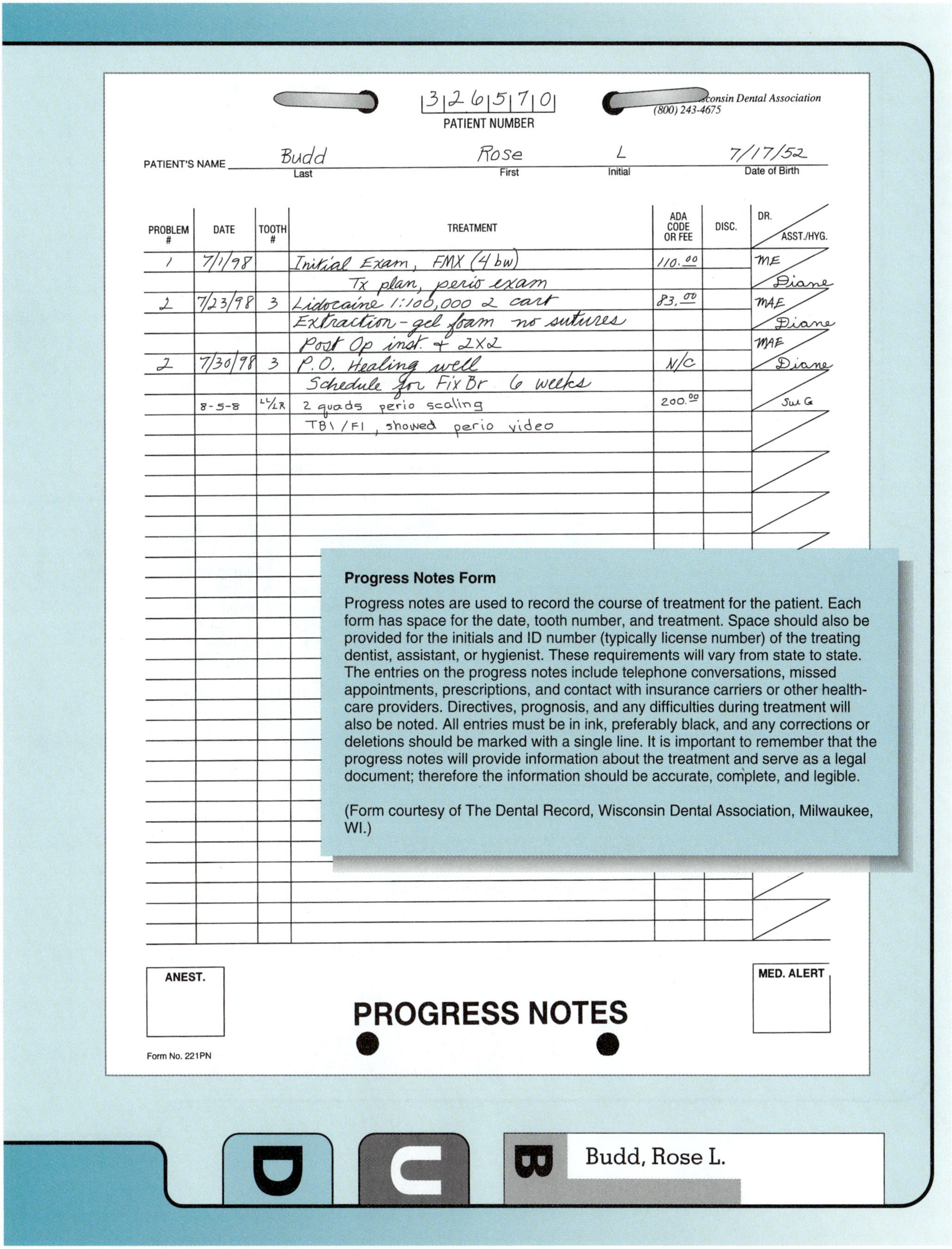

Wisconsin Dental Association
(800) 243-4675

3 2 6 5 7 0
PATIENT NUMBER

PATIENT'S NAME Budd (Last) Rose (First) L (Initial) 7/17/52 (Date of Birth)

PROBLEM #	DATE	TOOTH #	TREATMENT	ADA CODE OR FEE	DISC.	DR. / ASST./HYG.
1	7/1/98		Initial Exam, FMX (4 bw)	110.00		ME
			Tx plan, perio exam			Diane
2	7/23/98	3	Lidocaine 1:100,000 2 cart	83.00		MAE
			Extraction - gel foam no sutures			Diane
			Post Op inst. + 2X2			MAE
2	7/30/98	3	P.O. Healing well	N/C		Diane
			Schedule for Fix Br 6 weeks			
	8-5-8	LL/LR	2 quads perio scaling	200.00		Sue G
			TBI/FI, showed perio video			

ANEST.

MED. ALERT

PROGRESS NOTES

Form No. 221PN

Budd, Rose L.

Progress Notes Form

Progress notes are used to record the course of treatment for the patient. Each form has space for the date, tooth number, and treatment. Space should also be provided for the initials and ID number (typically license number) of the treating dentist, assistant, or hygienist. These requirements will vary from state to state. The entries on the progress notes include telephone conversations, missed appointments, prescriptions, and contact with insurance carriers or other health-care providers. Directives, prognosis, and any difficulties during treatment will also be noted. All entries must be in ink, preferably black, and any corrections or deletions should be marked with a single line. It is important to remember that the progress notes will provide information about the treatment and serve as a legal document; therefore the information should be accurate, complete, and legible.

(Form courtesy of The Dental Record, Wisconsin Dental Association, Milwaukee, WI.)

Fig. 26-10 **Example of a progress notes form.** (From Gaylor LJ: *The administrative dental assistant,* Philadelphia, 2000, Saunders.)

| 3 | 2 | 6 | 5 | 7 | 0 |

PATIENT NUMBER

PATIENT'S NAME Budd (Last) Rose (First) L (Initial) 7/17/52 (Date of Birth)

I hereby authorize Mary A. Edwards, DDS (DOCTOR'S NAME)

and whomever he/she may designate as his/her assistants, to perform upon me the following operation and/or procedures:

Extraction - #3
Fixed PFM Bridge — #2- #4
Four quadrants of perio scaling

I request and authorize him/her to do whatever he/she deems advisable if any unforeseen condition arises in the course of these designated operations and/or procedures calling, in their judgment, for procedures in addition to or different from those now contemplated.

I consent to the above treatment after having been advised of the risks, advantages and disadvantages of the treatments and the consequences if this treatment were withheld.

I consent to the above treatment plan after having been advised of the alternate plans of treatment available and the known material risks, advantages and disadvantages of the alternative treatment.

I further consent t… drugs that may be deem… the administration of any… cardiac arrest, and aspir… injury to blood vessels…

I am informed and f… In oral surgery, the mos… discomfort, stiff jaws, lo… loss or injury to adjacent… fractures, sinus exposur… ing in the jaw which mig…

I realize that in spit… sary and desired by me… acknowledge that no gu…

I have provided as… ics, drugs, medications… directed to me and permi…

Consent Form

This form outlines the work that will be done and describes reasonable results and alerts the patient to complications which could result from treatment. It also explains the responsibility the patient assumes in assuring that the treatment will be successful. The use of consent forms allows the patient to ask questions about the treatment and helps establish a partnership between the patient and the dental healthcare team. It is believed that these forms and the signatures help to reduce the number of malpractice suits. These forms should be designed with the assistance of an attorney who will check the form for legal content.

(Form courtesy of The Dental Record, Wisconsin Dental Association, Milwaukee, WI.)

I have had the opportunity to ask questions and receive answers to and responsive explanations for, all questions about my medical condition, contemplated and alternative treatment and procedures, and the risk and potential complications of the contemplated and alternative treatments and procedures, prior to signing this form.

Patient or Guardian's Signature Rose Budd Date 7/1/98

Dentist's Signature M Edwards Date 7/1/98

Witness's Signature Diane Feller Date 7/1/98

Form No. 243CF **CONSENT FORM**

Form 250SF **SIGNATURE ON FILE**

Form 260FA **FINANCIAL ARRANGEMENTS**

Form No. 231CL **CORRESPONDENCE LOG**

Fig. 26-11 Example of the informed consent form. (From Gaylor LJ: *The administrative dental assistant,* Philadelphia, 2000, Saunders.)

Standards and Criteria for Record-Keeping

All entries must be dated, legible, and completed in *black* ink.

The individual who documents the information must sign all entries.

Inaccurate entries should never be corrected by use of correction fluid or other methods of "blocking out" the original entry. Crossing through an entry should be done only to make corrections of errors in documentation and should be marked with a single line followed by the initials of the individual correcting the entry.

The patient's response to treatment (outcomes) should be routinely recorded.

All appointment cancellations, broken appointments, late arrivals, and changes of appointments should be documented, whether patient- or provider-generated.

All conversations with the patient or with other healthcare providers relating to the patient should be documented.

Evaluations and statements of "opinion" that the dentist is not professionally qualified to make should not be documented in the record (e.g., patient's mental health status). For example, instead of "Suspected drug abuser," document that "Patient requested narcotic meds after routine simple restorative procedure."

All individuals having access to the patient record must maintain the confidentiality of the information contained in the document. Information in the record may not be shared with anyone outside of the healthcare team without the patient's written authorization.

A patient's record must never be altered once there is a possibility of legal action by the patient.

The patient's treatment record is the property of the dentist and may not be removed from the dental practice. Original records and radiographs may not be given to anyone except through a court order.

Patients have a right to the information contained within their record and are entitled to receive a copy of their record. Release of a copy of the record, either in part or in its entirety, to anyone requires a written request from the patient.

Legal and Ethical Implications

The patient record is the most confidential document that exists between the dentist and the patient. The information that is shared between the dental healthcare team and the patient is private and must remain private.

The dental assistant must not share patient information, specific treatments, or patient discussions with anyone. Information discussed outside the office and then reported could have serious consequences for the dentist, the assistant, and the entire practice. All members of the dental team should be familiar with HIPAA.

Eye to the Future

The introduction of computer software specific to dentistry has minimized the use of the traditional patient record. Dental practices have switched to computerized patient records because of the advantage of storing more clinical information in less space with greater security than that offered by papers in a patient record. The computerized format virtually eliminates the problems of losing or misfiling a patient record.

The computerized record also can be displayed simultaneously on computer terminals in the business office and in the clinical area. The dentist has the option to review a printout of only the most important information pertaining to the patient's treatment plan.

Critical Thinking

1. What would make a document *not* legal in a court of law?
2. You are on the phone with a patient's insurance company. What form would you retrieve from the patient record to change insurance information?
3. How often should a patient update his or her medical-dental history?
4. What form would you use to chart existing restorations and present conditions?
5. How would you make a correction in the patient's progress notes?

27

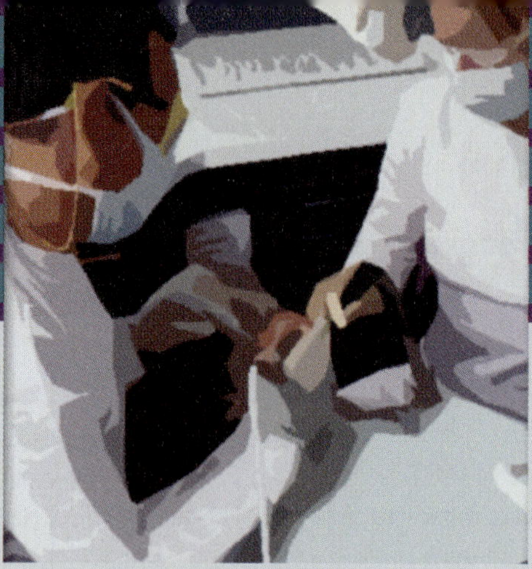

Vital Signs

Outline

KEY TERMS

Antecubital space (*an*-teh-**ku**-bi-tul) Small groove or fold in the inner arm, at or "in front of" *(ante)* the elbow *(cubitus).*

Arrhythmia (a-**rith**-me-a) Irregularity in the force or rhythm of the heartbeat.

Blood pressure (BP) Pressure exerted by the blood against the walls of the blood vessels.

Brachial (**bray**-kee-ahl) Relating to the arm *(brachium),* as in *brachial artery.*

Carotid (ka-**rot**-id) Relating to either of the two major arteries on each side of the neck that carry blood to the head.

Depth In respiration, the amount of air in a breath.

Diastolic (*di*-a-**stahl**-ik) Normal rhythmic relaxation and dilation of the heart chambers.

Electrocardiogram (e-*lek*-tro-**kahr**-de-o-*gram*) Instrument used in the detection and diagnosis of heart abnormalities. It generates a record of the electrical currents associated with heart muscle activity.

Korotkoff sounds (keh-**rot**-kof) Specific sounds heard when taking a blood pressure.

Metabolism (meh-**tab**-eh-*liz*-um) Physical and chemical processes that occur within a living cell or organism and are necessary for the maintenance of life.

Palpate (**pal**-pate) To examine or explore by touching.

Pulse Rhythmic throbbing of the arteries produced by the regular contractions of the heart.

Radial Relating to the radius (bone) or forearm *(antebrachium),* as in *radial artery.*

Rate A quantity measured, as in breaths and heartbeats.

Respiration Act or process of inhaling and exhaling; breathing.

Rhythm A sequence or pattern, as the heartbeat or breathing.

Sphygmomanometer (*sfig*-mo-ma-**nom**-eh-tur) Instrument for measuring blood pressure in the arteries.

Stethoscope Instrument used for listening to sounds produced within the body.

Systolic (sis-**tahl**-ik, sis-**tah**-lik) Rhythmic contraction of the heart, especially of the ventricles.

Temperature Degree of hotness or coldness of a body or an environment.

Thermometer Instrument for measuring temperature.

Tympanic (tim-**pan**-ik) Relating to or resembling a drum, as in the *tympanic membrane,* or eardrum.

Volume Quantity or amount, as in force of a heartbeat.

LEARNING OUTCOMES

On completion of this chapter, the student will be able to achieve the following objectives:

- Pronounce, define, and spell the Key Terms.
- List the four vital signs commonly taken in the dental office.
- Describe how metabolism affects a patient's vital signs.
- Discuss three types of thermometers.
- List the common pulse sites used for taking a pulse.
- Describe the characteristics of the pulse that you would look for in taking a patient's pulse.
- Describe the characteristics of respiration and how they affect a patient's breathing.
- Discuss the best way to obtain accurate readings of respiration.
- Explain the importance of taking a patient's blood pressure.
- Differentiate the Korotkoff sounds heard when taking a patient's blood pressure.

PERFORMANCE OUTCOMES

On completion of this chapter, the student will be able to meet competency standards in the following skills:

- Take an oral temperature reading with a digital thermometer.
- Take a patient's pulse.
- Take a patient's respiration.
- Take a patient's blood pressure.

Attentiveness toward a patient's immediate health should be the first priority of every healthcare provider. By taking a patient's vital signs on a routine basis, the dental team is obtaining a minimum level of wellness in determining a patient's health status. It is crucial that you gain the confidence in both the background knowledge and the practical applications of this essential task.

Obtaining vital signs includes the taking and recording of temperature, pulse, respiration, and blood pressure. If this is the patient's first visit, a 6-month recall, or an emergency situation, the clinical assistant will/should routinely take and record vital signs.

Having this baseline provides the dental team with added assurance of the patient's well-being and health status.

FACTORS AFFECTING VITAL SIGNS

The human body is influenced by both emotional and physical factors. Before a dental appointment, for example, the patient may drink a hot or cold beverage, which would alter the oral temperature. A patient may be fearful of an upcoming injection, resulting in his or her blood pressure and respiration being much higher than a previous reading.

If a patient were to come directly to a dental appointment from a workout at the gym, what changes would you expect in the patient's vital signs? If you predicted there would be an elevation in the patient's temperature, pulse, respiration, and blood pressure, you are correct. When there is an increase in metabolism (such as after strenuous exercise), vital signs will also typically increase.

One of your responsibilities as a dental assistant will be to recognize these situations and help the patient relax before taking vital signs. You may need to take these measurements more than once. If you think the patient would normally be calmer, you may need to provide reassurance, wait several minutes, and then repeat the procedure.

Recall

1. What are the four vital signs?

TEMPERATURE

Body **temperature** is the degree of hotness or coldness of the body's internal environment. The process of physical and chemical changes that takes place in the production of the body's heat is called **metabolism.** A healthy person's temperature will vary slightly throughout the day because of the amount of stimulus it encounters. A person's lowest body temperature occurs in the early morning hours, and the highest temperature occurs in the evening.

During an illness a person's metabolism increases in order to elevate the body's temperature. Most bacteria and viruses cannot survive in excess heat, and this is the body's way of defending against such diseases. Have you ever wondered why you become chilled when you have a fever? When fever is present, the blood vessels closest to the surface of the skin constrict, causing "goose bumps." The body's reaction to these goose bumps is to make you shiver. A chain reaction then begins, causing the body to produce internal heat for warmth.

Temperature Readings

The **thermometer** is the instrument used to measure the body's temperature. Temperature readings are calibrated in either the Fahrenheit (F) or the Celsius (C) scale. The Fahrenheit scale is the reading most frequently used in the United States, and the Celsius is most frequently used in Canada and Europe.

The average range of the oral temperature of a resting person is 97.6° to 99° F (36.4° to 37.3° C). Average body temperature is higher in infants and younger children than in adults.

Several areas of the body can be used to obtain a temperature reading. The thermometer can be placed under the tongue, in the ear, under the arm, or in the rectum. The temperature readings will vary according to the body site used (Box 27-1).

Types of Thermometers

Digital. Digital thermometers are popular because of their convenience (Fig. 27-1). These thermometers are battery-operated, and they function on the same theory as the glass thermometer except there is a timing system that shows a digital reading after 30 seconds rather than a line of mercury that expands ("rises") along a marked scale. It is important to remember the timed feature of the digital thermometer, because you may obtain an inaccurate reading if the battery is low.

A disposable plastic sheath slides over the probe before insertion. Most digital thermometers have a "beeping" sound to indicate completion. The reading will then appear on the digital screen. Procedure 27-1 reviews the use of a digital thermometer.

Tympanic

One of the newest techniques in taking a patient's temperature is by means of the ear canal (a **tympanic** reading). The ear canal is a protected cavity, so the tympanic temperature reading is not affected by an open mouth, hot or cold drinks, or nose congestion. The tympanic thermometer has a much smaller probe, which is gently placed in the ear canal (Fig. 27-2). An infrared signal is bounced off the eardrum, and an accurate reading is provided within 2 sec-

Box 27-1 Average Fahrenheit (F) Temperature Readings for Primary Body Sites

Site	Temperature (° F)
Oral	98.6
Rectal	99.6
Axillary (underarm)	97.6
Tympanic (ear)	98.6

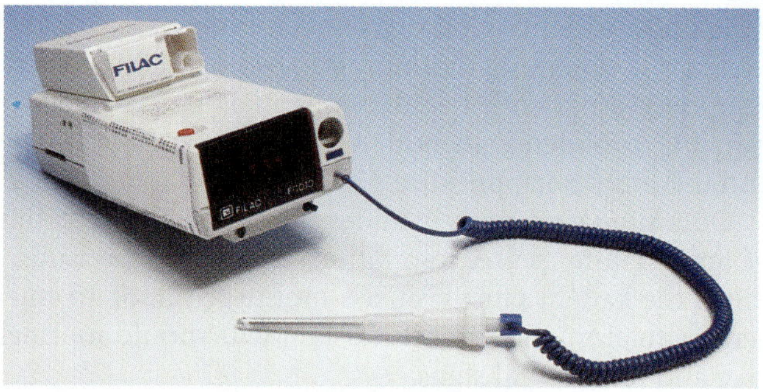

Fig. 27-1 Digital thermometer.

Procedure 27-1 Taking an Oral Temperature Reading with a Digital Thermometer

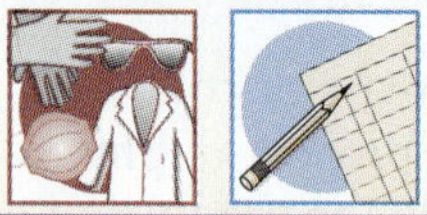

Equipment and Supplies

- Digital thermometer
- Probe cover
- Patient record for documenting temperature

PROCEDURAL STEPS

1. Wash hands and don gloves.
2. Place a new sheath over the probe of the digital thermometer.
3. Turn the thermometer on. When the display indicates that it is ready, gently place the tip under the patient's tongue.
4. Tell the patient to close his or her lips over the thermometer and to refrain from talking or removing it from the mouth.

   Purpose: Talking or removing the thermometer can alter the temperature reading.
5. Leave the thermometer in place until the display indicates a final reading; remove from the patient's mouth.
6. Record the reading in the patient's record.
7. Turn the thermometer off, remove the sheath, and disinfect the thermometer as recommended by the manufacturer.

Date	Temp 99°F	Signature

onds. The risk for spreading communicable diseases while taking a temperature tympanically is greatly reduced because the covered probe of the thermometer does not actually touch the eardrum. This approach has become very popular in children. The rapid measurement may be more accurate because of less patient movement.

Glass

The glass thermometer is a long glass tube with a small mercury bulb at the end that comes in contact with body tissue (Fig. 27-3). When it touches warm tissues of the body, the mercury expands and "rises" along a marked numeric scale. After 3 minutes the mercury stops expanding and registers its highest reading.

While mercury has proved useful in measuring devices such as thermometers, it is a toxic substance that can harm both humans and wildlife. Many states have banned the use of mercury thermometers because of these health hazards. In 1998, the American Hospital Association (AHA) signed an agreement with the U.S. Environmental Protection Agency (EPA) committing to the elimination of mercury from hospital waste streams. Furthermore, in July 2001, the American Academy of Pediatrics urged doctors and parents to stop using mercury thermometers.

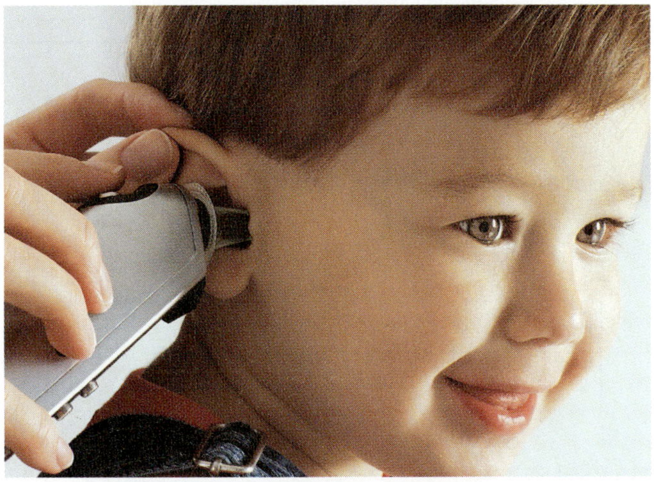

Fig. 27-2 Tympanic thermometer. (Courtesy WelchAllyn, Skaneateles Falls, NY.)

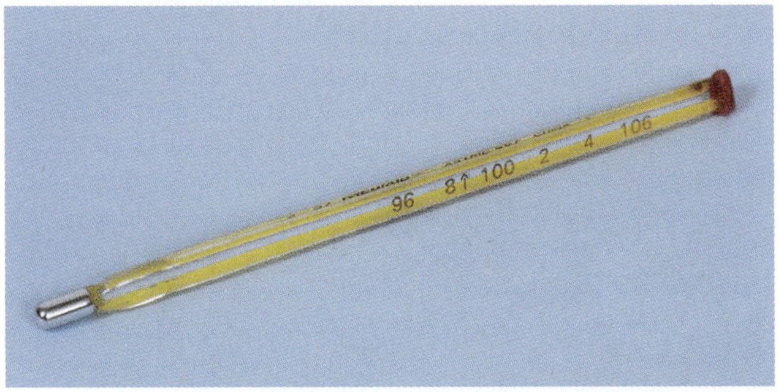

Fig. 27-3 Glass thermometer showing the mercury bulb.

Recall

2. What is the purpose of a thermometer?
3. What location on the body most often gives the highest temperature reading of the body?
4. Where is the tympanic thermometer placed?

PULSE

A **pulse** is the rhythmic expansion of an artery every time the heart beats. Every artery throughout the body has a pulse, although many pulses cannot be read because of their location. When an artery is close to the surface of the skin, you can push against it with your fingers as it rests on a tendon or bone and then feel the beating. The pulse can be felt with slight finger pressure in several areas of the body.

Radial Artery

The **radial** artery is located on the inner surface of the wrist (thumb side) and is the most common site for taking a patient's pulse in the dental office. To take the pulse, place your index and third finger lightly on the patient's wrist between the radius (bone on the thumb side) and the tendon (Fig. 27-4). This measures about 1 inch from the base of your thumb.

Brachial Artery

The **brachial** artery is located on the inner fold of the arm, also referred to as the **antecubital** area of the elbow (Fig. 27-5). This artery is used when taking a patient's blood pressure.

Carotid Artery

The **carotid** artery (Fig. 27-6) is located alongside the patient's larynx (Adam's apple). Taking the carotid pulse is common when performing cardiopulmonary resuscitation (CPR; see Chapter 31). Because CPR is an emergency

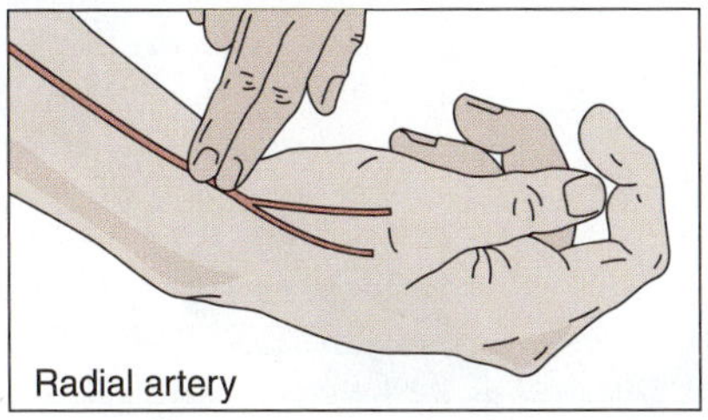

Fig. 27-4 Location of the radial artery. (From Kinn ME, Woods M: *The medical assistant: administrative and clinical,* ed 8, Philadelphia, 1999, Saunders.)

situation, it is important that you know how to find the carotid artery quickly.

To detect the carotid pulse, place two fingers alongside the patient's larynx on the side of the neck nearest you. Move your fingers slowly down the groove to the soft area above the clavicle (collarbone) and then **palpate** this area gently to determine a pulse.

Pulse Characteristics

When taking a patient's pulse, look for any distinct changes in the pulse. The following three characteristics must be noted in the patient record when documenting a patient's pulse:

- **Rate** is the number of beats that occur during the counting period.

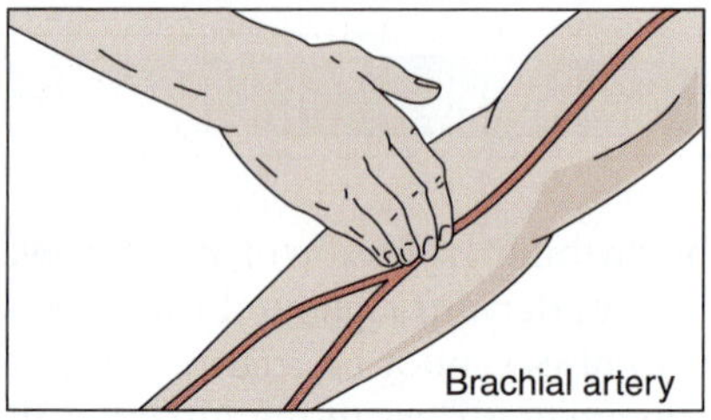

Fig. 27-5 Location of the brachial artery. (From Kinn ME, Woods M: *The medical assistant: administrative and clinical,* ed 8, Philadelphia, 1999, Saunders.)

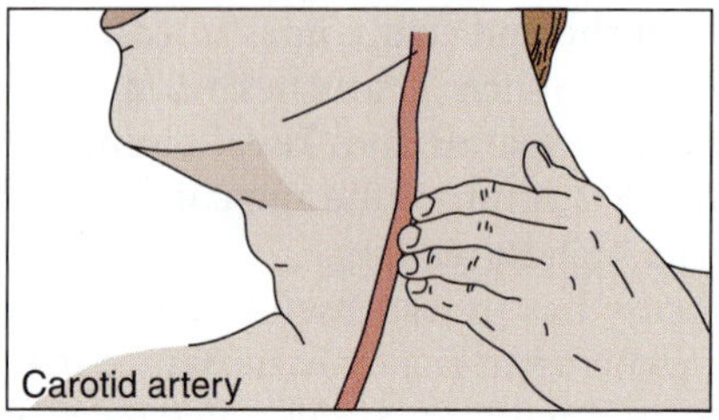

Fig. 27-6 Location of the carotid artery. (From Kinn ME, Woods M: *The medical assistant: administrative and clinical,* ed 8, Philadelphia, 1999, Saunders.)

Procedure 27-2 Taking a Patient's Pulse

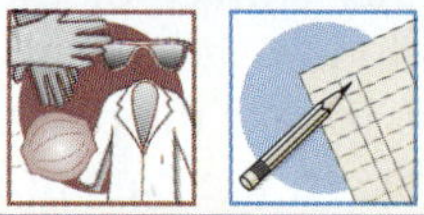

Equipment and Supplies

- Watch with second hand
- Patient record to document findings

PROCEDURAL STEPS

1. Seat the patient in an upright position.
2. Extend the patient's arm, resting it on his or her leg or on the arm rest of the chair. Have the arm at or below the heart level.
3. Place the tips of your index and middle fingers on the patient's radial artery.
   Note: Indicate in the patient's record whether you are using the right or left arm.

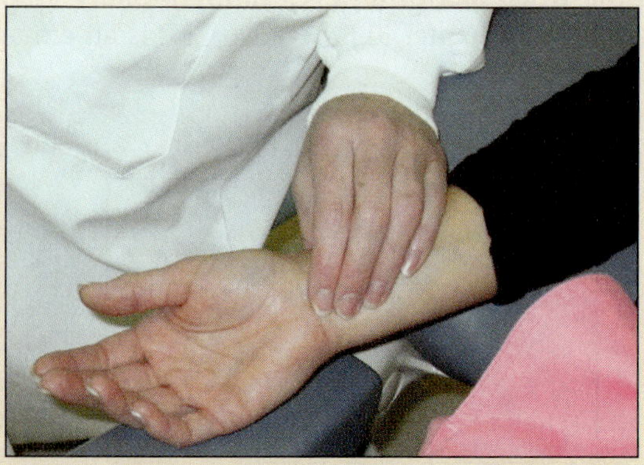

4. Feel for the patient's pulse before beginning to count.
   Purpose: This makes it easier to maintain one position during counting.
5. Count the pulse for 30 seconds; then multiply by 2 to compute the rate for a 1-minute reading.
6. Record the rate, along with any distinct changes in the rhythm.

Date	Pulse Rate - 77 (skipping but strong)	Signature

- **Rhythm** describes the pattern of the beats, such as an occasional skipping, speeding up, or slowing down of a beat.
- **Volume** is the force of the beat, such as a strong or weak beat.

Pulse Readings

When taking a patient's radial pulse, make sure the patient is positioned with his or her arm at the same level or lower than the heart. Make sure the arm is well supported and extended. The normal pulse rate in resting adults is 60 to 100 beats per minute. It is more rapid in a child, ranging from 70 to 120 beats.

A simple method of timing and counting pulse beats is to observe a watch or clock with a second hand while palpating the pulse. To minimize counting, you may count for 30 seconds and then double that number for the rate of 1 full minute. However, it is best not to count for less than 30 seconds, because it is difficult to detect any possible **arrhythmia** (irregularity) in the heartbeat in times shorter than 30 seconds.

Procedure 27-2 reviews taking a patient's pulse.

Recall

5. Which artery in the body has a pulse?
6. Which artery would you normally palpate when taking a patient's pulse?
7. What is the normal pulse rate for an adult?

RESPIRATION

Respiration is the process of inhaling and exhaling, or breathing. During respiration, oxygen is taken into the body, and carbon dioxide is released as a waste product. Breathing is an automatic response controlled by the body's nervous system. Respiration is an involuntary response and a voluntary function. Breathing is mostly under the control of the brain, which is why people can hold their breath for only a limited period. When the carbon dioxide level increases in the blood, the cells become starved for oxygen, and a stimulus is sent to the brain to breathe again.

Respiration Characteristics

A person's breathing is usually not noticeable unless that person is having trouble taking a breath. The following three characteristics are noted in the patient record when measuring a patient's respiration:

- **Rate** is the total number of breaths per minute.
- **Rhythm** refers to the breathing pattern (Fig. 27-7).
- **Depth** is the amount of air inhaled and exhaled during a breath.

Respiration Readings

The normal respiration rate for a relaxed adult is 10 to 20 breaths per minute. For children and teenagers, the rate ranges from 18 to 30 breaths. To obtain the respiratory rate, observe the number of times the patient's chest rises and falls (one count) for 30 seconds; then double the count to obtain the number of breaths for 1 minute.

If patients know that their breaths are being monitored, they usually change their breathing pattern. Therefore the best way to count a patient's respirations is to do it while your fingers are still positioned on the wrist as if taking the pulse. The patient will assume you are still taking the pulse, but you will refocus your eyes on the patient's chest and count the breaths instead. Procedure 27-3 reviews taking a patient's respiration.

Recall

8. Respiration is the process of doing what?
9. What breathing pattern is characteristic of an excessively rapid rate of breathing?
10. What is the normal respiration rate for an adult?

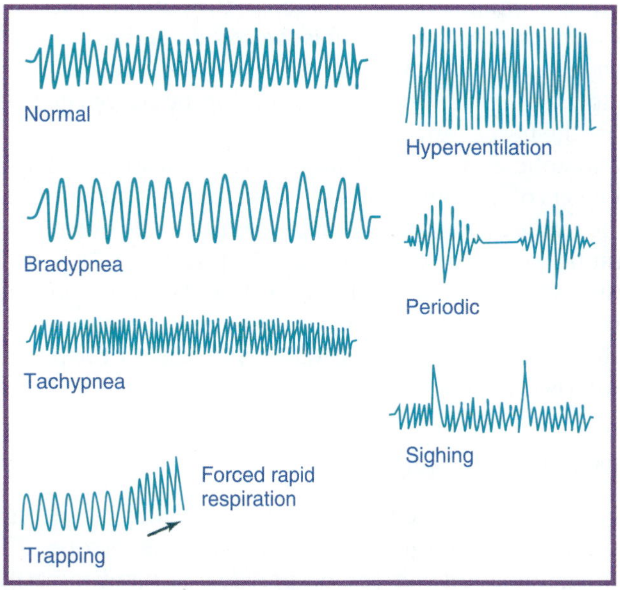

Fig. 27-7 Respiration patterns. ***Bradypnea*** **is an abnormally slow respiratory rate.** ***Tachypnea*** **is excessively short, rapid breaths, and** ***hyperventilation*** **is excessively long, rapid breaths.** (From Young AP, Kennedy DB: *Kinn's The medical assistant: an applied learning approach,* ed 9, St Louis, 2003, Saunders.)

Procedure 27-3 Taking a Patient's Respiration

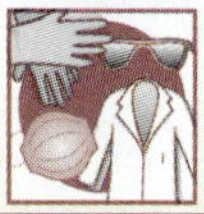
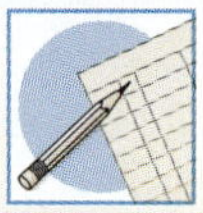

Equipment and Supplies

- Watch with second hand
- Patient record to document findings

PROCEDURAL STEPS

1. With patient seated, maintain the position you used while taking the pulse.

   Purpose: The patient should not be aware that you are observing his or her breathing.
2. Count the rise and fall of the patient's chest for 30 seconds; then multiply by 2 to compute the rate for a 1-minute reading.
3. Enter the rate, rhythm, and depth in the patient record.

Date	Respiration - 14 (slight sighing, depth—moderate)	Signature

BLOOD PRESSURE

Blood pressure (BP) refers to the amount of labor the heart has to exert to pump blood throughout the body. The heart produces two sounds for a blood pressure reading. The first sound *(systole)* indicates the **systolic** pressure, which is a *sharp* tapping sound and is the first and larger number recorded. This number reflects the amount of pressure required for the left ventricle of the heart to compress or push oxygenated blood out into the blood vessels. The last sound *(diastole)*, indicating the **diastolic** pressure, is a *soft* tapping sound and is the second and lower number recorded. This number reflects the heart muscle at rest, allowing the heart to take in blood to be oxygenated before the next contraction occurs.

Systolic and diastolic pressures are measured in millimeters of mercury (mm Hg) above atmospheric pressure. The reading is recorded with the systolic value over the diastolic value. For example, 129/78 ("129 *over* 78") indicates systolic pressure of 129 mm Hg and diastolic pressure of 78 mm Hg. Blood pressure readings for adults are classified according to normal values and stages of hypertension (Box 27-2).

Box 27-2 Blood Pressure Classifications for Adults

Category	Systolic (mm Hg)	Diastolic (mm Hg)
Normal	Less than 120	Less than 80
Prehypertension	120-139	80-89
Hypertension		
Stage 1	140-159	90-99
Stage 2 (moderate)	160+	100+

Blood Pressure Equipment

The instruments used when taking a patient's blood pressure are the sphygmomanometer and stethoscope. The **sphygmomanometer** (blood pressure cuff and meter) is used to measure blood pressure (Fig. 27-8). The sphygmomanometer must include specific parts to obtain a correct reading. The *cuff* is a cloth wrap that holds an inflatable rubber bladder. A *rubber bulb* is attached to the cuff with rubber tubing.

The **stethoscope** is used to amplify sounds (called *Korotkoff sounds,* named for the man who first described them) that occur within the artery (Fig. 27-9). **Korotkoff sounds** are a series of sounds produced by the blood rushing back into the brachial artery, which has been collapsed by the pressure of the blood pressure cuff. As the pressure in the cuff is slowly released, the stethoscope picks up a distinct thumping sound that grows louder and then softens to a murmur as the flow of blood causes the artery to expand to its former shape. Five phases of Korotkoff sounds occur during deflation of the blood pressure cuff (Box 27-3).

An *automated electronic blood pressure device* is used in many practices to simplify and speed the recording of a blood pressure (Fig. 27-10). As with the electronic thermometer, batteries operate the electronic blood pressure meter. Weak batteries may lead to an inaccurate reading. Use of the electronic device is similar to that of the sphygmomanometer without the stethoscope.

Blood Pressure Readings

A situation may arise in which it is necessary to take two or three blood pressure readings to obtain an accurate or av-

A

B

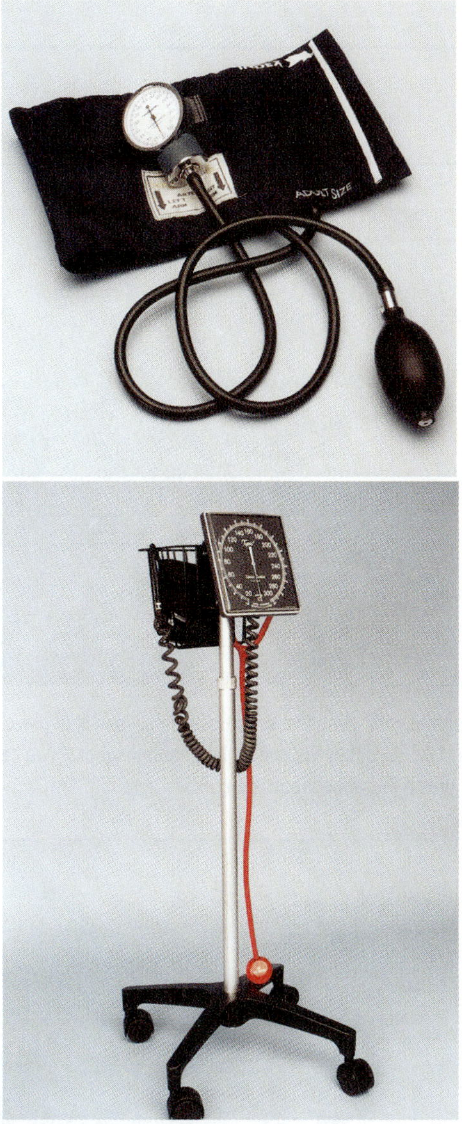

Fig. 27-8 **Types of sphygmomanometers. A, Aneroid (without liquid) dial system. B, Aneroid floor model.** (From Young AP, Kennedy DB: *Kinn's The medical assistant: an applied learning approach,* ed 9, St Louis, 2003, Saunders.)

erage reading. If this occurs, allow the deflated blood pressure cuff to remain on the patient for a minimum of 10 minutes before obtaining another reading. If taken too soon, the reading may be incorrect.

Medical Considerations

The stress and anxiety of a dental procedure can elevate a patient's blood pressure. Review the patient's health history and discuss the types of medication that he or she is taking. Many drugs have side effects that can interfere with dental treatment. A patient diagnosed with hypertension should be under the care of a physician during a treatment regimen. If there is a concern about a patient's medical status based on blood pressure readings, the patient may

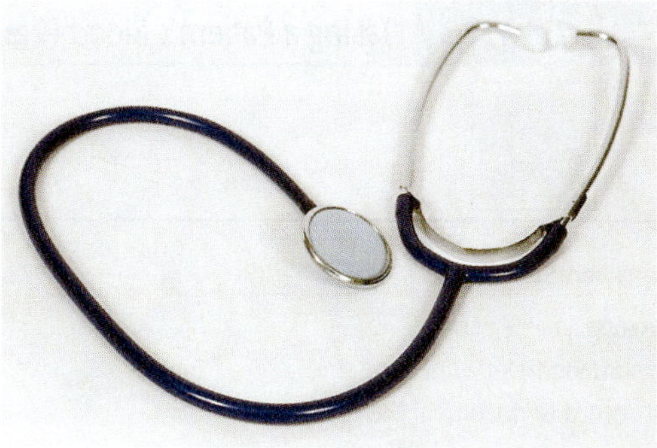

Fig. 27-9 **Stethoscope.**

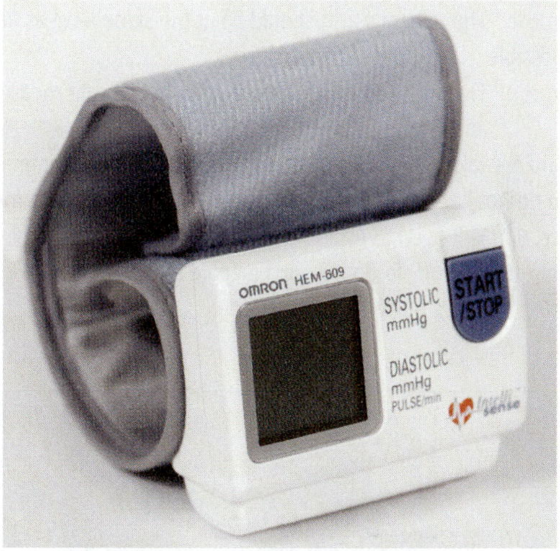

Fig. 27-10 **Automated electronic blood pressure device.**

Box 27-3 Five Phases of Korotkoff Sounds in Blood Pressure Measurement

Phase I: Blood is beginning to flow back into the artery and can be heard as a sharp tapping sound. *This is the systolic blood pressure reading.*

Phase II: The cuff deflates, and more blood flows. A swishing sound may be heard. This sound is softened and becomes prolonged into a murmur.

Phase III: A large amount of blood is flowing into the artery. A distinct, sharp tapping sound returns and continues rhythmically.

Phase IV: The blood is flowing easily, and the sound changes to a soft tapping. The sound becomes distinctly muffled and fainter.

Phase V: At this point the artery is fully open, and the sound disappears. *This is the diastolic blood pressure reading.*

Procedure 27-4 Taking a Patient's Blood Pressure

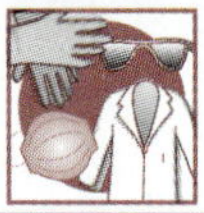

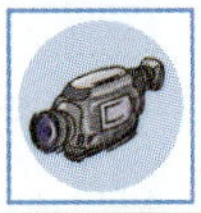

Equipment and Supplies

- Stethoscope
- Sphygmomanometer
- Patient record to document the findings

PROCEDURAL STEPS

1. Seat the patient with the arm extended at heart level and either supported on the chair arm or on a table.
   Purpose: The patient's arm should be at the same level as the heart.
2. If possible, roll up the patient's sleeve.
   Purpose: Tight clothing can interfere with an accurate measurement and reading.
3. If you are taking the patient's blood pressure for the first time and you do not have a previous blood pressure reading to use for reference, you will need to establish a basis to determine how high to pump up the cuff. To do this, first palpate the brachial artery to feel for the patient's pulse.

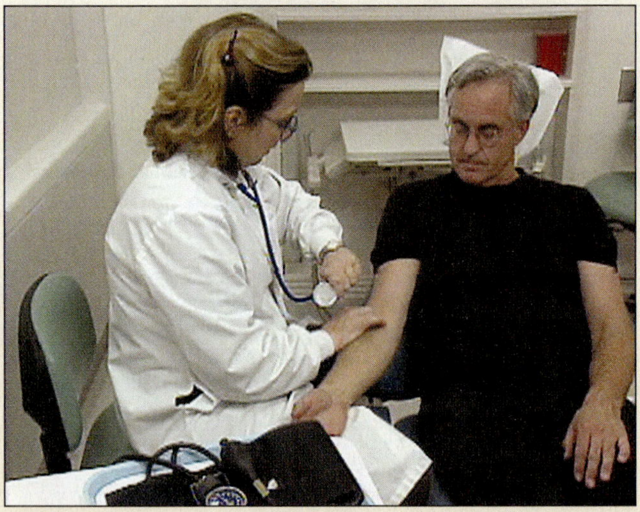

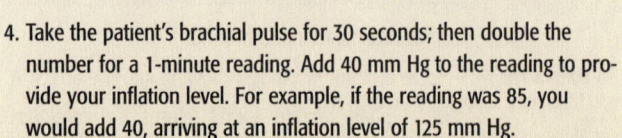

4. Take the patient's brachial pulse for 30 seconds; then double the number for a 1-minute reading. Add 40 mm Hg to the reading to provide your inflation level. For example, if the reading was 85, you would add 40, arriving at an inflation level of 125 mm Hg.
5. Expel any air from the cuff by opening the valve and pressing gently on the cuff.
6. Place the blood pressure cuff around the patient's arm approximately 1 inch above the **antecubital space,** making sure to center the arrow over the brachial artery.
   Purpose: Pressure must be applied directly over the artery for a correct reading.

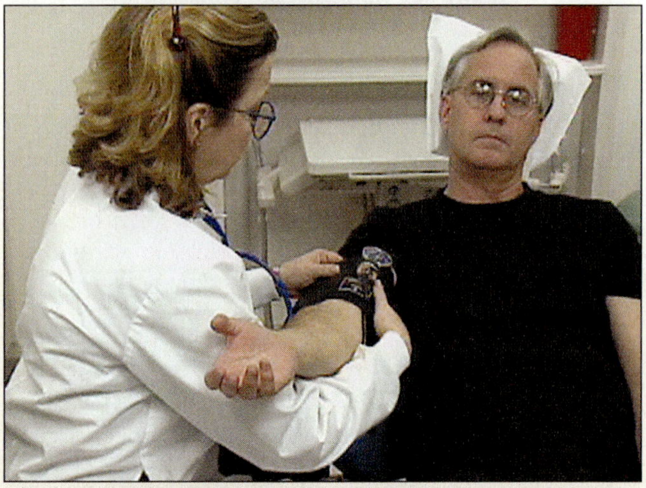

7. Tighten the cuff, using the Velcro closure to hold it in place.
   Note: Make sure that the cuff is tight enough so that you can squeeze only a finger between the cuff and arm.

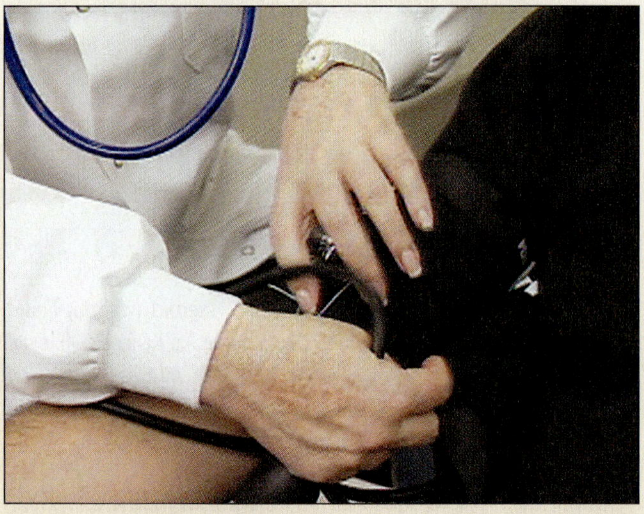

8. Place the earpieces of the stethoscope into your ears so that they are facing toward the front.
   Purpose: This position of the earpieces is more comfortable and blocks out distracting noises while you are taking blood pressure.

Procedure 27-4 Taking a Patient's Blood Pressure—cont'd

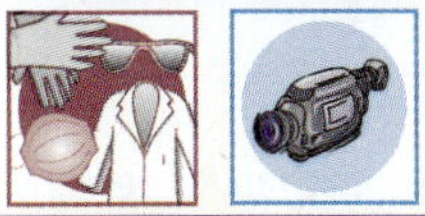

9. Place the stethoscope disc over the site of the brachial artery, using slight pressure with the fingers.

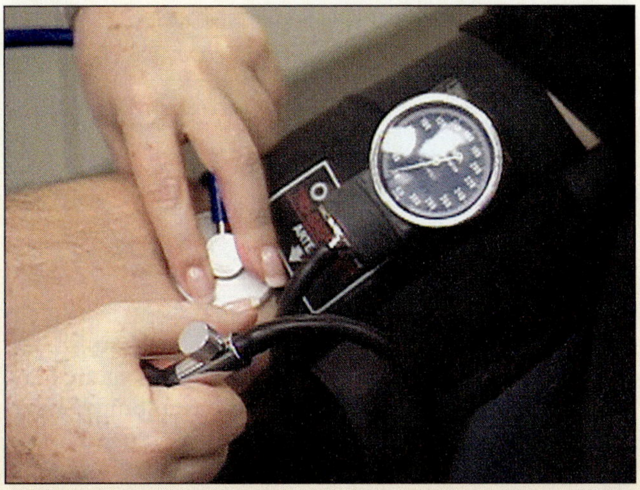

10. Grasp the rubber bulb with the other hand, locking the valve. Inflate the cuff to the noted reading.
   Note: You need to inflate the bulb *quickly.*
11. Slowly release the valve and listen through the stethoscope.
12. Note the first distinct thumping sound as the cuff deflates. *This is the systolic pressure reading.*
13. Slowly continue to release the air from the cuff until you hear the last sound. *This is the diastolic pressure reading.*

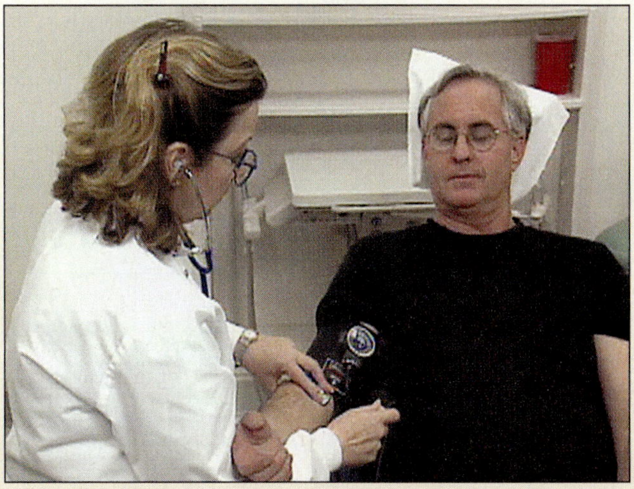

14. Record the reading, indicating which arm was used.
15. Disinfect the stethoscope earpieces and diaphragm as recommended by the manufacturer. Return the setup to its proper place.

Date	BP 117/68 R	Signature/Date

need to reschedule the appointment until after the dentist or surgeon has had the chance to speak directly to the patient's physician.

Procedure 27-4 reviews the steps in taking a patient's blood pressure.

Recall

11. Is the diastolic reading the first or last sound heard when taking a blood pressure?
12. What two instruments are used when taking a patient's blood pressure?
13. What is the term for the small groove or fold on the inner arm?
14. Who first described a series of sounds (now named for him) heard during the taking of a blood pressure?
15. What is the range of a normal blood pressure reading for an adult?

ELECTROCARDIOGRAM

The **electrocardiogram** (ECG or EKG) is a procedure that amplifies the electrical currents generated by the electrical impulses of the heart. This test is routinely completed in the diagnosis of heart disease. In dentistry, the ECG is used as a preventive measure when a patient is undergoing general anesthesia in a hospital or outpatient setting. The surgeon or dentist uses the ECG to follow the patient's cardiac activity during a procedure.

Wires with electrodes are attached to the patient. The machine amplifies many times the natural electrical currents generated by the electrical impulses of the heart. The pattern of the heartbeat is traced on graph paper. The ECG records a series of waves that move above or below a baseline. Each deflection corresponds to a particular part of the cardiac cycle (Fig. 27-11).

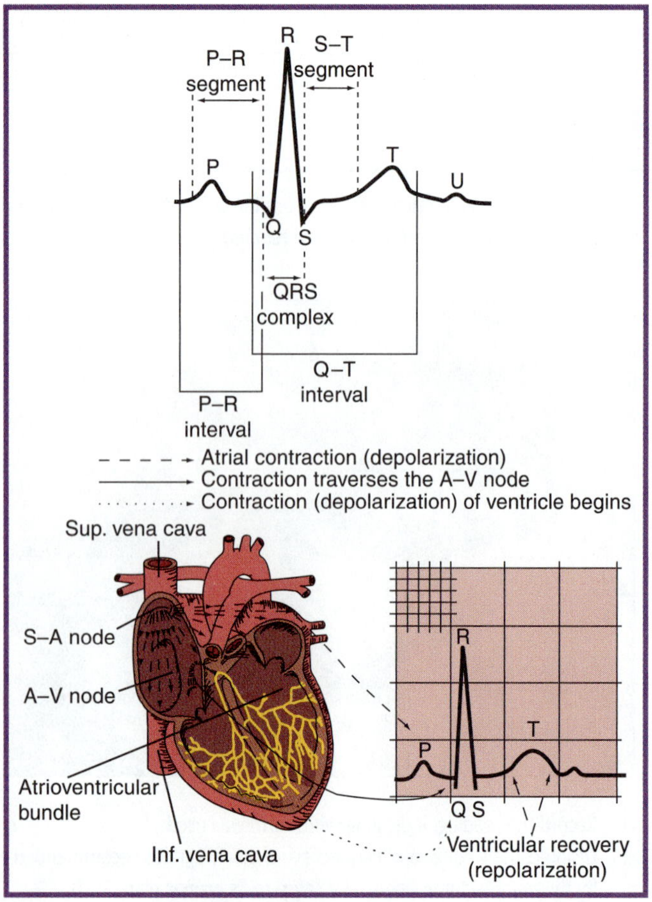

Stage	Heart Activity
P wave	Contraction of the artery
PR segment	Interval that reflects the time from the beginning of the arterial contraction to the beginning of the ventricular contraction
QRS complex	Contraction of the ventricle
ST segment	Interval that reflects the time between the ventricular contraction and the beginning of ventricular recovery
T wave	Ventricular recovery

Fig. 27-11 The cardiac cycle on the electrocardiogram. (From Kinn ME, Woods M: *The medical assistant: administrative and clinical,* ed 8, Philadelphia, 1999, Saunders.)

Patient Education

Many patients are knowledgeable about taking their temperature, pulse, and respiration. With new products on the market for taking blood pressure, many people, especially the older population, also have access to routine blood pressure monitoring. Increased awareness allows patients to better understand the importance of their vital signs to their overall health.

Legal and Ethical Implications

As easy as it is to take a patient's vital signs, more than 80 percent of dental offices do not complete this service on a routine basis. The main reason is lack of time in the schedule. However, it is crucial that you are aware of your patient's health before a dental procedure. If an emergency were to occur and you did not have a baseline of your patient's health (documented vital sign readings), the dental team would be liable for the type of emergency care provided.

Eye to the Future

Imagine a tiny implantable device that could be used to monitor a person's vital signs. This device is still in the early development stages, but a prototype named the Digital Angel will eventually be able to monitor a person's heart rate, breathing, and blood pressure. The device will trigger an alarm if the patient's health suddenly deteriorates, alerting emergency medical services for transport to a local hospital for immediate care.

Critical Thinking

1. How would you handle a pediatric patient who was continuously moving while you were trying to take vital signs?
2. Ms. Stewart is a new patient to your clinic, and you have just reviewed her medical-dental health history. Where would you take Ms Stewart to take her vital signs? In what order would you take them for optimum time efficiency?
3. After reviewing Ms. Stewart's medical history, you notice that she checked Yes next to hypertension. You take her blood pressure, and your reading is 143/95. Is this considered hypertensive? If so, what stage is her hypertension?
4. Your patient is overweight and slouching in the patient chair. What approach will you use to obtain an accurate respiration count?
5. Describe the three types of characteristics you are looking for when taking a patient's pulse.

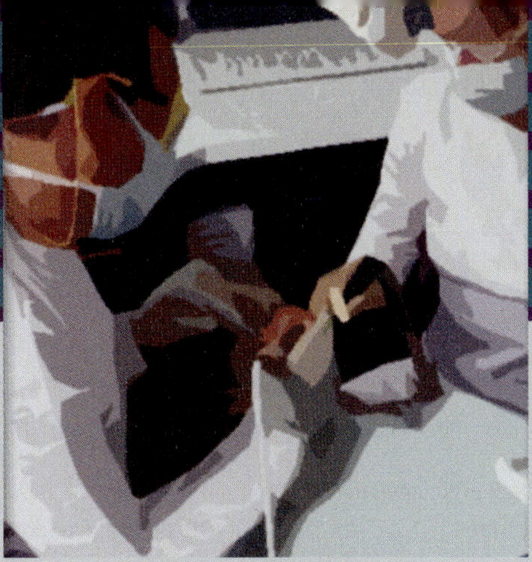

28 Oral Diagnosis and Treatment Planning

Outline

Examination and Diagnostic Techniques
- Visual Evaluation
- Palpation
- Instrumentation
- Radiography
- Intraoral Imaging
- Photography

Recording the Dental Examination
- Black's Classification of Cavities
- Tooth Diagrams
- Tooth-Numbering Systems
- Color Coding
- Abbreviations

Charting
- Restorative Materials
- Symbols

Clinical Examination of the Patient
- Soft Tissue Examination

Procedure 28-1: The Soft Tissue Examination
- Examination and Charting of Teeth
- Examination and Charting of Periodontium

Procedure 28-2: Charting of Teeth

Procedure 28-3: Periodontal Screening: Examination of the Gingival Tissues

The Treatment Plan
- Types of Plans
- Treatment Plan Presentation

Recording the Dental Treatment

Procedure 28-4: Recording the Completed Dental Treatment

Patient Education

Legal and Ethical Implications

Eye to the Future

Critical Thinking

KEY TERMS

Detection Act or process of discovering tooth imperfections or decay.

Extraoral Outside the oral cavity.

Furcation (fur-**kay**-shun) Area between two or more root branches.

Intraoral Within the oral cavity.

Mobility To have movement.

Morphologically (mor-fah-**lahj**-i-kul-lee), **morphologic** (mor-fah-**lah**-jik), **morphology** (mor-**fol**-eh-jee, mor-**fah**-leh-jee) Branch of biology that deals with the form and structure.

Palpation (pal-**pay**-shun) To touch or feel for abnormalities within soft tissue.

Probing Use of a slender, flexible instrument to explore and measure the periodontal pocket.

Restoration The use of a dental material to restore a tooth or teeth to a functional permanent unit.

Symmetric (si-**meh**-trik) Balanced or even on both sides.

LEARNING OUTCOMES

On completion of this chapter, the student will be able to achieve the following objectives:

- Pronounce, define, and spell the Key Terms.
- List and describe the examination and diagnostic techniques used for patient assessment.
- Discuss the role of the dental assistant in the clinical examination.
- List the six categories of Black's classification of cavities.
- Differentiate between an anatomic and a geometric diagram for charting.
- Explain the color coding of a chart diagram.
- Describe the pocket depth and bleeding index of the gingival tissues and how to record them.
- Describe the need for a soft tissue examination.
- Discuss the importance of a treatment plan.

PERFORMANCE OUTCOMES

On completion of this chapter, the student will be able to meet competency standards in the following skills:

- Chart the correct restorative material for either an existing restoration or a required treatment.
- Chart the correct symbol for either an existing restoration or a required treatment.
- Chart the periodontal examination correctly.

Sound dental care begins with a thorough examination of the head, neck, and oral cavity. For the dentist to make a correct diagnosis, he or she will first review the medical and dental history, continue with a thorough **extraoral** and **intraoral** examination, then conduct a review of radiographs and study models, and finally make a plan of treatment.

A patient will seek dental care for the following four reasons:

- As a new patient, to receive an examination and proceed with a plan of treatment and care.
- As an emergency patient, for a specific problem.
- For consultation with a specialist.
- As a returning patient, for continued assessment and care.

EXAMINATION AND DIAGNOSTIC TECHNIQUES

The examination of a patient involves many areas. The dentist cannot just look at a tooth or an area of soft tissue and determine its complete status. Currently in the field of dentistry, advanced technology allows the dentist to arrive at more accurate findings than ever before.

The techniques discussed in this chapter are effective in helping the dentist determine the patient's dental status. Once the required assessments are completed, the dentist will then recommend a treatment plan to the patient.

Visual Evaluation

The dentist must be able to distinguish between symptoms described by the patient and visual clues. The examination always begins with a visual evaluation of the soft tissue and oral cavity. This provides the dentist an overall assessment of the type of previous dental care, as well as any existing conditions that have been neglected. Specific examination areas include soft tissue, tooth structure, restorations, and missing teeth.

Soft tissue should appear light pink and uniform in color with no indications of swelling. If there are any unhealthy areas of soft tissue that appear reddened and not uniform in color, they should be noted in the soft tissue portion of the clinical examination form.

Tooth structure should appear uniform in color and **morphologically** sound and intact. The dentist uses the mouth mirror and dental light to look for any imperfections in the enamel. Unhealthy tooth structure may appear discolored, may be chipped, or may have an abnormal morphologic appearance. The dentist will also evaluate each **restoration** for discrepancies and complete coverage of tooth structure. Any missing teeth should also be noted.

After further investigation using additional techniques, the information is noted in the charting section of the clinical examination form. It is imperative to learn the names of the teeth and numbering system. You will need to acquire competence in this skill to chart in a clinical examination procedure (see later discussion).

Palpation

Palpation is an examination technique in which the examiner uses his or her fingers and hands to feel for texture, size, and consistency of hard and soft tissue (see Chapter 9 for a review of the basic anatomy and physiology of the head and neck). Procedure 28-1 provides a step-by-step process in this technique.

Instrumentation

Instrumentation is the application or use of tools or equipment to examine the teeth and surrounding tissues. The use of instruments enables the dentist or dental hygienist to further evaluate areas that were first detected visually.

The type of instruments selected for the dental setup should accomplish the following:

Detection

With the use of a sharp pointed explorer, the dentist can detect imperfections in the enamel surface, which may be the beginning of decay (Fig. 28-1). The dentist will also use an explorer to evaluate existing restorations for their stability and integrity.

Probing

The dentist or dental hygienist will use the dental probe to measure the sulcus for loss of gingival attachment or bone loss (Fig. 28-2).

Radiography

Radiographs have become indispensable tools for identifying decay, defective restorations, advanced periodontal conditions, pathology, developmental conditions, and other abnormalities. The dentist's decision to prescribe intraoral radiographs (Fig. 28-3) versus extraoral radiographs (Fig. 28-4) will depend on what the dentist needs to see and what would provide the maximal findings (see Chapters 38 to 42).

Intraoral Imaging

Intraoral imaging is similar to the use of a miniature video camera. This technique allows the dentist to use a computer monitor as a complement to a video camera system, with a display of live video on a monitor screen (Fig. 28-5). The intraoral camera provides the dentist with the following:

- Magnification of an image for better evaluation
- Easier access for areas that are difficult to view
- Images that can be photocopied for insurance verification
- Case simulation or case presentation
- Medical and legal documentation

Photography

Photography is a diagnostic tool for intraoral and extraoral structures. Photographs provide the dentist and patient with a visual means to identify and understand specific problems (Fig. 28-6). For more comprehensive treatment such as reconstructive or orthodontic procedures, a patient will have before-and-after photographs taken to see the changed results (see Chapter 60).

As the clinical assistant, your role in the dental examination procedure is to have the correct forms, instruments, and any additional supplies needed by the dentist ready for use.

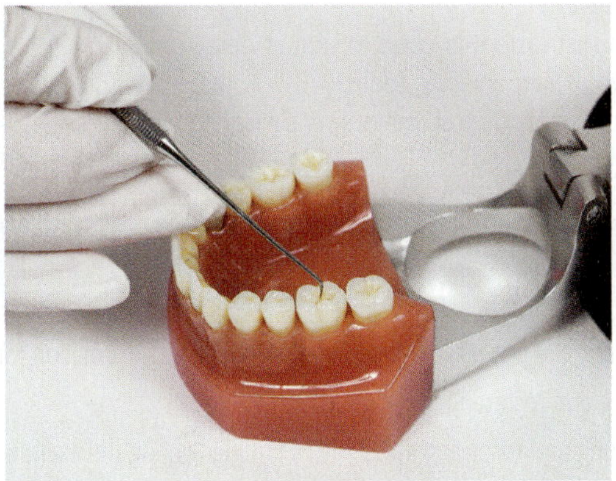

Fig. 28-1 Detecting decay.

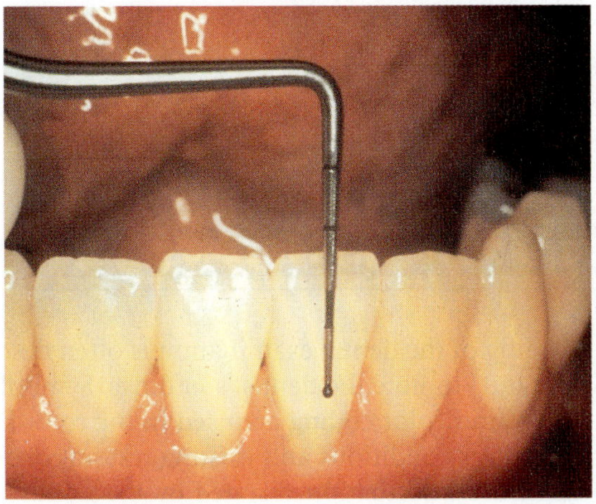

Fig. 28-2 Using a periodontal probe to measure the sulcus. (Courtesy Hu-Friedy.)

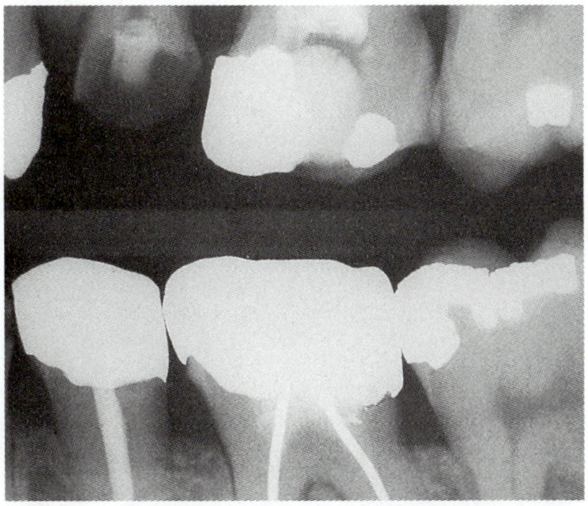

Fig. 28-3 Example of a bite-wing intraoral radiograph.

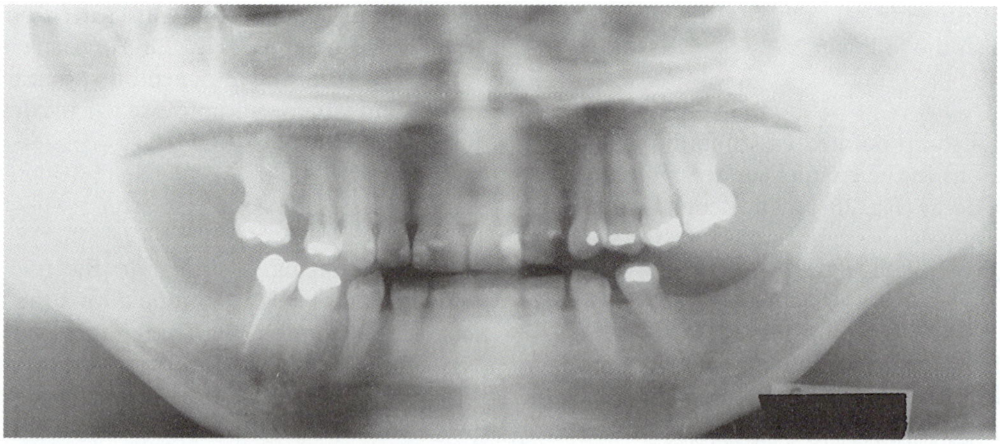

Fig. 28-4 Example of a Panorex extraoral radiograph.

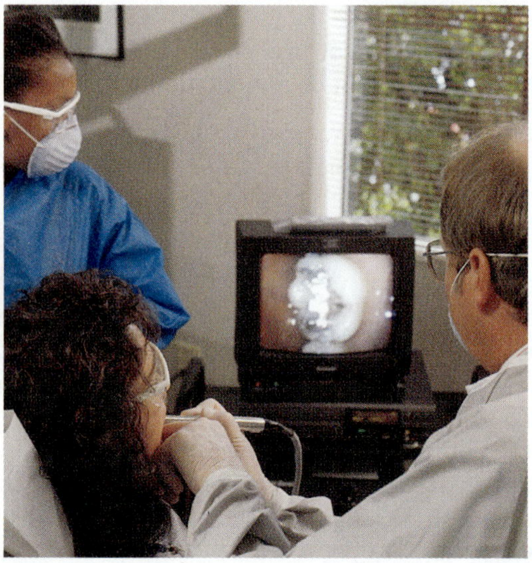

Fig. 28-5 An intraoral imaging system is used to diagnose and educate the patient.

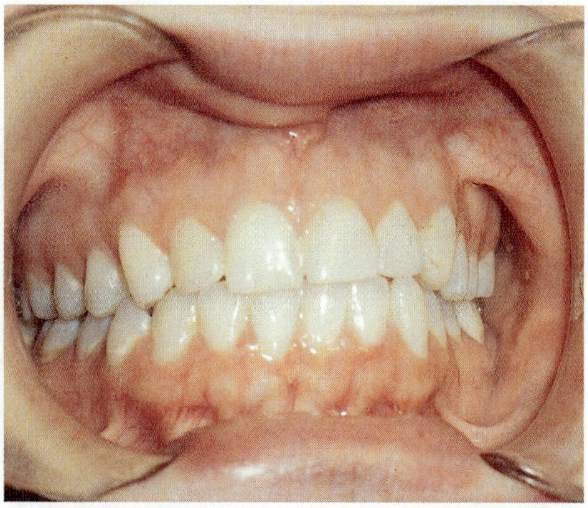

Fig. 28-6 Photographs are taken to provide a visual evaluation of the patient.

Recall

1. Identify four reasons why a patient seeks dental care.
2. What diagnostic techniques are used to evaluate a patient's oral conditions?
3. What instrument is used to detect decay?
4. Do you chart missing teeth?
5. Performing intraoral imaging is similar to what?

Role of the Dental Assistant in Patient Examination and Treatment Planning

- Assisting the patient in the completion of patient information forms
- Taking and recording vital signs
- Charting and recording the dentist's findings during the examination
- Exposing and processing intraoral and extraoral radiographs
- Taking preliminary impressions and fabricating (making) diagnostic models
- Taking intraoral and extraoral photographs
- Organizing the patient record
- Preparing the materials for treatment planning and case presentation

RECORDING THE DENTAL EXAMINATION

The recording of the dental examination is often described as "shorthand" to note the dentist's findings. Symbols, abbreviations, and color coding are used in the recording to indicate various conditions and existing restorations.

To chart the information dictated by the dentist accurately and quickly, the dental assistant must learn the dentist's preferred system for each of the areas described in this section.

Black's Classification of Cavities

Before you can master the charting methods, you need to understand the process of how a dentist decides the type of restoration needed from one tooth to many teeth. When a dentist detects a deviation from the normal, a decision is made to follow through with the best treatment for that area.

Dentists restore teeth according to a method developed by G.V. Black in the early 1900s. This standard classification system is universal to all dentists and is used to describe the location of decay and the best method for restoring the tooth. Black's original classification included Class I through Class V. Class VI was added later. Fig. 28-7 provides Black's classifications, surfaces involved, and a diagram of the cavity classification.

Classification	Location and Description	
Class I	Decay is diagnosed in the pits and fissures of the occlusal surfaces of molars and premolars, buccal or lingual pits of molars, and lingual pits of maxillary incisors. Because most of this type of decay is confined to a small area, the dentist will choose to restore these surfaces with composite (tooth-colored) resins.	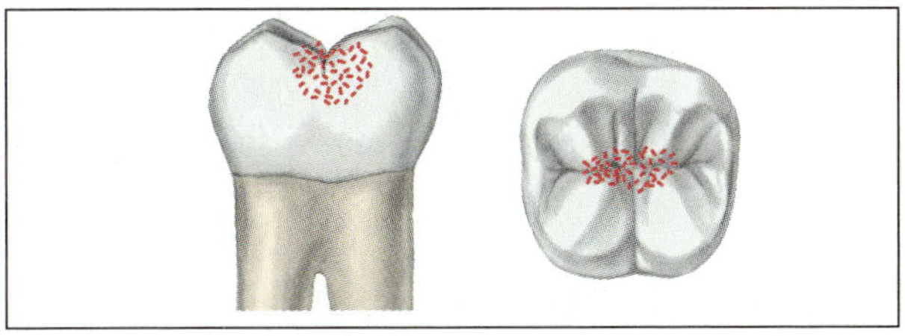
Class II	Decay is diagnosed in the proximal (mesial or distal) surfaces of premolars and molars. Because this surface area is harder to detect visually, a radiograph is used to detect the decay. The design of the restoration will most commonly include the occlusal surface and may possibly involve more than two surfaces. The type of dental material used to restore this classification is either silver amalgam (chosen for its strength) or newer composite (tooth-colored) resins designed for posterior teeth (chosen for esthetic appeal). If the tooth has extensive decay, the dentist may choose to crown the tooth with a gold or porcelain inlay, onlay, or crown.	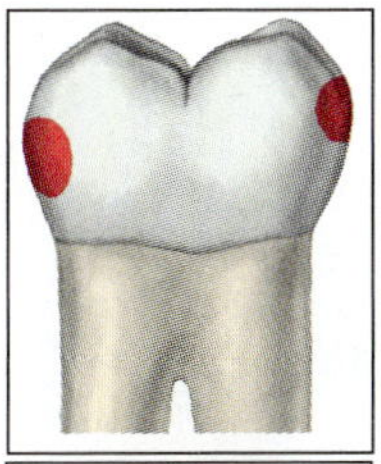
Class III	Decay is diagnosed in the proximal (mesial or distal) surfaces of incisors and canines. This decay is similar to that of Class II, except it involves anterior teeth. It is easier for the dentist to access these surfaces with less tooth structure affected. The type of dental material used to restore this classification is composite (tooth-colored) resins (for esthetic appearance).	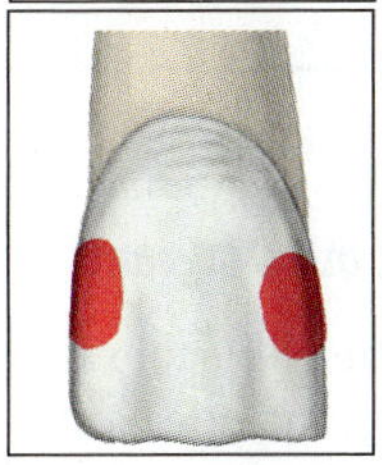
Class IV	Decay is diagnosed in the proximal (mesial or distal) surfaces of incisors and canines. The difference between Class IV and Class III decay is that Class IV involves the incisal edge or angle of the tooth. The type of dental material used to restore this classification is composite (tooth-colored) resins (for esthetic appearance). If the tooth has extensive decay, the dentist may choose to crown the tooth with a porcelain crown.	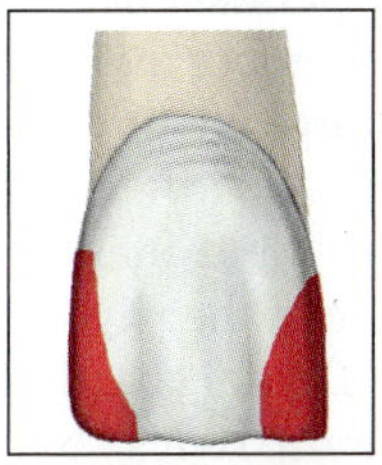
Class V	Decay is diagnosed in the gingival third of facial or lingual surfaces of any tooth. This is also referred to as a *smooth surface decay.* The type of dental material used to restore this classification depends on which teeth are affected. If the decay occurs in posterior teeth, the dentist may choose silver amalgam; if anterior teeth are involved, composite (tooth-colored) resin will most likely be used.	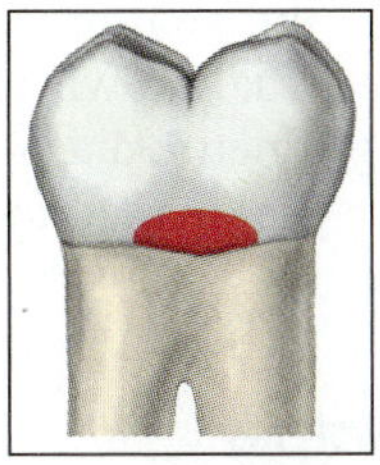 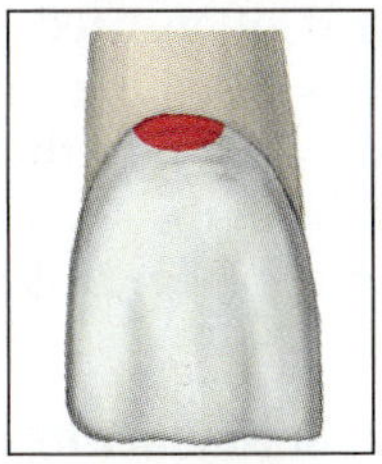
Class VI	Decay is diagnosed on the incisal edge of anterior teeth and the cusp tips of posterior teeth. Class VI decay is caused by abrasion (wear) and defects. The dental material is chosen based on which teeth are involved.	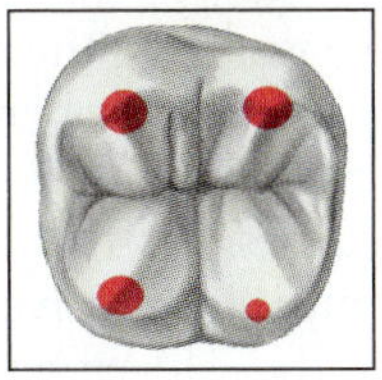

Fig. 28-7 Black's classification of cavities.

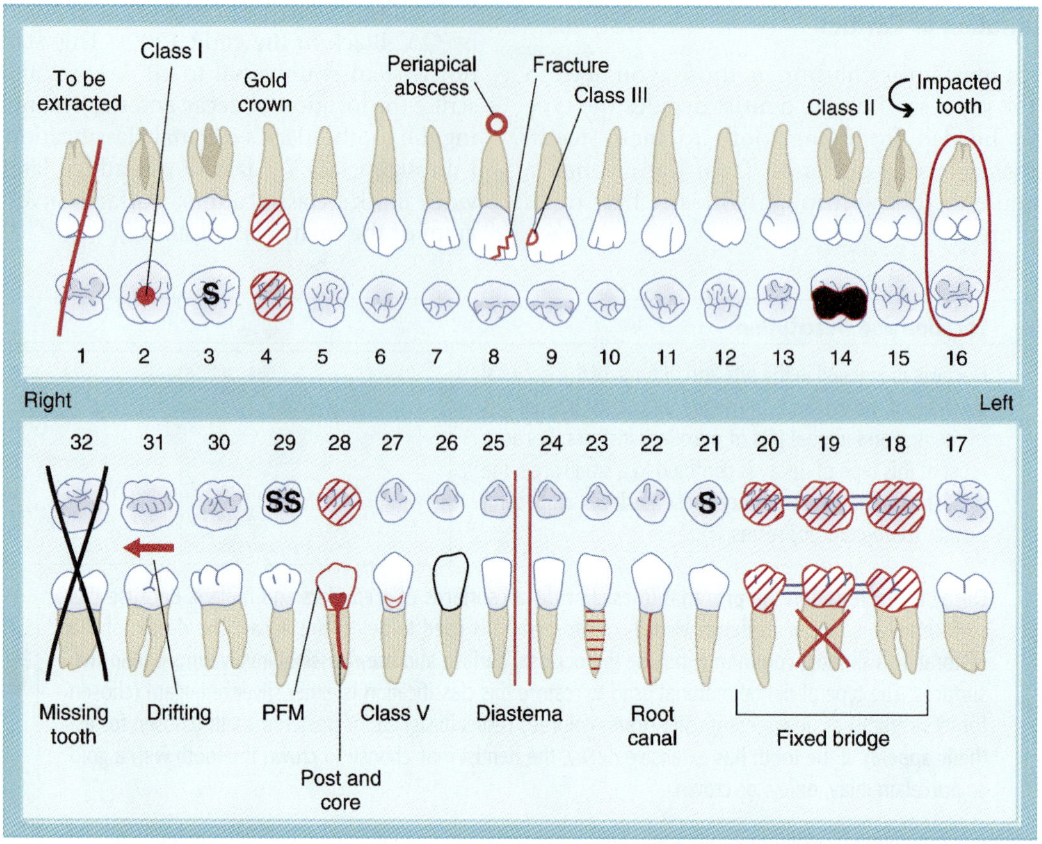

Fig. 28-8 Example of an anatomic diagram for charting conditions of the mouth (continued on page 427).

Tooth Diagrams

The clinical examination form used to complete the charting includes a diagram representing 20 primary teeth and 32 permanent teeth. When referring to the diagram, always remember that the teeth are presented from the perspective of looking into the patient's mouth. Thus the right side or right quadrants of the mouth are on the left side of the page, and the left side or left quadrants are on the right side of the page.

Dental charting systems are available in a variety of diagram styles, but anatomic and geometric designs are most often used. In the anatomic diagram the illustrations resemble the actual crown and root of the tooth (Fig. 28-8). In the geometric diagram, a circle represents each tooth. The circle is divided to represent each tooth surface (Fig. 28-9).

Tooth-Numbering Systems

To ensure that the recording is accurate, the teeth on the diagram are numbered in the sequence of a specified numbering system. The dentist selects the numbering system that best fits the dental practice, as well as the insurance companies involved.

The three most common numbering systems used for charting are described below:

Universal Numbering System

This numbering system (1-32) begins with the maxillary right third molar and concludes at the mandibular right third molar (Fig. 28-10, *A*).

International Standards Organization System/Fédération Dentaire Internationale System

This numbering system assigns a two-digit number to each tooth (the first number is the quadrant; the second number is the tooth) (Fig. 28-10, *B*).

Palmer Notation System

This numbering system uses a bracket to designate the four quadrants of the mouth (Fig. 28-10, *C*).

Color Coding

Color coding is used to represent and differentiate the treatment already completed and treatment that still needs to be completed. This method is used in both manual and computerized systems. By having this visual notation, it is easier to review the patient dental status each time the patient is seen in the dental office (Fig. 28-11).

Charting Symbol	Description
Amalgam	Outline the surfaces that are involved and color in area (refer to teeth 2 and 14).
Composite	Outline the surfaces involved (refer to teeth 9 and 27).
Porcelain fused to metal	Outline the coronal portion of the tooth and either add diagonal lines to indicate gold or use abbreviations if another metal is used (refer to tooth 28).
Gold	Outline the crown of the tooth and place diagonal lines (refer to tooth 4).
Sealant	Place an "S" on the occlusal surface (refer to teeth 3 and 21).
Stainless steel crown	Outline crown of tooth and place "SS" on occlusal surface (refer to tooth 29).
To be extracted	Draw a red diagonal line through the tooth. An alternative method is to draw two red parallel lines through the tooth (refer to tooth 1).
Missing tooth	Draw a black or blue "X" through the tooth. It does not matter if the tooth was extracted or it never erupted, just as long as the tooth is not visible in the mouth. If a quadrant, or arch, is edentulous, make one "X" over all teeth (refer to tooth 32).
Impacted or unerupted	Draw a red circle around the whole tooth, including the root (refer to tooth 16).
Decay	Depending on the caries classification, outline and color the area for amalgam (refer to tooth 2), or outline the area for composite (refer to tooth 9).
Recurrent decay	Outline the existing restoration in red to indicate decay in the area (refer to tooth 14).
Root canal	Draw a line through the center of each root involved (refer to tooth 22).
Periapical abscess	Draw a red circle at the apex of the root to indicate infection (refer to tooth 8).
Post and core	Draw a line through the root that requires a post; then continue the line into the gingival one third of the crown, making a triangle shape (refer to tooth 28).
Rotated tooth	If a tooth has rotated in its position, indicate the direction the tooth has turned by placing a red arrow to the side of the tooth (refer to tooth 15).
Diastema	When there is more space than normal between two teeth, draw two red vertical lines between the areas (refer to teeth 24 and 25).
Fixed bridge	Draw an "X" through the roots of the missing tooth or teeth involved. Then draw a line to connect each of the teeth that make up the bridge. The type of material used to make the bridge will determine whether you outline the crowns for porcelain, use diagonal lines for gold, or use a combination of the two (refer to teeth 18-20).
Full crown	Outline the complete crown if it is to be a porcelain crown, or outline and place diagonal lines if it will be a gold crown (refer to tooth 4).
Drifting	Place a red arrow pointing in the direction a tooth is drifting (refer to tooth 31).
Implant	In red, draw horizontal lines through the root or roots of a tooth (refer to tooth 23).
Bonded veneer	Veneers cover only the facial aspect of a tooth. Outline the facial portion only (refer to tooth 26).
Fractured tooth or root	If a tooth or a root is fractured, draw a red zigzag line where the fracture occurred (refer to tooth 8).

Fig. 28-8—cont'd Example of an anatomic diagram for charting conditions of the mouth (illustration on page 426).

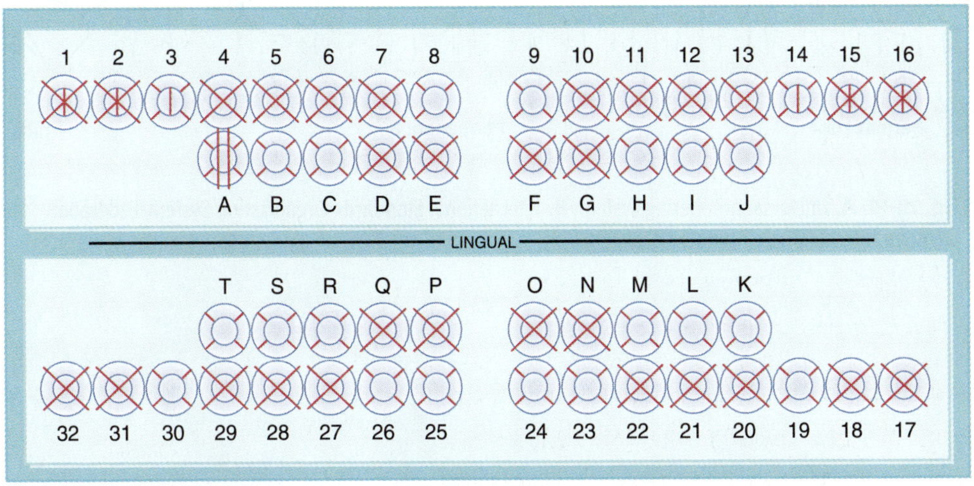

Fig. 28-9 Example of a geometric diagram for charting conditions of the mouth.

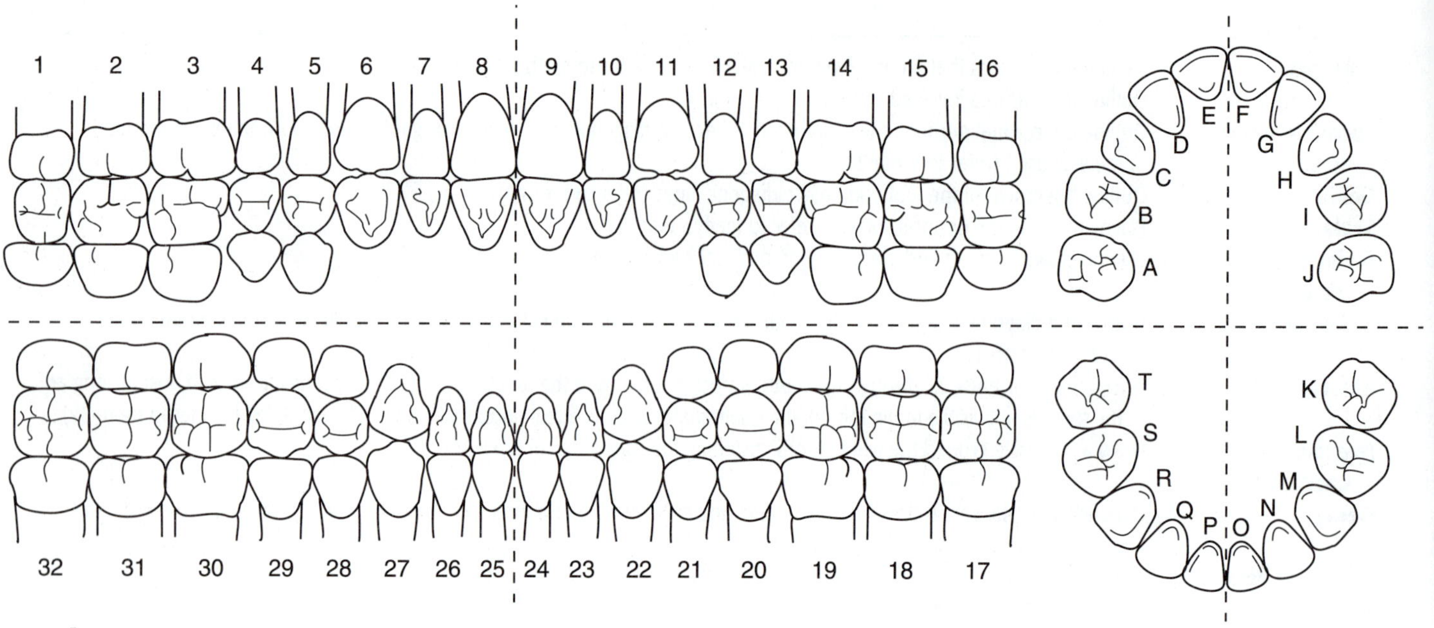

A

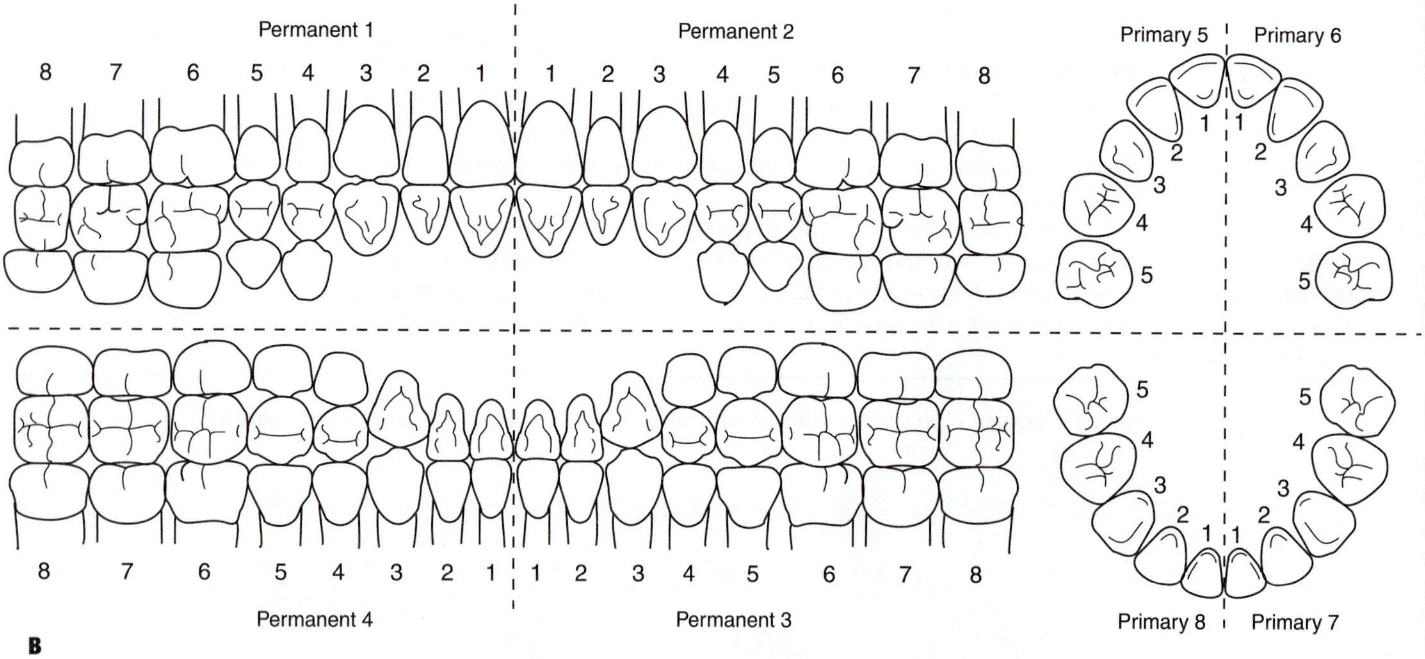

B

Fig. 28-10 **A,** Universal numbering system. **B,** International Standards Organization System/Fédération Dentaire Internationale numbering system.

continued

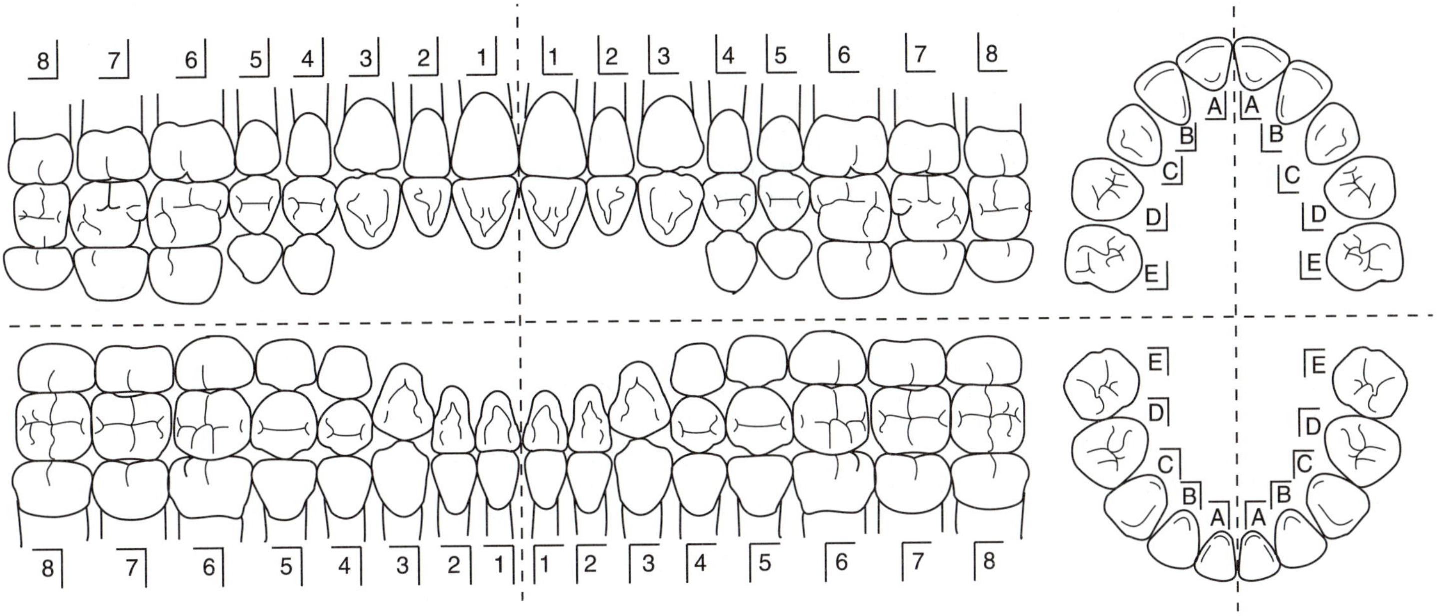

C

Fig. 28-10–cont'd C, Palmer notation system.

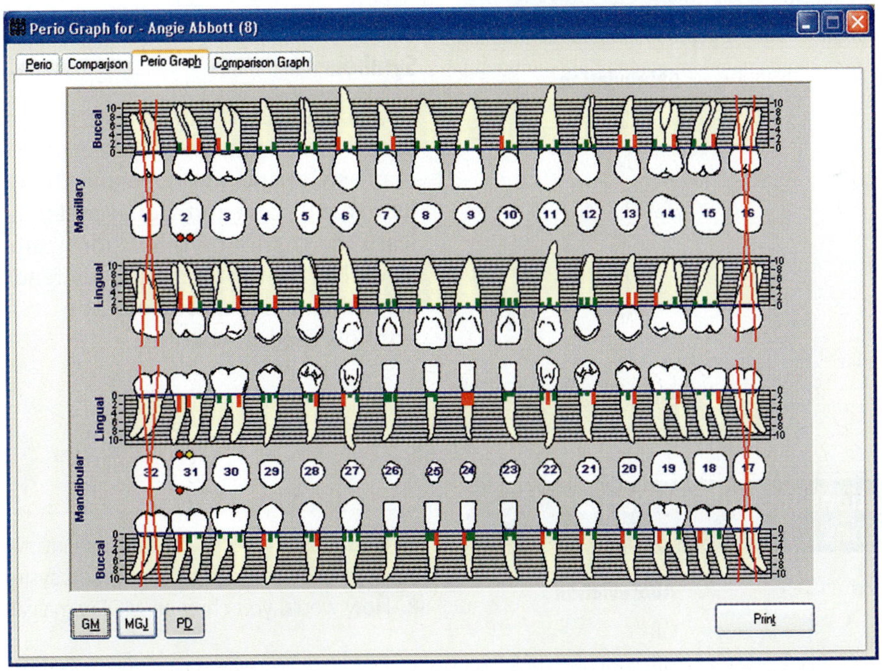

Fig. 28-11 Example of color coding, using red for existing problems and black or blue for treatment that is completed. (Courtesy Eaglesoft, a division of Patterson Dental, Inc.)

Black or *blue* symbols represent dental work already completed. This can indicate dental work completed by another dentist or during previous appointments with the current dentist. *Red* symbols indicate treatment that needs to be completed at future dental appointments. Once this work is completed, you will erase or mark over the red with a blue or black notation to indicate the work has been finished.

Abbreviations

Because of limited space in the progress notes or chart, it is best to abbreviate certain terms. Abbreviations are used to indicate a single surface or some combination of tooth surfaces.

For single-surface restorations, charting abbreviations are based on the names of the tooth surfaces (Box 28-1). For a review of tooth surfaces, see Chapter 11.

In multiple-surface restorations, two or more surfaces are involved. The combined surfaces become one name on which the abbreviation is based. The rule for combining two surfaces is to substitute the letter *"o"* for the *-al* ending of the first surface. For example, for distal and occlusal, the combined surfaces are referred to as disto-occlusal, or DO. If three surfaces are combined, the same rule applies—for example, mesio-occlusodistal, or MOD (Box 28-2). When referring to these combined surfaces, the letters of the abbreviations are pronounced separately, such as a "dee-oh" (D-O) or an "em-oh-dee" (M-O-D) restoration.

Box 28-1 Abbreviations for Single-Surface Restorations

Surface	Abbreviation
Buccal	B
Distal	D
Facial	F
Incisal	I
Lingual	L
Mesial	M
Occlusal	O

Box 28-2 Abbreviations for Multiple-Surface Restorations

Surface	Abbreviation
Occlusobuccal	OB
Distoincisal	DI
Distolingual	DL
Disto-occlusal	DO
Occlusolingual	OL
Mesioincisal	MI
Mesio-occlusal	MO
Mesio-occlusodistal	MOD
Mesio-occlusodistobuccolingual	MODBL

CHARTING

Now that you have become familiar with the clinical examination form, Black's classification of cavities, the anatomic diagram, the numbering system, and color coding, the next step is to learn the actual charting of dental materials and symbols that coordinate with the dental work that is completed or will be completed in a patient's mouth.

Restorative Materials

The anatomic diagram to be charted needs to convey what kind of dental material was used or will be used for each tooth. The best way to interpret this on a form is to have different patterns for each material.

Symbols

Charting symbols can be used on the tooth diagram of the dental record to represent the various treatments. There are many styles and ways of using charting symbols, and each dentist will have individual preferences. It is important to learn the charting symbols for treatment to be completed, as well as for treatment already rendered. See Fig. 28-8 for a review of the more common restorative materials and symbols used in charting.

Recall

6. What class in Black's classification involves premolars and molars?
7. What class in Black's classification system involves incisors?
8. How would you chart an MOD amalgam on tooth 4?

CLINICAL EXAMINATION OF THE PATIENT

The role of the clinical assistant is to escort the patient to the clinical area for the examination process. As the clinical assistant, you will follow a routine protocol for this procedure. The patient is seated in the dental treatment area, draped with a patient "napkin," and positioned for the dentist to begin the examination.

Soft Tissue Examination

The soft tissue examination involves a complete examination of the cheeks, mucosa, lips, lingual and facial alveolar bone, palate, tonsil area, tongue, and floor of the mouth. This examination requires the use of visual assessment and palpation. The purpose of this part of the examination is to detect any abnormalities in the head and neck area of a patient. Procedure 28-1 provides complete details of the soft tissue examination.

Procedure 28-1 The Soft Tissue Examination

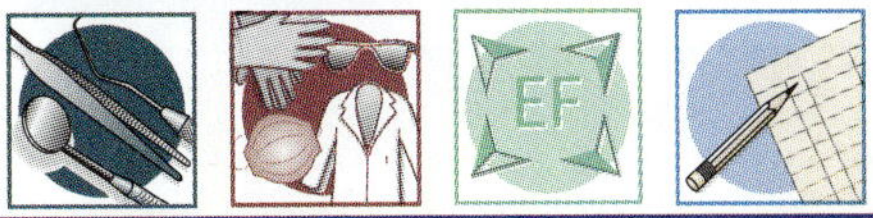

This procedure is legal for certified dental assistants to complete in many states.

Equipment and Supplies

- Gauze sponges (2 × 2 and 4 × 4)
- Tongue depressor (optional)
- Mouth mirror
- Patient record to document findings

PROCEDURAL STEPS

Patient Preparation

1. When escorting the patient to the treatment area, observe the patient's general appearance, speech, and behavior.
   Purpose: Unusual behavior or appearance must be immediately noted or called to the dentist's attention.
2. Seat the patient in the dental chair in an upright position. Drape the patient with a patient napkin.
3. Explain the procedure to the patient.
   Purpose: The patient who knows what to expect will be more comfortable and more willing to participate in the examination.

Extraoral Features

1. Examine the face, neck, and ears for asymmetry or abnormal swelling.
   Purpose: Both sides of the face should be **symmetric.**

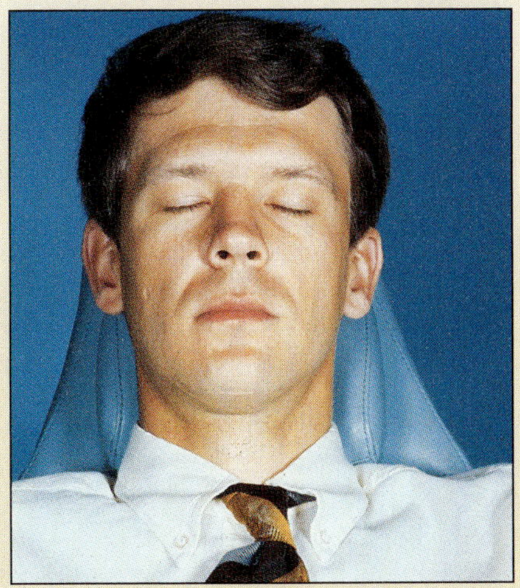

2. Look for abnormal tissue changes, skin abrasions, and discoloration.
   Purpose: Unusual bruising, scratches, or cuts may require further evaluation of the area.
3. Evaluate the texture, color, and continuity of the vermilion border, the commissures of the lips, the philtrum, and the smile line.
   Purpose: Lumps, dryness, and cracking of the tissues are deviations from normal and may require further evaluation of the area.
4. Document all findings in the patient record.

Cervical Lymph Nodes

1. Position yourself behind the patient so that you can easily place your fingers just below the patient's ears.
2. To examine the right side of the neck, use the left hand to steady the patient's head. The fingers and thumb of the right hand gently follow the chain of lymph nodes downward, starting in front of the right ear and continuing to the clavicle (collarbone).
   Purpose: You are looking for swelling, abnormal formation, and tenderness of the area.

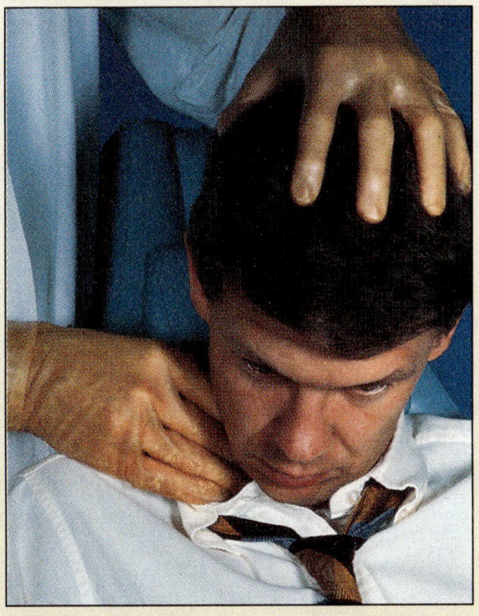

3. To examine the left side of the neck, use the right hand to steady the patient's head. The fingers and thumb of the left hand gently follow the chain of lymph nodes downward, starting in front of the left ear and continuing to the clavicle (collarbone).
4. Document all findings in the patient record.

continued

Procedure 28-1 The Soft Tissue Examination—cont'd

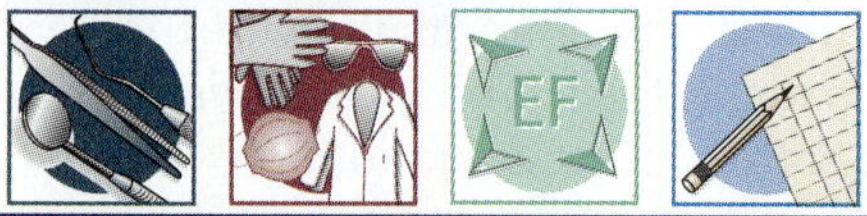

PROCEDURAL STEPS, cont'd

Temporomandibular Joint

1. To evaluate the temporomandibular joint (TMJ) movements in centric, lateral, protrusive, and retrusive movements, ask the patient to open and close the mouth normally and then to move the jaw from side to side.
2. To evaluate the movement of the TMJ further, gently place your fingers in the external opening of the ear. Ask the patient to open and close the mouth normally.

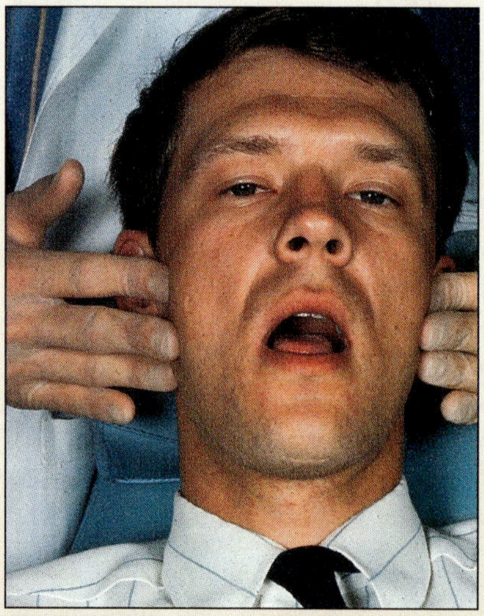

3. To determine whether there is noise in the TMJ during movement, listen as the patient opens and closes the mouth. A stethoscope placed on the joint may be used.
4. Note in the patient record any abnormalities or patient comments on pain, tenderness, or other problems related to opening and closing the mouth.

Indications of Oral Habits

1. Look for indications of oral habits such as thumb sucking, tongue-thrust swallow, mouth breathing, and tobacco use.
   Purpose: These habits can affect the patient's oral health.
2. Look for signs of other oral habits such as bruxism, grinding, and clenching. Indications include abnormal wear on the teeth and problems in the TMJ.

Interior of the Lips

1. Ask the patient to open his or her mouth slightly.
2. Examine the mucosa and labial frenum of the upper lip by gentle retraction of the lip with the thumbs and index fingers.
3. Examine the mucosa and labial frenum of the lower lip by gentle retraction of the lip with the thumbs and index fingers.
4. Palpate the tissues gently to detect lumps or similar abnormalities.

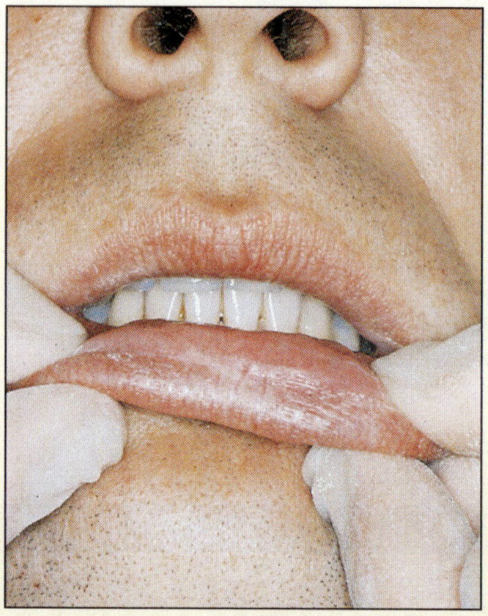

Oral Mucosa and Tongue

1. Palpate the tissue of the buccal mucosa gently by placing the thumb of one hand inside the mouth and the index and third fingers of the other hand on the exterior of the cheek.

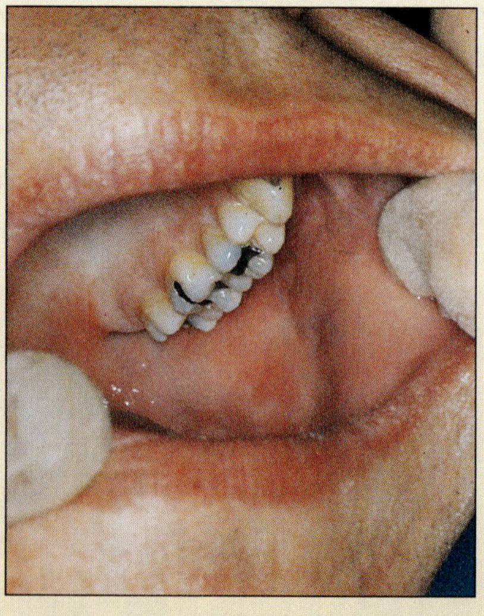

2. Examine the tissue covering the hard palate.

Procedure 28-1 The Soft Tissue Examination–cont'd

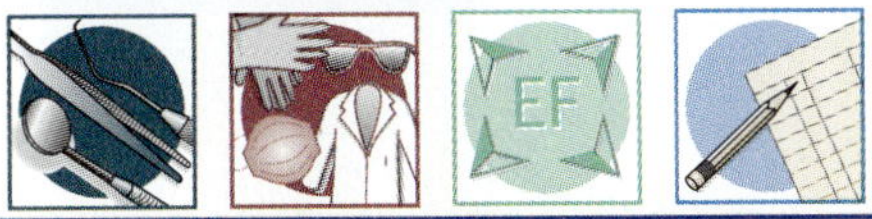

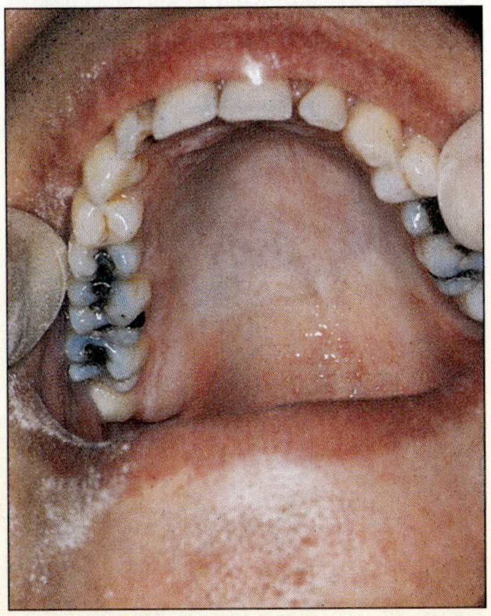

3. Examine the buccal mucosa and the opening of Stensen's duct visually. A warm mouth mirror may also be used to view the flow of saliva from the duct.
   Purpose: The mouth mirror is warmed to prevent fogging.
4. Ask the patient to extend the tongue and to relax it. Using sterile gauze, gently grasp the tip of the tongue and pull it forward.
5. Observe the dorsum (top) of the tongue for color, papillae, presence or lack of a coating, and abnormalities.
6. Gently move the tongue from side to side to examine the lateral (side) and ventral (underneath) surfaces.

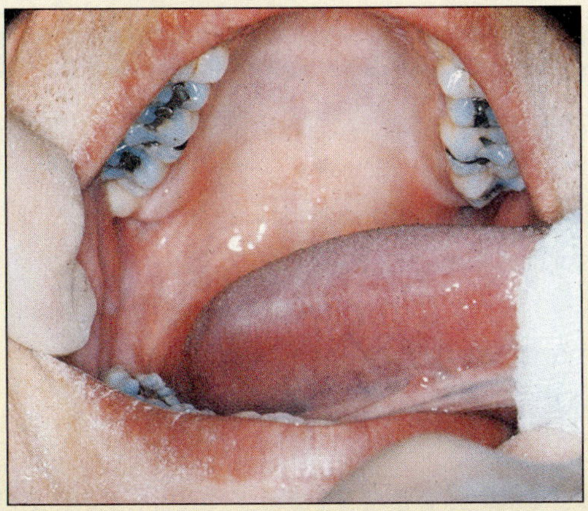

7. Use a warm mouth mirror to observe the posterior area.
   Caution: To avoid triggering the gag reflex, this mirror is placed very carefully and moved very little.
8. Examine the uvula, base of the tongue, and posterior area of the mouth by placing a mouth mirror or tongue depressor firmly at the base of the tongue.
   Caution: Firm but gentle placement reduces the possibility of triggering the gag reflex.

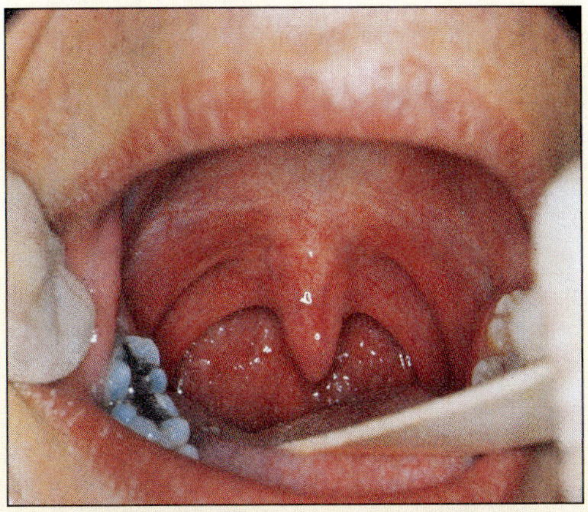

9. With the mouth mirror firmly depressing the base of the tongue, have the patient say "ahh."
   Purpose: The oropharynx expands, allowing a better view of the upper portion of the throat.

Floor of the Mouth

1. With the patient's mouth closed, palpate the soft tissues of the face above and below the mandible.
   Purpose: Tori and other abnormalities can be detected.
2. Gently palpate the interior of the floor of the mouth by placing the index finger of one hand on the floor of the mouth and placing the fingers of the other hand on the outer surface under the chin.

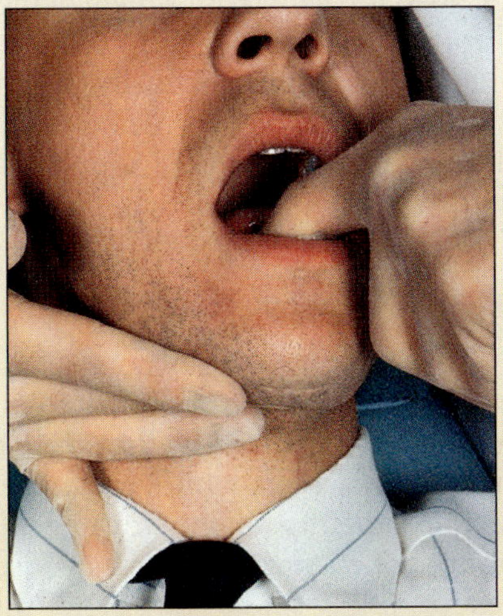

Procedure 28-1 The Soft Tissue Examination—cont'd

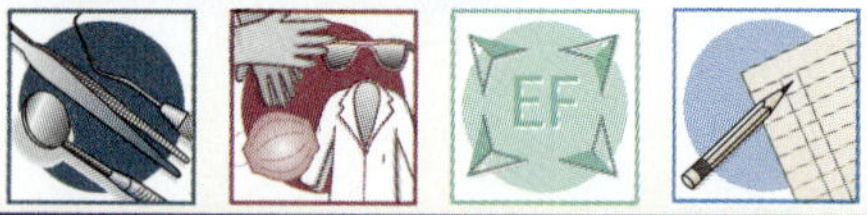

PROCEDURAL STEPS, cont'd

3. Instruct the patient to touch the tongue to the hard palate.
   Purpose: The floor of the mouth, lingual frenum, and salivary ducts can be visually examined.

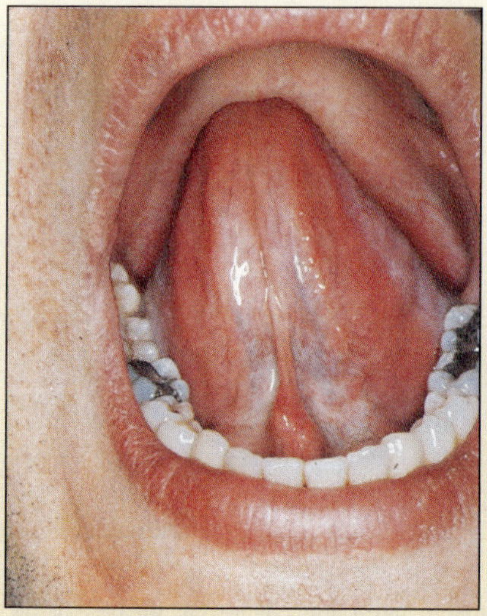

4. Observe the quantity and consistency of the flow of saliva. Depending on the patient's general health, diet, and medications, the saliva may vary in consistency from watery to thick and ropy.
5. Document all information accurately in the patient record.

Date	Extraoral examination; no changes since last exam	*Signature*

Examination and Charting of Teeth

A clinical examination of the teeth includes a thorough assessment of each tooth. Using instruments, the dentist examines each surface of each tooth and dictates the findings to the dental assistant, who records them in the clinical examination form of the patient's record. Regardless of whether findings are recorded manually or by computer, it is essential that all entries are recorded correctly and accurately. See Procedure 28-2 for complete details of the charting procedure.

Examination and Charting of Periodontium

The dental hygienist will generally complete this portion of the examination. One of the important roles of the dental hygienist is to assess the tissues that support the teeth, including the gingiva, cementum, periodontal ligament, and alveolar and supporting bone structures. The alveolar and supporting bone structure cannot be visually evaluated, so updated periapical radiographs are required for the examination process.

During this examination process, the dental hygienist notes specific conditions, using the mouth mirror, periodontal probe, and additional supplies. See Procedure 28-3 for details about how to conduct a periodontal screening.

Periodontal Findings to Be Recorded

- Overall health of the gingiva
- Signs and location of inflammation
- Location and amount of plaque and calculus
- Areas of unattached gingiva
- Areas of periodontal pockets measuring greater than 3 mm
- Presence of furcation involvement
- Mobility

Procedure 28-2 Charting of Teeth

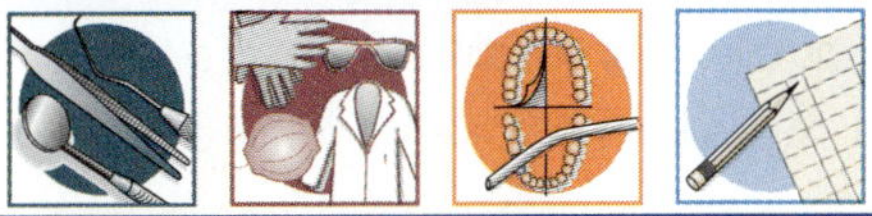

Equipment and Supplies

- Mouth mirror
- Explorer
- Cotton pliers
- Periodontal probe
- Gauze sponges (2 × 2)
- Dental floss
- Articulating paper
- Articulating paper holder
- Air-water syringe
- Colored pencils (red and blue/black)
- Eraser
- Clinical examination form

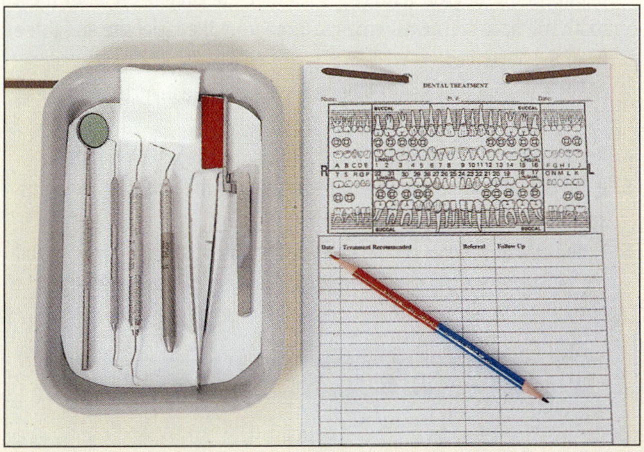

PROCEDURAL STEPS

Patient Preparation

1. The patient is already seated and draped with a patient napkin.
2. Reposition the patient in a supine position.
   Purpose: The dentist can use instruments more easily and has better intraoral vision with the patient in the supine position.

Examination of the Teeth and Occlusion

1. Ensure that colored pencils, an eraser, the clinical examination form, and a flat surface are readily available.
   Purpose: The more organized you are, the fewer errors and stops will be made.
2. Throughout the procedure, use the air syringe to clear the mouth mirror and adjust the operating light as necessary.
   Purpose: Better visualization is provided for the dentist as the teeth are examined.
3. Transfer the mirror and explorer to the dentist. The dentist will begin with tooth 1 and continue to 32. The dentist will examine every surface of each tooth.
4. Record the specific notations as the dentist calls them out.
5. The dentist will examine the patient's occlusion (bite). Place the articulating paper within the holder and transfer the instrument with the paper positioned correctly for that side of the mouth.
   Note: The holder is positioned closest to the cheek and the paper between the teeth.

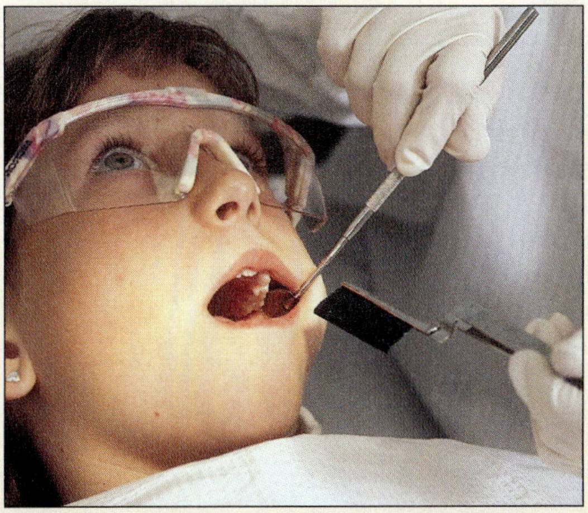

6. Any marks made by the paper will remain on the patient's occlusal and incisal surfaces.
   Purpose: The dentist will look for any abnormal markings to indicate improper occlusion.
7. At the completion of the procedure, rinse and dry the patient's mouth.
8. Document all information accurately in the patient record and sign.

Date	Intraoral exam. Patient has MO decay on tooth number 4.	
	Reschedule pt for a 2-unit appt.	*Signature/Date*

Description of Probing Scores

0: The colored area of the probe remains completely visible in the deepest sulcus in the sextant; no calculus or defective margins are detected.

1: The colored area of the probe remains completely visible in the deepest probing in the sextant; no calculus or defective margins are detected; bleeding occurs after gentle probing.

2: The colored area of the probe remains completely visible in the deepest probing in the sextant; supragingival or subgingival calculus and defective margins are detected.

3: The colored area of the probe remains partly visible in the deepest probing depth in the sextant.

4: The colored area of the probe completely disappears, indicating probing depth of more than 5.5 mm.

Procedure 28-3 Periodontal Screening: Examination of the Gingival Tissues

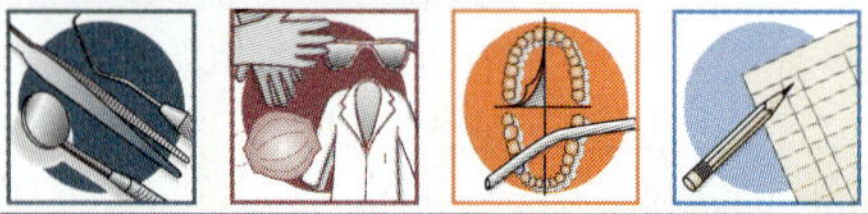

Equipment and Supplies

- Mouth mirror
- Air-water syringe
- Explorer
- Periodontal probe
- Dental floss
- Gauze sponges (2 × 2)
- Black ink pen
- Red pencil
- Clinical examination form

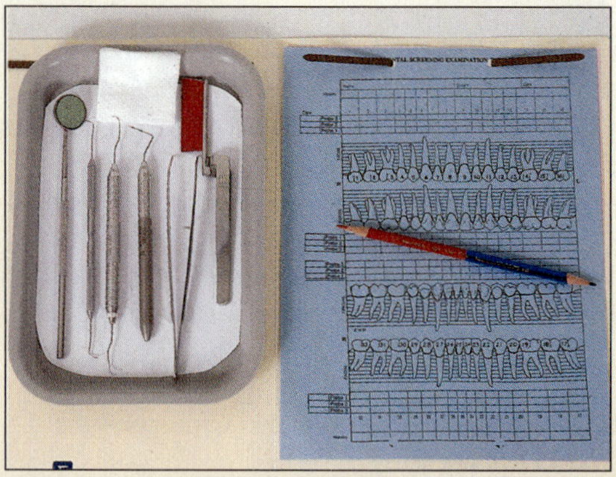

PROCEDURAL STEPS

1. The dentist or dental hygienist observes gingival status throughout the mouth using a mouth mirror. Provide a slight, continuous flow of air on the mirror from the air-water syringe.
   Purpose: This keeps the mirror from becoming fogged.
2. Transfer the periodontal probe.
   Purpose: The dental hygienist uses this instrument to determine the health of the gingiva, such as firmness of the tissue and presence of inflammation or bleeding.
3. The dental hygienist continues using the periodontal probe to measure depths of the gingival sulcus for each tooth. Beginning on tooth 1, each tooth will have six measurements: three from the facial site and three from the lingual site.
   Note: The dental hygienist follows a pattern or sequence when measuring the pocket depth.
4. Record each depth greater than 3 mm on the examination form.
5. If the dental hygienist notices bleeding during the **probing,** note this sign by circling the recorded reading.
6. Note additional items on the examination form as appropriate, including sensitivity, calculus, saliva changes, and **furcation** involvement.

Dental Mobility Scale

0: Normal

1: Slight mobility

2: Moderate mobility

3: Extreme mobility

7. If excessive bone loss is noticed on the radiograph, **mobility** may have resulted. Document any mobility on the examination form.
8. At the completion of the procedure, rinse and dry the patient's mouth.
9. Document all information accurately in the patient record and sign.

Date	Perio charting, distofacial of 14-16 recession w/pockets +5.	*Signature/Date*
	Refer to periodontist for consult.	

Using gentle pressure, the periodontal probe is inserted into the gingival sulcus until resistance is met. The probe is inserted into six specific sites for each tooth (mesiofacial, facial, distofacial, mesiolingual, lingual, and distolingual). The depth of insertion is read by noting the position of the markings on the probe while in the sulcus.

Recall

9. Which dental professional normally performs the periodontal examination and charting for a patient?

THE TREATMENT PLAN

After gathering sufficient information and reviewing it carefully, the dentist will diagnose the patient's dental conditions. On the basis of this diagnosis, the dentist may prepare one or more treatment plans for presentation to the patient.

A written treatment plan states that the dentist has made a thorough study of the patient's condition and is prepared to offer options to help the patient manage the dental treatment according to the patient's needs, priorities, and financial resources.

Types of Plans

Each treatment plan includes a description of the proposed treatment and an estimate of the fee involved. Many dentists prepare optional treatment plans for the patient's consideration. These plans can represent the following levels of care:

Level I: Emergency Care

The emergency care plan relieves immediate discomfort and provides relief to the patient.

Level II: Standard Care

The standard care plan restores the dentition to normal function. As needed, this includes restoring teeth with composite or amalgam restorations, saving teeth with endodontic treatment, conservatively treating periodontal problems, and replacing missing teeth with removable prostheses.

Level III: Optimum Care

The optimum care plan restores the dentition to maximum function and an esthetically pleasing result. When applicable, this includes restoring teeth with cast restorations (crowns, inlays, or onlays); treating periodontal, orthodontic, or endodontic problems; and replacing missing teeth with fixed and removable prosthodontic appliances or dental implants.

Treatment Plan Presentation

On completion of a thorough clinical examination, an appointment will be scheduled to present the treatment plan to the patient. The type of treatment to be rendered will determine the length of the presentation. Typically, a 30-minute to a 1-hour appointment is scheduled for the patient without interruptions.

Rather than seating the patient in a treatment room, the dentist conducts the case presentation in a private office. It is important to have available the diagnostic tools used to present the case. The dentist should have readied the patient chart, radiographs, diagnostic casts, and treatment plans. Other visual aids might include the following:

- Before-and-after photographs
- Diagnostic casts of similar cases
- Models of proposed appliances, such as full or partial dentures, dental implants, or fixed crowns and bridges

The patient is made comfortable, and the dentist takes care to present all information in terms that the patient can understand. The dentist then explains the findings regarding the patient diagnosis and prognosis.

Following the presentation, the dentist or finance manager will present the fee estimate for each treatment option. The patient is encouraged to ask questions and to discuss the advantages and disadvantages of each plan. When the patient makes a decision and accepts a treatment plan, he or she is giving informed consent for treatment. At this time the finance manager will explain the payment plans and make the necessary financial arrangements with the patient. When all these arrangements have been completed, the patient is scheduled for treatment.

RECORDING THE DENTAL TREATMENT

When a procedure is completed, a specific sequence is followed in recording treatment information in the patient dental record in the "Treatment Provided" section (Procedure 28-4).

At the end of the appointment, the dental record is completed with basic information about the visit, including the procedure or procedures performed, the tooth number or teeth numbers and surface or surfaces, and the fee charged for each procedure. All pertinent information, such as postoperative instructions, must be recorded in the dental record. The entry must be clear and concise and recorded in black ink.

Procedure 28-4 Recording the Completed Dental Treatment

Equipment and Supplies

- Black ink pen
- Patient's record

PROCEDURAL STEPS

1. In the Date column, record the date the treatment was provided, using numbers in a month/date/year format, such as 2/27/05.
2. In the Progress Notes column, record all areas of the dental procedure, such as the tooth, the surfaces of the tooth restored, the type and amount of anesthetic agent, the dental materials used, and the patient tolerance of the appointment.
3. If appropriate, describe the procedure that was performed with appropriate details, such as whether the tooth was prepared for a crown.
   Purpose: The treatment is documented, which serves as a reference for future appointments.
4. After entering the complete treatment, sign the entry.
   Note: Always make sure to have the dentist sign. This verifies the entry is accurate and was completed.
5. Return the completed dental record to the business office.
   Purpose: The patient returns to the business office area to make payment for services and schedule any additional appointments.

Patient Education

Diagnostic procedures are precise and often complex. These services provide the dentist and patient with a complete and accurate assessment of the patient's oral health condition. When properly informed, a patient is better prepared to continue with home oral health procedures.

It is important to have brochures, diagrams, and consumer information describing the types of dental conditions and available treatment for your patients. Patients prefer to have information they can take with them to review personally before making a final decision. When you work as a team, you are putting your patients first and providing them the best care.

Legal and Ethical Implications

The services and procedures described in this chapter are basic tasks that the dental assistant is required to perform every day. The techniques require knowledge and understanding of the clinical examination form and proper charting techniques. When you perform the charting for a patient, you are responsible for what has been documented. Remember the following:

- Understand the diagrams in the clinical examination form.
- Know the numbering system used in your office.
- Know the surfaces of teeth.
- Know charting symbols.

If you chart the wrong tooth or the wrong condition, you initiate a compromising legal situation.

Eye to the Future

With the increased intake of fluoridation in the population, dentists are finding it challenging to detect decay in areas of the teeth that are more difficult to examine. New devices are being designed using laser light energy (wavelength) that can be directed to a specific area of a tooth surface. When illuminated, the carious lesion will become fluorescent. The device will measure the laser fluorescence and calculate a value. The values will be used to determine a course of action ranging from no action, to preventive therapy, to monitoring of caries development, to placement of sealants, and finally, to restoration of the tooth.

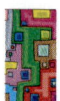

Critical Thinking

1. During what portion of the oral diagnosis examination is tooth mobility evaluated?
2. Describe two parts of the soft tissue examination that take place extraorally.
3. What instruments and supplies are included in the setup for the charting of the teeth?
4. When charting the periodontium, tooth 4 has recordings of 5 and 6 with bleeding. Are these charted? If so, how is the bleeding indicated on the chart?
5. With a charting form in front of you, chart the following conditions:
   a. Tooth 1 is missing.
   b. Tooth 2 has occlusal decay.
   c. Tooth 7 has a PFM crown.
   d. Tooth 11 has an MI composite.
   e. Tooth 13 has disto-occlusal decay.
   f. Tooth 16 is missing.
   g. Tooth 19 has a root canal.
   h. Tooth 21 has a sealant.
   i. Teeth 23 to 26 have a bridge to replace teeth 24 and 25.
   j. Tooth 29 has a periapical abscess.
   k. Tooth 32 is impacted.

29

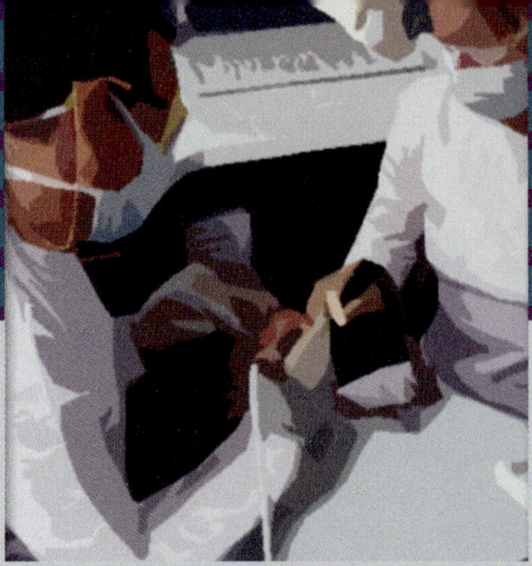

The Medically and Physically Compromised Patient

Outline

The Rights of All Patients
Role of the Dental Assistant
The Aging Population
- Stages of Aging
- Oral Health of the Aging
- Oral Health Conditions

The Medically Compromised Patient
Specific Illnesses of the Medically Compromised Patient
- Neurologic Disorders
- Cardiovascular Disorders
- Pulmonary Disorders
- Blood Disorders
- Musculoskeletal Disorders
- Endocrine Disorders
- Behavioral and Psychiatric Disorders

The Physically Compromised Patient
- The Wheelchair-Bound Patient
- The Vision-Impaired Patient
- The Hearing-Impaired Patient

Procedure 29-1: Transferring a Patient from a Wheelchair
Assistance from Organizations
Legal and Ethical Implications
Eye to the Future
Critical Thinking

KEY TERMS

Alzheimer's disease (**alts**-hi-merz) A form of progressive mental deterioration occurring in middle to older age.

Anemia (ah-**nee**-me-ah) A shortage of red cells or hemoglobin in the blood, resulting in paleness and weakness.

Angina (an-**ji**-nah) Severe chest pain associated with an insufficient supply of blood to the heart.

Arthritis (ar-**thri**-tis) Inflammation of a joint or many joints, resulting in pain and swelling.

Asthma (**az**-mah) Respiratory disease often associated with allergies and characterized by sudden recurring attacks of labored breathing, chest constriction, and coughing.

Atrophy (**a**-trah-fee) A wasting away or deterioration.

Bacteremia (bak-tah-**ree**-me-ah) Presence of bacteria in the blood.

Bronchitis (brahn-**ki**-tis) Inflammation of the mucous membranes of the bronchial tubes.

Cannula (**kan**-yuh-lah) Flexible tube inserted into a body opening.

Dementia (di-**men[t]**-shah) A mental disorder characterized by loss of memory, concentration, and judgment.

Diabetes mellitus (die-ah-**bee**-tez **me**-leh-tus, meh-**lie**-tus) Metabolic disorder characterized by high blood glucose and insufficient insulin.

Emphysema (em[p]-feh-**zee**-mah) Abnormal increase in the size of the air spaces in the lungs, resulting in labored breathing and an increased susceptibility to infection.

KEY TERMS—cont'd

Endocarditis (*en*-doe-kahr-**die**-tus) Inflammation of the endocardium.

Epilepsy (**eh**-pah-*lep*-see) Neurologic disorder with sudden recurring seizures of motor, sensory, or psychic malfunction.

Hemophilia (*heh*-meh-**fi**-lee-ah, *heh*-mo-**fil**-ee-ah) Blood coagulation disorder in which the blood fails to clot normally.

Hyperplasia (*hi*-per-**play**-zh[ee-]ah) Abnormal increase in the number of cells in an organ or a tissue.

Hyperthyroidism (*hi*-per-**thi**-roid-iz-em, *hi*-per-**thi**-roi-di-zem) Condition resulting from excessive activity of the thyroid gland.

Hypothyroidism (*hi*-poe-**thi**-roid-iz-em, *hi*-poe-**thi**-roi-di-zem) Condition resulting from severe thyroid hormone insufficiency.

Leukemia (lu-**kee**-me-ah) A progressive disease in which the bone marrow produces an increased number of immature or abnormal white cells.

Myocardial infarction (*mi*-oh-**kahr**-dee-ul in-**fark**-shun) Condition in which there is damage to the muscular tissue of the heart, commonly caused by obstructed circulation; also referred to as a *heart attack.*

Seizure A sudden attack, spasm, or convulsion, that occurs in specific disorders.

Stroke A sudden loss of brain function caused by a blockage or rupture of a blood vessel to the brain; also called *cerebrovascular accident.*

Xerostomia (*zir*-oh-**stoh**-me-ah) Loss of saliva production causing a dry mouth.

LEARNING OUTCOMES

On completion of this chapter, the student will be able to achieve the following objectives:

- Pronounce, define, and spell the Key Terms.
- Describe the stages of aging in the older population.
- Describe the orally related conditions affecting the older patient.
- Describe the importance of the medical history for the medically compromised patient.
- Describe the major medical disorders that can affect a patient's oral health.
- Describe the type of dental management a medically compromised patient would receive.

PERFORMANCE OUTCOMES

On completion of this chapter, the student will be able to meet competency standards in the following skill:

- Demonstrate the correct transfer of a wheelchair-bound patient.

With advances in medicine, people are living longer and surviving medical diseases that may have resulted in a disability or premature death in the past. Because of this progress, more individuals are also living longer with some type of medical or physical disorder.

It is the responsibility of the dentist and dental team to identify the challenges that face these patients. The dental team must provide dental care by seeking necessary consultations and modifying dental treatment according to the patient's needs.

Patients who enter your dental practice may be very ill, in pain, or physically challenged. Your job will be to use good judgment in helping these patients, which may mean bypassing some of the usual routines that take place during an appointment.

THE RIGHTS OF ALL PATIENTS

The *Americans with Disabilities Act* was designed to provide a national mandate for the elimination of discrimination against individuals with special needs. The act provides clear, strong, enforceable standards addressing discrimination against people with disabilities. *Disabilities* under this act include cancer, heart disease, diabetes, mental retardation, learning disabilities, and visual and hearing impairment, as well as acquired immunodeficiency syndrome (AIDS) and infection with human immunodeficiency virus (HIV).

The American Dental Association (ADA) has issued the following supporting statements:

- *Title I* eliminates employment discrimination policies in the hiring of a person with a disability.
- *Title II* states that a dental practice, clinic, or school must provide appropriate access for disabled persons.
- *Title III* opens public accommodations to disabled persons and provides them with access to equal goods and services.
- *Title IV* extends telecommunication services to hearing-impaired and speech-impaired persons.

ROLE OF THE DENTAL ASSISTANT

The dental assistant's role in caring for the medically and physically compromised patient can be divided into three major areas:

1. *Aiding the dentist in providing treatment.* The chairside assistant must be familiar with any specialized techniques

and equipment used in treating the medically and physically compromised patient. The efficiency of all dental team members is important to speed and ease in the treatment.

2. *Provide a source of information to the patient and the family.* Preventive dentistry is particularly important and may prove difficult for the physically and medically challenged patient. The assistant may be asked to work with the patient and family in developing and implementing a preventive program tailored to the needs of a patient.
3. *Making the patient more comfortable and reducing anxiety.* The patient may be particularly apprehensive because of extensive painful experiences with medical treatment. It is the dental team's job to help alleviate the anxiety and provide a comfortable environment.

THE AGING POPULATION

With a declining birthrate and increased longevity, the older population is the fastest-growing segment of the U.S. population. People age 65 and older make up at least 10 percent of the population in the majority of U.S. states (Fig. 29-1).

Stages of Aging

Aging refers to the irreversible and inevitable changes that occur with time. Most oral conditions developing in older adults were once believed to be a result of age, not disease. Current science teaches that this is not the case. In diagnosis and treatment planning, it is helpful to differentiate signs and symptoms caused by age from those caused by *disease.*

Older adults, or persons over 65, vary in their psychologic and physiologic stages. To identify their varying attitudes, characteristics, and needs more effectively, older persons can be divided into three categories, as follows:

1. *"Young-old" persons: ages 65 to 74.* Patients in this age group are better educated and more demanding of health services than in the past. This group has retained more of their natural teeth and expects to maintain them throughout their lives.
2. *"Old" persons: ages 75 to 84.* Persons in this age group are beginning to have multiple health problems. Some have maintained their natural teeth, but more of them have fixed and removable prostheses.
3. *"Old-old" persons: ages 85 and older.* Persons in this age group have fewer natural teeth and believe that tooth loss is an inevitable part of aging. This segment of the population tend to have medical conditions that are reflected in their oral health.

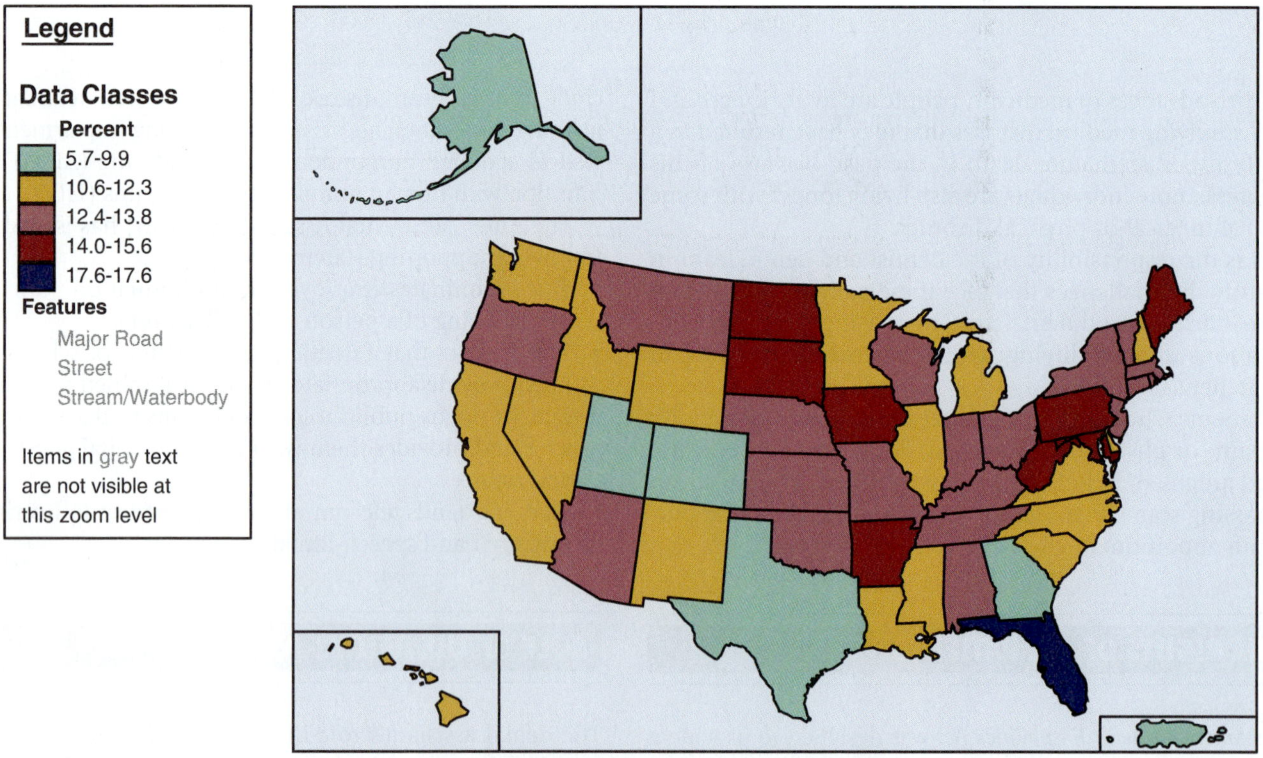

Source: U.S. Census Bureau, Census 2000 Summary File 1, Matrices P1, and P30.

Fig. 29-1 Percentages of Americans age 65 and older in each state. (From the U.S. Census Bureau 2000 Summary.)

Recall

1. What act protects people with special needs?
2. What is the fastest-growing segment of the population?

Oral Health of the Aging

Although the older population is faced with special health care problems, the goals of the dental team treating these patients are essentially the same as those for younger patients. Age itself is not a key factor in treatment planning; however, age-related oral changes, the prevalence of various oral diseases, multiple chronic diseases, and the greater use of prescription drugs can complicate treatment planning.

The condition of the mouth can affect self-esteem, esthetics, nutrition, social interaction, and personal comfort. General health can deteriorate because of problems with mastication, the mucosa, or the periodontium. These patients may have multiple chronic health conditions and may be taking several medications prescribed by different physicians.

Obtaining a current and complete medical and medication history is essential. The taking of the medical history is more important, more complex, and more time-consuming.

Along with the medical history, it is essential that a *medication profile* be completed for each patient. One of the hallmarks of disease is the list of prescriptions a patient is taking. These drugs not only indicate the patient's disease state but also have potential side effects and drug interactions that must be taken into consideration during treatment planning. A medication profile can indicate the severity of a patient's medical condition.

Oral Health Conditions

The most commonly reported oral-related health conditions affecting older patients are xerostomia, periodontal disease, tooth decay, dark and brittle teeth, and bone resorption.

Xerostomia

Also known as *dry mouth,* **xerostomia** is the result of disorders and medications that cause a decreased flow of saliva. Over 250 drugs have the potential to cause dry mouth as a side effect. In addition to drug side effects, xerostomia can also be a result of radiation treatment.

Periodontal Disease

Periodontal conditions are an increasing problem in the older population. Over 50 percent of older people may be affected by periodontal disease—with most of them unaware of it. As a larger number of older people retain their teeth, periodontal disease will increase (Fig. 29-2). Periodontal disease can be prevented with better oral hygiene care and more frequent visits to the hygienist.

Dental Decay

With age, often the gums recede, exposing the roots of the teeth. Unlike crowns, the roots of the teeth are not protected by enamel, so cavities can quickly develop on root surfaces (Fig. 29-3). Root caries can sometimes be prevented by diet adjustments and changes in the way teeth are brushed.

Dark and Brittle Teeth

As we age, teeth may darken and become more brittle. This is a result of deposits of secondary dentin that have gradually reduced the size of the pulp chamber. These teeth then become more susceptible to fracture (Fig. 29-4).

Bone Resorption

When teeth are missing or the patient is partially to fully edentulous, portions of the alveolar ridge are compro-

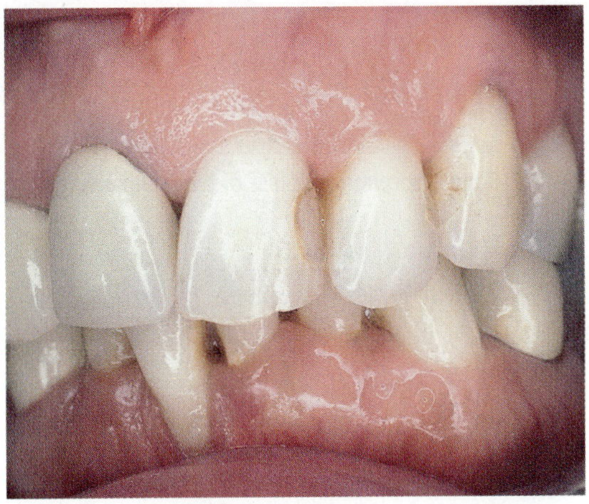

Fig. 29-2 Periodontal conditions of an older patient.

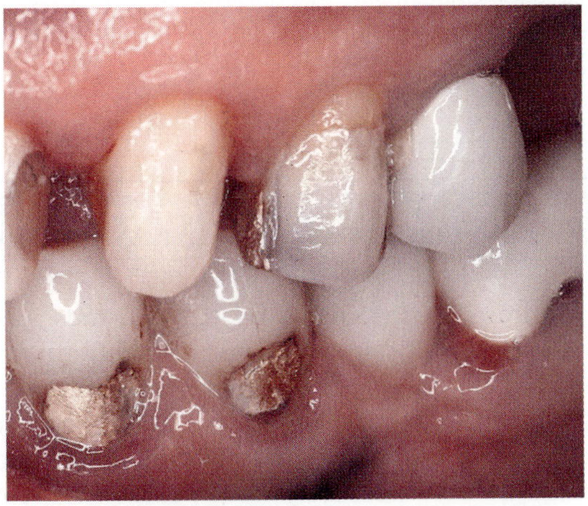

Fig. 29-3 Root caries of a tooth in an older patient.

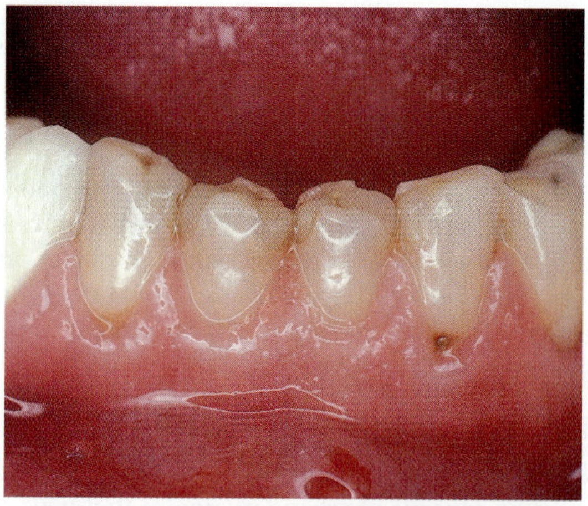

Fig. 29-4 Darkened teeth associated with secondary dentin and aging.

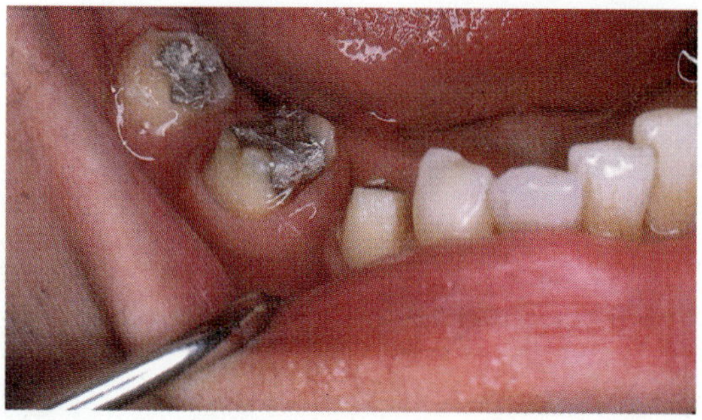

Fig. 29-5 Bone resorption with loss of teeth and alveolar ridge.

mised and lost (Fig. 29-5). Bone resorption can affect speech as well as a patient's diet (see Chapter 52).

Recall

3. What aging category would include a 76-year-old dental patient?
4. What is xerostomia?
5. What are four oral health conditions that affect the aging population?

THE MEDICALLY COMPROMISED PATIENT

The medically compromised patient demands a dental team that is aware of the necessary critical information regarding a patient in order to provide the safest and most thorough dental care available. Once an appropriate and accurate history is obtained from the patient, the information must be used effectively. Each patient should be assessed before treatment.

Patients can be categorized into five specific areas according to how treatment is to be provided:

1. *Category I* involves healthy patients who require no special modifications.
2. *Category II* involves patients with medical conditions who require scheduling changes or shorter appointments.
3. *Category III* involves patients with medical conditions that have lifelong implications; these patients require modifications in dental treatment planning, including alterations in anesthetic, types of dental materials, and patient positioning.
4. *Category IV* involves patients with medical conditions who require more significant modifications in dental treatment planning, including completion of dental needs within the operating room.
5. *Category V* involves patients with serious medical conditions who require only limited care to eliminate serious acute oral disease. This level is for patients who must be kept free of pain and discomfort.

SPECIFIC ILLNESSES OF THE MEDICALLY COMPROMISED PATIENT

Diseases do not only affect a specific body system; they can also affect other areas of the body, including the mouth. A basic understanding of how an illness or disease can affect oral function and help prevent unnecessary tooth loss or other complications is important for the dental assistant and dental team.

Symptoms of over 100 diseases show up in the mouth. Many illnesses indirectly affect the mouth by causing a person to be less capable of caring for his or her mouth. Also, medications prescribed to treat diseases can negatively affect the flow and consistency of saliva and the texture of the tongue or cause changes in the gums, which can result in diminished function and tooth loss.

Neurologic Disorders

Alzheimer's Disease

Alzheimer's disease is a brain disorder that is marked by deterioration of mental capacity **(dementia)** that begins at middle age. The patient shows loss of memory and impairment of judgment, comprehension, and intellect. Anxiety, depression, and emotional disturbances can occur as well. With time, the person becomes totally dependent and unable to perform any of the activities of daily living without help.

Seizures

A patient with a history of **seizures** can have an abrupt suspension of motor, sensory, behavioral or bodily function at any time. **Epilepsy,** *recurrent convulsive disorder,*

Treatment Plan Modifications for a Patient with Alzheimer's Disease

Have a thorough dental exam in the early stages of the disease. Dental treatment can be easily tolerated in the early stages.

Pay special attention to daily care of the mouth. This will allow the person to remain free of pain and be able to chew.

In the advanced stages of the disease, many patients cannot tolerate a denture and may need to have them permanently removed.

Patients may show signs of xerostomia resulting from a prescribed psychoactive drug. Regular oral hygiene and the use of fluoride supplements and salivary substitutes are important to preserve dental health.

Dental visits should be scheduled with an awareness of the patient's best time of day.

The presence of a familiar caregiver, such as a family member, in the treatment room often will allay the patient's fear.

and *epileptic seizures* are terms that are often used interchangeably to designate symptoms that can affect up to 1 percent of the general population. In about half the patients, no cause is found, although head injuries, brain tumors, lead poisoning, problems in brain development before birth, and certain genetic and infectious illnesses can cause epilepsy.

Petit mal seizures

This type of seizure lasts no longer than 30 seconds, usually 5 to 10 seconds. A petit mal seizure may be manifested in a variety of ways, such as a brief stare into space, a slight quivering of the trunk and limb muscles, drooping or nodding of the head, or upward rolling of the eyes or rapid blinking of the eyelids.

Grand mal seizures

Also known as *generalized seizures,* grand mal seizures have many causes and arise in all age groups. They may be preceded by an aura (a brief experience such as an unpleasant odor, visual or aural hallucinations, or strange sensations in the leg or arm) or by localized spasm or twitching of the muscles, followed by loss of consciousness.

Multiple Sclerosis

Multiple sclerosis is one of the most common neurologic diseases affecting adults between ages 30 and 50. As the disease advances, the patient has progressive weakening of the lower extremities, causing muscle weakness, unsteady gait, and paralysis. For the management of patients with multiple sclerosis, adrenal suppressants such as prednisone and muscle relaxants such as diazepam may be prescribed to control muscle spasms.

Specific Problems Related to Dental Care for a Patient with Epilepsy

Generalized seizures could occur in the dental office.

The drug phenytoin (Dilantin) is used to control epileptic seizures. A common side effect of this medication is **hyperplasia** (overgrowth) of the gingival tissue (see Chapter 17).

Treatment plan modifications for a patient with epilepsy

Maintain oral hygiene.

Perform surgical reduction of gingival hyperplasia.

Before treatment, question patients with a history of seizures about (1) skipping medications or meals, (2) stress and fatigue, (3) pain, and (4) alcohol consumption.

Treatment Plan Modifications for Patients with Multiple Sclerosis

Adrenal suppressants such as prednisone and muscle relaxants such as diazepam can be prescribed to help control muscle spasms during an appointment.

If a patient is wheelchair-bound, it may be more comfortable for the patient to remain in the wheelchair during dental treatment.

Stroke

A patient who has had a cerebrovascular accident, or **stroke,** has experienced a minor to severe loss of the central nervous system function caused by a sudden vascular lesion of the brain, such as hemorrhage, embolism, thrombosis, or ruptured aneurysm (Fig. 29-6). The clinical presentation of a patient can vary, depending on the area and extent of injury to the brain. The patient may have unilateral weakness or paralysis of the eyes and facial muscles, as well as slurring or loss of speech. Numbness, vertigo, visual disturbances, sweating, headache, and nausea often are present.

Recall

6. What is dementia?
7. What common side effect occurs from taking phenytoin?
8. What is another term for cerebrovascular accident?
9. What are two examples of neurologic disorders?

Specific Problems Related to Dental Care for a Stroke Patient

If paralysis occurs, a person could repeatedly bite his or her cheek or tongue and not feel it.

Patients may not be able to detect ulcers caused by dentures.

Food impaction could occur, resulting in decay and gum disease.

Treatment plan modifications for a patient with stroke

Schedule for the midmorning, with an average of 10 minutes added to the appointment for additional communication and explanation of instructions.

Modified oral hygiene aids may need to be introduced.

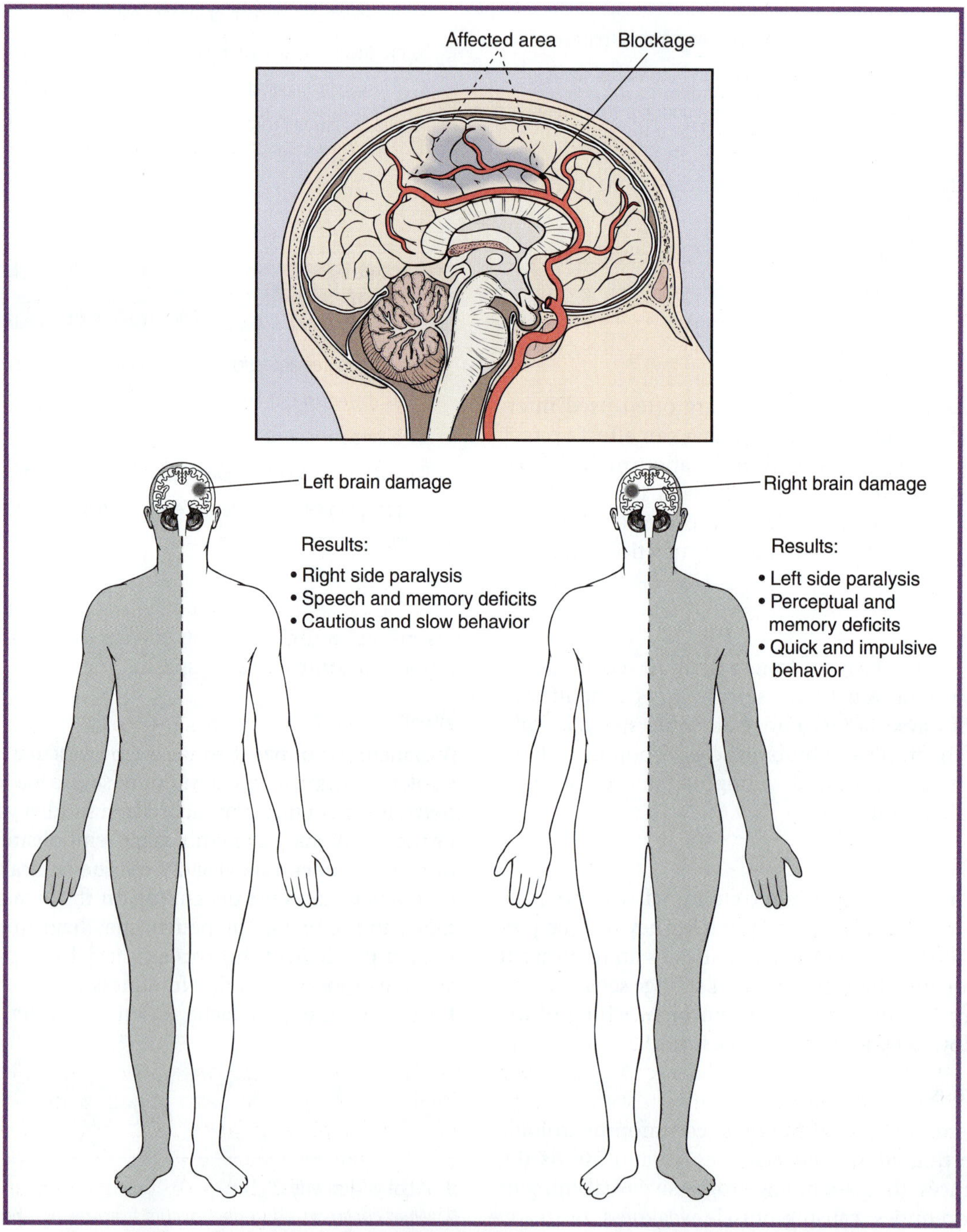

Fig. 29-6 Effects of a cerebrovascular accident (stroke). (From Frazier MS, Drzymkowski JA: *Essentials of human diseases and conditions,* ed 3, St Louis, 2004, Saunders.)

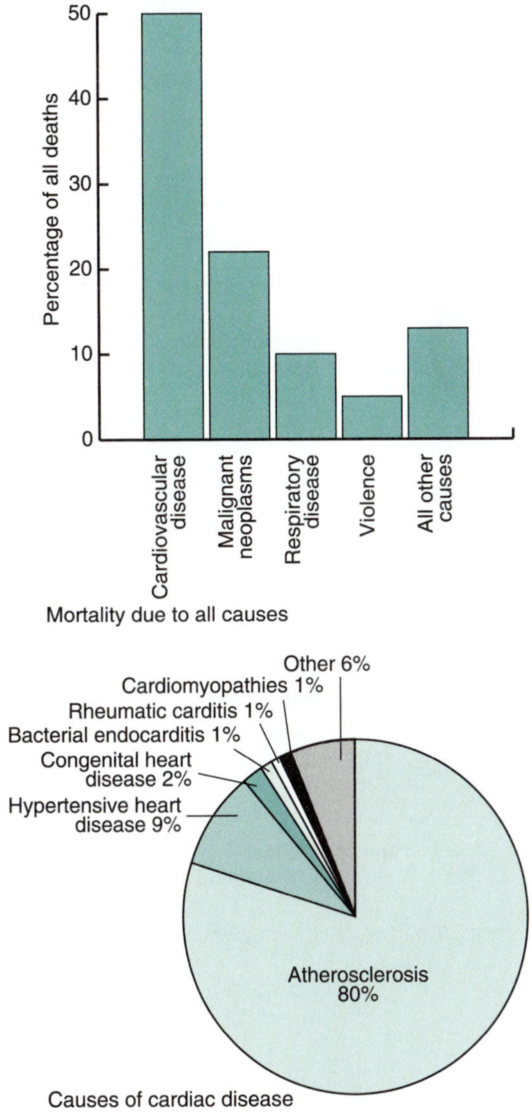

Fig. 29-7 Incidence of heart disease. (From Damjanov I: *Pathology for the health-related professions,* ed 2, Philadelphia, 2000, Saunders.)

Cardiovascular Disorders

It is estimated that 20 million Americans have some form of cardiovascular disease today. Heart disease continues to be one of the most serious threats to the health of individuals; it is the leading cause of death for men over the age of 40 and for women over the age of 65 (Fig. 29-7). Heart disease can manifest as any number of conditions, such as hypertension, stable or unstable angina, congestive heart failure, and **myocardial infarction.** The dentist must know how the patient's heart disease is being managed and what medications the patient is taking.

Congestive Heart Failure

Congestive heart failure is a condition in which the heart cannot pump enough blood to the body's other organs. People with heart failure cannot exert themselves because they become short of breath and tired. This lack of circulation throughout the body can result from any of the following:

- Narrowed arteries
- Scar tissue from a past heart attack interfering with the heart muscle
- High blood pressure
- Heart valve disease
- Heart defect
- Infection of the heart valve or muscle (endocarditis or myocarditis)

Treatment Plan Modifications for a Patient with Heart Disease

Avoid stressful, lengthy appointments

Obtain vital signs before treatment; consider monitoring throughout the procedure.

The dentist may use premedication and nitrous oxide to help relieve stress.

Consider the use of supplemental oxygen throughout the procedure.

The dentist may consider the use of prophylactic sublingual nitroglycerin immediately before treatment.

Epinephrine and other vasoconstrictors can be administered within limits to patients with mild to moderate cardiovascular disease.

Seated patients are more comfortable in a semisupine position rather than supine.

Hypertension

Also referred to as *high blood pressure,* hypertension is the result of the heart having to work harder as it pumps against resistance such as a blocked artery (Fig. 29-8). Stress is believed to be a major factor in hypertension. Age, heredity, smoking, and obesity are also contributing factors.

Most patients diagnosed with hypertension are on a program of drug therapy to help relieve the high blood pressure. In addition, patients will be instructed to limit salt intake, follow a particular diet, increase their exercise regimen, and reduce stress in their lives.

Angina

Angina pectoris is a coronary disease in which a decrease in blood supply to the heart muscle causes a sharp pain in the chest. **Angina** can be "stable," in which case the pain is usually predictable, or "unstable," in which case the pain is unpredictable. Patients diagnosed with angina usually have also been diagnosed with coronary atherosclerotic heart disease. Angina is a sign that a patient is at risk for a heart attack.

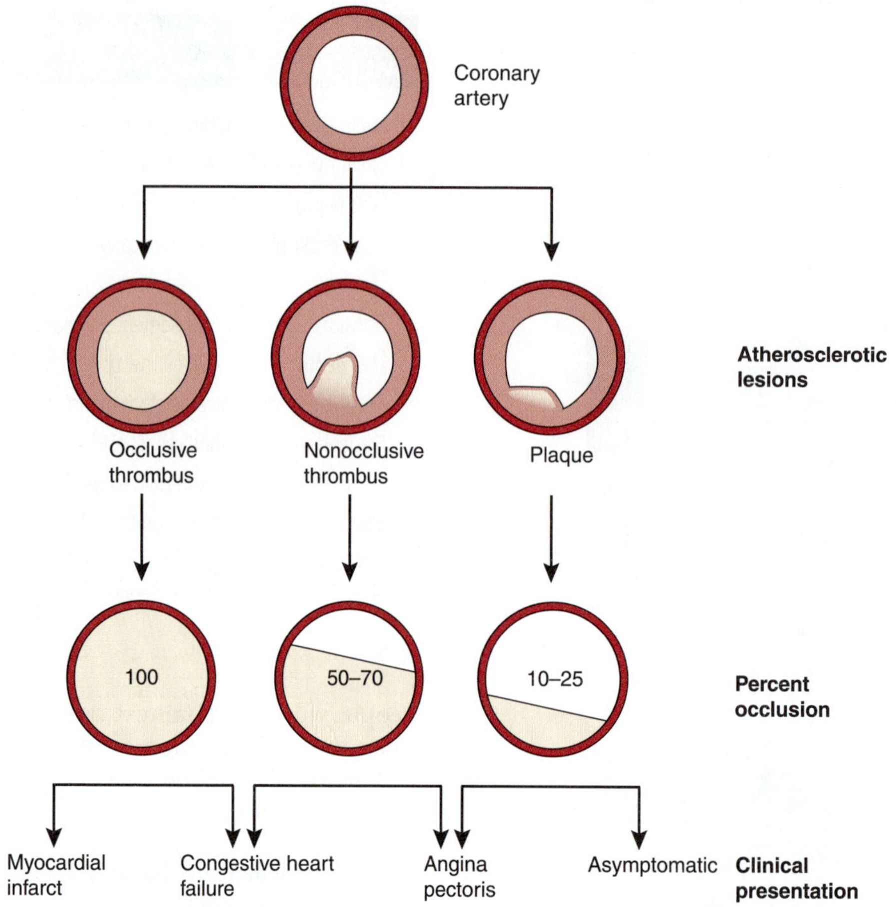

Fig. 29-8 Effects of a blocked artery. (From Kinn ME, Woods M: *The medical assistant: administrative and clinical,* ed 8, Philadelphia, 1999, Saunders.)

Patients with a history of angina pectoris should be on a program of drug therapy, exercise, weight control, restriction of salt, and cessation of smoking.

Endocarditis

The effects of cardiac disease and prosthetic replacements carry an increased risk for bacteria carried in the blood system **(bacteremia),** causing **endocarditis.** Infective endocarditis is a severe infection of the cardiac valves and supporting structures caused by bloodborne pathogens that gain entry to the bloodstream from such places as the mouth and gastrointestinal tract. Refer to Chapter 30 for information on antibiotic therapy when treating a patient requiring premedication.

Recall

10. What is the leading cause of death in the United States?
11. Is epinephrine recommended for use in patients with heart disease?
12. What is another term for hypertension?

Pulmonary Disorders

Pulmonary disorders affect the lungs and are characterized by airway obstruction. Patients can present with symptoms from several disease categories.

Allergies

It is estimated that 1 of every 4 people is allergic to something. An allergy is a condition in which the body reacts to an antigen. The common antigens are dust, mites, pollen, animal dander, food, and drugs. Most reactions are manageable by the patient taking either an over-the-counter medication or prescribed medication that reduces the symptoms of the allergy. If the reaction goes beyond patient management, the allergy becomes a life-threatening emergency (see Chapter 31).

Bronchial Asthma

Bronchial **asthma** often arises from allergies and is characterized by an increased hypersensitivity to various stimuli, resulting in bronchial edema and widespread narrowing of the bronchial airways.

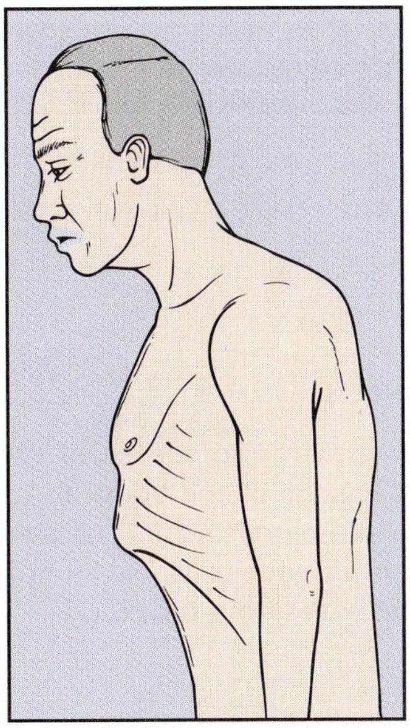

Fig. 29-9 **Appearance of a patient with chronic obstructive pulmonary disease (COPD).** (From Frazier MS, Drzymkowski JA: *Essentials of human diseases and conditions,* ed 3, St Louis, 2004, Saunders.)

Treatment Plan Modifications for a Patient with Asthma

Every effort should be made to minimize stress.

It is best to schedule short appointments and use sedation techniques.

The use of epinephrine and aspirin should be minimized. Epinephrine can enhance the side effects of bronchodilators, and aspirin may cause a laryngospasm or attack.

Chronic Obstructive Pulmonary Disease

Chronic obstructive pulmonary disease (COPD) is a general term for pulmonary diseases characterized by blocked airflow during respiration. Chronic **bronchitis** and **emphysema** are the two most common diseases classified as COPD.

Chronic bronchitis is a disorder resulting in irreversible narrowing of the bronchial airways as a result of chronic inflammation, increased mucus production, edema of the bronchial mucosa, and reduced ciliary activity (Fig. 29-9).

Emphysema is the irreversible enlargement of the size of the air spaces, resulting in labored breathing and an increased susceptibility to infection. This interferes with expiration, and the lungs become overinflated as a result of the trapping of air.

Recall

13. What organs do pulmonary disorders affect in the body?
14. What does the abbreviation *COPD* stand for?

Treatment Plan Modifications for a Patient with COPD

Minimize stress by keeping appointments short and scheduling them in the morning.

Consider using sedation techniques in low-risk to moderate-risk patients.

Consider using humidified oxygen by nasal **cannula.**

Avoid the use of nitrous oxide.

Do not treat patients in a fully reclined chair.

Avoid anticholinergic drugs, which dry bronchial secretions.

Do not schedule elective treatment during hot and humid weather.

Treatment Plan Modifications for a Patient with a Blood Disorder

The important factor for patients with a blood disorder is their *susceptibility to bacterial infections.*

Treatment modifications have to be made for any surgical procedure.

An antibiotic prophylaxis may need to be prescribed for high-risk procedures.

Blood Disorders

Blood disorders can involve the cellular elements of the body. The bone marrow can be susceptible to malignant cells, which can cause tumors of the bone marrow.

Red blood cells that are deficient in erythrocytes or hemoglobin can produce **anemia.** An excessive increase in white blood cells may indicate infection or **leukemia.** Excessive bleeding caused by a congenital lack of a protein substance necessary for blood clotting can occur in patients with **hemophilia.**

Musculoskeletal Disorders

Arthritis

The musculoskeletal system includes the bones, muscles, and joints. Older patients are more likely to have chronic progressive **arthritis** with stiffening of joints. This disorder causes the joints to become inflamed and painful (Fig. 29-10). Physicians prescribe aspirin and corticosteroids to reduce the symptoms of arthritis.

Muscular Dystrophy

Muscular dystrophy is a group of diseases characterized by progressive **atrophy** and weakness of the skeletal muscles with increasing disability and deformity. Muscular dystro-

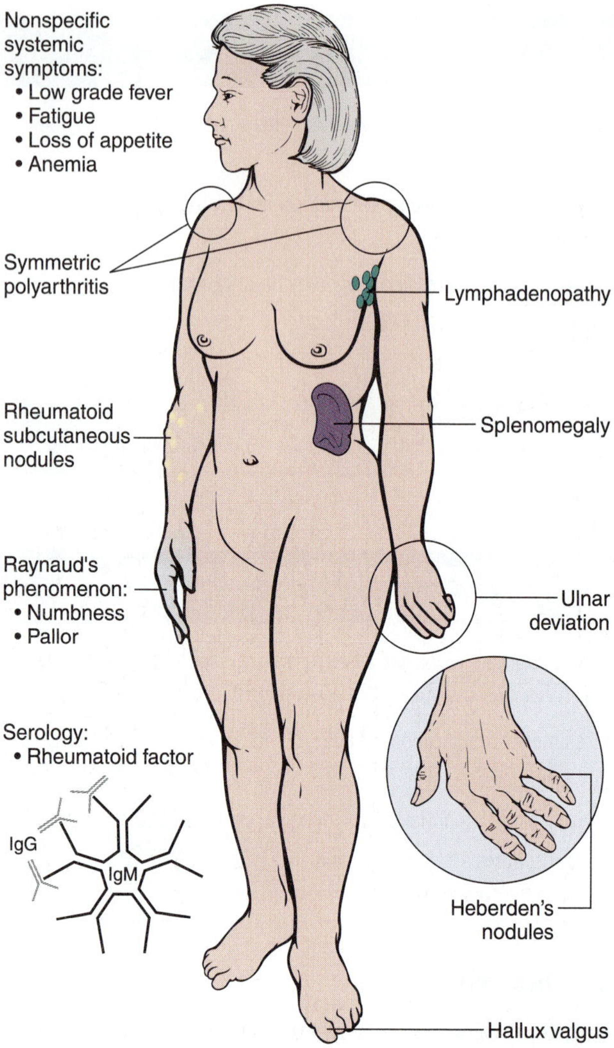

Fig. 29-10 Effects of rheumatoid arthritis on the body. (From Damjanov I: *Pathology for the health-related professions*, ed 2, Philadelphia, 2000, Saunders.)

Treatment Plan Modifications for a Patient with Arthritis

Schedule patients with arthritis in the morning and keep appointments short.

The disease can limit the ability to hold and use a toothbrush.

Arthritis of the jaw joints limits the ability to open the mouth or chew comfortably.

phy may eventually involve most of the striated muscles in the body. Atrophy of the muscles involved in respiration reduces the vital capacity of the lungs and interferes with the ability to cough.

The dentist and assistant must be aware of the diminished cough reflex of patients with muscular dystrophy and their inability to clear their throats by coughing.

Treatment Plan Modifications for a Patient with Muscular Dystrophy

Nitrous oxide, sedation, and general anesthesia should be avoided with these patients because of their impaired pulmonary (breathing) function.

Endocrine Disorders

The endocrine system is composed of glands located in many different regions of the body, all of which release hormones into the bloodstream. The *thyroid gland* regulates metabolism in body cells and stimulates passage of calcium into the bones from the blood.

Hyperthyroidism

A patient with an overactive thyroid gland has *Graves' disease,* the most common form of **hyperthyroidism.** The disorder affects women four to seven times more often than men. The average age of onset is before 40. Infection, physical or emotional stress, trauma, pain, or surgery may precipitate a *hyperthyroid crisis,* which can be fatal.

Treatment Plan Modifications for a Patient with Hyperthyroidism

An accurate and current patient history and medical consultation are essential.

Hyperthyroid patients who are not being treated are highly sensitive to epinephrine and other amine anesthetics.

Hypothyroidism

When the thyroid gland is underactive and produces fewer hormones, the patient is diagnosed with **hypothyroidism.** These patients are not in any danger from receiving dental care. Patients with mild hypothyroidism can receive depressants, sedatives, or narcotic analgesics before treatment, but may show signs of an exaggerated response to these drugs.

Patients who are not under a physician's care may be sensitive to narcotic analgesics, barbiturates, and tranquilizers because of the depressant effects of these drugs on the central nervous system.

Diabetes Mellitus

Diabetes mellitus (DM) is a disease characterized by a sustained high blood glucose level resulting from an absolute or a relative lack of insulin. Insulin insufficiency may be caused by a low output of insulin by the pancreas or by a decreased responsiveness to insulin. The disease is classified as follows:

Type 1 DM, in which the patient is *insulin-dependent.*
Type 2 DM, in which the patient is *non*–insulin-dependent.

Specific Problems Related to Dental Care for a Patient with Diabetes

The oral manifestations of patients with diabetes include acetone breath; dehydration of oral soft tissues due to xerostomia; red, swollen, and painful gingiva due to medication therapy; alveolar bone loss; toothaches; and delayed healing.

Treatment plan modifications for a patient with diabetes

Minimize stress by keeping appointments short and scheduling them in the midmorning.

Use sedation techniques such as nitrous oxide or oral diazepam.

Instruct patient to maintain normal dietary intake before dental appointments; the most common cause of hypoglycemia is failure to eat.

Minimize the risk for infection.

Recall

15. What disorder is associated with an overactive thyroid gland?
16. How is a patient with type 2 diabetes classified in relation to the need for insulin?

Behavioral and Psychiatric Disorders

Biologic, genetic, psychologic, and social components contribute to many types of behavioral and mental disorders. Psychiatric disorders will affect the treatment of dental patients because of the drugs prescribed, which influence the function of the brain.

Anxiety is a feeling that "all is not well," including a sense of impending disaster. Treatment may involve counseling, stress reduction therapy, and antianxiety medications.

Depression is a condition of general emotional rejection and withdrawal. The disorder may lead to a lack of interest in personal hygiene. Depression is most often treated with antidepressant agents.

Schizophrenia is a disturbance in thinking and perception, with delusions, hallucinations, and impaired reality testing. The therapy of choice involves antipsychotic agents and phenothiazines.

Treatment Plan Modifications for a Patient with a Psychiatric Disorder

Understand that xerostomia may result from the psychoactive drugs prescribed.

Regular hygiene and the use of fluoride supplements and salivary substitutes are important to preserve dental health.

Patient cooperation and informed consent may be problems, particularly in the patient with dementia.

THE PHYSICALLY COMPROMISED PATIENT

The patient who is physically challenged must adapt to a very fast-paced and mobile world. A wheelchair-bound, vision-impaired, or hearing-impaired patient entering the dental office can interrupt the daily routine if the office is not prepared. This patient may need more time for the appointment, and the dental unit may need to be arranged differently. However, the best way to prepare is through teamwork and communication.

Treatment Modifications for Hearing-Impaired Patients

Stand in front of patients so that they can see your face and follow your lip movements.

Do not shout. Speak slowly and distinctly.

Keep directions simple and provide visual demonstrations.

Keep a written copy of all instructions.

The Wheelchair-Bound Patient

A wheelchair provides mobility to persons who are paralyzed, have had an amputation, or have a debilitating disease that produces weakness in the lower half of the body. Many dental units now are designed to accommodate a wheelchair so that the patient may remain seated in the chair rather than having to be moved. If your office is not so equipped, you must follow a routine for transferring a patient into the dental chair (Procedure 29-1).

The Vision-Impaired Patient

The vision-impaired person has learned to rely on the sense of touch and verbal communication with others. For patients who cannot see their surroundings, all procedures should be thoroughly explained first (Fig. 29-11). The trip to the treatment area, positioning, and even smells from the dental materials must be discussed before treatment.

The Hearing-Impaired Patient

The patient who has impaired hearing should be treated with extra care and courtesy. Sometimes hearing-impaired patients show no visible evidence of hearing loss but may either not respond or respond inappropriately.

Procedure 29-1 Transferring a Patient from a Wheelchair

PROCEDURAL STEPS

1. Clear all items from the pathway of the wheelchair to the dental chair.
2. When entering the treatment room, determine whether it is best to go forward or to back the patient into the area.

   Purpose: You want the patient to be positioned the same way he or she would be seated in the dental chair.

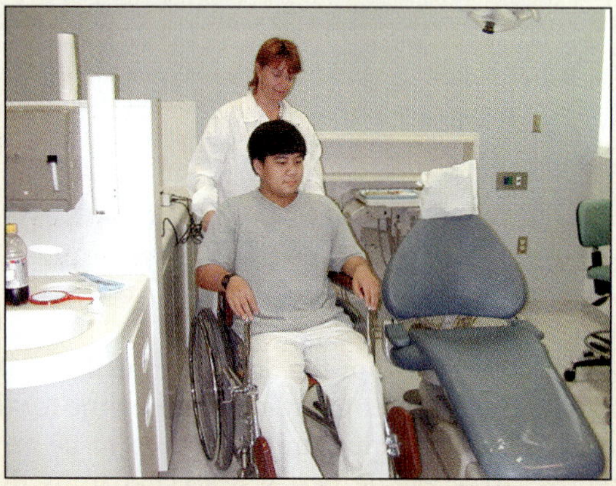

3. Move the wheelchair as close to the dental chair as possible so that it is at a 45-degree angle to the dental chair.

   Purpose: Allows the patient to move closer to the chair and not have to pivot as much.

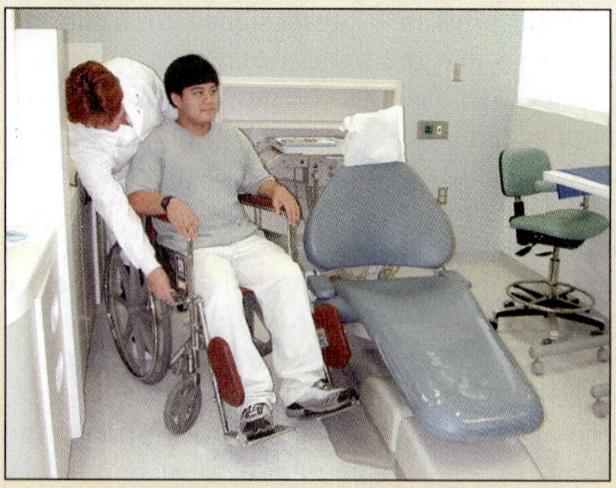

4. Lock the wheelchair and raise the footrests.
5. Bring patient to the edge of the wheelchair if possible.
6. Support the patient under the arms. If possible, have the patient push up with the hands from the wheelchair.
7. Help the patient stand slowly.
8. Pivot the patient so that the patient's backside is where the patient would be seated in the dental chair.

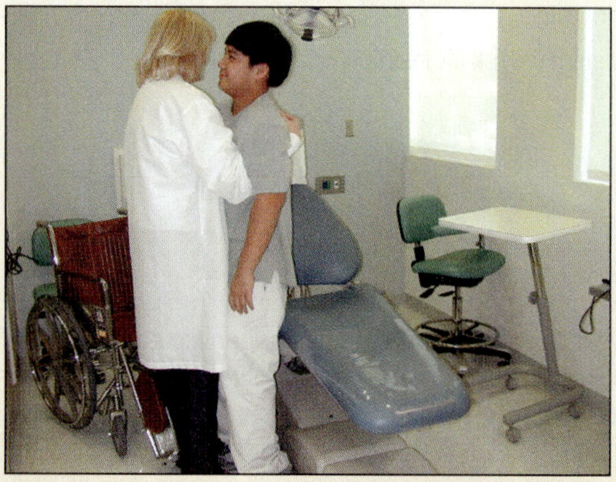

9. Instruct the patient to hold on to your arms as you slowly lower him or her down.
10. Swing the patient's legs over and onto the dental chair.

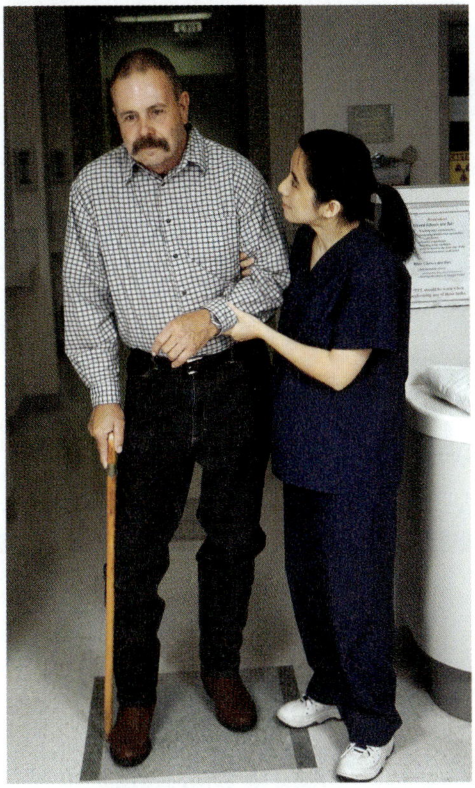

Fig. 29-11 Escorting a vision-impaired patient.

ASSISTANCE FROM ORGANIZATIONS

Many organizations can provide information to assist you in updating and educating the dental staff. To better prepare you, the patient, and the family, seek out guided assistance from these organizations.

The American Speech-Language-Hearing Association, for example, offers information on hearing loss and communication problems in older people and provides a list of certified audiologists and speech pathologists.

Organizations that Advocate for Medically and Physically Compromised Patients

ABLEDATA*–www.abledata.com
Alzheimer's Association–www.alz.org
American Cancer Society–www.cancer.org
American Council of the Blind–www.acb.org
American Diabetes Association–www.diabetes.org
American Heart Association–www.americanheart.org
American Speech-Language-Hearing Association–www.asha.org
Arthritis Foundation–www.arthritis.org
Cancer Information Service–www.cis.nih.gov
Hospice Hotline (800-658-8898)
National Association of Area Agencies on Aging–www.n4a.org
National Institute on Aging–www.nia.nih.gov
National Library Service for the Blind and Physically Handicapped–www.loc.gov/nls
National Meals-on-Wheels Foundation–www.nationalmealsonwheels.org
National Osteoporosis Foundation–www.nof.org

*National database that provides information on products for people with disabilities.

LEGAL AND ETHICAL IMPLICATIONS

All patients, whether they are healthy or present a compromising medical or physical condition, have the right to know about their treatment and alternative procedures available. Patients have rights regarding privacy of personal and medical information and informed consent. The dentist is accountable for obtaining a physical and medical background on every patient.

Eye to the Future

Medical advances occur daily. With preventive medicine, new findings, and new drugs, the compromised patient of today may be cured and rehabilitated tomorrow. The dentist and assistant are responsible for maintaining current information regarding medical issues that affect their patients.

Critical Thinking

1. One of your patients, Ms. Smith, has submitted an updated health history, and you notice she has checked "Yes" for having a blood disorder. When you inquire more information from her, Ms. Smith tells you that she has been tested positive for leukemia. What is one of your main considerations in how Ms. Smith will now be treated?
2. Mr. Jones, a patient of the practice, has diabetes but does not take insulin. How would you classify his type of diabetes? What dental considerations might apply to Mr. Jones?
3. You are preparing Mrs. Rodriguez for a dental procedure when she mentions that pollen has been bothering her lately. You review her medical-dental history and notice that she has asthma. What type of drugs should be minimized for an asthmatic patient such as Mrs. Rodriguez?
4. Provide three ways to manage a patient with coronary artery disease in the dental office.
5. Describe your thoughts and personal experiences about working with a medically or physically compromised patient.

30

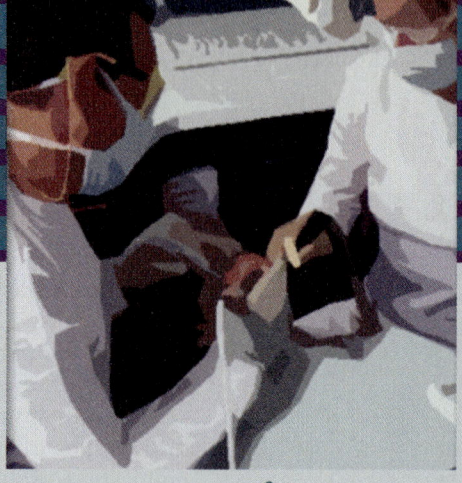

Principles of Pharmacology

Outline

Overview of Drugs
Dispensing of Drugs
- Prescriptions

Drug Reference Materials
- *Mosby's Drug Consult*
- Package Inserts

Drug Dosage and Forms
- Administration of Medications

Controlled Substances Act
- Schedule I Drugs
- Schedule II Drugs
- Schedule III Drugs
- Schedule IV Drugs
- Schedule V Drugs

Classification of Drugs
Antibiotic Prophylaxis
Adverse Drug Effects
- Drug Complications

Patient Education
Legal and Ethical Implications
Eye to the Future
Critical Thinking

KEY TERMS

Absorption Process by which the body takes in or receives (absorbs) a drug.

Distribution Action by which a drug is released throughout the body.

Dosage Amount of drug to be administered in a specific time, often according to body weight.

Dose A specified quantity of a drug or medicine.

Drug A substance used in the diagnosis, treatment, or prevention of a disease.

Ethical drug A drug that requires a prescription.

Excretion (ek-**skree**-shun) Action by which a drug leaves the body.

Generic (jeh-**nair**-ik) Sold without a brand name or trademark.

Inscription On a prescription, the name and quantity of a drug.

Metabolism (me-**tab**-eh-*liz*-um) Physical and chemical processes that occur within a living cell or organism and are necessary for the maintenance of life.

Patent medicine Drug that can be obtained without a prescription; also called *over-the-counter drug.*

Pharmacology A branch of medicine concerned with the uses, effects, and action of drugs.

Prescription A written order for a specific drug.

Prophylaxis (pro-fah-**lak**-sus) Administration of drugs to prevent disease or protect a patient.

Signature Instructions on a prescription explaining how to take a specific medicine.

Subscription Directions to the pharmacist for mixing the medication; this is seldom done by the pharmacist anymore.

Superscription The patient's name, address, date, and Rx symbol on a prescription.

Systemic (sis-**te**-mik) Referring to a drug that affects a specific system (or multiple systems) of the body.

LEARNING OUTCOMES

On completion of this chapter, the student will be able to achieve the following objectives:

- Pronounce, define, and spell the Key Terms.
- Differentiate between a drug's chemical, generic, and brand or trade name.
- List each part of a prescription.
- Describe the use of drug reference materials.
- Describe the stages a drug goes through in the body.
- Describe how medications are administered.
- Define the DEA and explain why drugs are categorized in five schedules of the Controlled Substance Act.
- Describe the effects of drug use.
- Describe the classification of prescription drugs and their effects.
- Cite the factors in determining the dosage of a drug.

Pharmacology is the science or branch of medicine that conducts research and development in the use and effects of drugs. A **drug** is a substance used in the prevention, diagnosis, or treatment of a disease. All drugs must be recognized and defined by the U.S. Food, Drug, and Cosmetic Act before they can be marketed to the public in the United States.

Your role in understanding pharmacology is to understand the classifications of drugs, the types of drugs, the terminology and use of prescriptions, and the drug reference materials when needed in a dental situation.

OVERVIEW OF DRUGS

Drugs are derived from many sources: *organic* drugs are derived from living organisms such as plants or animals, and *inorganic* drugs are synthesized in the laboratory or extracted from inorganic compounds. Most drugs today are derived from chemical sources, which makes them more pure in form than those derived from an original natural source that may be contaminated or polluted. Most manufacturing of drugs today takes place in a pharmaceutical laboratory.

A drug is identified by three names:

- *Chemical name,* which is the chemical formula of a drug.
- *Generic name,* which may be used by any company; *acetaminophen* is an example of a generic name.
- *Brand name,* or *trade name,* which is controlled by business firms as a registered trademark; for example, *Tylenol* is a brand name for acetaminophen.

Recall

1. Identify three sources of drugs.
2. What type of drug name is *Advil?*

DISPENSING OF DRUGS

Drugs are classified in two categories according to the way they are dispensed to patients: patent medicines and prescription drugs. **Patent medicines** are drugs that can be obtained without a prescription; these are also referred to as *over-the-counter drugs.* The U.S. Food and Drug Administration (FDA) regulates the sale of patent medicines and evaluates their safety and effectiveness for daily use. *Prescription drugs,* also termed **ethical drugs,** can be supplied to patients only by a pharmacist who has been provided a prescription from a physician or dentist. The term *ethical* is important in understanding that these types of drugs can be harmful to the patient if not used correctly (that is, it would not be ethical to prescribe or supply these drugs improperly). A patient taking these drugs must be under the guidance of a physician or dentist.

Prescriptions

A **prescription** is a written order by a physician or dentist for the preparation and administration of a medicine. Only a professional who is legally authorized to prescribe medications may write a prescription. A professional who is authorized to prescribe medications is issued a federal Drug Enforcement Agency (DEA) identification number.

Under no circumstances may a dental assistant prescribe medication. The dental assistant may dispense medicine only according to the explicit instructions and under the direct supervision of the dentist.

Prescription Terminology

Prescription pads should be kept in a locked drawer and should never be visible or available to use as notepaper. Individual state laws may regulate the format and information to be included on a prescription. In general, however, all prescriptions include the following four parts and use abbreviations (Fig. 30-1 and Box 30-1):

1. **Superscription**: patient name and address, the date, and the symbol Rx (Latin for "recipe")

2. **Inscription:** name and quantity of the drug
3. **Subscription:** directions for mixing the medication (no longer usually done by the pharmacist)
4. **Signature:** instructions for the patient on how to take the medicine, when to take it, and how much to take

Recording Prescriptions

The documentation of each drug prescribed must be recorded. The dentist will write the prescription in duplicate so that a copy can be retained in the patient record.

Box 30-1 Common Prescription Abbreviations

Abbreviation	Meaning
a.a.	of each
a.c.	before meals
a.m.	morning
b.i.d.	twice a day
disp.	dispense
h	hour
h.s.	at bedtime
NPO	nothing by mouth
p.c.	after meals
q.	every
q.d.	every day
q.i.d.	four times a day
t.i.d.	three times a day
t, tsp	teaspoon
T, tbs	tablespoon

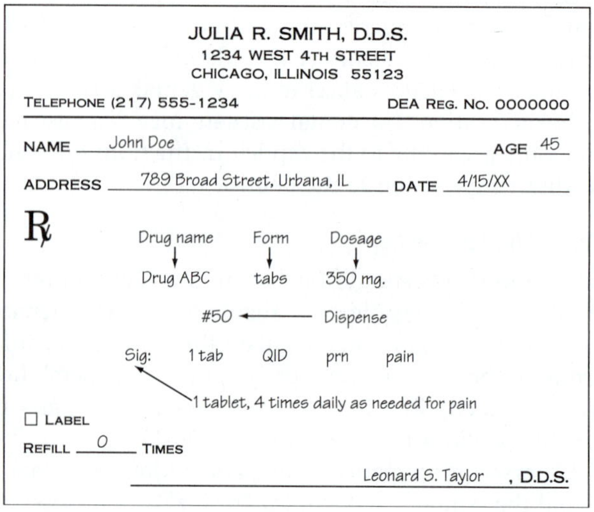
JULIA R. SMITH, D.D.S.
1234 WEST 4TH STREET
CHICAGO, ILLINOIS 55123
TELEPHONE (217) 555-1234 DEA REG. NO. 0000000
NAME John Doe AGE 45
ADDRESS 789 Broad Street, Urbana, IL DATE 4/15/XX
℞
Drug name Form Dosage
Drug ABC tabs 350 mg.
#50 Dispense
Sig: 1 tab QID prn pain
1 tablet, 4 times daily as needed for pain
☐ LABEL
REFILL 0 TIMES
Leonard S. Taylor , D.D.S.

Fig. 30-1 Example of a prescription pad. (Courtesy Colwell, a division of Patterson Companies, Inc., 1-800-637-1140.)

Telephone Guidelines

The following guidelines apply to the dental assistant regarding telephone interaction with a pharmacy:

- Narcotics cannot be ordered without a written prescription.
- It is illegal for a dental assistant to "call in" a prescription.
- When a pharmacist calls, notify the dentist immediately. Do not try to relay information between them.
- If the dentist is unable to come to the telephone, take the pharmacist's name and telephone number so that the dentist can return the call.
- Never attempt to evaluate a patient's reaction to a drug. Only the dentist or pharmacist is qualified to evaluate drug effects.

Recall

3. What agency regulates the sale of medicines?
4. Who is allowed to write prescriptions in the dental office?
5. What part of the prescription includes the name and quantity of the drug?
6. What does the abbreviation *b.i.d.* stand for?

DRUG REFERENCE MATERIALS

Your dentist must update his or her drug reference materials yearly. The pharmaceutical companies will either provide the latest information on existing drugs or introduce new agents that have gained approval from the FDA. Because of constant change in the industry, it is imperative that your dental office have several reference books on hand. An easier way to maintain current information is to have software programs that can be downloaded and updated or to have the ability to connect to the Internet for easy reference.

Mosby's Drug Consult

Mosby's Drug Consult is an annually updated source of information supplied by drug companies about their products (Fig. 30-2). This resource brings together the most current, complete, and impartial information on prescription pharmaceuticals available today. It is designed for ease of use and is organized in a way that serves the diverse needs of all healthcare professionals. *Mosby's Drug Consult* is an excellent resource for a dental office to have when you need to find information or identify a specific drug. It is available

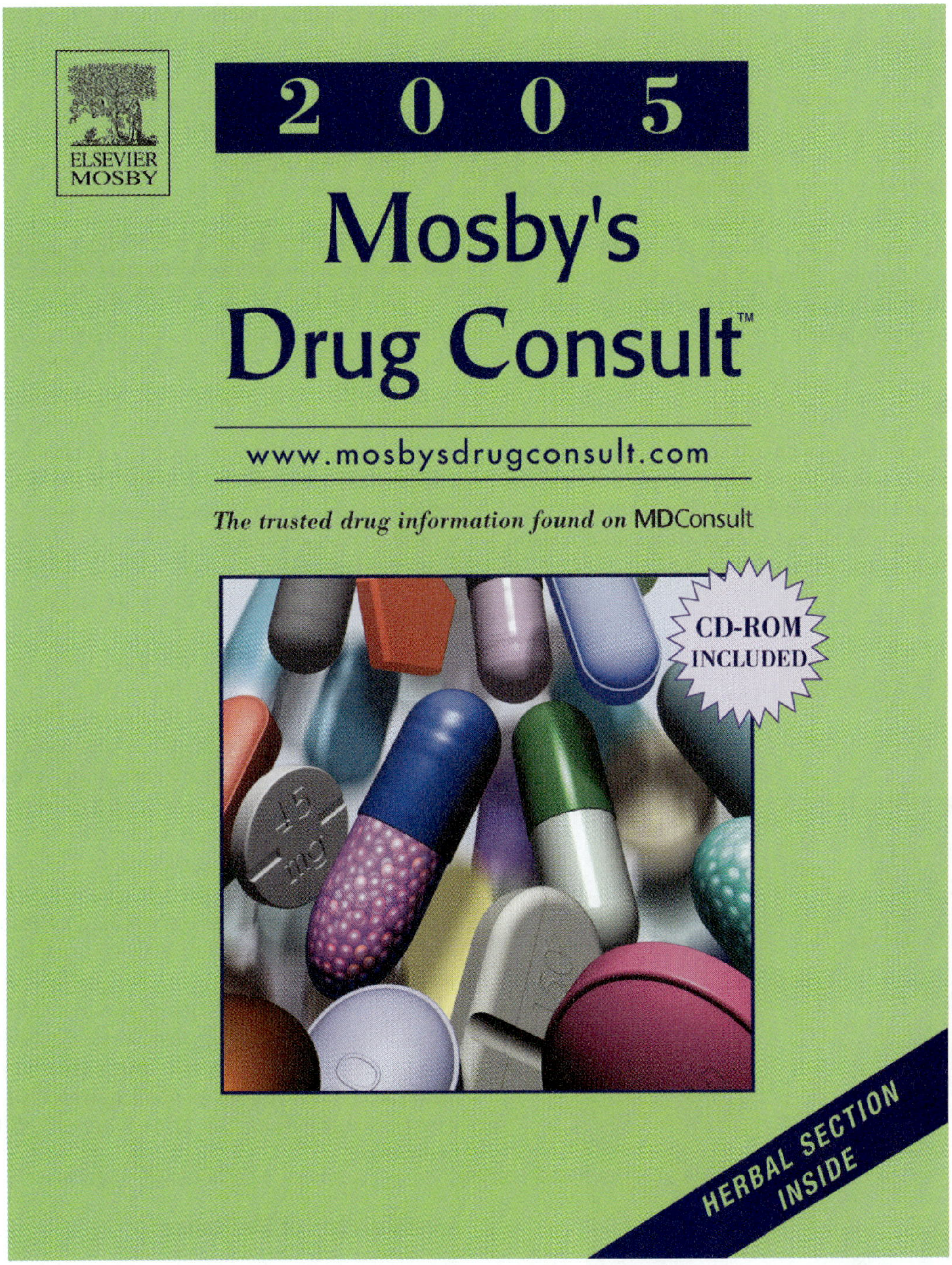

Fig. 30-2 Mosby's Drug Consult.

as a bound text, as well as in several electronic formats: as an uploadable CD-ROM, as a downloadable version for a PDA, or by Internet subscription.

When you first begin to search for a specific drug, you will see that *Mosby's Drug Consult* is divided into sections. A keyword index is located at the beginning of the resource for you to find the generic name of a drug (since drug information is listed by generic name). This index provides page numbers to find specific information on that drug. The information available on each generic drug includes the following: the category of drug, drug class, brand name(s), description, clinical pharmacology, indications and usage, contraindications, warnings, precautions, drug interactions, adverse reactions, dosage and administration, how the drug is supplied, product listing, indications for use, specific substances contained in the drug, contraindication to use, and side effects.

Package Inserts

Every prescription filled by a pharmacist includes an insert, or information sheet, that describes the drug for the patient (Fig. 30-3). Inserts contain the following information:

- How the drug will affect the body (e.g., relieve itchy, scratchy throat and eyes)
- For what condition the drug is being prescribed (e.g., allergies)
- Any side effects (e.g., drowsiness)
- Any adverse or long-term effects (e.g., possible liver damage)
- Special precautions to follow when taking the drug (e.g., do not drink alcohol)
- Contraindications to taking the drug (e.g., if taking blood pressure medication, consult physician)
- Dosage and route for the drug (e.g., take one tablet each day, orally)

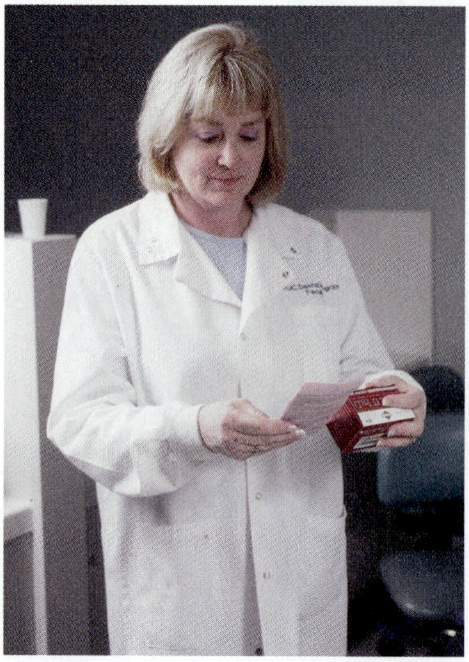

Fig. 30-3 Always review the package insert with your patient.

DRUG DOSAGE AND FORMS

The amount of a drug that a patient takes is called a **dose.** The manufacturer of the drug knows the exact time required for the drug to take effect and compiles the **dosage,** or the dose administered during a specified period, which is often determined according to body weight.

Specific factors are considered by the physician or dentist in determining the dosage of a drug:

- Age of the patient
- Weight of the patient
- Time of day the drug is to be taken
- Drug form
- Patient tolerance to the drug
- Other drugs the patient is taking

Drugs are manufactured in different forms. The way that a drug is taken or administered depends on the selected drug form. Drug forms include pills, capsules, liquids, drops, ointments, sprays, gases, and lotions.

If a drug is applied directly to the site of use, it is considered a *local-action drug,* or simply a *local drug.* This type of drug affects only the specific area of the body to which it is applied. An example is a first-aid antibiotic ointment, which would be applied directly to a cut or scrape to prevent infection.

If a drug is taken internally, it is considered a *systemic-action drug,* or simply a *systemic drug.* A **systemic** drug can affect the whole body by way of the circulatory system. An example is the antibiotic penicillin, which will eradicate an infection throughout the body when taken for the specified period.

Administration of Medications

Drugs can be applied or administered by several routes (Fig. 30-4). The way a drug is administered depends on how quickly or how slowly the drug will take effect. When a specific medication enters the body, the drug then undergoes four stages: **absorption, distribution, metabolism,** and **excretion** (Box 30-2).

Box 30-2 Stages of Drug Action in the Body

Action	Description
Absorption	The drug is absorbed from site of entry. (Sites of entry are described in Fig. 30-4.) The speed of absorption varies depending on the way a drug is administered. The slowest route of absorption is by mouth (orally).
Distribution	Once a drug has entered the bloodstream, the chemical compound of a drug attaches to the proteins within the blood. It is then circulated throughout the body to be released and take effect.
Metabolism	Once the chemical compound is released, the drug becomes metabolized and is then excreted through the liver or kidneys.
Excretion	The drug leaves the body by way of kidneys, liver, saliva, breast milk, and sweat.

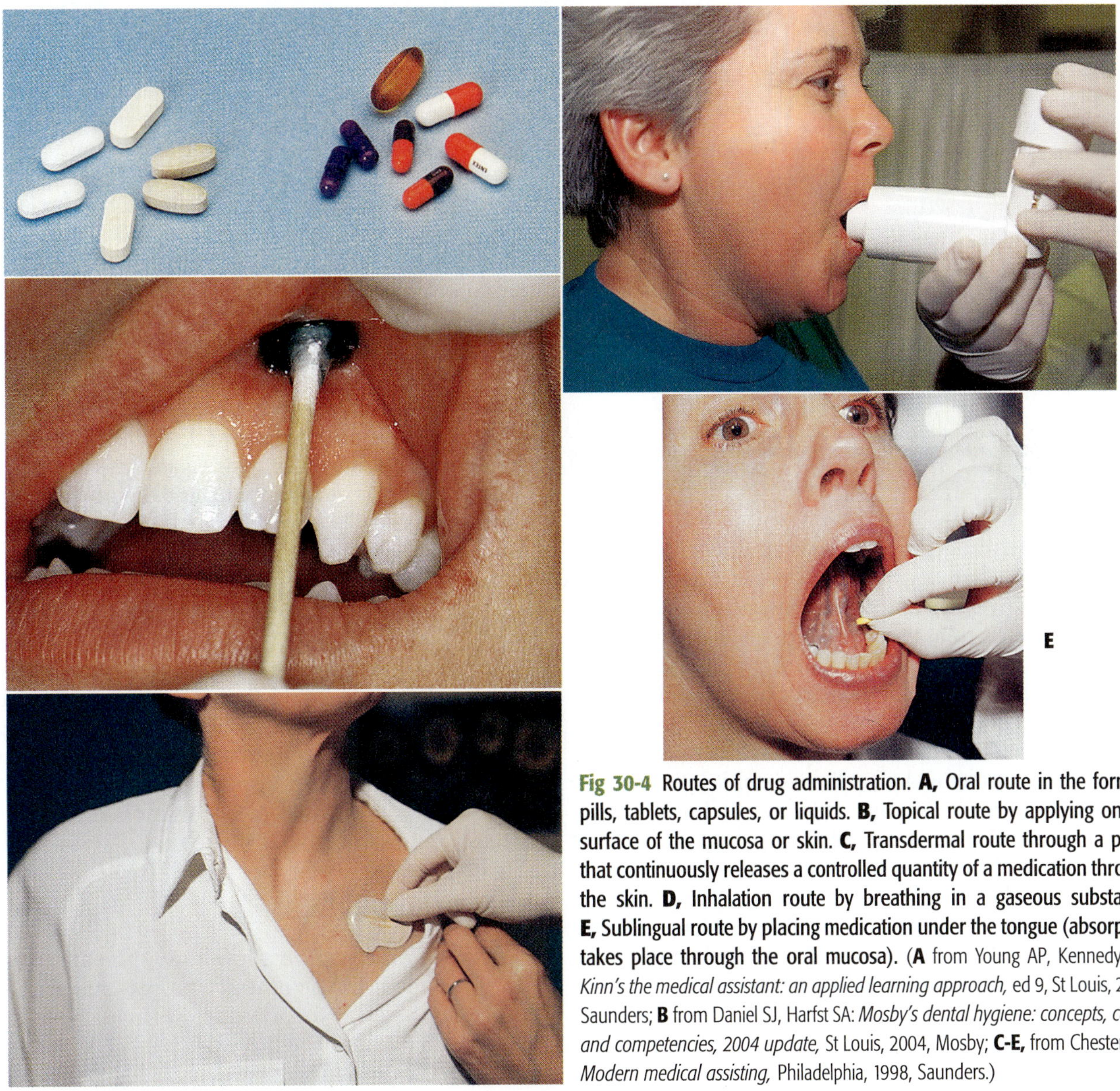

Fig 30-4 Routes of drug administration. **A,** Oral route in the form of pills, tablets, capsules, or liquids. **B,** Topical route by applying on the surface of the mucosa or skin. **C,** Transdermal route through a patch that continuously releases a controlled quantity of a medication through the skin. **D,** Inhalation route by breathing in a gaseous substance. **E,** Sublingual route by placing medication under the tongue (absorption takes place through the oral mucosa). (**A** from Young AP, Kennedy DB: *Kinn's the medical assistant: an applied learning approach,* ed 9, St Louis, 2003, Saunders; **B** from Daniel SJ, Harfst SA: *Mosby's dental hygiene: concepts, cases, and competencies, 2004 update,* St Louis, 2004, Mosby; **C-E,** from Chester GA: *Modern medical assisting,* Philadelphia, 1998, Saunders.)

continued

F

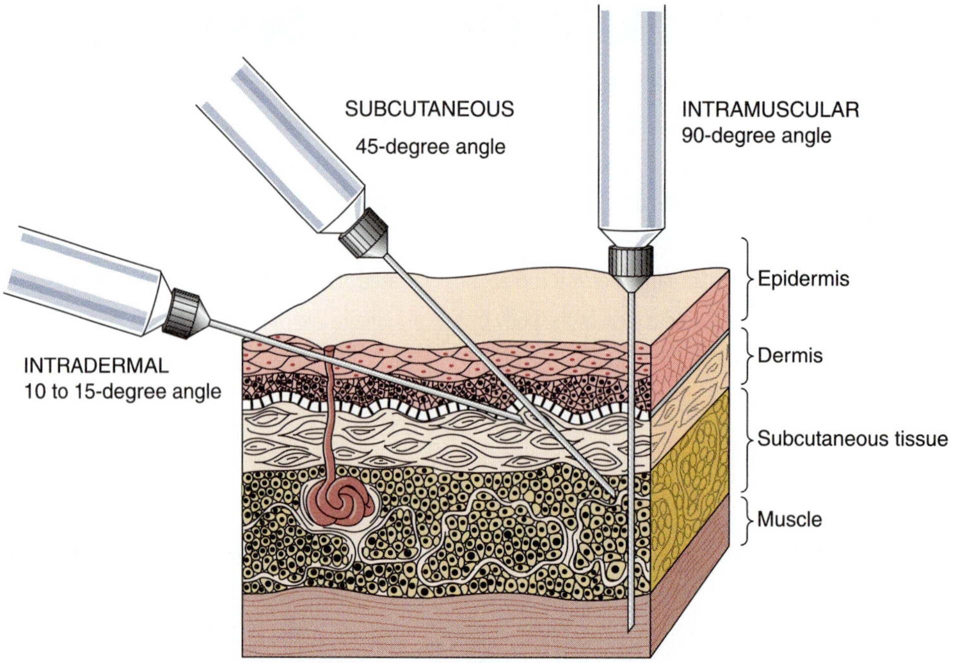

Fig 30-4—cont'd Routes of drug administration. **F,** Injection route. The type of drug determines how the injection is given: *subcutaneous*, directly under the skin; *intramuscular,* into a muscle; *intradermal*, into the skin; *intravenous*, into a vein. Note: Another method of administering drugs is rectally with suppositories or enemas. (**F,** from Chester GA: *Modern medical assisting,* Philadelphia, 1998, Saunders.)

Recall

7. Where is a sublingual drug administered?
8. Where is a subcutaneous drug administered?
9. What is the slowest route of absorption for a drug?

CONTROLLED SUBSTANCES ACT

The drugs and drug products covered under the *Federal Comprehensive Drug Abuse Prevention and Control Act* are divided into five schedules. The drugs included in this act, also referred to as *schedule drugs,* are classified based on their potential for abuse, medical usefulness, and the degree to which they may lead to physical and psychologic dependence.

Many individual states also have their own controlled substances act patterned after the federal law. Some state laws are more restrictive, but none may be less restrictive than the federal law. The dentist must comply with the provisions of the federal laws and those of the state in which he or she practices (always following the most restrictive guidelines when the laws differ). Under these laws, any professional who is authorized to prescribe these medications is issued a DEA identification number.

Schedule I Drugs

Schedule I drugs have no current accepted medical usefulness and have a high potential for abuse. Normally, Schedule I drugs cannot be prescribed. This includes certain derivatives (such as heroin), hallucinogenic substances (such as LSD and marijuana), depressants, and stimulants.

Schedule II Drugs

Schedule II drugs, although they have a high potential for abuse, can have accepted medical usefulness. Prescriptions for these drugs must be in writing and cannot be renewed. Schedule II drugs include opium and opium derivatives, cocaine, morphine, hydromorphone (Dilaudid), methadone, and barbiturates.

Schedule III Drugs

Schedule III drugs have less abuse potential than the drugs in Schedules I and II and also have accepted medical usefulness. Prescriptions for Schedule III drugs may be renewed. Schedule III drugs include some stimulants and depressants; the combination of Tylenol with codeine is an example of a common prescription included in this schedule.

Schedule IV Drugs

Schedule IV drugs have a low abuse potential and have accepted medical usefulness. The prescribing information is the same as for Schedule III drugs. A patient may have up to five refills of these drugs in a 6-month period. Examples of Schedule IV drugs include chlordiazepoxide (Librium), diazepam (Valium), and propoxyphene (Darvon).

Table 30-1 Classification of Drug Actions

Type of Drug	Action	Examples	Primary Use
Analgesic	Lessens the sensory function of the brain	Aspirin, acetaminophen, ibuprofen	Relief of pain
Anesthetic	Reduces level of pain	Bupivacaine, lidocaine	Local or general anesthesia
Antianxiety	Reduces anxiety and tension	Librium, Valium, Xanax	Produces a calming feeling
Antibiotic	Kills or inhibits the growth of microorganisms	Ceclor, tetracycline, amoxicillin	Treatment of a bacterial infection
Anticoagulant	Slows the clotting of blood	Heparin, Coumadin	Treatment of blood clots
Anticonvulsant	Reduces excessive stimulation of the brain	Dilantin, phenobarbital, Tegretol	Epileptic seizures
Antidepressant	Treats depression	Prozac, Tofranil, Elavil	Elevates mood
Antifungal	Slows the growth of fungus	Monistat, nystatin, Mycostatin	Treats fungal infections
Antihistamine	Counteracts the effects of histamine	Benadryl, Phenergan, Tagamet	Relief for allergies
Antihypertensive	Keeps arteries from constricting and slows heart rate	Tenormin, Cardura, Lopressor	Controls high blood pressure
Antiinflammatory	Reduces the inflammatory process	Advil, Motrin, cortisone, prednisone	Arthritis and other inflammatory diseases
Bronchodilator	Relaxes the smooth muscle of the bronchi	Albuterol, Ventolin	Asthma, bronchospasm
Contraceptive	Stops conception	Provera, Ovrette	Family planning
Decongestant	Relieves congestion in the nasal tissues	Neo-Synephrine, Sudafed, Afrin	Treats cold, respiratory and sinus congestion
Diuretic	Inhibits the reabsorption of sodium and chloride in the kidneys	Lasix, Dyazide, Dyrenium	Increases urinary output
Hemostatic	Coagulates blood	Gelfoam	Artificial clot
Hormone replacement	Replaces or compensates hormone deficiency	Humulin, Synthroid, estrogen	Maintains hormone level

Schedule V Drugs

Schedule V drugs have the lowest abuse potential and have accepted medical usefulness. Under federal law, these drugs are not required to be prescribed; however, they are available only under controlled circumstances. Some states do require that these drugs be dispensed only by prescription. Examples of Schedule V drugs include cough medicines with codeine.

CLASSIFICATION OF DRUGS

There is a vast variety of drugs on the market, with each drug producing a different effect. The most probable situations in which the dental assistant will need to know drug classification include the following: (1) when reviewing a patient's drug history, (2) when assisting in specific dental procedures that require premedication, (3) when assisting in a specific dental procedure requiring pain control, and (4) when assisting in a medical emergency.

Drugs are classified according to the body system they affect and their action on the body. Table 30-1 provides a glossary of the various types of drugs, along with drug actions, examples, and primary uses.

Recall

10. What type of schedule drug is Tylenol with codeine?
11. What is the term for the body's negative reaction to a drug?
12. An analgesic is used for what action?
13. What is an example of an antibiotic?
14. What type of drug slows the clotting of blood?
15. Would a patient be taking a diuretic to treat a cold?

ANTIBIOTIC PROPHYLAXIS

Antibiotic **prophylaxis** is the prescribing of antibiotics to uninfected patients in order to prevent bacterial colonization. The most common application in dentistry is for the prevention of infective endocarditis, a rare heart infection.

The bacterium *Streptococcus viridans* is abundant in the oral cavity, causing about 45 percent of all cases of endocarditis. Most cases are *not* caused by dental procedures but rather by poor oral health and poor hygiene, which result in frequent, transient bacteremia after brushing and chewing. The prophylactic antibiotic may decrease bacterial colonization or adherence to heart valves.

Other patient situations that may warrant prophylactic antibiotics are the presence of a prosthetic heart valve, surgically constructed systemic-pulmonary shunts, organic heart murmur, and mitral valve prolapse with valvular regurgitation.

The three types of antibiotics recommended by the American Heart Association for antibiotic prophylaxis are amoxicillin/penicillin, ampicillin, and clindamycin (Table 30-2).

Antibiotic Prophylaxis Recommendations

Prophylaxis Recommended for High-Risk to Moderate-Risk Cardiac Conditions

Dental extractions

Periodontal procedures, including surgery, scaling, root planing, probing, and recall maintenance

Dental implant placement and reimplantation of avulsed teeth

Endodontic instrumentation or surgery only beyond the apex

Subgingival placement of antibiotic fibers or strips

Initial placement of orthodontic bands, but not brackets

Intraligamentary local anesthetic injections

Prophylactic cleaning of teeth or implants where bleeding is anticipated

Prophylaxis Not Recommended

Restorative dentistry with or without retraction cord

Local anesthetic injections

Intracanal endodontic treatment, postplacement, and buildup

Placement of dental dams

Postoperative suture removal

Placement of removable prosthodontic and orthodontic appliances

Taking of oral impressions

Fluoride treatments

Taking of radiographs

Orthodontic appliance adjustment

Shedding of primary teeth

ADVERSE DRUG EFFECTS

When drugs are prescribed to prevent a disease, treat a condition, alleviate pain, or suppress fear, they can possibly also interfere with normal function or may even create a potentially life-threatening circumstance.

Adverse drug effects are the body's negative reaction to a drug. It is important to review the printed insert with the patient and cover any of the possible side effects that the drug could cause.

Drug Complications

An allergic reaction will occur if a drug triggers the immune response. Repeated exposure to the same drug can produce this type of allergic response. Reactions can range from a common rash to life-threatening anaphylactic shock. The most common cause of drug-induced anaphylaxis is penicillin.

Table 30-2 ***Recommended Doses and Regimens for Common Antibiotics***

Dental/Patient Situation	Agent	Regimen
Standard general prophylaxis	Amoxicillin	*Adults:* 2.0 g PO 1 hour before procedure
		Children: 50 mg/kg PO 1 hour before procedure
Unable to take oral medications	Ampicillin	*Adults:* 2.0 g IM or IV within 30 minutes before procedure
		Children: 50 mg/kg IM or IV within 30 minutes before procedure
Allergic to penicillin	Clindamycin	*Adults:* 600 mg PO 1 hour before procedure
		Children: 20 mg/kg PO 1 hour before procedure

Data from the American Heart Association.
PO, Orally; *IM,* intramuscularly; *IV,* intravenously.

Drug toxicity refers to toxin-induced cell damage and cell death. During the breakdown of a drug, biochemical damage may take place and harm the cell. This, in turn, may cause either the death or mutation of the cell.

Drug interaction takes place when an additional drug is introduced into the body system. The severity of interaction can range from minor reactions to life-threatening conditions. These types of reactions can be easily prevented by the dentist being knowledgeable of proper drug relationships and aware of all drugs a patient is taking.

Drug tolerance is the loss of a drug's effectiveness that occurs when a patient has taken the drug over time and no longer receives the drug's beneficial effects. When this occurs, the physician or dentist may need to increase the dosage or prescribe a different drug.

Drug addiction is physical dependence on a drug. If the person stops taking the drug, the body undergoes a withdrawal illness, displaying physical symptoms associated with stopping use of the drug.

Common Side Effects of Medications

- Hyperexcitability
- Insomnia
- Dizziness
- Drowsiness
- Central nervous system effects
- Gastrointestinal disturbances (nausea, vomiting, diarrhea)
- Changes in bleeding time
- Hypertension
- Hypotension and fainting
- Weight changes
- Appetite changes
- Edema
- Sexual dysfunction
- Sweating
- Opportunistic infections (yeast, fungal)
- Photosensitivity
- Loss of hair
- Blurred vision
- Cardiac arrhythmia
- Skin changes
- Respiratory difficulties

Patient Education

One of the most important informational tools for a patient is the medical history form, which provides a section on medications currently taken.

When first reviewing the medication history with the patient, emphasize the importance of your awareness of the type of medications being taken. Educate the patient about how some drugs can negatively interact with other types of drugs used in the dental office.

If patients are unsure of the names of drugs they are taking, ask them to bring their prescriptions with them on their next visit. You can then identify the drugs using *Mosby's Drug Consult* and list them in the patient record.

Legal and Ethical Implications

Under no circumstances may a dental assistant prescribe medication to a patient. The role of the dental assistant is to dispense medicine according to the direct instructions and under the direct supervision of the dentist.

It is your responsibility to become familiar with the drugs and medications that your dentist uses and prescribes. Develop the practice of referring to drug reference materials and researching any drug about which you are unsure.

Eye to the Future

In the twenty-first century, pharmaceuticals will continue to develop major advances in medications and how they are delivered. For example, the routes of drug administration are changing rapidly. Already, drugs can be delivered by means of a patch, which allows the active ingredients to be absorbed through the skin and into the blood.

Some patients with diabetes are using special insulin pumps that respond to their body's blood sugar level, releasing the right amount of hormone when needed. Other possibilities include microminiature "drug submarines" that carry minute packets of drugs along tiny blood vessels to the site where they are needed.

The way in which drugs are manufactured is changing as well. Advances in genetic engineering will eventually allow the manufacture of large amounts of drugs that are currently difficult and expensive to synthesize.

Critical Thinking

1. A patient has indicated on his medical history that he is taking Sudafed for the relief of allergy symptoms. Refer to *Mosby's Drug Consult* for contraindications to this and other medications.
2. Mrs. Greenville has called routinely over the last several months complaining of pain in a tooth that was restored with a Class III composite restoration. The dentist has reviewed Mrs. Greenville's patient record and radiographs, but sees no indication for pain. Mrs. Greenville has asked for the dentist to call in a prescription for pain medication until she can come back to the office. How would you handle this situation, and what possibly could be wrong?
3. You notice that a prescription pad is missing from the locked drawer. With whom do you discuss this?
4. An antibiotic has been prescribed for an adult patient scheduled for scaling and root planing. The patient indicates a history of mitral valve prolapse on the health history. Why has an antibiotic been prescribed?
5. Refer to *Mosby's Drug Consult* to determine the route of administration for the drug nitroglycerin.

31

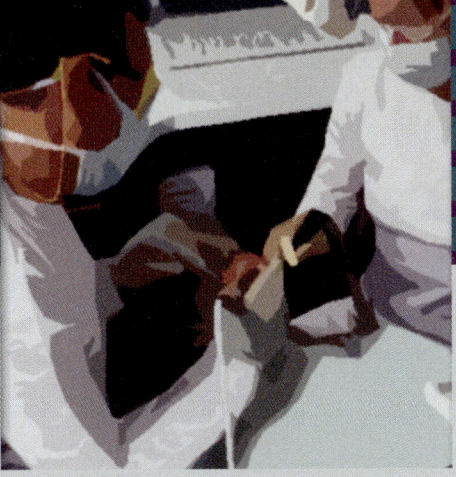

Assisting in a Medical Emergency

Outline

KEY TERMS

Acute Referring to a condition with a rapid onset.

Allergen (**al**-er-jen) A substance, such as pollen, that causes an allergy.

Allergy (**al**-er-jee) High sensitivity to a certain substance.

Anaphylaxis (*an*-ah-fah-**lak**-sis) Extreme hypersensitivity reaction to a substance that can lead to shock and life-threatening respiratory collapse.

Angina (an-**ji**-nah) Chest pain caused by inadequate oxygen to the heart.

Antibodies Immunoglobulins produced by lymphoid tissue in response to a foreign substance.

Antigen (**an**-ti-jen) A substance introduced into the body to stimulate the production of an antibody.

Aspiration (*as*-pah-**ray**-shun) The act of inhaling or ingesting, as of a foreign object.

Asthma (**az**-mah) Respiratory disease often associated with allergies and characterized by sudden recurring attacks of labored breathing, chest constriction, and coughing.

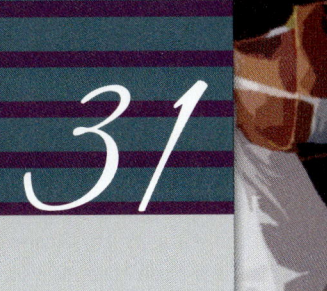

KEY TERMS, cont'd

Cardiopulmonary resuscitation (CPR) (*kar*-dee-oh-**pul**-mah-nare-ee ri-*suh*-sah-**tay**-shun) A planned action for restoring consciousness or life.

Convulsion (kun-**vul**-shun) An involuntary muscular contraction.

Epilepsy (**eh**-pah-*lep*-see) Neurologic disorder with sudden recurring seizures of motor, sensory, or psychic malfunction.

Erythema (*er*-ah-**thee**-mah) Skin redness, often caused by inflammation or infection.

Gait A particular way of walking, or *ambulating.*

Hyperglycemia (*hi*-per-gli-**see**-me-ah) Abnormally high blood glucose level.

Hypersensitivity State of being excessively sensitive to a substance, often with allergic reactions.

Hyperventilation Abnormally fast or deep breathing.

Hypoglycemia (*hi*-poe-gli-**see**-me-ah) Abnormally low blood glucose level.

Hypotension (*hi*-poe-**ten**-shun) Abnormally low blood pressure.

Myocardial infarction (*mi*-oh-**kahr**-dee-ul in-**fark**-shun) Condition in which there is damage to the muscular tissue of the heart, commonly caused by obstructed circulation; also referred to as *heart attack.*

Syncope (**sing**-keh-pee) Loss of consciousness caused by insufficient blood to the brain.

Ventricular fibrillation (ven-**tri**-kyeh-ler *fi*-breh-**lay**-shun) Abnormal cardiac rhythm that prevents the heart from pumping blood.

LEARNING OUTCOMES

On completion of this chapter, the student will be able to achieve the following objectives:

- Pronounce, define, and spell the Key Terms.
- Describe the preventive measures taken for a medical emergency.
- List the appropriate qualifications that a dental assistant must have for emergency preparedness.
- Describe the common signs and symptoms of an emergency and how to recognize them.
- List the basic items that must be included in an emergency kit.
- Discuss the use of a defibrillator in an emergency.
- Describe how to respond to specific emergencies.

PERFORMANCE OUTCOMES

On completion of this chapter, the student will be able to meet competency standards in the following skills:

- Accurately perform CPR on a simulated mannequin.
- Accurately perform the Heimlich maneuver on a mannequin.
- Demonstrate preparation and placement of oxygen.
- Demonstrate use of the automated external defibrillator.

A *medical emergency* is a condition or circumstance requiring immediate action for a person who has been injured or has suddenly become ill. When a medical emergency occurs, it is not possible to refer to a medical textbook for answers. You must be prepared to respond immediately. Your knowledge and skills could mean the difference between life and death.

At the time of a medical emergency, you might be the only person in the treatment area. If so, you would be responsible for initiating any first aid until the dentist or medical assistance arrives. If this is the case, it will be your responsibility to use well-chosen words of support, show a willingness to help, and demonstrate capable lifesaving skills.

PREVENTING A MEDICAL EMERGENCY

One of the most important ways to prevent a medical emergency is to *know your patient.* This means establishing open communication about the patient's health and having a completed or updated medical history before dental treatment is begun.

The front desk assistant (business assistant) is responsible for ensuring that patients update this information as they enter the office. Once they have received the forms, patients should indicate any changes in their health, even if they were seen as recently as the previous week. They should also verify that the information is accurate by dating and signing the form (see Chapter 26 for a review of a medical history update).

Most emergencies that occur in the dental office are caused by the combined *stress* of a person's daily life along with the visit to the dentist. If a patient has had a negative experience or is apprehensive about a specific procedure, this could alter the patient's stress level and create a medical problem. It is important to recognize the areas of dental treatment that are most stressful for the patient.

Recall

1. What is the best way to prevent an emergency?
2. What is the cause of most medical emergencies in the dental office?

EMERGENCY PREPAREDNESS

While the patient is in the dental office, the dentist is responsible for that individual's safety. If a medical emergency involving the patient arises, the dentist and staff are responsible for providing emergency care until more qualified personnel arrive. Emergency first-aid protocols must be established and routinely practiced in the dental office.

Successful management of medical emergencies in the dental office requires preparedness, prompt recognition, and effective treatment. Every member of the dental team must be prepared for emergencies when they occur in the dental office.

Ongoing observation of the patient is an important part of emergency preparedness. A calm, well-functioning staff is capable of handling an emergency in the dental office without complicating the seriousness of the situation by frightening the patient. To prevent added stress and complications, every staff member should know and practice his or her role in emergency protocols before any emergency arises. A standardized procedure for the management of emergencies must be established and followed.

Assigned Roles

In the management of an emergency, the combined efforts of trained persons are more efficient when each person takes on a specific, assigned role. It is the responsibility of the dentist to define these roles. Most often, dental team members are in charge of specific roles, as follows:

- Front desk staff (business assistant) will call emergency services and remain on the telephone at all times to obtain appropriate medical assistance (Fig. 31-1).
- The clinical assistant or dental hygienist will retrieve the oxygen unit and emergency drug kit (Fig. 31-2).
- The dentist, clinical assistant, or dental hygienist will remain with the patient to assist in assessment or with basic life support (Fig. 31-3).
- Additional dental team members will respond to the needs of other patients in the office.

Routine Drills

Training must be kept current at all times. A "mock emergency" should be created in the dental office monthly so that the dental team members can practice their roles, take on additional roles, and refine the office's emergency plan.

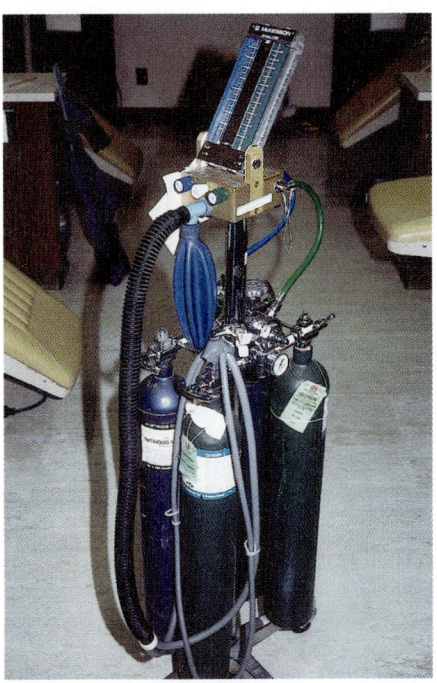

Fig. 31-1 It is important to have open communication with emergency personnel.

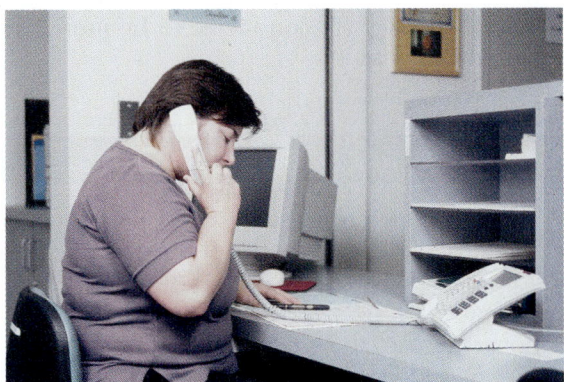

Fig. 31-2 Preparing oxygen for an emergency.

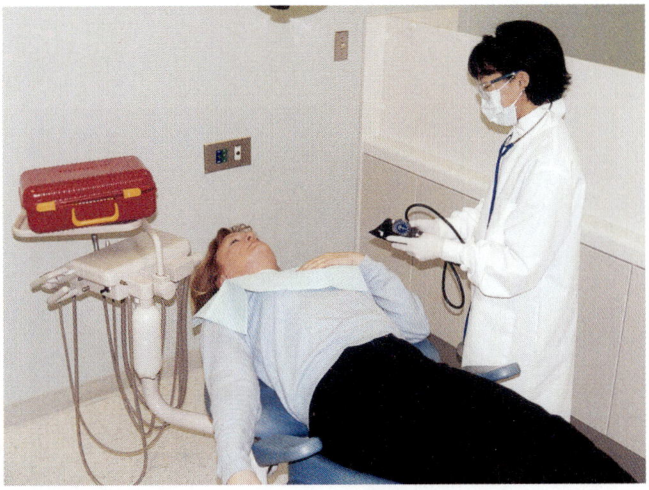

Fig. 31-3 The dental assistant has repositioned the patient and is assessing vital signs.

Emergency Telephone Numbers

A list of emergency numbers should be posted next to each telephone throughout the office. Maintaining a *current* list of these telephone numbers is an important part of emergency preparedness.

The list should include telephone numbers for local police, firefighters, and emergency medical services (EMS) personnel. In most areas, all three services can be reached by dialing 911 (Fig. 31-4). However, the ways in which these services respond to emergencies vary widely and depend on the geographic area and population served.

Two important factors in emergency preparedness are (1) the time it takes the local EMS personnel to reach the dental office and (2) the life support capabilities available on arrival (Fig. 31-5). Not all EMS personnel carry the same equipment or provide the same level of lifesaving care.

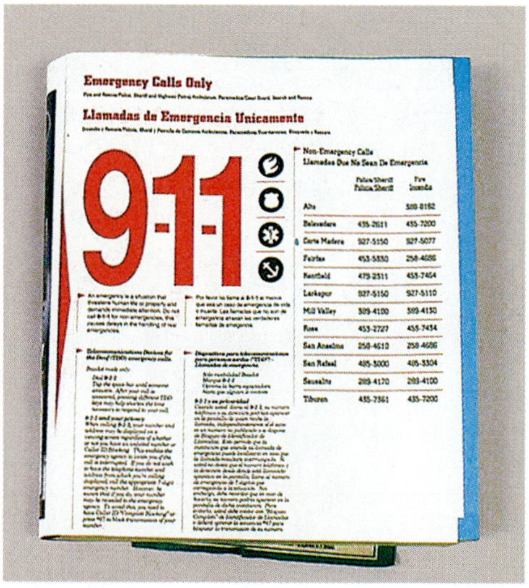

Fig. 31-4 Poster showing the most common number to dial for emergency services—911.

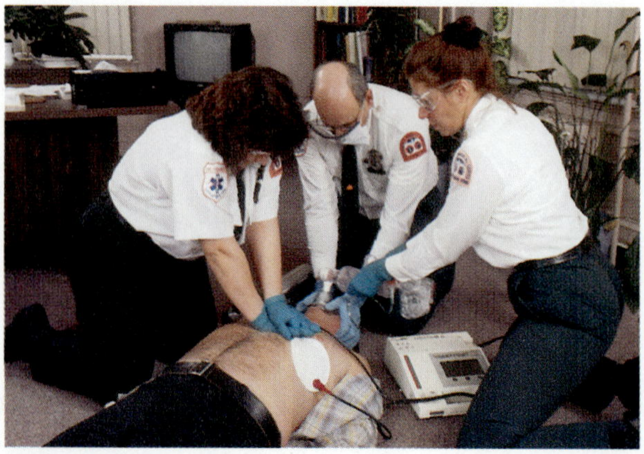

Fig. 31-5 EMS personnel on the scene. (From Henry MC, Stapleton ER: *EMT: prehospital care,* ed 3, St Louis, 2004, Mosby.)

A list of the telephone numbers of the nearest hospital, physicians, and oral surgeons should also be available. These professionals might be able to offer the life support needed while you are waiting for EMS personnel or another type of emergency response.

Recall

3. Who is responsible for a patient's safety in the dental office?
4. Who in the dental office would most likely be in charge of calling the emergency medical services?
5. Where should emergency phone numbers be kept?

RECOGNIZING A MEDICAL EMERGENCY

The dental staff must be aware that a medical emergency can occur at any time. For this reason, ongoing observation of the patient in the reception area, in the dental chair, or leaving the office cannot be overemphasized. The "alert" dental assistant observes the patient's general appearance and **gait** as he or she enters the clinical area.

Note the patient's response to routine questions. Slow responses and changes in speech patterns from a previous appointment should be noted for the dentist to evaluate. Recognition of a problem is critical.

Signs and Symptoms

When an emergency does occur, it is important to recognize it and to make notes in the patient's record of symptoms and signs. A *symptom* is what patients tell you regarding how they feel or what they are experiencing, such as, "I feel dizzy," "I'm having trouble breathing," or "My arm hurts."

A *sign* is what you observe in a patient, such as a change in skin color or an increased respiratory rate. Because signs are actually observed by you and/or another member of the dental team, they are considered to be more reliable than symptoms.

EMERGENCY CARE STANDARDS

It is imperative that each member of the dental team have the following knowledge and skills:

- Current credentials in basic life support (cardiopulmonary resuscitation, or CPR)
- Current credentials in the Heimlich maneuver (also known as *abdominal thrusts*)
- Ability to obtain and record vital signs accurately (see Chapter 27)

ABCDs of Life Support

In all emergency situations the rescuers must promptly initiate the ABCDs of basic life support: *a*irway, *b*reathing, *c*irculation, and *d*efibrillation, if necessary.

The *airway* must be opened and maintained. To establish an airway, tilt the patient's head back by pressing on the forehead and use the other hand to lift the chin. This is known as the *tilt-lift method.*

The rise and fall of the chest is evaluated to determine whether the patient is breathing. If the patient is not breathing, *rescue breathing* or the *Heimlich maneuver* must be started immediately. Circulation must be monitored to determine whether the heart is beating. If the heart is not beating, *external cardiac compression* is started immediately, followed by *external defibrillation* to restore circulation.

Cardiopulmonary Resuscitation

In an emergency in which the patient is not breathing and the heart is not beating, **cardiopulmonary resuscitation (CPR)** must be initiated immediately. CPR combines rescue breathing, which ensures adequate air is entering the lungs, with external cardiac compression to stimulate the heart. This emergency support system must be enacted immediately so that the flow of oxygen-carrying blood quickly reaches the brain. The cells of the brain, the most sensitive tissue in the body, are irreversibly damaged after 4 to 6 minutes without oxygen.

CPR for small children and infants is similar to that for adults, but a few changes must be made to adapt to their anatomy and smaller bodies. Emergency Procedure 31-1 reviews CPR for the adult, child, and infant.

Emergency Procedure 31-1 Performing Cardiopulmonary Resuscitation

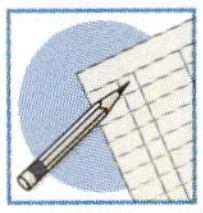

Equipment and Supplies

- Examination gloves
- CPR mouth barrier
- Mannequin approved by the American Heart Association (AHA) and equipped with a printout for demonstration of the proper technique (for instruction purposes and mock emergency drills).

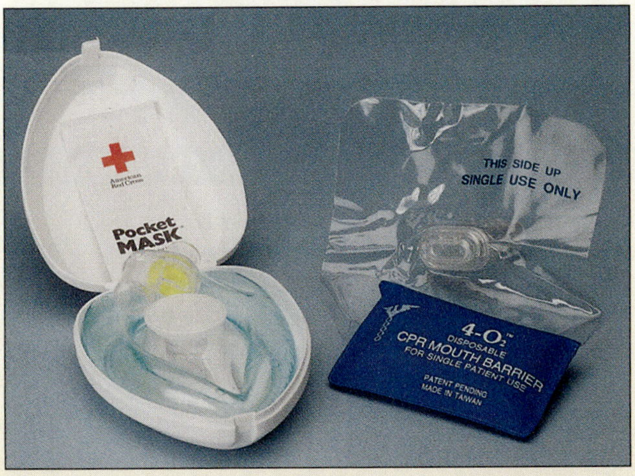

PROCEDURAL STEPS FOR CPR ON AN ADULT*

1. Approach the victim and check for signs of circulation, such as normal breathing, coughing, or movement in response to stimulation. Pinch or tap the victim and ask, "Are you OK?"
2. If there is no response, call for assistance and ask someone to call 911.
3. Tilt the victim's head and lift the chin. Look, listen, and feel for signs of breathing. Place your ear over the mouth and listen for breathing. Watch the rising and falling of the chest for evidence of breathing.

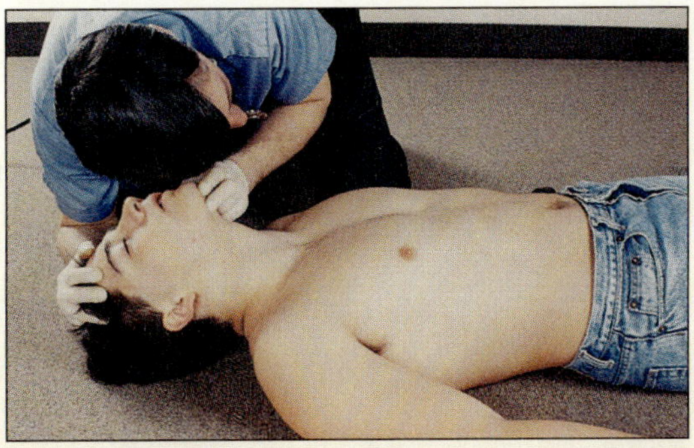

4. If there are no signs of breathing, place the CPR mouth barrier over the victim's mouth and begin rescue breathing by pinching the nose tightly with your thumb and forefinger.
   Purpose: To establish an airtight seal.

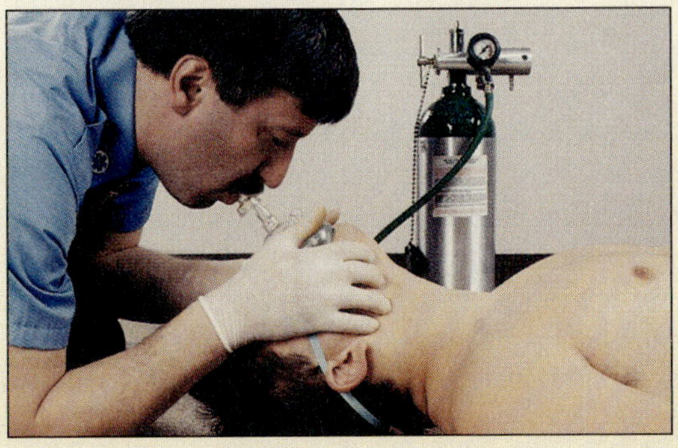

*From Young AP, Kennedy DB: *Kinn's the medical assistant: an applied learning approach,* ed 9, St Louis, 2003, Saunders.

Emergency Procedure 31-1 Performing Cardiopulmonary Resuscitation—cont'd

PROCEDURAL STEPS, cont'd

5. Give two full breaths.
6. Kneel at the victim's side opposite the chest. Move your fingers up the ribs to the point where the sternum and ribs join. Your middle finger should fit into the area, and your index finger should be next to it across the sternum.

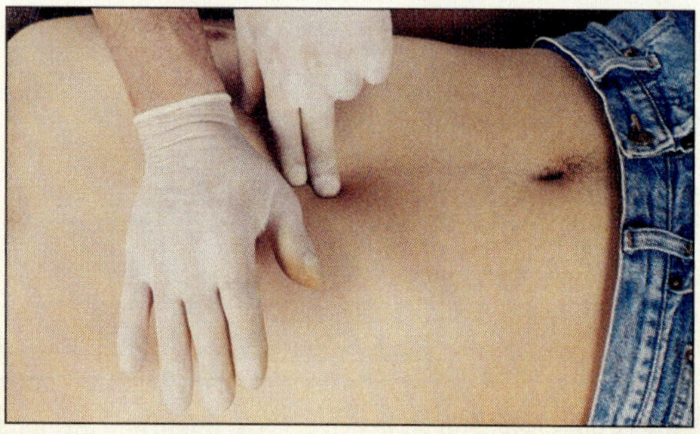

7. Place the heel of your hand on the chest midline over the sternum, just above your index finger.
8. Place your other hand on top of your first hand, and lift your fingers upward off the chest.

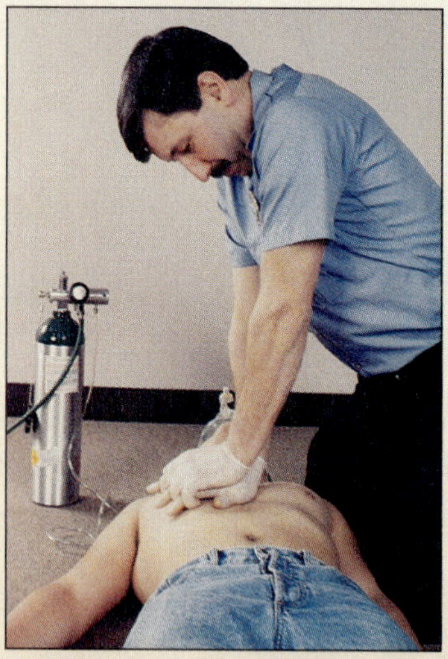

9. Bring your shoulders directly over the victim's sternum as you compress downward, and keep your arms straight.
10. Provide 15 compressions, making sure to depress the sternum 1 to 2 inches for an adult victim. Relax the pressure on the sternum after each compression, but do not remove your hands from the victim.
11. Complete three more cycles of 15 chest compressions and two breaths (15:2 ratio) regardless of whether one or two rescuers are present.

PROCEDURAL STEPS FOR CPR ON A CHILD[†]

CPR procedure for a child is essentially the same as for the adult, but you must follow a few specific technique adaptations:

1. For rescue breathing, give one breath every 3 seconds.
2. The hand position is the same as for adult chest compressions, but use the heel of only one hand and compress the sternum 1 to 1½ inches.

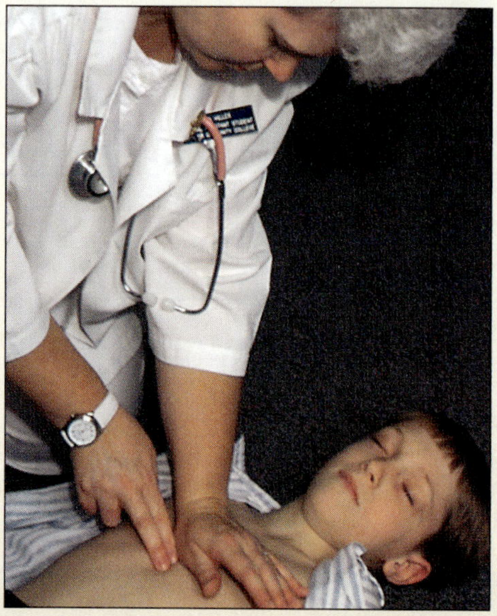

3. The ratio changes to five compressions to one breath (5:1 ratio).

PROCEDURAL STEPS FOR CPR ON AN INFANT[†]

1. For rescue breathing, give one breath every 3 seconds.
2. Breaths are given through both the nose and the mouth.
3. To complete chest compressions, place the middle fingers in the center of the chest between the nipples; then raise the index finger.

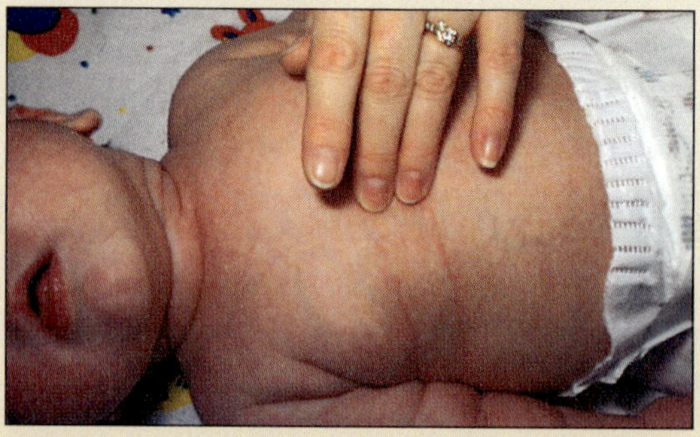

4. Compress the sternum ½ to 1 inch.
5. The ratio is five compressions to one breath (5:1).

[†]From Chester GA: *Modern medical assisting,* Philadelphia, 1998, Saunders.

Emergency Procedure 31-2 Responding to a Patient with an Obstructed Airway

Signs and Symptoms

- Patient grasping at throat, the universal sign of choking
- Ineffective cough
- High-pitched breathing sound
- Respiratory difficulty
- Change in skin color

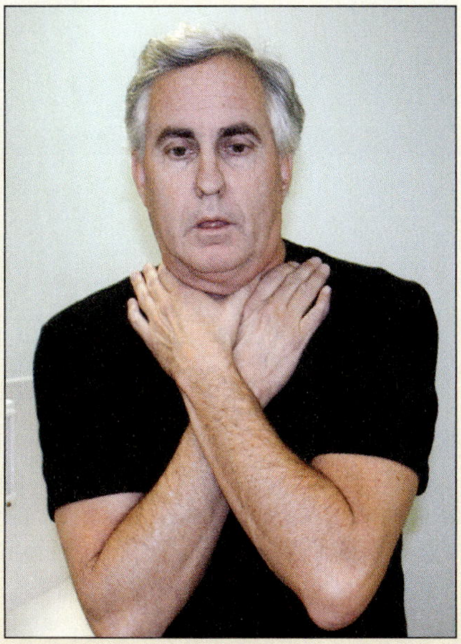

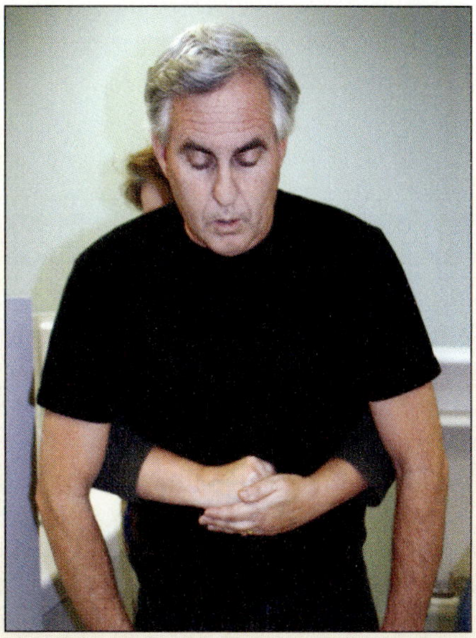

PROCEDURAL STEPS

Care of the Patient

1. If patient cannot speak, cough, or breathe, the airway is completely blocked. Immediately call for assistance and begin administering the Heimlich maneuver.
2. Make a fist with one hand and place thumb side of hand against the patient's abdomen, just above the navel and below the xiphoid process of the sternum.
3. Grasp the fist with the other hand and forcefully thrust both hands into the abdomen, using an inward and upward motion.
4. Repeat these thrusts until the object is expelled.

Responding to the Conscious Seated Patient

1. Do not try to move the patient out of the dental chair before administering the Heimlich maneuver.
   Purpose: Patient movement may cause the lodged item to be swallowed.
2. Place the heel of one hand at the patient's abdomen above the navel and well below the xiphoid process.
3. Place the other hand directly over the first hand. Administer a firm, quick, upward thrust into the patient's diaphragm.
4. Repeat this maneuver 6 to 10 times as needed until the object is dislodged or until advanced emergency assistance arrives.

Choking

A sudden coughing spasm or movement by the patient during a dental procedure may cause the accidental **aspiration** of a foreign object. The patient's discomfort is immediate; his or her hands go to the throat as spasms of coughing or choking occur.

The severity of the situation depends on (1) how tightly the item is lodged in the person's throat and (2) how much of the airway is blocked. The airway can become totally or partially blocked if the patient inhales a small object, such as a crown, debris, or tooth fragment. The three most important measures in preventing airway obstruction during dental treatment are:

- High-velocity suction
- Use of dental dam during routine treatment
- Placement of a *throat pack* (gauze placed at base of throat)

Emergency Procedure 31-2 reviews the steps to take in response to a choking patient.

Recall

6. What minimum credentials must you have for emergency care standards as a dental assistant?
7. What does the abbreviation *ABCD* stand for in emergency care?
8. What is the proper ratio of chest compressions to breaths for an adult victim when doing CPR?

EMERGENCY EQUIPMENT AND SUPPLIES

In most dental offices a drawer, tub, or portable standardized kit is used to store and organize emergency supplies (Fig. 31-6). The assistant may be assigned the responsibility for maintaining and updating these supplies.

If you do not have a standardized drug kit, the dentist will need to determine what emergency supplies and types of drugs should be maintained in the office. Table 31-1 lists the most common lifesaving drugs that would be included in a basic emergency kit, along with their brand name, use, route of administration, and precautions for use.

The maintenance of a drug kit includes the following:

- Routine check of supplies for quality to determine whether they are in *working condition* (rubber tubing, oxygen masks, tourniquets, intravenous lines, ventilation masks, blood pressure equipment)
- Weekly examination for *expiration* of drugs within the emergency kit. (Drugs past the expiration date should be replaced immediately.)
- Daily check of the oxygen tank or tanks

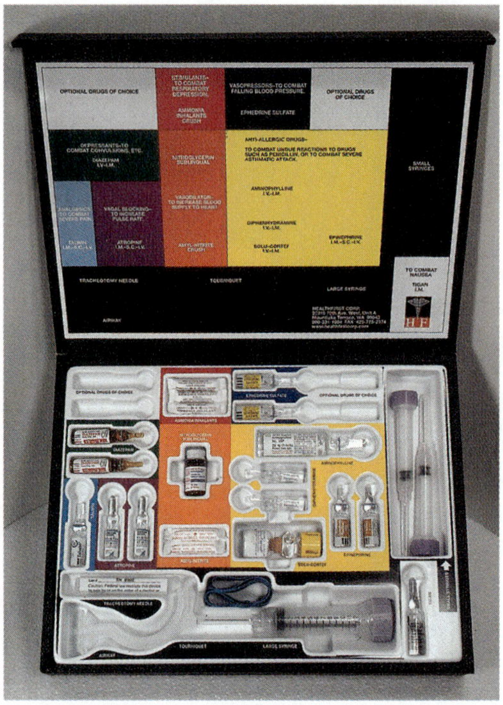

Fig. 31-6 Standardized color-coded basic emergency kit.

Table 31-1 ***Drugs Used in Medical Emergencies***

Drug	Brand or Common Name	Use	Route
Oxygen	N/A	Respiratory distress	Inhaled
Respiratory stimulant	Spirits of ammonia	Fainting	Inhaled
Epinephrine 1:1000	EpiPen	Allergic reaction	IM, IV, SC
Diphenhydramine	Benadryl	Allergic reaction	IV, deep IM
Chlorpheniramine	Chlor-Trimeton	Allergic reaction	IM, IV
Nitroglycerin	Nitrostat	Angina	Sublingually
Albuterol	Ventolin	Bronchospasm w/asthma	Inhaled
Diazepam	Valium	Seizures	IM, IV
Glucose	OJ, sugar, icing	Hypoglycemia	Orally
Morphine	Astramorph	Pain and anxiety	IM, IV, SC
Methoxamine	Vasoxyl	Blood pressure	IM, IV
Hydrocortisone	Solu-Cortef	Adrenocortical insufficiency, severe allergic reaction	IM, IV
Atropine	Atropair	Bradycardia	IM, IV, SC

IM, Intramuscular; *IV,* intravenous; *SC,* subcutaneous.

Oxygen

Oxygen is the most frequently used "drug" in a medical emergency. The ideal agent for resuscitation of a patient who is unconscious but still breathing is 100 percent oxygen. If the patient is not breathing, however, air must be forced into the lungs through rescue breathing or similar emergency measures.

A portable unit with tanks of oxygen may be stored where it can be moved quickly into a treatment room if needed. A reserve tank of oxygen should be available for the treatment of emergency situations. Remember, the oxygen cylinder is always color-coded green (Fig. 31-7). Emergency Procedure 31-3 reviews steps in preparing the oxygen system.

NOTE: If the dental office is equipped with a nitrous oxide–oxygen unit, the oxygen from these units can be used for emergency situations.

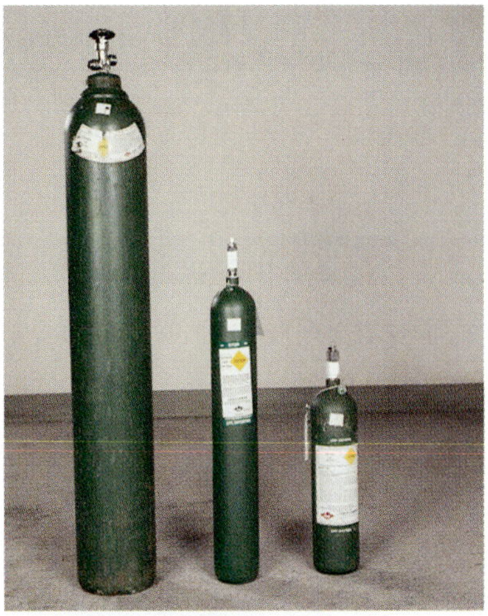

Fig. 31-7 Different sizes of oxygen cylinders. (From Henry MC, Stapleton ER: *EMT: prehospital care,* ed 3, St Louis, 2004, Mosby.)

Emergency Procedure 31-3 Preparing the Oxygen System

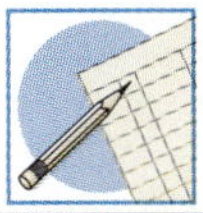

Equipment and Supplies

- Portable oxygen system
- Gauge regulator
- Tubing
- Face mask

PROCEDURAL STEPS

1. Confirm that the cylinder contains oxygen by checking the color and pin index grouping.

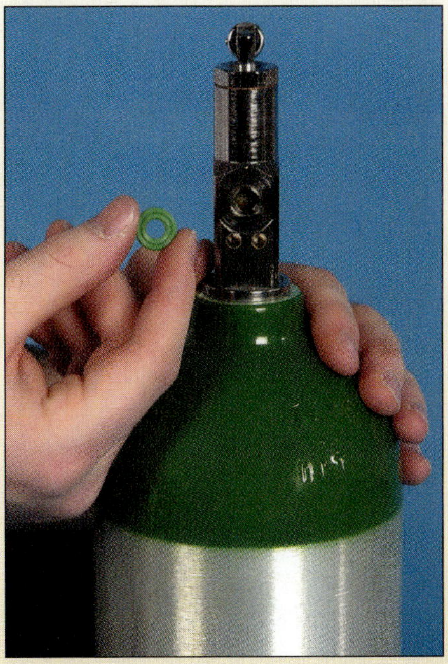

2. Open the main valve at the top of the cylinder slowly until gas starts to come out; then immediately close the valve.

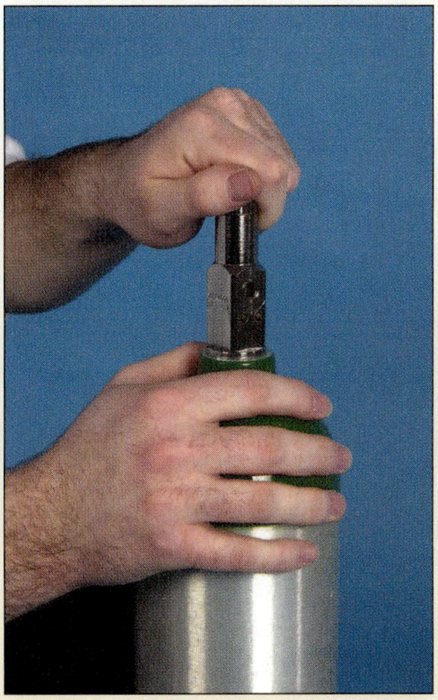

From Henry MC, Stapleton ER: *EMT: prehospital care,* ed 3, St Louis, 2004, Mosby.

continued

Emergency Procedure 31-3 Preparing the Oxygen System—cont'd

PROCEDURAL STEPS, cont'd

3. Attach the regulator by aligning the pin index into the cylinder holes.

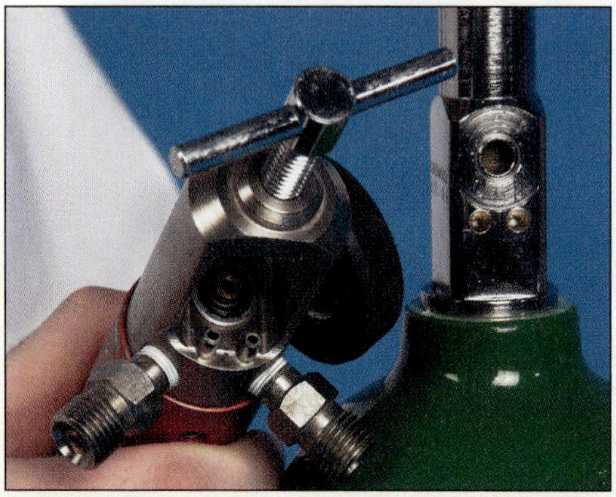

4. Tighten the clamp to ensure an adequate seal.
5. Open the valve two full turns. Check the pressure gauge to make sure that it is showing approximately 2000 pounds per square inch.
   Purpose: This much pressure is necessary for the oxygen to flow at a proper rate.

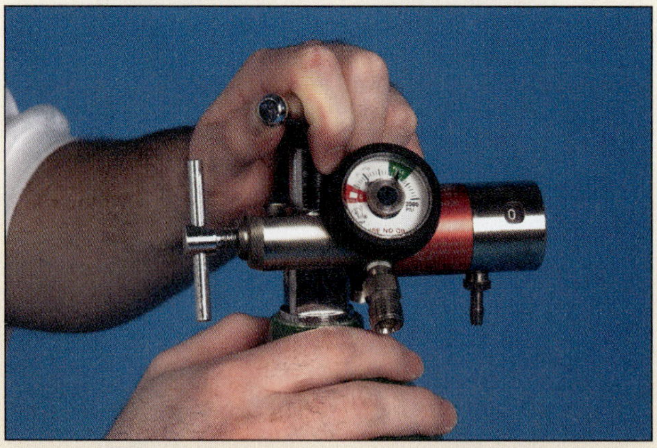

6. Attach the tubing if not already attached.

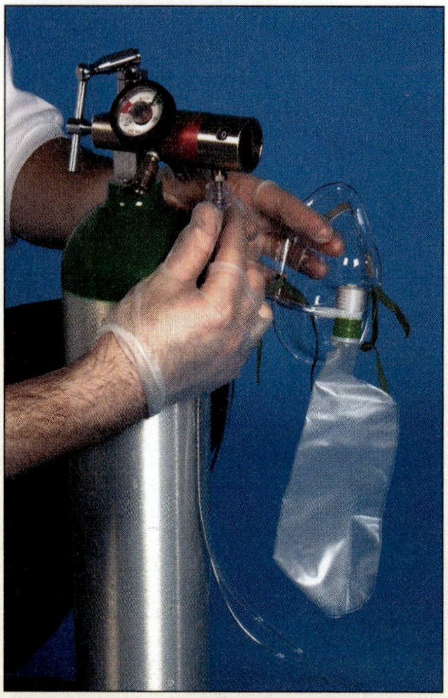

7. Position the mask comfortably over the patient's face.
   Note: Make sure that the mask is positioned so that it covers the nose and mouth and forms a good seal.

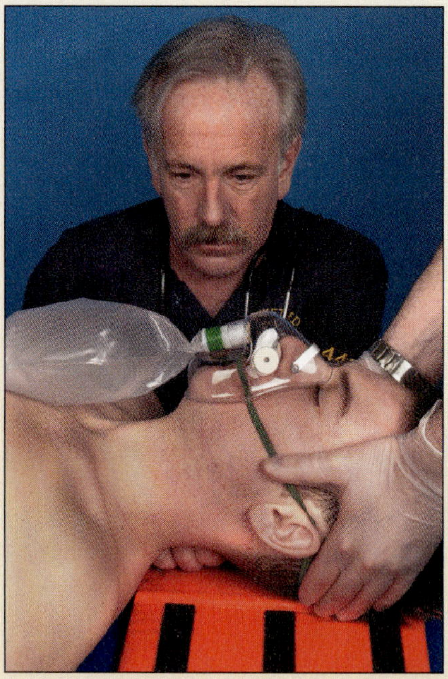

From Henry MC, Stapleton ER: *EMT: prehospital care,* ed 3, St Louis, 2004, Mosby.

Automated External Defibrillator

Most sudden cardiac arrest victims are experiencing what is called **ventricular fibrillation** (VF). VF is an abnormal, chaotic heart rhythm that prevents the heart from pumping blood. VF causes more cardiac arrests than any other rhythm (about 80 to 90 percent of cases).

You must defibrillate a victim immediately to stop VF and allow a normal heart rhythm to resume (Emergency Procedure 31-4). The sooner defibrillation begins, the better the victim's chances of survival. If defibrillation is provided within the first 5 minutes of a cardiac arrest, there is about a 50 percent chance that the victim's life can be saved. For each minute that passes during a cardiac arrest, however, the chance of successful resuscitation is reduced by 7 to 10 percent. After 10 minutes, there is very little chance of successful rescue.

Many places are now equipped with an automated external defibrillator (AED). The AED is attached to the patient, the power is turned on, and the device analyzes and defibrillates the patient without further input from the operator. A standard 110-volt current or battery powers this portable defibrillator. The monitor is equipped with a display and can print a copy of the victim's heart rate.

The AED is basically an advanced computer microprocessor that assesses the patient's cardiac rhythm and identifies any rhythm for which a shock is indicated. The shock is a massive jolt of electricity that is sent to the heart muscle to reestablish the proper rhythm of the heart. The AED (1) monitors the patient's heart rhythm, (2) distinguishes VF and other abnormal heart rhythms through a computed analysis, and (3) automatically defibrillates if needed.

Emergency Procedure 31-4 Operating the Automated External Defibrillator

Equipment and Supplies

- Examination gloves
- CPR equipment
- Defibrillator
- Electrode lines
- Paddles

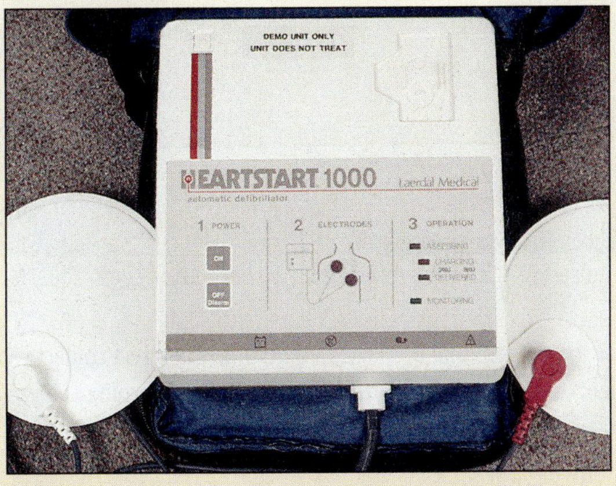

PROCEDURAL STEPS

1. Take infection control precautions by putting on examination gloves. Check for patient's responsiveness by tapping and shouting, pinching the muscles in the neck, or applying a sternal rub.

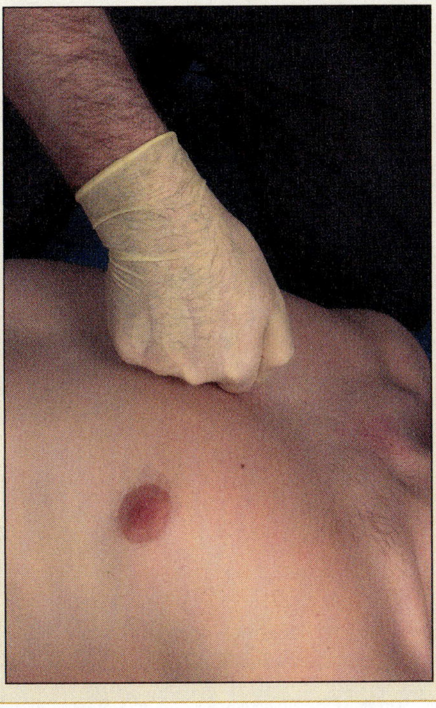

From Henry MC, Stapleton ER: *EMT: prehospital care,* ed 3, St Louis, 2004, Mosby.

continued

Emergency Procedure 31-4 Operating the Automated External Defibrillator–cont'd

PROCEDURAL STEPS, cont'd

2. Open the airway. Check for breathing in and provide two slow breaths.

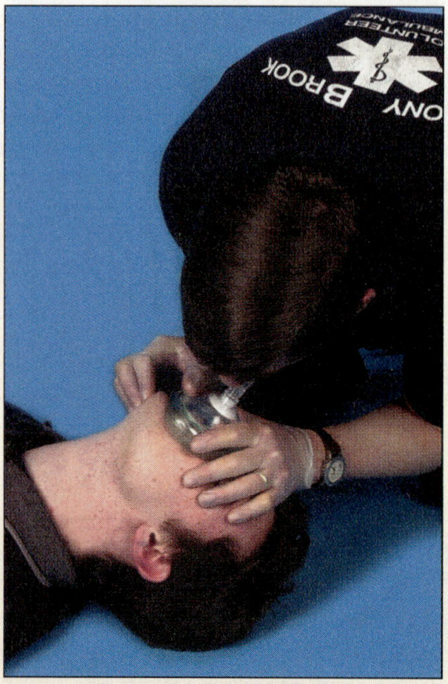

3. Check for signs of circulation.

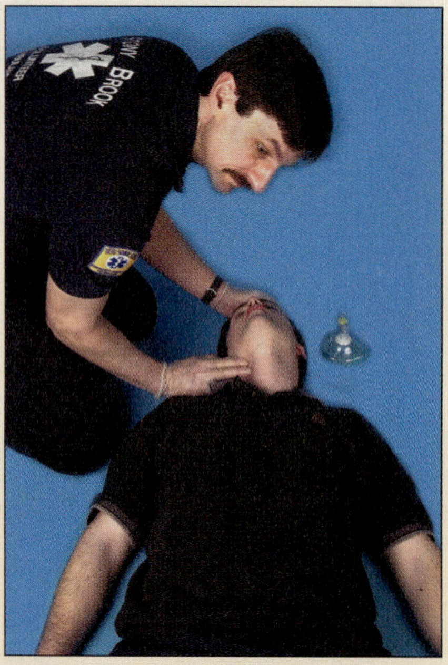

4. Position the defibrillator machine on the left side of the patient's head, close to the ear. Turn on the power by either lifting the top of the case or turning on the power switch.

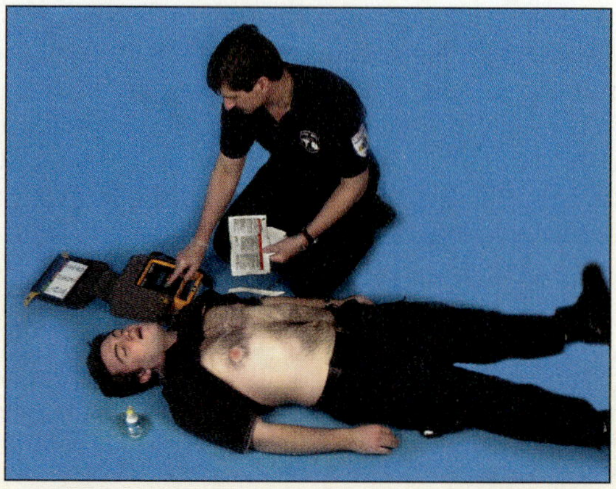

5. Attach the electrode lines to the paddles.
6. Attach the paddles to the patient, one at the left sternal border and the second on the right side above the nipple area.

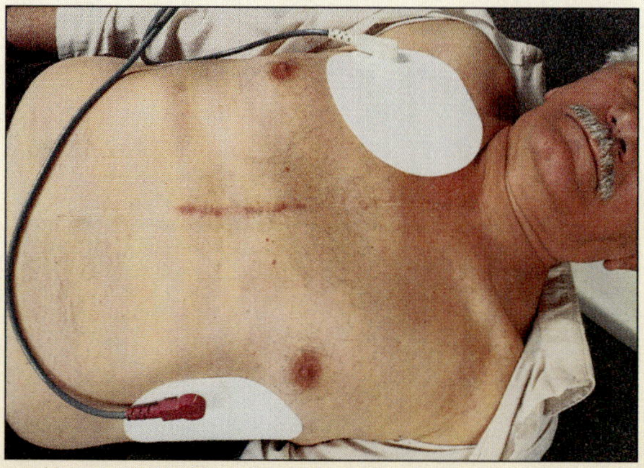

(From Aehlert B: *ACLS quick review study guide,* ed 2, St Louis, 2002, Mosby.)

7. Clear the patient (that is, make sure no one is in direct contact with the patient) and press the analyze button (or let the machine analyze automatically after attaching the pads).

From Henry MC, Stapleton ER: *EMT: prehospital care,* ed 3, St Louis, 2004, Mosby.

Emergency Procedure 31-4 Operating the Automated External Defibrillator—cont'd

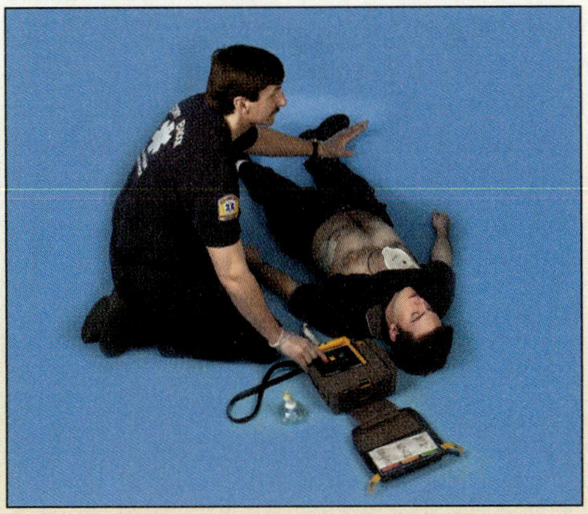

8. If the machine advises shock, confirm that everyone present is clear of the patient and deliver a shock.
9. Reanalyze the cardiac rhythm. If the machine advises shock, confirm that everyone is clear, and deliver a second shock. Complete this for three intervals if advised, and then reassess the patient's breathing and pulse.

Recall

9. What is the most frequently used "drug" in a medical emergency?
10. What does the abbreviation *AED* stand for?
11. What is the danger of ventricular fibrillation?

EMERGENCY RESPONSES

The diagnosis of a specific condition is *not* your responsibility. As a dental assistant, your responsibilities in relation to an emergency are (1) to recognize the symptoms and signs of a significant medical complaint and (2) to provide appropriate support in the implementation of emergency procedures.

During assessment of a medical emergency situation, the primary factor in determining the manner of treatment is the *physical change* in the patient. The physical changes most often seen during a dental office emergency are the following:

- *Unconsciousness,* the state of unresponsiveness to sensory stimulation
- *Altered consciousness,* with the patient conscious but acting strangely
- *Respiratory distress,* in which the conscious patient has difficulty breathing
- *Convulsions,* which are uncontrolled skeletal muscle contractions
- *Chest pain* in the conscious patient

Most emergencies in the dental office occur during or immediately after the administration of local anesthesia or at the onset of a procedure. The types of procedures during which medical emergencies most frequently arise in the dental office are *tooth extractions* and *endodontic treatment.* In these two procedures, adequate pain control may be difficult to achieve, and patient anxiety is high.

The remaining portion of this chapter discusses the most common medical emergencies occurring in the dental office.

Syncope

Syncope, commonly referred to as *fainting,* is one of the most frequent medical emergencies in the dental office. Syncope is caused by an imbalance in the blood distribution to the brain and the larger vessels within the body. This reduced blood flow to the brain causes the patient to lose consciousness.

Psychologic factors that can contribute to syncope include stress, apprehension, fear, and the sight of blood or certain instruments. Physiologic factors include remaining in one position for a long time, being in a confined environment, skipping meals or being hungry, and experiencing fatigue or exhaustion. The patient may complain of symptoms, and the signs may be noticed for several minutes before the patient actually loses consciousness.

Fainting is not harmful to the patient as long as someone is there to protect the person during unconsciousness. Even though quite common, syncope is one emergency that may be prevented by close observation of the patient.

Postural Hypotension

Postural **hypotension,** also referred to as *orthostatic hypotension,* is a level of altered unconsciousness that may lead to loss of consciousness. This emergency can occur when the patient assumes an upright position too quickly.

Postural hypotension results from insufficient blood flow to the brain and may occur in a patient immediately after a sudden change in positioning. Patients most often affected are those receiving nitrous oxide–oxygen or intravenous sedation and pregnant patients.

The duration of unconsciousness is very brief, usually lasting only seconds to minutes. If unconsciousness persists longer, other causes probably exist, and appropriate action must be taken immediately (Emergency Procedure 31-5).

The Pregnant Patient

While in a supine position, the pregnant patient may feel dizzy or lightheaded and may faint. This reaction results from the pressure of the enlarged uterus on the abdominal veins.

Unlike the procedure for postural hypotension, the patient should be turned onto her left side or moved into an upright sitting position. The change of position relieves the pressure on the involved blood vessels.

Emergency Procedure 31-5 Responding to the Unconscious Patient

SYNCOPE (FAINTING)

Signs and Symptoms

- Feeling of warmth or flushing (flushed)
- Nausea
- Rapid heart rate
- Perspiration
- Pallor (pale skin color)
- Lower blood pressure

Response Steps

1. Place the patient in a subsupine position with the head lower than the feet.
   Purpose: This position causes blood to flow away from the stomach and back toward the brain; this is frequently sufficient to revive the patient.

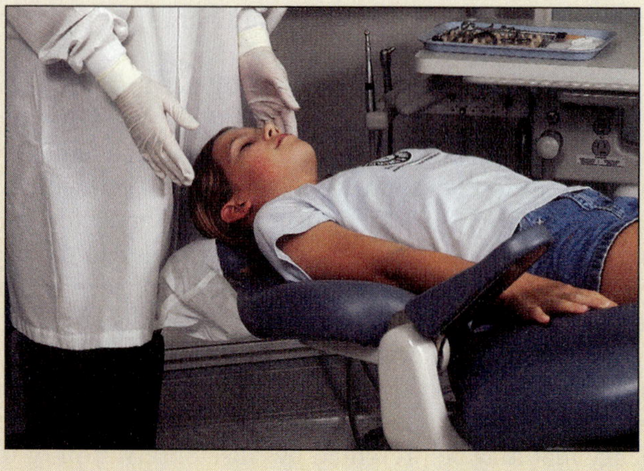

2. Call for emergency assistance (911).
3. Loosen any binding clothes on the patient.
4. Have an ammonia inhalant ready to administer by waving it under the patient's nose several times.
5. Have oxygen ready to administer.
6. Monitor and record patient's vital signs.

POSTURAL HYPOTENSION

Signs and Symptoms

- Low blood pressure
- Altered state of consciousness to possible loss of consciousness

Response Steps

1. Place the patient in a subsupine position with the head lower than the feet.
   Purpose: This position causes blood to flow away from the stomach and back toward the brain; this is frequently sufficient to revive the patient.
2. Establish an airway.
3. Slowly move the patient into an upright position.
4. If the patient does not respond immediately, call for emergency assistance (911).
5. Monitor and record vital signs.

Recall

12. When patients tell you how they feel, what is the term for such a "feeling"?
13. A patient who is unresponsive to sensory stimulation is in what state?
14. What is the medical term for fainting?

Cardiac Emergencies

Angina

The patient with **angina** feels severe *chest pain* because the heart muscle is deprived of adequate oxygen. Although painful, angina does not usually lead to death or permanent heart damage. However, such chest pain indicates that the person has some degree of coronary artery disease.

Because the signs and symptoms of angina and those of a myocardial infarction are very similar, it is important to distinguish angina, using the following criteria:

- Pain from angina usually lasts 3 to 8 minutes.
- Angina pain is relieved or eased promptly by the administration of a common drug, nitroglycerin.
- A patient with angina should specify this condition on the medical history.
- A patient with a history of angina usually carries some form of nitroglycerin to relieve the symptoms of an attack.
- Even if a patient has a history of angina, when an attack strikes, it is important to remember that the patient could be having a heart attack.

Acute Myocardial Infarction

During an **acute myocardial infarction,** commonly known as a *heart attack,* the muscles of the heart are damaged because of an insufficient oxygen supply. If this damage is severe enough, the patient will die; however, prompt medical treatment can help limit the damage to the heart.

Although other conditions have similar symptoms, any unexplained chest pain should be treated as a potential acute myocardial infarction (Emergency Procedure 31-6). Time is important, and the response of the dental team must be swift and prudent.

Cerebrovascular Accident

A cerebrovascular accident (CVA), commonly referred to as a *stroke,* is the interruption of blood flow to the brain. If blood flow is interrupted for a sufficient duration, damage to the brain may occur, resulting in the loss of brain function (Emergency Procedure 31-7). Most CVAs occur in older individuals who have other predisposing diseases, such as arteriosclerosis, heart disease, or uncontrolled high blood pressure.

Emergency Procedure 31-6 Responding to the Patient with Chest Pain

ANGINA ATTACK

Signs and Symptoms

- Tightness or squeezing sensation in the chest
- Pain radiating to the left shoulder
- Pain radiating to the left side of face, the jaws, and the teeth

Response Steps

1. Call for emergency assistance (911).
2. Position the patient upright.
3. If possible, have the patient self-medicate with personal nitroglycerin supply (tablets, spray, or topical cream). If this is not possible, obtain nitroglycerin from the office's emergency kit.
4. Administer oxygen.
5. Monitor and record vital signs.

ACUTE MYOCARDIAL INFARCTION (HEART ATTACK)

Signs and Symptoms

- Chest pain ranging from mild to severe
- Pain in the left arm, the jaw, and the teeth
- Shortness of breath and sweating
- Nausea and vomiting
- Pressure, aching, or burning feeling of indigestion
- Generalized feeling of weakness

Response Steps

1. Call for emergency assistance (911).
2. Initiate basic life support (CPR) if the patient becomes unconscious.
3. Medicate with nitroglycerin from the office's emergency kit.
4. Administer oxygen.
5. Monitor and record vital signs.

Emergency Procedure 31-7 Responding to the Patient Experiencing a Cerebrovascular Accident (Stroke)

Signs and Symptoms

- Paralysis
- Speech problems
- Vision problems
- Possible seizure
- Difficulty swallowing
- Headache
- Unconsciousness

Response Steps

1. Call for emergency assistance (911).
2. Initiate basic life support (CPR) if the patient becomes unconscious.
3. Monitor and record vital signs.

Hyperventilation

Hyperventilation, which is precipitated (initiated) by stress and anxiety, is an increase in the frequency or depth (or both) of respiration. As a result, the patient takes in too much oxygen. The patient usually remains conscious.

This medical emergency may occur when a patient is extremely anxious or apprehensive before dental treatment. To prevent or reduce hyperventilation, the dental team should be alert at all times and be prepared to help the patient deal with severe apprehension in a positive manner (Emergency Procedure 31-8).

Asthma Attack

Asthma is a pulmonary disorder characterized by attacks of sudden onset, during which the patient's airway narrows, causing difficulty in breathing and coughing and a wheezing sound. An allergic reaction, severe emotional stress, or respiratory infection may cause an asthma attack.

Patients with asthma usually carry an inhaler containing medication (bronchodilator) to relieve the first symptoms of an attack. It is essential that asthma be identified on the patient's medical history and that the patient brings the inhaler to each dental appointment (Emergency Procedure 31-8).

Recall

15. What is the medical term for chest pain?
16. What is the medical term for a stroke?

Allergic Reaction

An **allergy,** also referred to as **hypersensitivity,** is an altered state of reactivity in body tissues in response to specific antigens. An **antigen** is a substance that causes an immune response through the production of **antibodies.** An antigen that can trigger the allergic state is known as an **allergen.**

Although the patient's health history is the major factor in determining a risk for allergy, every new drug or dental material introduced to a patient can produce a reaction. Of particular concern is the increasing incidence of allergic reactions to the latex used in examination gloves and dental dams.

The two most important factors to consider when managing an allergic reaction are (1) the speed with which symptoms appear and (2) the severity of the reaction. A *localized* allergic response is usually slow to develop. The mild symptoms typically include itching, **erythema,** and hives.

The symptoms of **anaphylaxis** can be life-threatening and may develop very quickly. Without appropriate care, the patient could die within a few minutes (Emergency Procedure 31-9).

Epileptic Seizure

Epilepsy is a neurologic disorder characterized by recurrent episodes of seizures. In most patients, seizures or **convulsions** are controlled with medication. Under stressful conditions, however, a seizure can still occur. The two types of seizures of major concern are grand mal seizures and petit mal seizures.

A *grand mal seizure* is characterized by the temporary loss of consciousness accompanied by uncontrollable muscular contractions and relaxation. The seizure event has the following four phases:

- *Phase 1:* Before a grand mal seizure, the patient may experience a warning *aura* such as a peculiar smell, taste, vision, or sound. This can last several seconds or several hours.
- *Phase 2:* The patient loses consciousness and experiences a brief (10 to 20 second) period of generalized rigidity of the muscles. The patient may arch the back and emit a strange sound as air is expelled from the lungs.

Emergency Procedure 31-8 Responding to the Patient with a Breathing Problem

HYPERVENTILATION

Signs and Symptoms

- Rapid, shallow breathing
- Lightheadedness
- Tightness in the chest
- Rapid heartbeat
- Lump in the throat
- Panic-stricken appearance

Response Steps

1. Place the patient in a comfortable position.
2. Use a quiet tone of voice to calm and reassure the patient.
3. Have the patient breathe into a paper bag or cupped hands.

   Purpose: This response increases the carbon dioxide supply and restores the proper oxygen and carbon dioxide levels in the blood.

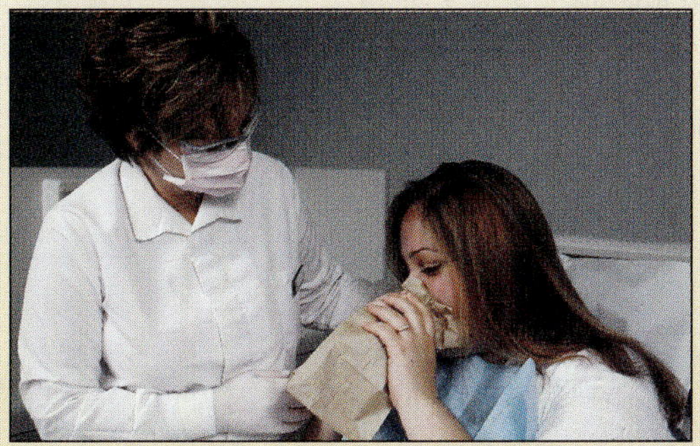

ASTHMA ATTACK

Signs and Symptoms

- Coughing
- Wheezing
- Increased anxiety
- Pallor
- Cyanosis (bluish skin around the nails)
- Increased pulse rate

Response Steps

1. Call for assistance
2. Position patient as comfortably as possible (upright is usually best).
3. Have patient self-medicate with inhaler.
4. Administer oxygen as needed.

Emergency Procedure 31-9 Responding to the Patient Experiencing an Allergic Reaction

LOCALIZED RASH

Signs and Symptoms

- Itching
- Erythema (skin redness)
- Hives

Response Steps

1. Call for emergency assistance (911).
2. Prepare an antihistamine for administration.
3. Be prepared to administer basic life support if necessary.
4. Refer the patient for medical consultation.

   Purpose: If the patient has an allergic reaction once, he or she may become increasingly hypersensitive and have a life-threatening response the next time.

ANAPHYLAXIS

Signs and Symptoms

- Feeling physically ill
- Nausea and vomiting
- Shortness of breath
- Heart arrhythmia (irregular heartbeats)
- Sudden drop in blood pressure
- Loss of consciousness

Response Steps

1. Call for emergency assistance (911).
2. Place the patient in a supine position.
3. Start basic life support (CPR) if patient becomes unconscious.
4. Prepare to administer epinephrine.
5. Administer oxygen.
6. Monitor and record vital signs.

- *Phase 3:* Muscle contractions may be violent or barely detectable. The respiratory, cardiovascular, and central nervous systems are stimulated simultaneously. The patient is in danger of self-injury.
- *Phase 4:* During this final phase, muscle contraction ends, leaving the affected systems "depressed."

These four phases can last from 10 to 30 minutes. During this time the patient sleeps deeply and may be difficult to awaken.

A *petit mal seizure* is a brief lapse of consciousness that may last only a few seconds. A patient may just stare or make no movement during the episode. The person will usually not collapse (Emergency Procedure 31-10).

Diabetes Mellitus

Diabetes mellitus is a metabolic disorder resulting from disturbances in the body's normal insulin mechanism. Most patients with diabetes manage the disease by balancing their food intake with their insulin therapy. When the balance shifts (either too much or too little food ingested), the insulin level changes, resulting in hyperglycemia or hypoglycemia (Emergency Procedure 31-11).

Hyperglycemia

Hyperglycemia results from an abnormal *increase* in the glucose (sugar) level in the blood. If untreated, hyperglycemia may progress to diabetic ketoacidosis and a life-threatening diabetic coma.

Hypoglycemia

Hypoglycemia results from an abnormal *decrease* in the glucose level in the blood. This condition can manifest itself rapidly. The most common causes of hypoglycemia are skipping a meal, taking too much insulin without adequate food intake, and exercising excessively without an appropriate adjustment of insulin and food intake.

Recall

17. A patient with asthma will usually carry what form of medication with them?
18. What type of allergic reaction can be life-threatening?
19. What condition results from an abnormal increase in blood glucose?

Emergency Procedure 31-10 Responding to the Patient Experiencing a Convulsive Seizure

GRAND MAL SEIZURE

Signs and Symptoms

- Unconsciousness
- Increased body temperature
- Rapid heart rate
- Increased blood pressure

Response Steps

1. Call for emergency assistance (911).
2. If a seizure occurs while the patient is in the dental chair, quickly remove all materials from the mouth and place the patient in a supine position.
   Purpose: The patient could inflict self-harm if something is in the mouth. Do not place anything in the patient's mouth during a seizure.
3. Protect the patient from self-injury during movements of the convulsion.
4. Initiate basic life support (CPR).
5. Monitor and record vital signs.
6. Prepare to use anticonvulsant (diazepam) from the drug kit.

PETIT MAL SEIZURE

Signs and Symptoms

- Intermittent blinking
- Mouth movements
- Blank stare
- Not responsive to surroundings; seems to be in his or her "own world"

Response Steps

1. Call for emergency assistance (911).
2. Prevent injury to patient.
3. Monitor and record vital signs.
4. Refer patient for medical consultation.

DOCUMENTATION OF AN EMERGENCY

When a medical emergency arises in the dental office, full documentation of the details is essential. After such an emergency, the dentist will make extensive notes in the patient's record explaining exactly what happened, the treatment provided, and the patient's condition at the time he or she left the office.

If an emergency is not fully resolved while the patient is in the office, the dentist may telephone the patient, the family, or the patient's physician the next day to inquire about the patient's health.

Emergency Procedure 31-11 Responding to the Patient Experiencing a Diabetic Emergency

HYPERGLYCEMIA

Signs and Symptoms

- Excessive urination
- Excessive thirst, dry mouth, and dry skin
- Acetone breath (fruity smell)
- Blurred vision and headache
- Rapid pulse
- Lower blood pressure
- Loss of consciousness

Response Steps

1. Call for emergency assistance (911).
2. If the patient is conscious, ask when he or she last ate, whether the patient has taken insulin, and whether he or she brought insulin along to the dental appointment.
   Purpose: If the patient has already eaten but has not taken insulin, the patient needs insulin immediately.
3. Retrieve the patient's insulin if it is available. If able, the patient should self-administer the insulin.
4. Provide basic life support (CPR) if the patient becomes unconscious.
5. Monitor and record vital signs.

HYPOGLYCEMIA

Signs and Symptoms

- Mood changes
- Hunger
- Perspiration
- Increased anxiety
- Possible unconsciousness

Response Steps

1. Call for emergency assistance (911).
2. If the patient is conscious, ask when he or she last ate, whether the patient has taken insulin, and whether he or she brought insulin along to the dental appointment.
3. If the patient is conscious, give a concentrated form of carbohydrate, such as a sugar packet, cake icing, or concentrated orange juice.
   Purpose: These substances will be absorbed rapidly into the bloodstream.

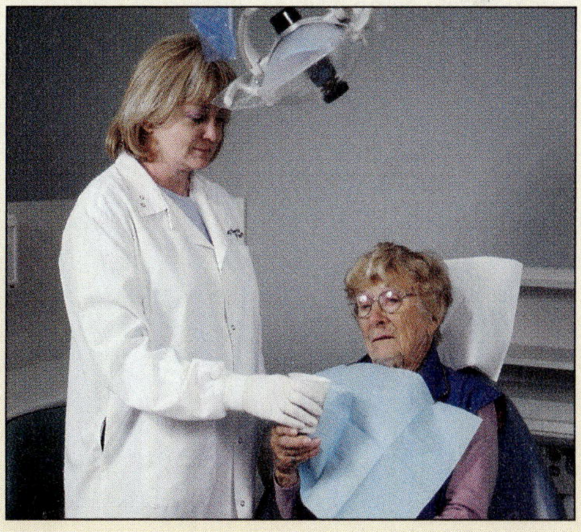

4. Provide basic life support (CPR) if the patient becomes unconscious.
5. Monitor and record vital signs.

Patient Education

Patients are more aware of their own health status today. Most patients are able to follow through with their personal care plan and know when to seek professional help.

On television and in newspapers, for example, you may see a report of a child saving a person's life because the child saw a TV show that discussed CPR or the Heimlich maneuver. The more the healthcare sector discusses the importance of individual awareness through workshops and patient education, the more our patients can help themselves or others in a time of need.

Eye to the Future

New technology is allowing individuals with serious medical conditions to live a normal life with confidence that the emergency medical system will be alerted when the need arises. Furthermore, the Internet has dramatically changed the way America communicates with individuals, emergency systems, and hospitals.

Advances in digital and compression technology mean that vast amounts of information can be stored on ever-smaller chips. Important applications of this technology include the creation of digital medical libraries and medical databases. The potential also exists to develop *electronic medical record systems* and credit-card–sized "smart cards" that store personal medical information.

Legal and Ethical Implications

As a professional dental assistant, you will often be asked for dental and medical advice from your patients, family, and friends. You must be very careful about what you say to people. You are not in the position to diagnose an illness, and you must not do so under any circumstance.

In the case of an emergency, however, the situation is different. You are protected under the "Good Samaritan Law," which states that if you try your best and do what is reasonably possible by others with the same training, the victim cannot legally hold you responsible if something goes wrong.

Critical Thinking

1. You are taking a patient to the treatment area and notice that she looks flushed and is perspiring. You decide to take her vital signs after seating her and note a rapid heart rate and a decrease in her blood pressure. What warning sign does this represent regarding a medical emergency?
2. What would be your response to the patient described in question 1?
3. The dentist has just finished giving the local anesthesia when a patient complains of shortness of breath and says he is "not feeling very well." What medical emergency would you suspect, and how should the dental team respond?
4. What should you keep in the dental office to have available for a patient with hypoglycemia?
5. Why would you not place anything in a patient's mouth during a grand mal seizure?

Part 7

Foundation of Clinical Dentistry

Before any professional can practice and perfect a skill, he or she must first understand how the skill is performed. As a clinical dental assistant, your role will be ever-changing because of the fast-changing technology of dentistry.

The chapters in this section will focus on the introductory level of knowledge and skill that the dental assistant must master when learning how dental care is delivered. Areas discussed are layout and design of the dental office, specific instruments and supplies used in most general dental procedures, and the importance of patient comfort during dental treatment.

32

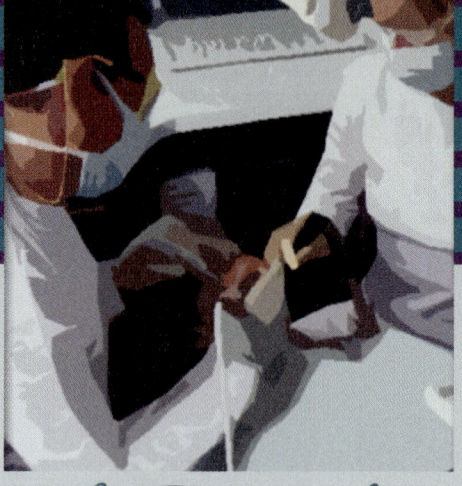

The Dental Office

Outline

KEY TERMS

Condensation (*kahn*-duhn-**say**-shun) Process by which liquid is removed from vapor.

Consultation room (*kahn(t)*-suhl-**tay**-shun) Meeting room or specified area where diagnostic and treatment information is discussed with the patient.

Dental operatory (**op**-er-ah-*tor*-ee) Dental treatment room and control center of the clinical area.

Rheostat (**ree**-uh-*stat*) Foot-controlled device used to operate dental handpieces.

Subsupine position (*sub*-**sue**-pine) Lying-down position in which the patient's head is lower than the feet (below the heart); used in emergency situations.

Supine position (**sue**-pine) Lying-down position in which the patient's head, chest, and knees are at the same level.

Triturate (**trich**-ur-ate, **tri**-chuh-*rate*) The process of mechanically mixing a material, as in using an amalgamator to mix an alloy and mercury to create dental amalgam.

Upright position Vertical seated position in which the back of the dental chair is upright at a 90° angle.

LEARNING OUTCOMES

On completion of this chapter, the student will be able to achieve the following objectives:

- Pronounce, define, and spell the Key Terms.
- Describe the six areas of the dental environment in a professional office.
- Discuss the important qualities of the reception area.
- Describe the goals in designing the dental treatment area.
- List the clinical equipment most commonly found in dental treatment areas.
- Discuss the basic function of the dental unit.

PERFORMANCE OUTCOMES

On completion of this chapter, the student will be able to meet competency standards in the following skills:

- Prepare the dental treatment area for patient care in the morning before seeing patients.
- Prepare the dental treatment area for patient care the next day.

OFFICE ENVIRONMENT

Patients often judge the quality of their care by the appearance of the office. A patient's first perception of a dental office will remain with that patient throughout further appointments. Attention to detail and organization in the way you receive, treat, and dismiss patients are important when creating a positive experience for the patient. All areas of the dental office must portray an organized and professional setting at all times.

Temperature

It is important to have the temperature in a room ideal for comfort. The ideal temperature for the reception area is 72° F. In the clinical areas, the temperature would be lowered to 68° to 70° F, because of the closer quarters and overhead and dental unit lights.

Air exchange should be constant throughout the office as well. Have you ever walked into a hospital and thought, "This smells like a hospital"? Distinguishing smells can also be associated with a dental office. These odors can be offensive to a patient if the air circulation is not appropriate.

Lighting

All areas of the office need to have appropriate lighting for the environment. In the reception area, more decorative lighting is preferable, such as table and floor lamps, which are sufficient for reading. The business, clinical, laboratory, and sterilization areas have fluorescent lighting, which is more uniform and radiates less heat. Additional lighting is provided in the clinical area for procedures and in the laboratory, as discussed in the Clinical Equipment section later in the chapter.

Wall and Floor Coverings

Key features in the design of a dental office include the use of colors that are calming, relaxing, and not too "busy" (Fig. 32-1). The wall covering may include paint, wallpaper, or both. In the selection of floor covering, a durable high-traffic carpet is suitable in the reception area, the administrative area, and the dentist's private office. A more suitable material for infection control, such as vinyl, is more appropriate in the clinical and laboratory areas.

Traffic Control

When a patient enters an office, furnishings should be arranged so that traffic flow is smooth to all areas of the office. Separate areas at the desk should be available for patients to check in and to check out. In the "back" of the office, the clinical, sterilization, and laboratory areas should be designed for easy entry in and out of areas for the dental team without causing chaos.

Sound Control

Specific sounds are associated with a dental office. Clinical areas should be arranged so that minimal sound is carried

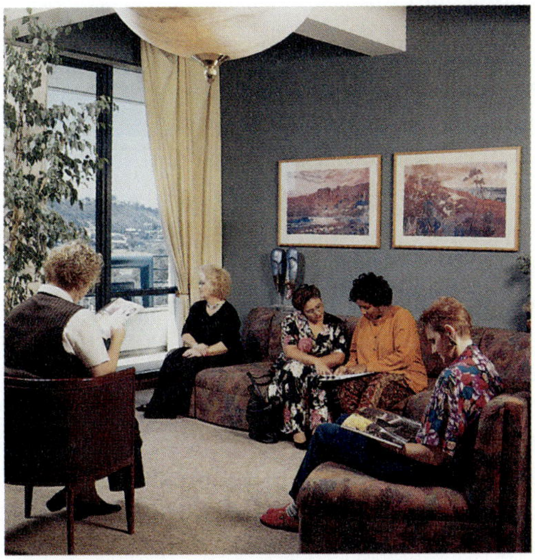

Fig. 32-1 Design of the dental office using calming colors. (From Kinn ME, Woods M: *The medical assistant: administrative and clinical,* ed 8, Philadelphia, 1999, Saunders.)

from one room to another. Music provides a distraction from the other sounds. Decide on music that will be relaxing and will provide a tranquil environment rather than constant percussion.

Privacy

Specific areas need to be private. The administrative area should project a professional regard for privacy, especially if the dentist is discussing financial matters with a patient or the business staff. The clinical areas require privacy to provide the patient and dental team with an area to complete treatment without interruptions. The dentist's office should also maintain privacy away from patient flow.

Recall

1. What is the ideal temperature for the reception area?
2. What type of flooring should be placed in the clinical area?

Specific Areas of the Dental Office

Although the size and types of practices vary greatly, the rooms or space usually found in most dental practices include:

- Reception area
- Administrative/business area
- Clinical treatment areas
- Sterilization center
- Dental laboratory
- Dentist's private office
- Dental staff lounge

RECEPTION AREA

The reception area is where patients are received, greeted pleasantly, and made to feel welcome (Fig. 32-2). This area should not be a "waiting area"; with proper scheduling, patients can be seen on time for their appointments.

Cleanliness should be of utmost concern daily. Have adequate seating for the patients and their families. Keep a selection of up-to-date magazines. Know the preferences of your patients, and have on hand what interests them. For example, if your office is in the business district, have business and financial magazines. Have a place to hang coats and umbrellas to help reduce clutter.

Remember to maintain a section of the reception area for children (Fig. 32-3). Items to keep in this area include books, toys, and comfortable seating for toddlers.

ADMINISTRATIVE AREA

The administrative area of the office is the hub for the management or the business side of the practice (Fig. 32-4). This area includes a desk, storage area for patient records and business materials, phone systems, computers, photocopier, calculators, and fax machines. More security measures are taken in this area because of the exchange of payment and the handling of insurance checks.

TREATMENT AREA

The actual dental treatment provided to the patient takes place in the **dental operatory**, also referred to as the *dental treatment area* (Fig. 32-5). This part of the dental office is the control center of the clinical area in the dental practice.

Most practices will have two or more dental treatment areas per dentist and one operatory for the dental hygien-

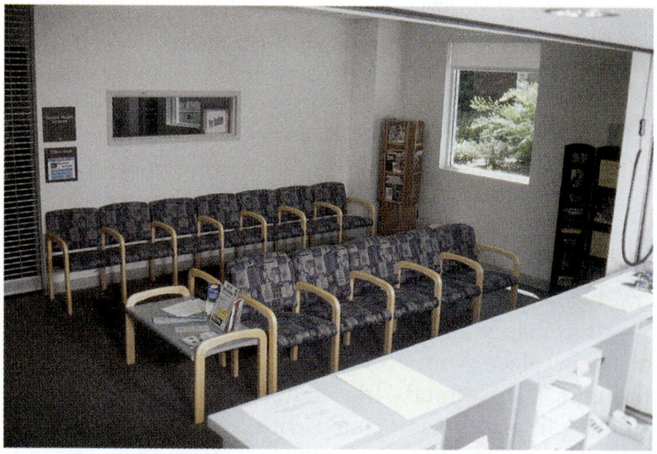

Fig. 32-2 Reception area of a dental office.

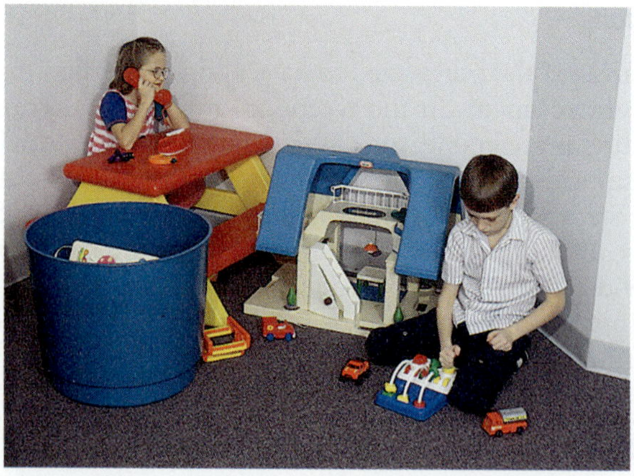

Fig. 32-3 Part of a reception area designed for children. (From Chester GA: *Modern medical assisting,* Philadelphia, 1998, Saunders.)

ist. To promote efficiency, the dentist will move from one room to another to deliver care. These rooms should be designed and furnished in a similar manner for easier access to items that may be kept in each room.

The design and arrangement of the treatment areas depend on the space available and the dentist's preferences regarding their style. The goal in designing the dental treatment area is to achieve the following:

- Comfort and mobility for the dental team
- Privacy and comfort for the dental patient
- Enhancement of the use of dental equipment through time management and efficient techniques

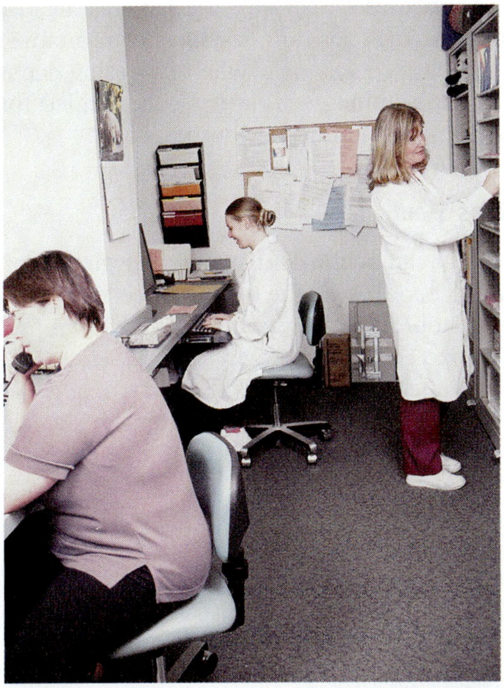

Fig. 32-4 **Organization and design of the business area.**

Recall

3. What are the important features of the reception area?
4. Where in the dental office are dental procedures performed?
5. What is another term for the treatment area?

CLINICAL EQUIPMENT

The basic equipment found in each treatment area includes a patient dental chair, stools for the dentist and assistant during a procedure, dental units, cabinetry for storage, an operating light, a wall-mounted radiograph unit, a radiograph view box, and a sink.

Patient Dental Chair

The patient dental chair is designed to provide patient comfort (Fig. 32-6). Chairs are available in sizes for adult practices as well as pediatric practices.

When the patient is properly seated, the patient's knees, bottom, and lumbar region of the back should be fully supported. The headrest holds the patient's head securely and comfortably in the appropriate position for the treatment being provided (Fig. 32-7). The headrest can be adjusted to accommodate positioning as well as height of the patient.

The arms of the chair comfortably support the patient's arms. Chair arms can be raised or moved aside when the patient is being seated or dismissed.

The dental chair has several controls to adjust for patient comfort and flexibility in positioning during dental

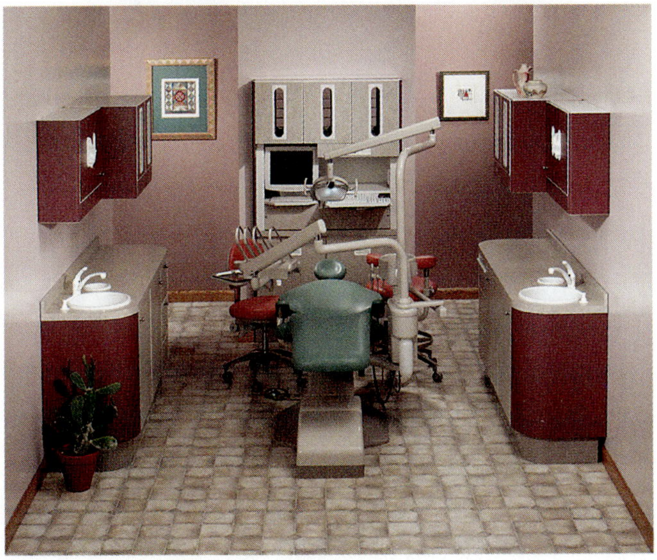

Fig. 32-5 **Dental treatment area.** (Courtesy A-dec.)

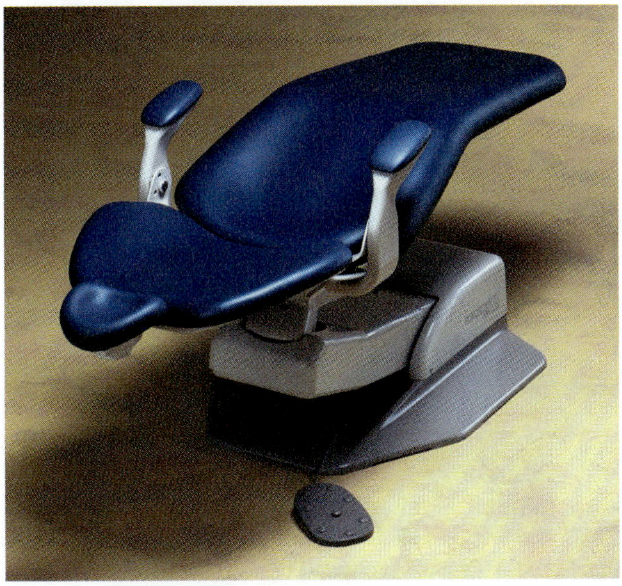

Fig. 32-6 **Patient dental chair.** (Courtesy A-dec.)

treatment. Patient chairs are designed to be seamless, with few visible mechanical parts to facilitate their cleaning and maintenance. Controls allow adjustment of the back of the chair to a lying-down or sitting-up position. The entire chair can also be adjusted to higher and lower positions for easier patient and oral access (Fig. 32-8).

Adjustment of the dental chair allows the patient to be placed in upright, supine, and subsupine positions. The area of the mouth being treated and the type of procedure determine the position selected.

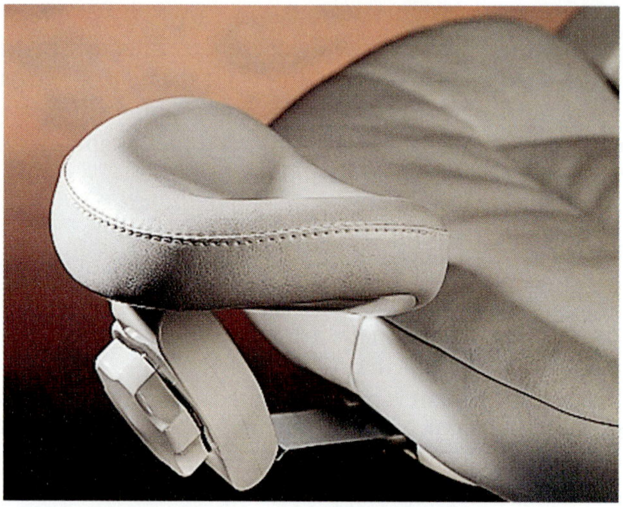

Fig. 32-7 Design of the headrest on a dental chair. (Courtesy A-dec.)

In the **upright position,** the back of the chair is positioned at a 90° angle. The upright position is used for patient entry and dismissal. It provides easy access for the operator when working on the patient's lower right side (for a right-handed operator). The upright position may also be used when radiographs are exposed and impressions taken (Fig. 32-9).

In the **supine position,** the patient is positioned as if lying down. Because of the contour of the patient chair, however, the patient will not appear flat. The patient's head and knees will be at approximately the same level. Most dental treatment is completed with the patient in the supine position (Fig. 32-10).

In the **subsupine position,** the patient's head is *lower* than the feet. This position is very uncomfortable for patients, so it is used very little when providing dental treatment. The subsupine position is recommended for emergency situations and unconscious patients.

Operator's Stool

The operator can be the dentist, dental hygienist, or dental assistant, depending on the dental procedure. This person requires a stool that can support the body for a prolonged period of fixed muscular activity (Fig. 32-11).

The operator's stool should provide a large seat and back with easily adjustable lumbar support. Seat cushioning should comfortably support the operator's body for

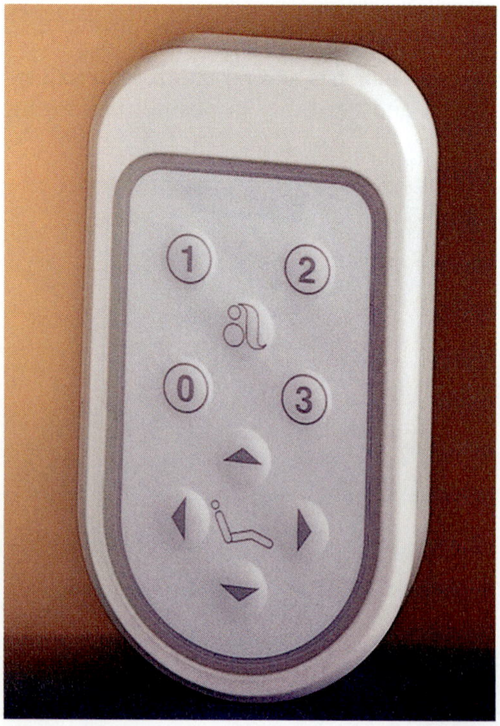

Fig. 32-8 Control buttons on a dental chair. (Courtesy A-dec.)

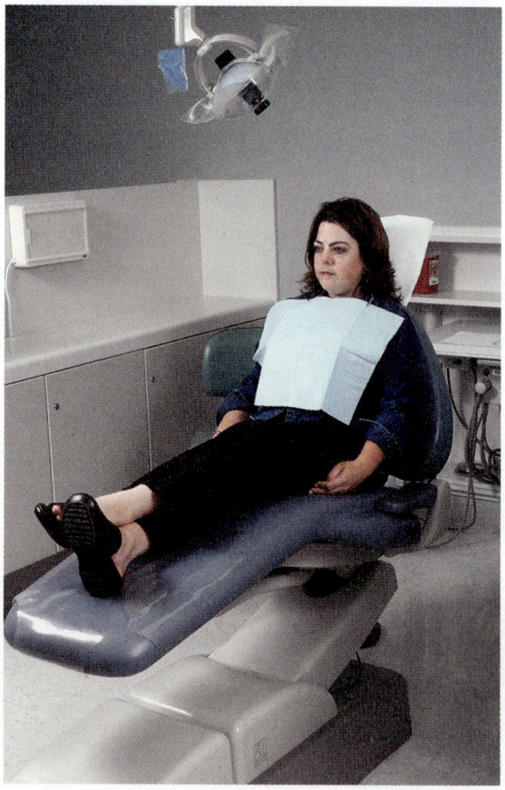

Fig. 32-9 Upright position of a patient in a dental chair.

an extended time. The ability of an operator's stool to adjust both higher and lower and to move easily around the patient's chair (without tilting for optimal access to the oral cavity) is extremely important to help reduce body and eye fatigue.

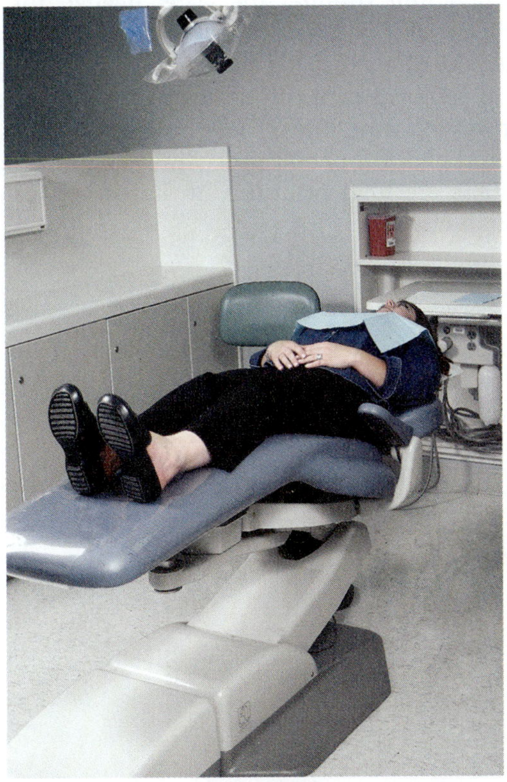

Fig. 32-10 Patient in a supine position in a dental chair.

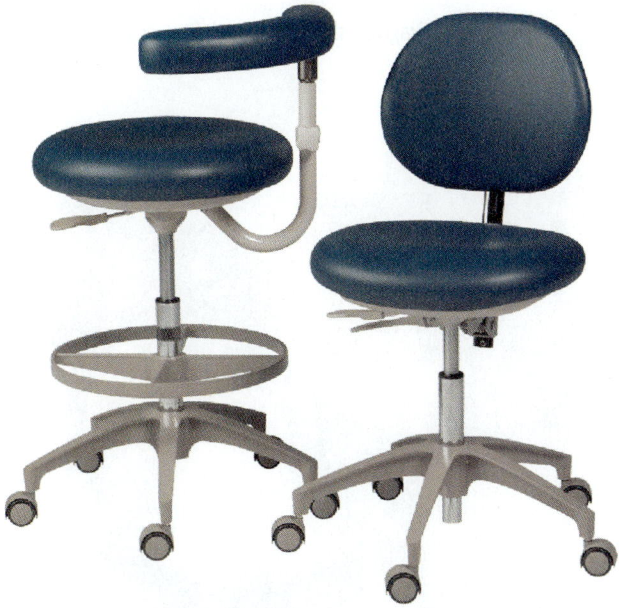

Fig. 32-11 *Left,* dental assistants' stool. *Right,* operators' stool. (Courtesy A-dec.)

Dental Assistant's Stool

The assistant's stool must provide stability, mobility, and comfort and should allow the assistant to assist with the proper fatigue-reducing posture. Regardless of the assistant's height or stature, the chair should allow the assistant to twist and turn to reach countertops and shelves.

The seating should be designed to minimize fatigue by providing an adjustable foot platform or foot ring, firm secure cushioning in the seat, and an abdominal support bar. This bar provides added support for the upper body and arm to allow unobstructed access to the oral cavity. The abdominal bar should be positioned for support, not for resting or leaning. With inappropriate use of the bar, the dental assistant can cause lower back pain by leaning over during the dental procedure (Fig. 32-11).

Dental Unit

The basic function of a dental unit is to provide the necessary electrical and air-operated mechanics to the hoses, attachments, and working parts of the unit (Fig. 32-12).

Dental units are supplied in a range of styles and equipment combinations. The type of dental units selected depends on 1) the space available, 2) the operator's preferred method of delivery, 3) whether the operator is left-handed or right-handed, and 4) whether the operator works primarily with or without a chairside assistant.

The attachments and controls of the dental unit are operated by initiating a master switch. Each attachment has its own control over how much air and water the particular device will receive.

Delivery Systems

The dental unit can be mounted on the floor, the wall, or most often the side of the dental chair.

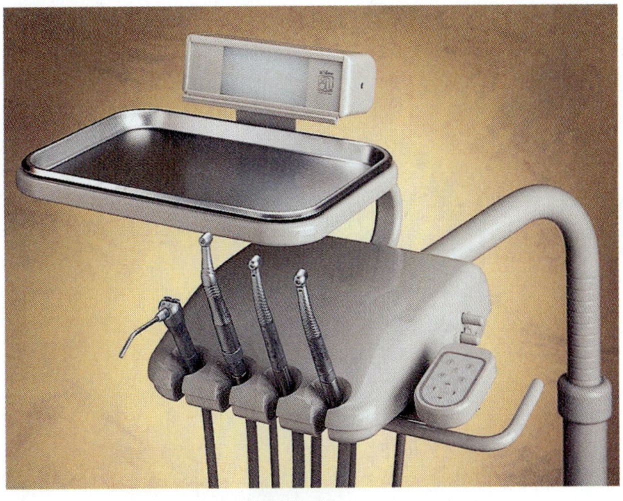

Fig. 32-12 Dental unit. (Courtesy A-dec.)

- *Front delivery* allows the dental unit to be positioned over the patient's chest. This provides the dentist with easy access to the dental handpieces without twisting of the body (Fig. 32-13).
- *Side delivery* allows the dental unit to be positioned at either side of the patient's chair. The unit provides separate sections for the dentist and assistant (Fig. 32-14).
- *Rear delivery* allows the dental unit and equipment to be positioned behind the dental chair near the back of the patient's head (Fig. 32-15).

Rheostat

The dental handpieces are attached to a specific hose in the dental unit. The dentist or operator will use a rheostat to operate and control the speed. A **rheostat** is a foot-controlled device that is placed on the floor near the operator (Fig. 32-16). With foot pressure, the slow-speed and high-speed handpiece can be controlled.

Waterlines

The dental unit supplies the water needed for dental procedures. This is crucial for keeping an area clean as well as cooled against the heat resulting from the mechanical removal of tooth structure. Several hoses are equipped with waterlines. These lines carry water that is used throughout a dental procedure. Maintenance and cleanliness are high priorities in the use of waterlines (see Chapter 24).

Fig. 32-13 Diagram showing front delivery system.

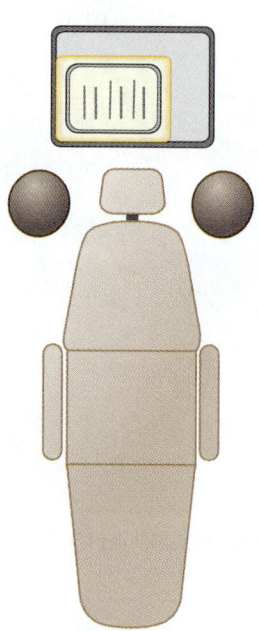

Fig. 32-15 Diagram showing rear delivery system.

Fig. 32-14 Diagram showing side delivery system.

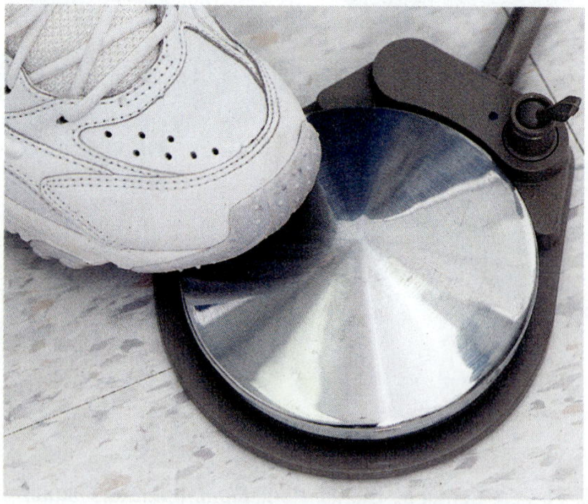

Fig. 32-16 A rheostat controls the handpieces of the dental unit.

Air-Water Syringe

The air-water syringe is attached to the dental unit and is a necessity for every procedure (Fig. 32-17). The air-water syringe functions in three ways:

- Delivers a stream of water
- Delivers a stream of air
- Delivers a combined spray of air and water

The tip of the air-water syringe, which is classified as *semicritical equipment* under infection-control policies, is replaced after every procedure. When using the device during patient care, the handle and tubing must be covered with a plastic barrier.

Operating Light

The operating light is used to illuminate the oral cavity during a procedure (Fig. 32-18). Halogen bulbs are used in most operating lights. The light is very bright, and care is taken to avoid shining it into the patient's eyes. The light is attached to a flexible arm that is either track-mounted from the ceiling or attached to the wall or dental chair.

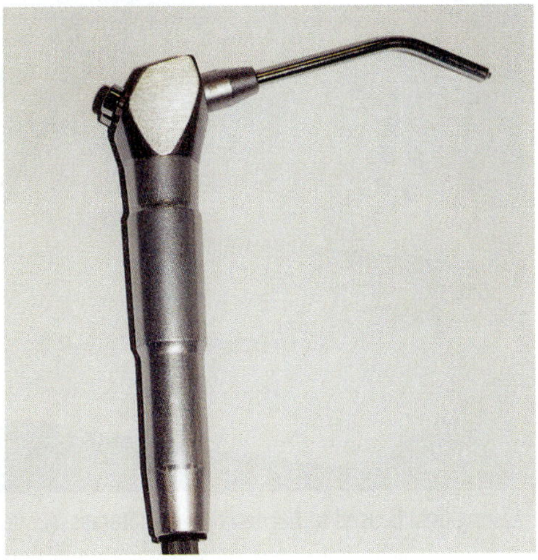

Fig. 32-17 Air-water syringe.

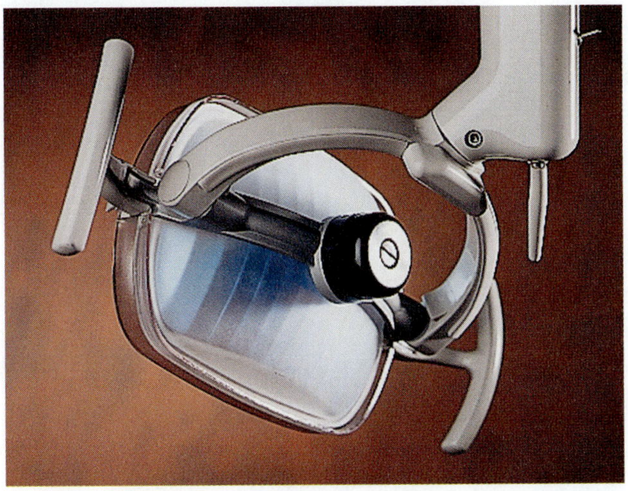

Fig. 32-18 Operating light. (Courtesy A-dec.)

After the patient is seated and the assistant is gloved, the assistant positions the light on the patient's chest approximately 25 to 30 inches (approximately arm's length) below the patient's chin. The light is turned on and then slowly adjusted upward to illuminate the oral cavity. When properly positioned, the light illuminates the area to be treated without projecting shadows of the operator's or assistant's hands onto the oral cavity.

The light becomes hot during use. Other than changing the removable barrier on the handle, the light is cleaned only when it has cooled. When the lens is cool, a mild disinfectant and a soft cloth are used to wipe it free of smudges and debris. NOTE: *Touching a warm lens with a damp cloth can cause the lens to crack.*

When the bulb of the operating light must be replaced, turn off the light and allow the old bulb to cool before removing it. If using a halogen bulb, follow the manufacturer's instructions. Extra bulbs should be kept in inventory to ensure immediate replacement as necessary. NOTE: *Halogen bulbs will break if touched with a bare hand.*

Recall

6. What patient chair position is used for most dental procedures?
7. Which two features on the dental assistant's stool are not part of the operator's stool?
8. What foot-controlled device is used to operate the dental handpiece?

Oral Evacuation System

Water is commonly used throughout a dental procedure; you must have some means to remove it. The dental unit contains two evacuation systems: the *saliva ejector* and *high-volume evacuator* (Fig. 32-19) (see Chapter 36).

The disposable *saliva ejector* has a less powerful suction system than the high-volume evacuator. The saliva ejector provides comfortable removal of the patient's excess fluids from the mouth. The saliva ejector is used in less-invasive procedures, such as routine cleanings, sealants, and fluoride application.

The assistant will use the *high-volume evacuator* (HVE) for most procedures. The system is more powerful than the saliva ejector and helps in maintaining a "clear field" for the dentist to work in. A new HVE tip is used for each patient. During use, the HVE handle and hose are covered with a protective plastic barrier.

Curing Light

The curing light is a wandlike attachment used to "harden or cure" light-cured dental materials. The curing light causes the chemical reaction that allows the material to harden. The components of the light are the protective shield handle and the trigger switch to turn it on and off (Fig. 32-20). If the curing light is not working at full strength or is not used correctly, the material will not set properly, and the results will be unsatisfactory.

Testing and Maintenance

The curing light should be tested periodically to determine whether the light is working at full strength. If a curing light does not reach the desired reading on the testing device, the light bulb must be changed before use.

Most curing lights use a halogen bulb. When it is necessary to replace it, do so according to the manufacturer's instructions, and do not touch the bulb with your hands. Test the new bulb before operation. Because the curing light is such an important part of productivity in the operatory, extra bulbs should always be available for replacement.

During use the curing light is protected with a plastic barrier. If additional cleaning and disinfection is necessary during treatment room preparation, the light should be cool before it is wiped with the solutions. *Note: A sudden change in temperature may damage the halogen bulb.*

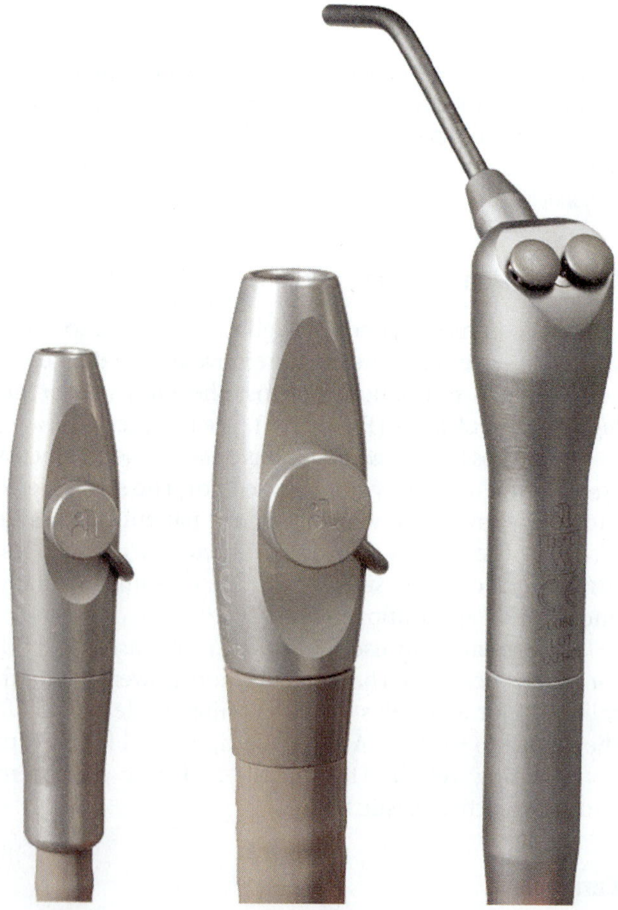

Fig. 32-19 Oral evacuation system that contains a saliva ejector, high-volume evacuator, and air-water syringe. (Courtesy A-dec.)

Amalgamator

An amalgamator is used to **triturate,** or mechanically mix, dental materials by vigorously shaking the capsule that holds the ingredients. The amalgamator may be mounted under a countertop or the edge of a mobile cabinet or stored in the top drawer of a mobile cabinet (Fig. 32-21).

Dental Radiograph Unit

Most dental treatment rooms include a dental radiograph unit (see Chapter 40). The master switch of the radiograph unit may safely be turned on at the beginning of the day and left on throughout the day. If the radiograph unit re-

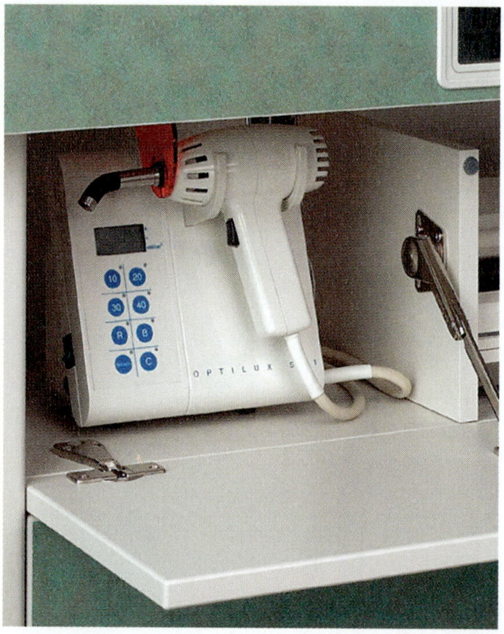

Fig. 32-20 Curing light is used to harden dental materials. (Courtesy A-dec.)

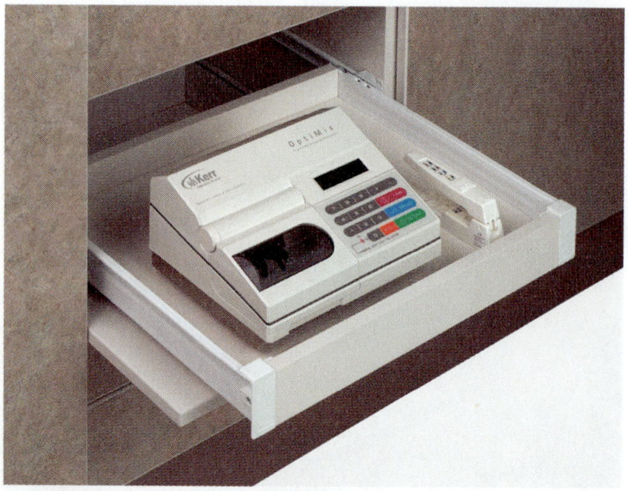

Fig. 32-21 Amalgamator. (Courtesy A-dec.)

quires maintenance, it first must be disconnected from its electrical source (Fig. 32-22).

NOTE: *Radiation is emitted from the radiograph unit only while the exposure timer switch is depressed.*

View Box for Radiographs

A view box, which is used to read and diagnose radiographs, is placed in the cabinetry or flush on the wall of the operatory. The view box consists of a bright white light source with a frosted-glass or plastic cover (Fig. 32-23).

The radiographs are mounted and then placed on the view box for evaluation. The light source shines through the radiograph, allowing for a better visual evaluation from the dentist.

Recall

9. What does the abbreviation HVE represent?
10. Where do you place dental materials to be triturated?

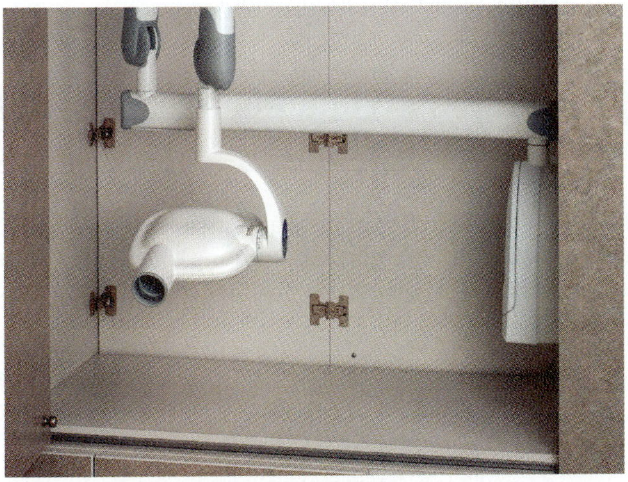

Fig. 32-22 Radiograph unit. (Courtesy A-dec.)

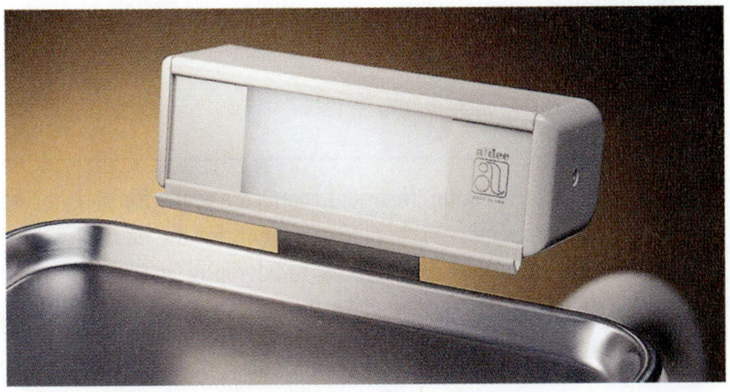

Fig. 32-23 View box. (Courtesy A-dec.)

CARE OF DENTAL EQUIPMENT

Dental equipment is expensive, complex, and delicate. It must be used carefully and maintained properly in accordance with the manufacturer's instructions.

The dental assistants working in the clinical area usually share responsibility for the routine care of this part of the office. However, one staff member may be assigned the responsibility of ensuring that preventive care is carried out on a routine basis. Larger practices may contract to have maintenance personnel provide this service.

Central Vacuum Compressor

A central vacuum compressor provides the suction needed for the oral evacuation systems. This equipment actually consists of two parts: the *compressor,* which creates the flow of air, and the *vacuum tank,* which screens the flow of air to create suction. The central vacuum compressor should be serviced regularly, in keeping with the manufacturer's instructions.

Central Air Compressor

A central air compressor is used to provide compressed air for the air-water syringe and air-driven handpieces. The capacity of the compressor depends on the number of dental units used in the practice. Because of the noise level and for safety reasons, the compressor system is placed outside the clinical setting.

The air compressor must receive routine service according to the manufacturer's instructions. This maintenance includes changing filters and occasionally checking for condensation in the lines. Trained maintenance personnel usually handle this service.

Condensation in the airlines could cause the presence of moisture, sediment, or algae. These contaminants can ruin handpieces and can cause debris to be ejected into the patient's mouth. If there is any indication of a condensation problem, the equipment should be serviced immediately.

Disposable traps are located on the dental unit and provide a filtering mechanism for the saliva ejector and HVE that catches debris drawn from the mouth. These traps are disposable and should be changed weekly. Utility gloves are worn, and cotton pliers or utility tongs should be used when handling these tight, contaminated screens (Fig. 32-24). Chapter 23 discusses removal of amalgam scrap from the traps.

CENTRAL STERILIZATION

The sterilization and supply center is where instruments are maintained, cleaned, sterilized, and stored in preparation

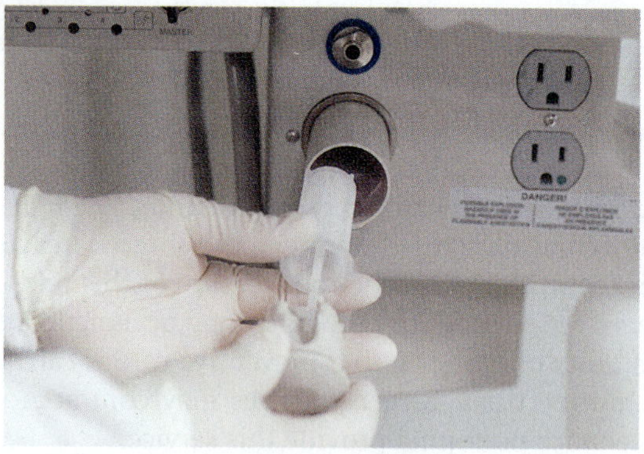

Fig. 32-24 Disposable traps must be changed weekly for proper functioning of the vacuum system.

for reuse. The sterilization center must be kept organized and clean at all times. The center is divided into two areas: the contaminated area and the clean area (see Chapter 21).

DENTAL LABORATORY

The dental laboratory is organized around workbenches and wall-mounted storage cabinets. In the laboratory, procedures such as pouring impressions, preparing diagnostic models, and creating custom impression trays are performed.

During work in the laboratory, infection control and safety are always major concerns. In addition, the entire laboratory must be kept organized and clean at all times. See Chapter 47 for a description of the major equipment found in the dental laboratory.

DENTIST'S PRIVATE OFFICE

The dentist maintains a private office for his or her personal use. Other staff members must respect the privacy of this area. The dentist will have a desk, personal items, phone system, computer system, comfortable chairs, and a side table.

This office can be used as a consultation room, or an additional area may be set up for this purpose. A **consultation room** is where the dentist discusses diagnoses and treatment plans with the patient.

DENTAL STAFF LOUNGE

A specific area in the dental office should be designated for the clinical and business staff to use during personal time. This area provides a table to use during lunchtime and possibly staff meetings. Additional items in this area would be a small refrigerator for personal use only and lockers or a locked cabinet for a purse and other personal items. It is also customary for the dentist to financially support a coffee service and food vendor.

MORNING AND EVENING ROUTINES FOR DENTAL ASSISTANTS

In most practices, clinical assistants assume the important responsibilities of evening and morning care of the clinical areas. Careful completion of all these steps helps ensure the smooth flow of patient care throughout the day.

Procedure 32-1 Performing the Morning Routine (Opening the Office)

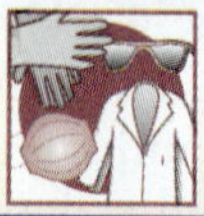

PROCEDURAL STEPS

1. Arrive 30 minutes before the first scheduled patient of the day.
   Purpose: This allows time to complete tasks so the day can start smoothly and on time.
2. Turn on the master switches for the central air compressor and vacuum units. Turn on the master switches for the dental and radiograph units.
3. Determine that the dental treatment rooms are ready for patient care.
4. Recheck the appointment schedule of patients for the day to be certain that instruments, patient records, radiographs, and laboratory cases are all available as needed for the planned treatments.
5. Set up the treatment room for the first patient.

Procedure 32-2 Performing the Evening Routine (Closing the Office)

PROCEDURAL STEPS

1. Complete the operatory room exposure-control cleanup and preparation protocols.
2. Wear appropriate personal protective equipment (PPE) while emptying waste receptacles and placing fresh plastic liners.
   Purpose: Waste must be disposed of safely (see Chapter 23).
3. Turn off all equipment.
4. Determine that the treatment area is adequately stocked for the next day.
5. Post appointment schedules for the next day in the treatment areas.
6. Check the appointment schedules to ensure that instruments, patient records, and laboratory work are ready for the next day.
7. Determine that all contaminated instruments have been processed and the sterilization center has been cleaned.
8. Determine that treatment rooms are ready for use.
9. Place any soiled PPE in the appropriate container.
   Purpose: Proper handling of contaminated PPE is an important part of exposure control.

The goal in the evening is to leave the office ready for patient care in the morning. Failure to complete these steps could result in loss of productive time for the dentist, inconvenience or discomfort for the patient, and unnecessary stress for everyone. Procedures 32-1 and 32-2 review steps in the morning and evening routines of the dental assistant.

Patient Education

When a patient enters the clinical areas of the dental office, the dental equipment can be foreign and possibly frightening. By educating your patients about their environment, not only will they feel more comfortable, but they may also ask questions about new dental procedures and techniques.

Eye to the Future

The design and layout of dental offices are keeping up with current interior design trends. You will see more adaptations of personal style than in the past. Offices are becoming more creative when patient comfort is of utmost importance. You might see a babbling brook running through the reception area to provide the relaxing sound of moving water. Many offices have murals on the ceiling of the dental treatment areas for the patient to view.

Additional items for the patient include personal headphones with a choice of music, and televisions with a selection of movies. Remember that the patient is the most important person in the office. Be sure that all of your patients are comfortable.

Critical Thinking

1. The reception area of your dental office was designed in the 1980s, and the furniture and colors are outdated. Your dentist asks you to help in the decision of remodeling. What qualities should you include when decorating the reception area?
2. Your dental office has an open bay structure where most of the clinical area is open. How could you provide a sense of patient privacy as well as sound control in this type of office design?
3. What features are important to consider when selecting an operator's stool?
4. The dental unit can be designed to come from different areas of the treatment area. Discuss the three delivery system setups for dental units.
5. Describe the difference between the operating light and the curing light.

33

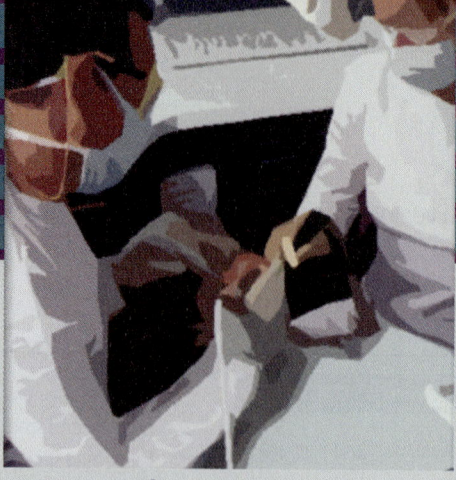

Delivering Dental Care

Outline

KEY TERMS

Delegate To authorize or entrust another person to perform a specific skill or procedure.

Direct supervision Level of supervision in which the dentist is physically present when the auxiliary performs delegated functions.

Expanded function Specific intraoral function delegated to an auxiliary that requires increased skill and training.

Four-handed dentistry Process by which the operator and assistant work together to perform clinical procedures in an ergonomically structured environment.

Fulcrum (**ful-**krum) Finger rest used when holding an instrument or handpiece for a specified time.

Grasp The correct way an instrument or handpiece is held.

Indirect supervision To oversee an assistant's work by being in the immediate area.

Indirect vision Viewing an object through the use of a mirror.

Operating zones Concept that uses the face of a clock to position the dental team, equipment, and supplies.

LEARNING OUTCOMES

On completion of this chapter, the student will be able to achieve the following objectives:

- Define and spell the Key Terms.
- Describe how to prepare the dental treatment area for a patient's arrival.
- Discuss the importance of preparing a dental treatment room for a procedure.
- Describe how the operator is positioned during treatment.
- Describe how the assistant is positioned during treatment.
- Explain instrument transfer.
- Specify three grasps used by the operator.
- Identify five areas in which the assistant must have competency when practicing expanded functions.

PERFORMANCE OUTCOMES

On completion of this chapter, the student will be able to meet competency standards in the following skills:

- Demonstrate admitting and seating the patient.
- Demonstrate instrument transfer using a selection of instruments.
- Demonstrate the proper use of a dental mirror.
- Demonstrate the correct grasp and use for hand instruments.
- Transfer instruments using the single-handed technique.
- Transfer instruments using the two-handed technique.
- Demonstrate the use of a dental instrument intraorally.

The clinical assistant has the responsibility of preparing the treatment area, assisting the dentist, and fulfilling the role of the operator when performing expanded functions. In order for a typical day to run smoothly and to provide the best patient care, the dentist and clinical assistant must be prepared and skilled in *four-handed dentistry.*

With advanced preparation of obtaining the patient record, knowing the upcoming procedure, and having the supplies and equipment ready, the daily routine of clinical care will be much less hectic and will ensure the smooth flow of patient care throughout the day. Failure to meet standards in these tasks will result in loss of production for the dentist, inconvenience or discomfort for the patient, and unnecessary stress for everyone.

KNOWING YOUR PATIENTS

Once a patient enters the reception area, it is essential that his or her presence be acknowledged immediately. One of the best ways to know your patients and be better prepared is to have a brief meeting or review of the day before patients arrive. Issues that should be discussed among the dental team include:

- Changes in the patient's health that could alter dental treatment
- Additional supplies or equipment that may be needed for the procedure
- Preparation for an apprehensive patient in the form of scheduling more time, using premedication, or preparing the setup for the use of nitrous oxide during the procedure
- Assignment of expanded functions to the dental assistant

REVIEWING THE PATIENT RECORD

Several areas of a patient record are reviewed at each patient visit. Administrative staff members discuss any changes in the patient's *personal information,* such as address or phone number change, and make any corrections as needed. Clinical staff will discuss any *medical alerts* or changes in medical status and update the health history form. The clinical assistant will refer to the progress notes for the planned treatment of the day.

PREPARING THE TREATMENT AREA

A treatment room preparation checklist should be completed before the patient is seated.

Treatment Room Preparation Checklist

- Is the treatment room clean, disinfected, and ready for the next patient?
- Are the patient's record, radiographs, and laboratory case in place?
- Are the appropriate sterile preset tray and other supplies in place and ready for use?
- Is the dental chair positioned to seat the patient?
- Has additional equipment been moved out of the path of entry for the patient and dental team?

GREETING AND SEATING THE PATIENT

As the clinical assistant, you will enter the reception area to greet and escort your patient to the designated clinical area. Remember that patients must be greeted in a courteous way. When you call your patients by their last name, make sure to establish eye contact, smile, and introduce yourself. Procedure 33-1 reviews the admitting and seating of a patient.

Procedure 33-1 Admitting and Seating the Patient

PROCEDURAL STEPS

1. Pleasantly greet the patient in the reception area by name. Introduce yourself, and request that the patient follow you to the treatment area.
2. Place the patient's personal items, such as a jacket or handbag, in a safe place away from the procedure.
3. Initiate conversation with the patient.
   Purpose: Chatting about things other than the treatment may help the patient feel more comfortable and relaxed.
4. Ask if the patient has any questions that you can answer about treatment for the day. If you do not know the answer, say so and offer to discuss this with the dentist.
   Purpose: Patients frequently ask the assistant questions about treatment that they are reluctant to ask the dentist. Willingness to answer these questions helps reassure the patient.
5. Ask the patient to sit on the side of the dental chair and then swing his or her legs onto the base of the chair.

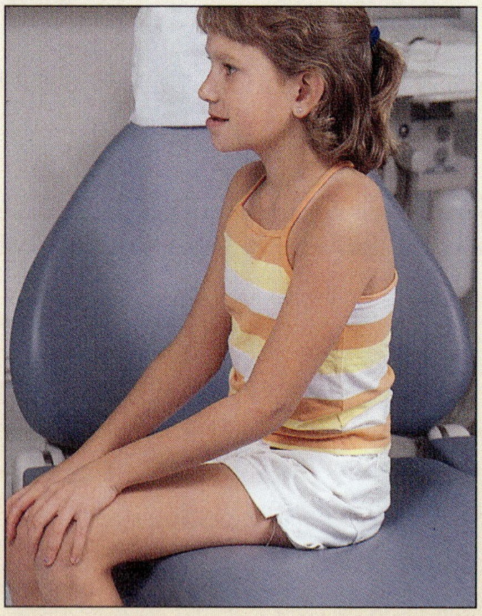

6. Lower or slide the chair arm into position.

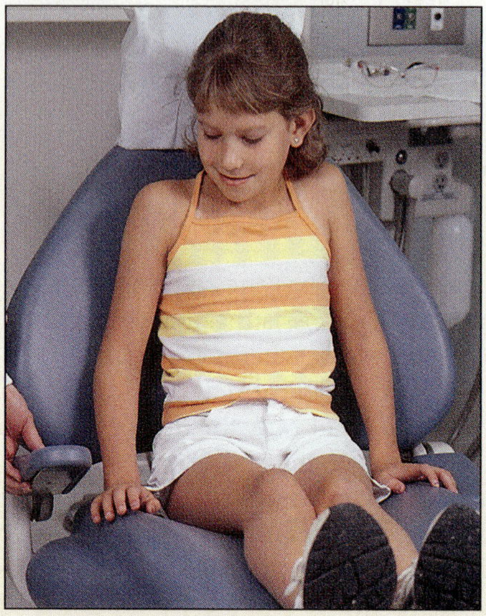

7. Place the disposable patient napkin over the patient's chest, and clasp the corners using a napkin chain.

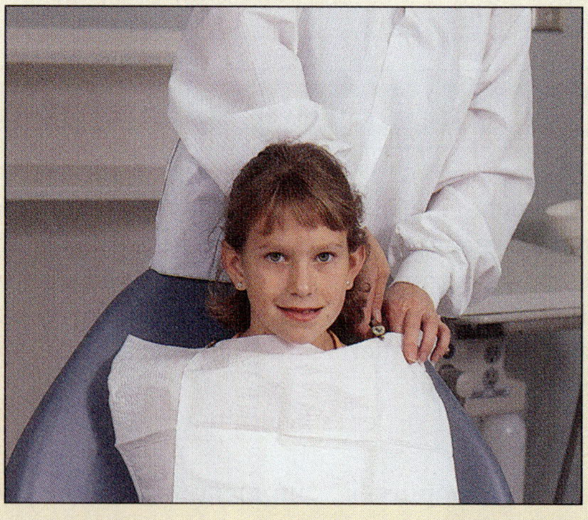

8. Inform the patient before adjusting the chair. Make the adjustments slowly until the patient and chair are in the proper position for the planned procedure.
   Note: Remember that the most common position for dental procedures is the supine position.

Procedure 33-1 Admitting and Seating the Patient—cont'd

PROCEDURAL STEPS, cont'd

9. Position the operating light over the patient's chest, and turn on.

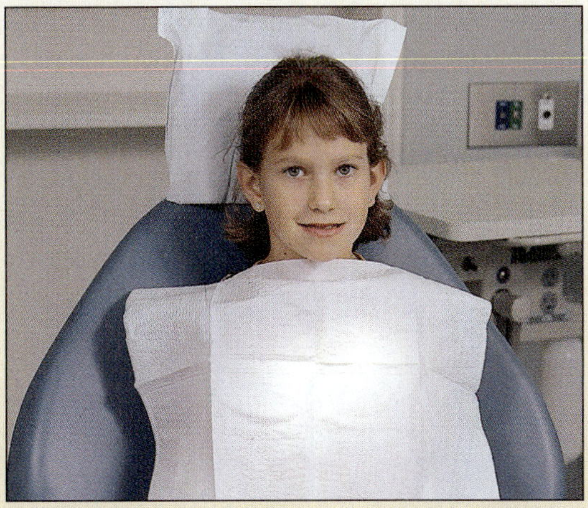

10. Review once again that all treatment room preparations are organized and set out.
11. Wash hands, and put on personal protective equipment.
12. You are now ready to position yourself and begin the procedure.

TEAM DENTISTRY

The theory of team dentistry, also referred to as *four-handed dentistry,* has been researched and introduced to dental students and dental assisting students for more than 50 years. In **four-handed dentistry,** the operator and assistant work together to perform clinical procedures in an ergonomically structured environment.

The main goal of this concept is to deliver the best and most effective care to your patient by increasing productivity.

Goals of Team Dentistry

To utilize ergonomically correct dental equipment.

To utilize preset trays for dental procedures.

To minimize stress and fatigue when performing dental procedures by following specific ergonomically correct positioning of the patient, dentist, and assistant (see Chapter 25).

To follow the principles of motion economy during the transfer of instruments and dental materials.

To use appropriate moisture-control techniques to maintain better visualization and working field in the mouth.

To delegate expanded functions of practice as legal within the state.

Recall

1. State two goals of the dental team that would simplify dental treatment in the dental office.

PRINCIPLES OF TEAM POSITIONING

Correct positioning of the dental team in the clinical area is essential. The dentist and dental assistant should develop positioning habits that allow access and visibility to all areas of the oral cavity, while maintaining a position that provides optimal comfort and support (Fig. 33-1).

Whenever the dentist and assistant must stretch to reach an instrument or gain access to an area of the mouth, stress is placed on the body. If this occurs daily, the accumulated strain will contribute to lower back pain, circulatory problems, and muscle aches and pain.

Positioning the Patient

Once the patient has been escorted to the treatment area and seated, he or she is then lowered to the supine position. The patient is then requested to slide up in the chair until the top of the head is even with the top of the headrest. The operator will then ask the patient to turn the head to the right or left to allow for easier access to a specific area in the mouth.

The operator makes final adjustments to the chair to establish the proper working distance. The distance between the patient's face and the operator's face should be approximately 12 to 14 inches (Fig. 33-2). When working in the mandibular area, the back of the chair is raised to a slightly more upright position for better vision.

Positioning the Operator

Access and vision are the most essential qualities for the operator. Chapter 32 describes the unique features of the operator's stool.

The positioning of the operator on the stool is important for comfort and support (Fig. 33-3).

The operator should practice the following guidelines:

- Seated as far back as possible, with front edge of stool just touching the backs of the knees
- Thighs parallel to floor, or knees slightly lower than the hips
- Feet kept flat on the floor and not crossed
- Backrest of chair positioned to support lower portion or small of the back
- Height of chair maintained to allow operator's forearms parallel to the floor when bent at the elbow

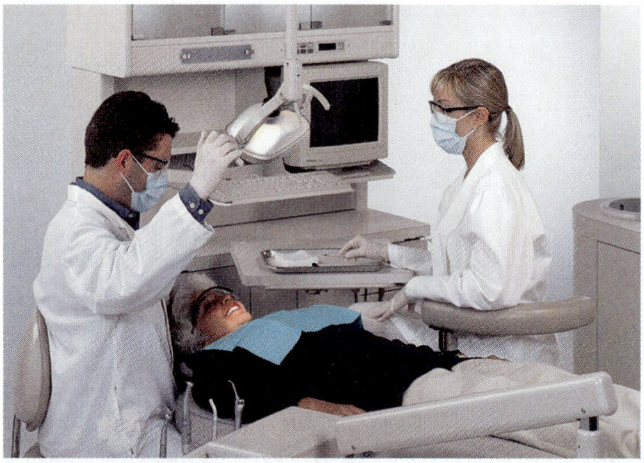

Fig. 33-1 The concept of four-handed dentistry is shown in the positioning of the patient and dental team. (Courtesy A-dec.)

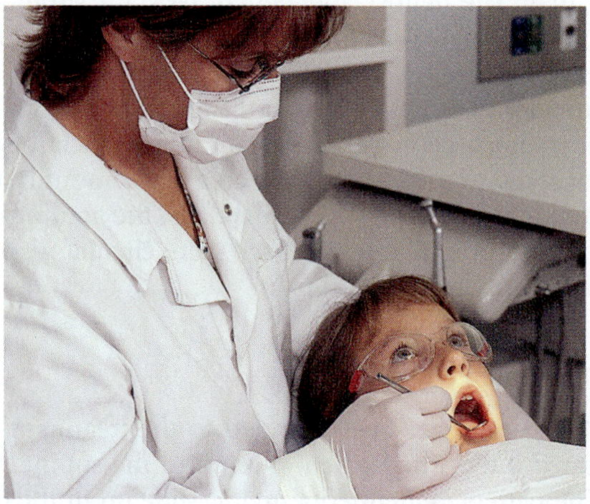

Fig. 33-2 Distance of the operator's face to the patient's face when positioned correctly.

Positioning the Dental Assistant

When assisting the dentist, the dental assistant not only has to anticipate what is needed, but also has to have *access* to the area of concentration (Fig. 33-4). Chapter 32 describes the features that are important to the dental assistant for comfort and support.

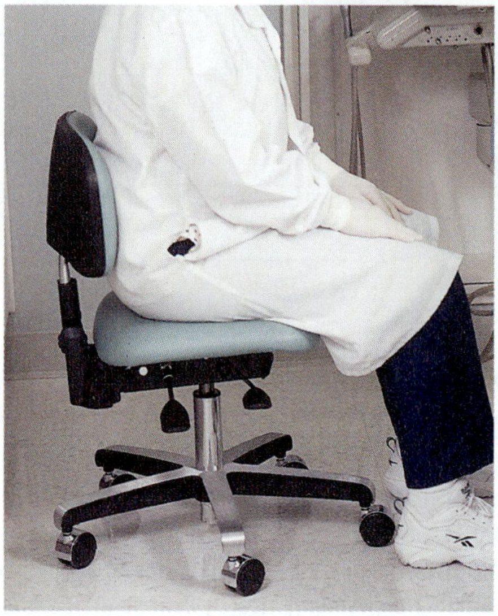

Fig. 33-3 Position of the operator when seated correctly.

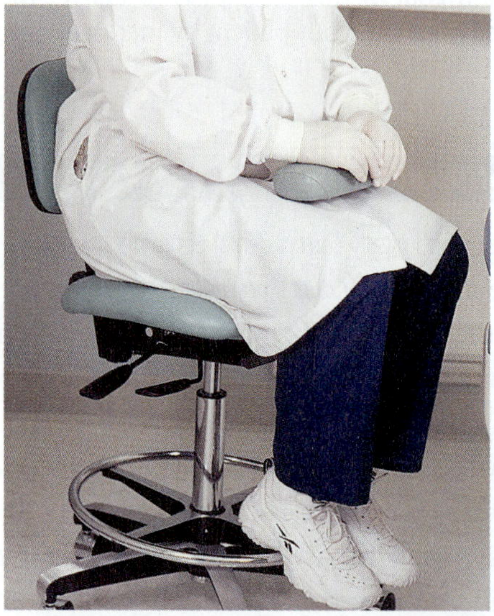

Fig. 33-4 Position of the dental assistant when seated correctly.

The assistant should practice the following guidelines for correct positioning on the stool:

- Seated well back on stool
- Feet resting on base or foot ring of stool
- Positioned as close as possible to dental chair
- Legs parallel to patient's chair
- Eye level four to six inches above that of operator

Recall

2. In relation to the operator, should the assistant be positioned lower or higher?
3. How should the operator maintain the forearms when working on a patient?

MOTION ECONOMY

If you ask members of the dental team in the business or clinical area what part of their body is most fatigued by the end of the day, they would most likely comment about their lower back. This is because of so much reaching, twisting, and turning while seated at their position.

Motions are classified into five categories according to their movement. By understanding early in your preclinical studies the need to eliminate or reduce Class IV and V motions, you will learn better habits and truly benefit ergonomically in the long run.

Classification of Motions

Class I: Movement of fingers only. Examples are picking up an instrument or a single object laying on a flat surface, or picking up a pencil or pen to write.

Class II: Movement of fingers and wrist. Examples are transferring an instrument using a pen grasp, or typing on a keyboard.

Class III: Movement of fingers, wrist, and elbow. Examples are using the slow-speed handpiece when performing coronal polishing and using the computer mouse.

Class IV: Use of the entire arm and shoulder. Examples are reaching for items in the mobile unit, moving the radiograph unit, and answering the phone.

Class V: Use of the entire upper torso. Examples are bending over to see intraorally, retrieving dental materials from a tub or drawer, and retrieving patient records.

OPERATING ZONES

This basic concept is utilized for practicing efficient and comfortable clinical dentistry and can be applied to any dental procedure. **Operating zones** are based on a "clock concept" and offer the best way to identify the working position of the dental team, dental equipment, and supplies needed to perform a procedure.

Visualize a circle placed over the dental chair. The patient's face is in the center of the circle, and the top of the patient's head is at the twelve o'clock position. The face of the clock is divided into four zones. The location of the zones will change depending on whether the operator is right-handed or left-handed. The operator's position varies within that zone depending on the treatment to be delivered (Figs. 33-5 and 33-6).

Operator's Zone

The operator's zone (right-handed—seven o'clock to twelve o'clock; left-handed—twelve o'clock to five o'clock) is the area where the person completing the procedure is seated. Most often the dentist is the operator. However, the dental assistant and dental hygienist can also be seated in the operator's position when working directly inside the oral cavity.

Transfer Zone

The transfer zone (right-handed—four o'clock to seven o'clock; left-handed—five o'clock to eight o'clock) is the area where instruments and dental materials are exchanged from the dental assistant to the dentist. This zone is directly over the patient's chest. In front delivery, the dental unit is located in the transfer zone within easy reach of the dentist and assistant.

Be sure that instrument transfer is not completed over the patient's face; this could be dangerous if an instrument were to fall.

Assistant's Zone

The assistant's zone (right-handed—two o'clock to four o'clock; left-handed—eight o'clock to ten o'clock) is the area where the dental assistant is positioned. The assistant's mobile cabinet or rear-delivery countertop is also positioned within this zone, holding the instrument tray, dental materials, and attached suction and air-water syringe unit.

Static Zone

The static zone (right-handed—twelve o'clock to two o'clock; left-handed—ten o'clock to twelve o'clock) is directly behind the patient. With rear delivery, the unit that holds the handpieces, air-water syringe, and additional countertop space would be positioned in the static zone.

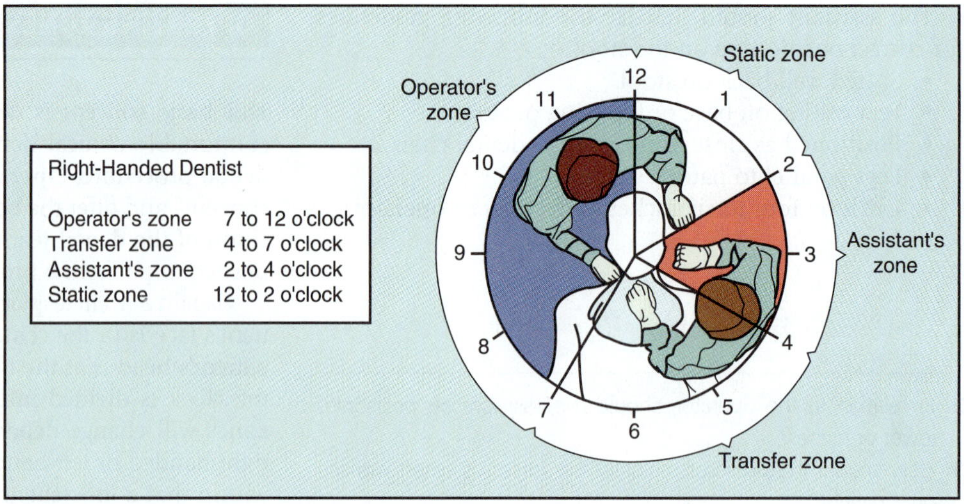

Fig. 33-5 Operating zones for a right-handed operator.

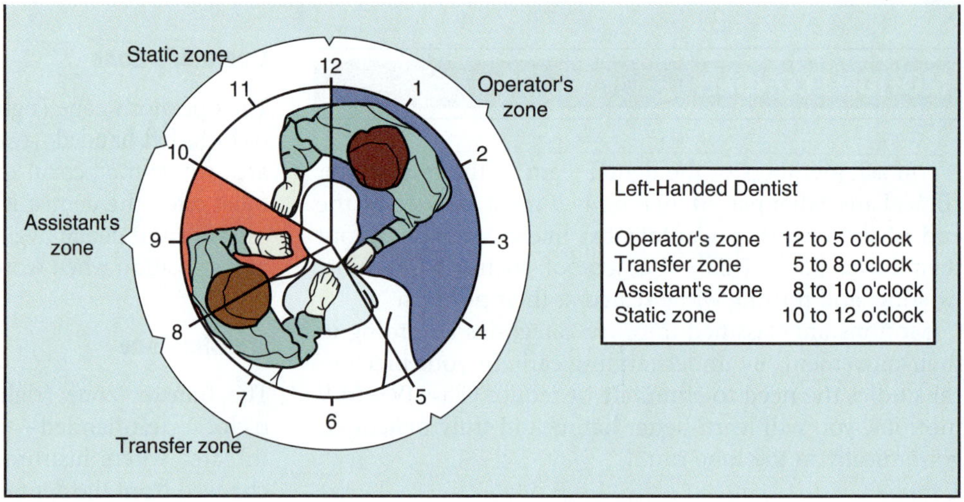

Fig. 33-6 Operating zones for a left-handed operator.

Portable equipment such as the nitrous oxide unit would be in the static zone.

Recall

4. When using the clock concept, where is the static zone for a right-handed operator?
5. Where are instruments exchanged during a procedure?
6. Besides the assistant, what may be located in the assistant's zone?

INSTRUMENT TRANSFER

Four-handed dentistry is based on the concept that a qualified chairside dental assistant is seated across from the dentist and they work as a team. This ergonomically sound way to practice dentistry uses the skills of the dental assistant along with work simplification techniques.

Instrument transfer, also referred to as *instrument exchange,* takes place in the transfer zone.

Team Objectives

Throughout the procedure, the dentist relies on the clinical assistant to have the supplies, instruments, and dental materials ready to be transferred into the dentist's hands. The smooth, efficient transfer of instruments and materials is a team effort that requires coordination, communication, and practice between the dentist and dental assistant.

Both the patient and the dental team benefit from a standardized operating sequence. The patient's time in the dental chair is decreased, and the dental team's productivity is increased, with less fatigue and stress. The techniques discussed in this chapter are based on assisting a right-handed dentist.

Objectives for Efficient Instrument Transfer

The assistant must understand the sequence of the procedure and anticipate when an instrument transfer will be required.

The assistant transfers dental instruments, the dental handpiece, and dental materials with the *left hand.* The right hand is kept free to suction and to ready the next materials and instruments.

The transfer of instruments should be accomplished with Class I, Class II, and Class III motions involving only the fingers, wrist, and elbow.

Instruments are transferred in the *position of use,* which refers to the working end of the instrument either pointing downward for mandibular areas or pointing upward for maxillary areas. Therefore the dentist does not need to reposition the instrument in his or her hand before use.

An instrument is transferred so that the dentist can grasp the instrument for its appropriate use.

The exchanged instrument must be positioned in the dentist's hand firmly so that the dentist can receive it without moving his or her eyes from the field of operation.

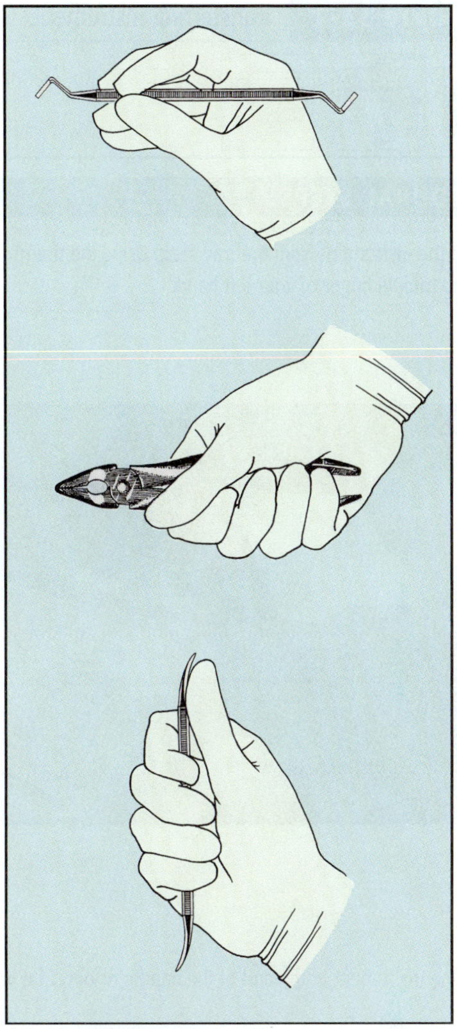

Fig. 33-7 Basic instrument grasps. **A,** Pen grasp. **B,** Palm grasp. **C,** Palm-thumb grasp.

Grasping an Instrument

The manner in which the operator grasps and holds an instrument depends on the type of instrument, how it is used, and which area of the mouth is being treated. An understanding of instrument **grasp** is essential to a smooth instrument transfer and exchange of instruments. The three basic grasps are as follows:

- *Pen grasp,* in which the instrument is held in the same manner as a pen (Fig. 33-7*A*)
- *Palm grasp,* in which the instrument is held securely in the palm of the hand (Fig. 33-7*B*)
- *Palm-thumb grasp,* in which the instrument is held in the palm, and the thumb is used to stabilize and guide the instrument (Fig. 33-7*C*)

Assistant's Transfer Technique

When transferring instruments during a procedure, the assistant uses a specific *single-handed technique* for efficiency. This single-handed transfer technique applies to hand instruments, dental handpieces, and air-water syringes (Procedure 33-2).

Variations in Instrument Exchange

Specific items and instruments need to be transferred differently because of their design or use.

Mirror and Explorer

When beginning a procedure, the dentist will always utilize the mouth mirror and explorer to inspect the area to be treated. The dental assistant delivers the mirror and explorer simultaneously, using a two-handed exchange. For the right-handed operator, the explorer is transferred with the left hand and the mirror with the right hand (Fig. 33-8).

The dentist signals the assistant by placing one hand on each side of the patient's mouth in position ready to receive the instruments.

Cotton Pliers

When cotton pliers are used to transfer small items to and from the oral cavity, a modification in the single-handed technique must be made.

The assistant delivers the pliers to the dentist while pinching together the "beaks" to avoid dropping the item held in the pliers (Fig. 33-9). Grasping the working end of the pliers makes retrieval of the cotton pliers eas-

Procedure 33-2 Transferring Instruments Using the Single-Handed Technique

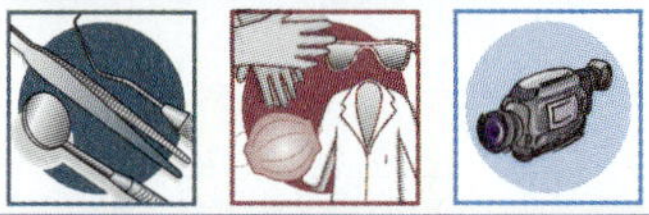

PROCEDURAL STEPS

1. Pick up the instrument from the tray setup using the thumb, index finger, and middle finger of your left hand.

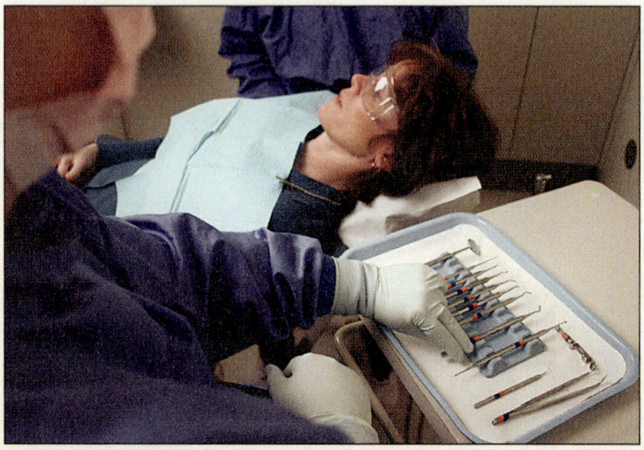

2. Grasp the instrument at the end of the handle or opposite the working end.

   NOTE: Most instruments have two ends (double-ended instruments).
3. Transfer the instrument from the tray into the transfer zone, ensuring that the instrument is parallel to the instrument in the dentist's hand.
4. Using the last two fingers of your left hand, retrieve the used instrument from the dentist, tucking in the instrument toward the palm.

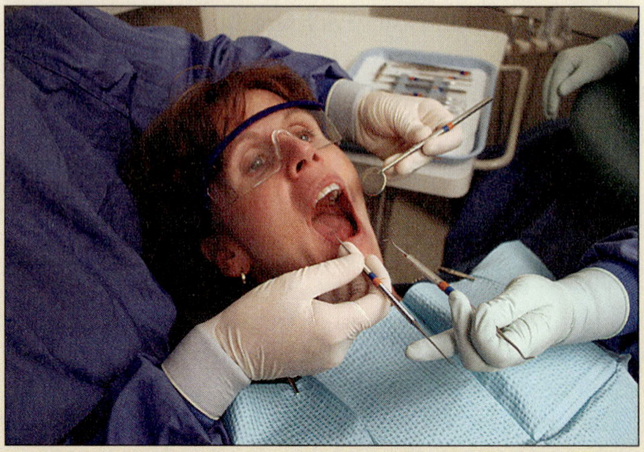

5. Position the new instrument firmly into the operator's fingers.

   NOTE: When placing the instrument, make sure the working end is positioned correctly for the proper area of the mouth.

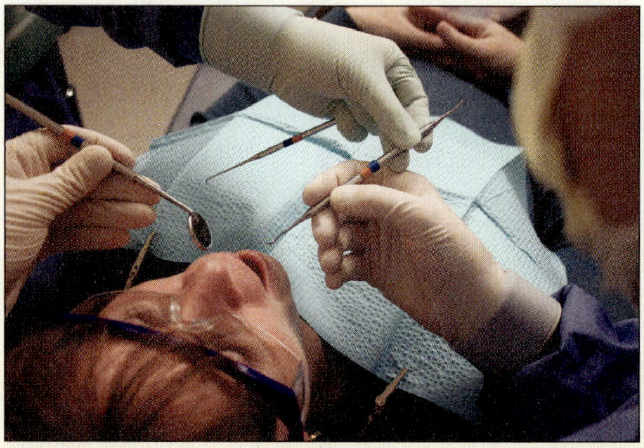

6. Place the used instrument back on the tray setup in its correct position of use.

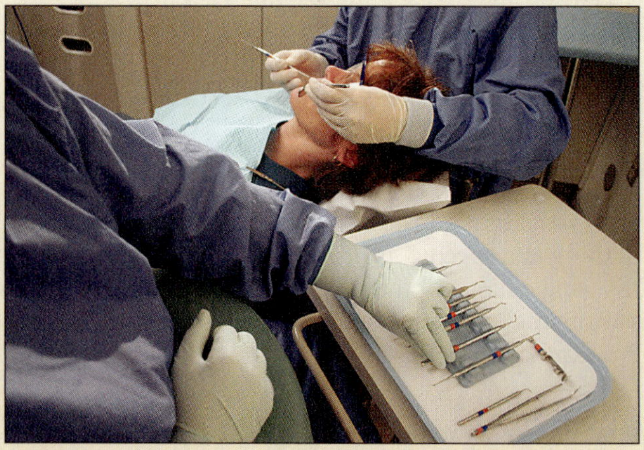

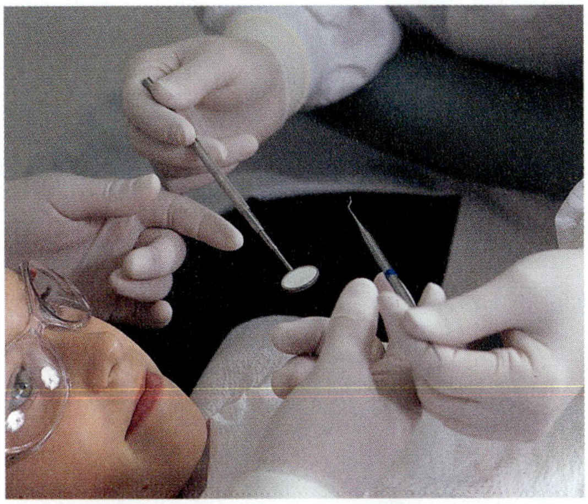

Fig. 33-8 The dentist prepares to receive the mirror and explorer by positioning the hand on either side of the patient's head.

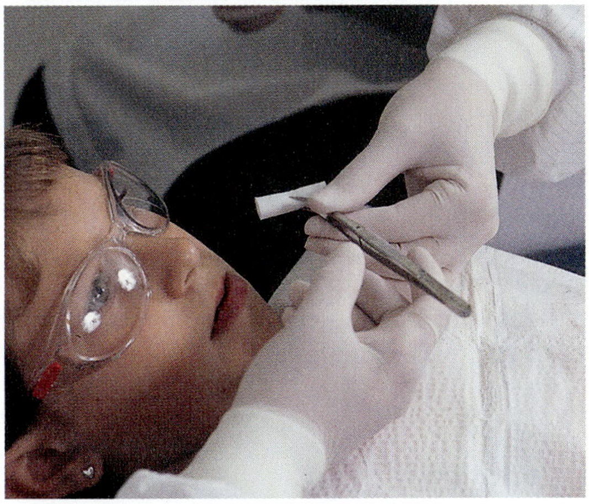

Fig. 33-9 The assistant transfers the cotton pliers, ensuring the ends are together so as not to drop the item.

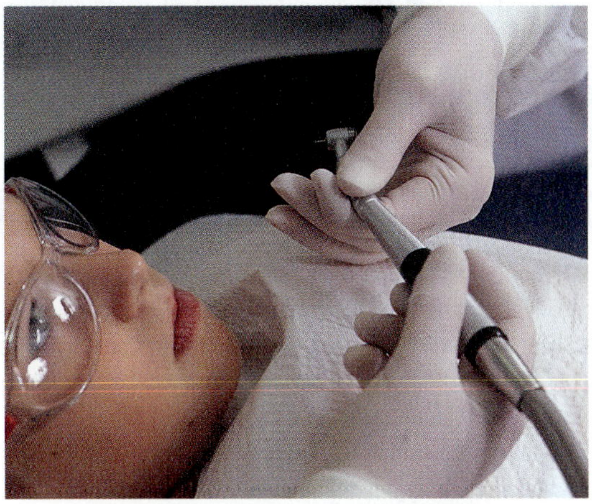

Fig. 33-10 Transferring the handpiece.

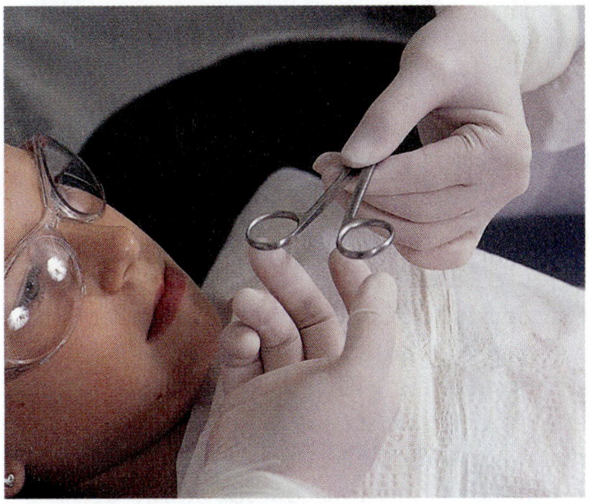

Fig. 33-11 Transferring scissors so that the dentist can grasp them correctly.

ier. This grasp also prevents the contents of the forceps from slipping out.

Handpiece

The handpiece can be exchanged for an instrument by using the same technique as when two instruments are transferred (Fig. 33-10). When exchanging the handpiece, take care to avoid tangling the hoses during the transfer.

Instruments with Hinges

Instruments with hinges are designed to have an open/closed use. The most common hinged instruments are the rubber dam forceps, surgical forceps, orthodontic pliers, and scissors.

These instruments are held at their hinge and transferred by directing their handles into the dentist's palm. The handles of scissors are positioned over the dentist's fingers (Fig. 33-11). Because hinged instruments are often heavier than other instruments and a steadier hand may be needed, a two-handed transfer technique is recommended (Procedure 33-3).

Recall

7. Should the assistant use one hand or both hands to transfer instruments?
8. Which hand is used primarily to transfer instruments to a right-handed dentist?

Procedure 33-3 Transferring Instruments Using Two-Handed Technique

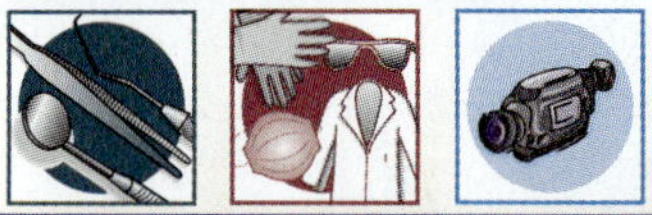

PROCEDURAL STEPS

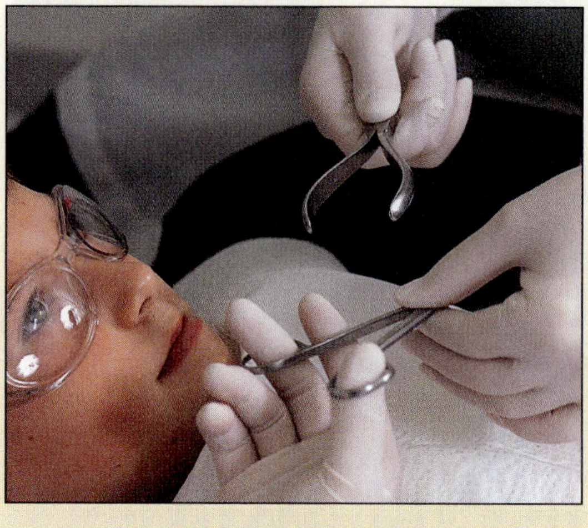

1. Using your right hand, grasp the instrument on the tray setup closer to the working end with your thumb and first two fingers.
2. With your left hand, retrieve the used instrument from the dentist, using the reverse palm grasp to hold the instrument before placing it back on the tray.
3. Deliver the new instrument to the dentist so that it is oriented with the working end in the appropriate position.
4. Return the used instrument to its proper position on the tray.

THE EXPANDED-FUNCTIONS DENTAL ASSISTANT

An **expanded function** refers to specific intraoral skill that is completed as a procedure or part of a procedure. The dentist delegates these expanded functions to the dental assistant. To **delegate** means to authorize another person to perform a specific skill or procedure.

The expanded function concept allows dentists to use time more effectively and efficiently. When specific legal expanded functions are delegated, studies have shown the following:

- Productivity increases in the dental office.
- Less stress is placed on the dentist.
- The dentist has more time available and can see more patients.
- Each member of the dental team can focus on specific tasks.
- The dental assistant has increased job satisfaction.

Credentialing

Most states require dental assistants to receive formal education before they can legally perform a specific expanded function in that state as an *expanded-functions dental assistant* (EFDA). The educational training typically includes lectures, laboratory or clinical practice, and a written examination requiring a passing grade. Training dental assistants for these functions occurs through the following approved programs:

- Accredited dental-assisting program
- Program approved by the state dental board but not accredited
- Specific course approved by the state dental board

After successfully completing all components, EFDAs are allowed to practice that function in the state where they work.

Dental Supervision

The dental practice act for each state will dictate if the expanded function must be under the direct or indirect supervision of the dentist. The dentist and assistant must remember that the dentist is the person *ultimately* responsible for the patient's care and well-being, even though a function is delegated to the EFDA.

With **direct supervision,** the dentist must be in the same treatment area as the EFDA for the assistant to perform the function.

With **indirect supervision,** the dentist must be in the dental office area, but not necessarily present in the same treatment room as the EFDA, and must be available to evaluate the assistant's expanded function.

WORKING AS THE OPERATOR

A dental assistant carrying out an expanded function assumes the role of operator. When this transition occurs, it is important for the dental assistant to become knowledgeable and competent in the areas of dental anatomy, operator positioning, mirror skills, using a fulcrum, understanding cavity preparations, adapting instrumentation, and applying dental materials.

Procedures often delegated to the dental assistant are described in their respective chapters. *The descriptions of these procedures are designed so that you can follow the sequence from laboratory to clinical situations.* Remember that you must acquire the appropriate background information before beginning the task.

Understanding Dental Anatomy

Many areas of dental anatomy are necessary components for understanding a dental procedure and a delegated function. (See Chapter 12 for a review of tooth morphology.) The dental assistant must have an in-depth knowledge of:

- Patient's occlusion of teeth to proper form and function
- Structures of teeth (enamel, dentin, cementum, pulp)
- Contours of each tooth
- Proximal contact area and its importance
- Pits and fissures of each tooth
- Periodontium and its importance

Following Guidelines for Operator Positioning

When working intraorally, it is important to follow the guidelines on positioning for the operator as listed earlier in the chapter. Continued neglect of your positioning will cause physical problems. Avoid positions that create unnecessary curvature of the spinal column or slumping of the shoulders.

See Chapter 25 for additional information on ergonomics of dentistry. Table 33-1 provides the suggested positioning of the operator for different areas of the mouth.

Developing Mirror Skills

Chapter 34 provides a review of the mouth mirror and its uses. The mouth mirror is a vital instrument when performing specific intraoral expanded functions.

Use of a mouth mirror for indirect vision of a specific area of the mouth is critical to maintain posture, reduce eyestrain, and complete specific functions. **Indirect vision** is viewing an object through the use of a mirror (Fig. 33-12). Much trial and error is involved in learning to use a mirror for indirect vision, because you are looking at the object reversed (mirror image).

Table 33-1 ***Suggested Positioning of the Operator and Patient According to Areas of the Mouth***

Mouth Area	Operator's Position	Type of Vision	Patient's Head Position
Maxillary right buccal	10-12 o'clock	Direct	Chin up and head turned away from operator
Maxillary right occlusal	11-12 o'clock	Indirect	Chin up and head turned toward operator
Maxillary right lingual	9 o'clock	Direct	Chin up and head turned toward operator
Maxillary anterior facial	11-12 o'clock	Direct	Chin up and head turned toward operator
Maxillary anterior lingual	11 o'clock	Indirect	Chin up and head straight forward
Maxillary left buccal	10 o'clock	Direct	Chin up and head turned toward operator
Maxillary left occlusal	11 o'clock	Indirect	Head turned slightly toward operator
Maxillary left lingual	9 o'clock	Direct	Head turned slightly toward operator
Mandibular right buccal	9-10 o'clock	Direct	Head turned away from operator
Mandibular right occlusal	9 o'clock	Direct	Chin down and head turned toward operator
Mandibular right lingual	9 o'clock	Direct	Chin down and head turned toward operator
Mandibular anterior facial	11-12 o'clock	Direct	Head straight forward
Mandibular anterior lingual	11-12 o'clock	Direct	Head straight forward
Mandibular left buccal	11 o'clock	Direct	Chin up and head turned toward operator
Mandibular left occlusal	11 o'clock	Direct	Chin up and head turned toward operator
Mandibular left lingual	9-10 o'clock	Direct	Chin up and head turned away from operator

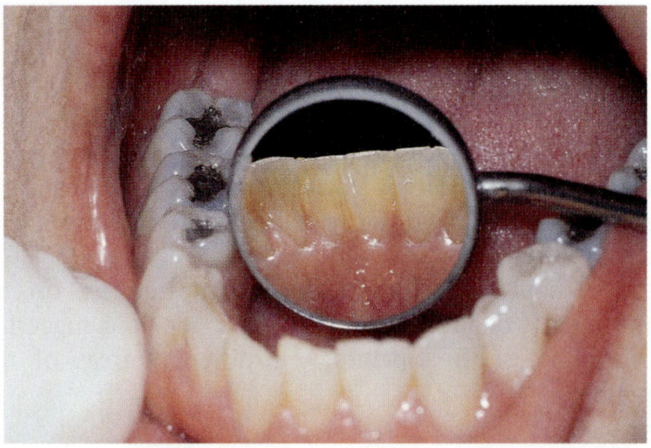

Fig. 33-12 Positioning the mirror to reflect image of the teeth correctly.

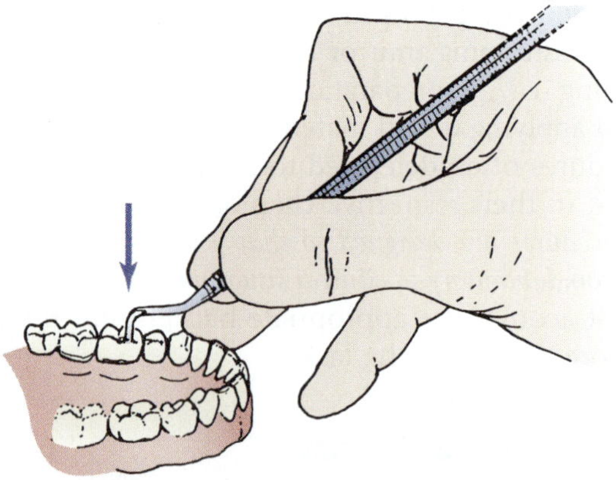

Fig. 33-13 Using a fulcrum to stabilize the hand and instrument. (From Baum L, Phillips R, Lund M: *Textbook of operative dentistry,* ed 3, Philadelphia, 1995, Saunders.)

Establish a Working Position

As the operator, you want to position yourself to have a "straight-on" visual effect. Once you are positioned, have the patient slightly tip the head back so the mandibular incisors are perpendicular to the floor. This allows you to position the mirror appropriately in relation to the tooth.

After you and the patient are situated properly, position the light. For the light to be used effectively for indirect vision, position it from your *nondominant* shoulder. That is, if you are right-handed, position the light from your left side.

Establish Preferred Mirror-to-Tooth Position

The mirror must be parallel to the working surface. Remember that you are looking at a mirror reflection, and any angle involved in the mirror will create distortion.

To create this parallel position, grasp the distal half of the mirror handle with the thumb, index finger, and middle finger. The farther away you hold the mirror, the more movement is available for you to position it (Procedure 33-4).

Using a Fulcrum

The operator needs more than a proper grasp when using an instrument or a handpiece in the mouth. When beginning to use specific instruments intraorally, you will discover the importance of *stabilizing your hand.*

A **fulcrum** is a "finger rest" that stabilizes the hand (Fig. 33-13). By stabilizing the hand, there is less possibility of slipping or traumatizing the tissue in the mouth. A good fulcrum should provide a stable resting area for the hand and allow the operator to use *wrist-forearm movement.*

A fulcrum that is established within the mouth is referred to as an *intraoral fulcrum.* Whenever possible, the fulcrum should be positioned on the same arch on which you are working, preferably in the same quadrant. The preferred way to position your finger or hand is with an intraoral fulcrum as close to the working area as possible.

Understanding Cavity Preparations

Several expanded functions delegated to dental assistants are associated with operative dentistry and the restoration of teeth. To know where to place dental materials and how to apply matrix bands and wedges, it is important to understand specific cavity terms and classifications (see Chapter 28).

Adapting Instrumentation

When performing an expanded function, the EFDA will use instruments to complete the function. When working with instruments, you need to be able to *adapt* the working end of the instrument to the tooth surface, and then go one step further by correctly moving the instrument.

Moving an instrument can be accomplished in two ways: (1) moving the hand, wrist, and forearm as one unit for more strength and (2) moving the fingers back and forth for a more confined or precise area (Procedure 33-5).

Applying Dental Materials

As a dental assistant, you have the skill to mix a dental material, and you know the material's appearance before the application. When you take on the function of placing a dental material in the mouth, you also need to know the application process.

Each dental material is unique in how it is used and where it is placed in the mouth. See the chapter that discusses the specific material, and review the assistant's role in its application.

Procedure 33-4 Using the Dental Mirror Intraorally

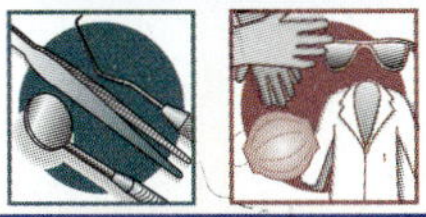

Equipment and Supplies

- Dental mirror
- Patient light

PROCEDURAL STEPS

1. Seat and position the patient in the dental chair in a supine position.
2. Turn on and position the dental light. Keep the light at arm's length away from the oral cavity, and have it coming slightly from your non-dominant shoulder.
   Purpose: The light is designed to illuminate the oral cavity. If the light is too close, it will not be as effective.
3. Position yourself as the operator.
   Note: Remember to follow the guidelines for the operator when seated.
4. Grasp the dental mirror in your left hand (for a right-handed operator) using a pen grasp.

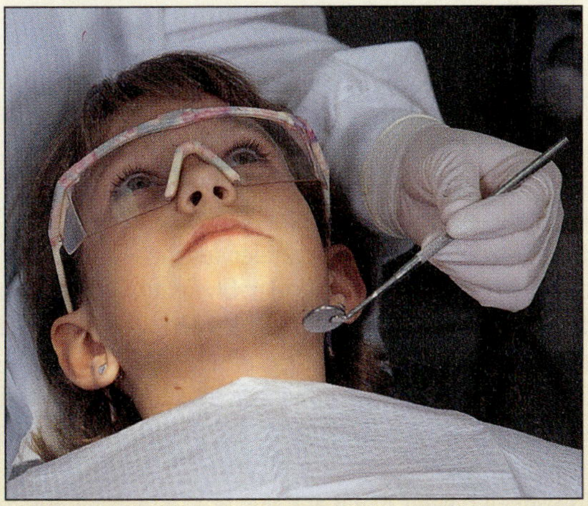

5. Position the dental mirror for indirect vision of the lingual aspect of the maxillary central incisors.

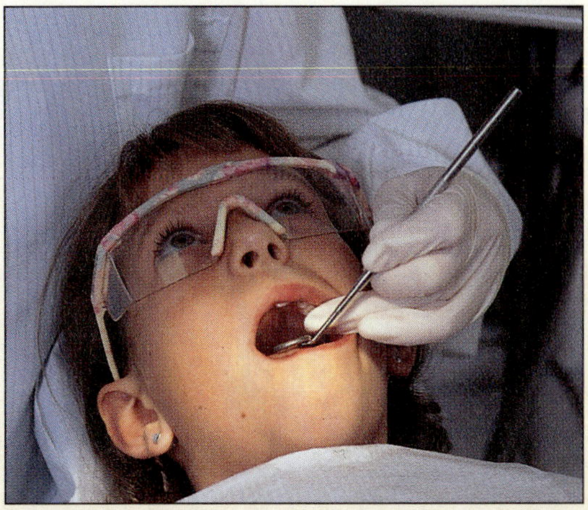

6. Position the dental mirror for light illumination on the lingual aspect of the mandibular central incisors.
7. Position the dental mirror for retraction to obtain better visualization.

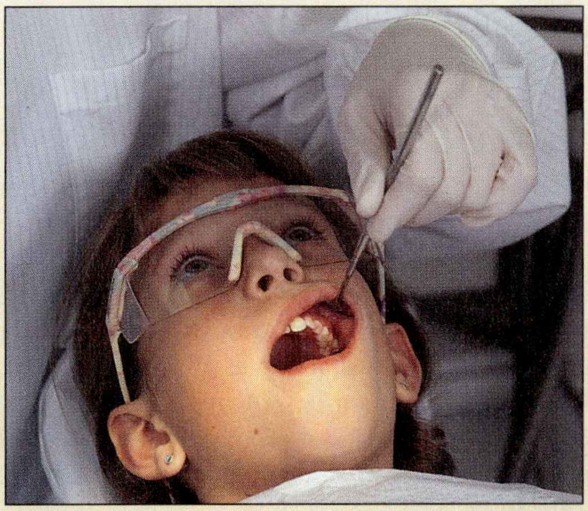

Evaluation of the Expanded Functions

An important aspect of acquiring additional responsibilities as a dental assistant is that *you are accountable for your work.* It is important that the dentist and dental assistant have the same expectations and goals in the evaluation process of delegated expanded functions.

You must attain the knowledge and skill of an expanded function not only through a course but also from the dentist with whom you practice. The dentist will have specific ways to make a temporary tooth, remove a matrix band, or place etchant. To learn the dentist's preferences, ensure open communication with the dentist when new expanded functions are delegated.

Procedure 33-5 Using an Instrument Intraorally

Equipment and Supplies

- Dental mirror
- Explorer
- Cotton pliers

PROCEDURAL STEPS

1. Seat and place the patient in the supine position.
2. Position yourself as the operator.
3. Adjust the dental light to illuminate the oral cavity.
4. Using a pen grasp, pick up the mirror with your nondominant hand, and the explorer with your dominant hand.

   Note: If you are right-handed, use your right hand to grasp the explorer.
5. Instruct your patient to open his or her mouth and turn toward or away from you, depending on the location of the mouth.
6. Establish a fulcrum close to the area that you will be exploring with your instrument.
7. Adapt the explorer to the most posterior tooth in the upper-right quadrant.

   Note: A well-adapted instrument prevents damage to the tooth and surrounding tissue.
8. Follow around the tooth with the mirror and explorer and examine all surfaces through visualization and touch.

Recall

9. What is indirect vision?
10. What is another term for a finger rest?

Patient Education

Do dental patients know your role in the dental office? You and the dentist are responsible for educating patients about the qualifications and responsibilities of the dental team. The best way is to display certificates, diplomas, and additional acknowledgments on the walls throughout the dental office.

Some offices provide a letter to new patients detailing the professional background of the dental staff. This approach assures the patient that the treatment team has a certain level of competence.

Legal and Ethical Implications

All the states have changed their dental practice laws to allow dental assistants to perform expanded functions. Confusion arises because each state varies considerably as to (1) what duties a dental assistant can perform in the state and (2) what educational requirements are needed to practice expanded functions.

Be sure that you work in an office that maintains a current state-approved expanded-functions list. Display all the credentials that you have earned.

As with all patient treatment, you are responsible for your interventions. The *ultimate* responsibility, however, lies with the dentist. All practices of the dental team should note that the dentist evaluated every procedure, critiqued the work, and communicated findings to the assistant, with documentation in the patient record.

Eye to the Future

What role will the dental assistant play in the future? It is predicted that a shortage of dentists will occur in this century, and that the dental assistant may take on many roles to compensate for that shortage.

The dental assistant may take on the role of *preventive assistant.* The EFDA may be responsible for assisting the dental hygienist in performing supragingival scaling, coronal polishing, application of sealants, and additional preventive procedures for patients.

The EFDA may also assume the role of *operative assistant.* These expanded functions might include simple and intermediate restorations, final impressions, and additional skills completed by the dentist.

As you will find, every state is different in what expanded functions are approved. Then you will find that every dental office varies in what functions the EFDA can perform. Stay informed about your profession by keeping up-to-date with new and approved expanded functions.

Critical Thinking

1. A patient is scheduled today for an extraction. She is very apprehensive about the procedure. What could be discussed among the dental team to help prepare for this patient?
2. Why do you think the team concept applies to dentistry? Is the team concept as prominent in medicine? Why or why not?
3. The operator is positioned a specific way to provide clinical care. Why is it so important to follow such guidelines?
4. At this point in your education, what role do you see for yourself as a clinical dental assistant? How can you contribute to the dental team in an office?
5. The dentist sees no problem in delegating expanded functions to you because you are a practicing dental assistant. However, you have been asked to complete some functions that you cannot legally perform in the state. How should you approach this problem?

34

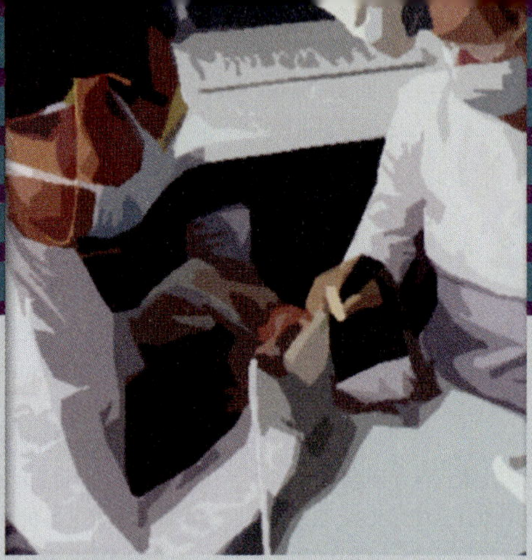

Dental Hand Instruments

Outline

Identifying Hand Instruments
- Instrument Number
- Instrument Design
- Black's Instrument Formula

Instrument Classification
- Instrument Sequence
- Examination Instruments

Procedure 34-1: Identifying Examination Instruments
- Hand Cutting Instruments
- Restorative Instruments

Procedure 34-2: Identifying Hand (Manual) Cutting Instruments

Procedure 34-3: Identifying Restorative Instruments
- Accessory Instruments and Items

Procedure 34-4: Identifying Accessory Instruments and Items
- Preset Cassettes (Trays)
- Storage Tubs
- Color-Coding Systems

Legal and Ethical Implications

Eye to the Future

Critical Thinking

KEY TERMS

Beveled (**bev**-uld) Characterized by an angle of a surface that meets another angle.

Blade Flat edge of instrument sharp enough to cut.

Handle Part of a dental instrument that the operator grasps.

Nib Blunt point or tip.

Plane Flat or level surface of the working end of an instrument.

Point Sharp or tapered end.

Serrated (*sur*-**ray**-ted) Having notchlike projections extending from a flat surface.

Shank Part of an instrument where the handle attaches to the working end.

Tactile (**tak**-t[uh]l) Having a sense of touch or feeling.

Working end Part of a dental instrument that is used on the tooth or when mixing dental materials.

LEARNING OUTCOMES

On completion of this chapter, the student will be able to achieve the following objectives:

- Define and spell the Key Terms.
- Describe the three parts of a dental hand instrument.
- Describe the instrument formula designed by G.V. Black.
- List the examination instruments and their uses.
- List the types of hand (manual) cutting instruments and their uses.
- List the types of restorative instruments and their uses.
- Describe additional accessory instruments and items used in general dentistry.
- Describe the use of preset trays and tubs in dentistry.
- Discuss the theory of placing an instrument in a specific sequence.

PERFORMANCE OUTCOMES

On completion of this chapter, the student will be able to meet competency standards in the following skills:

- Identify examination instruments.
- Identify hand (manual) cutting instruments.
- Identify restorative instruments.
- Identify accessory instruments and items.

A wide variety of dental instruments are used in dentistry today. This chapter describes the design and purpose of dental instruments that are most commonly used by dentists for general restorative procedures.

Dental supply companies manufacture many variations of instruments in order to accommodate personal preferences. As you study the instruments in this chapter, you will learn that each instrument is designed for specific areas of a tooth, as well as for the specific needs of the dentist.

IDENTIFYING HAND INSTRUMENTS

Each type of dental instrument has a specific purpose in a dental procedure. The knowledge and preparation of instruments are the responsibility of the clinical assistant when setting up for a procedure. The assistant sets up the instruments on the tray in a precise order of use, and is expected to transfer from the tray setup when the operator signals for a new instrument. Dentists will have a preference in how they refer to an instrument, whether by name or by a number.

Most hand instruments are made from stainless steel, carbon steel, plastic, or a specialized metal. Because instruments withstand constant use, they must be able to withstand sterilization procedures as indicated in Chapter 21.

Instrument Number

The dental manufacturer assigns a number to most instruments (Fig. 34-1). This number is a universal representation of that instrument. The dentist often refers to pliers and forceps by their number rather than by a name. When studying accessory and orthodontic pliers and surgical forceps, it is advantageous to learn both the number *and* name.

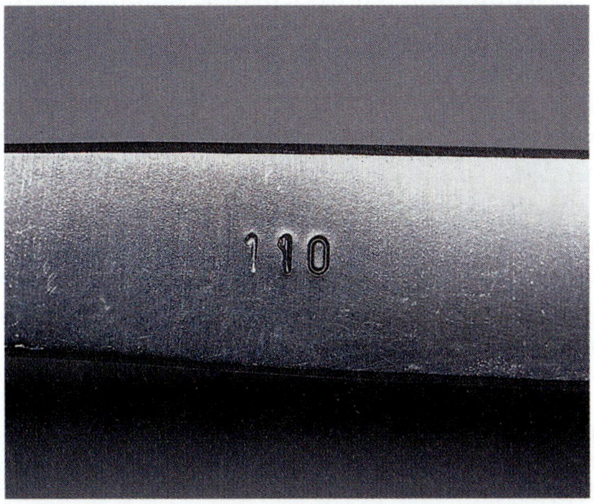

Fig. 34-1 Catalog or call number associated with Howe pliers.

Instrument Design

Hand instruments are designed with three specific parts: the handle, the shank, and the working end (Fig. 34-2).

Handle

The **handle** portion of the instrument is where the operator grasps or holds the instrument. Handles are manufactured in various shapes and sizes; some handles are round, and others are hexagonal. They may be smooth or may have a grooved pattern for a better grasp. Instruments are now designed to have a larger handle in circumference, as well as padding for a better grip. As seen on writing instruments, this new padding provides the operator with more control of the instrument and less fatigue on the fingers and hand muscles.

Shank

The **shank** refers to the part of the instrument that attaches the working end to the handle. The angles in the shank are designed so that an instrument can reach specific areas of the tooth. For example, instruments that are used interproximally have more angles in their shanks, whereas instruments used on the facial or buccal surfaces of a tooth have fewer angles.

The thickness and strength of the shank dictate the amount of pressure that can be applied to the instrument without breakage.

Working End

The **working end** refers to the portion of the instrument with a specific function. This end can have a **point, blade,** or **nib.** If the instrument has a nib, this area can be smooth or **serrated.**

Hand instruments are single or double ended. The *double-ended instrument* will have a shank and working end at both ends of the handle. Often, double-ended instruments are mirror images (reverse angles) of each other to allow adaptation to all surfaces of the tooth. These are referred to as *left and right instruments.*

Black's Instrument Formula

As you have learned, G.V. Black was significant in developing many aspects of the way dentistry is practiced today. Black designed a formula that described the angulations and dimensions of the working end of a hand instrument

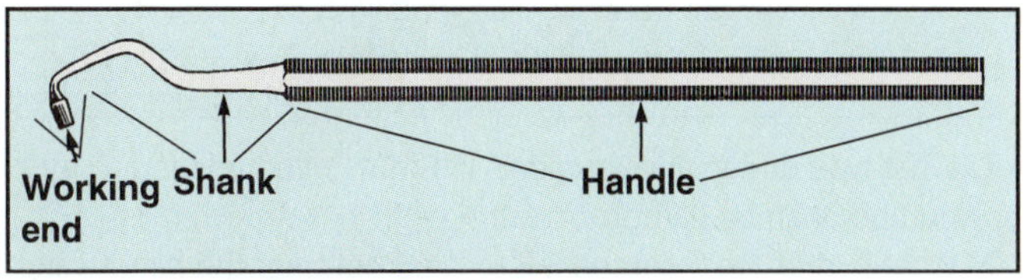

Fig. 34-2 Three parts of a dental hand instrument.

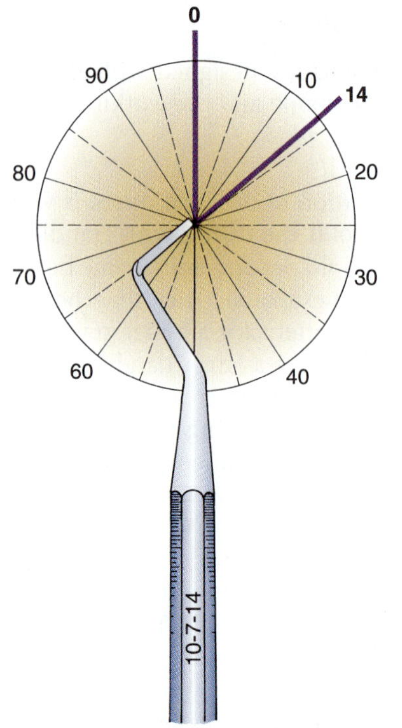

Fig. 34-3 **Black's instrument formula.** (From Baum L, Phillips RW, Lund MR: *Textbook of operative dentistry,* ed 3, Philadelphia, 1995, Saunders.)

Box 34-1 Numbers in G.V. Black's Instrument Formula

Sequence	Description
First number	Width of blade in tenths of millimeters (for example, if number is 10, width is 1 mm)
Second number	Length of blade in millimeters (for example, if number is 7, length is 7 mm)
Third number	Angle of blade in degrees in relation to handle (for example, if number is 90, working tip is [blade] at a 90-degree angle [right angle] to handle)

(Fig. 34-3). Hand cutting and scaling instruments have three sets of numbers that identify the blade's width, length, and angle. Box 34-1 describes the numbers and the formula used in the design of an instrument.

Recall

1. What type of dental instruments are more often referred to by a number than by name?
2. What part of the instrument is located between the handle and the working end?

INSTRUMENT CLASSIFICATION

The instruments used in restorative dental procedures are classified into four categories: *examination, hand, restorative,* and *accessory.* If you learn instruments by their classification, it will become easier to learn their names, uses, and sequencing for a procedure.

Classification of Hand Instruments

1. **Examination instruments** allow the operator to thoroughly examine the health status of the oral cavity.
2. **Hand cutting instruments** allow the operator to remove decay manually and to smooth, finish, and prepare the tooth structure for its final restoration.
3. **Restorative instruments** allow the operator to place, condense, and carve a dental material to the original anatomy of the tooth structure.
4. **Accessory instruments** are miscellaneous instruments and items that are used to complete a procedure.

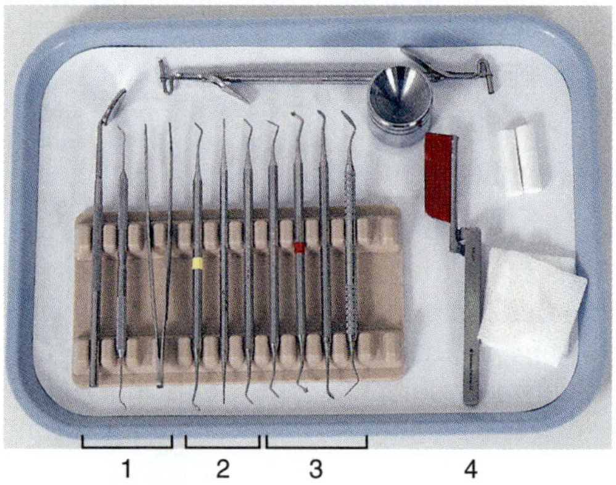

Instrument Sequence

A tray is set up from left to right. The rationale for this sequencing is based on how instruments are transferred and used throughout a dental procedure. Remember that the clinical assistant will use the *left hand* when transferring instruments. Therefore the most frequently used instruments will be closer to the dentist for ready availability.

Again, the basic setup will be first on the tray, followed by additional examination instruments, then hand cutting instruments and restorative instruments. Finally, any accessory items will be situated on the countertop in an organized and sequenced manner.

Examination Instruments

Examination instruments (Figure 34-4) are used in procedures ranging from the dentist checking a specific problem

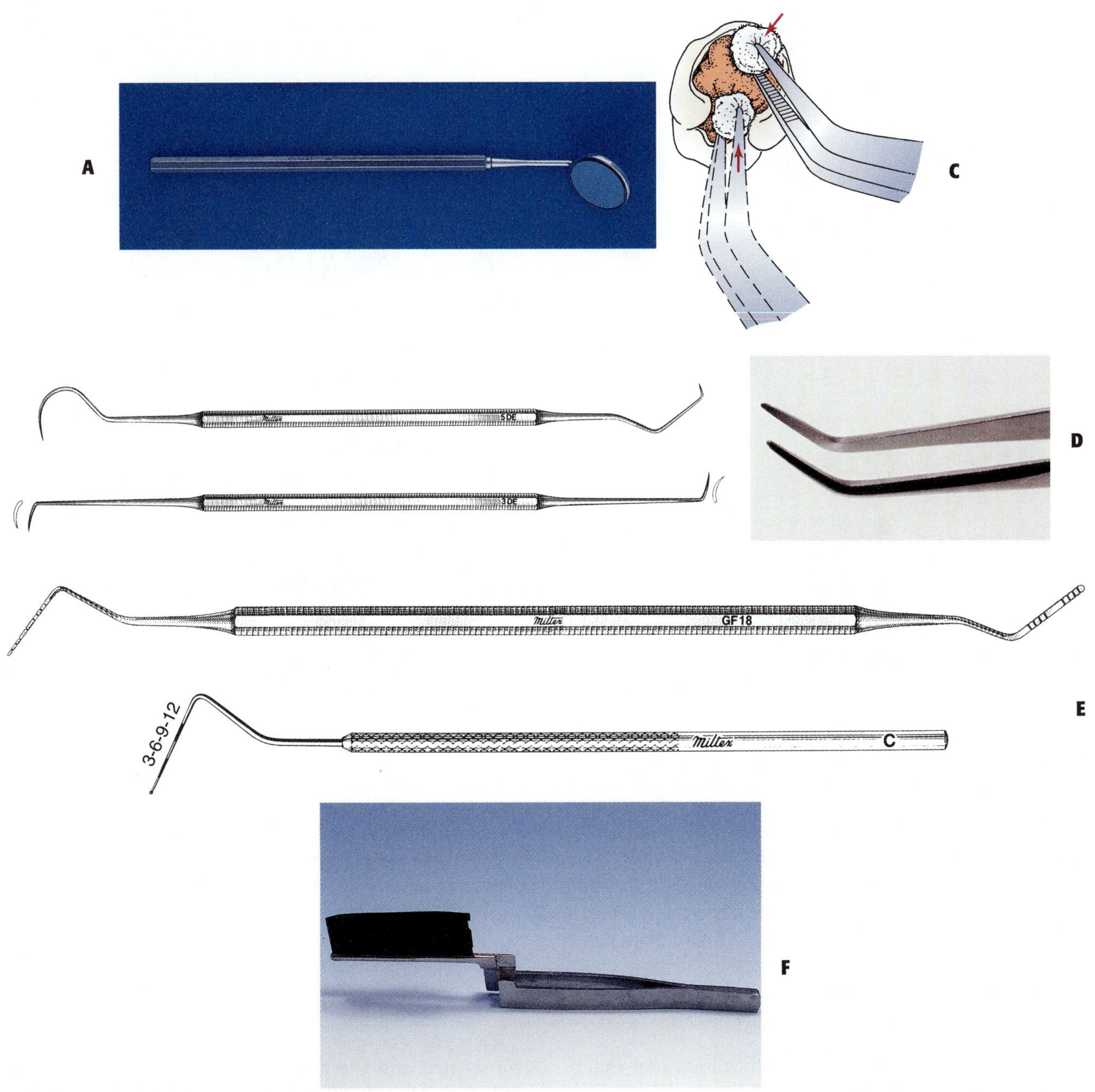

Fig. 34-4 Examination instruments. **A,** The *mouth mirror* is designed to have a straight handle, a slight angle to the shank, and a working end with a round metal disk and a mirror on one side. The mirror can have a flat or a concave (indented) surface. Mouth mirrors are used for a variety of purposes (see Figure 34-4). **B,** *Explorers* are multifunctional instruments that are included in the setup for every procedure. Many shapes of explorers are available, but all explorers have a thin, flexible, wirelike working end with a sharp point at the tip. Common types of explorers are the *right angle, pig tail,* and *shepherd's hook.* This thin tip enables the operator to use **tactile** sensitivity to distinguish areas of calculus or decay from discrepancies on the surface of the teeth. **C,** *Cotton pliers* are used to carry, place, and retrieve small objects, such as cotton pellets, gingival retraction cord, matrix bands, and wedges to and from the mouth. **D,** With *nonlocking* cotton pliers, the handles must be held closed with the fingers. With *locking* pliers, the handles can be locked in a closed position, and the tips do not open until the lock is released. The tips of the cotton pliers are available with plain or serrated points, or *beaks.* **E,** The *periodontal probe* is used to measure the sulcus or pocket depth of the periodontium of each tooth. This measurement provides the clinician with the overall gingival health of that area. The working end of the instrument has calibrated markings in millimeters, which are easier to read. Some probes are color-coded to enhance reading (see Chapter 55). **F,** *Articulating paper* is a carbon paper varying in thickness and color. It is used to check a patient's "bite" with a new restoration, crown, bridge, or denture. This mark must appear equal in distribution across the occlusal surface of the tooth. If one area appears lighter or darker, the patient's bite is incorrect and must be adjusted. The metal articulating paper holder is used to hold and carry the paper to the mouth. (**C** from Baum L, Phillips RW, Lund MR: *Textbook of operative dentistry,* ed. 3, Philadelphia, 1995, Saunders. **E** courtesy Miltex, Inc, York, Pennsylvania.)

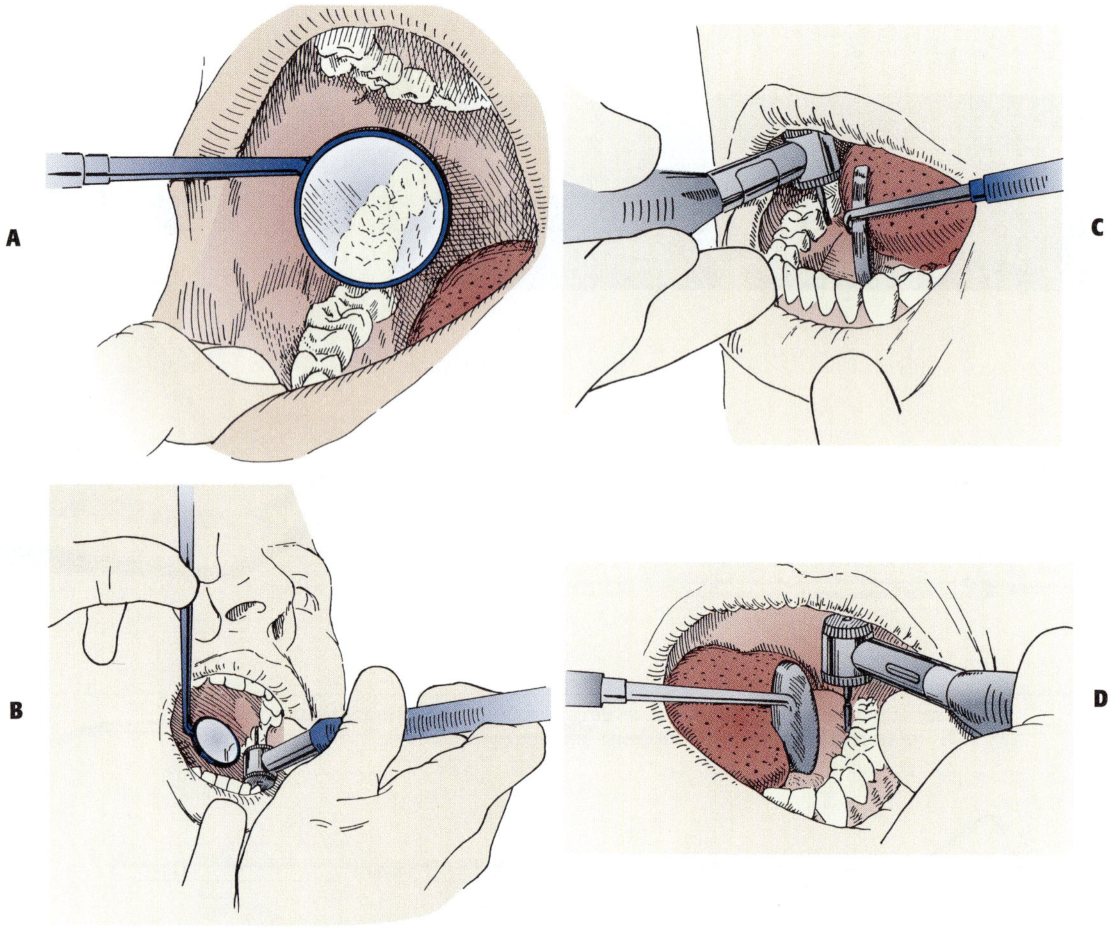

Fig. 34-5 Uses for the mouth mirror. **A,** *Indirect vision* allows the operator to see areas of the mouth that are not visible with direct vision. **B,** *Light reflection* directs light into areas of the mouth that are not directly accessible with the operating light. **C,** *Retraction* maintains a clear operating field by keeping the tongue or cheek out of the way during a procedure. **D,** *Tissue protection* helps guard the tongue or cheek against accidental injury from a dental bur.

area to the dental team providing a thorough oral examination. Figure 34-4 describes the examination instruments along with their use. Figure 34-5 provides descriptions of the four major uses of the mouth mirror. Procedure 34-1 reviews steps in identifying examination instruments.

Basic Setup

The mouth mirror, double-ended explorer, and cotton pliers will be set up for every procedure. These instruments are referred to as the *basic setup* (Fig. 34-6).

When preparing the tray setup from left to right, the mirror, explorer, and cotton pliers are the first three instruments, followed by additional examination instruments, hand cutting instruments, restorative instruments, and accessory instruments.

The mirror and explorer are transferred simultaneously using a two-handed transfer. It is best to position the explorer first and the mirror second on the tray. This setup will prevent crossover of your hands when transferring the two instruments to the dentist (Fig. 34-7).

Recall

3. What classification of instruments is used to remove decay manually?
4. What are the four uses of the mouth mirror?
5. What is the main feature of the working end of an explorer?
6. What instruments make up the basic setup?
7. What instrument is used to measure the sulcus of a tooth?

Procedure 34-1 Identifying Examination Instruments

Equipment and Supplies

- Mouth mirror
- Explorer
- Cotton pliers
- Periodontal probe
- Articulating paper
- Articulating paper holder

PROCEDURAL STEPS

1. Carefully examine the instrument.
2. Consider the general classification of the instrument.
3. Write the complete name of each instrument or item, spell it correctly, and give its uses.

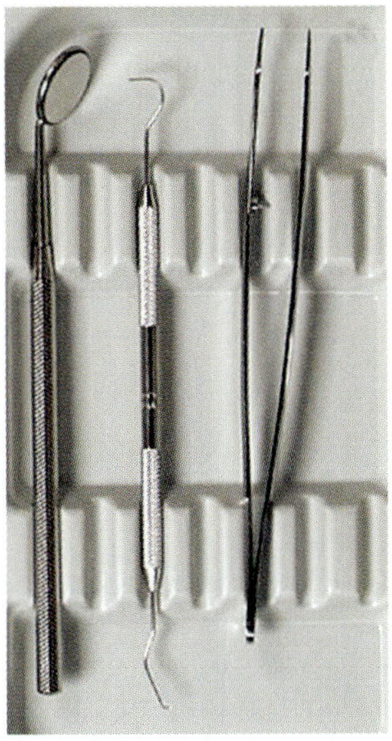

Fig. 34-6 Basic setup that includes mouth mirror, explorer, and cotton pliers. (Courtesy A-dec.)

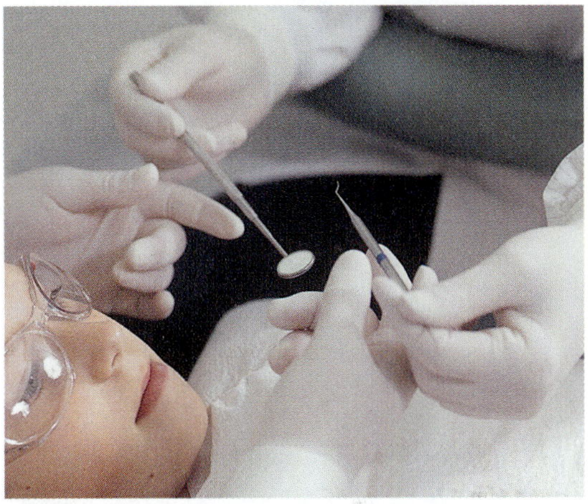

Fig. 34-7 Transferring mirror and explorer simultaneously to operator.

Hand Cutting Instruments

Hand cutting instruments are the next group of instruments placed on the tray setup after the examination instruments. These instruments allow the dentist to manually remove decayed tooth structure, smooth cavity walls and floors of the preparation, and place any bevels or retention grooves to hold the dental material in the tooth. Figure 34-8 shows the evacuator, hoe, chisel, hatchet, and gingival margin trimmer and their uses.

Dentists have a specific preference as to what instruments they want in this section. Most dentists use rotary instruments and manual cutting instruments interchangeably throughout a procedure. Procedure 34-2 reviews steps in identifying hand cutting instruments.

Procedure 34-2 Identifying Hand (Manual) Cutting Instruments

Equipment and Supplies

See Figure 34-8 for examples of instruments.

- Excavators
- Hoe
- Chisels
- Hatchets
- Gingival margin trimmer

PROCEDURAL STEPS

1. Carefully examine the instrument.
2. Consider the general classification of the instrument.
3. Write the complete name of each instrument, with its correct spelling and uses.

Recall

8. What are the two most common excavators used in restorative dentistry?

Restorative Instruments

Restorative instruments are used primarily to place, condense, and carve the restorative dental material back to its normal anatomy of that tooth. Figure 34-9 describes the restorative instruments most commonly used. Most dentists will use these instruments in a specific sequence. The instruments selected for the tray setup depend on the dentist's preference. Procedure 34-3 reviews steps in identifying restorative instruments.

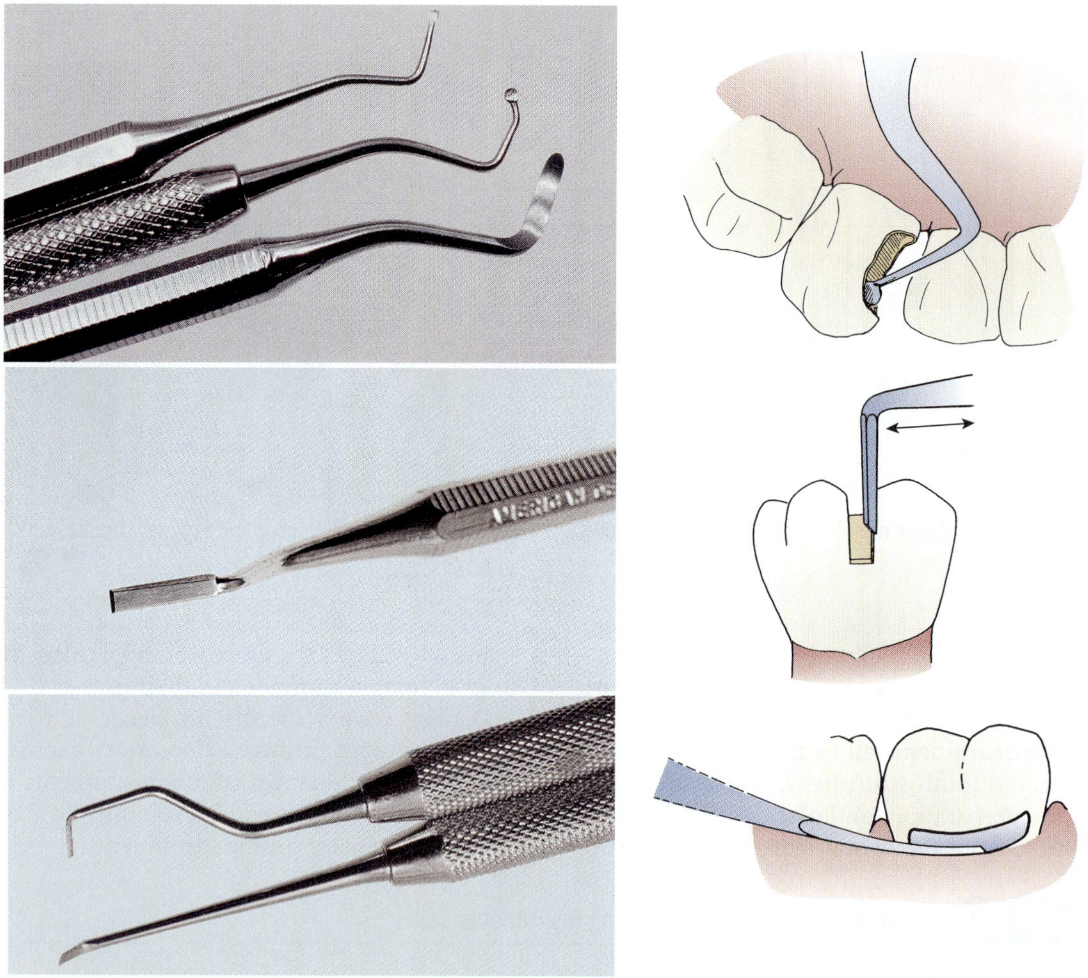

A B C D E F

Fig. 34-8 Hand (manual) cutting instruments. **A,** The *excavator* is one of the most versatile instruments on the tray setup. Excavators have a working end that is circular or elongated. The two most common excavators used are the *spoon* excavator and the *black spoon.* **B,** The *spoon excavator* is used for the removal of soft dentin, debris, and decay from the tooth. **C,** The hoe is similar in appearance to the garden tool. The blade is almost perpendicular to the handle. **D,** The *hoe* is used to prepare the tooth and to *plane* the walls and floors of the tooth preparation in a push-pull action. **E,** The *chisel* has a straight or angled shank and a single-**beveled** cutting edge. Common types are the *straight* chisel, *bin-angle* chisel, "Wedelstaedt" chisel, and *angle-former* chisel. **F,** Chisels are mainly used to cut the enamel margin of the tooth preparation, form sharp lines and point angles, and place retention grooves. (**B, D,** and **F** from Baum L, Phillips RW, Lund MR: *Textbook of operative dentistry,* ed 3, Philadelphia, 1995, Saunders.)

continued

Procedure 34-3 Identifying Restorative Instruments

Equipment and Supplies

- Amalgam carrier
- Condensers
- Burnishers
- Carvers
- Amalgam knife
- Composite placement instruments
- Plastic instrument

PROCEDURAL STEPS

1. Carefully examine the instrument.
2. Consider the general classification of the instrument.
3. Write the complete name of each instrument, spell it correctly, and give its uses.

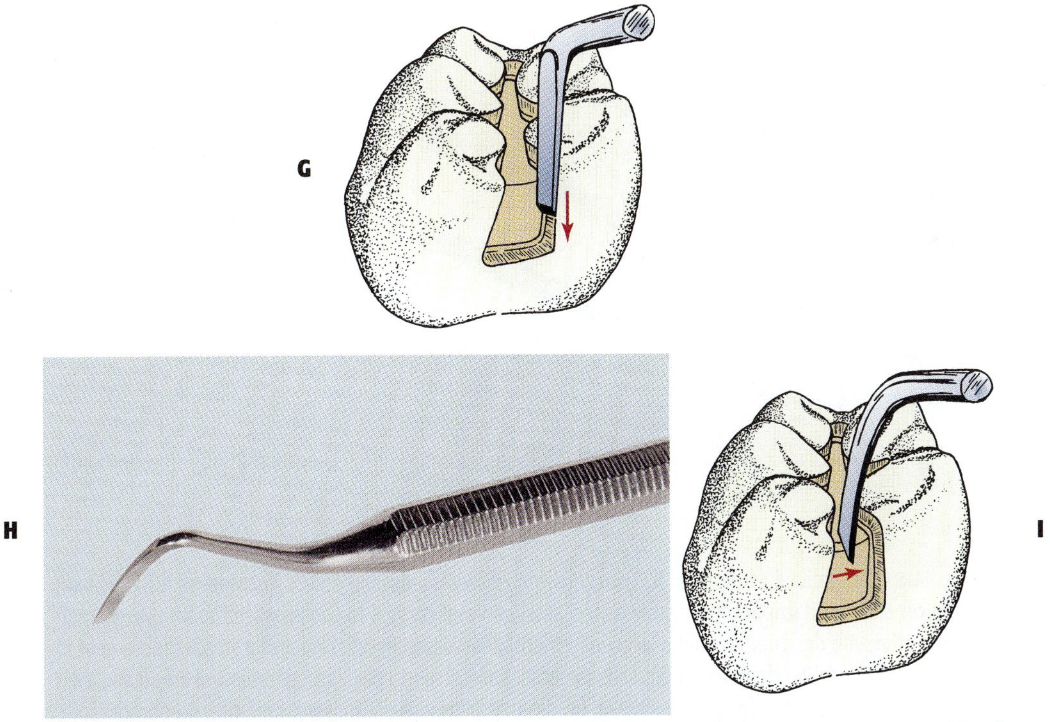

Fig. 34-8—cont'd Hand (manual) cutting instruments. **G,** *Hatchets* are similar in appearance to wood hatchets. The cutting edge is parallel with the long axis of the handle. Hatchets are used for cutting enamel and to smooth the walls and floors of the tooth preparation. **H,** The *gingival margin trimmer* is a variety of chisel that has been modified so that the blade is curved slightly for mesial or distal access into the preparation. **I,** Gingival margin trimmers are used to cut enamel and place bevels along the gingival enamel margins of the preparation. (**G** and **I** from Baum L, Phillips RW, Lund MR: *Textbook of operative dentistry,* ed 3, Philadelphia, 1995, Saunders.)

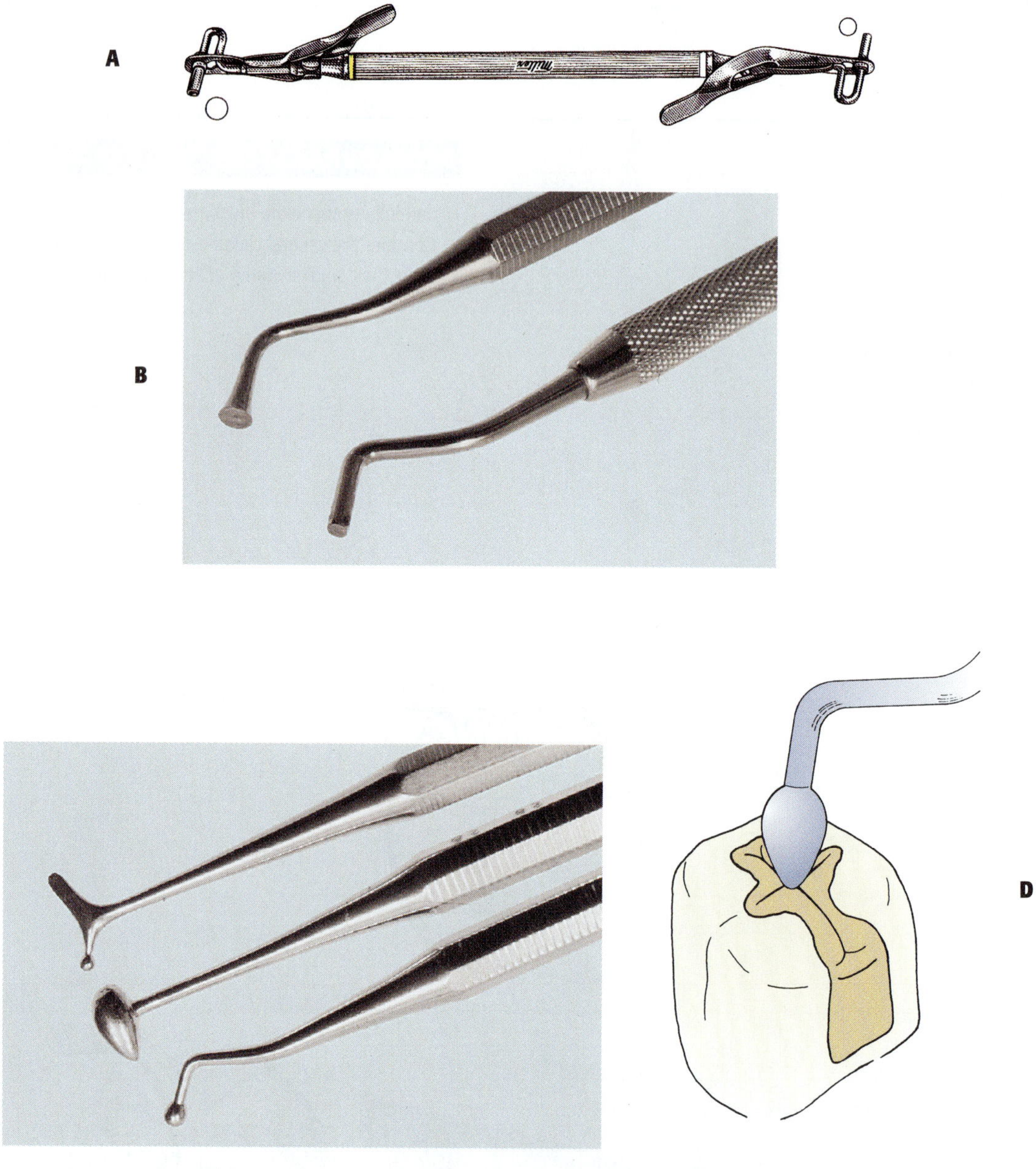

Fig. 34-9 Restorative instruments. **A,** The *amalgam carrier* is a double-ended instrument designed with wells on either end to pack the freshly mixed amalgam and carry it to the prepared tooth. Most amalgam carriers are designed to hold a large increment of amalgam in one end and a smaller increment in the opposite end. The dental assistant uses the amalgam carrier to pack an increment of amalgam, then either transfers the carrier to the dentist or directly places the amalgam into the prepared tooth. **B,** *Condensers* have a flat working end that can be smooth or serrated and come in varying sizes to accommodate the size of the preparation. To enable the operator to reach all areas of the preparation, the shank of the instrument is angled. The amalgam condenser, also known as a plugger, is used to condense (pack down) the freshly placed amalgam into the preparation. **C,** A *burnisher* is an instrument with a smooth working end. The rounded working end is available in many shapes to accomplish different tasks. Common types include the ball, football, T-ball, and beavertail. Burnishers are routinely used to smooth the surface of a freshly placed amalgam restoration. (**A** courtesy Miltex, Inc, York, Pennsylvania; **D** from Baum L, Phillips RW, Lund MR: *Textbook of operative dentistry,* ed 3, Philadelphia, 1995, Saunders.)

continued

E

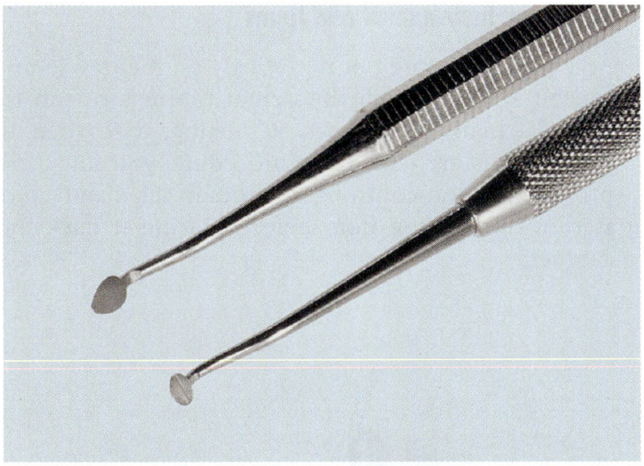

G

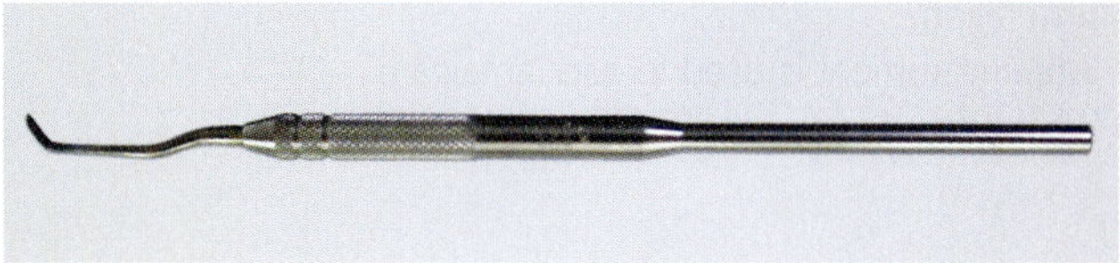

F

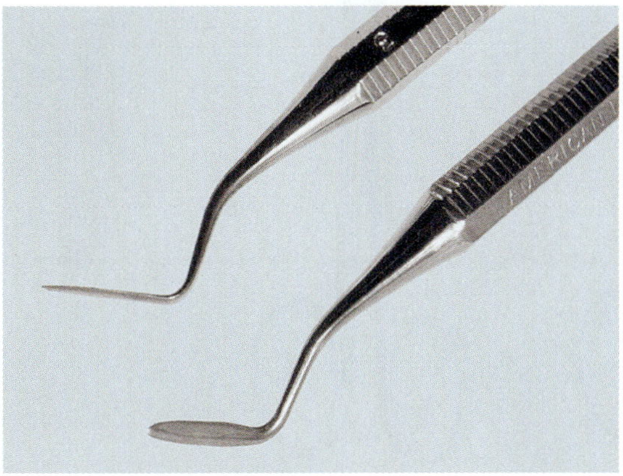

H

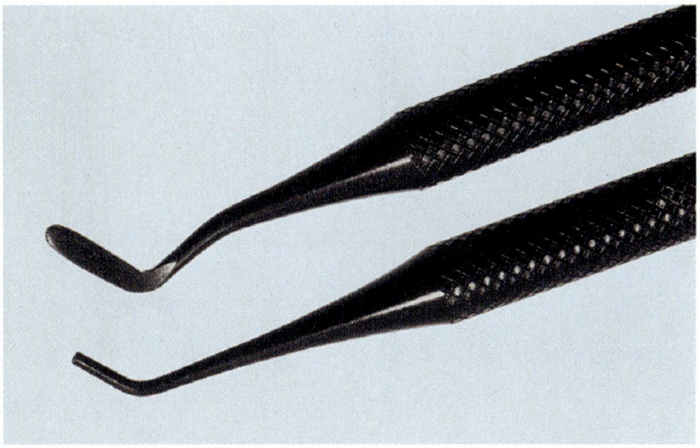

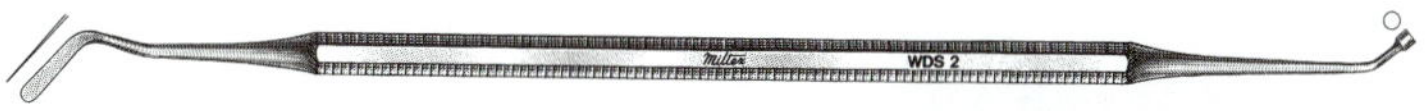

I

Fig. 34-9–cont'd Restorative instruments. **E,** *Carvers* are designed with a sharp edge on the working end to remove excess material, contour surfaces, and carve anatomy back into the amalgam or intermediate restoration before it hardens. Various styles of carvers are available. A discoid-cleoid carver is especially useful for carving of the occlusal surfaces. **F,** The *Hollenback carver* is used for contouring or removing excess material interproximally. **G,** The *amalgam knife* is designed with a sharp edge for the removal of excess restorative material along the margin where the material and tooth structure meet. The knife has several angles in the shank and working end to enable the operator to reach specific areas of a tooth, most often interproximal areas. **H,** The *composite placement instrument* is designed specifically for the placement of composite restorative materials. A composite is a tooth-colored material used for anterior restorations (see Chapter 43). Composite placement instruments are made from anodized aluminum or Teflon. These materials prevent the composite material from being scratched. These instruments do not discolor the composite material, as do stainless steel instruments. **I,** The *FP 1* is a double-ended instrument made from a hard plastic or stainless steel. One end is a "paddle" for carrying dental materials to the prepared tooth structure. The other end is a nib, which resembles a condenser. (**G** courtesy Boyd L: *Dental Instruments,* ed 2, St Louis, 2005, Mosby; **I** courtesy Miltex, Inc, York, Pennsylvania).

Recall

9. What instrument would you transfer to the dentist to carve anatomy back into the interproximal portion of an amalgam restoration?

10. What instrument is used to pack amalgam?

11. What type of instrument is discoid/cleoid?

Accessory Instruments and Items

Accessory items are not necessarily on the tray setup but can be "pulled" from the dental cabinets or tub to be used for many procedures. Remember that when additional items are used for a procedure, you must follow proper infection-control guidelines in the disinfection or sterilization of the item before placing it back in the cabinet.

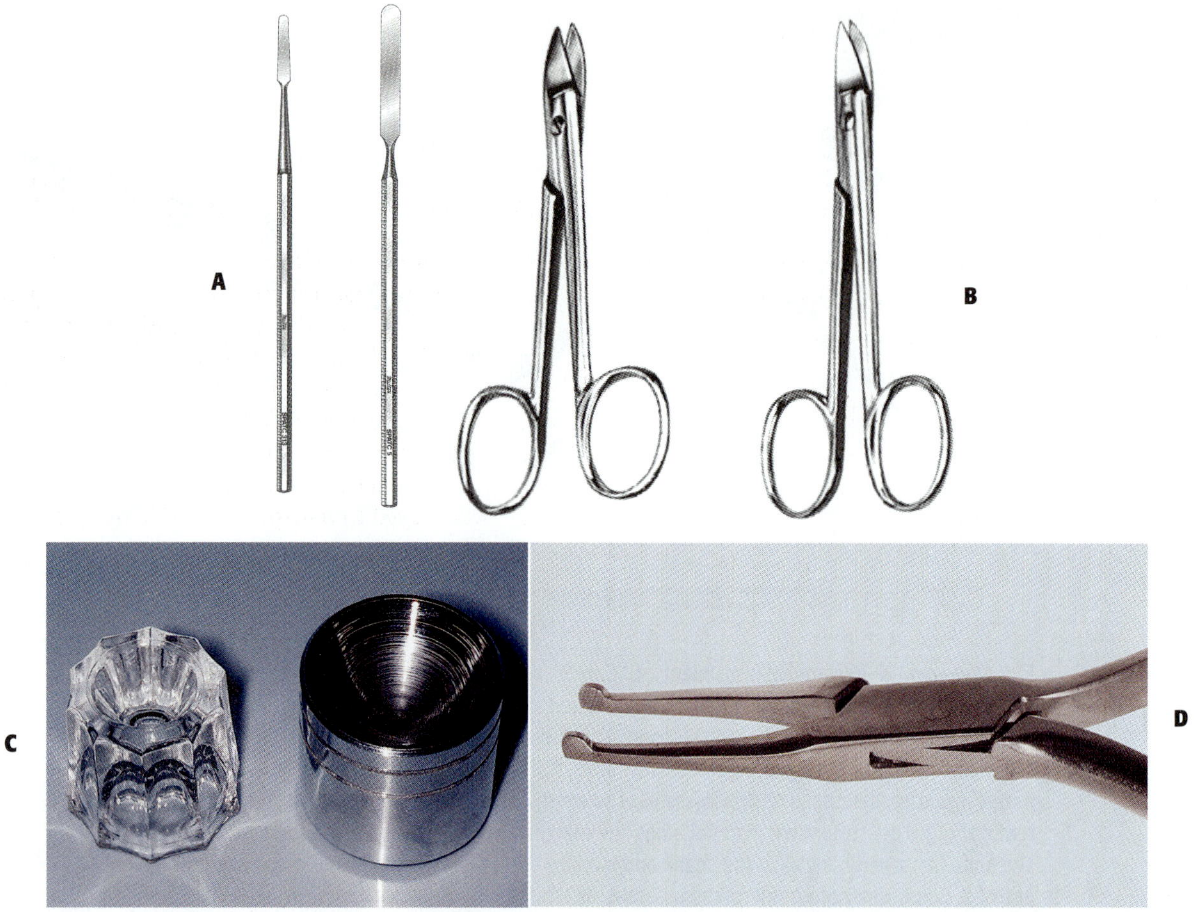

Fig. 34-10 Accessory instruments and items. **A,** *Spatulas* are used for most procedures when a dental material is involved. Two types of spatulas are usually required for a dental procedure. *Cement* spatulas are single-ended, made of stainless steel, come in two sizes (#15, #24), and are used to mix liners, bases, and cements. *Impression* spatulas are larger and have a wider blade. The handles are made of metal or wood and allow you to have a better grip when mixing an impression material. **B,** The *scissors* most often associated with restorative dental procedures are *crown and bridge* scissors, available with either curved or straight blades. They are useful for many tasks, such as cutting dental dam material, retraction cord, and stainless steel crowns. **C,** The *dappen dish* is a small glass dish with different sizes of wells on either side *(left).* Its primary function is to hold certain liquid dental materials during a procedure. The amalgam well is made of metal and is weighted with a nonskid base *(right).* The newly mixed amalgam is placed in the well, then picked up in the carrier for transfer to the dentist. **D,** *Howe pliers,* also referred to as *110 pliers,* are versatile pliers that can be used in many procedures for many tasks. Their design is straight with beaks that have a flat rounded end, making them useful for holding items. Howe pliers are useful for carrying cotton products to and from the oral cavity, removing the matrix band, and placing and removing the wedge.

Procedure 34-4 Identifying Accessory Instruments and Items

Equipment and Supplies

- Cement spatulas
- Impression spatulas
- Scissors
- Dappen dish
- Amalgam well
- Howe pliers

PROCEDURAL STEPS

1. Carefully examine the instrument or item.
2. Consider the general classification of the instrument.
3. Write the complete name of each instrument or item, spell it correctly, and give its uses.

Figure 34-10 introduces some of the most common accessory instruments that are used in a restorative procedure. Procedure 34-4 reviews steps in identifying accessory instruments and items.

Recall

12. What type of scissors is placed on the restorative tray setup?
13. What is another term for Howe pliers?
14. Where is the freshly mixed amalgam placed before transporting it in the amalgam carrier?

Preset Cassettes (Trays)

Hand instruments and related accessories for a given procedure are prepared, stored, and transported together as a *preset tray* or *preset cassette* (Fig. 34-11).

A dental practice will have sufficient trays or cassettes for most common procedures to allow adequate sterilization and preparation time before the tray is needed again. The sterile tray or cassette is taken to the treatment area for preparation before seating the patient.

Storage Tubs

Supplies and dental materials for specific procedures can be stored in a covered plastic tub within each operatory (Fig. 34-12). The combination is known as the *tub and tray system.*

Color-Coding Systems

Color-coding is one of the most convenient and efficient ways to organize instruments and supplies for specific procedures. The ways in which color-coding can be used are limited only by the user's creativity.

The instrument tray and the tub of related materials can be used to indicate the procedure. For example, if blue is the color chosen to indicate composite restorations, each of the instruments has a blue band, the tray has a blue label, and a blue tub is used to transport the related materials.

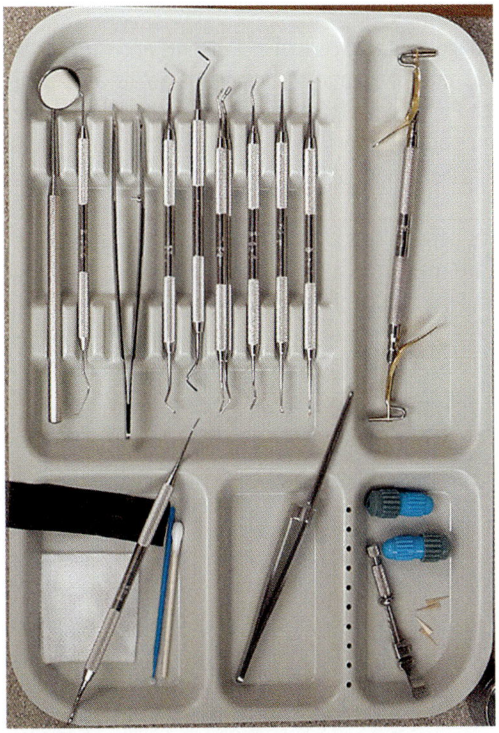

Fig. 34-11 Preset restorative tray. (Courtesy A-dec.)

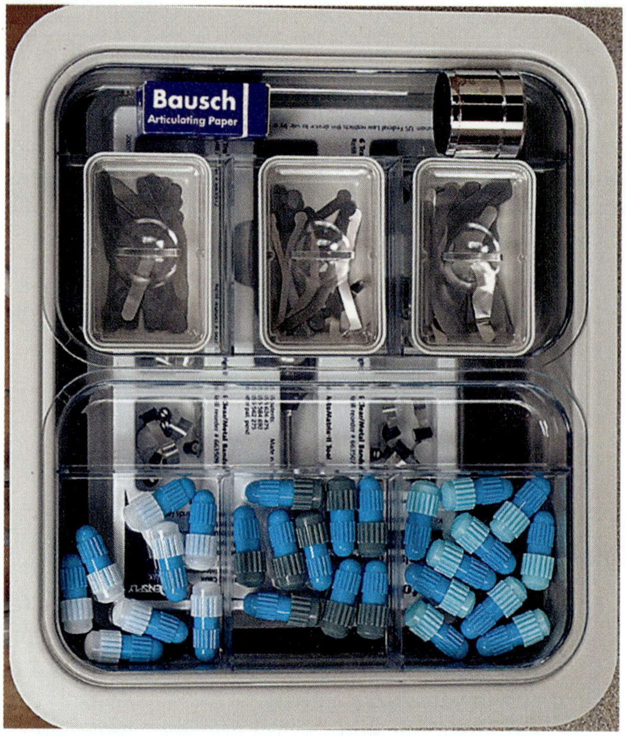

Fig. 34-12 Storage tub holding additional items needed for a procedure. (Courtesy A-dec.)

Legal and Ethical Implications

The management and care of instruments and supplies for a procedure is one of your most important duties as a patient care provider. By carefully following infection-control guidelines in the way you package, sterilize, and store instruments, you are protecting patients and clinical staff from a possible infectious disease.

Many patients are knowledgeable enough to ask how instruments are maintained. Be certain that you can assure your patients and provide the best answer.

Eye to the Future

Because of more awareness and concern in the transmission of infectious diseases, you will find that more and more instruments are made from disposable material. This technology has pros and cons. The positive aspects are less transmission of disease and less time spent between patients in the sterilization center. The negative concerns involve the handling of more contaminated waste.

Critical Thinking

1. Give the four instrument classifications, and describe how the dentist would sequence the instruments for the restoration of a tooth.
2. You have just seated your next patient. The dentist sits down and extends her hands on either side of the patient's face. What is she doing, and how do you respond?
3. You are sitting down to assist the dentist in a composite procedure. You notice that the enamel hatchet is missing from the setup. Is there anything else that the dentist could use in place of a tooth preparation instrument?
4. You are given the following instruments for an amalgam tray: condenser, spoon excavator, mirror, carrier, cotton pliers, burnisher, explorer, discoid/cleoid carver, periodontal probe, Hollenback carver, and hatchet. Place them in order in relation to their classification and use.
5. What accessory instrument or item would you pull from the cabinet or tub for an amalgam procedure?

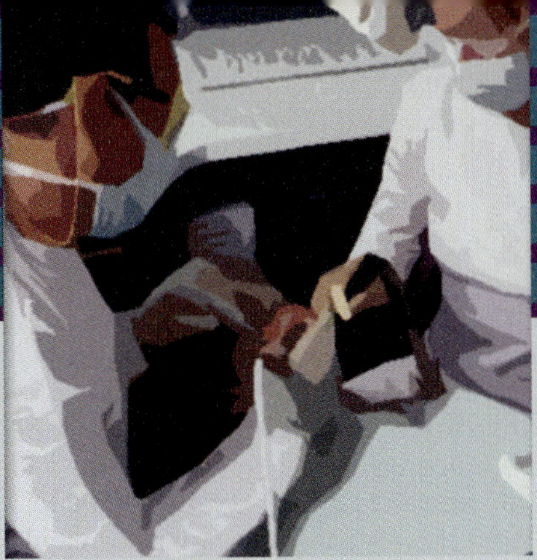

35

Dental Handpieces and Accessories

Outline

KEY TERMS

Console (**kahn**-sole) Freestanding cabinet that holds contents or control devices, such as the laser handpiece.

Flutes Blades on the working end of a finishing rotary instrument, which resemble pleats.

Mandrel (**man**-druhl) Metal shaft on which a sandpaper disk or other abrasive materials are mounted.

Rotary (**roh**-teh-ree) Part or device that rotates around an axis.

Shank Part of an instrument in which the handle attaches to the working end.

Torque (**tork**) Twisting or turning force.

Ultrasonic (*uhl*-treh-**sah**-nik) Referring to mechanical radiant energy of water and sound vibrations used to break down materials or tissue.

LEARNING OUTCOMES

On completion of this chapter, the student will be able to achieve the following objectives:

- Pronounce, define, and spell the Key Terms.
- Discuss the historical importance of the dental handpiece.
- Describe the low-speed handpiece and its use in dentistry.
- Describe the attachments used on the low-speed handpiece.
- Describe the high-speed handpiece and its uses.
- Review other handpieces used in dentistry.
- Describe rotary instruments and how they are used.
- List the parts of a bur.
- Give the composition, shape, and use of the carbide and diamond burs.

PERFORMANCE OUTCOMES

On completion of this chapter, the student will be able to meet competency standards in the following skills:

- Identify dental handpieces and correctly attach them to the dental unit.
- Identify accessories and correctly attach them to the low-speed handpiece.
- Identify rotary cutting instruments and correctly attach them to the appropriate dental handpiece or attachment.

If you understand the concept of the home power tool, in which a drill and bit are used to create an outline or finish a piece of wood, then you will understand the dental handpiece and its attached rotary instruments. A **rotary** is a part or device that rotates around an axis. When attached to a specific handpiece, these rotary instruments operate at different speeds to accomplish different functions in the cutting, polishing, and finishing of tooth structure in the restoration process.

EVOLUTION OF ROTARY EQUIPMENT

Rotary instruments were introduced to dentistry in the 1940s to complement the use of hand instruments in the cutting, grinding, and polishing procedures of operative dentistry. A significant advancement in the creation of the dental handpiece was the addition of electricity as a power source for rotary instruments.

The first dental handpiece was operated by a long belt running over a series of pulleys then back to the motor, continuously moving the inserted rotary instrument (Fig. 35-1). From the 1940s through the 1950s, development of diamond cutting burs and the invention of tungsten carbide burs greatly improved the way dentists could cut into and remove hard tooth structure. Further study of diamond and carbide burs showed that these rotary instruments performed better at higher speeds. The air-driven turbine handpiece was introduced to dentistry in the 1950s.

DENTAL HANDPIECES

Dental handpieces are the most frequently used devices in restorative dentistry. The two most common types of dental handpieces are the low-speed and high-speed handpiece. The dental unit provides the power to the handpiece, rotating the bur, which completes the actual cutting or polishing of tooth structure and castings.

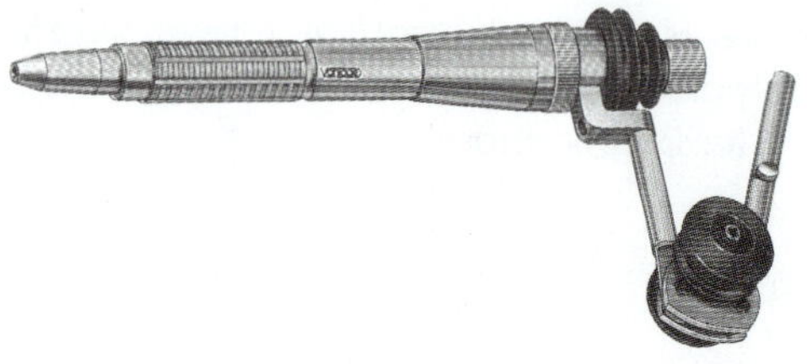

Fig. 35-1 Belt-driven handpiece. (Courtesy Miltex Inc, York, Pennsylvania.)

Low-Speed Handpiece

The low-speed handpiece, often referred to as the *straight handpiece* because of its straight-line design, is one of the most versatile handpieces used by the dental team (Fig. 35-2).

The low-speed handpiece is designed in two sizes: standard length and "shorty" (small). Available speeds range from 10,000 to 30,000 rotations per minute (rpm). The rotary instrument *(bur)* can be positioned to operate with a forward or backward movement.

To adapt the low-speed handpiece for clinical and laboratory procedures, a variety of attachments, or *sleeves,* are used that fit onto the handpiece.

Straight Attachment

The straight attachment slides onto the low-speed motor and locks into place (Fig. 35-3). This straight attachment is

Uses of the Low-Speed Handpiece

Clinical

- Removal of soft decay and fine finishing of a cavity preparation
- Finishing and polishing of restorations
- Coronal polishing and removal of stains
- Porcelain adjustments
- Root canal treatment

Laboratory

- Trimming and contouring of temporary crowns
- Trimming and relining of removable partials and dentures
- Trimming and contouring of orthodontic appliances

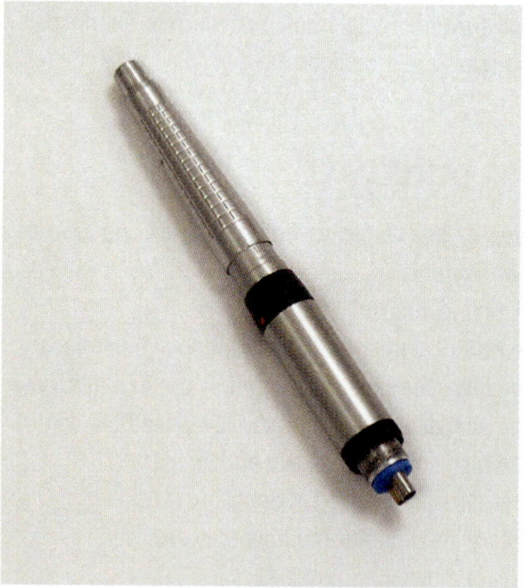

Fig. 35-2 Low-speed handpiece.

most commonly used for laboratory procedures or for trimming removable prostheses outside of the mouth.

Contra-Angle Attachment

The contra-angle attachment slides directly onto the low-speed motor and locks into place (Fig. 35-4). The angle of this attachment is designed to allow the operator intraoral access with easier adaptation to tooth surfaces. This attachment holds latch-type rotary instruments, endodontic files, prophylaxis cups, and mandrels (see later in chapter for discussion).

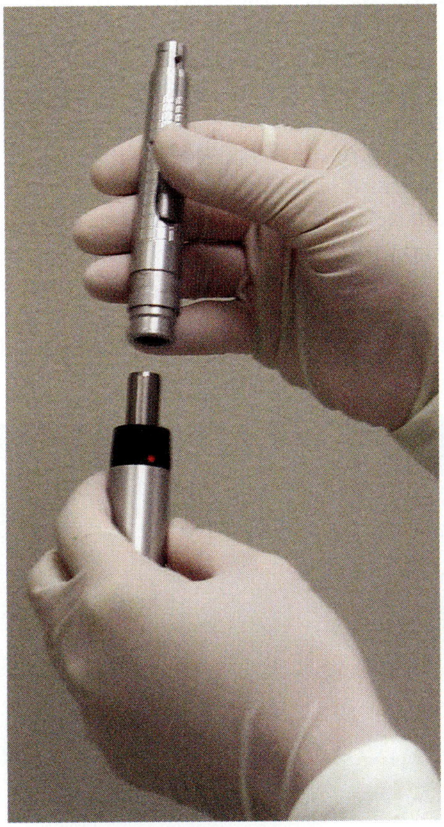

Fig. 35-3 Straight attachment slides onto the slow-speed motor.

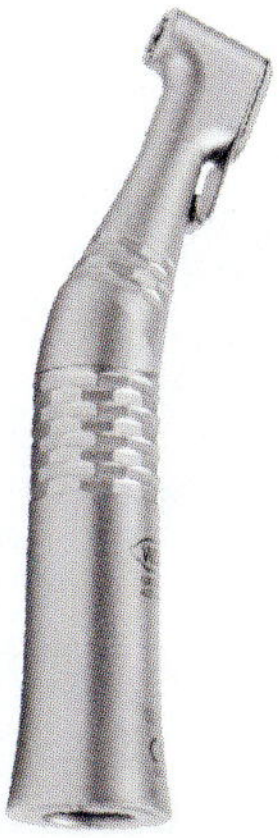

Fig. 35-4 Contra-angle attachment. (Courtesy A-dec.)

Prophylaxis Angle

Prophylaxis attachments, or "prophy angles," are used during polishing procedures to hold the prophy cup and bristle brush. The most common type of prophy angle is the *plastic disposable* prophy angle, which is discarded after a single use (Fig. 35-5). This attachment is available with a rubber cup or bristle brush already in place.

Recall

1. How did the first dental handpiece operate?
2. What are the two most common types of dental handpiece?
3. How fast does the low-speed handpiece rotate?
4. Which attachment is used to hold a latch-type bur?

High-Speed Handpiece

The dentist uses the high-speed handpiece in every restorative procedure. The rotary instrument in the high-speed handpiece rapidly removes pathologic tooth structure caused by decay or faulty restoration. Refinement of the

Uses of the High-Speed Handpiece

- Removal of decay
- Removal of an old or faulty restoration
- Reduction in the crown portion of the tooth in preparation for a crown or bridge
- Preparation of the outline and retention grooves for a new restoration
- Finishing and polishing of restorations
- Sectioning of a tooth during surgery

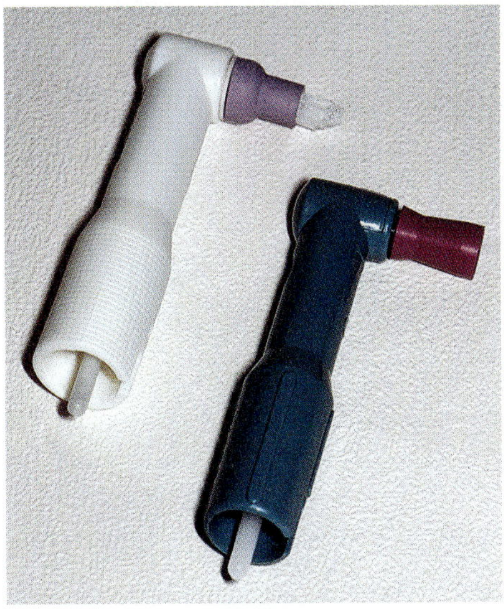

Fig. 35-5 Disposable prophy cup and brush.

preparation and removal of soft decay are then accomplished using the low-speed handpiece and hand cutting instruments.

Unlike the low-speed handpiece, the high-speed handpiece does not have attachments. The only additional item placed in this handpiece would be the rotary instrument itself. The high-speed handpiece operates from air pressure and reaches speeds up to 450,000 rpm (Fig. 35-6).

Water Coolant System

The extremely high speed of the bur or stone attached to the high-speed handpiece can generate frictional heat on a tooth, possibly causing damage to the pulp. To protect against pulp damage, the high-speed handpiece is equipped with a water coolant system. The tooth and bur are constantly sprayed with cool water during use. The water spray also helps remove debris from the tooth preparation to allow the operator better visibility.

Bur Adaptation

Burs for high-speed handpieces have a different locking system than those for low-speed handpieces. High-speed handpieces operate with a *friction-grip* device.

Many high-speed handpiece designs are on the market, and the method of inserting and removing burs from the handpiece varies according to the manufacturer's design. Regardless of the manufacturer, all high-speed handpieces use the friction-grip method to hold burs, stones, and polishing devices. Some older handpieces require the use of a bur-changing device. Others have a release built into the head of the handpiece, and a bur-changing device is not required.

Fiberoptic Lighting

High-speed handpieces are equipped with a fiberoptic light mounted in the head of the handpiece. Light ports near the bur deliver the proper amount of light directly onto the operating site (Fig. 35-7).

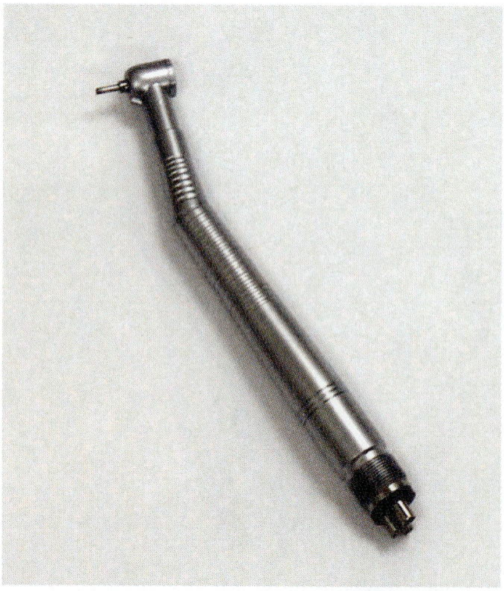

Fig. 35-6 High-speed handpiece.

Recall

5. How fast does the high-speed handpiece operate?
6. How is the tooth kept cool and clean during the use of the high-speed handpiece?
7. What type of bur locking system is on the high-speed handpiece?

Ultrasonic Handpiece

The **ultrasonic** handpiece uses mechanical radiant energy of water and sound vibrations to create a pulsating effect on a tooth surface. The ultrasonic handpiece is used primarily for the prophylaxis procedure (Fig. 35-8). The dentist will request it to be set up for removing bonding materials from a tooth surface after orthodontic appliances are removed.

The ultrasonic handpiece is attached to the dental unit and powered by electricity. The attachments for the ultrasonic handpiece are designed similarly to hand (manual)

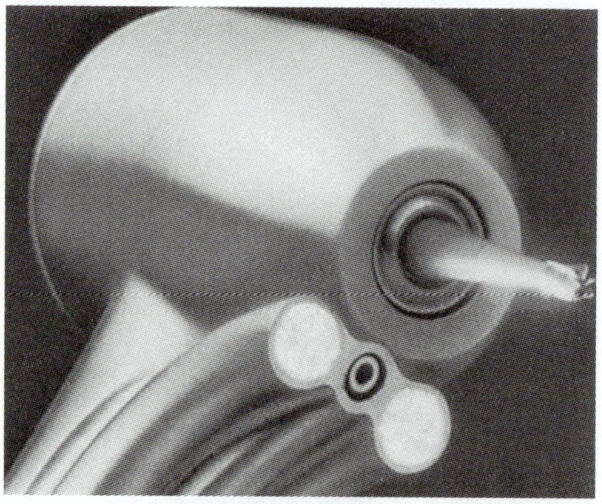

Fig. 35-7 A fiberoptic light provides better illumination of an area for the operator.

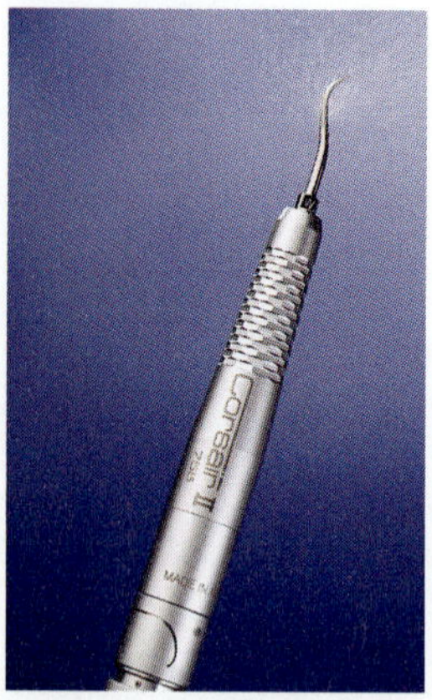

Fig. 35-8 Ultrasonic handpiece. (Courtesy A-dec.)

scaling instruments. A specific tip is selected depending on the surface and location of its use. When activated, the ultrasonic handpiece delivers a pulsating spray of water, causing the calculus and stain or the bonding agent to break down for easier removal.

Laser Handpiece

Instead of rotary instruments, the laser handpiece uses a beam of laser light to cauterize soft tissue or vaporize decayed tooth structure (Fig. 35-9). The laser handpiece resembles the standard handpiece and has many similar qualities, such as water and air to cool the tooth and keep the area clean. The laser, however, is operated through a fiberoptic cable extending from the **console** to the laser handpiece.

Using a laser handpiece has many benefits over the traditional handpiece or surgical instruments. Laser treatment is usually painless, so anesthesia is unnecessary. Dentists do not have to wait for the patient to "get numb" before proceeding.

Disadvantages of using the laser at this time include (1) the laser cannot be used on teeth with restorations already in place, and (2) laser procedures can take longer than conventional methods.

Precautions in the Care and Handling of Laser Handpieces*

Do not sharply bend or twist the fiberoptic cable. The cable could break and burn during use, resulting in injury to the user or patient.

Do not touch the exposed fiberoptic cable. Dirt and fingerprints can damage the cable.

Do not touch the end of the fiberoptic cable connector. The end connector contains a small optical fiber that may degrade if contaminated.

Keep the connecting parts clean.

*Follow these precautions to avoid damage to the fiberoptic cables and laser handpiece.

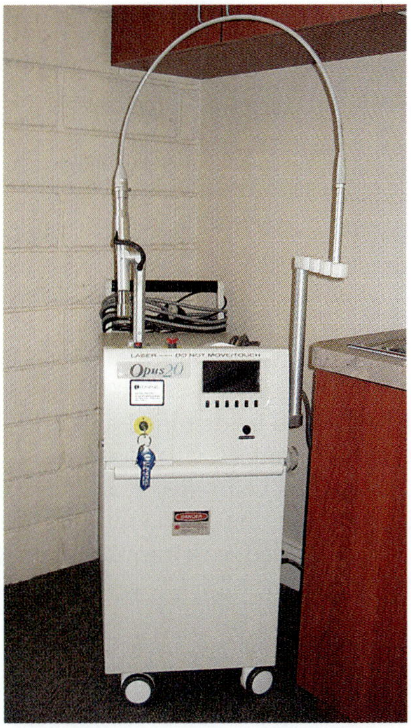

Fig. 35-9 Laser unit.

Air Abrasion Handpiece

The air abrasion unit, a small version of the sandblaster, was introduced to dentistry in the 1940s. This unit was designed to remove stains and tooth decay. Air abrasion was not widely recognized by the dental community and seemed to fade out of use. Air abrasion technology has been brought back into the dental practice, however, and has become a patient-friendly approach to restorative dental treatment.

The air abrasion technique allows high-pressure delivery of aluminum oxide particles through a small probe (Fig. 35-10). This unique technology is able to remove enamel, dentin, and restorative materials without compromising healthy tooth structure. Dentists can now conservatively remove diseased enamel and dentin without the use of local anesthesia.

Although not meant to replace conventional rotary instruments, air abrasion is shifting the way teeth are prepared and treated toward a more conservative approach. The air abrasion technique is most effective when used for the following:

- Sealants
- External stain removal
- Class I through class VI preparations
- Endodontic access
- Crown margins
- Preparation of tooth surface for cementation of cast restoration (crown, veneer)

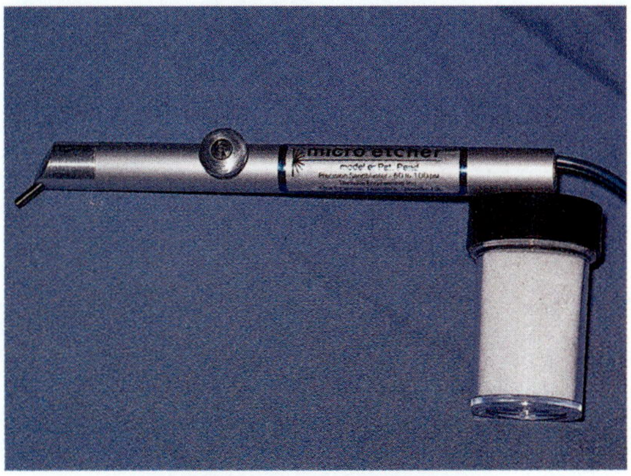

Fig. 35-10 Air abrasion handpiece.

Laboratory Handpiece

The laboratory handpiece is designed for the dental laboratory. This handpiece operates at speeds up to 20,000 rpm and uses laboratory burs of various shapes and sizes. The laboratory handpiece provides greater torque than handpieces used intraorally. **Torque** is a twisting or turning force. The increased torque is better suited to the heavier pressure required during grinding and polishing procedures that take place outside the mouth.

Procedure 35-1 reviews the steps in the identification and the attachment of the various dental handpieces.

Recall

8. On the high-speed handpiece, what helps to illuminate the working field?
9. What type of handpiece resembles a sandblaster?

Handpiece Maintenance

Problems with dental handpieces most often result from improper cleaning and lubrication. Inadequate cleaning of the handpiece before sterilization can result in the collection of debris in the internal parts of the handpiece.

Debris creates wear similar to sludge within an automobile engine. Excessive lubrication is as damaging as inadequate lubrication. Handpieces are also available with ceramic bearings or heads that require no lubrication. If inappropriate cleaning solutions or techniques are used, the working life of the handpiece is significantly shortened. It is imperative to follow the manufacturer's directions for the maintenance of each handpiece.

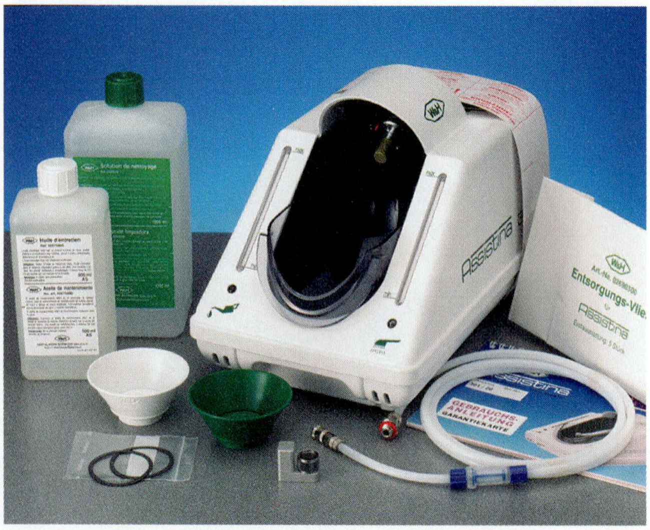

Fig. 35-11 **Lubrication system.** (Courtesy A-dec.)

Failure to do so can result in voiding of the handpiece warranty.

Some types of handpieces require lubrication *before* sterilization, some require lubrication *after* sterilization, and others require lubrication both *before and after* sterilization. You must carefully follow the manufacturer's instructions for the handpiece being sterilized (Fig. 35-11).

General Considerations for Handpiece Sterilization

Wear personal protective equipment (PPE), and follow Universal Precautions. The used handpiece is contaminated and must be handled with appropriate care.

Use mild soap and water, or water alone, to clean debris from the external surface of the handpiece. Disinfectants are neither necessary nor cost-effective because the handpiece will be sterilized. In addition, disinfectants could damage the handpiece.

Clean the internal components of the handpiece according to the manufacturer's instructions. Some manufacturers recommend ultrasonic cleaning; others do not.

Ensure that handpieces are dry before being packaged. Dryness is important to avoid corrosion with autoclave use.

Wrap the handpiece for sterilization according to the type of sterilization and the manufacturer's care instructions.

Sterilize the handpiece according to the manufacturer's instructions. Most manufacturers recommend autoclaving or chemical vapor sterilization.

After sterilization, wipe the light port on the fiberoptic handpieces with an alcohol swab to remove any excess lubricant. The light will be dimmed if any lubricant remains.

Before attaching the sterile handpiece, flush the air and water lines on the handpiece hose for 30 to 60 seconds. Flushing reduces any bioburden that may be sprayed into the patient's oral cavity.

Handpiece Sterilization

The dental handpiece is identified as a *critical instrument* (one that comes in contact with blood, saliva, and tissue) that *must* be sterilized before reuse. Dental handpieces require special considerations for sterilization because blood and saliva may be sucked back into the internal portions of the handpiece.

Sterilization Procedure Sheets

A dental office may acquire handpieces made by different manufacturers over time as handpieces are replaced or new models become available. Sterilization instructions vary

Procedure 35-1 Identifying and Attaching Dental Handpieces

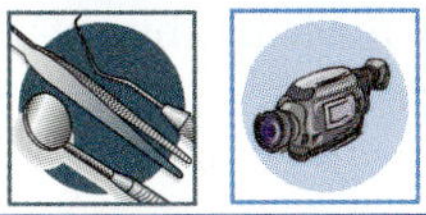

Equipment and Supplies

- Low-speed handpiece
- Straight attachment
- Contra-angle attachment
- Prophylaxis attachment
- High-speed handpiece
- Ultrasonic handpiece

PROCEDURAL STEPS

1. Identify and attach the low-speed handpiece to the dental unit, ensuring that the receptors are aligned and the handpiece fits correctly onto the correct line.

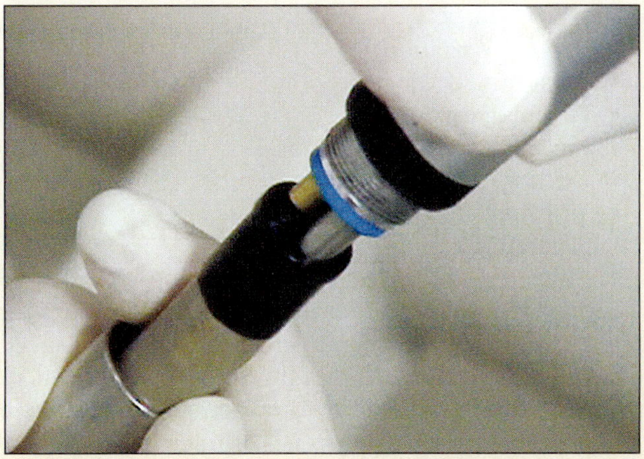

2. Identify and attach the contra-angle attachment onto the straight attachment of the low-speed handpiece, ensuring that the attachment is locked.

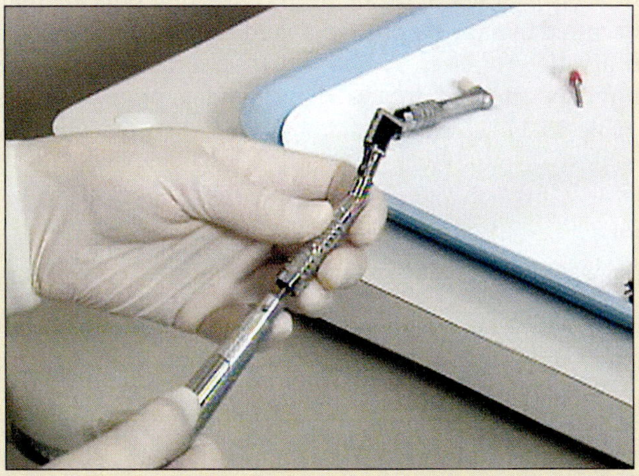

3. Identify and attach the prophylaxis-angle attachment onto the straight attachment of the low-speed handpiece, ensuring that the attachment is locked.

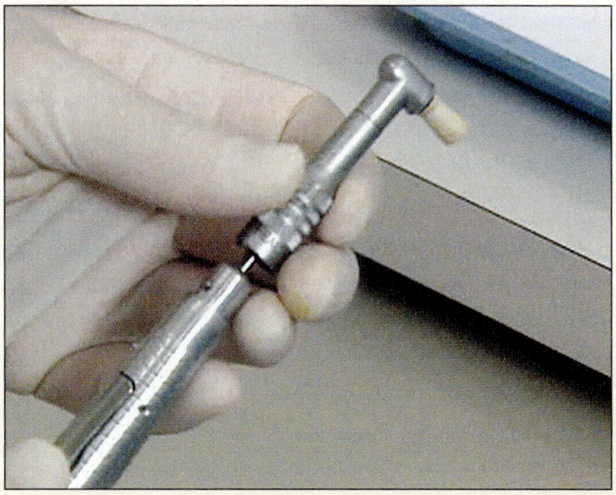

4. Identify and attach the high-speed handpiece to the dental unit, ensuring that the receptors are aligned and the handpiece fits correctly onto the correct line.

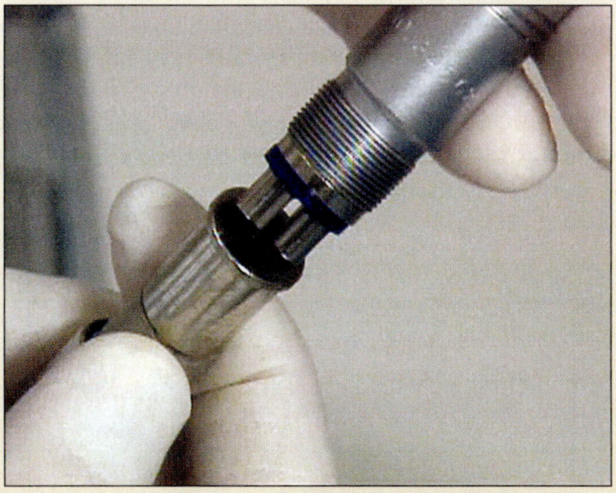

5. Identify and attach the ultrasonic handpiece to the dental unit, ensuring that the receptors are aligned and the handpiece fits correctly onto the correct line.

not only between manufacturers but also between different models made by the same manufacturer.

The use of a sterilization procedure sheet is one way to avoid errors in handpiece sterilization. This practice is particularly helpful if several team members are involved in the process. Sterilization procedure sheets can be created for the dental office by using the information found in each manufacturer's instruction book.

ROTARY CUTTING INSTRUMENTS

Rotary cutting instruments are accessories intended for use with the dental handpiece. Hundreds of different types of rotary instruments are available, and each is designed for a specific use. As with hand instruments, dentists have their preference and will only select a few rotary instruments. Rotary instruments have three basic parts: the shank, neck, and head (Fig. 35-12).

Shank Types

The **shank** of the bur is the portion that fits into the handpiece. Shank length varies according to the specific function of the bur and the handpiece to which it is attached. Rotary instruments are manufactured in three basic shank styles.

- *Straight shank* The long, straight shank is used in the straight-line attachment, which fits on the low-speed handpiece. Straight shanks are held in place by a mechanism within the straight attachment.
- *Latch-type shank* The latch-type shank has a small groove at the end that mechanically locks into the contra-angle attachment, which fits on the low-speed handpiece.
- *Friction-grip shank* The friction-grip shank is short and smooth and has no retention grooves in the end. The shank is held in the high-speed handpiece by the creation of friction that grips the entire shank.

Neck

The neck of the rotary instrument is the narrow portion that connects the shank and the head.

Head

The head of the rotary instrument is the cutting, polishing, or finishing portion. The head is manufactured in a large variety of sizes, shapes, and materials.

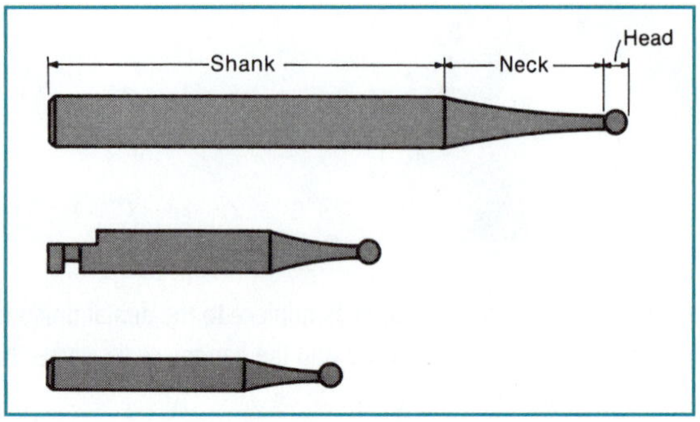

Fig. 35-12 **Bur parts and types of shanks: A, Long straight lab. B, Latch-type. C, Friction grip.** (From Robinson D, Bird D: *Essentials of dental assisting,* ed 3, Philadelphia, 2001, Saunders.)

DENTAL BURS

The term *bur* is applied to all rotary instruments that have a sharp cutting head. Blades make up these cutting surfaces. Burs are needed in restorative dentistry for the following procedures:

- Tooth preparation
- Excavating decay
- Finishing cavity walls
- Finishing restoration surfaces
- Drilling out old fillings
- Finishing crown preparations
- Separating crowns and bridges
- Adjusting and correcting acrylic temporary crowns

Earlier burs were made primarily of steel, but dentists found that using steel burs on enamel at high speeds caused these burs to dull rapidly. Since the late 1940s, a tungsten carbide material has replaced the steel bur for cavity preparation. Tungsten carbide is stiffer and stronger than steel and stays sharp much longer.

Bur Shapes

When discussing the "shape" of a bur, you are referring to the *contour* or *design* of the head of the bur. Burs are manufactured in a variety of shapes, and each shape is available in a variety of sizes. A bur will have a name, a series of numbers attached to the shape, and a purpose of use (Table 35-1).

Recall

10. What type of shank fits into the contra-angle attachment?
11. Restorative burs are made from what material?
12. What design of bur is a 33½?

Table 35-1 *Burs for Restorative Dentistry*

Type of Bur	Series of Numbers	Use	Example
Round 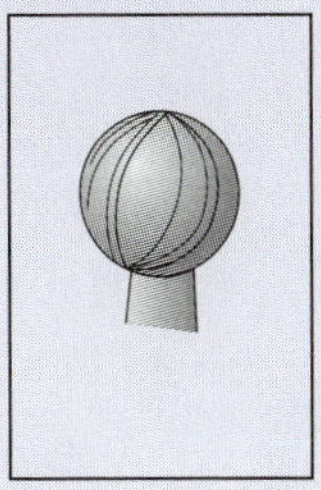	¼, ½, 1-8, 10	• Initial entry into tooth structure • Extends preparation • Retention • Removes decay	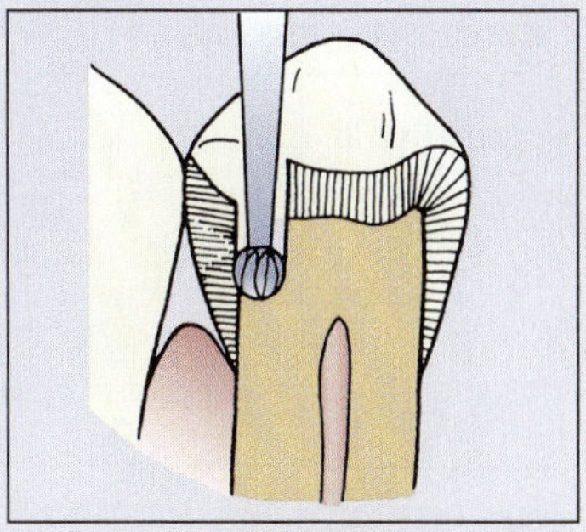
Inverted cone 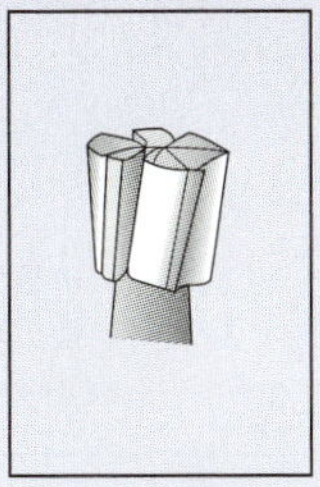	33½, 34-39, 36L, 37L	• Removes decay • Establishes retentive grooves	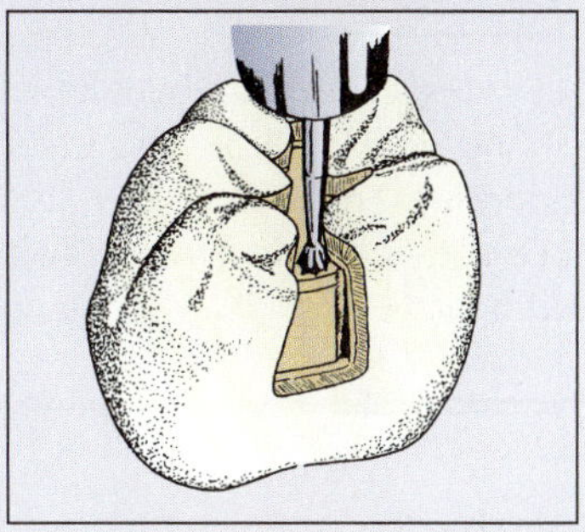
Straight fissure plain cut 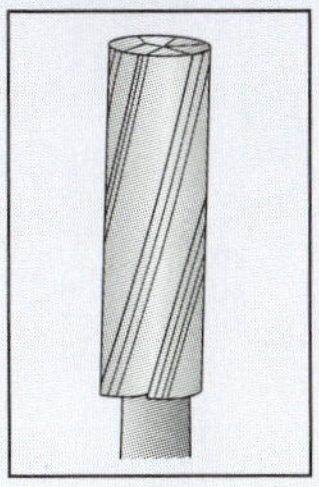	55-60, 57L, 58L	• Initial entry into tooth • Helps in forming the internal walls of the preparation	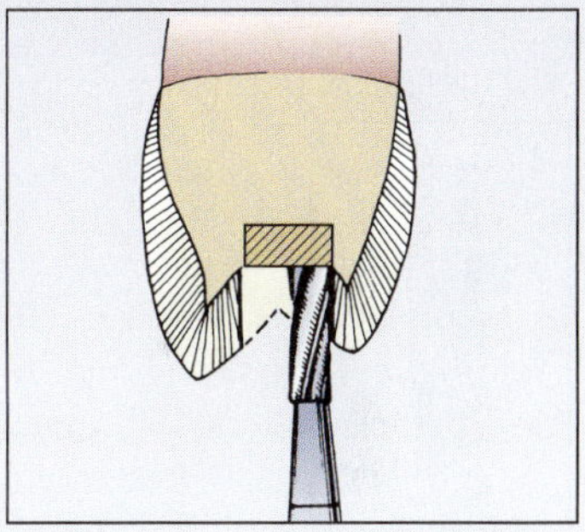
Straight fissure cross cut 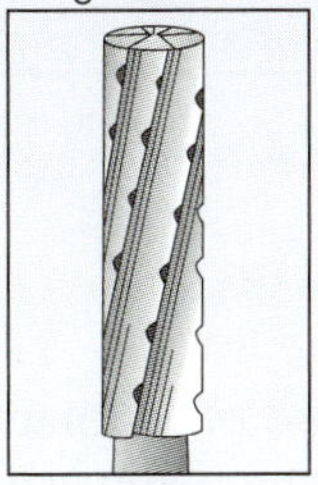	556-560, 567L, 568L	• Helps in forming the internal walls of the preparation	
Tapered fissure plain cut 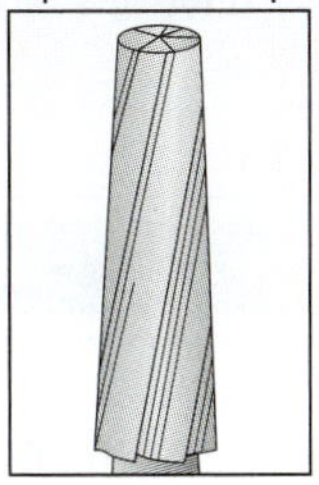	169-172, 169L, 170L, 171L	• Helps in providing angles to the walls of the prepared tooth	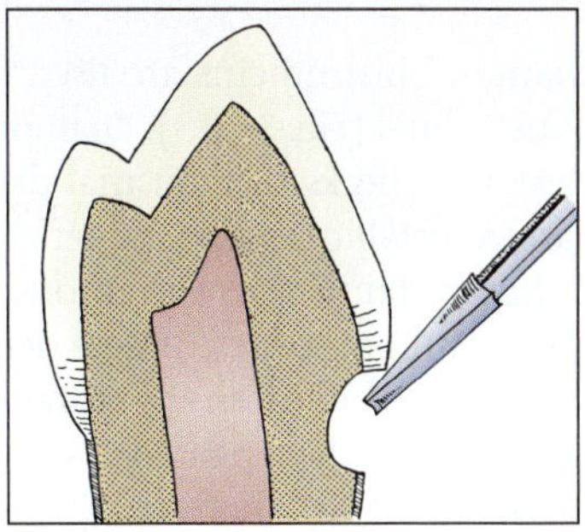

Illustrations in first column from Finkbeiner BL, Johnson CS: Mosby's comprehensive dental assisting, *St Louis, 1995, Mosby.*
Illustrations in last column from Baum L, Phillips RW, Lund MR: Textbook of operative dentistry, *ed 3, Philadelphia, 1995, Saunders.*

continued

Table 35-1 ***Burs for Restorative Dentistry—cont'd***

Type of Bur	Series of Numbers	Use	Example
Tapered fissure cross cut 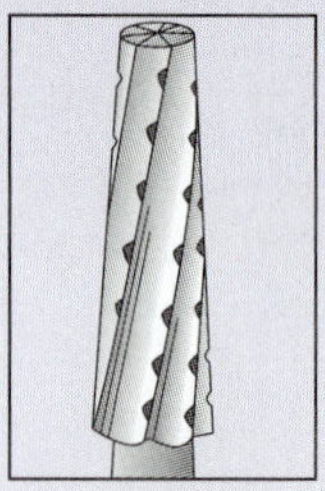	699-703, 699L, 700L, 701L	• Helps in providing angles to the walls of the prepared tooth	
Pear 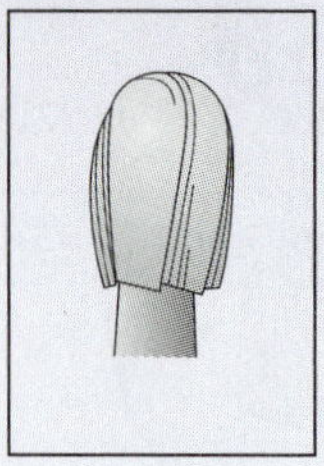	330-333, 331L	• Initial entry into tooth structure • Extends preparation	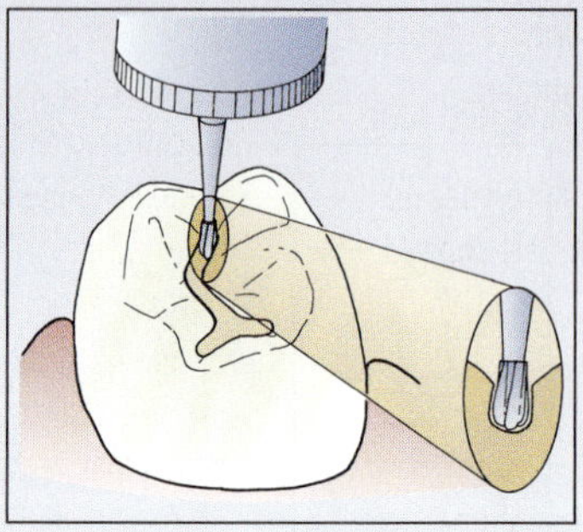
End cutting 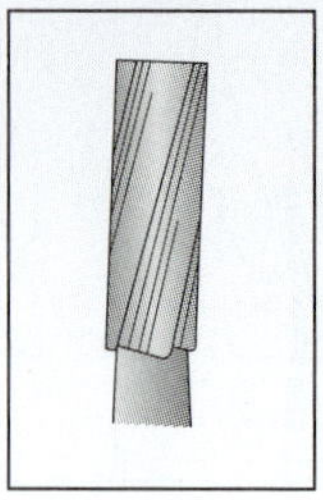	957, 958	• Initial entry into tooth structure • Creates a shoulder for the margin of a crown preparation	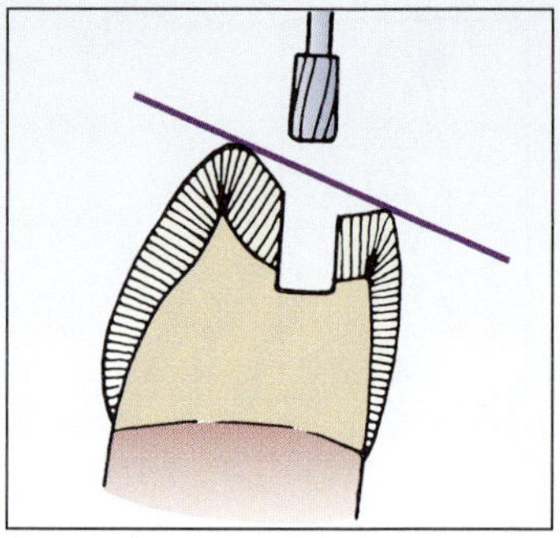

Illustrations in first column from Finkbeiner BL, Johnson CS: Mosby's comprehensive dental assisting, *St Louis, 1995, Mosby.*
Illustrations in last column from Baum L, Phillips RW, Lund MR: Textbook of operative dentistry, *ed 3, Philadelphia, 1995, Saunders.*

DIAMOND ROTARY INSTRUMENTS

Diamond instruments are used for many of the same functions as burs (Fig. 35-13). Diamond instruments have a metal base, with flecks of industrial diamonds embedded into the base. A metallic bonding material holds the bits onto the base.

Many dentists use diamond rotary instruments as an important part of restorative dentistry. This is because their *cutting ability* shortens preparation time and increases productivity. With repeated use and sterilization, however, *debonding* of the diamond particles occurs, decreasing the cutting efficiency of the diamond.

Diamond burs are manufactured in a range of *grit* (coarseness) classifications to allow selection of the proper grit and cutting rate for each phase of restorative dentistry. To identify the various grits, some manufacturers use a letter designation at the end of the bur number to indicate the grit or cutting rate. Others have a color-coded band on the bur.

FINISHING ROTARY INSTRUMENTS

A finishing bur is similar in appearance to the cutting bur, except the number of blades, or **flutes,** in the working end of a finishing bur is increased. The greater the number of cutting surfaces on the head of a bur, the greater the polishing capability.

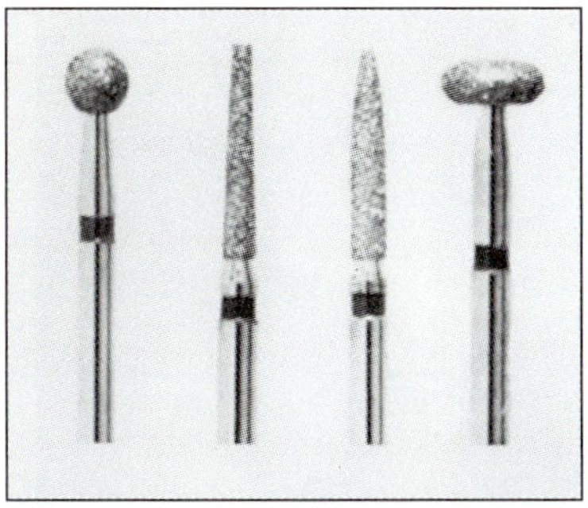

Fig. 35-13

Design	**Purpose**
Round	Provide access to pulp chamber
Tapered cylinder	Adjust and shape occlusal and lingual surfaces
Cylinder	Prepare crown
	Smooth and finish cavity walls
Flame-shaped	Extend small fissures
Wheel-shaped	Make subgingival finish lines (bevels) in crown preparation
	Reduce lingual surface for anterior crown preparations
	Make gross reductions of incisal edges
Disc-shaped	Adjust and shape occlusal surfaces
	Remove tooth structure
	Cut through fixed prostheses

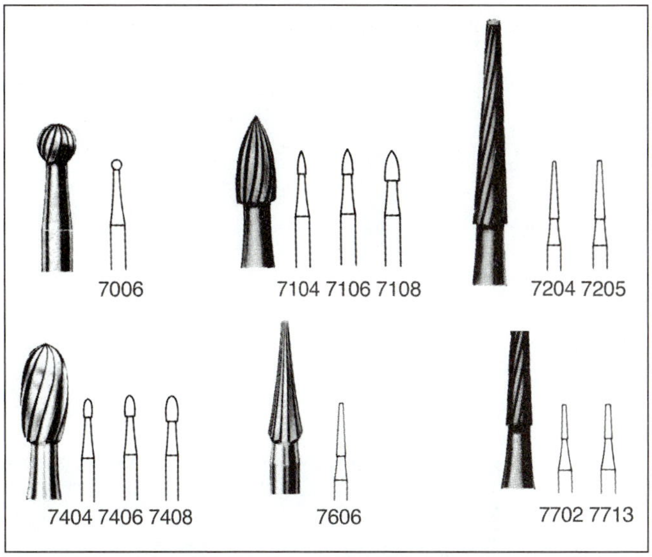

Fig. 35-14 **Finishing burs.** (Courtesy Miltex, Inc, York, Pennsylvania.)

In your studies of esthetic materials, you will find that these materials require a final stage of polishing with a finishing bur. The designs of a finishing bur resemble the carbide bur. The most common finishing bur shapes are round, tapered, and flame-shaped (Fig. 35-14).

ABRASIVE ROTARY INSTRUMENTS

Abrasive rotary instruments are the most varied of the rotary instruments. Many types of abrasive material are applied to many shapes to create a flexible working surface that can be adapted to the contour of the tooth or restoration. The abrasive materials are made in shapes ranging from discs and stones to points and strips (Fig. 35-15).

Accessories

Abrasive discs and wheels are supplied separately and not attached to a shank. Because of this, a **mandrel** (a metal shaft on which a sandpaper disc or other abrasive materials are mounted) is used to attach these abrasives to the dental handpiece (Fig. 35-16).

Mandrels are designed according to the different types of shank so that they may be used in both low-speed and high-speed handpieces.

LABORATORY ROTARY INSTRUMENTS

Laboratory burs are easy to distinguish from dental burs because of their size. Laboratory burs have a longer shank and a larger head than dental burs.

Laboratory burs are used in the low-speed handpiece for functions such as cutting and polishing of acrylic. The *acrylic bur* is the most common bur used in the laboratory. As with other types of burs, the heads of the acrylic bur come in various shapes for a specific use (Fig. 35-17).

Procedure 35-2 reviews steps in the identification and attachment of burs for rotary dental instruments.

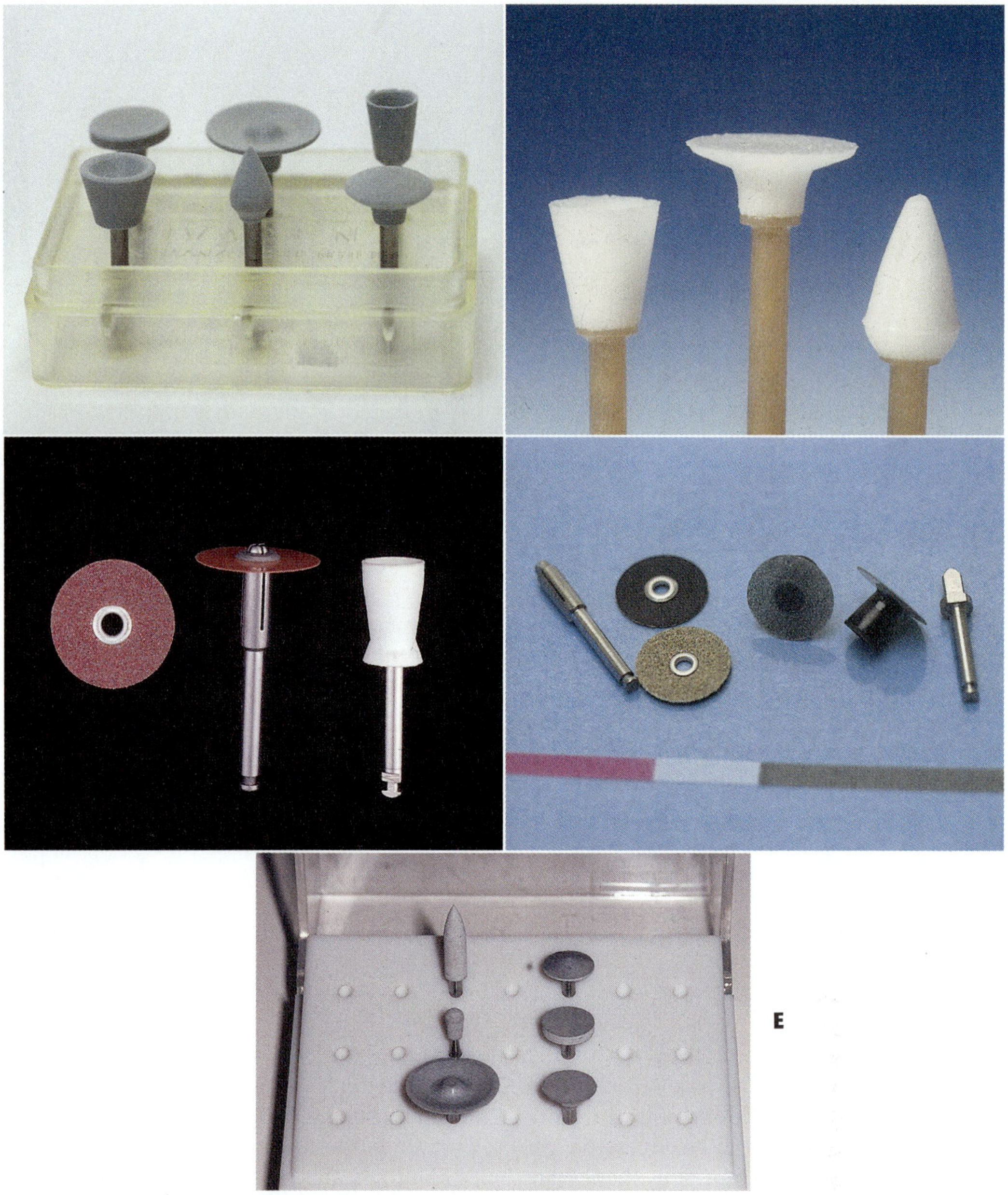

Fig. 35-15 Abrasive materials for rotary instruments. **A,** *Silicon carbide* produces a moderately rough surface. It is available in wheels, points, and stones, and the color varies from gray-green to black. It is used for polishing metal restorations. **B,** *Garnet* is a reddish abrasive most often adhered to discs. It produces a coarse to medium-fine finish. It is used in the beginning stages of finishing a restoration. **C,** *Cuttlebone* is most often adhered to discs and points. It is used for final finishing and polishing of the restoration. **D,** *Sandpaper* is sand particles adhered to flexible paper discs or strips as a medium abrasive. It is used for finishing and polishing a restoration. **E,** *Carborundum* particles adhered to disc. As with carborundum on burs, it is used to cut or separate one structure from another.

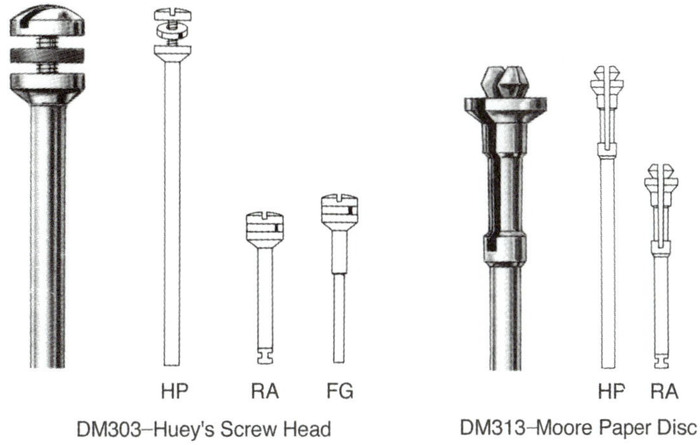

Fig. 35-16 Types of mandrels. (Courtesy Miltex, Inc, York, Pennsylvania.)

Procedure 35-2 Identifying and Attaching Burs for Rotary Cutting Instruments

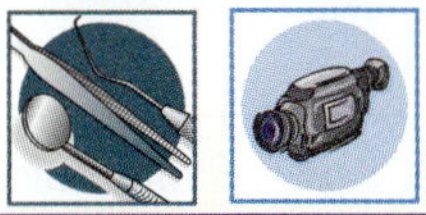

Equipment and Supplies

- Various types of dental rotary instruments, including carborundum, diamond, finishing, abrasives, and laboratory burs.
- Low-speed handpiece
- High-speed handpiece
- Contra-angle attachment
- Mandrel

PROCEDURAL STEPS

1. Identify specific dental burs, such as carborundum, diamond, finishing, and abrasion burs, by their name and number sequence.
2. Attach latch-type burs to the contra-angle attachment on the low-speed handpiece, ensuring that the bur is locked in place.

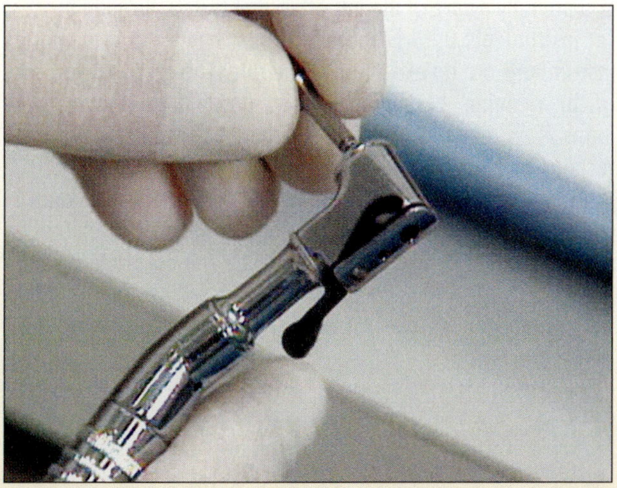

3. Attach friction-grip bur to the high-speed handpiece, ensuring that the bur is locked in place.
4. Attach abrasive discs to the mandrel correctly by screwing to tighten or by positioning the metal opening onto the mandrel, ensuring that the disc is securely locked.

Recall

13. What gives the diamond bur its advantage?
14. Finishing burs are used on what type of dental material?
15. What is used to hold a disc in the handpiece?

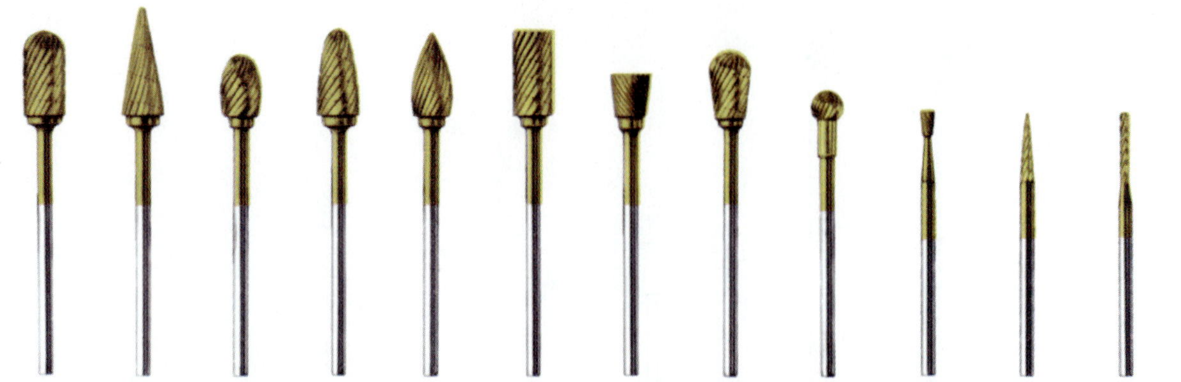

Fig. 35-17 Varying shapes of a laboratory acrylic bur. (Courtesy Miltex, Inc, York, Pennsylvania.)

Legal and Ethical Implications

You are fully aware of the importance of the sterilization process for instruments used intraorally. Dental handpieces and rotary instruments are no exception to the rule. The care that you take in the cleaning, packaging, and sterilization process of these items is an essential step in preventing the transmission of infectious diseases.

Great emphasis has been placed on the internal makeup of dental handpieces and the way infectious blood and bioburden remain inside a contaminated handpiece and on a rotary instrument. Steps taken to decrease the patient's risk of infection reflect both the legal guidelines for dentistry and the philosophy of the dental practice.

Eye to the Future

Patients will have their teeth prepared, finished, and polished exclusively by lasers and air abrasion handpieces in the future. Technologic advancements will allow these handpieces to be used without patient anesthesia.

New technology will dramatically change the roles of the dental team. The dental assistant and dental hygienist will perform more traditional and conservative dental treatment while the dentist focuses on more advanced and serious problems.

Critical Thinking

1. You are setting up the dental hygiene room for a patient. What dental handpieces and accessories would be assembled for a prophylactic procedure?
2. While setting up the treatment room in preparation for a restorative appointment, you notice that the #2 round bur has dried blood on it. What do you do with the bur, and what caused this?
3. The dentist has just completed restoring tooth #7. Because this is an anterior tooth, how would the dental material be finished and polished?
4. A patient who received a new denture yesterday has returned in pain. The dentist tells the patient that the denture must be adjusted to fit better. Describe how you would set up the low-speed handpiece with a laboratory-type acrylic bur.
5. It is 11 A.M., and you have a patient seated for a restorative procedure. You notice that you have depleted the supply of clean handpieces because of the emergency patients seen earlier. What do you do?

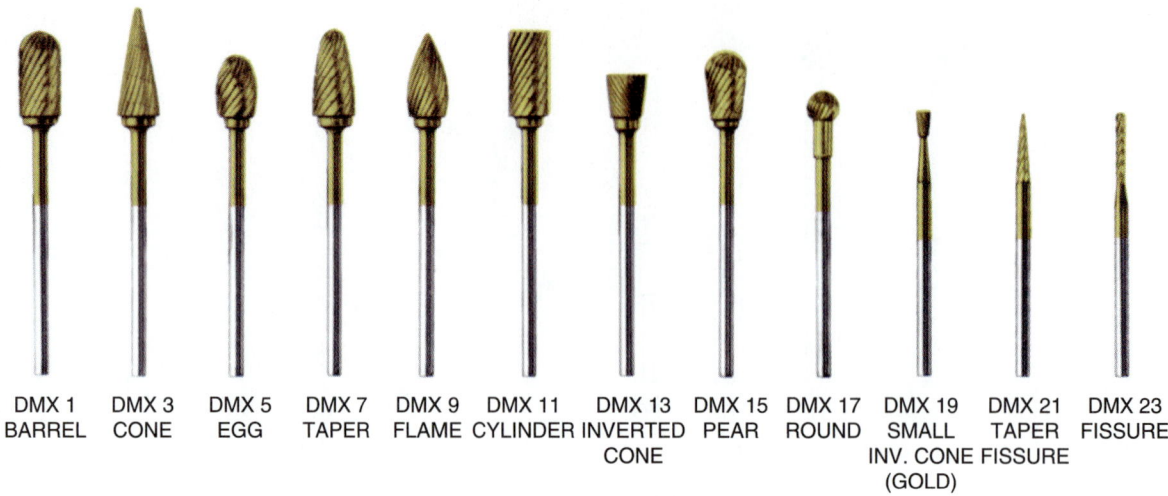

36

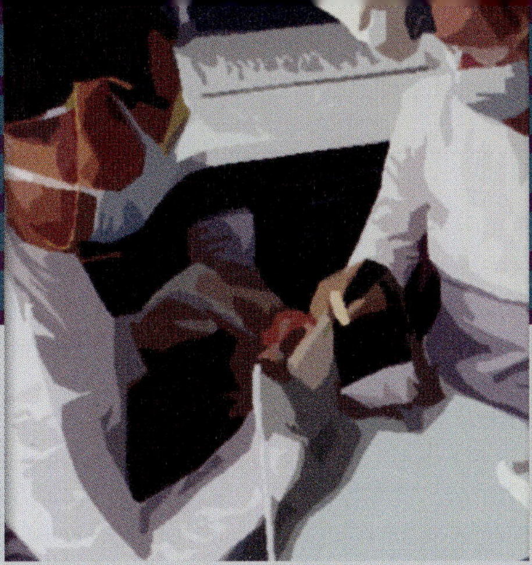

Moisture Control

Outline

KEY TERMS

Aspirate (**as**-puh-**rate**) To draw back or to draw within.

Beveled (**be**-vuld, **bev**-uld) Characterized by an angle of a surface that meets another angle.

Bow Rounded part of clamp that extends through the dental dam.

Exposed Pertaining to selected teeth visible through the dam; *isolated.*

Invert (in-**vert**) To reverse the position, order, or condition. To turn inside out or upside down.

Isolated Pertaining to selected teeth visible through the dam; *exposed.*

Jaws Part of a clamp that is shaped into four prongs to help stabilize the clamp on the tooth.

Malaligned (*mal*-eh-**lined**) Displaced out of line, especially teeth displaced from normal relation to the line of the dental arch; also called *malposed.*

Septum (**sep**-tuhm) Dental dam material located between the holes of the punched dam.

Stylus (**sti**-lus) Sharp, pointed tool used for cutting.

Universal Pertaining to the same clamp that can be placed on the same type of tooth in the opposite quadrant.

Winged clamp Type of dental dam clamp with extensions to help retain the dental dam.

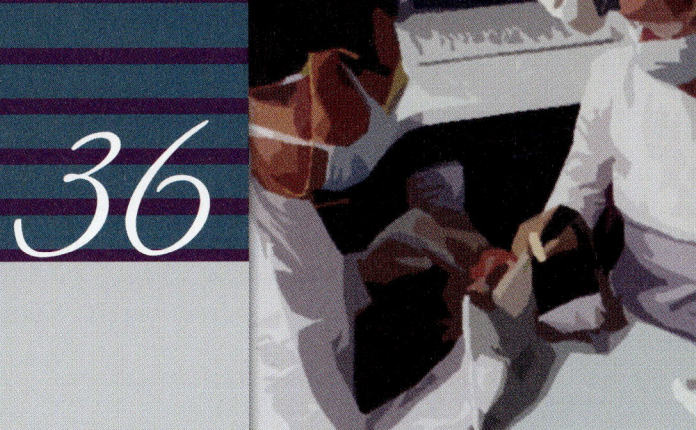

LEARNING OUTCOMES

On completion of this chapter, the student will be able to achieve the following objectives:

- Define and spell the Key Terms.
- List isolation techniques used to decrease moisture during a dental procedure.
- Describe the two types of oral evacuation systems used in dentistry.
- Describe the grasp and positioning of the high-volume evacuator tip.
- Discuss the use of the air-water syringe.
- Describe the dental dam and its role in moisture control.
- List the equipment and supplies for dental dam application.
- Describe the special preparation and placement of the dental dam.

PERFORMANCE OUTCOMES

On completion of this chapter, the student will be able to meet competency standards in the following skills:

- Perform the grasp and positioning of the high-volume evacuator during a procedure.
- Perform limited-area and full-mouth rinses.
- Place cotton rolls for isolation.
- Identify the equipment and supplies used for dental dam application.
- Have the dental dam prepared correctly for a procedure.
- Place the dental dam as an expanded function.
- Remove the dental dam as an expanded function.

When assisting in a dental procedure, one of the most important responsibilities of the chairside dental assistant is to maintain moisture control during a procedure. The assistant keeps the operating field free of excess water, saliva, blood, tooth fragments, and excess dental materials.

This chapter describes several moisture-control techniques and their incorporation into the dental procedure.

ORAL EVACUATION SYSTEMS

The term *oral evacuation* describes the process of removing excess fluid and debris from the mouth. The use of an oral evacuator completes this process before, during, and after a dental procedure. The two types of evacuators most often used in a dental procedure are the *saliva ejector* and the *high-volume evacuator.*

Saliva Ejector

The saliva ejector is a small, straw-shaped oral evacuator that is used during less-invasive dental procedures (Fig. 36-1). The main function of the ejector's vacuum is to remove liquids from the mouth; it is not powerful enough to remove solid debris.

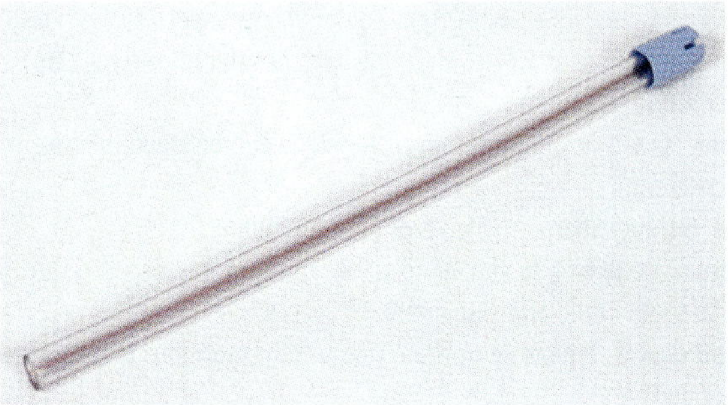

Fig. 36-1 Saliva ejector.

The saliva ejector is made from soft plastic tubing that can be shaped for easy placement in the oral cavity. The ejector can be used (1) by holding it throughout the procedure, using repeated sweeps of the mouth to remove fluids or (2) by positioning the suction in the mouth during a procedure.

To place the saliva ejector in a stationary position, bend and form the tubing into the shape of a candy cane (Fig. 36-2). This shape allows the saliva ejector to be positioned under the tongue, where most fluids will accumulate. When placing the saliva ejector, insert a cotton roll to act as a buffer for the saliva ejector so that it will not traumatize oral tissues. When positioning the saliva ejector for a procedure, place it

Indications for Using the Saliva Ejector

Preventive procedures, such as prophylactic placement of sealants or fluoride treatments

Control of saliva and moisture accumulation under the dental dam

Cementation of crown and bridge prostheses

Orthodontic bonding procedures

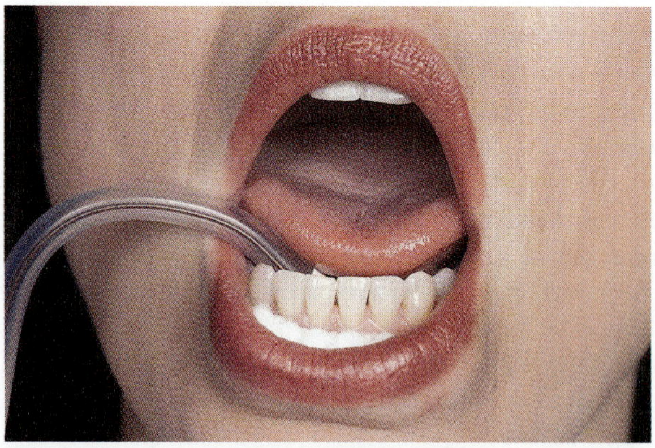

Fig. 36-2 Saliva ejector placed under the tongue for a procedure.

opposite the side on which the dentist is working to reduce the number of items in the operating field.

High-Volume Evacuator

The high-volume evacuator (HVE) is used to remove saliva, blood, water, and debris during a dental procedure. The HVE system, also known as the *oral evacuator,* works on a vacuum principle that is similar to that of a household vacuum cleaner. It is able to take up water and debris, because a high volume of air is moved into the vacuum hose at a low pressure to create the strong suction. The HVE has the three main purposes:

- To keep the mouth free of saliva, blood, water, and debris
- To retract the tongue and cheek away from the field of operation
- To reduce the bacterial aerosol caused by the high-speed handpiece

Suction Tips

Oral evacuation tips for the HVE system are designed to accommodate different types of procedures (Fig. 36-3).

Operative suction tips are larger in circumference and are designed with a straight or slight angle in the middle. Each end has a **beveled** (having a surface angle that meets another angle) working end so that the tip can be positioned parallel to the site for better suction. Most HVE tips are made of a durable plastic and are disposed of after a single use. Tips also are available in stainless steel or reusable plastic, but must be sterilized before reuse.

Surgical suction tips are much smaller in circumference. This design is critical to placement within the surgical site, which is typically more limited in size and visibility. The concern in a surgical procedure is the removal of blood, tissue, and debris rather than a large amount of water and fluid. Surgical tips are made of stainless steel and are part of the surgical setup. Refer to Chapter 56 for further discussion.

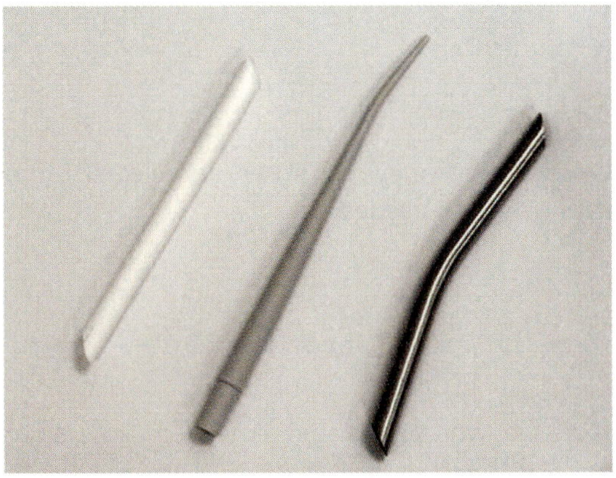

Fig. 36-3 High-volume evacuator suction tips.

Grasping the Evacuator

The HVE may be held in the *thumb-to-nose grasp* or the *pen grasp* (Fig. 36-4). Either method provides the dental assistant with control of the tip, which is necessary for patient comfort and safety.

Positioning the Evacuator

Depending on the resistance of the tissue to retract and the area being treated, you may want to alternate between positioning of the evacuator. When assisting a right-handed dentist, the assistant grasps the evacuator in the right hand. When assisting a left-handed dentist, the assistant grasps the evacuator in the left hand. The hand not holding the suction is free to operate the air-water syringe or participate in the transfer of instruments to the dentist as needed. HVE positions in this chapter are for a right-handed dentist (Procedure 36-1).

As a dental assistant, you must understand your role in placing and operating the oral evacuation system (Fig. 36-5). The timing of when suction is used, when the HVE is positioned, and when suction is removed from the mouth is critical to the efficient and effective performance of the procedure.

Specific guidelines for positioning the high-volume evacuator are:

- Place the evacuator before the dentist positions the handpiece and mouth mirror.
- Position the suction tip on the surface of the tooth that is closest to you.
- Position the tip close to the tooth being treated.
- Position the bevel of the suction tip so that it is parallel to the tooth surface.
- Keep the edge of the suction tip even with or slightly beyond the occlusal surface or incisal edge.

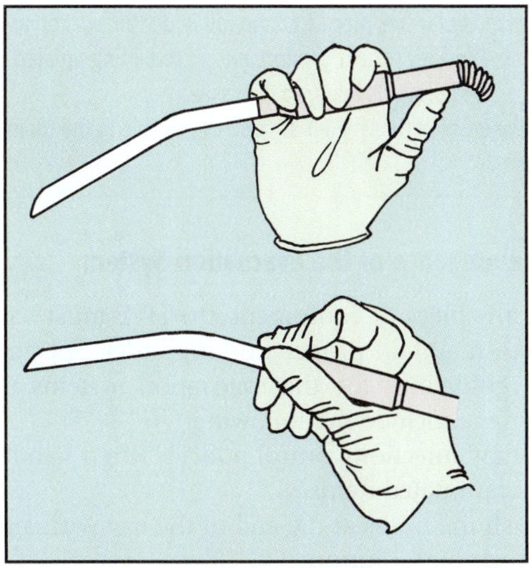

Fig. 36-4 Grasps used for operating the high-volume evacuator. *Top,* thumb to nose grasp; *bottom,* pen grasp.

Procedure 36-1 Positioning the High-Volume Evacuator during a Procedure

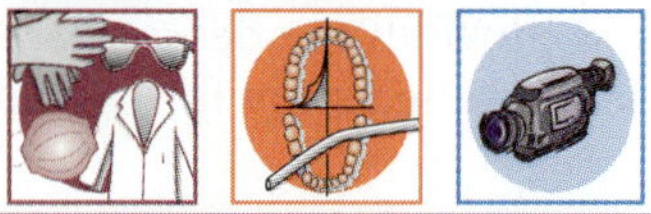

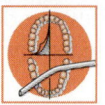

Equipment and Supplies

- Sterile HVE tip
- Plastic barrier cover for HVE handle and hose
- Cotton rolls

PROCEDURAL STEPS

1. Place the HVE tip in the holder by pushing the end of the tip into the holder through the plastic barrier.
   Purpose: Leaves the opposite end exposed and ready for use.
2. If necessary, use the HVE tip or a mouth mirror to gently retract the cheek or tongue.

POSTERIOR PLACEMENT

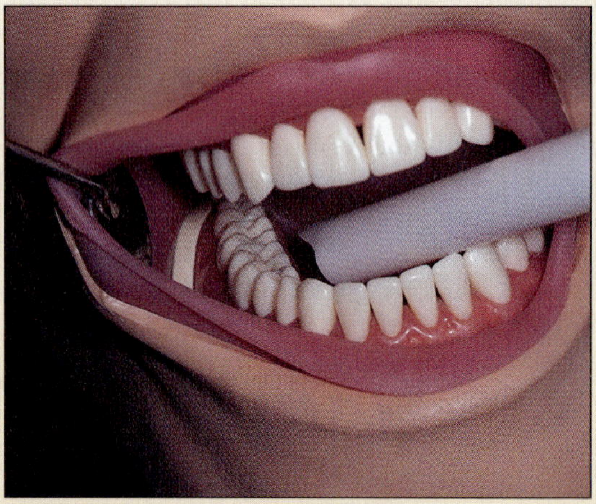

1. For a mandibular site, place a cotton roll under the suction tip.
   Purpose: Provides patient comfort, aids in stabilizing tip placement, and prevents injury to the tissues.
2. Place the bevel of the HVE tip as close as possible to the tooth being prepared.
   Purpose: Suction will draw the water into the tip immediately after it leaves the tooth being prepared.
3. Position the bevel of the HVE tip parallel to the buccal or lingual surface of the tooth being prepared.
4. Place the upper edge of the HVE tip so that it extends slightly beyond the occlusal surface.
   Purpose: Suction will catch the water spray from the handpiece as it leaves the tooth being prepared.

ANTERIOR PLACEMENT

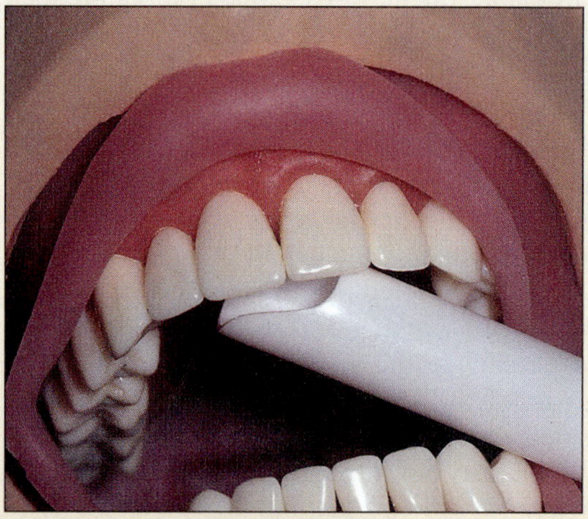

1. When the dentist is preparing the tooth from the *lingual* aspect, position the HVE tip so that it is parallel to the facial surface and slightly beyond the incisal edge.
2. When the dentist is preparing the tooth from the *facial* aspect, position the HVE tip parallel to the lingual surface and slightly beyond the incisal edge.

Daily Maintenance of the Evacuation System

As with any piece of equipment, the HVE must have daily upkeep to maintain proper working order. Specific maintenance guidelines for the evacuation systems and air-water syringe include the following:

- Follow infection-control policies when handling contaminated items.
- Flush the hoses at the end of the day with an antimicrobial solution.
- Check the disposable traps weekly, and replace if needed.
- Open the saliva ejector hoses, and clean or replace the screens as needed.

Recall

1. What are the two types of evacuators used in operative dental procedures?
2. What is the main function of the saliva ejector?
3. What are operative suction tips made of?

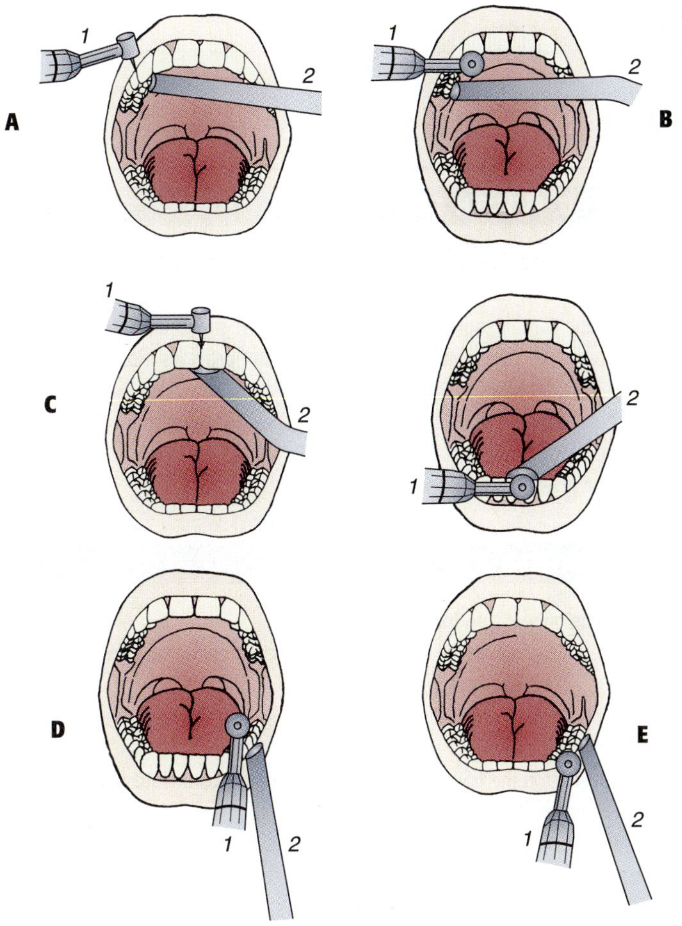

Fig. 36-5 Operator and assistant positions in high-volume evacuation. **A,** Maxillary right buccal/mandibular occlusal surface. *1,* Operator's position with handpiece is buccal or occlusal; *2,* Assistant's position with suction tip is lingual. **B,** Maxillary lingual/mandibular right surface. *1,* Operator's position with handpiece is lingual; *2,* Assistant's position with suction tip is lingual. **C,** Maxillary central incisors/mandibular central incisors. *1,* Operator's position with handpiece is facial or lingual; *2,* Assistant's position with suction tip is lingual or facial. **D,** Maxillary lingual/mandibular left occlusal surface. *1,* Operator's position with handpiece is lingual; *2,* Assistant's position with suction tip is buccal. **E,** Maxillary left buccal/mandibular left buccal surface. *1,* Operator's position with handpiece is buccal; *2,* Assistant's position with suction tip is buccal.

RINSING THE ORAL CAVITY

Frequent rinsing of the oral cavity maintains a clear operating field for the dentist and keeps the patient comfortable. Rinsing also removes debris from the patient's mouth before dismissal. The two basic types of rinsing procedures used in dentistry are limited-area rinsing and complete mouth rinsing, also referred to as a full-mouth rinse (Procedure 36-2).

Limited-Area Rinsing

This is performed frequently throughout a procedure as debris accumulates during the preparation and restoration of a tooth. This rinsing must be accomplished quickly and efficiently without causing any delay in the procedure. Limited-area rinsing is frequently accomplished when the dentist exits the mouth and pauses for inspection.

Full-Mouth Rinsing

The full-mouth rinse is used when the patient's entire mouth needs freshening. Complete mouth rinsing may be done after a long restorative procedure, after the dental prophylaxis, or before patient dismissal following any dental procedure.

The saliva ejector can be used as an alternative to the HVE in the complete mouth rinse procedure when the assistant performs this alone.

Air-Water Syringe

To complete the rinsing process, the air-water syringe is used for convenience and accuracy. As described in Chapter 32, the air-water syringe is connected to the dental unit and provides a means of air, water, or a combination through a small sterile tip. The attached disposable tip can be positioned for the maxillary and mandibular arches by directing the end toward the specific arch.

Recall

4. What type of rinsing technique is performed throughout a procedure?

Guidelines for Using the Air-Water Syringe

Direct the syringe tip toward the tooth being treated.

Keep a close distance between the operative site and the syringe tip. Being too far away from the working site will cause aerosol to be splattered.

Use the air on the mouth mirror continuously when indirect vision is involved.

When you hear the handpiece stop, rinse and dry the site.

When completing a limited-area or full-mouth rinse, move the tip while spraying the area.

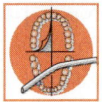

Procedure 36-2 Performing a Mouth Rinse

Equipment and Supplies

- HVE tip
- Saliva ejector
- Air-water syringe

PROCEDURAL STEPS

1. Decide which oral evacuation system would be best for the rinsing procedure.
2. Grasp the air-water syringe in your left hand and the HVE or saliva ejector in your right hand.

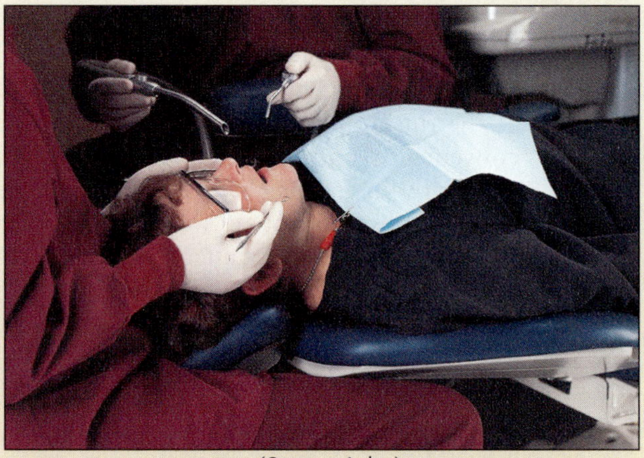

(Courtesy A-dec.)

LIMITED-MOUTH RINSE

1. Turn on the suction, and position the tip toward the site for a limited-area rinse.
2. Spray the combination of air and water onto the site to be rinsed.
   Purpose: The combination of the air and water provides more force to clean the area thoroughly.
3. Suction all fluid and debris from the area, being sure to remove all fluids.
4. Dry the area by pressing the air button only.

FULL-MOUTH RINSE

1. Have the patient turn toward you.
   Purpose: Turning the head allows the water to pool on one side, making it easier for you to suction.
2. Turn on the HVE or saliva ejector and position it in the vestibule of the patient's left side.
   Note: Position the tip carefully so that it does not come into contact with soft tissue.
3. With the HVE or saliva ejector tip positioned, direct the air-water syringe from the patient's maxillary right across to the left side, spraying all surfaces.
4. Continue down to the mandibular arch, following the same sequence from right to left.
   Purpose: This pattern of rinsing forces the debris to the posterior mouth, where the suction tip is positioned for easier removal of fluids and debris.

ISOLATION OF TEETH

For optimum results in a dental procedure, a tooth, quadrant, or even the entire arch must be kept dry and isolated from its normal environment. For ideal conditions of a dental procedure, the following features should characterize the isolation technique:

- Easy to apply
- Protective of the soft and hard tissues
- Comfortable for the patient
- Retraction provides better visualization for the operator
- Prevention of moisture contamination
- Isolation of the area of concern

Various techniques are used to isolate a specific area of the mouth. The three most common isolation methods use (1) cotton roll isolation, (2) dry angles, and (3) the dental dam. The clinical situation will dictate which isolation technique is best suited for the procedure.

Cotton Roll Isolation

Cotton roll isolation is the use of tightly formed absorbent cotton preshaped to be positioned close to the salivary gland ducts to absorb the flow of saliva and close to the working field to absorb excess water (Fig. 36-6). Cotton roll isolation is the most common type of isolation used for short procedures, such as examinations, application of sealants, cementation of castings, and simple restorations (Procedure 36-3).

Cotton Roll Holders

Cotton roll holders are designed to hold multiple cotton rolls in a more secure manner for the mandibular quadrant (Fig. 36-7). Holders are especially important when the operator is working alone, without an extra hand to maintain isolation.

A metal prong is slid into each cotton roll. The rolls are then seated with one roll positioned on the buccal side and the other on the lingual side. A sliding bar is attached to the base of the holder. After being positioned under the

Using Cotton Rolls

Advantages

Easy application

No additional equipment is required

Cotton rolls are available in a variety of sizes and are flexible for easy adaptability to areas of the mouth

Disadvantages

Does not provide complete isolation

Does not protect the patient from aspiration

If removed improperly, a dry cotton roll may stick to the oral mucosa and cause injury

Cotton rolls must be replaced frequently because of saturation

Limited retraction

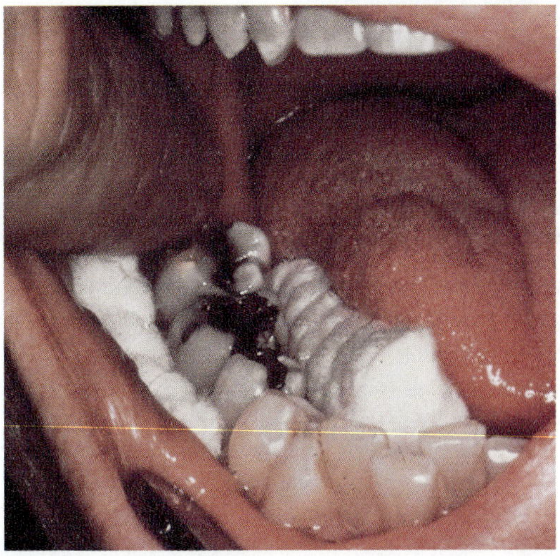

Fig. 36-6 Cotton roll isolation in the mandibular quadrant.

Procedure 36-3 Placing and Removing Cotton Rolls

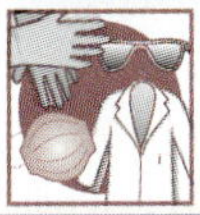

Equipment and Supplies

- Basic setup
- Cotton rolls
- Air-water syringe

MAXILLARY PLACEMENT

1. Have the patient turn toward you with the chin raised.
   Purpose: Provides better visualization and easier placement of cotton roll.

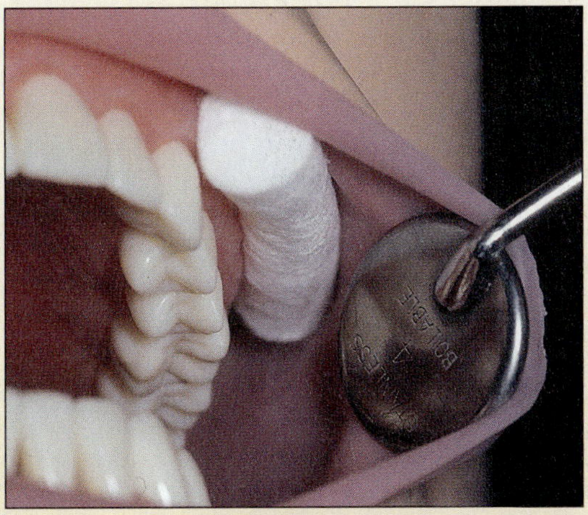

2. Using the cotton pliers, pick up a cotton roll so that it is positioned evenly with the beaks of the cotton pliers.
3. Transfer the cotton roll to the mouth, and position it securely in the mucobuccal fold closest to the working field.
   Note: Once you place the cotton roll with the pliers, you may want to use your finger to push the cotton roll farther into the mucobuccal fold.

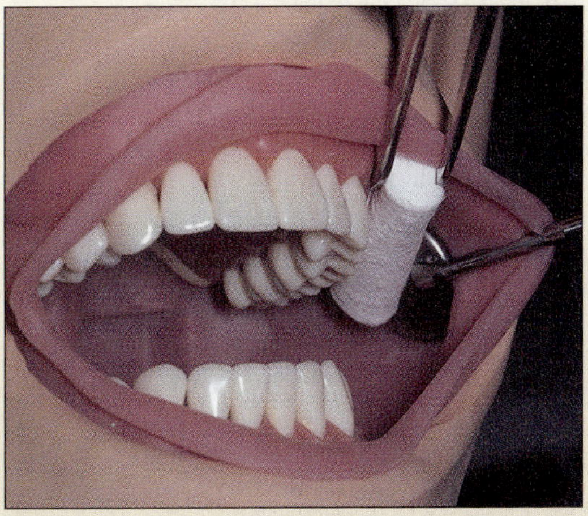

4. This placement can be used for any location on the maxillary arch.

continued

Procedure 36-3 Placing and Removing Cotton Rolls—cont'd

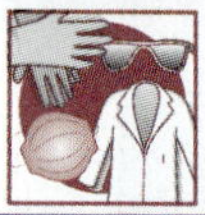

MANDIBULAR PLACEMENT

1. Have the patient turn toward you with the chin lowered.
   Purpose: Provides better visualization and ease in the placement of the cotton roll.
2. Using the cotton pliers, pick up a cotton roll so that it is positioned even with the beaks of the pliers.

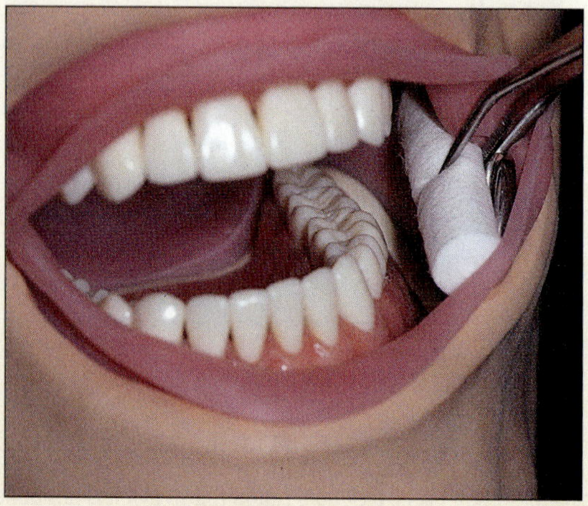

3. Transfer the cotton roll to the mouth, and position it securely in the mucobuccal fold closest to the working field.
4. Carry the second cotton roll to the mouth, and position it in the floor of the mouth between the working field and the tongue.
   Note: Have the patient lift the tongue during placement and then relax, to help secure the cotton roll in position.

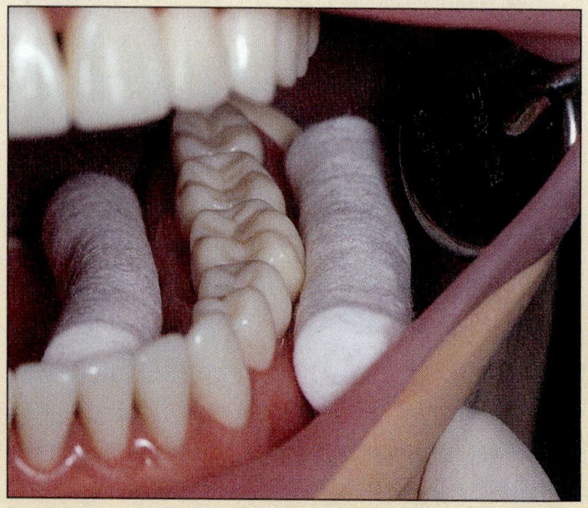

5. If you are placing cotton rolls for the mandibular anterior region, bend the cotton roll before placement for better fit.

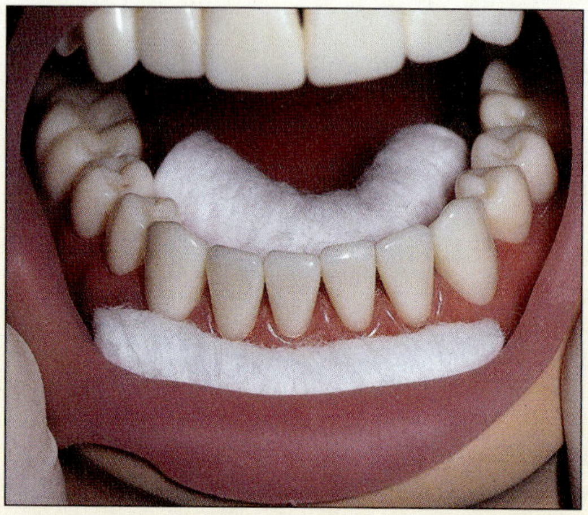

6. If using a saliva ejector for the procedure, place it after the cotton roll is in position in the lingual vestibule.

COTTON ROLL REMOVAL

1. At the completion of a procedure, remove the cotton roll before the full-mouth rinse. If the cotton roll is dry, moisten it with water from the air-water syringe.
   Purpose: Dry cotton rolls will adhere to the oral mucosa lining, and tissues may be damaged when a dry cotton roll is pulled away from the area.
2. Using cotton pliers, retrieve the contaminated cotton roll from the site.
3. If appropriate for the procedure, perform a limited rinse.

chin, the bar is slid upward to secure the cotton roll holder in place.

Dry-Angle Isolation

An additional isolation technique involves the use of a triangular absorbent pad called the *dry angle.* This pad helps isolate posterior areas in both the maxillary and mandibular arches. The pad is placed on the buccal mucosa over Stensen's duct, which is from the parotid gland and located opposite the maxillary second molar (Fig. 36-8). These pads block the flow of saliva as well as protect the tissues in this area.

Follow the manufacturer's instructions for placement, and if necessary, replace pads if they become soaked before the procedure is completed. To remove, use water from the air-water syringe to wet the pad thoroughly before separating it from the tissues.

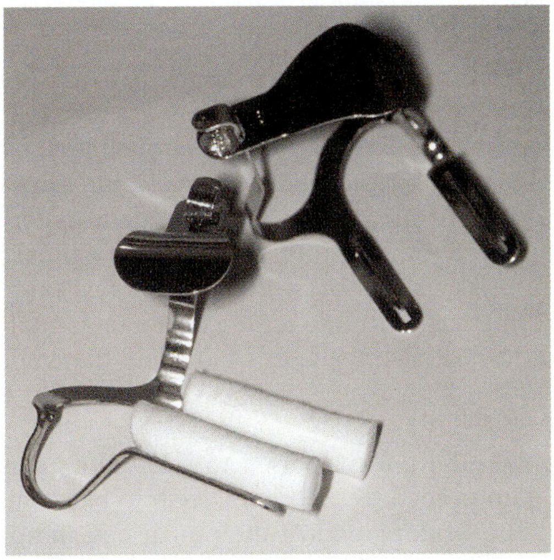

Fig. 36-7 Cotton roll holder.

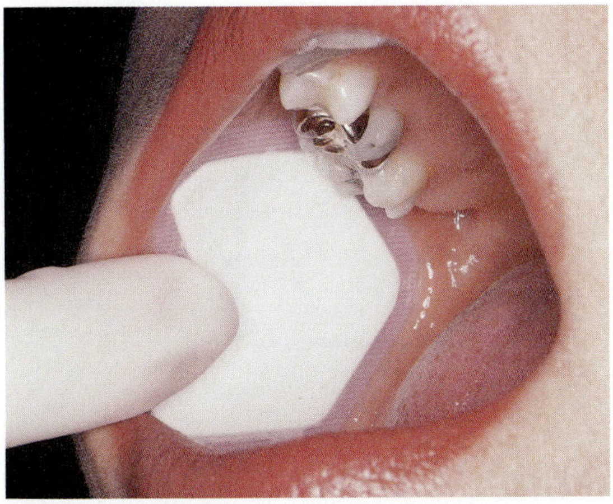

Fig. 36-8 Dry angle placement in the buccal mucosa.

Recall

5. What three means of isolation are most often used in dentistry?
6. What type of isolation is commonly chosen for shorter procedures?
7. Why is it important to wet a cotton roll before removal?

THE DENTAL DAM

The dental dam is a thin, stretchable latex material that becomes a barrier when appropriately applied to selected teeth. When the dam is in place, only the selected teeth are visible through the dam. These teeth are referred to as being **isolated** or **exposed.**

The dental dam is regularly placed after the local anesthetic has been administered. An efficient dental team can place the dam in about 2 minutes. The expanded-functions dental assistant (EFDA) working alone can complete this procedure in about 3 to 5 minutes.

Dental Dam Equipment

Dental Dam Material

The dental dam is made of either latex or latex-free material (see Chapter 19 for specific information on latex aller-

Indications for the Use of the Dental Dam

- Serves as an important infection-control barrier for the preparation of teeth.
- Safeguards the patient's mouth against contact with debris, dental materials, or other liquids during treatment.
- Protects the patient from accidentally **aspirating** or swallowing debris, such as small fragments of a tooth or scraps of restorative material.
- Protects the tooth from contamination by saliva or debris if pulpal exposure accidentally occurs.
- Protects the oral cavity from exposure when an infected tooth is opened during endodontic treatment.
- Provides the moisture control that is essential for the placement of restorative materials.
- Improves access by retracting the lips, tongue, and gingiva from the field of operation.
- Provides better visibility due to the contrasting colors of the dam and the tooth.
- Increases dental team efficiency by discouraging patient conversation, and reducing time required for treatment.

gies). The type of dental dam selected for each application is based on the operator's choice of size, color, and thickness (Fig. 36-9).

Size

The dental dam is available in a continuous roll or in two precut sizes. The 6-by-6–inch size is used for applications on the posterior teeth in the permanent dentition. The 5-by-5–inch size is used for primary dentition or anterior application on the permanent dentition.

Color

The dental dam is available in a wide range of colors from light to dark, including green, blue, and pastels. Scented and flavored dams also are available. The brighter colors are widely used and have good patient acceptance, but some dentists prefer a darker color because it provides contrast to tooth structure and reduces glare.

Thickness

The usual dam thicknesses or gauges are thin (light), medium, and heavy. *Thin* is most frequently used for endodontic applications. Since only one tooth is isolated, less stretch is required. *Medium* is widely used in operative procedures because of its ease of handling and ability to isolate selected teeth. *Heavy* is selected when tissue retraction and extra resistance to tearing is important. Examples of this would be in placement over a crown, fixed bridge, or teeth with tight contacts.

Dental Dam Frame

A frame or holder is necessary to stabilize and stretch the dam so that it fits tightly around the teeth and is out of the operator's way. Plastic and metal frames are available, and both can be sterilized for reuse (Fig. 36-10).

The *plastic U-shaped frame* is placed *under* the dam (next to the patient's face). Because this frame is *radiolucent* (does not block radiographs), it is not necessary to remove when radiographs are required during treatment.

The *Young frame* is a stainless steel U-shaped holder with sharp projections on its outer margin. The Young frame is placed on the *outside* of the dam, and the dam is stretched over the projection of the frame. This approach increases patient comfort by holding the dam away from the patient's face.

The *Ostby frame* is a round plastic frame with sharp projections on its outer margin. It also is placed *outside* the dam, and the dam is stretched over the projections of the frame.

Dental Dam Napkin

The disposable dental dam napkin can be used and is placed between the patient's face and the dam. The primary purpose of the napkin is to increase patient comfort by absorbing moisture. The napkin also protects the patient's face from direct contact with the dam, reducing the risk of the patient developing a latex sensitivity.

Lubricants

When the dam is placed, two types of lubricants may be selected. One lubricant is placed on the patient's lips to ensure patient comfort. Some operators use zinc oxide ointment for this purpose; others use petroleum jelly.

The second lubricant is *water-soluble* and is placed on the *underside* of the dam to help the dam material slide over the teeth and through the interproximal spaces. Petroleum jelly should not be used for this purpose because it interferes with the setting of certain dental materials and breaks down the latex in the dam material.

Dental Dam Punch

The dental dam punch is used to create the holes in the dental dam needed to expose the teeth to be isolated (Fig. 36-11). The working end of the punch has an adjustable **stylus** (cutting tip) that makes the hole as it strikes an opening in the punch plate. The *punch plate* is a rotary plat-

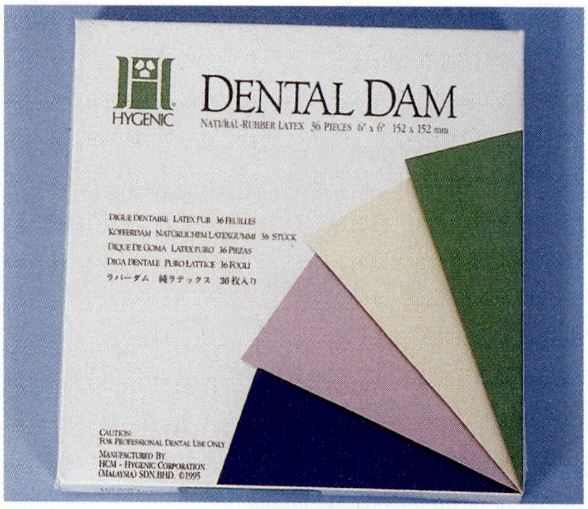

Fig. 36-9 Dental dam material.

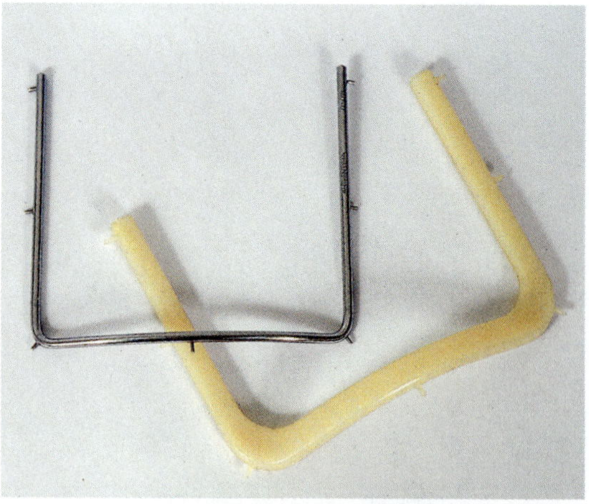

Fig. 36-10 Dental dam frames.

form with five or six holes of different sizes cut into the face of the plate. These holes are approximately 1 mm deep with sharp edges to accommodate the stylus.

The position of the punch plate is rotated to produce holes of different sizes. When the punch plate is turned, a slight click may be heard as the plate falls into position. This click indicates that the stylus is positioned directly over the hole in the punch plate. The correct position of the stylus is checked by slowly lowering the stylus point over the hole in the punch plate. If the stylus is not placed properly, it may be dulled or broken.

In addition, the holes may not be punched cleanly. If the holes have ragged edges, they may tear easily as the dam is placed over the crown of the tooth. The holes also may irritate the gingiva and may allow leakage of moisture around the tooth.

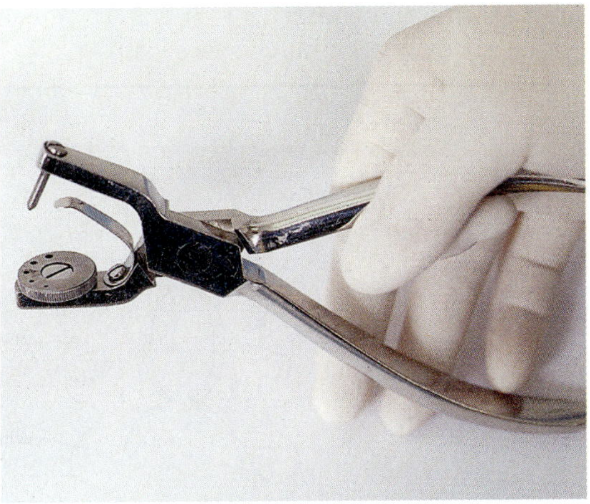

Fig. 36-11 Dental dam punch.

Size of holes on punch plate

The holes on the punch plate are graduated in size and are numbered 1 to 5, with 1 being the smallest size. Each size has specific recommended uses. Figure 36-12 provides recommended uses for each size of hole.

Dental Dam Stamp and Template

The *dental dam stamp* and inkpad are used to mark the dental dam with predetermined markings for the average adult and pediatric arches (Fig. 36-13).

The use of a *dental dam template,* which has holes where the teeth should be marked, provides more flexibility when one or more teeth in the arch are out of alignment. The template is placed on the dental dam, and a pen is used to mark through the template to indicate the location of the punch holes.

Dental Dam Forceps

Dental dam forceps are used in the placement and removal of the dental dam clamp (Fig. 36-14). The beaks of the forceps fit into holes on the jaws of the clamp (Fig. 36-15).

The handles of the forceps work with a spring action. A sliding bar keeps the handles of the forceps in a fixed position while the clamp is being held and positioned on the tooth. The handles are squeezed to release the clamp. The beaks of the forceps are turned toward the arch being treated. This permits the operator to place or remove the clamp without having to rotate the forceps to put them into position.

Dental Dam Clamps

The dental dam clamp is the primary means of anchoring and stabilizing the dental dam. The clamps are made of

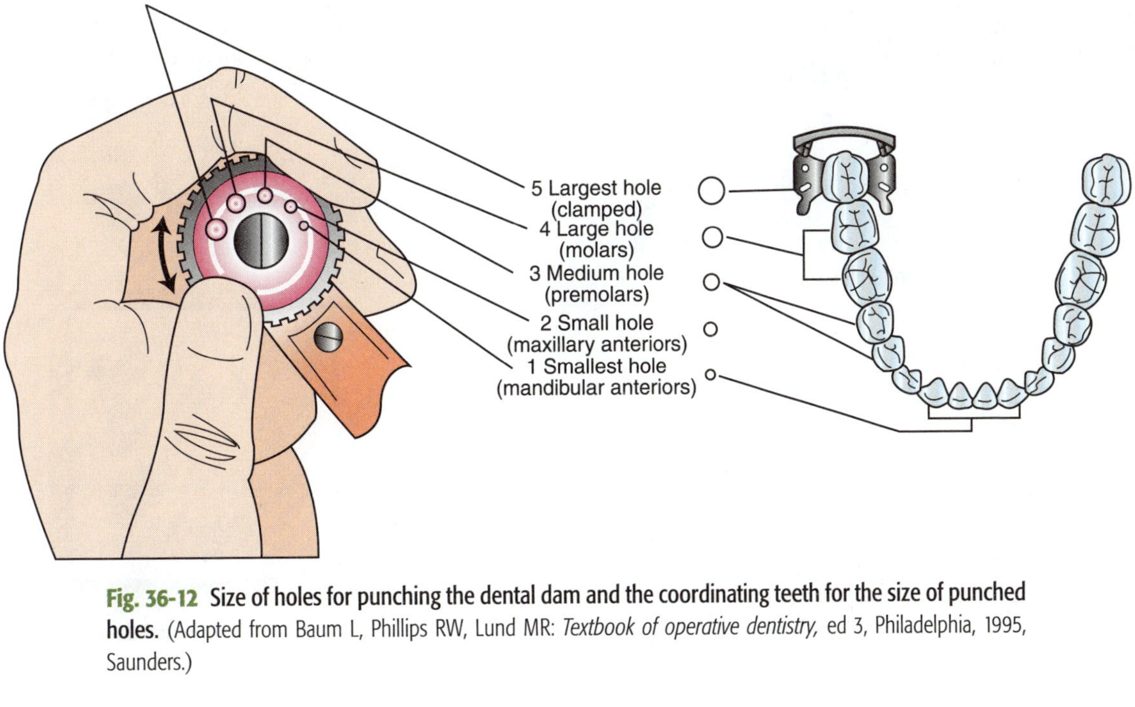

Fig. 36-12 Size of holes for punching the dental dam and the coordinating teeth for the size of punched holes. (Adapted from Baum L, Phillips RW, Lund MR: *Textbook of operative dentistry,* ed 3, Philadelphia, 1995, Saunders.)

chrome or nickel-plated steel, and are designed to hold the dental dam secure at the end nearest the tooth being treated. The opposite end of the dental dam application will also be stabilized, and this is accomplished by using another clamp, a dental dam stabilizing cord, or dental floss or tape. This technique is also known as *ligating* the dam.

Parts of the dental dam clamp

Parts of the clamp important to identify are the bow and the jaws (Fig. 36-16). The **bow** is the rounded portion of the clamp that extends through the dental dam. The clamp is always positioned on the tooth so the bow is located on the distal aspect.

The **jaws** encircle the tooth and are shaped into four prongs. All four prongs must be firmly seated on the tooth to create the facial-to-lingual balance necessary to stabilize the clamp. A hole is located on each side of the jaw of the clamp. The beaks of the dental dam forceps fit into these holes to allow for placement and removal of the clamp.

A **winged clamp** is designed with extra extensions to help retain the dental dam. Wingless clamps have names beginning with the letter *W. Wingless* clamps do *not* have extra projections to engage the dam.

Fitting the dental dam clamp

Dental dam clamps are available in many sizes and designs to accommodate different needs (Fig. 36-17).

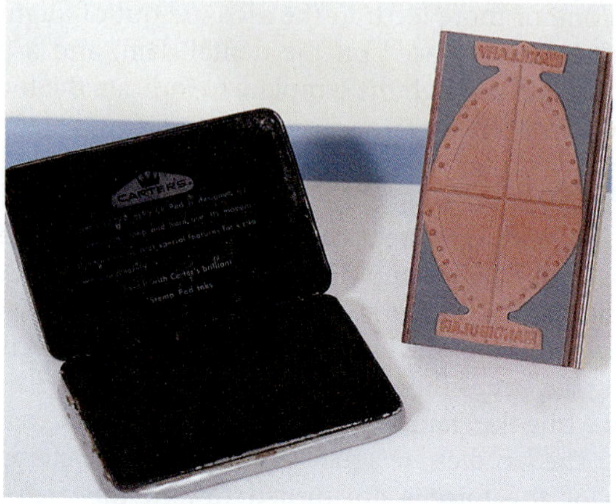

Fig. 36-13 Dental dam stamp.

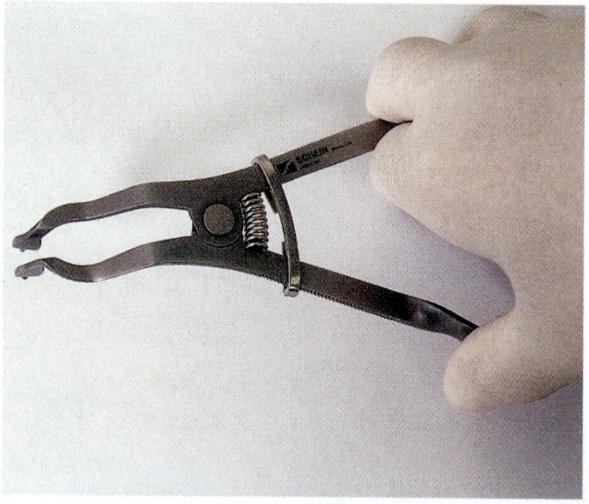

Fig. 36-14 Dental dam forceps.

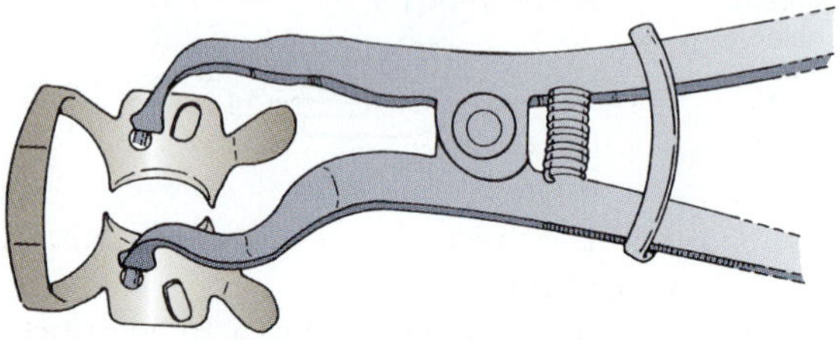

Fig. 36-15 **Positioning the beaks of the dental dam forceps into the clamp properly.** (From Baum L, Phillips RW, Lund MR: *Textbook of operative dentistry,* ed 3, Philadelphia, 1995, Saunders.)

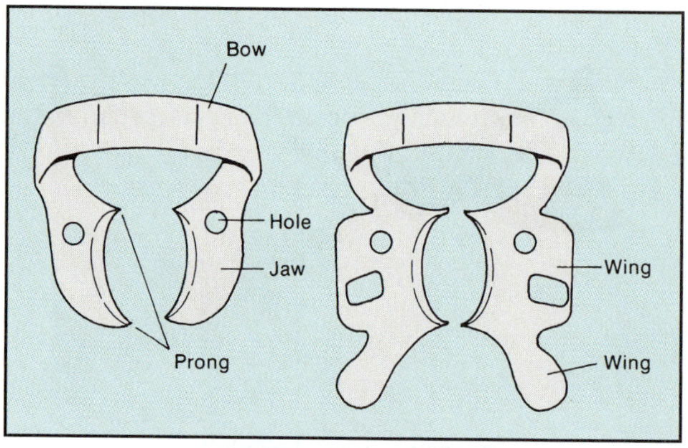

Fig. 36-16 Parts of the dental dam clamp.

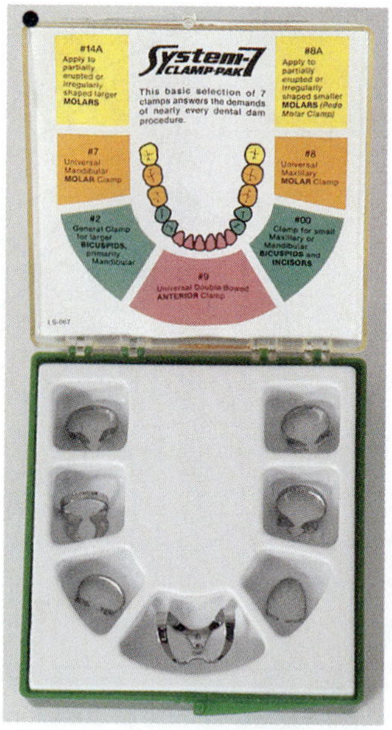

Fig. 36-17 Types of dental dam clamps.

The jaws of the clamps are designed to fit on the *cervical area* of the tooth below the height of contour and at, or slightly below, the cementoenamel junction. The *height of contour* is the widest point on the facial and lingual contours of the tooth (Fig. 36-18).

The clamp must be positioned with all four prongs firmly in place on the tooth *before* the clamp forceps are loosened. If the clamp is not placed properly, it may spring off the tooth and could possibly injure the patient, dentist, or assistant.

Posterior dental dam clamps are for the maxillary and mandibular posterior teeth. These clamps are **universal,** meaning that the same clamp can be placed on the same type of tooth in the opposite quadrant. Clamps 7 and W7 are universal mandibular molar clamps, and clamps 8 and W8 are universal maxillary molar clamps.

Anterior dental dam clamps, such as clamps 9 and W9, are designed to (1) retract the gingiva on the facial surface, (2) improve visibility for the restoration of cervical class V cavities, and (3) permit isolation of an anterior tooth during endodontic treatment.

Pediatric dental dam clamps for primary teeth are designed to accommodate the smaller size and shape of the primary teeth or partially erupted permanent teeth. The clamps for primary teeth are sizes 00, W00, and 2.

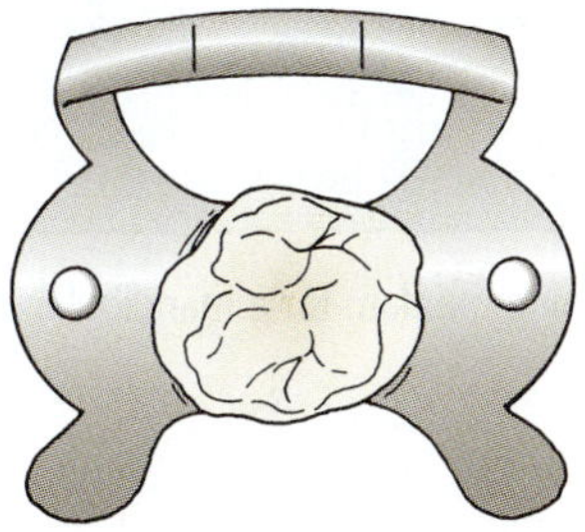

Fig. 36-18 Positioning the clamp on the tooth.

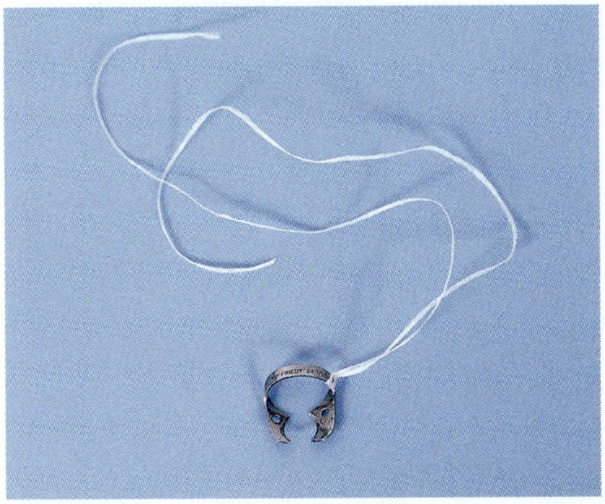

Fig. 36-19 Ligature placed on the bow of the clamp for protective reasons.

Ligatures on clamps

Dental floss or dental tape should *always* be attached to the bow of the dental dam clamp as a ligature *before* the clamp is placed in the patient's mouth. *This is an important safety step that must not be omitted.* The ligature makes it possible to retrieve a clamp should it accidentally become dislodged and then inhaled or swallowed by the patient (Fig. 36-19).

The ends of this ligature are always kept out of the patient's mouth on the outside of the dental dam material and within easy reach. During treatment, the ligature may be attached to the dam frame to keep it available yet out of the operator's way.

Dental Dam Stabilizing Cord

The dental dam stabilizing cord is a disposable latex cord and is an alternative to the conventional clamp method of securing the dental dam. The cord is available in three sizes: extra small, small, and large.

During insertion, the cord is stretched so that it becomes narrow and slips easily between the teeth. Once placed and released, the cord resumes its original shape and holds the dam tightly in place. The *size* of the cord selected depends on the amount of contact space available. The *length* of the cord depends on the application.

Recall

8. What is the term for teeth that are visible through the dam?
9. What piece of equipment stabilizes and stretches the dam away from the tooth?
10. If you are unable to slide the dam interproximally, what could be placed on the underside of the dam to help in the application?

DENTAL DAM PREPARATION

Each application of the dam is preplanned to accommodate the dentist's preferences, the tooth or teeth involved, and the procedure to be performed. The following six factors must be included in the planning for the holes to be punched in the dental dam:

- Maxillary or mandibular arch
- Shape of the arch
- Any irregularities, such as missing teeth, a fixed prosthesis, or malpositioned teeth
- Teeth to be isolated
- Identification of the anchor tooth and location of the keypunch hole
- Size and spacing of the other holes to be punched

The *anchor tooth* holds the dental dam clamp, and the *keypunch hole* covers the anchor tooth.

Maxillary Arch Application

In preparation for maxillary application, the dam material is stamped or marked, and the holes are punched. Because the holes for the maxillary anterior teeth are punched one inch down from the upper edge of the dam, it is helpful to stamp or mark the extension in back of the punch plate of the dental dam punch to indicate 1 inch (Fig. 36-20). This mark automatically designates the margin of dam for these holes. If the patient has a mustache or a very thick upper lip, it is necessary to allow slightly more than a 1-inch margin from the edge.

Mandibular Arch Application

In preparation for a mandibular application, the dam is stamped or marked, and the holes are punched, leaving a 2-inch margin from the edge (Fig. 36-21). Because of the small size of the mandibular teeth, the holes are punched closer together than for posterior teeth. Extra care should be taken when punching holes for anterior teeth. Use a water-soluble lubricant if there is crowding or tight contacts in this area.

Curve of the Arch

It may be necessary to make adjustments to accommodate an extremely narrow or wide arch. Failure to do this will increase the difficulty with inversion of the edges of the holes in the dam.

Bunching and stretching on the lingual aspect of the dental dam occur if the curve of the arch is punched too flat or too wide. *Folding and stretching* of the dam on the facial aspect occur if the arch is punched too curved or too narrow.

Malaligned Teeth

If a tooth or teeth are **malaligned** within the dental arch, special consideration of their position is taken *before* the dental dam is punched.

If the tooth is *lingually malposed,* the hole-punch size remains the same, but the hole is placed about 1 mm lingually from the normal arch alignment (Fig. 36-22).

If the tooth is *facially malposed,* the hole-punch size remains the same, but the hole is placed about 1 mm facially from the normal arch alignment.

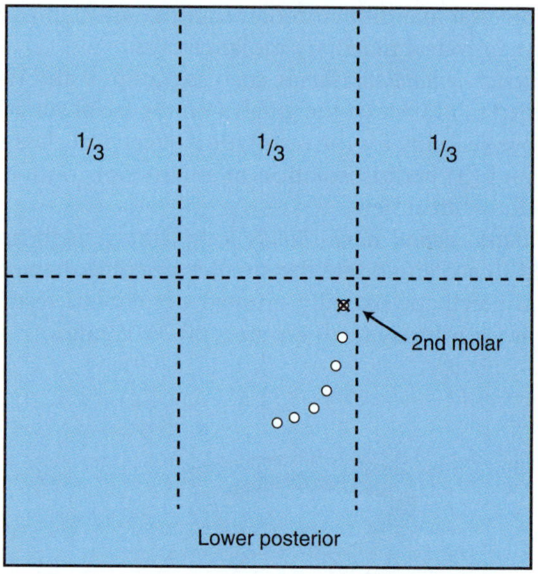

Fig. 36-21 Punching the dam for a mandibular application.

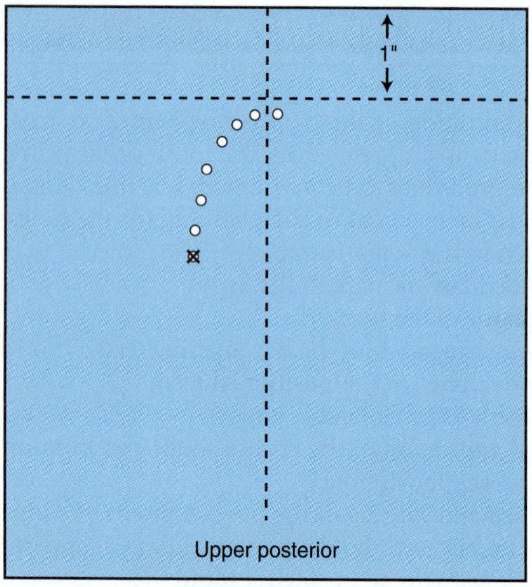

Fig. 36-20 Punching the dam for a maxillary application.

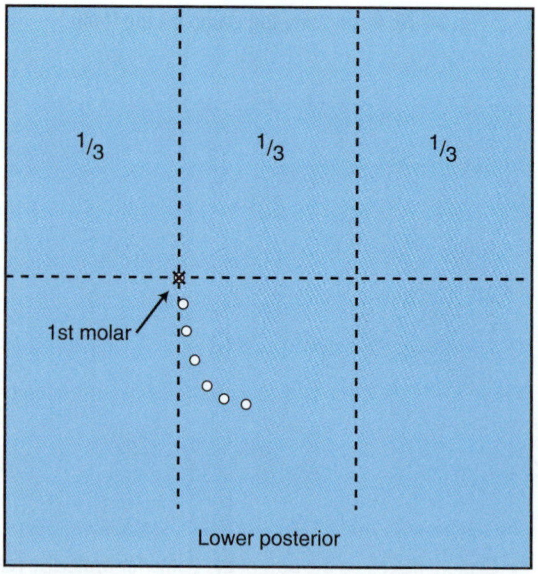

Fig. 36-22 Punching the dam for a malaligned tooth.

Teeth to be Isolated

Single-tooth isolation is typically used for selected restorative procedures and for endodontic treatment. Some dentists isolate only the tooth to be treated, and others prefer to have two teeth isolated so that the second tooth acts as an anchor tooth to hold the clamp. During treatment in the posterior area, this second tooth provides more stability and better visibility.

For *multiple-tooth isolation,* many dentists expose three or four teeth. However, for optimum stability, it is desirable to have six to eight teeth isolated to counteract the pull on the dam that is created by the curvature of the teeth in the arch. At least one tooth posterior to the tooth being treated should be isolated.

When maxillary anterior teeth are to be isolated, maximum stability is achieved by isolating the six anterior teeth (canine to canine).

Keypunch Hole

As mentioned, the anchor tooth holds the dental dam clamp, and the keypunch hole is punched in the dental dam to cover the anchor tooth. The largest size hole (#5) is necessary for the keypunch because it must also accommodate the clamp.

The selection of the anchor tooth and the location of the keypunch hole are important considerations in the application of the dental dam. For maximum stability and ease of access, the keypunch hole is placed one or two teeth distal to the tooth that is receiving treatment.

Hole Sizing and Spacing

The size of each hole selected on the dental dam punch must be appropriate for the tooth to be isolated. A correctly sized hole allows the dam to slip easily over the tooth and fit snugly in the cervical area. This is important to prevent leakage around the dam.

In general, the holes are spaced with 3.0 to 3.5 mm between the *edges,* not the centers, of the holes. This allows adequate spacing between the holes to create a septum that can slip between the teeth without tearing or injuring the gingiva.

The **septum** is the dental dam material between the holes of the punched dam. During application, this portion of the dam is passed between the contacts.

DENTAL DAM PLACEMENT AND REMOVAL

There are two methods of dental dam placement. The main difference between the two is the sequencing in the placement of the clamp and dental dam. The remaining steps are the same.

In the *one-step method,* the dam and clamp are placed at the same time. In the *two-step method,* first the clamp is placed and then the dental dam material is stretched over it.

Troubleshooting Hole Size and Spacing

If the holes are *too large,* the dam will not fit tightly around the tooth. This may allow saliva to leak through the hole.

If the holes are *too small,* the dam will not slip easily over the tooth. This may cause the dam to stretch or tear and leave gingiva exposed.

If the holes are *too close,* the dam may tear or stretch. The stretched holes may leave the gingiva exposed and may cause leakage.

If the holes are *too far apart,* there is excess material between the teeth. This may block the dentist's vision or catch in instrumentation.

Procedure 36-4 Preparation, Placement, and Removal of the Dental Dam

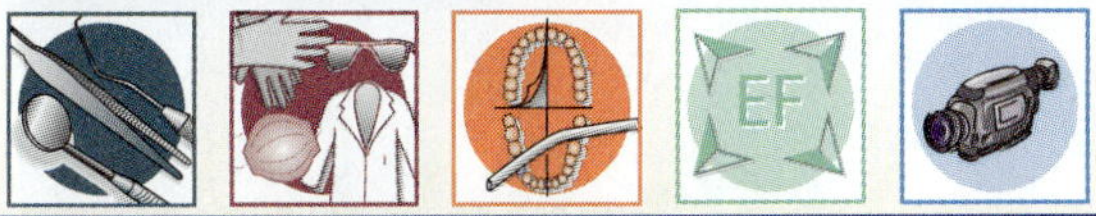

Equipment and Supplies

- Basic setup
- Precut 6-by-6–inch dental dam
- Dental dam stamp and inkpad *or* template and pen
- Dental dam punch
- Dental dam clamp or clamps with ligature attached
- Dental dam clamp forceps
- Young frame
- Dental dam napkin

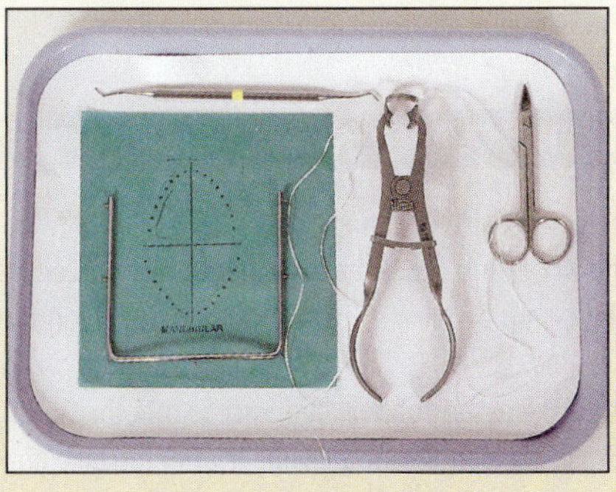

continued

Procedure 36-4 Preparation, Placement, and Removal of the Dental Dam—cont'd

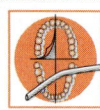

Equipment and Supplies, cont'd

- Dental tape or waxed floss
- Cotton rolls
- Lubricant for patient's lips
- Lubricant for dam
- Black spoon
- Crown and bridge scissors

PATIENT PREPARATION

1. Check the patient's record for contraindications and to identify the area to be isolated. Inform the patient of the need to place a dental dam, and explain the steps involved.
2. Administer local anesthetic. The operator will determine which teeth are to be isolated, and note whether there are any malposed teeth to be accommodated.
3. Apply lubricating ointment to the patient's lip with a cotton roll or cotton tip applicator.
   Note: The patient's comfort is of concern throughout the placement and removal of the dental dam.
4. Use the mouth mirror and explorer to examine the site where the dam is to be placed. It should be free of plaque and debris.
   Purpose: If the dam is placed in an area with plaque and debris, the dam could push the plaque and debris into the sulcus and irritate the gingival tissues.
   Note: If debris or plaque is present, selective coronal polishing is performed on these teeth before the application of the dental dam.
5. Floss all contacts involved in the placement of the dental dam.
   Purpose: Any tight contacts may tear the dam.

PUNCHING THE DENTAL DAM

1. Use a template or stamp to mark on the dam the teeth to be isolated.
2. Correctly punch the marked dam according to the teeth to be isolated. Be sure to use the correct size of punch hole for the specific tooth.
3. If teeth have tight contacts, lightly lubricate the holes on the tooth surface (undersurface) of the dam.
   Purpose: This eases placement of the dam over the contact area of the teeth.

PLACING THE CLAMP AND FRAME

1. Select the correct size of clamp.
   Note: The W7 clamp has been selected for this procedure.
2. Secure the clamp by tying a ligature of dental tape on the bow of the clamp.
3. Place the beaks of the rubber dam forceps into the holes of the clamp. Grasp the handles of the rubber dam forceps, and squeeze to open the clamp. Turn upward, and allow the locking bar to slide down to keep the forceps open for placement.
4. Place yourself in the operator's position, and adjust your patient for easier access.
5. Retrieve the rubber dam forceps. Position the lingual jaws of the clamp first, then the facial jaws. During placement, keep an index finger on the clamp to prevent the clamp from coming off before it has been stabilized on the tooth. Check the clamp for fit.
   Purpose: Lingual jaw placement serves as a fulcrum for placement of the facial jaws.

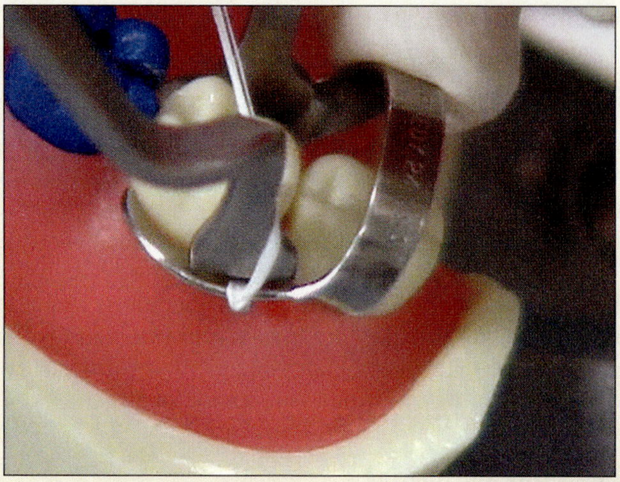

6. Transfer the dental dam to the site; stretch the punched hole for the anchor tooth over the clamp.

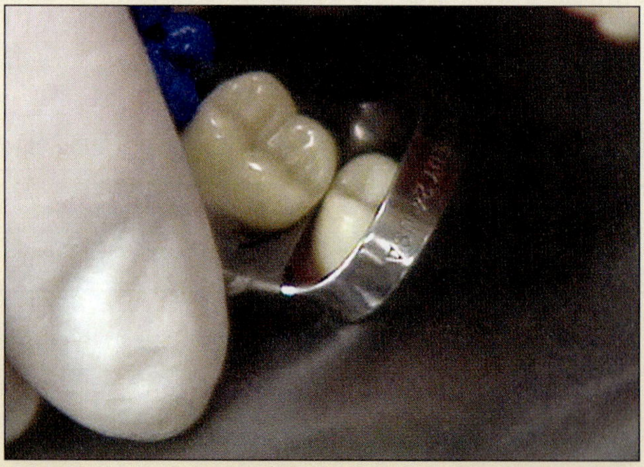

7. Using cotton pliers, retrieve the ligature and pull it through so that it is exposed and easy to grasp if necessary.
8. Position the frame over the dam, and slightly pull the dam, allowing it to hook onto the projections of the frame.
   Purpose: Ensures a smooth and stable fit.

Procedure 36-4 Preparation, Placement, and Removal of the Dental Dam—cont'd

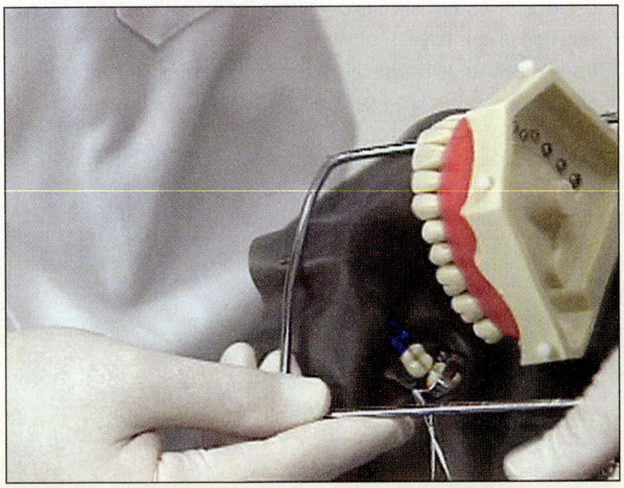

9. Fit the last hole of the dam over the last tooth to be exposed at the opposite end of the anchor tooth.
   Purpose: This stabilizes the dam and aids in locating the remaining punch holes for the teeth to be isolated.
10. Using the index fingers of both hands, stretch the dam on the lingual and facial surfaces of the teeth so that the dam slides through each contact area.
11. With a piece of dental tape or waxed floss, floss through the contacts, pushing the dam below the proximal contacts of each tooth to be isolated.
   Note: Slide the floss through the contact rather than pulling it back through the contact. This will keep the dam in place.

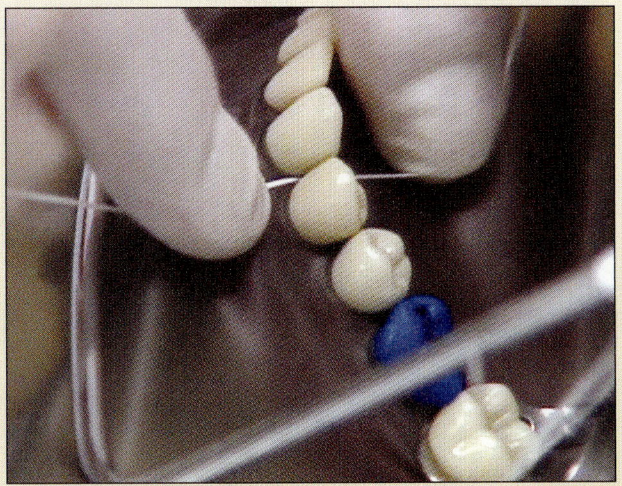

12. If the contacts are extremely tight, use floss or a wooden wedge placed into the interproximal area to separate the teeth slightly.
13. A ligature is placed to stabilize the dam at the *opposite* end of the anchor tooth.

INVERTING THE DAM

1. **Invert,** or reverse, the dam by gently stretching it near the cervix of the tooth.
   Purpose: Inverting the dam creates a seal to prevent the leakage of saliva.
2. Apply air from the air-water syringe to the tooth being inverted to help in turning the dam material under.
   Purpose: When the tooth surface is dry, the margin of the stretched dam usually inverts into the gingival sulcus as the dam is released.

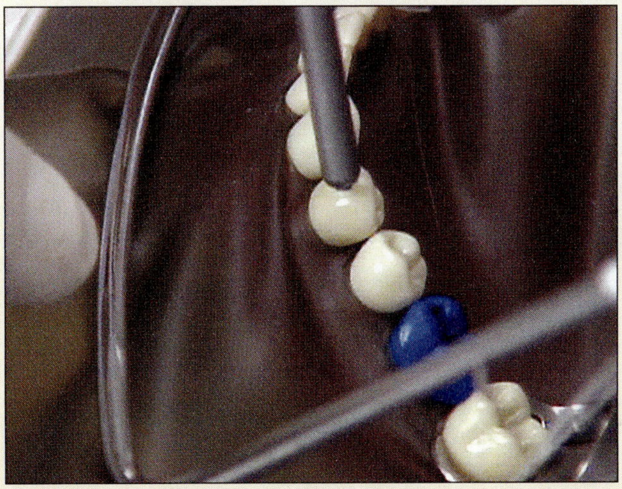

3. A black spoon or beaver tail burnisher can be used to invert the edges of the dam.
4. When all punched holes are properly inverted, the dental dam application is complete.
5. If necessary for patient comfort, a saliva ejector may be placed under the dam. This is positioned on the floor of the patient's mouth on the side *opposite* the area being treated.
6. If the patient is uncomfortable and has trouble breathing only through the nose, cut a small hole in the palatal area of the dam by pinching a piece of dam with cotton pliers and cutting a small hole near the palatal area.

REMOVING THE DAM

1. If a ligature was used to stabilize the dam, remove it first. If a saliva ejector was used, remove it.
2. Slide your finger under the dam parallel to the arch, and pull outward so that you are stretching the holes away from the isolated teeth.

continued

Procedure 36-4 Preparation, Placement, and Removal of the Dental Dam—cont'd

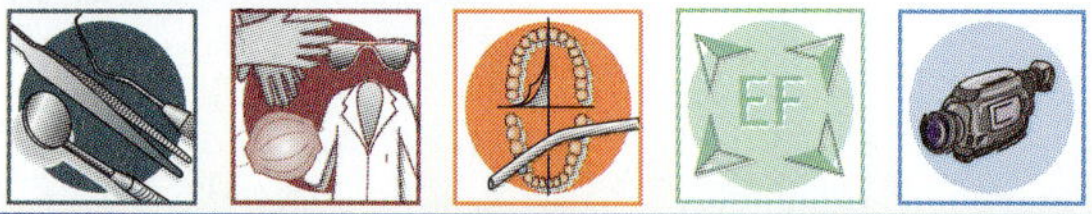

REMOVING THE DAM—cont'd

Working from posterior to anterior, use the crown and bridge scissors to cut from hole to hole, creating one long cut.

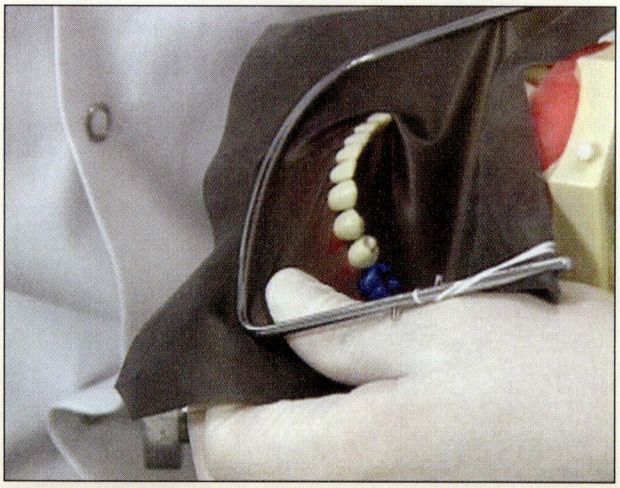

3. When all septa are cut, the dam is pulled lingually to free the rubber from the interproximal space.
4. Using the dental dam forceps, position the beaks into the holes of the clamp, and open the clamp by squeezing the handle. Gently slide the clamp from the tooth.
5. Remove both the dam and the frame at one time.

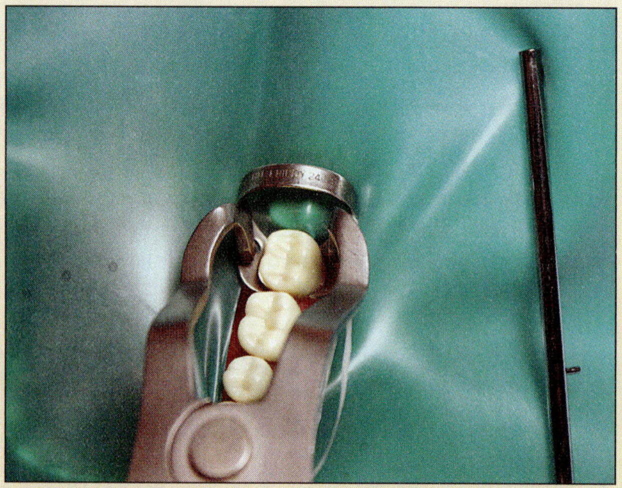

6. Use a tissue or the dam napkin to wipe the patient's mouth, lips, and chin free of moisture.
7. Inspect the dam to ensure that the entire pattern of the torn septa of the dental dam has been removed.

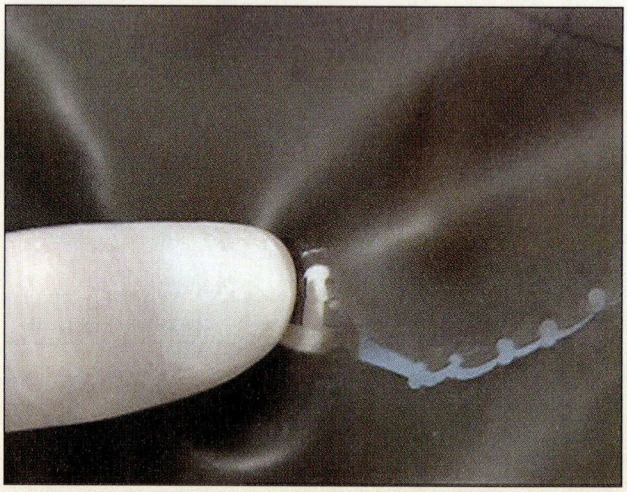

8. If a fragment of the dental dam is missing, use dental floss to check the corresponding interproximal area of the oral cavity.
   Purpose: Fragments of the dental dam left under the free gingiva can cause gingival irritation.

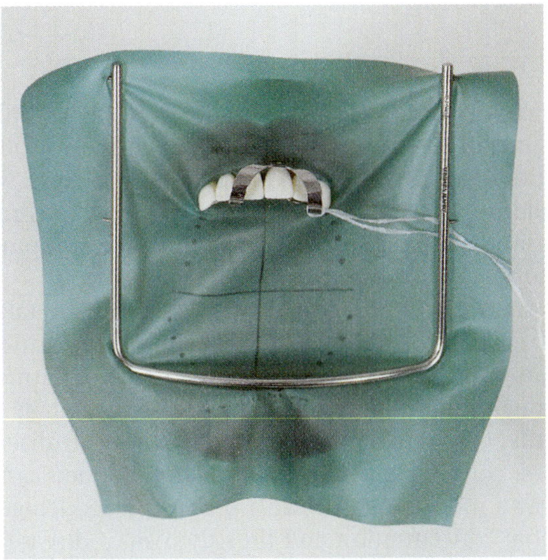

Fig. 36-23 Maxillary anterior dam application.

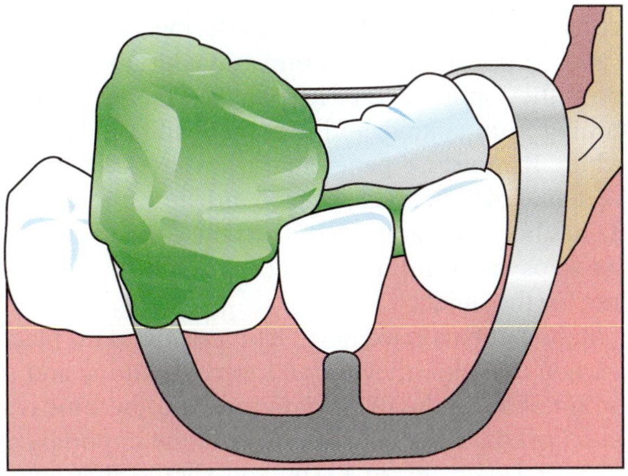

Fig. 36-24 Compound wax used to stabilize anterior clamp. (Adapted from Baum L, Phillips RW, Lund MR: *Textbook of operative dentistry,* ed 3, Philadelphia, 1995, Saunders.)

SPECIAL APPLICATIONS FOR THE DENTAL DAM

Anterior Teeth

When the dam is to be applied for anterior teeth, the isolation and application procedures change. The isolation of anterior teeth is typically from canine to canine. When the isolation is complete, a dental dam clamp is not required. The dental dam will remain secure by placing dental tape or stretching a small corner of dental dam interproximally between the canine and first premolar on each side (Fig. 36-23).

A cervical or anterior clamp as seen in Figure 36-23 may be required if the gingival third of a tooth is to be restored, and if the gingival tissue must be retracted for better exposure. The jaws of this type of clamp are positioned lightly on the cementum of the root just below the carious lesion.

Stabilizing the Cervical Clamp

Occasionally, additional stabilization of the cervical clamp is necessary. Softened stick compound may be used for this purpose (Fig. 36-24). A heat source such as a butane torch or Bunsen burner is needed, with the steps in stabilization as follows:

- Soften red or green stick compound by holding it over a flame until the tip bends. Then place the tip in hot water for five seconds.
- Twist off approximately one inch of the tip, and shape it into a cone.
- Very carefully reheat the cone of compound in the flame. Then place the softened compound under the bow of the clamp (occlusal surface), away from the area to be treated.
- Repeat this procedure for the second bow on the opposite side of the clamp.
- On completion of treatment, remove the compound before removing the dam and clamp.

Fixed Bridge

A fixed bridge is a prosthetic device that is cemented in place to replace one or more adjacent missing teeth. Because the units of the bridge are joined together, it is not possible to place the dental dam septum between them. For this reason, placement of a dental dam on fixed bridgework requires a specialized technique.

When punching the dental dam, punch a hole for each fully crowned tooth, but *do not* punch a hole for the teeth that are replacing the missing teeth. A clamp is placed on the distal aspect of the bridge, and in some situations a second clamp is placed on the mesial portion. The remainder of the application and the removal are performed as usual.

Recall

11. The hole sizes on the rubber dam punch range from 1 to 5. Which is the smallest size?

12. For what purpose would you use an anterior dental dam clamp?

Patient Education

Patients are not aware of how much saliva, water, and debris accumulates in the mouth during a procedure. It is your responsibility to inform and educate the patient about the importance of keeping the mouth open, refraining from talking, and remaining still during a procedure. If moisture penetrates an exposed tooth, or if the dental material is exposed to moisture, the operative site has been contaminated. Then the dental team must take steps backward in the procedure, which causes lost time for the office.

Many patients have never had a dental dam placed, or when they did, they found it very confining and uncomfortable. As the EFDA, your role is to become competent in educating the patient about the importance of the dental dam. As an EFDA, you should then master the skill in placement that will provide complete isolation of tooth or teeth, as well as comfort for the patient.

Eye to the Future

You now understand the importance of practicing infection control in your daily care of patients. You follow infection-control policies in (1) the way you dress, with the addition of PPE, (2) how you disinfect the clinical environment, and (3) how you sterilize the equipment and supplies used intraorally.

In the near future your dental office will be taking moisture control one step further, by having patients use an oral antiseptic before any dental treatment. Therapeutic antiseptics are being prescribed daily for patients with susceptibility to infection or disease. Phenol, chlorhexidine, and *Sanguinaria* products can be used as a mouthwash before a procedure, reducing the bacterial concentration and thus the risk of disease for the patient and dental team.

Legal and Ethical Implications

If you assist with a coughing patient who suddenly swallows the crown, or a patient who has swallowed a bur from the handpiece, you will understand the importance of the dental dam. The dental dam provides much more than moisture control for the patient and dental team. By using the dental dam, you are protecting the health of the patient as well as the tooth or teeth being treated.

If you are practicing in a state where the placement and removal of the dental dam is an *expanded function,* follow all guidelines for proper placement, which includes attaching a ligature to the clamp for safe and quick removal.

Critical Thinking

1. You are an EFDA, and the dentist has requested that you place sealants on the patient's mandibular first permanent molars. What isolation technique would you use for this procedure, and why?
2. The dentist is preparing tooth #4 for a disto-occlusal amalgam. Where will you place the high-volume evacuator during this procedure?
3. The dentist is halfway through preparing tooth #4 and pulls out to examine the extent of the remaining decay. What would you do at this moment?
4. You will be assisting in a composite procedure today on tooth #24. How will you punch the dental dam for this procedure?
5. What size holes would be punched for the isolation of teeth #18 through #22, with the anchor tooth being #18?

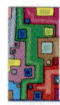

37

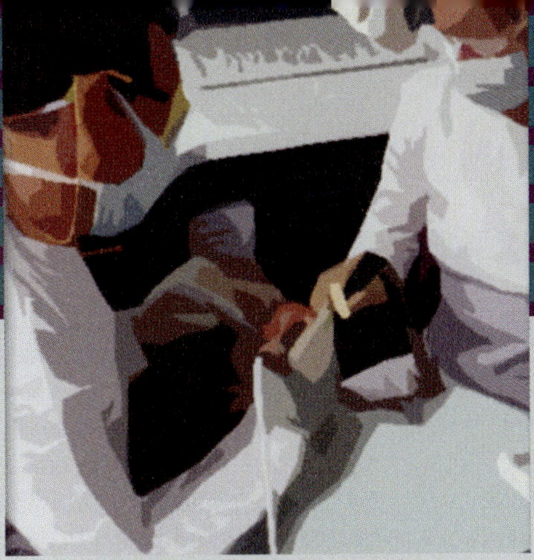

Anesthesia and Pain Control

Outline

KEY TERMS

Analgesia (*a*-nul-**jee**-zee-ah; *a*-nul-**jee**-zhuh) Stage of anesthesia in which the patient is relaxed and conscious.

Anesthesia (*a*-nuhs-**the**-zee-ah, *a*-nuhs-**the**-zhuh) Temporary loss of feeling or sensation.

Anesthetic Medication that produces the temporary loss of feeling or sensation.

Aspirate (**as**-puh-*rate*) To draw back or to draw within.

Diffuse (di-**fyuz**) To spread from an area of high concentration to one of low concentration.

Duration (duh-**ray**-shun) Time from induction to complete reversal of anesthesia.

Gauge Standard dimension or measurement of the thickness of an injection needle.

Induction (in-**duhk**-shun) Time from injection to effective anesthesia.

KEY TERMS, cont'd

Innervation (*i*-ner-**vay**-shun) Supply or distribution of nerves to a specific body part.

Lumen (lu-**mun**) The hollow center of the injection needle.

Oximetry (ok-**sim**-uh-tree) Measurement of oxygen concentration in the blood.

Permeate (**per**-me-ate) To spread or flow throughout.

Porous (**pore**-us) An object with minute openings that allow the passage of gas or fluid.

Systemic toxicity (sis-**te**-mik *tahk*-**sis**-i-tee) Relating to a system, or typically the entire body.

Tidal volume Amount of air inhaled and exhaled with each breath.

Titrate (**tie**-trate) To determine the concentration of a substance.

Titration The process of determining the exact amount of a drug or substance that would be used to achieve a desired level of sedation.

Vasoconstrictor (**vay**-zoh-kun-**strik**-tor) Type of drug that constricts (narrows) blood vessels; used to prolong anesthetic action.

LEARNING OUTCOMES

On completion of this chapter, the student will be able to achieve the following objectives:

- Define, pronounce, and spell the Key Terms.
- Discuss the importance of pain control in dentistry.
- Describe the composition and application of topical anesthetics.
- Discuss the composition and application of local anesthetic agents.
- Describe nitrous oxide/oxygen sedation and its use in dentistry.
- Discuss the importance of reducing the dental team's exposure to nitrous oxide.
- Discuss intravenous sedation and its use in dentistry.
- Discuss general anesthesia and its use in dentistry.

PERFORMANCE OUTCOMES

On completion of this chapter, the student will be able to meet competency standards in the following skills:

- Demonstrate the placement of a topical anesthetic agent.
- Demonstrate the preparation and management of the local anesthetic setup.
- Assist during the administration of local anesthesia.
- Assist in the administration and monitoring of nitrous oxide/oxygen sedation.

A wide variety of anxiety and pain-control procedures has allowed the dental profession to extend oral healthcare to millions of individuals who would otherwise remain untreated. *Anxiety and pain control* is defined as the practice of various psychological, physiological, and chemical approaches to the prevention and treatment of preoperative, operative, and postoperative anxiety and pain.

The methods of pain control most often used in dentistry to alleviate or reduce anxiety and pain are:

- Local anesthetic agents
- Inhalation sedation
- Antianxiety agents
- Intravenous sedation
- General anesthesia

LOCAL ANESTHETIC AGENTS

Topical Anesthesia

Anesthetics are drugs that produce the temporary loss of feeling or sensation. The primary use of topical anesthesia in dentistry is to provide a numbing effect in the area where an injection is to take place. Topical anesthetic agents provide a temporary numbing effect on nerve endings located on the surface of the oral mucosa. The drugs in topical anesthetics are concentrated to allow penetration of the mucous membranes and action at the nerve endings.

Topical anesthetic agents are available in the form of ointments, liquids, sprays, and patches that are applied directly on the affected area (Fig. 37-1). For topical anesthetic ointments to have optimum effectiveness, the ointment must remain on the site of injection for 3 to 5 minutes.

The liquid and spray topical anesthetic agents are applied to larger surface areas of the oral tissues. These anesthetics are useful when applied at the back of the throat in patients with a strong gag reflex who need to have an impression or intraoral radiographs taken.

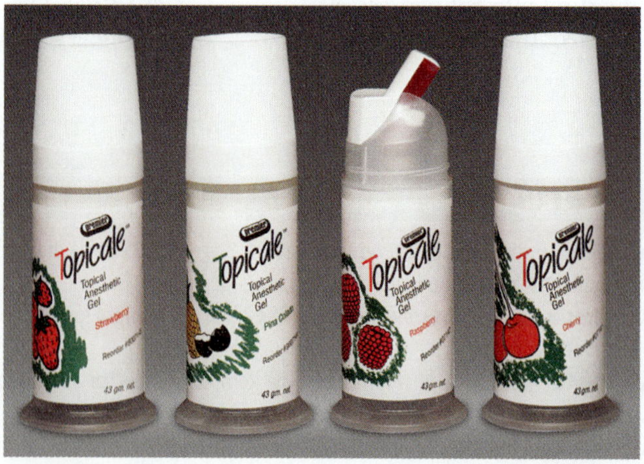

Fig. 37-1 Topical anesthetic. (Courtesy Premier Dental Products.)

The topical patch is a new product that when placed will provide topical anesthesia within 10 seconds. The patch is used for injections, as well as for the alleviation of discomfort from denture sores and oral ulcers (Fig. 37-2). See Procedure 37-1: Applying a Topical Anesthetic.

Recall

1. Why are topical anesthetics used in dentistry?

Local Anesthesia

Local anesthetics were first discovered in the mid-1800s and have greatly reduced pain during dental care. Local anesthetic agents are the most frequently used form of pain control in dentistry. This method of anesthesia provides a safe, effective, and dependable method of anesthesia of suitable duration for virtually all forms of dental treatment.

Method of Action

Local anesthesia is obtained by injecting an anesthetic solution near a nerve where treatment is to take place. The local anesthetic agent temporarily blocks the ability of the nerve membrane to generate an impulse. When this anesthetic solution attaches to specific receptors within the nerve, it slows down neuron conductance, causing the patient to feel numbness in that area.

After the injection is completed, the anesthetic **diffuses,** or spreads, into the nerve and blocks its normal action. To obtain complete anesthesia after the injection, the nerve must be sufficiently **permeated** by a concentration of the anesthetic base to inhibit conduction in all fibers. The action of local anesthesia is reversed as the bloodstream carries away the solution.

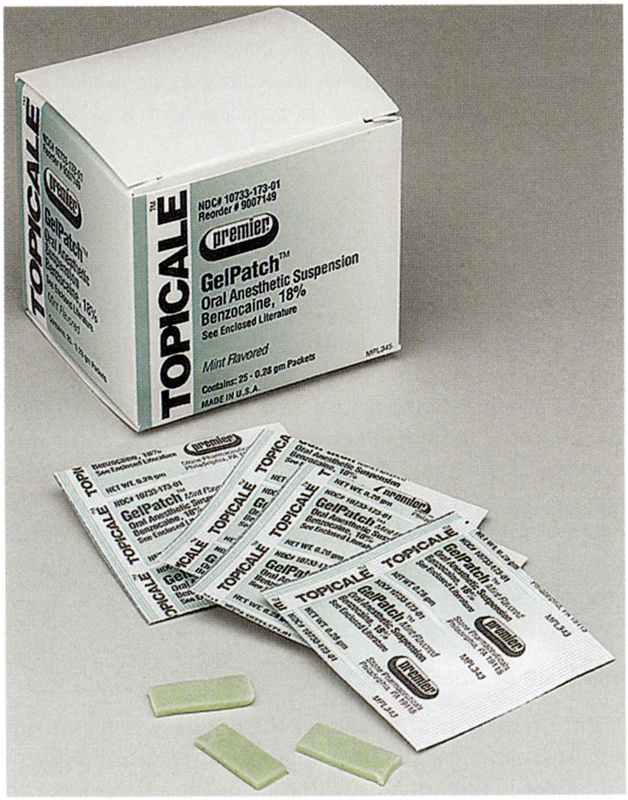

Fig. 37-2 Topical gel patch. (Courtesy Premier Dental Products.)

Chemical Composition of Anesthetics

Local anesthetic solutions for dental use come under two chemical groups, the *amides* and *esters.* The amides were first introduced to clinical practice in the 1940s, and have maintained the standards by which all other local anesthetics are measured. The ester-type anesthetic solutions are mainly used as topical anesthetics. The difference between the two groups is how they are metabolized by the body. The amide local anesthetics are metabolized by the liver, and the ester local anesthetics are metabolized primarily in the plasma.

Each local anesthetic cartridge contains a combination of the following ingredients:

- *Local anesthetic drug.* The choice depends on the procedure, health of the patient, and dentist's preference.
- *Sodium chloride,* which makes the solution that is isotonic with body tissues.
- *Distilled water,* which supplies added volume of solution.

Vasoconstrictors in Anesthetics

To slow down the intake of an anesthetic agent and increase the duration of action, a **vasoconstrictor** can be added to the local anesthetic agent. The action of a vasoconstrictor can:

- Prolong the effect of the anesthetic agent by decreasing the blood flow in the immediate area of the injection.
- Decrease bleeding in the injected area during surgical procedures.

Characteristics of Local Anesthetics

Nonirritating to the tissues in the area of the injection

Associated with minimal toxicity (causes the least possible damage to the body systems)

Rapid onset (takes effect quickly)

Able to provide profound anesthesia (completely eliminates the sensation of pain during a procedure)

Sufficient duration (remains effective long enough for the procedure to be completed)

Completely reversible (leaves the tissue in its original state after the patient's recovery from anesthesia)

Sterile or capable of being sterilized by heat without deterioration

Procedure 37-1 Applying a Topical Anesthetic

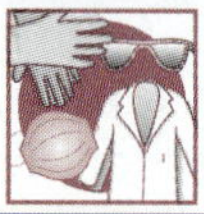

Equipment and Supplies

- 2- × 2-inch gauze squares
- Topical anesthetic ointment
- Sterile cotton-tipped applicator

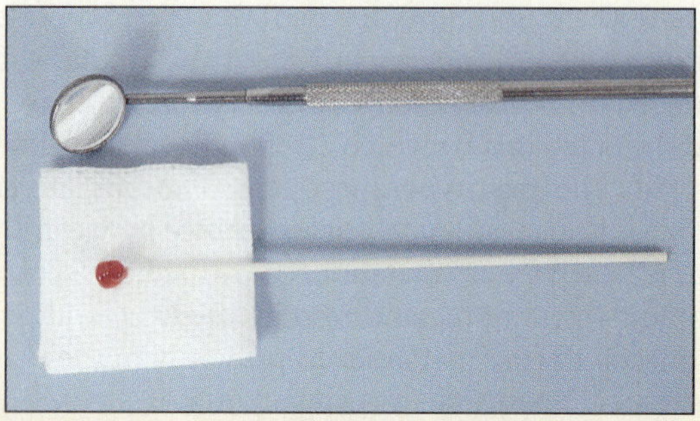

PROCEDURAL STEPS

Preparation

1. Place a small amount of topical ointment on the cotton-tipped applicator, and then replace the cover of the ointment.
   Note: Never insert the same applicator into the ointment after it has been used and contaminated.
2. Explain the procedure to the patient.
   Purpose: Patients are more comfortable and less anxious when they are well informed and know what to expect.
3. Determine the injection site, and gently dry the site with gauze squares.
   Purpose: Drying the site allows the ointment to penetrate the surface area better and not become diluted by saliva, which would decrease its effectiveness.

Placement

1. Place the ointment directly on the injection site.

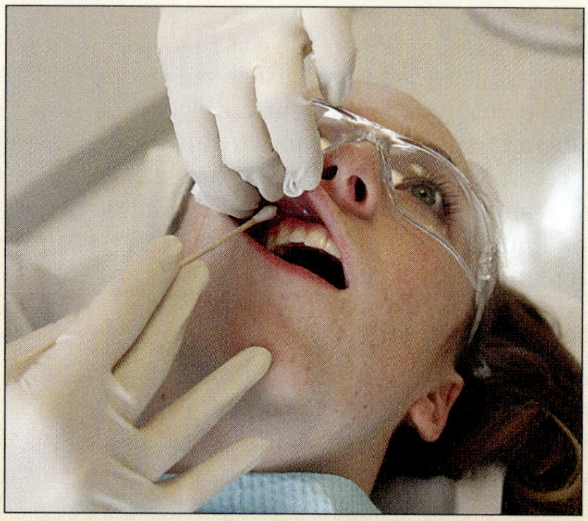

2. Repeat above steps if multiple injections are to be given.
3. Allow the applicator to remain on the site for three to five minutes.
4. Remove the applicator just before the dentist gives the injection.
   Purpose: The site should not be wet with saliva, which would decrease the effect of the ointment.

Major vasoconstrictors used with local anesthetic agents are *epinephrine, levonordefrin,* and *Neo-Cobefrin.* A very small quantity of vasoconstrictor is added to the local anesthetic solution, usually in the ratio of vasoconstrictor to anesthetic solution of 1:20,000; 1:50,000; 1:100,000; or 1:200,000 (Fig. 37-3). With the concentration levels of a vasoconstrictor, the smaller the ratio, the higher the percentage of vasoconstrictor. In most situations it is desirable to use as high a ratio as possible.

Contraindications to Vasoconstrictors

Because a vasoconstrictor may cause strain on the heart as the local anesthetic solution is absorbed into the body, the use of an anesthetic solution *without a vasoconstrictor* is recommended for patients with a history of heart conditions. Such conditions include unstable angina (heart-related chest pain), recent myocardial infarction (heart attack), recent coronary artery bypass surgery, untreated or uncontrolled severe hypertension (high blood pressure), and untreated or uncontrolled congestive heart failure.

The vasoconstrictor action also may interact with other drugs that the patient is taking. Therefore the dentist must be aware of the patient's current medication intake and always update and review the patient's medical history.

Before preparing a syringe, always check with the dentist as to the type of local anesthetic solution and the desired vasoconstrictor/anesthetic solution ratio.

Time Span of Anesthetics

An important consideration for the dentist when choosing a local anesthetic is the time span of pain control required. **Induction** is the length of time from the injection of the anesthetic solution to complete and effective conduction

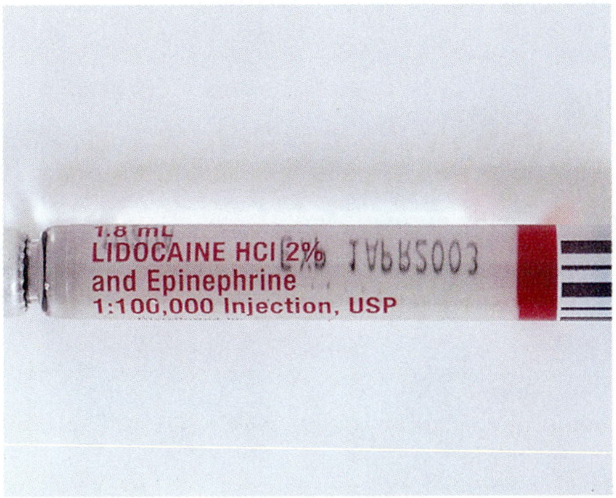

Fig. 37-3 Local anesthetic cartridge showing vasoconstrictor solution.

Box 37-1 Routinely Used Dental Anesthetics

Agent

Short duration

Lidocaine HCl

Prilocaine (infiltration)

Mepivacaine HCl

Intermediate duration

Lidocaine HCl with epinephrine 1:50,000

Lidocaine HCl with epinephrine 1:100,000

Mepivacaine HCl with levonordefrin 1:20,000

Prilocaine HCl (block)

Prilocaine HCl with epinephrine 1:200,000

Articaine with epinephrine 1:100,000

Long duration

Bupivacaine with epinephrine 1:200,000

Modified from Malamed SF: *Handbook of local anesthesia,* ed 5, St Louis, 2004, Mosby.

blockage. **Duration** is the length of time from induction until the reversal process is complete.

Depending on the procedure, the dentist may select a local anesthetic agent on the basis of its duration, as follows:

- A short-acting local anesthetic agent can last from 60 to 180 minutes.
- An intermediate-acting local anesthetic agent lasts from 120 to 240 minutes. (Most local anesthetic agents are in this group and are used for dental procedures.)
- A long-acting local anesthetic agent lasts from 240 to 540 minutes.

Box 37-1 lists routinely used dental anesthetics.

Recall

2. What is the most frequently selected form of pain control used in dentistry?
3. To create a numbing effect, where does a local anesthetic need to be injected?
4. What is added to a local anesthetic to prolong its effect?

INJECTION TECHNIQUES

The location and **innervation** (nerve supply) of the tooth or teeth to be anesthetized determine the topical anesthetic placement and the type of injection. Figure 37-4 reviews specific sites of maxillary and mandibular injections.

Infiltration Anesthesia

Infiltration is achieved by injecting the solution directly into the tissue at the site of the dental procedure. Infiltration anesthesia is generally used for the maxillary teeth because of the **porous** nature of the alveolar cancellous bone. This type of bone structure allows the solution to diffuse through the bone and reach the apices of the teeth.

Infiltration anesthesia may also be used as a secondary injection to block gingival tissues surrounding the mandibular teeth. Infiltration of a local anesthetic solution containing a vasoconstrictor is used to minimize localized bleeding.

Block Anesthesia

Because of the dense, compact nature of the *mandibular* bone, anesthetic solution does not diffuse easily through it. Therefore block anesthesia is the type of injection frequently required for most mandibular teeth. The solution is injected near a major nerve, and the entire area served by that nerve branch is numbed.

Inferior alveolar nerve block, often referred to as a *mandibular block,* is obtained by injecting the anesthetic solution near, but not in, the branches of the inferior alveolar nerve close to the mandibular foramen. The nerve and blood supplies are close to each other, and the dentist must be careful not to inject directly into a blood vessel (see later discussion). The patient will experience numbness over half of the lower jaw, including the teeth, tongue, and lip.

Incisive nerve block is given when only the mandibular anterior teeth or premolars require anesthesia. The incisive block injection is given at the site of the mental foramen. The branch of this nerve continues within the mandibular canal to the apices of the anterior teeth.

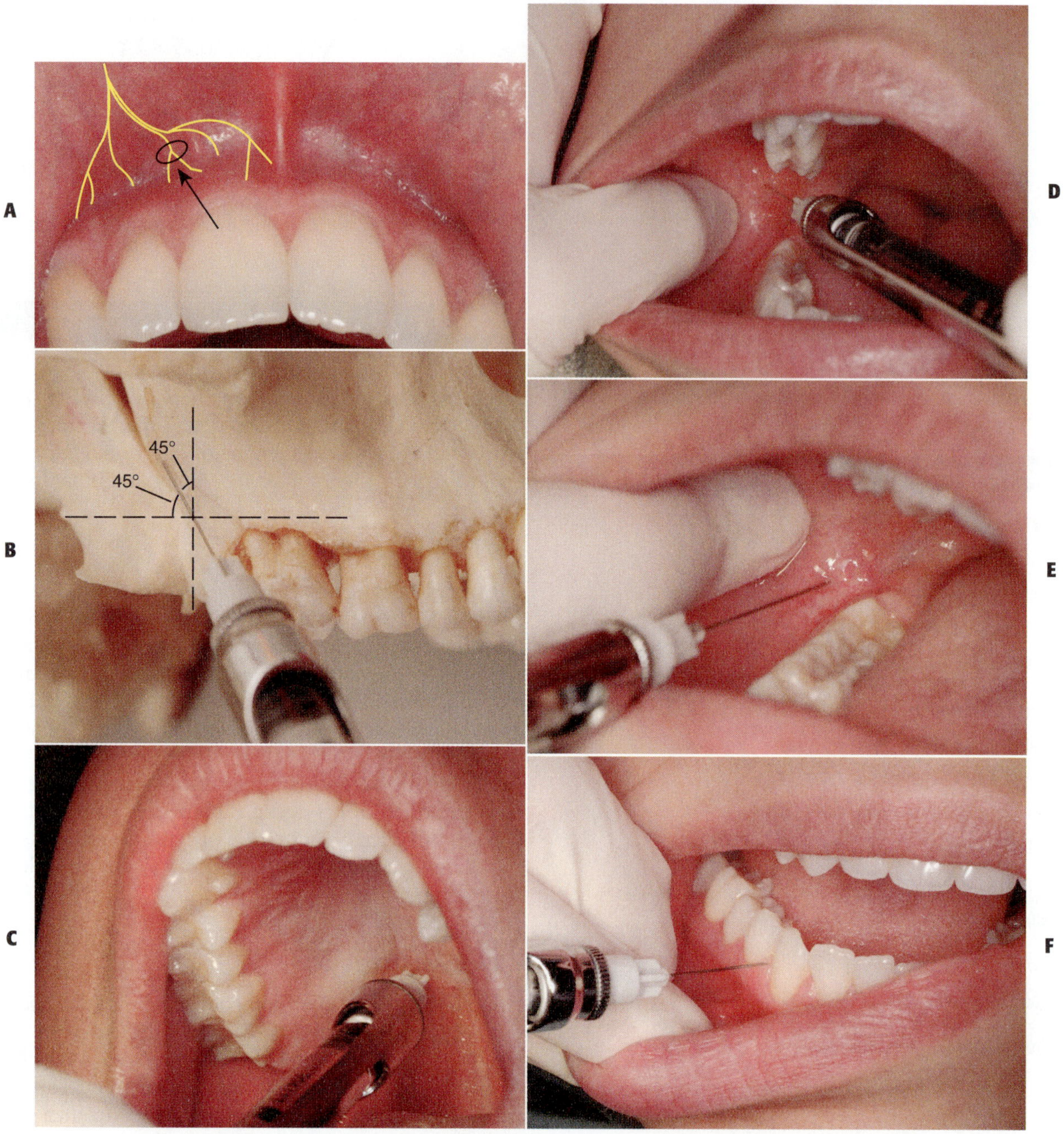

Fig. 37-4 Maxillary and mandibular injection sites. **A,** Maxillary infiltration injection. **B,** Maxillary nerve block injection. **C,** Maxillary greater palatine nerve block injection. **D,** Mandibular inferior nerve block injection. **E,** Mandibular buccal nerve block injection. **F,** Mandibular incisive nerve block. (From Malamed SF: *Handbook of local anesthesia,* ed 5, St Louis, 2004, Mosby.)

Periodontal Ligament Injection

An alternative infiltration technique involves injection of the anesthetic solution under pressure directly into the periodontal ligament and surrounding tissues. Periodontal ligament injection is generally an *adjunct* (addition) to conventional techniques. This type of injection may be completed by using either a conventional syringe or a special periodontal ligament injection syringe (Fig. 37-5).

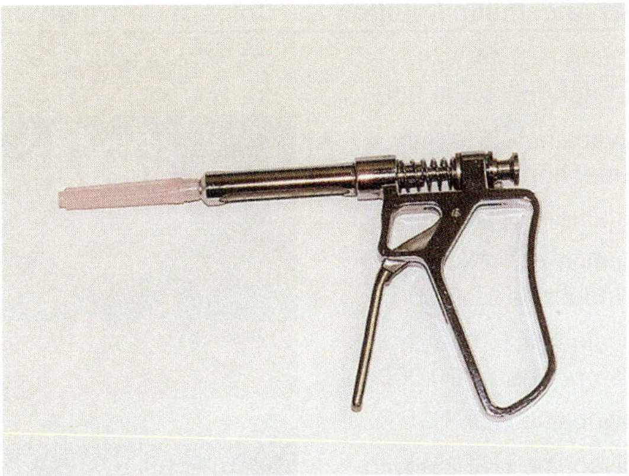

Fig. 37-5 Lig-a-Jet syringe, used to give periodontal ligament injections.

LOCAL ANESTHESIA SETUP

Anesthetic Syringe

Figure 37-6, *A* provides a diagram of the type of syringe used in the administration of local anesthesia. It is made up of the following parts:

Thumb Ring, Finger Grip, and Finger Bar. These parts allow the dentist to control the syringe firmly and to aspirate effectively with one hand.

Harpoon. The harpoon is a sharp hook that locks into the rubber stopper of the anesthetic cartridge so that the stopper can be retracted by pulling back on the piston rod. This action makes aspiration possible.

Piston Rod. This rod pushes the rubber stopper of the anesthetic cartridge and forces the anesthetic solution out through the needle.

Barrel of the Syringe. The barrel firmly holds the anesthetic cartridge in place. The cartridge is loaded through the open side of the barrel. A window on the other side allows the dentist to watch for blood during aspiration.

Threaded Tip. The hub of the needle is attached to the syringe on the threaded tip. The cartridge end of the needle passes through the small opening in the center of the threaded tip, puncturing the rubber diaphragm of the anesthetic cartridge.

Anesthetic Cartridges

Local anesthetic solutions are supplied in glass Carpules. These cartridges have a rubber or silicone stopper at one end and an aluminum cap with a rubber diaphragm at the other end (Fig. 37-6, *B*). Cartridges are supplied in "blister packs" already sterilized and in a sealed environment (Fig. 37-7).

Color-Coding of Local Anesthetic Cartridges

A color-coding system designed by the American Dental Association Council on Scientific Affairs created standard-

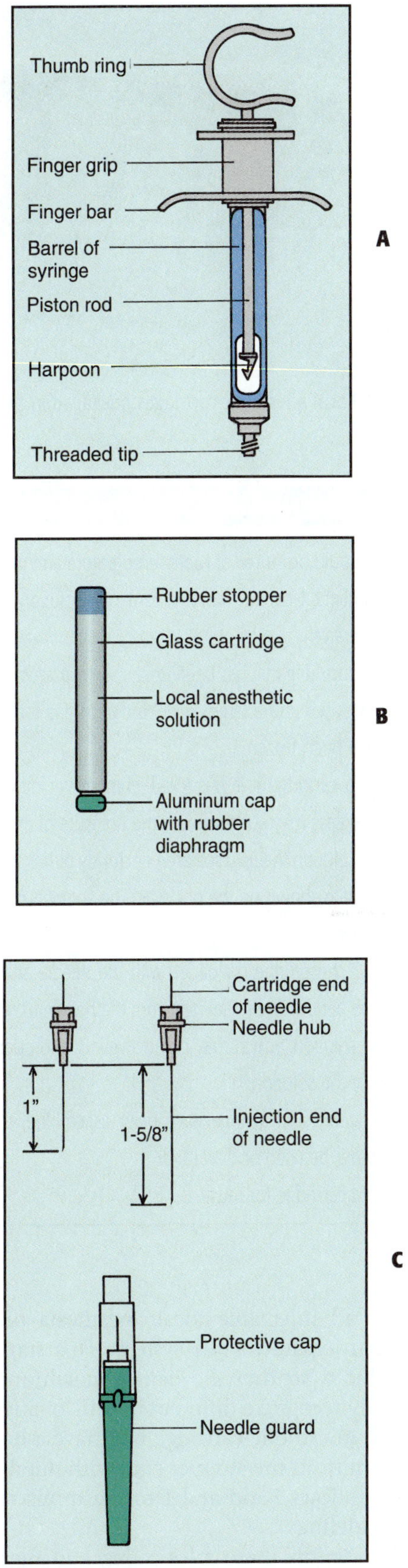

Fig. 37-6 **A,** Aspirating syringe. **B,** Anesthetic cartridge. **C,** Disposable needle.

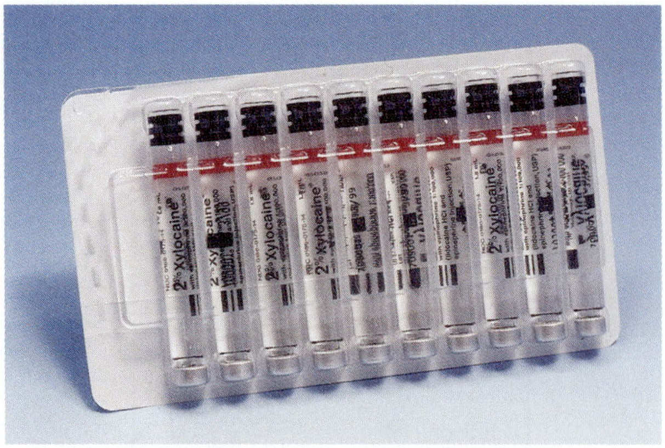

Fig. 37-7 Local anesthetic cartridges packaged in blister packs.

Local Anesthetic Solution	Color of Cartridge Band
Articaine HCl 4% with epinephrine 1:100,000	Gold
Bupivacaine 0.5% with epinephrine 1:200,000	Blue
Lidocaine HCl 2%	Light blue
Lidocaine HCl 2% with epinephrine 1:50,000	Green
Lidocaine HCl 2% with epinephrine 1:100,000	Red
Mepivacaine HCl 3%	Tan
Mepivacaine HCl 2% with levonordefrin 1:20,000	Brown
Prilocaine HCl 4%	Black
Prilocaine HCl 4% with epinephrine 1:200,000	Yellow

Fig. 37-8 Anesthesia color codes. (From Malamed SF: *Handbook of local anesthesia,* ed 5, St Louis, 2004, Mosby.)

Guidelines for Handling Anesthetic Cartridges

Cartridges should be stored at room temperature and protected from direct sunlight. Heat and sun may cause the solution to deteriorate and be less effective.

Never use a cartridge that has been frozen. An *extruded* (pushed out) rubber stopper and a large air bubble are signs that the solution may have been frozen.

Do not use a cartridge if it is cracked, chipped, or damaged in any way. The glass may shatter under the pressure of injection.

Never use a solution that is discolored or cloudy or has passed the expiration date shown on the package. The solution may no longer be effective.

Do not leave the syringe preloaded with the needle attached for an extended period. The metal ions from the needle may be released into the solution, which may cause swelling and edema after injection of the solution.

Once the needle and syringe have been assembled, the cartridge must either be used or discarded.

Never save a cartridge for reuse.

ization for all injectable local anesthesia products that chose to participate in this system. This standardization was introduced so that the dental practitioner could be able to easily recognize different brands of anesthetic (Fig. 37-8). Each anesthetic cartridge will have a band of color placed 3 mm from the stopper end, with durable black lettering that follows Food and Drug Administration (FDA) labeling guidelines.

Learn to identify these color codes, and always take care to select the ratio specified by the dentist. Also, always take the precaution of double-checking the patient's record before selecting an anesthetic solution.

Disposable Needle

The sterile needle used for the injection is protected by a two-part plastic covering (Fig. 37-6, *C*). The two parts are sealed together to ensure sterility. The needle should not be used if this seal is broken.

The *cartridge end* of the needle is the shorter end of the needle. It fits through the threaded tip of the syringe and punctures the rubber diaphragm or the anesthetic cartridge. The protective plastic cap covers the cartridge end of the needle.

The *needle hub* is made of self-threading plastic or prethreaded metal. It is used to attach the needle to the threaded tip of the syringe.

The *injection end* of the needle is protected by the needle guard and is either 1 inch or $1\frac{5}{8}$ inches in length. Most often, the 1-inch *short needle* is used for infiltration anesthesia, and the $1\frac{5}{8}$-inch *long needle* is used for block anesthesia. This end of the needle is *beveled* (angled). Before the injection, the needle is turned so that the beveled angle is toward the bone. This angle enables the dentist to deposit the solution next to the bone without actually contacting the bone.

The **lumen** is the hollow center of the needle through which the anesthetic solution flows. The **gauge** refers to the thickness or size of the needle. Gauges are numbered as follows:

- The *larger* the gauge number, the *thinner* the needle
- The *smaller* the gauge number, the *thicker* the needle

Because a longer needle needs more strength, these needles are generally used in a smaller gauge number. The most frequently used gauge numbers are 25, 27, and 30. See Procedure 37-2: Assembling the Local Anesthetic Syringe.

Procedure 37-2 Assembling the Local Anesthetic Syringe

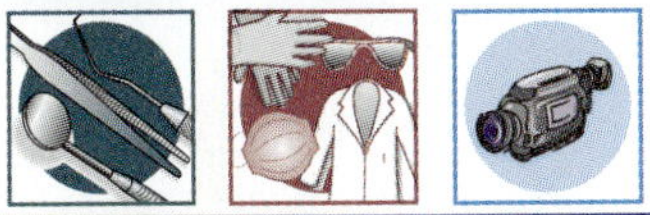

Equipment and Supplies

- Sterile syringe
- Sealed disposable needle or needles
- Sterile local anesthetic cartridges

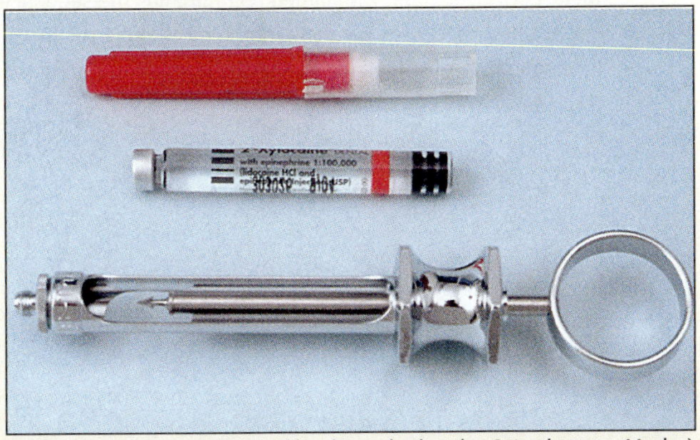

(From Malamed SF: *Handbook of local anesthesia,* ed 5, St Louis, 2004, Mosby.)

PROCEDURAL STEPS

Selecting the Anesthetic

1. The location of the injection will determine the needle length. The dentist determines the type of anesthetic solution.
   Purpose: These choices depend on the patient's medical/dental history and the procedure.
2. Organize supplies, and position the items at chairside out of the patient's view.
3. Wash hands before preparing the syringe.

Loading the Anesthetic Cartridge

1. Hold the syringe in one hand, and use the thumb ring to pull back the plunger.

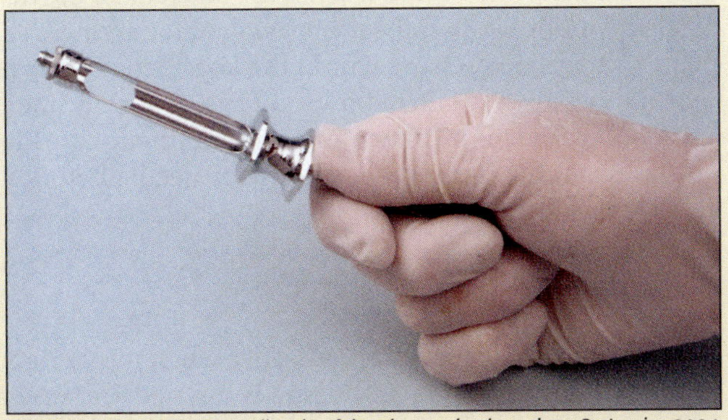

(From Malamed SF: *Handbook of local anesthesia,* ed 5, St Louis, 2004, Mosby.)

2. With the other hand, load the anesthetic cartridge into the syringe. The stopper end goes in first, toward the plunger.

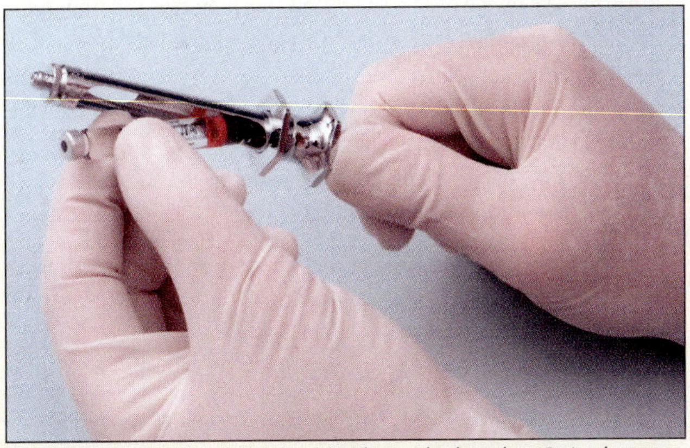

(From Malamed SF: *Handbook of local anesthesia,* ed 5, St Louis, 2004, Mosby.)

3. Release the thumb ring, and allow the harpoon to engage into the stopper.
4. Use gentle finger pressure to engage the piston forward until the harpoon is engaged into the stopper.
   Note: DO NOT hit the piston with the palm of your hand in an effort to engage the harpoon. This leads to the fracturing of glass cartridges.

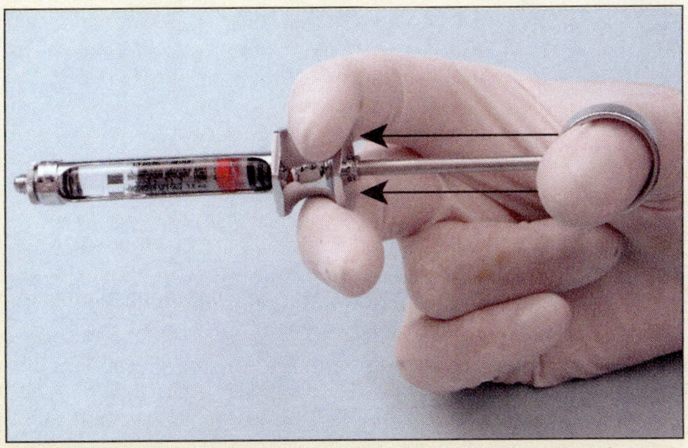

(From Malamed SF: *Handbook of local anesthesia,* ed 5, St Louis, 2004, Mosby.)

4. To check that the harpoon is securely in place, gently pull back on the plunger.
   Purpose: The harpoon must be securely engaged so that the dentist can aspirate during the injection.

continued

Procedure 37-2 Assembling the Local Anesthetic Syringe—cont'd

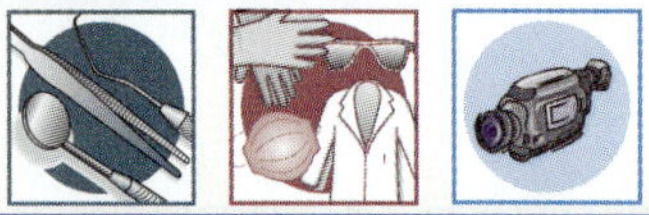

PROCEDURAL STEPS

Placing the Needle on the Syringe

1. Break the seal on the needle and remove the protective cap from the needle. The protective guard (clear plastic) is removed at this time. The needle guard is not yet removed.
2. Screw the needle into position on the syringe. Take care to position the needle so that it is straight and firmly attached.
   Purpose: If the needle is not positioned correctly, the anesthetic solution may leak or may not flow properly.

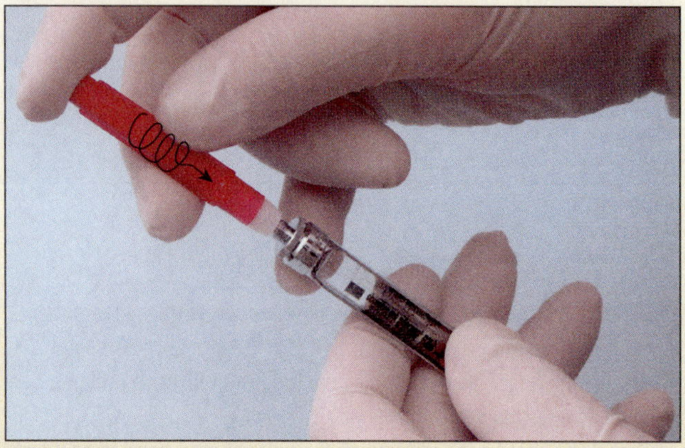

(From Malamed SF: *Handbook of local anesthesia,* ed 5, St Louis, 2004, Mosby.)

3. Place the prepared syringe on the tray ready for use and out of the patient's sight.
   Note: It has been common teaching for years that the needle be attached to the syringe prior to the placement of the anesthetic cartridge. Stanley Malamed recommends the sequence stated above because it virtually eliminates the possibility of a broken cartridge or leakage of anesthetic solution during the procedure.

Recall

5. What type of injection technique does the dentist most frequently use for maxillary teeth?

6. How many lengths of needles are used in dentistry, and for what are they used?

COMPLICATIONS AND PRECAUTIONS

Injection into a Blood Vessel

Local anesthetic solution injected directly into a blood vessel can alter the function of vital organs, notably the heart. To be certain that the solution is not being injected into a vessel, the dentist always **aspirates** (draws back or draws within) before depositing any local anesthetic solution using an aspirating-type syringe. The dentist inserts the needle into the mucosa and advances it to the desired depth. When the tip of the needle reaches the target area, the dentist slowly pulls back on the thumb ring of the syringe. This creates a negative pressure within the anesthetic cartridge.

If the needle has entered a blood vessel, a thin line of red blood cells will be drawn into the anesthetic cartridge. In this event, the dentist repositions the needle before injecting the solution.

Infected Areas

Local anesthetic agents are not effective when injected into an area where a tooth or soft tissue is infected. Because of an increase of lymphocytes (white blood cells) to combat the infection in the area, the anesthetic solution cannot reach the nerves. Injection into an infected area also carries the risk of spreading the infection.

Toxic Reactions

Localized Reactions

Local anesthetic solutions are generally tolerated by the tissues but still may produce a variety of local tissue changes. In some sensitive individuals, even slight contact with solutions containing local anesthetic agents can cause *contact dermatitis,* which is an inflammation of the tissues caused by an allergic reaction to the anesthetic solution.

Systemic Reactions

Although local anesthetic solutions are remarkably safe in their use, the importance of their **systemic toxicity** cannot be ignored. Manifestations of these toxic actions are variable and depend on the following:

- Individual patient physiology
- Local anesthetic solution
- Rate of injection
- Rate of absorption
- Quantity of anesthetic injected
- Other drugs in the patient's system

Temporary Numbness

Because local anesthesia effectively blocks all pain sensation, the patient must be cautioned against biting the tongue, cheek, or lip when numb. This temporary numbness disappears as the effect of the anesthetic agent wears off.

Because the brain is not receiving normal nerve sensations, the numb area may feel swollen when it is not. The patient may complain that the lip feels "fat."

Paresthesia

Paresthesia is a condition in which numbness lasts after the effects of the local anesthetic solutions should have worn off. Paresthesia may be caused by the following:

- Use of contaminated anesthetic solution, most often contamination with alcohol or sterilizing solution used to disinfect the anesthetic cartridge before use
- Trauma (injury) to the nerve sheath during the injection or surgery
- Hemorrhage (bleeding) into or around the nerve sheath

Paresthesia may be temporary or permanent. Most paresthesia is resolved in about eight weeks without treatment. Paresthesia is permanent only if the damage to the nerve is severe.

See Procedure 37-3: Assisting in the Administration of Local Anesthesia.

Procedure 37-3 Assisting in the Administration of Local Anesthesia

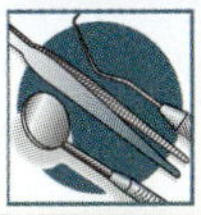
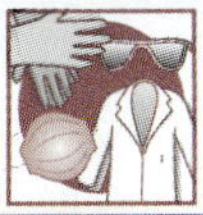
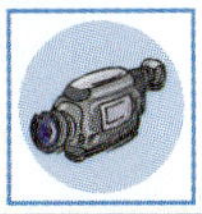
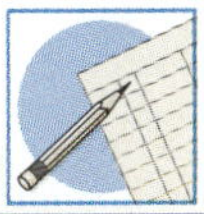

Equipment and Supplies

- Topical anesthetic ointment
- Sterile cotton-tipped applicators
- Sterile gauze sponges
- Sterile assembled local anesthetic syringe

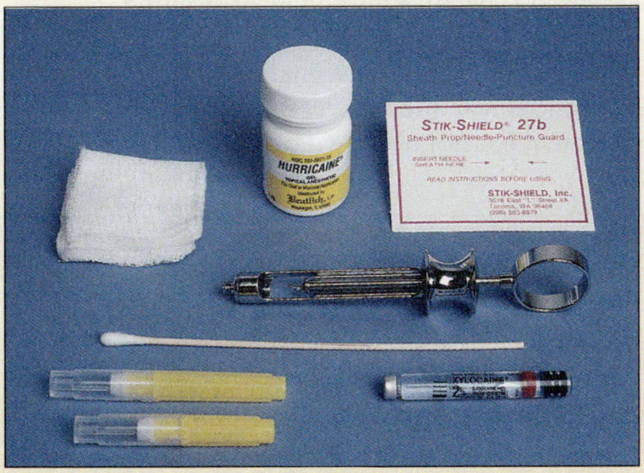

PROCEDURAL STEPS

1. Apply topical anesthetic to the appropriate area of injection (see Procedure 37-1).
2. Loosen the needle guard.
3. Transfer the syringe to the operator by placing the thumb ring over the dentist's thumb.

   Note: This exchange takes place just below the patient's chin and out of the patient's line of vision.

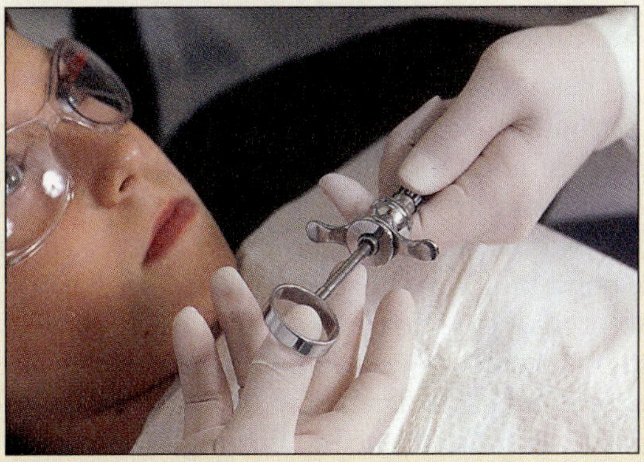

continued

Procedure 37-3 Assisting in the Administration of Local Anesthesia—cont'd

PROCEDURAL STEPS, cont'd

4. While the dentist is giving the injection, monitor the patient for any adverse effects, and project a calming and relaxed manner.
5. The dentist will replace the needle guard on the syringe by using a one-handed scoop technique or a recapping device.
   Purpose: This prevents the possibility of a needlestick injury.

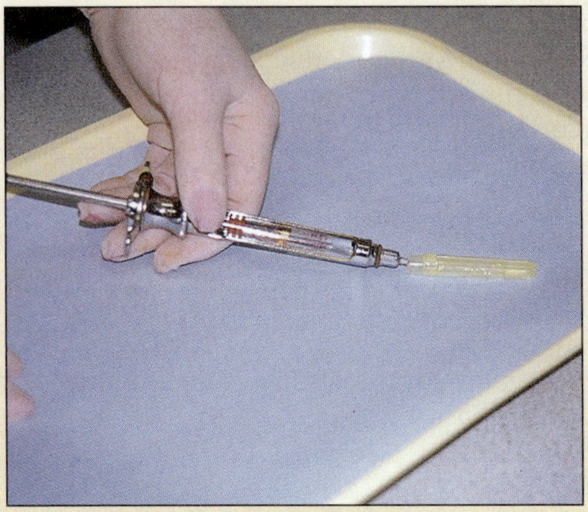

6. After the injection is completed, have the patient turn toward you. Rinse the patient's mouth using the air-water syringe and either the high-volume evacuator or saliva ejector.
7. Continue monitoring the patient throughout the procedure for any adverse effects.
8. At the completion of the procedure, instruct the patient about the numbness, and not to bite his or her lip or cheek.
9. Before leaving the dental treatment area, remove the used needle with the needle guard still in place, and dispose of it in the sharps container.
10. Remove the anesthetic cartridge and dispose of it with the medical waste. Place the syringe on the tray to be returned to the sterilization center.

Recall

7. Should a patient with an abscess receive local anesthesia? Why or why not?
8. What is paresthesia?

ELECTRONIC ANESTHESIA

An electronic anesthesia system is an innovative, noninvasive form of anesthesia. The system is designed to block pain electronically by using a low current of electricity. Contact pads target a specific electronic waveform directly to the nerve bundle at the root of the tooth.

The patient is seated and positioned with hand pads placed on the back of each hand. The area of the operative site is determined, isolated, and dried. The third pad, the *intraoral receptor,* is attached to the lingual side 3 to 5 mm from the gingival margin. As instructed, the patient has control in activating the unit and gradually increasing the level of the pain-blocking signal.

This alternative psychological and physiological approach to local anesthesia benefits the patient for the following reasons:

- No needles
- No postoperative numbness or swelling
- Chemical-free method of anesthesia
- No risk of cross-contamination
- Reduced fear and anxiety in patients
- Patient control over own comfort level

INHALATION SEDATION

Inhalation sedation, also referred to as nitrous oxide/oxygen (N_2O/O_2) analgesia, may be the safest type of sedation method used in dentistry. The use of nitrous oxide in dentistry dates back to 1844, when Horace Wells (the first dentist) used these gases on his patients.

N_2O/O_2 sedation produces stage I anesthesia/analgesia by using a combination of nitrous oxide and oxygen gases. The patient inhales these gases through a nosepiece and feels the effect almost immediately. N_2O/O_2 sedation produces a pleasant, relaxing experience for the patient and is associated with easy onset, minimal side effects, and rapid recovery.

Chemical Makeup

Nitrous oxide is a tasteless, sweet-smelling, colorless gas that is housed in a blue-colored cylinder. The cylinder stores the nitrous oxide liquid/gas combination in equilibrium at 650 lb to 900 lb per square inch (psi), with only the gas being delivered to the patient.

Advantages of Nitrous Oxide Use

- Administration is relatively simple and easily managed by the dentist.
- Although special training is required for the dentist and dental assistant, the services of an anesthetist or other special personnel are not necessary.
- This type of sedation has an excellent safety record, and the side effects are minimal.
- The patient is awake and able to communicate at all times.
- Recovery is rapid and complete within a matter of minutes.
- N_2O/O_2 sedation may be used with patients of all ages.

Contraindications to Nitrous Oxide Use

No absolute medical contraindications exist to N_2O/O_2 analgesia, but certain conditions make it a poor choice for some patients.

Pregnancy

No evidence indicates that enough nitrous oxide crosses the placenta to damage the fetus. However, N_2O/O_2 analgesia is usually administered to a pregnant patient *only* after the first trimester and *only* with the permission of her obstetrician.

Nasal Obstruction

Nasal obstruction can prevent the patient from obtaining the benefit of nitrous oxide.

Emphysema and Multiple Sclerosis

Patients with emphysema or multiple sclerosis may have breathing difficulties while receiving N_2O/O_2 sedation. The increased oxygen delivery during administration may lower the stimulus to breathe as often as necessary.

Emotional Instability

The altered perception of reality produced by N_2O/O_2 analgesia may intensify a patient's emotional instability.

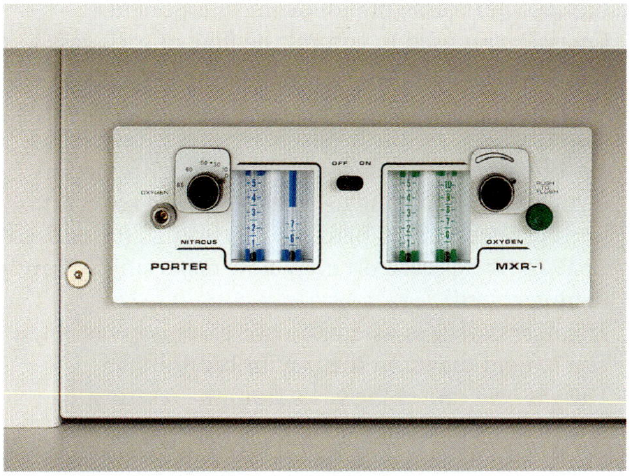

Fig. 37-9 Nitrous oxide system stabilized as part of the dental unit. (Courtesy A-dec.)

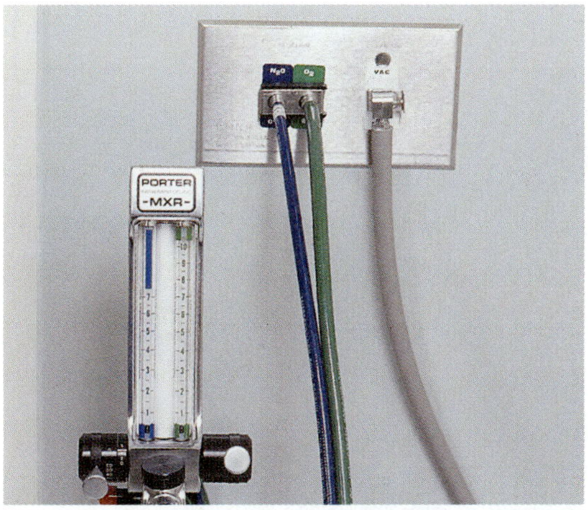

Fig. 37-10 Portable nitrous oxide system unit.

Equipment

The dental office may be equipped with built-in N_2O/O_2 equipment in the treatment area (Fig. 37-9). An alternative is the use of a portable unit that is moved from room to room as needed (Fig. 37-10).

In most states, ordering of a new supply of these gases involves the dentist's signature and license number. It is also necessary to comply with Occupational Safety and Health Administration (OSHA) and state requirements for safe installation and storage of these supplies.

Gas Tanks

The N_2O and O_2 gases are dispensed in steel cylinders, and are color-coded green for oxygen and blue for nitrous oxide (Fig. 37-11). Cylinders should be stored in an upright position, away from a heat source, and chained to the wall (or portable unit) to prevent them from falling on the valve stem, which could cause them to explode.

Gas devices include the following components:

- *Control valves* used to control the flow of each gas.
- The *flow meter* indicates the rate of flow of the gas. Current flow meters employ a fail-safe mechanism that stops the flow of nitrous oxide whenever the percentage of oxygen drops below 30 percent. This mechanism also prevents the delivery of N_2O in concentrations greater than 70 percent. This feature, introduced in 1976, is standard on every flow meter unit currently manufactured.
- The *reservoir bag* is where the two gases are combined. The patient draws on the bag for breathing.
- The *gas hose* carries the gases from the reservoir bag to the mask or nosepiece.

Masks, also referred to as *nosepieces,* are the nasal inhalers through which the patient breathes the gases. Masks are supplied in sizes for adults and children (Fig. 37-12). They are available in a disposable variety that is discarded after a single use and in rubber that can be sterilized or disinfected for reuse.

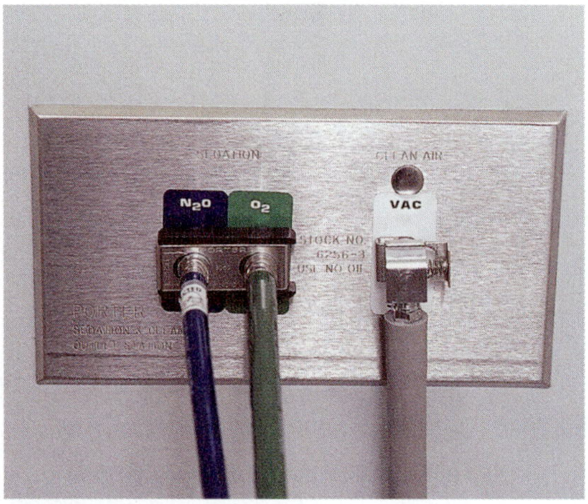

Fig. 37-11 Nitrous oxide gas lines are color-coded blue, and oxygen gas lines are color-coded green.

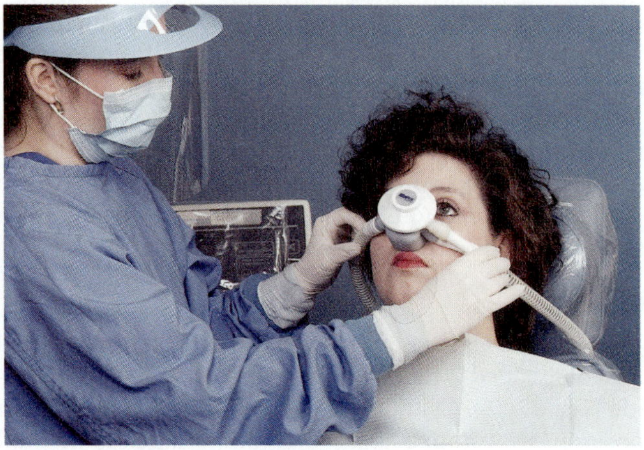

Fig. 37-12 Nasal mask used for inhalation.

Scavenger System

A scavenger system is essential to protect you and other dental personnel from the occupational risks of nitrous oxide. Scavenger systems should have an evacuation flow rate of 45 liters per minute (L/min) and incorporate a scavenging nasal mask, or *hood* (Fig. 37-13).

Members of the dental team use a scavenger system to reduce the amount of N_2O that escapes into the atmosphere, which is then inhaled. The use of a scavenger system is recommended to reduce the N_2O released into the treatment room.

Reducing Exposure to Nitrous Oxide

Nitrous oxide is used only during patient treatment. N_2O is never administered unnecessarily or used for recreational purposes, which can lead to the abuse of this substance.

Nitrous oxide is a toxic substance. Over a period of months, with large amounts unscavenged in the atmosphere, N_2O can produce harmful side effects to dental personnel (see Chapter 23). For dental professionals, the safest maximum allowable amount of N_2O in the dental environment is 50 parts per million (ppm). To reduce N_2O hazards to dental personnel, you should take the following steps:

- Use a scavenger system.
- Use a patient mask that fits well so that gas does not leak around the edges.
- Discourage patients from talking while receiving N_2O/O_2.
- Vent gas outside the building.
- Routinely inspect equipment and hoses for leaks.
- Use an N_2O monitoring badge system.

Patient Assessment and Monitoring

Always review the patient's medical history before administering N_2O/O_2 analgesia. Keep in mind that the sedative effects of N_2O/O_2 may enhance the effects of medications either directly or indirectly.

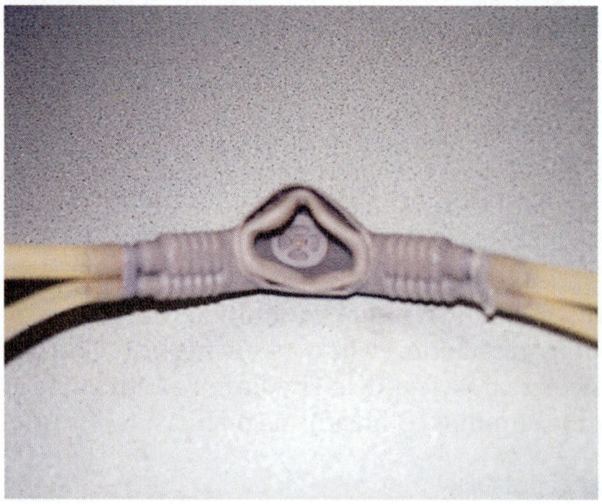

Fig. 37-13 Scavenger system attached to mask and evacuation unit to redirect unused nitrous oxide gas.

The vital signs of blood pressure, pulse, and respiration should be recorded before, during, and after the administration of N_2O/O_2 analgesia. The preoperative readings provide a baseline against which preoperative and postoperative readings can be compared. Postoperative readings are used to confirm the patient's recovery or identify adverse responses.

Patient Education

Before N_2O/O_2 administration begins, the patient should be informed about what to expect. The dentist or the assistant should describe (1) the process of gas administration, (2) proper use of the mask and the importance of nasal breathing, and (3) the sensations of warmth and tingling that the patient will experience. Reassure patients that they will remain conscious, aware, and in control of their actions.

Administration

Under the dental practice act in some states, the dental assistant is permitted to aid in monitoring the administration of N_2O/O_2 only under the direct supervision of the dentist. To ensure the patient's safety, it is vital to understand the process and the assistant's role in its administration.

N_2O/O_2 sedation should begin with the administration of 100 percent oxygen. Start with pure O_2 while establishing the patient's tidal volume, and then slowly **titrate,** or determine the concentration of, the N_2O until the desired results are achieved. Patients can respond differently to N_2O from one appointment to the next. The dosage at one appointment may seem excessive or insufficient for the patient at a later visit. There is no set dosage regimen, only the goal of **titration** to the patient's needs.

Patients should refrain from talking or mouth breathing. This can expel N_2O into the air that the dental team can inhale and can reduce the concentration of N_2O inhaled by the patient.

The N_2O/O_2 analgesia should end with the administration of 100 percent oxygen for three to five minutes. Assess the patient afterward for dizziness, headache, or lethargy, and continue 100 percent oxygen if such symptoms exist.

After the patient once again feels normal, obtain postoperative vital signs and compare them to the preoperative recordings. Do not let patients drive themselves home if you believe they pose a risk to themselves or others. See Procedure 37-4: Assisting in the Administration and Monitoring of Nitrous Oxide/Oxygen Sedation (Expanded Function).

Recall

9. Who was the first dentist to use nitrous oxide on his patients?
10. What color code is used for nitrous oxide?
11. How is the dental team at risk for overexposure to nitrous oxide?
12. What is given to the patient before and after N_2O/O_2 sedation?

Procedure 37-4 Assisting in the Administration and Monitoring of Nitrous Oxide/Oxygen Sedation (Expanded Function)

Equipment and Supplies

- N_2O/O_2 system
- Scavenger-type masks (adult and child sizes)
- Equipment for measuring vital signs

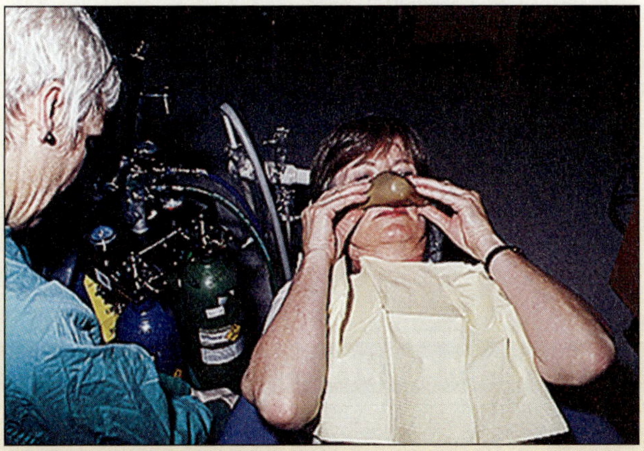

(From Darby M, Walsh M: *Dental hygiene theory and practice,* ed 2, St Louis, 2003, Saunders.)

PROCEDURAL STEPS

1. Check the tanks for adequate supply of gases. Select and place the appropriate size of mask on the tubing.
2. Seat the patient, update the medical history, and take and record vital signs.
3. Review the use of nitrous oxide with the patient.
   Purpose: Informing the patient before administration helps to eliminate fear of the unknown.
4. Place the patient in a supine position.
5. Have the patient put on the mask, and adjust the fit.

continued

Procedure 37-4 Assisting in the Administration and Monitoring of Nitrous Oxide/Oxygen Sedation (Expanded Function)—cont'd

PROCEDURAL STEPS, cont'd

6. Tighten the tubing once it is comfortable to the patient.
   Purpose: To eliminate the need for the patient to hold the mask in place, and to prevent leakage from around the mask.
7. If the mask pinches or causes discomfort, place gauze square under the edge.

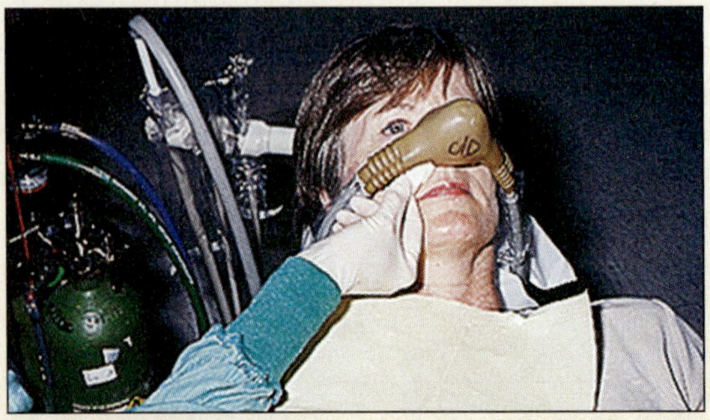

(From Darby M, Walsh M: *Dental hygiene theory and practice,* ed 2, St Louis, 2003, Saunders.)

Administration

1. At the dentist's instructions, begin adjusting the flow meter for O_2 flow only. The patient is given 100 percent oxygen for at least one minute.
   Purpose: To assist the dentist in determining the patient's **tidal volume.**

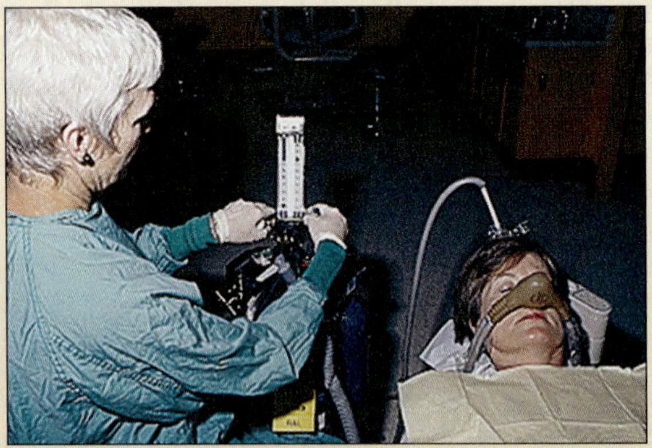

(From Darby M, Walsh M: *Dental hygiene theory and practice,* ed 2, St Louis, 2003, Saunders.)

2. At the dentist's direction, adjust N_2O flow in increments of 0.5 to 1 L/min, and reduce O_2 flow by a corresponding amount.
   Note: Most machines perform this function automatically.
3. At 1-minute intervals, the previous step is repeated until the dentist determines that the patient has reached the baseline reading.
   Purpose: This slow process minimizes the risk of administering too much N_2O.
4. Note the patient's baseline level.
5. Monitor the patient closely throughout the procedure.

Oxygenation

1. Toward the end of the procedure, N_2O is depleted and 100 percent O_2 administered, as directed by the dentist.
   Purpose: Oxygenation of patients for a minimum of 5 minutes helps to prevent *diffusion hypoxia,* which creates a feeling of lightheadedness.
2. After oxygenation is complete, remove the mask. *Slowly* position the patient upright.
   Purpose: Bringing the patient upright too quickly may cause postural hypotension (fainting).

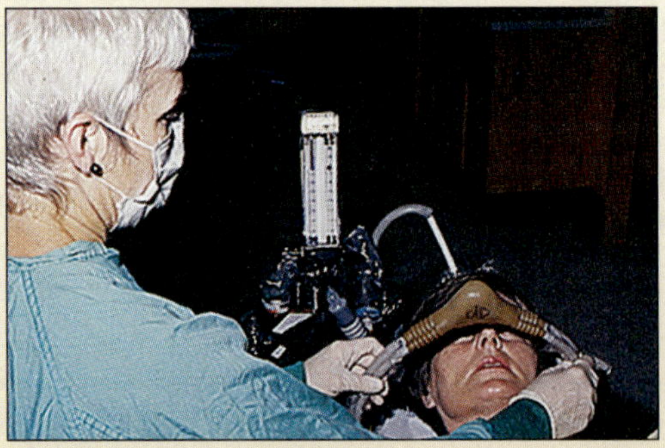

(From Darby M, Walsh M: *Dental hygiene theory and practice,* ed 2, St Louis, 2003, Saunders.)

3. Record the patient's baseline level of N_2O and O_2 and response during analgesia.
   Purpose: This documentation provides a legal record of care and serves as a reference for future care and administration of N_2O/O_2 sedation (analgesia).

ANTIANXIETY AGENTS

Drugs that are administered for the relief of anxiety are termed *antianxiety drugs,* or *anxiolytics.* In larger doses, these drugs can produce sleep, sedation, and anesthesia. Antianxiety agents can be administered orally, intravenously, or by inhalation (gases). Before administering any form of agent, the dentist is required to have specialized training in the choice of agents and the mode of delivery.

Sedatives may be used in the following situations:

- Patients are very nervous about a procedure.
- A procedure will be long or difficult.

- Mentally challenged patients are receiving treatment.
- Very young children are undergoing extensive treatment.

The types of sedatives commonly prescribed to dental patients are *secobarbital* (Seconal), *chlordiazepoxide* (Librium), and *diazepam* (Valium). With these types of drugs, the patient will be asked to take the drug orally 30 to 60 minutes before the appointment. Patients must be informed that these drugs induce drowsiness and that they should not drive themselves to the appointment. *Chloral hydrate* (Noctec) is a sedative often used for sedation of children, and it produces the same type of effect.

INTRAVENOUS SEDATION

Intravenous (IV) conscious sedation results in a minimally depressed level of consciousness. The patient maintains the ability to keep an open airway and to respond appropriately to physical or verbal stimulation. Specific antianxiety drugs are administered intravenously (directly into a vein) throughout the procedure at a slower rate, providing a deeper stage I analgesia.

The process of starting, monitoring, and removal of IV sedation is completed only by an individual trained and certified in this area. The oral and maxillofacial surgeon and the periodontist are the two dental specialists who most often receive this additional training. Specialty offices employ registered nurses to administer and monitor IV sedation procedures.

Patient Management and Monitoring

Before the administration of IV conscious sedation, a physical examination is performed and a pertinent history and signed consent are obtained. Parental or guardian informed consent is required for children. Baseline vital signs, level of consciousness, and motor function; **oximetry** (blood oxygen concentration) results; and the electrocardiogram are completed and recorded. The patient's weight should be recorded for dose determination.

During intravenous conscious sedation, IV access must be maintained continuously. All patients are monitored throughout the procedure as well as in the recovery phase. Physiologic measurements should be taken and recorded at least every 15 minutes. These measurements include, but are not limited to, level of consciousness, respiratory function, oximetry, blood pressure, heart rate, and cardiac rhythm. Supplemental oxygen, suction, and a defibrillator must be available immediately and used as needed in an emergency situation.

Recall

13. Is the patient conscious during intravenous sedation?

GENERAL ANESTHESIA

Another way to administer antianxiety agents is through general anesthesia. General anesthesia is a controlled state of unconsciousness characterized by loss of protective reflexes, including the ability to maintain an airway independently and to respond appropriately to physical stimulation or verbal command. This method provides a controlled state of loss of consciousness, or stage III general anesthesia.

General anesthesia is achieved by using a combination of gases, N_2O/O_2, halothane or enflurane mixtures, and IV agents such as thiopental and methohexital.

General anesthesia is most safely administered in a hospital setting or another facility with the necessary equipment for administration and the management of an emergency. *Anesthesiologists* are physicians who specialize in this form of anesthesia.

Four Stages of Anesthesia

Specific antianxiety agents or a combination of agents can produce different levels of consciousness and unconsciousness. These levels are termed *stages* of anesthesia.

Stage I: Analgesia is the stage during which a patient is relaxed and fully conscious. The patient is able to keep the mouth open without assistance and is capable of following directions. The patient experiences a sense of euphoria and a reduction in pain. Vital signs are normal. Depending on the agent, the patient can move into different levels of analgesia.

Stage II: Excitement is the stage during which the patient is less aware of the immediate surroundings and may start to become unconscious. The patient may become excited and unmanageable. Nausea and vomiting may occur. Excitement is an undesirable stage.

Stage III: General anesthesia is the stage of anesthesia that begins when the patient becomes calm after stage II. The patient feels no pain or sensation. The patient soon becomes unconscious. This stage of anesthesia can be achieved only under the guidance of an anesthesiologist in a controlled environment such as a hospital setting.

Stage IV: Respiratory failure or cardiac arrest occurs when the lungs and heart slow down or stop functioning. If this stage is not reversed quickly, the patient will die.

Patient Preparation

The patient must have a preoperative physical examination, laboratory tests, or both performed before administration of the general anesthetic agent. The patient or legal guardian must sign a consent form before the anesthesia and procedure can be performed.

Patient Education

The dentist reviews the procedure as well as the risks of and probable reactions to the general anesthesia. Most surgical procedures are scheduled in the early morning because patients must not eat or drink 8 to 12 hours before receiving general anesthesia (NPO status). The patient must have a driver for transport home after the procedure.

Patient Recovery

Once the procedure is completed, the patient is monitored closely until normal reflexes return. The patient should respond to name and be able to move the limbs, turn the head, and speak coherently. The patient should not be left alone while regaining consciousness.

Recall

14. Is the patient conscious during general anesthesia?
15. In what environment is general anesthesia most often administered?

DOCUMENTATION OF ANESTHESIA AND PAIN CONTROL

Maintaining accurate records is an essential aspect of pain and anxiety analgesia. Always document the following measures and observations:

- Review of patient's medical history
- Preoperative and postoperative vital signs
- Tidal volume if using inhalation sedation
- Time anesthesia began and ended
- Peak concentration administered
- Postoperative time (minutes) for patient recovery
- Adverse events or patient complaints

Record this information in the progress notes section of the patient record or on a separate form.

Patient Education

Many patients are hesitant to discuss their fears resulting from a story by another dental patient who had a bad experience or based on what they think will occur during a dental procedure. It is important for the patient to be aware of the type of pain and anxiety control measures that are provided for patients. *Good communication* is the key to the patient being well informed, feeling confident about the dental care, and becoming a knowledgeable and compliant patient at future appointments.

LEGAL AND ETHICAL IMPLICATIONS

Some degree of risk is always associated with the use of any drug, even when administered by trained individuals. The dentist and the dental team have a responsibility to minimize risk to patients undergoing dental treatment by following these guidelines:

- Use only sedation methods with which they are thoroughly familiar.
- Limit the use of sedation methods only to patients who require them.
- Conduct a comprehensive preoperative evaluation of the patient.
- Monitor the patient continuously.
- Document all records of drugs used, dosage, vital signs, reactions, and recovery.
- Treat high-risk patients in an appropriate setting.

Eye to the Future

An alternative to sedative drugs is the use of acupuncture. *Acupuncture* originated in China more than 3000 years ago and is becoming a method of pain control in the dental office. Needles are inserted at various *acupuncture points* on the body as a means of reducing aches, pains, stress, and anxiety related to dental treatment.

Critical Thinking

1. You are assisting in a restorative procedure. The dentist will be placing an amalgam in tooth #14. The dentist has indicated that a short-acting anesthetic agent will be used. How long does a short-acting anesthetic agent last?
2. Describe where you will place the topical anesthetic for tooth #14 and what type of injection the dentist will perform for this area of the mouth.
3. The dentist has completed anesthesia and transfers the syringe back to you. What is wrong with this scenario, and how do you handle it with the patient in the chair?
4. A five-year-old child is scheduled to have a tooth restored with a stainless steel crown. The patient record already notes that there is pulpal damage, which means the tooth will require a pulpotomy. The pediatric patient is very apprehensive about the visit and what to expect. Describe additional anxiety and pain-control measures that the dentist could use along with local anesthesia.
5. A patient is scheduled to have her third molars extracted. What type of pain control might the surgeon select to prolong the anesthesia and decrease the bleeding around the surgical site?
6. You are scheduled to assist in a procedure that includes the monitoring of N_2O/O_2 sedation. You check all the equipment and review the procedure with the patient. You notice that the patient seems to have a cold. When you inquire about this, the patient indicates that his allergies have been acting up. How will this affect the administration of N_2O?

Part 8

Dental Radiology

Quality diagnostic radiographs are essential in the practice of dentistry. Dental radiography involves the use of x-radiation to create radiographs necessary to identify and diagnose conditions that may otherwise go undetected. The images that are produced using x-radiation are seen either on film or on a digital display. The role of the dental assistant is to expose and process the images, manage the patient, maintain proper infection control and quality control, and *always* follow radiation safety procedures. Producing diagnostic-quality radiographs with minimal exposure is your professional responsibility.

The chapters in this section will provide you with the information you need to understand radiation and how to use it safely in the dental office to produce radiographs that are of the best possible diagnostic quality. Each chapter provides a balance of theory and technique.

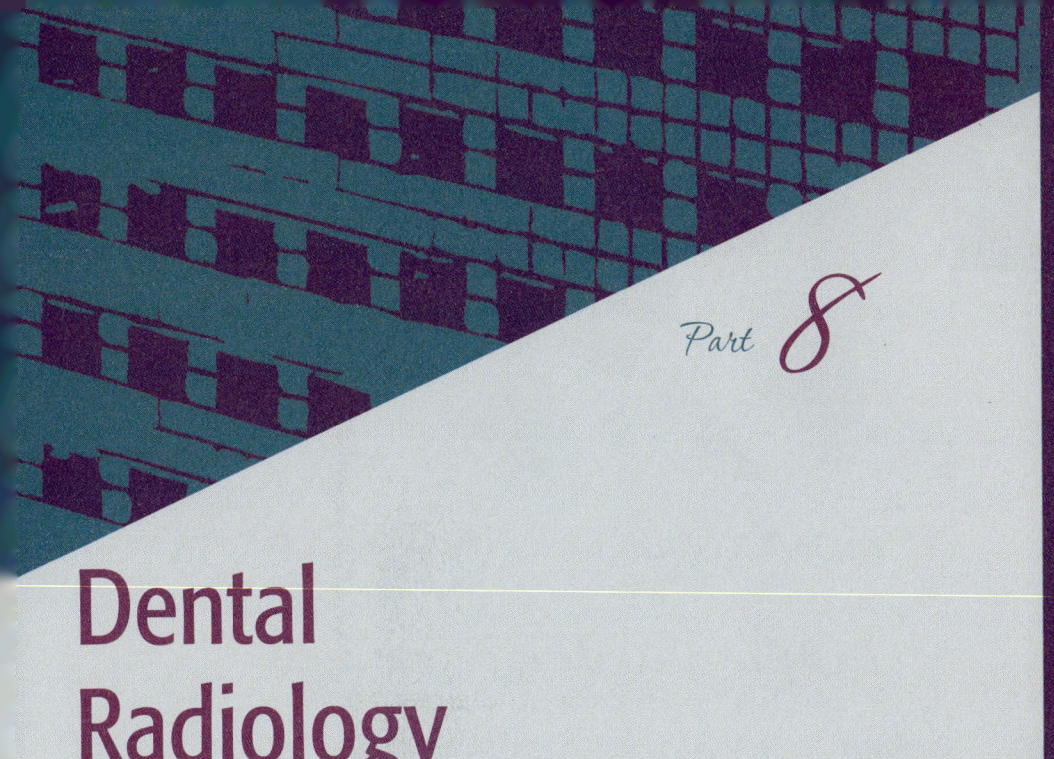

38

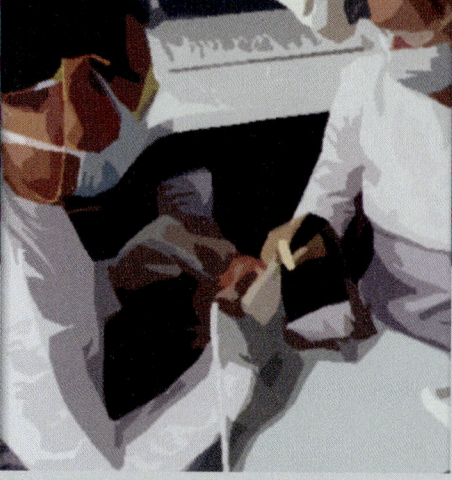

Foundations of Radiography, Radiographic Equipment, and Radiologic Safety

Outline

Discovery of X-Radiation
- Pioneers in Dental Radiography

Radiation Physics
- Atomic Structure
- Ionization
- Properties of Radiographs

The Dental X-Ray Machine
- Tubehead
- X-Ray Tube
- Position Indicator Device (PID)
- Extension Arm
- Control Panel

X-Ray Production

Types of Radiation

Characteristics of Radiograph Beam
- Radiolucent and Radiopaque Characteristics
- Contrast
- Density
- Geometric Characteristics

Radiation Effects
- Tissue Damage
- Biologic Effects
- Critical Organs

Radiation Measurement
- Maximum Permissible Dose

Radiation Safety
- Protective Devices
- Patient Protection
- Pregnancy
- Operator Protection and Monitoring
- Equipment Monitoring
- Pediatric Patients
- ALARA Concept

Patient Education

Legal and Ethical Implications

Eye to the Future

Critical Thinking

KEY TERMS

ALARA concept Concept of radiation protection that states all exposures should be kept "*as low as reasonably achievable.*"

Anode (**a**-node) The positive electrode in the x-ray tube.

Atom The basic unit of matter.

Cathode (**ka**-thode) The negative electrode in the x-ray tube.

Central ray X-rays at center of beam.

Contrast The differences in degrees of blackness on a radiograph.

Control panel The portion of the x-ray unit that contains the master switch, the indicator light, the selector buttons, and the exposure button.

Density The overall darkness or blackness of a radiograph.

KEY TERMS, cont'd

Dental radiography (*ray*-dee-**ah**-greh-fee) Process of making radiographs of the teeth and adjacent structures by exposure to radiographs.
Distortion Change in the size of an image on a radiograph caused by incorrect vertical angulation.
Dose (of radiation) The amount of energy absorbed by tissues.
Electron A negatively charged particle in the atom.
Energy The ability to do work.
Extension arm Flexible arm that is attached to the x-ray tubehead.
Genetic effects (juh-**neh**-tik) Effects of radiation that are passed on to future generations through genetic cells.
Ion (**eye**-on) An electrically charged particle.
Ionization (**eye**-eh-nuh-**zay**-shun) Process by which electrons are removed from atoms, causing the harmful effects of radiation in humans.
Ionizing radiation (**eye**-ah-*nize*-ing) Radiation that produces ionization, resulting in harmful effects.
Kilovoltage peak (kVp) (**ki**-luh-*vole*-tij) Highest voltage of radiograph tube used during a radiograph exposure.
Latent period (**lay**-tunt) Time between exposure to ionizing radiation and appearance of symptoms.
Lead apron Device used to protect the reproductive and blood-forming tissues from scatter radiation.
Magnification The proportional enlargement of a radiographic image.
Master switch, indicator light, selector buttons, exposure button Components of control panel.
Matter Anything that occupies space and has form or shape.
Milliampere (mA) (*mi*-lah-**am**-peer) One one-thousandth (1/1000) of an ampere, a unit of measurement used to describe the intensity of an electric current.
Penumbra (puh-**num**-bruh) The blurred or indistinct area that surrounds an image.
Photon (**fo**-tahn) A minute (tiny) bundle of pure energy that has no weight or mass.
Primary beam The most penetrating beam produced at the target of the anode.
Primary radiation Same as primary beam.
Radiation Forms of waves of energy emission through space or a material.
Radiograph (**ray**-dee-oh-*graf*) Image produced on photosensitive film by exposing the film to radiation and then processing it.
Radiology (*ray*-dee-**ah**-luh-jee) The science or study of radiation as used in medicine.
Scatter radiation A form of secondary radiation that occurs when an x-ray beam has been deflected from its path by interaction with matter.
Secondary radiation X-radiation that is created when the primary beam interacts with matter.
Sharpness A measure of how well the radiograph reproduces the fine details or outlines of an object.
Somatic effects (so-**ma**-tik) Effects of radiation that cause illness and are responsible for poor health (such as cancer, leukemia, and cataracts) but are not passed on to offspring.
Thyroid collar A flexible lead shield that is placed securely around the neck.
Tubehead The part of the x-ray unit that contains the x-ray tube, the high-voltage and low-voltage transformers, and insulating oil.
Tungsten target A focal spot in the anode.
X-radiation High-energy ionizing electromagnetic radiation.

LEARNING OUTCOMES

On completion of this chapter, the student will be able to achieve the following objectives:

- Pronounce, define, and spell the Key Terms.
- Describe the uses of dental radiographs.
- Name the highlights in the history of dental radiography.
- Describe the discovery of x-radiation.
- Explain what happens during ionization.
- Describe the properties of x-radiation.
- Explain how radiographs are produced.
- Label the parts of the dental x-ray tubehead and tube.
- Describe the effect of the kilovoltage on the quality of the x-ray beam.
- Describe how the milliamperage affects the quality of the x-ray beam.
- Identify the range of kilovoltage and milliamperage required for dental radiography.
- Discuss the effects of radiation exposure on the human body.
- Discuss the risks versus benefits of dental radiographs.
- Identify the critical organs that are sensitive to radiation.
- Discuss the ALARA concept.
- Describe the methods of protecting the patient from excess radiation.
- Describe the measures used to protect the operator from excess radiation.

The dental assistant must have a thorough knowledge and understanding of the importance and uses of dental radiographs. Dental radiographs are a necessary component of a comprehensive dental examination, as well as a part of the dental patient's permanent record.

Radiographs enable the dentist to see conditions that are not visible in the oral cavity and to identify many conditions that might otherwise remain undetected. Many dental diseases and conditions have no clinical signs or symptoms and are typically discovered *only* through the use of dental radiographs.

To understand how radiographs are produced, the dental assistant must first understand the fundamental concepts of atomic structure and have a working knowledge of ionizing radiation and the properties of radiographs. These will be discussed later in this chapter.

Radiation, which is used to produce dental radiographs, has the ability to cause damage to all types of living tissues.

Uses of Dental Radiographs

1. Detect dental caries in the early stages.
2. Identify bone loss in the early stages.
3. Locate abnormalities in the surrounding hard and soft tissues.
4. Evaluate growth and development.
5. Provide information during dental procedures (such as root canal therapy).
6. Document a patient's condition at a specific time.

Any exposure to **radiation,** *no matter how small,* has the potential to cause harmful biologic changes in the operator and patient. The dental assistant must thoroughly understand the principles of safety when dealing with radiation.

This chapter provides a brief history of **dental radiography** and introduces you to radiation physics and the characteristics of radiation. You will learn the guidelines for radiation safety and the methods to protect the patient and yourself as the operator.

DISCOVERY OF X-RADIATION

Wilhelm Conrad Roentgen (*rent*-guhn), a Bavarian physicist, discovered the x-ray on November 8, 1895 (Fig. 38-1, *A*). This monumental discovery revolutionized diagnostic capabilities and changed the practice of medicine and dentistry forever.

Before discovering the x-ray, Roentgen had experimented with the production of cathode rays (streams of electrons). He used a Crookes tube (vacuum tube), an electrical current, and special screens covered with a material that glowed *(fluoresced)* when exposed to x-rays (Fig. 38-1, *B*). While working in a darkened laboratory with a vacuum tube, Roentgen noticed a faint green glow *(fluorescence)* coming from some screens across the room. He realized that something was causing the glow and knew he had discovered a powerful and unknown ray. He named his discovery the "x-ray." (The symbol *x* is used in mathematics to represent the unknown.)

In the following weeks, Roentgen continued experimenting with the unknown rays. He replaced the fluorescent screens with photographic plates. He demonstrated that shadowed images could be permanently recorded on the photographic plate by placing objects between the tube and the plate. Roentgen placed his wife's hand on a photographic plate and exposed it to the unknown rays for 15 minutes. When he developed the photographic plate, the outline of the bones in her hands could be seen, representing the first radiograph of the human body (Fig. 38-2).

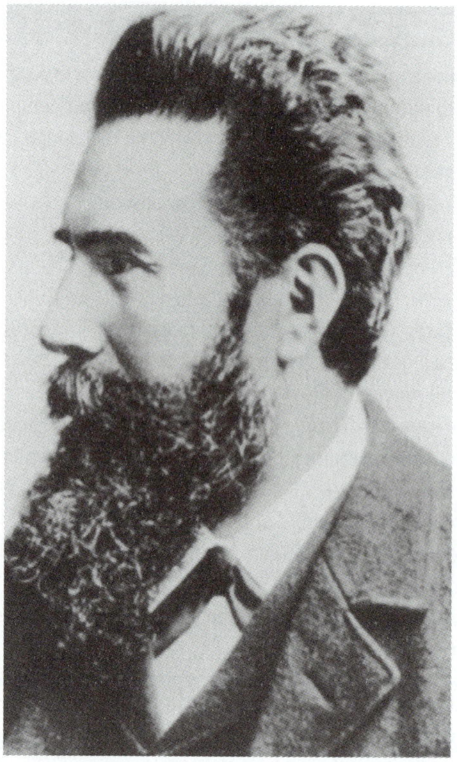

A

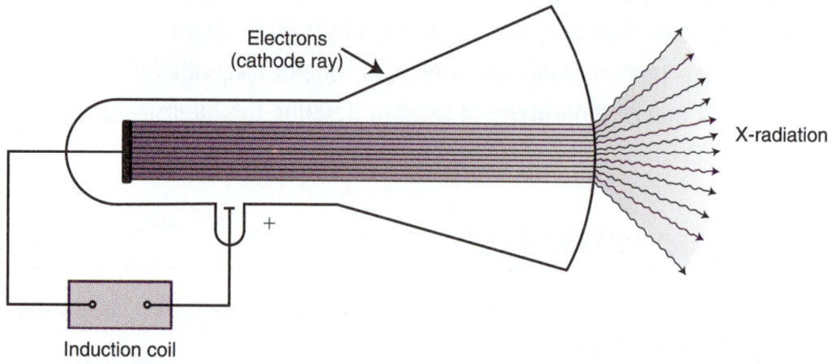

B

Fig. 38-1 A, Wilhelm Conrad Roentgen (1845-1923), discoverer of x-rays. B, Crookes tube, which Roentgen worked with at the time of his discovery of x-rays in 1895. (From Frommer HH, Stabulus JJ: *Radiology for the dental professional,* ed 8, St Louis, 2005, Mosby.)

To honor Wilhelm Roentgen for his discovery, for many years, x-rays were referred to as *roentgen rays,* **radiology** was referred to as *roentgenology,* and **radiographs** were known as *roentgenographs.* During his lifetime, Roentgen was awarded many honors and distinctions, including the first Nobel Prize ever awarded in physics in 1901.

Pioneers in Dental Radiography

Although Roentgen discovered the x-ray, others later helped to develop the field of dental radiography (Table

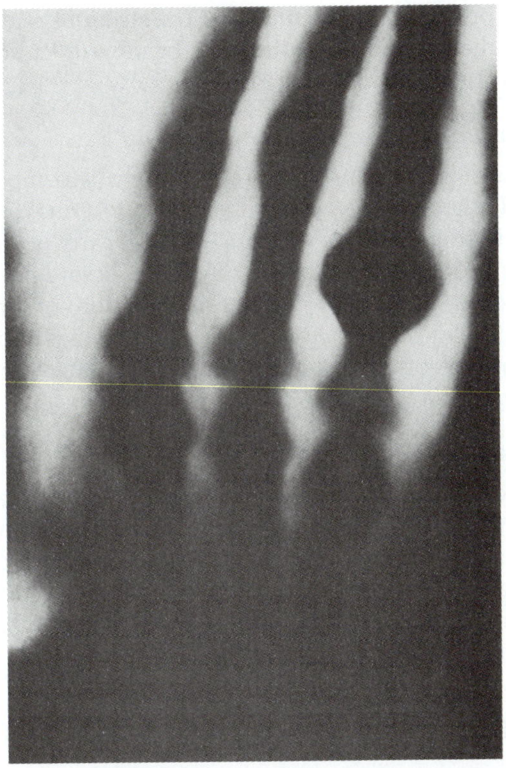

Fig. 38-2 First radiograph of the human body, showing the hand of Roentgen's wife. (From Goaz PW, White SC: *Oral radiology and principles of interpretation,* ed 2, St Louis, 1987, Mosby.)

38-1). In fact, many of the early pioneers died from overexposure to x-rays. At the time x-rays were discovered, no one knew about the hidden dangers that resulted from using these penetrating rays.

In 1895, German dentist Otto Walkhoff made the first *dental* radiograph. He placed a glass photographic plate wrapped in black paper and rubber in his mouth and submitted to 25 minutes of x-ray exposure. Also in 1895, a New York physician made the first dental radiograph in the United States using a skull.

New Orleans dentist C. Edmund Kells is credited with the first practical use of radiographs in dentistry in 1896. During his many experiments, Dr. Kells exposed his hands to x-rays every day for years. This overexposure to **x-radiation** caused numerous cancers to develop on his hand. His dedication to the development of dental radiography eventually cost Dr. Kells his fingers, later his hand, and then his arm. After enduring much pain and faced with the prospect of becoming a burden to his family, he committed suicide in 1928.

Dental radiography has progressed from these early discoveries to its current status as an invaluable science. New technology continues to improve dental imaging capabilities.

Table 38-1 Highlights in the History of Dental Radiography

Year	Event	Individual/Group
1895	Discovery of x-radiation	W.C. Roentgen
1896	First dental radiograph	O. Walkhoff
	First U.S. dental radiograph (skull)	W.J. Morton
	First U.S. dental radiograph (live patient)	C.E. Kells
1901	First paper on dangers of x-radiation	W.H. Rollins
1904	Introduction of bisecting technique	W.A. Price
1913	First dental text*	H.R. Raper
	First prewrapped dental films	Eastman Kodak
	First x-ray tube	W.D. Coolidge
1920	First machine-made film packets	Eastman Kodak
1923	First dental x-ray machine	Victor Radiograph
1925	Introduction of bite-wing technique	H.R. Raper
1933	Proposal of rotational panoramics concept	
1947	Introduction of long-cone paralleling technique	F.G. Fitzgerald
1948	Introduction of panoramic radiography	
1955	Introduction of D-speed film	
1957	First variable-kilovoltage dental x-ray machine	General Electric
1978	Introduction of dental xeroradiography	
1981	Introduction of E-speed film	
1987	Introduction of intraoral digital radiography	
1999	Oral and maxillofacial radiology recognized as a dental specialty	American Dental Association
2001	Introduction of F-speed intraoral film	Eastman Kodak

**Modified from Haring JI, Jansen L:* Dental radiography: principles and practice, *ed 2, Philadelphia, 2000, Saunders.*

RADIATION PHYSICS

All things in the world are composed of energy and matter. **Energy** is defined as the ability to do work. Although energy cannot be created or destroyed, it can change form. **Atoms** are the basic form of *matter,* and they contain energy. **Matter** is anything that occupies space and has form or shape.

Matter has many forms, including solids, liquids, and gases. Matter is composed of atoms grouped together in specific arrangements called *molecules* (Figs. 38-3 and 38-4). A molecule is the smallest particle of substance that retains the property of the original substance. The fundamental unit of matter for discussion in this chapter is the atom.

Atomic Structure

The *atom* consists of two parts: a central nucleus and orbiting electrons. An atom is identified by the composition of its nucleus and the arrangement of its orbiting electrons. At present, 105 different atoms exist. The arrangement within the atom is similar to that of the solar system: the atom has a nucleus (sun) at its center, and the electrons (planets) revolve (orbit) around the nucleus. The electrons remain stable in their orbit unless disturbed or moved. Radiographs can disturb the orbiting electrons.

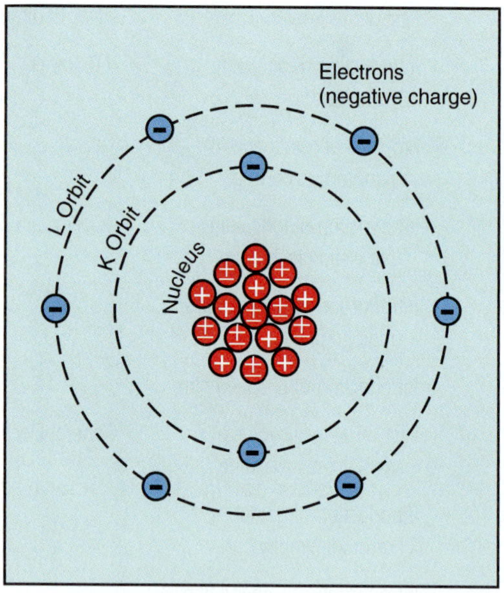

Fig. 38-3 Diagrammatic representation of an oxygen atom.

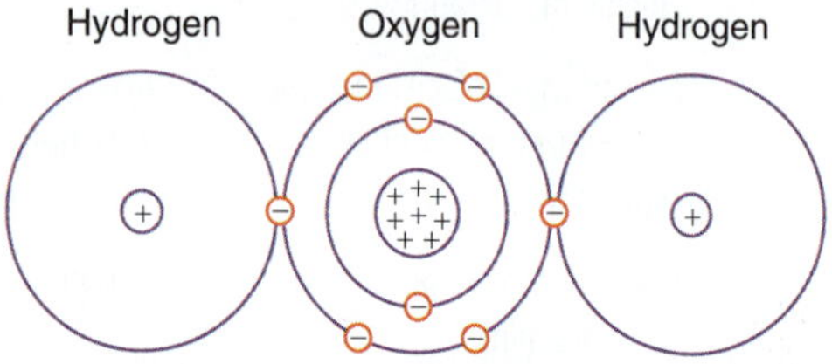

Fig. 38-4 A molecule of water (H_2O) consists of two atoms of hydrogen connected to one atom of oxygen. (From Haring JI, Jansen L: *Dental radiography: principles and techniques,* ed 2, Philadelphia, 2000, Saunders.)

Nucleus

The nucleus, or dense core of the atom, is composed of particles known as *protons* and *neutrons.* Protons carry positive electrical charges, whereas neutrons carry no charge.

Dental x-rays do not affect the tightly bound nucleus of the atom and are only changed in direction, or scattered. Dental x-rays *cannot make atoms radioactive;* that is, patients do not give off x-rays after the x-ray machine stops producing x-rays.

Electrons

Electrons are tiny, negatively charged particles that have very little mass. The orbital path of an electron around the nucleus is called an *electron shell.* Each shell can contain only a specific number of electrons. The electrons are maintained in orbit by electron binding energy, a force similar to gravity.

Ionization

The electrons remain stable in their orbit around the nucleus until radiograph photons collide with them. A **photon** is a minute (tiny) bundle of pure energy that has no weight or mass.

Ions are atoms that gain or lose an electron and become electrically unbalanced. X-rays have enough energy to produce ions because of a process called **ionization.** In this process, electrons are removed from the orbital shells of

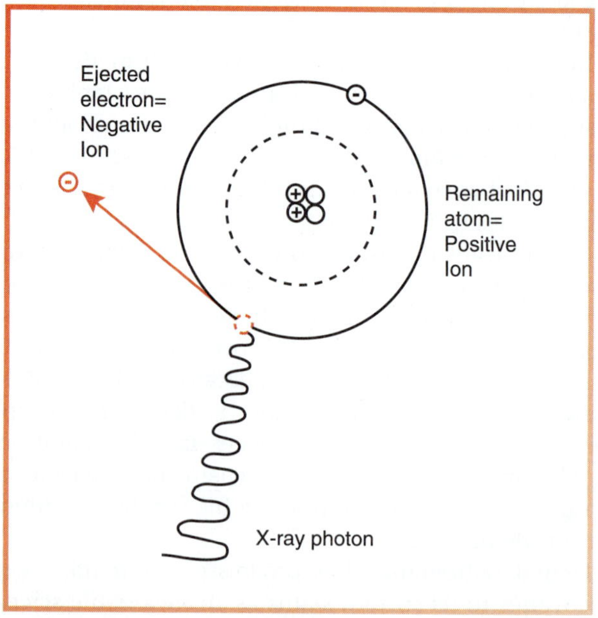

Fig. 38-5 Ionization occurs when an electron is removed from the orbital shell of the electronically stable atom. (From Haring JI, Jansen L: *Dental radiography: principles and techniques,* ed 2, Philadelphia, 2000, Saunders.)

the electrically stable atoms through collisions with x-ray photons (Fig. 38-5).

Properties of Radiation

The dental assistant must be familiar with the unique characteristics of x-rays (Box 38-1). X-rays are a form of energy that can penetrate matter. X-rays belong to a group classified as *electromagnetic radiation* (Fig. 38-6). Visible light, radar, radio, and television waves are also classified as electromagnetic radiation. Electromagnetic radiation is made up of photons that travel through space at the speed of light in a straight line with a wavelike motion.

The *shorter* the wavelength of the x-ray, the *greater* its energy. Because of their high energy, short wavelengths can penetrate matter more easily than longer wavelengths, making shorter wavelengths especially useful in dentistry (Fig. 38-7).

Recall

1. Who discovered x-rays?
2. Who was the first person to make practical use of x-rays in dentistry?
3. What is ionization?

Box 38-1 Characteristics of X-Rays

Invisible and undetectable by the senses
No mass or weight
No charge
Travel at speed of light
Travel in short-wavelength, high-frequency waves
Travel in straight line and can be deflected or scattered
Absorbed by matter
Cause ionization
Can cause certain substances to fluoresce
Can produce image on photographic film
Cause changes in living cells

Modified from Haring JI, Jansen L: *Dental radiography: principles and techniques,* ed 2, Philadelphia, 2000, Saunders.

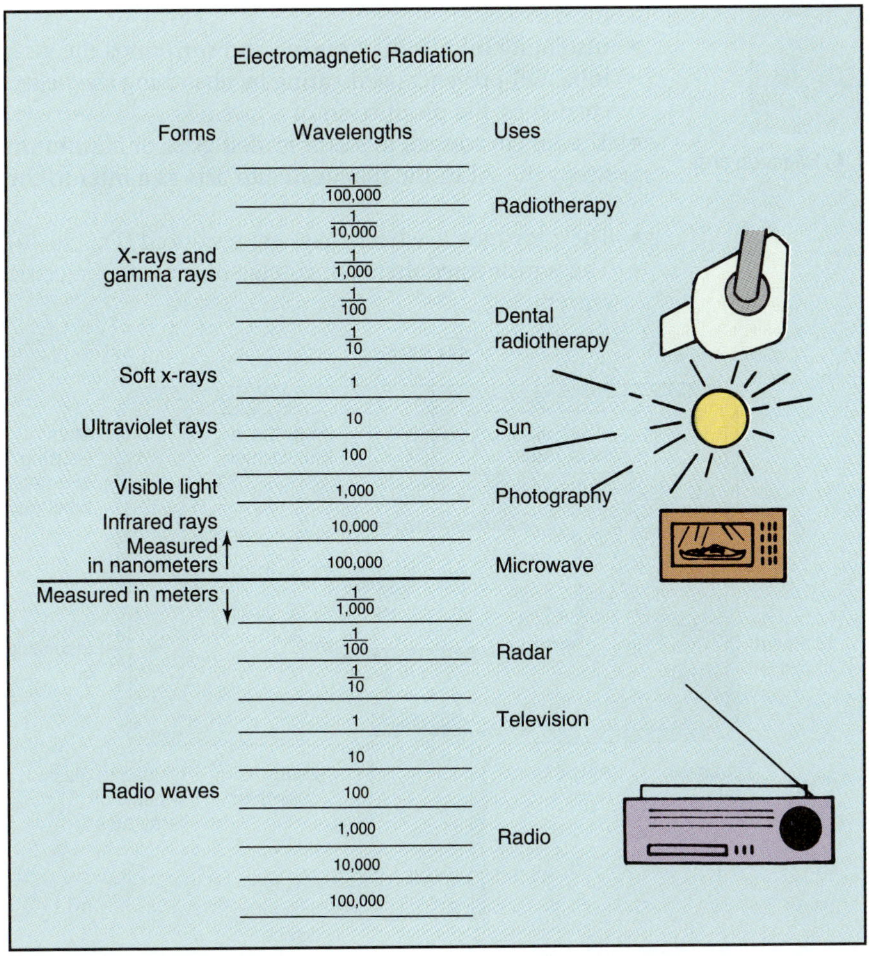

Fig. 38-6 Electromagnetic spectrum, showing the various wavelengths of radiation typically used.

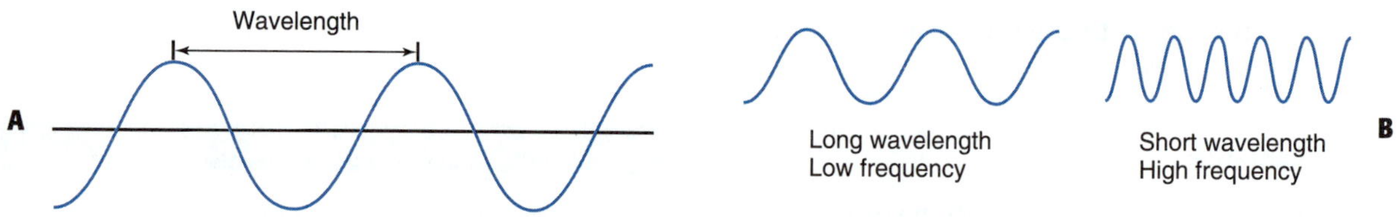

Fig. 38-7 A, **Wavelength is the distance between the crest (peak) of one wave and the crest of the next. B, The shorter the wavelength, the greater the energy and penetration. The longer the wavelength, the less the energy and penetration.** (From Haring JI, Jansen L: *Dental radiography: principles and techniques,* ed 2, Philadelphia, 2000, Saunders.)

THE DENTAL X-RAY MACHINE

Depending on the age and manufacturer, dental x-ray machines may vary slightly in size and appearance, but all machines have three primary components: the **tubehead,** an **extension arm,** and the **control panel** (Fig. 38-8).

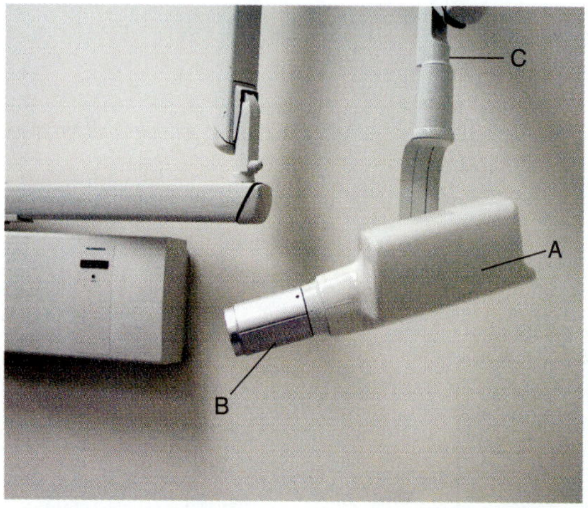

Fig. 38-8 Dental x-ray machine. **A,** Tubehead. **B,** PID. **C,** Extension arm.

Tubehead

The x-ray tubehead is a tightly sealed, heavy metal housing that contains the radiograph tube. The components of the tubehead are as follows (Fig. 38-9):

- The housing is the metal body that contains the x-ray tube.
- Insulating oil fills the housing and surrounds the x-ray tube. Oil prevents overheating by absorbing the heat created by the production of x-rays.
- The tubehead seal, made of leaded glass or aluminum, keeps the oil in the tubehead and acts as a filter to the x-ray beam.
- The x-ray tube is where x-rays are produced (Fig. 38-10).
- The transformer alters the voltage of incoming electric current.

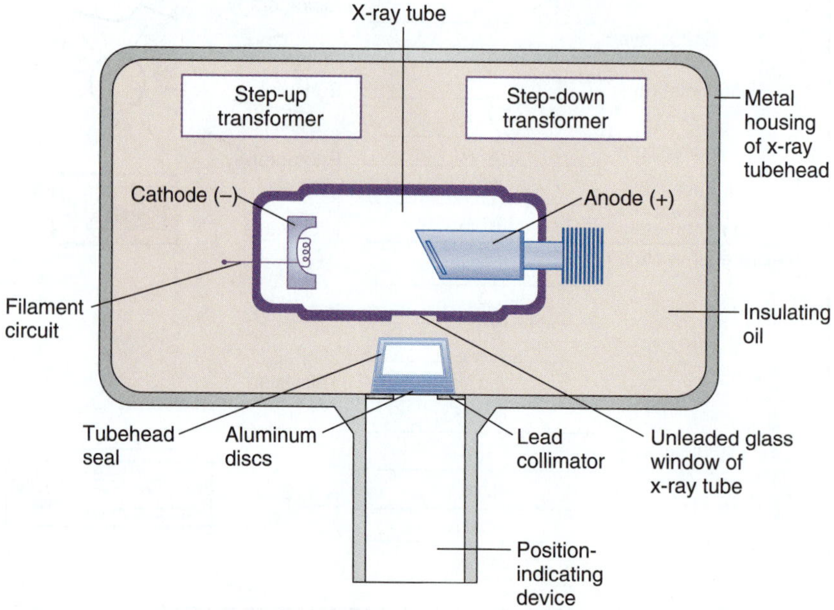

Fig. 38-9 **Diagram of the dental x-ray tubehead.** (From Haring JI, Jansen L: *Dental radiography: principles and techniques,* ed 2, Philadelphia, 2000, Saunders.)

- The lead collimator is a metal disc with a small opening in the center. It is located inside the position indicator device (PID), in the path of the x-ray beam. The small opening forms the size and shape of the x-ray beam as it leaves the tubehead (Fig. 38-11, *A*). The collimator limits the size of the x-ray beam to a circular 2-inch opening at the PID. When the size and shape of the beam are changed to a rectangle, only slightly larger than the film, the amount of tissue exposed to radiation can be reduced by more than one half (Fig. 38-12).

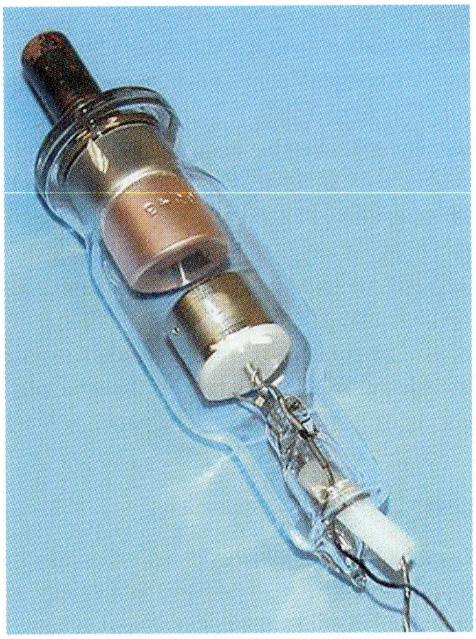

Fig. 38-10 **X-ray tube.** (Courtesy Xintek.)

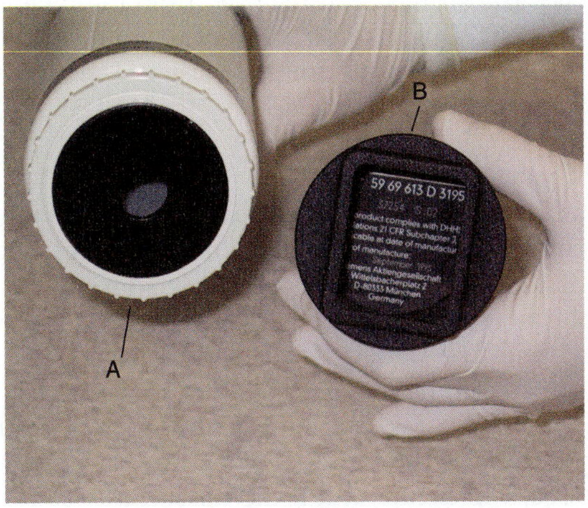

Fig. 38-11 **A,** Collimator. **B,** Filter.

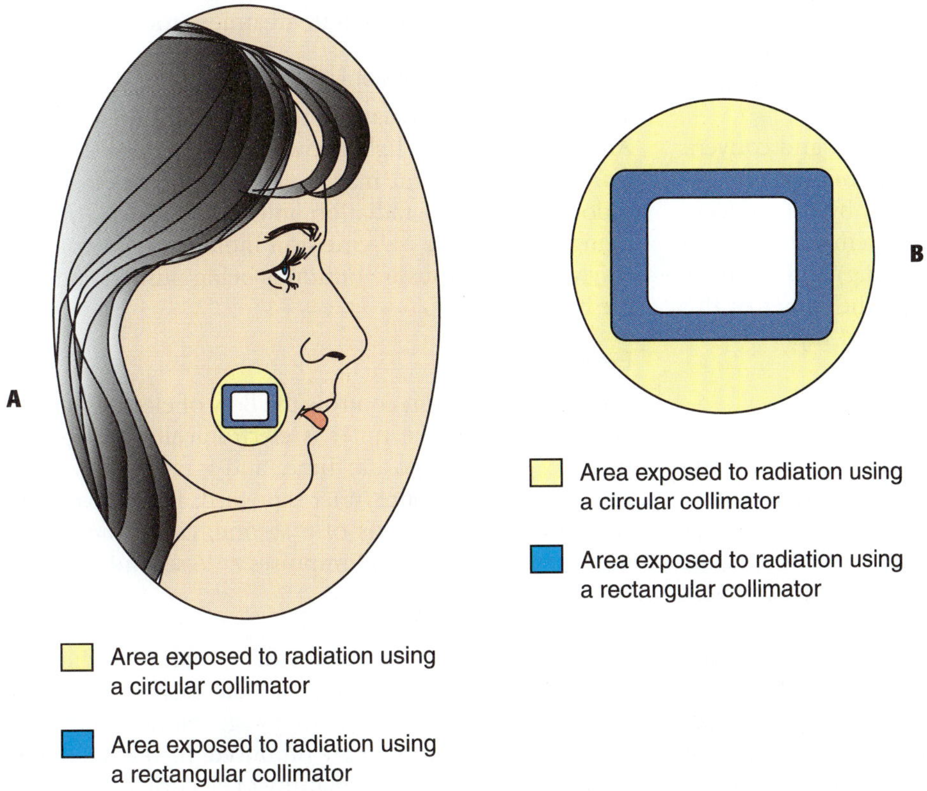

Fig. 38-12 **A** and **B,** Rectangular collimation.

- The aluminum filter is a 0.5-mm–thick sheet located inside the PID, in the path of the x-ray beam to filter out the nonpenetrating, longer wavelength radiographs (Fig. 38-11, *B*). For further discussion, see Chapter 39.
- The PID is the open-ended lead-lined cylinder that extends from the opening of the metal housing.

X-Ray Tube

The x-ray tube is the heart of the x-ray generating system. It is made of glass and is about 6 inches long and 1 inch in diameter. The air has been removed from the tube to create a vacuum. This vacuum environment allows the electrons to flow with minimum resistance between the electrodes (cathode and anode).

Cathode

The **cathode,** or *negative (–) electrode,* consists of a tungsten filament in a focusing cup made of molybdenum. The purpose of the cathode is to supply the electrons necessary to generate x-rays. Electrons are generated in the x-ray tube at the cathode. The hotter the filament becomes, the more electrons are produced.

The *focusing cup* keeps the electrons suspended in an electron cloud at the cathode. When the exposure button is pressed, the circuit within the tubehead is completed, and the electrons rapidly cross from the cathode to strike the anode.

Anode

The **anode,** or *positive (+) electrode,* acts as the target for the electrons. It is composed of a **tungsten target** (a small block of tungsten) embedded in the larger copper stem. The copper around the target conducts the heat away from the target, thus reducing wear on the target.

The tungsten target serves as a focal spot and converts the bombarding electrons into x-ray photons. The oil absorbs about 99% of the x-rays generated by this process, and this energy is given off as heat. The remaining 1% exits the tubehead through the port (opening) as a divergent beam toward the patient. The x-rays at the center of this beam are known, collectively, as the **central ray.**

Position Indicator Device (PID)

The lead-lined PID is used to aim the x-ray beam at the film in the patient's mouth. The open end of the PID is placed against the patient's face during film exposure. The PID may be cylindrical or rectangular. The rectangular PID limits the size of the beam to that of a dental film (see Chapter 39).

PIDs used in dentistry are usually 8, 12, or 16 inches long. The length selected is determined by the radiographic technique being used. However, a long (12- to 16-inch) PID is more effective in reducing exposure to the patient than a short (8-inch) PID because there is less *divergence* (spreading out) of the beam.

Extension Arm

The wire between the tubehead and the control panel is enclosed in the hollow extension arm. The arm also has an important function in positioning the tubehead.

The tubehead is attached to the extension arm by means of a yoke that can be turned 360 degrees horizontally. *Horizontally* means to move in a side-to-side motion. *Vertically* means to move in an up-and-down motion. These movements are necessary to align the tubehead and the film.

The extension arm folds up and can be swiveled from side to side. Never leave the extension arm in an extended position when the machine is not in use, because the weight of the tubehead can cause it to become loose. If the tubehead is loose, it can *drift* (slip out of position) after it is positioned for an exposure. This movement can cause a *cone cut* (central ray positioned off the film). If the tubehead drifts, the arm should be repaired immediately. The dental assistant or the patient must *never* hold the tubehead to keep it in place during exposure.

Control Panel

The control panel is located on a wall outside of the x-ray area to prevent radiation exposure to the operator while exposing the film (Fig. 38-13). The control panel contains the **master switch,** an **indicator light, selector buttons,** and an **exposure button.** The selector button is used to select the exposure time, milliamperage (mA), and kilovoltage (kV), thereby regulating the x-ray beam. A single, centrally located control panel may be used to operate several tubeheads located in separate treatment rooms.

Master Switch and Indicator Lights

The master switch is used to turn the machine on and off. An orange indicator light shows when the master switch is on. The x-ray machine may be safely left on all day because it does not produce radiation unless the exposure button is being pushed. The red emission indicator light comes on *only* when the exposure button is being pushed and x-rays are being emitted.

Exposure Button

The exposure button controls the flow of electricity to generate the x-rays. The timer is electronically controlled to provide precise exposure time, and x-rays are generated *only* while the exposure timer is pressed. The exposure time is measured in fractions of a second, called *impulses* (60 impulses = 1 second; 30 impulses = $\frac{1}{2}$ second).

Milliamperage Selector

The milliamperage (mA) of a dental x-ray machine is a measure of the electric current that passes through the tungsten filament. The milliamperage selector controls the number of electrons that are produced. Increasing the milliamperage increases the quantity of electrons available for

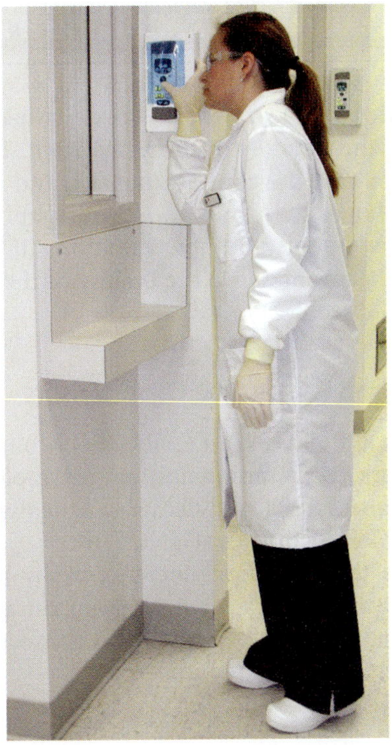

Fig. 38-13 The operator stands at the central panel located outside the x-ray room.

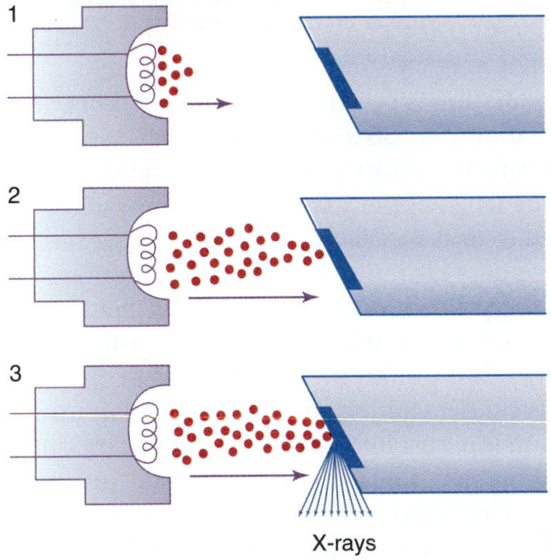

Fig. 38-14 The production of dental radiographs occurs in the x-ray tube. **1,** When the filament circuit is activated, the filament heats up, and thermionic emission occurs. **2,** When the exposure button is activated, the electrons are accelerated from the cathode to the anode. **3,** The electrons strike the tungsten target, and their kinetic energy is converted to x-rays and heat. (From Haring JI, Jansen L: *Dental radiography: principles and techniques,* ed 2, Philadelphia, 2000, Saunders.)

the production of x-rays. This will be discussed in more detail later in this chapter.

Kilovoltage Selector

The **kilovoltage peak (kVp)** selector is used to control the penetrating power of the x-ray beam. Dental x-ray machines generally operate at 70 or 90 kVp. The effects of kilovoltage settings are discussed later in this chapter.

Recall

4. What are the primary components of a dental x-ray machine?
5. What is the negative electrode inside the x-ray tube?
6. What is the positive electrode inside the x-ray tube?
7. What is usually found on a control panel?

X-RAY PRODUCTION

When the x-ray machine is plugged into the wall outlet and the machine is turned on, the electric current enters the control panel and the following events occur in an *instant:*

1. The current travels from the control panel to the tubehead through electrical wires in the extension arm.
2. The current travels through the step-down transformer to the filament of the cathode. The purpose of the step-down transformer is to decrease the voltage from the incoming 110 or 220 volts to 3 to 5 volts.
3. The filament circuit uses the 3 to 5 volts to heat the tungsten filament in the cathode portion of the x-ray tube. The heating of the filament results in thermionic emission. *Thermionic emission* is the release of electrons from the tungsten filament when the electric current passes through it and heats it up. The electrons stay in an electron cloud around the tungsten filament within the focusing cup, until the high-voltage circuit is activated by pushing the exposure button.

Then, after the exposure button is engaged, x-rays are produced in an instant in the following way (Fig. 38-14):

1. Pushing the exposure button activates the high-voltage circuit. The electrons in the cloud are shot across the x-ray tube to the anode. The molybdenum cup in the cathode directs the electrons to the tungsten target in the anode.
2. The electrons speed from the cathode to the anode. When the electrons strike the tungsten target, their energy of motion *(kinetic energy)* creates x-rays and heat. Less than 1% of the energy is converted to x-rays, with 99% lost as heat.
3. The heat is carried away from the copper stem and absorbed by the insulating oil in the tubehead.
4. The x-rays travel through the unleaded glass window of the tube, the tubehead seal, and the aluminum filter. The aluminum filter removes the longer-wavelength x-rays from the beam.
5. The x-ray beam then travels through the collimator, where its size is restricted; it then travels down the PID and exits at the opening.

TYPES OF RADIATION

The x-radiation is described as primary, secondary, or scatter radiation (Fig. 38-15).

Primary radiation is made up of the x-rays that come from the target of the x-ray tube. Primary radiation is often referred to as the *useful beam,* or **primary beam.**

Secondary radiation refers to x-radiation that is created when the primary beam interacts with matter. For example, secondary radiation is created when the x-rays of the primary beam contact the patient's tissues. Secondary radiation is *less* penetrating than primary radiation. Secondary radiation is *not* useful radiation, because it produces fog on the radiograph, damaging the diagnostic quality.

Scatter radiation is a form of secondary radiation that occurs when an x-ray beam has been deflected from its path by interaction with matter. Scatter radiation is deflected in all directions by patient tissues and travels to all parts of the patient's body and to all areas of the dental operatory. Scatter radiation is dangerous to both the patient and the operator.

Recall

8. During the production of x-rays, how much energy is lost as heat?
9. What are the three types of radiation?

CHARACTERISTICS OF RADIOGRAPH BEAM

Characteristics of the x-ray beam are described as the *quality, quantity,* and *intensity* of the x-ray beam. These characteristics determine the contrast, density, and image detail, the qualities necessary for a good radiograph. The dental assistant must understand how variations in the character of the x-ray beam influence the quality of the resulting radiographs (Table 38-2).

Radiolucent and Radiopaque Characteristics

Structures that radiation can easily pass through appear *radiolucent* (dark) on a radiograph. For example, air spaces, soft tissues, abscesses, tooth decay, and the dental pulp appear as radiolucent images (Fig. 38-16).

Structures that radiation does not easily pass through appear *radiopaque* (white or light gray) on a radiograph. Metal restorations, tooth enamel, and dense areas of bone are examples of radiopaque images.

Contrast

The image on a radiograph appears in a range of shades from black to white with multiple shades of gray (Fig. 38-17). This range is referred to as the *gray scale.*

The range of shades of gray to black to white is called **contrast.** The ideal contrast of a film clearly shows the radiopaque white of a metal restoration, the radiolucent

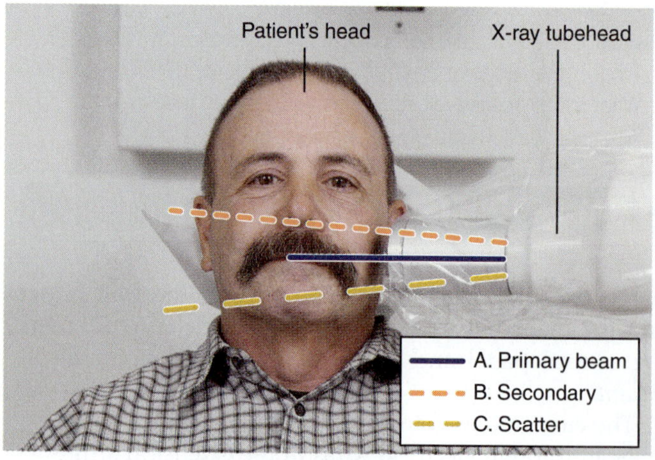

Fig. 38-15 Types of radiation interaction with the patient. **A,** Primary. **B,** Secondary. **C,** Scatter.

black of air, and the many shades of gray between these extremes. *Higher* kilovoltage produces more penetrating radiographs and *lower* radiographic contrast, as follows:

- A 90-kVp setting requires less exposure time and produces a radiograph that has low contrast (more shades of gray).
- A 70-kVp setting requires a slightly longer exposure time and produces a radiograph with high contrast (fewer shades of gray).

The amount of contrast in a film is often the dentist's preference. Some dentists prefer radiographs with more contrast, whereas others prefer low contrast.

Table 38-2 X-Ray Beam Factors' Influence on Density and Contrast of Radiographs

Factor	Effect
Milliamperage (mA)	
↑	Increased density
↓	Decreased density
Kilovoltage peak (kVp)	
↑	Long-scale contrast; low contrast
	Increased density
↓	Short-scale contrast; high contrast
	Decreased density
Time	
↑	Increased density
↓	Decreased density

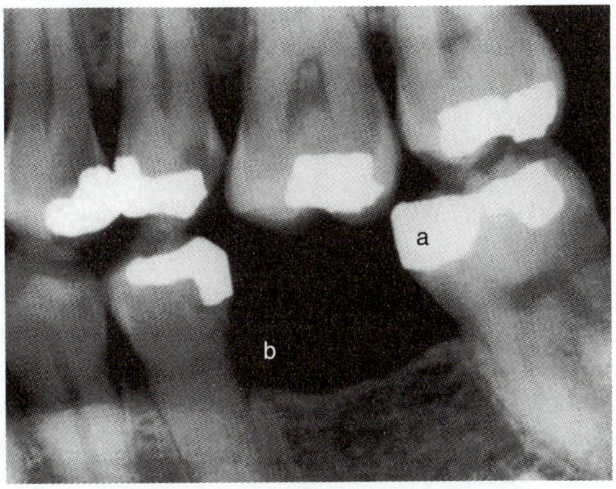

Fig. 38-16 Bite-wing radiograph showing radiopaque (white, *a*) area of amalgam restoration and radiolucent (black, *b*) area of air and cheek tissue.

Density

Density is the overall blackness or darkness of a film. A radiograph with the correct density enables the dentist to view black areas (air spaces), white areas (enamel, dentin, and bone), and gray areas (soft tissues). The degree of density is controlled by the *milliampere seconds (mAs)*.

The mAs control the amount of time given to the exposure of the radiograph. If the radiograph is not exposed for a sufficient amount of time or with a low **milliampere (mA)** setting, the resulting radiograph will not have the correct overall density or will be light in appearance (see Table 38-2). Other factors that influence the density of a radiograph include the following:

1. *Distance from the x-ray tube to the patient.* If the operator lengthens the source-film distance without changing the exposure settings, the resulting radiographs will be light or less dense.
2. *Developing time and temperature.* If the processing time is too long, the radiograph will appear dark.

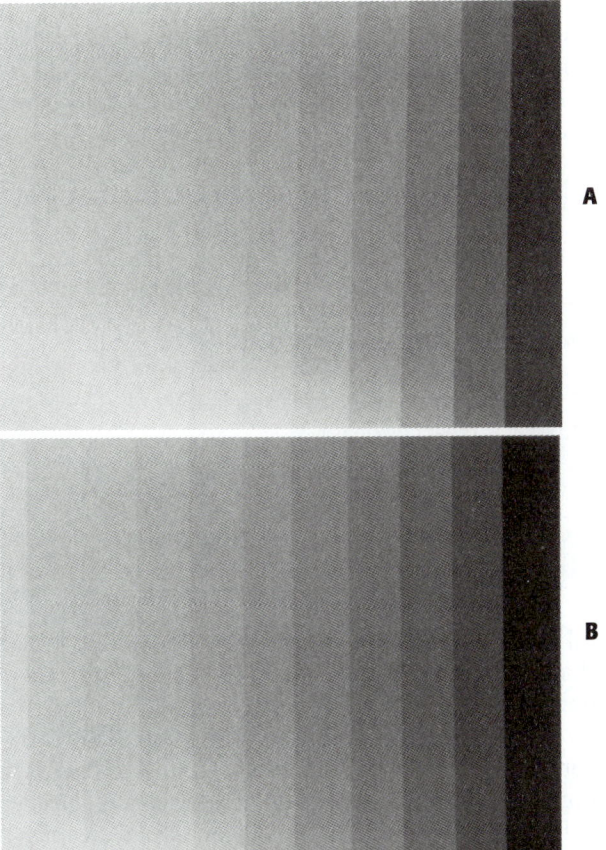

Fig. 38-17 A, A radiograph produced with lower kilovoltage exhibits high contrast. Many light and dark areas are seen. **B,** A radiograph produced with higher kilovoltage exhibits low contrast. Many shades of gray are seen instead of black and white. (From Haring JI, Jansen L: *Dental radiography: principles and techniques,* ed 2, Philadelphia, 2000, Saunders.)

3. *Body size of the patient.* A patient who is very small or thin requires less radiation than a husky, heavy-boned person.

Geometric Characteristics

Three geometric characteristics affect the quality of the radiograph: sharpness, magnification, and distortion.

Sharpness refers to how well the radiograph reproduces the fine details or distinct outlines of an object. Sharpness is sometimes referred to as *detail, resolution,* or *definition* and is similar to the "fine tuning" adjustment on a television. The fuzzy or blurred area that surrounds an image is termed **penumbra.** The sharpness of an image is influenced by the following factors:

1. *Focal spot size.* A small focal spot results in a sharper image than a machine with a larger focal spot size.
2. *Film composition.* Fast film speeds result in less sharp detail because of the large crystal size.
3. *Movement.* Any movement of the patient or the film, no matter how slight, will degrade the sharpness of the image.

Distortion refers to the disproportional change in the size of images on radiographs that is caused by excessive or insufficient vertical angulation. Elongation and foreshortening of images are discussed in Chapter 41.

Magnification refers to the proportional enlargement of a radiographic image.

Recall

10. What does the term *radiolucent* mean?
11. What does the term *radiopaque* mean?
12. What exposure factors control contrast?
13. What is meant by density?

RADIATION EFFECTS

All **ionizing radiation** is harmful and produces biologic changes in living tissues. Although the amount of x-radiation used in dental radiography is small, biologic changes do occur. Thus the dental assistant must know how the harmful effects of radiation occur and how to discuss radiation risks with patients. The entire x-ray area is considered a radiation hazard area, and a radiation hazard area sign must be posted in sight of all personnel and patients (Fig. 38-18).

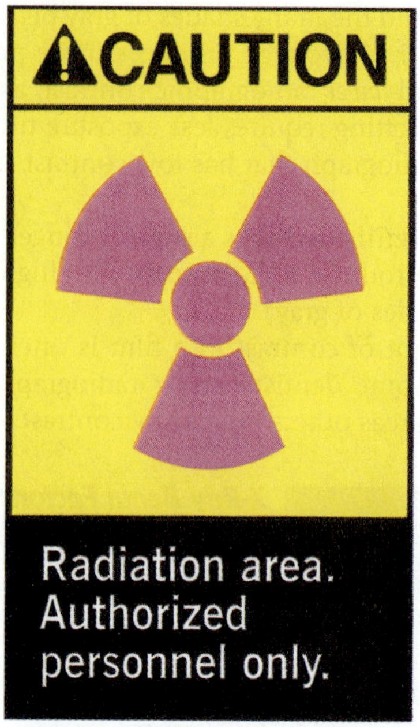

Fig. 38-18 Sign indicating a radiation hazard area.

Tissue Damage

In dental radiography, not all x-rays pass through the patient and reach the dental film; the patient's tissues absorb some x-rays. When the energy from the x-ray photon is absorbed, chemical changes result in biologic damage.

Ionization

Ionization results in the harmful effects of x-rays in humans. Ionization can cause a disruption of cellular metabolism and permanent damage to living cells and tissues (see earlier discussion). The atoms that lose electrons become positive ions; as such, they are unstable structures capable of interacting with and damaging other atoms, tissues, or chemicals.

Biologic Effects

Exposure to radiation can bring about changes in body chemicals, cells, tissues, and organs. The effects of the radiation may not become evident for many years after the time the x-rays were absorbed. This time lag is called the **latent period.**

Cumulative Effects

Exposure to radiation has a cumulative effect over a lifetime. When tissues are exposed to x-rays, some damage occurs. Although tissues can repair some damage, the tissues do not return to their original state. The cumulative effect of radiation exposure can be compared with cumulative effect from repeated exposure over the years to the rays of the sun (Table 38-3).

Acute and Chronic Radiation Exposure

Acute radiation exposure occurs when a large **dose** of radiation is absorbed in a short period, such as in a nuclear accident. Chronic radiation exposure occurs when small

Table 38-3 Disorders of Critical Organs Resulting from Cumulative Radiation Exposure

Critical Organ	Disorder
Lens of the eye	Cataracts
Bone marrow	Leukemia
Salivary gland	Cancer
Thyroid gland	Cancer
Skin	Cancer
Gonads	Genetic abnormalities

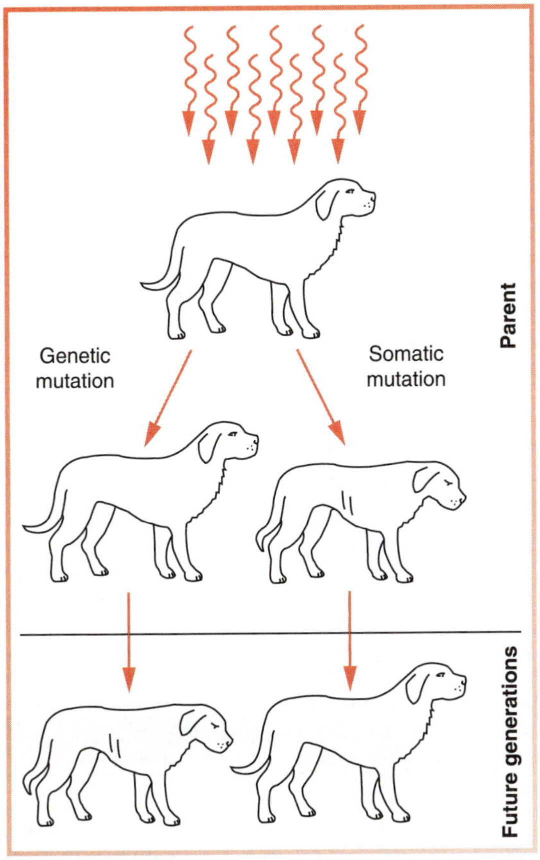

Fig. 38-19 **Comparison of somatic and genetic effects of radiation.** (From Haring JI, Jansen L: *Dental radiography,* ed 2, Philadelphia, 2000, Saunders.)

amounts of radiation are absorbed repeatedly over a long period. The effects of chronic radiation exposure may not be observed until years after the original exposure.

Genetic and Somatic Effects

Table 38-4 compares the relative radiation sensitivity (high to low) of cells and tissues. Note that the skin, eye, and

Table 38-4 Relative Radiation Sensitivity of Cells and Tissues

Radiation Sensitivity	Cell/Tissue
High	Small lymphocyte
	Bone marrow
	Reproductive cells
Fairly high	Skin
	Lens of eye
	Oral mucosa
Medium	Connective tissue
	Small blood vessels
	Developing bone and cartilage
Fairly low	Mature bone and cartilage
	Salivary gland
	Thyroid gland
	Kidney
	Liver
Low	Muscle tissue
	Nerve tissue

Modified from Miles DA, et al: Radiographic imaging for dental auxiliaries, *ed 2, Philadelphia, 1994, Saunders.*

oral mucosa, all of which might be affected by dental radiographs, have a "fairly high" sensitivity to radiation.

X-rays affect both genetic and somatic cells. *Genetic* cells are the reproductive cells (sperm and ova). Damage to genetic cells *is* passed on to succeeding generations. These changes from **genetic effects** are referred to as *genetic mutations.*

All other cells in the body belong to the group of *somatic* tissue (*somatic* refers to the body). X-rays can damage somatic tissue, but the damage from **somatic effects** is *not* passed on to future generations (Fig. 38-19).

Critical Organs

Although the risk associated with dental x-rays is minimal, some tissues and organs are exposed to more radiation when dental radiographs are exposed. The following organs are more sensitive to radiation and are thus termed *critical organs:*

- *Skin.* Because it is exposed during dental radiographic procedures, skin is considered a critical organ. The effects of radiation on skin can be seen as a reddening, or erythema, similar to sunburn. This effect requires moderate to high doses of radiation, not used in normal dental radiography.

- *Thyroid gland.* If a thyroid collar were not used, the radiation dose to the thyroid gland could be significant. In adults, thyroid tissue is considered fairly resistant to radiation, but the thyroid gland in children is radiation-sensitive.
- *Lens of the eye.* High doses of radiation to the lens of the eye can cause cataracts (a cloudiness of the lens). However, many experts no longer consider the lens of the eye a critical organ in dental radiography because of the low dose. Using the paralleling technique reduces exposure to the eye (see Chapter 40).
- *Bone marrow.* Significant radiation-induced changes in bone marrow can result in leukemia. Bone marrow sites are active in the mandible and skull, and this should be a consideration in dental radiography.

Recall

14. What is the name of the process that results in the harmful effects of x-rays?
15. What is the name of the time period between x-ray exposure and the appearance of symptoms?
16. What is meant by genetic effects?

RADIATION MEASUREMENT

Radiation can be measured in a manner similar to time, distance, and weight. Just as distance can be measured in miles or kilometers, and time can be measured in hours or minutes, the International Commission on Radiation Units and Measurements has established special units for the measurement of units of radiation.

Two sets of systems are used to define the way in which radiation is measured. The older system is referred to as the *traditional system,* or *standard system.* The newer system is the metric equivalent known as the *Systeme Internationale (SI).*

The traditional units of radiation measurement include (1) the *roentgen* (R), (2) the *radiation absorbed dose* (rad), and (3) the *roentgen equivalent in [hu]man* (rem). The SI units include (1) *coulombs* per kilogram (C/kg), (2) the *gray* (Gy), and (3) the *sievert* (Sv). Both systems are presented in Table 38-5.

Maximum Permissible Dose

The maximum permissible dose (MPD) of whole-body radiation for persons occupationally exposed to radiation is 5000 millirem (mrem), or 5.0 rem, per year, which equals approximately 100 mrem per week. This amount of radiation to the whole body is associated with minimal risk for injury. For non–occupationally exposed persons, the MPD is 500 mrem, or 5.0 millisieverts (mSv), per year.

Table 38-5 ***Equivalent Traditional and SI Units of Radiation Measurement***

Measurement	Traditional System	SI System
Radiation exposure	1 roentgen (R)	1 coulomb per kilogram (C/kg)
Absorbed dose	100 radiation absorbed doses (rad)	1 gray (Gy)
Dose equivalence	100 roentgen equivalents in [hu]man (rem)	1 sievert (Sv)

Dental personnel should strive for an occupational dose of *zero* by adhering to strict radiation protection practices. Zero exposure is not difficult to achieve when radiation safety precautions are taken. Dental personnel should also not exceed the *maximum accumulated lifetime dose,* calculated as follows:

$$(N - 18) \times 5000 \text{ mrem/year}$$

In this formula, *N* is the operator's age.

Recall

17. What are the two systems of radiation measurement?
18. What is the maximum permissible dose of radiation for occupationally exposed persons?

RADIATION SAFETY

We are exposed to radiation every day of our lives. *Background radiation* comes from natural sources such as radioactive materials in the ground and cosmic radiation from space (Table 38-6).

Exposure from medical or dental sources is an additional radiation risk. Because of concerns, patients frequently say, "I've heard x-rays are bad for me. Do you really have to take them?" The dental assistant should anticipate this patient reaction and be prepared to explain to the patient the risks and diagnostic benefits of dental radiation.

When dental radiographs are prescribed and properly taken, the benefit of disease detection far outweighs the risk for biologic damage from receiving small doses of ra-

Table 38-6 Radiation Sources and Whole-Body Exposure

Source	EXPOSURE Millirems/Year	Sieverts/Year
Natural		
Radon	200.00	0.002
Cosmic	27.00	0.00027
Terrestrial	28.00	0.00028
Internal	39.00	0.00039
Artificial		
Medical/dental	53.00	0.00053
Consumer products	9.00	0.00009
Other		
Occupational	<1.00	<0.00001
Nuclear fuel cycle	<1.00	<0.00001
Fallout	<1.00	<0.00001

Modified from Haring JI, Jansen L: Dental radiography: principles and techniques, *ed 2, Philadelphia, 2000, Saunders.*

Table 38-7 Absorbed Doses from Intraoral X-Rays

Film*	Dose (millirad)
Bite-Wing	
E speed, 4 films, round	19.5
E speed, 4 films, rectangular	3.1
Full-Mouth Survey	
E speed, 20 films, round	51.4
E speed, 20 films, rectangular	16.1

Modified from Underhill TE et al: Radiologic risk estimation from dental radiology, Oral Surg Oral Med Oral Pathol *66:1-120, 1988.*
**All with 16-inch position indicator device.*

diation (Table 38-7). However, when radiographs must be retaken because of poor operator technique, the patient is exposed to unnecessary additional radiation.

The decision to expose new radiographs must be based on how recently previous films were obtained and the clinical need for additional films. Radiographs should never be taken on a "routine basis."

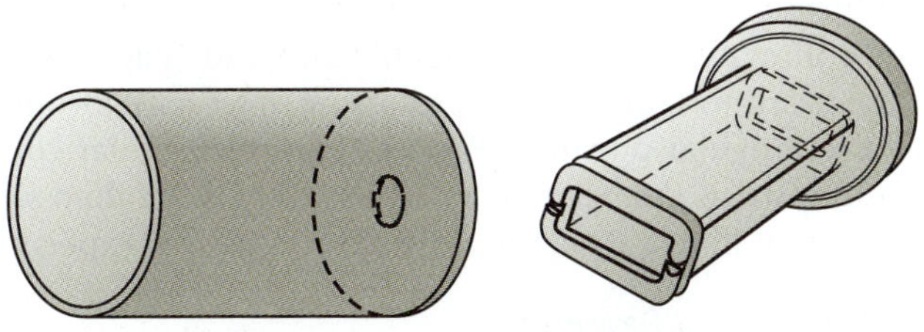

Fig. 38-20 **Aluminum discs are placed in the path of the x-ray beam to filter out the low-energy, long wavelengths that are harmful to the patient.** (From Haring JI, Jansen L: *Dental radiography: principles and techniques,* ed 2, Philadelphia, 2000, Saunders.)

Dentist's Responsibilities for Dental Radiography

1. Prescribe only radiographs that are required for diagnostic purposes.
2. Ensure that all radiographic equipment is maintained in safe working condition.
3. Ensure that there is appropriate shielding to protect staff and patients from the effects of radiation.
4. Require that all personnel who obtain radiographs be properly trained, credentialed, and appropriately supervised while exposing radiographs.
5. Use only techniques that will produce diagnostic-quality radiographs with minimal radiation exposure to the patient and operator.
6. Follow the state's radiographic licensing requirements, rules, and regulations.
7. Participate in obtaining informed consent from patient and family.
8. Review the patient's record to determine when radiographs were last taken.

Protective Devices

Other measures that provide further patient protection include the use of properly operating radiographic equipment. The x-ray tubehead must be equipped with appropriate aluminum filters, lead collimators, and PIDs. Equipment should be checked on a regular basis by state or federal regulating agencies. Faulty or malfunctioning equipment should be repaired immediately.

Aluminum Filtration

The purpose of the aluminum filter is to remove the low-energy, long-wavelength, least penetrating x-rays from the beam (Fig. 38-20). These x-rays are harmful to the patient and are not useful in producing a diagnostic-quality radiograph.

X-ray machines operating at 70 kVp or greater must have aluminum filtration of 2.5 mm. This is a federal requirement.

Collimator

The collimator, used to restrict the size and shape of the x-ray beam to reduce patient exposure, may have a round or a rectangular opening (Fig. 38-21). A rectangular collimator restricts the beam to an area slightly larger than size 2 intraoral film and significantly reduces patient exposure.

Position Indicator Device

The PID, used to direct the x-ray beam, has a round or rectangular shape available in two lengths: *short* (8-inch) and *long* (16-inch).

Patient Protection

With the use of proper radiation protection measures, the amount of x-radiation to the patient can be minimized. Patient protection begins with understanding and practicing general guidelines for obtaining radiographs in pediatric, adolescent, and adult patients.

Lead Apron and Thyroid Collar

A lead apron and a thyroid collar must be used on *all* patients for *all* exposures (Fig. 38-22). This rule applies to all patients regardless of age or gender or the number of films being exposed.

The **lead apron** should cover the patient from the neck and extend over the lap area to protect the reproductive and blood-forming tissues from scatter radiation. Many states mandate the use of a lead apron.

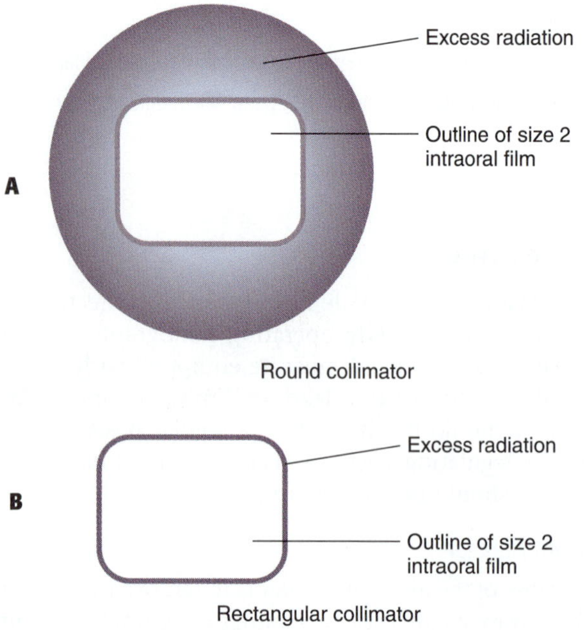

Fig. 38-21 A, The x-ray beam produced by a circular collimator is 2 inches in diameter, which is much larger than size 2 intraoral film. **B,** The beam produced by a rectangular collimator is just slightly larger than size 2 intraoral film. (From Haring JI, Jansen L: *Dental radiography: principles and techniques,* ed 2, Philadelphia, 2000, Saunders.)

The **thyroid collar** is a flexible lead shield that is placed securely around the patient's neck to protect the thyroid gland from scatter radiation. The collar may be a separate shield or part of the lead apron. The lead protects the highly sensitive thyroid gland from scatter radiation. A low rate of exposure to dental x-rays has *not* been shown to cause thyroid disease, but the use of collars further minimizes the patient's exposure to x-radiation.

Lead aprons and thyroid collars must *not be folded* when stored. Folding eventually cracks the lead and allows radiation leakage. Instead, the lead apron and thyroid collar should be hung up or laid over a rounded bar.

Fast-Speed Film

The size of the silver bromide crystals is the main factor in determining the film speed: the larger the crystals, the faster the film. A fast film requires less exposure to produce a quality radiograph.

Fast-speed film is the most effective method of reducing a patient's exposure to x-radiation. Fast film is available for both intraoral and extraoral radiography (see Chapter 39).

Film-Holding Devices

The use of a film-holding instrument keeps the patient's hands and fingers from being exposed to x-radiation (Fig. 38-23). Film holders also hold the film in a stable position and assist the operator in properly positioning the film and PID. The individual types of film holders are discussed in Chapter 39.

Exposure Factor

Using the proper exposure factors also limits the amount of x-radiation exposure to the patient. Adjusting the selectors for kilovoltage peak, milliamperage, and time controls the exposure factors. A setting of 70 to 90 kVp keeps patient exposure to a minimum. On some dental units the

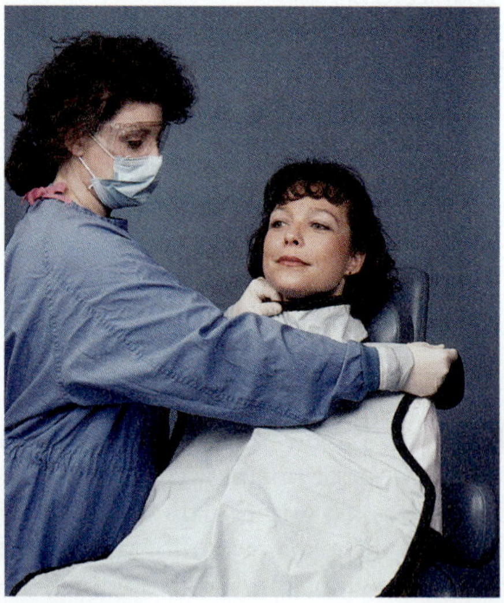

Fig. 38-22 The lead apron and thyroid collar must be large enough to cover the seated patient from the neck to above the knees.

kVp and mA settings are preset by the manufacturer and cannot be adjusted.

Proper Technique

Using the correct techniques is necessary to ensure the diagnostic quality of films and reduce the amount of exposure to a patient. Films that are nondiagnostic must be retaken; this results in additional radiation exposure to the patient. Retakes are a major cause of unnecessary radiation to patients and must be avoided.

Pregnancy

The manual *Guidelines for Prescribing Dental Radiographs,* issued by the American Dental Association (ADA) and U.S. Food and Drug Administration (FDA), states that dental radiographic procedures "do not need to be altered because of pregnancy." When a lead apron is used during dental radiographic procedures, the amount of radiation received in the pelvic region is nearly zero. The embryo or fetus receives no detectable exposure with the use of a lead apron.

Although scientific evidence indicates that dental x-ray procedures can be performed during pregnancy, many dentists and pregnant patents prefer to postpone such x-ray procedures because of the patient's concern.

Recall

19. What is the purpose of the collimator?
20. What is the purpose of the aluminum filter?
21. What precautions should be taken when handling the lead apron?
22. What is the most effective measure in reducing a patient's exposure to radiation?

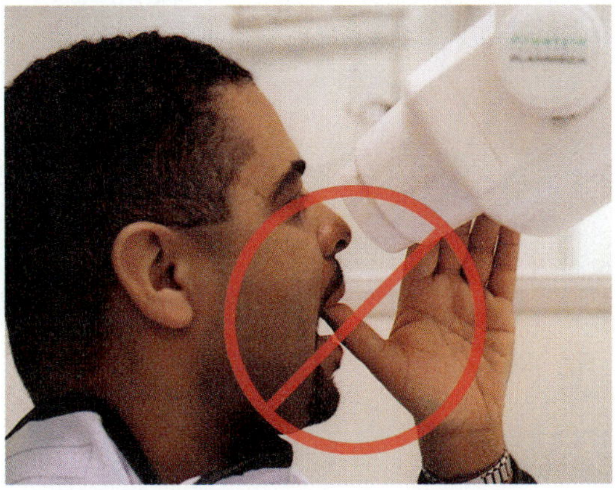

Fig. 38-23 The patient's fingers are unnecessarily exposed to radiation when film holders are not used.

Operator Protection and Monitoring

The dental assistant must use proper operator protection measures to avoid occupational exposure to radiation, including primary radiation, leakage radiation, and scatter radiation. The assistant must carefully follow the safety guidelines and use radiation monitoring devices.

A dental assistant who fails to follow the rules of radiation protection may suffer the results of chronic radiation exposure. By following these rules, dental personnel can keep their radiation exposure to zero (Fig. 38-24).

Radiation Monitoring

Radiation monitoring can be used to protect the operator by identifying occupational exposure to radiation. Both equipment and dental personnel can be monitored. Three types of monitoring devices are used to determine the amount of radiation exposure to personnel: (1) film badge, (2) pocket dosimeter (pen style), and (3) thermoluminescent device (TLD).

The *film badge* is most commonly used to measure the amount of occupational exposure. The badge contains a

Rules of Radiation Protection

1. Never stand in the direct line of the primary beam.
2. Always stand behind a lead barrier or a proper thickness of drywall. If a lead barrier is not available, stand at right angles to the beam.
3. Never stand closer than 6 feet from the x-ray unit during an exposure, unless you are behind a barrier.

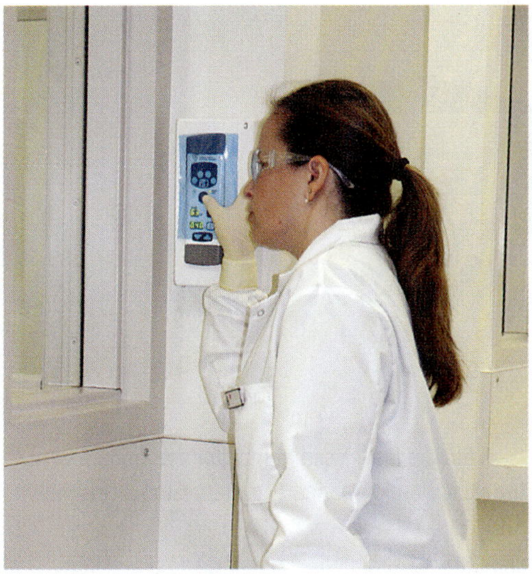

Fig. 38-24 For safety, the dental assistant must stand out of the path of the primary beam.

film packet, similar to dental film, that is embossed with the wearer's name and identification number (Fig. 38-25).

The badge is worn at all times while the employee is at work. At the end of the reporting period, usually every 3 to 4 weeks, the badge is returned to the monitoring service company. The company processes the badge and prepares a report that is returned to the dental office. The report contains the radiation exposure results for the reporting period and the accumulated quarterly, yearly, and lifetime exposures of the individual.

Film badges should not be worn outside the office, especially in bright sunlight. Film badges must be removed when the wearer is having medical or dental x-ray films taken because the badges are intended to measure only *occupational* exposure.

Equipment Monitoring

Dental x-ray machines must be monitored for *leakage* radiation, or any radiation (except for the primary beam) that is emitted from the tubehead. If an x-ray tubehead has a faulty seal, leakage radiation results. Dental x-ray equipment can be monitored through a film device available from the manufacturer or the state health department.

Pediatric Patients

If the patient is a child who is unable to cooperate, the patient may be seated on the parent's lap in the dental chair. Both parent and child are covered with the lead apron, and the parent holds the film in place (Fig. 38-26).

Having the parent hold the film is acceptable because this is a single exposure for the parent. If the assistant were to hold the film in this manner, he or she would have repeated exposures and would suffer the cumulative effects of radiation.

ALARA Concept

The **ALARA concept** states that all exposure to radiation must be kept to a minimum, or "*a*s *l*ow *a*s *r*easonably *a*chievable." Every possible method of reducing exposure to radiation should be used to minimize risk.

The radiation protection measures detailed in this chapter should be used to minimize patient, operator, and staff exposure, thus keeping radiation exposure "ALARA."

Recall

23. What is the purpose of personnel monitoring?
24. What is the purpose of equipment monitoring?
25. What is the ALARA concept?

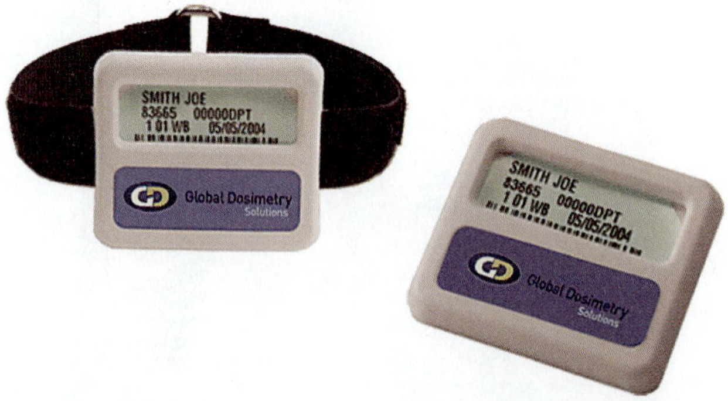

Fig. 38-25 A film badge is used to monitor the amount of radiation that reaches the dental radiographer. (Courtesy Global Dosimetry Solutions, Irvine, CA.)

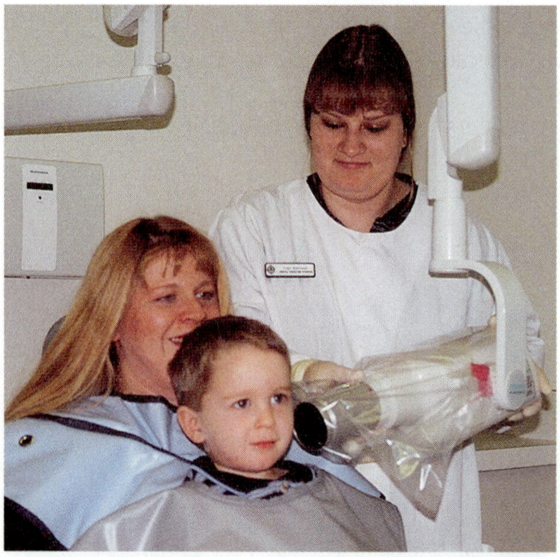

Fig. 38-26 Child sitting on parent's lap for dental x-ray.

Patient Education

Patients often have questions and concerns about radiation. As a dental assistant, you must be prepared to answer their questions and educate them about the importance of radiographs. The following examples are comments *you* can make to patients during informal discussions:

- "The doctor orders radiographs based on your individual needs."
- "Our office takes every step possible to protect you from unnecessary radiation."
- "We use a lead apron and thyroid collar to protect your body from stray radiation."
- "We use a high-speed film that requires only minimal amounts of radiation."
- "We use film holders so that your fingers are not exposed to radiation."
- "Do you have any questions before we begin?"

Legal and Ethical Implications

Although the risks of radiation exposure involved in dental radiography are not significantly greater than other everyday risks in life, it is important that dental professionals do everything possible to protect patients from unnecessary exposure to x-radiation.

Every patient's dental condition is different, and consequently, every patient should be evaluated for dental radiographs on an individual basis. Radiographic examinations should not be based on a standard number of radiographs, and radiographs should not be taken at predetermined times. For example, the dentist who prescribes a set number of radiographs (such as four bite-wing views) at a set interval (such as every 6 months) for every patient is not considering the special needs of each patient.

Eye to the Future

Dental manufacturers are continually striving to develop products that will minimize exposure to radiation. The new F-speed film has already cut previous exposure times in half, and new dental x-ray machines are operating at lower settings.

Other imaging machines that do not require the use of radiation are currently used in medicine and will soon be available for dentistry as well.

Critical Thinking

As a dental assistant, how would you answer the following patient questions regarding dental x-rays?

1. Are dental x-rays really necessary?
2. Should I have x-rays every 6 months?
3. Why do you use a lead apron?
4. Should x-rays be taken during pregnancy?
5. Why do you leave the room when x-rays are taken?
6. Are dental x-rays safe?

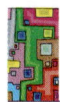

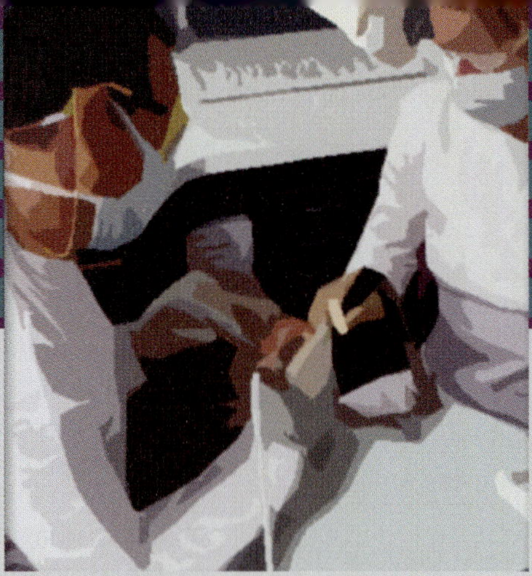

39 Dental Film and Processing Radiographs

Outline

KEY TERMS

Automatic processor Device that automates all film processing steps.

Beam alignment device Assists in the positioning of the PID.

Bite-wing Radiographic view that shows the crowns of both arches on one film.

Calcium tungstate Common type of phosphor.

Cassette Holder for extraoral films during exposure.

Cephalometric film Shows the bony and soft tissue areas of the facial profile.

Duplicating film Film designed for use in film duplicating machines.

Emulsion (ee-**mul**-shun) A layer on the x-ray film that contains the radiograph-sensitive crystals.

Extraoral film Film designed for use in cassettes.

Film holder Device used to position and hold dental x-ray films.

Film speed The sensitivity of the emulsion on the film to radiation.

Intensifying screen Device used to convert x-ray energy into visible light, which in turn exposes screen film.

Intraoral film Film designed for placement in the patient's mouth.

Label side Colored side of the film that faces the tongue.

Latent image (**lay**-tunt) The invisible image on the x-ray film after exposure but before processing.

Occlusal Radiographic view that shows large areas of the maxilla or mandible.

Panoramic film Provides a wide view of the upper and lower jaws.

Periapical (*pehr*-ee-**a**-pi-kul) Radiographic view that shows the crown, root tip, and surrounding structures.

Processing A series of steps that changes exposed film into a radiograph. The steps include developing, rinsing, fixing, washing, drying.

Radiograph (**ray**-dee-oh-*graf*) Image produced on photosensitive film by exposing the film to radiation and then processing it.

Tube side Solid-white side of the film that faces the x-ray tube.

LEARNING OUTCOMES

On completion of this chapter, the student will be able to achieve the following objectives:

- Pronounce, define, and spell the Key Terms.
- Identify the types of dental x-ray film holders and devices.
- Describe the composition of a dental x-ray film.
- Describe the care and maintenance of the processing solutions, equipment, and equipment accessories used in manual and automatic film processing.
- List and identify the component parts of an automatic film processor.
- Describe common time and temperature errors during film processing.
- Describe chemical contamination errors during film processing.
- Describe film handling errors that can occur during film processing.
- Describe some common lighting errors during film processing.
- State the types of and indications for the three types of dental radiographs.
- Identify the five basic sizes of intraoral dental film.
- Explain the purpose of an intensifying screen.
- Describe the process for duplicating radiographs.
- Discuss the requirements necessary for the darkroom.

The dental assistant is the individual who is most often responsible for processing film. Therefore, the dental assistant must thoroughly understand the procedures and techniques necessary to process films into high-quality diagnostic dental radiographs. It is also important to use the correct terminology. *Film* is the correct term to use *before* it has been processed. The *film* is in the packet; the *film* is placed in the bite-block; the *film* is exposed and processed. *After* the film has been processed, it becomes a **radiograph.**

In addition to manual and automatic film processing, you will learn about various types of x-ray film and film holders and how to duplicate dental radiographs. You will also learn how to recognize common errors in film processing and how to prevent them from occurring.

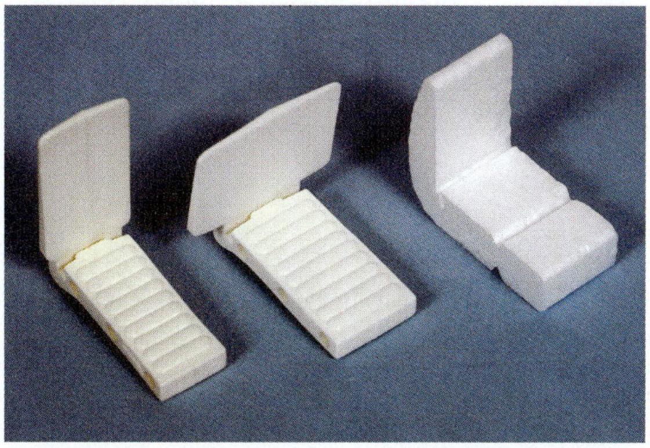

Fig. 39-1 Plastic- and Styrofoam-type disposable bite-block film holders.

DENTAL FILM HOLDERS

A **film holder** is a device used to position and hold dental x-ray films in the patient's mouth. The use of a film holder keeps the patient's fingers from being exposed to x-radiation. Film holders also assist the operator in properly positioning the film and the position indicator device (PID). When using a rectangular PID, a film holder is absolutely necessary to avoid *cone cuts,* or clear areas of the film that are not exposed to radiation (see Chapter 38).

Various types of intraoral film holders are currently available. A basic-style film holder is the disposable polystyrene (Styrofoam) bite-block with a backing plate and a slot for film retention (Fig. 39-1). The EeZee-Grip (formerly, the Snap-A-Ray) is a double-ended instrument that holds the film between two serrated plastic grips that can be locked into place (Fig. 39-2). Other devices include the Endoray (Fig. 39-3) and Uni-bite devices made by Rinn.

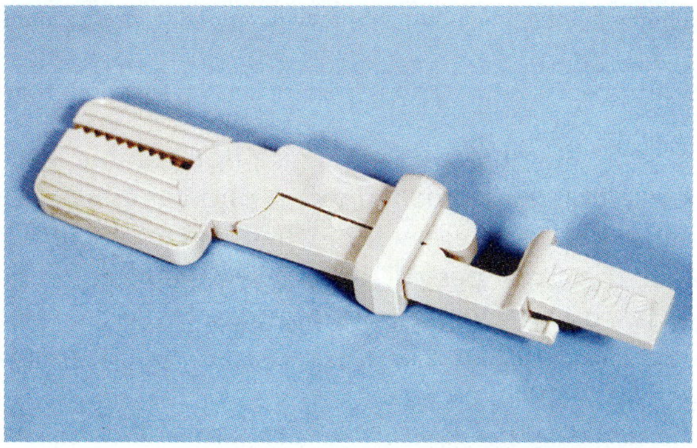

Fig. 39-2 The EeZee-Grip film holder (formerly the Snap-A-Ray).

Devices used to align the beam are available from several manufacturers. The **beam alignment device** assists in the positioning of the PID in relation to the tooth and film. Rinn XCP instruments use color-coded plastic bite-blocks, plastic aiming rings, and metal indicator arms (Fig. 39-4).

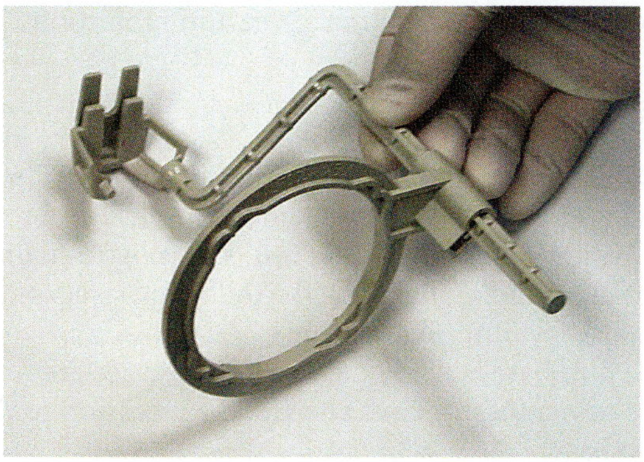

Fig. 39-3 The Endoray is designed to be used for radiographs of teeth with endodontic instruments in the canal.

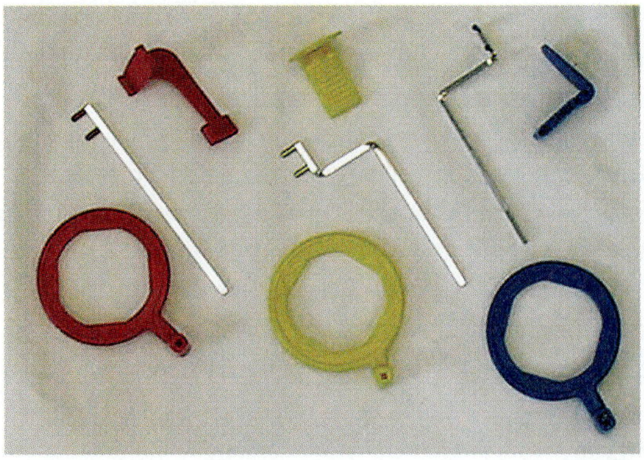

Fig. 39-4 Rinn XCP instruments are color-coded for easier assembly. The *red* instruments are for bite-wing placement, *yellow* for posterior placement, and *blue* for anterior placement.

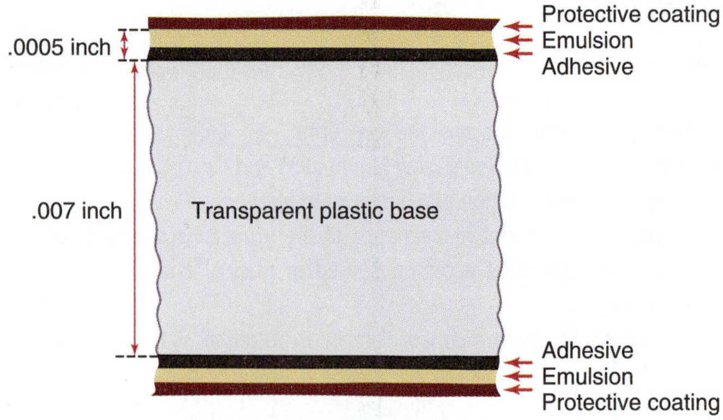

Fig. 39-5 Cross-sectional diagram of film base and emulsion. (From Frommer H, Stabulus JJ: *Radiology for the dental professional,* ed 8, St Louis, 2005, Mosby.)

Recall

1. How does the use of film holders protect the patient from unnecessary radiation?
2. What makes up the basic type of film holder?
3. What is the purpose of a beam alignment device?

DENTAL FILM

Film used in dental radiography is photographic film that has been adapted for dental use. A photographic image is produced on dental x-ray film when it is exposed to radiographs that have passed through teeth and adjacent tissues. The concept is similar to an image being recorded on photographic film after being exposed to light through the shutter and lens of a camera.

The dental assistant must understand the composition of x-ray film and latent image formation. The assistant must also be familiar with the types of film used in dental radiography, as well as film storage and protection.

Film Composition

Intraoral film consists of a semiflexible acetate film base coated on both sides with an emulsion of silver bromide, silver halide, and silver iodide that is sensitive to radiation. Beginning with the film base, the following layers make up a dental x-ray film (Fig. 39-5):

- The film base is made of clear cellulose acetate.
- The thin adhesive layer attaches the emulsion to the film base.
- The gelatin suspends the emulsion of microscopic silver crystals over the film base. During film processing the gelatin absorbs the processing solutions and allows the chemicals to react with the silver halide crystals.
- The silver halide crystals absorb radiation during x-ray exposure and store energy from the radiation (Fig. 39-6).
- The protective layer is a thin transparent coating that protects the emulsion surface.

Latent Image

When the radiation interacts with the silver halide crystals in the film emulsion, the image on the film is produced. The image is not visible before processing and is called the **latent image.**

An example of another type of latent image is *fingerprints.* If you touch an item, you leave your fingerprints even though you cannot see them on the object. When the item is treated, however, your fingerprints become visible.

Film Speed

Film speed refers to the amount of radiation required to produce a radiograph of standard density (darkness). The film speed is determined by the following:

- Size of the silver halide crystals
- Thickness of the emulsion
- Presence of special radiosensitive dyes

The film speed determines how much exposure time is required to produce the image on the film. For example, a fast film requires less radiation. The fast film responds more quickly because the silver halide crystals in the emulsion are larger; the *larger* the crystals, the *faster* the film speed. This same principle applies to film speed on photographic film.

Film speed is classified by the American National Standards Institute (ANSI), using the letters A through F. Only D, E, and F speeds are used in intraoral dental radiography. *F speed* is the newest and fastest film currently available and reduces radiation exposure to the patient by

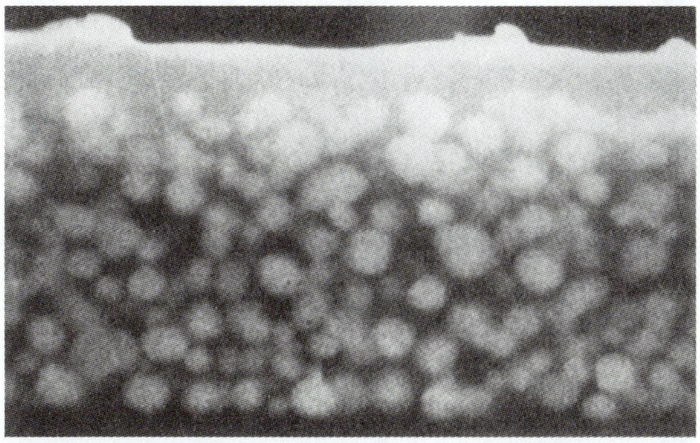

Fig. 39-6 Scanning electron micrograph of unprocessed emulsion of Kodak Ultra Speed dental film (5000 × magnification). Note white-appearing, unexposed silver bromide grains. (Courtesy Eastman Kodak, Rochester, NY.)

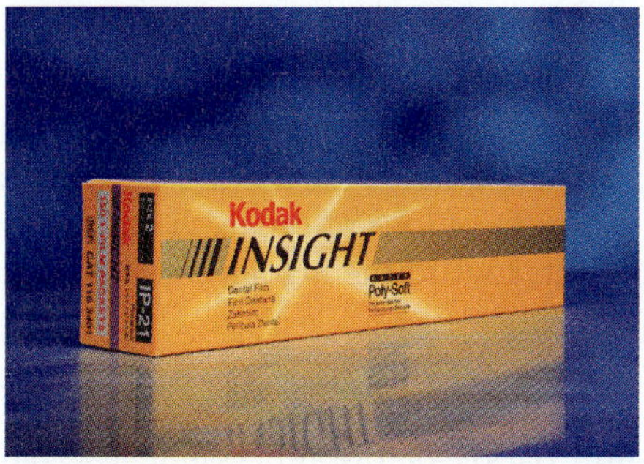

Fig. 39-7 Insight is the new F-speed film available from Kodak. (Courtesy Eastman Kodak, Rochester, NY.)

20 to 60 percent compared with E-speed and D-speed film, respectively (Fig. 39-7).

The film speed is clearly indicated on the label side of the intraoral film packet as well as on the outside of the film box or container.

TYPES OF FILM

The three types of x-ray film used in dental radiography are intraoral film, extraoral film, and duplicating film.

Intraoral Film

An intraoral film is placed *inside* the mouth (*intra*orally) during x-ray exposure. Intraoral radiographs are used to examine the teeth and supporting structures. Intraoral x-ray film has emulsion on *both sides* of the film instead of only one side because it requires less radiation to produce an image.

Film Packet

Film is sealed in a film packet to protect it from light and moisture. The terms *film packet* and *film* are often used interchangeably (Fig. 39-8).

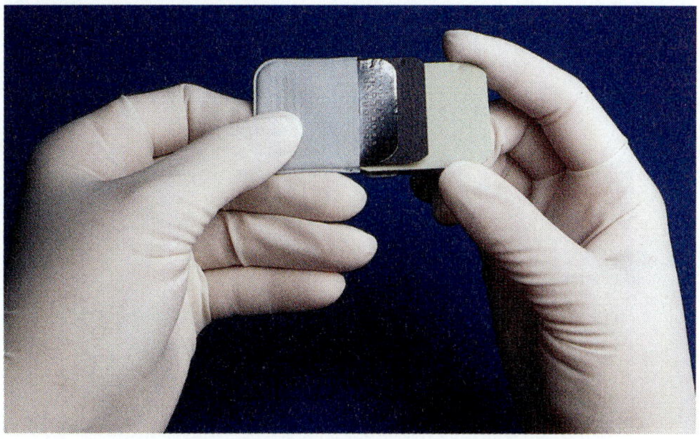

Fig. 39-8 Contents of a dental film packet: lead foil, radiograph film, and black paper.

Intraoral film packets are typically available in boxes of 25, 100, or 150 films. The film packet may contain one film (one-film packet) or two films (two-film packet). A two-film packet (also referred to as a *double film packet*) produces two identical radiographs with the same amount of radiation necessary to produce a single radiograph. The two-film packet is used when duplicate radiographs are necessary, such as for insurance claims and referrals to a specialist.

Packet information

The boxes of film are labeled with the (1) type of film, (2) film speed, (3) number of films per individual packet, (4) total number of films in the box, and (5) film expiration date.

On one corner of the film packet is a small raised bump known as the *identification dot*. This bump or dot is used to determine the left side from the right side when placing the film. The dot is also important when mounting radiographs (see Chapter 41).

Wrapper and lead sheet

The black paper film wrapper inside the film packet is a protective sheet that covers the film and shields it from light. Always make certain the black paper wrapper is removed before processing the film.

The lead foil sheet is a single piece of foil included in the film packet, behind the film and wrapped in black protective paper. The thin lead foil sheet is positioned *behind* the film to shield the film from back-scattered (secondary) radiation that results in film fog (Fig. 39-9).

Package positioning

If the film packet is inadvertently positioned in the mouth backward and then exposed, a *herringbone* pattern will be visible on the radiograph. This pattern is caused by the embossed pattern on the lead foil (Fig. 39-10).

Package disposal

In many states the lead foil from radiograph packets is considered a hazardous waste and must not be disposed of

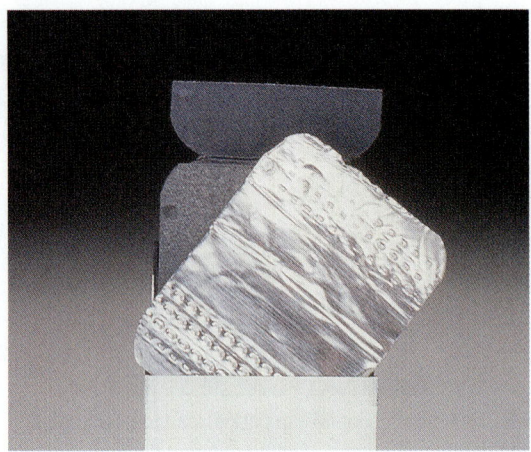

Fig. 39-9 The lead foil insert in this package has a raised diamond pattern across both ends.

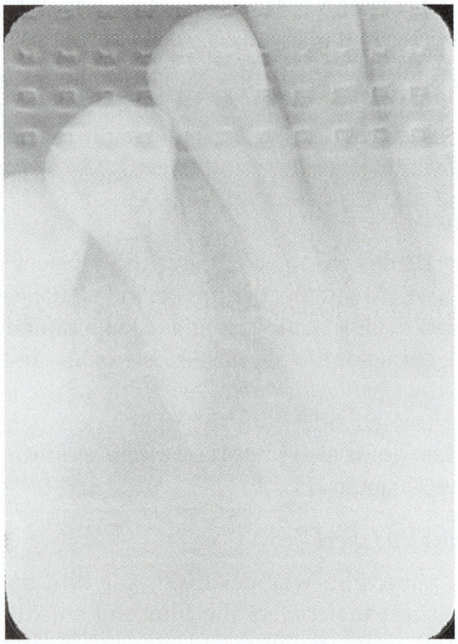

Fig. 39-10 A radiograph that was positioned backward in the mouth will have a herringbone pattern on it. (From Haring JI, Jansen L: *Dental radiology: principles and techniques,* ed 2, Philadelphia, 2000, Saunders.)

with the regular trash. Check with the department of environmental health in your state. Recycling programs are available for the lead foil from radiograph packets.

Outer Packet

The outer packet wrapping is a soft vinyl or paper wrapper that seals the film packet, protective black paper, and lead foil sheet. The outer wrapper protects the film from exposure to light and saliva.

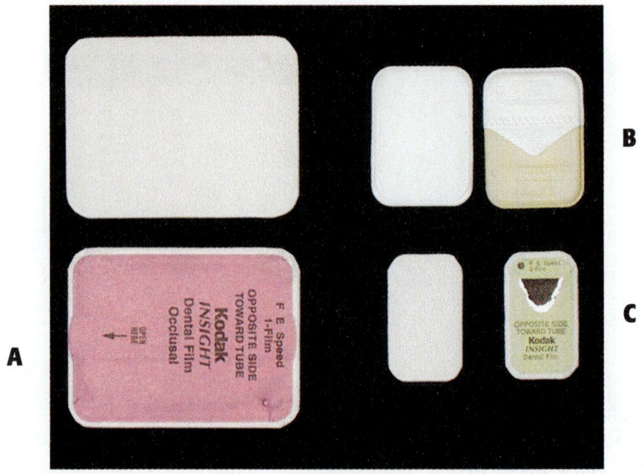

Fig. 39-11 The white side of the film packet faces the tube. **A,** Size 4 occlusal film. **B,** Size 2 film. **C,** Size 1 film.

Tube side

The **tube side** is solid white and has the raised bump on one corner. When placed in the mouth, the white side (tube side) of the film faces toward the teeth and tubehead, and raised dot points toward the incisal/occlusal surface.

Label side

The **label side** of the film packet has a flap that is used to open the film packet before processing. The label side is the color-coded side to identify films. Color codes are used to distinguish between one-film and two-film packets and between film speeds. When placed in the mouth, the color-coded side of the packet faces toward the tongue.

Film Sizes

Intraoral film packets come in five basic sizes (Fig. 39-11), as follows:

1. Child size (#0): children younger than 3 years
2. Narrow anterior (#1): anterior views on adults and children
3. Adult size (#2)
4. Preformed **bite-wing** (#3): infrequently used
5. **Occlusal** (#4)

Full-mouth radiographic surveys for adults usually involve film sizes #1 and #2. Adult bite-wing examinations normally use #2 film.

Recall

4. What are the five components of intraoral film?
5. What is a latent image?
6. How can you tell which side of the film is placed toward the tube?
7. What number film is used for adult radiographs?
8. What size film is used for occlusal radiographs?

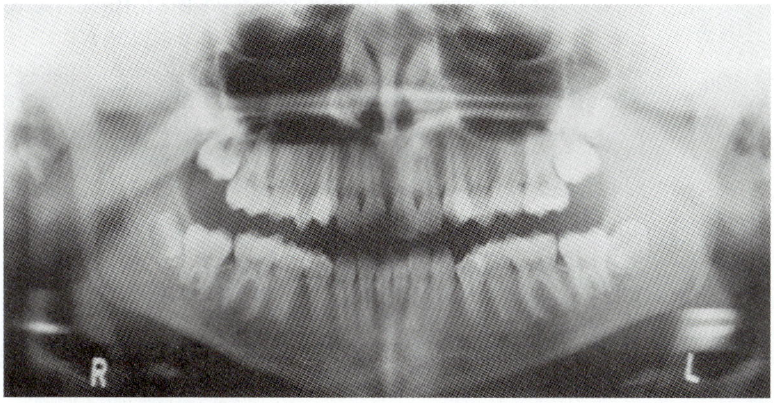

Fig. 39-12 **Panoramic x-ray film.** (Courtesy Eastman Kodak, Rochester, NY.)

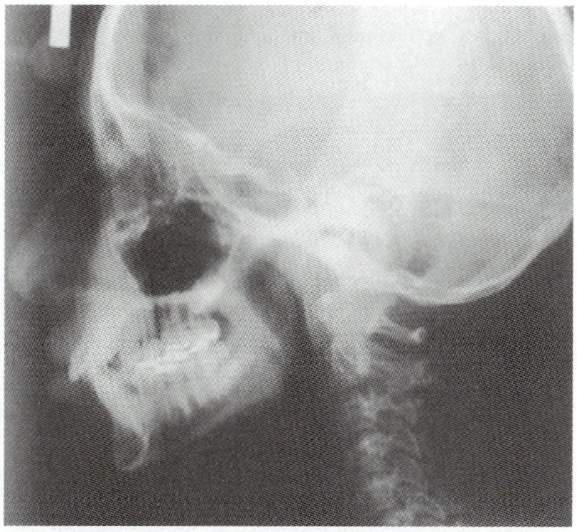

Fig. 39-13 **Cephalometric radiograph.** (Courtesy Eastman Kodak, Rochester, NY.)

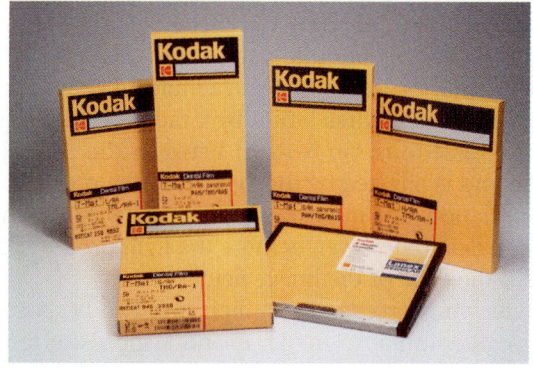

Fig. 39-14 **Boxes of extraoral x-ray film.** (Courtesy Eastman Kodak, Rochester, NY.)

Extraoral Film

An **extraoral film** is placed *outside* the mouth (*extra*orally) during x-ray exposure. Extraoral films are used to examine large areas of the head or jaws.

Common extraoral films include the panoramic and cephalometric films. A **panoramic film** shows a panoramic (wide) view of the upper and lower jaws on a single radiograph (Fig. 39-12). A **cephalometric film** shows the bony and soft tissue areas of the facial profile (Fig. 39-13).

Film Packaging

Extraoral radiography uses a film-screen system, which means that the film is used with intensifying screens, as discussed later.

Extraoral film is supplied in boxes of 50 or 100 films. Extraoral film used in dental radiography is available in 5- × 7- and 8- × 10-inch size. Boxes of extraoral film are labeled with the (1) type of film, (2) film size, (3) total number of films enclosed, and (4) film expiration date.

Extraoral film is not supplied in film packets. The film is stacked in the box much like a deck of cards. Important note: Extraoral film boxes must be opened in the darkroom and the film then placed into a film cassette. The film in the box is not protected with paper wrappers as is intraoral film. If the box is opened where light is present, all the film in the box will be exposed and ruined (Fig. 39-14).

Film Cassette

A **cassette** is a plastic or metal case used to hold the film and protect it from exposure to light. The cassette also holds the film in tight contact with the intensifying screen. Cassettes are available in rigid and flexible styles (Fig. 39-15).

Extraoral film does not have a raised dot on it. Therefore, to distinguish the patient's left from the right as on intraoral films, the front of the cassettes must be marked with the letter *L* (left side) or *R* (right side). After exposure the letter will be superimposed on the radiograph. The front side of the cassette is typically constructed of plastic to permit the passage of the radiograph beam, whereas the back side is made of metal to reduce scatter radiation. *The front side of the cassette must always face the patient during exposure.*

Intensifying Screen

An intensifying screen is mounted on the front and back of the inside surfaces of a rigid-type film cassette (Fig. 39-16). The flexible-type film cassette uses removable intensifying screens.

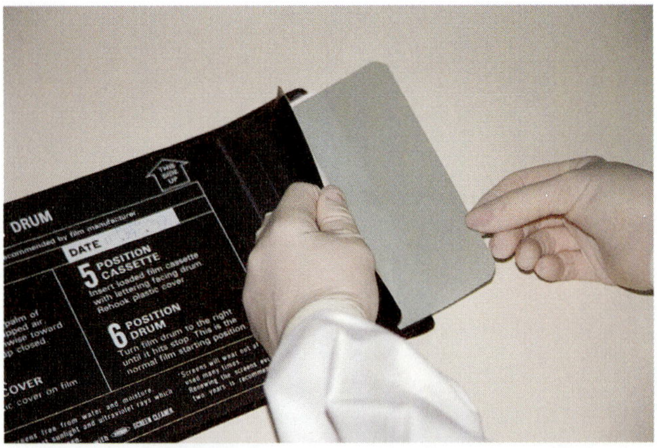

Fig. 39-15 The dental assistant removes a film from a flexible film cassette.

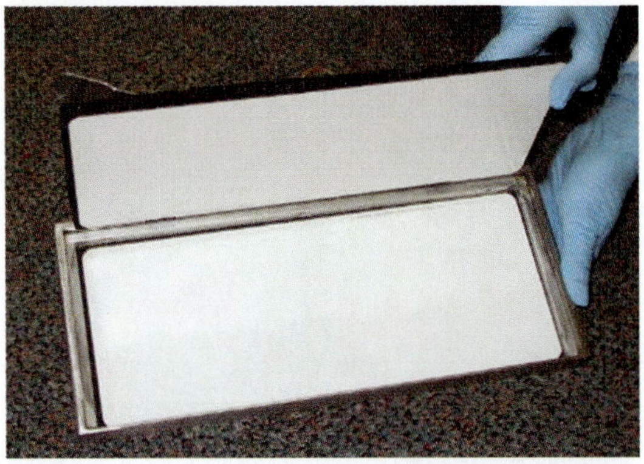

Fig. 39-16 Rigid-type film cassette with an intensifying screen.

An **intensifying screen,** as the name implies, is a device that intensifies or increases the effect of the radiation and thus decreases the amount of exposure time needed. The intensifying screen is coated with a material called *phosphor* that gives off light when struck by x-radiation. The film inside the cassette is sandwiched between the intensifying screens and is affected by the light from the phosphor *and* the x-radiation. The intensified beam results in a slight loss of image detail, however, because the light produces a *halo* effect at the edge of the image field.

Intensifying screens vary in their speed and exposure requirements, similar to the D, E, and F speeds of intraoral film. The speed of the screen depends on the type of phosphor and the size of the crystal; the larger the crystal, the faster the screen, but the poorer the definition. One type of screen uses a common type of phosphor called **calcium tungstate,** which produces a *blue light.*

The other type of phosphors are called the rare earth elements, which produce a *green light.* The rare earth element screens are four times more efficient in converting x-ray energy into light than calcium tungstate screens and therefore are faster and require less exposure time. Be certain to use the appropriate film for the type of intensifying screen.

When film is placed in and removed from the cassette, care must be taken not to scratch the intensifying screen. If an intensifying screen is badly scratched and the phosphor is removed, a white streak will appear on any films taken with this cassette.

Film Types

The two types of film that may be used in extraoral radiography are screen film and nonscreen film.

Screen film is sensitive to the light emitted from the intensifying screen; this means that the film is more sensitive to the light emitted by the phosphor in the intensifying screen than it is to radiation. The use of screen-type film and intensifying screens *reduces* the amount of radiation to the patient. The two types of screen film used in extraoral radiography are as follows:

- *Green-sensitive* film is used with cassettes that have rare earth intensifying screens.
- *Blue-sensitive* film is used with cassettes that have calcium tungstate intensifying screens.

Nonscreen film is an extraoral film that does *not* require the use of intensifying screens for exposure. A nonscreen extraoral film is exposed directly to x-rays; the emulsion is sensitive to direct x-ray exposure rather than to fluorescent light. A nonscreen extraoral film requires more exposure time than a screen film and is *not recommended* for use in dental radiography.

Recall

9. What are the two types of extraoral film cassettes?
10. What is an intensifying screen?
11. How does extraoral film react differently from intraoral film?

Duplicating Film

Duplicating radiographs may be necessary when referring patients to specialists, for insurance claims or legal purposes, or when patients change dentists and request that copies of their records be sent to the new dentist. Film duplication creates an identical copy of an intraoral or extraoral radiograph. Special duplicating film and a duplicating machine are needed to duplicate radiographs (Fig. 39-17). (See Procedure 39-1: Duplicating Dental Radiographs.)

Duplicating film is used only in a darkroom setting and is *never* exposed to x-rays. Duplicating film is sensitive to light and has emulsion on one side only. The emulsion side of the film appears dull, whereas the side without emulsion appears shiny. Duplicating film is available in all **periapical** sizes, as well as 5- × 12- and 8- × 10-inch sheets.

The duplicating machine produces white light to expose the film. Because the film is light-sensitive, the duplication process is performed in the darkroom with the safelight.

Procedure 39-1 Duplicating Dental Radiographs

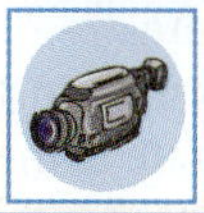
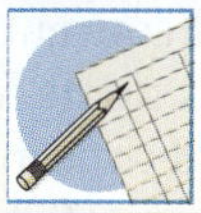

Goal

To duplicate a set of dental radiographs.

Equipment and Supplies

- Darkroom environment
- Duplicating film
- Duplicating machine
- Radiograph label
- Pen

PROCEDURAL STEPS

1. Turn on the safelight and turn off the white light.
2. Place the radiographs on the duplicator machine glass.
3. Open the box of duplicating film and remove one film.
4. Place the duplicating film on top of the radiographs with the emulsion side against the radiographs and close the lid.
5. Turn on the light in the duplicating machine for the manufacturer's recommended time.
   Purpose: The light passes through the radiographs and strikes the duplicating film.
6. Remove the duplicating film and radiographs from the machine.
7. Process the duplicating film as you would other film, using either manual or automatic techniques.
8. Return the original radiographs to the patient's file.
9. Document the duplication in the patient's record.

Date	Procedure	Operator
8/15/05	Duplicated FMX and mailed to Delta Dental Insurance	PJL

Note: The longer the duplicating film is exposed to light, the lighter the duplicate films will become. This is the opposite of x-ray films, which become darker when exposed to light.

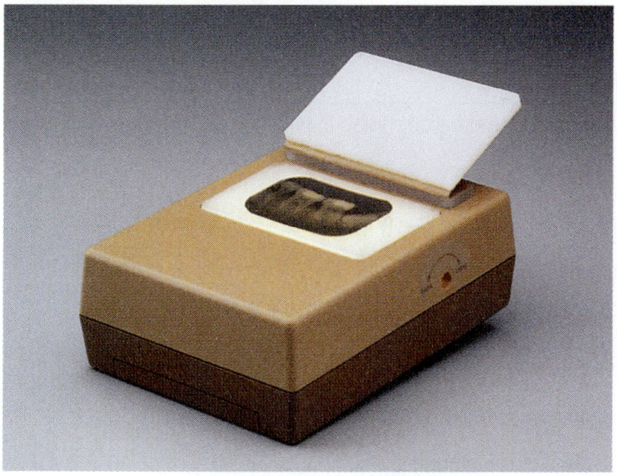

Fig. 39-17 Example of a film duplicator.

Film Storage

All dental films should be stored according to the manufacturer's instructions; this includes protecting them from light, heat, moisture, chemicals, and scatter radiation. Optimum temperature for film storage ranges from 50° to 70° F, and relative humidity levels range from 30 to 50 percent.

To avoid exposure to stray radiation, film should not be kept in the treatment room or near the radiograph unit.

The box of x-ray film is marked with an expiration date. If expired film is accidentally used, the radiographs produced may be fogged and may not be of diagnostic quality. This effect is also known as *age fog.*

Always check the expiration date on the box when new film is purchased. If the expiration date on the box indicates that the film will soon be out of date, you should immediately return the box to the dental supplier. Always rotate the supply of film by using the oldest packages first.

Recall

12. When might it be necessary to duplicate x-rays?
13. What precautions should be taken when storing x-ray film?
14. How can you find the expiration date of a package?

FILM PROCESSING

Processing is a series of steps that change the latent image on the exposed film into a radiograph by producing a visible image on the film. Proper processing is just as important as the exposure technique in producing diagnostic-quality radiographs. Radiographs that are nondiagnostic because of poor processing techniques must be retaken, exposing the patient to unnecessary radiation.

In many practices, intraoral films are processed in an automatic processor. In some dental offices, however, it is still necessary to know how to process the film manually. Whichever method of processing is used, the steps are the same. Both manual and automatic methods are discussed in this chapter.

Five Steps in Processing

1. Developing is the first step in processing films. A chemical solution called *developer* is used. The purpose of the developer is to reduce the exposed silver halide crystals chemically into black metallic silver. The developer solution also softens the film emulsion during this process (Table 39-1).
2. Rinsing the films is necessary to remove the developer from the film so that the development process stops.
3. Fixing uses an acidic solution to remove the unexposed silver halide crystals from the film emulsion. The fixer also hardens the film emulsion during this process.

   Films that are not properly fixed will fade and turn brown in a short time. Leaving films in the fixer for a long period (such as over a weekend) can remove the image from the film (Table 39-2).
4. Washing follows fixation. A water bath is used to wash the film.
5. Drying the film is the final step in film processing.

Processing Solutions

Film processing solutions are available in three forms: powder, ready-to-use liquid, and liquid concentrate.

Both the powder and the liquid concentrate forms must be mixed with distilled water. The liquid concentrate is the most widely used form and the preference of many dental offices; it is easy to mix and occupies little storage space (Fig. 39-18). Always follow the manufacturer's recommendation for preparing solutions.

Fresh chemicals produce the best radiographs. To maintain freshness, film processing solutions must be replenished daily and changed every 3 to 4 weeks. More frequent changing of solutions may be necessary when large numbers of films are processed. "Normal" use is defined as 30 intraoral films per day.

Recall

15. What are the five steps in processing dental radiographs?
16. Which is the most widely used form of processing solution?
17. How often should processing solutions be replenished?

Table 39-1 ***Developer Composition***

Ingredient	Chemical	Function
Developing agent	Hydroquinone	Converts exposed silver halide crystals to black metallic silver
		Slowly generates black tones and contrast
	Elon	Converts exposed silver halide crystals to black metallic silver
		Quickly generates gray tones
Preservative	Sodium sulfite	Prevents rapid oxidation of developing agents
Accelerator	Sodium carbonate	Activates developer agents
		Provides necessary alkaline environment for agents
		Softens gelatin of film emulsion
Restrainer	Potassium bromide	Prevents developer from developing unexposed silver halide crystals

From Haring JI, Jansen L: Dental radiography: principles and techniques, *ed 2, Philadelphia, 2000, Saunders.*

Table 39-2 ***Fixer Composition***

Ingredient	Chemical	Function
Fixing agent	Sodium thiosulfate, ammonium thiosulfate	Removes all unexposed, undeveloped silver halide crystals from emulsion
Preservative	Sodium sulfite	Prevents deterioration of fixing agent
Hardening agent	Potassium alum	Shrinks and hardens gelatin in emulsion
Acidifier	Acetic acid, sulfuric acid	Neutralizes alkaline developer and stops further development

From Haring JI, Jansen L: Dental radiography: principles and techniques, *ed 2, Philadelphia, 2000, Saunders.*

The Darkroom

A well-organized darkroom facilitates the processing of dental x-ray films. The ideal darkroom is the result of careful planning. The darkroom should (1) have adequate working space, proper lighting, and good ventilation; (2) be kept clean at all times; and (3) be equipped with the necessary devices and supplies.

Requirements for a Film Processing Darkroom

- Infection-control items (gloves, disinfectant, spray, paper towels)
- Container with a biohazard label for contaminated film packets or barriers (see Chapter 23)
- Recycling container for lead foil pieces, which should not be thrown in the trash
- "Light-tight room" with no cracks around doors or corners that would allow light leaks
- Processing tanks for the developer and fixer solution and a circulating water bath
- Running water supply with mixing valves to adjust the temperature
- Both a safelight and a source of white (normal) light
- Accurate timer
- Accurate floating thermometer to indicate the temperature of the solutions
- Stirring rod or paddle to mix the chemicals and equalize the temperature of the solutions
- Safe storage space for chemicals
- Film hangers
- A film-drying rack and a film dryer

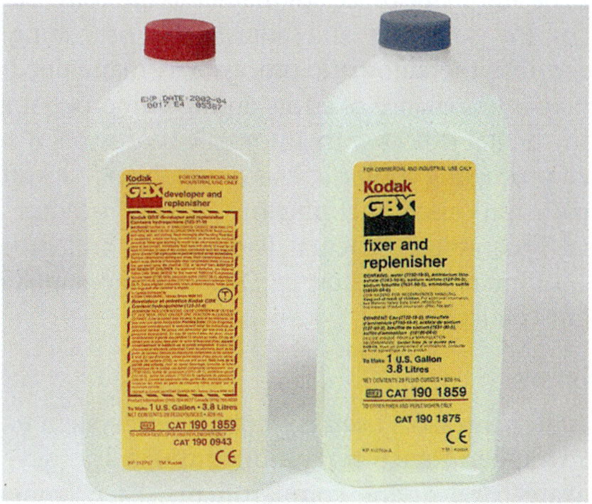

Fig. 39-18 Concentrated solutions of film developer and fixer. (Courtesy Eastman Kodak, Rochester, NY.)

Lighting

The darkroom must be completely dark. The term *light-tight* is often used to describe the darkroom. To be light-tight, no light leaks can be present.

Any white light that "leaks" into the darkroom, such as from around the door, is termed a *light leak.* When you are in the darkroom with the light turned off, no white light should be seen. If you see *any* light leaks around the door, such as through a vent or keyhole, it must be corrected with weather stripping or black tape. X-ray film is *extremely* sensitive to visible white light. Any leaks of white light can cause film fog. A fogged film appears dull gray, lacks contrast, and is nondiagnostic.

Two types of lighting are essential in a darkroom: room lighting and "safelighting."

Room lighting

The darkroom must have an overhead white light that provides adequate lighting when performing tasks such as cleaning, restocking materials, and mixing chemicals.

Safelighting

A *safelight* is a low-intensity light in the red-orange spectrum. Safelighting provides enough illumination in the darkroom to process films safely without exposing or damaging the film.

A safe distance must be maintained between the light and the working area. Also, exposure to the safelight must be kept as short as possible by working quickly. Unwrapped films that are left too close to the safelight or exposed to the safelight for more than 2 to 3 minutes appear fogged. A safelight must be placed at least 4 feet away from the film and working area (Fig. 39-19).

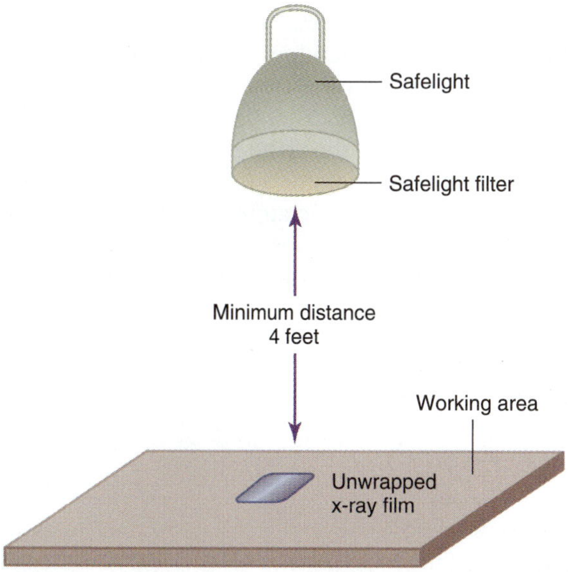

Fig. 39-19 A distance of at least 4 feet must separate the safelight from the working area. (From Haring JI, Jansen L: *Dental radiography: principles and techniques,* ed 2, Philadelphia, 2000, Saunders.)

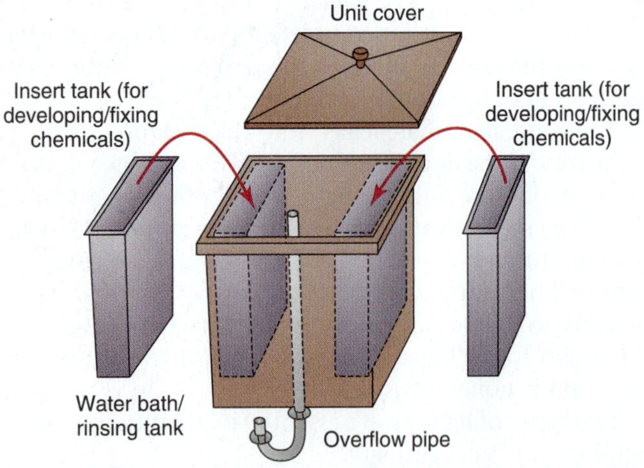

Fig. 39-20 Processing tanks showing developing and fixing tanks inserts in bath of running water. (From Haring JI, Jansen L: *Dental radiography: principles and techniques,* ed 2, Philadelphia, 2000, Saunders.)

Table 39-3 *Processing Temperatures and Times*

Solution Temperature (° F [° C])	TIME IN PROCESSING STEP (MINUTES)			
	Developer	Rinse	Fixer	Wash
65 (18.5)	6	½	10-12	20
68 (20.0)	5	½	10	20
70 (21.0)	4½	½	9-10	20
72 (22.0)	4	½	8-9	20
75 (24.0)	3	½	6-7	20
80 (26.5)	2½	½	5-6	20

Modified from Haring JI, Jansen L: Dental radiography: principles and techniques, *ed 2, Philadelphia, 2000, Saunders.*

Of the many types of safelights available, some are made only for intraoral films, others only for extraoral films, and some for both intraoral and extraoral films. A good universal safelight filter for *both* extraoral screen films and intraoral films is the GBX-2 safelight filter by Kodak. Recommendations for specific safelights and filters are provided on the film package.

Processing Tanks

Manual processing is a method that is used to develop, rinse, fix, and wash dental radiograph films. The essential piece of equipment required for manual processing is a processing tank. The processing tank is divided into compartments to hold the developer solution, water bath, and fixer solution. A processing tank has two insert tanks and one master tank (Fig. 39-20).

The temperature of the circulating water in the master tank controls the temperatures of the developer and fixer solutions. The water temperature is controlled through a mixing valve, which functions similarly to those found in bathroom showers. The optimum temperature for the water bath is 68° F.

Recall

18. What is a safelight?
19. What is the minimum distance between the safelight and the working area?
20. What is the optimum temperature for the water in the manual processing tanks?

Automatic Processor

Automatic film processing is a fast and simple method used to process dental radiograph films (Fig. 39-21). Other than opening the film packet, the **automatic processor** automates all film processing steps.

Advantages of automatic film processing include the following:

1. Less processing time is required.
2. Time and temperatures are automatically controlled.
3. Less equipment is used.
4. Less space is required.

Automatic film processing requires only 4 to 6 minutes to develop, fix, wash, and dry a film, whereas manual processing and drying techniques require approximately 1 hour. In addition, the automatic processor maintains the correct temperature of the solutions and adjusts the processing time. Provided that the automatic processor is maintained properly, there is less chance of errors during film processing.

Many dental offices with automatic processors maintain manual processing equipment as a standby or backup if the automatic processor malfunctions. (See Procedure 39-2: Manual Processing of Dental Radiographs and Procedure 39-3: Automatic Processing of Dental Radiographs Using Daylight Loader.)

Components

Automatic processors use a roller transport system to move the unwrapped dental x-ray film through the developer, fixer, water, and drying compartments. Each component has its own special function (Fig. 39-22), as follows:

- The processor housing covers all the component parts of the automatic processor.

Procedure 39-2 Manual Processing of Dental Radiographs

Goal

To process dental radiograph films using a manual tank.

Equipment and Supplies

- Fully equipped darkroom
- Surface barriers or disinfecting solution for counters
- Exposed films
- Film rack
- Timer
- Pencil
- Film dryer (optional)

PROCEDURAL STEPS

Preparation

1. Follow all the infection-control steps discussed in Chapter 40.
2. Stir the solutions with the corresponding paddle.
   Purpose: The chemicals are heavy and tend to settle to the bottom of the tank. Do not interchange mixing paddles, or cross-contamination will occur.
3. Check the temperature of the solutions and refer to the processing chart to determine the times (Table 39-3).
   Purpose: The temperature of the solution determines the processing time.
4. Label the film rack with the patient's name and date of exposure.
5. Turn on the safelight; then turn off the white light.
6. Wash hands and put on gloves.
7. Open the film packets and allow the films to drop onto the clean paper towel. Take care not to touch the films.
   Purpose: The films have not been contaminated. Films that have been touched become contaminated and may remain contaminated even after processing.

Processing

1. Attach each film to the film rack so that the films are parallel and not touching each other.

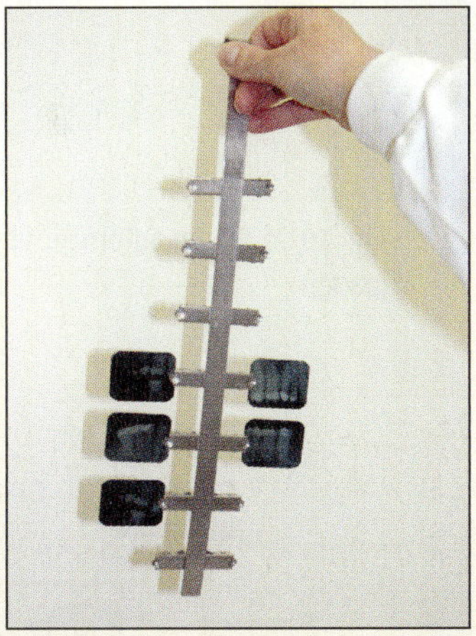

2. As you immerse the film rack in the developer solution, agitate (jiggle) the rack slightly.
   Purpose: Agitating the film rack prevents air bubbles from forming on the film.
3. Start the timer. The timer is set according to the recommendations stated on the processing chart (for example, 5 minutes if the solution is 68° F).
4. When the timer goes off, remove the rack of films and rinse it in the circulating water in the center tank for 20 to 30 seconds. Let the excess water drip off the films.
   Purpose: Water dripping from the racks into the fixer will dilute it.
5. Insert the rack of films into the fixer tank, and set the timer for 10 minutes.
   Purpose: For permanent fixation the film is kept in the fixer for a minimum of 10 minutes. However, films may be removed from the fixing solution after 3 minutes for viewing; this is a wet reading. The films must be returned to the fixer to complete the process.
6. Return the rack of films to the center tank of circulating water for at least 20 minutes.
   Purpose: Incomplete washing will cause the films to eventually turn brown.
7. Remove the rack of films from the water and place it in the film dryer. If a film dryer is not available, it is recommended to hang the films to air-dry.
   Purpose: Films may be air-dried at room temperature in a dust-free area or placed in a heated drying cabinet. Films must be completely dried before they can be handled for mounting and viewing.
8. When the films are completely dry, remove them from the rack and mount and label (see Chapter 41).

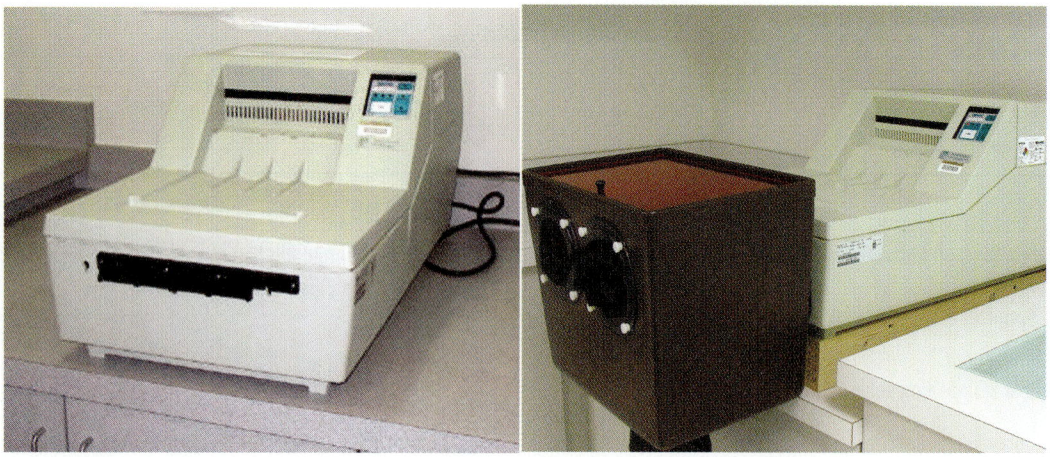

Fig. 39-21 **A,** An automatic film processor. **B,** An automatic film processor equipped with a daylight film loader.

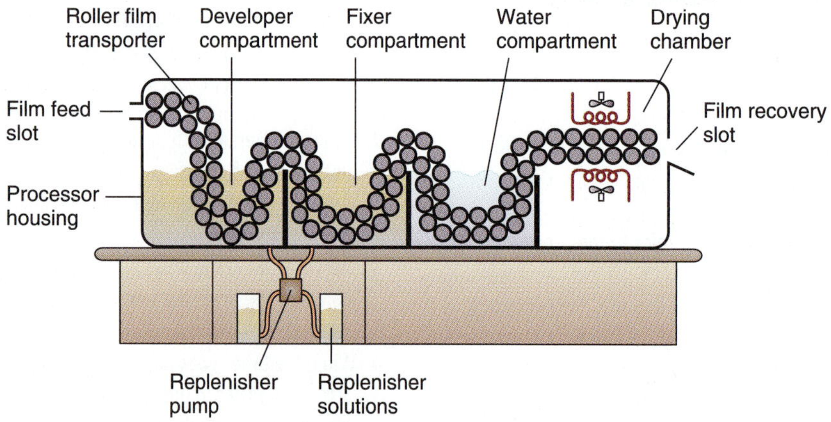

Fig. 39-22 **Component parts of the automatic processor.** (From Haring JI, Jansen L: *Dental radiography: principles and techniques,* ed 2, Philadelphia, 2000, Saunders.)

- The film feed slot is where the unwrapped films are inserted into the automatic processor.
- The roller film transporter is a system of rollers that rapidly moves the film through the developer, fixer, water, and drying compartments. The rollers are turned by motor-driven gears or belts.
- The developer compartment holds the developer solution. The developer used in an automatic processor is a specially formulated solution designed to react at temperatures between 80° and 95° F. Because of the high temperatures, development occurs rapidly.
- The fixer compartment holds the fixer solution. The film is transported directly from the developer into the fixer without a rinsing step. The fixer used in an automatic processor is a specially formulated, highly concentrated chemical solution that contains additional hardening agents.

NOTE: *The chemicals used in manual processing should* never *be used in an automatic processor.*

- The water compartment holds circulating water. Water is used to wash the films after fixation. Some units have a plumbed water system that provides continuous fresh water. Other models require the water to be changed manually.
- The drying chamber holds heated air and dries the wet film.

Processing Solutions

Levels of solutions in the automatic processor must be checked at the beginning of each day and replenished as necessary. Failure to add replenisher results in exhausted solutions and poor-quality radiographs.

Processing solutions in the automatic processor should be replaced every 2 to 6 weeks, depending on the number

Procedure 39-3 Automatic Processing of Dental Radiographs Using Daylight Loader

Equipment and Supplies

- Automatic x-ray processor with daylight loader
- Exposed dental films
- Chemical disinfection spray
- Two disposable cups or containers for lead foil and film packets
- Paper towel

PROCEDURAL STEPS

1. At the beginning of the day, turn on the machine and allow the chemicals to warm up according to the manufacturer's recommendations.
   Purpose: The heating unit must warm the chemicals to the correct temperature so that the films will be of diagnostic quality.
2. Follow the infection-control steps discussed in Chapter 40.
   Purpose: The film packets are contaminated because they have been in the patient's mouth.
3. Wash and dry hands.
4. Open the lid on the daylight loader and place a paper towel over the bottom. Then place two disposable cups on the towel.
   Purpose: The paper towel will act as a surface barrier on the bottom of the daylight loader. One disposable cup is for the lead foil in the film packet; the other is to dispose of the paper towel, film packets, and gloves.
5. Put on gloves and slide gloved hands through the sleeves of the daylight loader.
6. Remove the film from its packet, and check to be sure that the black paper has not stuck to the film. If the black paper is left on the film, or if double film packets have not been separated, the films will be ruined, and the automatic processor could jam.
7. Feed the film into the machine.
   Purpose: Open the film packets and feed films in one at a time to avoid having films overlap during loading.
8. While the film is feeding into the machine, remove the lead foil from the packet and place it in one of the disposable cups. Then drop the empty packet onto the paper towel.
9. Keep the films straight as they are fed slowly into the machine. Allow at least 10 seconds between insertion of each film into the processor and the insertion of the next film. Place films in alternate film slots when possible.
10. After the last film is inserted into the machine, carefully remove gloves and drop them into the center of the paper towel. Touching only the corners and underside of the paper towel, wrap the paper towel over the contaminated film packets and gloves. Place the wrapped paper towel into the second cup.
    Purpose: Handling the paper towel only by the corners and underside will help eliminate cross-contamination during film processing procedures.
11. Remove the cup containing the lead foil and take it to the recycling container.
12. Remove the processed radiographs from the film recovery slot on the outside of the automatic processor. Allow 4 to 6 minutes for the automated process to be completed.
    Note: When processing extraoral films, carefully remove the film from the cassette. Handle all films by the edges only to avoid fingerprints and scratches on the films.

of films processed and the replenishment schedule. Follow the manufacturer's recommendations carefully. Some units have pumps that add replenisher solutions automatically to maintain proper solution concentration and levels. Other models require the operator to replenish the solutions.

Recall

21. What is the major advantage of automatic film processing?
22. How often should the levels of solution in the automatic processor be checked?
23. Are manual processing solutions and automatic processing solutions interchangeable?

PROCESSING ERRORS

Processing errors may result in nondiagnostic radiographs. Films must be free from processing errors to be of diagnostic quality. Poor-quality radiographs may result from the following:

- Time and temperature errors (Table 39-4)
- Chemical contamination errors (Table 39-5)
- Film-handling errors (Table 39-6)
- Lighting errors (Table 39-7)

Many processing errors can be attributed to one or more errors. The dental assistant must be able to recognize the appearance of common processing errors and must know the proper solutions as well as the actions to prevent a recurrence (Fig. 39-23).

Table 39-4 ***Time and Temperature Errors and Solutions***

Example	Appearance	Error	Solution
Underdeveloped film	Light	Inadequate development time	Check development time
		Developer solution too cool	Check developer temperature
		Inaccurate timer or thermometer	Replace faulty timer or thermometer
		Depleted developer solution	Replenish developer with fresh solution as needed
Overdeveloped film	Dark	Excessive developing time	Check development time
		Developer solution too hot	Check developer temperature
		Inaccurate timer or thermometer	Replace faulty timer or thermometer
		Concentrated developer solution	Replenish developer with fresh solution as needed
Reticulation of emulsion	Cracked	Sudden temperature change between developer and water bath	Check temperature of solutions and water bath Avoid extreme temperature changes

Modified from Haring JI, Jansen L: Dental radiography: principles and techniques, *ed 2, Philadelphia, 2000, Saunders.*

Table 39-5 ***Chemical Contamination Errors and Solutions***

Example	Appearance	Error	Solution
Developer spots	Dark spots	Developer contacts film before processing	Use clean work area in darkroom
Fixer spots	White spots	Fixer contacts film before processing	Use clean work area in darkroom
Yellow-brown stains	Yellowish brown color	Exhausted developer or fixer	Replenish chemicals with fresh solutions as needed
		Insufficient fixation time	Ensure adequate fixation time
		Insufficient rinsing	Rinse for at least 20 minutes

Modified from Haring JI, Jansen L: Dental radiography: principles and techniques, *ed 2, Philadelphia, 2000, Saunders.*

Table 39-6 ***Film Handling Errors and Solutions***

Example	Appearance	Error	Solution
Developer cut-off	Straight white border	Undeveloped part of film from low level of developer	Check developer level before processing; add solution if needed
Fixer cut-off	Straight black border	Unfixed part of film from low level of fixer	Check fixer level before processing; add solution if needed
Overlapped films	White or dark areas	Two films in contact during processing	Separate films to prevent contact during processing
Air bubbles	White spots	Air trapped on film surface after film placed in solution	Gently agitate film racks after placing in processing solutions
Fingernail artifact	Black crescent-shaped marks	Film emulsion damaged by operator's fingernail during rough handling	Gently handle films only by the edges
Fingerprint artifact	Black fingerprint	Film touched by fingers contaminated with fluoride or developer	Wash and dry films thoroughly before processing
Static electricity	Thin, black, branching lines	Occurs when film pack is opened quickly	Open film packs slowly
		Occurs when film pack is opened before operator touches conductive object	Touch a conductive object before unwrapping film
Scratched film	White lines	Soft emulsion removed from film by sharp object	Use care when handling films and film racks

Modified from Haring JI, Jansen L: Dental radiography: principles and techniques, *ed 2, Philadelphia, 2000, Saunders.*

Table 39-7 ***Lighting Errors and Solutions***

Example	Appearance	Error	Solution
Light leak	Black (exposed area)	Accidental exposure of film to white light	Examine film packs for defects before using
			Never wrap films in presence of white light
Fogged film	Gray; lack of detail and contrast	Improper "safelighting"	Check filter and bulb wattage of safelight
		Light leaks in darkroom	Check darkroom for light leaks
		Outdated (expired) films	Check expiration date on the box of film
		Improper film storage	Store films in cool, dry area
		Contaminated solutions	Avoid contamination by covering tanks after each use
		Solution too hot	Check temperature of developer

Modified from Haring JI, Jansen L: Dental radiography: principles and techniques, *ed 2, Philadelphia, 2000, Saunders.*

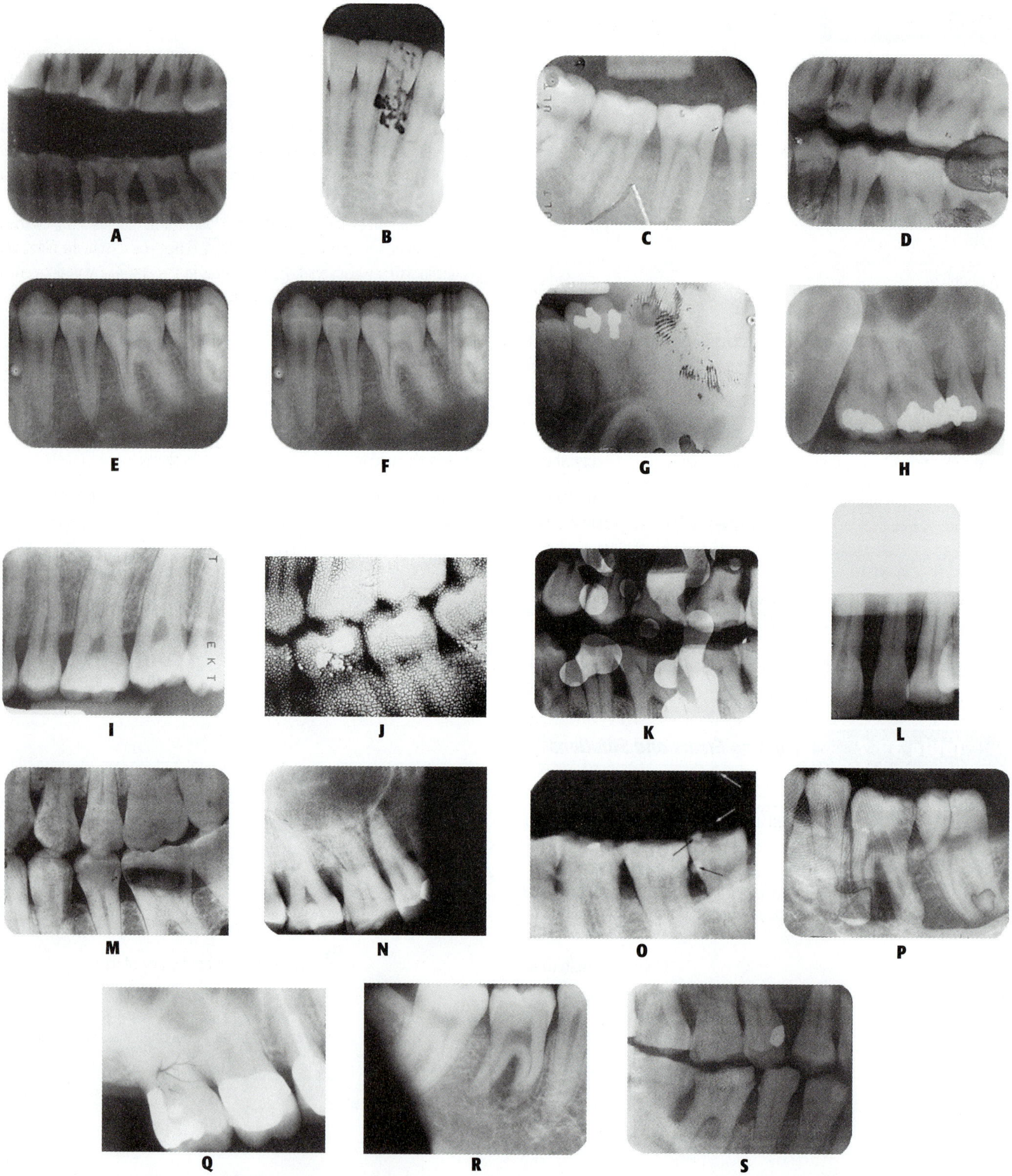

Fig. 39-23 Radiograph processing errors. **A,** Overdevelopment. **B,** Developer splash. **C,** Scratched film. **D,** Water spots. **E,** Solution too low. **F,** Roller marks. **G,** Fingerprints. **H,** Overlapped films. **I,** Underdeveloped. **J,** Reticulation. **K,** Fixer spots. **L,** Developer cut-off. **M,** Number of errors. **N,** Fixer cut-off. **O,** Air bubbles. **P,** Black fingerprint. **Q,** Static electricity. **R,** Exposure to light. **S,** Fogged film. (Radiographs from Haring JI, Jansen L: *Dental radiography: principles and techniques,* ed 2, Philadelphia, 2000, Saunders.)

Legal and Ethical Implications

The importance of properly processing dental radiographs must never be overlooked. The dental assistant is usually the team member responsible for this important procedure. In addition to processing films, the dental assistant must keep the darkroom area clean, follow infection-control procedures, and change the processing solutions.

When errors in processing ruin a radiograph and make it necessary to retake the film, the patient is exposed to unnecessary additional radiation.

Eye to the Future

The dental radiography techniques of the future will be based on methods that further reduce the amount of radiation exposure to the patient. Techniques might include even faster dental radiograph film or perhaps imaging techniques that do not involve the use of radiation at all.

Digital radiography has already eliminated the need for processing radiographs (see Chapter 42). More changes undoubtedly will occur in dental imaging techniques.

Critical Thinking

1. Jason Weber is a 4-year-old patient in your office, and you are going to take bite-wing radiographs on him. What size film do you think you will need?
2. As a dental assistant, one of your responsibilities in the office is to maintain the automatic film processor. The office is moderately busy and processes about 25 films a day. What would be your schedule of solution replenishment?
3. Nancy is a new dental assistant in your office, and she just finished manually processing some dental radiographs. When you look at the films, you notice that they are very light. You exposed the films, so you are certain that the exposure factors were correct. What could have gone wrong?

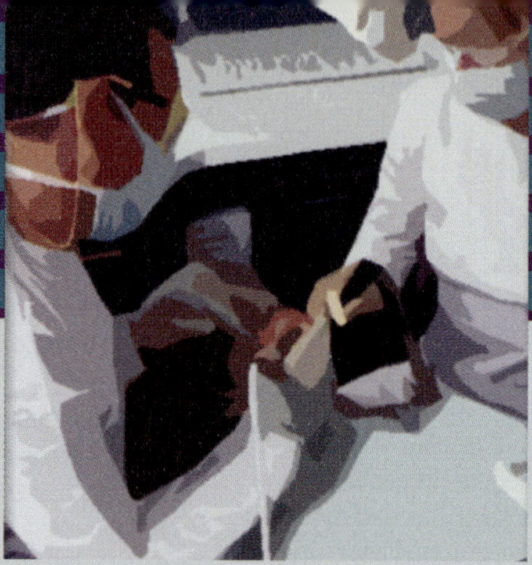

40 Legal Issues, Quality Assurance, and Infection Control

Outline

Legal Considerations
- Federal and State Regulations
- Licensure Requirements
- Risk Management
- Informed Consent
- Liability
- Patient Records
- Patient Refusal
- Patient Education

Quality Assurance in the Dental Office
- Quality Control Tests
- Quality Administration Procedures

Infection Control
- Centers for Disease Control and Prevention Guidelines
- The Radiography Operatory
- Equipment and Supplies
- Procedures During and After X-Ray Film Exposure

Procedure 40-1: Practicing Infection Control During Film Exposure
- Procedures During X-Ray Film Processing

Procedure 40-2: Practicing Infection Control in the Darkroom

Procedure 40-3: Practicing Infection Control with Use of Daylight Loader

Legal and Ethical Implications

Eye to the Future

Critical Thinking

KEY TERMS

Artifact An image on a radiograph that is not an actual structure but is caused by the technique.

Disclosure Process of informing the patient about a procedure; for example, the procedure for taking x-rays.

Informed consent Permission granted by a patient after being informed about the details of a procedure.

Liable Accountable or legally responsible.

Quality assurance A plan to ensure that the dental office produces consistent, high-quality images with a minimum of exposure to patients and personnel.

Quality control tests Specific tests used to ensure quality in dental x-ray equipment, supplies, and film processing.

Stepwedge Device constructed of layered aluminum steps to demonstrate the film densities and contrasts.

Viewbox An illuminated boxlike device used to view radiographs.

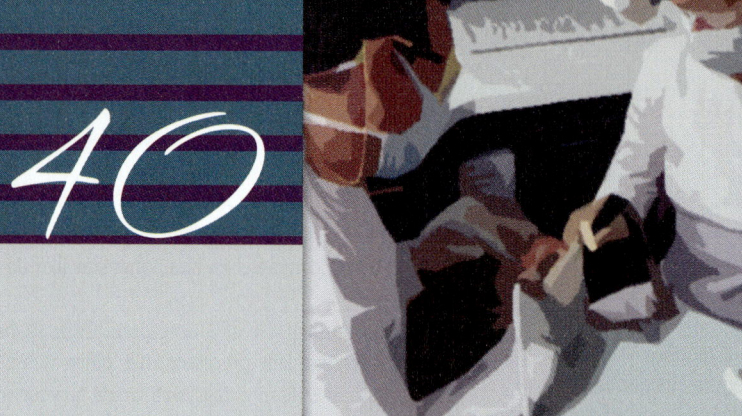

LEARNING OUTCOMES

On completion of this chapter, the student will be able to achieve the following objectives:

- Pronounce, define, and spell the Key Terms.
- Describe the components of informed consent with regard to dental radiographs.
- Describe the types of laws affecting the practice of dental radiography.
- Describe the Consumer-Patient Radiation Health and Safety Act.
- Identify the individual that "owns" the dental radiographs.
- Name the eight annual tests recommended for x-ray equipment.
- Describe the components of a quality assurance program.
- Describe quality control tests for processing solutions.
- Explain the use of a stepwedge.
- Discuss the purpose of a reference radiograph.
- Explain the infection-control requirements for preparing a radiography operatory.
- Implement the CDC guidelines for infection control in dental radiology.

As a dental assistant, it is your responsibility to understand the laws that apply to you when you are exposing dental radiographs.

Federal and state regulations control the use of dental radiographic equipment. Individual state requirements also determine the educational qualifications of dental personnel who expose dental radiographs.

To ensure the highest quality for radiographs and the least risk for exposure to patients and personnel, a *quality assurance program* is necessary. **Quality assurance** means regular testing to detect equipment malfunctions, planned monitoring, and scheduled maintenance. Regular testing of equipment also helps to ensure compliance with state and federal regulations.

When radiographs are taken, there is always the potential to cross-contaminate equipment and environmental surfaces if good infection control is not practiced.

In this chapter you will learn the details and the step-by-step infection-control procedures necessary in dental radiography. Refer to Part 4 for a detailed discussion of disinfection, sterilization, and other general infection-control measures.

LEGAL CONSIDERATIONS

There are three major categories of legal considerations regarding the use of radiographs in dentistry: (1) federal and state *regulations* regarding x-ray equipment and its use, (2) *licensure* for individuals exposing radiographs, and (3) *risk management* for avoiding potential lawsuits.

Federal and State Regulations

The use of dental radiograph equipment is regulated by both *federal* and *state* regulations. All dental x-ray machines manufactured or sold in the United States after 1974 must meet federal regulations. These include safety specifications for minimum filtration and accuracy of the milliamperage, time, and kilovoltage settings.

All x-ray equipment is also subject to state, county, or city radiation health codes. These codes may include regulations concerning barriers, film speeds, position of the operator, and film processing. Many states require x-ray machines to be registered and charge a fee for this registration. In addition, most states have laws that require inspections of dental x-ray equipment on a regular basis, such as every 5 years. Be certain that you understand the requirements in your area.

Licensure Requirements

The Consumer-Patient Radiation Health and Safety Act is a federal law that requires all persons who take dental radiographs to be properly trained and certified. It is then up to the individual state to determine the policy regarding training and certification of individuals exposing radiographs.

Thus requirements for certification in radiography for dental assistants vary from state to state. Some states require Dental Assisting National Board (DANB) certification, and other states may require an additional examination. Because each state deals with dental radiography differently, it is your responsibility to become informed about the specific requirements in your particular state.

Recall

1. What federal act requires persons who take radiographs to be trained and certified?

Risk Management

Risk management involves following policies and procedures that will reduce the chance of a malpractice lawsuit against the dentist. Key areas of risk management include *patient consent, patient records, liability issues,* and *patient education,* as discussed in the following sections.

In today's society, people tend to file more malpractice lawsuits than in the past. Thus the dental assistant should always practice risk management. For example, the assistant must be careful not to make casual negative comments about the radiograph equipment or its operation. Statements made without thinking, such as "The timer must be off," "This thing never works right," or "The solutions are weak," are unnecessary and can make the patient feel uncomfortable. Remember, statements made by anyone at the time of an alleged negligent act are admissible as evidence in court.

Informed Consent

It is the dentist's responsibility to discuss the need for radiographs and treatment procedures with the patient, but the dental assistant may participate in the process of obtaining **informed consent.** Patients must give their informed consent for dental radiographs in addition to other procedures. In order for patients to give informed consent, they must be provided with the following information in *lay terms:*

1. Risks and benefits of radiographic procedures
2. Person who will be exposing the radiographs
3. Number and type of radiographs that will be taken
4. Consequences of not having the radiographs
5. Alternative diagnostic aids that may provide the same information as the radiographs

The process of informing the patient about the nature and purpose of dental radiographs is termed **disclosure.** After disclosure the patient may give informed consent or may refuse the radiographs. If the dentist has *not* obtained informed consent from a patient before exposure of dental radiographs, a patient may legally claim malpractice or negligence.

Liability

Under state laws the supervising dentist is legally responsible, or **liable,** for the actions of the dental auxiliary personnel. Known as the *respondeat superior* doctrine, this means that the employer is responsible for the actions of the employee.

Even though dental assistants work under the supervision of a licensed dentist, they can still be held legally liable for their *own* actions. Most often the dentist is the only person sued for negligence or malpractice, but in some cases the dentist and the dental assistant have been sued for the actions of the dental assistant. You must be aware of the laws in your state and practice accordingly.

Patient Records

Dental radiographs are a part of the patient's dental record and are considered to be a legal document. The dental record must accurately reflect all aspects of patient care. Documentation of dental radiographs must include the following information:

1. Informed consent
2. Number and type of radiographs exposed
3. Rationale for exposing the radiographs
4. Diagnostic interpretation

It is important to document the exposure of dental radiographs. The number of films exposed and the quality of the radiographs may be important issues in a malpractice suit. If poor-quality radiographs are used in court, it reflects poorly on the dentist.

Ownership of Dental Radiographs

Radiographs are the property of the dentist, even though the patient or the patient's insurance company paid for them, because dental radiographs are a part of the patient's *dental records.*

However, patients have a right to reasonable access to their records. When patients transfer to another dentist, it is reasonable to have a copy of their records, including x-rays, forwarded to the new dentist. Patients may request a copy of their radiographs; this request should be written and signed by the patient. The dentist should be informed of the patient's request and an entry made in the chart stating when and to whom the duplicate radiographs were sent. A reasonable fee may be charged for duplication. *Never* give or send the original radiographs to a patient. If a lawsuit should occur, there would be no defense without the radiographs.

Dental radiographs and other dental records should be retained indefinitely. Statute of limitation laws vary, and the question of when to destroy or discard a patient record may not always have a simple answer. Patient records must be stored carefully so that they do not become damaged.

Patient Refusal

On occasion, patients may refuse dental radiographs. This refusal presents a difficult situation because the dentist must decide whether an accurate diagnosis can be made without radiographs and whether treatment can be provided. In most cases a lack of radiographs compromises the patient's diagnosis and treatment. The use of dental radiographs is now the accepted *standard of care.*

Every effort should be made to educate the patient about the importance of dental radiographs. No document can be signed that totally releases the dentist from liability for treating a patient without taking radiographs. Even if the patient suggests signing a release or waiver that would release the dentist from liability, such a document would be considered invalid if an injury were to result. Legally, a patient cannot consent to negligent care. It should be recorded in the patient's record if a patient refuses recommended radiographs. The dentist must then make the decision as to whether to proceed without radiographs or not.

Patient Education

As a dental assistant, you should understand and be sensitive to the patient's concern and fears about exposure to radiation during dental radiographs. The patient often feels more comfortable confiding these fears to the dental assistant rather than to the dentist.

The dental assistant can explain to the patient the importance of radiographs in detecting diseases and planning treatment. The dental assistant can inform patients of the federal and state laws enacted for their protection. In addition, you can give patients educational materials on the subject (e.g., American Dental Association pamphlets, such as *Dental Radiograph Examinations, Your Dentist's Advice,* and *The Benefits of Radiograph Examinations,* or the U.S. Food and Drug Administration's *Radiographs: Get the Picture on Protection*). These educational materials can also be placed in the reception room. Furthermore, the dental assistant can remind patients that the dose from four bitewing films is about the same as 1 day's worth of natural background radiation.

Recall

2. What type of consent is necessary before exposing radiographs on a patient?
3. Under state laws, who is allowed to prescribe dental radiographs?
4. Who legally owns a patient's dental radiographs?

QUALITY ASSURANCE IN THE DENTAL OFFICE

Quality assurance (QA) is a way of ensuring that everything possible is being done to produce high-quality diagnostic radiographs. QA includes *quality control tests* that monitor dental radiograph equipment, supplies, and film processing. It also involves *quality administration procedures* that include keeping schedules of maintenance and record-keeping logs.

The benefits of a QA program far outweigh the time, effort, and costs. Fewer retakes mean time and cost savings for both patients and operators.

Quality Control Tests

Quality control tests are specific tests used to monitor dental x-ray equipment, supplies, and film processing. The American Academy of Dental Radiology recommends a number of annual tests for dental radiograph machines. These tests are designed to identify minor malfunctions, including (1) variations in the radiation output, (2) inadequate collimation, (3) tubehead drifting, (4) errors in the timer, and (5) inaccurate kilovoltage and milliamperage readings.

Types of Quality Control Tests

Dental radiograph film: Test each new box for freshness.
Dental x-ray machine: Calibrate equipment regularly.
Cassettes and screens: Clean and examine for scratches.
Safelighting: Check for light tightness.
Automatic processor: Follow manufacturer's recommendations meticulously regarding maintenance.
Manual processor: Replenish daily and change every 3 to 4 weeks.

X-Ray Machine Quality Control Steps

1. Test output of radiographs.
2. Test size of focal spot.
3. Test tubehead for stability.
4. Test timer for accuracy.
5. Test milliamperage.
6. Test kilovoltage.

Dental X-Ray Machines

Regulations require that dental x-ray machines be inspected periodically. Some state and local regulatory agencies provide inspections of dental x-ray equipment without charge as part of their registration and licensing procedures. Dental x-ray machines must also be *calibrated,* or adjusted for accuracy, at regular intervals. A qualified technician must check the x-ray machine performance and perform the calibration of dental x-ray equipment.

The dentist, the dental assistant, or the manufacturer's service representative can perform annual tests for dental x-ray machines. The tests are easy to perform and require only basic test materials and test logs to record the results. You can obtain a free pamphlet called *Quality Control Tests for Dentistry* from Eastman Kodak (Rochester, NY). This easy-to-follow pamphlet describes step-by-step procedures for performing each of the tests.

Dental X-Ray Film

You should check each box of film while opening it. Even though the film may not be expired, the box may have been improperly stored before reaching your office. Follow these easy steps to test the film for freshness:

1. In the darkroom, unwrap one unexposed film from the newly opened box.
2. Process the film using fresh chemicals.
3. Check the results.

a. If the processed film appears clean with a slight blue tint, the film is fresh and has been properly stored and handled. This film is safe for use.
b. If the processed film appears fogged, the film has been improperly stored or exposed to radiation. This film must not be used.

Screens and Cassettes

The intensifying screens inside the extraoral cassette should be periodically checked for dirt and scratches. Screens should be cleaned monthly with a commercially available cleaner. After cleaning, an antistatic solution should be applied to the screen to prevent static electricity affecting the film quality. Screens that appear visibly scratched should be replaced.

Cassettes should be checked for worn closures, light leaks, and warping, which may result in fogged and blurred radiographs; these cassettes must be repaired or replaced. Follow these easy steps to test the cassette for adequate film-screen contact:

1. In the darkroom, insert one film between the screens in the cassette.
2. Place a wire mesh test object on top of the loaded cassette.
3. Using a 40-inch target-film distance, direct the central ray perpendicular to the cassette.
4. Expose the film using 10 mA, 70 kVp, and 15 impulses.
5. Process the exposed film.
6. View the film on a viewbox in a dimly lit room at a distance of 6 feet.
7. Check the results.
   a. If the wire mesh image seen on the film exhibits a uniform density, good film-screen contact has taken place. The cassette and screen are safe to use.
   b. If the wire mesh image seen on the film exhibits varying densities, poor film-screen contact has taken place. Areas of poor film-screen contact appear darker than good contact areas. If the film-screen contact is poor, the cassette should be repaired or replaced.

Recall

5. What is meant by quality assurance?
6. What are quality control tests?

Viewboxes

A properly functioning **viewbox** is necessary for the interpretation of dental radiographs (Fig. 40-1). The viewbox contains fluorescent bulbs that emit light through an opaque plastic or Plexiglas front. The viewbox should emit a uniform and subdued light when functioning properly.

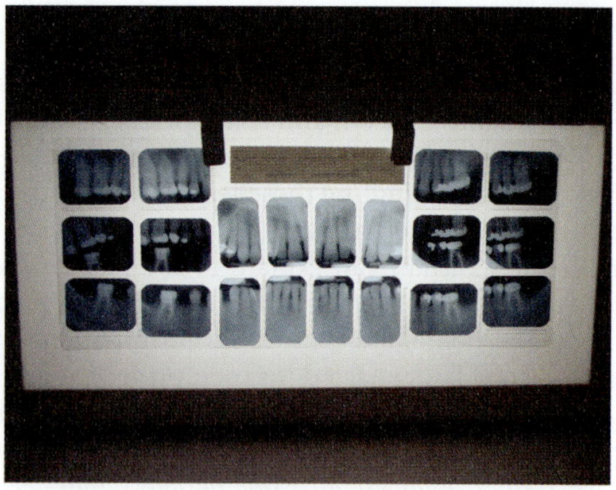

Fig. 40-1 Viewbox with clean Plexiglas and new bulb.

The viewbox should be periodically checked for dirt and discoloration of the Plexiglas surface. The surface of the viewbox should be wiped clean daily. Permanently discolored Plexiglas or blackened fluorescent bulbs must be replaced.

Darkroom Lighting

Check the darkroom for light leaks every 6 months. Follow these easy steps to test the darkroom for light leaks:

1. While standing in the darkroom, turn off all the lights, including the safelight.
2. Once your eyes become accustomed to the darkness, look around the room for any signs of white light. Check around the door, the seams on the walls and ceilings, the vent area, and the keyhole for light leaks.
3. Check the results.
   a. If the darkroom has no visible light leaks, the room is safe for processing films.
   b. If light leaks are present, they must be corrected with weather stripping or black electrical tape before proceeding with film processing.

Safelight test

The "light-tightness" of the darkroom must be confirmed before you can test the effectiveness of the safelight. Follow these easy steps for the *coin test* to check the safelight:

1. Turn off all the lights in the darkroom, including the safelight.
2. Unwrap one unexposed film. Place the film on a flat surface at least 4 feet away from the safelight. Place a coin on top of the film (Fig. 40-2, *A*).
3. Turn on the safelight. Allow the film and coin to be exposed to the safelight for 3 to 4 minutes.
4. Remove the coin and process the film as usual.
5. Check the results.
   a. If no image is visible on the film, the safelight is functioning and it is safe to process other films.

A

B

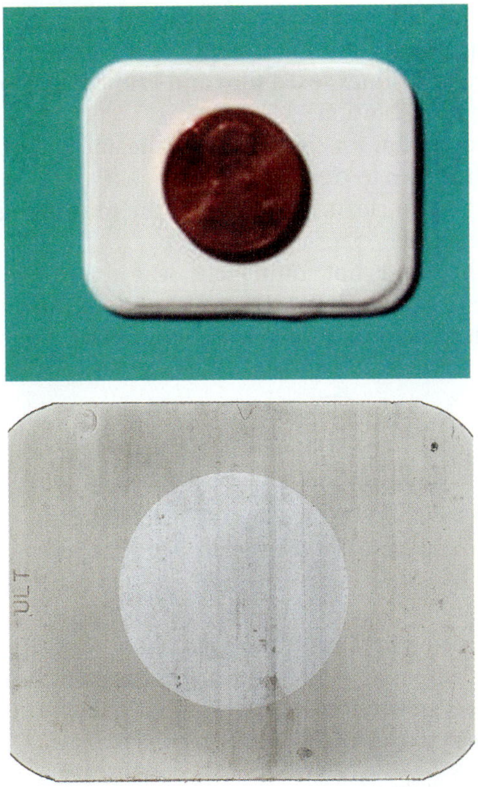

Fig. 40-2 **A,** Unexposed film with coin on it. **B,** Radiograph showing outline of coin.

b. If the image of the coin and a fogged background appear on the processed film, the safelight is not safe to use with that type of film (Fig. 40-2, *B*). Safelighting problems must be corrected before proceeding with film processing.

Film Processing

Perform quality control procedures routinely, because film processing is one of the most critical areas in a quality control program and must be monitored on a daily basis.

Manual processing

With the manual system, the thermometer and timer must be checked for accuracy. The temperature and levels of the water bath, developer, and fixer solutions must also be checked. Always strictly follow the processing time and temperature recommendations of the solution manufacturer.

Automatic processing

With automatic equipment, you must check the water circulation system, the solution levels, the replenishment system, and temperatures. Always follow the manufacturer's procedure and maintenance directions carefully. Each day, you should process two test films in the automatic processor. Follow these steps to verify the functioning of the automatic processor:

1. Unwrap two unexposed films; expose one to light.
2. Process both films in the automatic processor.
3. Check the results.
   a. If the unexposed film appears clear and dry and if the film exposed to light appears black and dry, the automatic processor is functioning properly.
   b. If the unexposed film does not appear clear and dry or if the exposed film does not appear completely black and dry, the automatic processor must be checked. Corrections must be made before processing patient films.

Processing solutions

The processing solutions are the most critical component in the quality control of film processing. As discussed in Chapter 39, you must replenish the processing solutions daily and change them every 3 to 4 weeks, as recommended by the manufacturer.

As an alternative to using the calendar to determine the freshness of solutions, you can use quality control tests to monitor the strength of the developer and fixer solutions. You should check the processing solutions each day *before* any patient films are processed.

Developer Strength. As the developer loses strength, the time-temperature chart is no longer accurate. An easy way to check the strength of the developer solution is to compare film densities against a standard. You can do this by using a reference radiograph or stepwedge radiograph.

Reference Radiograph. A reference radiograph is processed under ideal conditions and then used to compare the film densities of radiographs that are processed daily. Use the following steps to create a reference radiograph:

1. Expose fresh film, using correct exposure factors.
2. Process the film using fresh chemicals at the recommend time and temperature.
3. View the reference radiograph and the daily radiographs side by side on a viewbox.
4. Check the results.
   a. If the densities seen on the reference radiograph match the densities seen on the daily radiographs, the developer solution strength is adequate. You may process patient films.
   b. If the densities seen on the daily radiograph appear *lighter* than those seen on the reference film, the developer solution is either weak or cold.
   c. If the densities seen on the daily radiograph appear *darker* than those seen on the reference radiograph, the developer solution is either too concentrated or too warm.
   d. Weakened or concentrated developer solution must be replaced. If the developer solution is too warm or too cold, the temperature must be adjusted before processing patient films.

Stepwedge Radiograph. A **stepwedge** is a device constructed of layered aluminum steps. When a stepwedge is placed on top of a film and then exposed to radiographs, the different steps absorb varying amounts of radiation. When the film is processed, different densities are seen on the dental radiograph as a result of the stepwedge.

Use the following steps to create stepwedge radiographs:

1. Use a total of 20 fresh films (one for each work day in the month). Place an aluminum stepwedge on top of one film.
2. Expose the film. Then expose the remaining films using the same exposure factors.
3. Using fresh chemicals, process only *one* of the exposed films. This processed radiograph will exhibit different densities as a result of the stepwedge, and it becomes the *standard stepwedge radiograph.*
4. Store the remaining 19 exposed films in a cool dry area protected from x-radiation.
5. Each day, after the chemicals have been replenished, process one of the exposed stepwedge films.
6. Compare the *standard stepwedge radiograph* and the daily radiograph side by side on a viewbox. Compare the densities seen on the daily radiograph with the densities seen on the standard radiograph (Fig. 40-3).
7. Check the results.
   a. Use the middle density seen on the standard stepwedge radiograph for comparison. If the density seen on the standard radiograph matches the density seen on the daily radiograph, the developer solution strength is adequate for processing patient films.
   b. If the density on the daily radiograph differs from that on the standard stepwedge radiograph by more than two steps, the developer solution is depleted and must be changed before processing patient films.

Fixer Strength. When the fixer solution loses its strength, the film takes a longer time to "clear," or become transparent, in the unexposed areas. When the fixer is at full strength, a film should clear within 2 minutes. Follow these steps to monitor the strength of the fixer:

1. Unwrap one unexposed film and immediately place it in the fixer solution.
2. Check the film for clearing. Note the amount of time the film takes to clear.
   a. If the film clears in 2 minutes, the fixer strength is adequate.
   b. If the film is not completely clear in 3 to 4 minutes, the fixer is depleted. The fixer solution must be replaced before processing patient films.

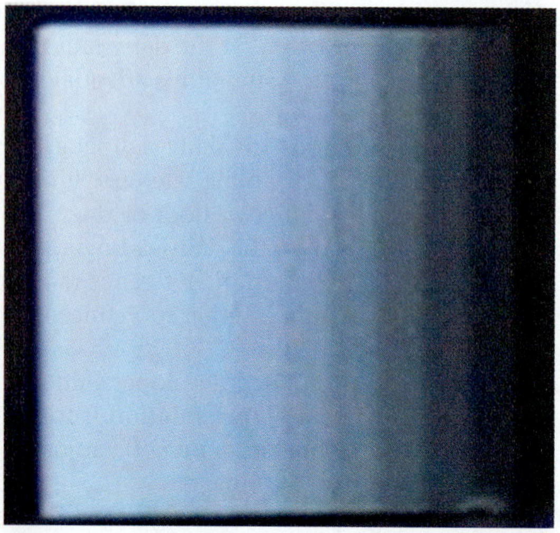

Fig. 40-3 Radiograph of a stepwedge.

Recall

7. When should you check a box of film for freshness?
8. Should you use a film cassette that has scratches?
9. What is one of the most critical areas in a quality control program?
10. What is the purpose of the coin test?
11. How often should processing solutions be replenished?
12. Why are the reference radiograph and stepwedge used?
13. How can you tell when the fixer loses its strength?

Quality Administration Procedures

Quality administration deals with the management of the QA program in the dental office. Although the dental assistant may be responsible for performing the quality control tests, the dentist is ultimately responsible for overall QA.

Description

A detailed, *written description* of the QA plan should be available to all staff members. Each staff member involved in the QA program must understand the quality standards as well as the importance of maintaining quality control of radiographic procedures.

Monitoring

A *written* monitoring schedule should be posted in the office. This schedule should describe all quality control tests and the frequency of testing for all dental radiograph equipment, supplies, and film processing.

Administrative Quality Control Steps

1. Develop and maintain a written description of the quality assurance plan.
2. Assign specific duties to staff members and ensure that each individual is thoroughly trained to perform those assigned duties.
3. Maintain records of monitoring and maintenance.
4. Review the plan periodically and revise it as necessary.

Maintenance

A *record-keeping log* of all quality control tests should be maintained and should include the specific test performed, date performed, and test results. A *processing solutions log* that lists the dates of solution replacement/replenishment and processor or tank cleaning should be kept as well.

Evaluation

A *written plan* for the periodic evaluation and revision of the existing QA program should also be a part of the quality administration plan.

Training

In-service training should be provided to all staff members to upgrade and improve their radiograph exposure techniques and processing procedures.

Recall

14. What is the purpose of a quality administration program?

15. Which staff members need to be aware of the quality administration program?

INFECTION CONTROL

Dental radiography presents unique infection-control problems because of the potential for cross-contamination of equipment and environmental surfaces with blood and saliva. Think of the many opportunities for cross-contamination in the procedure: you place the film into the mouth, then move to the exposure controls outside the operatory, and then return to remove the film from the mouth, and then walk to the processing area. Some dentists prefer that the patient remain in the x-ray room until the films are processed to determine the need for retakes; other dentists have the dental assistant dismiss the patient before the films are processed.

Centers for Disease Control and Prevention Guidelines

The Centers for Disease Control and Prevention (CDC) has recognized dental radiology as a potential source of cross-contamination and included recommendations for dental radiology in the *Guidelines for Infection Control in Dental Health-Care Settings—2003.*

Checklist for Infection Control in Dental Radiography

I. Before Exposure
- A. Treatment Area *(covered or disinfected)*
  1. X-ray machine
  2. Dental chair
  3. Work area
  4. Lead apron
- B. Equipment and Supplies *(prepared before seating patient)*
  1. Film
  2. Film-holding devices
  3. Cotton rolls
  4. Paper towel
  5. Disposable container
- C. Patient Preparation *(performed before putting on gloves)*
  1. Adjust chair.
  2. Adjust headrest.
  3. Place lead apron.
  4. Remove personal objects.
- D. Radiographer Preparation *(completed before exposure)*
  1. Wash hands.
  2. Put on gloves.
  3. Prepare film-holding devices.

II. During Exposure
- A. Film Handling
  1. Dry exposed film with paper towel.
  2. Place dried film in disposable container.
- B. Film-Holding Devices
  1. Transfer device from work area to mouth.
  2. Transfer device from mouth back to work area.

  Note: Do not place device on uncovered countertop.

III. After Exposure
- A. Before Glove Removal
  1. Dispose of all contaminated items.
  2. Place film-holding devices in designated area for contaminated equipment.
- B. After Glove Removal
  1. Wash hands.
  2. Remove lead apron.

Modified from Haring JI, Jansen L: *Dental radiography: principles and techniques,* ed 2, Philadelphia, 2000, Saunders.

The Radiography Operatory

The radiography operatory and darkroom are not usually associated with the spatter of blood or saliva. Transmission of infectious diseases is still possible, however, because the radiographic equipment, operatory surfaces, film holders, and film packets are contaminated.

CDC Guidelines for Dental Radiology

1. Wear gloves when exposing radiographs and handling contaminated film packets. Use other personal protective equipment (PPE) (e.g., protective eyewear, mask, and gown) as appropriate if spattering of blood or other body fluids is likely. (IA, IC)
2. Use heat-tolerant or disposable intraoral devices whenever possible (e.g., film holding and positioning devices). Clean and heat-sterilize heat-tolerant devices between patients. (IB)
3. Transport and handle exposed film in an aseptic manner to prevent contamination of the developing equipment. (II)
4. The following apply for digital radiography sensors:
   a. Use FDA-cleared barriers. (IB)
   b. Clean and heat-sterilize, or high-level–disinfect, between patients, barrier-protected semicritical items. If an item cannot tolerate these procedures, then, at a minimum, protect with an FDA-cleared barrier and clean and disinfect with an EPA-registered hospital disinfectant with intermediate-level (i.e., tuberculocidal claim) activity, between patients. Consult the manufacturer for methods of disinfection and sterilization of digital radiography sensors and for protection of associated computer hardware. (IB)

See Chapter 19 to review the CDC rankings.
Adapted from *Guidelines for Infection Control in Dental Health Care Settings–2003,* Department of Health & Human Services, Centers for Disease Control and Prevention, Atlanta, Ga.

Surfaces Likely to Be Contaminated During X-Ray Procedures

X-ray tubehead	Dental chair controls
PID	Operatory counter surfaces
X-ray control panel	Darkroom equipment
Exposure button	Sleeves on automatic processors
Lead apron	

Your first step in preparation of the operatory is to determine the surfaces to be covered or disinfected with a high-level surface disinfectant. In general, surfaces that cannot be easily cleaned and disinfected should be protected by *barriers,* usually plastic or foil. Surface barriers are preferred on electrical switches because of the possibility of the cleaner and disinfectant causing an electrical short (Fig. 40-4).

X-Ray Machine

The tubehead, position indicator device (PID), control panel, and exposure button must be covered or carefully disinfected (Fig. 40-5).

Lead Apron

The lead apron should be considered contaminated and wiped with a disinfectant after each use.

Dental Chair

The back and arms of the chair, the headrest, and the headrest adjustment controls must be covered or disinfected. Once the radiography operatory is set up, you can set up the film and film holders.

Work Area

The work area where the x-ray film and film holders are placed during exposure should be disinfected. Then a barrier, such as a paper sheet, paper towels, or plastic cover, should be placed (Fig. 40-6).

Once the procedure is completed, discard the barriers. If the counter surfaces are not protected by barriers, they should be cleaned and disinfected.

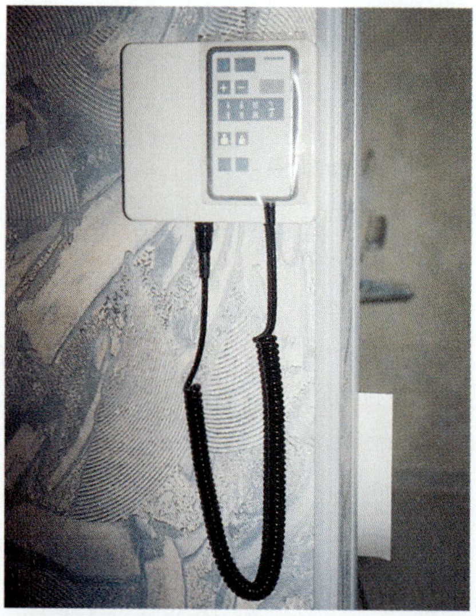

Fig. 40-4 X-ray equipment with barriers in place.

Equipment and Supplies

Before beginning the procedure, gather all necessary supplies to decrease the chance of cross-contamination. For example, think about the type of film-holding devices, cotton rolls, and bite-wing tabs that you may need.

Note: If you need additional supplies during the procedure, use overgloves (food handler's gloves) or ask for assistance.

Film

Dispense the film from a central area in a disposable container, such as a paper cup.

Film Packets

Once films are removed from the mouth, they are obviously contaminated and should only be handled with gloved hands. One technique to minimize contamination of the film packet by saliva is to place a clear-plastic barrier envelope over the film packet. Some films available commercially are enclosed in a clear-plastic barrier packet (Fig. 40-7). The barrier-protected film packets are exposed and brought to the processing area. The barriers are contaminated and must be removed carefully without touching the inner packet so that the packet can be handled with bare hands.

Film-Holding Devices (Film Holders)

Film-holding instruments and bite-blocks that are placed in the patient's mouth are *semicritical items* and should be sterilized before reuse. The alternative is to use disposable film holders and discard them after a single use.

Sterilized film-holding devices should remain packaged until the patient is seated and can view the opening of the package. Patients appreciate knowing that proper infection-control procedures are in place throughout the office.

Miscellaneous Items

Other supplies include cotton rolls that can be used to stabilize film placement and paper towels that can be used to wipe saliva from exposed films. A disposable container, such as a paper cup labeled with the patient's name, is also necessary to collect the exposed films. All miscellaneous items should be dispensed from a central supply area.

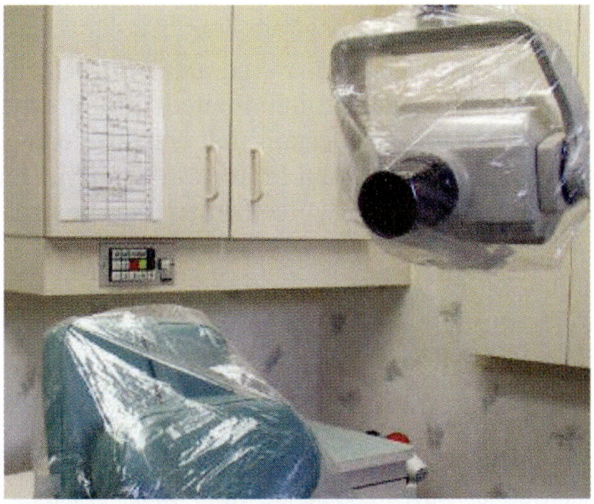

Fig. 40-5 Radiography operatory with barriers in place.

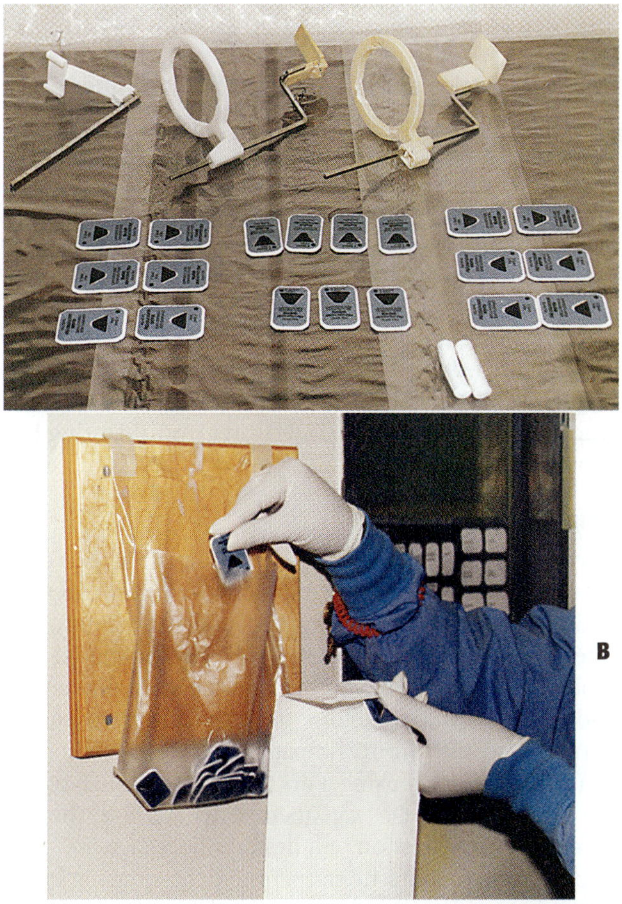

A

B

Fig. 40-6 **A,** Plastic surface barrier is placed over the work surface. **B,** After each exposure, the dental assistant wipes the film dry using a paper towel and then places the exposed film into a plastic bag that has been taped to the wall. (Courtesy University of California, School of Dentistry, Oral Radiology Department; photographs by Thomas Cao.)

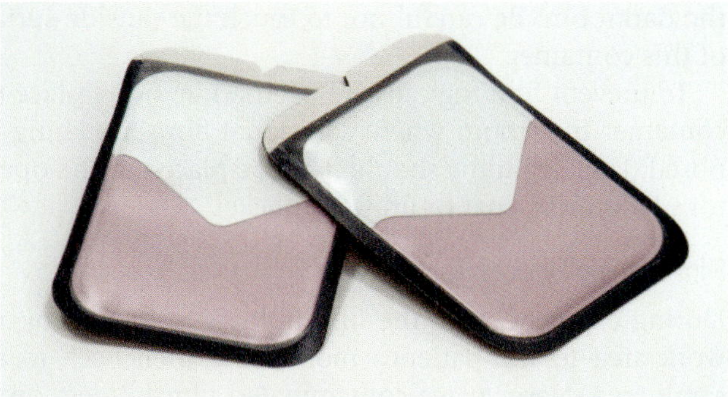

Fig. 40-7 Protective barrier on x-ray film.

Recall

16. What unique infection control problems occur in dental radiography?
17. What surfaces must be covered with barriers?
18. What precautions should be taken when handling contaminated film?
19. When should the packages containing the film-holding device be opened?

Procedures During and After X-Ray Film Exposure

Operator Preparation

Always wear gloves and protective clothing while exposing radiographs and handling the contaminated films (Fig. 40-8). You should also wear a mask and eyewear if there is likelihood of spattering of blood or other body fluids. Masks are also indicated if you or the patient has a cough or cold.

After putting on gloves, be careful not to touch any surfaces that are not covered. The best approach is to develop a sequence in which you touch as few surfaces as possible (Procedure 40-1: Practicing Infection Control During Film Exposure).

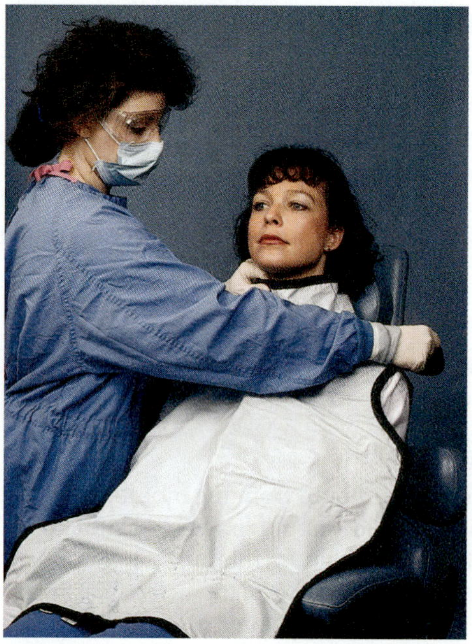

Fig. 40-8 While wearing the appropriate personal protection, the operator places the lead apron on the patient.

Drying of Exposed Film

The contaminated film packet is the major source of cross-contamination during radiographic procedures. When you remove the film packet from the patient's mouth, it is coated with saliva (or occasionally contaminated with blood). For this reason, you must *always* wear gloves while handling contaminated film packets. After you remove each exposed film from the patient's mouth, wipe saliva from the film packet using a dry 2- × 2-inch gauze sponge or a paper towel. Do *not* attempt to sterilize the film packet. Heat sterilization will destroy the image.

Some film manufacturers permit light spraying of the film packets with a disinfectant spray. However, immersion of the packet in a disinfecting solution can result in the solution's seeping into the emulsion and damaging the image.

Collection of Contaminated Films

Once the film is dried, place it in a disposable container (plastic bag or paper cup) that is labeled with the patient's name. This container will be used to transport the films to the darkroom. Be careful not to touch the outside surface of this container.

To prevent film fog caused by radiation, never place the container in a room where additional films are being exposed. Exposed films should *never* be placed in the operator's laboratory coat or uniform pocket.

Film-Holding Devices

During exposure, take the film holders from the covered work area to the patient's mouth and then back to the same area. Never place contaminated film holders on an uncovered surface.

Disposal of Contaminated Items

When you finish all the exposures, all contaminated items must be discarded and any uncovered surfaces must be disinfected. Handle contaminated radiography items in the same manner as other contaminated dental instruments. You must wear gloves while disposing of contaminated items, including the disposable surface coverings. All covered surfaces should be carefully uncovered; the actual surfaces should not be touched by gloved hands.

While wearing gloves, remove the contaminated film holder from the treatment area and place it in the area designated for contaminated instruments.

Handwashing

After removal and disposal of all contaminated items, remove your gloves and wash your hands.

Surface Disinfection

Clean and disinfect any uncovered areas in the radiography operatory that were contaminated during exposure; use a hospital-grade disinfectant that is registered and approved by the Environmental Protection Agency (EPA). Be sure to wear utility gloves while disinfecting the surfaces.

Recall

20. What PPE should the operator wear while exposing radiographs?
21. What type of gloves should be worn while disinfecting the radiography operatory?

Procedure 40-1 Practicing Infection Control During Film Exposure

Goal

To perform all infection control practices during film exposure.

Equipment and Supplies

- Barriers for the operatory
- Paper towels
- Radiograph film (sizes as necessary)
- Packaged film-holding device
- Film barriers *(optional)*
- Lead apron with thyroid collar
- Disposable container for exposed films (labeled with patient's name)
- Surface cleaner or disinfectant

PROCEDURAL STEPS

1. Wash and dry hands.
2. Place surface barriers on equipment and work area.

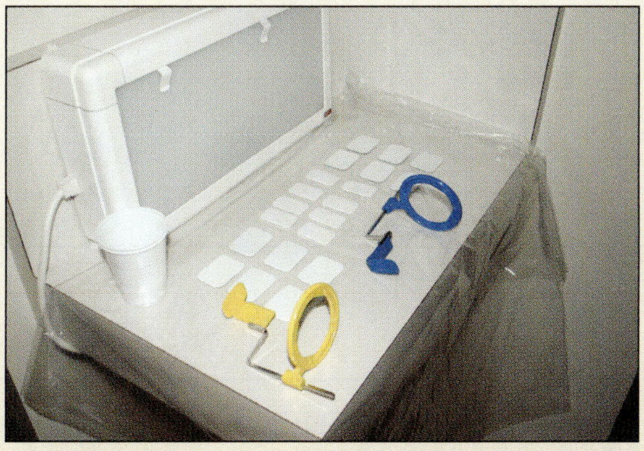

3. Set out the packaged film-holding device, film, labeled container for exposed film, paper towel, and other miscellaneous items you might need.

   Purpose: Once gloved, you should not have to leave the operatory area for additional materials.

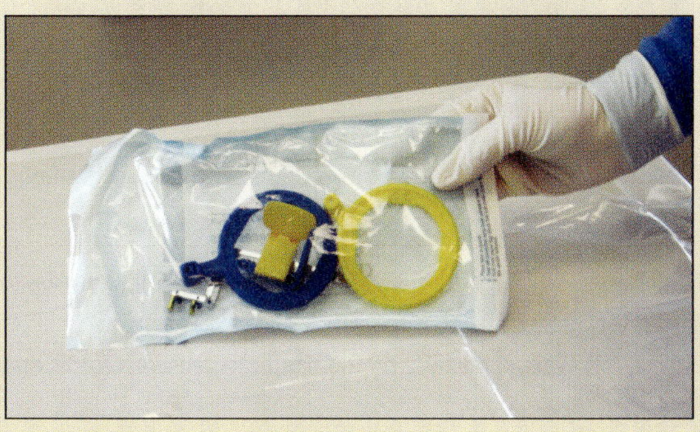

4. Seat the patient and place the lead apron.
5. Wash and dry hands and don gloves.
6. After each exposure, wipe the excess saliva from the film using a paper towel.
7. Place each exposed film into the container, being careful not to touch the external surface.

   Purpose: Your contaminated gloves will contaminate the outer surface of the container.

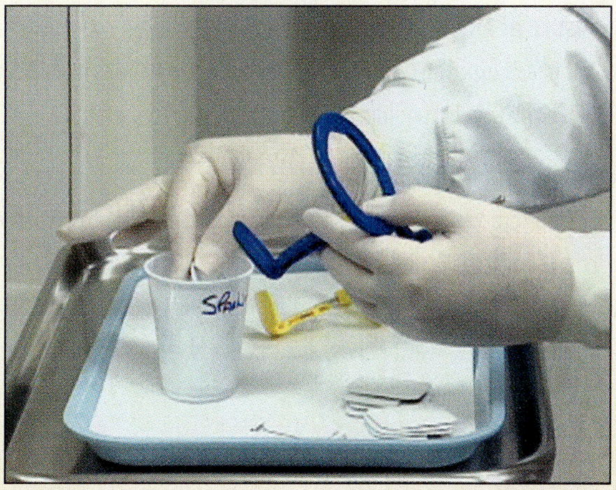

8. After the exposures are complete, remove the lead apron and dismiss the patient.

   Note: To remove the lead apron and still maintain aseptic technique, you can wear overgloves to remove the apron, or you can take off your gloves and remove the apron barehanded. If you remove the lead apron while gloved, you must disinfect the lead apron.
9. While still gloved, remove barriers, taking care not to touch the surfaces underneath.

   Purpose: You must wear gloves while removing barriers, because they are contaminated. If you touch a surface underneath the barrier while you are removing it, that surface will become contaminated and must then be disinfected.
10. Dispose of barriers and paper towels.
11. Place the film-holding device on a tray to be returned to the instrument processing area.
12. Wash and dry hands.
13. Take the exposed films to the processing area.

Infection Control Steps in Dental Radiography

Treatment Area

1. Place barriers or disinfect the x-ray machine, dental chair, work area, and lead apron.
2. Before seating the patient, gather film, film holders, cotton rolls, paper towels, and disposable cup.

Preparation of Patient and Operator

1. Before gloving, seat the patient and adjust the chair and headrest. Ask the patient to remove objects from the face and mouth. Place the lead apron.
2. Wash hands, put on gloves, and assemble film-holding devices.

Exposure of Films

1. After each exposure, dry the film and place it in the disposable cup.
2. Never place a film-holding device on uncovered surfaces.

After Exposure of Films

1. Before removing gloves, dispose of contaminated items (such as cotton rolls).
2. Place film-holding device in area for contaminated instruments.
3. Remove gloves, wash hands, and remove the lead apron.

Procedures During X-Ray Film Processing

After the films have been exposed, specific infection-control procedures must be followed during transport of the films to the darkroom, during film handling, and during automatic and manual film processing.

Transporting Film

You should never touch the disposable container with your gloved hands. Only after your gloves have been removed, your hands washed and dried, the patient dismissed, and the area cleaned and disinfected should you carry the container with contaminated films to the darkroom.

Procedures 40-2 and 40-3 review infection-control steps to follow in the darkroom and when using daylight film loaders.

Recall

22. What precautions must be taken when transporting films to the darkroom?

Procedure 40-2 Practicing Infection Control in the Darkroom

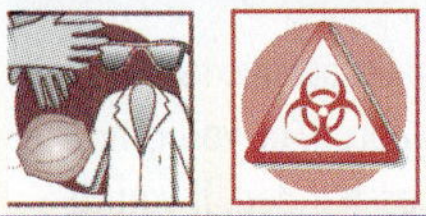

Goal

To practice infection-control measures when in the darkroom.

Equipment and Supplies

- Paper towels
- Clean gloves
- Clean paper cup
- Container for lead foil

PROCEDURAL STEPS

1. Place a paper towel and a clean cup on the counter near the processor.
   Purpose: The paper towel provides a barrier for the work surface, and the cup is used to discard the opened film packets.

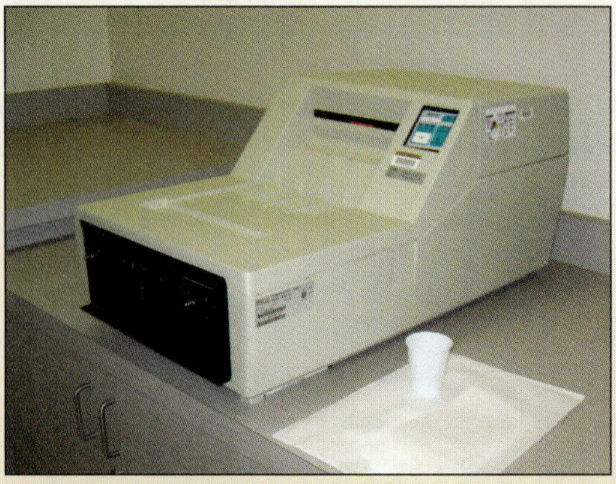

2. Wash hands and put on a new pair of gloves, preferably the type that does not contain powder.
   Purpose: Powder remaining on the hand can cause **artifacts** on the exposed film.

Procedure 40-2 Practicing Infection Control in the Darkroom—cont'd

3. Turn on the safety light; then turn off the white light. Open the film packets and allow each exposed film to drop onto the paper towel. Be careful that the unwrapped films do not come into contact with the gloves.
   Purpose: The film must remain free from contamination. A contaminated film may remain contaminated even after processing.

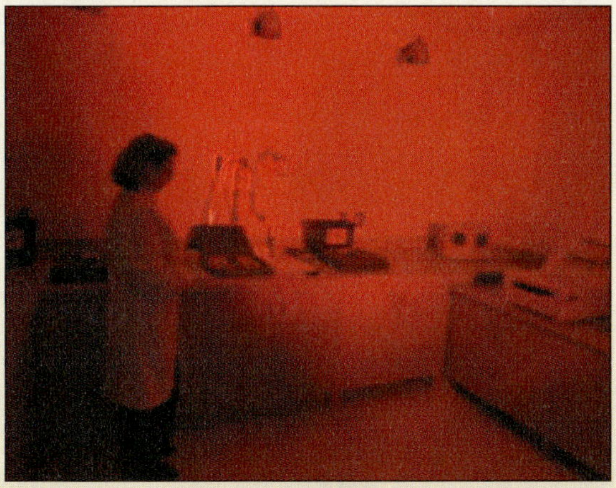

4. Remove the lead foil from the packet and place into the foil recycling container.
   Purpose: Lead foil is considered an environmental hazard and should not be discarded with the general waste.
5. Place the empty film packets into the clean cup.
6. Discard the cup. Remove your gloves by turning them inside out; then discard them.
7. Place the films into the processor or on developing racks with bare hands.

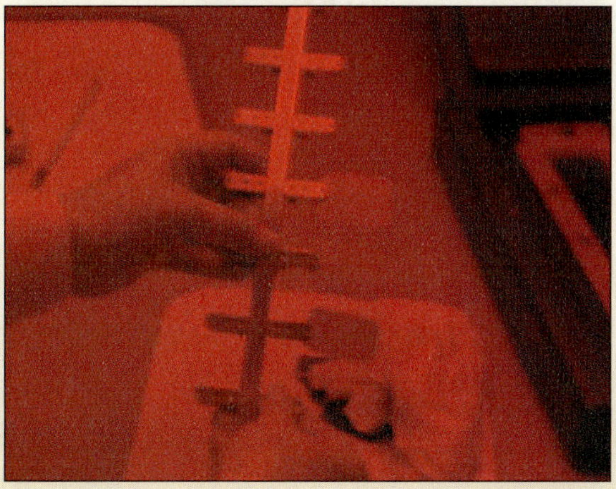

Note: If you used films with plastic barriers, you would have already removed the protective barrier in the operatory with gloved hands. You would then open the packets with your bare hands and feed the films into the processor.

Procedure 40-3 Practicing Infection Control with Use of Daylight Loader

Goal

To practice infection-control measures when using the daylight loader in processing dental radiograph films.

Equipment and Supplies

- Paper towels
- Clean gloves
- Clean cup
- Container for lead foil

PROCEDURAL STEPS

1. Wash and dry your hands; then place a paper towel or piece of plastic as a barrier to cover the bottom of the daylight loader.

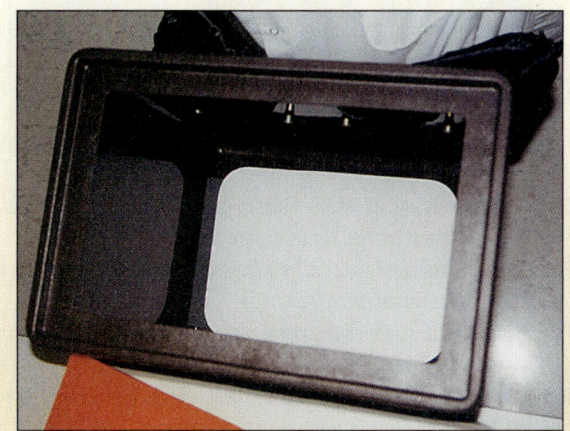

continued

Procedure 40-3 Practicing Infection Control with Use of Daylight Loader–cont'd

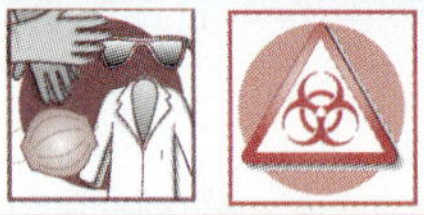

2. Place the following into the bottom of the daylight loader: the cup containing the contaminated film, a clean pair of gloves, and a second empty paper cup. Then close the top.

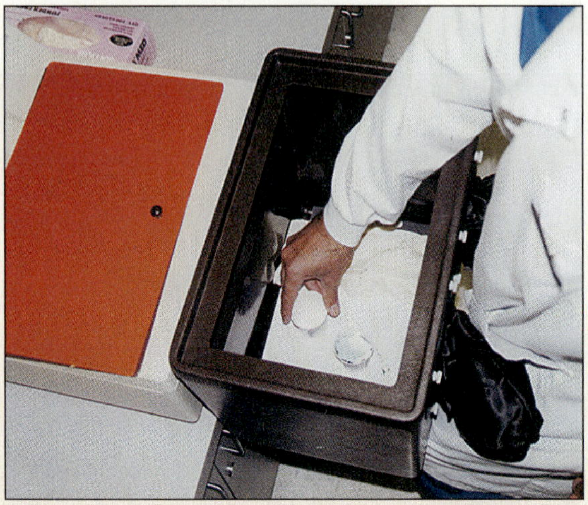

3. Put your clean hands through the sleeves of the daylight loader; then put on the gloves.
   Purpose: Clean hands prevent contamination of the sleeves. Contaminated gloves should never be placed through the sleeves of the daylight loader.

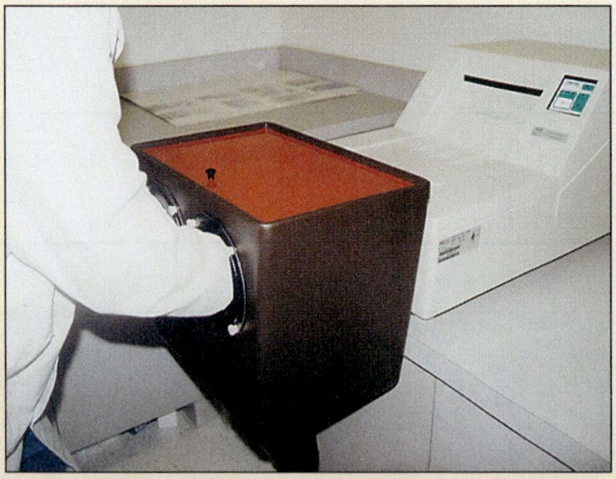

4. Open the packets and allow the films to drop onto the clean barrier.
   Purpose: The clean barrier keeps dust or powder from the film.
5. Place the contaminated packets into the second cup, and place the lead foil into the foil container.
   Purpose: The cup confines the contaminated film packets and makes disposal easier.
6. After you open the last packet, remove your gloves by turning them inside out. Insert the films into the developing slots.
   Purpose: The film remains uncontaminated and eliminates the question of whether organisms can survive in the solutions.

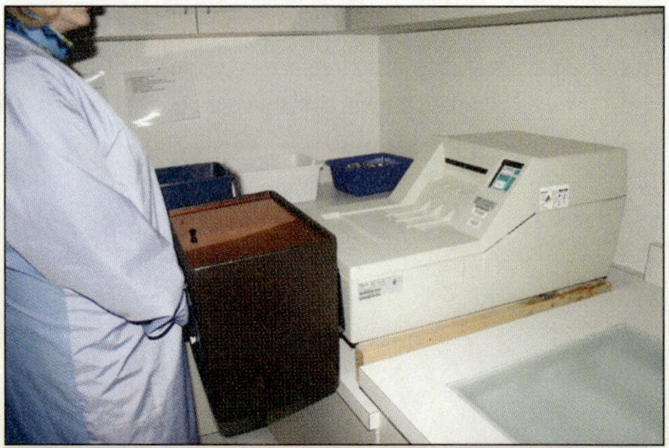

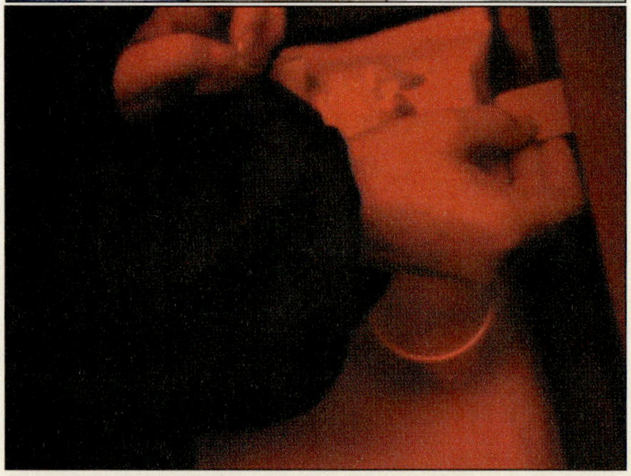

7. After you insert the last film, pull your ungloved hands through the sleeves.
8. Open the top of the loader; then carefully pull the ends of the barrier over the paper cup and used gloves and discard.

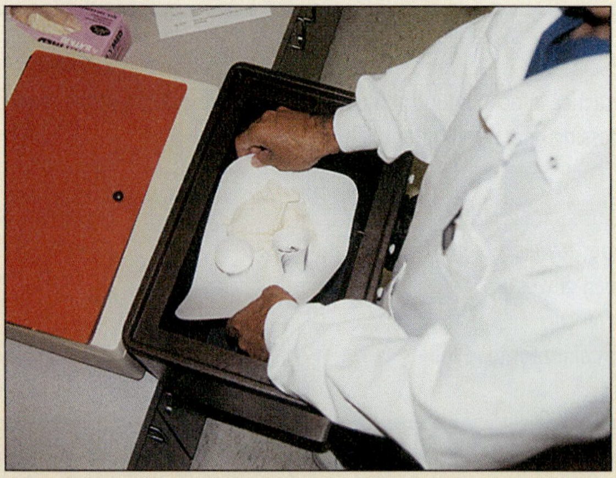

Note: Be careful not to touch the contaminated parts of the barrier with your bare hands.

Legal and Ethical Implications

Dental malpractice results when the dental practitioner is negligent in the delivery of dental care. Because dental radiographs are an essential part of diagnosis and treatment planning, negligence may result from radiograph-related action or inaction of the dental practitioner. For example, a patient of Dr. Daniels refused x-rays, and Dr. Daniels decided to treat the patient anyway. Later, the patient developed an abscess, resulting from undetected caries under a filling. Dr. Daniels could be held liable in this case, because she should not have treated the patient without radiographs. Treating a patient without the diagnostic aid of radiographic examination may result in significant harm to a patient. Harm for which the dentist could be held liable may include stress, embarrassment, loss of income, and expenses incurred in seeking additional treatment.

Eye to the Future

The Internet and World Wide Web have changed the way information is communicated. Patients are exposed to increasing amounts and sources of information, and many patients have heard or read about the harmful effects of radiation. Media coverage often highlights the dangers of radiation and casts doubt on the benefits of dental radiographs. Such reports are misleading and often poorly researched. Many times, these reports cause patients to avoid or refuse radiographs out of a fear of exposure to x-radiation.

As new information becomes available and with improved communications, the dental assistant must continue to educate patients now and in the future about the importance, benefits, and relative safety of dental radiographs.

Critical Thinking

1. You are the person in your office assigned the responsibility of replenishing and maintaining the radiograph solutions. What tasks will you have to perform, and how often will you need to do them?
2. You are using a stepwedge film to evaluate the quality of the developer solution. You notice that the middle density on the daily film is much lighter than the middle density on the stepwedge film. What is the problem, and how do you solve it?
3. Mrs. Colton, a patient in your office, stops by one morning and asks to pick up her radiographs because she is moving to another city. Kathy, the receptionist, explains to Mrs. Colton that her films need to be duplicated, which will take some time. Mrs. Colton becomes angry and wants her films immediately, saying, "Those radiographs belong to me. I paid for them, and I want them." What should Kathy tell Mrs. Colton?

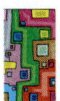

41

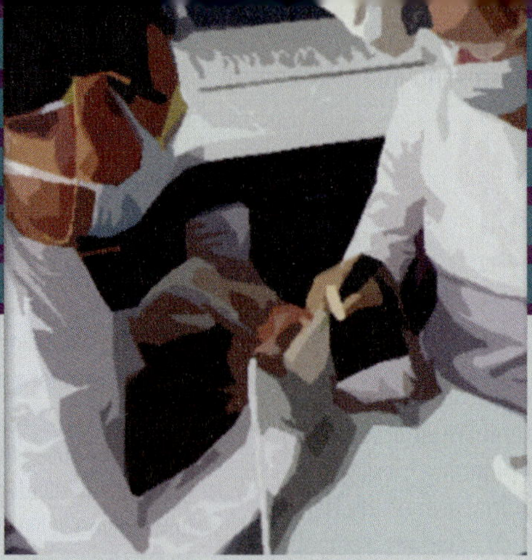

Intraoral Radiography

Outline

KEY TERMS

Angulation Alignment of central ray of x-ray beam in horizontal and vertical planes.

Bisecting (bisection of the angle) **technique** Intraoral technique of exposing periapical films.

Bite-wing film Type of radiograph used in the interproximal examination.

Central ray X-ray at center of beam.

Contact area Area of the mesial or distal surfaces of a tooth that touches adjacent tooth in the same arch.

Crestal bone Coronal portion of alveolar bone found between the teeth.

Developmental disability Impairment of mental or physical functioning that usually appears before adulthood and lasts indefinitely.

Diagnostic quality Referring to radiographs with the proper images and necessary density, contrast, definition, and detail for diagnostic purposes.

Interproximal Between two adjacent surfaces.

Intersecting Cutting across or through.

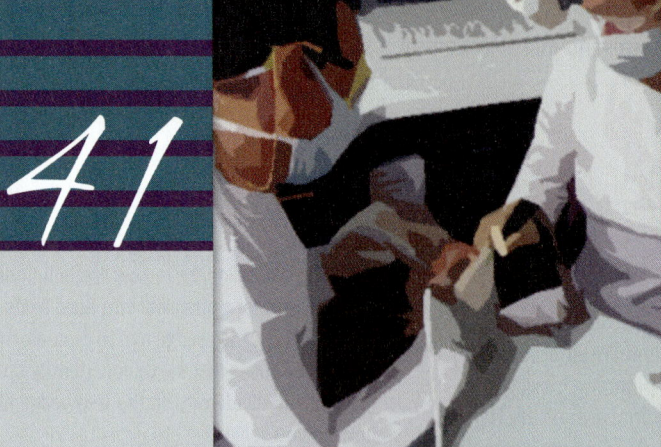

KEY TERMS, cont'd

Long axis of the tooth Imaginary line dividing the tooth longitudinally (vertically) into two equal halves.

Occlusal technique Used to examine large areas of the upper or lower jaw.

Parallel Moving or lying in the same plane, always separated by the same distance.

Paralleling technique Intraoral technique of exposing periapical films.

Perpendicular Intersecting at or forming a right angle.

Physical disability Impairment in certain function(s) of the body, such as vision, hearing, or mobility.

Right angle Angle of 90 degrees formed by two lines perpendicular to each other.

LEARNING OUTCOMES

On completion of this chapter, the student will be able to achieve the following objectives:

- Pronounce, define, and spell the Key Terms.
- Describe how to prepare a patient for dental x-rays.
- Name the two primary types of projections used in an intraoral technique and describe the differences.
- Explain the advantages and disadvantages of the paralleling and bisecting techniques.
- Explain the basic principle of the paralleling technique.
- Explain why a film holder is necessary with the paralleling technique.
- State the five basic rules of the paralleling technique.
- Label and identify the parts of the Rinn XCP instruments.
- Explain the recommended vertical angulation for all bite-wing exposures.
- Explain the basic rules for the bite-wing technique.
- Describe the appearance of opened and overlapped contact areas on a dental radiograph.
- Explain the procedural principles of the bisecting technique.
- Identify the film size used in the bisecting technique.
- Describe the correct vertical angulation.
- Describe incorrect vertical angulation.
- Identify the types of film holders that can be used with the bisecting technique.
- Explain the technique for exposing occlusal radiographs.
- Describe techniques for managing the patient with a hypersensitive gag reflex.
- Describe techniques for managing patients with physical and mental disabilities.

PERFORMANCE OUTCOMES

On completion of this chapter, the student will be able to meet competency standards in the following skills:

- Mount and label a full series of dental radiographs.
- Expose a full series of radiographs using the bisecting angle technique.
- Expose a full series of radiographs using the paralleling technique.
- Expose and mount a series of bite-wing radiographs.
- Expose a maxillary and mandibular occlusal radiograph.

It is possible for every dental assistant to be successful in producing quality dental radiographs—radiographs that are free from distortion, have the correct density and contrast, and can be used for the detection of dental disease. You can create such radiographs by carefully following the steps in *film placement, exposure,* and *processing* (Fig. 41-1).

Your patients will come in a variety of sizes, physical and mental abilities, types of dentitions, and personalities. Often you will take x-rays on patients with special needs. For example, you will explain x-rays to a 6-year-old patient differently than to an adult. Also, your technique will vary if the patient has a palate that is very high and narrow. This chapter provides guidelines about various situations you are likely to encounter in your career.

Even the most skilled operators can make errors; the ability to recognize the errors and know the steps to take to prevent their recurrence is most important. This chapter explains common technique errors and how to prevent them. In addition, you will learn to recognize and use normal anatomic landmarks in mounting radiographs.

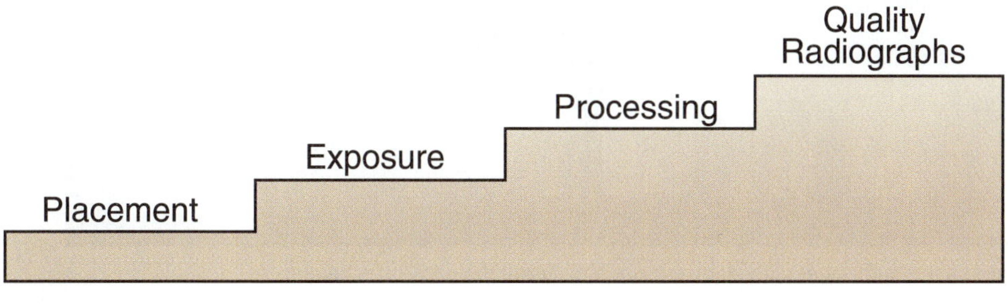

Fig. 41-1 Steps to quality radiographs.

FULL-MOUTH SURVEY

No dental examination can be complete without dental radiographs, and in almost all cases, the full mouth survey is the preferred technique.

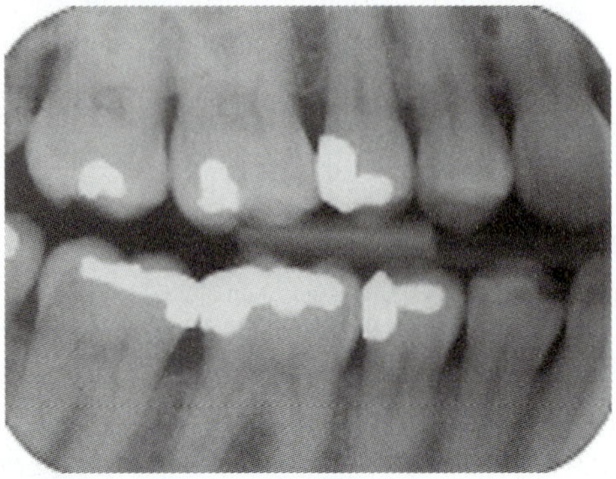

Fig. 41-2 Bite-wing radiograph. Note that only the crowns and alveolar ridge are visible, but not the roots.

An intraoral *full-mouth survey (FMX)* contains both *periapical* and *bite-wing* radiographs. The bite-wing radiograph shows the upper and lower teeth in occlusion. Only the crowns and a small portion of the root are seen. This radiograph is used for detecting **interproximal** decay, periodontal disease, recurrent decay under restorations, and the fit of metallic fillings or crowns (Fig. 41-2). The periapical radiograph shows the entire tooth from occlusal surface or incisal edge to about 2 to 3 mm beyond the apex to show the periapical bone. This radiograph is used to diagnose pathologic conditions of the tooth, root, and bone, as well as tooth formation and eruption (Fig. 41-3, *A* and *B*). Periapicals are essential in endodontics and oral surgical procedures.

For the average adult, a full-mouth series consists of 18 to 20 films, generally 14 periapical projections and four to six bite-wing views. The number may vary, however, depending on the dentist's preference and the number of teeth present. For example, in the patient without teeth, 14 periapical views are enough to cover the edentulous

A

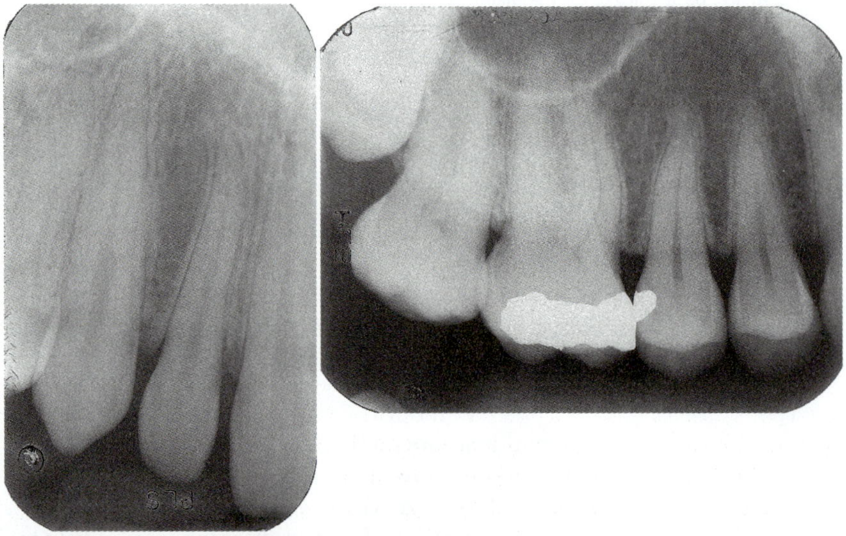

B

Fig. 41-3 **A**, Anterior periapical. **B,** Posterior periapical. Note that the entire tooth and surrounding bone are visible in the radiograph.

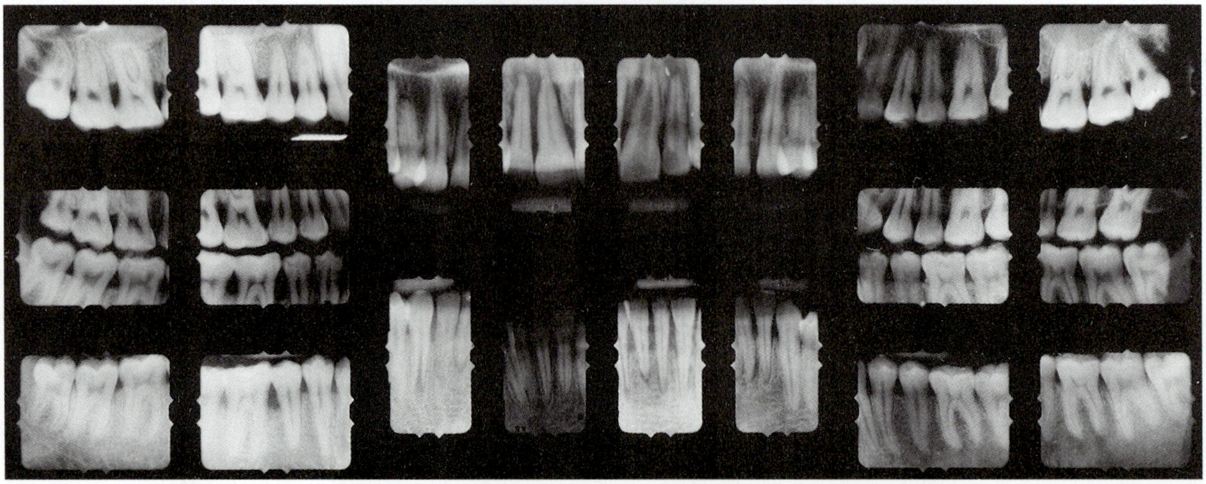

Fig. 41-4 Mounted full-mouth series with eight anterior films using the parallel technique.

arches; bite-wings are not necessary. For the patient with a full dentition, the number of periapical films varies depending on whether the paralleling or bisecting technique is used.

The *anterior* area is the region in which the number of films varies. The size of the film to be used depends on which technique you use. With the **bisecting technique,** three anterior films are taken on each arch (maxillary and mandibular) using size #2 film. For the **paralleling technique** you would use three or four size #1 films on each arch (Fig. 41-4).

Recall

1. What is the difference between a bite-wing and a periapical radiograph?
2. What are the two techniques for exposing radiographs?

INTRAORAL X-RAY TECHNIQUES

The two basic techniques for obtaining periapical x-rays are the paralleling technique and the bisecting *(bisection of the angle)* technique. The American Academy of Oral and Maxillofacial Radiology and the American Association of Dental Schools recommend the use of the *paralleling technique* because it provides the most accurate image with the least amount of radiation exposure to the patient. In some situations, however, such as a small mouth, shallow palate, or tori, the operator may need to use the bisecting technique. This chapter provides step-by-step procedures on how to produce diagnostic-quality radiographs using both techniques (Fig. 41-5).

PARALLELING TECHNIQUE

The paralleling technique is also known as the *extension-cone paralleling (XCP), right-angle,* or *long-cone* technique. To use the paralleling technique competently, you must understand the terminology, including **parallel** (Fig. 41-6), **intersecting, perpendicular, right angle, long axis of the tooth** (Fig. 41-7), and **central ray,** in addition to the five basic rules.

Five Basic Rules

The following basic rules *must* be followed when using the paralleling technique:

1. *Film placement.* The film must be positioned so that it will cover the correct teeth to be examined.
2. *Film position.* The film must be positioned parallel to the long axis of the tooth. The film, in the film holder, must be placed away from the teeth and toward the middle of the mouth (Fig. 41-8).
3. *Vertical angulation.* The central ray of the x-ray beam must be directed perpendicular (at a right angle) to the film and the long axis of the tooth.

Guidelines for Film Placement

1. The white side of the film always faces the teeth.
2. The anterior films are always placed vertically.
3. The posterior films are always placed horizontally.
4. The identification dot on the film is always placed in the slot of the film holder (dot in the slot).
5. The film holder is always positioned away from the teeth and toward the middle of the mouth.
6. The film is always centered over the areas to be examined.
7. The film is always placed parallel to the long axis of the teeth.

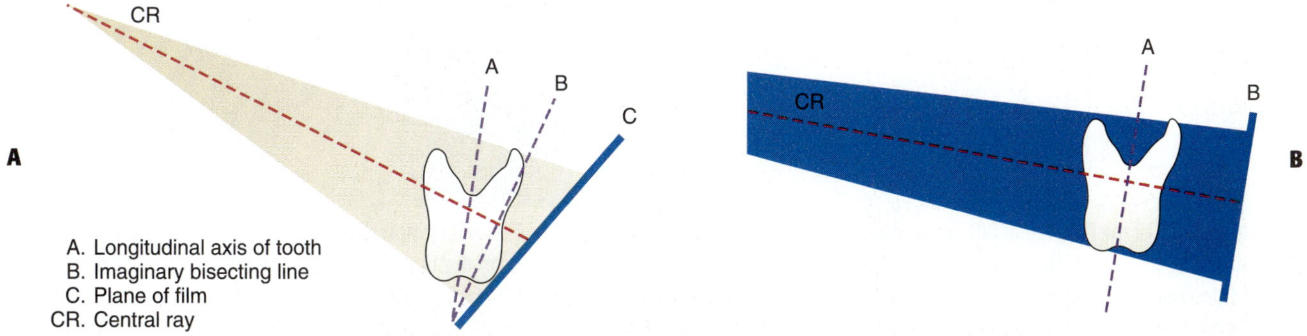

Fig. 41-5 Intraoral x-ray techniques. **A,** Bisecting angle technique. **B,** Paralleling technique.

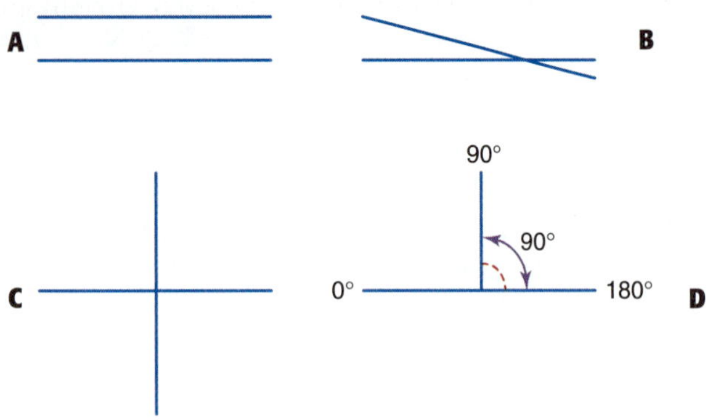

Fig. 41-6 **A,** Parallel lines are always separated by the same distance and do not intersect. **B,** Intersecting lines cross one another. **C,** Perpendicular lines intersect one another to form right angles. **D,** Right angle measures 90 degrees and is formed by two perpendicular lines. (From Haring JI, Jansen L: *Dental radiography: principles and techniques,* ed 2, Philadelphia, 2000, Saunders.)

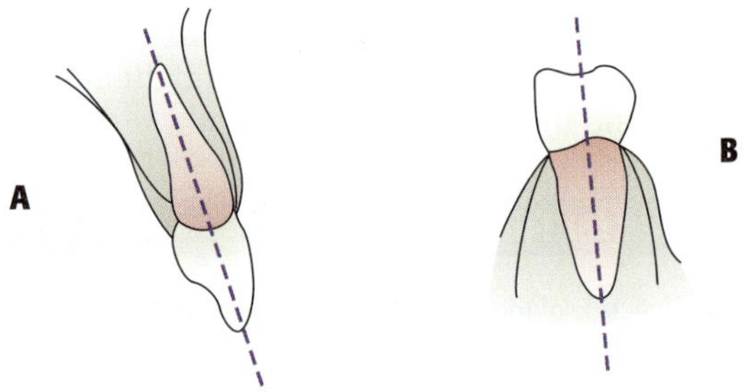

Fig. 41-7 **A,** Long axis of maxillary incisor divides the tooth into two equal halves. **B,** Long axis of mandibular premolar divides the tooth into two equal halves. (From Haring JI, Jansen L: *Dental radiography: principles and techniques,* ed 2, Philadelphia, 2000, Saunders.)

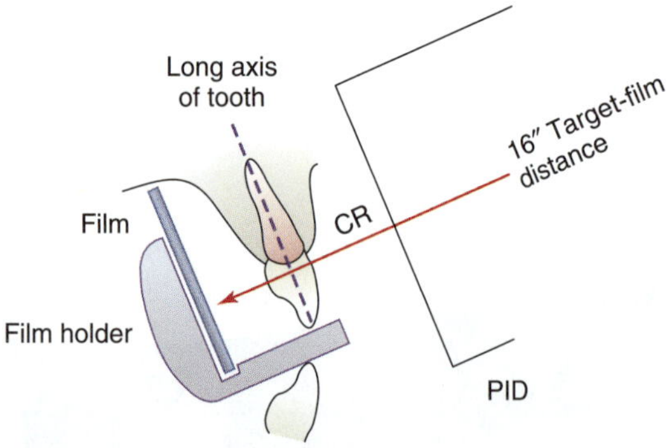

Fig. 41-8 Position of the film, teeth, PID, and central ray of the x-ray beam in the paralleling technique. The film and long axis of the tooth are parallel. The central ray (CR) is perpendicular to the tooth and film. An increased film distance (16 inches) is required. (From Haring JI, Jansen L: *Dental radiography: principles and techniques,* ed 2, Philadelphia, 2000, Saunders.)

4. *Horizontal angulation.* The central ray of the x-ray beam must be directed through the **contact areas** between the teeth (Fig. 41-9).
5. *Central ray.* The x-ray beam must be centered on the film to ensure that all areas of the film are exposed. Failure to center the x-ray beam results in a partial image, or *cone cut* (Fig. 41-10).

Patient Preparation

The patient having dental x-rays should be seated after the room has been prepared and the infection-control procedures completed (Procedure 41-1: Preparing the Patient for Dental X-Rays).

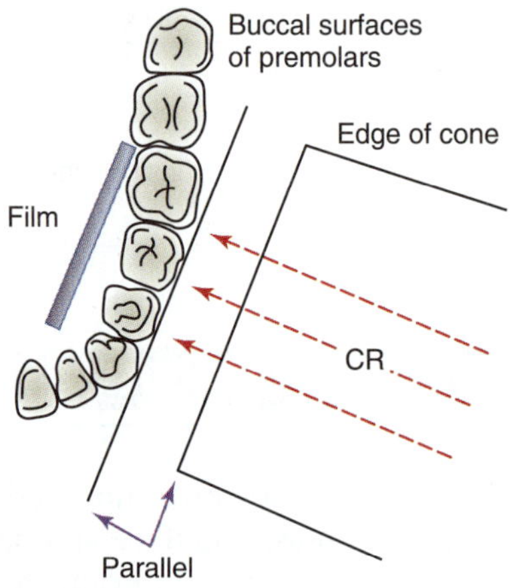

Fig. 41-9 In this diagram, x-rays pass through the contact areas of the premolars because the central ray is directed through the contacts and perpendicular to the film. If the central ray (CR) is not directed through the contacts, overlap of the premolar contacts occurs. (From Haring JI, Jansen L: *Dental radiography: principles and techniques,* ed 2, Philadelphia, 2000, Saunders.)

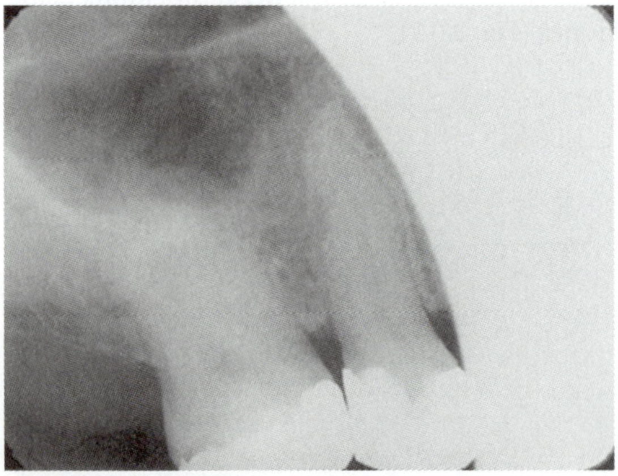

Fig. 41-10 This radiograph demonstrates a cone cut, that is, a clear unexposed area on the film. The PID was positioned too far distally, so the anterior portion of the film received no exposure. (From Haring JI, Jansen L: *Dental radiography: principles and techniques,* ed 2, Philadelphia, 2000, Saunders.)

Exposure Sequence for Film Placement

You should plan an **exposure sequence,** or a definite order, for periapical film placement when you are taking radiographs. If you work without a planned exposure sequence, you are more likely to omit an area or expose the same area twice.

Anterior Exposure Sequence

When exposing periapical films with the paralleling technique, *always* start with the anterior teeth (canines and incisors), for the following reasons:

- The size of anterior film (#1) is small and easier for patients to tolerate.
- Patients more easily adapt to the anterior film holder.
- Patients are less likely to gag with anterior film placement. Once the gag reflex is stimulated, the patient may gag on subsequent films that would normally be tolerated (see later discussion).

When using size #1 film, a total of seven or eight anterior film placements are used in the paralleling technique: four maxillary exposures and three mandibular exposures (Fig. 41-11). Some operators will choose to expose four maxillary and four mandibular anterior films. If size #2 film is used instead, there are six anterior film placements: three maxillary and three mandibular exposures. The authors recommend the use of #1 film.

The recommended anterior exposure sequence for the Rinn XCP instruments is as follows:

1. Assemble the anterior XCP instrument (Procedure 41-2).
2. Begin with the maxillary right canine (tooth #6).
3. Expose all the maxillary anterior teeth from *right* to *left*.
4. End with the maxillary left canine (tooth #11).
5. Move to the mandibular arch.
6. Begin with the mandibular left canine (tooth #22).

Procedure 41-1 Preparing the Patient for Dental X-Rays

Goal

To follow the basic steps in preparing a patient for intraoral x-ray procedures.

Equipment and Supplies

- Lead apron with thyroid collar
- Plastic container for prosthetic devices

PROCEDURAL STEPS

1. Explain the x-ray procedure to the patient. Ask whether the patient has any questions.

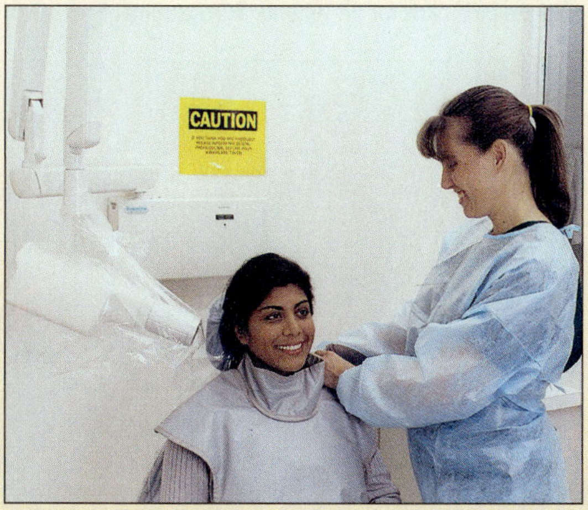

2. Adjust the chair so that the patient is positioned upright. The level of the chair must be adjusted to a comfortable working height for the operator.
3. Adjust the headrest to support and position the patient's head. The patient's head must be positioned so that the upper arch is parallel to the floor and the midsagittal (midline) plane is perpendicular to the floor.
4. Place and secure the lead apron with the thyroid collar on the patient.
5. Ask the patient to remove all objects from the mouth, including dentures, retainers, chewing gum, and any pierced-tongue or pierced-lip objects. Place any objects into a plastic container.
   Purpose: Objects in the mouth can cause artifacts on the radiograph.

7. Expose all the mandibular anterior teeth from *left* to *right*.
8. Finish with the mandibular right canine (tooth #27).

There is no wasted movement or shifting of the PID when you work from right to left in the maxillary arch and then from left to right in the mandibular arch. You may find an exposure sequence that works better for you. The most important thing is to always use the same sequence. This allows you to keep track of the last exposure if you are interrupted (Procedure 41-3).

Text continues on p. 652

A

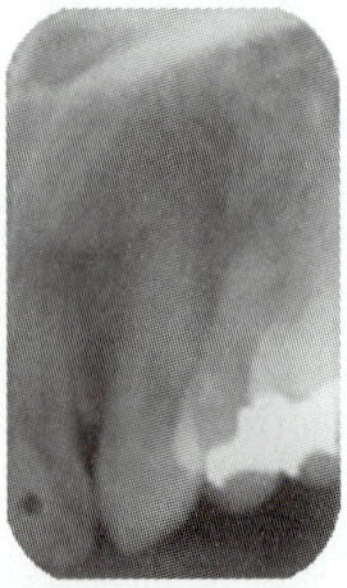

- Entire crown and tooth of canine, including apex and surrounding structures.
- Interproximal alveolar bone and mesial contact of canine.
- Lingual cusp of first premolar usually obscures distal contact of canine.

B

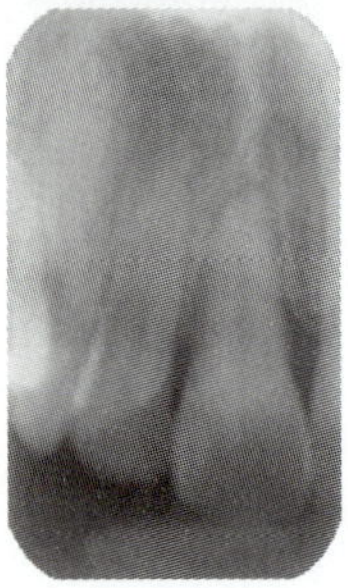

- Entire crown and roots of one lateral and one central incisor, including apices of teeth and surrounding structures.
- Interproximal alveolar bone between central and lateral contact area, mesial and distal contact areas, and surrounding regions of bone.
- Mesial contacts of adjacent central incisor and adjacent canine.

C

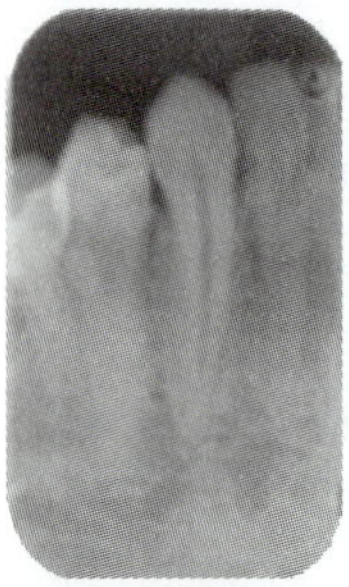

- Entire crown and root of canine, including apex and surrounding structures.
- Interproximal alveolar bone and mesial and distal contacts.

D

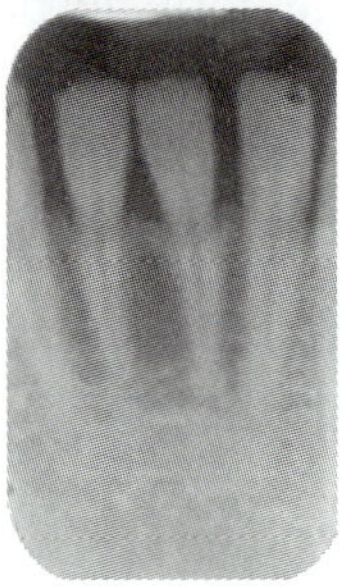

- Entire crown and roots of four mandibular incisors, including apices of teeth and surrounding structures.
- Contacts between central incisors and between central and lateral incisors.
- In most cases, not necessary to see distal contacts of lateral incisors.

Fig. 41-11 Anterior periapical film placement showing structures visible on the radiograph. **A,** Maxillary canine exposure. **B,** Maxillary incisor exposure. **C,** Mandibular canine exposure. **D,** Mandibular incisor exposure. (Radiographs from Haring JI, Jansen L: *Dental radiography: principles and techniques,* ed 2, Philadelphia, 2000, Saunders.)

Procedure 41-2 Assembling XCP (Extension-Cone Paralleling) Instruments

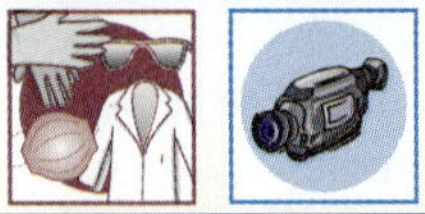

Goal

To assemble the Rinn XCP instruments for all areas of the mouth in preparation for radiographic surveys.

Equipment and Supplies

- Rinn XCP instruments

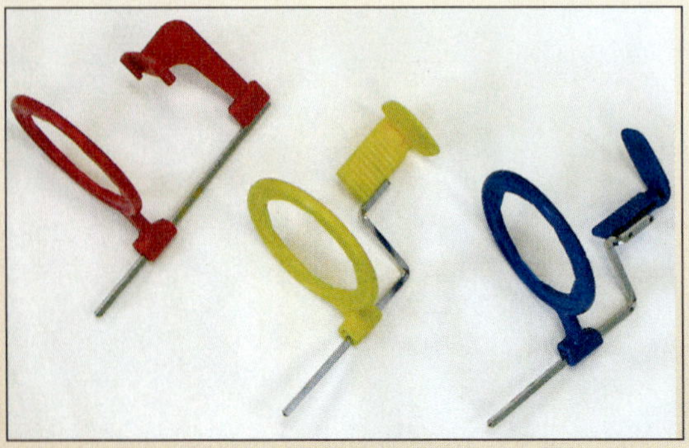

PROCEDURAL STEPS

Anterior Assembly

1. Lay out the blue parts for the anterior XCP instrument.

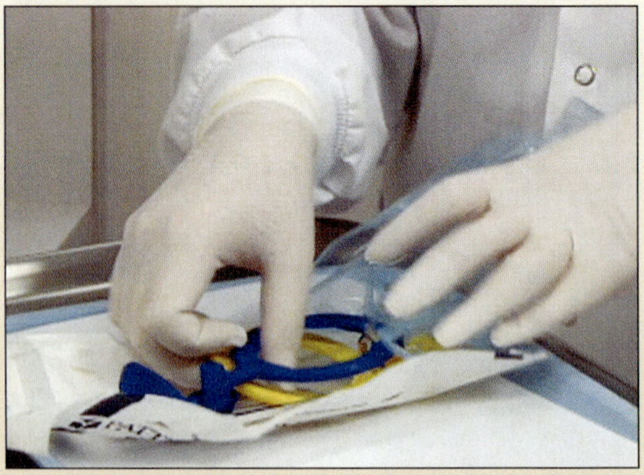

Procedure 41-2 Assembling XCP (Extension-Cone Paralleling) Instruments–cont'd

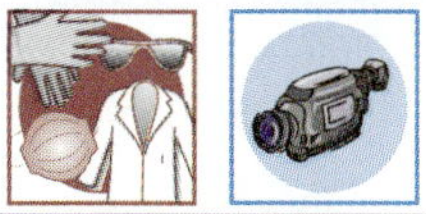

2. Assemble the anterior XCP instrument by inserting the two prongs of the blue anterior indicator arm into the openings in the blue anterior bite-block.

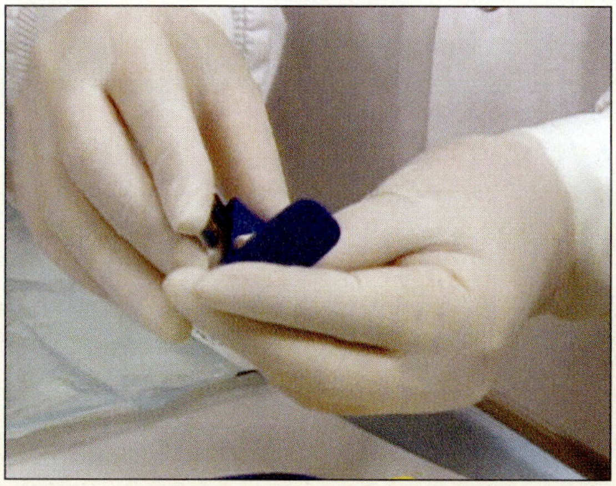

3. Insert the anterior indicator arm into the opening on the blue anterior aiming ring.

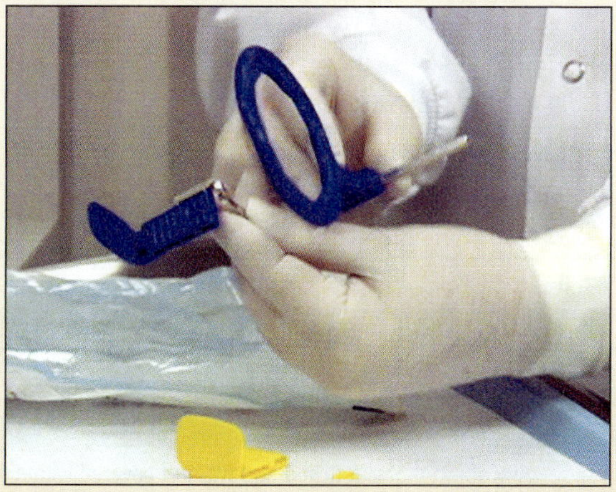

4. Flex the plastic backing of the blue bite-block to open the film slot for easy insertion of the anterior film packet.

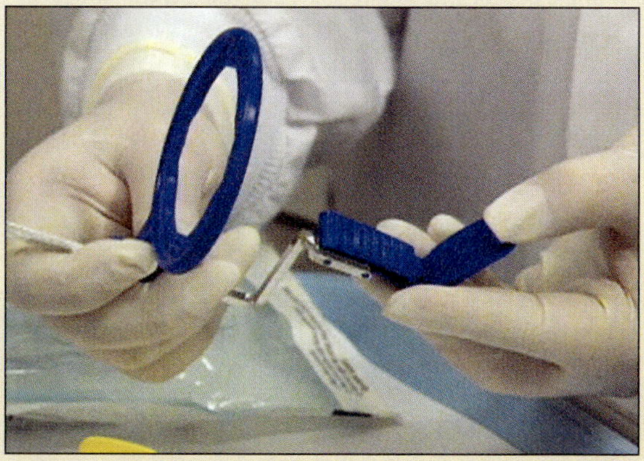

5. The blue anterior XCP instrument is correctly assembled when the film is seen centered in the middle of the aiming ring.

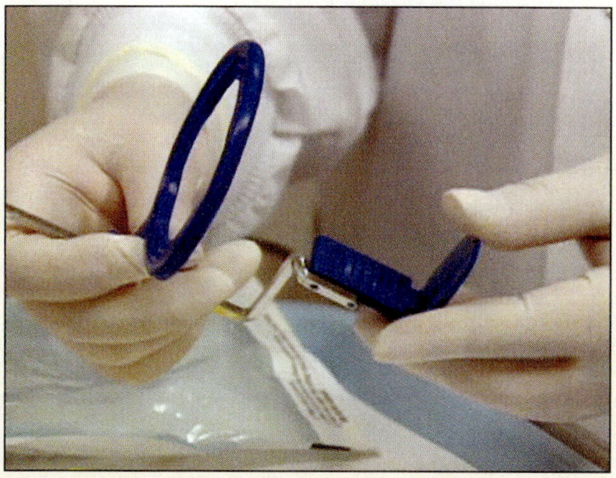

Posterior Assembly

1. Lay out the yellow parts for the posterior XCP instrument.
2. Assemble the yellow posterior XCP instrument by inserting the two prongs of the yellow posterior indicator arm into the openings in the yellow posterior bite-block as shown.

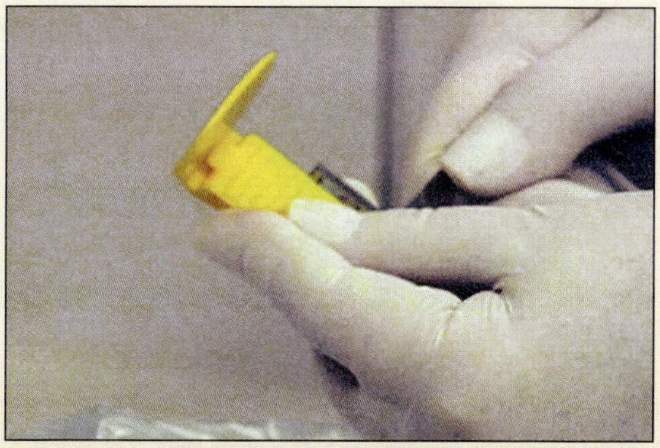

3. Insert the yellow posterior indicator arm into the opening on the yellow posterior aiming ring as shown.

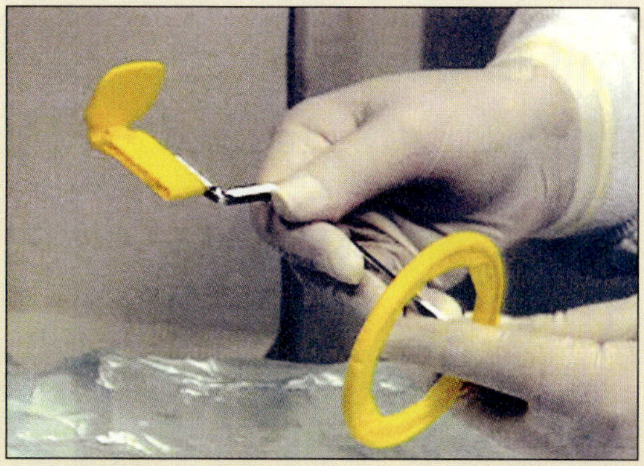

continued

Procedure 41-2 Assembling XCP (Extension-Cone Paralleling) Instruments—cont'd

Posterior Assembly, cont'd

4. Flex the plastic backing of the yellow bite-block to open the film slot for easy insertion of the posterior film packet.

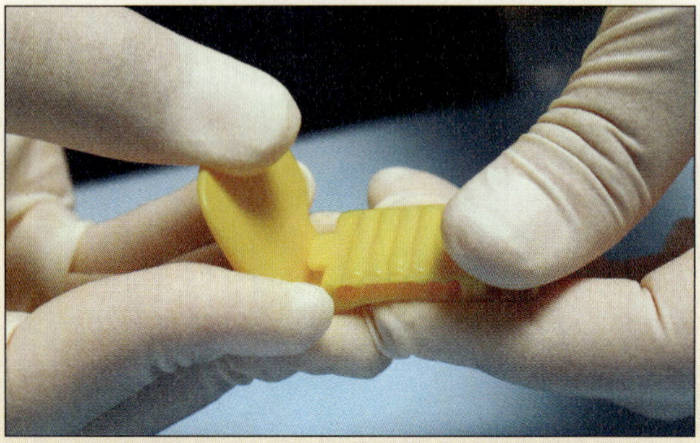

5. The posterior XCP instrument is correctly assembled when the film is seen centered in the middle of the aiming ring.

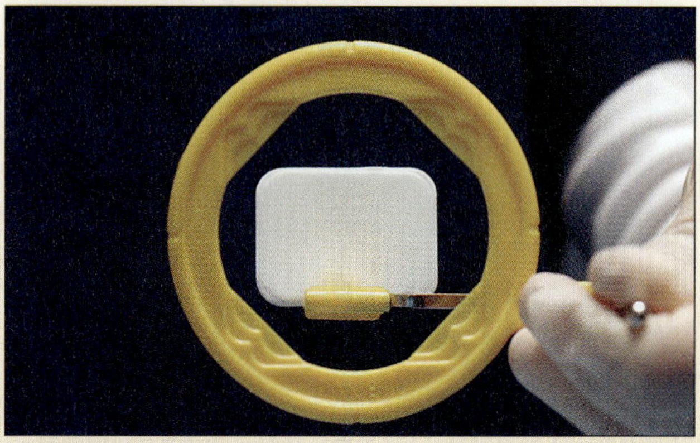

Procedure 41-3 Producing a Full-Mouth Radiographic Survey Using the Paralleling Technique

Goal

To follow the proper steps to produce a full-mouth survey using the paralleling technique.

Equipment and Supplies

- Appropriate number and size of radiographic films
- Appropriate infection-control materials (paper cup, barriers, paper towel, and impervious surface cover)
- Lead apron and thyroid collar
- Sterile packaged XCP instruments
- Cotton rolls
- Patient chart

PROCEDURAL STEPS

Preparation Before Seating Patient

1. Prepare the operatory with all infection-control barriers.
   Purpose: Any object that is touched and was not covered with a barrier must be disinfected after the patient is dismissed.
2. Determine the number and type of films to be exposed through a review of the patient's chart, directions from the dentist, or both.

Procedure 41-3 Producing a Full-Mouth Radiographic Survey Using the Paralleling Technique—cont'd

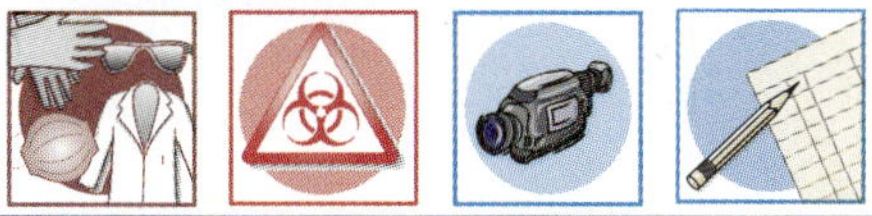

3. Label a paper cup with the patient's name and the date. Place it outside the room where the radiograph machine will be used.
   Purpose: This is the transfer cup for storing and moving exposed films.

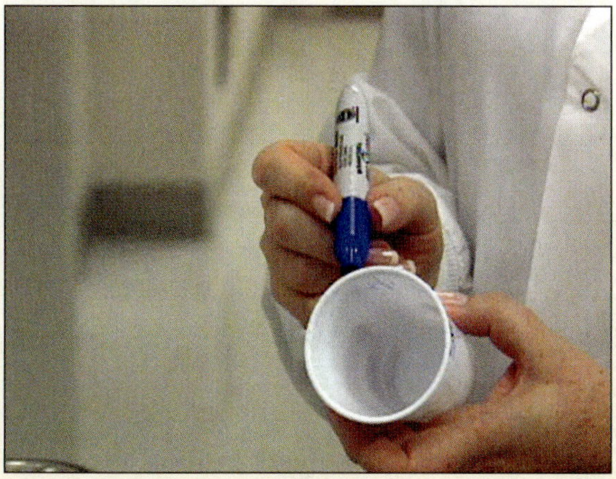

4. Turn on the x-ray machine and check the basic settings (kilovoltage, milliamperage, exposure time).
5. Wash and dry your hands.
6. Dispense the desired number of films and store them outside the room where the x-ray machine is being used.
   Purpose: To prevent fogging caused by scatter radiation.

Positioning Patient

1. Seat the patient comfortably in the dental chair, with the back in an upright position and the head supported.
2. Ask the patient to remove eyeglasses and bulky earrings.
   Purpose: These objects may cause radiopaque images to be superimposed on the radiographs.

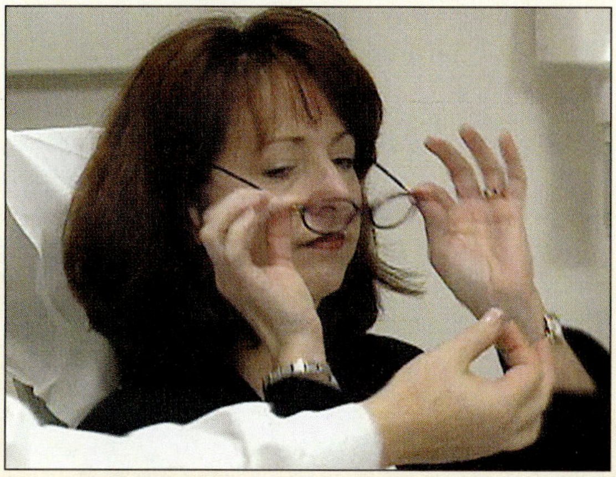

3. Ask the patient to remove prosthetic appliances or objects from the mouth.
   Note: Always wear gloves when handling a prosthetic appliance.
4. Position the patient so that the occlusal plane of the jaw being x-rayed is parallel to the floor when the mouth is open.
5. Drape the patient with a lead apron and thyroid collar.
6. Wash and dry hands and put on clean examination gloves.
7. Open the package and assemble the sterile film-holding instruments.
   Purpose: Allowing the patient to observe you washing your hands, putting on clean gloves, and opening the sterile package of instruments assures the patient that appropriate infection-control measures are being taken.

continued

Procedure 41-3 Producing a Full-Mouth Radiographic Survey Using the Paralleling Technique—cont'd

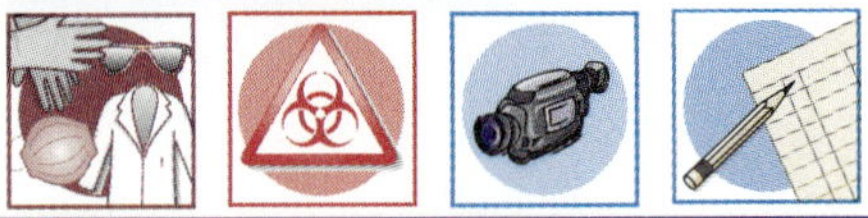

Maxillary Canine Region

1. Insert the #1 film packet vertically into the anterior bite-block.
2. Position the film packet with the canine and first premolar centered. Position film as far posterior as possible.
3. With the film-holding instrument and film in place, instruct the patient to close the mouth slowly but firmly.
4. Position the localizing ring and PID; then expose the film.

   Note: The image of the lingual cusp of the first premolar is usually superimposed on the distal surface of the canine because of the curvature of the maxillary arch. This contact area must be "opened" on the view of the premolar region.

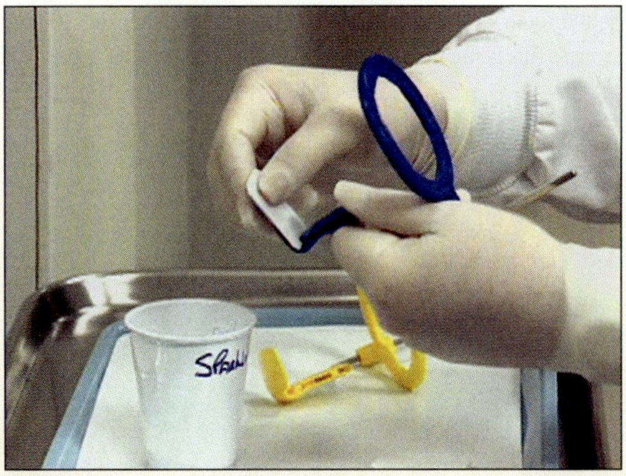

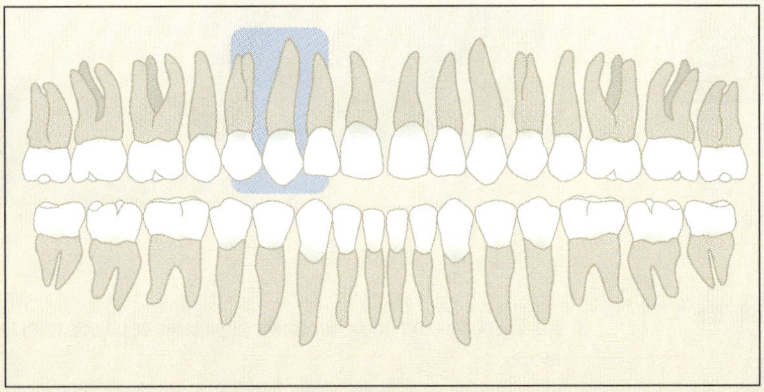

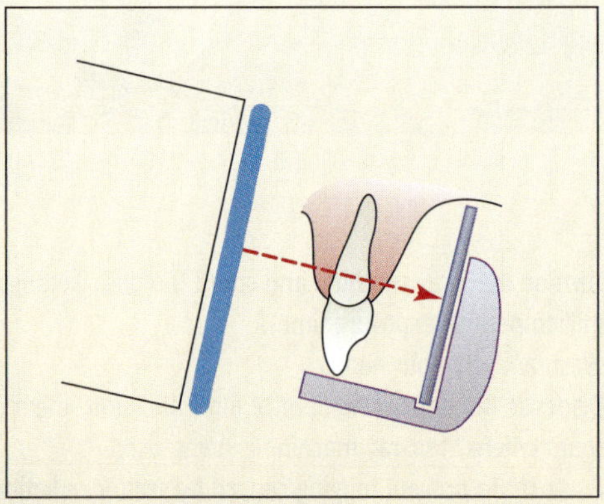

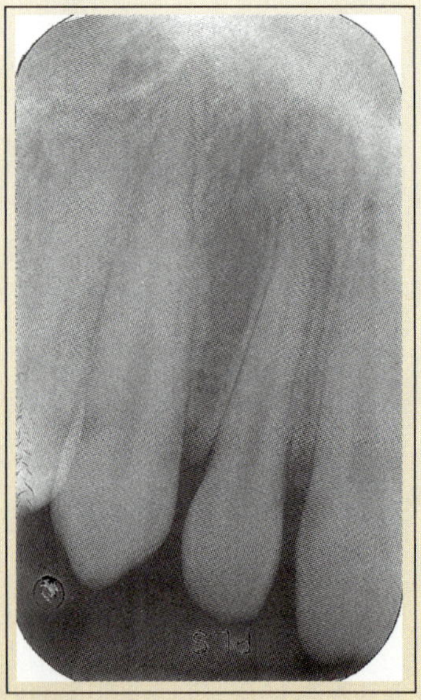

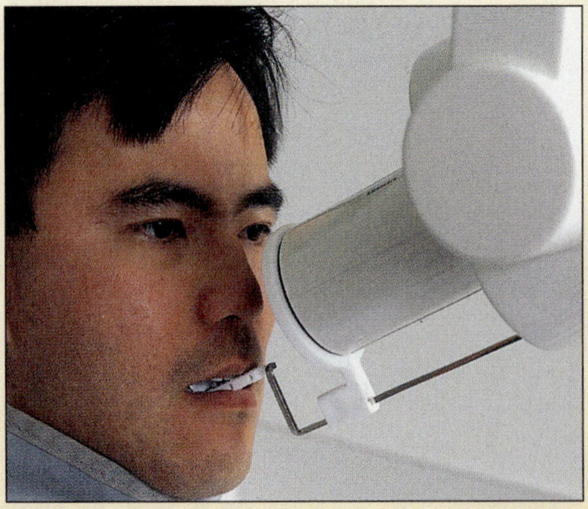

Procedure 41-3 Producing a Full-Mouth Radiographic Survey Using the Paralleling Technique—cont'd

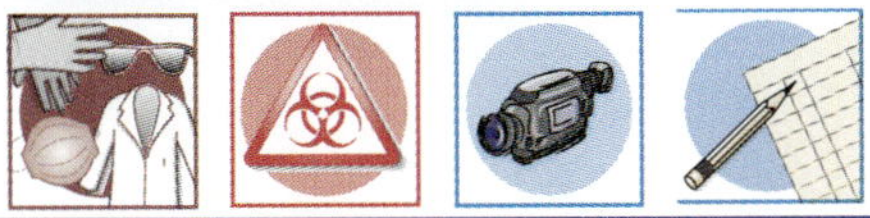

Maxillary Central/Lateral Incisor Region

1. Insert the #1 film packet vertically into the anterior block.
2. Center the film packet between the central and lateral incisors. Position the film as posterior in the mouth as possible.
3. With the instrument and film in place, instruct the patient to close the mouth slowly but firmly.
4. Position the localizing ring and PID; then expose the film.

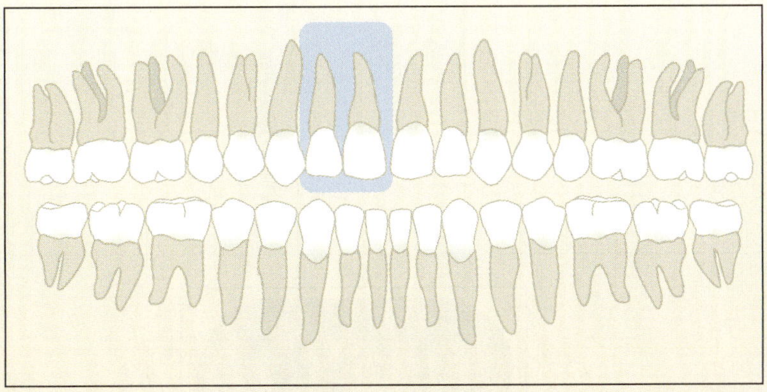

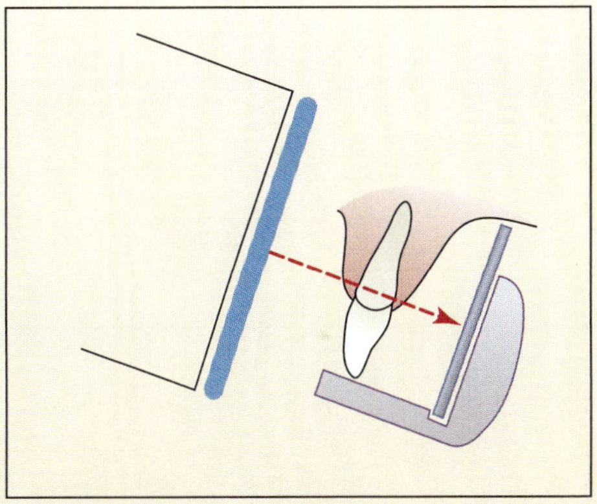

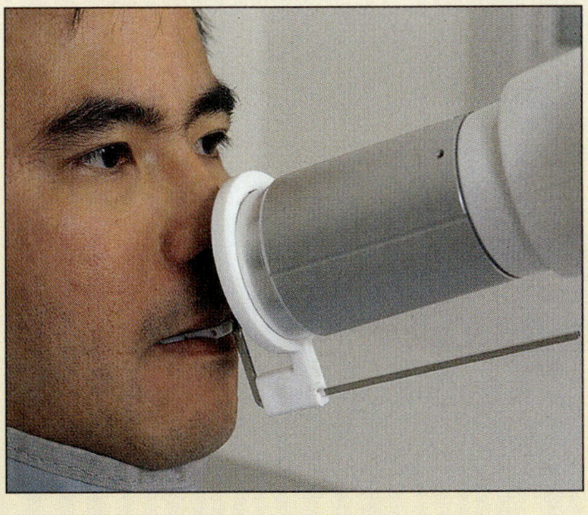

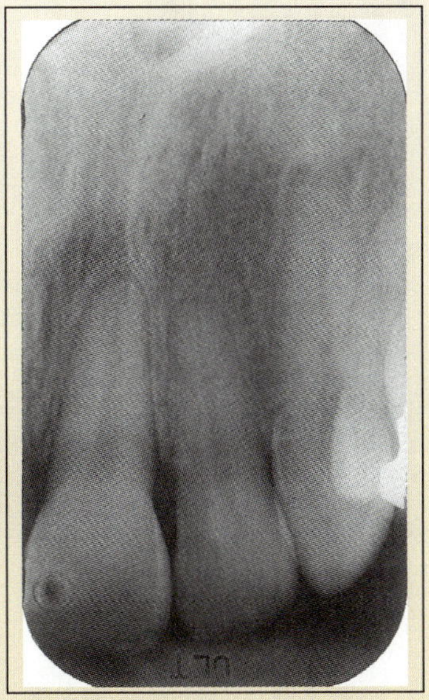

continued

Procedure 41-3 Producing a Full-Mouth Radiographic Survey Using the Paralleling Technique—cont'd

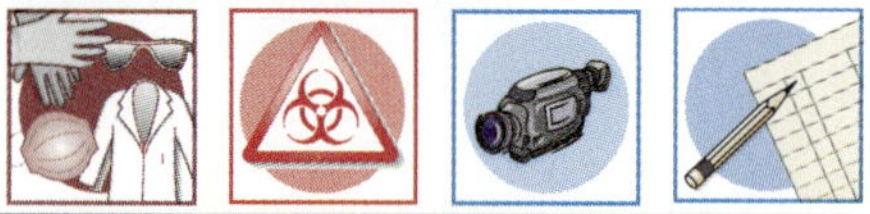

Mandibular Canine Region

1. Insert the #1 film packet vertically into the anterior bite-block.
2. Center the film on the canine. Position the film as far in the lingual direction as the patient's anatomy will allow.

   Note: A cotton roll may be placed between the maxillary teeth and bite-block to prevent rocking of the bite-block on the canine tip and to increase patient comfort.
3. With the instrument and film in place, instruct the patient to close the mouth slowly but firmly.
4. Position the localizing ring and PID; then expose the film.

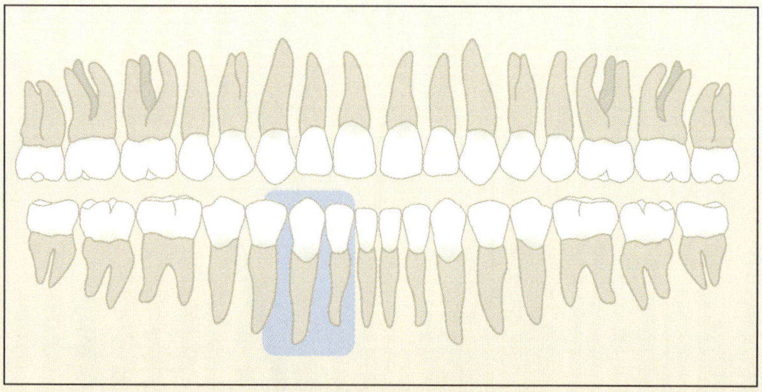

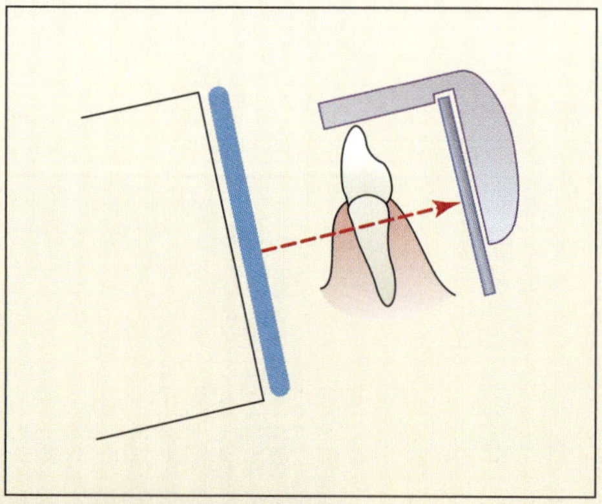

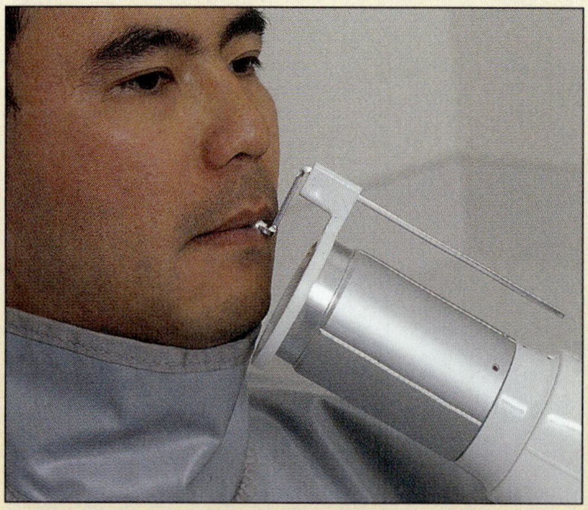

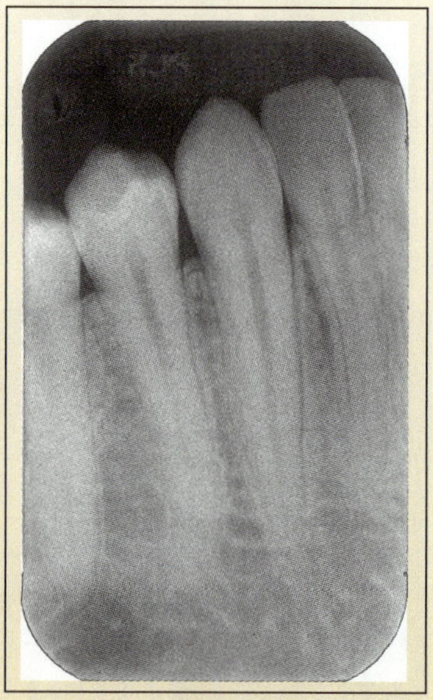

Procedure 41-3 Producing a Full-Mouth Radiographic Survey Using the Paralleling Technique—cont'd

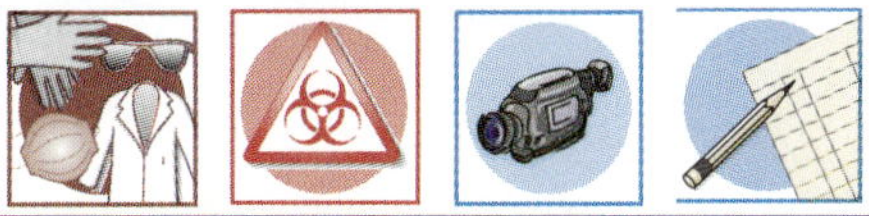

Mandibular Incisor Region

1. Insert the #1 film packet vertically into the anterior bite-block.
2. Center the film packet between the central incisors. Position the film as far in the lingual direction as the patient's anatomy will allow.
3. With the instrument and film in place, instruct the patient to close the mouth slowly but firmly.
4. Slide the localizing ring down the indicator rod to the patient's skin surface.
5. Position the localizing ring and PID; then expose the film.

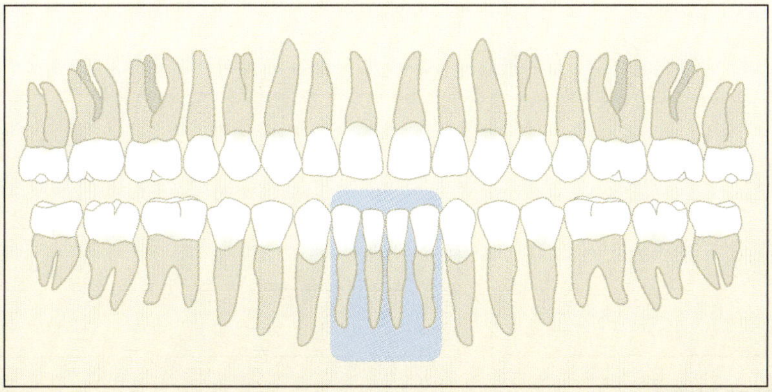

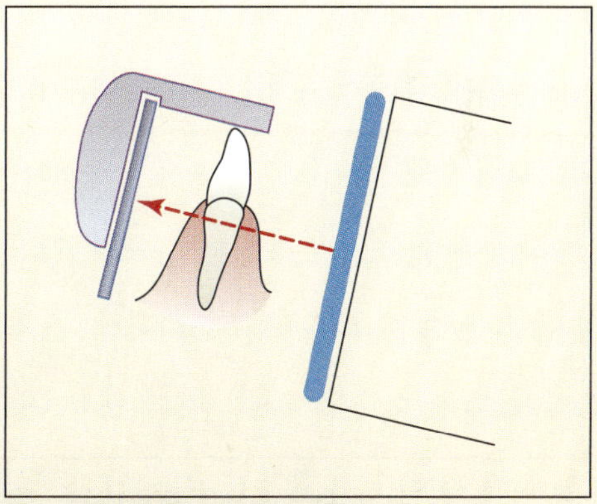

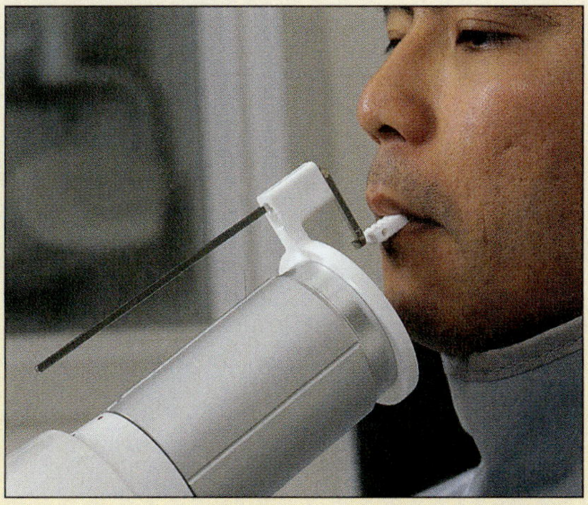

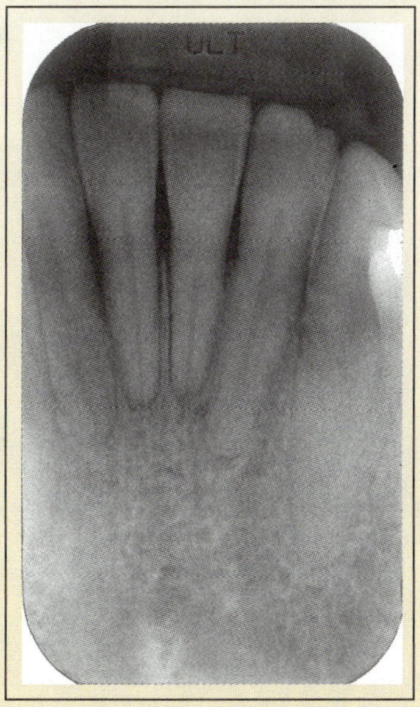

continued

Procedure 41-3 Producing a Full-Mouth Radiographic Survey Using the Paralleling Technique—cont'd

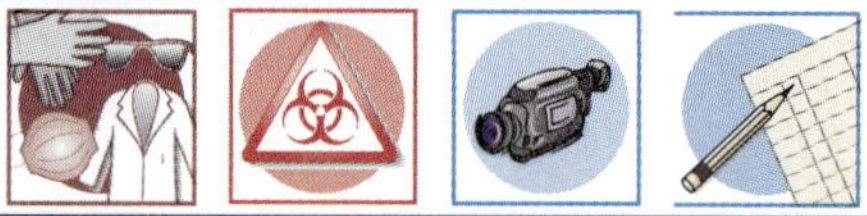

Maxillary Premolar Region

1. Insert the film packet horizontally into the posterior bite-block, pushing the film packet all the way into the slot.
2. Center the film packet on the second premolar. Position film in the mid-palate area.
3. With the instrument and film in place, instruct the patient to close the mouth slowly but firmly.
4. Position the localizing ring and PID; then expose the film.

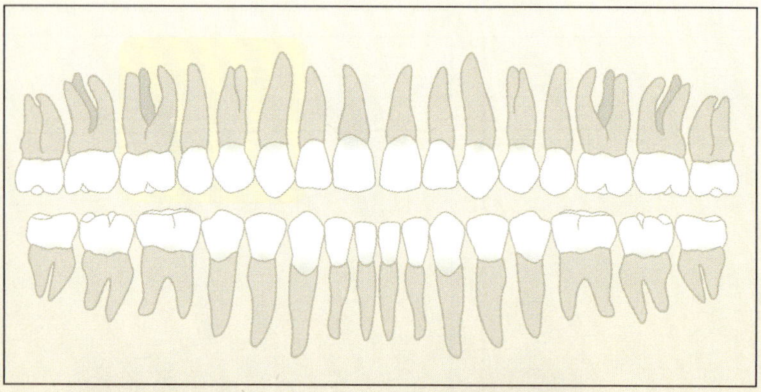

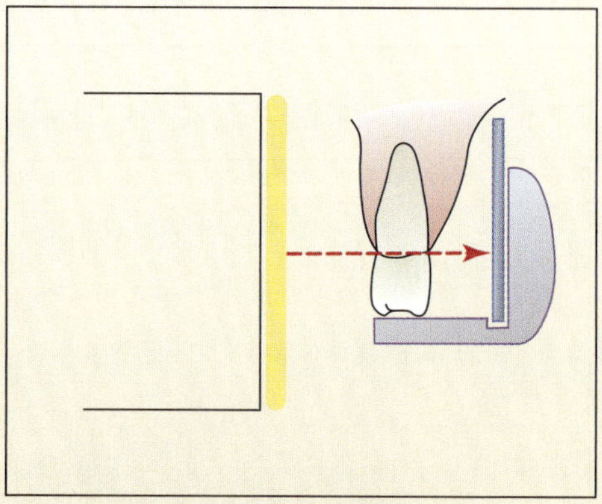

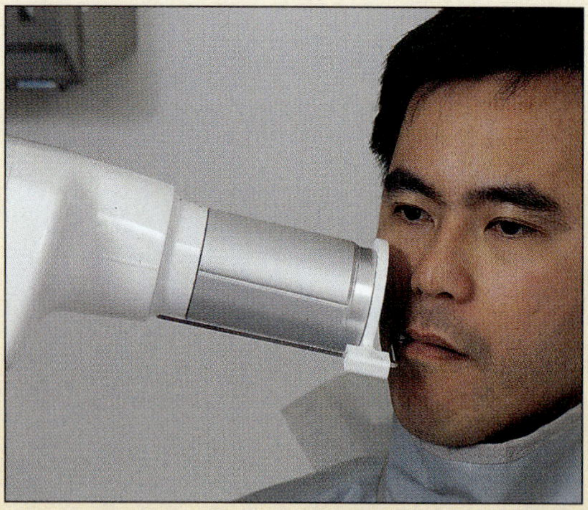

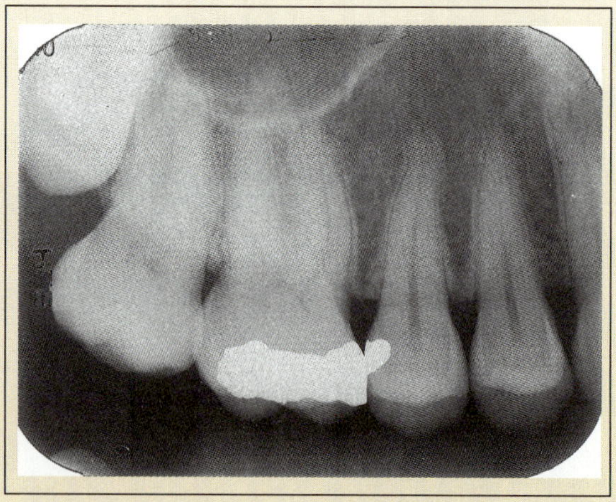

Procedure 41-3 Producing a Full-Mouth Radiographic Survey Using the Paralleling Technique—cont'd

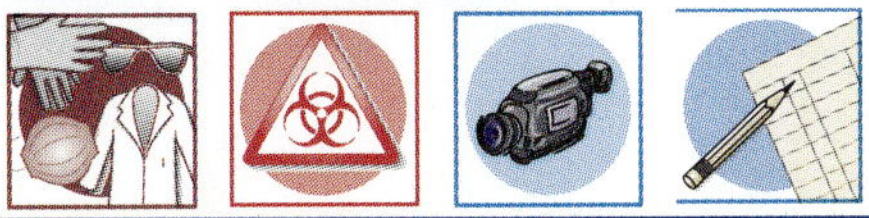

Maxillary Molar Region

1. Insert the film packet horizontally into the posterior bite-block.
2. Center the film packet on the second molar. Position the film in the midpalate area.
3. With the instrument and film in place, instruct the patient to close the mouth slowly but firmly.
4. Position the localizing ring and PID; then expose the film.

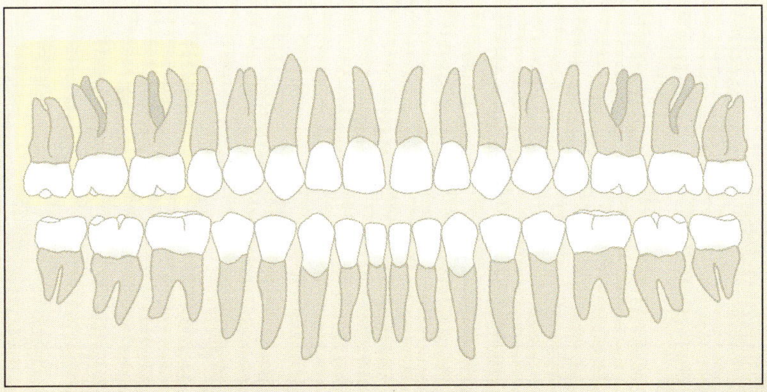

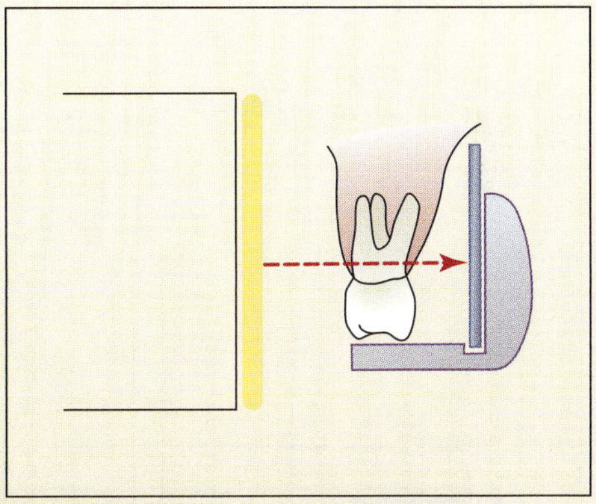

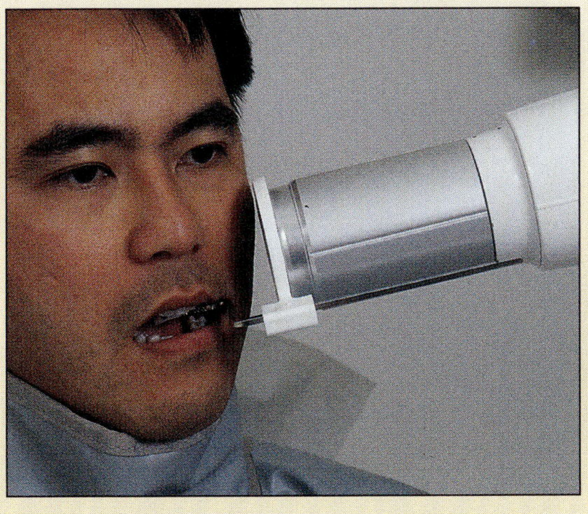

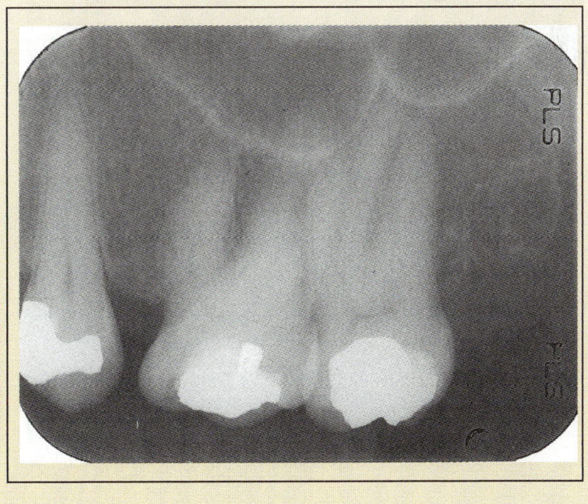

continued

Procedure 41-3 Producing a Full-Mouth Radiographic Survey Using the Paralleling Technique—cont'd

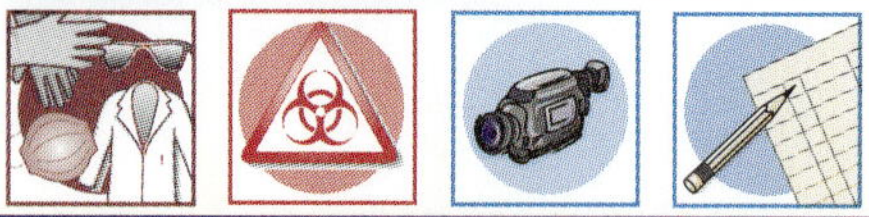

Mandibular Premolar Region

1. Insert the #2 film horizontally into the posterior bite-block.
2. Center the film on the contact point between the second premolar and first molar. Position the film as far lingual as the patient's anatomy will allow.
3. With the instrument and film in place, instruct the patient to close the mouth slowly but firmly.
4. Slide the localizing ring down the indicator rod to the patient's skin surface.
5. Position the localizing ring and PID; then expose the film.

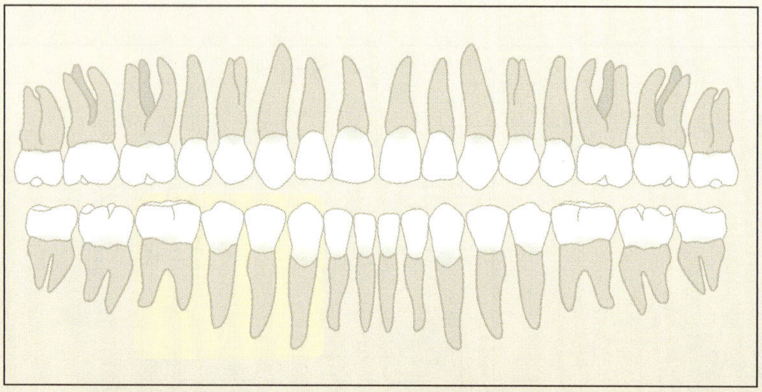

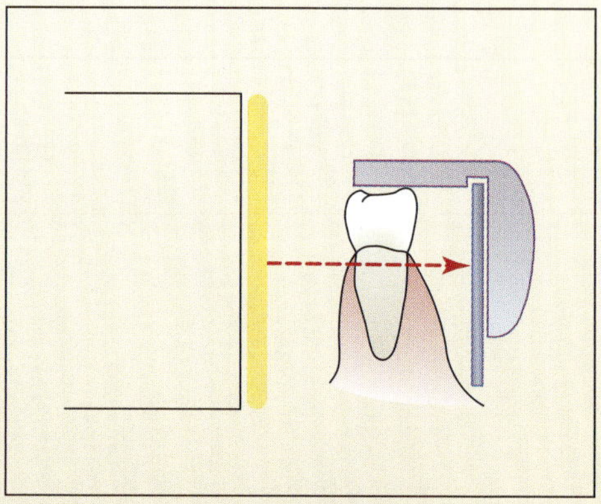

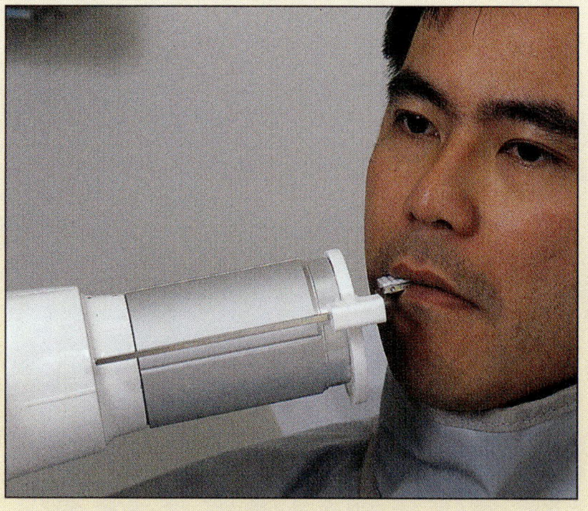

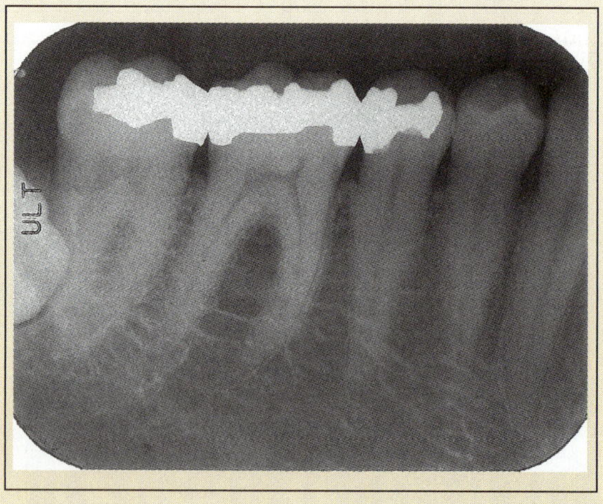

Procedure 41-3 Producing a Full-Mouth Radiographic Survey Using the Paralleling Technique—cont'd

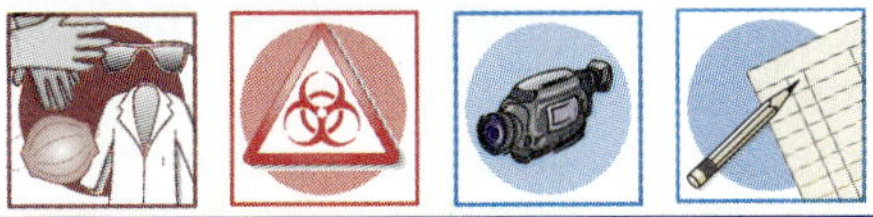

Mandibular Molar Region

1. Insert the #2 film horizontally into the posterior bite-block.
2. Center the film on the second molar. Position the film as far lingual as the tongue will allow.

   NOTE: This position will be closer to the teeth than that for the premolar and anterior views.
3. With the instrument and film in place, instruct the patient to close the mouth slowly but firmly.
4. Slide the localizing ring down the indicator rod to the patient's skin surface.
5. Position the localizing ring and PID; then expose the film.

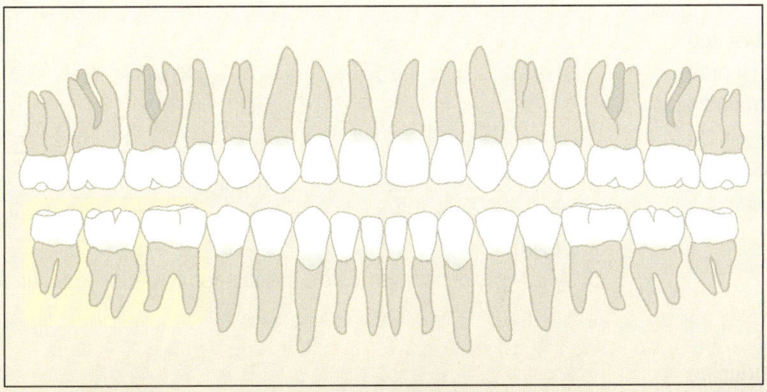

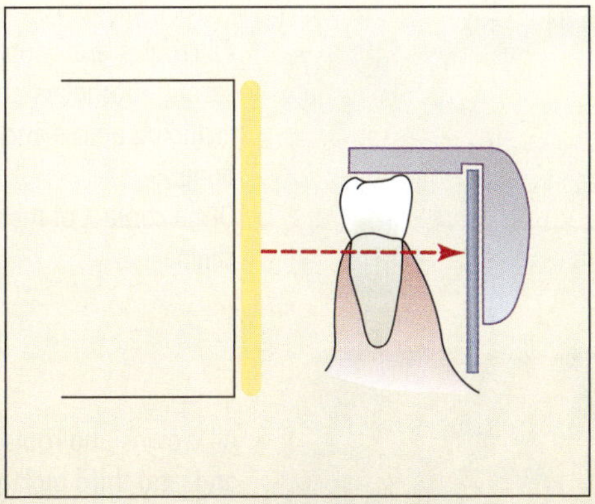

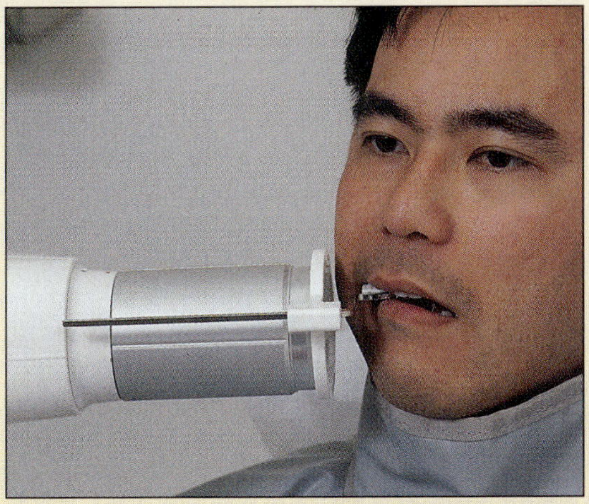

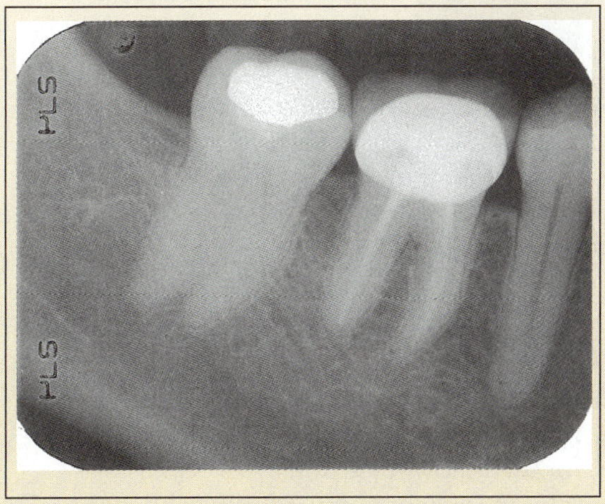

A

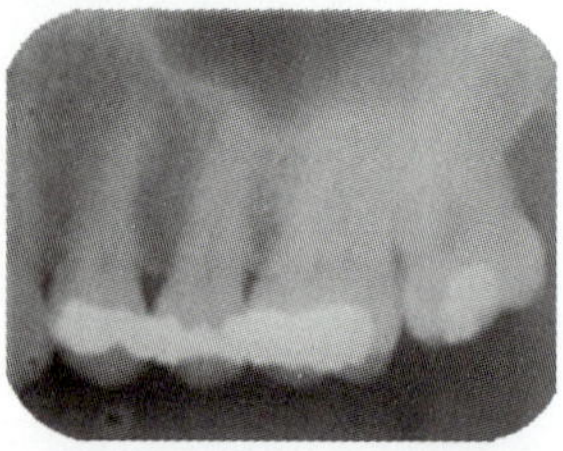

- All crowns and roots of first and second premolars and first molar, including apices, alveolar crests, contact areas, and surrounding bone

B

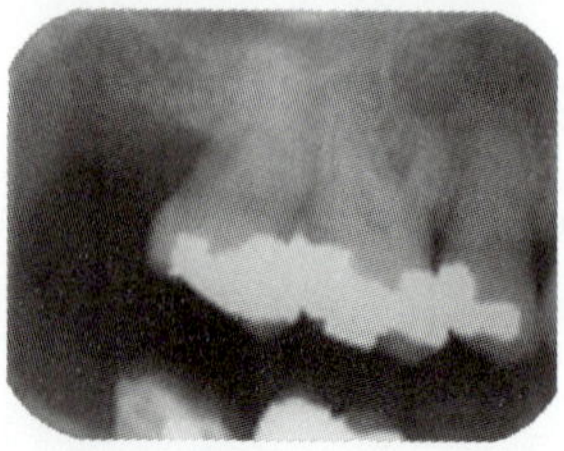

- All crowns and roots of first, second, and third molars, including apices, alveolar crests, contact areas, surrounding bone, and tuberosity region

C

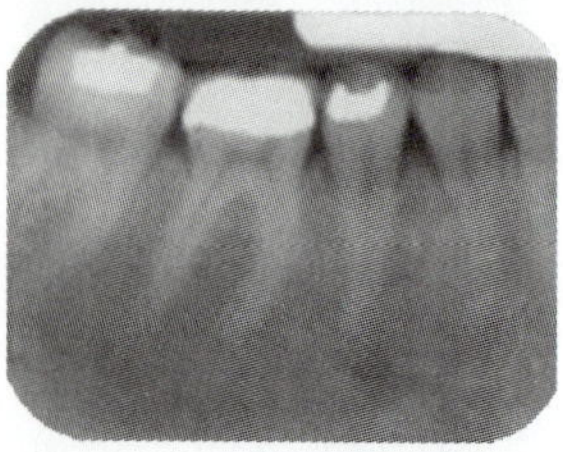

- All crowns and roots of first and second premolars and first molar, including apices and surrounding bone
- Distal contact of mandibular canine

D

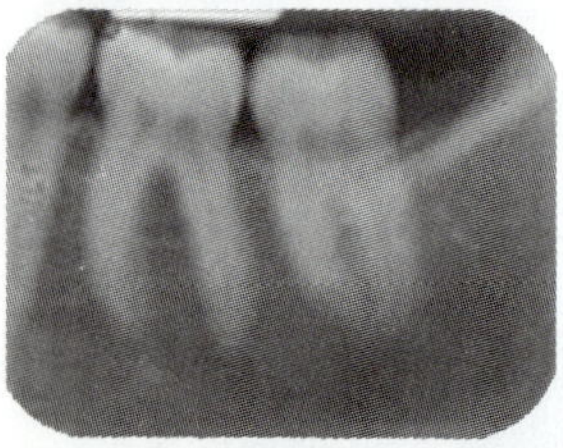

- All crowns and roots of first, second, and third molars, including apices and surrounding bone

Fig. 41-12 **Posterior periapical film placement showing structures visible on the radiograph. A, Maxillary premolar exposure. B, Maxillary molar exposure. C, Mandibular premolar exposure. D, Mandibular molar exposure.** (Radiographs from Haring JI, Jansen L: *Dental radiography: principles and techniques,* ed 2, Philadelphia, 2000, Saunders.)

Posterior Exposure Sequence

After you have completed the anterior teeth, begin the posterior teeth. *Always* begin with the premolar film before the molar film, for the following reasons:

- Premolar film placement is easier for the patient to tolerate than molar placement.
- Premolar exposure is less likely to evoke the gag reflex.

With the paralleling technique, eight posterior film placements are used: four maxillary exposures and four mandibular exposures (Fig. 41-12).

The recommended posterior exposure sequence for the XCP instruments is as follows:

1. Begin with the maxillary right quadrant.
2. Assemble the posterior XCP instrument for this area (see Procedure 41-2).
3. Expose the premolar film (teeth #4 and #5) first, then the molar film (teeth #1, #2, and #3).
4. Without reassembling the XCP instrument, move to the mandibular left quadrant.
5. Expose the premolar film (teeth #20 and #21) first, then the molar film (teeth #17, #18, and #19).
6. Move to the maxillary left quadrant and reassemble the posterior XCP instrument for this area.
7. Expose the premolar film (teeth #12 and #13) first, then the molar film (teeth #14, #15, and #16).
8. Finish with the mandibular right quadrant.
9. Expose the premolar film (teeth #28 and #29) first; then end with the exposure of the molar film (teeth #30, #31, and #32).

Film Placement

There are specific teeth that must be on each radiograph for every projection (see Figs. 41-11 and 41-12).

Recall

3. Why is an exposure sequence important?
4. When exposing films, in which area of the mouth should you begin?
5. Which projection should be the first for posterior exposures?

BISECTING TECHNIQUE

Another method of exposing periapical films is the bisecting technique, also known as the *bisecting-angle, bisection of the angle,* or *short-cone* technique. Although the bisecting technique was first used with a short cone, this technique can be used with either a short or long PID.

The American Academy of Oral and Maxillofacial Radiology recommends the paralleling technique as the technique of choice for periapical radiographs. Therefore the bisecting technique should be used as an alternative method in special circumstances when it is not possible to use the paralleling technique. Such special circumstances include patients with very small mouths, children, and patients with low or flat palatal vaults.

The bisection of the angle technique is based on the geometric principle of equally dividing a triangle. Unlike the paralleling technique, in which you move the film away from the teeth to make the film and teeth parallel, the bisecting technique places the film *directly against* the teeth to be radiographed. Thus the film and the teeth are not parallel, but at an angle.

With the bisecting technique, the angle formed by the long axes of the teeth and the film is bisected into two equal parts, and the x-ray beam is directed perpendicular to the bisecting line (Fig. 41-13).

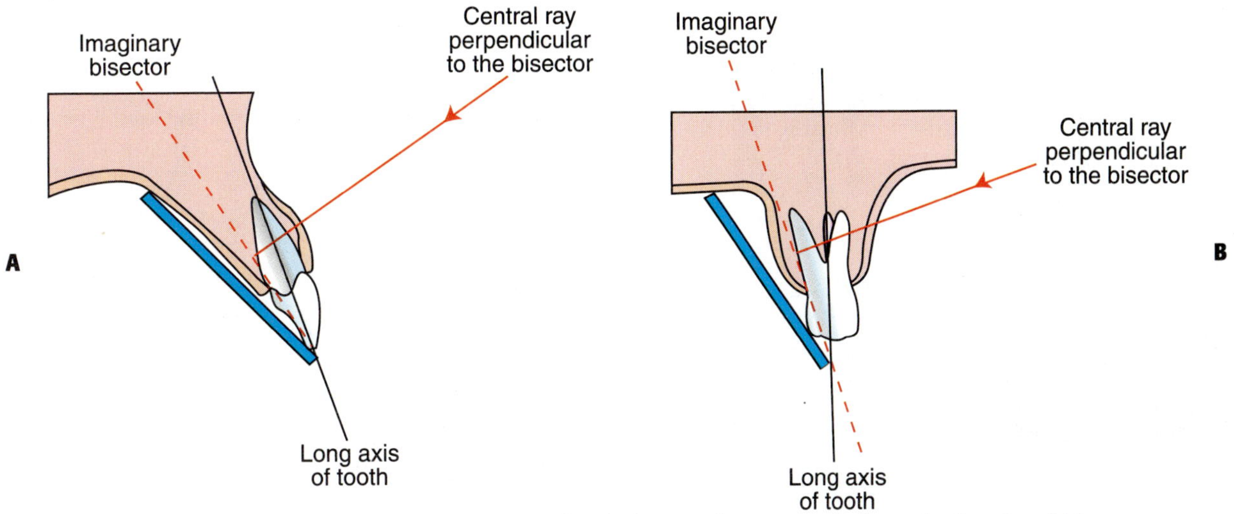

Fig. 41-13 **A,** A diagram of an anterior tooth with the central ray perpendicular to the "imaginary" bisector of the angle between the long axis of the tooth and the film plane. **B,** A posterior tooth using the bisecting angle concept. (From Miles D, et al: *Radiographic imaging for dental auxiliaries,* ed 3, Philadelphia, 1999, Saunders.)

The major disadvantage of this technique is that the image on the film is dimensionally distorted.

Film Holders

When the bisecting technique is being used, you may see operators asking the patient to hold the film with his or her fingers to stabilize the film in the mouth. This practice is *not* recommended. Holding the film exposes the patient's hand and finger to unnecessary radiation.

Available types of film holders include the following:

- The BAI (bisecting-angle instrument; Rinn) includes plastic bite-blocks, plastic aiming rings, and metal indicator arms.
- The Stabe bite-block (Rinn) is a disposable bite-block that can be used with the paralleling technique or the bisecting technique. With the bisecting technique, the scored front section is removed and the film placed *as close as possible* to the teeth (Fig. 41-14).
- The EeZee-Grip film holder (Rinn), previously called the Snap-A-Ray, is a film-holding device used in either the paralleling or the bisecting technique.

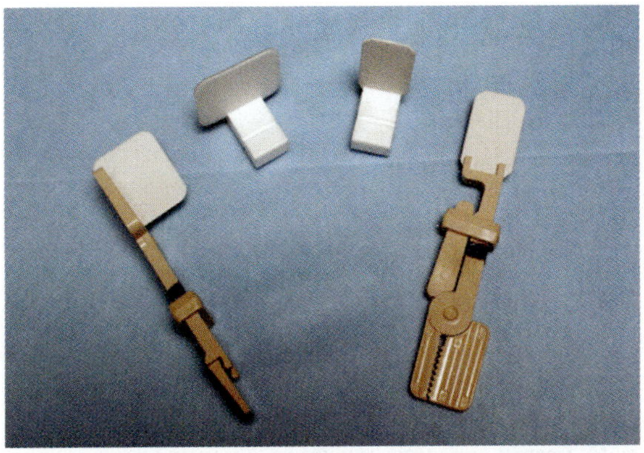

Fig. 41-14 EeZee-Grip (Rinn) film holder (posterior), Stabe anterior, Stabe posterior, and EeZee-Grip (Rinn) film holder (posterior).

Angulation of Position Indicator Device

In the bisecting technique, the angulation of the PID is *critical.* **Angulation** is a term used to describe the alignment of the central ray of the x-ray beam in the horizontal and vertical planes. Angulation can be changed by moving the PID in either a horizontal or a vertical direction. The BAI instruments with aiming rings dictate the proper PID angulation. However, when the finger-holding method or the EeZee-Grip method is used, the operator must determine both the horizontal and the vertical angulation.

Horizontal Angulation

Horizontal angulation refers to the positioning of the tubehead and direction of the central ray in a horizontal, or side-to-side, plane. The horizontal angulation *remains the same* whether you are using the paralleling or bisecting technique (Fig. 41-15).

Correct horizontal angulation

With correct horizontal angulation, the central ray is directed perpendicular to the curvature of the arch and through the contact areas of the teeth (Fig. 41-16).

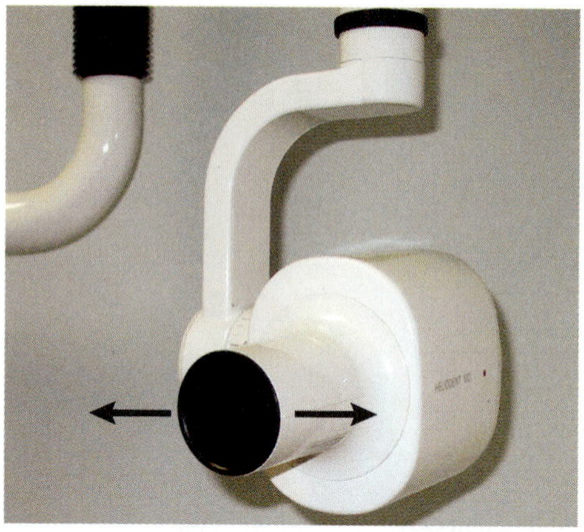

Fig. 41-15 The arrows indicate movement in a horizontal direction.

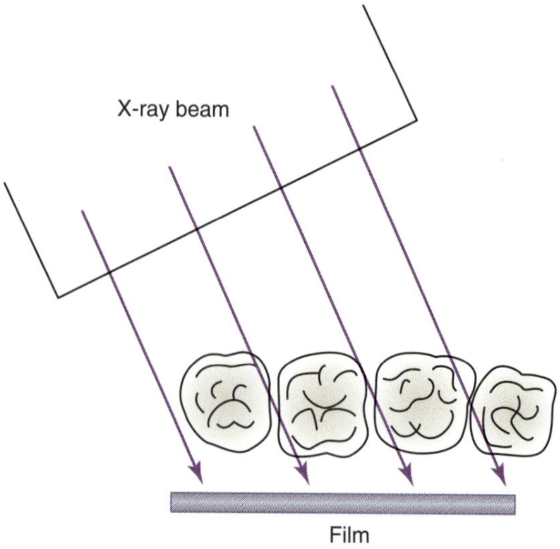

Fig. 41-17 Incorrect horizontal angulation. (From Haring JI, Jansen L: *Dental radiography: principles and techniques,* ed 2, Philadelphia, 2000, Saunders.)

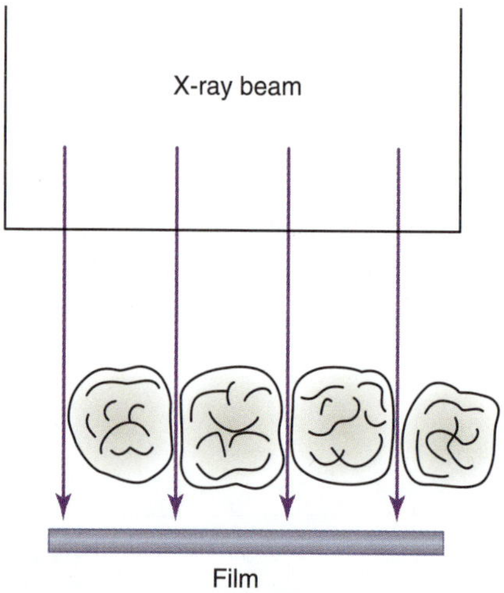

Fig. 41-16 Correct horizontal angulation. (From Haring JI, Jansen L: *Dental radiography: principles and techniques,* ed 2, Philadelphia, 2000, Saunders.)

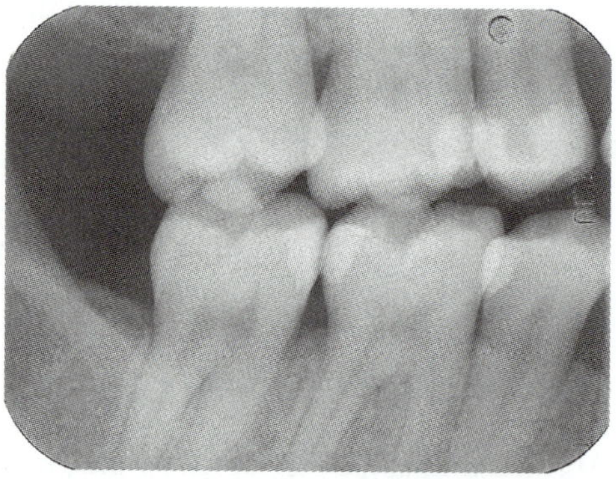

Fig. 41-18 Overlapped contact areas.

Incorrect horizontal angulation

Incorrect horizontal angulation results in overlapped (unopened) contact areas (Fig. 41-17). A film with overlapped contact areas cannot be used to examine the interproximal areas of the teeth (Fig. 41-18).

Vertical Angulation

Vertical angulation refers to the positioning of the PID in a vertical, or up-and-down, plane (Fig. 41-19). Angulation is measured in degrees according the markings on the outside of the tubehead. Vertical angulation differs according to the x-ray technique being used, as follows:

1. With the paralleling technique, the vertical angulation of the central ray is directed perpendicular to the film and the long axis of the tooth.
2. With the bisecting technique, the vertical angulation is determined by the imaginary bisector; the *central ray is directed perpendicular to the imaginary bisector.*
3. With the bite-wing technique, the vertical angulation is predetermined; the central ray is directed at +10 degrees to the occlusal plane (see later discussion).

Correct vertical angulation

Correct vertical angulation results in a radiographic image that is the same length as the tooth (Table 41-1).

Incorrect vertical angulation

Incorrect vertical angulation results in an image that is not the same length as the tooth being x-rayed. The image appears either longer or shorter. *Elongated* or *foreshortened images* are not diagnostic.

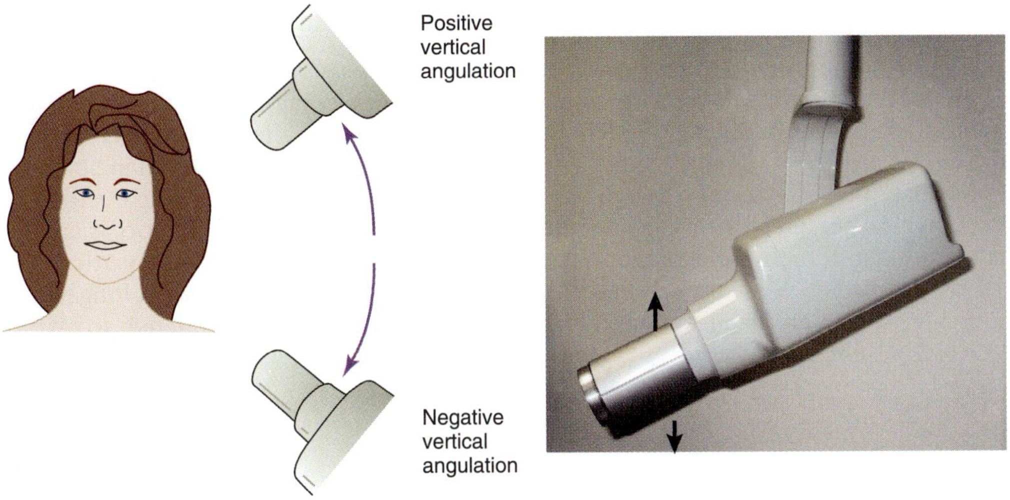

Fig. 41-19 Vertical angulation of the position indicator device refers to PID placement in an up-and-down (head-to-toe) direction.

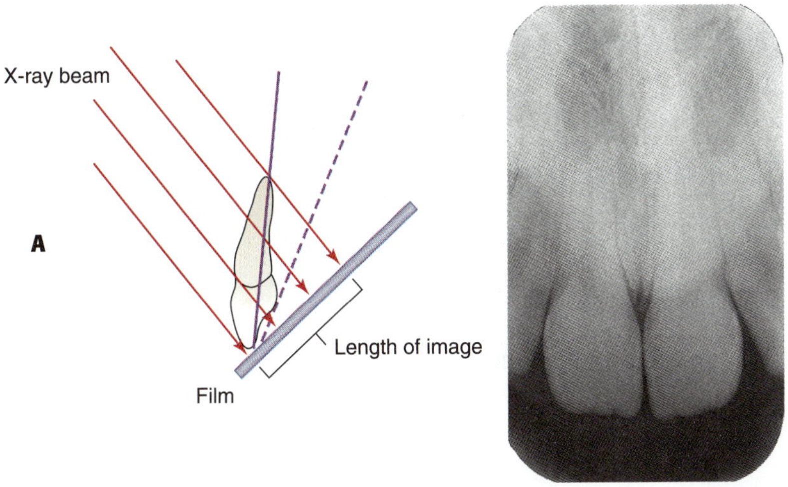

Fig. 41-20 **A,** If the vertical angulation is too steep, the image on the film is *shorter* than the actual tooth. **B,** Foreshortened images. (From Haring JI, Jansen L: *Dental radiography: principles and techniques,* ed 2, Philadelphia, 2000, Saunders.)

To better understand this concept, think of the sun and your own shadow. When the sun (central beam) is high in the sky, your shadow is short. When the sun (central ray) is low in the sky, your shadow appears longer than you actually are.

Foreshortened images

On a foreshortened image, the teeth appear too short. Foreshortening of images results from *excessive* vertical angulation (Fig. 41-20).

Elongated images

On elongated images, the teeth appear too long. Elongation of images is caused by *insufficient* vertical angulation, or vertical angulation that is too "flat" (Fig. 41-21).

Film Size and Placement

In the bisecting technique the film is placed close to the crowns of the teeth to be x-rayed and extends at an angle into the palate or floor of the mouth. The film packet should extend beyond the incisal or occlusal aspect of the teeth by about 1/8 inch. Film holders for the bisection of the angle technique, including some with alignment indicators, are available commercially.

Table 41-1 ***Recommended Vertical Angulation Ranges for Bisecting Technique****

Dentition	Maxillary (Degrees)	Mandibular (Degrees)
Canines	+45 to +55	−20 to −30
Incisors	+40 to +50	−15 to −25
Premolars	+30 to +40	−10 to −15
Molars	+20 to +30	−5 to 0

From Haring JI, Jansen L: Dental radiography: principles and techniques, *ed 2, Philadelphia, 2000, Saunders.*

Patient Positioning

The patient's midsagittal plane should be perpendicular to the floor. This means that the patient's head is upright for maxillary films and tipped back slightly for the mandibular arch.

Size #2 film is used in both the anterior (in a vertical position) and posterior (in a horizontal position) regions. Only three films are needed in the maxillary anterior region because all four maxillary incisors can be imaged on the #2 film if the arch is wide. If the arch is narrow, it may be necessary to use four #1 films.

Beam Alignment

The x-ray beam is directed to pass between the contacts of the teeth being x-rayed in the horizontal dimension, just as it is in the paralleling technique. The vertical angle, however, must be directed at 90 degrees to the imaginary bisecting line. Too much vertical angulation produces images that are too *short* (foreshortened; see Fig. 41-20), and too little vertical angulation results in images that are too *long* (elongated; see Fig. 41-21). The beam must be centered to avoid cone cutting (Procedure 41-4).

Text continues on p. 665

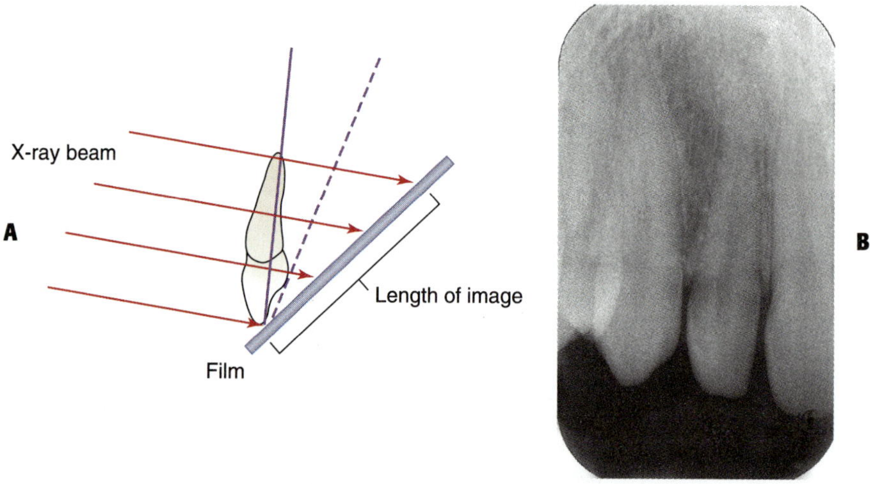

Fig. 41-21 A, If the vertical angulation is too flat, the image on the film is *longer* than the actual tooth. **B,** Elongated images. (From Haring JI, Jansen L: *Dental radiography: principles and techniques,* ed 2, Philadelphia, 2000, Saunders.)

Procedure 41-4 Producing a Full-Mouth Radiographic Survey Using the Bisecting Technique

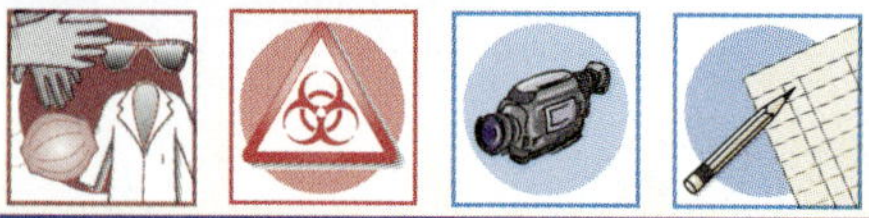

Goal

To produce a full mouth series of radiographs using the bisecting technique.

Equipment and Supplies

- Appropriate number and size of x-ray films
- Appropriate infection-control materials (paper cup, barriers, paper towel, and impervious surface cover)
- Lead apron and thyroid collar
- Sterile packaged EeZee-Grip instruments
- Cotton rolls
- Patient chart

PROCEDURAL STEPS

Preparation Before Seating Patient

1. Prepare the operatory with all infection-control barriers.
   Purpose: Any object that is touched and was not covered with a barrier must be disinfected after the patient is dismissed.
2. Determine the number and type of films to be exposed through a review of the patient's chart, directions from the dentist, or both.
3. Label a paper cup with the patient's name and the date, and place it outside the room where the radiograph machine will be used.
   Purpose: This is the transfer cup for storing and moving exposed films.
4. Turn on the x-ray machine and check the basic settings (kilovoltage, milliamperage, exposure time).
5. Wash and dry hands.
6. Dispense the desired number of films and store them outside the room where the x-ray machine is being used.
   Purpose: This prevents fogging caused by scatter radiation.

Procedure 41-4 Producing a Full-Mouth Radiographic Survey Using the Bisecting Technique—cont'd

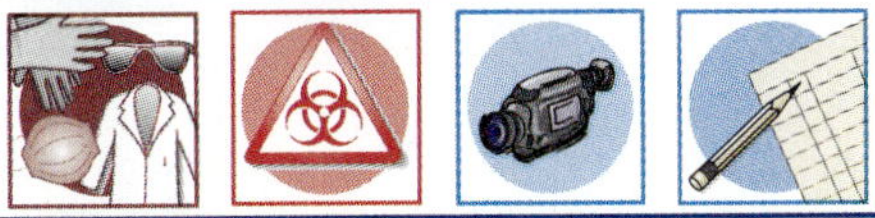

Maxillary Canine Exposure

1. Position the patient so that the occlusal plane is positioned parallel to the floor and the sagittal plane of the patient's face is perpendicular to the floor.
2. Center the film packet on the canine.
3. Position the lower edge of the film holder to the occlusal plane so that it extends about ⅛ inch below the incisal edge of the canine.
4. Instruct the patient to exert light but firm pressure on the lower edge of the film holder.
5. The vertical angulation will range from +45 to +55 degrees.
6. Establish the correct horizontal angulation by directing the central ray between the contacts of the canine and first premolar.
7. Center the PID over the film to avoid cone cutting.
8. Expose the film.

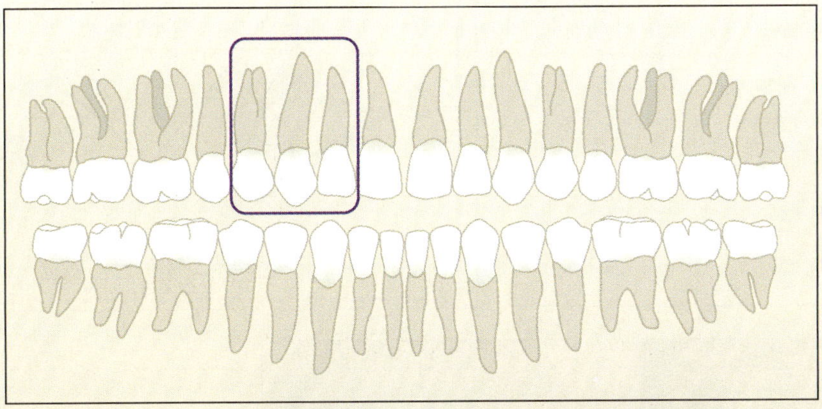

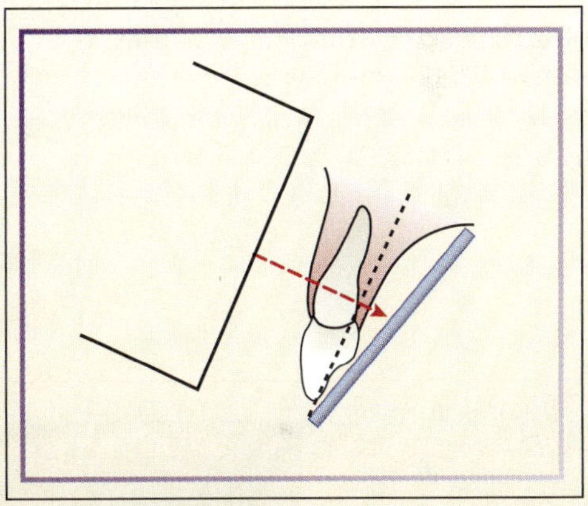

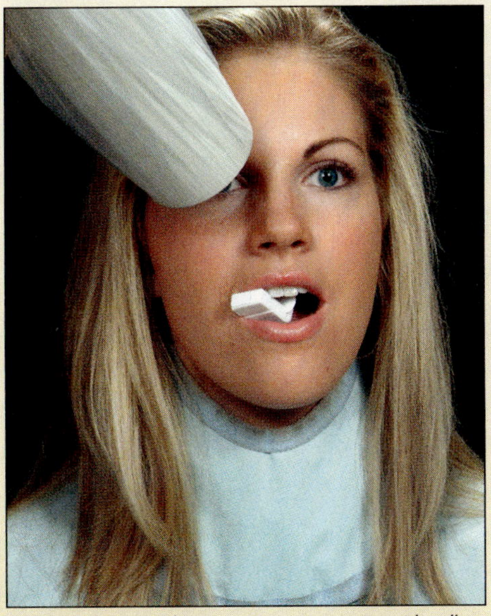

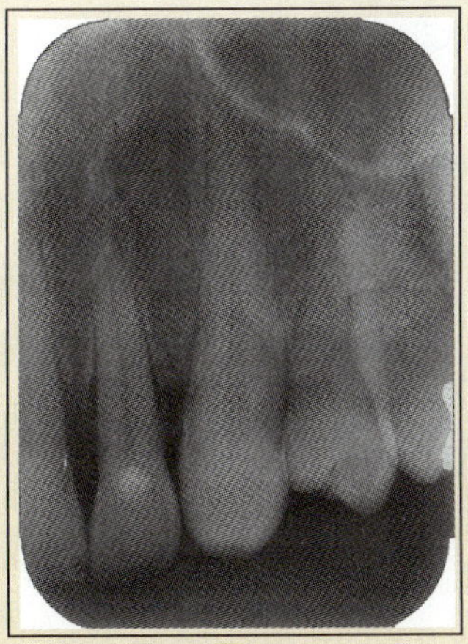

(From Haring JI and Jansen Howerton L: *Dental radiography: principles and techniques*, ed 3, St. Louis, 2006, Saunders.)

continued

Procedure 41-4 Producing a Full-Mouth Radiographic Survey Using the Bisecting Technique—cont'd

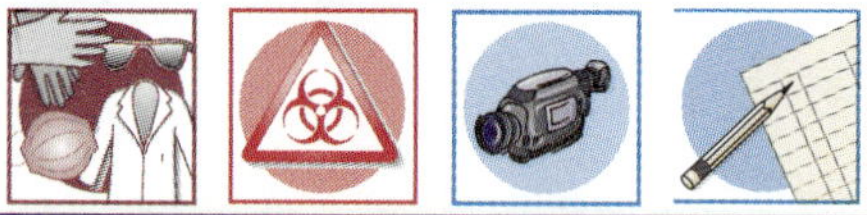

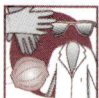

Maxillary Incisor Exposure

1. Position the patient so that the occlusal plane is parallel to the floor and the sagittal plane of the patient's face is perpendicular to the floor.
2. Place the film packet vertically into the film holder.
3. Position the edge of the film holder on the incisal edge of the incisors. Position the film packet as close as possible to the lingual surface of the incisors.
4. Instruct the patient to bite lightly on the edge of the film holder.
5. The vertical angulation will range from +40 to +50 degrees.
6. Establish the correct horizontal angulation by directing the central ray between the contacts of the central incisors.
7. Center the PID over the film to avoid cone cutting.
8. Expose the film.

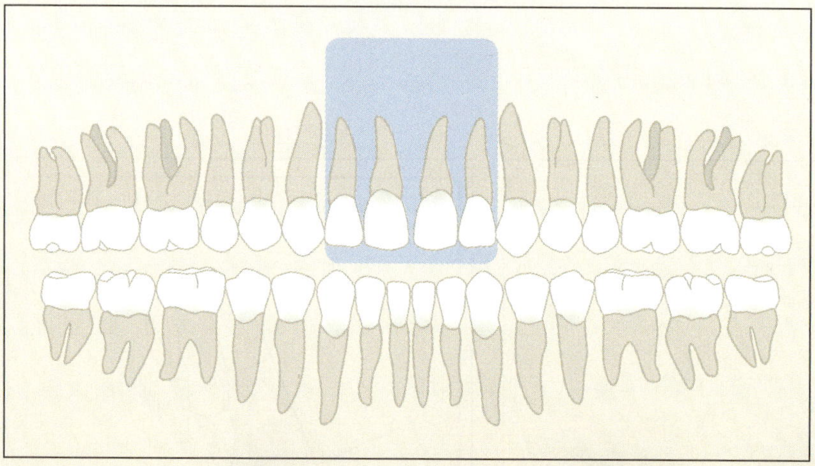

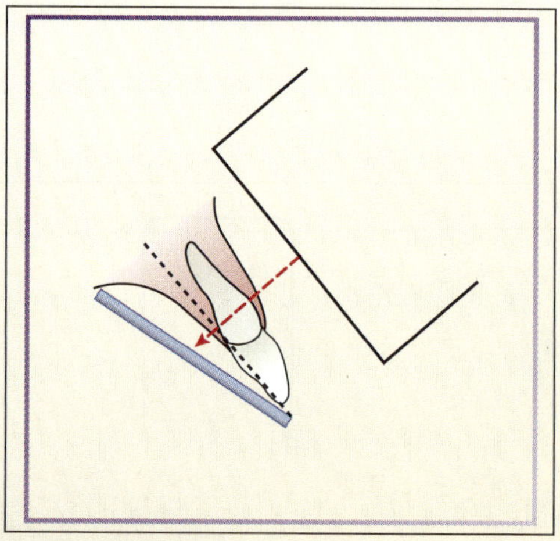

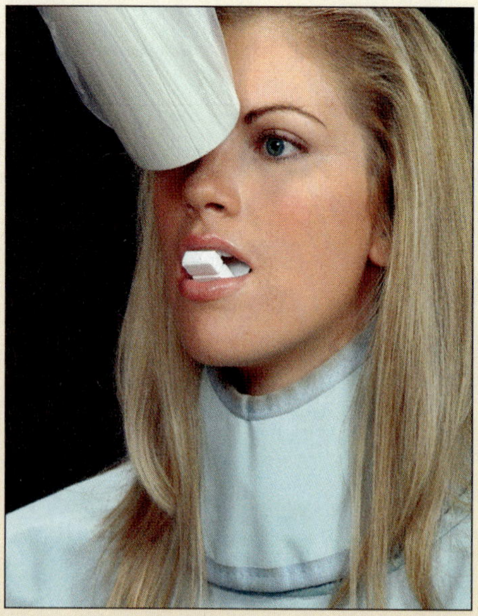

(From Haring JI and Jansen Howerton L: *Dental radiography: principles and techniques*, ed 3, St. Louis, 2006, Saunders.)

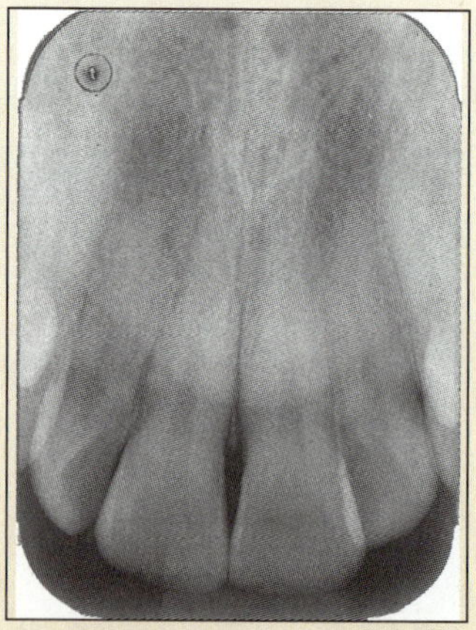

Procedure 41-4 Producing a Full-Mouth Radiographic Survey Using the Bisecting Technique–cont'd

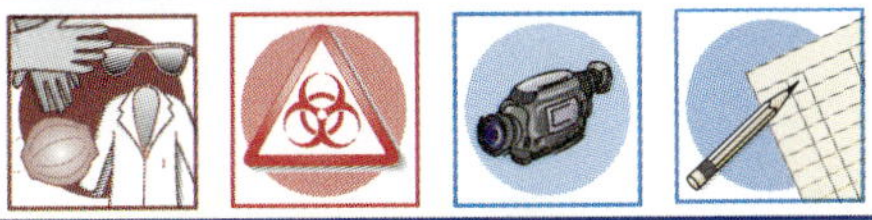

Mandibular Canine Exposure

1. Position the patient so that when the mouth is open, the maxillary occlusal plane is parallel to the floor and the sagittal plane of the patient's face is perpendicular to the floor.
2. Place the film packet horizontally into the film holder.
3. Position the edge of the film holder on the incisal edge of the canine.
4. Instruct the patient to bite lightly but firmly on the edge of the film holder.
5. The vertical angulation will range from −20 to −30 degrees
6. Establish the correct horizontal angulation by directing the central ray between the contacts of the canine and first premolar.
7. Center the PID over the film to avoid cone cutting.
8. Expose the film.

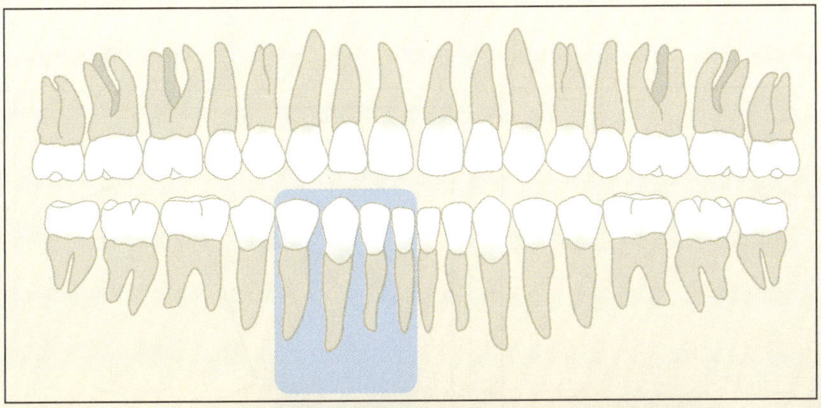

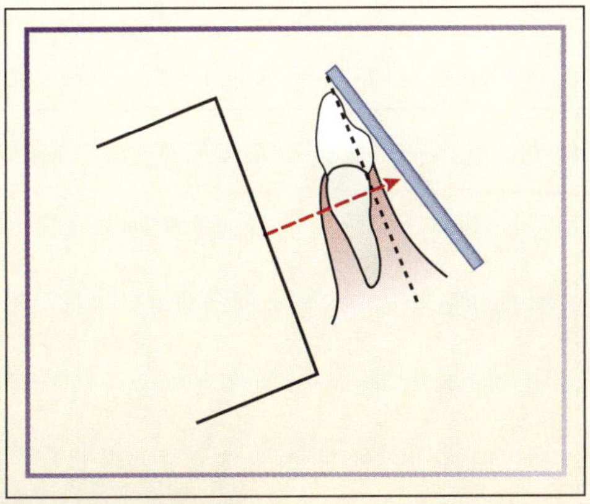

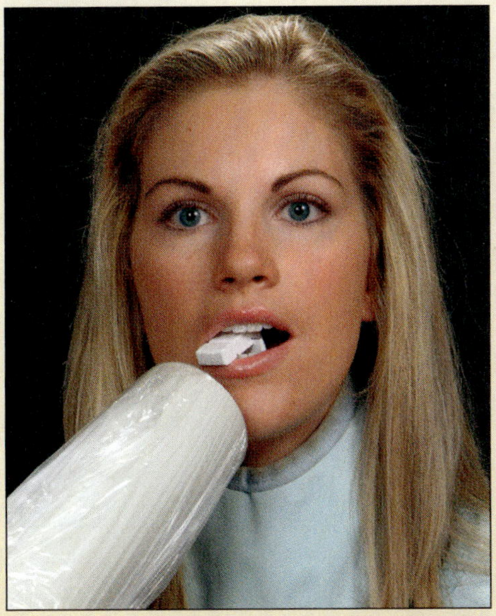

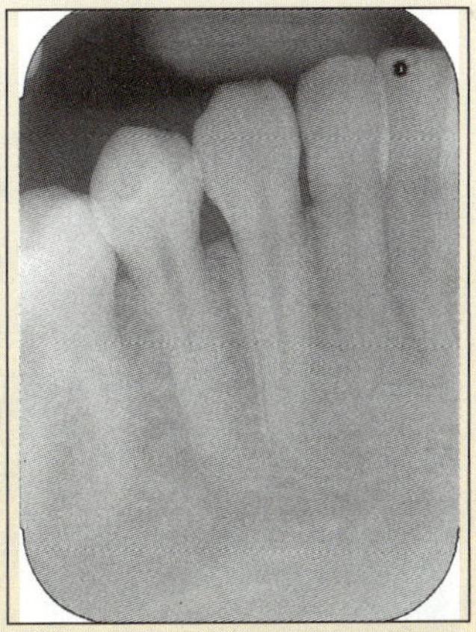

(From Haring JI and Jansen Howerton L: *Dental radiography: principles and techniques*, ed 3, St. Louis, 2006, Saunders.)

continued

Procedure 41-4 Producing a Full-Mouth Radiographic Survey Using the Bisecting Technique—cont'd

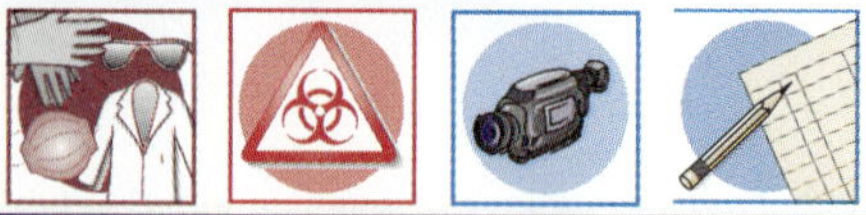

Mandibular Incisor Exposure

1. Position the patient so that when the mouth is open, the mandibular occlusal plane is parallel to the floor and the sagittal plane of the patient's face is perpendicular to the floor.
2. Place the film packet vertically into the film holder.
3. Center the film packet on the contact between the two central incisors and against the lingual surfaces of the incisors.
4. Instruct the patient to bite lightly but firmly on the edge of the film holder.
5. The vertical angulation will range from −15 to −25 degrees.
6. Establish the correct horizontal angulation by directing the central ray between the contacts of the central incisors.
7. Center the PID over the film to avoid cone cutting.
8. Expose the film.

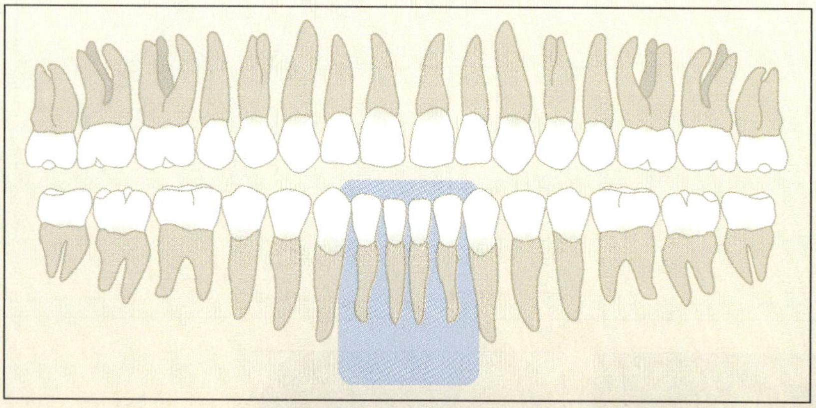

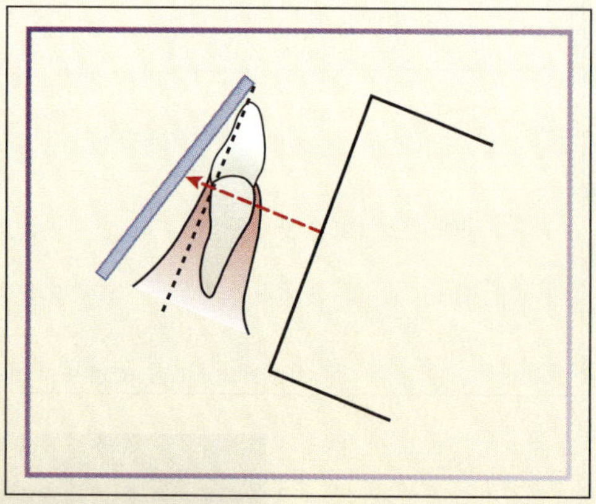

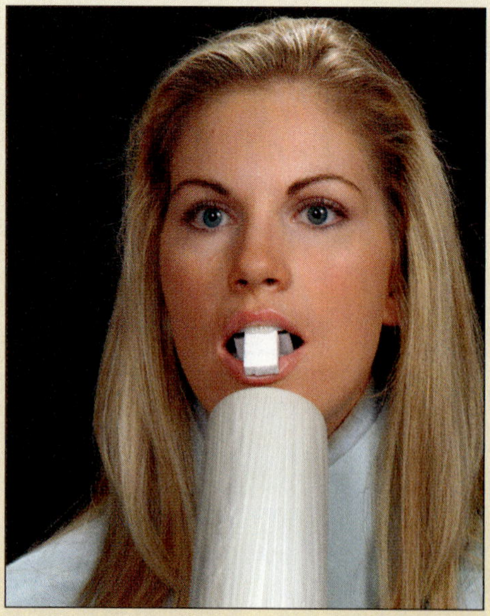

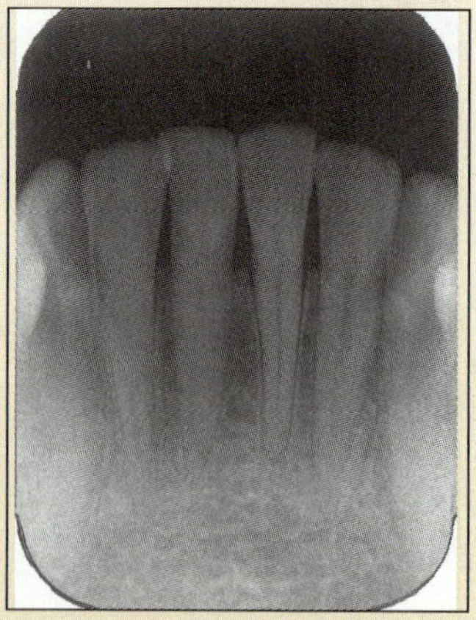

(From Haring JI and Jansen Howerton L: *Dental radiography: principles and techniques*, ed 3, St. Louis, 2006, Saunders.)

Procedure 41-4 Producing a Full-Mouth Radiographic Survey Using the Bisecting Technique—cont'd

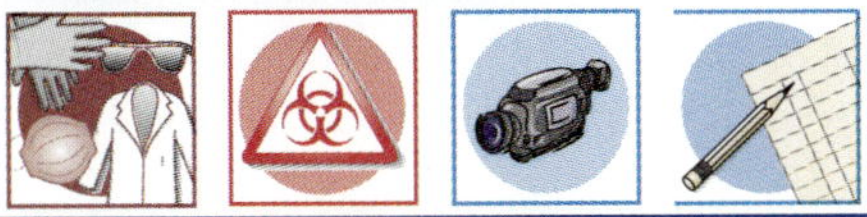

Maxillary Premolar Exposure

1. Position the patient so that when the mouth is open, the maxillary occlusal plane is parallel to the floor and the sagittal plane of the patient's face is perpendicular to the floor.
2. Place the film packet horizontally into the film holder.
3. Center the film packet on the second premolar and against the lingual surfaces of the teeth. Avoid shaping the packet to the arch.
4. The central ray is directed at the most anterior part of the cheekbone. The vertical angulation will range from +30 to +40 degrees.
5. Establish the correct horizontal angulation by directing the central ray between the contacts of the premolars.
6. Center the PID over the film to avoid cone cutting.
7. Expose the film.

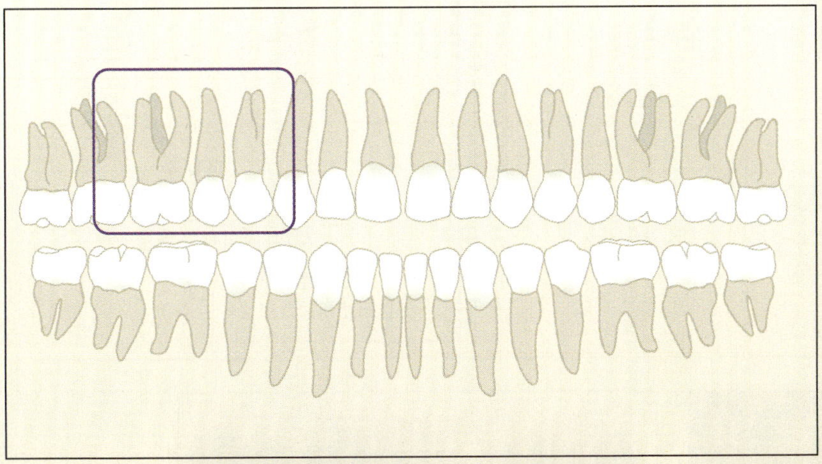

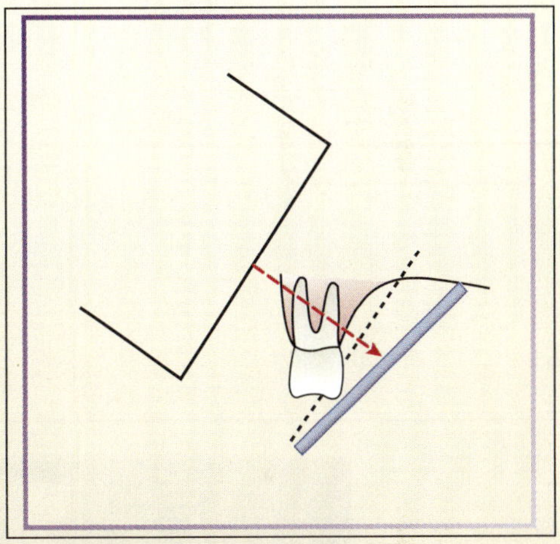

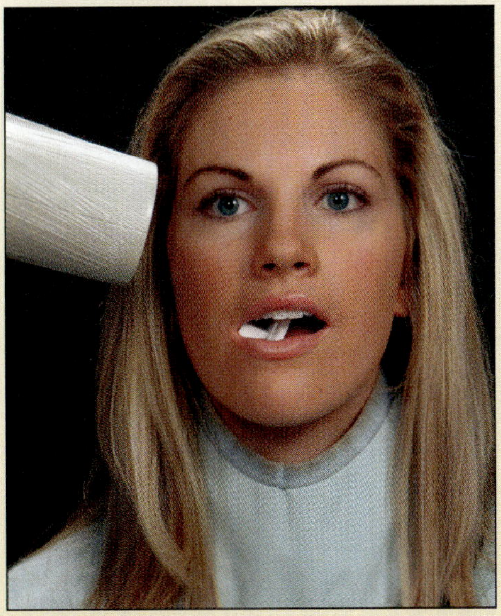

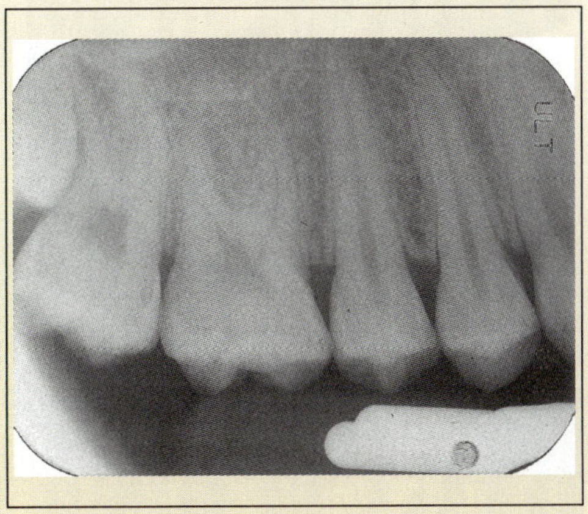

(From Haring JI and Jansen Howerton L: *Dental radiography: principles and techniques*, ed 3, St. Louis, 2006, Saunders.)

continued

Procedure 41-4 Producing a Full-Mouth Radiographic Survey Using the Bisecting Technique—cont'd

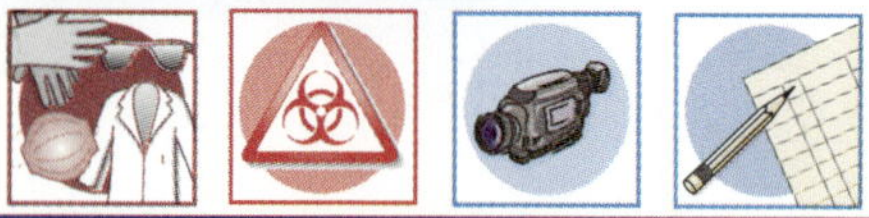

Maxillary Molar Exposure

1. Position the patient so that when the mouth is open, the maxillary occlusal plane is parallel to the floor and the sagittal plane of the patient's face is perpendicular to the floor.
2. Place the film packet horizontally into the film holder.
3. Center the film packet on the second molar, and place it against the lingual surfaces of the teeth.
4. The central ray is directed through the zygomatic arch at the center of the film. The distal edge of the PID should not be distal to the outer corner of the eye. The vertical angulation will range from +20 to +30 degrees.
5. Establish the correct horizontal angulation by directing the central ray between the contacts of the molars.
6. Center the PID over the film to avoid cone cutting.
7. Expose the film.

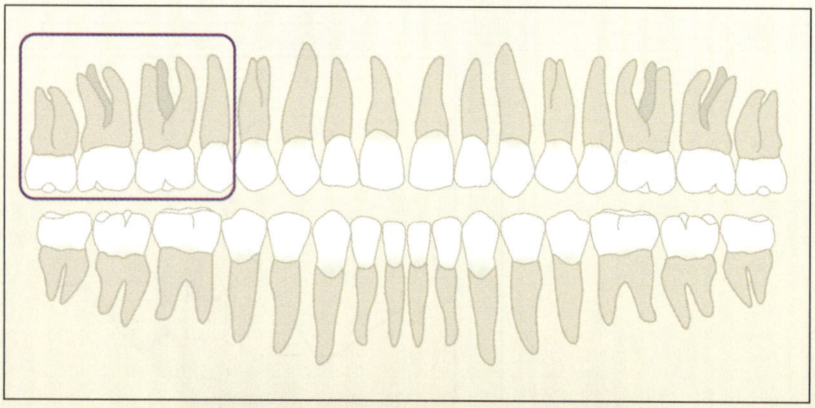

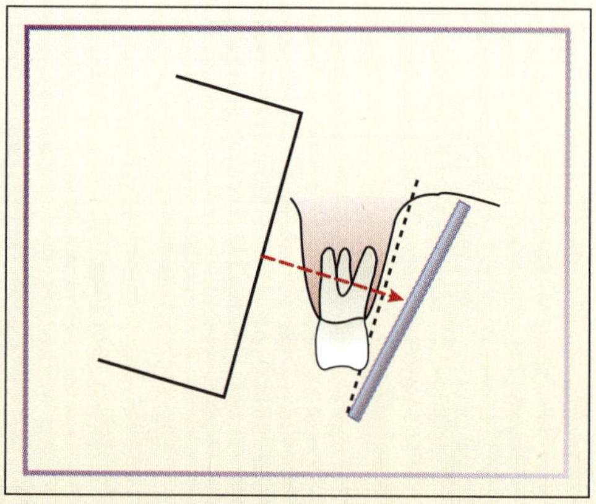

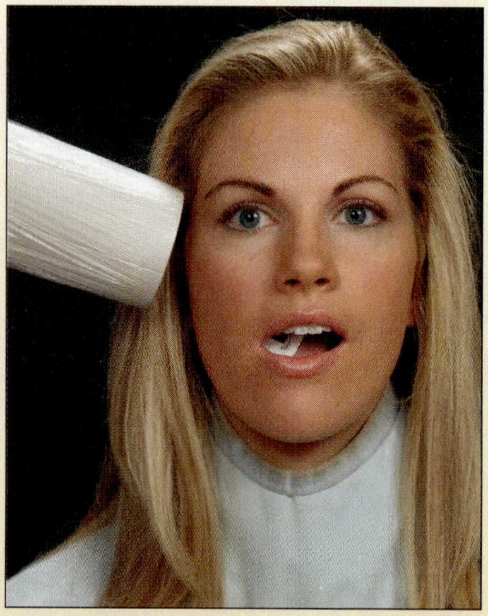

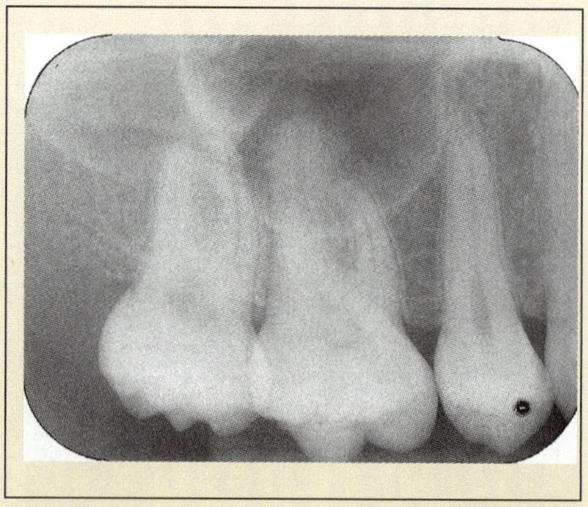

(From Haring JI and Jansen Howerton L: *Dental radiography: principles and techniques*, ed 3, St. Louis, 2006, Saunders.)

Procedure 41-4 Producing a Full-Mouth Radiographic Survey Using the Bisecting Technique–cont'd

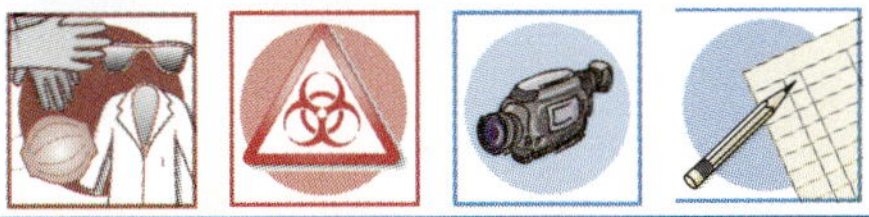

Mandibular Premolar Exposure

1. Position the patient so that when the mouth is open, the mandibular occlusal plane is parallel to the floor and the sagittal plane of the patient's face is perpendicular to the floor.
2. Place the film packet horizontally into the film holder.
3. Center the film packet on the second premolar; the front edge of the film should be aligned with the mesial aspect of the canine. Position the film packet against the lingual surfaces of the teeth.
4. Instruct the patient to bite gently but firmly on the film holder.
5. The central ray is directed at the mental foramen, aimed at the center of the film packet. The vertical angulation will range from −10 to −15 degrees.
6. Establish the correct horizontal angulation by directing the central ray between the contacts of the premolars.
7. Center the PID over the film to avoid cone cutting.
8. Expose the film.

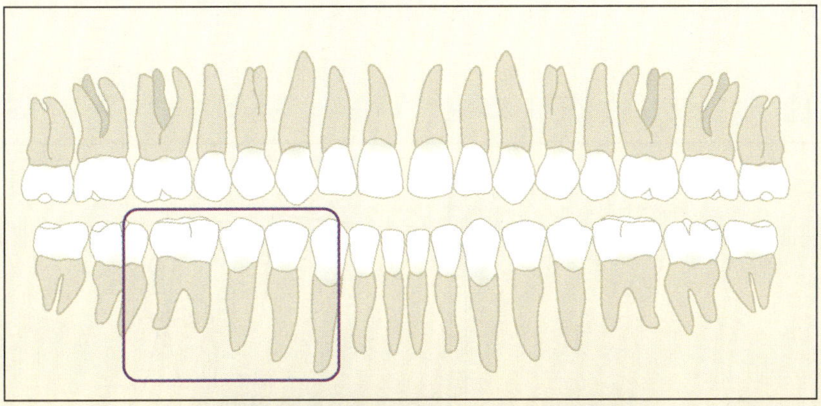

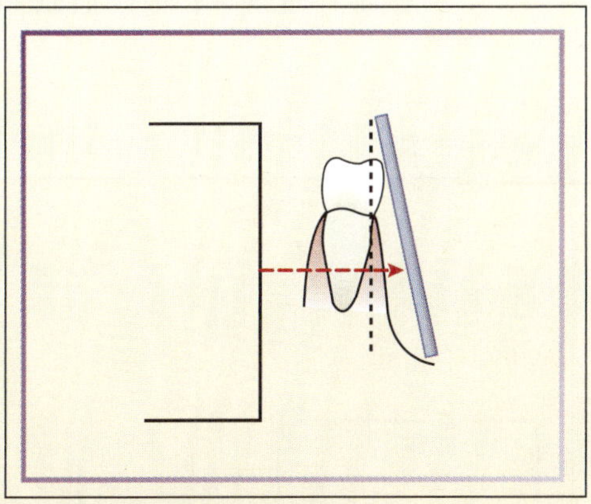

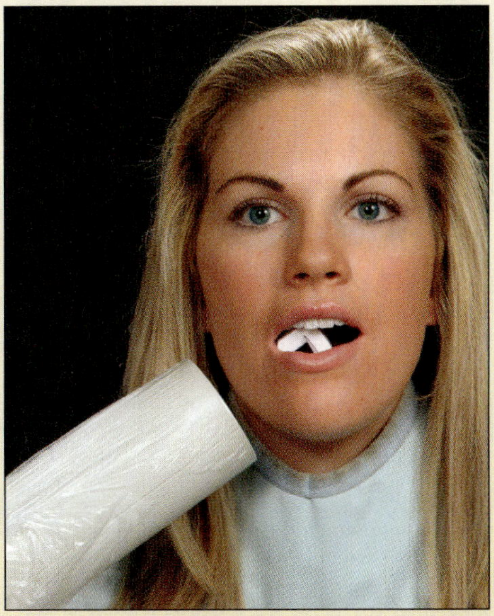

(From Haring JI and Jansen Howerton L: *Dental radiography: principles and techniques*, ed 3, St. Louis, 2006, Saunders.)

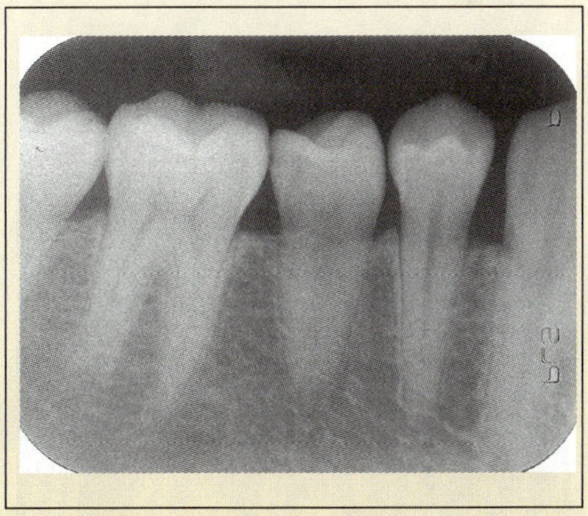

continued

Procedure 41-4 Producing a Full-Mouth Radiographic Survey Using the Bisecting Technique—cont'd

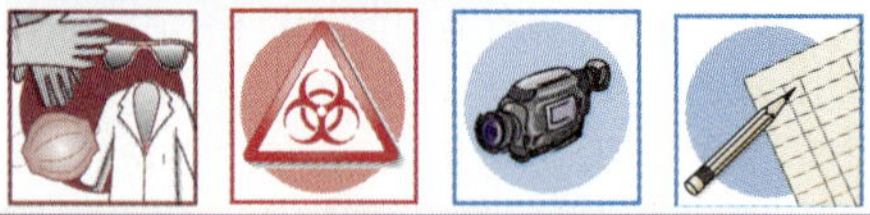

Mandibular Molar Exposure

1. Position the patient so that when the mouth is open, the mandibular occlusal plane is parallel to the floor and the sagittal plane of the patient's face is perpendicular to the floor.
2. Place the film packet horizontally into the film holder.
3. Center the film holder and film packet on the second molar; the front edge of the film should be aligned with the midline of the second premolar.

   Note: Because of the anatomy of the area, the film packet is almost parallel to the long axis of the tooth; therefore most molars radiographed with the bisecting technique are actually parallel films.
4. Instruct the patient to bite gently but firmly on the film holder.

   Note: You may have to ask the patient to raise the chin so that the occlusal surfaces are parallel to the floor.
5. The central ray is directed at the roots of the molars. The vertical angulation will range from −5 to 0 degrees.
6. Establish the correct horizontal angulation by directing the central ray between the contacts of the molars.
7. Center the PID over the film to avoid cone cutting.
8. Expose the film.

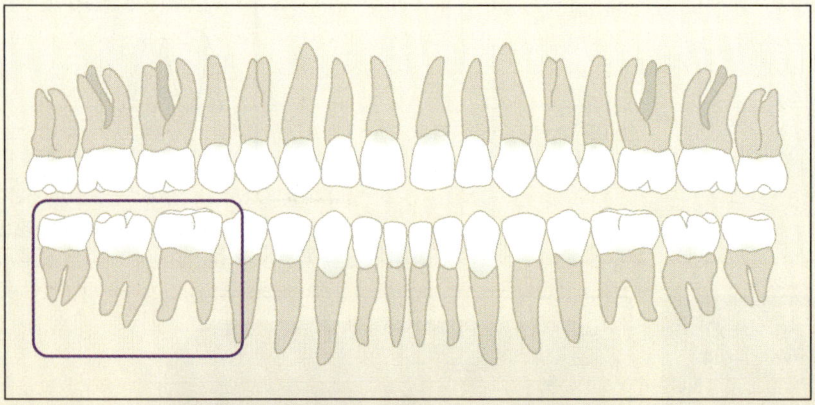

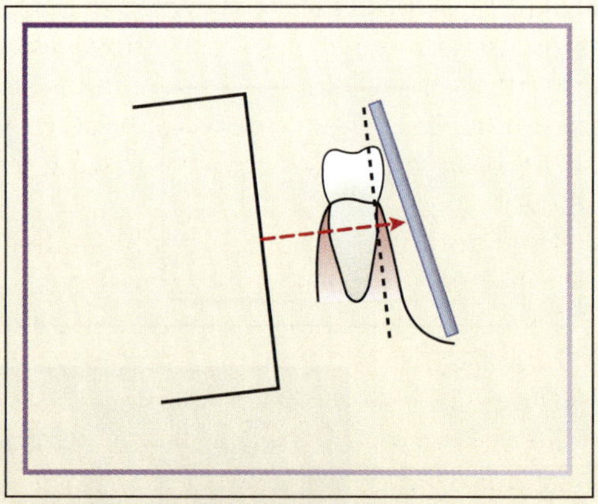

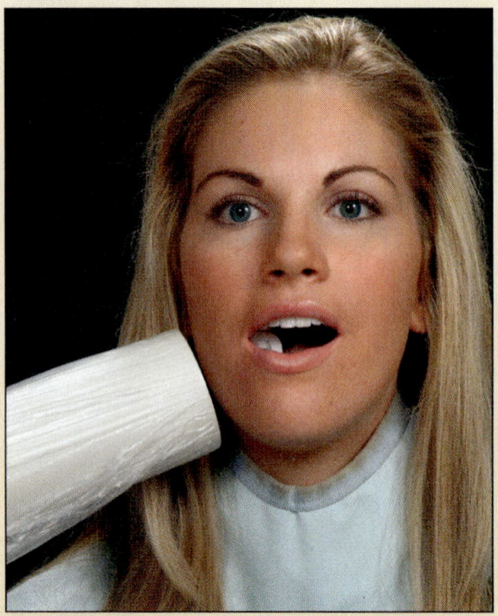

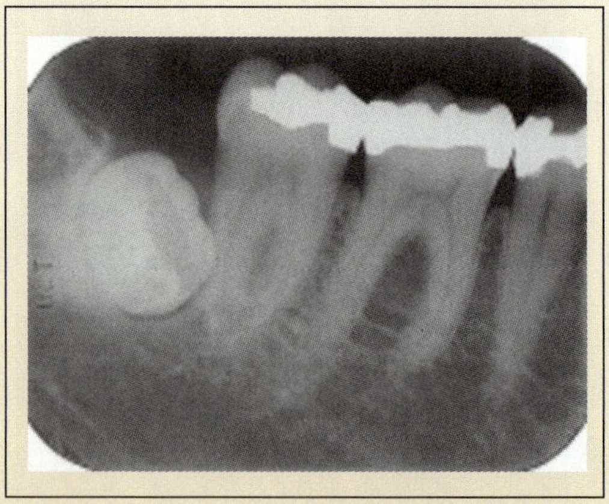

(From Haring JI and Jansen Howerton L: *Dental radiography: principles and techniques*, ed 3, St. Louis, 2006, Saunders.)

Recall

6. Why is it not recommended to have the patient hold the film during exposure?
7. What type of film holders can be used in the bisecting technique?
8. What error occurs when the horizontal angulation is incorrect?
9. What two errors occur when the vertical angulation is incorrect?
10. In the bisecting technique, how is the film placed in relation to the teeth?

BITE-WING TECHNIQUE

A **bite-wing film** shows the crowns and interproximal areas of the maxillary and mandibular teeth and the areas of **crestal bone** on one film. Bite-wing radiographs are used to detect interproximal caries (tooth decay) and are particularly useful in detecting early carious lesions that are not clinically evident. Bite-wing radiographs are also useful in examining the crestal bone levels between the teeth.

The basic principles of the bite-wing technique are as follows:

1. The film is placed in the mouth parallel to the crowns of both the upper and the lower teeth.
2. The film is stabilized when the patient bites on the bite-wing tab or bite-wing film holder.
3. The central ray of the x-ray beam is directed through the contacts of the teeth, using +10 degrees of vertical angulation (Fig. 41-22).

Film Holder and Bite-Wing Tab

In the bite-wing technique, either a film holder or a bite-wing tab is used to stabilize the film (Fig. 41-23).

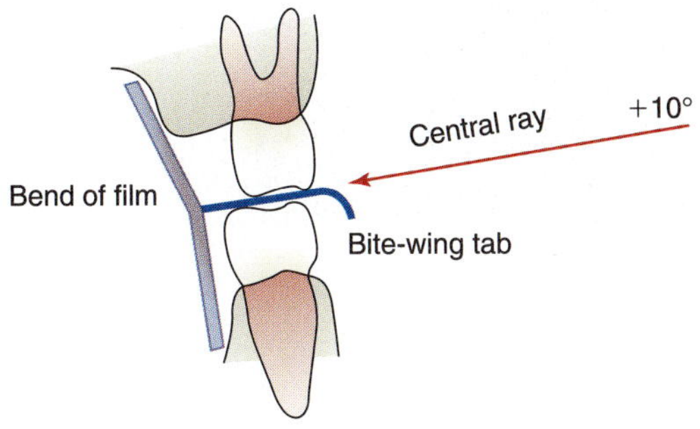

Fig. 41-22 Vertical angulation of +10 degrees is used to compensate for the slight bend of the upper portion of the film and the tilt of the maxillary teeth. (From Haring JI, Jansen L: *Dental radiography: principles and techniques,* ed 2, Philadelphia, 2000, Saunders.)

Angulation of Position Indicator Device

The angulation of the PID is critical in the bite-wing technique. The film-holding instruments and aiming rings provide the proper angulation. When a bite-wing tab is used, however, the operator must determine both the horizontal and the vertical angulation. Even a slight error will result in a film that is not diagnostic.

Exposure for Film Placement

Bite-wing films are always parallel films regardless of the technique used for the periapical radiographs. The number of bite-wing films necessary is based on the curvature of the arch and the number of teeth present in the posterior areas. The curvature of the arch often differs in the premolar and molar areas. If the curvature of the arch differs, it is impossible to open *all* the posterior contact areas on one bite-wing film. Consequently, two bite-wing films are usually exposed on each side of the arch.

Because the curvature of the arch differs in most adult patients, a total of four bite-wing films are exposed: one right premolar, one right molar, one left premolar, and one left molar. The film is positioned (with either a bite tab or a film-holding device) parallel to the crowns of both upper and lower teeth, and the central ray is directed perpendicular to the film.

The *premolar* bite-wing radiograph should include the distal half of the crowns of the canines, both premolars, and often the first molars on both maxillary and mandibular arches. The *molar* film should be centered over the second molars (Procedure 41-5).

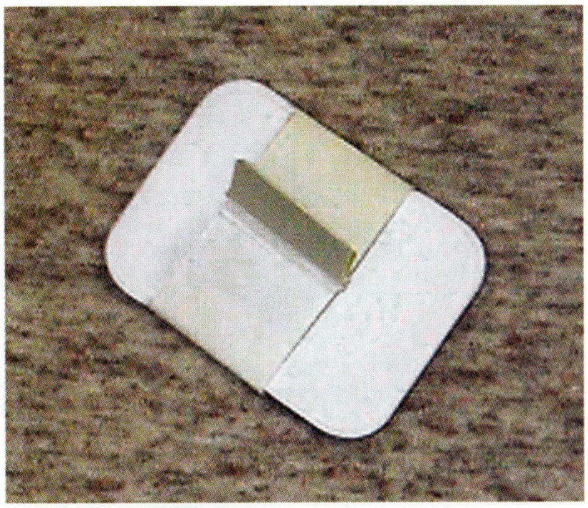

Fig. 41-23 Bite-wing tab and film holder.

Procedure 41-5 Producing a Four-Film Radiographic Survey Using the Bite-Wing Technique

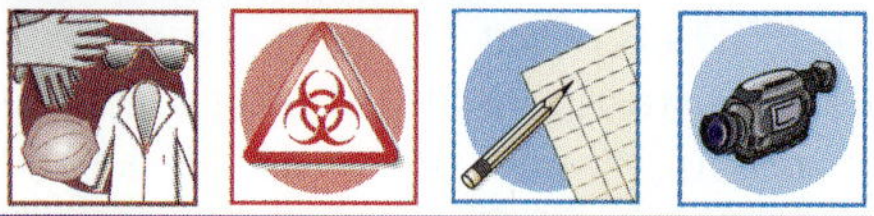

Goal

To produce a four-film series of radiographs using the bite-wing technique.

Equipment and Supplies

- Four size #2 films
- Paper cup
- Lead apron and thyroid collar
- Bite-wing tab or film-holding device

PROCEDURAL STEPS

Premolar Bite-Wing Exposure

1. Set vertical angulation at +10 degrees.
   Purpose: A positive angulation means that the PID points downward. This places the beam so that it is nearly perpendicular to both upper and lower halves of the film.
2. Position the patient so that the occlusal plane is parallel to the floor. If necessary, ask the patient to lower or raise the chin.
3. Position the film in the patient's mouth by placing the lower half between the tongue and mandibular teeth. Position the film with the anterior border at the middle of the canine.
4. Hold the film in place by pressing the tab over the occlusal aspect of the mandibular teeth.
   Purpose: To prevent the film from slipping out of position.
5. Ask the patient to close the mouth slowly. Take care not to allow the patient to close on the fingertip of your glove.
6. Do not pull the film too tightly against the lower teeth as the patient closes the mouth.
   Purpose: This can cause the film to push against the lingual aspect of the maxillary alveolar ridge and force the film down into the floor of the mouth.
7. Stand in front of the patient to set the horizontal angulation. To better visualize the curvature of the arch, place your index finger along the premolar area. Align the open end of the PID parallel with your index finger and the curvature of the arch in the premolar area.

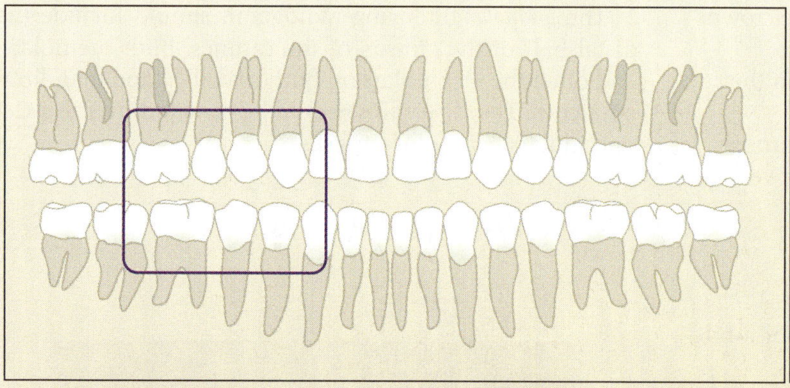

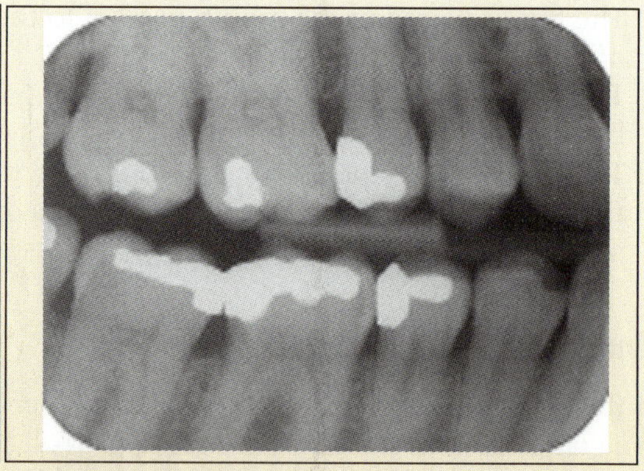

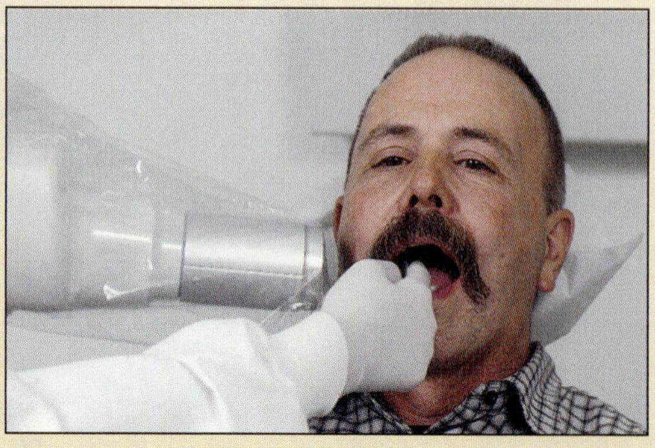

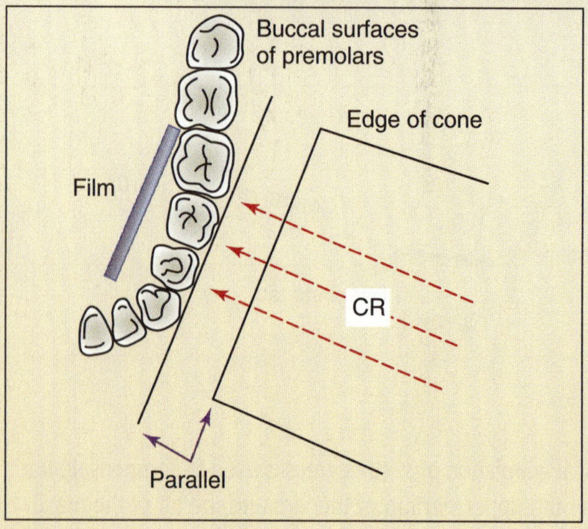

Procedure 41-5 Producing a Four-Film Radiographic Survey Using the Bite-Wing Technique—cont'd

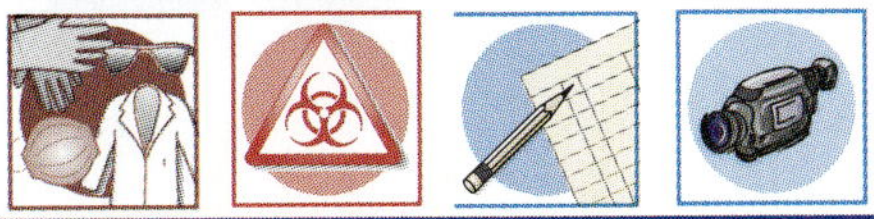

Molar Bite-Wing Exposure

1. Set vertical angulation at +10 degrees.
   Purpose: A positive angulation means that the PID points downward. This places the beam so that it is nearly perpendicular to both upper and lower halves of the film.
2. Position the patient so that the occlusal plane is parallel with the floor. If necessary, ask the patient to lower or raise the chin.
3. Position the film in the patient's mouth by placing the lower half between the tongue and mandibular teeth. Center the film on the second molar; the front edge of the film should be aligned with the middle of the mandibular second premolar.
4. Hold the film in place by pressing the tab over the occlusal aspect of the mandibular teeth.
   Purpose: To prevent the film from slipping out of position.
5. Ask the patient to close the mouth slowly. Take care not to allow the patient to close on the fingertip of your glove.
6. Do not pull the film too tightly against the lower teeth as the patient closes the mouth.
   Purpose: This can cause the film to push against the lingual aspect of the maxillary alveolar ridge and force the film down into the floor of the mouth.
7. Stand in front of the patient to set the horizontal angulation. To better visualize the curvature of the arch, place your index finger along the premolar area. Align the open end of the PID parallel with your index finger and the curvature of the arch in the molar area.
   Purpose: Different film placement and horizontal angulations are needed to open the proximal contact areas.

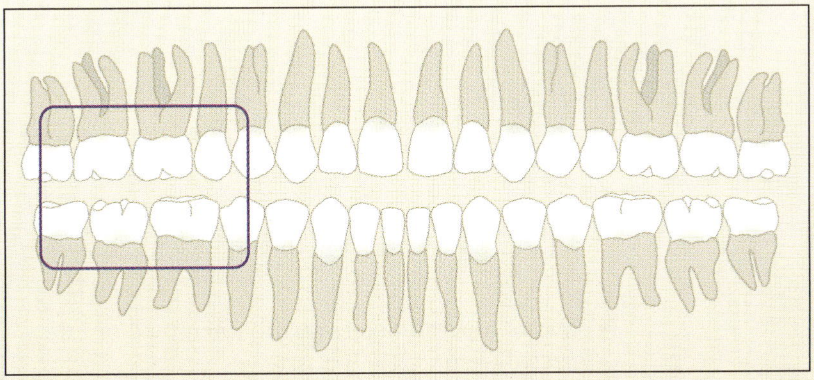

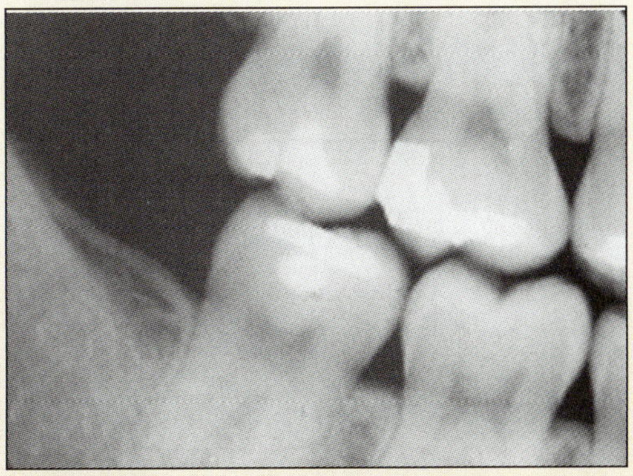

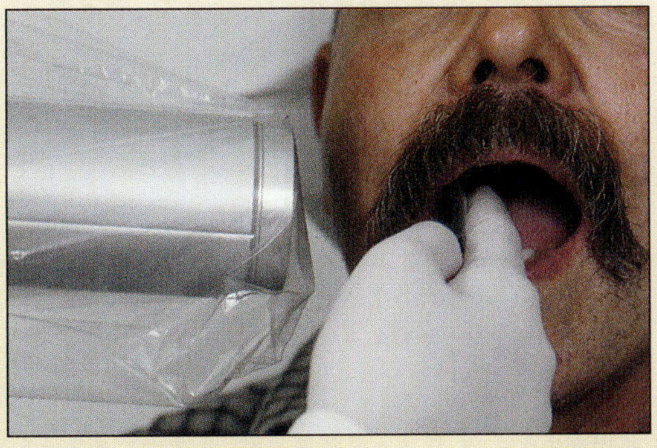

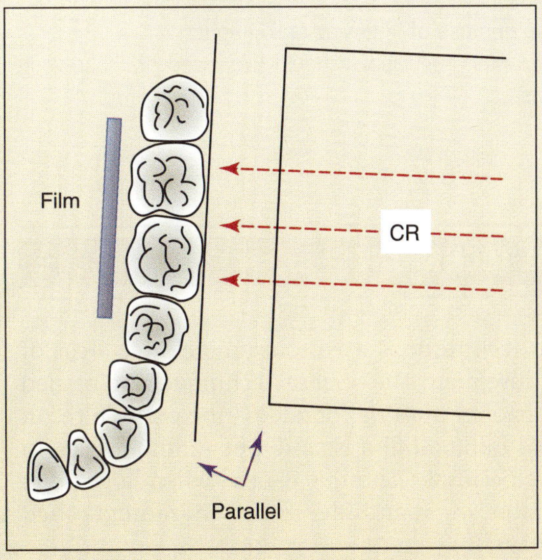

continued

Procedure 41-5 Producing a Four-Film Radiographic Survey Using the Bite-Wing Technique—cont'd

8. Make certain that the PID is positioned far enough forward to cover both the maxillary and the mandibular canines to avoid a cone cut.
   Purpose: To check for a cone cut, stand directly behind the tubehead and look along the side of the PID. No portion of the film should be visible; the film should be covered by the PID.
9. Direct the central ray through the contact areas.
10. Expose the film.

Recall

11. What is the purpose of bite-wing radiographs?
12. What horizontal angulation should be used for bite-wing radiographs?

OCCLUSAL TECHNIQUE

The **occlusal technique** is used to examine large areas of the upper or lower jaw. The occlusal technique is so named because the patient bites or "occludes" the entire film. In adults, size #4 intraoral film is used, but #2 film is used in children. The occlusal technique is used when large areas of the maxilla or mandible must be radiographed (Procedure 41-6).

Occlusal radiographs can be used for the following purposes:

- Locate retained roots of extracted teeth
- Locate supernumerary (extra) unerupted or impacted teeth
- Locate salivary stones in duct of the submandibular gland
- Locate fractures of the maxilla and mandible
- Examine the area of a cleft palate
- Measure changes in the size and shape of the maxilla or mandible

The basic principles of the occlusal technique follow:

1. The film is positioned with the white side facing the arch being exposed.
2. The film is placed in the mouth between the occlusal surfaces of the maxillary and mandibular teeth.
3. The film is stabilized when the patient gently bites on the surface of the film.

Recall

13. What size film is used in the occlusal technique?
14. When are occlusal radiographs indicated?

Procedure 41-6 Producing Maxillary and Mandibular Radiographs Using the Occlusal Technique

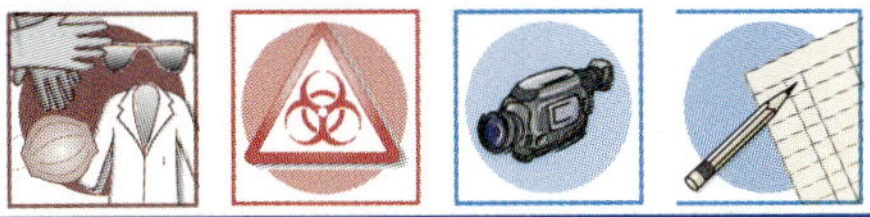

Goal

To follow the steps of the occlusal technique in producing diagnostic-quality maxillary and mandibular x-ray films.

Equipment and Supplies

- Two #4 films
- Paper cup
- Lead apron and thyroid collar

PROCEDURAL STEPS

Maxillary Occlusal Technique

1. Ask the patient to remove prosthetic appliances or objects from the mouth.
2. Place the lead apron and thyroid collar.
3. Position the patient's head so the film plane is parallel to the floor and the midsagittal plane is perpendicular to the floor.
4. Place the film packet in the patient's mouth with the white side of the film on the occlusal surfaces of the maxillary teeth. The long edge of the film is placed in a side-to-side direction.
5. Place the film as far posterior as possible.
6. Position the PID so that the central ray (CR) is directed at +65 degrees through the center of the film. The top edge of the PID is placed between the eyebrows on the bridge of the nose.

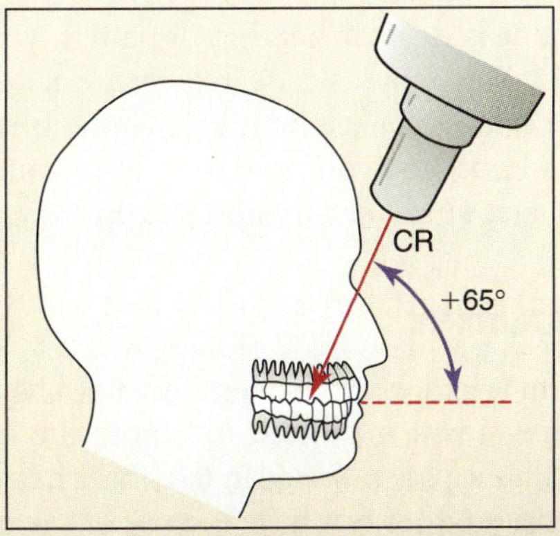

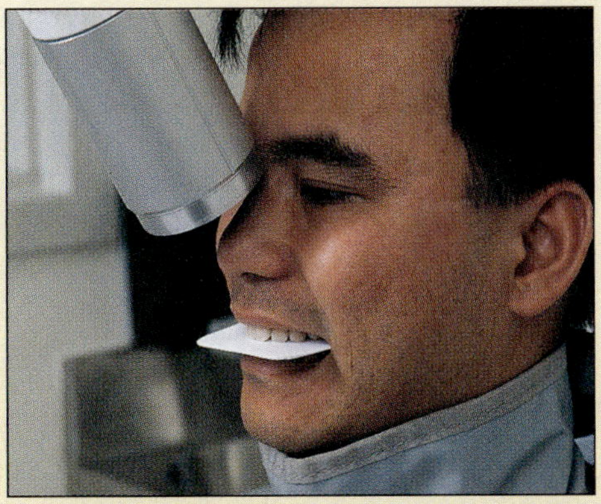

7. Press the x-ray machine activating button and make the exposure.

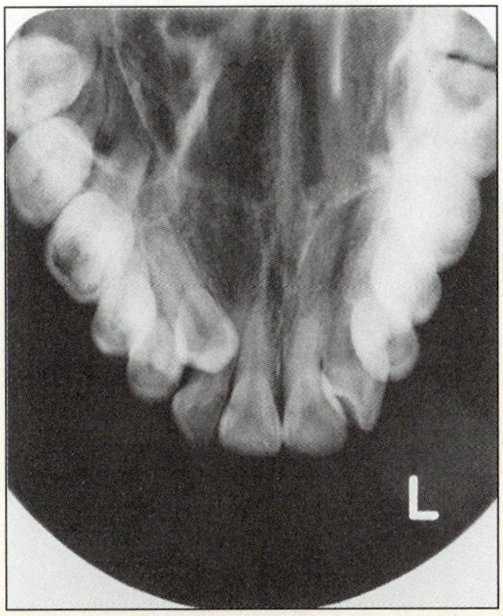

8. Document the procedure.

Mandibular Occlusal Technique

1. Recline the patient and position the head with the midsagittal plane perpendicular to the floor.
2. Place the film packet in the patient's mouth with the white side of the film on the occlusal surfaces of the mandibular teeth. The long edge of the film is placed in a side-to-side direction.
3. Position the film as far posterior on the mandible as possible.
4. Position the PID so that the CR is directed at a 90-degree angle to the center of the film packet. The PID should be centered about 1 inch below the chin.

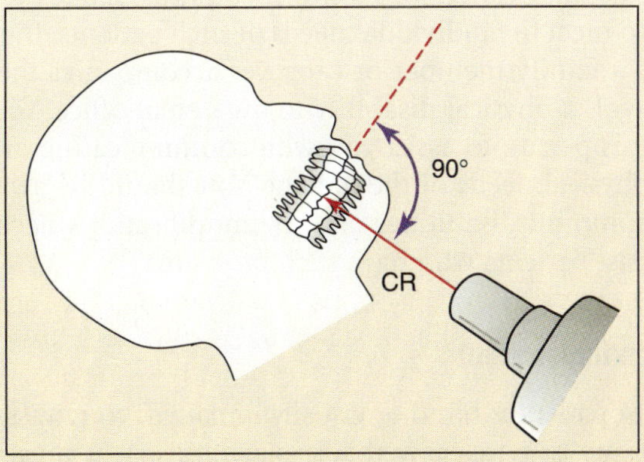

continued

Procedure 41-6 Producing Maxillary and Mandibular Radiographs Using the Occlusal Technique—cont'd

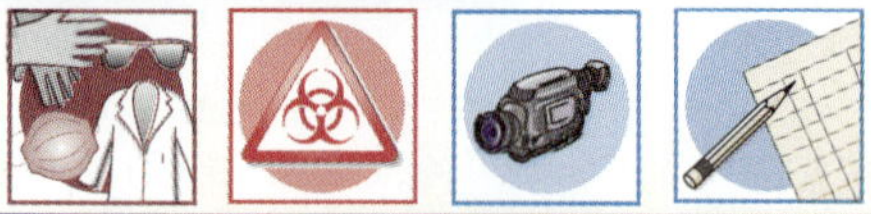

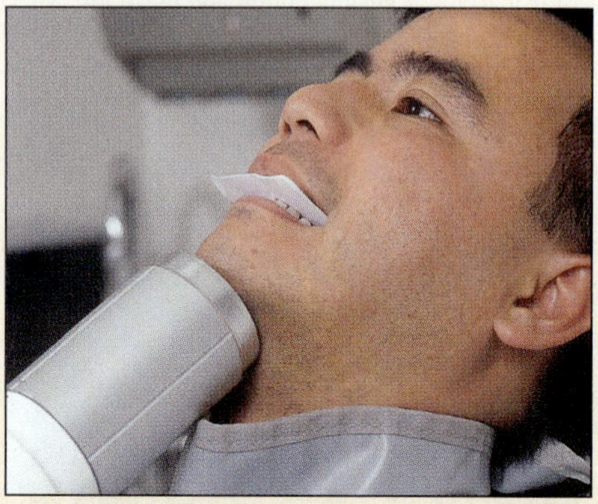

5. Press the x-ray machine activating button and make the exposure.

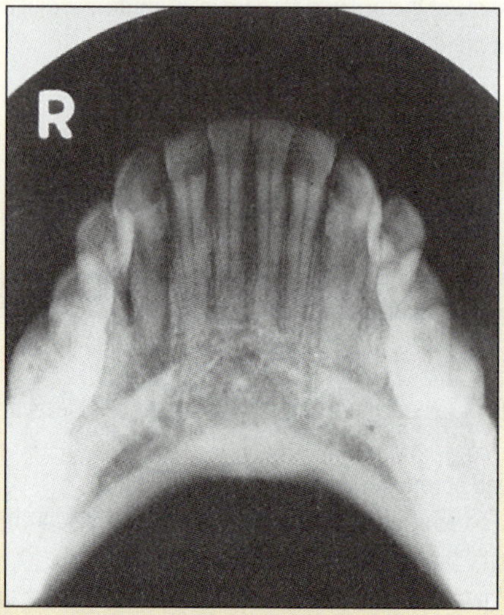

6. Document the procedure.

PATIENTS WITH SPECIAL MEDICAL NEEDS

Radiographic examination techniques must often be modified to accommodate patients with special needs. You must be prepared to alter your radiographic technique to meet the specific need of the individual patient.

A person with a **physical disability** may have problems with vision, hearing, or mobility. You must make every effort to meet the individual needs of such patients. In many cases a family member or caregiver accompanies the person with a physical disability to the dental office. You can ask this person to assist you with communicating or with the physical needs of the patient. You should be aware of the common disabilities and the modifications necessary to assist patients who have such problems.

Vision Impairment

If your patient is blind or visually impaired, you must communicate using clear verbal explanations. You must keep your patient informed of what you are doing and explain each procedure *before* performing it. You must *never* gesture to another person in the presence of a person who is blind. Blind persons are sensitive to this form of communication and perceive that you are "talking behind their backs."

Hearing Impairment

If your patient is deaf or hearing-impaired, you have several options. You may ask a caregiver to act as an interpreter, use gestures, or use written instructions. If the patient can read lips, you will need to remove your mask, face the patient, and speak clearly and slowly.

Mobility Impairment

If your patient is in a wheelchair and does not have the use of the lower limbs, you may need to expose the necessary radiographs with the patient seated in the wheelchair (Fig. 41-24).

If your patient does not have the use of the upper limbs and a film holder cannot be used to stabilize the films in the mouth, you may ask the patient's caregiver to assist with holding the film. This person must wear a lead apron and thyroid collar during the exposure of the films. In this case, give the caregiver specific instructions on how to hold the film or patient.

Remember, regardless of the situation, you must *never* hold a film for a patient during an exposure.

Developmental Disabilities

A **developmental disability** is a substantial impairment of mental or physical functioning that occurs before adulthood

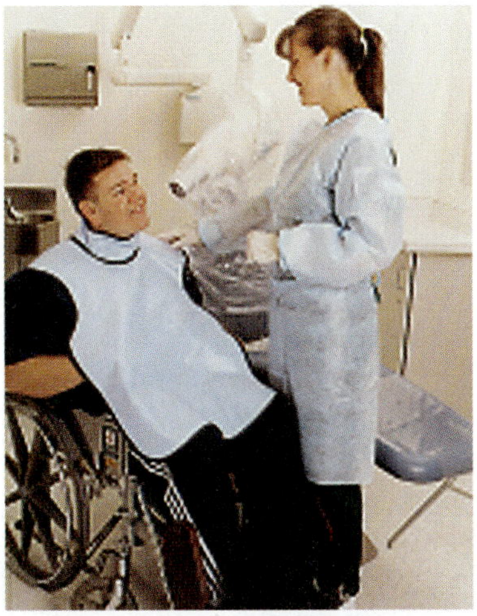

Fig. 41-24 Wheelchair-bound patient having x-rays taken.

Guidelines for Dental Treatment of Patients with Disabilities

1. Do *not* ask personal questions about the patient's disability.
2. *Do* offer assistance, for example, to push a wheelchair or direct a person who is blind. Often a blind patient may prefer to hold your arm rather than having you hold the patient's arm.
3. *Do* talk directly to the person with a disability. It is rude to talk to the caregiver instead of the patient. For example, instead of asking the caregiver, "Can Mrs. Jones get out of her wheelchair?" speak directly to Mrs. Jones.

and lasts indefinitely. Examples of such developmental disabilities include autism, cerebral palsy, epilepsy, and mental impairment. You must make every effort to meet the individual needs of the patient with a developmental disability.

A person with a developmental disability may have problems with *coordination* or *comprehension* of instructions. As a result, you may have difficulties in obtaining intraoral films. If coordination or comprehension is a problem, mild sedation may be useful.

It is important that you recognize situations in which the patient *cannot tolerate* intraoral film exposure. Intraoral films should *not* be attempted in these patients; such exposure results only in nondiagnostic films and needless radiation exposure of the patient. In patients who cannot tolerate intraoral film exposure, extraoral films such as lateral jaw and panoramic x-rays may be used.

Recall

15. What physical disabilities may affect dental patients?
16. Under what circumstance would you hold a film for a patient?

PATIENTS WITH SPECIAL DENTAL NEEDS

Dental x-rays are indicated for a variety of patient needs. Often, you may need to modify the basic x-ray techniques to accommodate patients with special dental needs, including edentulous, endodontic, and pediatric patients.

Edentulous Patient

Edentulous means "without teeth." Radiographs on edentulous patients may be required for the following reasons:

- Detect retained root tips, impacted teeth, and lesions (cysts, tumors)
- Identify objects embedded in bone
- Observe the amount and health of the bone

The radiographic examination of an edentulous patient may include a panoramic radiograph (see Chapter 42), periapical radiographs, or a combination of occlusal and periapical radiographs (Fig. 41-25).

Radiographic images must be taken in all areas of the arches, whether or not teeth are present. For edentulous patients, either the bisecting or the paralleling technique may be used. Because no teeth are present, the distortion inherent in the bisecting technique does not interfere with the diagnostic intrabony conditions.

For *partially edentulous* patients, film-holding instruments can be used by substituting a cotton roll for the space normally occupied by the crowns of the missing teeth and then following the standard exposure procedures.

Pediatric Patient

In children, radiographs are useful for (1) detecting conditions of the teeth and bones, (2) showing changes related to caries and trauma, and (3) evaluating growth and development (see Chapter 57).

You must explain the x-ray procedures you are about to perform in terms that the child can easily understand. For example, you can refer to the tubehead as a "camera," the lead apron as a "coat," and the radiograph as a "picture."

Exposure factors (milliamperage, kilovoltage, exposure time) must be reduced because of the smaller size of the pediatric patient. The shorter exposure time will reduce the effect of blurring if the child moves. All exposure factors should be set according to the recommendations of the equipment and film manufacturer (Fig. 41-26).

As described in Chapter 39, size #0 film is recommended for use in the pediatric patient with a primary dentition because of the small size of the mouth. In the child with mixed dentition, size #1 or #2 film may be used.

Always remember that management of children requires you to be confident, patient, and understanding.

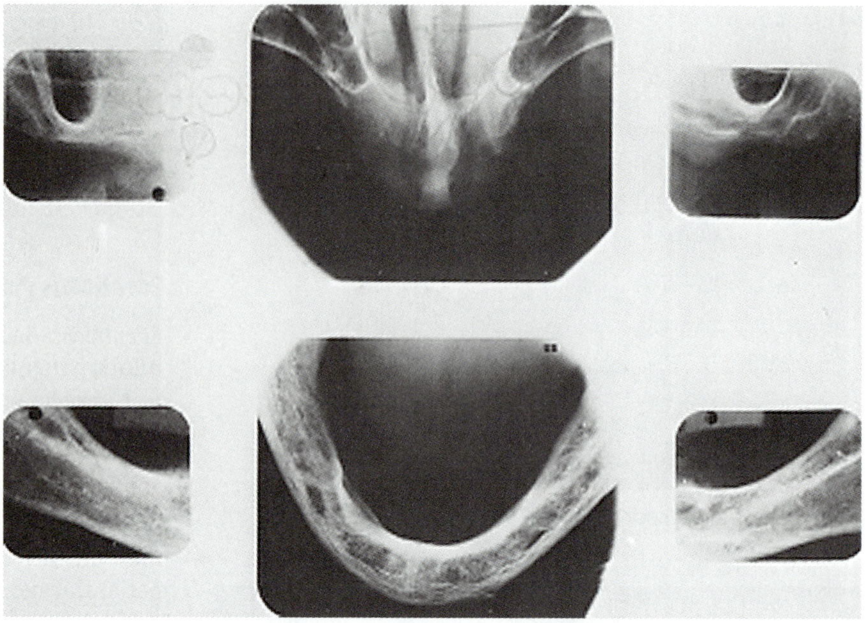

Fig. 41-25 Mixed occlusal-periapical edentulous survey.

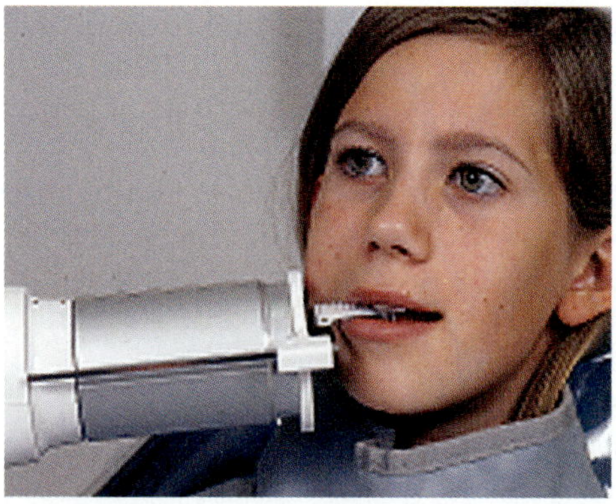

Fig. 41-26 Extension-cone paralleling (XCP) instruments can also be used for the pediatric patient, but the exposure time is reduced.

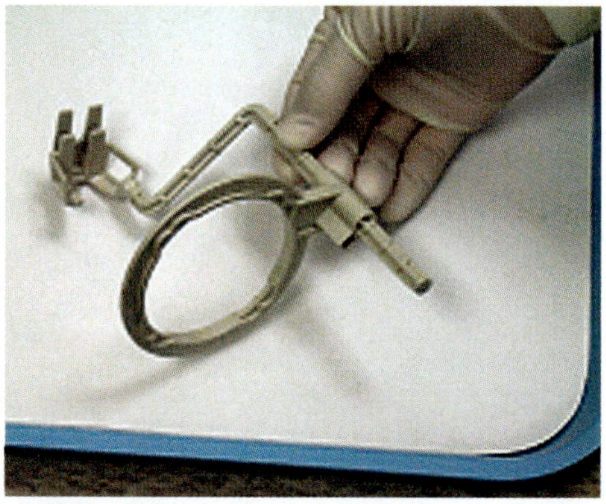

Fig. 41-27 EndoRay II film holder is designed for use during endodontic procedures when x-rays must be taken while instruments are in the canal.

Endodontic Patient

It often is difficult to obtain accurate radiographs during *endodontic* ("root canal") treatment because of the rubber dam clamp, endodontic instruments, or filling material extending from the tooth. The EndoRay film holder can be used to aid in positioning the film during this portion of the root canal procedure (Fig. 41-27). This holder fits around a rubber dam clamp and allows space for endodontic instruments and filling materials to protrude from the tooth.

A diagnostic quality endodontic film must have the following qualities:

- The tooth is centered on the film.
- At least 5 mm of bone beyond the apex of the tooth is visible.
- The image is as anatomically correct as possible.

The preoperative diagnostic film and the postoperative film should be taken with the standard paralleling technique and using a film-holding device. The bisecting technique is *not* recommended for preoperative diagnostic x-rays because of the inherent dimensional distortion.

Gagging Patient

On occasion, you will have a patient with a *hypersensitive gag reflex*. To help prevent the gag reflex, you must convey a confident attitude. If the patient senses nervousness, a *psychogenic stimulus* may result and cause the gag reflex.

In addition, be patient, tolerant, and understanding. Explain the procedure and then compliment the patient as each exposure is completed. As the patient becomes more confident with the procedure, the less likely the patient is to gag.

Guidelines for Dental Radiography of Pediatric Patients

1. *Show and tell.* Most children are curious. The "show and tell" approach best prepares the child for the x-ray procedure.
2. *Be self-assured.* Most children will respond well to the authority of a self-assured and capable operator. Be patient with the child.
3. *Reassure the child.* Most children are afraid of the unknown. A frightened child is not a cooperative patient, so you must reassure the child that everything will be safe.
4. *Demonstrate actions.* Show children exactly what you want them to do. For example, if you want them to open wide or move their tongue, demonstrate this action first, and then ask them to do the same thing.
5. *Request assistance.* If the child cannot sit still or hold the film in the mouth, you can ask the accompanying adult to help. The adult can hold the film or the child during the x-ray exposure. Be sure that the adult and the child are wearing lead aprons and thyroid collars.
6. *Postpone films* (if indicated). If a child is particularly frightened or uncooperative and the procedure is not an emergency, it is often better to postpone the x-rays rather than force the child to undergo the procedure. It may be better to try again on the second or third visit to the office, rather than instilling fear of the dental office in the child.

Exposure Sequencing

As discussed earlier, exposure sequencing plays an important role in preventing the gag reflex. Anterior films are easier for the patient to tolerate and are less likely to elicit the gag reflex. With posterior film placements, you should always expose the premolar film before the molar film.

The maxillary molar film placement is the one most likely to cause the gag reflex. For the patient with a hypersensitive gag reflex, you should expose the maxillary molars last.

Film Placement

Avoid the palate

When you place films in the maxillary posterior, do not slide them along the palate. This elicits the gag reflex. Instead, position the film lingual to the teeth and then firmly bring the film into contact with the palatal tissues in one decisive motion.

Demonstrate film placement

In the areas that are most likely to elicit the gag reflex, rub a finger along the tissues near the intended area of film placement while telling the patient, "This is where the film will be positioned." Then quickly position the film. This technique demonstrates where the film will be placed and desensitizes the tissues in the area.

Guidelines to Reduce Gag Reflex in Dental Patients

1. *Never* ask a patient about the gag reflex. The power of suggestion can trigger it.
2. *Reassure the patient.* If the patient begins to gag, remove the film quickly. Reassure the patient that such a response is not unusual. Patients may feel embarrassed. Remain calm and in control.
3. *Suggest breathing techniques.* Instruct the patient to "breathe deeply" through the nose during film placement and exposure. For the gag reflex to take place, respiration must cease; therefore, if the patient is breathing, the gag reflex cannot occur.
4. *Distract the patient.* You can instruct the patient to do one of the following during film placement and exposure: (a) bite as hard as possible on the film holder or (b) raise a leg or arm in the air. These actions help to divert the patient's attention and lessen the likelihood of eliciting the gag reflex.
5. *Reduce tactile stimuli.* You can try one of the following techniques before placing and exposing the film: (a) give the patient a cup of ice water to drink or (b) place a small amount of ordinary table salt on the tip of the tongue. These techniques help to "confuse" the sensory nerve endings and lessen the likelihood of stimulating the gag reflex.
6. *Consider use of topical anesthetic.* In the patient with a severe gag reflex, a topical anesthetic may be used. A spray or gel may be used to numb the areas that elicit the gag reflex. You should instruct the patient to exhale while the anesthetic is sprayed on the soft palate and posterior tongue.

   NOTE: Caution must be used to ensure that the patient does *not* inhale the spray, because inflammation of the lungs may occur. The topical anesthetic spray takes effect after 1 minute and lasts for approximately 20 minutes.

   NOTE: Topical anesthetic sprays should *not* be used in patients who are allergic to benzocaine.

   Not all states allow dental assistants to place topical anesthetic. Check the regulations in your state/province before you apply topical anesthetics.

Extreme Cases

At times, you may encounter a patient with an *uncontrollable* gag reflex. In such patients, intraoral films are impossible to obtain, and you must use extraoral radiographs such as panoramic or lateral jaw films.

A

Cause: Unexposed
Correction: Be sure machine is on. Listen for exposure sound.

B

Cause: Exposed to white light
Correction: Do not unwrap film in light. Check darkroom for light leaks.

C

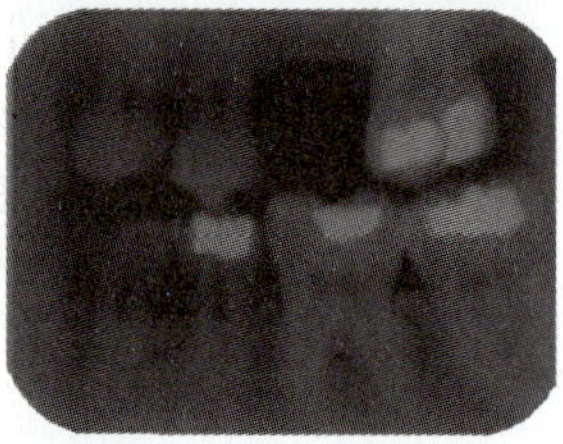

Cause: Overexposed
Correction: Check exposure settings, and decrease as necessary.

D

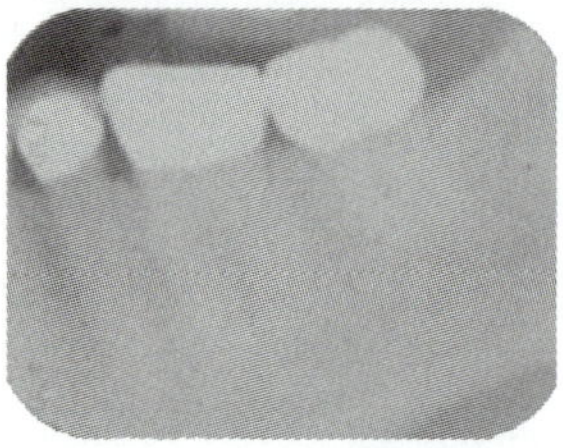

Cause: Underexposed
Correction: Check exposure settings, and increase as necessary.

E

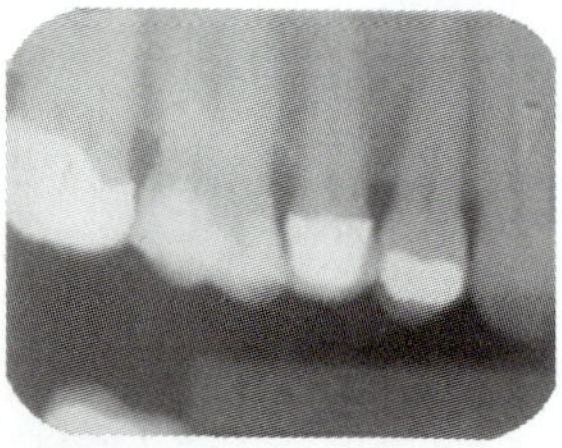

Cause: Incorrect film placement
Correction: No more than ⅛ inch of film extends beyond incisal/occlusal surfaces.

F

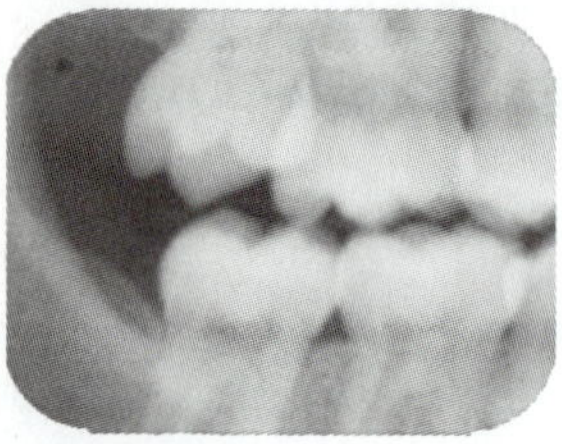

Cause: Incorrect horizontal angulation
Correction: Direct central ray through interproximal spaces.

G

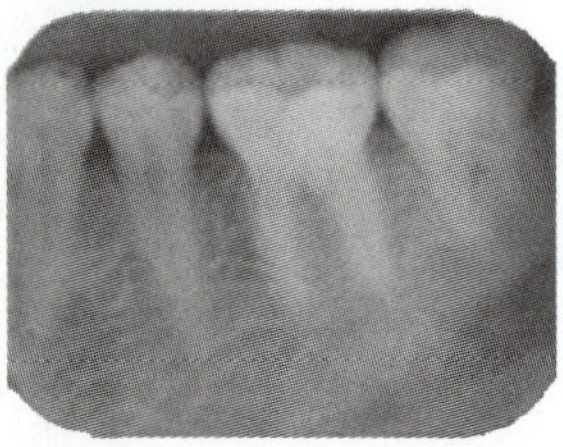

Cause: Vertical angulation too steep
Correction: Use XCP instruments to avoid excessive angulation.

H

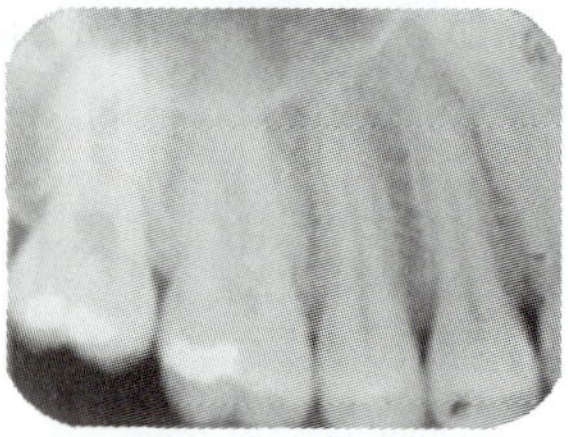

Cause: Vertical angulation too flat
Correction: Use XCP instruments to avoid insufficient angulation.

I

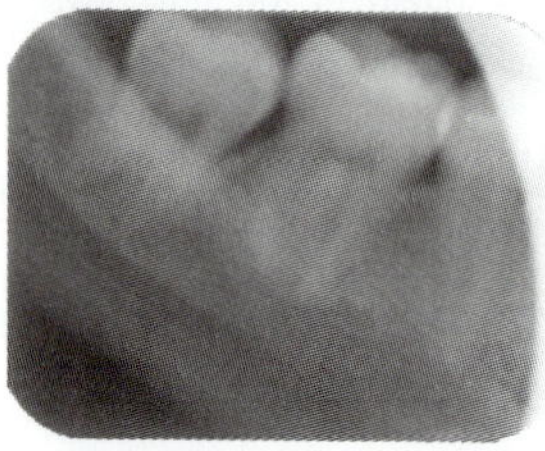

Cause: PID not properly aligned
Correction: Always check film for bending before exposure.

J

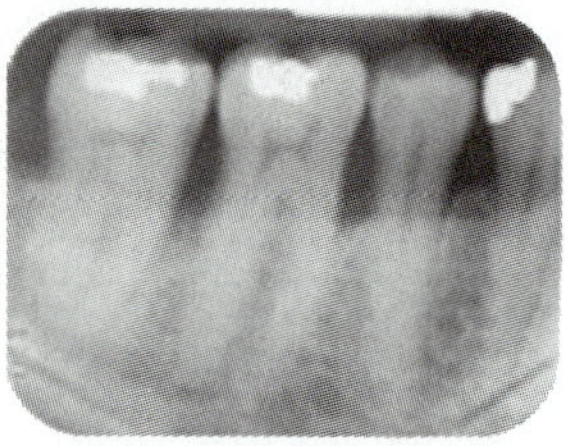

Cause: Film excessively bent
Correction: Always check film for bending before exposure.

K

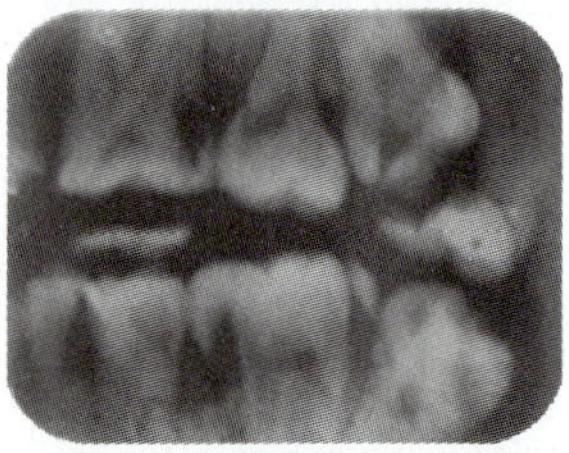

Cause: Film exposed twice
Correction: Always separate exposed and nonexposed films.

L

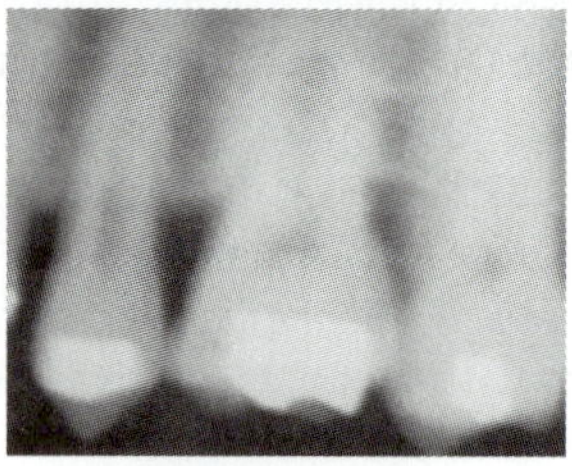

Cause: Patient movement
Correction: Stabilize patient's head before exposure. Instruct patient not to move.

M

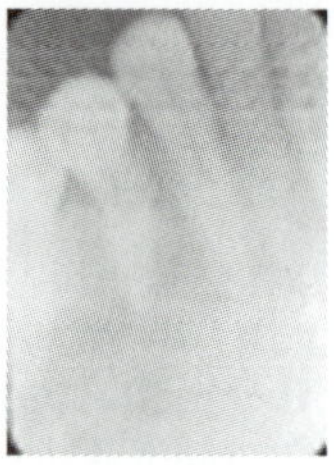

Cause: Film placed in mouth backwards
Correction: Check film placement; white side always faces PID.

Fig. 41-28 Radiographic exposure errors. **A,** Clear. **B,** Black. **C,** Dark. **D,** Light. **E,** No apices. **F,** Overlapped contacts. **G,** Foreshortened image. **H,** Elongated image. **I,** Cone cut. **J,** Distorted image with dark lines on corners. **K,** Double image. **L,** Blurred image. **M,** Light image with herringbone pattern. *XCP,* Extension-cone paralleling; *PID,* position indicator device. (Radiographs from Haring JI, Jansen L: *Dental radiography: principles and techniques,* ed 2, Philadelphia, 2000, Saunders.)

Recall

17. For partially edentulous patients, how can you modify the technique for using a bite-block?
18. When exposing films on a pediatric patient, how can you best describe the tubehead to the patient?
19. What changes must be made in the exposure factors when exposing radiographs on a pediatric patient?
20. What size of film is recommended for a pediatric patient with all primary dentition?
21. Why is the exposure sequence especially important when taking x-rays on a patient with a severe gag reflex?

RADIOGRAPHIC TECHNIQUE ERRORS

The purpose of dental radiographs is to benefit the patient. However, only radiographs of **diagnostic quality** benefit the patient. Diagnostic-quality radiographs are those that have been properly *placed, exposed,* and *processed;* errors in any one of these three areas may result in nondiagnostic films. Nondiagnostic films must be retaken, which results in additional exposure of the patient to ionizing radiation.

You must be able to recognize film errors, identify their causes, and know what steps are necessary to correct such problems (Fig. 41-28).

MOUNTING DENTAL RADIOGRAPHS

Recognizing Anatomic Landmarks

To mount dental radiographs correctly, the dental assistant must be able to recognize the normal anatomic landmarks on intraoral radiographs (Fig. 41-29).

Processed radiographs are arranged in anatomic order in holders, called mounts, to make it easier for the dentist to view the films. The mount must always be labeled with the patient's name and the date that the radiographs were exposed. The dentist's name and address should also be on the mount.

Selecting the Mount

Mounts are available in many sizes, with different numbers and sizes of *windows* (openings) to accommodate the number and sizes of exposures in the patient's radiographic survey. The mounts most often used for radiographic surveys are available in black, gray, and clear plastic.

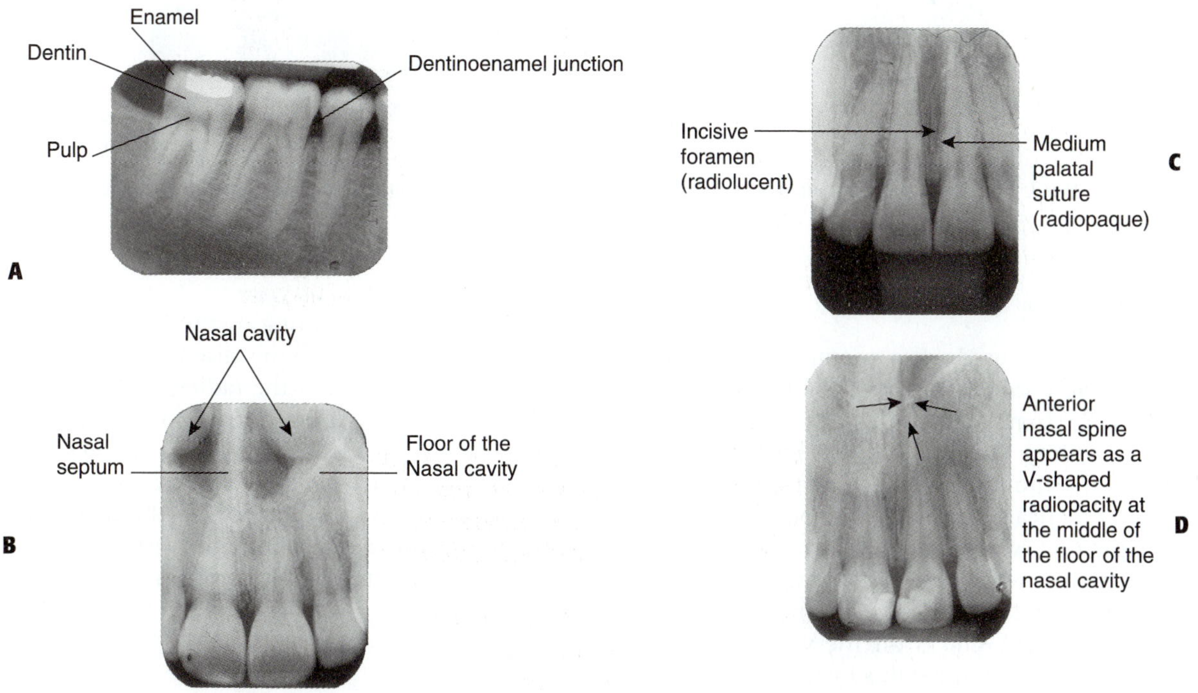

Fig. 41-29 Radiographic landmarks of normal anatomy. **A,** Structures of the tooth. **B-D,** Maxillary structures.

continued

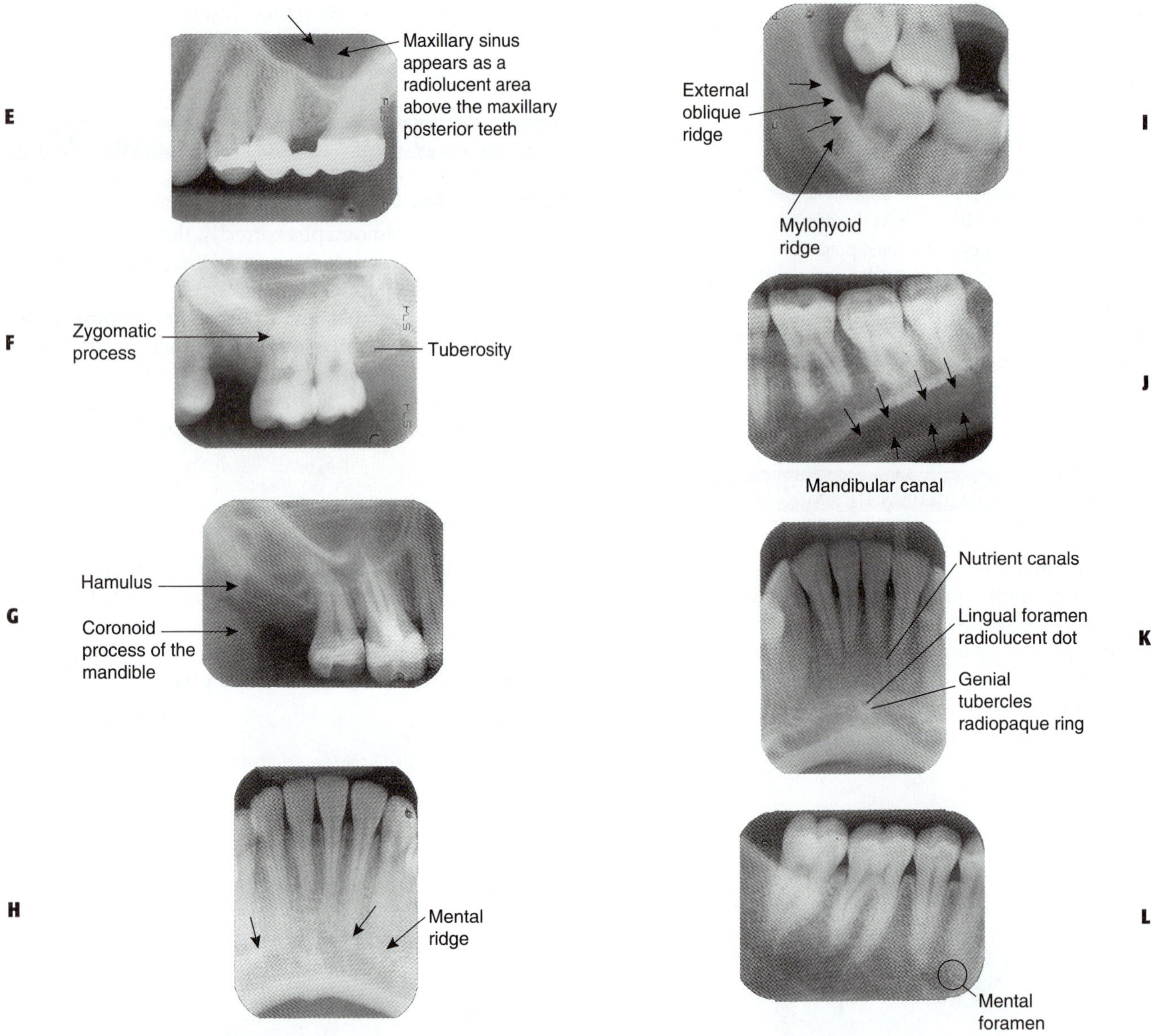

Fig. 41-29, cont'd Radiographic landmarks of normal anatomy. **E-G,** Maxillary structures. **H-L,** Mandibular structures.

Methods of Mounting

Two methods can be used when mounting radiographs. Both methods rely on identification of the raised (*embossed*) dot on the film.

In the first method, the *labial mounting method*, the films are placed in the mount with the raised dots facing up (*convex*). The American Dental Association (ADA) recommends this method of mounting radiographs. The radiographs are viewed as if the viewer is looking directly at the patient; thus the patient's left side is on the viewer's right, and the patient's right side is on the viewer's left (Fig. 41-30). Procedure 41-7 outlines this method.

In the second mounting method, the radiographs are placed in the mount with the raised dots facing down (*concave*). With this method the radiographs are viewed as if the viewer is inside the patient's mouth and looking out; that is, the patient's left side is on the viewer's left, and the patient's right side is on the viewer's right.

Note: It is *critical* to know how the dentist prefers to have the radiographs mounted. Mistakes in mounting radiographs have resulted in errors in the treatment of the dental patient.

Procedure 41-7 Mounting Dental Radiographs

Goal

To mount a full-mouth series of dental radiographs.

Equipment and Supplies

- Appropriate size of film mount
- Pencil
- Viewbox
- Paper towel
- Processing for full-mouth series of radiographs

PROCEDURAL STEPS

1. Place a clean paper towel over the work surface in front of the viewbox.
   Purpose: To keep the films clean.
2. Turn on the viewbox.
3. Label and date the film mount.

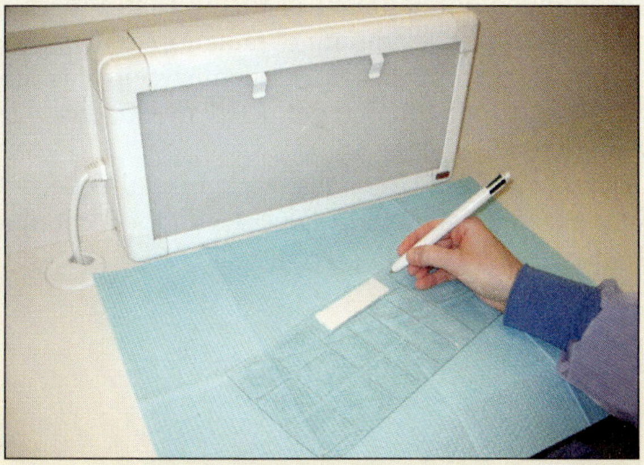

4. Wash and dry the hands.
   Purpose: To prevent finger marks on the radiographs.
5. Identify the embossed dot on each radiograph; place the film on the work surface with the dot facing up.
   Purpose: The ADA recommends mounting with the dot up.
6. Sort the radiographs into three groups: bite-wing, anterior periapical, and posterior periapical views.
7. Arrange the radiographs on the work surface in anatomic order. Use your knowledge of normal anatomic landmarks to distinguish maxillary from mandibular radiographs.
8. Arrange all maxillary radiographs with the roots pointing upward and all mandibular radiographs with the roots pointing downward.
9. Place each film in the corresponding window of the film mount. The following order for film mounting is suggested:

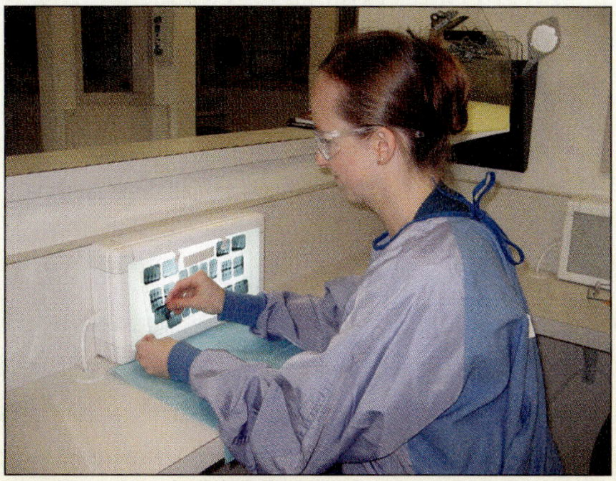

   a. Maxillary anterior periapical films
   b. Mandibular anterior periapical films
   c. Bite-wing films
   d. Maxillary posterior periapical films
   e. Mandibular posterior periapical films
10. Check the mounted radiographs to ensure that (a) the dots are all oriented properly, (b) the films are arranged properly in anatomic order, and (c) the films are secure in the mount.

Recall

22. What is the definition of a diagnostic-quality radiograph?
23. When mounting radiographs, what is the recommendation of the ADA concerning placement of the raised dot?
24. Why is it important for the dental assistant to recognize anatomic landmarks?
25. Why is it important to avoid retakes?

Guidelines for Mounting Radiographs

1. Handle films only by the edges.
2. Learn the normal anatomy of the maxilla and mandible.
3. Label and date the film mount *before* mounting the films. Include the patient's full name, date of exposure, and dentist's name.
4. Mount films immediately after processing.
5. Use clean, dry hands.
6. Use the order of the teeth to distinguish the right side from the left.
7. Use a definite order for mounting films. For example, start with the maxillary anterior periapical films, proceed to mandibular anterior periapical and bite-wing views, and finish with maxillary and mandibular posterior periapical views.
8. Mount bite-wing radiographs with the curve of Spee (occlusal plane between the maxillary and mandibular teeth) directed *upward* toward the distal. The result resembles a smile.

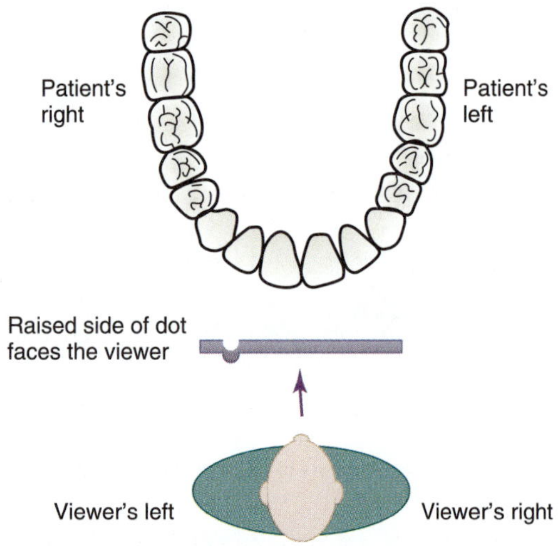

Fig. 41-30 With the labial mounting method, radiographs are viewed as if the dental radiographer were looking directly at the patient. (From Haring JI, Jansen L: *Dental radiography: principles and techniques,* ed 2, Philadelphia, 2000, Saunders.)

Legal and Ethical Implications

Public awareness of the harmful effects of x-radiation has caused dental patients to question the value and necessity of having dental x-rays. The dental assistant should be prepared to explain to the patient the amount of risk that is associated with dental radiographs. Radiographs should never be exposed on a patient unless the patient understands the need for the radiographs and has given consent.

To avoid retakes and unnecessary radiation to the patient, the dental assistant must be competent in performing various x-ray techniques.

Eye to the Future

The focus of dental radiography in the future will be on the continued development of methods and machines to further reduce the amount of radiation to the patient. The new F-speed film is an excellent step in this direction. Digital radiography, discussed in Chapter 42, is leading the way today.

Dental professionals must recognize the need for lifelong learning to remain current with the technologic advances in dental radiography.

Critical Thinking

1. Mr. Li Trung is a 65-year-old patient in your office who needs a full-mouth survey of dental radiographs. You notice that Mr. Trung has a very small mouth and a very shallow palate. What technique would you use to expose his radiographs? Why?
2. Mrs. Jackson has brought her 14-year-old son Jamal into your office for an examination. During the examination the dentist explains to Mrs. Jackson that Jamal's maxillary canine teeth have not erupted into the mouth and may be impacted in the palate. What type of radiograph will the dentist most likely request? Why?
3. As you begin to mount a set of bite-wing radiographs, you notice that the contacts on the right premolar film are overlapped. What common error occurred during the exposure of this film? What type of correction is needed on the retake?

42

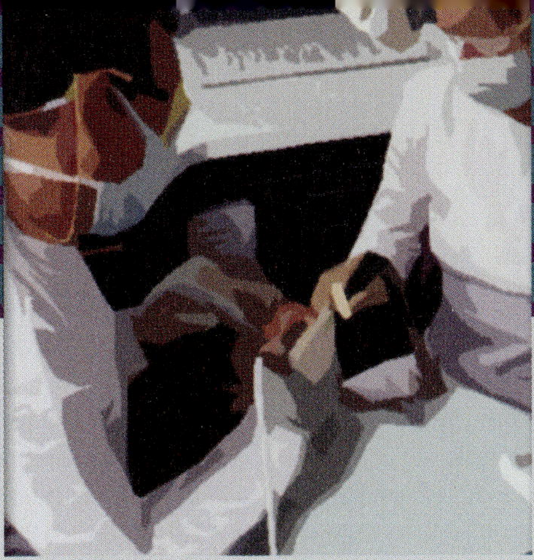

Extraoral and Digital Radiography

Outline

KEY TERMS

Cephalostat Special device that allows the operator to easily position both film and patient.

Charge-coupled device (CCD) Image receptor found in the intraoral sensor.

Digital radiography Filmless imaging system that uses a sensor to capture images, then converts the images into electronic pieces and stores them in a computer.

Digitize (di-jeh-*tize*) To convert an image into a digital form that, in turn, can be processed by a computer.

Exposure controls Feature that allows the operator to adjust the milliamperage and kilovoltage settings.

Extraoral radiographs Radiographs taken when large areas of the skull or jaw must be examined.

Focal trough (trof) Imaginary three-dimensional horseshoe-shaped zone used to focus panoramic radiographs.

Frankfort plane Imaginary plane that passes through the top of the ear canal and the bottom of the eye socket.

Grid Device used to reduce the amount of scatter radiation that reaches an extraoral film.

Midsagittal plane Imaginary line that divides the patient's face into right and left sides.

Sensor Small detector that is placed intraorally to capture a radiographic image.

Temporomandibular (*tem*-pah-ro-man-**dib**-u-lar) Joint on each side of the head that allows for movement of the mandible.

Tomography (toe-**mah**-greh-fee) Radiographic technique that allows imaging of one layer or section of the body while blurring images from structures in other planes.

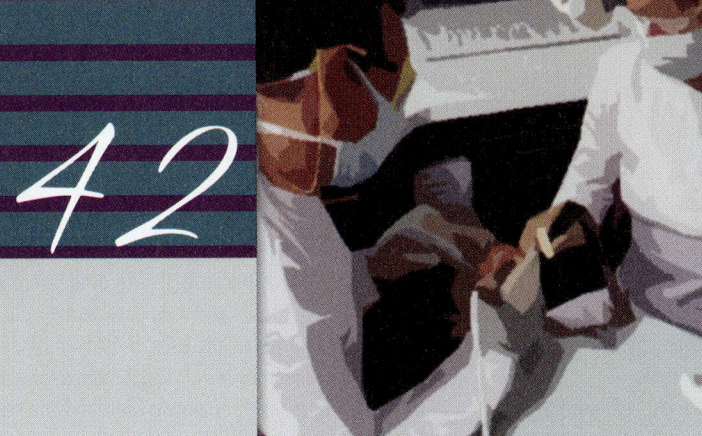

LEARNING OUTCOMES

On completion of this chapter, the student will be able to achieve the following objectives:

- Pronounce, define, and spell the Key Terms.
- Describe the purpose and uses of panoramic radiography.
- Describe the equipment used in panoramic radiography.
- Describe the steps for patient positioning in panoramic radiography.
- Discuss the advantages and disadvantages of panoramic radiography.
- Describe the errors caused during patient preparation and positioning during panoramic radiography.
- Describe the equipment used in extraoral radiography.
- Identify the specific purpose of each of the extraoral film projections.
- Describe the purposes and uses of extraoral radiography.
- Describe the purposes and uses of digital radiography.
- Discuss the fundamentals of digital radiography.
- List and describe the equipment used in digital radiography.
- List and discuss the advantages and disadvantages of digital radiography.

Extraoral radiographs are taken when large areas of the skull or jaw must be examined or when patients are unable to open their mouths for film placement. (*Extraoral* means "outside the mouth.") Extraoral films are very useful for evaluating large areas but are not recommended for detection of subtle changes, such as dental caries or early periodontal changes. This is because extraoral radiographs do not show details as well as intraoral films.

There are many types of extraoral radiographs. Some types are used to view the entire skull, whereas other types focus on the maxilla and mandible. This chapter discusses the various extraoral radiographic techniques and their advantages and disadvantages.

Digital radiography is changing the way dental radiography is practiced. You probably use some form of digital imaging already. Fax machines, home video cameras, and digital video discs (DVDs) all use digital technology. This chapter discusses the various types of digital imaging used in dentistry, including their advantages and disadvantages.

Recall

1. When are extraoral radiographs needed?

PANORAMIC RADIOGRAPHY

Panoramic radiographs allow the dentist to view the entire dentition and related structures on a single film. Depending on the type of equipment used, a panoramic dental radiograph can be made with the patient standing or sitting. Regardless of the type of machine, you must follow the manufacturer's instructions carefully.

The images on a panoramic film are not as well defined or clear as the images on intraoral films (Fig. 42-1). Therefore bite-wing films are used to supplement a panoramic film to detect dental caries or periapical lesions.

Basic Concepts

In panoramic radiography, both the film and the tubehead rotate around the patient, producing a series of individual images. When these images are combined on a single film, an overall view of the maxilla and mandible is created (Fig. 42-2).

The movement of the film and the tubehead produces an image through a process known as **tomography** (*tomo-* means "section"). Tomography is a radiographic technique that allows the imaging of one section, or layer, of the body while blurring images from structures in other planes. In panoramic dental radiography, this image conforms to the shape of the dental arches.

Focal Trough

The **focal trough,** also known as the *image layer,* is an imaginary three-dimensional curved area or space, shaped like a horseshoe (Fig. 42-3). When the patient's jaws are positioned within this area, the resulting radiograph is reasonably clear and well defined. If the jaws are positioned outside of this area, the images on the radiograph appear blurred or indistinct. Imagine this trough as an area of ideal focus.

Panoramic Radiographs in Dentistry

Are used to:

Locate impacted teeth

Observe tooth eruption patterns

Detect lesions in the jaw

Detect features in the bone

Provide an overall view of the mandible and maxilla

Are *not* used to:

Substitute for intraoral films

Diagnose dental caries

Diagnose periodontal disease

Diagnose periapical lesions

The size and shape of the focal trough vary with the manufacturer of the panoramic unit. Panoramic x-ray units are designed to accommodate the average jaw. The quality of the resulting radiograph depends on how the patient's jaws are positioned within the trough and how closely the patient's jaws conform to the focal trough, which is designed for the average jaw.

Each manufacturer provides specific instructions about patient positioning to ensure that the teeth are positioned within the focal trough. When the jaws are outside this area, the resulting images are distorted. Proper positioning is important and is discussed later in this chapter.

Equipment

Panoramic radiography requires the use of a panoramic x-ray unit, screen-type film, intensifying screens, and cassettes (see Chapter 39).

A number of different panoramic x-ray units are available. Although each manufacturer's panoramic unit is slightly different, all machines have similar components. The main components of the panoramic unit include the panoramic x-ray tubehead, head positioner, and exposure controls (Fig. 42-4).

Tubehead

The panoramic x-ray tubehead is similar to an intraoral tubehead in that it has a filament to produce electrons and a target to produce radiographs. The *collimator* used in the panoramic x-ray machine is a lead plate with an opening shaped like a narrow vertical slit.

Unlike the intraoral tubehead, the vertical angulation of the panoramic tubehead is not adjustable. In addition, the tubehead of the panoramic unit always rotates *behind* the patient's head as the film rotates in front of the patient.

A

B

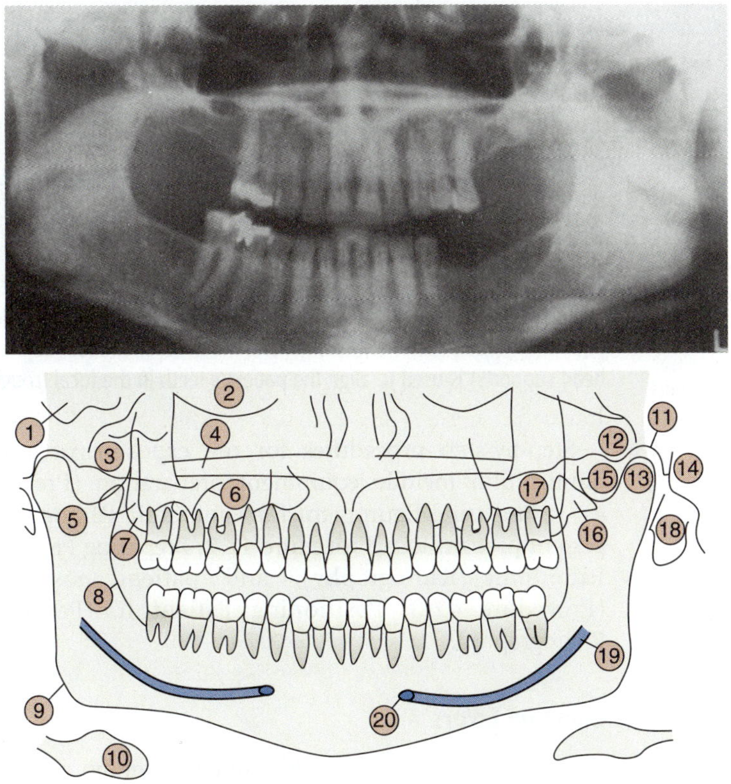

Fig. 42-1 A, Panoramic radiograph. **B,** Panoramic anatomy. (From Haring JI, Jansen L: *Dental radiography: principles and techniques,* ed 2, Philadelphia, 2000, Saunders.)

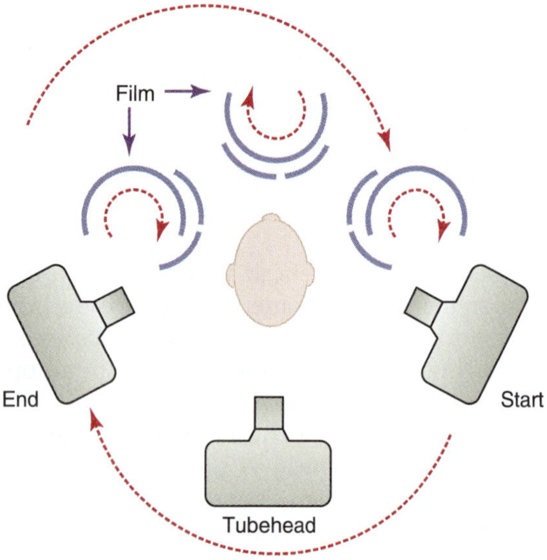

Fig. 42-2 **The film and x-ray tubehead move around the patient in opposite directions in panoramic radiography.** (From Haring JI, Jansen L: *Dental radiography: principles and techniques,* ed 2, Philadelphia, 2000, Saunders.)

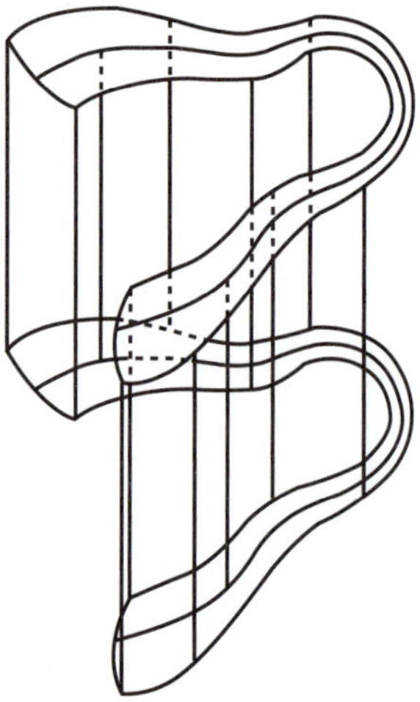

Fig. 42-3 **Example of an image layer, or focal trough.** (From Haring JI, Jansen L: *Dental radiography: principles and techniques,* ed 2, Philadelphia, 2000, Saunders.)

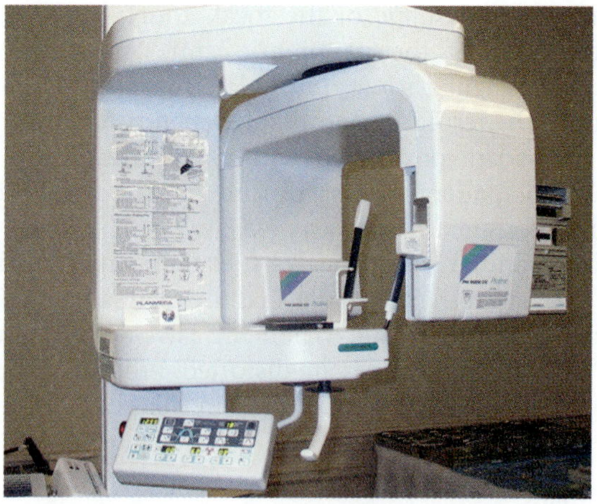

Fig. 42-4 **Main components of a panoramic unit.**

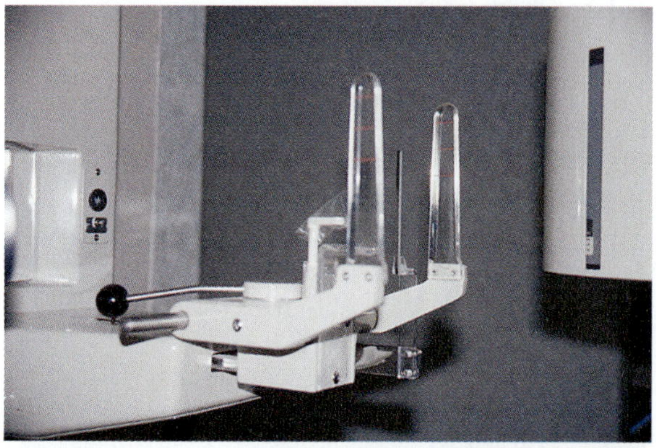

Fig. 42-5 **Head positioner (notched bite-block, forehead rest, and lateral head supports) is used to align the patient's teeth in the focal trough.**

Head Positioner

Each panoramic unit has a head positioner used to align the patient's teeth as accurately as possible. Each head positioner consists of a chin rest, notched bite-block, forehead rest, and lateral head supports or guides (Fig. 42-5). Each panoramic unit is unique, and the operator must follow the manufacturer's instructions to position the patient correctly in the focal trough.

Exposure Controls

The **exposure controls** allow the milliamperage and kilovoltage settings to be adjusted to accommodate patients of different sizes. However, *the exposure time cannot be changed.*

Step-by-step procedures for the exposure of a panoramic film include equipment preparation (Procedure 42-1: Preparing Equipment for Panoramic Radiography), patient preparation (Procedure 42-2: Preparing Patient for Panoramic Radiography), and patient positioning (Procedure 42-3: Positioning Patient for Panoramic Radiography).

Common Errors

To produce a diagnostic panoramic radiograph and minimize patient exposure, you must avoid mistakes. To do this, you must be able to recognize the following common patient preparation and positioning errors and understand what you can do to prevent such errors from occurring.

Patient Preparation Errors

Ghost images

If all metallic or radiodense objects, including eyeglasses, earrings, necklaces, removable partial dentures, orthodontic retainers, and hearing aids, are not removed from the patient before the exposure of a panoramic film, a "ghost"

Procedure 42-1 Preparing Equipment for Panoramic Radiography

Goal

To prepare the equipment necessary for a panoramic radiograph.

Equipment and Supplies

- Extraoral film
- Cassette
- Infection-control barriers

PROCEDURAL STEPS

1. Load the panoramic cassette in the darkroom under safelight conditions. Handle the film by its edges only to avoid fingerprints.
   Purpose: The panoramic film is sensitive to light, and the remainder of the film in the box will be ruined if exposed to light.
2. Place all infection-control barriers and containers.
3. Cover the bite-block with a disposable plastic barrier. If the bite-block is not covered, it must be sterilized before it is used on the next patient.
   Purpose: The bite-block is considered a semicritical item and must be either disposable or sterilized.
4. Cover or disinfect (or both) any part of the machine that comes in contact with the patient.
   Purpose: Parts of the machine touching the patient but not used intraorally are considered noncritical items and must be disinfected with a high-level disinfectant.

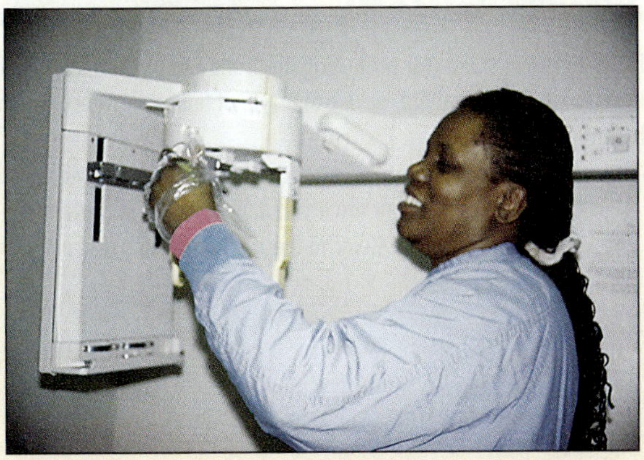

5. Set the exposure factors (kilovoltage, milliamperage) according to the manufacturer's recommendations.
6. Adjust the machine to accommodate the height of the patient; align all movable parts properly.
7. Load the cassette into the carrier of the panoramic unit.

Procedure 42-2 Preparing Patient for Panoramic Radiography

Goal

To prepare a patient for a panoramic x-ray.

Equipment and Supplies

- Double-sided lead apron (or style recommended by the manufacturer)
- Plastic container

PROCEDURAL STEPS

1. Explain the procedure to the patient. Give the patient the opportunity to ask questions.
   Purpose: The patient has the right to be informed and give consent to the procedure.
2. Ask the patient to remove all objects from the head and neck area; this includes eyeglasses, earrings, lip-piercing and tongue-piercing objects, necklaces, napkin chains, hearing aids, hairpins, and complete and partial dentures. Place objects in a container.
   Purpose: If not removed, these objects will appear on the radiograph and could superimpose diagnostic information.

continued

Procedure 42-2 Preparing Patient for Panoramic Radiography—cont'd

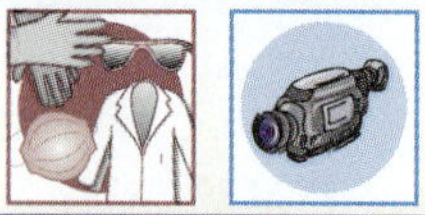

PROCEDURAL STEPS, cont'd

3. Place a double-sided (for protecting the front and back of the patient) lead apron on the patient, or use the style of lead apron recommended by the manufacturer.
   Note: A thyroid collar is not recommended for all panoramic units because it blocks part of the beam and obscures important anatomic structures. Refer to the manufacturer's instructions for the unit you use.

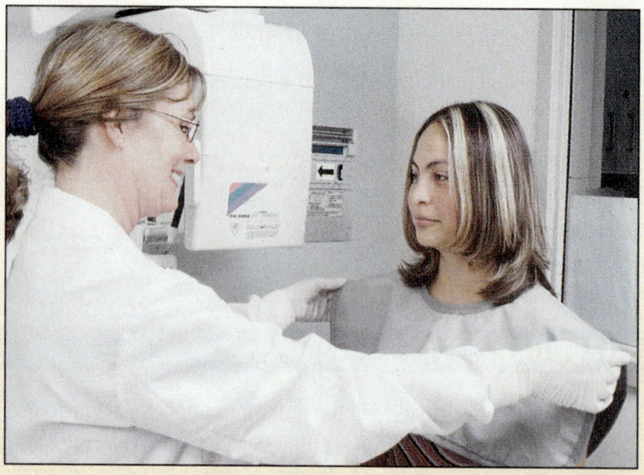

Procedure 42-3 Positioning Patient for Panoramic Radiography

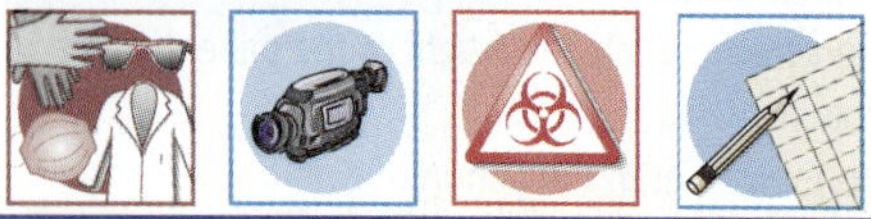

Goal

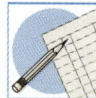

To position the patient for a panoramic radiograph.

PROCEDURAL STEPS

1. Instruct the patient to sit or stand "as tall as possible" with the back straight and erect.
   Purpose: The spinal column is very dense; if the spine is not straight, a white shadow appears over the middle of the radiograph and obscures diagnostic information.
2. Instruct the patient to bite on the plastic bite-block and then slide the upper and lower teeth into the notch (groove) on the end of the bite-block.
   Purpose: The groove aligns the teeth in the focal trough.

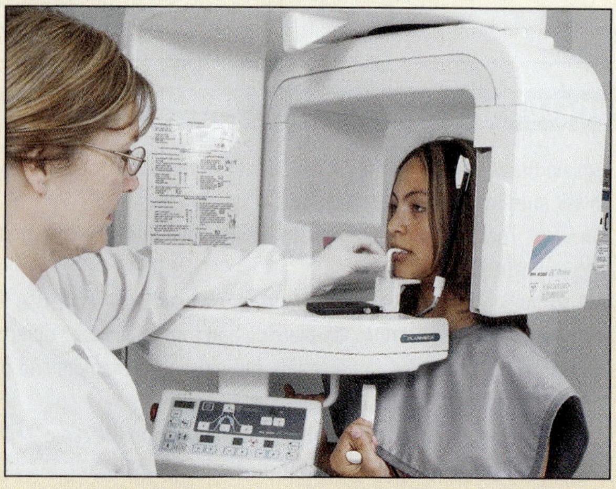

3. Position the **midsagittal plane** (the imaginary line that divides the patient's face into right and left sides) perpendicular to the floor.
   Purpose: If the patient's head is tipped or tilted to one side, a distorted image will result.
4. Position the **Frankfort plane** (the imaginary plane that passes through the top of the ear canal and the bottom of the eye socket) parallel with the floor.
   Purpose: The occlusal plane will be positioned at the correct angle.

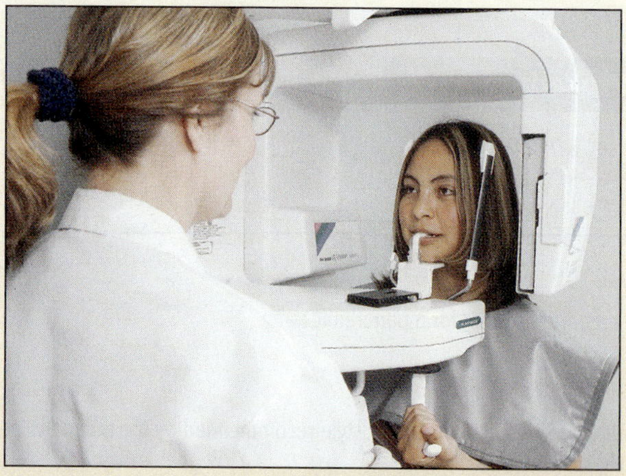

5. Instruct the patient to position the tongue on the roof of the mouth and then to close the lips around the bite-block.
   Purpose: If the tongue is not placed on the roof of the mouth, a radiolucent shadow will be superimposed over the apices of the maxillary teeth.

Procedure 42-3 Positioning Patient for Panoramic Radiography—cont'd

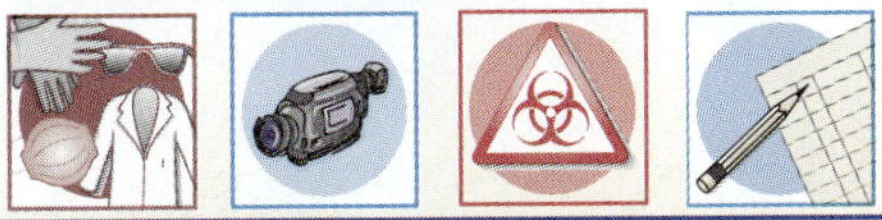

6. After the patient has been positioned, instruct him or her to remain still while the machine rotates during exposure.

   Purpose Any movement of the patient will result in a blurred image on the radiograph.

7. Expose the film and proceed with film processing as described in Chapter 39.
8. Document the procedure.

Date	Procedure	Operator
1/25/05	Exposed panoramic radiograph	DLB

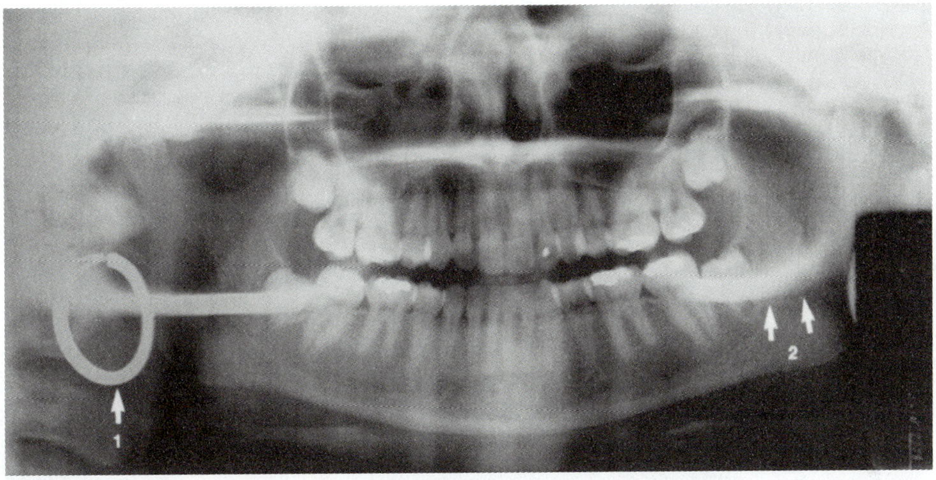

Fig. 42-6 **Large hoop earrings *(1)* and "ghost" images *(2)*. The ghost image of the earring appears on the opposite side of the film and is enlarged and laterally distorted.** (From Haring JI, Jansen L: *Dental radiography: principles and techniques,* ed 2, Philadelphia, 2000, Saunders.)

image results. A ghost image looks similar to the real object except that it appears on the opposite side of the film.

For example, if an earring was on the patient's left side, the ghost image on the radiograph would appear on the right side and slightly higher than the real object. In addition, the ghost image of the earring would appear blurred and larger (Fig. 42-6).

Solution. The patient must be instructed to remove all radiodense objects in the head and neck region before being positioned for a panoramic radiograph.

Lead apron artifact

If the lead apron is incorrectly placed or a lead apron with a thyroid collar is used during exposure of panoramic films, a radiopaque cone-shaped artifact results and interferes with the diagnostic information (Fig. 42-7).

Solution. Use a lead apron *without* a thyroid collar, and place the lead apron low around the neck of the patient so that it does not block the x-ray beam.

Patient Positioning Errors

Lips and tongue

The patient's lips must be closed on the bite-block during the exposure of a panoramic film. If they are not, the result is a dark radiolucent shadow that obscures the anterior teeth. Also, the tongue must be in contact with the palate during the exposure of a panoramic film. If it is not, the result is a dark radiolucent shadow that obscures the apices of the maxillary teeth (Fig. 42-8).

Solution. The patient must be instructed to close the lips around the bite-block. The patient must also be instructed to swallow and then raise the tongue up to the palate during the exposure of the film.

Chin too high (positioning of Frankfort plane)

If the Frankfort plane is incorrect and the patient's chin is positioned too high or is tipped upward (Fig. 42-9), the following problems will occur:

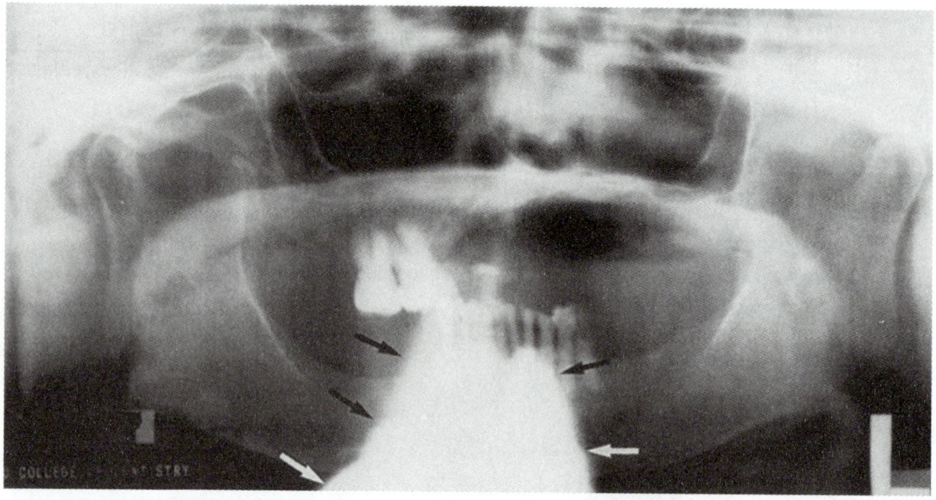

Fig. 42-7 **On a panoramic radiograph, a lead apron artifact appears as a large cone-shaped radiopacity obscuring the mandible.** (From Haring JI, Jansen L: *Dental radiography: principles and techniques,* ed 2, Philadelphia, 2000, Saunders.)

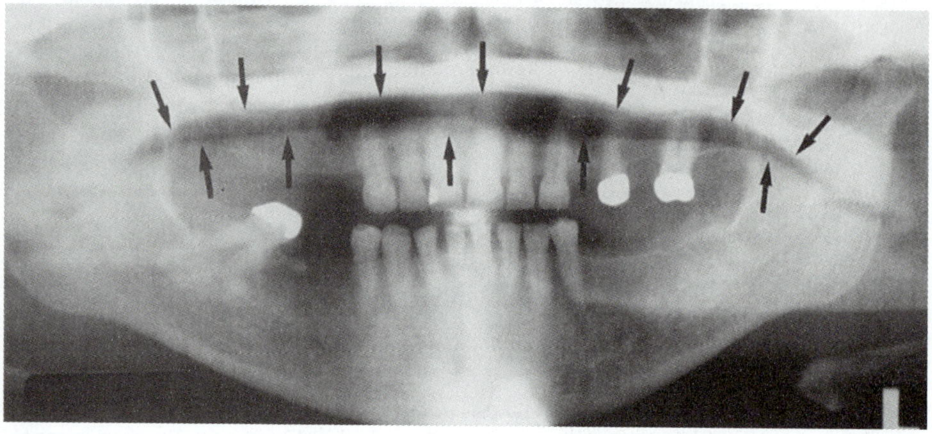

Fig. 42-8 **If the tongue is not placed on the roof of the mouth, a radiolucent shadow will be superimposed over the apices of the maxillary teeth.** (From Haring JI, Jansen L: *Dental radiography: principles and techniques,* ed 2, Philadelphia, 2000, Saunders.)

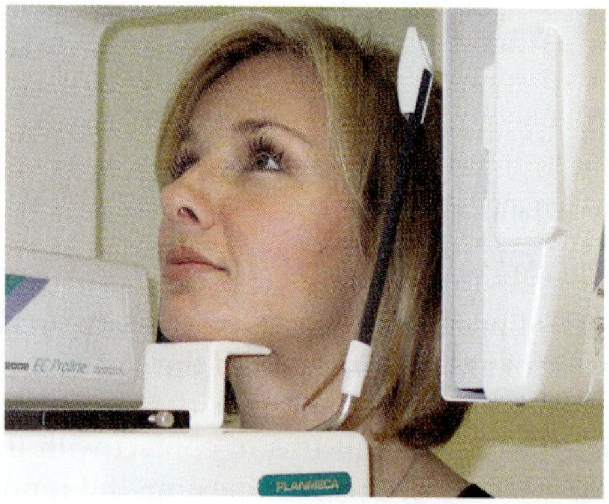

Fig. 42-9 **Patient's head is incorrectly positioned; the chin is tipped upward.**

- The hard palate and floor of the nasal cavity appear superimposed over the roots of the maxillary teeth.
- Detail in the maxillary incisor region is lost.
- The maxillary incisors appear blurred and magnified.
- A "reverse smile line" (curved downward) is apparent on the radiograph (Fig. 42-10).

Solution. Position the patient so that the Frankfort plane is parallel to the floor.

Chin too low

If the Frankfort plane is incorrect and the patient's chin is positioned too low or is tipped downward (Fig. 42-11), the following will occur:

- The mandibular incisors appear blurred.
- Detail in the anterior apical regions is lost.
- The condyles are not visible.
- An "exaggerated smile line" (curved upward) is apparent on the radiograph (Fig. 42-12).

Solution. Position the patient so that the Frankfort plane is parallel to the floor (Fig. 42-13).

Posterior to focal trough

If the patient's anterior teeth are positioned too far back on the bite-block, or posterior to the focal trough (Fig. 42-14), the anterior teeth appear "fat" and out of focus on the radiograph (Fig. 42-15).

Solution. Position the patient so that the anterior teeth are placed in an end-to-end position in the groove on the bite-block.

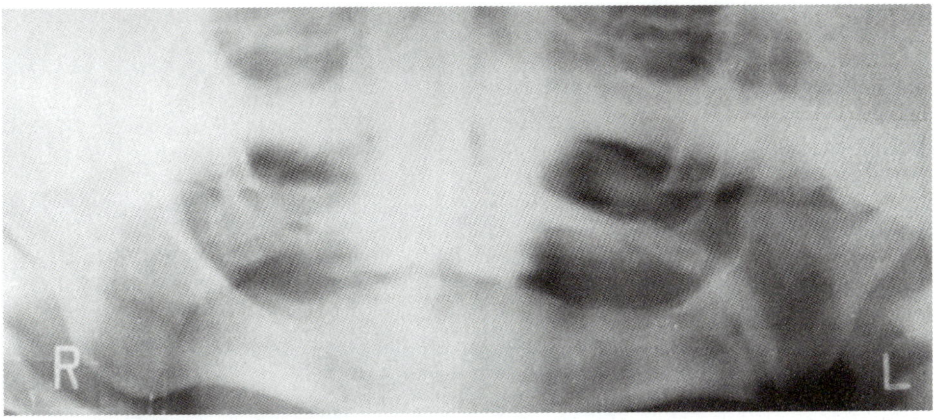

Fig. 42-10 **"Reverse smile line" is seen on a panoramic film when the patient's chin is tipped upward.** (From Haring JI, Jansen L: *Dental radiography: principles and techniques,* ed 2, Philadelphia, 2000, Saunders.)

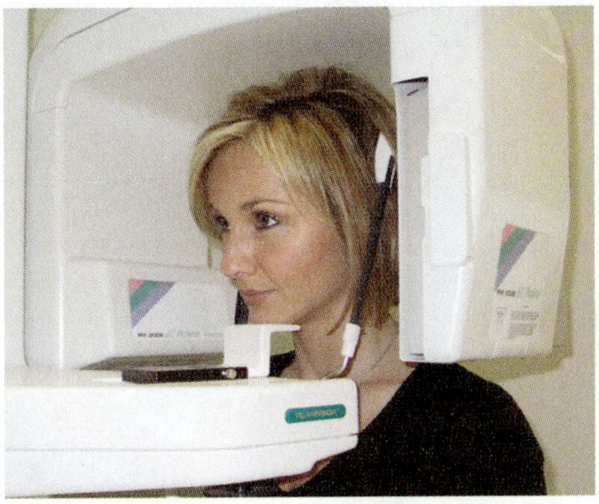

Fig. 42-11 **Patient's head is incorrectly positioned; the chin is tipped downward.**

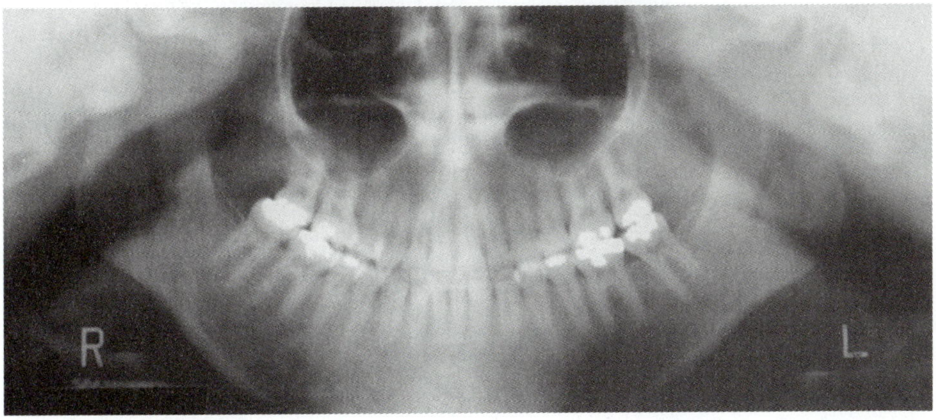

Fig. 42-12 **"Exaggerated smile" is seen on a panoramic film when patient's chin is tipped downward.** (From Haring JI, Jansen L: *Dental radiography: principles and techniques,* ed 2, Philadelphia, 2000, Saunders.)

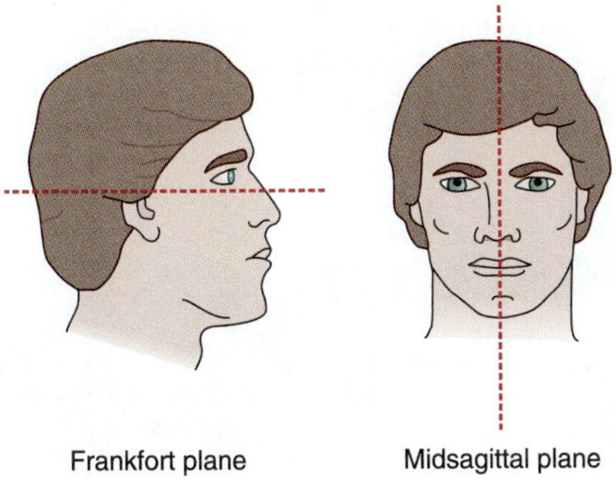

Fig. 42-13 **Frankfort and midsagittal planes. The Frankfort plane passes through the floor of the orbit and the external auditory meatus. The midsagittal plane divides the tooth in half into right and left sides.** (From Haring JI, Jansen L: *Dental radiography: principles and techniques,* ed 2, Philadelphia, 2000, Saunders.)

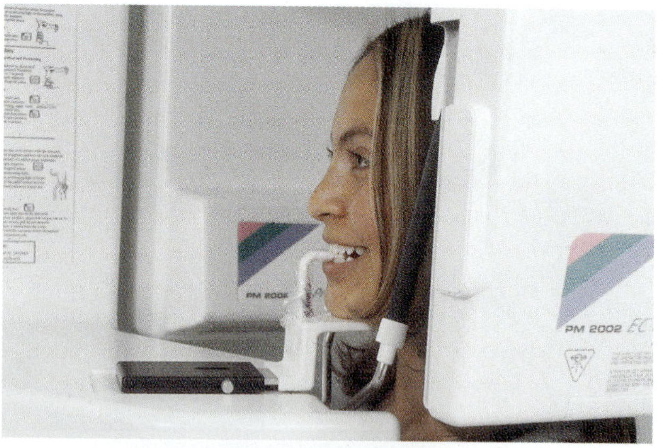

Fig. 42-14 Patient is biting too far back on the bite-block.

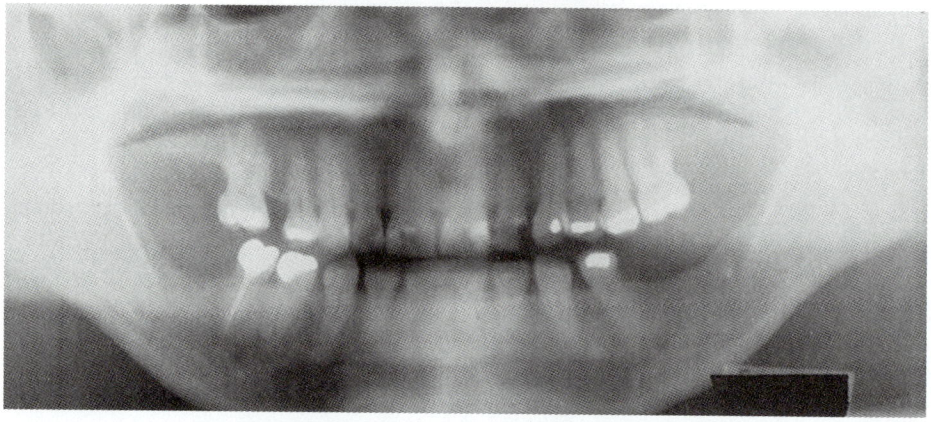

Fig. 42-15 **Anterior teeth appear widened and blurred on a panoramic film when the patient is positioned too far back on the bite-block.** (From Haring JI, Jansen L: *Dental radiography: principles and techniques,* ed 2, Philadelphia, 2000, Saunders.)

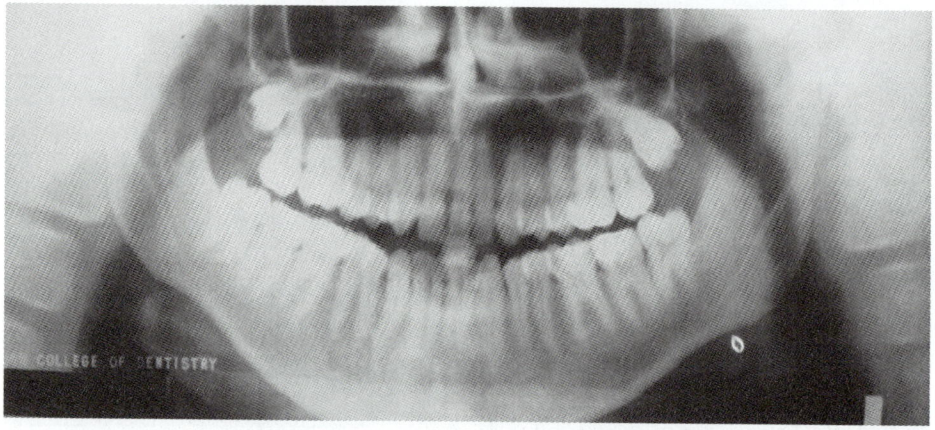

Fig. 42-16 **Anterior teeth appear narrowed and blurred on a panoramic film when the patient is positioned too far forward on the bite-block.** (From Haring JI, Jansen L: *Dental radiography: principles and techniques,* ed 2, Philadelphia, 2000, Saunders.)

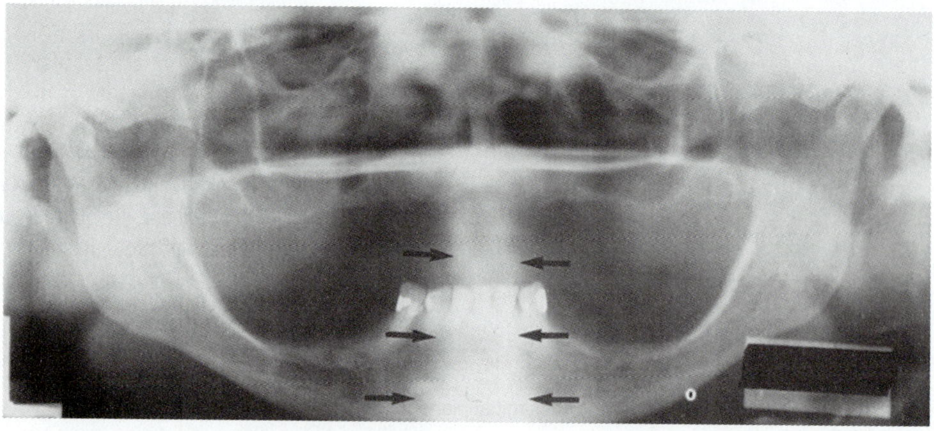

Fig. 42-17 **If the patient is not standing erect, superimposition of the cervical spine *(arrows)* may be seen on the center of the panoramic film.** (From Haring JI, Jansen L: *Dental radiography: principles and techniques,* ed 2, Philadelphia, 2000, Saunders.)

Anterior to focal trough

If the patient's anterior teeth are not positioned in the groove on the bite-block and are too far forward, or anterior to the focal trough, the teeth will appear "skinny" and out of focus (Fig. 42-16).

Solution. Position the patient so that the anterior teeth are placed in an end-to-end position in the groove on the bite-block.

Spine not straight

If the patient is not standing or sitting with a straight spine, the cervical spine appears as a radiopacity in the center of the film and obscures diagnostic information (Fig. 42-17).

Solution. The patient must be instructed to stand or sit "as tall as possible" with a straight back.

Advantages and Disadvantages

As with all radiographic techniques, panoramic radiography has both advantages and disadvantages (Table 42-1).

Table 42-1 ***Advantages and Disadvantages of Panoramic Radiography***

Advantages	
Field size	The entire maxilla and mandible can be seen on one panoramic film.
Ease of use	Learning how to expose a panoramic radiograph is relatively quick and easy.
Patient acceptance	Most patients prefer the panoramic radiograph because they do not have to hold uncomfortable film in their mouths.
Less radiation exposure	The patient receives less radiation exposure as compared with the FMX.
Disadvantages	
Image sharpness	The images seen on a panoramic radiograph are not as sharp as those seen on an intraoral film.
Focal trough limitations	Structures must be within the focal trough or they will appear out of focus.
Distortion	Even when proper technique is used, there will always be some overlapping of the teeth and distortion of the images.
Cost of equipment	Compared with the cost of an intraoral radiograph unit, a panoramic unit is more expensive

Guidelines for Exposing Panoramic Radiographs

1. Use a plastic barrier on the bite-block.
2. Use the manufacturer's recommendations for exposure factors.
3. Explain the procedure to the patient.
4. Place the proper type of lead apron.
5. Ask the patient to remove all radiolucent objects.
6. Ask the patient to sit or stand as straight as possible.
7. Ask the patient to place the anterior teeth in the groove on the bite-block.
8. Position the patient with the midsagittal plane perpendicular to the floor.
9. Position the patient with the Frankfort plane parallel to the floor.
10. Ask the patient to close the lips on the bite-block and to swallow and place the tongue against the roof of the mouth.
11. Ask the patient to remain still during the exposure.

Recall

2. What types of film are needed to supplement a panoramic radiograph? Why?
3. What is a focal trough?

EXTRAORAL RADIOGRAPHY

The extraoral radiograph provides an overall image of the skull and jaws. In some cases an extraoral film is used because the patient has swelling or severe pain and is unable to tolerate the placement of intraoral films.

Extraoral radiographs may be used alone or in conjunction with intraoral films. As in the panoramic radiograph, the images seen on an extraoral film are not as well defined or as sharp as the images seen on an intraoral radiograph. Extraoral radiographs are used for the following reasons:

- To identify trauma or fractures
- To determine the size and area of large lesions
- To identify temporomandibular joint disorders
- To detect diseases of the jaws
- To identify the location of impacted teeth
- To determine jaw growth and development

Equipment

A standard intraoral x-ray machine may be used for a variety of extraoral projections, including transcranial and lateral jaw. Special head positioning and beam alignment devices are attached to the intraoral x-ray machine for use in positioning the patient's head (Fig. 42-18).

Some panoramic x-ray units may also be fitted with special devices known as *cephalostats.* The **cephalostat** includes a film holder and head positioner that allow the operator to easily position both the film and patient (Fig. 42-19).

Film and Intensifying Screens

Most extraoral exposures use screen film placed in a cassette that has an intensifying screen. An occlusal film (size #4) may be used for some extraoral radiographs, such as lateral jaw or transcranial projections. An occlusal film is a *nonscreen film* and does not require a cassette; however, it requires more radiation than a screen film (see Chapter 39).

Grid

A **grid** is a device used to reduce the amount of *scatter radiation* that reaches an extraoral film during exposure. As discussed in Chapter 39, scatter radiation causes film fog and reduces film contrast. A grid decreases film fog and increases the contrast of the radiographic image.

A grid is composed of a series of thin lead strips embedded in plastic that permits the passage of the x-ray beam. The grid is placed between the patient's head and the film. During exposure, the grid permits the passage of the beam between the lead strips. When certain x-rays interact with the patient's tissues, scatter radiation is produced, which is then directed at the grid and film at an angle. As a result, scatter radiation is absorbed by the lead strips and does not reach the surface of the film to cause film fog (Fig. 42-20).

Despite the benefits of grid use, an increased exposure time must be used to compensate for the lead strips found in the grid. Therefore, a grid should be used only when improved image quality and high contrast are necessary to minimize radiation to the patient.

Procedures

Step-by-step procedures for the exposure of an extraoral film include the same equipment preparation, patient preparation, and patient positioning as for panoramic radiographs (see Procedures 42-1 to 42-3). Before exposing an extraoral film, infection-control procedures must be completed (see Chapter 40). If an extraoral x-ray unit with

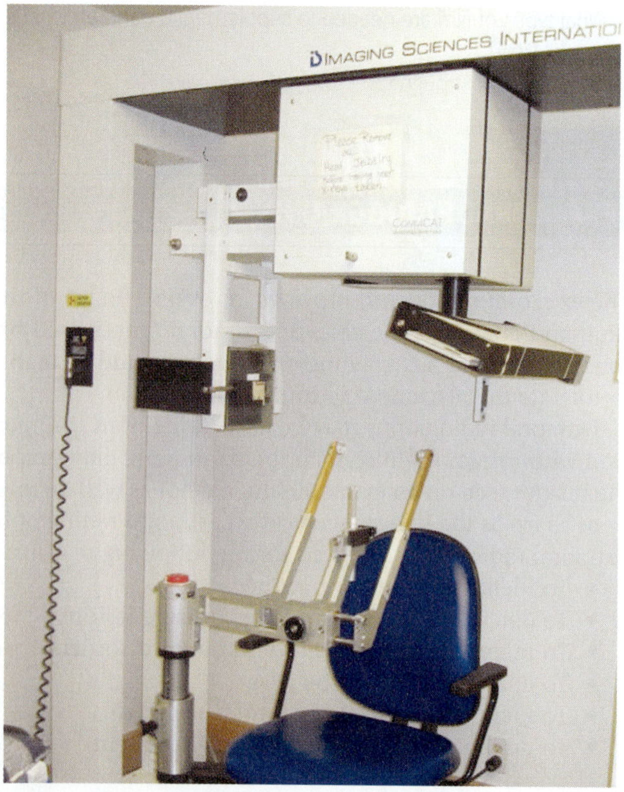

Fig. 42-18 This radiographic unit can be used with most intraoral tubeheads. It is equipped with a collimator to allow accurate beam alignment and a head positioner to allow for proper patient positioning. (From Haring JI, Jansen L: *Dental radiography: principles and techniques,* ed 2, Philadelphia, 2000, Saunders.)

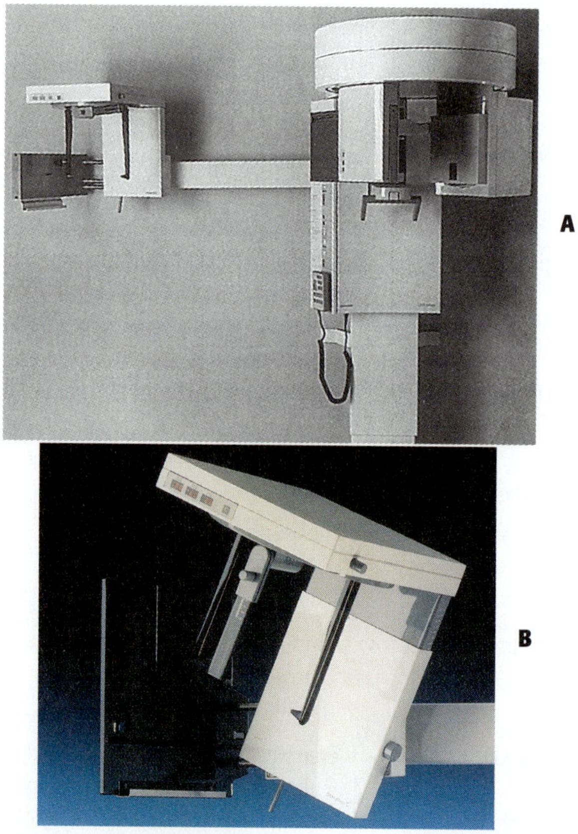

Fig. 42-19 A, Extraoral radiographic unit with cephalostat. B, Example of a cephalostat. (From Haring JI, Jansen L: *Dental radiography: principles and techniques,* ed 2, Philadelphia, 2000, Saunders.)

a cephalostat is used, the ear rods must be wiped with a disinfectant between patients.

Lateral Jaw Radiography

Lateral jaw radiography is used to view the posterior region of the mandible. It is very useful in children, patients with limited jaw opening, and patients who cannot tolerate intraoral film placement. A lateral jaw radiograph is *not* as useful as a panoramic radiograph because more diagnostic information is obtained with the panoramic radiograph.

Lateral jaw radiography does not require the use of a special x-ray unit; a standard intraoral radiograph machine can be used. Two lateral jaw projection techniques are used: the *body* of the mandible and the *ramus* of the mandible.

Body of Mandible

This projection is used to evaluate impacted teeth, fractures, and lesions located in the body of the mandible. This projection shows the mandibular premolar and molar regions as well as the inferior border of the mandible (Fig. 42-21).

Film placement

The cassette is placed flat against the patient's cheek and is centered over the body of the mandible. The cassette must be positioned parallel with the mandibular body. The patient must hold the cassette in position with the thumb placed under the edge of the cassette and the palm against the outer surface of the cassette.

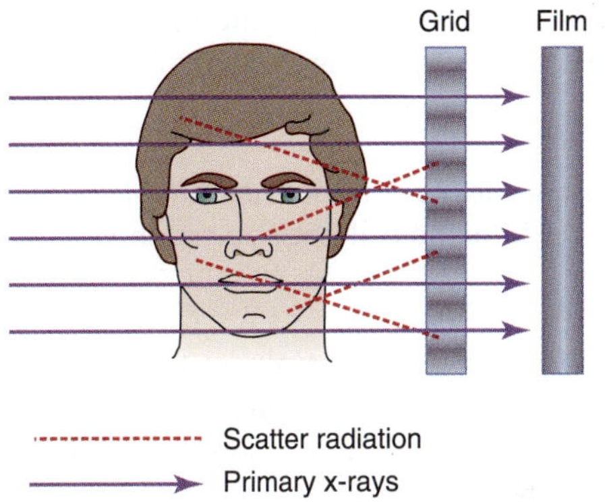

Fig. 42-20 **A grid decreases the amount of scatter radiation that reaches the extraoral film.** (From Haring JI, Jansen L: *Dental radiography: principles and techniques,* ed 2, Philadelphia, 2000, Saunders.)

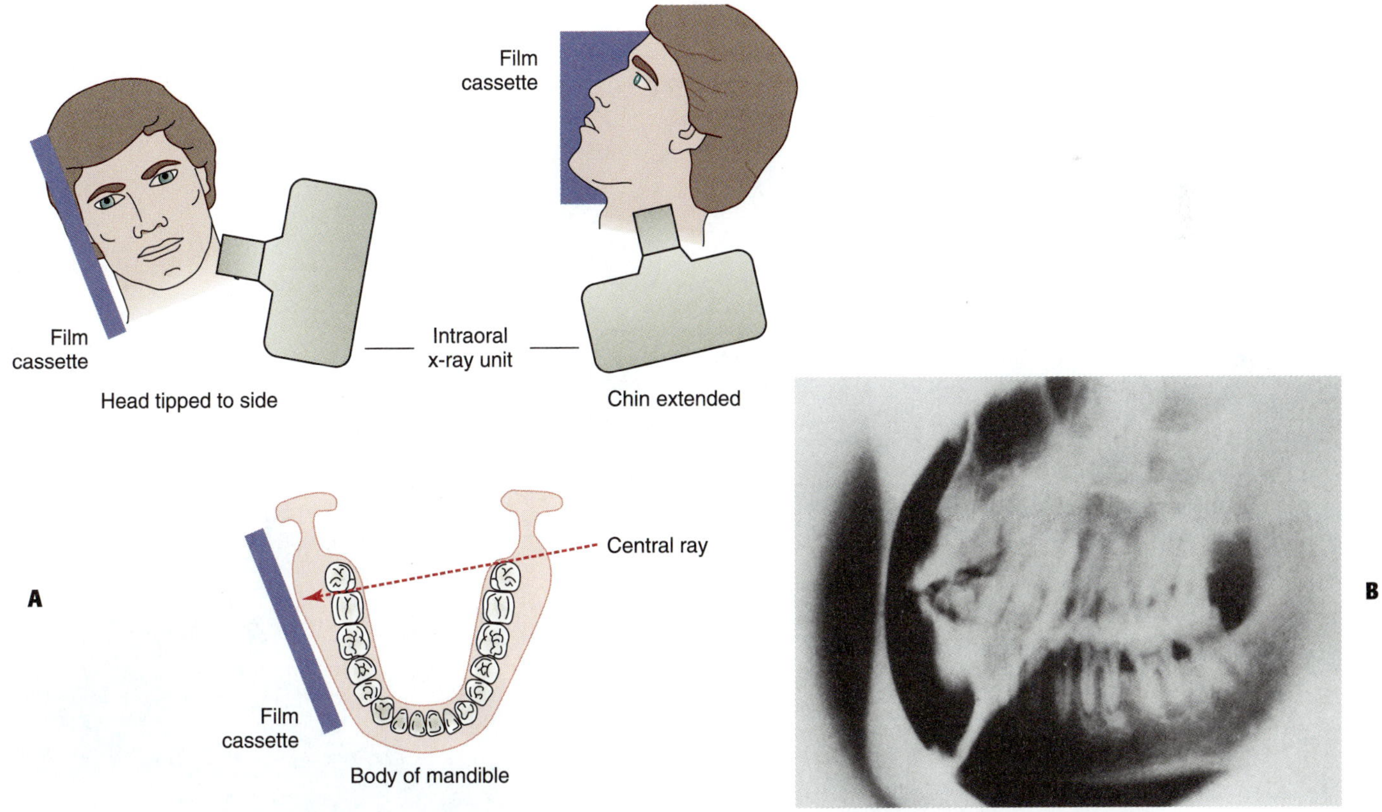

Fig. 42-21 **A, For the lateral jaw projection of the body of the mandible, proper patient and film positioning is shown as viewed from the front and side of the patient. B, Lateral jaw radiograph of mandibular body.** (From Haring JI, Jansen L: *Dental radiography: principles and techniques,* ed 2, Philadelphia, 2000, Saunders.)

Head position

The head is tipped approximately 15 degrees toward the side being radiographed. The chin is extended and elevated slightly.

Beam alignment

The central ray is directed to a point just below the inferior border of the mandible on the side *opposite* the cassette. The beam is directed upward at −15 to −20 degrees and centered on the body of the mandible. The beam must be directed *perpendicular* to the horizontal plane of the film.

Exposure factors

The exposure factors for the mandibular body projection vary with the film, intensifying screens, and equipment used.

Ramus of Mandible

This projection is used to evaluate third molars, large lesions, and fractures that extend into the ramus of the mandible. This view shows the ramus from the angle of the mandible to the condyle (Fig. 42-22).

Film placement

The cassette is placed flat against the patient's cheek and is centered over the ramus of the mandible. The cassette is positioned parallel with the ramus of the mandible. The patient must hold the cassette in position with the thumb placed under the edge of the cassette and the palm placed against the outer surface of the cassette.

Head position

The head is tipped approximately 15 degrees toward the side being radiographed. The chin is extended and elevated slightly.

Beam alignment

The central ray is directed to a point posterior to the third molar region on the side *opposite* the cassette. The beam is directed upward at −15 to −20 degrees and centered on the ramus of the mandible. The beam must be directed *perpendicular* to the horizontal plane of the film.

Exposure factors

The exposure factors for this projection vary with the film, intensifying screens, and equipment used.

Skull Radiography

Skull radiography is used most often in oral surgery and orthodontics. Although some skull films can be exposed

A

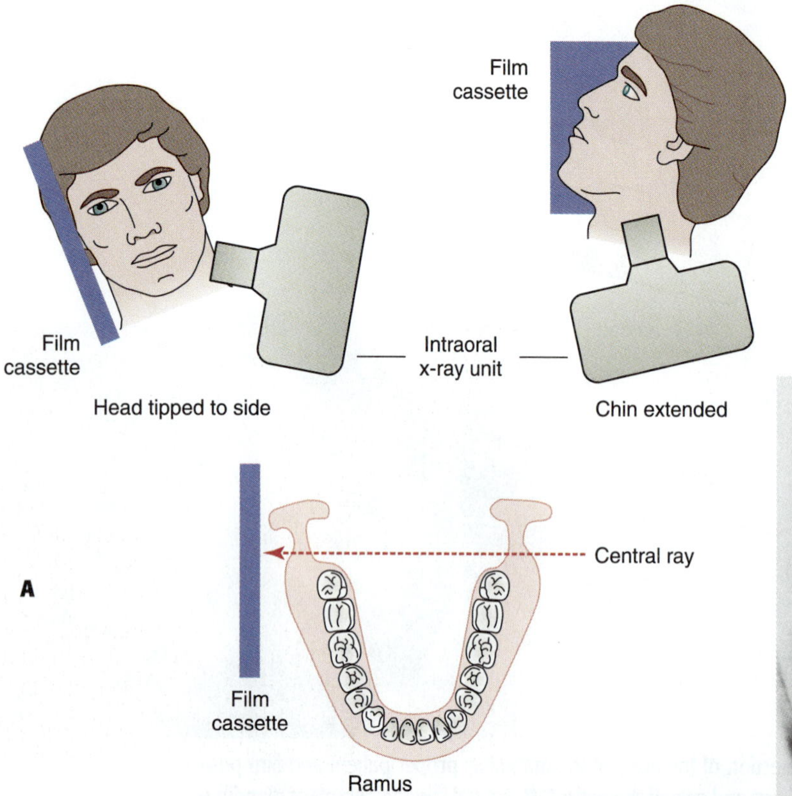

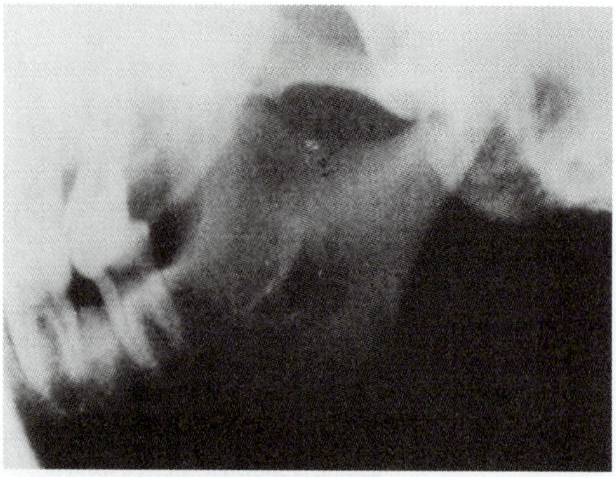

B

Fig. 42-22 A, For the lateral jaw projection of the ramus of the mandible, proper patient and film positioning is shown as viewed from the front and side of the patient. **B,** Lateral jaw radiograph of mandibular ramus. (From Haring JI, Jansen L: *Dental radiography: principles and techniques,* ed 2, Philadelphia, 2000, Saunders.)

using a standard intraoral radiograph machine, most require the use of an extraoral unit and cephalostat.

Skull radiographs may be difficult to interpret because of the numerous anatomic structures that exist in that area. Often these structures appear superimposed over one another. In many cases, multiple exposures may be necessary to obtain a clear view of the area in question. The most common skull radiographs used in dentistry include the following:

- Lateral cephalometric projection
- Posteroanterior projection
- Waters projection
- Submentovertex projection
- Reverse Towne projection

Lateral Cephalometric Projection

The lateral cephalometric projection is used to evaluate facial growth and development, trauma, disease, and developmental abnormalities. This projection shows the bones of the face and skull, as well as the soft tissue profile (Fig. 42-23).

Posteroanterior Projection

The posteroanterior projection is used to evaluate facial growth and development, trauma, disease, and developmental abnormalities. This projection shows the frontal and ethmoid sinuses, the orbits, and the nasal cavities (Fig. 42-24).

Waters Projection

The Waters projection is used to evaluate the sinus area. This view shows the frontal and ethmoid sinuses, the orbits, and the nasal cavity (Fig. 42-25).

Submentovertex Projection

The submentovertex projection is used to identify the position of the condyles, show the base of the skull, and evaluate fractures of the zygomatic arch. This projection also shows the sphenoid and ethmoid sinuses and the lateral wall of the maxillary sinus (Fig. 42-26).

Reverse Towne Projection

The reverse Towne projection is used to identify fractures of the condylar neck and ramus (Fig. 42-27).

Temporomandibular Joint Radiography

The **temporomandibular** joint (TMJ) is the *jaw joint.* This area can be very difficult to examine radiographically because of the multiple adjacent bony structures.

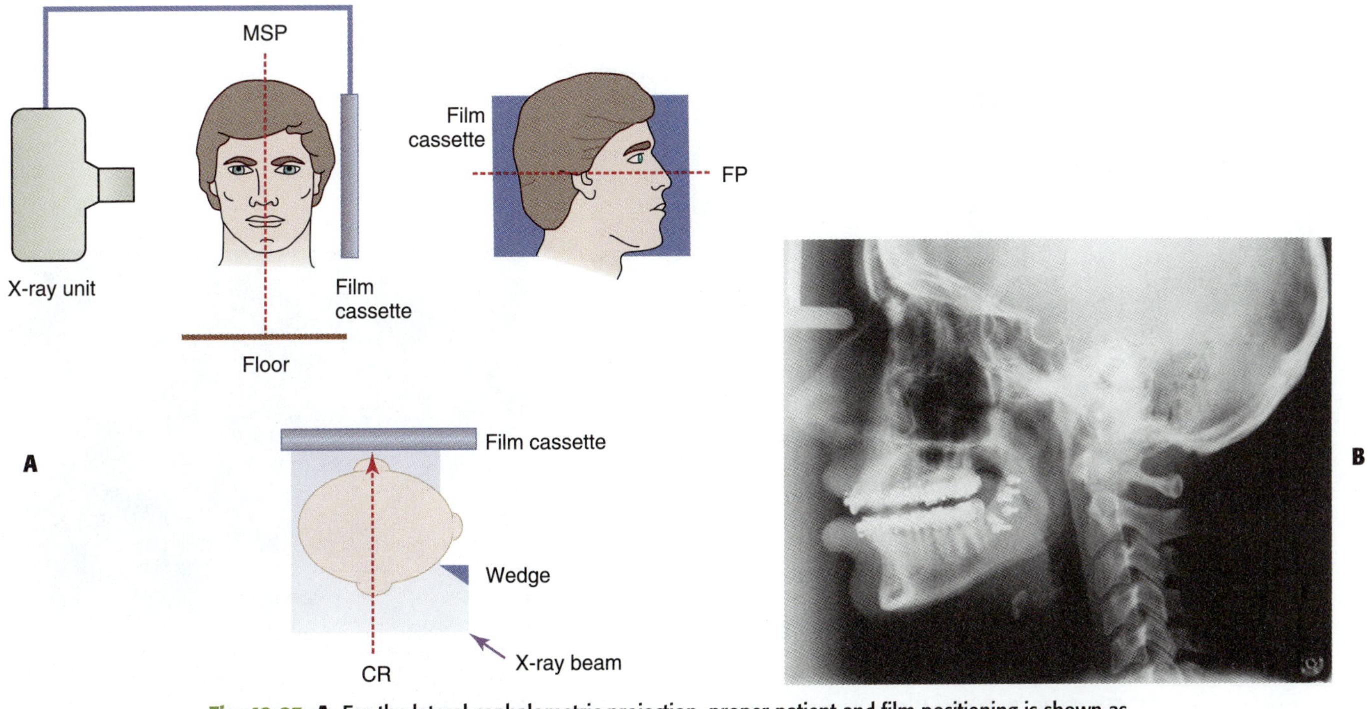

Fig. 42-23 A, For the lateral cephalometric projection, proper patient and film positioning is shown as viewed from the front, side, and top of the patient. MSP, Midsagittal plane; FP, Frankfort plane; CR, central ray. **B,** Lateral cephalometric radiograph. (From Haring JI, Jansen L: *Dental radiography: principles and techniques,* ed 2, Philadelphia, 2000, Saunders.)

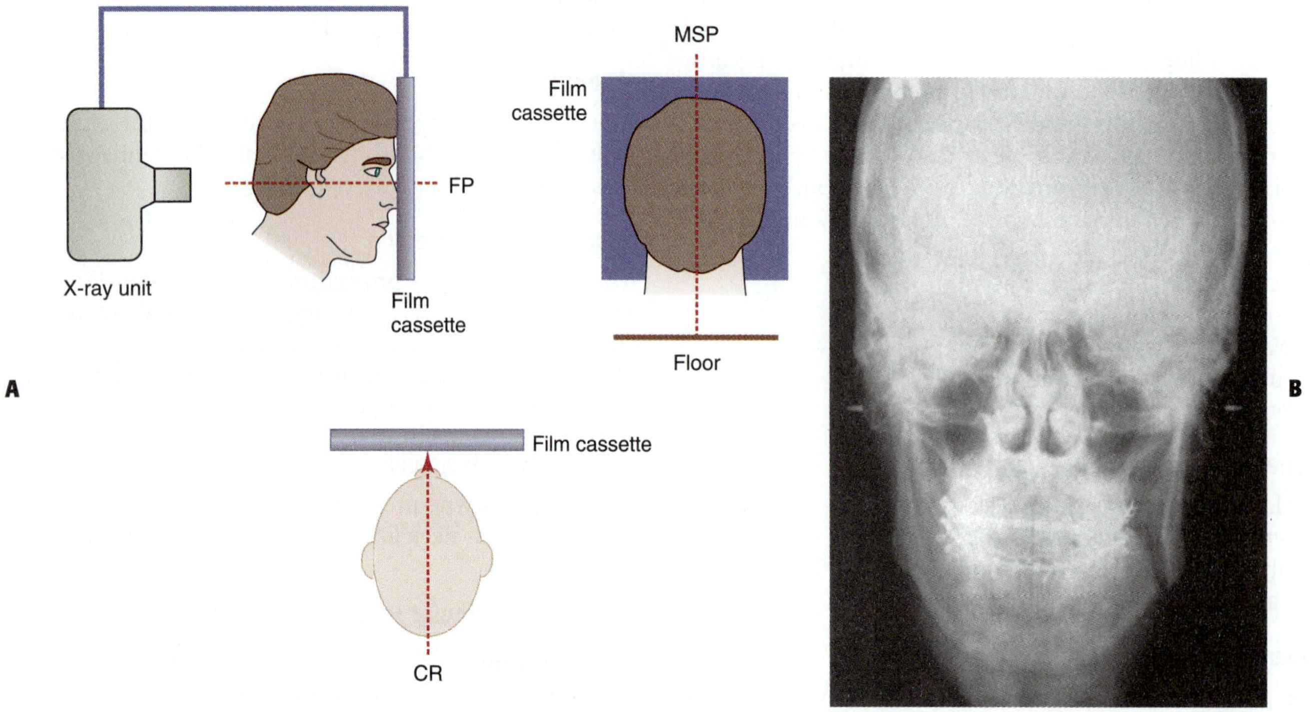

Fig. 42-24 **A,** For the posteroanterior skull projection, proper patient and film positioning is shown as viewed from the side, back, and top of the patient. *MSP,* Midsagittal plane; *FP,* Frankfort plane; *CR,* central ray. **B,** Posteroanterior skull radiograph. (From Haring JI, Jansen L: *Dental radiography: principles and techniques,* ed 2, Philadelphia, 2000, Saunders.)

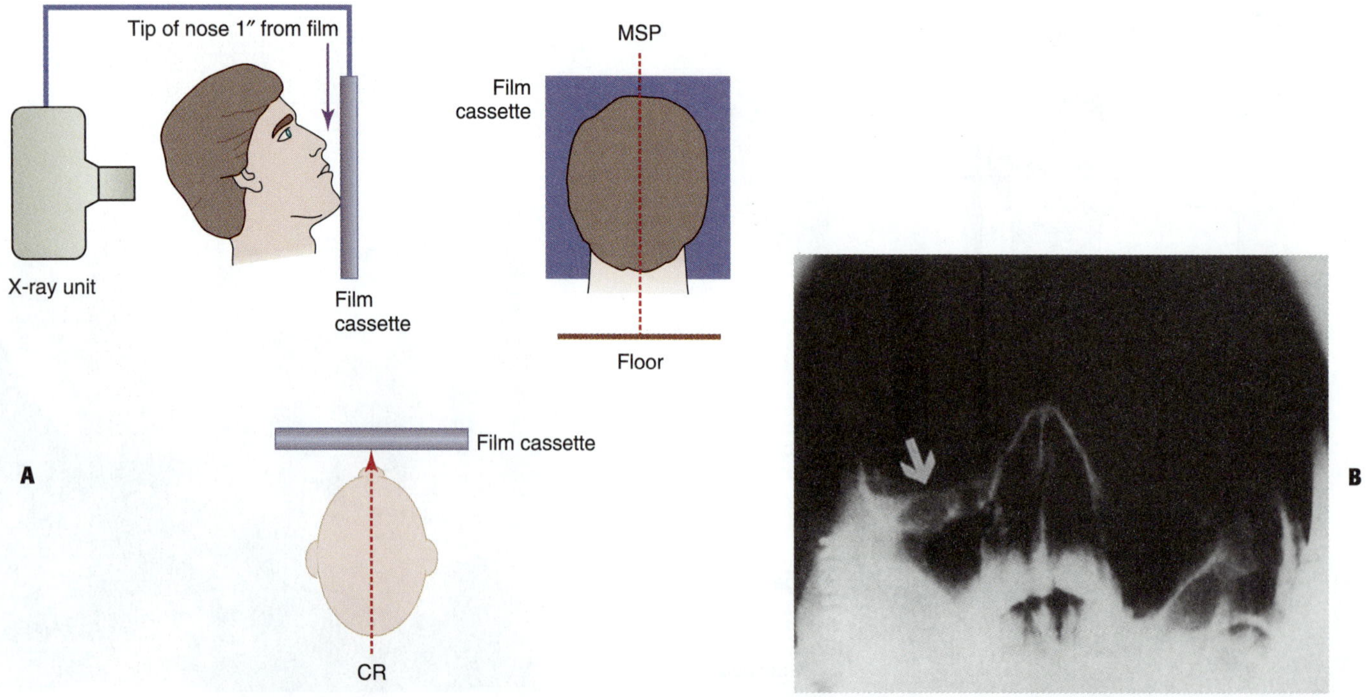

Fig. 42-25 **A,** For the Waters projection, proper patient and film positioning is shown as viewed from the side, back, and top of the patient. *MSP,* Midsagittal plane; *CR,* central ray. **B,** This case of chronic maxillary sinusitis secondary to an oroantral fistula is represented by a thickening of the lining membrane *(arrow).* (From Haring JI, Jansen L: *Dental radiography: principles and techniques,* ed 2, Philadelphia, 2000, Saunders.)

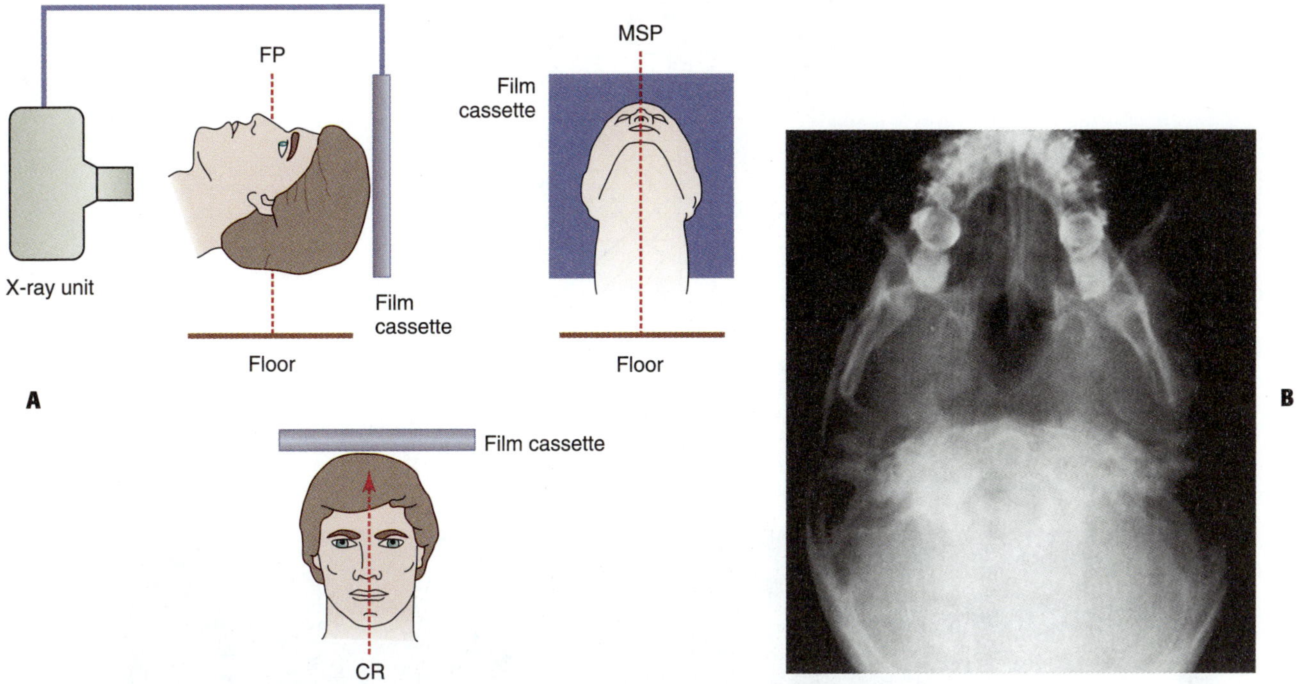

Fig. 42-26 **A,** For the submentovertex projection, proper patient and film positioning is shown as viewed from the side, front, and top of the patient. *MSP,* midsagittal plane; *FP,* Frankfort plane; *CR,* central ray. **B,** Submentovertex radiograph. (From Haring JI, Jansen L: *Dental radiography: principles and techniques,* ed 2, Philadelphia, 2000, Saunders.)

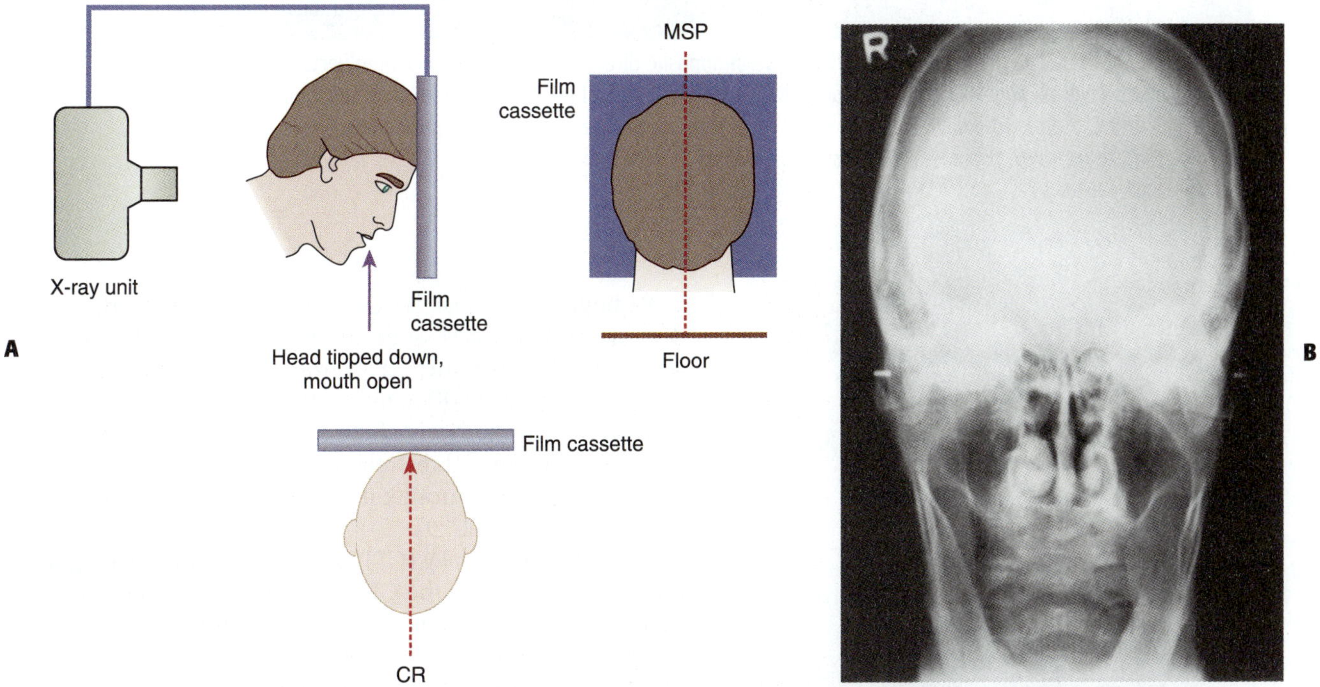

Fig. 42-27 **A,** For the reverse Towne projection, proper patient and film positioning is shown as viewed from the side, back, and top of the patient. *MSP,* midsagittal plane; *CR,* central ray. **B,** Reverse Towne radiograph. (From Haring JI, Jansen L: *Dental radiography: principles and techniques,* ed 2, Philadelphia, 2000, Saunders.)

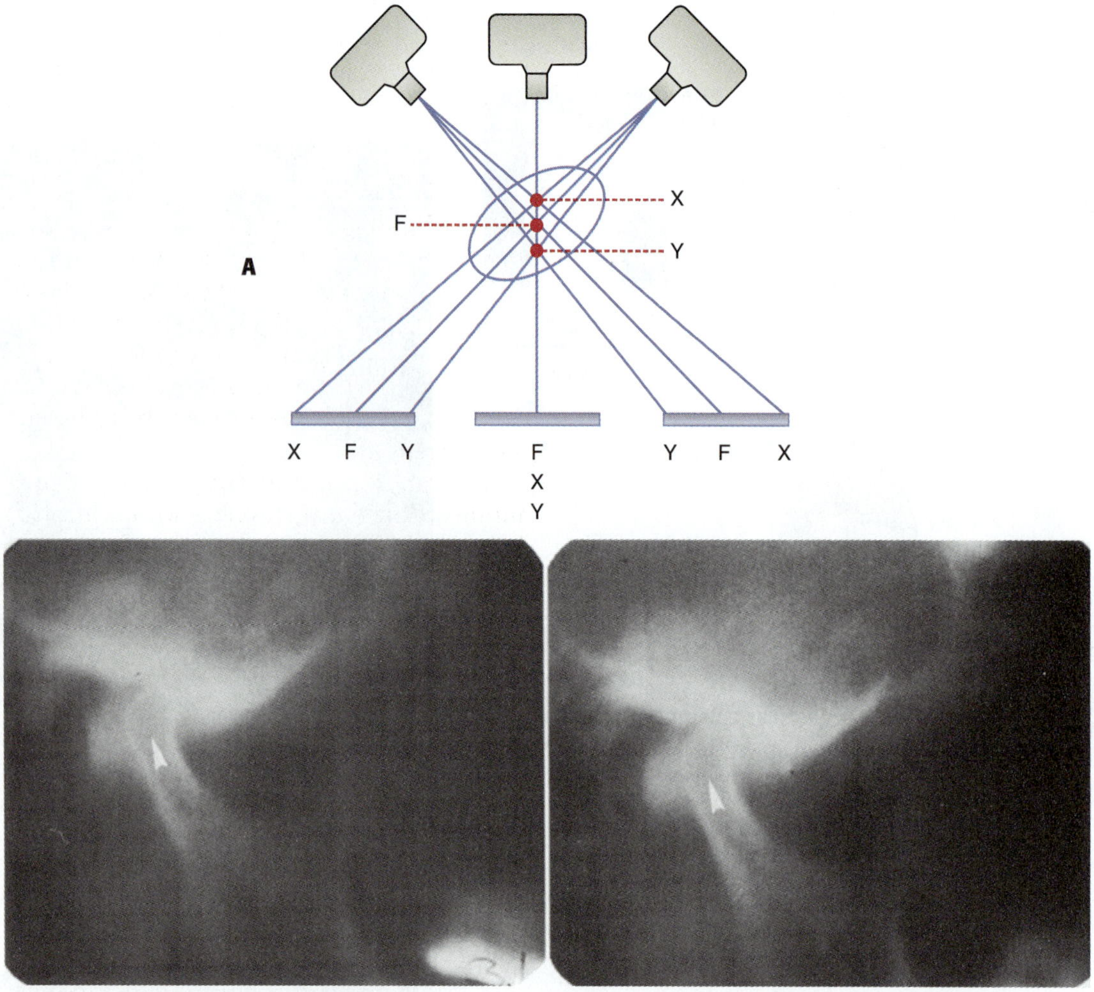

Fig. 42-28 **A,** As the tubehead and film move in opposite directions around the patient, objects in the image layer (F) appear sharp on the film. Objects on either side of the image layer (*X* < *Y*) are blurred. **B** and **C,** Corrected axial CT images show decreased joint space and posterior positioning of the left condyle *(arrows).* (From Haring JI, Jansen L: *Dental radiography: principles and techniques,* ed 2, Philadelphia, 2000, Saunders.)

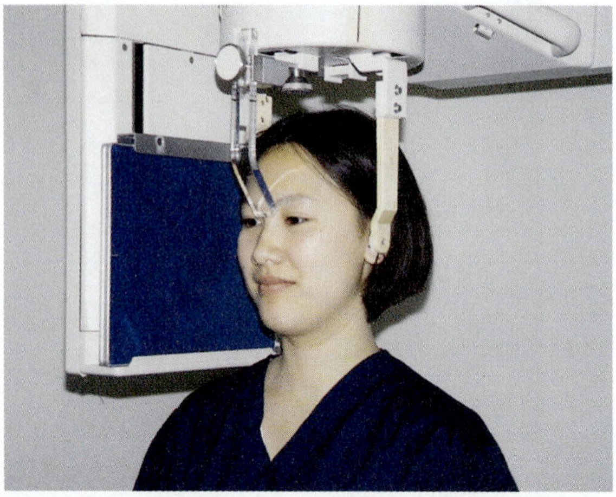

Fig. 42-29 Patient positioned for a transcranial radiograph of the temporomandibular joint.

Radiography *cannot* be used to examine the articular disc and other soft tissues of the TMJ. Instead, special imaging techniques such as arthrography and *magnetic resonance imaging* (MRI) must be used (Fig. 42-28). Radiographic projections of the TMJ, however, can be used to show the bone and the relationship of the jaw joint. For example, changes in bone can be seen on transcranial TMJ radiographs (Fig. 42-29).

Computed tomography (CT) provides the best imaging of the TMJ. In addition, the CT scan can be used to estimate joint space and evaluate the extent of movement of the condyle when the mouth is open. Most dental offices do not purchase such specialized radiographic equipment because of the high cost. As a result, dental patients who require CT of the TMJ are usually referred to a specialized radiographic imaging facility.

Recall

4. What is the purpose of extraoral radiographs?
5. What is the name of the device that may be added to a panoramic unit to allow the operator to easily position the film and patient?
6. What is the purpose of a grid?
7. What type of imaging is best for soft tissues of the TMJ?

DIGITAL RADIOGRAPHY

Advances in computer technology have led to a unique "filmless" imaging system known as **digital radiography.** Since its introduction to dentistry in 1987, digital radiography has greatly influenced how dental disease is recognized and diagnosed. The use of digital radiography is rapidly increasing in both general and specialty dental practices.

Digital radiography is used to record x-ray images. Unlike the conventional dental radiography, there is no film or processing chemistry used. Rather, digital radiography uses an electronic sensor (instead of film) to record the images and then sends this information to a computer that **digitizes** (converts to numbers) these electronic impulses. This allows the computer to produce a diagnostic image on a monitor almost instantaneously (Fig. 42-30).

Several companies now produce digital imaging systems for dentistry. This section describes only the basic principles and types of digital imaging, the digital equipment, and the advantages and disadvantages of the system.

Basic Concepts

The purpose of digital radiography is to produce images that can be used in the diagnosis of dental disease. The digital images are diagnostically equal to film-based images and allow the dentist to identify many conditions that may otherwise go undetected. As with film-based radiographic procedures, digital radiography allows the dentist to obtain detailed information about the teeth and supporting structures.

The term *digital radiography* refers to a method of capturing an x-ray image using a sensor, breaking the image into electronic pieces, and storing it in a computer. The resulting image is displayed on a computer screen rather than on film that must be processed in a darkroom. With digital radiography, the term *image* (not *radiograph* or *radiograph film*) is used to describe the pictures that are produced.

A **sensor** is used in place of intraoral dental film (Fig. 42-31). When the x-ray beam strikes the sensor, an electronic charge is produced on the surface of the sensor. This electronic signal is digitized, or converted into "digital" form. The digital sensor in turn transmits this information to the computer. Software in the computer is used to store the image electronically.

The digital image is displayed within seconds and can then be manipulated to enhance the appearance for interpretation and diagnosis. Digital images are not limited to

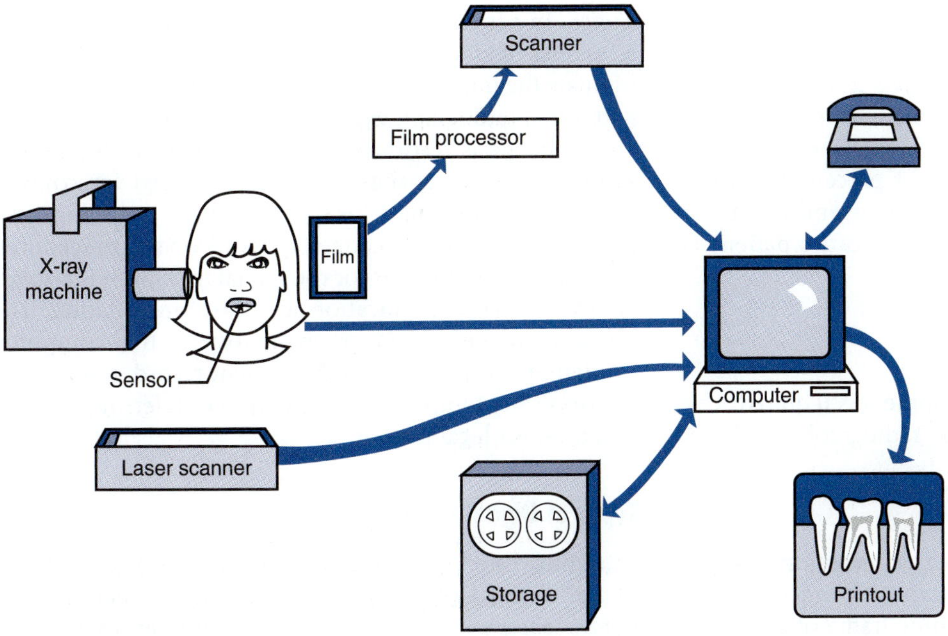

Fig. 42-30 Diagram of a digital imaging system. (From Frommer HH, Stabulus JJ: *Radiology for the dental professional,* ed 8, St Louis, 2005, Mosby.)

A

B

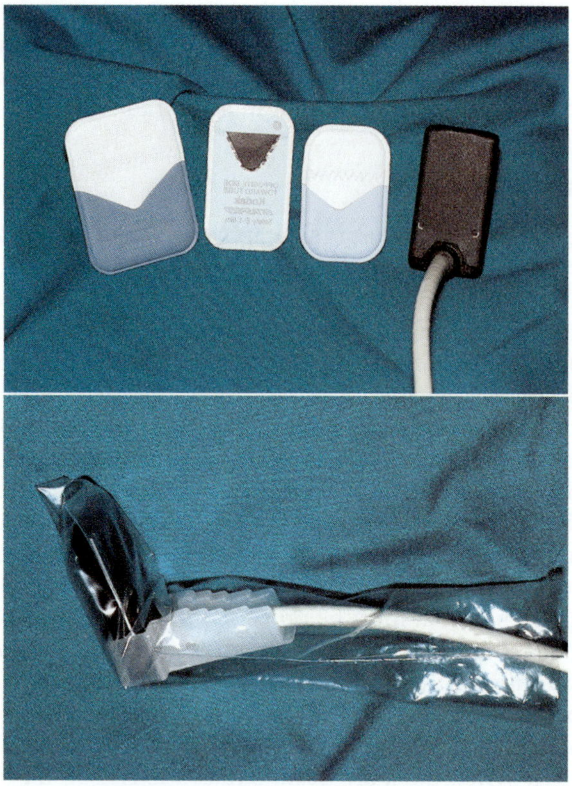

Fig. 42-31 **A,** Size of the electronic sensor is compared with sizes #0, #1, and #2 of traditional intraoral film. **B,** Electronic sensor is protected with a plastic barrier and is ready for positioning into the patient's mouth in the same manner as for a traditional film and holder. (Courtesy Michael Danford, Santa Rosa, Calif.)

intraoral images; panoramic and cephalometric images may also be obtained (Fig. 42-32).

Radiation Exposure

Digital radiography requires much *less x-radiation* than conventional radiography because the sensor is *more sensitive* to x-rays than conventional film. Exposure times for digital radiography are 50 to 80 percent less than those required for radiography using conventional film. With less radiation, the absorbed dose to the patient is significantly lower.

Equipment

For digital radiography, special equipment is required. The essential components include the radiograph machine, intraoral sensor, and computer.

Radiograph Machine

Most digital radiography systems use a conventional dental radiograph machine. However, the exposure timer must be calibrated to allow exposures in a time frame of a second.

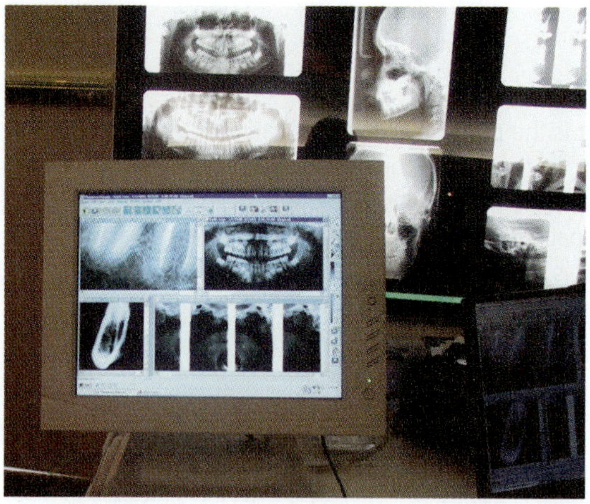

Fig. 42-32 All types of radiographs may be produced in digital format.

A standard x-ray unit that is adapted for digital radiography can still be functional for conventional radiography.

Intraoral Sensor

Intraoral sensors used in digital radiography may be wired or wireless. *Wired* means that the imaging sensor is held by a fiberoptic cable to a computer that records the generated signal. The cable in wired systems varies in length from 8 feet to 35 feet; the shorter the cable, the more limited the range of motion will be. *Wireless* means that the sensor is *not* linked by a cable. The concept of wireless is similar to a remote control for a television.

Computer

The computer stores the incoming electronic signal and converts it from the sensor to shades of gray that are viewed on the computer monitor. The computer is capable of creating 256 shades of gray, referred to as a pixel's *gray-scale resolution.* In comparison, the human eye can appreciate only 32 shades of gray. This technology allows the dentist to manipulate the image to enhance contrast and density without additional radiograph exposure to the patient.

The image is recorded on the computer in 0.5 to 120 seconds, much less time than that required for conventional film processing. This speed of image recording is extremely useful during certain types of dental procedures, such as surgical implants or root canal therapy. It is also excellent for patient education and case presentation. The image may be stored permanently in the computer, printed on a hard copy for the patient record, transmitted electronically to insurance companies or referring dentists, and used for legal purposes.

Types of Digital Imaging

Currently, three methods are available to obtain a digital image: *direct digital imaging, indirect digital imaging,* and *storage phosphor imaging.* The main differences between these methods are in how the image is obtained and in what size receptor plates are available. Once the image is obtained, the systems do not vary greatly in how they display, adjust, store, or transmit the image.

Direct Digital Imaging

In the direct technique an intraoral sensor is placed into the mouth of a patient and exposed to x-rays. The sensor may be either the wired or wireless type. The sensor captures the image and then transmits the image to the computer. Within seconds of exposing the sensor to the x-rays, the image appears on the computer screen. Software is then used to enhance the image. This is probably the most frequently used method.

Indirect Digital Imaging

The essential components in the indirect system include an existing radiograph, a **charge-coupled device (CCD)** camera, and a computer. A CCD is a solid-state detector used in devices such as fax machines and home video cameras. In digital radiography a CCD is an image receptor found in the intraoral sensor.

With indirect imaging an existing radiograph is digitized using the CCD camera and is then displayed on the computer. This concept is similar to scanning an image, such as a photograph, to a computer screen. Indirect digital imaging is inferior to direct digital imaging because the resultant image is similar to a "copy" of the image versus the "original."

Storage Phosphor Imaging

This is a *wireless* method in which a reusable imaging plate is used instead of a sensor with a fiberoptic cable. The phosphor-coated plates are flexible and the same size as traditional films; they are placed into the mouth similar to intraoral films. The phosphor plate is similar to an intensifying screen, converting x-ray energy into light.

In the storage phosphor technique, after the exposure is made, the plate is removed from the mouth and placed into an electronic processor, where a laser scans the plate and produces an image that is then transferred to the computer screen. No chemicals are used in the "processing." Because of the laser setup, this type of digital imaging is *slower* than direct digital imaging.

As the name *storage phosphor technique* indicates, the image is *stored* in the phosphor on the sensor. In theory, the image is similar to an image being stored on a computer disk; to be viewed, it must be put into the computer.

Procedures

Step-by-step procedures for the use of digital radiography systems vary by manufacturer. It is *critical* to refer to the manufacturer's instruction booklet for information concerning the operation of the system, equipment preparation, patient preparation, and exposure factors. Only general guidelines on sensor preparation and placement are discussed here.

Sensor Preparation

The technique for placement of the intraoral sensor in the mouth of the patient is similar to the technique used in conventional film placement. Although the numbers and sizes of sensors may vary with different manufacturers, each sensor is sealed and waterproofed. For infection-control purposes, the sensor must be covered with a disposable barrier because it *cannot* be sterilized (Fig. 42-33).

Sensor Placement

The sensor is held in the mouth by special film-holding devices. The *paralleling technique* is the preferred exposure method because of the dimensional accuracy of the images (see Chapter 41). Paralleling technique film holders must be used to stabilize the sensor in the mouth. As with conventional intraoral film, the sensor is centered over the area of interest (Fig. 42-34).

Advantages and Disadvantages

As with any intraoral radiographic technique, digital radiography has both advantages and disadvantages (Table 42-2).

Recall

8. In digital radiography, what replaces the intraoral film?
9. How are sensors sterilized?
10. Which exposure technique is preferred when using digital radiography?

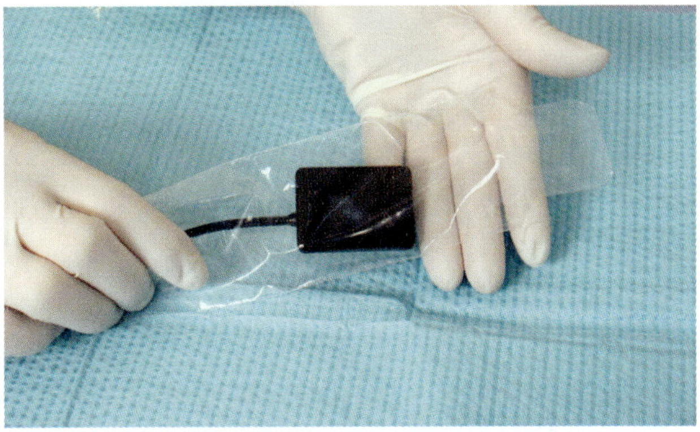

Fig. 42-33 Sensor being prepared for use.

Table 42-2 ***Advantages and Disadvantages of Digital Radiography***

Advantages	
Gray-scale resolution	Gray-scale resolution is excellent, which is important because an accurate diagnosis is often based on contrast.
Reduced radiation exposure to the patient	Digital radiography systems require 50% to 80% less exposure than conventional radiographic units.
Faster viewing of images	Images are almost immediately ready for viewing.
Lower equipment and film costs	Costs for x-ray film and processing solutions are eliminated. In addition, there are no environmental concerns related to disposal of processing chemicals.
Patient education	Patients can see and understand conditions within the teeth. Digital radiography can also increase the patient's willingness to accept treatment plans.
Disadvantages	
Initial set-up costs	Digital radiography systems require an initial investment estimated at $10,000, depending on the type of computer and other auxiliary features.
Quality of images	Not everyone agrees, but the images appear to be satisfactory to diagnose dental disease.
Sensor size	Some patients find the sensors bulky and complain about the thickness. In addition, some patients tend to gag more frequently than when traditional film is used.
Infection control	The sensor must be protected with disposable control barriers because the digital sensor cannot be heat sterilized.

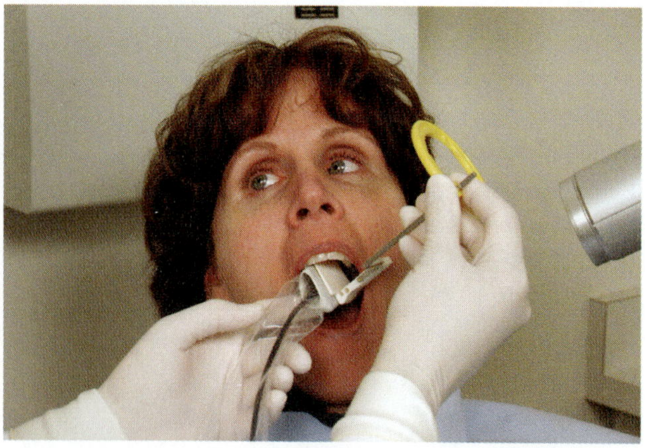

Fig. 42-34 Sensor being placed in patient's mouth.

Legal and Ethical Implications

When digital radiography first appeared on the market, there was a great deal of concern about the legal implications of the capability of manipulating the digital image. Unethical practitioners could alter images to justify unwarranted procedures or alter treatment records. In addition, jurors may not consider digital images as "hard" evidence because of the possibility that they had been altered.

Today, companies are producing software that will not allow an altered image to be saved (except as a copy). For example, Eastman Kodak's Digital Science Dental Scanning System includes a warning feature that appears if the original image is not the same as the image displayed on the monitor. There is also another technique, called *digital watermarking,* that embeds an invisible ID into the image, making fraudulent modifications too difficult to accomplish. Because of these advances, most insurance companies today are not concerned about accepting digital images.

Eye to the Future

A revolutionary new advanced dental imaging system called the CB MercuRay is now available. This system uses digital ConeBeam X-Ray. The ConeBeam technology provides excellent image quality with less radiation than an ordinary CT scan. The digital x-ray scanner rotates around the head in just 10 seconds, providing three-dimensional imaging of hard and soft tissues. This system has uses for dental implants, impacted teeth, pathology, orthodontics, endodontics, and periodontics, as well as sinus, airway, and TMJ assessment.

At this time, there are only a few of these machines in the United States. Further research using this technology will allow for more accurate diagnosis and treatment planning. Additional information about the CB MercuRay can be obtained from Hitachi Medical Systems America, Inc., by phone (800-800-3106) or online (www.hitachimed.com).

Critical Thinking

1. Mr. Robert Herrera is a patient in your office and is scheduled for a panoramic radiograph. He is relieved when the receptionist tells him that he will not need to have films placed in his mouth. How will you explain to him the need for supplemental bite-wing films? What will you say to the receptionist?
2. After processing Mr. Herrera's panoramic film, you notice that the anterior teeth appear very wide and distorted. What could have been the problem? What are you going to tell Mr. Herrera?
3. Do you agree or disagree that digital radiographs are the "wave of the future"? Why?

Part 9

Dental Materials

The clinical use of dental materials is an essential component for most dental procedures. The role of the dental assistant in the preparation and application of dental material is an integral part of this process.

The chapters in this section will provide you with a level of background knowledge and skill necessary to become competent as a dental assistant in clinical practice. The dental materials presented in the following chapters will guide and develop your skill level when you work in the general and specialized areas of dentistry.

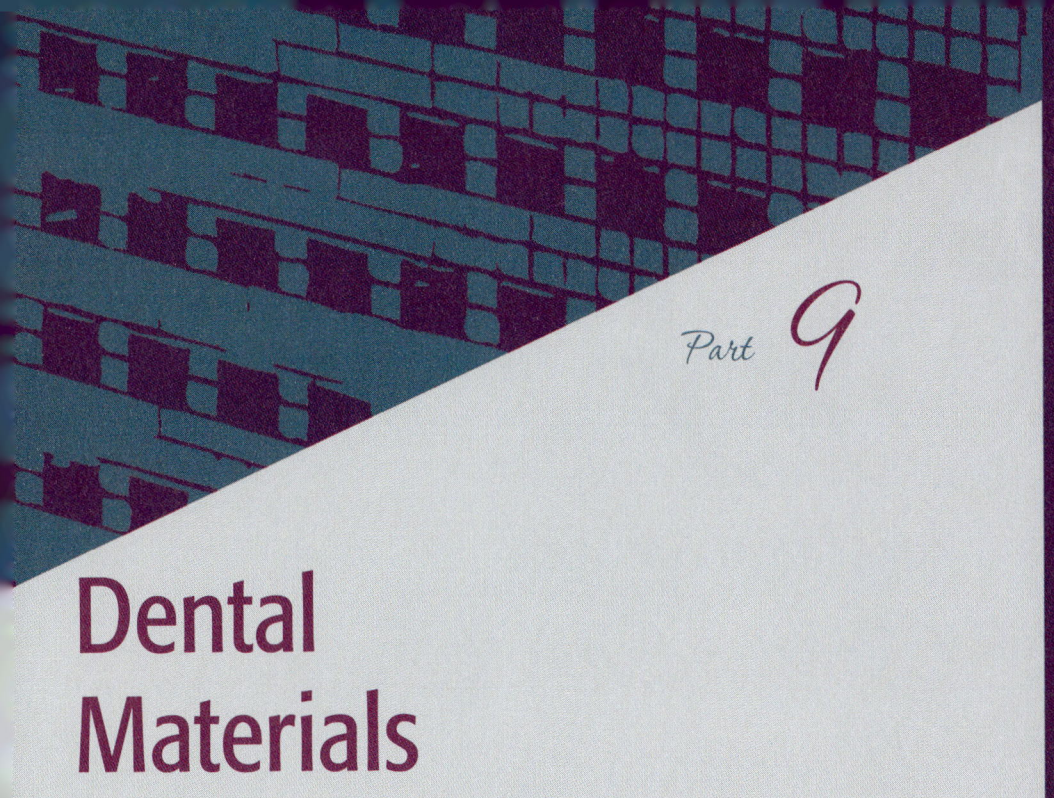

43

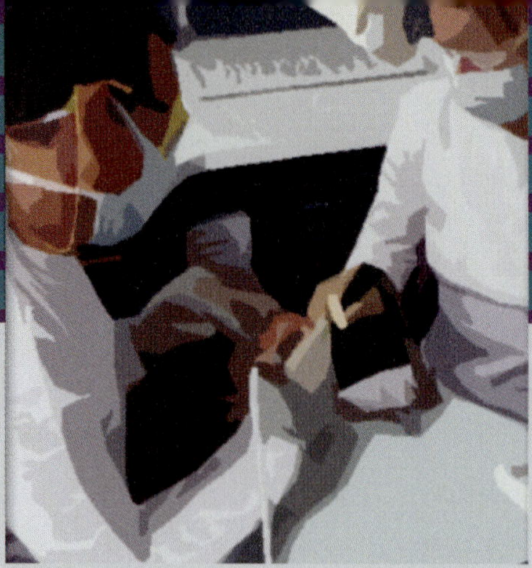

Restorative and Esthetic Dental Materials

Outline

KEY TERMS

Adhere To stick or glue two items together.

Alloy Mixture of two or more metals.

Amalgam (ah-**mal**-gum) Mixture of an alloy with mercury.

Auto-cured Hardened or set by a chemical reaction of two materials.

Ceramic Hard, brittle, heat- and corrosive-resistant material such as clay.

Coupling agent Agent that strengthens resin by bonding filler to the resin matrix.

Cured Preserved or finished by a chemical or physical process.

Dual-cured Prepared, preserved, or finished by a chemical or physical process.

Esthetic (es-**the**-tik) Artistically pleasing and beautiful appearance; also spelled *aesthetic.*

Filler Inorganic material that adds strength and other characteristics to composite resins.

Force To cause a physical change through energy and strength.

Galvanic (gal-**va**-nik) An electrical current that takes place when two different or dissimilar metals come together.

Gold A soft, yellow, corrosive-resistant metal used in the making of indirect restorations.

Irregular Not straight, uniform, or symmetrical.

Malleability (*ma*-lee-ah-**bi**-leh-tee) The ability of a material to withstand permanent deformation under compressive stress without permanent damage.

Matrix (**may**-triks) Foundation binding a substance together; continuous phases (organic polymer) in which particles of filler are dispersed in composite resin.

Microleakage (**my**-cro-*leak*-age) Microscopic leakage at the interface of the tooth structure and the sealant or restoration.

Palladium (puh-**lay**-dee-um) Soft, steel-white, tarnish-resistant metal that occurs naturally with platinum.

KEY TERMS, cont'd

Pestle (**pe**-sul, **pes**-tul) An object that moves vertically, pounding or pulverizing a material.

Platinum (**plat**-i-num) Silver-white noble metal that does not corrode in air.

Porcelain (**por**-su-lun) Hard, white, translucent ceramic made by firing and then glazing.

Restorative (ri[reh]-**stor**-eh-tiv) Having the ability to restore or bring back a natural appearance.

Retention (ri-**ten[t]**-shun) The result of adhesion, mechanical locking, or both.

Spherical (**sfer**-i-kul) Round in shape.

Strain The distortion or change produced as a result of stress.

Stress The internal reaction or resistance to an externally applied force.

Trituration (*tri*-chuh-**ray**-shun) To mix together, as in the process of mixing an alloy with mercury to form an amalgam.

Viscosity (vis-**kah**-suh-tee) Physical property of fluids for resistance to flow.

Wetting Covering or soaking something with a liquid.

LEARNING OUTCOMES

On completion of this chapter, the student will be able to achieve the following objectives:

- Pronounce, define, and spell the Key Terms.
- Discuss how a dental material is evaluated before being marketed to the profession.
- List the properties of dental materials and ways that they affect their application.
- Discuss the difference between direct and indirect restorative materials.
- Describe the factors that affect how dental materials are manufactured for the oral cavity.
- Describe the properties of amalgam and its application in restoring teeth.
- Describe the properties of composite resin materials and their application in restoring teeth.
- Describe the properties of glass ionomers and their application in restoring teeth.
- Describe the properties of temporary restorative materials and their application in restoring teeth.
- Discuss the use of tooth-whitening products.
- Describe the properties of gold alloys and their application in restoring teeth.
- Describe the properties of porcelain and its application in restoring teeth.

PERFORMANCE OUTCOMES

On completion of this chapter, the student will be able to achieve competency standards in the following skills:

- Mix and transfer amalgam.
- Prepare composite resin material.
- Mix intermediate restorative material.
- Prepare acrylic resin for provisional coverage.

Dental materials fulfill an important role in the way dentistry is delivered today. Selection of the most appropriate dental material depends on the extent of decay, type of defect in the tooth, condition of the entire mouth, whether the restoration will be visible, and cost factors. The most common dental restorative materials used in today's dentistry are:

- Amalgam
- Composite resins
- Glass ionomers
- Temporary materials
- Tooth-whitening products
- Gold alloys
- Ceramic castings

Restorative is a term used to describe the ability to replace or bring something back to its natural appearance and function. **Esthetic** is a term used for an artistically pleasing appearance.

The types of dental materials introduced in this chapter are restorative and esthetic materials that are most often used by the general dentist. An understanding of these frequently used dental materials provides you with the necessary knowledge to recognize the types of procedures practiced by the general dentist.

As a clinical dental assistant, it is essential that you learn the general characteristics of each dental material discussed, selection criteria for each material, and the preparation of the restorative and esthetic materials for a procedure. It is the dental assistant's responsibility to retrieve the setup for each material and to be attentive to the manufacturer's recommended proportions and mixing techniques.

STANDARDIZATION OF DENTAL MATERIALS

When a new dental material is developed, the product must undergo a strict evaluation and assessment before being marketed to the profession. The Council on Dental

Criteria for a New Dental Material

Must *not* be poisonous or harmful to the body
Must *not* be harmful or irritating to the tissues of the oral cavity
Must help protect the tooth and tissues of the oral cavity
Must resemble the natural dentition as closely as possible so as to be esthetically pleasing
Must be easily formed and placed in the mouth to restore the mouth's natural contour
Must conform and function despite limited access, wet conditions, and poor visibility

Materials, Instruments and Equipment was formed as a subcommittee by the American Dental Association (ADA) in combination with federal organizations to ensure that standards and strict specifications are followed by dental material manufacturing companies when developing new dental materials.

Recall

1. What professional organization evaluates a new dental material?

PROPERTIES OF DENTAL MATERIALS

The type of dental materials used to restore a tooth must respond to and withstand specific factors associated with oral conditions. The following characteristics enhance the ability of dental materials to withstand the oral environment and allow for easy application.

Mechanical Properties

The average biting and chewing force in the posterior area of the mouth of persons with their natural teeth is approximately 170 pounds (77 kg). This is approximately 28,000 pounds of pressure per square inch (psi) on a single cusp of a molar tooth. Materials used in restoring the occlusal surfaces of teeth must have sufficient strength to withstand these forces.

A **force** is any push or pull on matter. In turn, this type of force creates a stress and a strain. **Stress** is the *reaction within* the material that can cause distortion. **Strain** is the *change* produced within the material that occurs as the result of stress.

Types of Stress and Strain

Tensile stress pulls and stretches the material. A tug-of-war is an example of tensile stress (Fig. 43-1, *A*).

Compressive stress pushes the material together. Chewing is an example of compressive stress (Fig. 43-1, *B*).

Shear stress is the breakdown of the material as a result of something sliding over the two areas. Cutting with scissors is an example of shear stress (Fig. 43-1, *C*).

Thermal Change

When a person drinks hot coffee and then eats ice cream, the temperature in the mouth can change from 150° to 100° F (66° to 38° C) within seconds. These thermal changes are of major concern for two reasons: (1) contraction and expansion and (2) the need to protect the pulp from thermal shock.

Contraction and Expansion

When temperature changes occur, each type of dental material will contract or expand at its own rate. It is essential that the tooth structure and the restorative material have, as nearly as possible, the same rate of contraction and expansion. Significantly different rates of contraction and expansion can cause the dental material to pull away from the tooth, which can cause **microleakage** or a faulty restoration.

Electrical Properties

The electrical current (also referred to as **galvanic** action) in the oral cavity is created when two different or dissimilar metals are present in the oral cavity (Fig. 43-2). Conditions that allow these electrical currents include the following:

- Saliva contains salt, which makes it a good conductor of electricity
- Two metallic components of different composition acting as the battery (two restorations or a metal object such as a fork placed in the mouth)
- Galvanic action, or shock, which is the coming together of all these conditions

Corrosive Properties

Corrosion is the type of reaction within a metal when it comes into contact with corrosive products. Certain foods contain metallic forms that will cause corrosion of a dental material (Fig. 43-3). Most corrosion, however, is only surface discoloration and can be easily removed with the use of polishing agents.

Solubility

Solubility is the degree to which a substance will dissolve in a given amount of another substance. For example, sand

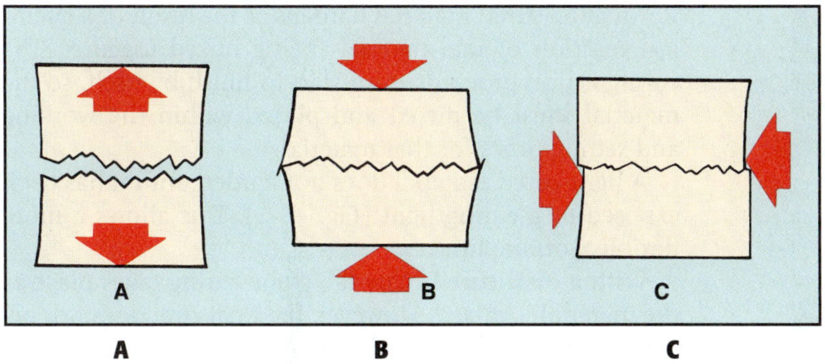

Fig. 43-1 Types of stress and strain. **A,** Tensile stress. **B,** Compressive stress. **C,** Shear stress.

has *low* solubility because it does not dissolve easily; sugar has *high* solubility because it does dissolve easily. Solubility of a material placed in the mouth is a concern (Fig. 43-4). A material that dissolves easily in the oral environment is of limited use because it will wash away and leave the tooth structure exposed.

Application Properties

For a dental material to have specific mechanical properties, steps must occur in the application of the dental material. Techniques used in the application help create this effect.

Flow

When removing decay and preparing healthy tooth structure to receive a permanent filling material, dental material must be pliable enough to be placed in the preparation. Dental materials are designed to have a certain amount of flow for placement, to be able to fit in corners, boxes, and pits of the tooth.

Adhesion

Adhesion is the force that causes unlike materials to **adhere** to each other. Adhesion between the dental material and the tooth structure is a major concern. Without proper adhesion, microleakage may occur, and the restoration may be lost. The characteristics of dental materials that affect adhesion are wetting, viscosity, surface characteristics, and film thickness.

Wetting is the ability of a liquid to flow over the surface and to come into contact with the small irregularities that may be present. For example, water has *high* wetting ability because it flows easily.

Viscosity is the property of a liquid that causes it *not* to flow easily. A liquid with high viscosity, such as heavy syrup, does not flow easily and is not effective in wetting a surface.

Surface characteristics also influence the wetting ability of the material. A liquid flows more easily on a rough surface than on a very smooth surface. For example, water usually flows easily on a rough surface; however, on a waxed surface, it beads up and does not flow as readily.

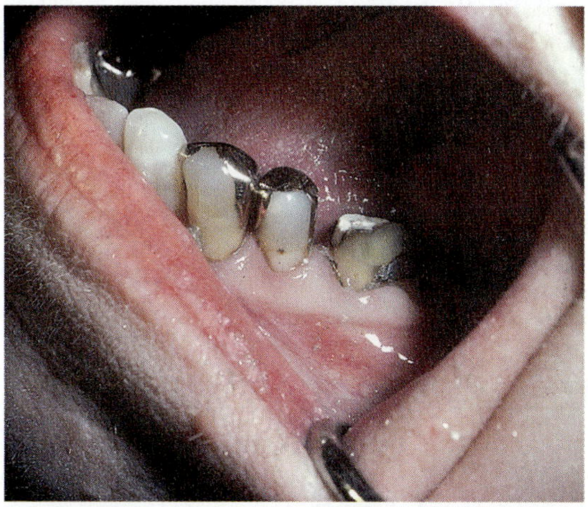

Fig. 43-2 A galvanic action can occur when different types of metals touch each other.

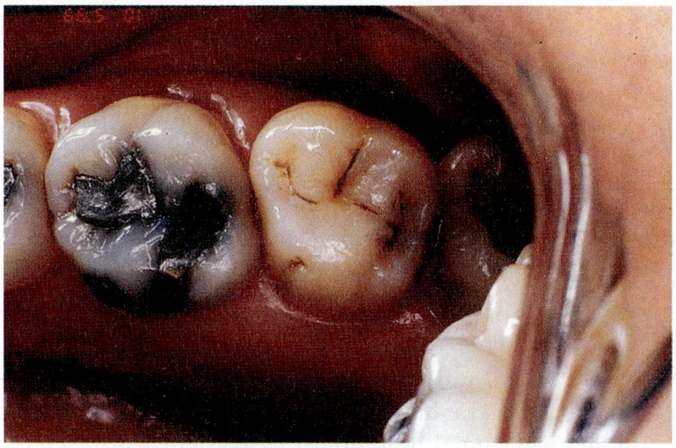

Fig. 43-3 Corrosion can occur on certain metals.

For adhesion to take place, the materials being joined must be in close contact with each other, which requires a *thin film thickness.* In general, the thinner the film, the stronger the adhesive junction. For example, the ideal film thickness for cementing a permanent restoration is 25 mm or less.

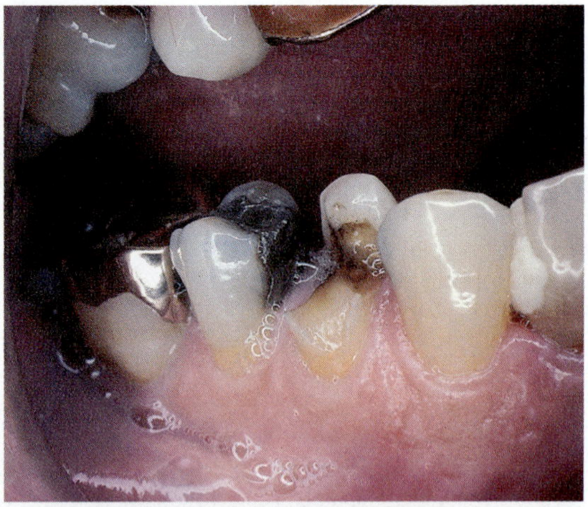

Fig. 43-4 **Dental materials must withstand solubility of saliva in the oral cavity.**

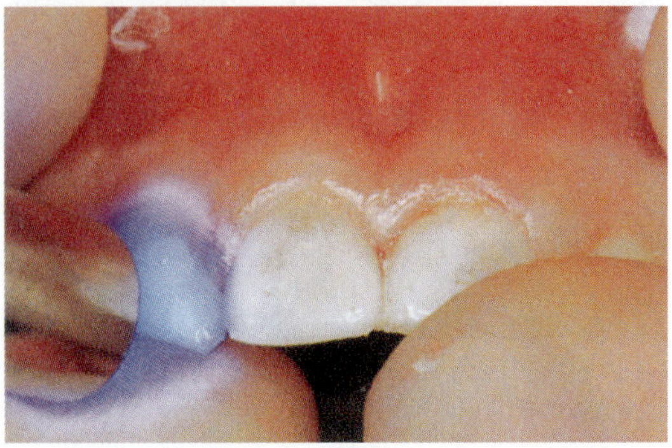

Fig. 43-5 **Light curing of a composite resin.** (From Duggal MS, et al: *Restorative techniques in paediatric dentistry,* Philadelphia, 1995, Saunders.)

Retention

Retention is the ability to hold two things firmly together when they will not adhere to each other. For example, amalgam and cast metals do not adhere directly to tooth structure. Retention is an extremely important concept in dentistry because dental restorations, casting, and appliances must be held in place by using materials and methods that are not harmful to the body.

Because amalgam and tooth structure do not adhere to each other, a traditional cavity preparation includes a retention form. The dentist uses a bur or hand cutting instrument to create this retention form, creating a crevice into which the material can lock. Although this holds the amalgam in place, microleakage may occur between the material and the tooth if a bonding material is not placed to create a seal.

Curing

Curing most dental materials is the process of placing a paste type material in the tooth preparation for adaptation. After the material is in place, it is then **cured** to stay in place and perform its function.

An **auto-cured** material hardens as the result of a chemical reaction of the materials being mixed together. The curing action proceeds from start to finish by itself, so the material must be mixed and placed within the working and setting times for that material.

A light-cured material does not harden until it has been exposed to a curing light (Fig. 43-5). This allows a more flexible working time.

With a **dual-cured** material, some curing takes place as the material is mixed. However, the final cure does not occur until the material has been exposed to a curing light.

Recall

2. What type of reaction does a dental material undergo when distortion occurs?
3. What happens to a dental material when exposed to hot and cold?
4. What is a source of galvanic action?
5. What are the four properties that must be considered in the application of a dental material?
6. How does an auto-cured material harden or set?

DIRECT RESTORATIONS

Dental restorative materials that are applied to a tooth or teeth while the material is pliable and can be adapted, carved, and finished are classified as *direct restorations.* The materials included in these types of restorative procedures are amalgam, composite resins, glass ionomers, intermediate restorative materials, and tooth-whitening products.

Amalgam

For more than 150 years, billions of dental amalgam fillings have been used to restore decayed teeth. **Amalgam** is the name that is given to silver fillings (Fig. 43-6). Actually, silver fillings consist of a number of different metals, with silver being the predominant metal. These metals are in powder form and are mixed with mercury, forming a soft, pliable mixture. When placed into a tooth, condensed, carved, and allowed to harden, the mixture becomes a permanent amalgam restoration.

Dental amalgam is a safe, affordable, and durable material that is used predominantly to restore premolars and molars.

Indications for Dental Amalgam

- Primary and permanent teeth
- Stress-bearing areas of the mouth
- Small to moderate-sized cavities in the posterior teeth

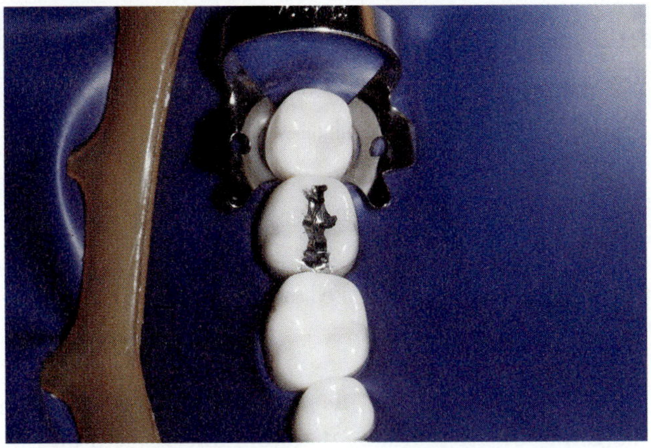

Fig. 43-6 **Example of class II amalgam restorations.**

- With severe destruction of tooth structure
- As a foundation for cast-metal, metal-ceramic, and ceramic restorations
- When a patient's commitment to personal oral hygiene is poor
- When moisture control is problematic
- When cost is an overriding patient concern

Contraindications to Dental Amalgam

- When esthetics is particularly important, such as in the anterior teeth
- With patients who have a history of allergy to mercury or other amalgam components
- When a large restoration is needed, and the cost of other restorative materials is not a significant factor in the treatment decision

Composition of Dental Amalgam

Dental amalgam is the end result of mixing approximately equal parts of mercury (43 to 54 percent) and an amalgam **alloy** powder (57 to 46 percent) (Fig. 43-7). The alloy powder is a combination of metals. Amalgam alloy powder is composed of the following metals:

- *Silver,* which gives it its strength
- *Tin,* for its workability and strength
- *Copper,* for its strength and corrosion resistance
- *Zinc,* to suppress oxidation

The main differences in the composition and classification of dental amalgam alloy powders are based on (1) alloy particle shape and size, (2) copper content, and (3) zinc content.

High-Copper Alloys

High-copper alloys, frequently used in dentistry, are named this because they contain a higher percentage of copper than previous alloys. High-copper alloys are classified according to their particle shape: **spherical** (round particles) or **irregular** (rough, lathe-cut particles) (Fig. 43-8). These particle shapes influence the trituration and working char-

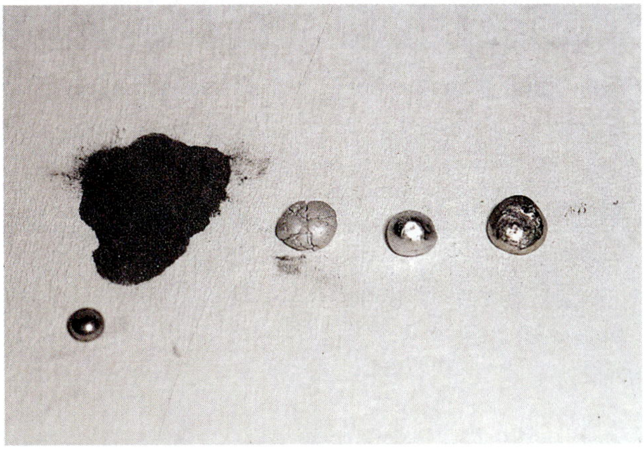

Fig. 43-7 **The mercury and alloy powder are in their purest form before trituration.** (From Hatrick CD, Eakle WS, Bird WF: *Dental materials: clinical applications for dental assistants and dental hygienists,* St Louis, 2003, Saunders.)

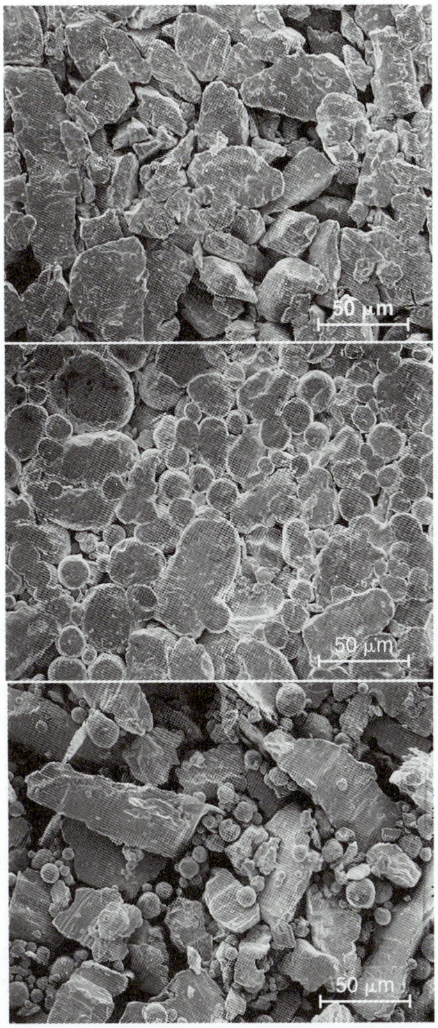

A

B

C

Fig. 43-8 **Microscopic view of alloy powder particles. A, Irregular. B, Spherical. C, Mixed.** (From Roberson T, et al: *Sturdevant's art and science of operative dentistry,* ed 4. St Louis, 2002, Mosby.)

Examples of Amalgam Alloys

High-Copper Alloys	Low-Copper Alloys
Dispersalloy	Dentalloy
Tytin	Velvalloy
Sybraloy	Spheralloy
Cupralloy	Micro II
Phasealloy	
Aristalloy CR	
Indiloy	
Valiant	
Valiant PhD	

Hygiene Guidelines When Using Amalgam

Do *not* allow mercury to contact your skin.

Protect against spillage during trituration.

Keep lid closed during trituration.

Do *not* discard scrap amalgam into waste containers.

Collect all scrap amalgam and store under water or under photographic fixer solution in a closed container.

acteristics (condensing and carving) of the resulting amalgam mixture.

A high-copper alloy is made up of 40 to 70 percent silver, 8 to 28 percent copper, and 15 to 30 percent tin. The percentages are expressed as percentages of the composition by weight.

Mercury-to-Alloy Ratios

The appropriate mercury-to-alloy ratio is very important. The ratio must contain just enough mercury to make the mix workable without containing an excessive amount of mercury. A 1:1 mercury:alloy ratio, also known as the *Eames technique,* is widely used. This ratio is one portion of mercury to one portion of alloy by weight.

Nonmercury Alloys

A nonmercury alloy called *Galloy* is composed of gallium, indium, and tin and has been approved by the ADA. *Gallium,* which is the alloy base ingredient, is a soft, silver-hued metal that liquefies at 86° F. The combination of gallium with indium and tin provides a strong, durable seal. Galloy is sensitive to moisture, which can cause corrosion and expansion. It is recommended that this material be placed after the tooth is lined with a resin and that an application of sealant be placed over the restoration.

Controversial Issues in Mercury

Mercury in dental amalgam has been under much controversy for many years. The controversy has evolved in the following two directions: (1) harm to patients from the mercury within the amalgams placed in their teeth and (2) the toxicity level of mercury vapors affecting dental personnel exposed over a long period of time.

When mercury is combined with other materials in dental amalgam, its chemical nature changes so that it is essentially harmless. The amount released in the mouth under the pressure of chewing and grinding is extremely small and no cause for alarm. In fact, this amount is less than what patients are routinely exposed to in food, air, and water. The ADA firmly supports the use of dental amalgams for the permanent restoration of teeth and believes this is the best dental material for the purpose of posterior restorations.

Dental personnel exposed to mercury vapors daily should be aware of toxic effects. An increase in exposure can result in tremors, kidney dysfunction, depression, and central nervous system disorders.

The Application of Dental Amalgam

Preparation

Amalgam is supplied by the manufacturer in sealed single-use capsules with the proper ratio of alloy powder in one side of the capsule and mercury on the other side, separated by a thin membrane. This ensures an accurate ratio and reduces the possibility of exposure to any of the materials. Immediately after use, the capsule is reassembled and discarded with nonregulated waste.

Capsules are available in 600 mg of alloy, which is the appropriate amount of material for a small or single-surface restoration, or 800 mg of alloy, which is used for a larger restoration (Fig. 43-9). If more than this amount of amalgam is required, additional capsules are placed with the setup and triturated as needed. (See Procedure 43-1: Mixing and Transferring of Amalgam.)

Trituration

Also known as *amalgamation,* **trituration** is the process by which the mercury and alloy powder are mixed together to form the mass of amalgam needed to restore the tooth. The preloaded capsule of amalgam alloy and mercury contains a **pestle,** which aids in the mixing process.

Before placement of the capsule in the amalgamator, many types of capsules require the use of an activator, which breaks the separating membrane (Fig. 43-10). The activated capsule is placed in the amalgamator, and the cover is closed to prevent mercury vapors from escaping during trituration.

The amalgamator is set to operate for the length of time specified in the manufacturer's directions (Table 43-1). In a proper mix the mass of amalgam is free of dry alloy particles and holds together as one unit. The mix is placed from the capsule into an amalgam well; the pestle

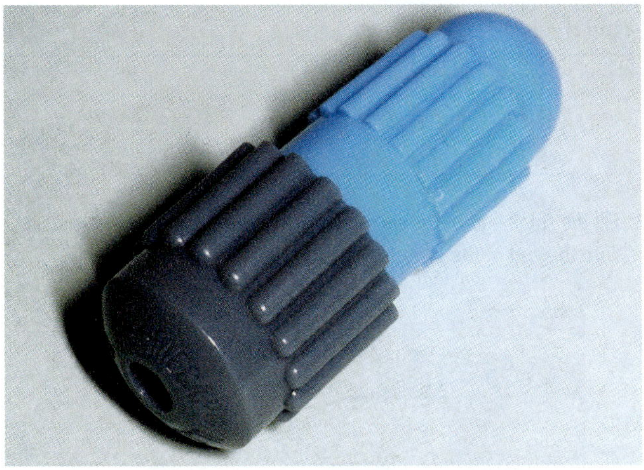

Fig. 43-9 Precapsulated amalgam.

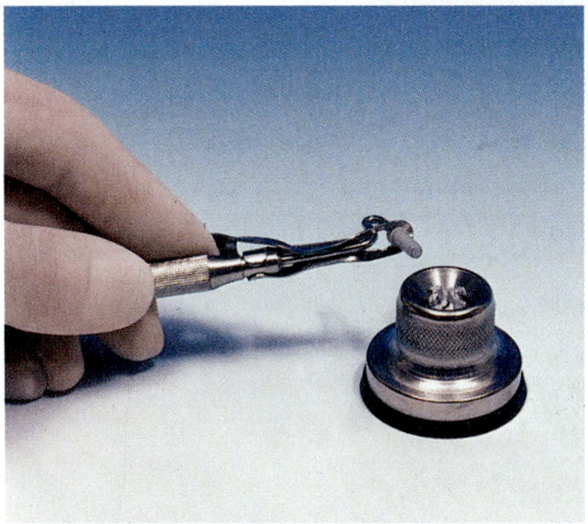

Fig. 43-11 Packing the amalgam in the carrier for placement.

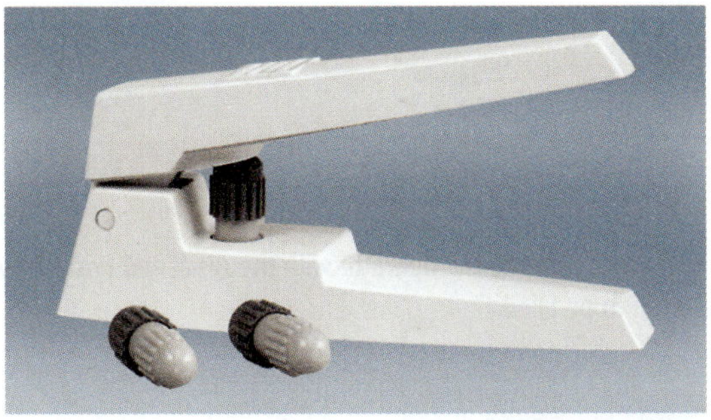

Fig. 43-10 Activator used to break the separating membrane in the capsule.

Table 43-1 ***Amalgamation Time***

Type of Amalgam	Setting	Time (Seconds)
Dispersalloy	M-2	13
Tytin	M-2	4-5
Sybraloy	M-2	13
Spheralloy	M-2	15
Valiant	M-2	13
Valiant PhD	M-2	15
Velvalloy	M-2	20

Procedure 43-1 Mixing and Transferring Dental Amalgam

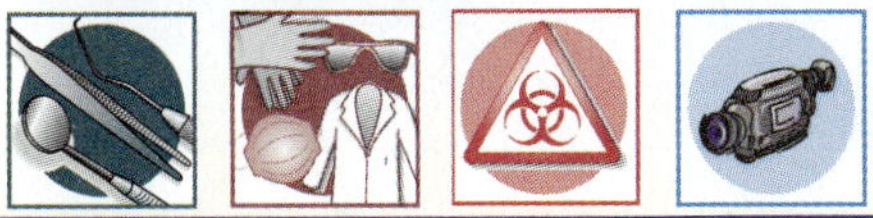

Equipment and Supplies

- Amalgam capsule
- Capsule activator
- Amalgamator
- Amalgam well or cloth
- Amalgam carrier

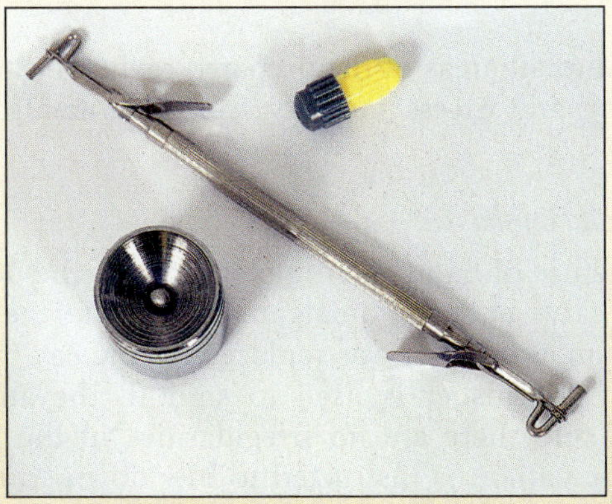

PROCEDURAL STEPS

1. Activate the capsule using the activator, if required, for type of amalgam.
   Purpose: This breaks the separating membrane to allow the mercury and alloy powders to mix.

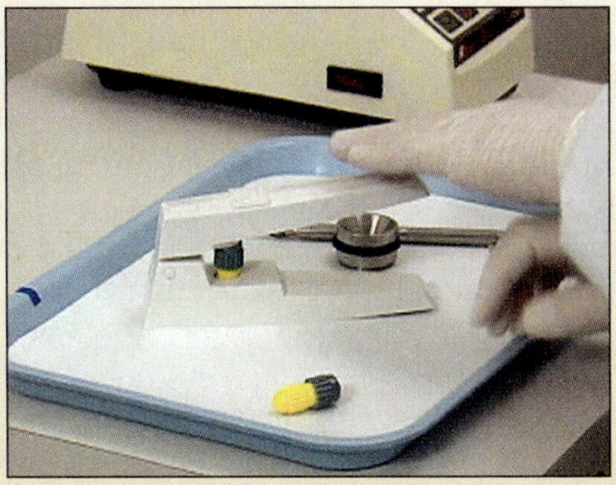

continued

Procedure 43-1 Mixing and Transferring Dental Amalgam—cont'd

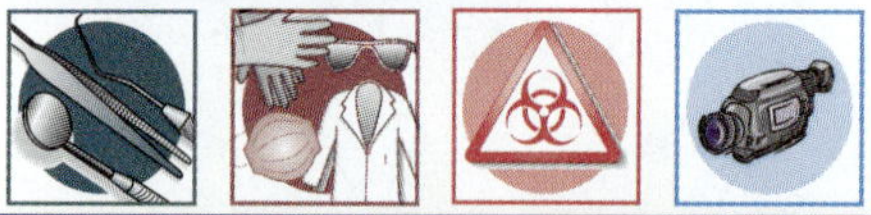

PROCEDURAL STEPS, cont'd

2. Place the capsule in the amalgamator.

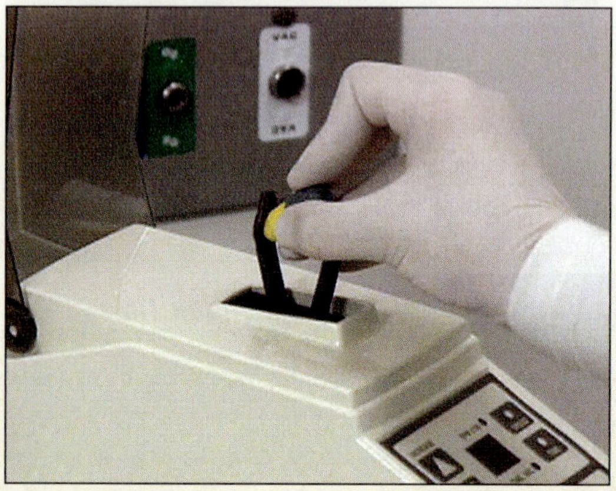

3. Adjust the settings on the amalgamator.
4. Close the cover on the amalgamator and begin trituration.
5. Remove the capsule, twist it open, and dispense amalgam in the well or amalgam cloth.

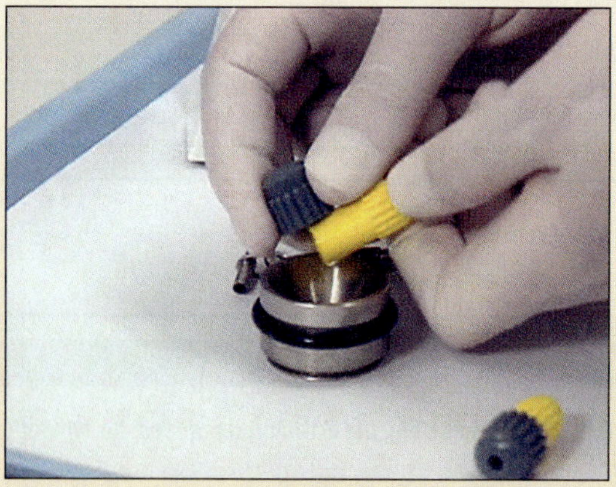

6. Fill the small end of the carrier first; then transfer the carrier, making sure the end of the carrier is directed toward the preparation.

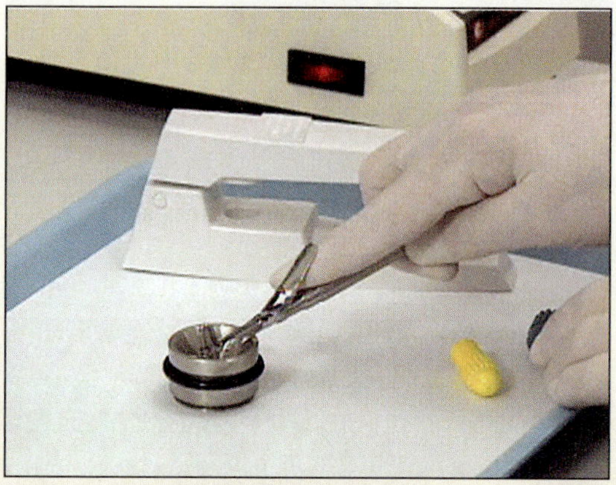

7. Transfer the carrier to the operator with the small end facing toward the tooth to be filled.

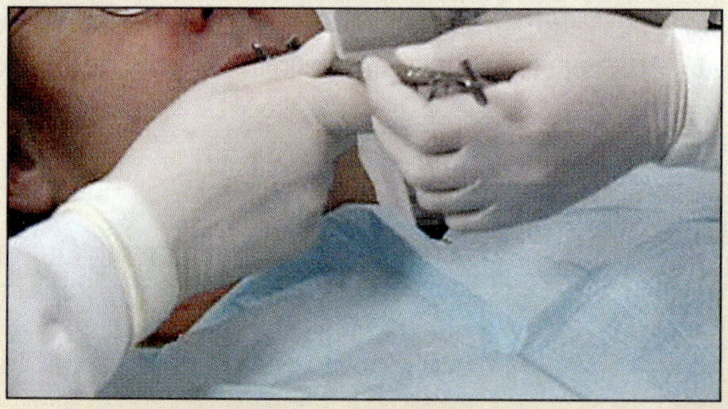

8. Continue this process until the preparation is overfilled.

is removed, and the mix is loaded into the amalgam carrier (Fig. 43-11).

Amalgam is soft, pliable, and easily shaped when it is first triturated. At this stage, amalgam can be placed and condensed to fit the prepared tooth. Once it hardens, amalgam forms a very strong restoration that can withstand the mechanical properties mentioned.

Condensation

The amalgam is placed in increments in the prepared tooth, and each increment is condensed immediately. The purpose of condensation is to compact the amalgam tightly into all areas of the prepared cavity and to aid in removing any excess mercury from the amalgam mix (Fig. 43-12).

Carving and finishing

With the use of hand carving instruments, the dentist is able to carve back the amalgam material to the tooth's normal anatomy that was replaced during cavity preparation. A burnisher is used to smooth the amalgam, making sure there are no irregularities in the restoration. The patient is instructed to bite down so that the dentist can check how the new restoration occludes with

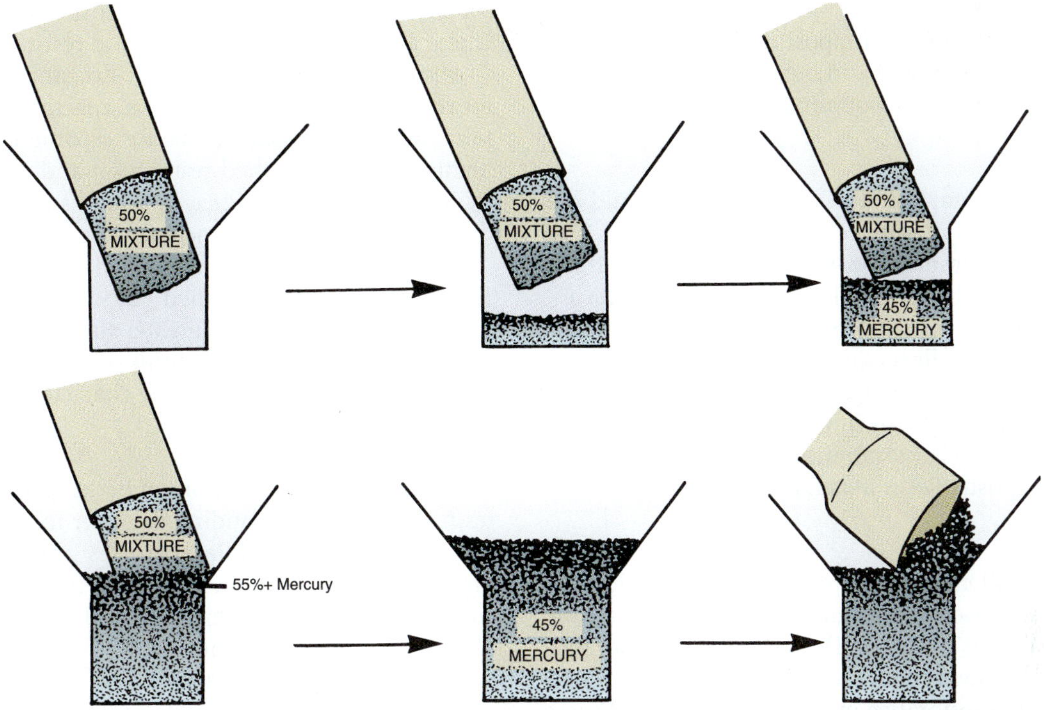

Fig. 43-12 Increments of amalgam placed. (From Baum L, Phillips RW, Lund MR: *Textbook of operative dentistry,* ed 3, Philadelphia, 1995, Saunders.)

the opposing tooth and then make any final carvings (Fig. 43-13).

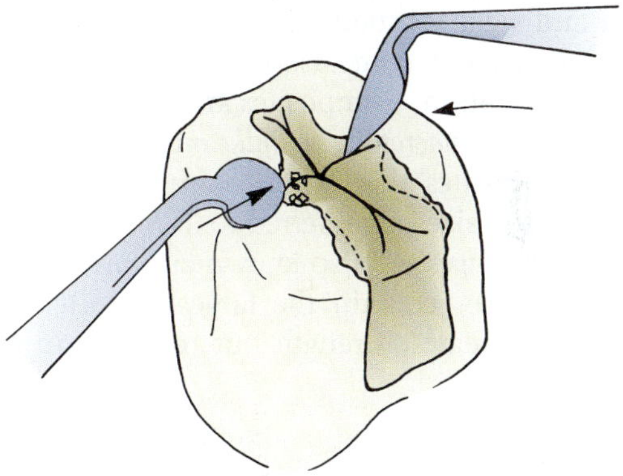

Fig. 43-13 Carving an amalgam restoration. (From Baum L, Phillips RW, Lund MR: *Textbook of operative dentistry,* ed 3, Philadelphia, 1995, Saunders.)

Recall

7. What metals make up the alloy powder in amalgam?
8. Is dental amalgam placed in anterior teeth?
9. What does copper provide to amalgam restorations?
10. Where do you dispose of amalgam scraps?
11. How is the amalgam triturated?
12. How long do you triturate Sybraloy?

Composite Resins

Composite resins are becoming the most widely accepted materials of choice by dentists and patients (Fig. 43-14). Composite resins are placed mainly in anterior teeth because of their esthetic qualities, but with new advances in their makeup, they are increasingly being placed in posterior teeth as well.

Composite resins are not as strong as amalgams or gold alloy restorations, but they are designed to meet the needs of a specific area of a tooth or mouth. This tooth-colored material is designed to have the following qualities:

- Withstand the environments of the oral cavity
- Be easily shaped to the anatomy of a tooth
- Match the natural tooth color
- Be bonded directly to the tooth surface

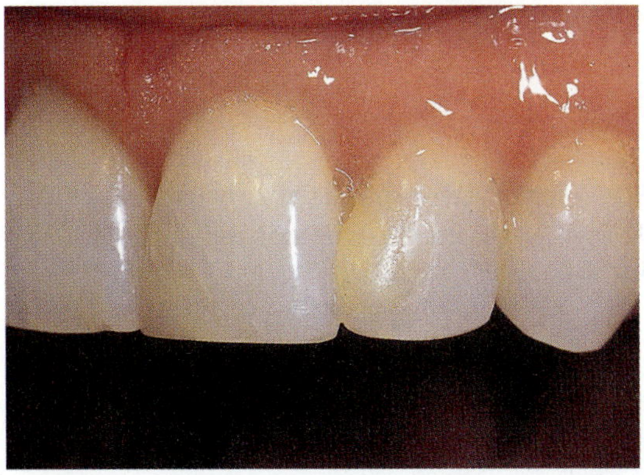

Fig. 43-14 Class III composite restoration on tooth #10. (Courtesy Premier Dental Products.)

Composition of Composite Resins

The major composition of composite resins is a chemical makeup, which includes: (1) an organic resin **matrix,** (2) inorganic **fillers,** and (3) a **coupling agent.**

Resin matrix

The resin matrix component of composite is a fluid-like material dimethacrylate, also referred to as *BIS-GMA*. This fluid, which is the monomer, is used to make synthetic resins. BIS-GMA is the foundation of resins. By itself, it is not strong enough to be used as a restorative dental material. The addition of fillers and coupling agents allows the polymerization to take place. Additional additives included in this process are the initiator, accelerator, retarder, and ultraviolet, (UV) light stabilizers. (See Procedure 43-2: Preparing Composite Resin Materials.)

Filler

The inorganic fillers used in composite resins include *quartz* (a hard rock-forming mineral), glass, *silica* (white colorless crystalline compound) particles, and colorants. These fillers add the strength and other characteristics necessary for use as a restorative material. The ability of these materials to reflect light aids in creating an esthetically pleasing restoration. The amount of filler, particle size, and types of fillers are important factors in determining the strength and wear-resistant characteristics of the material (Fig. 43-15). These factors also influence the polished finish of the restoration. Composites are classified by particle size as *megafill, macrofill, midifill, minifill, microfill,* and *nanofill.* Composites that have a combination or mixed range of particle sizes are referred to as *hybrids.*

Macrofilled composites, also known as *conventional or traditional composites,* contain the largest of filler particles, providing the greatest strength but resulting in a duller, rougher surface. Macrofilled composites are used in areas where greater strength is required to resist fracture.

Microfilled composites contain inorganic fillers that are much smaller than those of a macrofilled composite. Microfilled composite resins are capable of producing a highly polished finished restoration and are used primarily in anterior restorations, in which smoothness and esthetics are the primary concerns.

Hybrid composites contain a mixed range of particle sizes. The hybrids can be polished smoother than the macrofilled composites yet have greater strength than the microfilled composites. Hybrid composites also have high wear resistance and excellent shading characteristics.

Coupling agent

The coupling agent is important because it strengthens the resin by chemically bonding the filler to the resin matrix. To achieve this, the filler particles are coated with an organosilane compound. The *silane* portion of the molecule bonds to the quartz, glass, and silica filler particles. The *organic* portion bonds with the resin matrix, thus bonding the filler to the matrix.

Commercial Examples of Composite Resins

Aurafil	Prisma-Fil
Command	Prodigy
Durafil	Profile
Estilux	Silar
Finesse	Silux
Herculite	Visar

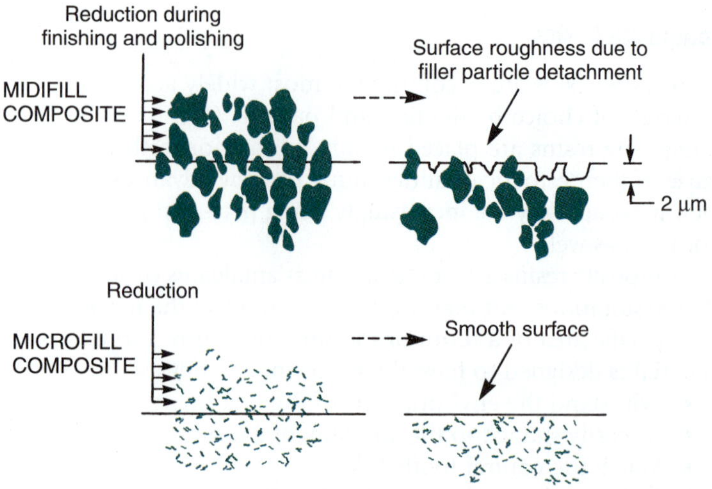

Fig. 43-15 Effect of particle size on surface finish of composite. (From Roberson T, et al: *Sturdevant's art and science of operative dentistry,* ed 4. St Louis, 2002, Mosby.)

The Application of Composites

Important differences in the technique between an amalgam restoration and a composite restoration include the following:

- The cavity preparation for a composite resin is designed to hold the resin by means of a bonding system rather than retention within the preparation.
- Specific dental materials cannot be used with composite resins.
- The matrix system varies and is different with composite resins.
- Placement of composite resin is accomplished by increments and then *light-cured* before additional increments are added.

Application

Resins are supplied in a single-paste, lightproof syringe. Light-cured resins do not require mixing and are used directly as they come from the syringe. This paste contains both the photoinitiator and the amine activator and will not polymerize until exposed to the curing light.

The material is supplied in a kit that includes varying shades of the composite resin, along with an etching and bonding system that works specifically for the application process of that material (Fig. 43-16). Color matching is one of most critical aspects when working with composite resins. If a correct shade is not selected, it will be apparent to the patient after the restoration is in place. A shade guide is always used when determining the correct shade for application (Fig. 43-17).

Polymerization

Polymerization is the process in which the resin material is changed from a plastic state (in which it can be molded or shaped) into a hardened restoration. Polymerization occurs through auto-curing or light-curing.

The *light-curing process* uses a high-intensity blue light source that provides an effective curing of resins. The blue light source is a combination of tungsten and a halogen lighting system. The exact curing time depends on the following:

- Composite manufacturer's instructions (most often, 20 to 60 seconds)
- Thickness and size of the restoration (when larger quantities of the material are being placed, each increment is cured before the next is placed)
- Shade of the restorative material used (the darker the shade, the longer the required curing time)

Procedure 43-2 Preparing Composite Resin Materials

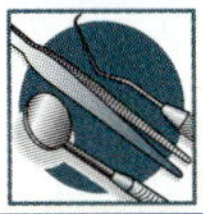
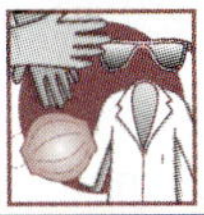

Equipment and Supplies

- Shade guide
- Composite resin material
- Treated paper pad or material dispenser
- Composite instrument
- 2- × 2-inch alcohol gauze pads
- Curing light

PROCEDURAL STEPS

1. Select the shade of the tooth.
   Purpose: Composites come in varying shades; with the use of a shade guide, you can select the color that most resembles the patient's natural tooth color.
   Note: Make sure to use natural lighting for this decision. Fluorescent lighting can change the natural appearance.
2. Once the shade is selected, express the needed amount for the restoration onto the treated pad or in the light-protected well.
   Note: Most often, you need a very small amount, so do not waste the material.
3. Transfer the composite instrument and material to the transfer zone for the dentist.
4. The dentist may ask for the liquid bonding resin or alcohol gauze to be available during placement of material increments.
   Purpose: These will aid in the flow of the material.
5. Have the curing light readied during placement of the material. It is best when the material can be light-cured as increments are placed.
   Purpose: This completes the final setting of the material.

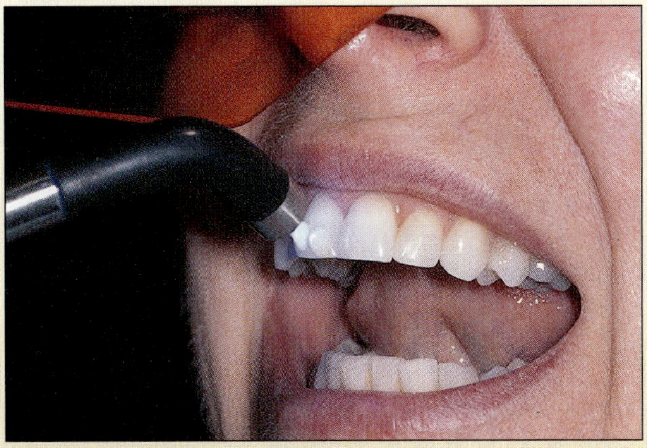

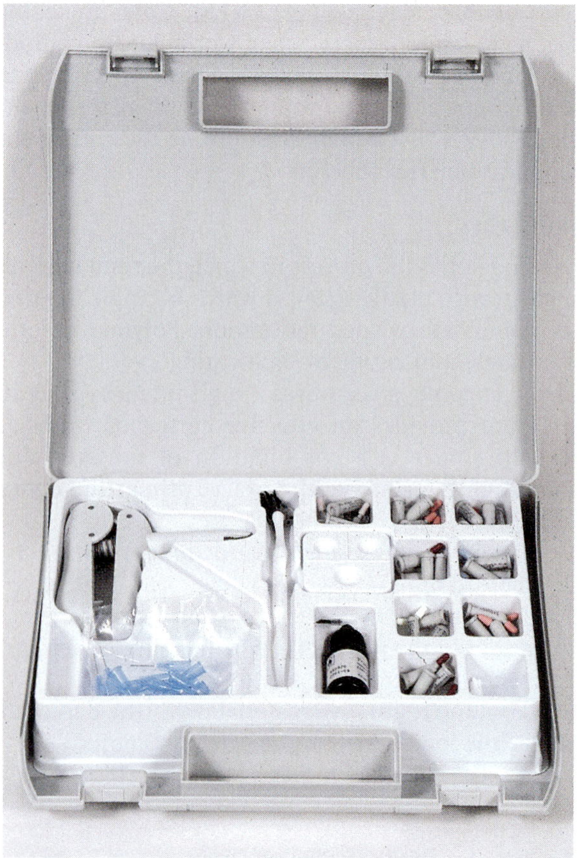

Fig. 43-16 Composite resin kit.

Finishing and polishing

The finishing and polishing of composite resins are much different from the completion steps in the amalgam procedure. Because composite materials go from the soft pliable state to being completely hardened by polymerization, the dentist is not able to carve or make adjustments with hand instruments.

Recall

13. What is the common term used for dimethacrylate?

14. What filler type of composite resin is the strongest and used most often for posterior restorations?

15. When composite resins are being light-cured, what factors might require a longer curing time for the material?

16. What item is used to determine the color of composite for a procedure?

17. What is the final step in finishing a composite resin?

Glass Ionomers

Glass ionomers represent one of the most versatile dental materials available. The ability of glass ionomers to alter chemical properties allows them to be used as restorative

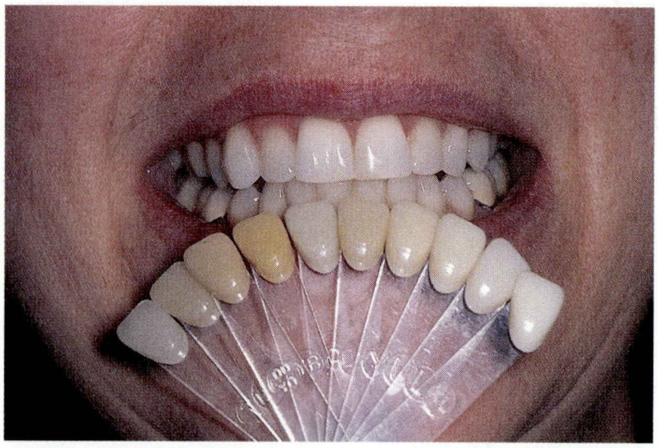

Fig. 43-17 **Use of a shade guide for color matching.** (From Hatrick CD, Eakle WS, Bird WF: *Dental materials: clinical applications for dental assistants and dental hygienists,* St Louis, 2003, Saunders.)

Steps in Finishing a Composite Resin

1. Reduction of the material is completed by the use of a white stone or a finishing diamond.
2. Fine finishing is done with carbide finishing burs, then with diamond burs.
3. Polishing the resin begins with the medium discs and finishes with the superfine discs.
4. Finishing strips assist in the polishing of the interproximal surfaces.
5. Polishing paste applied to a rubber cup completes the step.

materials, liners, bonding agents, and permanent cements. (Chapters 44 and 45 describe the materials used as liners, bonding agents, and cements.)

Because glass ionomers have the ability to bind chemically (not mechanically) to teeth, the need to prepare the tooth structure is not as extensive as in the preparation for an amalgam or composite resin. The most unique feature of glass ionomers is the release of *fluoride* after its final setting. This provides the added advantage of stopping or preventing decay from around a restoration. This type of material is especially desirable for the following applications:

- Primary teeth
- Final restorations in nonstressed areas
- Intermediate restorations
- Core material for buildups
- Provisional (longer-term temporary) restorations

In the term *glass ionomer,* the word *glass* actually refers to a combination of glass, ceramic particles, and a glassy matrix. From this special glass combination, the material derives its translucency and prolonged fluoride release. *Ionomer* refers to ion–cross-linked polymers, such as acrylic acid, tartaric acid, and maleic acid (common materials found in most dental cements). The type of polymer and its molecular weight ensure excellent adhesion and resistance to acid erosion.

Cautions for Placing Glass Ionomers

Avoid water contamination and contact of the material.

Be aware that when the material's glossy appearance has disappeared, the setting stages have begun.

Protect the matrix band from the material; the material will adhere to the metal band.

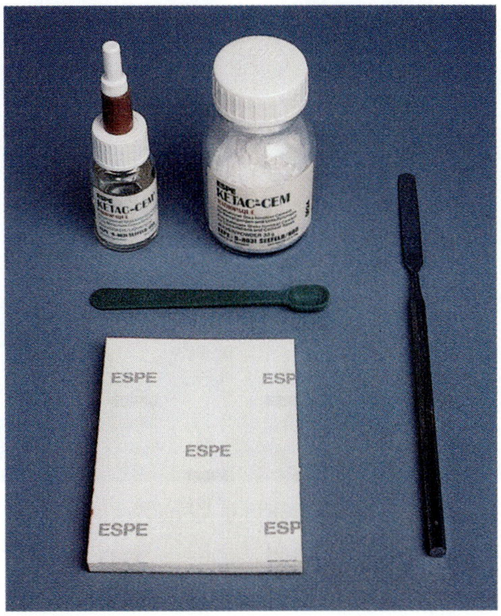

Fig. 43-18 Setup for mixing glass ionomer liquid and powder.

Metal Reinforcement

The blend of spherical silver-tin alloy with glass ionomer produces a strong, abrasion-resistant dental material. The glass component provides a desirable balance between working and setting time together with sustained fluoride release. The particles are a polymer of *acrylic acid,* which provides toughness and resistance to acid erosion. The level of metal addition also provides an optimal level of radiopacity. This product is extremely versatile in its clinical application for core buildups; for repair of fractured cusps and amalgam fillings in class I, II, and V cavities; as a base; and as an abutment for overdentures.

Fabrication and Application

When supplied as a powder and liquid, glass ionomers are manually mixed together on a treated paper pad, incorporating the powder into the liquid in several increments (Fig. 43-18). The material must be completely mixed in less than 45 seconds.

Glass ionomers are also supplied in light-protected tubes. The material is dispensed onto a treated paper pad for placement, and then allowed to auto-cure for 10 to 15 minutes (Fig. 43-19). The metal glass ionomers are supplied as a liquid or paste system or in a premeasured capsule and mixed or triturated for application.

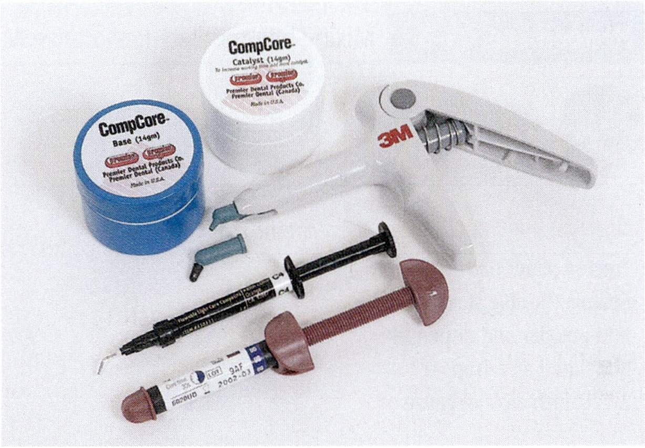

Fig. 43-19 Glass ionomers are supplied in tubes, cartridges, and tubs. (From Hatrick CD, Eakle WS, Bird WF: *Dental materials: clinical applications for dental assistants and dental hygienists,* St Louis, 2003, Saunders.)

Temporary Restorative Materials: Intermediate and Provisional

Temporary restorations are placed by the dentist in various dental situations. The type of material selected for a temporary restoration is designed to maintain or restore function and keep the patient comfortable for a limited period of time. Temporary restorative materials are used for the following reasons:

- Reduce sensitivity and discomfort of a tooth to determine its diagnosis
- Maintain the function and esthetics of a tooth until a permanent restoration can be placed
- Protect the margins of a prepared tooth that will receive a permanent casting at a later time
- Prevent shifting of the adjacent or opposing teeth because of open space

The type of temporary restorative material selected depends on the location and amount of the tooth structure that needs to be restored. If a tooth has lost a filling or has a small pit within the enamel, an intermediate restorative material would be selected. If a cusp is gone or the dentist has prepared the tooth for a cast restoration involving the gingival margin, a provisional coverage material would be selected.

Intermediate Restorative Materials

An intermediate restoration is frequently recommended by the dentist as a short-term restoration. The material most often used for this situation is *intermediate restorative material, or IRM* (Fig. 43-20). IRM is a reinforced zinc oxide–eugenol composition. The *eugenol* has a sedative effect on the pulp, and fillers are added to improve the strength and durability of the material.

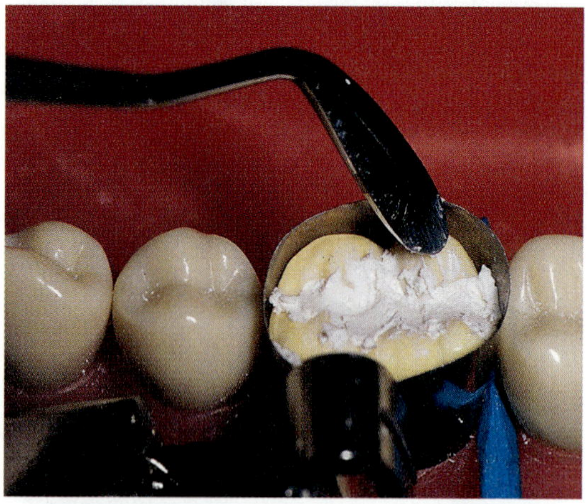

Fig. 43-20 Placement of IRM into a molar.

Common uses of IRM include:

- Restoration of primary teeth (when permanent teeth are 2 years or less from eruption)
- Restorative emergencies
- Caries management programs

IRM is supplied as a powder and liquid, which is mixed manually on a treated paper pad, or from premeasured capsules that are activated and then triturated.

Because the application of an intermediate restoration is not considered permanent, it is a procedure that can be performed as an expanded function of the dental assistant in most states. Chapter 48 provides the skill process for this advanced function. (See Procedure 43-3: Mixing Intermediate Restorative Materials.)

Provisional Restorative Materials

A provisional restorative material is designed to cover the major portion, if not the entire clinical portion, of a tooth or several teeth for a longer period of time. Because of so much coverage, this material has to withstand biting forces and the daily wear and tear of oral conditions (Fig. 43-21).

Procedure 43-3 Mixing Intermediate Restorative Materials

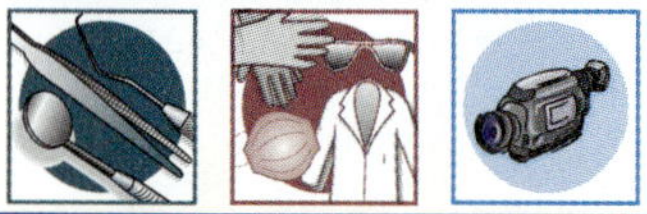

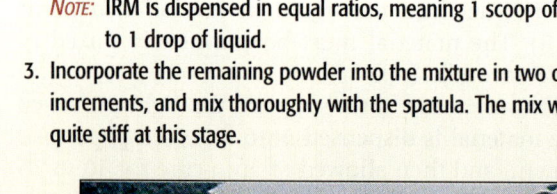

Equipment and Supplies

- Treated paper pad
- Spatula (flexible stainless steel)
- IRM powder and dispenser
- IRM liquid and dropper
- 2-× 2-inch alcohol gauze

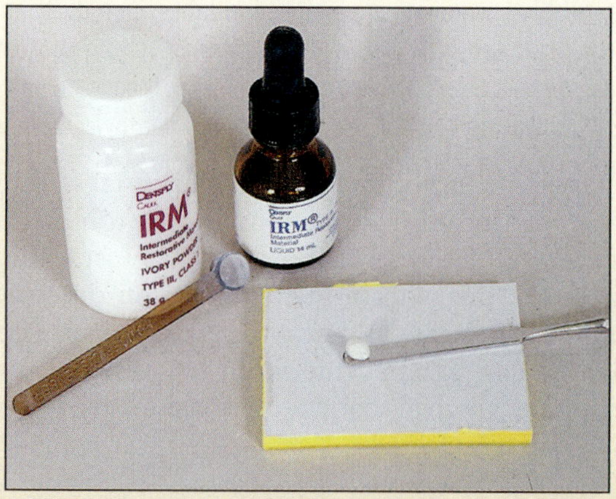

PROCEDURAL STEPS

1. Shake the powder before dispensing; then measure the powder onto the mixing pad.
   Purpose: When the powder is fluffed, it will not be as packed, thus creating a drier mix.
2. Make a well in half the powder; then dispense the liquid into the mix. Recap the containers.
   Note: IRM is dispensed in equal ratios, meaning 1 scoop of powder to 1 drop of liquid.
3. Incorporate the remaining powder into the mixture in two or three increments, and mix thoroughly with the spatula. The mix will be quite stiff at this stage.

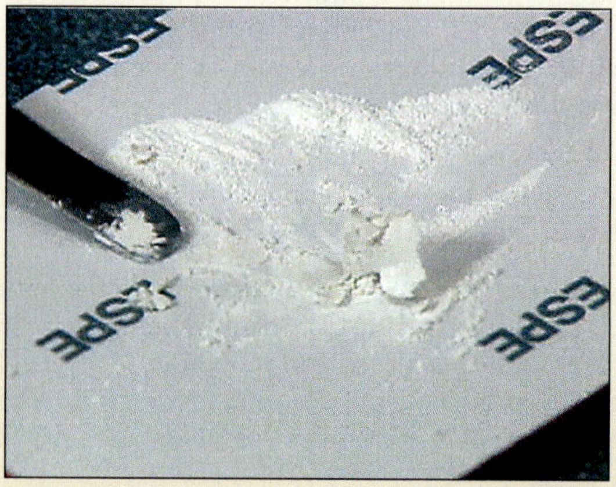

4. Wipe the mix back and forth on the mixing pad for 5 to 10 seconds. The resulting mix should be smooth and adaptable. The mix must be completed within 1 minute.
5. Clean and disinfect the equipment immediately.

An auto-cured acrylic (methylmethacrylate) or light-cured composite resin (different properties from composite restorative material) is selected (Fig. 43-22). The material is placed in an alginate impression or a vacuum-formed tray and seated over the prepared tooth and allowed to cure. The occlusion is adjusted, and the temporary is polished and cemented in place with temporary cement.

Because the application of a provisional restoration is not considered permanent, it is a procedure that can be performed by the expanded-function dental assistant in most states. Chapter 51 provides the skill process for this expanded function. (See Procedure 43-4: Mixing Acrylic Resin for Provisional Coverage.)

Tooth-Whitening Materials

Tooth whitening, also referred to as *bleaching*, is one of the fastest and most cost-effective ways of restoring the esthetic appearance of teeth. You can find whitening products used as ingredients in everyday items such as toothpaste, fluoride, toothbrushes, mouth rinses, and even chewing gum.

Composition of Whitening Materials

Most tooth-whitening products are made from a peroxide-based ingredient. Peroxide-based solutions come in different concentrations (10, 16, and 22 percent). Peroxide-based whitening products work deep within the tooth to remove staining and discoloration that have come from years of accumulated stain and aging. Teeth become dis-

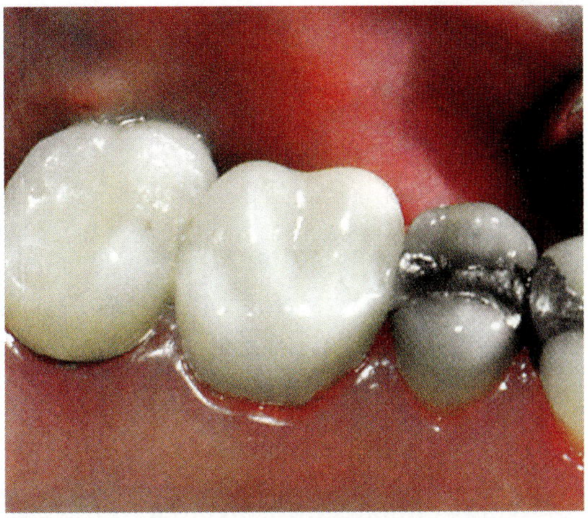

Fig. 43-21 Examples of provisional coverage materials.

Procedure 43-4 Mixing Acrylic Resin for Provisional Coverage

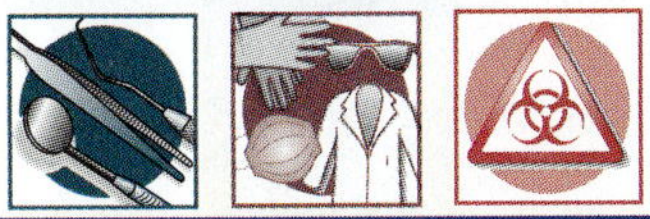

Equipment and Supplies

- Self-curing acrylic resin (liquid and powder)
- Dropper
- Spatula (small metal)
- Dappen dish or disposable dish available with material

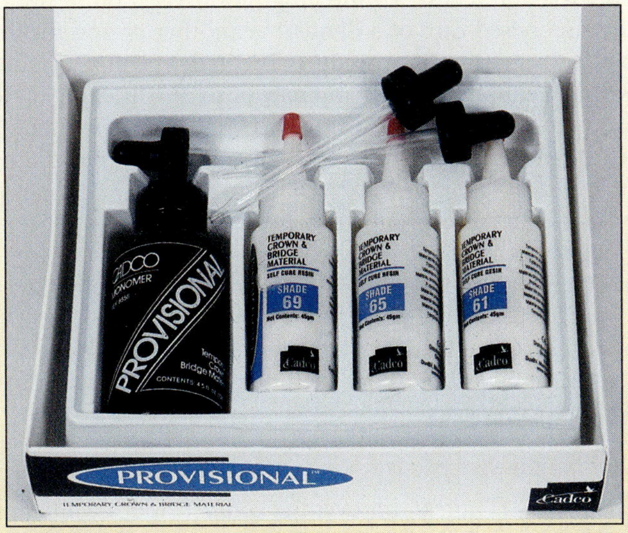

PROCEDURAL STEPS

1. Using the dropper, dispense liquid monomer in the mixing container. The recommended amount is 10 drops of liquid per tooth.
   Note: Cover the monomer container immediately. This material is volatile.
2. Dispense the selected shade of self-curing powder (polymer) into the liquid quickly until the liquid is overfilled. Quickly turn over the dish onto a paper towel, removing excess powder that was not absorbed by the liquid.
3. Use a small spatula to blend the powder and liquid to a homogeneous mix.
4. Allow the material to sit untouched until the mix loses some of its shine and changes to a doughlike state.
5. The material is ready to be placed in the impression or tray.

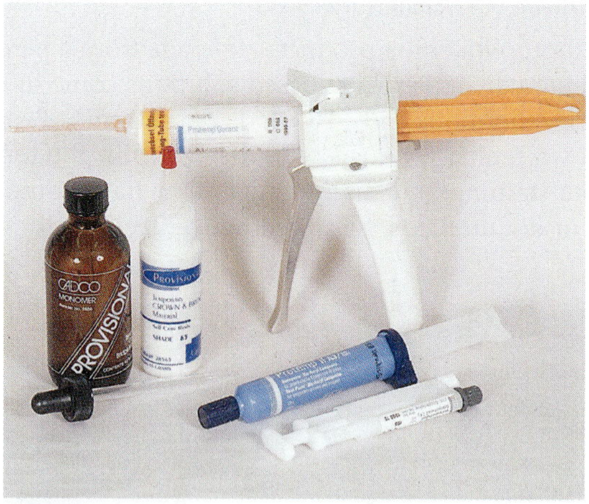

Fig. 43-22 **Acrylic resin is supplied as liquid/powder, tubes, and automix cartridges.** (From Hatrick CD, Eakle WS, Bird WF: *Dental materials: clinical applications for dental assistants and dental hygienists,* St Louis, 2003, Saunders.)

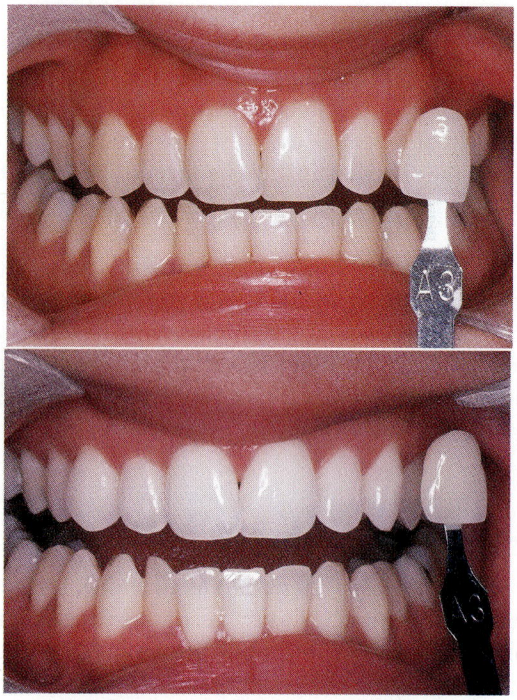

Fig. 43-23 **Before and after the use of a whitening product.**

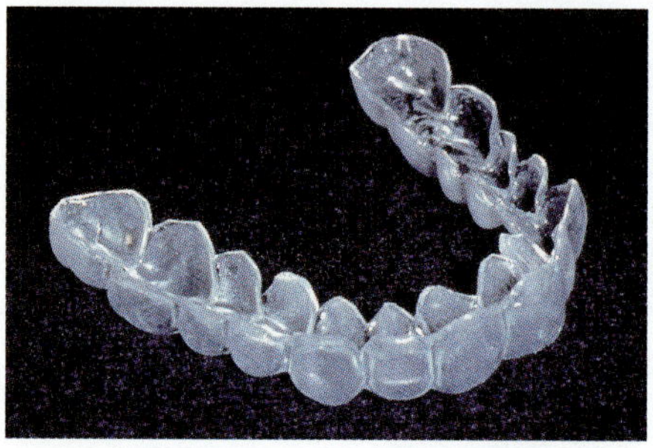

Fig. 43-24 **Custom tray used to hold the whitening gel.**

Commercial Examples of Bleaching Products

Contrast p.m.	Nupro Gold
Dental Lite	Opalescence
Illumine	Prestige
Nite White	Zaris

colored and stained for many reasons, most commonly aging, consumption of staining substances (coffee, tea, colas, and tobacco), trauma, use of tetracycline (antibiotic), excessive fluoride, nerve degeneration, and old restorations.

When the peroxide-based product contacts the teeth, it allows oxygen to enter the enamel and dentin and then whitens the colored substances. The structure of the tooth is not altered; the tooth is simply made lighter and whiter (Fig. 43-23).

Treatment Options

In-office treatment

Professionally applied tooth whitening can be accomplished by the dentist in as little as one hour. Results vary, but patients usually see their teeth whitened up to five shades lighter. The in-office tooth-whitening process requires that the dental team follow specific criteria in the application:

- Complete isolation of teeth involved (includes use of the dental dam, or a light-reflective resin barrier)
- Whitening agent at a higher concentration applied to facial surfaces of teeth
- Light or laser source used to enhance the application

At-home treatment

The decision to use a whitening product at home (under the supervised care of a dentist) is another option for the patient wanting this procedure. The patient will see results within a couple of weeks and may observe whitening up to six shades lighter with this process. At-home whitening treatment requires that the patient follow specific criteria of application:

- Having a custom-fitted tray made in the dental office to hold the peroxide-based gel (Fig. 43-24).
- Having a supply of peroxide-based gel for application for the suggested period of time.
- Usage regimens vary. Some products are used twice a day for 2 weeks; others are intended for overnight use for 1 to 2 weeks.

Over-the-counter options

There are a variety of over-the-counter tooth-whitening products available today. Most of the products that are man-

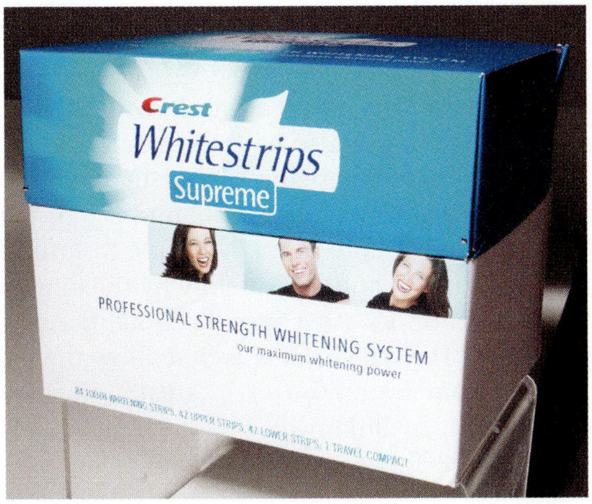

Fig. 43-25 Strips used for whitening. (Courtesy Procter and Gamble.)

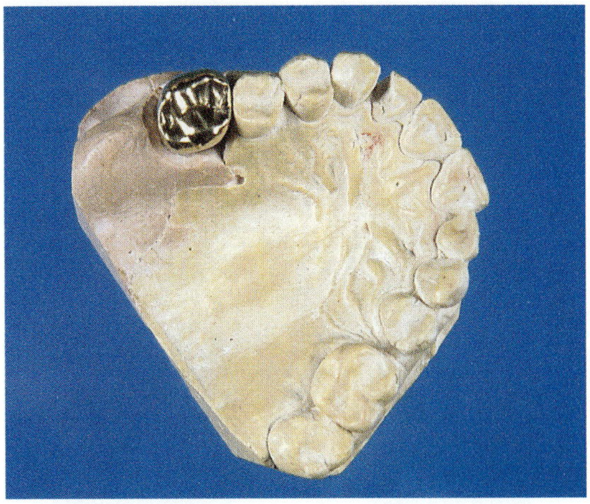

Fig. 43-26 Gold crown.

ufactured by the larger oral health companies are safe, reliable, and effective. However, these products will not achieve the dramatic improvements that are available from the dentist-applied or dentist-supervised products (Fig. 43-25).

Recall

18. What are some of the most common uses of glass ionomer materials?
19. What will contaminate the setting of glass ionomers?
20. What does the abbreviation *IRM* stand for?
21. What temporary restorative material would be selected for a class II cavity preparation?
22. What material would you use to prepare for provisional coverage?
23. How many drops of monomer are recommended per tooth when mixing acrylic resin?

INDIRECT RESTORATIONS

The types of dental restorations that the dental laboratory technician creates in the dental laboratory are classified as indirect restorations. These restorations, also referred to as castings, are fabricated by the dental laboratory technician and are ready to be tried-in and cemented.

When the dentist receives the casting from the lab, the patient has already been scheduled for the delivery appointment. At that time, the dentist will make any minor adjustments, then finish and polish the restoration.

Indirect restorative materials include gold alloys and ceramic castings. The finished castings are then either bonded or cemented into place.

Gold–Noble Metal Alloys

Gold in its purest form has the ability to resist tarnish and etching when exposed to the harsh conditions in the mouth, but it is much too soft for use in cast dental restorations. However, gold can be combined with other metals to form an alloy, thus acquiring the characteristics and hardness required of an indirect restoration (Fig. 43-26).

One way of describing the alloys used in indirect restorations is on the basis of their noble and base metal content.

Noble metals used for cast restorations are **gold** (Au), **palladium** (Pd), and **platinum** (Pt). All other metals in the alloys that are not classified as noble metals are considered to be base metals. A *base metal* is a metal of relatively low value and with inferior properties such as lack of resistance to corrosion and tarnish. Iron, tin, and zinc are examples of base metals.

Gold alloys are described according to their hardness, **malleability,** and adaptability. Using this descriptive system, the four types of gold alloys are as follows:

1. Soft, *type I alloys* are used for casting inlays subject to slight stress during mastication.
2. Medium, *type II alloys* can be used for almost all types of cast inlays and possibly posterior bridge abutments.
3. Hard, *type III alloys* are acceptable for inlay, full crowns, three-quarter crowns, and anterior or posterior bridge abutments.
4. Extra hard, *type IV alloys,* also known as *partial denture alloys,* are designed for cast-removable partial dentures.

Ceramic Castings

Ceramic is a type of material similar to that used in the dishes or pottery in your home. Ceramics are *compounds,* a combination of metallic and nonmetallic elements. As with dishes and pottery, ceramic castings are made of a claylike material with a *glaze* that has metallic components

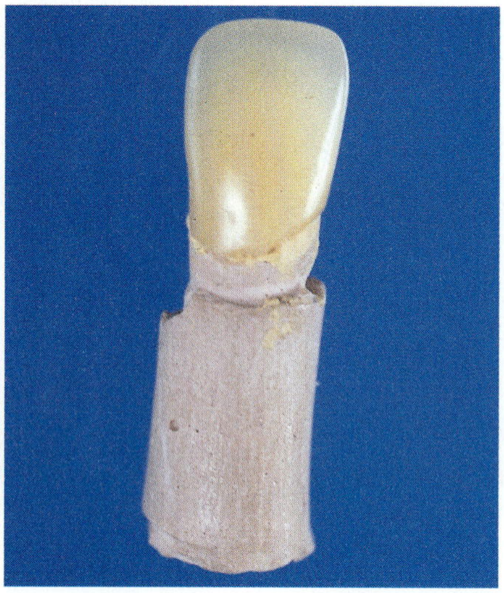

Fig. 43-27 Porcelain crown.

to make it durable and able to withstand temperature change. A ceramic material is adhered to a metal casting, creating the "best of both worlds" in strength and esthetics. Combinations of ceramic-metal restorations include the following:

- Porcelain fused to metal (PFM)
- Porcelain bonded to metal (PBM)
- Ceramco-metal (C/M)
- Porcelain-metal (P/M)

Porcelain

The type of ceramic most often used in dentistry is **porcelain.** This type of ceramic combines strength, translucence, and the ability to match the natural tooth color (Fig. 43-27). Because laboratory fabrication techniques incorporate heat and pressure, these restorations are stronger than direct restorations, such as composite resins, which are created in the mouth. The ceramic porcelain is fused to the metal backing shell, glazed, and fired to produce a highly smooth surface that is extremely hard and similar to enamel.

Porcelain material is chosen for the following reasons:

- The shading of colors matches tooth color well.
- Porcelain improves the esthetic appearance of anterior teeth.
- The material has the strength of metal.
- Porcelain is a good insulator.
- The material has a low coefficient of thermal expansion.

Recall

24. What are the three noble metals used in dentistry?
25. What type of restoration is made in the dental laboratory?

Patient Education

Most patients are concerned not only with the appearance of their teeth, but also with the safety and quality of the dental materials being placed in their mouth. When scheduling a patient for a temporary or permanent restoration, be sure to include time to inform patients of their needs and to explain why the dentist has made the decision to use a specific dental material for the procedure. Having visual aids that allow the patient to view different restorations can greatly alleviate the patient's fear of the unknown.

Legal and Ethical Implications

As with any procedure, it is important to indicate in the patient's record what material was used during the restoration. If a patient has any negative medical reaction to a specific material or a problem associated with the restoration that requires attention, the dentist will have a record of what might be causing the problem. This also provides the patient with a sense of assurance that the dentist is following through to provide complete treatment.

Eye to the Future

In the near future, the new term for restoration may be regeneration. This may sound like something from *Star Trek,* but decayed or missing teeth soon will be *regrown,* either in the mouth or in the laboratory. A group of scientists are currently working on a cavity treatment that will stimulate the growth of dentin. The new treatment eventually will be applied to the cavity before it is filled, thus helping the tooth to heal itself.

Critical Thinking

1. An emergency patient has been scheduled today because of a lost "filling." The dentist examines tooth #5 and requests that a radiograph be taken. You are asked to place a temporary restoration. Which temporary dental material would you most likely use to replace the lost filling?
2. A patient has discussed her concern over the large amount of amalgam fillings in her mouth, and she fears that the mercury may be harming her health. She has scheduled an appointment to discuss this with the dentist. If you were the dentist, how would you respond to this patient?
3. In regard to direct restorative dental materials, which dental material would you say is the most versatile, and why?
4. Tooth whitening has become one of the procedures most requested by patients. Why is this procedure so popular with patients, and why is it best to have the dentist involved in the process?
5. What is the difference between composite resins and ceramics?

44

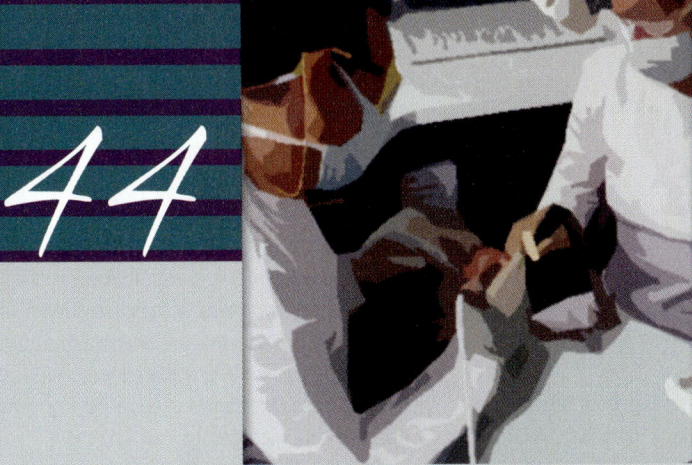

Dental Liners, Bases, and Bonding Systems

Outline

KEY TERMS

Desiccate (**de**-si-kate) To remove all moisture from an item; to dry out.

Etchant (**eh**-chunt) Chemical agent used in etching.

Etching (**ech**-ing) Process of cutting into a surface by the use of an acid product.

Eugenol (**yu**-jeh-nol) Colorless liquid made from clove oil and used for its soothing qualities.

Hybrid (**hi**-brid) Material that produces a similar outcome to its natural counterpart.

Insulating Preventing the passage of heat or electricity.

Micromechanical (*my*-kro-mi-**ka**-ni-kul) Describes the means by which a material and structure lock onto one another through minute cuttings.

Obliterating (uh-**bli**-tur-ate-ing) Removing or eliminating something completely.

Polymerize (pah-**li**-meh-rize) To subject a material to the bonding process of two or more monomers.

Retention (ri-**ten[t]**-shun) The result of adhesion, mechanical locking, or both.

Sedative (**se**-dah-tiv) Having a soothing effect.

Smear layer Very thin layer of debris on newly prepared dentin.

Thermal (**thur**-mul) Relating to heat.

LEARNING OUTCOMES

On completion of this chapter, the student will be able to achieve the following objectives:

- Pronounce, define, and spell the Key Terms.
- Discuss how the sensitivity of a tooth determines what type of dental material is selected for a procedure.
- Discuss how and why cavity liners are used in restoring tooth structure.
- Discuss how and why varnishes are used in restoring tooth structure.
- Discuss how and why dentin sealers are used in restoring tooth structure.
- Discuss how and why dental bases are used in restoring tooth structure.
- Describe the etching process of a tooth and its importance in the bonding of tooth and material.
- Describe the bonding systems and how they provide a better adherence of dental materials to the tooth structure.

PERFORMANCE OUTCOMES

On completion of this chapter, the student will be able to achieve competency standards in the following skills:

- Apply calcium hydroxide to a prepared tooth surface.
- Apply dental varnish to a prepared tooth surface.
- Apply dentin sealer to a prepared tooth surface.
- Mix and place three types of bases on a prepared tooth surface.
- Apply etchant material.
- Apply a bonding system to the prepared tooth structure.

A classification of supplementary dental materials is incorporated in a restorative and esthetic procedure for the health and well-being of the tooth. This chapter explains and guides you in the use of liners, varnish, dentin sealers, bases, and bonding materials that provide added protection to the pulp and surrounding structures in the final restoration process.

When dentists begin preparing a tooth, they are not 100 percent certain as to the extent of the disease in the tooth's structure until the tooth is accessed by the use of a rotary and hand cutting instrument. If the decay has extended into the dentin and extends close to the pulp, it becomes a moderately deep or deep preparation. At this time, the tooth would require the use of a liner, varnish, dentin sealer, base, bonding agent, or a combination of the five before the permanent restoration is placed.

Table 44-1 summarizes the use of the supplementary materials discussed in this chapter and the order in which they would be placed for specific procedures.

PREPARED TOOTH STRUCTURES

The type of additional materials selected by the dentist will determine how the tooth will be prepared. If you look at existing restorations in your mouth, you will see a specific outline or design of the restoration. These cavity designs are for the sole purpose of creating strength within the tooth, which determines how well the tooth will hold the restoration in place. The more natural tooth structure remaining, the easier it is to hold in the restorative material.

Table 44-1 ***Supplementary Dental Materials and Application in Order of Use***

Type of Restorative Material	Shallow Preparation	Moderately Deep Restoration	Deep Restoration
Amalgam	1. Dentin sealer	1. Base	1. Liner
	2. Bonding system	2. Dentin sealer	2. Base
		3. Bonding system	3. Dentin sealer
			4. Bonding system
Composite resin	1. Bonding system	1. Bonding system	1. Liner
			2. Bonding system
Gold inlays/onlays		1. Base	1. Liner
			2. Base
Ceramic	1. Bonding system	1. Bonding system	1. Liner
			2. Bonding system

If the tooth structure is weak, however, or has little foundation, the dentist must rely on dental materials for their retaining properties.

PULPAL RESPONSES

As mentioned in earlier chapters, if decay has progressed through the enamel and into the dentin, the patient may have more sensitivity and discomfort even after placement of a permanent restoration. The patient can experience sensitivity immediately, a month after placement, or even several months after placement. The dentist must decide at this point of the procedure what additional materials will be placed to provide medication and protection against a pulpal response. The pulp responds differently to different stimuli.

Types of Pulpal Stimuli

- Physical stimuli include **thermal** changes from hot and cold or electrical energy created by other metals coming into contact with the tooth.
- Mechanical stimuli include vibration from a handpiece when the tooth is being prepared, as well as traumatic occlusion, which occurs when a person's "bite" does not occlude properly and added pressure is placed on a specific area.
- Chemical stimuli occur as a result of acidic materials coming into contact with pulpal tissues.
- Biological stimuli occur as a result of bacteria from saliva coming into contact with pulpal tissues.

DENTAL LINERS

A dental liner does exactly what its name implies: it lines the deepest portion of the dental preparation to provide pulpal protection or dentinal regeneration. This thin barrier protects the pulpal tissue from irritation caused by physical, mechanical, chemical, and biological elements. The health and condition of the tooth being restored determine what lining agent the dentist selects.

Calcium Hydroxide

Calcium hydroxide is a frequently selected type of cavity liner because of its unique characteristics:

- It protects the pulp from chemical irritation through its sealing abilities.
- It stimulates the production of reparative or secondary dentin.
- It is compatible with all types of restorative materials.

Application

The expanded-functions dental assistant (EFDA) can place dental liners if the function is legal in the state in which the assistant is practicing. Because of the variations of cavity preparations, you must be certain of where the liner is to be placed. Knowledge of pulpal anatomy will aid you in your placement.

Liners are available as a two-paste system (base and catalyst) and as a light-cured material. A liner is placed only on *dentin* and must be avoided on enamel or in retentive grooves (Fig. 44-1). (See Procedure 44-1: The Application of Calcium Hydroxide [Expanded Function].)

Recall

1. What is the function of a dental liner?
2. On what tooth structure is a liner placed?
3. What are the three unique qualities of calcium hydroxide?

Examples of Commercial Dental Liners

- Cavitec
- Dycal
- Hydrex
- Life
- Pulprotex
- Temrex
- Timeline
- Ultrabend
- ZOE

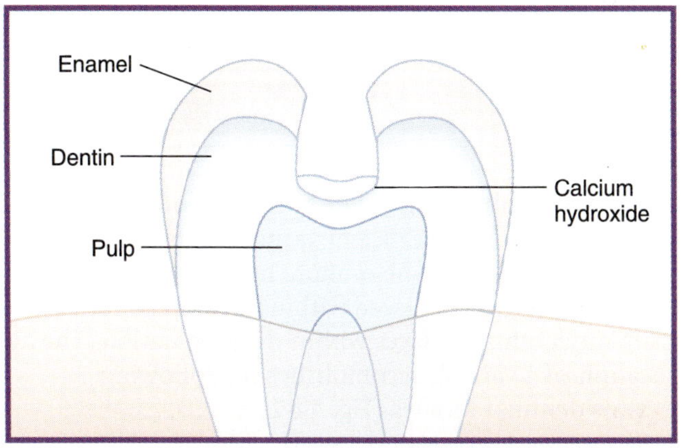

Fig. 44-1 Placement of a liner.

Procedure 44-1 The Application of Calcium Hydroxide (Expanded Function)

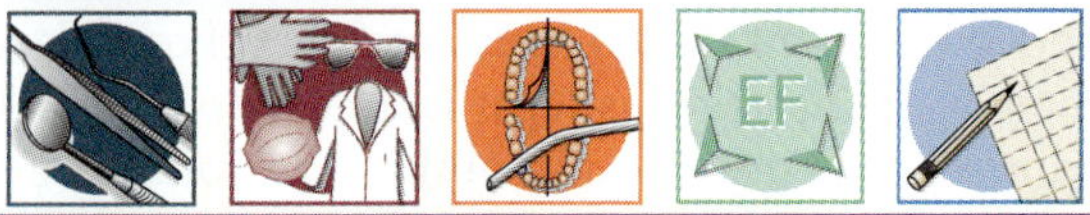

Equipment and Supplies

- Small paper mixing pad
- Small spatula
- Calcium hydroxide applicator
- Calcium hydroxide base and catalyst paste (from the same manufacturer)
- 2- × 2-inch gauze pads

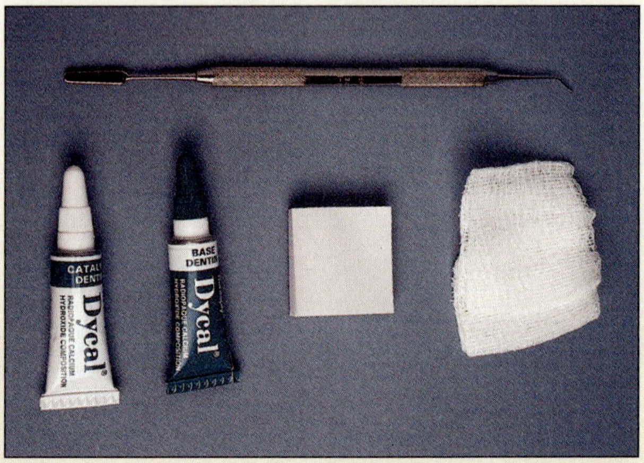

PROCEDURAL STEPS

1. Dispense small, equal amounts of the catalyst and base pastes onto the paper mixing pad.
   Purpose: The area to be covered will be 0.5 to 1 mm, depending on the size of the cavity preparation.
2. Using a circular motion, quickly mix (10 to 15 seconds) the material over a small area of the paper pad with the spatula.

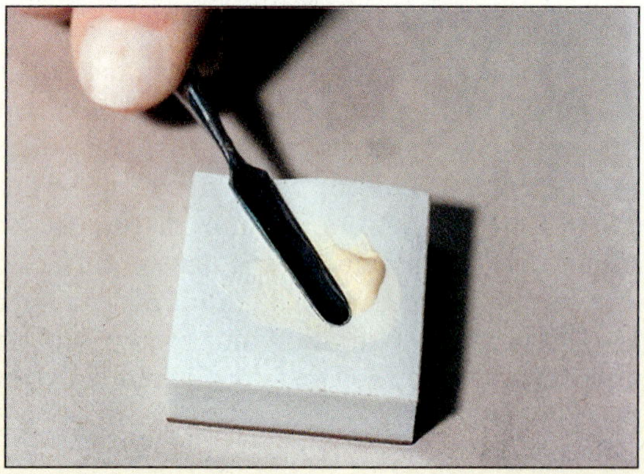

3. Use gauze to clean the spatula.
4. With the tip of the applicator, pick up a small amount of the material, and apply a thin layer at the deepest area of the preparation.
5. Use an explorer to remove any material from the enamel before drying.

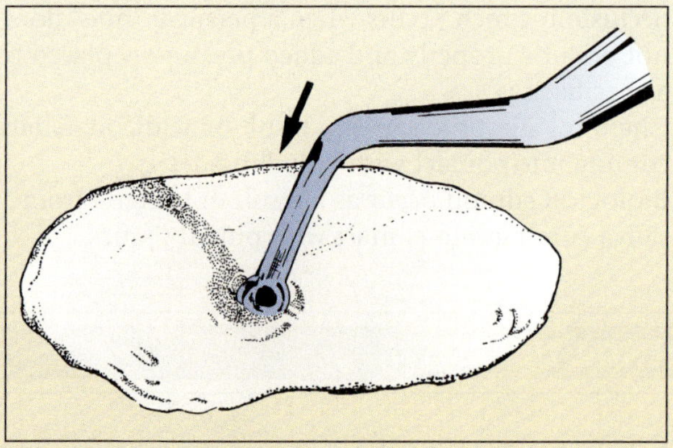

6. Clean and disinfect equipment.

VARNISH

If you are familiar with refinishing furniture, you should understand the significance of varnish. A dental varnish is a liquid consisting of one or more resins in an organic solvent. This material is placed within the preparation specifically on dentinal surfaces within the preparation. The application of a varnish accomplishes the following:

- Seals dentinal tubules (Fig. 44-2)
- Reduces leakage around a restoration
- Acts as a barrier to protect the tooth from highly acidic cements such as zinc phosphate

Application

The EFDA can place dental varnish if the function is legal in the state in which the assistant is practicing. The varnish is always placed *after* the application of the liner (Fig. 44-3). Because dental varnish interferes with the bonding and setting reaction of composite resins and glass ionomer restorations, the use of varnish is contraindicated with these materials. (See Procedure 44-2: The Application of Dental Varnish [Expanded Function].)

Varnish is applied with a small disposable applicator or with a cotton pellet held in sterile cotton pliers. When using cotton pliers, care must be taken not to contaminate the remaining liquid or the bottle.

Procedure 44-2 The Application of Dental Varnish (Expanded Function)

Equipment and Supplies

- Micro brush applicators (2)
- Cotton pliers and cotton pellets (2)
- Dental varnish

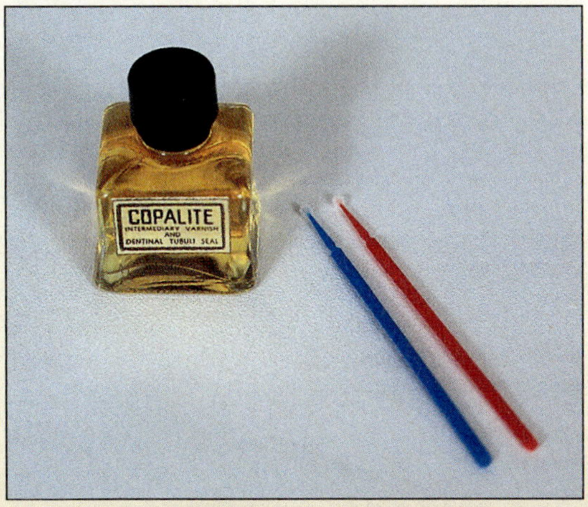

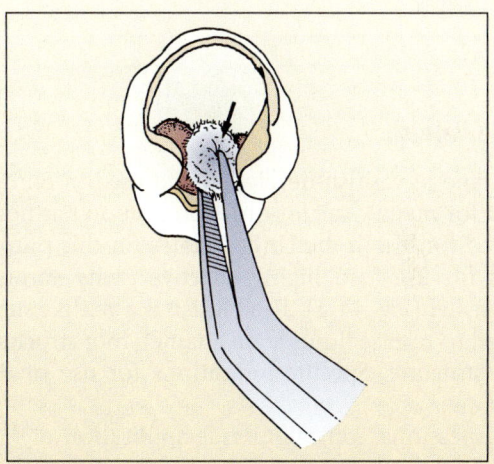

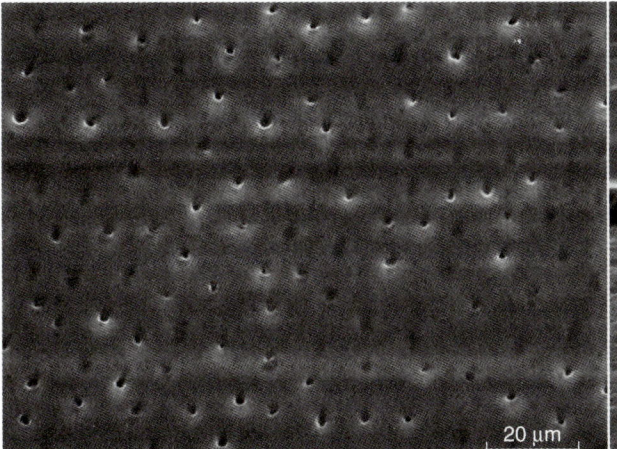

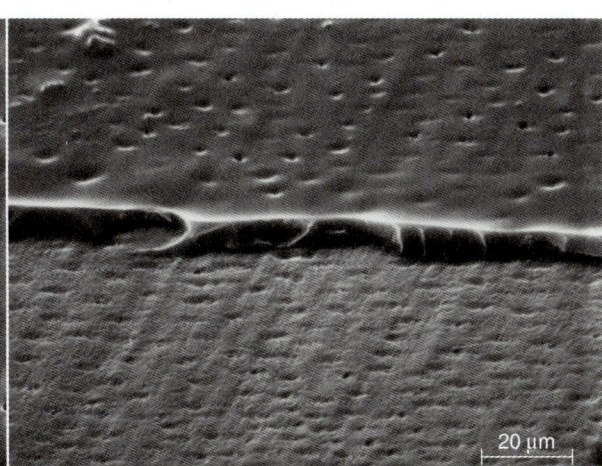

PROCEDURAL STEPS

1. Retrieve a new applicator or cotton pellets in cotton pliers.
2. Open the bottle of varnish and place the tip of the applicator or cotton pellet into the liquid.
3. Replace the cap on the bottle immediately.
   Purpose: When varnish is exposed to air, evaporation causes this liquid to thicken. If it becomes too thick, a thinning agent must be added.
4. Place a thin coating of the varnish on the walls, floor, and margin of the cavity preparation. Allow to air-dry.

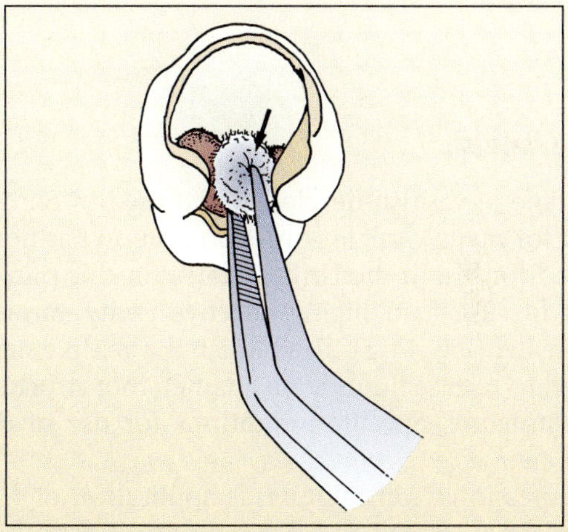

5. Apply a second coat; repeat steps 1 through 4.

A B

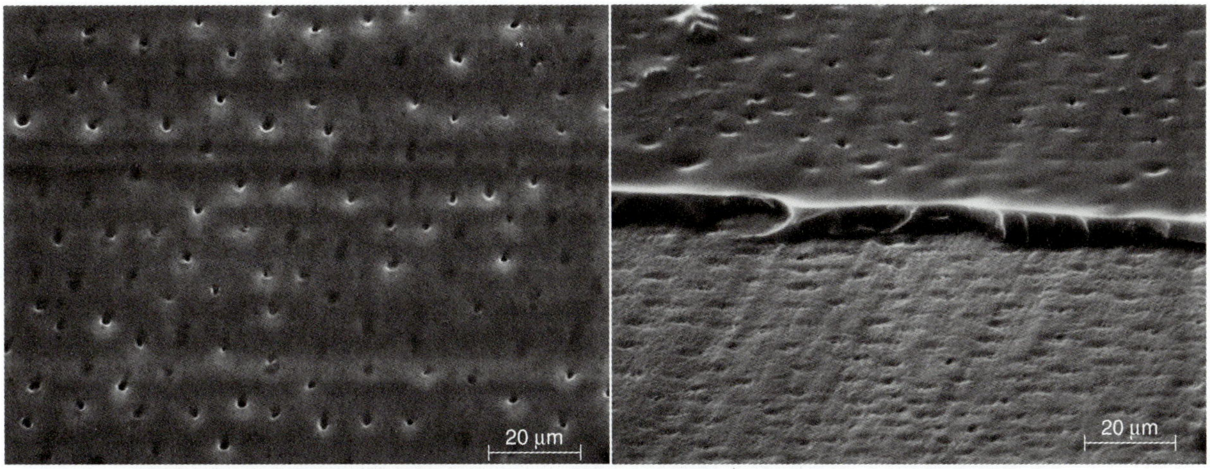

Fig. 44-2 Microscopic view of dentin structure with exposed dentinal tubules. **A,** Showing one layer of varnish. **B,** Two layers of varnish sealing the dentinal tubules. (From Roberson T, et al: *Sturdevant's art and science of operative dentistry,* ed 4. St Louis, 2002, Mosby.)

Examples of Commercial Varnishes

- Caulk varnish
- Cavaseal
- Chembar
- Coplite
- Handiliner
- Hydroxyline
- Repelac
- Tubilitec
- Varnall

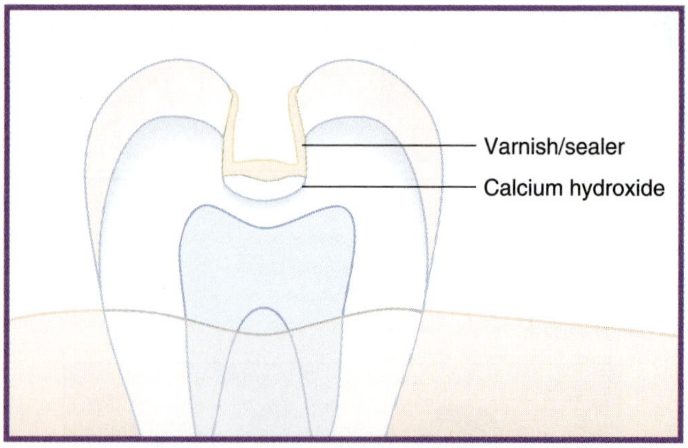

Fig. 44-3 Location for placement of cavity varnish.

Fluoride Varnish

A new type of varnish developed and used in Europe and Canada for many years for caries prevention has now been approved for use in the United States for this purpose, as well as for use as a highly effective cavity varnish and dentin sealer (Fig. 44-4). The varnish is a gel-like substance designed to release fluoride on enamel, root structure, and dentin structure. Specific indications for use of fluoride varnish are:

- Professional topical fluoride application
- Treatment of hypersensitive cervical areas
- Orthodontic patients
- Cavity varnish
- Dentin sealant

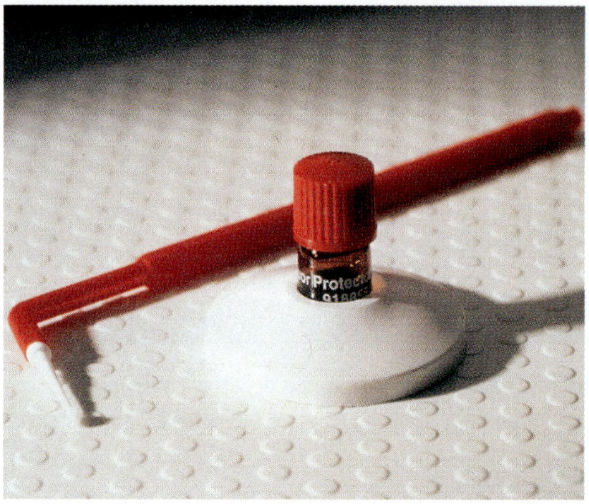

Fig. 44-4 Fluoride varnish currently used in the United States. (Courtesy Ivoclar.)

Recall

4. What is the main ingredient in varnish?
5. Can varnish be placed under all restorative materials? If not, with which materials is it contraindicated?

DENTIN SEALER

A method to treat or prevent the hypersensitivity that patients may experience from a newly placed restoration is to apply a dentin sealer, also referred to as a *desensitizer.* A dentin sealer is an agent that is used instead of a varnish. The dentin sealer is designed to seal the dentinal tubules, thus preventing oral fluids from seeping in between the tooth and restoration, which could eventually cause sensitivity. No surface layer is formed when using a dentin sealer, which makes the material ideal for use under *all* indirect restorations.

Application

The EFDA can place dentin sealer if the function is legal in the state in which the assistant is practicing. Because the dentin sealer contains HEMA and glutaraldehyde, it is very important that this material be used sparingly and that no material is allowed to contact soft tissue. (See Procedure 44-3: Application of Dentin Sealer [Expanded Function].)

Recall

6. What is the other name used for dentin sealer?
7. What does the dentin sealer *seal*?

Procedure 44-3 The Application of Dentin Sealer (Expanded Function)

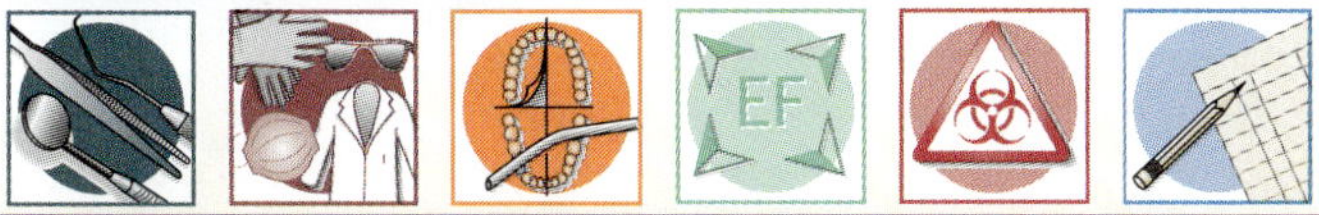

Equipment and Supplies

- Basic setup
- Dentin sealer material
- Microbrush applicator
- Air-water syringe
- Oral evacuation system

PROCEDURAL STEPS

1. Provided that the tooth and tissues are not sensitive, rinse the area with water, but avoid over-drying.
2. Apply the dentin sealer with the applicator over all areas of the dentin.
   Purpose: To assist with the delivery of the solution to all the affected dentinal tubules.
3. Wait 30 seconds; then dry thoroughly (*do not rinse*).
4. Repeat application if sensitivity has been a problem with the patient.

Examples of Commercial Cement Bases

Zinc oxide–eugenol
IRM
ZOE
ZOE 2200

Zinc phosphate
Dropsin
Fleck's Extraordinary
HyBond SP
Modern Tenacin
Zinc Cement Improved

Polycarboxylate
Carboxylon
Chemit
Durelon
Durelon Fast Set
Hybond
PC Cement
Polybond
Poly-F Plus
Tylok

Glass ionomer
ASPA
Chembond
Dentin Cement LC
Fuji Lining LC
Ketac-Bond
Vitrebond
Zionomer

Resin modified glass ionomer
Fuji Duet
Vitremer Cement

DENTAL BASES

When a posterior tooth ends up becoming a moderately deep to deep preparation, the dentist will most likely choose to place a base under the permanent restoration. A base is an additional layer in the restoration process in order to protect the pulp. A base is designed to provide pulpal protection in the following three ways:

1. *Protective bases* are placed when it is necessary to protect the pulp before the restoration is placed. Without this protection, there may be postoperative sensitivity and damage to the pulp.
2. *Insulating bases* are placed in a deep cavity preparation to protect the tooth from thermal shock. (*Thermal shock* occurs when sudden temperature changes occur within the tooth.)
3. *Sedative bases* help soothe a pulp that has been damaged by decay or has been irritated during the process of removing the decay.

Types of Materials Used

Different types of cement products are used to form these specialized bases under permanent restorations.

Zinc oxide–eugenol (ZOE) would be selected for use as an **insulating** base and as a **sedative** base. The unique quality of this material is the eugenol in the liquid. With its oil from cloves, **eugenol** has a soothing effect on a painful, irritated pulp. However, ZOE cannot be used under composite resins, glass ionomers, or other resin restorations. The eugenol in the liquid delays the setting of the resin materials. (See Procedure 44-4: Mixing and Placing Zinc Oxide–Eugenol [ZOE] Cement as a Base [Expanded Function].)

Zinc phosphate cement is an excellent thermal insulator because it has a thermal conductivity rate similar to that of dentin. Because the phosphoric acid in the liquid can be irritating to the pulp, it would be necessary to place a cavity liner *under* the zinc phosphateinsulating base. (See Procedure 44-5: Mixing and Placing Zinc Phosphate as a Base [Expanded Function].)

Procedure 44-4 Mixing and Placing Zinc Oxide–Eugenol (ZOE) Cement as a Base (Expanded Function)

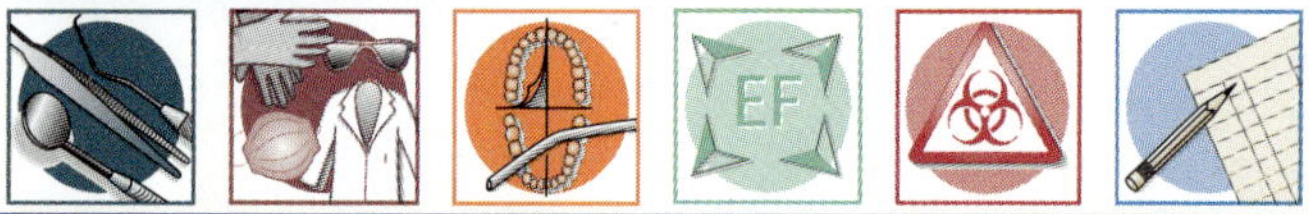

Equipment and Supplies

- Basic setup
- Treated paper pad
- Spatula (flexible stainless steel)
- Zinc oxide powder and dispenser
- Eugenol liquid and dropper
- Plastic instrument (for placement)
- Amalgam condenser (for condensation)
- 2- × 2-inch gauze pads

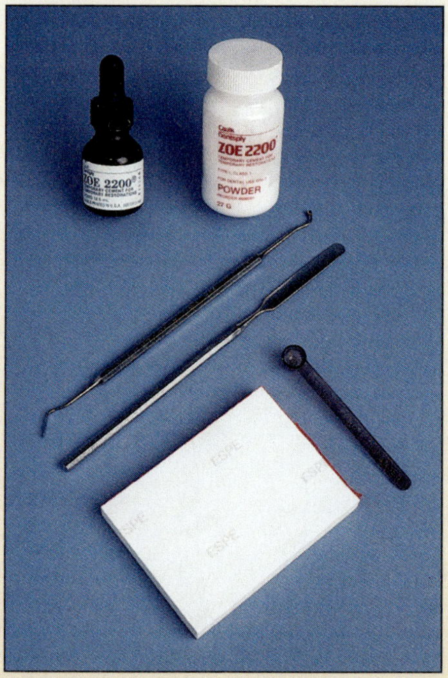

PROCEDURAL STEPS

1. Examine the preparation.
2. Measure the powder onto the mixing pad. Replace the cap immediately.
3. Dispense the liquid near the powder on the mixing pad. Replace the cap immediately.
4. Incorporate half the powder into the liquid; mix with the spatula for 20 to 30 seconds.
5. Incorporate the remaining portion into the mixture. Continue mixing for an additional 20 to 30 seconds. The material should be thick and putty-like.
6. Pick up half the material with your spatula and roll it into a small ball. Do this with the other portion as well.
   Purpose: To make the material easier to place in the cavity preparation.
7. Pick up the material by placing the condenser into the material; then carry it to the preparation.
8. Use a light tapping stroke to adapt the material into place.

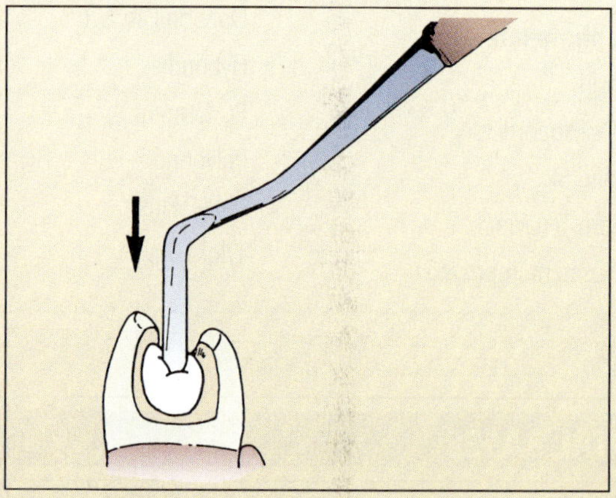

(From Baum L, Phillips RW, Lund MR: *Textbook of operative dentistry,* ed 3, Philadelphia, 1995, Saunders.)

9. Ensure that the entire pulpal floor is covered with the base.

Polycarboxylate cements are selected for the material's protective and insulating qualities. Polycarboxylate is nonirritating to the pulp, and can be placed under all types of direct and indirect restorations. (See Procedure 44-6: Mixing and Placing Polycarboxylate Cement as a Base [Expanded Function].)

Application

The EFDA can place a base if the function is legal in the state in which the assistant is practicing. A base material is much thicker than a liner, varnish, or sealer, so it actually provides a buffer between the pulp and the restorative material. The entire pulpal floor is covered with the base to a thickness of 1 to 2 mm (Fig. 44-5).

Recall

8. What does an insulating base do for a tooth?
9. What effect does eugenol have on the pulp?
10. Where is a base applied in the preparation?
11. What dental instrument is used to adapt a base into place?

Procedure 44-5 Mixing and Placing Zinc Phosphate Cement as a Base (Expanded Function)

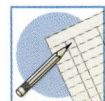

Equipment and Supplies

- Basic setup
- Glass slab (cool)
- Spatula (flexible stainless steel)
- Zinc phosphate powder and dispenser
- Zinc phosphate liquid and dropper
- Plastic instrument (for placement)
- Amalgam condenser (for condensation)
- 2- × 2-inch gauze pads

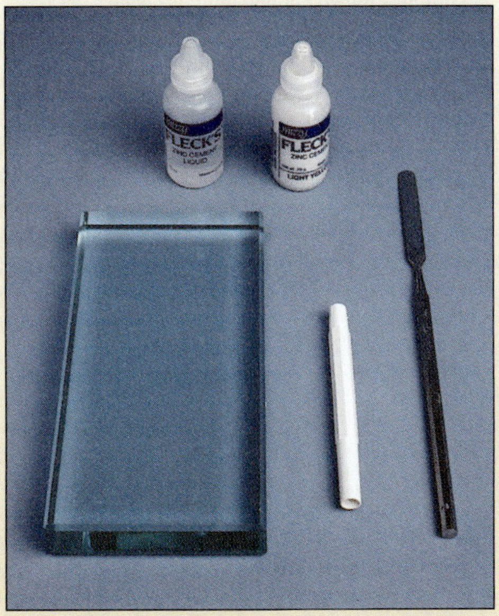

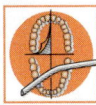

PROCEDURAL STEPS

1. Examine the preparation.
2. Dispense the powder and the liquid onto the slab. Use the powder-to-liquid ratio recommended to produce the desired thick, putty-like mix.

   Note: This requires more powder in proportion to the amount of liquid.
3. Mix to the desired consistency.
4. Form the completed mix into a small ball.
5. Pick up the material by placing the condenser into the material; then carry it to the preparation.
6. Using a light tapping stroke, adapt the material into place.
7. Ensure that the entire pulpal floor is covered with the base.
8. Have excess powder available for use when condensing the material into the tooth.

   Purpose: This powder will prevent the instrument from sticking to the material.

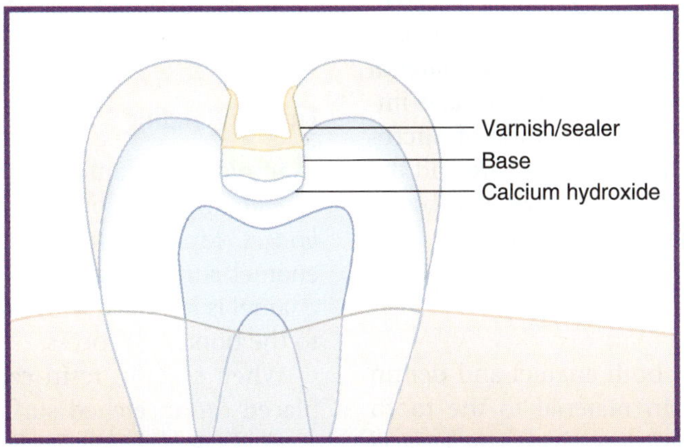

Fig. 44-5 Location for placement of a base.

Procedure 44-6 Mixing and Placing Polycarboxylate Cement as a Base (Expanded Function)

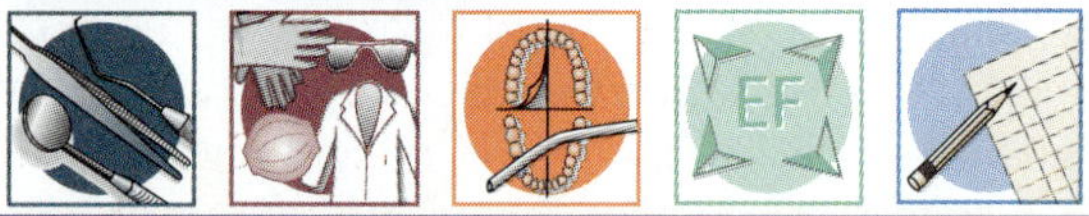

Equipment and Supplies

- Basic setup
- Treated paper pad
- Spatula (flexible stainless steel)
- Polycarboxylate powder and dispenser
- Polycarboxylate liquid (in squeeze bottle or calibrated syringe)
- Plastic instrument (for placement)
- Amalgam condenser (for condensation)
- 2- × 2-inch gauze pads

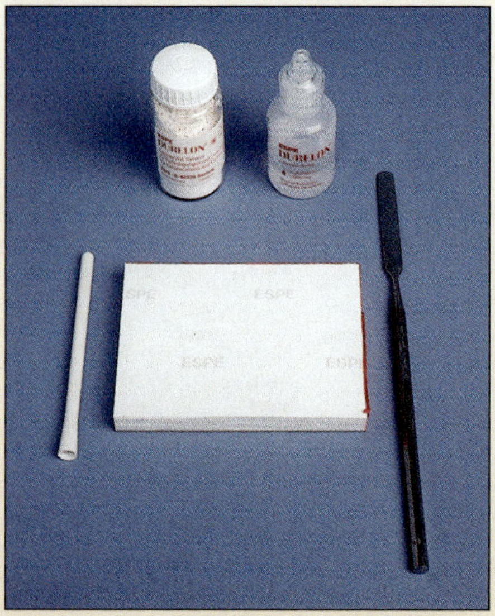

PROCEDURAL STEPS

1. Examine the preparation.
2. Dispense the powder and liquid onto the pad.
   Note: When used for a base, the liquid portion is decreased to make a thicker consistency.
3. Incorporate all the powder into the liquid, with total mixing time not to exceed 45 seconds.
4. Form the completed mix into a small ball.
5. Pick up the material by placing the condenser into the material; then carry it to the preparation.
6. Using a light tapping stroke, adapt the material into place.
7. Ensure that the entire pulpal floor is covered with the base.
8. Clean and disinfect the equipment immediately.
   Note: This cement must set for approximately 5 minutes before the placement of the permanent restoration.

DENTAL BONDING

Many of the **retention** problems with dental materials have improved with the application of a bonding material. Dental bonding, also referred to as *dental adhesion,* is a process of a solid and/or liquid contact of one material with another at a single margin. Bonding systems have improved retaining properties through the creation of **micromechanical** retention between the tooth structure and the restoration. With bonding materials, it is now possible to bond restorative materials to enamel and dentin.

Etching Systems

The use of **etchant** is critical on both enamel and dentin surfaces for bonding of the resin material to the tooth structure. Acid **etching** is a technique in which a *maleic acid* etchant or a *phosphoric acid* etchant is placed on either the enamel or the dentin to remove the smear layer in preparation for bonding (Fig. 44-6). Acid etchant is supplied in either liquid or gel form.

Whether using the etchant liquid or gel, it is important to understand the application process.

Enamel Bonding

Examples of enamel bonding include the placement of *sealants,* bonded orthodontic *brackets,* and resin-bonded *bridges.* Most of these are attached directly to the intact enamel surface. For resin-bonded *veneers,* a thin layer of enamel is removed with the use of rotary instruments prior to the bonding process.

When sealant, resin cement, or restorative material is placed on an etched surface, it flows in and around the enamel tags (Fig. 44-7). The material hardens in this location to form a strong mechanical bond with the enamel.

Dentin Bonding

Unlike enamel, dentin consists of a range of organic substances, and bonding of dental materials can be more difficult. A major factor in the success of bonding to dentin is the removal of the **smear layer,** which is a very thin layer (5 to 10 mm) of debris composed of fluids and tooth components remaining on the dentin after the cavity preparation (Fig. 44-8). During the preparation of a tooth for a restoration, thousands of dentinal tubules are cut. The open ends of these tubules can transmit fluids and microorganisms to the pulp of the tooth, which can result in postoperative sensitivity, pain, or even damage to the pulp. Unlike enamel, a slight amount of moisture must be maintained on the dentin so as not to **desiccate** (dry out) the tooth. If dentin is completely dried, the tooth structure could be harmed.

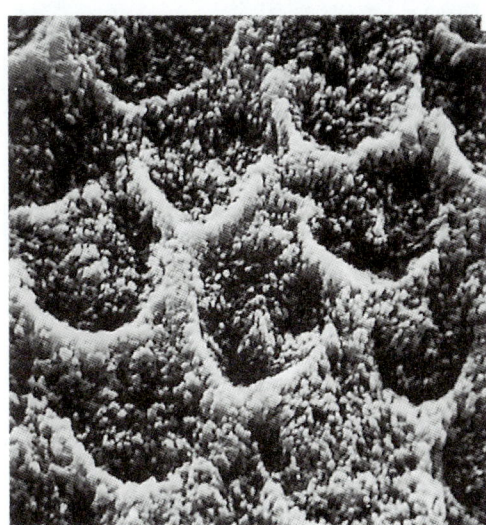

Fig. 44-6 **Microscopic view of enamel tags after etching.** (From Phillips RW, Moore BK: *Elements of dental materials for dental hygienists and dental assistants,* ed 5. Philadelphia, 1994, Saunders.)

The smear layer, which has been described as "nature's bandage," protects the tooth by **obliterating** the openings of the dentinal tubules. However, before dentin bonding, the smear layer must be removed and these tubules opened. As part of the bonding process, the tubules are sealed with the bonding material, and the protection is restored to the tooth.

Application

The EFDA can apply the etchant and place the bonding material if the function is legal in the state in which the assistant is practicing. (See Procedure 44-7: Applying an Etchant Material [Expanded Function] and Procedure 44-8: Applying a Bonding System [Expanded Function].) Bonding applications are available as self-curing, dual-cured, and light-cured systems. Some systems use one application, whereas others require the mixing of two liquids. Each bonding system is different, and the material from one system is not interchangeable with that of another. It is essential that the manufacturer's instructions be followed exactly for each product.

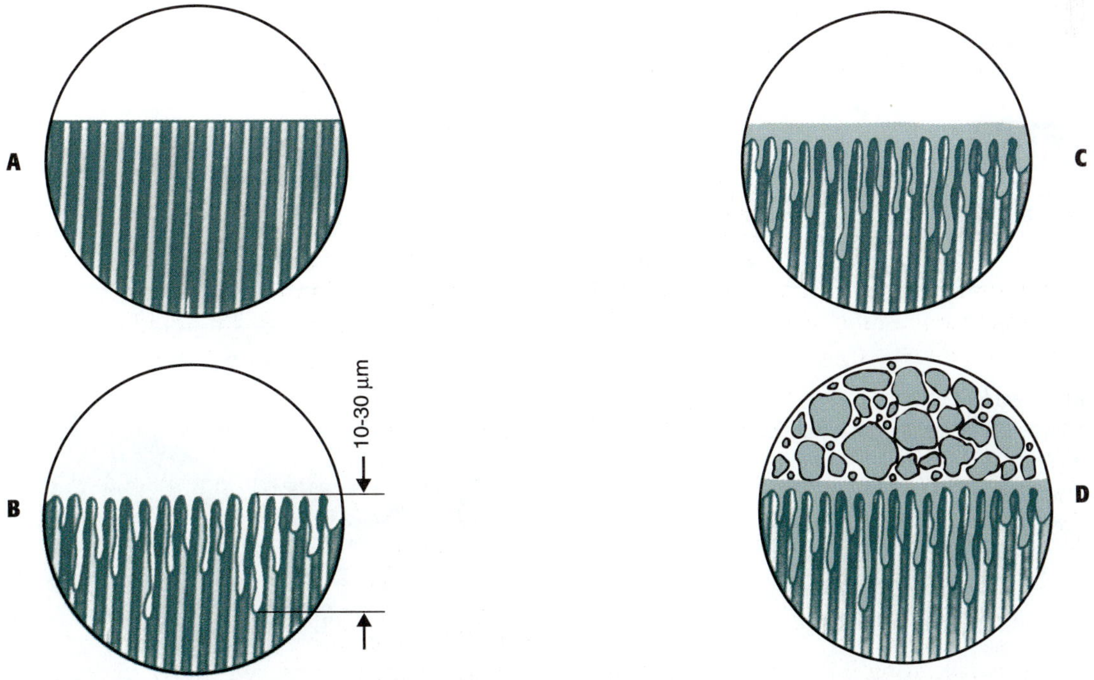

Fig. 44-7 **Process of bonding. A, Enamel rods unetched. B, Enamel rods etched. C, Bonding agent mechanically bonding to tooth. D, Resin chemically bonding to bonding agent.** (From Roberson T, et al: *Sturdevant's art and science of operative dentistry,* ed 4. St Louis, 2002, Mosby.)

A

B

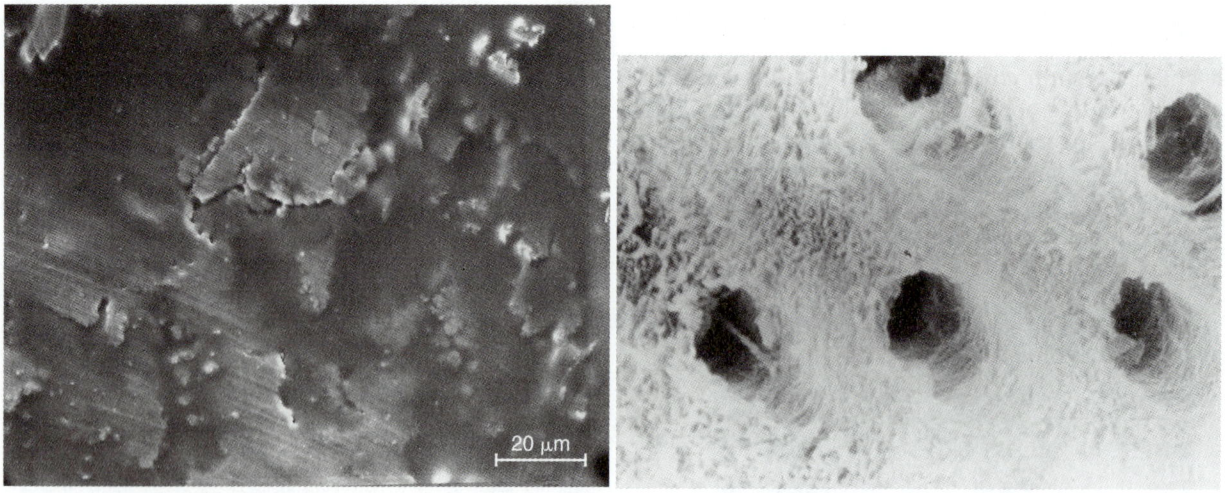

Fig. 44-8 **Microscopic view in various stages of etching. A, Unetched dentin with smear layer. B, Over-etched dentin.** (From Roberson T, et al: *Sturdevant's art and science of operative dentistry,* ed 4. St Louis, 2002, Mosby.)

The following general description outlines what occurs in the bonding system. However, specifics vary according to the brand, and the manufacturer's instructions must always be followed. The etchant removes the smear layer, and then the bonding component is allowed to flow into these small defects and into the partially opened tubules. Once this material is placed, it will be allowed either (1) to harden and act as a **hybrid** layer or (2) to remain in a liquid state while the restoration is being placed to bond together the tooth and the dental material.

Guidelines for Clinical Application of Bonding Products

- Perform the steps in the bonding process precisely.
- Avoid expiration, contamination, and thickening of liquids.
- Remove any plaque or debris before the bonding process.
- Avoid over-drying teeth; these products work best on a slightly moist tooth structure.
- Note that too much primer is better than too little; multiple layers work best.

Procedure 44-7 Applying an Etchant Material (Expanded Function)

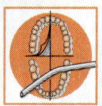

Equipment and Supplies

- Basic setup
- Cotton rolls/dental dam for isolation
- Applicator (cotton pellets for liquid etchant and syringe tip for gel)
- Etchant material
- High-velocity evacuator
- Air-water syringe
- Timer

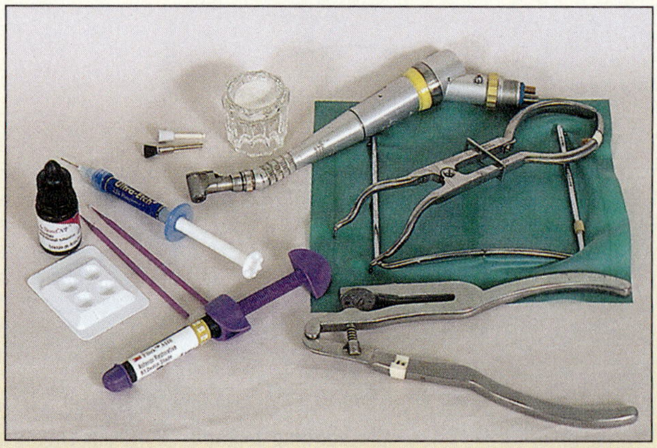

Procedure 44-7 Applying an Etchant Material (Expanded Function)—cont'd

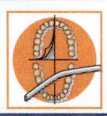

PROCEDURAL STEPS

1. The prepared tooth must be isolated from contamination. Either a dental dam or cotton rolls are placed before the etching process begins.
   Purpose: Saliva must not contaminate the preparation.
2. The surface of the tooth structure must be clean and free of any debris, plaque, or calculus before etching.
   Purpose: Debris on the surface may interfere with the etching process.
3. After cleaning, the surface is carefully dried but not desiccated.
   Purpose: Too much drying of the tooth structure will harm the tooth.
4. The etchant is selected. Most manufacturers supply a gel etchant in a syringe that can be applied to enamel or dentin.
   Purpose: The gel allows the etchant to be carefully placed *only* where it is needed.

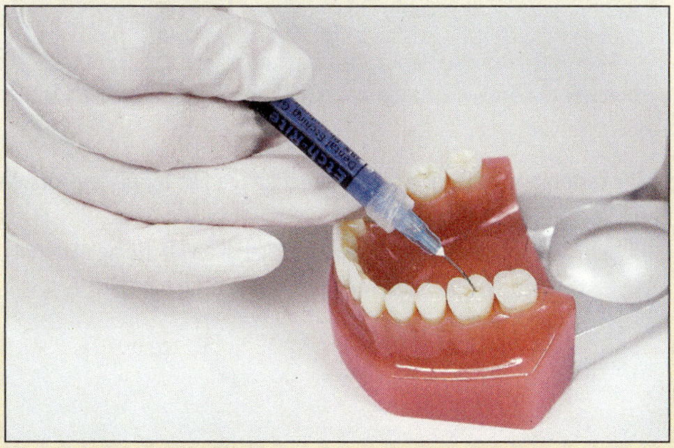

5. The tooth structure is etched for the time recommended by the manufacturer; this usually ranges from 15 to 30 seconds.
   Purpose: The exact time depends on the material and the use. For example, etching time for placing sealants is not the same as the etching time for bonding orthodontic brackets.
6. After etching, the surface is thoroughly rinsed and dried for 15 to 30 seconds.
7. An etched surface has a frosty-white appearance. If the surface does not have this appearance or has been contaminated with moisture, it is necessary to repeat the etching process.

Procedure 44-8 Applying a Bonding System (Expanded Function)

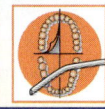

Equipment and Supplies

- Bonding agent
- Applicator device or brush
- Air-water syringe
- Oral evacuation system
- 2- × 2-inch gauze pads

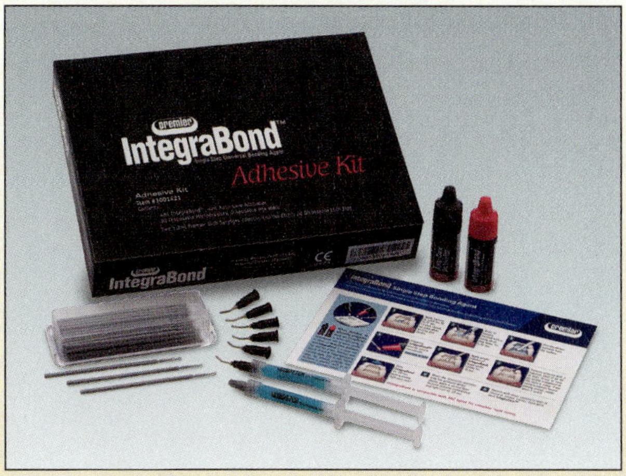

continued

Procedure 44-8 Applying a Bonding System (Expanded Function)—cont'd

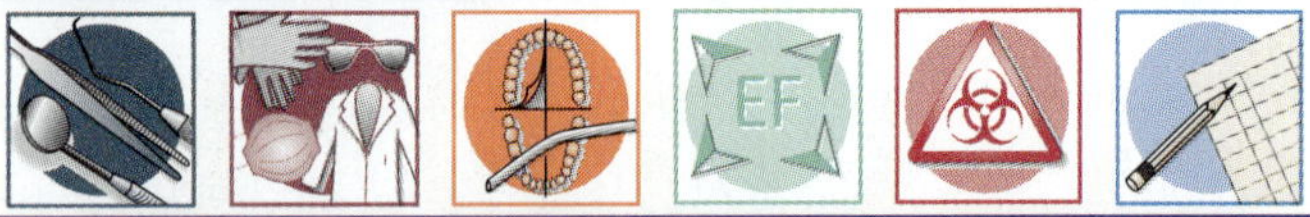

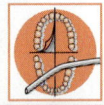

PROCEDURAL STEPS

1. If a metal matrix band is used, the band is prepared with either cavity varnish or wax before placement around the tooth.

   Purpose: This prevents the bonding resin and amalgam from adhering to the surface (see Chapter 49 for the application of a matrix).

   Caution: No varnish should come in contact with the tooth, because this will interfere with the bonding effects of the resin primers.
2. The cavity preparation and the enamel margins should be etched according to the manufacturer's directions.
3. A primer is applied to the entire preparation in one or multiple coats, depending on the manufacturer's directions.
4. The dual-cured adhesive resin is placed in the entire cavity preparation and lightly air-thinned. The resin should appear unset or partially set.

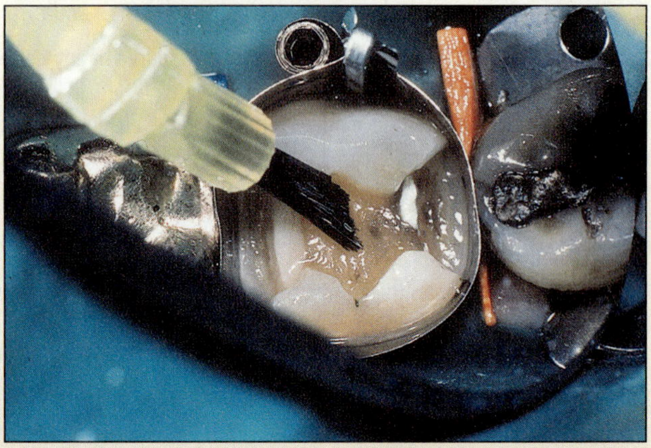

5. The restorative material is mixed and then readied for placement into the cavity preparation.

   Purpose: To integrate the restorative material and bonding material at the preparation walls before the resin has time to **polymerize** (set).

- Ensure that the bonding solution covers all surfaces.
- Avoid any contamination with saliva, blood, or debris, which will require the entire procedure to be redone.
- Allow as much time as possible for the bond to mature before completing the restoration and removing the cotton rolls or dental dam.

Recall

12. What is the purpose of a dental bonding material?
13. What is an example of enamel bonding?
14. What must be removed from the tooth structure for bonding material to reach dentin?
15. Which material is applied first—the bonding or etchant material?

Patient Education

If a patient comes to you with concern over the sensitivity or discomfort he or she is experiencing, you must know how to discuss and interpret these sensations with the patient. You also must be able to distinguish these problems for the dentist.

A patient may experience many types of sensitivities from a dental procedure. You have to become the "detective" in this process and ask the following specific questions about the type of discomfort the patient is experiencing:

- How long has this been bothering you?
- Is there a certain time of day that it seems to bother you the most?
- Do hot or cold beverages bother you?
- When you bite down, does it bother you?
- Does air that you breathe in your mouth bother you?

By understanding the materials discussed in this chapter, you will have a better knowledge of how dental liners, bases, and bonding systems are important in eliminating the discomfort and sensitivity that a patient may experience from tooth restoration.

Legal and Ethical Implications

If the dentist and dental team do not treat a patient's sensitivity or discomfort from a dental procedure as a serious concern, a problem—and perhaps even a legal issue—will arise. You must follow through with a patient who is experiencing discomfort by bringing the patient into the office and completing any diagnostic evaluations to determine the source of the problem. Too often dental professionals say to patients, "It is common to experience discomfort or sensitivity from a procedure." With the materials and techniques currently available, however, patients should be pain-free after their dental experience.

Eye to the Future

One area of dentistry that is ever-changing is the application of evolving dental materials. It is difficult to believe that these products are even easier to mix and use today than they were just a few years ago. Companies are now providing materials in easy-to-use packets, syringes, capsules, and applicators; soon the whole process of restorative materials and supplemental materials will be supplied as a single application. This approach will save an enormous amount of time for the dental team and reduce the steps required in the restorative procedure.

Critical Thinking

1. You are assisting in a composite restorative procedure on tooth #12. The preparation is moderately deep and has extended into the dentin. The dentist indicates that she will be using a sealer. Your office has varnish and dentin sealer. Which one of the two would you use for this procedure, and why?
2. Three types of base materials are discussed in this chapter. You are assisting in a procedure that requires a base that is nonirritating and provides protection and insulation. Which one of the three would most likely be selected?
3. You are assisting in an amalgam procedure on tooth #30. The preparation becomes very deep. Describe the supplemental materials that would be set out for this procedure and give the order in which they would be placed.
4. Describe how the design of a preparation relates to the type of supplemental materials used in restorative dentistry.
5. Are any of the procedures in this chapter considered an "expanded function" for dental assistants in your state? If so, what additional techniques do you find that are important for you as the operator?

45

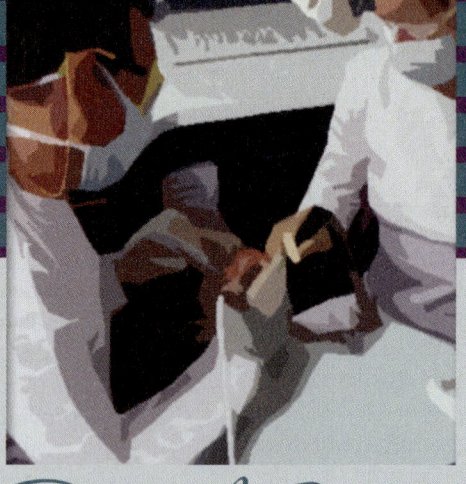

Dental Cements

Outline

Classification of Dental Cements
- Luting Agents

Variables Affecting Final Cementation
- Mixing Time
- Humidity
- Powder/Liquid Ratio
- Temperature

Types of Cements
- Zinc Oxide–Eugenol Cement

Procedure 45-1: Mixing Zinc Oxide–Eugenol (ZOE) for Permanent Cementation

Procedure 45-2: Mixing ZOE for Temporary Cementation
- Zinc Phosphate Cement

Procedure 45-3: Mixing Zinc Phosphate for Permanent Cementation
- Polycarboxylate Cement

Procedure 45-4: Mixing Polycarboxylate for Permanent Cementation
- Glass Ionomer Cement

Procedure 45-5: Mixing Glass Ionomer for Permanent Cementation
- Composite Resin Cement

Procedure 45-6: Mixing Composite Resin for Permanent Cementation

Cement Removal

Procedure 45-7: Removing Cement from Permanent or Temporary Cementation (Expanded Function)

Patient Education

Legal and Ethical Implications

Eye to the Future

Critical Thinking

KEY TERMS

Dissipate (**di**-sah-pate) To cause something to scatter, or become dispersed, and gradually disappear.

Exothermic (*ek*-so-**thur**-mik) Characterized by the released heat from a chemical reaction.

Luting agent (**lut**-ing) Cement-like substance used to seal a surface.

Provisional Pertaining to temporary coverage made for crown or bridge preparations and worn during cast preparation.

Retard (re-**tard**) To slow down a process.

Spatulate (**spa**-chu-late) To mix using a spatula-like instrument.

LEARNING OUTCOMES

On completion of this chapter, the student will be able to achieve the following objectives:

- Pronounce, define, and spell the Key Terms.
- Describe luting cements and differentiate between permanent and temporary cements.
- Discuss the factors that influence luting cements.
- List the five cements discussed in the chapter and identify their similarities and differences.

PERFORMANCE OUTCOMES

On completion of this chapter, the student will be able to achieve competency standards in the following skills:

- Mix and prepare zinc oxide–eugenol for cementation.
- Mix and prepare two-paste zinc oxide–eugenol (Tempbond) for temporary cementation.
- Mix and prepare polycarboxylate for cementation.
- Mix and prepare glass ionomer for cementation.
- Mix and prepare composite resin for cementation.
- Remove cement from permanent and temporary cementations.

CLASSIFICATION OF DENTAL CEMENTS

Dental cements are a category of dental materials routinely used when working with indirect restorations. The American Dental Association (ADA) and the International Standards Organization (ISO) have classified dental cements into three types according to their properties and their intended use in dentistry:

- *Type I* is a luting agent that includes permanent and temporary cements.
- *Type II* involves the restorative materials such as glass ionomers (previously discussed in Chapter 43) to be used as a restorative material.
- *Type III* includes liners and bases placed within the cavity preparation (previously discussed in Chapter 44).

Luting Agents

A **luting agent** is classified as a type I dental cement that acts as an adhesive to hold the indirect restoration to the tooth structure. Luting agents are designed to be either permanent or temporary.

Permanent Cements

Permanent cements are used as luting agents for the long-term cementation of cast restorations such as inlays, crowns, bridges, laminate veneers, and orthodontic fixed appliances. As discussed in Chapter 43, permanent indirect restorations, such as those produced from gold and ceramic, are designed and cast by the dental laboratory technician.

Once completed in the laboratory, cast restorations are delivered to the dentist for the cementation appointment. Because these types of restorations are seated over the tooth preparation, their hollow, shell-like structure requires a luting agent to be applied for adhesion (Fig. 45-1). Because castings need to fit so precisely, the cement must have qualities that do not interfere with a proper fit.

Temporary Cements

Temporary cements are used when the dentist needs to remove the indirect restoration at a later time, when the tooth is sensitive or is exhibiting other symptoms that might require removing the cast restoration, or when temporary cementation of provisional coverage is required while the patient waits for a short period until the laboratory technician completes the cast restoration (see Chapter 51). **Provisional** coverage is a temporary coverage placed to protect the tooth until the permanent restoration is ready to be cemented.

VARIABLES AFFECTING FINAL CEMENTATION

A number of factors can influence the performance of luting cements. Cementing errors are the result of improper technique, humidity, and/or incorrect temperature.

Mixing Time

Make sure to follow the manufacturer's directions for mixing time, working time, and delivery time. Any delay between completion of the mix and seating will result in

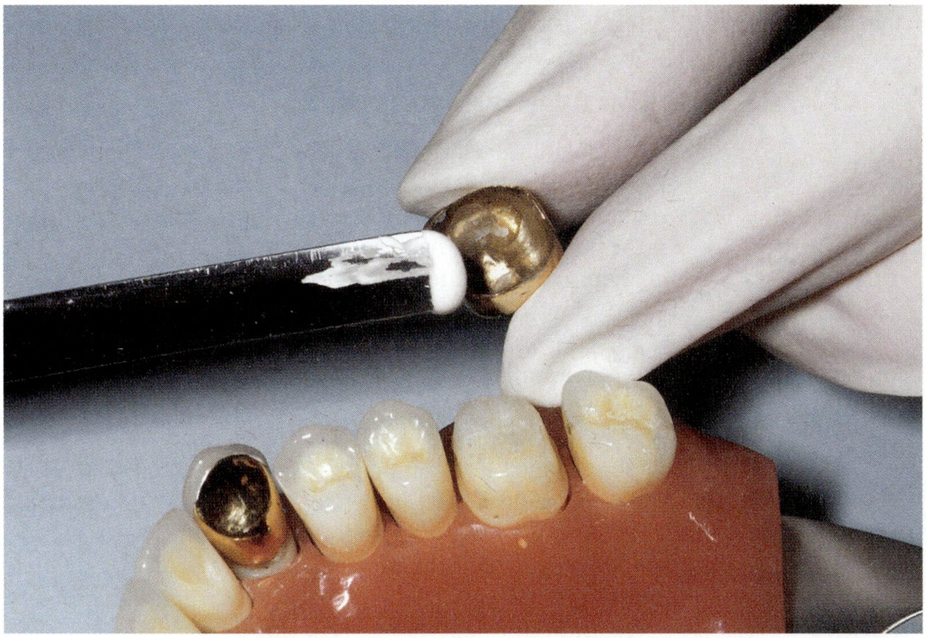

Fig. 45-1 Casting ready to be cemented.

an initial setting process, and the casting may not seat completely.

Regardless of the type of dental cement used, basic guidelines must be followed.

Guidelines for Mixing Dental Cements

- Before mixing, read and carefully follow the manufacturer's directions for the type of cement being mixed.
- Determine the use of the cement (restorative, liner, base, cement); then measure the powder and liquid according to the manufacturer's instructions.
- Place the powder toward one end of the glass slab or paper pad and the liquid toward the opposite end (the space between allows room for mixing).
- Divide the powder into increments. Each manufacturer uses a slightly different system for sectioning the powder. Some manufacturers divide the powder into equal parts, whereas others divide the powder into progressively smaller increments. When increment sizes vary, use the smaller increments first.
- Incorporate each powder increment into the liquid; then mix thoroughly. The mixing time per increment also varies.

Humidity

If the clinical area is warm or if it is a humid day, premature exposure of the cement to these environmental conditions can create a loss of water from the liquid or addition of moisture to the powder. Always dispense the powder first, *then* the liquid, to minimize the loss of water from evaporation.

Powder-to-Liquid Ratio

Incorporating too much or too little powder will alter the cement's consistency. Be sure to fluff the powder in the bottle before dispensing the powder in the measuring scoop. Always hold the bottle or vial upright to ensure consistent-sized drops when dispensing liquid (Fig. 45-2).

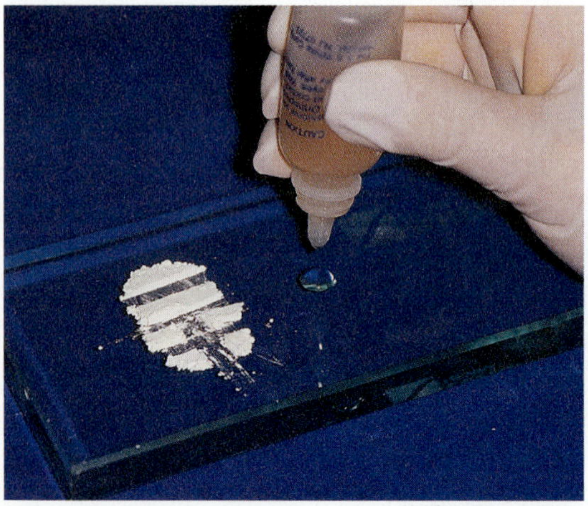

Fig. 45-2 Hold the bottle upright when dispensing the liquid of a cement.

Temperature

Some types of cements put off an **exothermic** reaction. In such cases, it may be beneficial to cool the glass slab in the refrigerator before mixing the cement. If the glass slab is kept in the refrigerator, make sure to thoroughly wipe the slab dry before dispensing the material.

Recall

1. What is another name used for permanent cement?
2. When is temporary cement used instead of permanent cement?
3. What variable affects the addition or loss of water in a dental cement?

TYPES OF CEMENTS

Some types of cements are supplied in more than one of the three types of classifications mentioned earlier. Selection of cements for a specific procedure requires knowledge of the chemical and physical properties of the particular cement type.

The types of cements described in this chapter are designed to be versatile in their properties, uses, and mixing techniques. Each dental cement has distinct characteristics, with the dentist deciding which type of cement will be used, depending on the type of indirect restoration.

Zinc Oxide–Eugenol Cement

Zinc oxide–eugenol (ZOE) cement is one of the most versatile cements available. As you learned in Chapter 44 regarding ZOE as a base, the eugenol in ZOE does not irritate the pulp. Eugenol has a soothing effect on pulp, and ZOE is often used on patients when postoperative sensitivity may be a concern (see Procedure 45-1 and Procedure 45-2).

ZOE type I lacks strength and long-term durability. For this reason, type I is used for temporary cementation or provisional coverage.

ZOE type I is supplied as a two-paste system (Tempbond) for temporary cement (Fig. 45-3). These pastes are dispensed in equal lengths on a paper pad and mixed according to the manufacturer's directions.

ZOE type II has reinforcing agents added. For this reason, type II is used for permanent cementation of cast restorations or appliances (Fig. 45-4).

Chemical Makeup of Zinc Oxide–Eugenol Cement

Liquid: eugenol, water, acetic acid, zinc acetate, and calcium chloride
Powder: zinc oxide, magnesium oxide, and silica

ZOE has a pH level close to 7.0, which makes it less acidic than most other cements. ZOE is one of the least irritating of all dental cements. The eugenol has a very strong odor, however, and may be offensive to some patients. Take care when using a eugenol product because of its irritating qualities to the oral mucosa. Try not to let the liquid come into direct contact with tissue.

Application

Because the eugenol is an oil-based liquid, ZOE is mixed on an oil-resistant paper pad that will not absorb any of the liquid. When a slower set is required, a glass slab can be used. The thickness of the mix is determined by the powder-to-liquid ratio, as recommended by the manufacturer. For use as a luting agent, a thinner mix is necessary. The normal mixing time ranges from 30 to 60 seconds. The normal setting time in the mouth ranges from 3 to 5 minutes.

Examples of Commercial ZOE Cement

ZOE 2200	Tempbond
Zogenol	Fynal

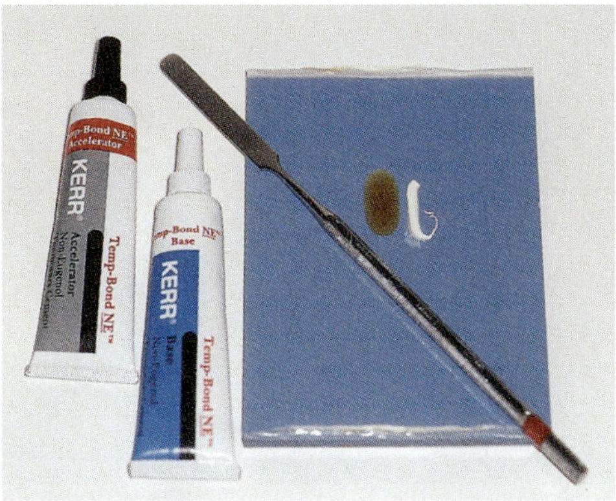

Fig. 45-3 ZOE type I cement for temporary cementation.

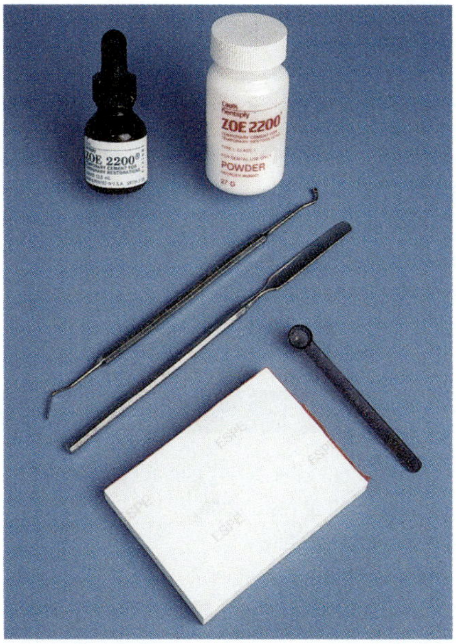

Fig. 45-4 ZOE type II cement for permanent cementation.

Procedure 45-1 Mixing Zinc Oxide–Eugenol (ZOE) for Permanent Cementation

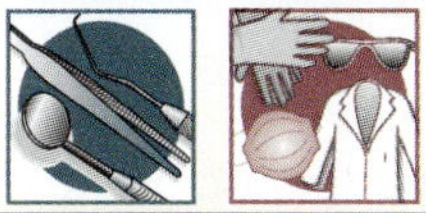

Equipment and Supplies

- Treated paper pad
- Spatula (flexible stainless steel)
- Zinc oxide powder and dispenser
- Eugenol liquid and dropper
- 2- × 2-inch gauze pads

PROCEDURAL STEPS

1. Measure the powder and place it onto the mixing pad. Replace the cap on the powder immediately.
2. Dispense the liquid near the powder on the mixing pad. Replace the cap on the liquid container immediately.

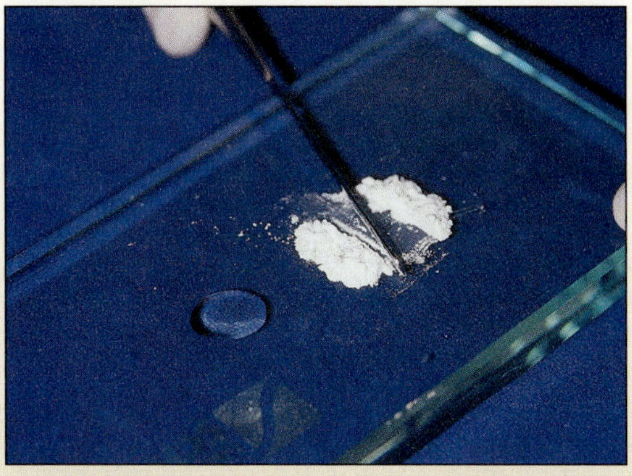

(From Hatrick CD, Eakle WS, Bird WF: *Dental materials: clinical applications for dental assistants and dental hygienists,* St Louis, 2003, Saunders).

continued

Procedure 45-1 Mixing Zinc Oxide–Eugenol (ZOE) for Permanent Cementation–cont'd

PROCEDURAL STEPS, cont'd

3. Incorporate the powder and liquid all at once; then mix with the spatula for 30 seconds.
4. Initially, the mix is putty-like, but with additional mixing for 30 seconds, it will become more fluid for loading into a casting.
5. Clean and disinfect the equipment immediately.

Procedure 45-2 Mixing ZOE for Temporary Cementation

Equipment and Supplies

- Treated paper pad
- Spatula (flexible stainless steel)
- ZOE eugenol catalyst paste
- ZOE accelerator paste
- 2- × 2-inch gauze pads

PROCEDURAL STEPS

1. Measure the pastes onto the mixing pad at equal lengths, approximately ½ inch per unit of restoration.
2. Replace the caps immediately.
3. Incorporate the two pastes together.
4. Mix while wiping the material over an area of the mixing pad.
5. The material should be smooth and creamy and completed within 20 to 30 seconds.

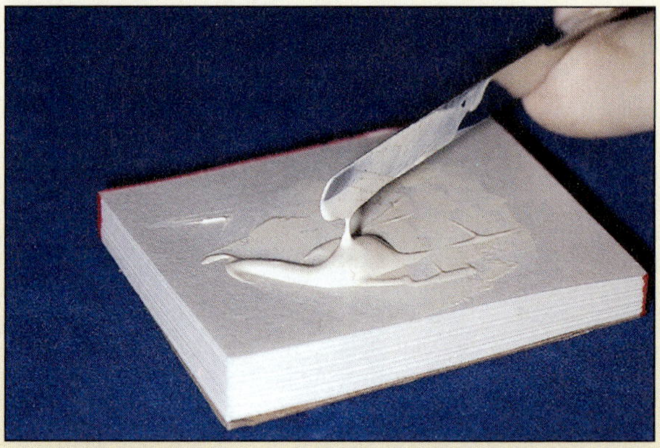

6. Immediately fill the temporary coverage with the cement.
   Purpose: Because the material has weaker properties than does permanent cement, fill the provisional rather than line it.
7. Clean and disinfect the equipment immediately.

Recall

4. What type of ZOE is used for permanent cementation?
5. On what mixing surface is ZOE mixed?
6. How is Tempbond supplied?

Zinc Phosphate Cement

Zinc phosphate, one of the oldest dental cements in use, is classified as two types (Fig. 45-5).

Type I (fine-grain) zinc phosphate cement is used for the permanent cementation of cast restorations such as crowns, inlays, onlays, and bridges. This material creates a very thin film layer, which is necessary for accurate cementation of castings.

Type II (medium-grain) zinc phosphate cement is recommended for use as an insulating base for deep cavity preparations (see Chapter 44).

When using zinc phosphate, remember that the phosphoric acid can be irritating to the pulp. Because of the irritating factors, a liner, sealer, or desensitizer should be placed first to reduce the sensitivity to the phosphoric acid (see Procedure 45-3).

Chemical Makeup of Zinc Phosphate Cement

Liquid: 50 percent phosphoric acid in water, and buffered with aluminum phosphate, and zinc salts to control the pH.
Powder: 90 percent zinc oxide and 10 percent magnesium oxide.

Application

During the mixing and setting process, zinc phosphate cement gives off an exothermic reaction. To **dissipate** this heat before cementation on the prepared tooth, the cement must be **spatulated** over a wide area of a cool, dry,

Procedure 45-3 Mixing Zinc Phosphate for Permanent Cementation

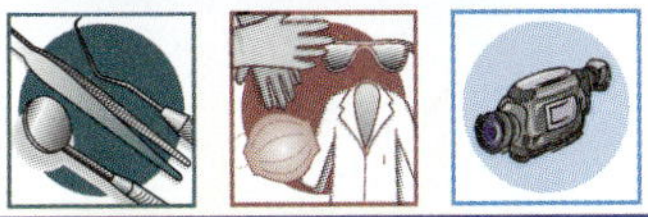

Equipment and Supplies

- Glass slab (cool)
- Spatula (flexible stainless steel)
- Zinc phosphate powder and dispenser
- Zinc phosphate liquid and dropper
- 2- × 2-inch gauze pads

PROCEDURAL STEPS

Preparing the Mix

1. Dispense the powder toward one end of the slab and the liquid at the opposite end.
2. Recap the containers.
   Purpose: These materials are damaged by prolonged exposure to air.
3. Divide the powder into small increments as directed by the manufacturer.
4. Incorporate each powder increment into the liquid.
   Note: When increment sizes vary, the smaller increments are used first. Mixing time per increment also varies; the time is approximately 15 to 20 seconds.

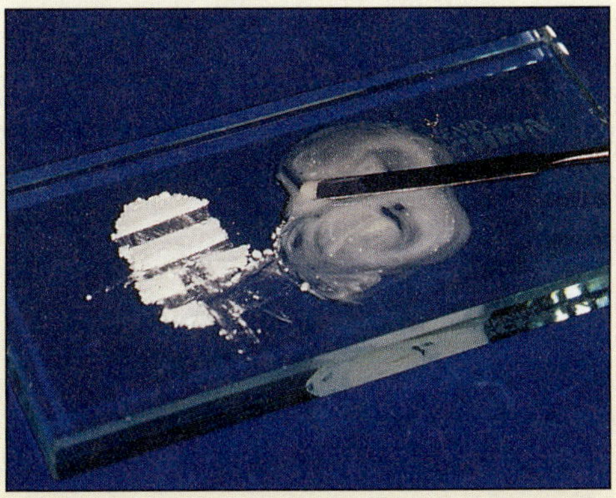

5. Spatulate the mix thoroughly, using broad strokes or a figure-8 movement over a large area of the slab.
   Purpose: This aids in dissipating the heat generated during mixing.

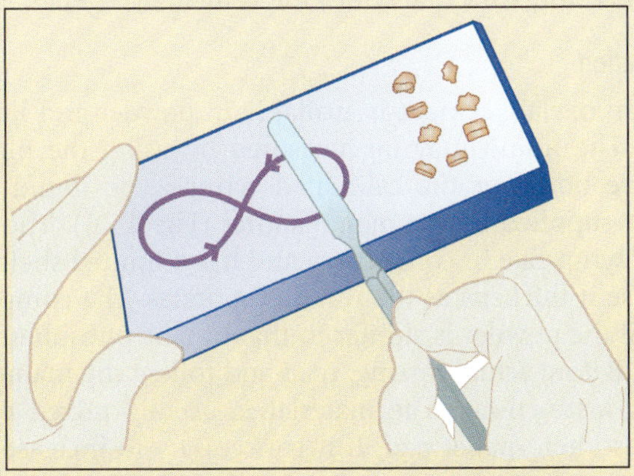

6. Test material for appropriate cementation consistency. The cement should string up and break about 1 inch from the slab. Total mixing time is approximately 1 to 2 minutes.

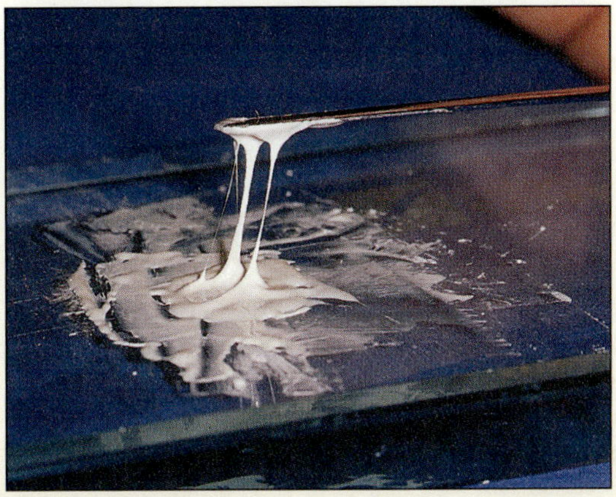

Placing Cement in the Casting

In addition to preparing and mixing the material, the assistant will have the important responsibility of placing the cement in the casting.

7. Hold the casting with the inner portion facing upward.
8. Retrieve the cement onto the spatula. Scrape the edge of the spatula along the margin to cause the cement to flow from the spatula into the casting.

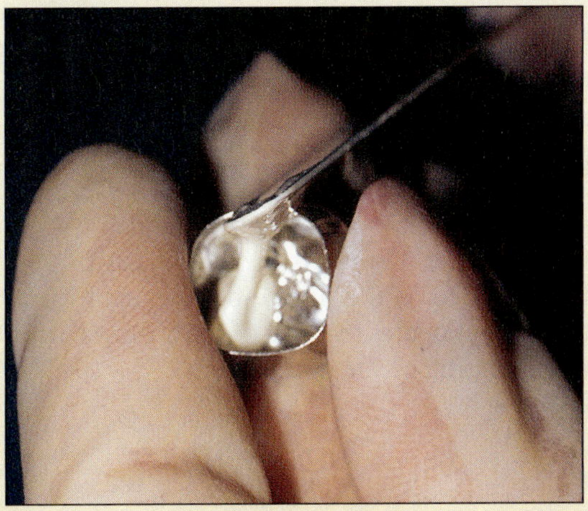

9. Place the tip of the spatula or a black spoon into the bulk of the cement; move the material so that it covers all internal walls with a thin lining of cement.
10. Turn the casting over in your palm and transfer to the dentist.
    Purpose: By having the outer portion of the casting facing up, the dentist can rotate it safely to obtain a better grasp for seating it.
11. Transfer a cotton roll so that the patient can bite down on it to help seat the crown and displace the excess cement.
12. Clean and disinfect the equipment immediately.

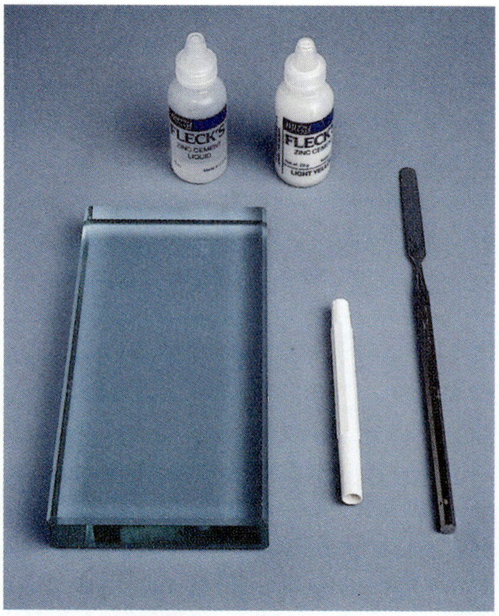

Fig. 45-5 Zinc phosphate type I cement for permanent cementation.

Examples of Commercial Zinc Phosphate Cement

Modern Tenacin	Lang-C B
Fleck's Extraordinary	Elite
Smith's Zinc Cement	

thick glass slab. The temperature of the glass slab is an important variable in the mixing time for zinc phosphate cement. The ideal slab temperature is 68° F. This temperature allows a longer working time and permits a maximum amount of powder to be incorporated into the liquid without making the mix too thick.

The powder is divided into increments varying in size, and each increment is spatulated slowly and thoroughly before the next increment is added. It is critical that the powder be added to the liquid in very small increments. This method dissipates the heat of the chemical action and **retards** the setting of the cement.

Recall

7. What is the main component in the liquid form of zinc phosphate cement?
8. How do you dissipate the heat from zinc phosphate in the mixing process?
9. What size of powder increment is first brought into the liquid of zinc phosphate when mixing?
10. Do you "fill" or "line" a crown with permanent cement?

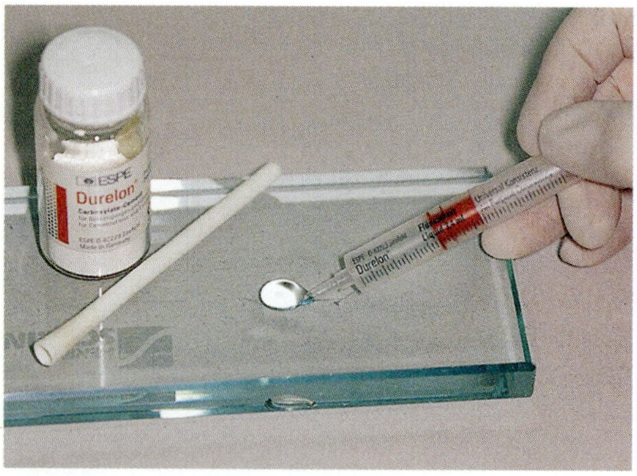

Fig. 45-6 Powder and calibrated syringe of polycarboxylate cement.

Examples of Commercial Polycarboxylate Cement

Tylok	Carboxylon
Durelon	Poly-F
Chemit	

Polycarboxylate Cement

Polycarboxylate cement, also known as *polyacrylic cement*, is used as permanent cement for cast restorations, stainless steel crowns, and orthodontic bands. As discussed in Chapter 44, polycarboxylate also maintains its versatility as a nonirritating base under both composite and amalgam restorations and also as an intermediate restoration (see Procedure 45-4).

Chemical Makeup of Polycarboxylate Cement

Liquid: polyacrylic acid, itaconic acid, maleic acid, tartaric acid, and water
Powder: zinc oxide

When properly mixed, polycarboxylate cement is similar to zinc phosphate cement in solubility and tensile strength. The pH increases rapidly as the material sets, and after 24 hours the cement is similar to that of zinc phosphate cement. Polycarboxylate cement is less irritating to the pulp than zinc phosphate cement, and the pulpal reaction is similar to that with ZOE cement.

Application

Polycarboxylate cement is available in powder and liquid form. The liquid may be measured by using the plastic squeeze bottle or the calibrated syringe-type liquid dispenser supplied by the manufacturer (Fig. 45-6). The liquid is syrup-like in consistency and has a limited shelf life because it thickens as the water evaporates. The composition of the powder is similar to that of zinc phosphate cement. Before actual mixing, read and follow the manufacturer's instructions. The material is usually mixed on a nonabsorbent paper pad. If it is necessary to increase the working time, however, a cool, dry glass slab is used.

Procedure 45-4 Mixing Polycarboxylate for Permanent Cementation

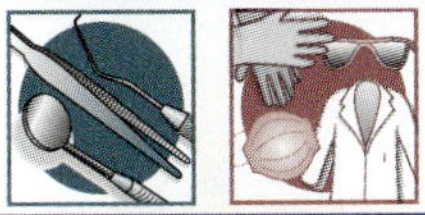

Equipment and Supplies

- Treated paper pad
- Spatula (flexible stainless steel)
- Polycarboxylate powder and dispenser
- Polycarboxylate liquid (in plastic squeeze bottle or calibrated syringe)
- 2- × 2-inch gauze pads

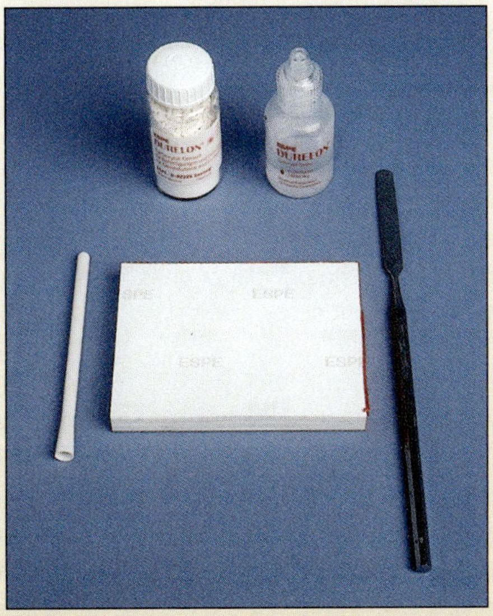

PROCEDURAL STEPS

1. Gently shake the powder to fluff the ingredients. Measure the powder onto the mixing pad and immediately recap the container.
2. Dispense the liquid; then recap the container.
3. Use the flat side of the spatula to incorporate all the powder quickly into the liquid at one time. The mix must be completed within 30 seconds.
4. A correct mix should be somewhat thick and have a shiny, glossy surface.

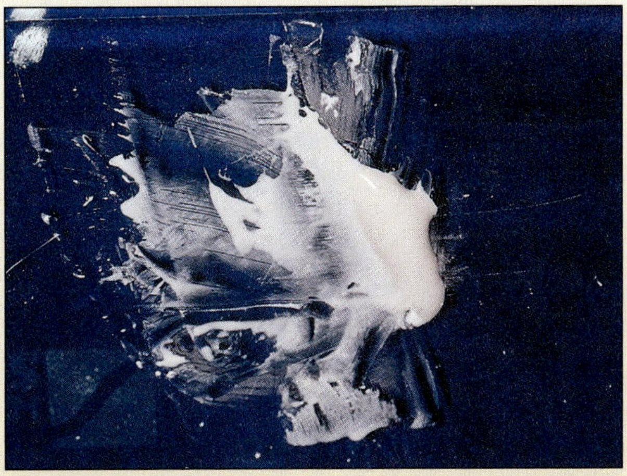

5. Clean and disinfect the equipment immediately.

Recall

11. In what two forms is the polycarboxylate cement supplied?
12. How should polycarboxylate cement appear after the mixing process?

Glass Ionomer Cement

Glass ionomer cement is one of the most versatile types of cement used in dentistry. This type of cement adheres to enamel, dentin, and metallic materials. Glass ionomer cements are supplied in special formulations according to their use (See Procedure 45-5).

Type I is for the cementation of metal restorations and direct-bonded orthodontic brackets.

Type II is designed for restoring areas of erosion near the gingiva, as discussed in Chapter 43.

Type III is used as liners and dentin bonding agents, as discussed in Chapter 44.

Glass ionomer cement has the following benefits, which explain its popularity:

- The powder is an acid-soluble calcium. The slow release of fluoride from this powder aids in inhibiting recurrent decay.
- The cement causes less trauma or shock to the pulp than many other types of cement.
- The cement has a low solubility in the mouth.
- The cement adheres to a slightly moist tooth surface.
- The cement has a very thin film thickness, which is excellent for ease of seating.
- Glass ionomer cement can be formulated for use as a dentin substitute or base material.

Chemical Makeup of Glass Ionomer Cement

Liquid: itaconic acid, tartaric acid, maleic acid, and water
Powder: zinc oxide, aluminum oxide, and calcium

Examples of Commercial Glass Ionomer

Cement	Biobond
Aspa	Aquacem
Ionomer	Rely-X
Fuji	Dyract
Ketac-Cem	Permacen
Vitrebond	

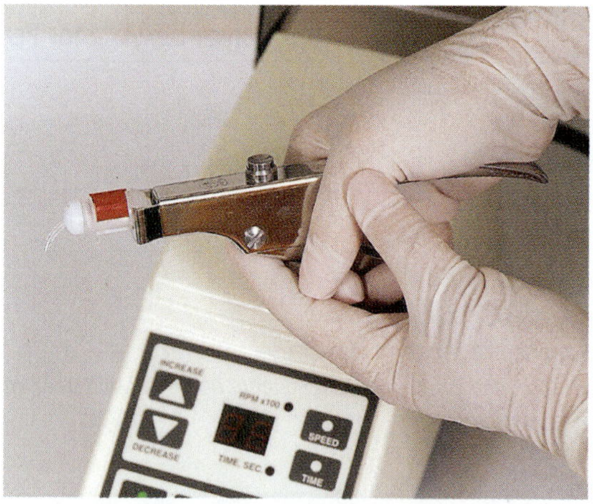

Fig. 45-7 Premeasured capsules of glass ionomer permanent cement.

Application

Glass ionomers are available in self-curing and light-cured formulas. The cements are supplied in bottles of powder and liquids, which can be mixed manually on a paper pad or a cool, dry, glass slab. The use of the glass slab increases the working time of the cement. Glass ionomer material is also supplied in premeasured capsules, which are triturated and expressed through a dispenser (Fig. 45-7). The capsules have the advantages of (1) being more convenient to use, (2) requiring less mixing time, and (3) producing consistent mixes because of the controlled powder-to-liquid ratio.

Recall

13. Can glass ionomer cements be used for restorations?

14. What ingredient in the powder of glass ionomer cement helps in inhibiting recurrent decay?

Procedure 45-5 Mixing Glass Ionomer for Permanent Cementation

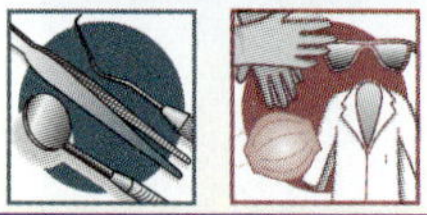

Equipment and Supplies

- Paper mixing pad
- Spatula (flexible stainless steel)
- Glass ionomer powder and dispenser
- Glass ionomer liquid and dropper
- 2- × 2-inch gauze pads

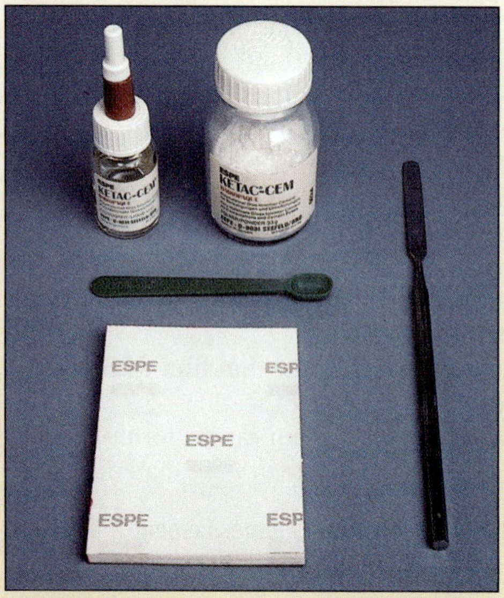

PROCEDURAL STEPS

1. Dispense the manufacturer's recommended proportion of the liquid on one half of the paper pad.
2. Dispense the manufacturer's recommended proportion of the powder on the other half of the pad; this is usually divided into two or three increments.
3. Incorporate the powder and liquid, following the recommended mixing time. The material should have a glossy appearance.
4. Clean and disinfect the equipment immediately.

Composite Resin Cement

A newer classification of cement material is *composite resin cements,* which have been designed especially for the following indications:

- Cementation of ceramic or resin inlays and onlays
- Ceramic veneers
- Orthodontic bands
- Direct bonding of orthodontic brackets
- All metal castings

Chemical Makeup of Composite Resin Cement

Composite resin cements have physical properties comparable to those of composite resins, including thin film thickness and virtual insolubility in the mouth. An important aspect in using composite resin cements is that the tooth must be free of all plaque and debris and either prepared by etching or treated with a bonding system before cementation.

Application

Composite resin cements are supplied (1) as a powder and liquid mix, (2) in a syringe-type applicator as a base and catalyst, and (3) in a versatile light-cured/dual-cured system (Fig. 45-8). Recommended portions of either application are dispensed onto a paper pad and mixed rapidly with a spatula (see Procedure 45-6).

Recall

15. Can resin cements be used under metal castings?

16. What is important to complete in the composite resin cementation procedure before applying the composite resin cement?

Commercial Resin Cements

Comspan	Opal Luting
Panavia	Compolute
Enforce	Nexus

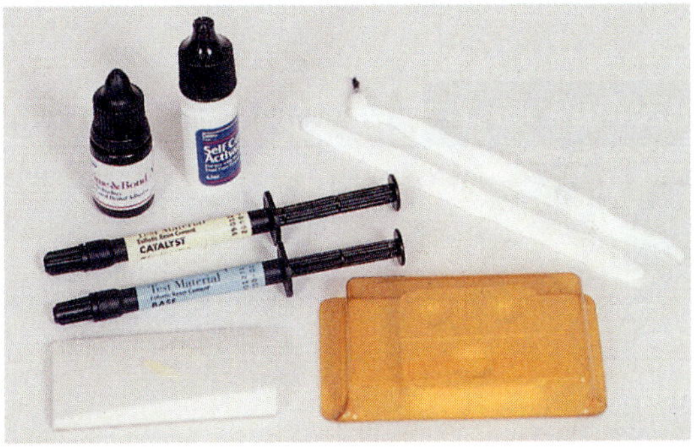

Fig. 45-8 Examples of composite resin cements supplied in variable systems.

Procedure 45-6 Mixing Composite Resin for Permanent Cementation

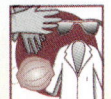

Equipment and Supplies

- Basic setup
- Etching system
- Cotton pellets
- Applicators
- Bonding system
- Applicators
- Resin cement (supplied in powder/liquid or syringe type)
- Mixing pad
- Spatula
- 2- × 2-inch gauze pads

PROCEDURAL STEPS

1. Apply etchant to enamel and dentin for 15 seconds; then rinse. Blot excess water with a moist cotton pellet, leaving tooth moist.
   Purpose: During this procedure, you do not want the tooth completely dry.
2. Apply a bond adhesive to enamel and dentin; then dry gently. Avoid excess adhesive on all prepared surfaces.
3. Light-cure each surface for 10 seconds.
4. The dentist will roughen the internal surface of the crown with a diamond or by air abrasion.
5. Apply primer to etched porcelain or roughened metal surfaces. Dry for 5 seconds.
6. Dispense a 1:1 ratio of powder-to-liquid onto a mixing pad; then mix for 10 seconds. Apply a thin layer of cement to the bonding surface of the restoration.
7. Once the crown is seated, margins may be light-cured for 40 seconds or allowed to self-cure for 10 minutes from the start of the mixing.
   Note: For porcelain and precured composite crowns, margins must be light-cured for 40 seconds.

CEMENT REMOVAL

Once the dentist has completed the cementation of an indirect restoration, the patient is asked to bite down for a few minutes on a cotton roll for the initial setting process. The material selected will determine the correct time to remove excess cement from around the margins, interproximal spaces, and adjacent areas covered with excess cement (Fig. 45-9). If excess cement is not removed from in and around the gingival margin and sulcus of a tooth, the cement can irritate the area and can cause additional problems, such as inflammation and discomfort.

Cement removal may be an *expanded function* for dental assistants in the state in which you are practicing. Therefore it is extremely important that you understand your role as an operator with knowledge of (1) instruments used in the process (explorer, mouth mirror, excavator), (2) proper use of a fulcrum, and (3) use of dental floss in and around the embrasure areas (see Procedure 45-7).

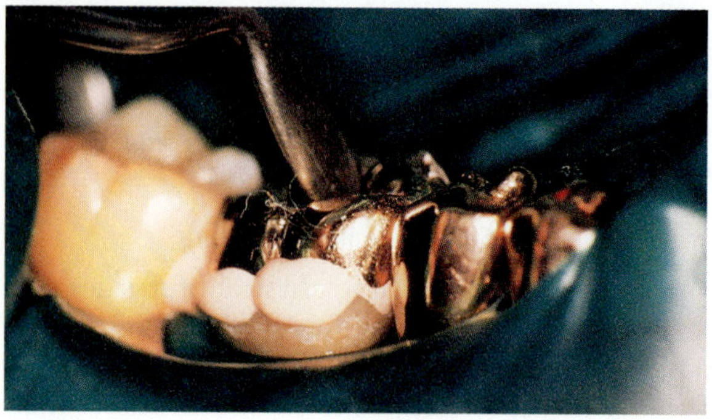

Fig. 45-9 Excess cement must be removed after setting process.

Procedure 45-7 Removing Cement from Permanent or Temporary Cementation (Expanded Function)

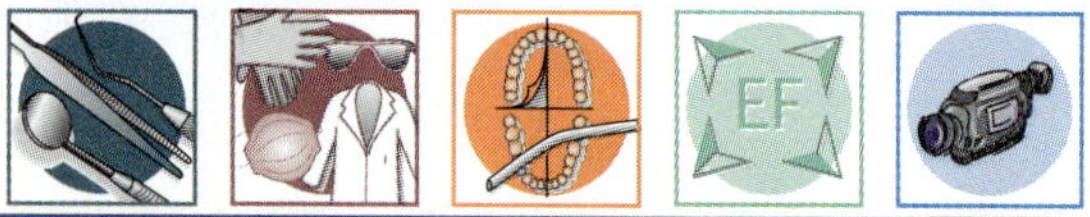

Equipment and Supplies

- Basic setup
- Spoon excavator
- Dental floss
- 2- × 2-inch gauze

PROCEDURAL STEPS

1. After cement has completed its initial setting, remove the cotton rolls from the area.
2. Using your explorer, examine the material to ensure the proper set.
3. With a firm fulcrum, take the edge of the explorer and carefully move the instrument in a horizontal direction, pulling the excess material away from the tooth.
   Purpose: Pulling the material down away from the casting will stretch or weaken the material directly under the margins.

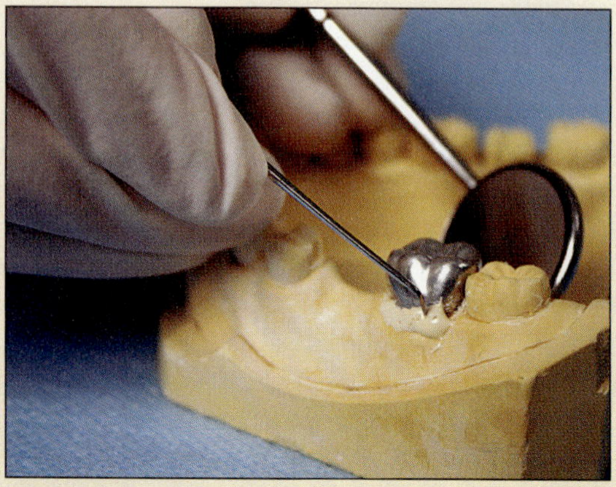

4. With the tip of the instrument at the gingival edge of the crown, use overlapping strokes to remove the bulk of the cement.
5. Follow along the margin to remove small pieces still adhering to the surface.
6. Tie a knot in the middle of the dental floss and pass it through the contact on both sides to remove excess cement from the interproximal area.
   Purpose: The knot adds extra mass in removing the cement from this space.

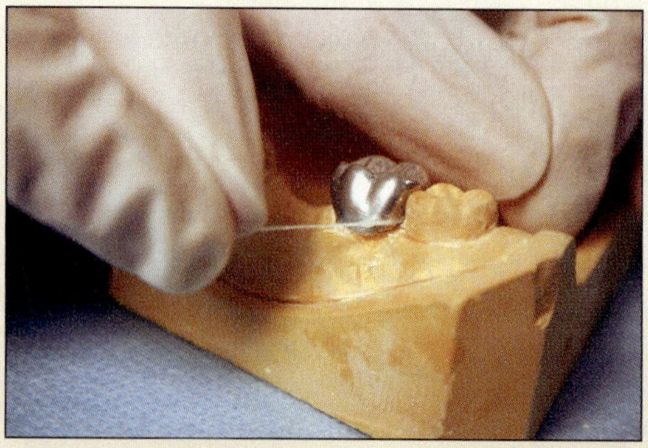

7. After removing the excess cement, thoroughly rinse and dry the area for evaluation of the procedure.

Patient Education

Cementation of an indirect restoration can be a stressful and demanding process for the dentist and dental assistant if the procedural steps do not go smoothly. Patients must be able to express how the indirect restoration feels to their "bite," as well as the overall feeling within their mouth. When preparing the cement for the cementation, remind your patient of the importance of keeping the mouth open and not getting the area wet. Explain how the material will react during the setting phase.

Your role in preparing the cement must be exact in the mixing and delivery steps so that the restoration is seated properly. Explain to the patient that as with many dental materials, cement requires 24 hours to complete its final setting. Advise the patient to take care when chewing sticky or hard foods on the side of the restoration during this period.

Legal and Ethical Implications

When an indirect restoration has been placed with permanent cement, the tooth that has been restored is considered to be a final restoration. This means that the dentist has done everything possible to treat this tooth. Is this correct?

No, the above statement is not correct. Many other treatments could have been provided to the patient, such as extraction, root canal therapy, or implants. Just because the tooth has undergone a final restoration procedure does not mean that the tooth will not need future work. The patient needs to understand that when a restoration, crown, or bridge is placed the tooth may still require further treatment, and that the dentist has not provided inadequate care to the patient.

Eye to the Future

The future of dental cements and adhesives will include biogenetics research into human tissue made from dentin and enamel cells. These materials will be designed to be so similar to actual tooth structure that when they are applied to an indirect restoration, the tooth and restoration will become one over time.

Critical Thinking

1. You are mixing permanent cement and notice halfway through the mixing process that the material is becoming very stiff. What factors may be associated with this setting of the mix?
2. You are a clinical assistant in an orthodontic office. What types of procedures in this specialty use permanent cements? What three types of cements listed in this chapter are typically used in an orthodontic practice?
3. What is the difference between preparing ZOE for permanent cementation and for temporary cementation?
4. You are preparing to mix dental cement for the permanent cementation of a bridge. You notice that after you have incorporated half the powder into the liquid, the cement is starting to thicken. Should you (a) stop mixing and use the material at this point, (b) keep incorporating all of the powder, or (c) start over? Why did you select your answer?
5. One cement presented in this chapter requires procedural steps before cementing an indirect restoration that are different from the steps for the other materials discussed. What material has this unique characteristic, and why are these initial steps taken for this cement?

46

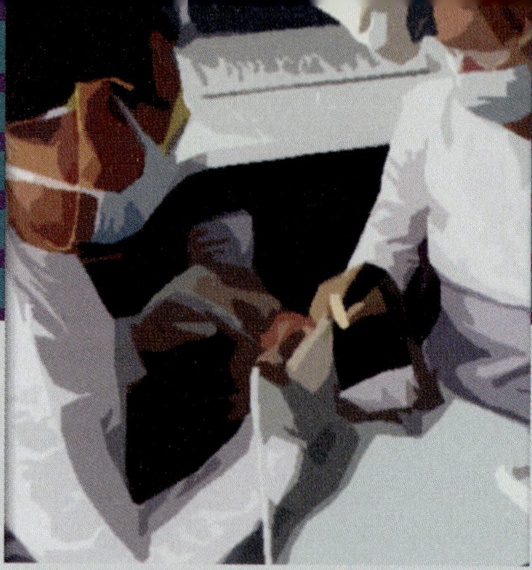

Impression Materials

Outline

Classification of Impressions
- Preliminary Impressions
- Final Impressions
- Bite Registrations

Impression Trays
- Characteristics
- Stock Trays
- Custom Trays
- Tray Adhesives

Hydrocolloid Materials
- Irreversible Hydrocolloid: Alginate

Procedure 46-1: Mixing Alginate Impression Material

Procedure 46-2: Taking a Mandibular Preliminary Impression (Expanded Function)

Procedure 46-3: Taking a Maxillary Preliminary Impression (Expanded Function)
- Reversible Hydrocolloid

Elastomeric Materials
- Characteristics
- Form of Materials
- Curing Stages and Types
- Mixing of Materials
- Types of Elastomeric Materials

Procedure 46-4: Mixing a Two-Paste Final Impression Material

Procedure 46-5: Preparing an Automix Final Impression Material

Occlusal (Bite) Registration
- Wax Bite Registration
- Polysiloxane Bite Registration Paste

Procedure 46-6: Taking a Wax Bite Registration
- Zinc Oxide–Eugenol Bite Registration Paste

Procedure 46-7: Mixing Polysiloxane Material for a Bite Registration

Procedure 46-8: Mixing Zinc Oxide–Eugenol Bite Registration Material

Patient Education

Legal and Ethical Implications

Eye to the Future

Critical Thinking

KEY TERMS

Agar (**a**-gar) Gelatin-type material derived from seaweed.

Alginate (**al**-jeh-nate) Irreversible hydrocolloid material used for taking preliminary impressions.

Base Foundation or the basic ingredient of a material.

Border molding Closer adaptation of impression edges to the mucobuccal fold.

Catalyst (**ka**-tul-ust) Substance that modifies or increases the rate of a chemical reaction.

Centric (**cen**-trik) Having an object centered, such as the maxillary teeth centered over mandibular teeth in correct relation.

Colloid (**kol**-loid, **kah**-loid) A suspension of particles in a dispersion medium such as water. Its two phases are sol and gel.

Elastomeric (i-*las*-tuh-**mer**-ik) Material having elastic properties from rubber.

Extrude (ik-**strude**) To push or force out.

Hydro- Prefix meaning "water."

Imbibition (*im*-bah-**bi**-shun) Absorption of water, causing an object to swell.

Occlusal registration (ah-**klu**-sul, a-**klu**-zul) Reproduction of a patient's bite using wax or elastomeric material.

Syneresis (seh-**ner**-eh-sus) Loss of water, causing something to shrink.

Tempering (**tem**-p[uh-]ring) Bringing a material to a desired consistency.

Viscous, Viscosity (vis-**kah**-suh-tee) Physical property of fluids for resistance to flow.

LEARNING OUTCOMES

On completion of this chapter, the student will be able to achieve the following objectives:

- Pronounce, define, and spell the Key Terms.
- List the three types of impressions taken in a dental office.
- Describe the types of impression trays and their characteristics of use.
- Discuss hydrocolloid impression materials and their uses, mixing techniques, and application.
- Discuss elastomeric impression materials and their uses, mixing techniques, and application.
- Describe the importance of an occlusal registration and its use in a procedure.

PERFORMANCE OUTCOMES

On completion of this chapter, the student will be able to achieve competency standards in the following skills:

- Mix alginate impression material at a competent level.
- Take a maxillary and mandibular preliminary impression at competency level.
- Competently mix a paste final impression material.
- Competently prepare an automix impression material.
- Take a wax bite.
- Prepare and assist in a closed bite registration procedure.

In various dental procedures, impression materials are used to obtain an impression of the teeth and the surrounding oral tissues. Impressions are a *negative* reproduction of those structures, and the stone or plaster model created from the impression is the *positive* reproduction of the structures. The type of impression material selected for a procedure depends on how the impression will be used.

As the clinical assistant, you will be responsible for knowing what type of impression tray to prepare, what material to set up, and the proper mixing sequence to use for the procedure. Your role in the procedure will be either as a dental assistant to help in the taking of the impression or as an expanded-functions dental assistant (EFDA) to participate in the actual taking of the impression.

CLASSIFICATION OF IMPRESSIONS

The three classifications of impressions used in dental procedures are *preliminary, final,* and *occlusal (bite) registration.* The type of dental material selected by the dentist to take these impressions depends on what will be constructed from the impression. This chapter describes the hydrocolloid and elastomeric impression materials, as well as the bite registration materials regularly used for dental procedures.

Preliminary Impressions

Preliminary impressions are taken either by the dentist or the EFDA and are used to create a reproduction of the teeth and surrounding tissues. A preliminary impression is used for:

- Diagnostic models
- Custom trays
- Provisional coverage
- Orthodontic appliances
- Pretreatment and posttreatment records.

Final Impressions

Final impressions are taken by the dentist and are used to produce the most accurate reproduction of the teeth and surrounding tissue. A final impression provides the dentist and dental laboratory technician the essential information needed for the creation of indirect restorations, partial or full dentures, and implants.

Bite Registrations

Bite registrations are taken by the dentist or dental assistant to produce a reproduction of the occlusal relationship of the maxillary and mandibular teeth when the mouth is occluded. This provides the dentist and laboratory technician with an accurate registration of the patient's centric relationship between the maxillary and mandibular arches.

Recall

1. Is an impression a negative or positive reproduction?
2. Of the three classifications of impressions, which can the EFDA legally take?
3. Which of the three classifications of impressions is used for occlusal relationship?

IMPRESSION TRAYS

Impression trays are used to hold the material for taking impressions. These trays must be sufficiently rigid to (1) carry the impression material into the oral cavity, (2) hold the material close to the teeth, (3) avoid breaking during removal, and (4) prevent warping the completed impression.

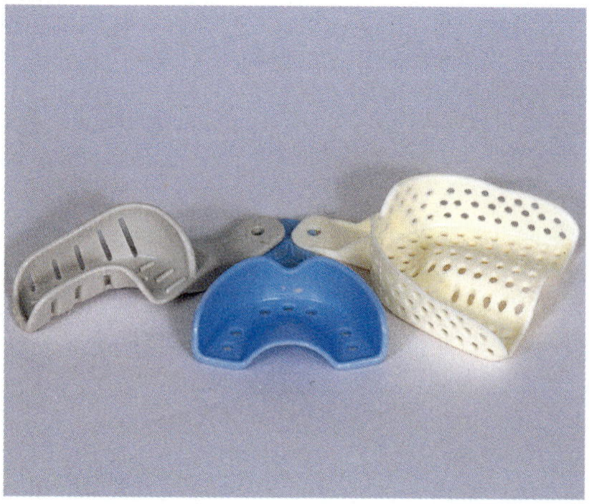

Fig. 46-1 Examples of quadrant, section, and full-arch impression trays.

Characteristics

Impression trays are supplied in one of the following ways (Fig. 46-1):

- *Quadrant trays,* which cover half of an arch
- *Section trays* used to cover the anterior portion of the arch
- *Full-arch trays,* which cover the entire arch

An impression tray is also characterized by whether the surface of the tray is perforated or smooth. When a *perforated* surface tray is used, the impression material oozes through the holes of the tray, creating a mechanical lock to hold the material in place. When a *smooth* surface tray is used, there is no mechanical lock, so the interior of the tray is painted or sprayed with an adhesive to hold the impression material securely in the tray.

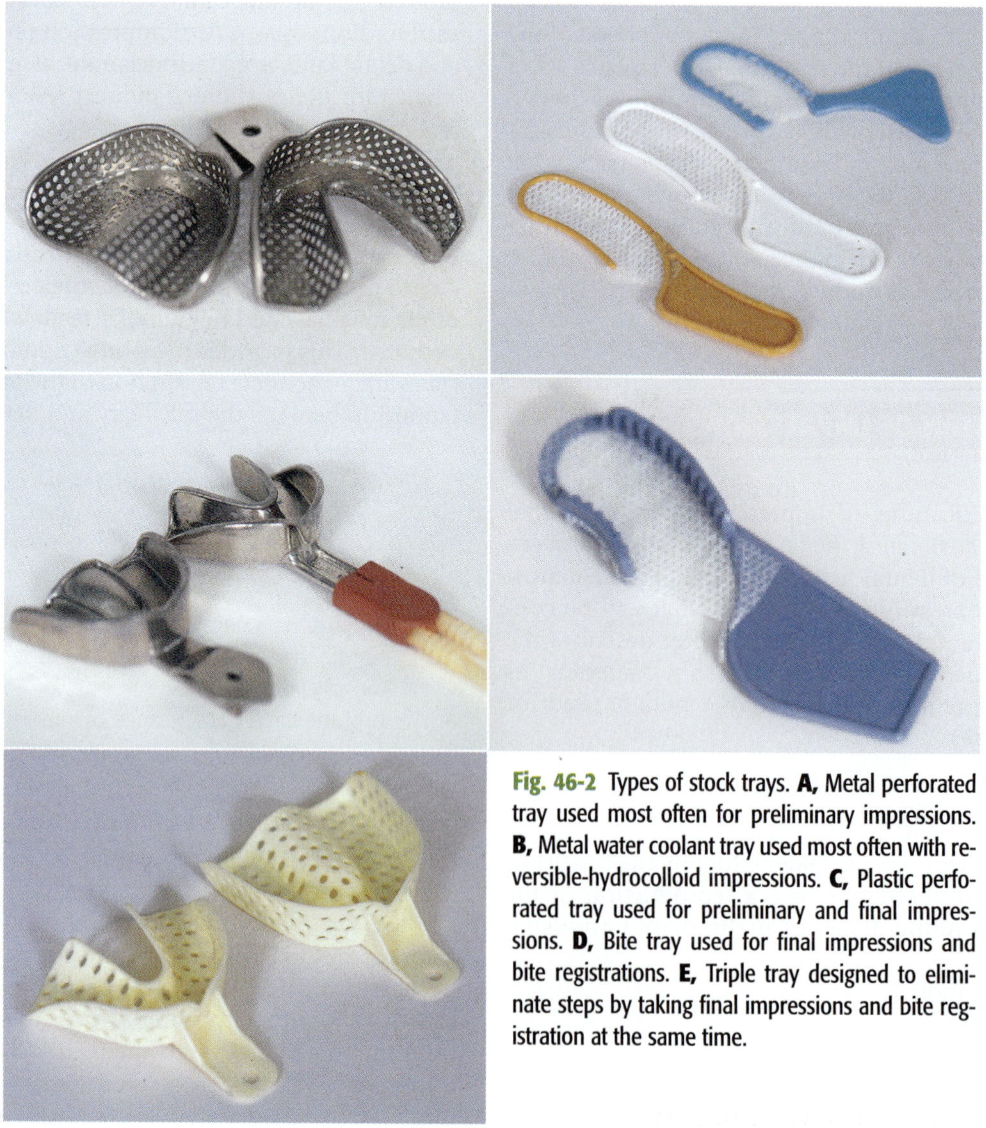

A

B

C

D

E

Fig. 46-2 Types of stock trays. **A,** Metal perforated tray used most often for preliminary impressions. **B,** Metal water coolant tray used most often with reversible-hydrocolloid impressions. **C,** Plastic perforated tray used for preliminary and final impressions. **D,** Bite tray used for final impressions and bite registrations. **E,** Triple tray designed to eliminate steps by taking final impressions and bite registration at the same time.

Impression trays are of two basic types: stock trays and custom trays.

Stock Trays

Stock trays are manufactured several ways and are available in a range of sizes and styles. Fig. 46-2 illustrates the different types of stock trays that you would most often use in a dental procedure.

Selection

Impression trays are selected for size by trying the tray in the patient's mouth before taking the impression. The correct tray accomplishes the following:

- Is comfortable for the patient
- Extends slightly beyond the facial surfaces of the teeth
- Extends approximately 2 to 3 mm beyond the third molar, retromolar, or tuberosity area of the arch
- Is sufficiently deep to allow 2 to 3 mm of material between the tray and the incisal or occlusal edges of the teeth

Adaptation

If necessary, the depth or length of the tray can be extended by adding utility wax to the border of the tray. This addition might be necessary if the tray does not completely cover the third molars (Fig. 46-3). For a patient with an unusually high palate, softened utility wax can be added to the palate area of the impression tray.

Custom Trays

A custom tray is constructed to fit the mouth of a specific patient. The dental assistant or laboratory technician constructs the custom tray in the lab. Box 46-1 describes the three types of custom trays most often used in dentistry.

The custom tray is created in the dental laboratory from a diagnostic model made from a preliminary impression of the arch *before* the dentist has prepared the teeth. Chapter 47 describes the construction of a custom tray using an acrylic resin, light-cured resin, or thermoplastic resin technique.

Tray Adhesives

Because there are no porous openings in a smooth tray to create a mechanical lock, an adhesive is applied to the tray before loading it with an impression material.

It is important that an adhesive be dry before the impression material is loaded into the tray. If the adhesive has not had time to dry, the impression will pull away from the tray, causing deformity in the impression. Paint the tray with the adhesive at least 15 minutes before use (Fig. 46-4).

Box 46-1 Types of Custom Trays*

Type	Use
Acrylic resin custom tray	Primarily for final impressions
Light-cured resin custom tray	Primarily for final impressions
Thermoplastic custom tray	Fabricating provisional coverage Bleaching tray

*All designed from a diagnostic model.

Adhesives for Specific Impression Materials

VPS adhesives (*blue* color)–used with polyvinyl siloxane (polysiloxane) and polyether impression materials

Rubber base adhesives (*brown* color)-used with rubber base impression materials

Silicone adhesives (*orange-pink* color)–used with silicone impression materials

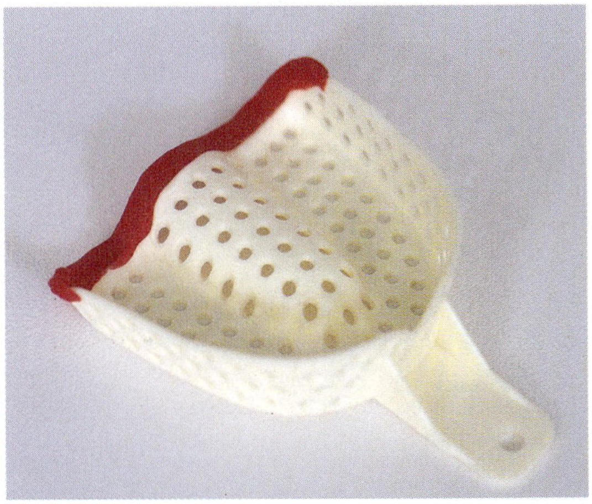

Fig. 46-3 Extending impression tray with utility wax.

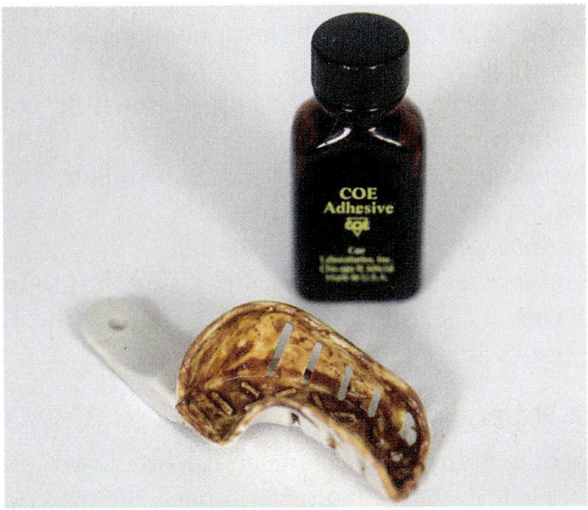

Fig. 46-4 Impression tray with adhesive applied.

Recall

4. Which type of impression tray covers half the arch?
5. Which type of tray allows impression material to lock on mechanically?
6. Which type of impression tray is most often used for taking final impressions?
7. What is used to extend the length of a tray?

HYDROCOLLOID MATERIALS

Hydrocolloid (***hydro***- meaning water and ***colloid*** meaning a gelatinous substance) is a material used to obtain preliminary and final impressions. Depending on the type of hydrocolloid, the physical change from *sol (solution)* to *gel (solid)* can be *irreversible* (changed by chemical factors) or *reversible* (changed by thermal factors).

Irreversible Hydrocolloid: Alginate

Hydrocolloid impression materials that cannot return to the sol state after they become a gel are irreversible *hydrocolloids.* The change in this physical state results from a chemical change in the material. Cake mix is an example of an irreversible change. When water is added to the powder in a cake mix, a chemical reaction occurs. It is impossible to remove the water and return the mixture to powder.

Alginate is the irreversible hydrocolloid most widely used for preliminary impressions.

Composition and Chemistry

The main components of alginate are:

- *Potassium alginate,* which is derived from seaweed, is used as a thickening agent. This ingredient is used in some ice creams for the same reason.
- *Calcium sulfate* reacts with the potassium alginate to form the gel.
- *Trisodium phosphate* is added to slow down the reaction time for mixing.
- *Diatomaceous earth* is a filler and adds bulk to the material.
- *Zinc oxide* adds bulk to the material.
- *Potassium titanium fluoride* is added so as not to interfere with the setting and surface strength of the product used when making the model.

Physical Phases

Hydrocolloid impression materials have two physical phases. First, in the *sol* (solution) phase, the material is in a liquid or semiliquid form. Second, in the *gel* (solid) phase, the material is semisolid, similar to a gelatin dessert. The gel strength of hydrocolloid is not as great as that of elastomeric impression materials. The hydrocolloids have difficulty withstanding tensile fracture *(tearing)* and elastic strain *(stretching)*.

Strength

It is important for alginate to be sufficiently strong to resist tearing when the impression is being removed from the patient's mouth. The strength of the material continues to increase even after it appears to be set. Therefore, leaving the impression in the mouth for the full length of time recommended by the manufacturer is important to achieve maximum strength.

Packaging and Storage

Alginate can be purchased in a variety of ways. Containers about the size of a coffee can are the most common form of packaging. Premeasured packages are more expensive than other types of packaging, but they save time by eliminating the need for measurement of the powder (Fig. 46-5). Alginate can deteriorate very quickly if exposed to elevated temperatures and moisture, resulting in the material failing to set or setting too rapidly. The shelf life of alginate is approximately 1 year.

Most alginate impression materials must be "poured up" within 1 hour of taking the impression, a requirement dictated by the environment. Because so much of the material is made from water, a slight change in the surroundings can distort the impression and cause *dimensional* change.

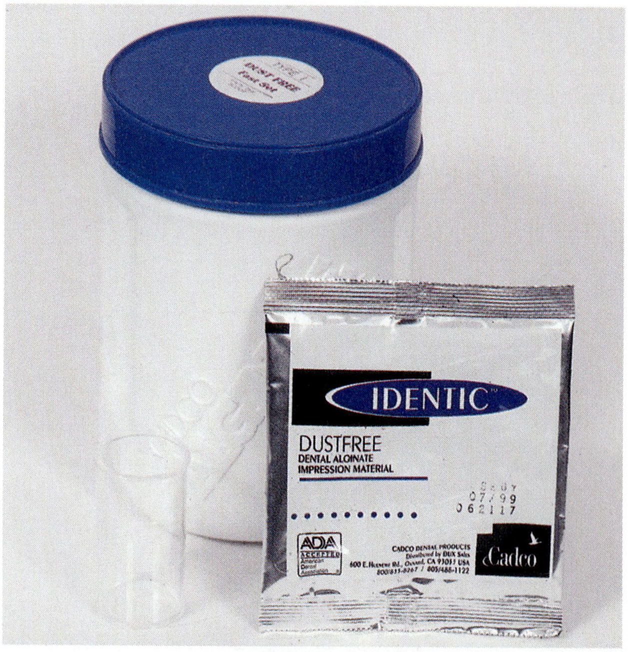

Fig. 46-5 Packaging of alginate.

If an alginate impression is stored in water or in a very wet paper towel, the alginate will absorb additional water and expand. This condition is called **imbibition.**

If an alginate impression remains in the open air, moisture will evaporate from the material, causing it to shrink and distort. This condition is called **syneresis.**

Storage of the disinfected impression in a plastic biohazard bag covered with a slightly moistened towel will provide an atmosphere close to 100 percent relative humidity, which causes the least amount of distortion.

Types of Setting

Alginate is available in two settings, *normal set* and *fast set.* The types of alginate refer to the working time and setting time. Normal-set alginate has a working time of 2 minutes and a setting time of up to $4\frac{1}{2}$ minutes after mixing. Fast-set alginate has a working time of $1\frac{1}{4}$ minutes and a setting time of 1 to 2 minutes.

Working time is the time allowed for mixing the alginate, loading the tray, and positioning the tray in the patient's mouth.

Setting time is the time required for the chemical action to be completed, after which the impression is ready to be removed from the patient's mouth.

There is no difference in the completed impression between the two setting types of alginates. The decision as to which type to use is based on time-related factors, which include the following:

- Difficulty in seating the impression tray (normal set allows more time for insertion and placement of the tray)
- Whether or not the operator is working alone (normal set allows the operator more time to mix the alginate, load the impression tray, and seat the tray in the mouth)
- Patients with a severe gag reflex (fast set allows the tray to be removed from the mouth much sooner)

Procedure 46-1 Mixing Alginate Impression Material

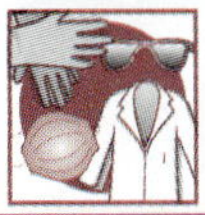

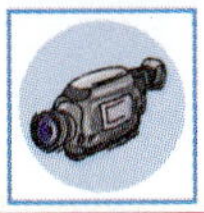

Equipment and Supplies

- Alginate
- Powder measure
- Water measure
- Medium-size rubber bowl
- Beavertail-shaped wide-blade spatula

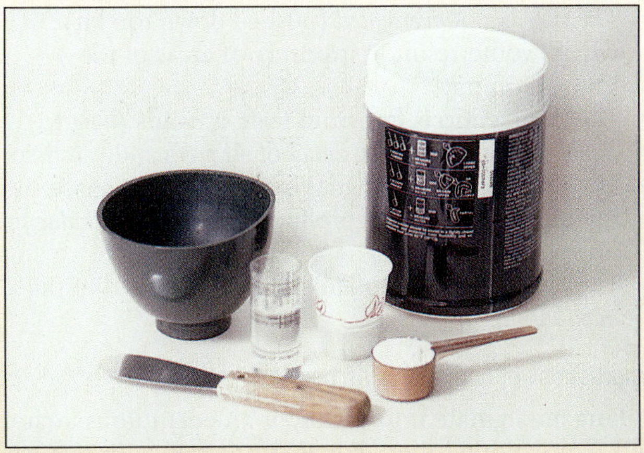

PROCEDURAL STEPS

1. Place the appropriate amount of water into the bowl.
2. Shake the can of alginate to "fluff" the contents. After fluffing, carefully lift off the lid to prevent the particles from flying into the air.
   Purpose: Alginate is fluffed because the material tends to settle and pack down in the can, making the measurement inaccurate. When using preweighed packages, fluffing is not necessary.
3. Sift the powder into the water and use the spatula to mix with a stirring action to wet the powder until it has all been moistened.
4. Firmly spread the alginate between the spatula and the side of the rubber bowl.

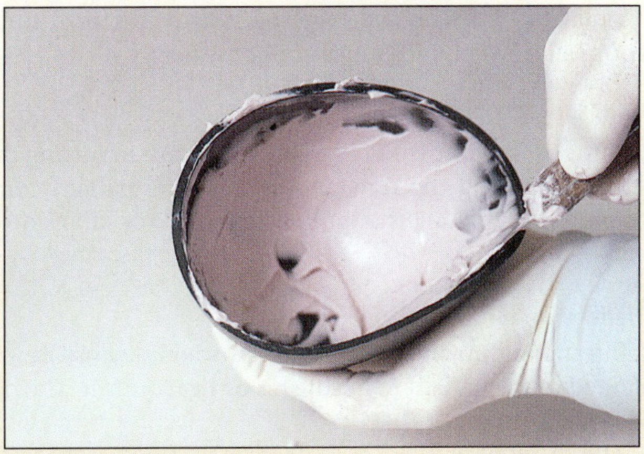

5. Mix with the spatula for the appropriate time. The mixture should appear smooth and creamy.
   Purpose: Inadequate mixing of alginate causes the mix to contain air bubbles and a grainy texture, which may produce an unsatisfactory impression.
6. Wipe the alginate mix into one mass on the inside edge of the bowl.

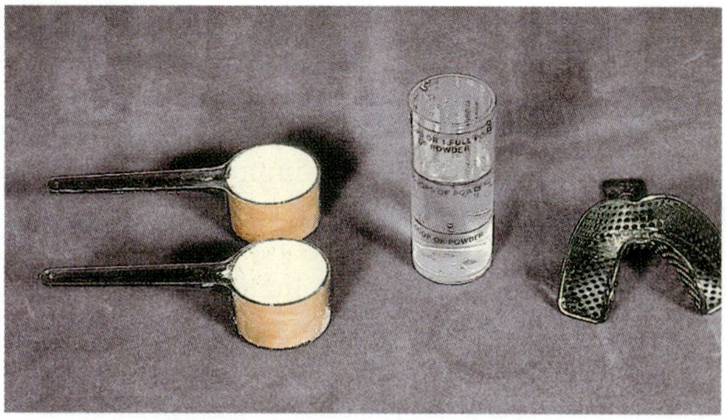

Fig. 46-6 A plastic scoop and plastic cylinder are supplied with alginate.

Altering setting time

Room-temperature water (21° C, or 70° F) should be used when mixing alginate. Cooler water will increase the setting time if additional time is needed for the procedure. Warmer water will shorten the setting time of the procedure.

Water-to-Powder Ratio

It is important to accurately measure the alginate powder and the water with which it is to be mixed. To help ensure accuracy, the manufacturer supplies a plastic scoop for dispensing the bulk powder and a plastic cylinder for measuring the water (Fig. 46-6). The water-to-powder ratio for mixing alginate is clearly marked on these measures. The ratio is one scoop of powder to 1 "measure" of water (see Procedure 46-1).

An adult *mandibular impression* generally requires two scoops of powder and 2 measures of water.

An adult *maxillary impression* generally requires three scoops of powder and 3 measures of water.

Taking an Alginate Impression

It is important for the EFDA to be competent in mixing the alginate, loading the tray, and keeping the patient comfortable while taking the impression (see Procedures 46-2 and 46-3).

Explain procedure to patient

Before taking an impression, the procedure must be explained to the patient to ensure his or her comfort. The patient needs to know that:

- The material will feel cold, there is no unpleasant taste, and the material will set quickly.
- Breathing deeply through the nose will help the patient relax and be more comfortable.
- The patient can use some type of hand signals to communicate any discomfort.

Evaluating alginate impression

An acceptable alginate impression must meet specific criteria (Fig. 46-7):

- The impression tray should be centered over the central and lateral incisors.

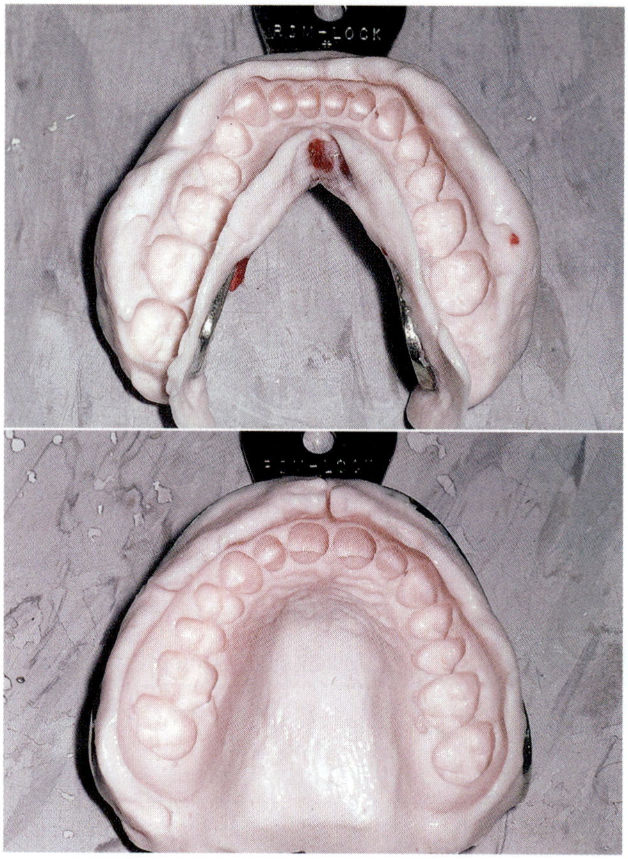

Fig. 46-7 How an impression must appear.

- There is a complete "peripheral roll," which includes all the *vestibular* areas.
- The tray is not *overseated* (pushed down too far), which would result in exposure of areas of the impression tray.
- The impression is free from tears or voids *(holes)*.
- There is sharp anatomic detail of all teeth and soft tissues.
- The *retromolar area*, lingual frenum, tongue space, and mylohyoid ridge are reproduced in the *mandibular* impression.
- The *hard palate* and tuberosities are recorded in the *maxillary* impression.

Impressions of Edentulous Arches

Taking an alginate impression of an edentulous arch differs from taking other alginate impressions in two ways: (1) the height of the teeth is missing, and (2) it is important to include more extensive tissue details. An edentulous tray is used to take this impression. This tray is not as deep as other trays used for alginate impressions. In addition, attaching sticky wax or similar material to the edges will modify the borders of the tray. This modification allows **border molding,** also known as *muscle trimming*, to achieve closer adaptation of the edges of the impression of the tissues in the mucobuccal fold.

Procedure 46-2 Taking a Mandibular Preliminary Impression (Expanded Function)

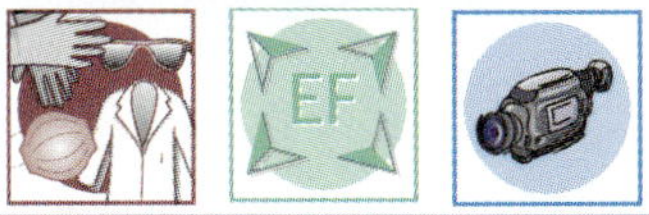

Equipment and Supplies

- Alginate powder
- Alginate measure scoop (provided by the manufacturer)
- Water measure (provided by the manufacturer)
- Room-temperature water
- Rubber bowl
- Wide-blade spatula
- Sterile impression trays
- Tray adhesive (used on nonperforated trays)
- Utility wax (if tray needs to be extended)
- Saliva ejector
- Precaution (biohazard) bag

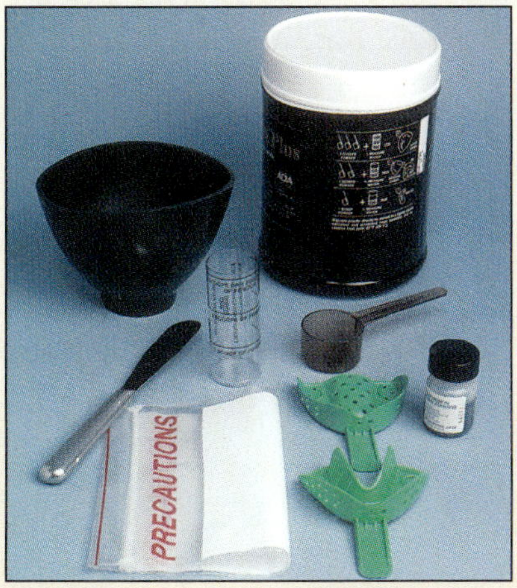

PREPARATION

1. Gather all necessary supplies.
2. Seat and prepare the patient.
3. Explain the procedure to the patient.
4. Select and prepare the mandibular impression tray.
5. Take two measures of room-temperature water with two scoops of alginate. Mix the material as specified in Procedure 46-1.

LOADING THE MANDIBULAR IMPRESSION TRAY

1. Gather half the alginate in the bowl onto the spatula, then wipe alginate into one side of the tray from the lingual side. Quickly press the material down to the base of the tray.
   Purpose: To remove any air bubbles trapped in the tray.

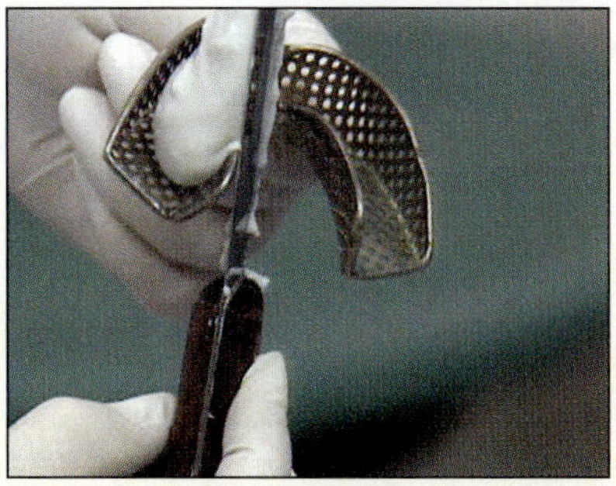

2. Gather the remaining half of the alginate in the bowl onto the spatula; then load the other side of the tray in the same way.
3. Smooth the surface of the alginate by wiping a moistened finger along the surface.

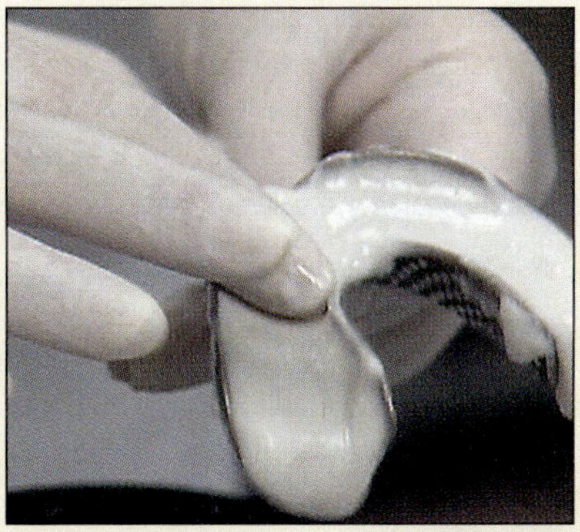

SEATING THE MANDIBULAR IMPRESSION TRAY

1. Place additional material over the occlusal surfaces of the mandibular teeth.
   Purpose: To place extra material in the fissures and interproximal surfaces to create less discrepancy in the anatomy of the impression.
2. Retract the patient's cheek with the index finger.
3. Turn the tray slightly sideways when placing it into the mouth.
4. Center the tray over the teeth.

continued

Procedure 46-2 Taking a Mandibular Preliminary Impression (Expanded Function)—cont'd

SEATING THE MANDIBULAR IMPRESSION TRAY, cont'd

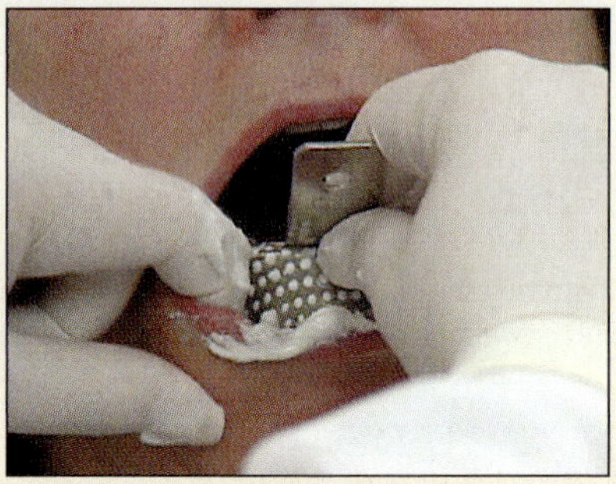

5. Press down the posterior border of the tray first.
   Purpose: To form a seal.
6. Push down the anterior portion of the tray and ask the patient to lift the tongue to the roof of the mouth and then relax it.
   Purpose: To allow the alginate to form an impression of the lingual aspect of the alveolar process.
7. Instruct the patient to breathe normally while the tray is in place.
8. Observe the alginate around the tray to determine when the material has set.
   Note: When set, the material should not register a dent when pressed with a finger.

REMOVING THE MANDIBULAR IMPRESSION

1. First, place your fingers on the top of the impression tray.
   Purpose: To protect the maxillary teeth from damage during removal of the mandibular tray.
2. Gently break the seal between the impression and the peripheral tissues by moving the inside of the patient's cheeks or lips with the finger.
3. Grasping the handle of the tray with your thumb and index finger, use a firm lifting motion to break the seal.
4. Snap up the tray and impression from the dentition.
5. Have the patient rinse with water to remove any excess alginate material.
6. Evaluate the impression for accuracy.
7. Rinse, disinfect, wrap in a slightly moistened towel, and place the impression in the appropriate precaution bag before pouring up.

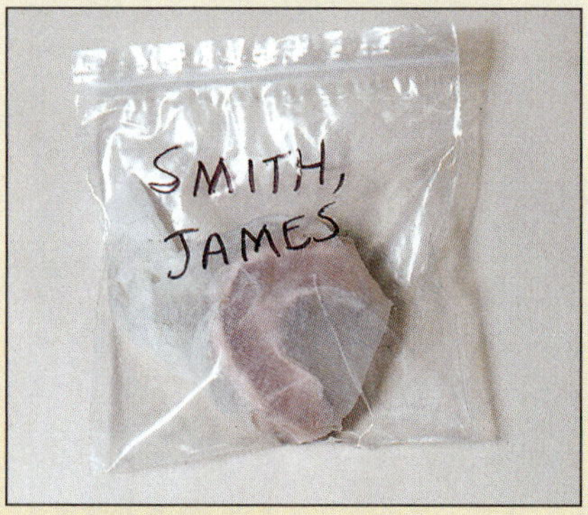

Procedure 46-3 Taking a Maxillary Preliminary Impression (Expanded Function)

Equipment and Supplies

- Maxillary tray
- Other equipment and supplies are the same as for a mandibular impression (see Procedure 46-2). If the same bowl and spatula are being reused, make certain they are clean and dry before beginning the next mix. For a maxillary impression, 3 measures of water are mixed with 3 scoops of powder.

PREPARATION

1. The preparation of the material is the same as in Procedure 46-2.

Procedure 46-3 Taking a Maxillary Preliminary Impression (Expanded Function)—cont'd

LOADING THE MAXILLARY IMPRESSION TRAY

1. Load the maxillary tray in one large increment, using a wiping motion to fill the tray from the posterior end.
   Purpose: To help prevent the formation of air bubbles in the material.

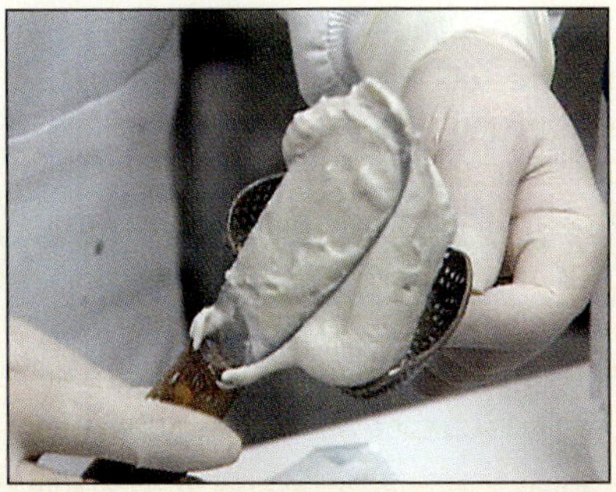

2. Place the bulk of the material toward the anterior palatal area of the tray.
   Purpose: To prevent the alginate from flowing beyond the tray and into the throat during tray placement.
3. Moisten fingertips with tap water and smooth the surface of the alginate.

SEATING THE MAXILLARY IMPRESSION TRAY

1. Use index finger to retract the patient's cheek.
2. Turn the tray slightly sideways to position the tray into the mouth.

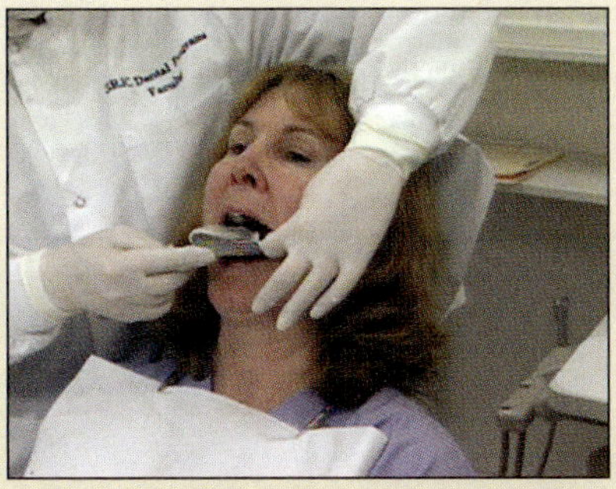

3. Center the tray over the patient's teeth.
4. Seat the posterior border (back) of the tray up against the posterior border of the hard palate to form a seal.
   Purpose: To prevent the excess material from going toward the back of the mouth.
5. Direct the anterior portion of the tray upward over the teeth.
6. Gently lift the patient's lips out of the way as the tray is seated.
   Purpose: This retraction allows the material to flow into the vestibular areas.
7. Check the posterior border of the tray to ensure that no material is flowing into the patient's throat. If necessary, wipe excess material away with a cotton-tipped applicator.
   Purpose: This technique helps to prevent triggering the gag reflex when the material touches the soft palate area.
8. Hold the tray firmly in place while the alginate sets.

REMOVING THE MAXILLARY IMPRESSION

1. To avoid injury to the impression and the patient's teeth, place a finger along the lateral borders of the tray to push down and break the palatal seal.
2. Use a straight, downward snapping motion to remove the tray from the teeth.
3. Instruct the patient to rinse with water to remove any excess alginate impression material.

CARING FOR ALGINATE IMPRESSIONS

1. Gently rinse the impressions under cold tap water to remove any blood or saliva.
   Purpose: Bioburden will interfere with the setting of the gypsum products.
2. Spray the impression with an approved disinfectant.
3. If the impression must be stored before pouring, wrap it in a damp paper towel and store the impression in a covered container or plastic bag labeled with the patient's name.

BEFORE DISMISSING THE PATIENT

1. Examine the patient's mouth for any remaining fragments of alginate and remove them using an explorer and dental floss.
2. Use a moist facial tissue to remove any alginate from the patient's face and lips.

Border molding is performed after the impression tray is in place. The dentist uses the fingers to gently massage the area of the face over these borders. This action shapes the wax-covered edges of the tray so that these edges more closely approximate the tissues.

Recall

8. What is the organic substance of hydrocolloid materials?
9. Why would you select a fast-set alginate over a normal-set alginate?
10. What is the water-to-powder ratio for taking a maxillary impression?
11. What does the prefix hydro- mean?

Reversible Hydrocolloid

Hydrocolloid impression materials that change physical states from a sol to a gel and then back to a sol are called *reversible hydrocolloids.* A change in temperature causes the reversible hydrocolloid material to transform from one physical state to another.

Ice cream is a good example of a reversible hydrocolloid. When ice cream is frozen, it is in the gel state. When left at room temperature, the ice cream melts and turns into a *sol* (solution) state. When returned to the freezer, the ice cream again becomes a *gel* (solid).

Reversible hydrocolloid material is approximately 85 percent water and 13 percent **agar.** As with alginate, agar is an organic substance derived from seaweed. Additional chemical modifiers are added to aid in the handling characteristics.

In order for the reversible hydrocolloid to change from one consistency to another, a specialized conditioning bath is used. The following three compartments maintain water at three different temperatures (Fig. 46-8):

1. The first bath is for *liquefying* the semisolid material. Immersing the tube of material in a special water bath called a *hydrocolloid conditioner* at 212° F (100° C) liquefies the material. After liquefying, the preset thermostat automatically cools the temperature to 150° F (65.5° C).
2. The second bath becomes a *storage* bath that cools the material, readying it for the impression. At this temperature the tubes are waiting for use.
3. A third temperature in a separate bath is kept at 110° F (44° C) for **tempering** the material after it has been placed in the tray.

Tray Material

Reversible hydrocolloid material is packaged in plastic tubes. Each tube has enough material to fill a full-arch, water-cooled tray (Fig. 46-9).

Application of Reversible Hydrocolloid Impression Material

The dentist and dental assistant must coordinate the following steps to ensure that the impression will be as accurate as possible:

1. A stock water-cooled tray is selected, making sure that the tray does not impinge on any of the teeth or soft tissues.
2. Plastic stops are placed in the tray, to help keep the tray from sticking to the teeth.
3. Tubing is connected to the tray and to the water outlet for drainage.
4. The material is liquefied and moved to the storage bath (second bath).
5. The light-bodied material is placed in the syringe; the heavy-bodied material is placed in the tray and moved to the tempering bath (third bath).
6. The light-bodied material is expressed around the prepared tooth, and the dentist seats the tray.

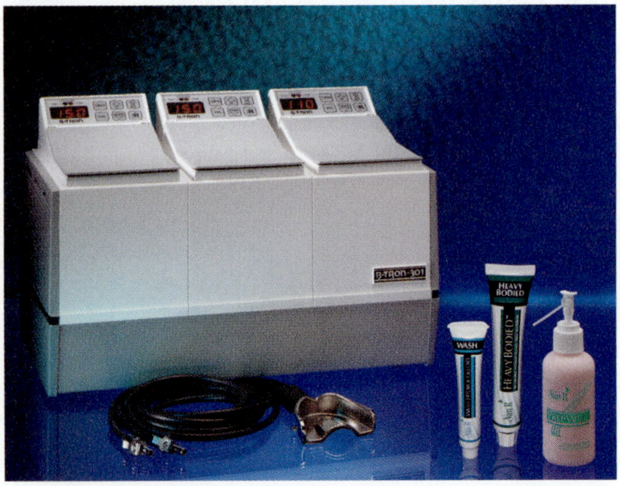

Fig. 46-8 Conditioning bath for reversible hydrocolloid.

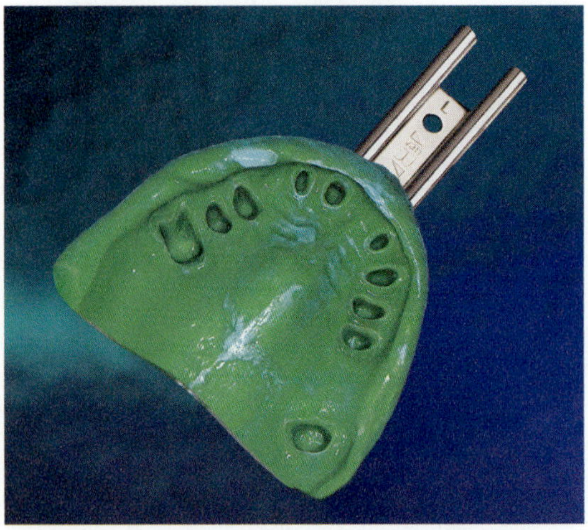

Fig. 46-9 Reversible hydrocolloid tray material.

The material needs enough viscosity to keep the material from flowing out of the tray when dispensed at 150° F (65.5° C). An impression tray is filled and then immersed in the 110° F (43.3° C) bath for a few minutes to further increase viscosity and reduce the temperature to a comfortable level for the patient.

Syringe Material

A conventional hydrocolloid is dispensed directly onto prepared and surrounding teeth. It is less **viscous** than tray material. The hydrocolloid is packaged in plastic or glass cartridges that fit a syringe, or it comes in preloaded syringes or preformed sticks that refill special hydrocolloid inlay syringes.

The syringe material is liquefied and placed in the same 150° F (65.5° C) storage bath as the tray material. Requiring easy flow, the syringe material is never tempered at 110° F (43.3° C). As the small stream flows through the dispensing needle, it cools to a comfortable temperature. If tempered, the syringe material would be too thick for accurate placement and would gel too quickly, preventing the proper displacement of contaminating fluids and bubbles.

Recall

12. What is another name for irreversible hydrocolloid?
13. Do you mix irreversible hydrocolloid on a paper pad or in a mixing bowl?
14. Before taking an impression with reversible hydrocolloid, where is the material kept?

ELASTOMERIC MATERIALS

Elastomeric impression materials are used when an extremely accurate impression is essential (Fig. 46-10). The term **elastomeric** means having elastic or rubberlike qualities. This rubbery quality makes it possible to remove the impression after it has set without creating any distortion or tearing.

Characteristics

Elastomeric impression materials are self-curing and supplied as a **base** and a **catalyst.** The base is packaged as a paste in a tube, in a cartridge, or as putty in a jar. The catalyst, also known as the *accelerator,* is packaged as a paste in a tube, in a cartridge, or as a liquid in a bottle with a dropper top.

These materials are supplied with the appropriate base and catalyst in the same package, and they should always be used together. If the base from one box is mixed with the catalyst from another, the material may not set properly or may lack important characteristics.

Form of Materials

Elastomeric impression materials are generally supplied in three forms: light bodied, regular, and heavy bodied.

Light-Bodied Material

Light-bodied material, also referred to as *syringe-type* or *wash-type* material, is used because of its ability to flow in and around the details of the prepared tooth. A special syringe, or *extruder,* is used to apply the light-bodied material immediately around the prepared teeth.

Regular and Heavy-Bodied Material

Regular and *heavy-bodied* materials, also referred to as *tray-type* materials, are much thicker than light-bodied impression materials and are used to fill the tray. Their stiffness helps to force the light-bodied material into close contact with the prepared teeth and surrounding tissues to ensure a more accurate impression and details of a preparation.

Curing Stages and Types

The curing reaction *(polymerization),* as the elastomeric material changes from a paste into a rubberlike material, begins as soon as the base and the catalyst are brought together. The change occurs in a three-stage process: initial set, final set, and final cure.

Initial Set

Initial set results in stiffening of the paste without the appearance of elastic properties. The material may only be *manipulated* during this first stage. The mix must be completed within the limited working time specified by the manufacturer.

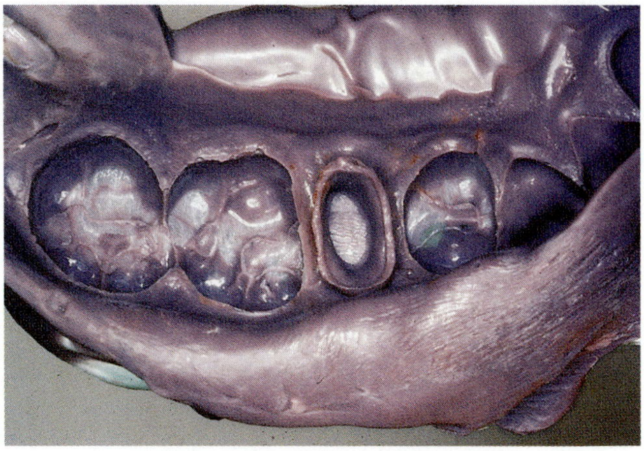

Fig. 46-10 Example of a final impression.

Final Set

Final set begins with the appearance of elasticity and proceeds through a gradual change to a solid, rubbery mass. The material must be in place in the mouth before the elastic properties of the final set begin to develop.

Final Cure

Final cure occurs within 1 to 24 hours. Only slight dimensional change is noted in the detail of the impression during this time.

Mixing of Materials

Many different mixing techniques are available for use with impression materials. The most common sequence, however, involves preparing the light-bodied material *first,* then the heavy-bodied material.

Paste System

When working with an elastomeric material in a paste system, *timing* is the most important reason for having everything prepared and ready to mix when the dentist signals the go-ahead. Make sure that you have enough material placed out for the type of tray you are using (see Procedure 46-4).

Automix System

Automix systems are designed by manufacturers to complete the mixing process for the procedure. The unique automix system device provides a homogeneous mix with the appropriate amount of material without waste. The extruder

Basic Impression Technique

1. The material selected depends on the dentist's preference and the type of impression required for the procedure.
2. The dentist prepares the tooth (or teeth) for the impression.
3. The light-bodied material is prepared, loaded into the syringe, and transferred to the dentist.
4. The dentist places the light-bodied material over and around the prepared teeth and onto the surrounding tissues.
5. The heavy-bodied material is prepared and loaded into the tray and transferred to the dentist.
6. When the impression material has reached final set, the impression is removed and inspected for accuracy.
7. The impression is disinfected, placed in a biohazard bag, labeled, and readied for the laboratory technician.

Procedure 46-4 Mixing a Two-Paste Final Impression Material

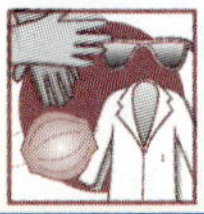

Equipment and Supplies

- Stock or custom tray with appropriate adhesive
- Large, stiff, tapered spatulas (2)
- Large paper pads (2)
- Light-bodied base and catalyst
- Heavy-bodied base and catalyst
- Impression syringe with sterile tip
- 2- $\times$ 2-inch gauze pads

PROCEDURAL STEPS

Preparing Light-Bodied Syringe Material

1. Dispense approximately $1\frac{1}{2}$ to 2 inches of equal lengths of the base and catalyst of the light-bodied material onto the top third of the pad, making sure that the materials are not too close to each other.
   Purpose: Some paste materials tend to start spreading on the pad, and it is important to prevent a premature reaction.
2. Wipe the tube openings clean with gauze; recap immediately.
   Purpose: Cleaning the top of the tube and the threads prevents the cap from becoming messy and sticking.
3. Place the tip of the spatula blade into the catalyst and base; then mix in a swirling direction for approximately 5 seconds
4. Gather the material onto the flat portion of the spatula. Place it on a clean area of the pad, preferably the center.
   Purpose: By beginning the mix on a clean area of the pad, you will obtain a more homogenous mix.
5. Spatulate smoothly, wiping back and forth and trying to use only one side of the spatula during the mixing process.
   Purpose: Material is lost by using both sides of the blade.

Procedure 46-4 Mixing a Two-Paste Final Impression Material—cont'd

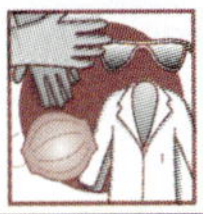

6. To obtain a more homogeneous mix, pick the material up by the spatula blade and wipe it onto the pad.
   Purpose: To pull the material from the bottom to the top of the mix.

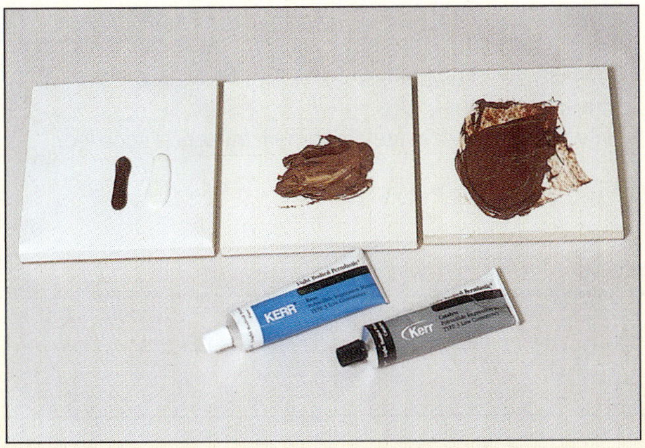

7. Gather the material together and take your syringe tube and begin "cookie cutting" the material into the syringe. Insert the plunger and express a small amount of the material to make sure it is in working order.

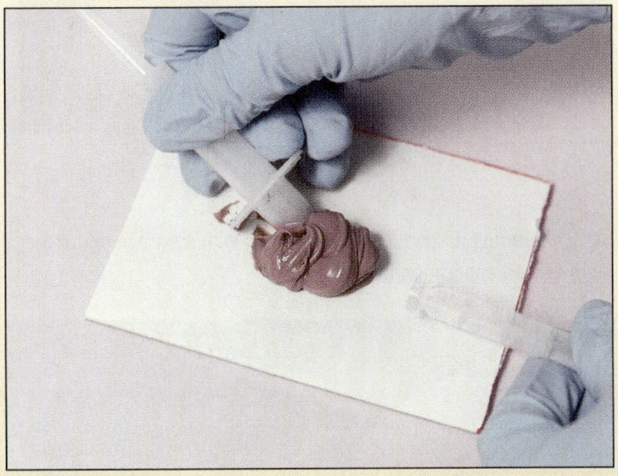

8. Transfer the syringe to the dentist, making sure the tip of the syringe is directed toward the tooth.

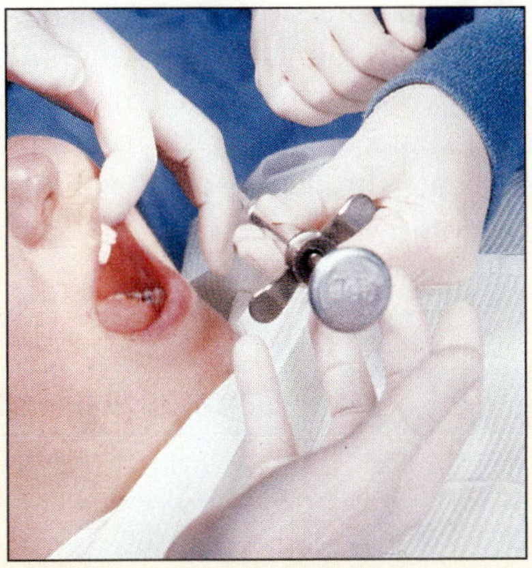

Preparing Heavy-Bodied Tray Material

1. Dispense approximately 3 to 4 inches of equal lengths of the base and catalyst of the heavy-bodied material on the top third of the pad for a quadrant tray.
   Note: The amount of material placed depends on whether you are using a quadrant tray or a full-arch tray.
2. Place the tip of the spatula blade into the catalyst and base; then mix in a swirling direction for approximately 5 seconds.
3. Gather the material onto the flat portion of the spatula and place it on a clean area of the pad, preferably the center.
   Purpose: Starting the mix on a clean area of the pad results in a more homogeneous mix.
4. Spatulate smoothly, wiping back and forth and trying to use only one side of the spatula during the mixing process.
   Purpose: Material is lost by using both sides of the blade.
5. To get a more homogeneous mix, pick the material up by the spatula blade and wipe it on the pad.
   Purpose: To pull the material from the bottom to the top of the mix.
6. Gather the bulk of the material with the spatula and load it into the tray. The best way to complete this without incorporating air is to use the flat side of the spatula and follow around the outside rim of the tray, "wiping" the material into the tray.
7. Using the tip of the spatula, spread the material evenly from one end of the tray to the other without picking up the material.
   Purpose: When you pull the material in an upward direction, you are incorporating air into the mixture.
8. Retrieve the syringe from the dentist and transfer the tray, making sure the dentist is able to grasp the handle of the tray properly.

is used to automatically mix and dispense elastomeric impression materials. The unit can be used with either light-bodied or heavy-bodied material and is operated with a trigger-like handle. The extruder is loaded with dual cartridges consisting of a tube of catalyst and a tube of base material (see Procedure 46-5).

Types of Elastomeric Materials

The four types of elastomeric impression materials most often used in dental practices are *polysulfide, polyether, silicone,* and *polysiloxane* (polyvinyl siloxane). Although similar in some aspects, each material has slightly different properties and characteristics. Of particular concern with these materials are the dimensional stability and permanent deformation.

Dimensional stability is the ability of the material to keep its shape after it has been removed from the mouth.

Deformation is the ability of the material to resist permanent change caused by stresses during removal from the mouth.

Permanent deformation means the material was changed and will not regain its previous shape.

Recall

15. Is an elastomeric material used for preliminary impressions or final impressions?

16. In which three ways are elastomeric materials supplied?

Procedure 46-5 Preparing an Automix Final Impression Material

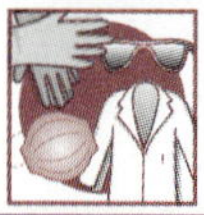

Equipment and Supplies

- Stock or custom tray with appropriate adhesive
- Extruder units (2)
- Extruder mixing tips (2)
- Light-bodied mixing tip
- Cartridge of light-bodied material
- Cartridge of heavy-bodied material
- 2- × 2-inch gauze pads

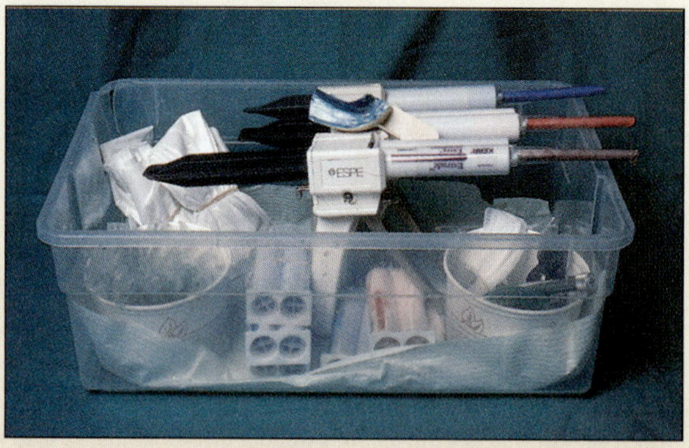

PROCEDURAL STEPS

1. Load the extruder with dual cartridges of the base and the catalyst of light-bodied material.
2. Remove the caps from the tube and **extrude** (force or push out) a small amount of unmixed material onto the gauze pad.
   Purpose: To ensure that no air bubbles are in the mix and to remove any hardened material that might remain.

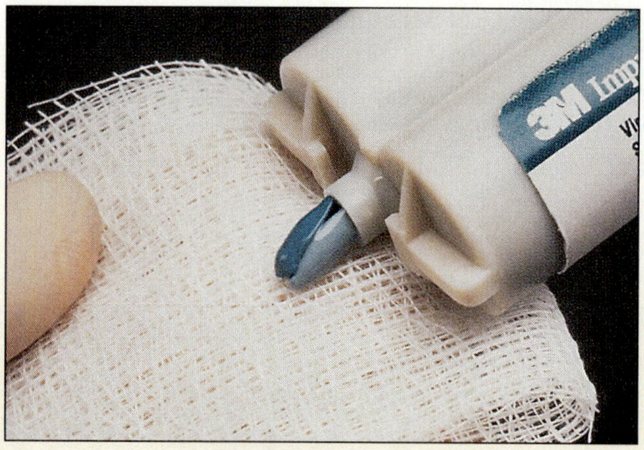

(Courtesy 3M ESPE, St Paul, Minn.)

3. Attach a mixing tip on the extruder, along with a syringe tip for the light-bodied application by the dentist.

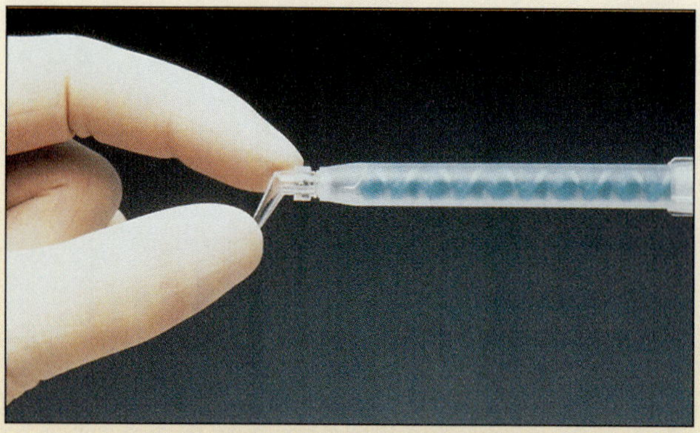

(Courtesy 3M ESPE, St Paul, Minn.)

Procedure 46-5 Preparing an Automix Final Impression Material—cont'd

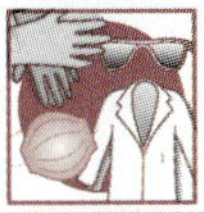

4. When the dentist signals readiness, begin squeezing the trigger until the material has reached the tip.
5. Transfer the extruder to the dentist, making sure that the tip is directed toward the area of the impression.
6. The dentist places the light-bodied material over and around the prepared teeth and onto the surrounding tissues.

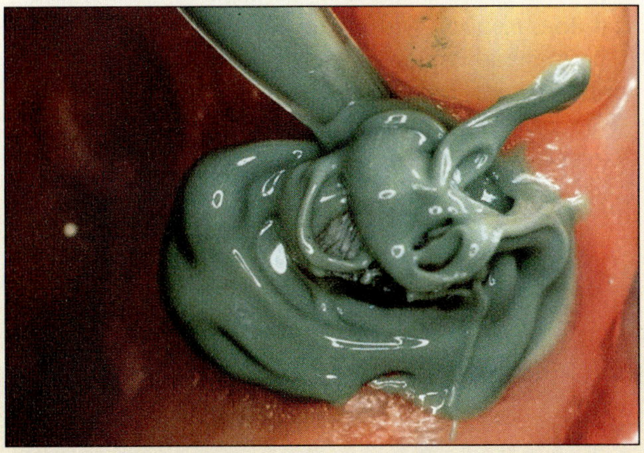

7. Place the heavy-bodied cartridges in the extruder, making sure to express a small amount (same as with the light-bodied material). Attach the mixing tip to the cartridge.
8. At the dentist's "ok" begin squeezing the trigger, mixing the heavy-bodied material.
9. Load the impression tray with heavy-bodied material, making sure not to trap air into the material.
   Note: Begin expressing the material at one end of the tray and follow through to the other end without taking the tip out of the material.
10. Transfer the tray, making sure the dentist is able to grasp the handle of the tray.
11. When the impression materials have reached final set, the impression is removed and inspected for accuracy by the dentist.

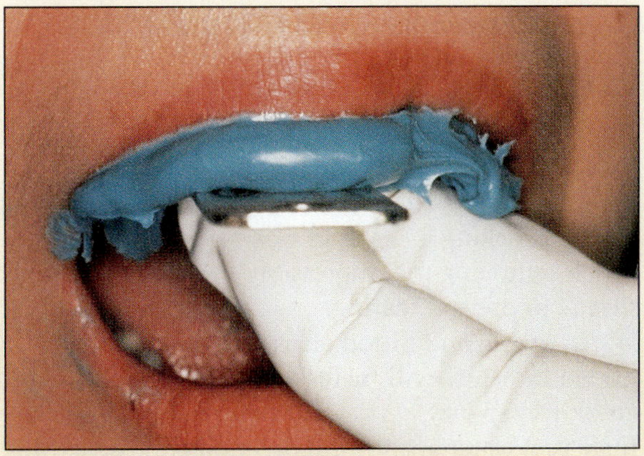

(Courtesy 3M ESPE, St Paul, Minn.)

12. The impression is disinfected, placed in a precaution bag, labeled with the patient's name, and taken to the laboratory.

Polysulfide

Polysulfide, also referred to as *rubber base,* is a final impression material that has been used in dentistry as a final impression material for many years (Fig. 46-11). Polysulfide impression materials are available in light-bodied, regular, and heavy-bodied forms.

The material is supplied as a two-paste system: the base and the catalyst. Disadvantages of rubber base material are its strong odor and the fact that it easily stains clothing.

Chemical makeup of polysulfide impression material

Base: mercaptan polysulfide
Cross-linking agent: sulfur and/or lead peroxide
Catalyst: copper hydroxide, zinc peroxide, or organic hydroperoxide
Filler: zinc sulfate, lithopone, or calcium sulfate dihydrate

Polysulfide material has a relatively long working and setting time. Its stiffness is low, which allows this material to maintain some flexibility on removal from the mouth and separation from the cast.

Guidelines for mixing polysulfide impression material

- Dispense pastes at the top of the mixing pad.
- Mix pastes with the tip of the spatula to incorporate the material first.
- Transfer material to a fresh surface of the pad.
- Refer to the excess mixed material on the pad to monitor setting time.
- Water, saliva, and blood affect polysulfide material.
- Impressions should be removed quickly after setting; do not rock tray.
- Adhesive must be thin and dry before adding impression material.
- Wait 20 to 30 minutes before pouring the impression for the stress relaxation to occur in the material.
- Be careful of glove powder contamination of impression.

Polyether

Polyether impression material provides better mechanical properties than polysulfide and less dimensional change than silicone (Fig. 46-12). Because the set material is quite stiff, a third component called a thinner (or body modifier) is included. The thinner is added to the mix to reduce the thickness of the mix and the finished impression.

Chemical makeup of polyether impression material

Base: polyether
Cross-linking agent: sulfate
Catalyst: glycol-based plasticizers
Filler: silica

Polyether material is supplied as a two-paste system (the base and the catalyst) and as cartridges. The tubes are *not* the same size; however, dispensing equal lengths delivers the correct amount of each material.

Guidelines for mixing polyether impression material

- Excellent impression accuracy and dimensional stability are necessary.
- Material is very stiff, which makes it difficult to remove without rocking.
- When removing the impression, break seal and rock *slightly* to prevent tearing.
- Water, saliva, and blood affect polyether material.
- Added moisture will increase the impression's marginal discrepancy.
- Increased water absorption occurs if you use a thinning agent.
- Impressions can be dispensed from an automated extruder and mixer.

Silicone

Condensation silicone is a material that is odor-free, nonstaining, and relatively easy to mix (Fig. 46-13). The deformation is much less than that of polysulfide, but the dimensional stability is superior.

Chemical makeup of silicone impression material

Base: polydimethyl siloxane
Cross-linking agent: alkyl orthosilicate or organo hydrogen siloxane
Catalyst: organo tin compounds
Filler: silica

Condensation silicone materials are supplied with the base as a paste in a tube and the catalyst as a liquid in a bottle or smaller tube of paste.

Guidelines for mixing silicone impression material

- The material has a limited shelf life.
- The tray requires a special tray adhesive.
- No syneresis or imbibition occurs, but silicone material does respond with shrinkage over time.
- The material is more flexible, so there is more chance for distortion during removal.
- Wait 20 to 30 minutes before pouring of models for stress relaxation to occur.

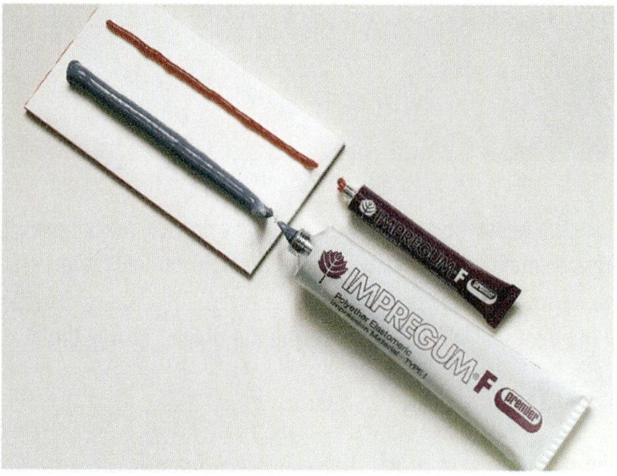

Fig. 46-12 **Polyether material.** (Courtesy Premier Dental Products, Morristown, Pa.)

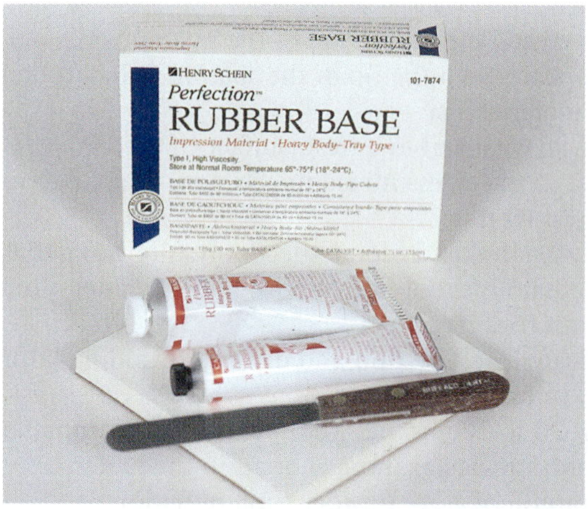

Fig. 46-11 Polysulfide material.

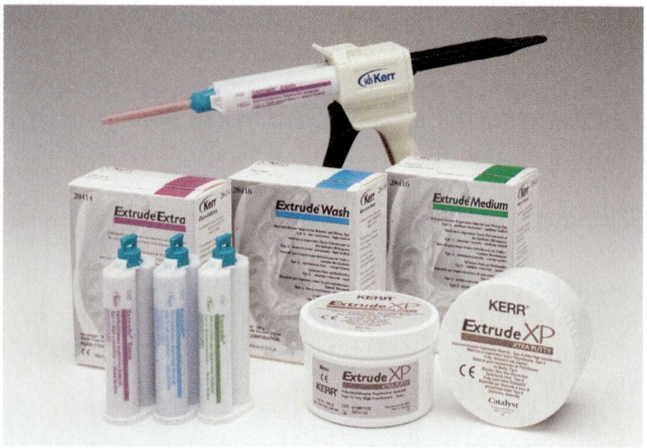

Fig. 46-13 Silicone material.

Polysiloxane

Polysiloxane *(polyvinyl siloxane)* material has high dimensional stability and low tear resistance, making it easy to handle when taking final impressions (Fig. 46-14). There is no taste or odor to the material, making it acceptable to patients.

Chemical makeup of polysiloxane impression material

Base: silica-based polymers
Catalyst: chloroplatinic acid
Filler: silica

Polysiloxane impression material is available in light-bodied, regular, and heavy-bodied forms. It is supplied in cartridges and in putty consistencies for single-impression or double-impression techniques.

Guidelines for mixing polysiloxane impression material

- For dimensional stability, polysiloxane is the best impression material.
- Pouring of the model can be delayed up to 7 to 10 days.
- Stiffness of the material makes removal of the tray difficult.
- Material is dispensed using an automixer and mixing tips.

Recall

17. What material does the dentist first apply to the teeth, the heavy-bodied or the light-bodied form?
18. What is another term for polysulfide?
19. How is light-bodied material placed around a prepared tooth?
20. What system completes the mixing of final impression material for you?

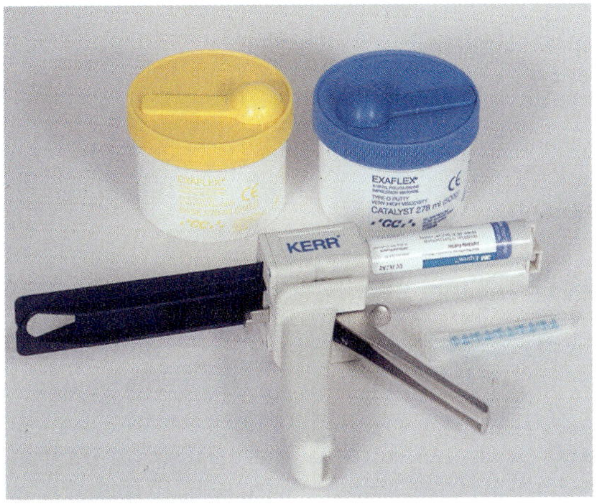

Fig. 46-14 Polysiloxane (polyvinyl siloxane) material.

OCCLUSAL (BITE) REGISTRATION

In addition to having an accurate impression of the prepared teeth, the dentist and laboratory technician need an accurate registration of the normal **centric** relationship of the maxillary and mandibular arches (Fig. 46-15). This relationship is recorded as the **occlusal registration,** most often referred to as the bite registration.

Wax Bite Registration

A wax bite registration is used to show the occlusal relationship of the maxillary and mandibular teeth (Fig. 46-16). It is particularly useful when the diagnostic casts are trimmed. The most common technique employs a softened baseplate wax (see Procedure 46-6).

Polysiloxane Bite Registration Paste

One of the most popular materials used for bite registrations is polysiloxane. This material is supplied as a paste system and as cartridges (see Procedure 46-7). Polysiloxane

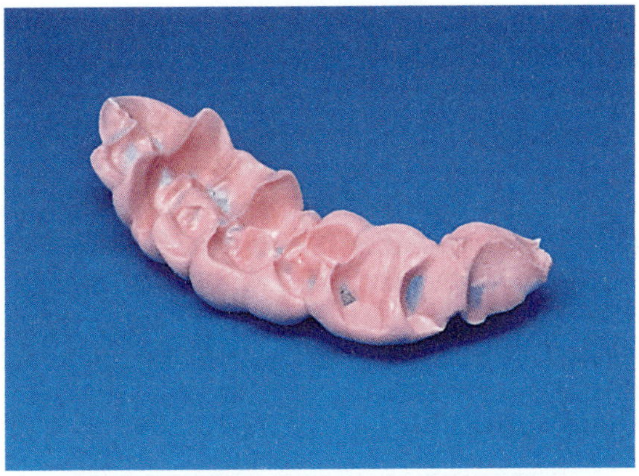

Fig. 46-15 Example of a bite registration. (Courtesy 3M Dental Products, St Paul, MN.)

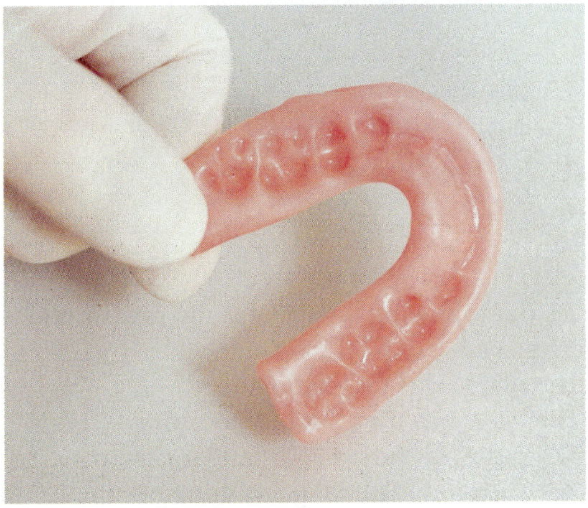

Fig. 46-16 Wax bite registration.

Procedure 46-6 Taking a Wax Bite Registration

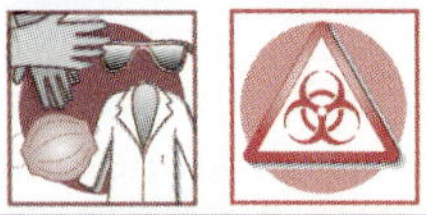

Equipment and Supplies

- Baseplate wax
- Laboratory knife
- Heat source (warm water, Bunsen burner, or torch)

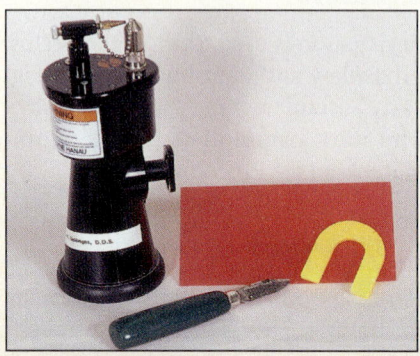

PROCEDURAL STEPS

1. Explain the procedure to the patient. Reassure the patient that the wax placed will be warm, not hot.
2. Have the patient practice opening and closing the mouth normally.
   Purpose: To ensure that the correct position will be recorded in the wax. When the wax is in place, the patient may close the teeth together instead of biting directly into the wax, resulting in an inaccurate bite registration.
3. Place the wax over the biting surfaces of the teeth and check the length. If the wax extends so far beyond the last tooth that the patient is uncomfortable, remove the wax from the patient's mouth. Use the laboratory knife to shorten the length of the wax.
4. Use a heat source to soften the wax.

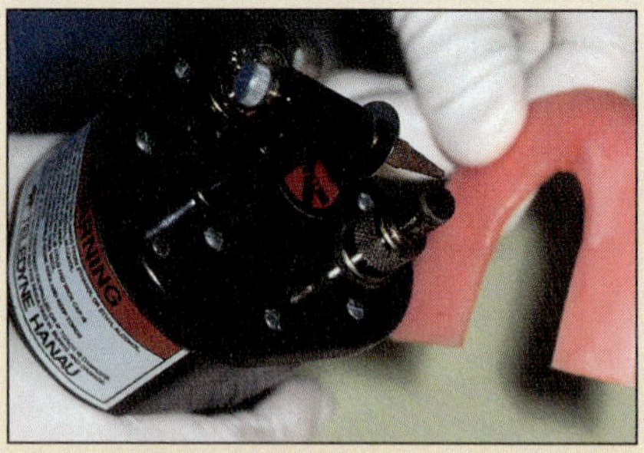

5. Place the softened wax against the biting surfaces of the teeth.
6. Instruct the patient to bite gently and naturally into the wax.

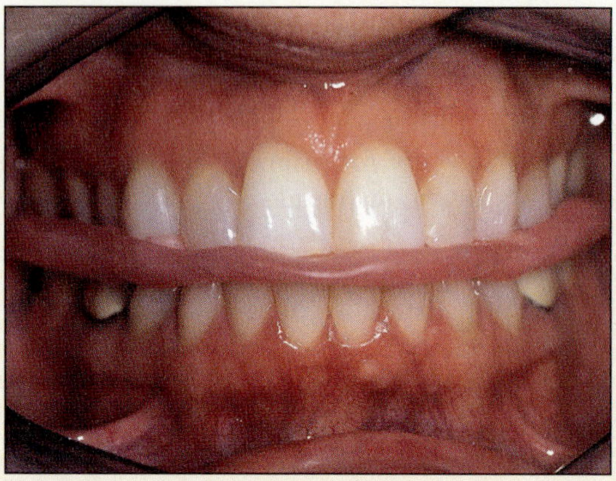

7. Allow the wax to cool.
   Note: The wax will cool quickly and may be removed from the mouth in 1 to 2 minutes.
8. Remove the wax bite registration carefully to avoid distortion.
9. Write the patient's name on a piece of paper and keep it with the wax bite registration.
10. Store the wax bite registration with the impressions or casts until it is needed during the trimming of the casts.

provides the following benefits for the dentist and laboratory technician:

- The material is fast-setting.
- The paste has no resistance to biting forces.
- The paste has no odor or taste for the patient.
- Polysiloxane material gains dimensional stability over time.
- The material is convenient to use.

Zinc Oxide–Eugenol Bite Registration Paste

When a more durable material is needed for a bite registration, a zinc oxide–eugenol (ZOE) material may be selected. ZOE paste has little to no resistance to bite closure and is a fast-setting material. The material is supplied in a paste system, which is dispensed onto a paper pad, mixed, and placed onto a gauze tray for the patient to bite into (see Procedure 46-8).

Procedure 46-7 Mixing Polysiloxane Material for a Bite Registration

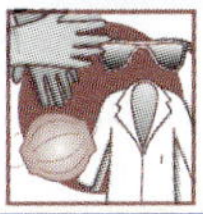

Equipment and Supplies

- Extruder unit
- Cartridge of bite registration material (base and catalyst)
- Mixing tip
- Tray

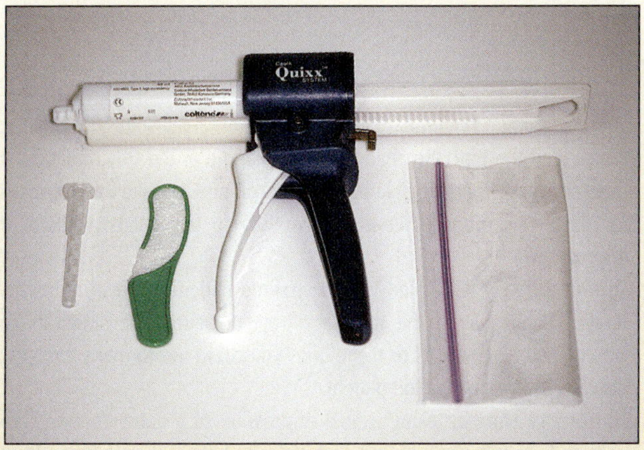

(From Hatrick CD, Eakle WS, Bird WF: *Dental materials: clinical applications for dental assistants and dental hygienists,* St Louis, 2003, Saunders.)

PROCEDURAL STEPS

1. Mix the material and dispense it using an extruder.

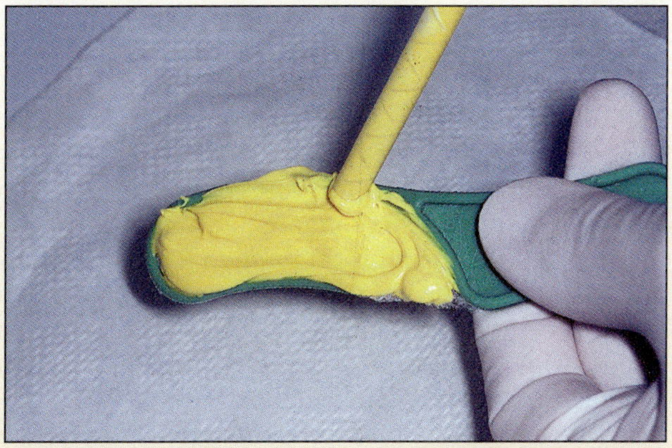

(From Hatrick CD, Eakle WS, Bird WF: *Dental materials: clinical applications for dental assistants and dental hygienists,* St Louis, 2003, Saunders.)

2. Extrude the material directly onto the tray, making sure to fill both sides of the tray.
3. Instruct the patient to close in proper occlusion.
4. After the material has set (about 1 minute), remove the impression, which is checked for accuracy.
5. Rinse, disinfect, and dry the impression; then send it to the laboratory with the written prescription and other impressions.

Procedure 46-8 Mixing Zinc Oxide–Eugenol Bite Registration Material

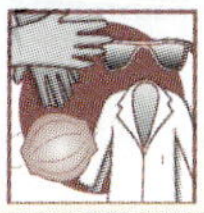

Equipment and Supplies

- ZOE bite registration material (base and catalyst)
- Mixing pad
- Heavy spatula
- Bite tray
- 2- × 2-inch gauze pads

PROCEDURAL STEPS

1. Dispense 1 to 2 inches of base and catalyst paste onto the pad.
2. Mix the material thoroughly for 45 seconds.
3. Gather half the material on the spatula; then wipe the material onto one side of the gauze tray. Gather the remaining half and wipe onto the other side of the tray.

   Purpose: It is important to have material on both sides of the tray to ensure that you have the patient's bite from the maxillary and the mandibular arches.
4. Place the tray in the patient's mouth over the desired areas and have the patient bite down. The material should set within 1 minute.
5. Have the patient open the mouth; then remove the tray.
6. Rinse, dry, and disinfect the bite registration. Send it to the laboratory with the written prescription and other impressions.

Recall

21. What material is most often used for a bite registration?
22. What type of tray is used when using ZOE bite registration paste?
23. Do you cool or warm the wax before placing the tray in the patient's mouth for a bite registration?

Patient Education

As you complete this chapter, you should have a clearer understanding of the importance and versatility of impressions in dentistry. It is common to hear patients express anxiety or discomfort when having an impression taken. Patients tend to lose their sense of control when a tray with impression material is placed in their mouth. Also, the procedure can be uncomfortable if patients are not used to breathing through their nose or if they have an oversensitive gag reflex.

Be prepared to explain the impression procedure to your patient. With your confidence and skill, the patient will have a much easier time allowing the dental team to complete this important procedure.

Legal and Ethical Implications

The reason that the expanded-functions dental assistant can take preliminary impressions is that these impressions are used for procedures that will not permanently alter a patient's dentition. Final impressions, though, are used solely for the making of indirect restorations, partials, dentures, and implants. All of these procedures do alter a patient's dentition and are the full responsibility of the dentist. Always check with your state board in regard to your legal qualifications in taking preliminary impressions.

Eye to the Future

With advances in biomechanics and computer technology, impression materials will soon be a "thing of the past." The use of computers in dentistry will allow dentists to construct indirect restorations, partial dentures, or implants completely in the dental laboratory within their office. Time and effort will instead be spent on enhancing and increasing patient care, and the waiting time for construction of the restoration will be virtually eliminated.

Critical Thinking

1. You are taking a preliminary impression on an 8-year-old girl. While you are seating the tray, the child grabs the handle of the tray and says she does not want "that thing" in her mouth. You need to take this impression for diagnostic models. What can you say to this child to obtain the impression?
2. You have finally convinced your 8-year-old patient to have impressions taken. When seating the maxillary tray, however, she starts to gag. Describe some concepts or techniques you could use to make this procedure a positive one for the patient.
3. You are assisting in taking a final impression of a patient's mandibular arch and are using an automix material. You have just transferred the syringe material and are readying the heavy-bodied material for the tray. While preparing the tray, the cartridge runs out of material before the tray is completely filled. What could have prevented this? What should you do?
4. Your dentist has a habit of "getting behind" with patients. You have worked with this dentist for 12 years, and you know exactly what steps are taken for every procedure. Because he is behind, the dentist asks whether you would mind seeing the next patient and taking the final impression. He notes that by the time you get the tray in, he will be in the room to take the impression out. Do you feel confident in following through? What do you think about this request by the dentist?
5. When you assist the dentist in taking a final impression, you must always obtain a bite registration as well. Explain why the dental laboratory technician needs a reproduction of the opposing arch for designing an indirect restoration.

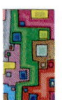

47

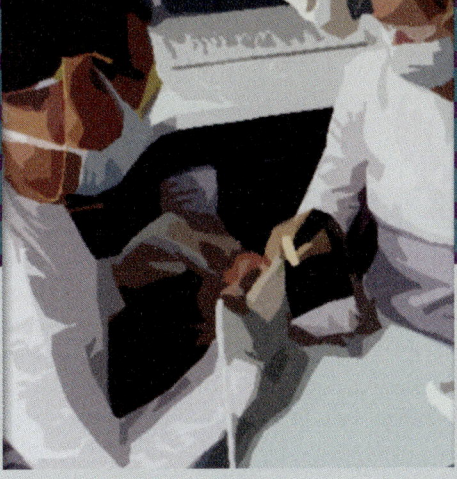

Laboratory Materials and Procedures

Outline

Safety in the Dental Laboratory
- Physical Safety
- Chemical Safety
- Biohazards

Dental Laboratory Equipment
- Heat Sources
- Model Trimmer
- Vacuum Former
- Vibrator
- Laboratory Handpiece
- Sandblaster
- Articulator
- Dental Lathe
- Specialized Spatulas and Bowls

Dental Models
- Gypsum Products

Procedure 47-1: Mixing Dental Plaster

Pouring Dental Models
- Double-Pour Method
- Box-and-Pour Method
- Inverted-Pour Method
- Trimming and Finishing Dental Models

Procedure 47-2: Pouring Dental Models Using Inverted-Pour Method

Procedure 47-3: Trimming and Finishing Dental Models

Custom Impression Trays
- Criteria for Creating Custom Impression Trays
- Acrylic Resin Tray Materials

Procedure 47-4: Constructing an Acrylic Resin Custom Tray
- Light-Cured Resin Tray Materials

Procedure 47-5: Creating a Light-Cured Custom Tray
- Vacuum-Formed Thermoplastic Resin

Procedure 47-6: Constructing a Vacuum-Formed Custom Tray

Dental Waxes
- Boxing Wax
- Utility Wax
- Sticky Wax
- Inlay Casting Wax
- Casting Wax
- Baseplate Wax
- Bite Registration Wax

Patient Education

Legal and Ethical Implications

Eye to the Future

Critical Thinking

KEY TERMS

Anatomic portion (*a*-neh-**tah**-mik) The structural portion of a dental model created from the alginate impression.

Articulator (ahr-**tik**-u-lay-*ter*) Dental laboratory device that simulates the movements of the mandible and temporomandibular joint.

Crystallization (*kris*-tah-lah-**zay**-shun) Chemical process in which crystals form a structure.

Die An accurate replica of the prepared portion of a tooth used in the laboratory during the fabrication of a cast restoration.

Dihydrate (di-**hi**-drate) Relating to gypsum products and indicating two parts of water to one part of calcium sulfate.

Dimensionally stable (dah-**mench**-nah-lee) Resistant to change in width, height, and length.

Facebow Portion of articulator used to measure the upper teeth compared to the temporomandibular joint.

Gypsum (**jip**-sum) Mineral used in the formation of plaster of paris and stone.

continued

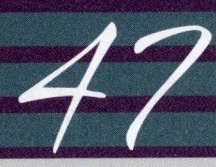

KEY TERMS, cont'd

Hemihydrate (*he*-mi-**hi**-drate) Removal of one-half part water to one part of calcium sulfate, forming the powder product of gypsum.

Homogeneous (*ho*-mah-jee-**ne**-us) (also known as homogenous) Having a uniform quality and consistency throughout.

Lathe **(layth)** Machine used for cutting or polishing dental appliances.

Model Replica of the maxillary and mandibular arches made from an impression.

Monomer (**ma-**nah-mur) A molecule that, when combined with other molecules, forms a polymer.

Polymer (**pah**-leh-mur) Compound of many molecules.

Slurry (**slur**-ee) Mixture of gypsum and water used in the finishing of models.

Volatile (**vah-**leh-tul) Evaporates easily and is very explosive.

LEARNING OUTCOMES

On completion of this chapter, the student will be able to achieve the following objectives:

- Pronounce, define, and spell the Key Terms.
- Discuss the safety precautions that should be taken in the dental laboratory.
- List the types of equipment found in a dental laboratory and their uses.
- Describe dental models and how they are used in dentistry.
- Discuss gypsum products and their role in making dental models.
- Describe the three types of custom impression trays and their use in dentistry.
- Describe the types of dental waxes and their use in dentistry.

PERFORMANCE OUTCOMES

On completion of this chapter, the student will be able to achieve competency standards in the following skills:

- Mix dental stone.
- Pour a set of dental models using the inverted-pour method.
- Trim and finish a set of dental models.
- Construct an acrylic resin custom tray.
- Construct a light-cured custom tray.
- Construct a vacuum-formed custom tray.

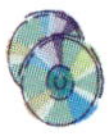

The dental laboratory is a separate area of the dental office (away from the patient treatment area) where the dentist and clinical staff complete the following procedures:

- Pour up preliminary impressions
- Trim and finish diagnostic models
- Prepare custom trays
- Polish provisionals, partial or full dentures, and indirect restorations

Some specialty practices, such as pediatric dentistry, orthodontics, and fixed and removable prosthodontics, have more extensive laboratories. Having more equipment and expertise in the laboratory allows the dentist or private dental laboratory technician to handle larger cases and keep overhead costs to a minimum. If a case cannot be handled in the laboratory, it is sent to a commercial dental laboratory (Fig. 47-1).

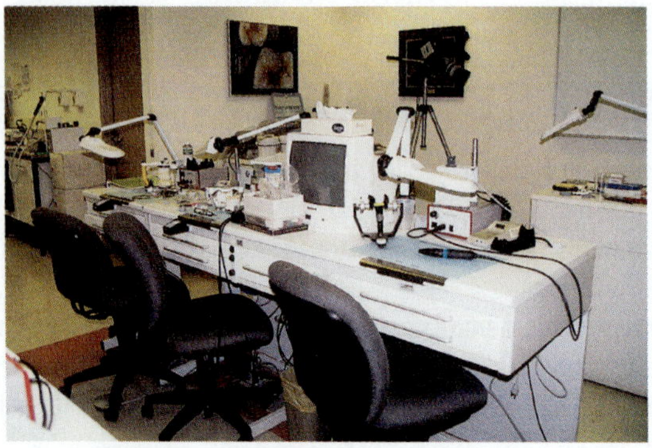

Fig. 47-1 Commercial dental laboratory.

SAFETY IN THE DENTAL LABORATORY

When working in the laboratory, you must also make safety your first concern. It is essential to follow safety precautions and infection control procedures. Remember, items that are brought into the laboratory from the treatment room area are contaminated, and exposure control is just as important here as when you are with the patient.

Laboratory Rules

1. No eating, drinking, or smoking.
2. Keep all cosmetics away from the area.
3. Wear personal protective equipment (PPE) when working in the lab.
4. Keep hair back.
5. Report all accidents to the dentist immediately.
6. Follow the manufacturer's instructions for equipment operation.
7. Clean the work area before and after every procedure.

Physical Safety

When working around electrical equipment or items that produce high heat, become familiar with the location of the fire extinguisher and fire escape routes. Keep all equipment in good working order, and always follow the manufacturer's directions when handling equipment.

Chemical Safety

Dental materials in the laboratory area may include corrosive, toxic, or carcinogenic substances. Take care in the handling and use of these materials and take special precaution to not to come in direct contact with chemicals that could be inhaled, absorbed, or ingested. (See Chapter 23 on exposure to and protection from hazardous chemicals).

Biohazards

Biohazards are usually associated with the treatment area and sterilization center. However, impressions and other items brought into the laboratory can also harbor blood and saliva that could be infectious. The laboratory area and contaminated items must also be disinfected before and after each use when dealing with biohazards.

Recall

1. Where would the dental laboratory be located in a dental office?
2. What specialty practices might have a more extensive laboratory setup?
3. What is an example of a contaminated item in the dental laboratory?

DENTAL LABORATORY EQUIPMENT

The dental laboratory is generally equipped with a countertop and cabinets to provide adequate work areas and safe storage for the supplies and equipment used in the laboratory (Fig. 47-2).

Wall-mounted bins are used to store bulk supplies of plaster, stone, and investment materials. These bins protect the materials from moisture contamination and make it easy to remove gypsum products as needed. After retrieving the material, the bin should be re-covered immediately.

Work pans are open plastic containers with identification labels that are used to hold the laboratory work in progress for an individual patient. Pans may be color-coded to indicate the type of procedure.

Heat Sources

A heat source is often required in the laboratory to heat wax or other materials. A *propane* or *butane* torch is used for this purpose. If a gas line has been installed into the laboratory, rubber hosing will be attached to a *Bunsen burner* and then to the gas outlet. Remember to turn the handle completely *on* or completely *off*. Otherwise, gas can escape and create a very dangerous environment.

Model Trimmer

The model trimmer is a machine used to trim stone or plaster models (Fig. 47-3). The model trimmer has an abrasive grinding wheel that is used to grind away excess plaster or stone. The wheels work more effectively if the wheel is kept clean, not allowing stone or plaster to build up. Models are placed on the work surface and held in place by firm pressure with your hands or with a holding device that can be attached.

To control the dust level from the cast and to facilitate cutting, a gentle stream of water continuously runs on the wheel when in use. The used water drains directly into a sink equipped with a plaster trap that catches the grindings and prevents them from clogging the drain.

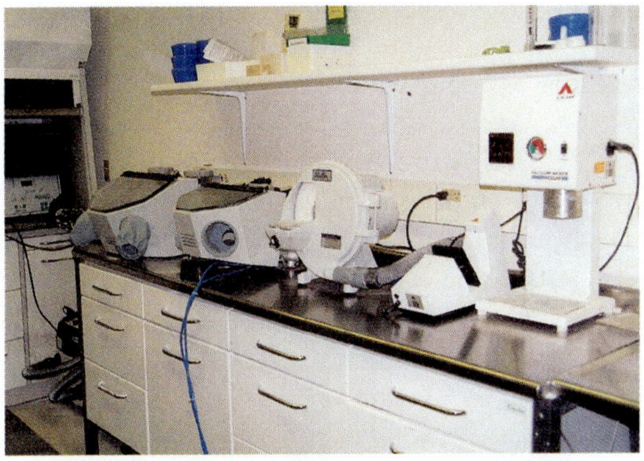

Fig. 47-2 Dental laboratory within a dental office.

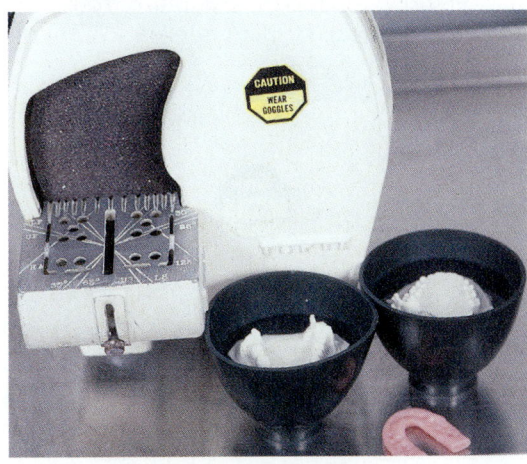

Fig. 47-3 Model trimmer.

Vacuum Former

A vacuum former is a small electrical appliance used to construct custom trays for bleaching, mouth guards, and positioners for orthodontics (Fig. 47-4). The upper part of the unit is a heating element that warms and softens a sheet of thermoplastic resin. The work surface has holes that allow the vacuum to pull and shape the warmed plastic around the model.

Vibrator

A vibrator is used to remove air from the mix of plaster or stone and to aid in the flow of material when pouring up a diagnostic model (Fig. 47-5). The vibrator has a flat working surface that vibrates the bowl or tray. To help keep the vibrator clean, a disposable cover is placed on the vibrator work surface before it is used. After use, this cover is discarded.

Laboratory Handpiece

A low-speed laboratory handpiece is used for many tasks, such as trimming custom impression trays, adjusting dentures, and polishing provisional and indirect restorations. The laboratory handpiece and burs are discussed further in Chapter 35.

Sandblaster

A sandblaster is a hand-held unit that sprays sand at a high speed, creating an etching or pitting on a surface area of metals, porcelain, or acrylic. These elevations in the surface area create added retention through surface roughening. Sandblasting is suitable for the repair of crowns, dentures, and appliances, as well as for the cementation of crowns, bridges, and inlays.

Articulator

An **articulator** is a machine that works as close as is practical to the way in which the mouth works (Fig. 47-6). Dental **models** are prepared and placed on the articulator for examination and diagnosis or to construct dental appliances. Special records are taken to position the dental models accurately on the articulator.

The **facebow,** which is a portion of the articulator, records the measurement from the upper teeth to the temporomandibular joint. The *centric relation* or *bite record* is a measurement of where the teeth are positioned when the joints are aligned correctly and before the teeth actually come into contact.

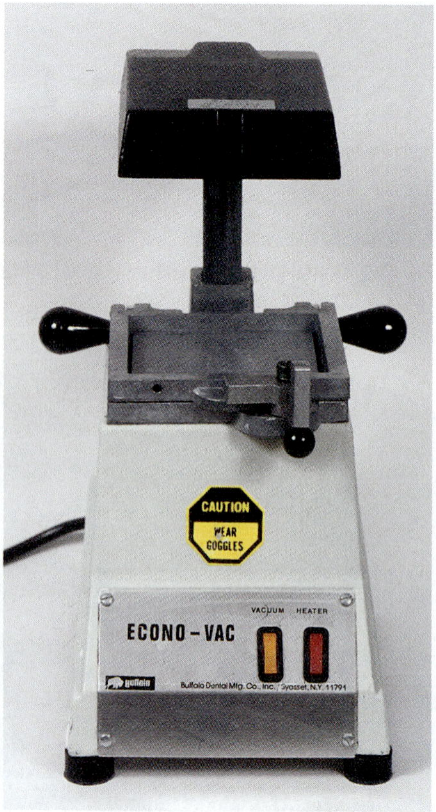

Fig. 47-4 Vacuum former.

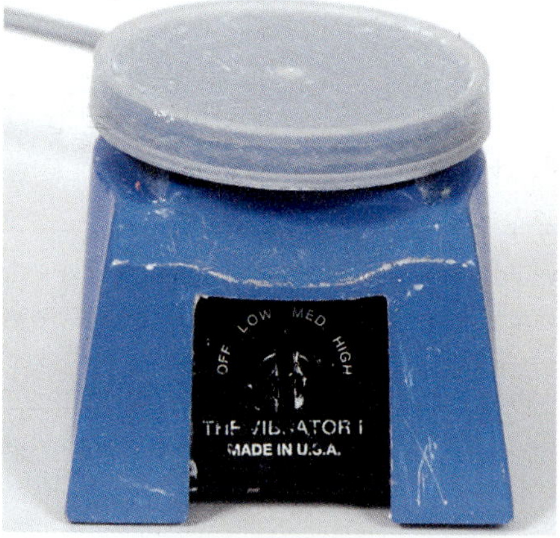

Fig. 47-5 Vibrator.

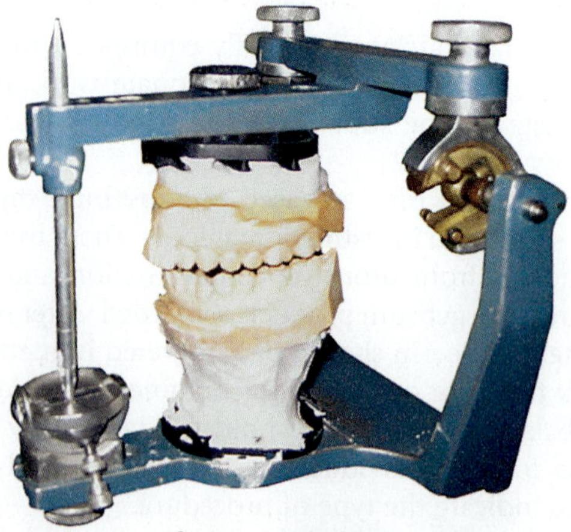

Fig. 47-6 Articulator.

Dental Lathe

The dental **lathe** is used to polish or trim custom trays, provisional coverage, dentures, and indirect restorations. The lathe is designed with a protective plastic see-through shield that is brought down over the work area. The lathe has a revolving threaded extension from each end of the motor. Attachments such as an abrasive grinding wheel or rag wheel are placed on these extensions. After each use, these items must be sterilized before reuse.

Pumice and other polishing agents are used during polishing. A protective pan behind and under the wheel is used to hold the pumice and catch the spatter.

Specialized Spatulas and Bowls

A few specialized instruments are often used in the dental laboratory. As with any instruments, these must be sterilized and stored properly after each use.

Wax Spatulas

A wax spatula is a double-ended instrument used in waxing a pattern or when working with wax for a partial or full denture. The #7 wax spatula is the most common spatula used in the laboratory.

Mixing Spatulas

Several types of mixing spatulas may be found in the laboratory. The type of spatula chosen depends on the strength of the dental material being mixed.

Rubber Bowls

Rubber bowls are used in the mixing of alginate in the treatment area and are also used in the mixing of stone or plaster in the laboratory setting. Make sure to have an adequate supply of rubber bowls in the office.

Recall

4. What piece of equipment is used to grind away plaster or stone?
5. What piece of equipment does the dentist use to determine centric relation on a diagnostic model?
6. What is the most common wax spatula size used in the laboratory?

DENTAL MODELS

Dental models, also referred to as *study casts,* are accurate three-dimensional reproductions of the teeth and surrounding soft tissue of the patient's maxillary and mandibular arches (Fig. 47-7). A model is created from an alginate impression. The alginate impression is taken to the laboratory and then poured in a gypsum product to create the completed model.

Because these models show a three-dimensional view of conditions, they prove to be a valuable diagnostic tool. The dentist can use these models to study the patient's mouth from angles impossible during the clinical examination. Dental models are used for the following procedures in dentistry:

- Diagnosis for planning a fixed or removable prosthetic device
- Diagnosis of orthodontic treatment
- Visual presentation of dental treatment
- Production of custom trays
- Creation of orthodontic appliances
- Making of provisional coverage
- Making of mouth guards

Gypsum Products

Gypsum products are used extensively in dentistry to make dental models. Many characteristics and properties affect the use of gypsum.

Chemical Properties

Gypsum is a mineral that is mined from the earth. In its unrefined state, gypsum is the **dihydrate** form of calcium sulfate, meaning two parts of water to every one part of calcium sulfate. Heating during the manufacturing process removes the water, and the gypsum is converted into a powdered **hemihydrate,** indicating only one-half-part water to one part of calcium sulfate.

Setting Reactions

When the gypsum powder is mixed with water, the hemihydrate crystals dissolve in water to form clusters known as the *nuclei of crystallization.* These nuclei are so close together that as the gypsum crystals grow during the setting process, they intermesh and become entangled with each other. The more intermeshing of crystals, the greater the strength, rigidity, and hardness of the final product.

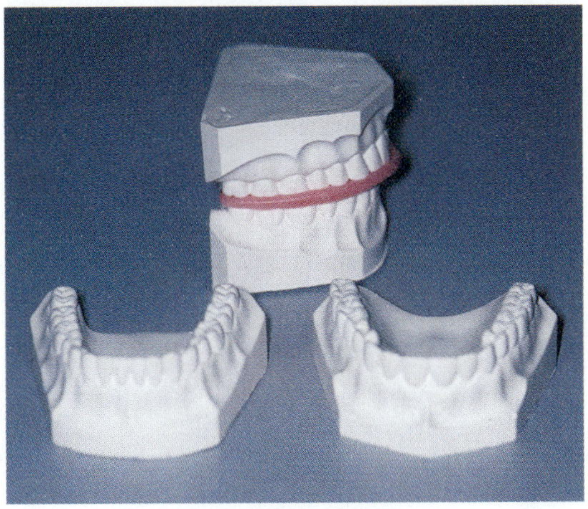

Fig. 47-7 Dental models.

Forms

Three forms of gypsum products are typically used in pouring up casts: *model plaster, dental stone,* and *high-strength stone.* These materials consist of hemihydrate crystals, with the size, shape, and porosity of the hemihydrate crystals differing for each material. The differences in the hemihydrate crystals determine the characteristics and water-to-powder ratios for each type of gypsum product.

Model plaster

Also commonly referred to as *plaster of paris,* model plaster is used primarily for pouring preliminary impressions and making diagnostic models. The crystals in plaster are irregular in shape and very porous, similar in appearance to a sponge. Because of the porous and irregular crystals, model plaster requires the most water for mixing, which produces a weaker cast.

Dental stone

Dental stone is used when a more durable diagnostic cast is required or for use as a working model in the making of dentures. The crystals in dental stone are uniform in shape and less porous than those in plaster. The resulting cast is much stronger and denser than one made from plaster.

High-strength stone

Also known as *densite* or *improved dental stone,* high-strength stone has a strength, hardness, and dimensional accuracy that make it ideal for the dental laboratory technician to create the **dies** used in the production of crowns, bridges, and indirect restorations. The crystals in high-strength stone are smooth and very dense and require the least amount of water for mixing.

Water-to-Powder Ratio

The water-to-powder ratio has a dramatic effect on the setting time and strength of any gypsum product. The exact water-to-powder ratio depends in part on the intended use of the finished product. Each gypsum product has an optimal ratio specified by the manufacturer. These ratios should be carefully observed because deviations will

Procedure 47-1 Mixing Dental Plaster

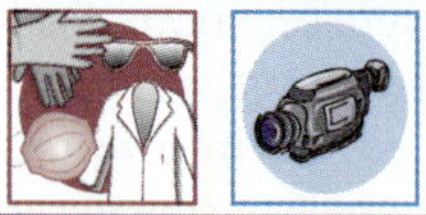

Equipment and Supplies

- Flexible rubber mixing bowl (clean and dry)
- Metal spatula (stiff blade with a rounded end)
- Scale
- Plaster (100 g)
- Water-measuring device
- Room-temperature water (70° F)
- Vibrator with a disposable cover

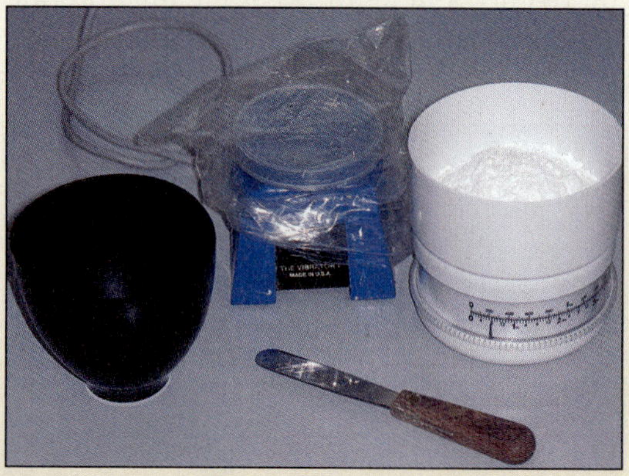

PROCEDURAL STEPS

1. Measure 45 ml of room-temperature water into a clean rubber mixing bowl.
2. Place the paper towel on the scale and make necessary adjustments.
3. Weigh out 100 g of dental plaster.
4. Add the powder to the water in steady increments. Allow the powder to settle into the water for about 30 seconds.
   Purpose: To prevent trapping of air bubbles.
5. Use the spatula to incorporate the powder slowly into the water. A smooth and creamy mix should be achieved in about 20 seconds.
   Purpose: To avoid spilling the powder.

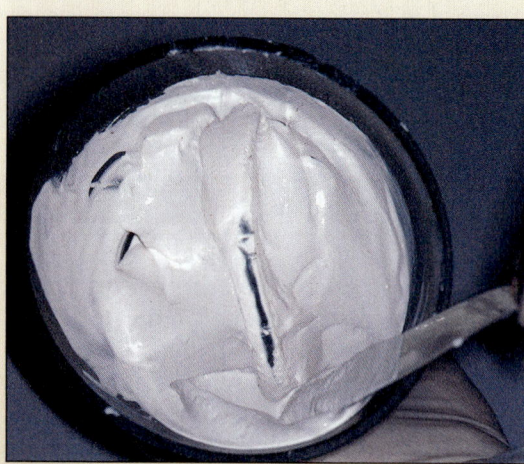

Procedure 47-1 Mixing Dental Plaster—cont'd

6. Turn the vibrator to low or medium speed and place the bowl of plaster mix on the vibrator platform.
   Purpose: To reduce the air in the mix.
7. Lightly press and rotate the bowl on the vibrator. Air bubbles will rise to the surface.
8. Complete mixing and vibration of the plaster in *no longer than* 2 minutes.

change both the consistency of the material and the properties of the set cast (Box 47-1).

When *too little* water is used, the mix will be difficult to mix and will have a shorter working time. If additional water is added to thin the mixture, the **crystallization** (setting) process will be disturbed, and the model will not have the desired strength.

When *too much* water is used, the mix will be thin and runny and will take longer to set; this creates a model that will be considerably weaker. If additional powder is added after the stirring begins, the continued stirring will break up the crystals that have begun to form. The result is a cast that is weak and brittle.

Measuring the water and powder in each mix *must be exact.* The water is measured by volume with a measuring device such as a large syringe or a milliliter-graduated cylinder. The powder is measured by weight with the use of a scale. The scale is adjusted for this weight *before* the powder is weighed. If a scale is not available, the powder may be measured by volume (see Procedure 47-1).

Recall

7. What is another term for a dental model?
8. What dental materials are used to make dental models?
9. What are the three forms of gypsum?
10. What is the water-to-powder (g/ml) ratio of plaster?
11. When mixing gypsum materials, do you add the "powder to the water" or the "water to the powder"?
12. What are gypsum materials mixed in?

Box 47-1 Recommended Water/Powder Ratios for Gypsum Products

Gypsum Product	Mixing Water
Model plaster (100 g)	45 to 50 ml
Dental stone (100 g)	30 to 32 ml
High-strength stone (100 g)	19 to 24 ml

POURING DENTAL MODELS

A model consists of two parts: the **anatomic portion,** which is created from the alginate impression, and the *art portion,* which forms the base of the cast (Fig. 47-8). Three different pouring methods are used to create the base portion (Fig. 47-9).

Double-Pour Method

The anatomic portion of the cast is poured first. Then a second mix of plaster or stone is used to prepare the art portion. A free-form base may be created by hand or by the use of a commercial rubber mold.

Box-and-Pour Method

The impression is surrounded with a "box" made of wax. The completed box should extend at least ½ inch above the palatal area of the maxillary impression and ½ inch above the tongue area of the mandibular impression.

Inverted-Pour Method

The inverted-pour approach consists of mixing one large mixture of plaster or stone and pouring both portions of the model in a single step (see Procedure 47-2).

Recall

13. What are the two parts of a dental model?

Trimming and Finishing Dental Models

When models are to be used for a case presentation or as part of the patient's permanent record, they must have a professional appearance. This is accomplished by trimming the models to a *geometric standard.* The wax bite registration is used to articulate the casts during the trimming process (see Procedure 47-3).

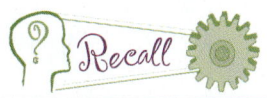

Procedure 47-2 Pouring Dental Models Using Inverted-Pour Method

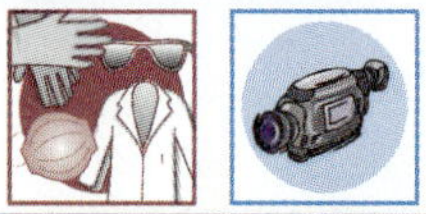

Equipment and Supplies

- Maxillary and mandibular impression
- Glass slab or tile
- Laboratory spatula
- Laboratory knife and cutters
- 150 g of plaster (additional is needed for the base)
- 60 ml of water (additional water needed for the base)
- Flexible rubber bowl
- Vibrator

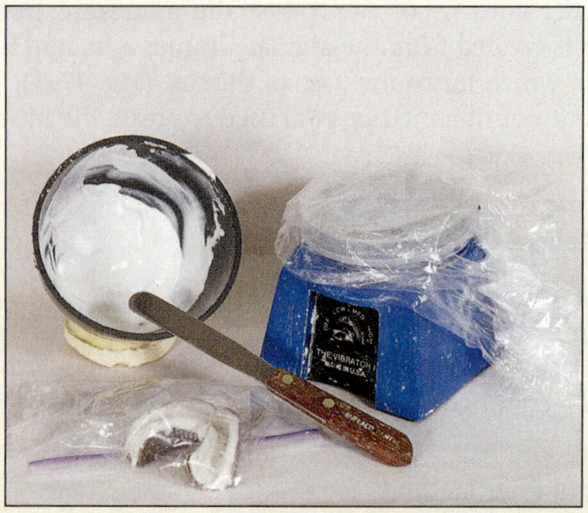

PROCEDURAL STEPS

Preparing the Impression

1. Use a gentle stream of air to remove excess moisture from the impression. Be careful not to dry out the impression too much.
   Purpose: Over-drying could cause distortion of the material.
2. Use your laboratory knife or laboratory cutters to remove any excess impression material that will interfere with the pouring of the model.

Pouring the Mandibular Model and Base

1. Mix the plaster; then set the vibrator at low to medium speed.
   Note: A separate mix is made for each impression.
2. Hold the impression tray by the handle and place the edge of the base of the handle on the vibrator.
3. Dip the spatula into the plaster mix, picking up a small increment (about ½ tsp).
4. Place that small increment in the impression near the most posterior tooth. Guide the material as it flows lingually.
   Purpose: The flowing action pushes out the air ahead of it and eliminates air bubbles.

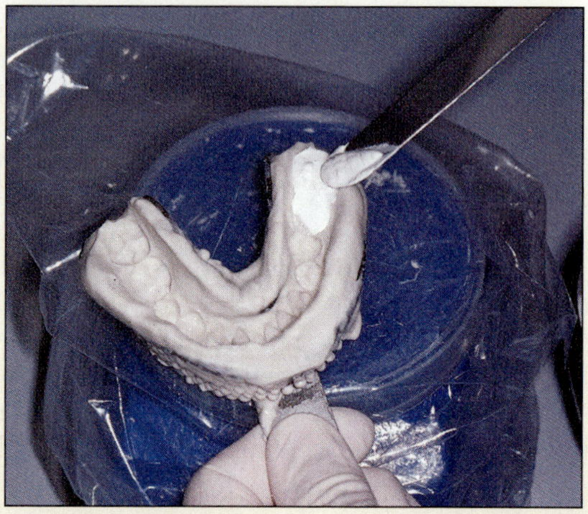

5. Continue to place small increments in the *same area* as the first increment and allow the plaster to flow toward the anterior teeth.
6. Turn the tray on its side to provide the continuous flow of material forward into each tooth impression.
7. Once all of the teeth in the impression are covered, begin to add larger increments until the entire impression is filled.

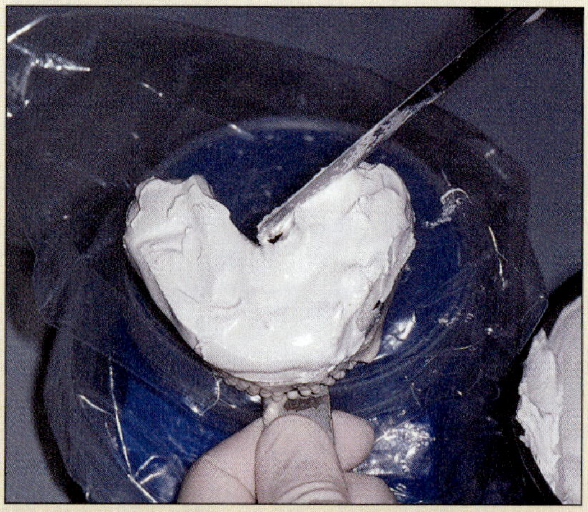

Procedure 47-2 Pouring Dental Models Using Inverted-Pour Method—cont'd

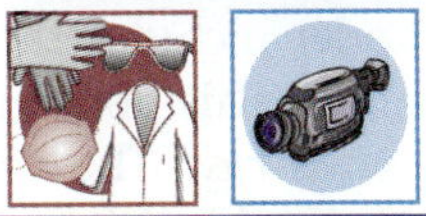

8. Place the additional material onto a glass slab (or tile); shape the base to approximately 2 by 2 inches by 1 inch thick.
   Note: Commercial rubber molds are available for making bases. These molds provide symmetry to the cast and reduce the need for trimming.

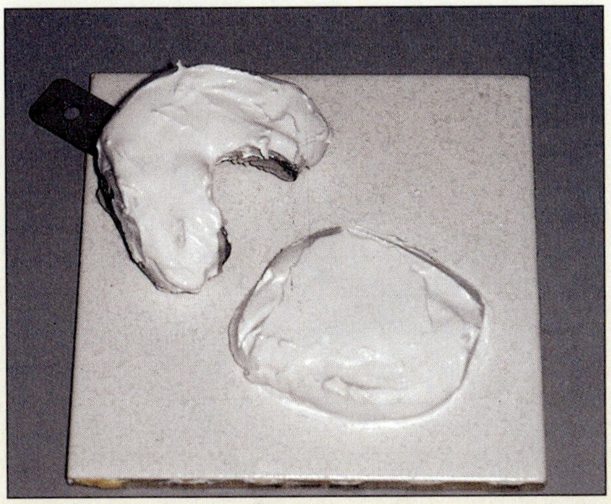

9. Invert the impression onto the new mix. Do not push the impression into the base.
   Purpose: When the poured impression is inverted onto the new mix, the fresh material tends to flow excessively. This can result in a base that is too large and too thin.
10. Holding the tray steady, use a spatula to smooth the plaster base mix up onto the margins of the initial pour. Be careful not to cover the impression tray with material, or you will have difficulty in removing the cast from the impression.

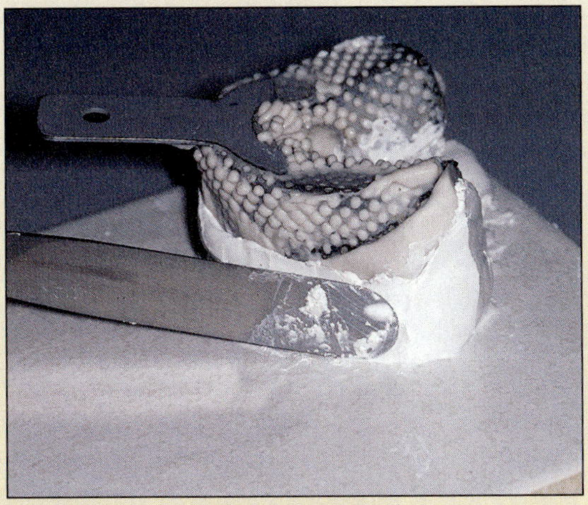

Pouring the Maxillary Cast

1. Repeat steps 3 through 5, using clean equipment for the fresh mix of stone.
2. Place the small increment of plaster in the posterior area of the impression. Guide the material as it flows down into the impression of the most posterior tooth.
3. Continue to place small increments in the *same area* as the first increment and allow the plaster to flow toward the anterior teeth.
4. Rotate the tray on its side to provide the continuous flow of material into each tooth impression.
5. Once all the teeth in the impression are covered, begin to add larger increments until the entire impression is filled.
6. Place the mix onto a glass slab (or tile) and shape the base to approximately 2 by 2 inches by 1 inch thick.
   Note: Commercial rubber molds are available for making bases. These molds provide symmetry to the cast and reduce the need for trimming.
7. Invert the impression onto the new mix. Do not push the impression into the base.
   Purpose: When the poured impression is inverted onto the new mix, the fresh material tends to flow excessively. This can result in a base that is too large and too thin.
8. Holding the tray steady, use a spatula to smooth the stone base mix up onto the margins of the initial pour. Be careful not to cover the impression tray with plaster, or you will have difficulty in removing the cast from the impression.
9. Place the impression tray on the base so that the handle and occlusal plane of the teeth on the cast are parallel with the surface of the glass slab (or tile).
   Purpose: To help form a base with uniform thickness.

Separating the Cast from the Impression

1. Wait 45 to 60 minutes after the base has been poured before separating the impression from the model.
2. Use the laboratory knife to gently separate the margins of the tray.
3. Apply firm, straight, upward pressure on the handle of the tray to remove the impression.
4. If the tray does not separate easily, check to see where the tray is still attached to the impression. Again, use the laboratory knife to free the tray from the model.
5. Pull the tray handle straight up from the model.
   Note: Never wiggle the impression tray from side to side while it is on the cast. This can cause the teeth on the cast to fracture.
6. The models are ready for trimming and polishing.

Recall

14. When pouring an impression, where do you begin placing the gypsum material in the maxillary impression?
15. How long should you wait before you separate the model from the impression?

Anatomic and Art Portions

The anatomic portion of the dental model includes the teeth, oral mucosa, and muscle attachments. This portion makes up two thirds of the overall trimmed cast. The art portion of the model forms the base and should make up one third of the overall trimmed cast.

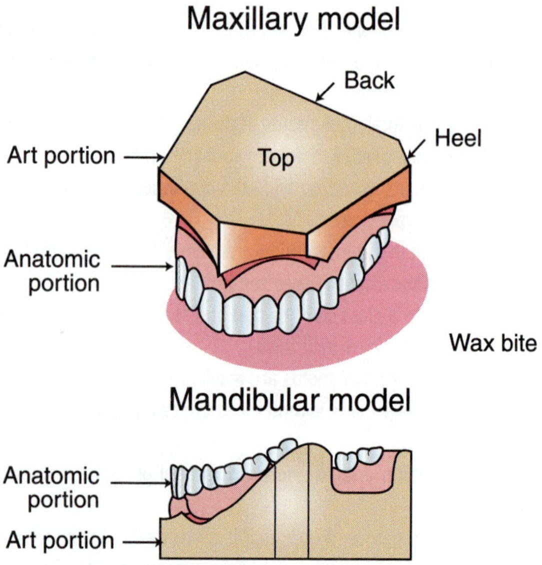

Fig. 47-8 Anatomic and art portions of a dental model.

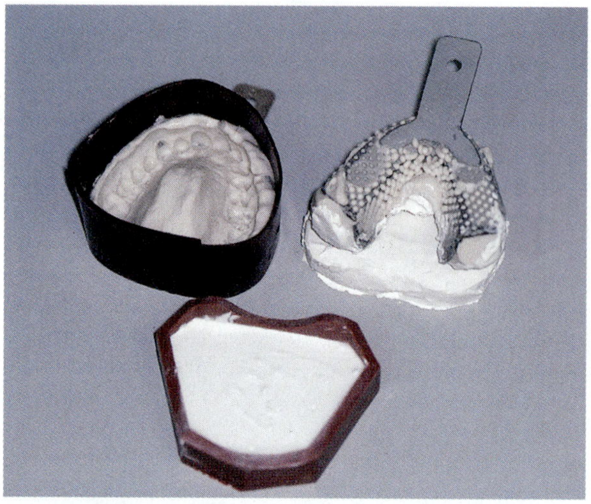

Fig. 47-9 Examples of pouring methods. *Upper left,* boxed; *upper right,* inverted; *lower middle,* double-pour.

Procedure 47-3 Trimming and Finishing Dental Models

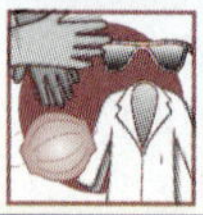

Equipment and Supplies

- Poured stone maxillary and mandibular dental model
- Wax bite registration
- Pencil
- Ruler
- Laboratory knife
- Model trimmer

PROCEDURAL STEPS

Preparing the Model

1. Soak the art portion of the model in a bowl of water for at least 5 minutes.
   Purpose: To make the trimming much easier.

Trimming the Maxillary Model

1. Place the maxillary model on a flat countertop with the teeth setting on the table.
2. Use your pencil to measure up 1¼ inches from the counter and draw a line around the model.

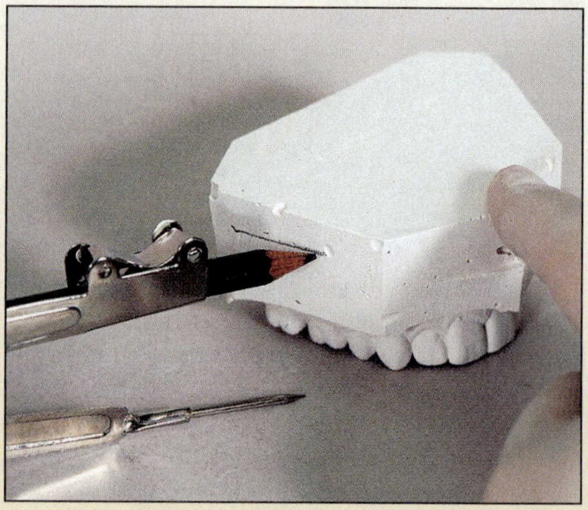

Procedure 47-3 Trimming and Finishing Dental Models—cont'd

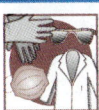

3. Turn on the trimmer, hold the model firmly against the trimmer, and trim the bottom of the base to the line that you drew.
4. Draw a line ¼ inch behind the maxillary tuberosities. With the base flat on the trimmer, remove excess plaster in the posterior area of the model to the marked line.
5. To trim the sides of the model, draw a line through the center of the occlusal ridges on one side of the model. Measure out ¼ inch from this line and draw a line parallel to the previous line drawn.
   Note: If you need to measure out beyond ¼ inch so that the mucobuccal fold is not trimmed away, do so.
6. Repeat these measurements on the other side of the model.
7. Trim the sides of the cast to the lines drawn.

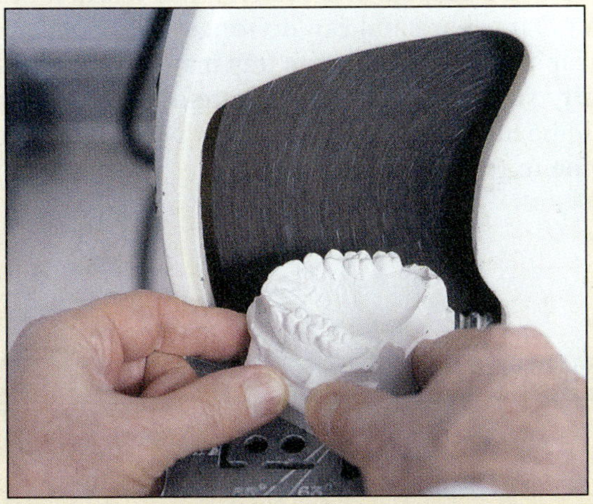

8. Draw a line behind the tuberosity that is perpendicular to the opposite canine and trim to that line. This completes the maxillary heel cuts.
9. The final cut is made from drawing a line from the canine to the midline at an angle. Complete this on both sides and trim to the line.

Trimming the Mandibular Model

1. Occlude the mandibular model with the maxillary model, using the wax bite.
2. With the mandibular base on the trimmer, trim the posterior portion of the mandibular model until it is even with the maxillary model.

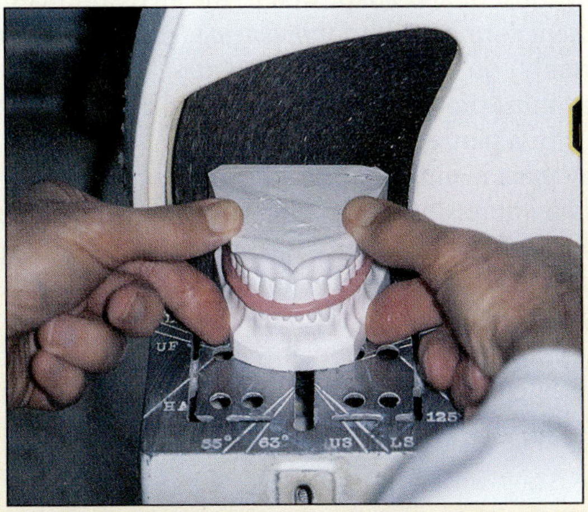

3. Place the models upside down (maxillary base on the table), measure 3 inches from the surface up, and mark a line around the base of the mandibular model.
4. Trim the mandibular model base to the line drawn.
5. With the models in occlusion with the wax bite, place the mandibular model on the trimmer, and trim the lateral cuts to match the maxillary lateral cuts.
6. Trim the back and heel cuts to match the maxillary heel cuts.
7. Check that the mandibular anterior cut is rounded from the mandibular right canine to the mandibular left canine.
8. The models are now ready to be finished.

Finishing the Model

1. Mix a **slurry** of gypsum and fill in any voids.
2. Using a laboratory knife, remove any extra gypsum that occurs as beads on the occlusion or model.

Polishing Plaster Models

Many dental offices use the dental model for the presentation of the diagnosis and treatment plan. It is important for the model to have a professional-quality appearance.

To create a more polished look to a plaster model, soak the model in a soapy solution for 24 hours, allow it to dry, and then polish it with a soft cloth. An alternative to the solution is a commercial model gloss spray that can be used for the same purpose.

Recall

16. Which of the two models (maxillary or mandibular) do you begin measuring and trimming first?
17. What area on the maxillary and mandibular model is trimmed differently?
18. What should be placed between the two models when trimming them together?

CUSTOM IMPRESSION TRAYS

As discussed in Chapter 46, custom impression trays are made specifically for a patient. Custom trays are created by the dental assistant in the dental laboratory before the patient returns for his or her appointment.

Criteria for Creating Custom Impression Trays

- Tray must be sufficiently rigid to hold and support the material during tray placement and removal.
- Tray must fit and adapt well to the arch and maintain patient comfort without *impinging* (pressing uncomfortably) on the surrounding tissues.
- Tray must provide accurate adaptation to an edentulous or a partially edentulous arch.
- Tray must maintain an even distribution of 3 to 4 mm of the impression material between itself and the teeth.
- The completed maxillary tray must cover the teeth and hard palate and extend slightly beyond the gingival margin (but not into the mucobuccal fold).
- The completed mandibular tray must cover the teeth and extend beyond the gingival margin (but not into the mucobuccal fold).

The primary materials used to construct custom trays are *self-curing acrylic resin, light-cured resin,* and *thermoplastic material.* Regardless of the material used in the construction of the tray, a diagnostic model must be prepared first, followed by specific guidelines (Box 47-2).

Acrylic Resin Tray Materials

Self-curing acrylic resin provides a strong and easily adaptable material to create a custom tray. The major disadvantage of this material is the hazards of working with the liquid monomer, which is very **volatile.** The vapor is highly flammable, it is hazardous if inhaled in large concentrations, and it may be irritating to the skin. This material must be handled with great care.

When using a self-curing resin, polymerization begins when the **monomer** and **polymer** are mixed together. The material reaches an initial cure stage within minutes; during this time it becomes harder and gives off heat, but it can still be shaped. The material has reached final set when (1) it is hard and can no longer be shaped and (2) the heat has diminished. The tray material is not **dimensionally stable** for 24 hours. Therefore the custom tray should be made 24 hours before the patient is scheduled to come in (see Procedure 47-4).

Box 47-2 Elements and Guidelines for Creating a Custom Impression Tray

Elements	Guidelines and Description
Undercuts	The first step in cast preparation is to fill all undercuts with wax or other molding material.
	Air bubbles in the cast, the shape of the arch and ridge, carious lesions, fractured teeth, and deep interproximal spaces and malposed teeth may cause undercuts.
Outlining the tray	The margins of the cast where the finished tray will be seated are outlined in pencil.
	The outline, which designates the area to be covered by the tray, extends over the attached gingiva to the mucogingival junction and 2 to 3 mm beyond the last tooth in the quadrant.
Spacer	A spacer is placed on the cast to create room in the tray for the impression material.
	Baseplate wax, a folded moist paper towel, or commercial nonstick molding material may be used for this purpose.
	To create the spacer, cut a length of baseplate wax, warm it, and place it on the cast over the area of the tray. A warmed plastic instrument is used to *lute* the wax to the cast.
Spacer stops	Spacer stops are placed to prevent the tray from seating too deeply onto the arch or quadrant.
	Spacer stops also allow for an adequate quantity of impression material around the preparations.
	Spacer stops are triangular or round holes that are cut out of the spacer with a laboratory knife or wax spatula. These cutouts will form bumps on the tissue side of the tray. (The *tissue side* is the inner surface of the completed tray.)
	An *edentulous tray* requires a minimum of four stops: one each on the crest of the alveolar ridge in the area of the first or second molar. Additional stops may be placed on the crest of the ridge in the area of each canine.
	A tray to take an impression of prepared natural teeth, as for a crown or bridge, has the stops placed near, but not on, the prepared teeth.

Box 47-2 Elements and Guidelines for Creating a Custom Impression Tray—cont'd

Elements	Guidelines and Description
Separating medium	The prepared cast, spacer, and immediate surrounding area are painted with a separating medium so that the completed tray can be readily separated from the cast.
Handle	A handle adapted to the tray will allow easier placement in and removal from the patient's mouth.
	The handle is *always* placed at the anterior of the tray, as near the midline as possible, facing outward and parallel to the occlusal surfaces of the teeth.
	The handle is formed from a piece of scrap acrylic that was cut away from the tray.
	The end of the handle and the area where it will be attached to the tray are moistened with tray resin liquid.
Spacer removal	After the tray has been formed, it is necessary to remove the spacer and clean the tissue side of the tray. A small, stiff brush, such as a toothbrush, is used to remove most of the wax at this time.
	The remainder of the spacer is removed, and the interior of the tray is cleaned after the tray reaches its final set.
Finishing	It is *not* necessary to remove rough areas on the *tissue* side of the tray; this surface will be covered with impression material.
	If the outer edges of the tray are rough, however, it is necessary to smooth them so they do not injure the tissues of the patient's mouth.
	A laboratory knife can be used to smooth minor rough areas.
	An acrylic bur in a straight handpiece can be used to remove major rough areas. An alternative is to use the laboratory lathe to smooth the edges.
	The tray is given a final rinse and disinfected according to manufacturer's instructions.

Procedure 47-4 Constructing an Acrylic Resin Custom Tray

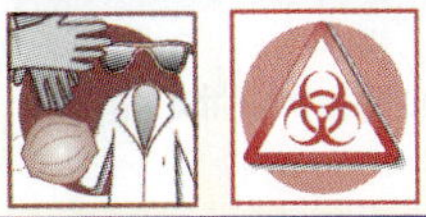

Equipment and Supplies

- Diagnostic model
- Pencil
- Tray resin (monomer and polymer)
- Measures for liquid and powder
- Baseplate wax
- Separating medium with brush
- Heat source
- Laboratory knife
- Laboratory spatula
- Tongue blade
- Wax spatula #7
- Glass jar with lid or smooth-surface paper cup
- Petroleum jelly

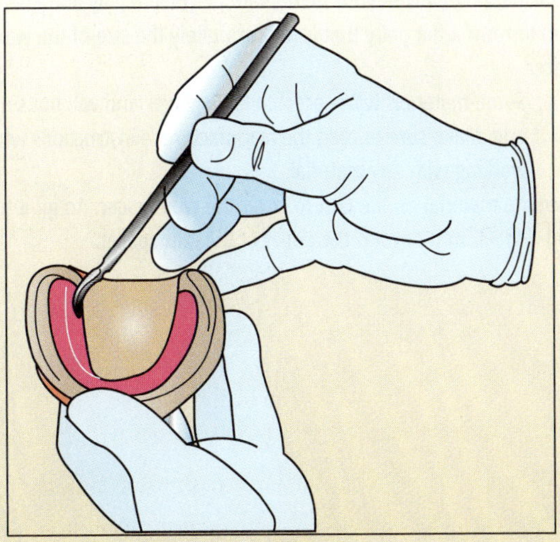

PROCEDURAL STEPS

Preparing the Model

1. Fill the undercuts on the diagnostic model.
2. Outline the tray in pencil.
3. Place the baseplate wax spacer, trim it, and lute the wax to the cast.

continued

Procedure 47-4 Constructing an Acrylic Resin Custom Tray—cont'd

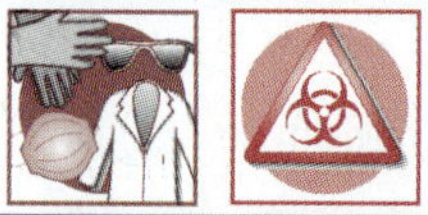

PROCEDURAL STEPS, cont'd

4. Cut the appropriate stops in the spacer.
5. Paint the spacer and surrounding area with separating medium.

Mixing the Acrylic Resin

1. Use the manufacturer's measuring devices to measure the powder into the mixing container. Then add an equal part of liquid and recap the container immediately.
   Purpose: The fumes are toxic.
2. Use the tongue blade to mix the powder and liquid. A **homogeneous** mix should be obtained within 30 seconds. The mix will be thin and sticky.
3. Set the mix aside for 2 to 3 minutes to allow polymerization. If the manufacturer specifies a covered container, place the cover during this time.

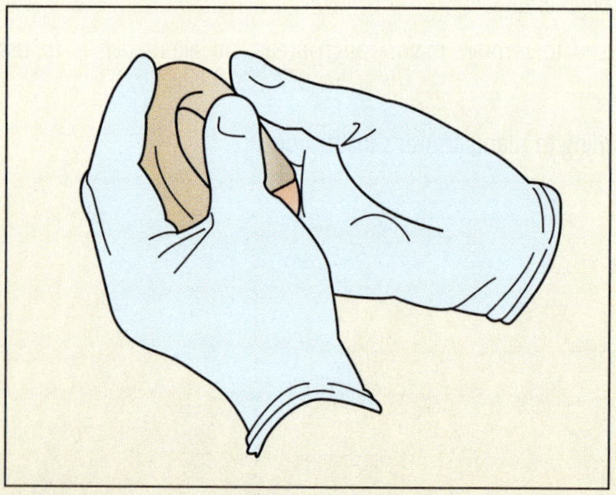

Forming the Tray

1. When the mix has reached a "doughy" stage, remove it from the container with the spatula.
2. Lubricate the palms of your hands with petroleum jelly and knead the resin to form a flat patty that is approximately the size of the wax spacer.
   Note: Some materials will react with latex gloves and will not set properly. Make sure to read the manufacturer's instructions when working with any material.
3. Place the material on the cast to cover the wax spacer. Adapt it to extend 1 to 1.5 mm beyond the edges of the wax spacer.
4. Use an instrument or laboratory knife to trim away the excess tray material quickly while it is still soft.
   Purpose: The material is easier to cut away at this stage.

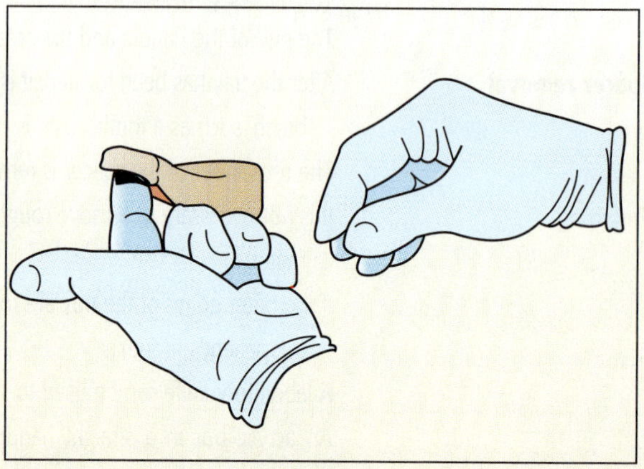

Creating the Handle

1. Use the excess material to shape the handle.
2. Place a drop of monomer on the handle and on the tray, where they will join.
3. Attach the handle so that it extends out of the mouth and is parallel with the occlusal surfaces of the teeth.
4. Hold the handle in place until it is firm.

Finishing the Tray

1. After the initial set (7 to 10 minutes), remove most of the spacer and return the tray to the cast.
2. Clean the wax completely from the inside of the tray after the tray resin has reached final cure.
3. Finish the edges; then clean and disinfect the tray.

Light-Cured Resin Tray Materials

This premixed, prefabricated tray material is a visible light-cured material that does *not* contain methylmethacrylate monomer (the hazardous material associated with the acrylic resin material). Light-cured resin has very low shrinkage, which provides excellent adaptation of the cast. This material may be used for any impression situation, including dentulous, edentulous, or partially edentulous impressions.

With light-cured resins, a curing light acts as the catalyst to bring about polymerization, which allows the material to remain workable until it has been exposed to the light again. Once exposed, the resin polymerizes and hardens very quickly (see Procedure 47-5).

Procedure 47-5 Creating a Light-Cured Custom Tray

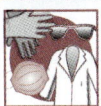

Equipment and Supplies

- Diagnostic model
- Pencil
- Prefabricated tray material
- Baseplate wax
- Separating medium with brush
- Scalpel or laboratory knife
- Curing light system
- Barrier coating

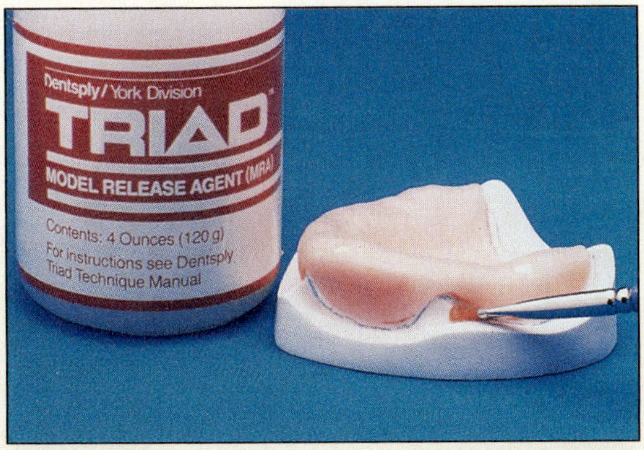

PROCEDURAL STEPS

1. A model is completed before tray construction.
2. Use a pencil to outline the vestibular area and posterior tray border on the stone model.
3. Paint separating medium on the model before placement of the material.
   Note: The material is supplied in uniform precut sheets and stored in a dark container to prevent premature curing.
4. Adapt precut sections of the custom tray material for use on the maxillary model with full palatal coverage and on the mandibular model without full palatal coverage.
5. Mold the sheet of tray material to conform to the study model, using your thumb and forefinger with minimal pressure.
   Note: Be sure to push material through the "occlusal stop" areas of the tray so that acrylic will be in contact with the occlusal surfaces.
6. Trim away excess tray material with a laboratory knife.
   Note: If desired, the excess material can be used to form a handle on the tray.
7. Place the model and tray in a light-curing unit. Cure the tray for 2 minutes.

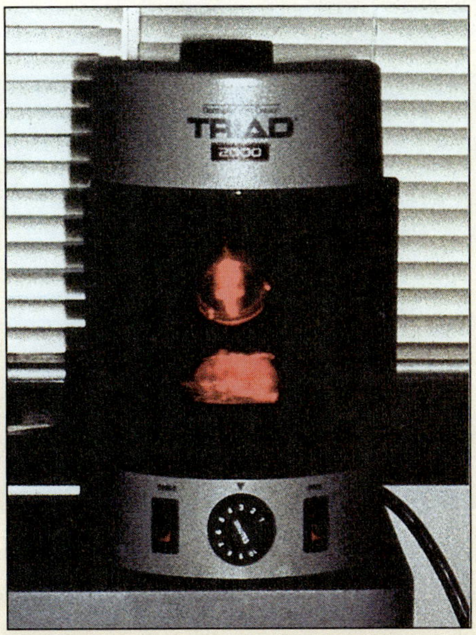

8. After curing, place the model and tray in cool water to solidify the wax spacer and facilitate separation of the tray from the model.
9. Use the acrylic extruded through the holes in the spacer to create the occlusal stops on the inside of the tray.
10. Remove the wax spacer from the tray using a #7 wax spatula.
11. Place the tray in hot water to remove any remnants of wax from the inside.
12. Trim the borders of the tray using an acrylic laboratory bur.
13. Use a thin acrylic bur to perforate the custom tray.
    Note: Perforations and tray adhesives ensure a solid lock of the impression material to the custom tray.
14. Using a laboratory acrylic bur, trim the borders of the edentulous tray to 2 mm short of the vestibule to allow for border molding material.

Vacuum-Formed Thermoplastic Resin

The vacuum former uses heat and a vacuum to shape a sheet of thermoplastic resin to a diagnostic model. The vacuum former is a versatile machine. The major differences in this technique, compared with the acrylic resin and light-cured resin applications, are the model preparation and the weight and type of plastic used (see Procedure 47-6).

When constructing an *impression tray,* you will use a rigid, heavy-gauge plastic that requires a spacer and a handle.

When constructing *provisional coverage,* you will use a lighter-gauge plastic that does not require a spacer or handle.

When constructing a *vital bleaching tray,* you will use a lighter-gauge plastic that does not require a spacer or a handle.

When constructing a *mouth guard,* you will use a heavier-gauge, flexible plastic that does not require a spacer but does require an attachment for the strap.

Procedure 47-6 Constructing a Vacuum-Formed Custom Tray

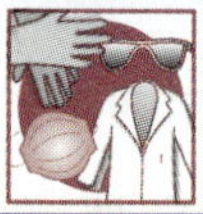
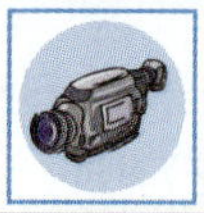

Equipment and Supplies

- Diagnostic model
- Thermoplastic resin material
- Crown and bridge scissors
- Vacuum former

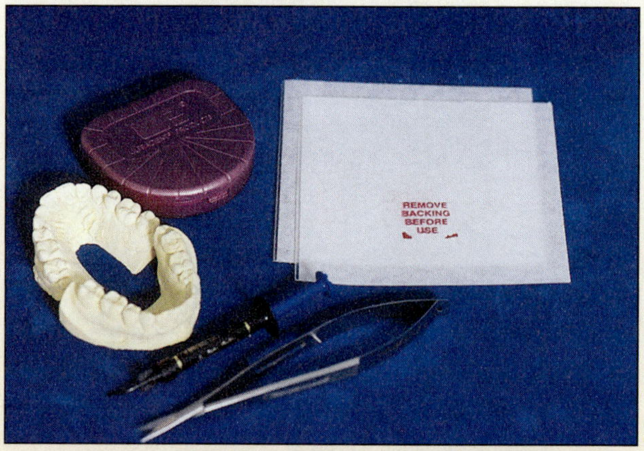

Procedural Steps

1. Trim the model so that it extends 3 to 4 mm past the gingival border.

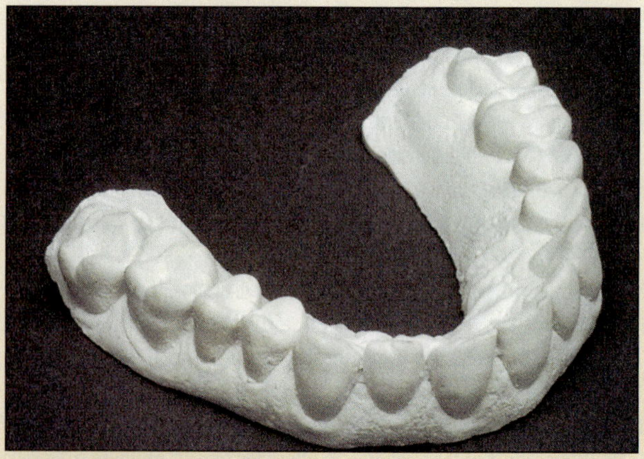

2. To extend the tray from the teeth for the purpose of holding bleaching solution, place a spacer's material on the facial surfaces of the teeth on the model.
   Note: Some materials will require the tray to be light-cured.
3. Using a vacuum former, heat a tray sheet until it sags ½ to 1 inch.

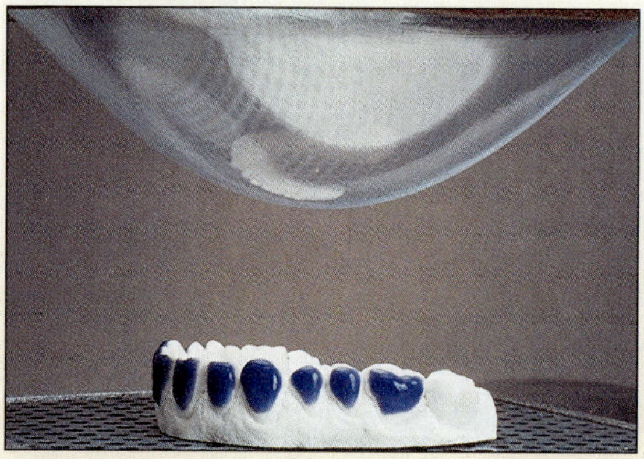

4. Lower the sheet over the model and turn on the vacuum for 10 seconds.
5. Remove the sheet after allowing it to cool completely.
6. Using your scissors, cut the excess material from the tray.
7. Use small, sharp scissors to trim the tray approximately 0.5 mm away from the gingival margin.
   Purpose: You want to avoid the tray irritating the patient's gingiva.

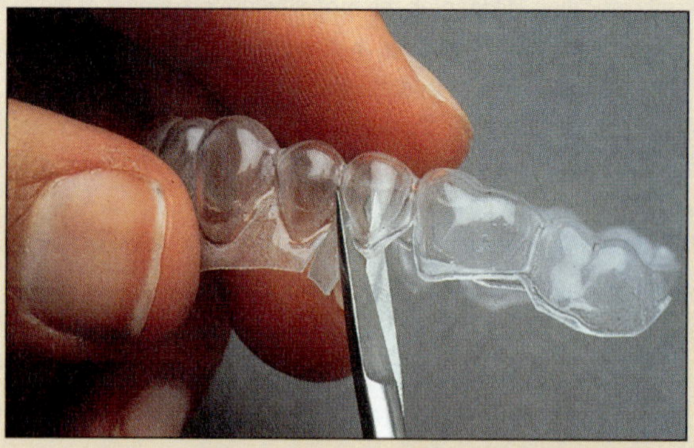

Procedure 47-6 Constructing a Vacuum-Formed Custom Tray—cont'd

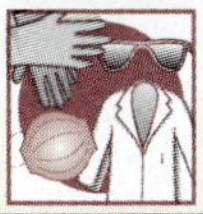
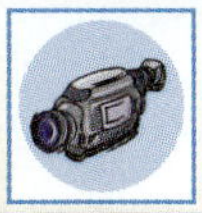

8. Place the tray onto the original model, and check gingival extensions.
9. If necessary, apply a thin coat of petroleum jelly to the facial surface. Using a low flame, gently heat and readapt the margins on the model so that the entire tooth is covered, taking care to avoid overlapping onto the gingiva.
10. After readaptation of all the margins, retrim excess material. If any areas appear to be too short or if accidental perforation occurs, simply reheat the tray and stretch the material by pushing it in the desired direction.
11. Leave the tray on the model until the delivery appointment, at which time it should be washed in cold, soapy water and then cold-sterilized.

Recall

19. Of the three types of custom trays discussed, which technique uses a more hazardous material?
20. Which type of custom tray is made for a vital bleaching procedure?
21. In which two forms is acrylic resin supplied?
22. Which type of material is used for a vacuum-formed custom tray?
23. What is the purpose of a spacer?
24. How are undercuts corrected on a model when preparing a custom tray?

DENTAL WAXES

Dental waxes have specific purposes in a clinical procedure, as well as in the laboratory area. These waxes can be made from *natural* products, such as beeswax, gum, fats, fatty acids, and oils, or from *synthetic* products, which are made to have certain qualities that cannot be attained from natural sources.

Boxing Wax

Boxing wax is a soft, pliable wax with a smooth, shiny appearance. It is supplied in long, narrow strips measuring 1 to 1½ inches wide by 12 to 18 inches long (Fig. 47-10).

Boxing wax is often used to form a wall or box around a preliminary impression when pouring it up, producing a cleaner model without the need to trim as much material.

Utility Wax

Utility wax is a soft, pliable wax with a slightly tacky consistency. This type of wax is supplied in different forms depending on its use. Utility wax can be purchased in strips, sticks, or rope form (Fig. 47-11). It is made of beeswax, petrolatum, and other soft waxes. Uses of utility wax include extending the borders of an impression tray and covering brackets in orthodontic treatment when they are irritating the cheek or lips.

Sticky Wax

Sticky wax is a very brittle wax, but when it is heated, it becomes very tacky and is useful in creating a wax pattern or joining acrylic resin together. This type of wax is supplied in sticks or blocks. Its main ingredients are beeswax and resin.

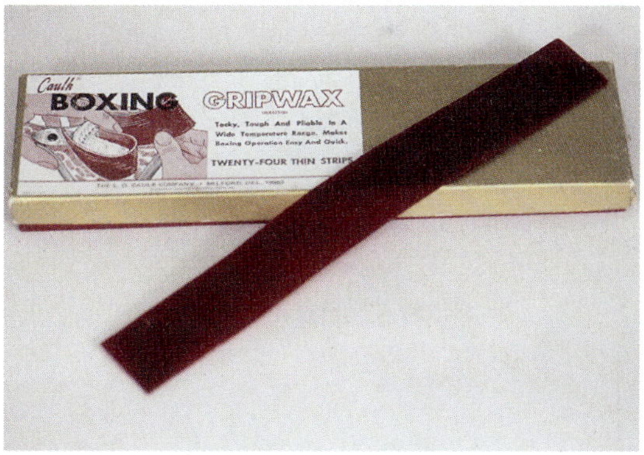

Fig. 47-10 Boxing wax.

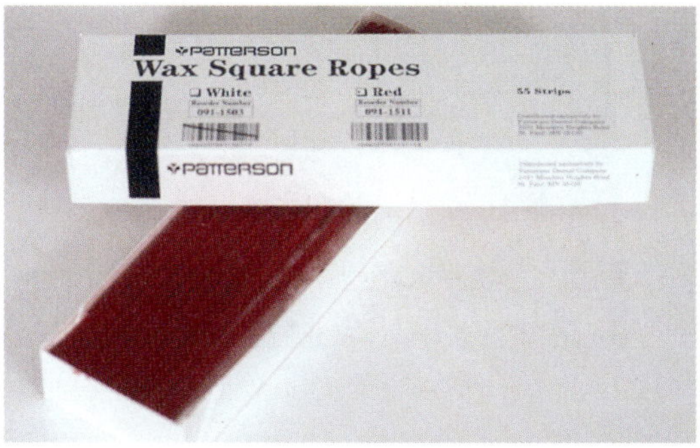

Fig. 47-11 Utility wax.

Inlay Casting Wax

Inlay wax is a hard, brittle wax made from paraffin wax, carnauba wax, resin, and beeswax (Fig. 47-12). The dental laboratory technician uses this wax to create a pattern of the indirect restoration on a model.

Inlay waxes are classified according to how they flow (hardness), as follows:

Type A is a hard wax used for indirect wax patterns.

Type B is a medium inlay wax and can be used for wax patterns directly in the mouth in a cavity preparation.

Type C is a soft inlay wax used for indirect waxing techniques in the dental laboratory.

Casting Wax

Like inlay wax, casting waxes are used for single-tooth indirect restorations and fixed bridges and for casting metal portions of a partial denture. The wax is supplied in sheets of various thicknesses. The makeup of casting wax is paraffin, ceresin, beeswax, and resins.

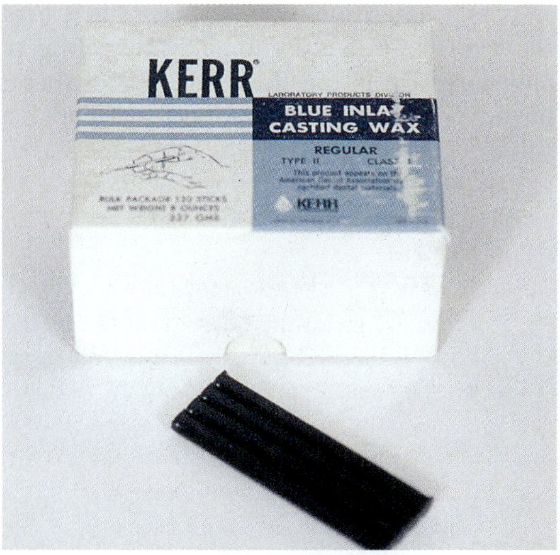

Fig. 47-12 Inlay casting wax.

Baseplate Wax

Baseplate wax is used to record the occlusal rims, for the initial arch form for setting denture teeth, and for denture wax-up. It is hard and brittle at room temperature. Baseplate wax is supplied in sheets and is made from paraffin or ceresin with beeswax and carnauba wax (Fig. 47-13).

The American Dental Association (ADA) classifies baseplate wax as the following three types:

Type I is a softer wax used for denture construction.

Type II is a wax of medium hardness used in moderate climates.

Type III is a harder wax for use in tropical climates.

Bite Registration Wax

Bite registration waxes are soft and very similar to casting waxes. After the wax is softened under warm water, the patient is instructed to bite down so that the wax forms an imprint of the teeth.

Bite wafers are another example of bite registration wax (Fig. 47-14). This wax is preformed in a horseshoe shape with a thin sheet of aluminum foil between the layers.

Recall

25. What type of wax is used to form a wall around a preliminary impression when pouring it up?

26. To extend an impression tray, what type of wax would you use?

27. What type of wax would you use to obtain a patient's bite impression?

28. What is the most common wax used to create a pattern for an indirect restoration?

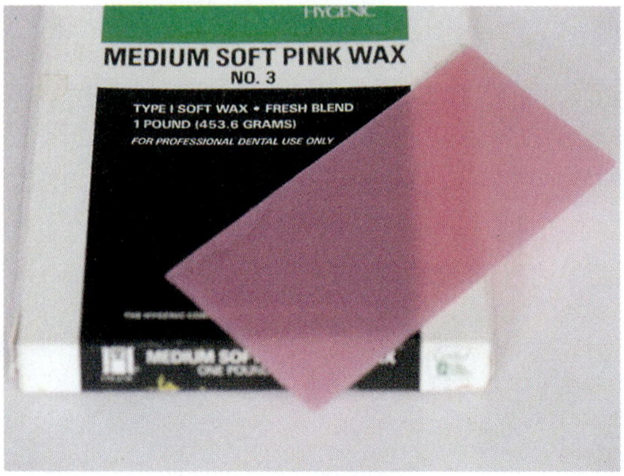

Fig. 47-13 Baseplate wax.

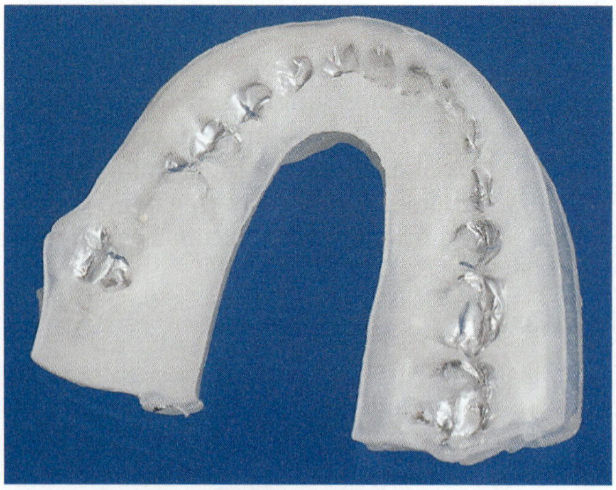
Fig. 47-14 Bite registration wax.

Patient Education

Dental models can be one of the most useful tools in explaining and educating patients about their own mouth. The dentist will use these models when presenting a treatment plan for fixed and removable prosthodontics, pediatrics, orthodontics, surgical procedures, and implants.

Because of their importance, your role in pouring, trimming, and polishing diagnostic models will benefit the patient greatly. Remember that your expertise in this procedure represents your skills as well as the dentist's expertise.

Eye to the Future

As dentistry becomes more sophisticated, dentists will seek more highly skilled dental assistants for the performance of laboratory procedures to provide the optimum treatment for their patients. Dental schools are teaching fewer laboratory skills to dental students, which in turn makes dentists more dependent on the skills and knowledge of the dental assistant and dental laboratory technician. As a dental assistant, it will be important for you to take a more active role in keeping up with procedures and materials used in the dental laboratory setting.

Legal and Ethical Implications

As a clinical dental assistant, you may find that your artistic and creative abilities promote interest in a hands-on role with laboratory procedures. If you find that making custom trays, trimming and finishing dental models, and performing additional laboratory functions are areas of interest, you might consider furthering your skills by taking continuing education courses in these areas.

The more responsibility that you obtain in the laboratory setting, the more aware you must be of the legal limitations in what procedures a dental assistant can perform in your state.

Critical Thinking

1. You are preparing a preliminary impression to be poured with plaster. How would you ready the impression before pouring it up?
2. You have measured the water and weighed the plaster correctly for a maxillary impression and base. A few seconds after you begin mixing, you notice that the mix is very dry. You know you measured correctly. Offer reasons why this happened.
3. It has been approximately 30 minutes since you poured up the maxillary impression and base. As you remove the impression from the model, two anterior teeth break off. Discuss possible reasons why this happened.
4. In your own words, describe the trimming process of the maxillary and mandibular model.
5. The dentist has asked you to prepare a vital bleaching tray. What types of procedures are involved in the making of a bleaching tray?

Part 10

Assisting in Comprehensive Dental Care

Practicing as a clinical dental assistant is one of the most challenging and rewarding professions in dentistry. The diversity of clinical responsibilities is unlimited in both the general and specialized settings.

The chapters in this section are intended to provide a level of knowledge and skill that will prepare you for clinical dentistry. As you progress and demonstrate competence in the general and specialized areas of dentistry, you will be better prepared for graduation, the Dental Assisting National Board, and a career in dental assisting.

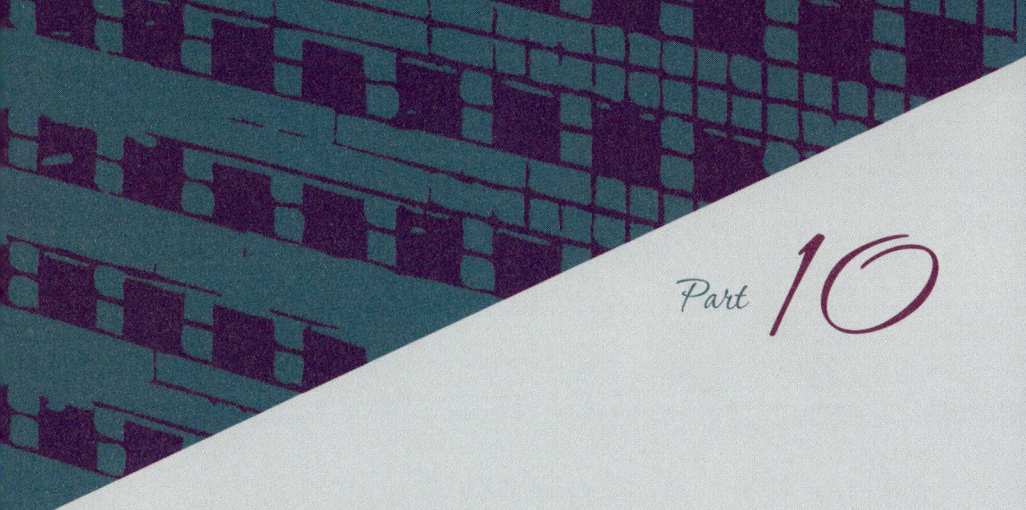

48

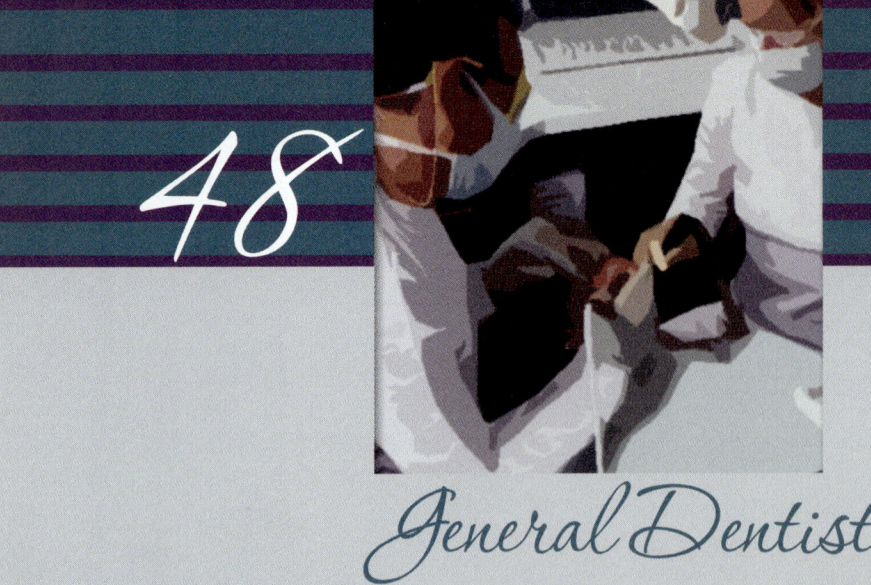

General Dentistry

Outline

Cavity Preparation
- Terminology
- Initial Preparation
- Final Preparation

Permanent Restorations
- Class I Restorations
- *Procedure 48-1: Assisting in a Class I Restoration*
- Class II Restorations
- *Procedure 48-2: Assisting in a Class II Amalgam Restoration*
- Class III and IV Restorations
- *Procedure 48-3: Assisting in a Class III or IV Restoration*
- Class V Restorations
- *Procedure 48-4: Assisting in a Class V Restoration*

Complex Restorations
- Retention Pins

Intermediate Restorations
- *Procedure 48-5: Placing and Carving an Intermediate Restoration (Expanded Function)*

Veneers
- *Procedure 48-6: Assisting in the Placement of a Veneer*

Tooth Whitening
- Treatment Options
- Abuse of Whitening Products
- Assistant's Role and Patient Instructions in Tooth Whitening

Patient Education

Legal and Ethical Implications

Eye to the Future

Critical Thinking

KEY TERMS

Axial wall (**ak**-see-ul) Internal surface of a cavity preparation positioned in the same vertical direction as the pulp within the tooth.

Cavity Pitted area in a tooth caused by decay.

Cavity preparation Process of decay removal and tooth design in the preparation for restoring a tooth.

Cavity wall Internal surface of a cavity preparation.

Convenience form Cavity preparation step that allows the dentist easier access when restoring a tooth.

Diastema (*di*-uh-**stee**-muh) A space between two teeth.

Esthetic dentistry (es-**theh**-tik) Type of dentistry that improves the appearance of teeth by camouflaging defects and whitening teeth.

Line angle Junction of two walls in a cavity preparation.

Operative dentistry Common term used when describing restorative and esthetic dentistry.

Outline form Design and initial depth of sound tooth structure used by the dentist when restoring a tooth.

Pulpal wall (**puhl**-puhl) Surface of the cavity preparation perpendicular to the pulp of a tooth.

Resistance form (ri-**zis**-tun[t]s) Shape and placement of cavity walls in the preparation of tooth restoration.

Restoration The use of a dental material to restore a tooth or teeth to a functional permanent unit.

Restorative dentistry (ri-**stor**-ah-tiv) Type of dentistry that restores teeth by removing decay and restoring defects.

Retention form (ri-**ten**[t]-shun) The shaping of the cavity walls to aid in retaining the restoration.

Retention (retentive) pin Basis of a stronger system used to retain and support a tooth restoration.

Veneer (vuh-**nir**) Thin layer of composite resin or porcelain bonded or cemented to a prepared facial surface.

LEARNING OUTCOMES

On completion of this chapter, the student will be able to achieve the following objectives:

- Define, spell, and pronounce the Key Terms.
- Describe the process and principles of cavity preparation.
- Discuss the differences in assisting with an amalgam versus a composite restoration.
- Discuss why retention pins would be selected for a complex restorative procedure.
- Describe the need for placement of an intermediate restoration.
- Describe the procedure of composite veneers.
- Describe tooth-whitening procedures and the role of the dental assistant.

PERFORMANCE OUTCOMES

On completion of this chapter, the student will be able to achieve competency standards in the following skills:

- Prepare the setup and assist in a class I restoration.
- Prepare the setup and assist in a class II restoration.
- Prepare the setup and assist in a class III restoration.
- Prepare the setup and assist in a class IV restoration.
- Prepare the setup and assist in a class V restoration.
- Prepare the setup and place and carve an intermediate restoration (*expanded function*).

Restorative and esthetic dentistry, also referred to as **operative dentistry,** is an integral part of general dentistry, and one of the primary responsibilities of the general dentist. This chapter presents the background knowledge and describes the techniques necessary for the clinical dental assistant to learn in restorative and esthetic procedures such as amalgam restorations, composite resin restorations, intermediate restorations, resin veneers, and tooth-whitening procedures.

Restorative dentistry is indicated when teeth must be restored to their original structure by the use of direct and indirect restorative materials. Specific conditions that determine the need for restorative dentistry include:

- Initial or recurring decay **(cavities)**
- Replacement of failed restorations
- Abrasion or wearing away of tooth structure
- Erosion of tooth structure

Esthetic dentistry is primarily devoted to improving the appearance of teeth by either restoring imperfections with direct and indirect restorative materials, or with the use of whitening techniques. Specific conditions that initiate a need for esthetic treatment include the following:

- Discoloration due to extrinsic or intrinsic staining
- Anomalies caused by developmental disturbances
- Abnormal spacing between teeth
- Trauma

CAVITY PREPARATION

In order for the dental team to restore a tooth to its normal function and still maintain its esthetic appearance, the dentist masters a technique that involves specific steps to complete the process of restorative dentistry. When preparing a tooth for a permanent **restoration,** the dentist has the necessary knowledge about the direction of the enamel rods, the thickness of the enamel, the body of the dentin, the size and position of the pulp, and the crown of the tooth as it relates to the gingiva.

Terminology

The understanding of the terminology of cavity preparation aids in the sequencing of the steps by enabling the assistant to have dental instruments, dental accessories, and dental materials ready at the appropriate times throughout a procedure. This specific terminology refers to anatomic structures as they relate to cavity preparation, which is especially helpful for the expanded-functions dental assistant (EFDA) in the application of dental materials and intermediate restorations.

Cavity preparation is the process of removing unhealthy tooth structure while leaving a limited amount of healthy tooth structure for the tooth to maintain a restoration. The principles of cavity preparation are divided into two stages, each with several steps. The dentist follows these steps in an exact order so that ideal results are achieved.

Initial Preparation

Cavity preparation involves the initial design and extension of the preparation's external walls to a limited depth. This is completed in order to gain access to the decay or defect and reach sound tooth structure. The steps in initial cavity preparation are as follows:

1. The dentist decides on an **outline form** (design) and initial depth of sound tooth structure (Fig. 48-1).
2. The dentist determines the primary **resistance form,** which is the shape and placement of cavity walls (Fig. 48-2).

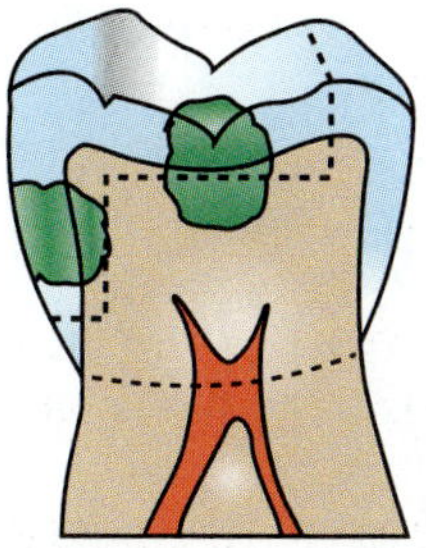

Fig. 48-1 Outline form of a cavity preparation.

Terminology in Understanding Cavity Preparation

Cavity wall: Internal surface of the tooth prepared for the restoration.

Internal wall: Cavity wall/surface that does not extend to the external tooth surface.

External wall: Surface of the tooth preparation that extends to the external tooth surface, named according to the tooth surface involved: distal, mesial, facial, lingual, and gingival.

Axial wall: Internal wall/surface of the prepared tooth that runs parallel to the long axis of the tooth.

Pulpal wall: Internal wall/surface of a prepared tooth that is perpendicular to the long axis of the tooth; also known as the *pulpal floor.*

Line angle: Angle formed by the junction of two walls/surface in a cavity preparation (similar to the angle formed where two walls of a room meet to form a corner). To identify a line angle, the names of the two involved walls/surfaces are combined. For example, the angle formed by the *mesial* and *lingual* walls is called the *mesiolingual line angle;* the suffix *-al* of mesial is dropped and the letter *o* added. The two terms are then combined to form the term *mesiolingual.* It is important not to confuse the names of these angles with the names used to describe the surfaces involved in the restoration itself.

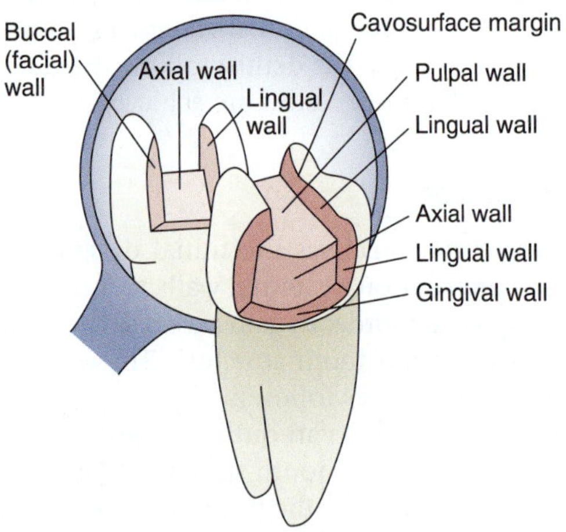

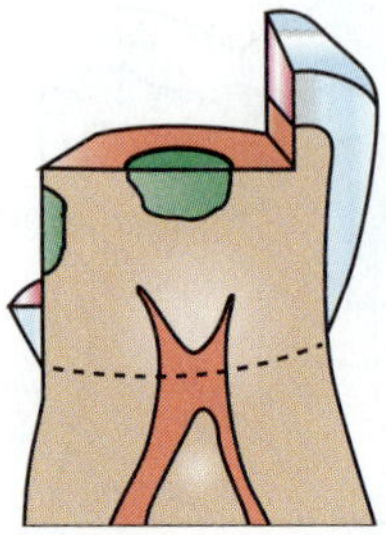

Fig. 48-2 Resistance form of a cavity preparation.

3. The dentist knows where to place **retention form,** which will resist displacement or removal of the restoration (Fig. 48-3).
4. The dentist will follow **convenience form,** which provides accessibility in preparing and restoring the tooth (Fig. 48-4).

Final Preparation

After the tooth has been readied with the initial cavity preparation, the dentist continues the procedure with the steps in the final cavity preparation:

1. Remove of any remaining enamel in the preparation, infected dentin, or old restorative material (or a combination).
2. Insert additional resistance and retention notches, grooves, and coves to provide strength in the maintenance of the restoration.
3. Place protective dental materials, which could include lining agents, bases, and desensitizing or bonding agents for pulpal protection and better retention.

Recall

1. What is restorative and esthetic dentistry often referred to as?
2. What is a common term used to describe decay?
3. Which step in the initial preparation allows the dentist to determine the shape and placement of the cavity walls?
4. What wall of a cavity preparation is perpendicular to the long axis of the tooth?

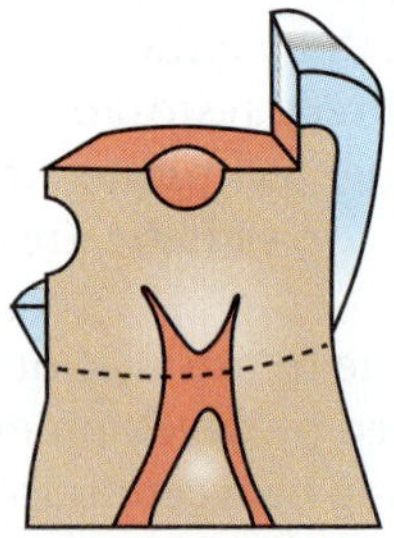

Fig. 48-3 Retention form placed in the cavity preparation.

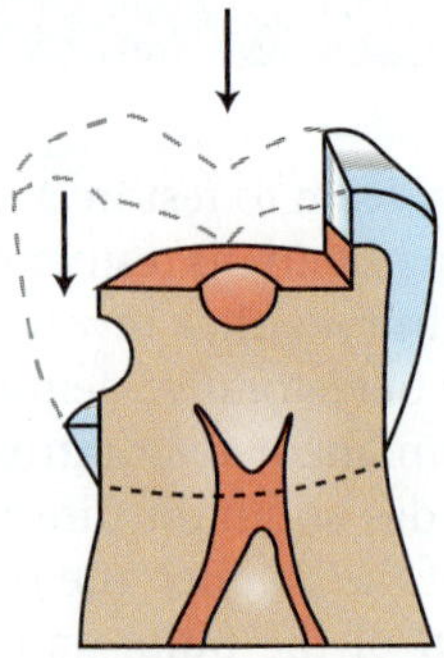

Fig. 48-4 Convenience form is used for easy access to tooth decay.

PERMANENT RESTORATIONS

Before treatment begins, the following preparatory steps are taken to ensure patient comfort and safety:

- Inform the patient about the upcoming procedure and what to expect during the treatment. The patient must always give informed consent before the dentist continues with the procedure.
- Position the patient correctly for the dentist and the type of procedure.
- Explain each step to the patient as the procedure progresses.

The dental assistant has the following responsibilities throughout a restorative dental procedure:

- Be familiar with the procedure and anticipate the dentist's needs.
- Prepare the setup for the restorative procedure.
- Provide moisture control and better visualization for the dentist by using high-velocity suction and air-water syringe.
- Transfer dental instruments and accessories.
- Mix and transfer dental materials.
- Perform any expanded functions.
- Maintain patient comfort and appropriate infection-control precautions.

Permanent restorations can be everything from a small conservative restoration to an extensive multisurface foundation. With the exception of steps added to the procedures by involving supplementary accessories and dental materials, restorative procedures will follow a standardized plan.

Class I Restorations

The class I cavity, or *lesion,* is typically small and involves the pits and fissures of teeth. Because the anatomic features of posterior teeth accumulate plaque and debris, it is difficult for the patient to keep this area clean. Therefore the pits and fissures are very susceptible to decay. Class I decay involves the following areas of concern:

- Occlusal pits and fissures of premolars and molars (Fig. 48-5, *A*)
- Buccal pits and fissures of mandibular molars (Fig. 48-5, *B*)
- Lingual pits and fissures of maxillary molars (Fig. 48-5, *C*)
- Lingual pits of maxillary incisors, most frequently near the cingulum (Fig. 48-5, *D*)

Tooth Preparation

The occlusal or lingual class I cavity preparation is a simple preparation for the dentist. The outline of the cavity preparation involves the pit, groove, or fissures that are decayed. The dentist uses a bur to open the enamel, taking care not to create any sharp angles or corners within the preparation. This preparation should be smooth throughout the internal structure.

Steps in a Restorative Procedure

1. Evaluate the tooth to be restored (see Chapter 28).
2. Obtain local anesthesia (see Chapter 37).
3. Determine the type of moisture control to be used during the procedure (cotton roll, dry angles, dental dam; see Chapter 36).
4. Prepare the tooth for the restoration (including the use of dental hand instruments and dental handpieces with rotary instruments; see Chapters 34 and 35).
5. Determine the type of dental materials to be used (see Chapters 43 and 44).
6. Apply the dental materials.
7. Burnish, carve, or finish the dental material.
8. Check the occlusion of the restoration.
9. Finish and polish the restoration.

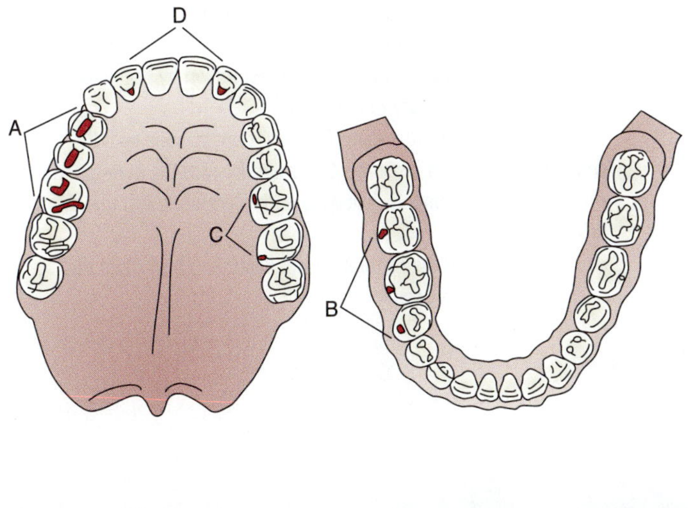

Fig. 48-5 Class I restorations. **A,** Occlusal pits and fissures of premolar/molar. **B,** Buccal pits and fissures of mandibular molars. **C,** Lingual pits and fissures of maxillary molars. **D,** Lingual pits of maxillary incisors.

The restoration's location in the mouth will determine the type of permanent restorative material used. Because class I lesions are small restorations and most likely will not interfere with occlusal forces, the dentist usually selects *composite resin* material for the permanent restoration.

Special Considerations

Because most class I restorations occur on the occlusal surface, the dentist must evaluate the patient's occlusion before replacing tooth structure. An easy way for the dentist to review how the tooth occludes with an opposing tooth is to mark the occlusion with *articulating paper* before beginning the restorative process (see Procedure 48-1).

Procedure 48-1 Assisting in a Class I Restoration

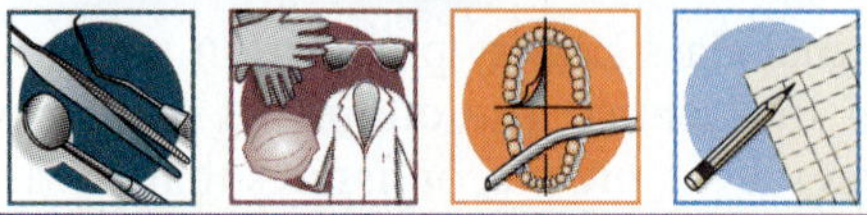

Equipment and Supplies

- Restorative tray (basic setup, hand cutting instruments, composite placement instrument, amalgam carrier, condensers, burnishers, carvers, articulating paper holder)
- Local anesthetic setup
- Dental dam setup
- High-volume oral evacuator (HVE) tip
- Saliva ejector
- High-speed and low-speed handpieces
- Burs, assorted (dentist's choice)
- Cotton pellets, cotton rolls, 2- × 2-inch gauze
- Dental liners, base, sealers, bonding agents
- Permanent restorative material (composite or amalgam)
- Dental floss

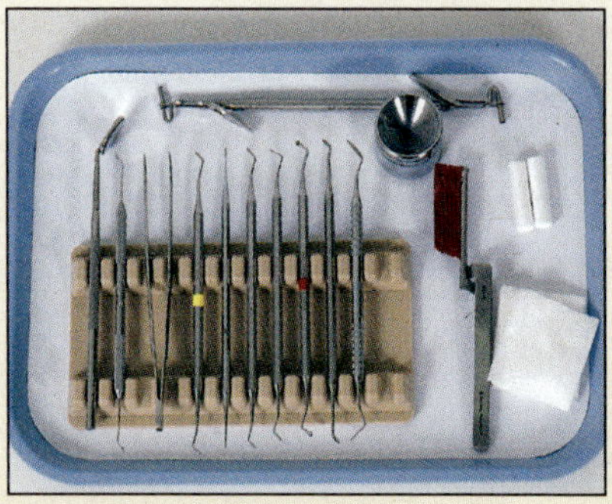

PROCEDURAL STEPS

Preparing the Tooth

1. Transfer the mouth mirror and explorer to the dentist.
   Purpose: The dentist will examine the tooth to be prepared.
2. Assist in administration of the topical and local anesthetic agent.
3. Place and secure cotton rolls or dental dam.

Preparing the Cavity

1. Transfer the mirror and the high-speed handpiece with a cutting bur to the dentist.
2. During cavity preparation, use the HVE and air-water syringe, adjust the light, and retract the patient's cheek as necessary to maintain a clear field for the dentist.
   Purpose: With efficient placement and use of the HVE and air-water syringe, the dentist will maintain a clear operating field, with comfort to the patient.
3. Transfer the explorer, excavators, and hand cutting instruments as needed throughout the cavity preparation.

Placing Dental Materials

1. Rinse and dry the preparation for the dentist to evaluate.
2. If a base, liner, or sealer is required, mix and transfer these materials in proper sequence.
3. After the tooth is etched and primed, prepare and transfer the bonding material to the dentist before insertion of the permanent material.
4. If using amalgam, activate the capsule, place in the amalgamator, close the cover, and mix according to recommended time.
5. If using composite, place a small amount of universal color material on a paper pad and cover it from the light.

Placing Permanent Material

1. With amalgam, fill the smaller end of the amalgam carrier and transfer the carrier to the dentist for placement, having the condenser in the transfer position ready for use.
2. Assist as the process of placing and condensing the amalgam is repeated until the preparation is slightly overfilled.
3. When the preparation is slightly overfilled, exchange the condenser for the burnisher so that the dentist can burnish the surface and margins of the restoration.
   Purpose: This strengthens the finished restoration by burnishing the excess mercury to the surface.
4. With composite, carry the material to the transfer zone with the composite placement instrument. The dentist adds the material to the preparation in increments, following each placement with the curing light.
   Note: The depth of the restoration will determine how often the curing light is used.

Procedure 48-1 Assisting in a Class I Restoration—cont'd

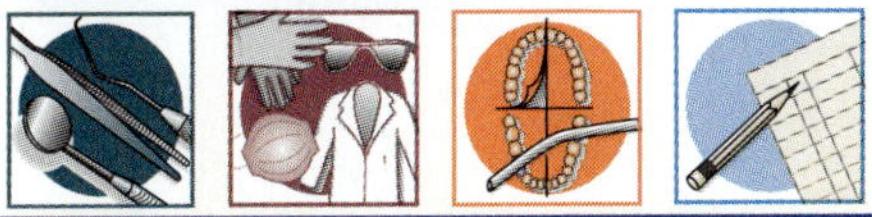

Final Carving or Finishing

1. For amalgam, transfer the carvers until the carving is complete.
2. For composite, transfer the high-speed handpiece with finishing burs.
3. Keep the tip of the HVE close to the restoration during the carving and finishing process.
   Purpose: To remove all particles as soon as possible. This step is especially important when a dental dam is not used.

Occlusal Adjustment

1. Remove the cotton rolls or the dental dam, and rinse and dry the area.
2. Place articulating paper to check the occlusion, instructing the patient to close teeth together *very* gently.
   Note: Heavy blue marks will appear on any high spots on the new restoration. If the patient bites too hard, the restoration may fracture.
3. Assist with transfers or as necessary while the dentist uses a carver or finishing bur to remove any remaining high spots.
   Note: This step is repeated as often as necessary to bring the new restoration into proper occlusion.
4. Transfer a moistened cotton pellet or cotton roll to gently clean the surface of the restoration.
   Purpose: To remove any remaining small surface irregularities.

Postoperative Instructions

1. Caution the patient not to chew on a new amalgam restoration for a few hours.
   Purpose: Amalgam takes several hours to reach its maximum strength, and biting on it could cause the restoration to fracture.

Date	Tooth	Surface	Charting Notes
7/20/05	3	O	1 carpule Xylocaine w/o epi, cotton roll isolation, liner, Sybralloy, Pt tolerated procedure fine. OK T. Clark, CDA/L. Stewart, DDS

Class II Restorations

The class II lesion is an extension of the class I cavity into a proximal surface(s) of premolars and molars. The proximal surfaces of a tooth can be more difficult to keep decay free, especially if a patient is not disciplined at routine flossing. Class II decay involves the following areas:

- Two-surface restoration of a posterior tooth (Fig. 48-6*A*)
- Three-surface restoration of a posterior tooth (Fig. 48-6*B*)
- Multisurface restoration (four or more surfaces) of a posterior tooth (Fig. 48-6*C*)

Tooth Preparation

Because of the difficulty in reaching the proximal surfaces with a handpiece or hand instrument, the dentist will involve the occlusal surface in the preparation and restoration of the tooth. A class II restoration can be *conservative,* involving two surfaces of the tooth, or *comprehensive,* involving four or more surfaces with the removal of a cusp. The decay may extend from the enamel into the dentin, which would also require additional retention placed in the cavity preparation and the use of bonding materials.

Amalgam or composite resin can be used as a direct restorative material for a class II procedure. The dentist most often selects *amalgam* for its strength and qualities required for a class II restoration.

Special Considerations

The outline of a class II preparation involves the removal of one or both of the proximal surfaces. Because there is no wall or tooth structure to hold the material in place, a *matrix system* must be used for this procedure. (See Chapter 49 and Procedure 48-2.)

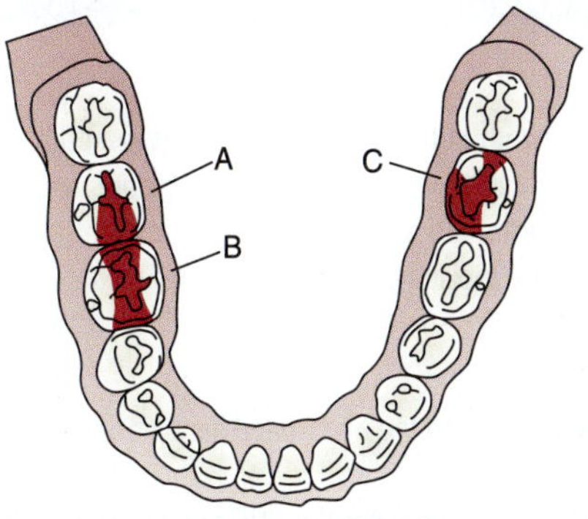

Fig. 48-6 Class II restorations. **A,** Two-surface restoration. **B,** Three-surface restoration. **C,** Multisurface restoration. (From Baum L, et al: *Textbook of operative dentistry,* ed 3, Philadelphia, 1995, Saunders.)

Procedure 48-2 Assisting in a Class II Amalgam Restoration

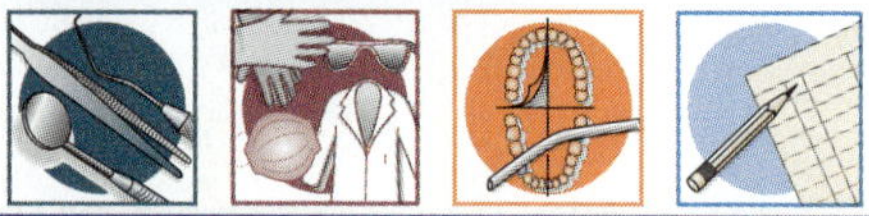

Equipment and Supplies

- Restorative tray (basic setup, hand cutting instruments, composite placement instrument, amalgam carrier, condensers, burnishers, carvers, articulating paper holder)
- Local anesthetic setup
- Dental dam setup
- High-volume oral evacuator (HVE) tip
- Saliva ejector
- High-speed and low-speed handpieces
- Burs, assorted (dentist's choice)
- Matrix setup
- Dental liners, base, sealers, bonding agents
- Premeasured amalgam capsules
- Dental floss
- Articulating paper
- Cotton pellets, cotton rolls, 2- × 2-inch gauze
- Dental floss

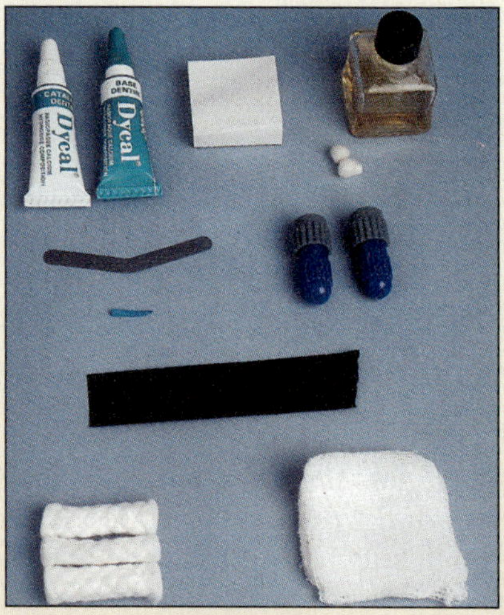

PROCEDURAL STEPS

Preparing the Tooth

1. Transfer the mouth mirror and explorer to the dentist.
   Purpose: The dentist examines the tooth to be prepared.
2. Assist in administration of the local anesthetic agent.
3. Place and secure moisture-control techniques (cotton roll, dental dam).

Preparing the Cavity

1. Transfer the mirror and the high-speed handpiece with cutting bur to the dentist.
2. During cavity preparation, use the HVE and air-water syringe, adjust the light, and retract the patient's cheek as necessary to maintain a clear field for the dentist.
   Purpose: With efficient placement and use of the HVE and air-water syringe, the dentist will maintain a clear operating field, with comfort to the patient.
3. Transfer the explorer, excavators, and hand cutting instruments as needed throughout the cavity preparation.

Placing the Base and Cavity Liner (Expanded Function)

1. After examination, rinse and dry the preparation. Mix and place any necessary cavity liners or bases.

Placing the Matrix Band and Wedge (Expanded Function)

1. Assist in placing the preassembled universal (Tofflemire) retainer and matrix.
2. Assist in placing the wedge or wedges in the proximal box using cotton pliers or #110 pliers.

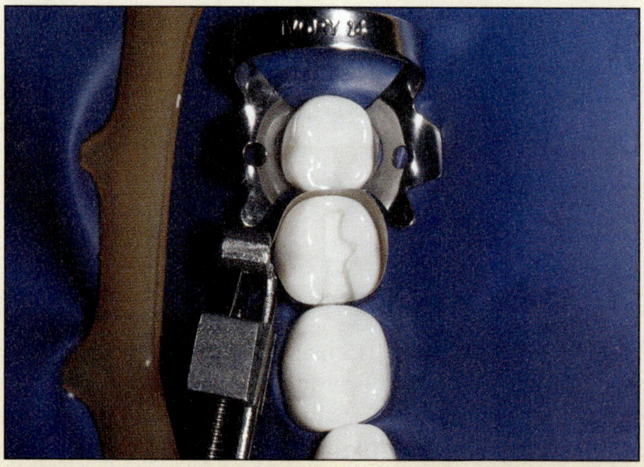

Placing the Bonding Agent (Expanded Function)

1. After the tooth is etched and primed, assist the dentist in preparing and placing the bonding material.

Mixing the Amalgam

1. Activate the capsule, place in the amalgamator, close the cover, and set the timer for the time recommended by the manufacturer.
2. At the signal from the dentist, start the amalgamator.
3. Open the capsule, and remove the pestle with cotton pliers. Drop the amalgam into the amalgam well.
4. Reassemble and discard the capsule.
   Purpose: To prevent mercury vapor from escaping into the air.

Procedure 48-2 Assisting in a Class II Amalgam Restoration–cont'd

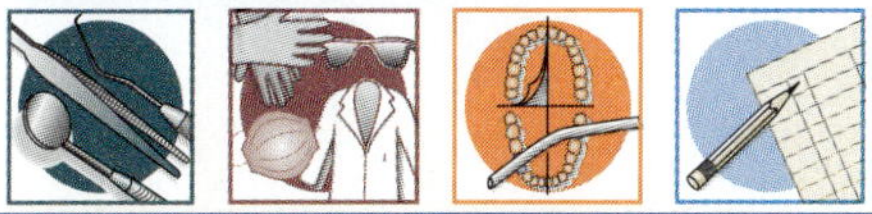

Placing and Condensing the Amalgam

1. Fill the smaller end of the amalgam carrier, and transfer the carrier to the dentist.
2. Assist when necessary as the dentist exchanges the carrier for a condenser and begins condensing the first increments of amalgam with the smaller end of the condenser.

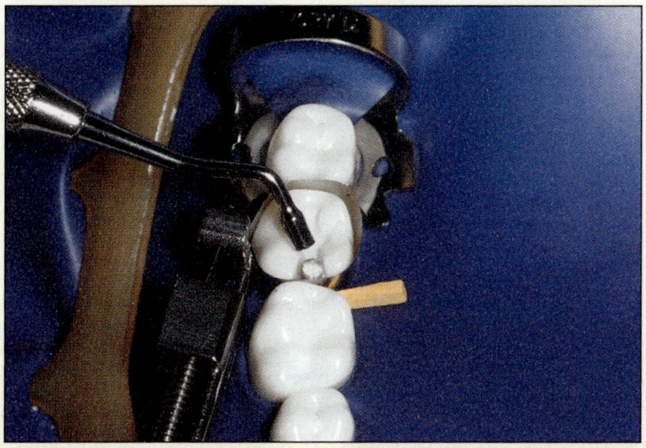

3. Assist as the process of placing and condensing the amalgam is repeated until the cavity is slightly overfilled.
4. When the cavity preparation is slightly overfilled, exchange the condenser for the burnisher so that the dentist can burnish the surface and margins of the restoration.
   Purpose: This strengthens the filled restoration by burnishing the excess mercury to the surface.

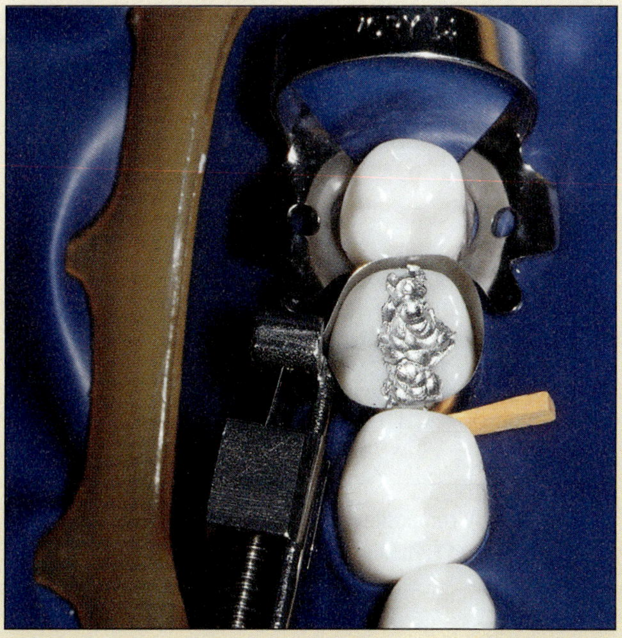

Initial Carving

1. Assist while the dentist uses an explorer and discoid/cleoid carver to remove the excess amalgam on the occlusal surface, from between the matrix band, and the marginal ridge of the tooth.
   Purpose: This prevents the restoration from fracturing during removal of the matrix band.

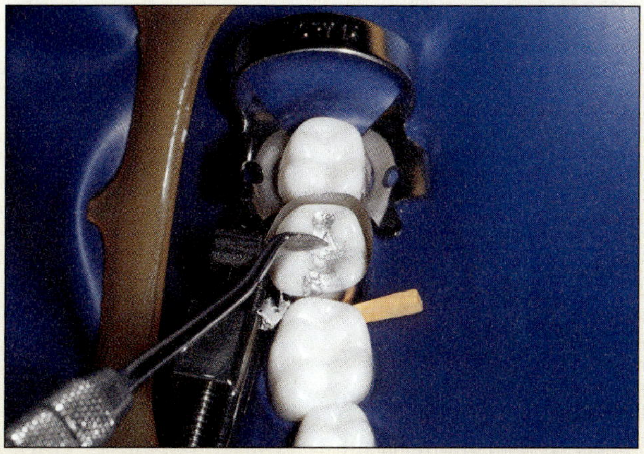

2. Assist in removing the Tofflemire retainer, matrix band, and wedge.

Final Carving

1. Transfer the amalgam carvers until the carving is complete.
2. Keep the tip of the HVE close to the restoration during the carving process.
   Purpose: To remove all amalgam particles as soon as possible.
   Note: This step is especially important when a dental dam is not used.

Occlusal Adjustment

1. Remove moisture-control materials (cotton rolls, dental dam).
2. Place articulating paper on the teeth to be checked, and instruct the patient to close the teeth together *very* gently.
   Note: Heavy blue marks will appear on any high spots on the new restoration. If the patient bites too hard, the restoration may fracture.

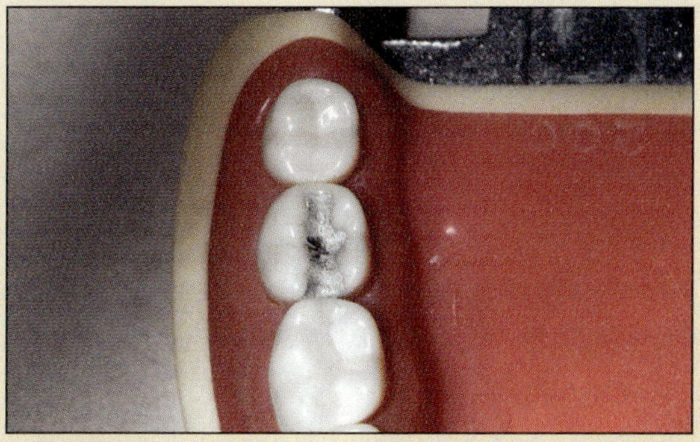

continued

Procedure 48-2 Assisting in a Class II Amalgam Restoration—cont'd

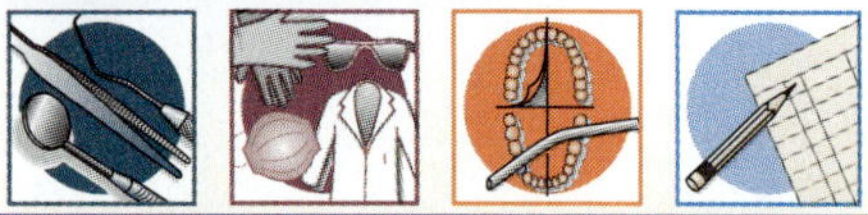

3. Assist with transfers as the dentist uses an amalgam carver to remove any remaining high spots.
   Note: This step is repeated as often as necessary to bring the new restoration into proper occlusion.
4. Transfer a moist cotton pellet in cotton pliers to rub gently the surface of the amalgam.
   Purpose: To remove any remaining small surface irregularities.

Postoperative Instructions

1. Caution the patient not to chew on the new restoration for a few hours.
   Purpose: Amalgam takes several hours to reach its maximum strength, and biting on it could cause the restoration to fracture.

Date	Tooth	Surface	Charting Notes
7/20/05	3	MO	1 carpule Xylocaine w/o epi, dam isolation, liner/bonding/Sybralloy, Pt tolerated procedure fine. T. Clark, CDA/L. Stewart, DDS

Class III and IV Restorations

A class III lesion affects the interproximal surface (mesial and distal) of incisors and canines (Fig. 48-7). The class IV cavity involves a larger surface area, which includes the incisal edge and the interproximal surface of incisors and canines (Fig. 48-8).

Tooth Preparation

The anatomy of these teeth is such that the dentist is able to access the anterior interproximal surface without affecting other surfaces of the tooth. If possible, the dentist will enter the tooth from the lingual surface to reduce the size of the restoration from the facial aspect. If the decay has moved subgingivally, special precautions are used in keeping the area isolated and dry during the restorative process.

Because incisors and canines are so visible, esthetics is a concern. The dentist will select *composite resin* when restoring the class III or IV cavity. It is important to pay special attention in the shade selection of the composite resin material. Use natural lighting, and involve the patient in the selection.

Special Considerations

It is advisable to use a dental dam during the preparation and restoration of class III and IV lesions. This isolation provides better retraction of gingival tissue and maintains a drier environment. The dentist will pay close attention to the contouring of a class III and IV restoration, being sure to reproduce the correct contours and contact. To help in the contouring process, a *Mylar matrix system* is used in the restoration process. (See Chapter 49 and Procedure 49-3.)

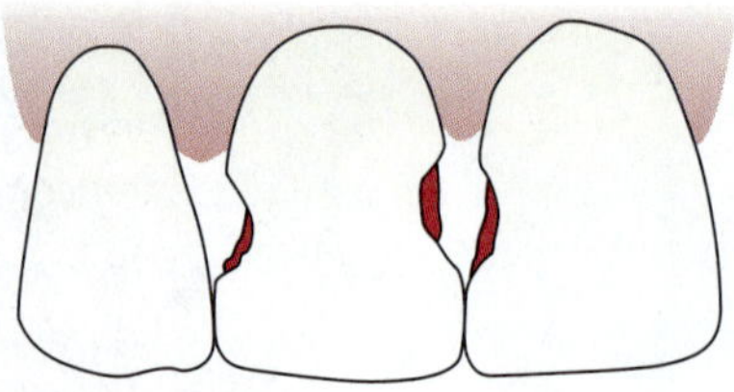

Fig. 48-7 Class III composite restoration. (From Baum L, et al: *Textbook of operative dentistry,* ed 3, Philadelphia, 1995, Saunders.)

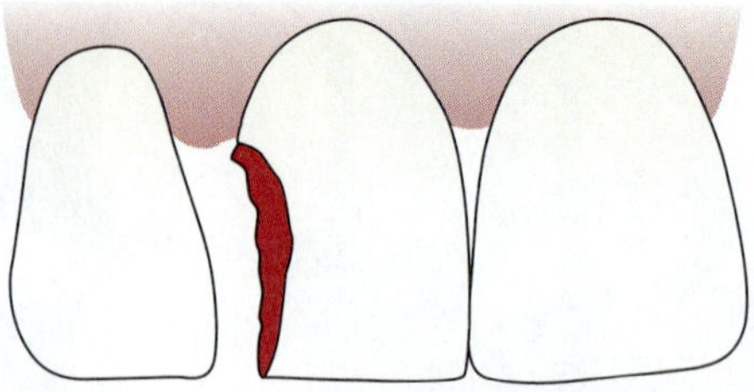

Fig. 48-8 Class IV composite restoration. (From Baum L, et al: *Textbook of operative dentistry,* ed 3, Philadelphia, 1995, Saunders.)

Procedure 48-3 Assisting in a Class III or IV Restoration

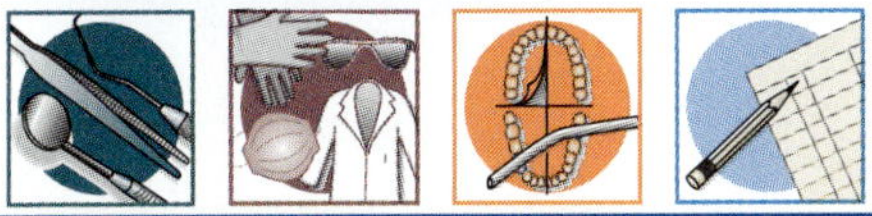

Equipment and Supplies

- Restorative tray (basic setup, hand cutting instruments, composite placement instrument, amalgam carrier, condensers, burnishers, carvers, articulating paper holder)
- Composite shade guide
- Local anesthetic setup
- Dental dam setup
- HVE tip
- Saliva ejector
- High-speed and low-speed handpieces
- Burs, assorted (dentist's choice)
- Mylar matrix setup
- Dental liners, base, sealers, bonding agents
- Composite material
- Curing light with protective shield
- Finishing burs and diamonds
- Dental floss
- Articulating paper
- Cotton pellets, cotton rolls, 2- × 2-inch gauze
- Dental floss
- Abrasive strips
- Articulating paper
- Polishing kit (disc and mandrel)
- Polishing paste

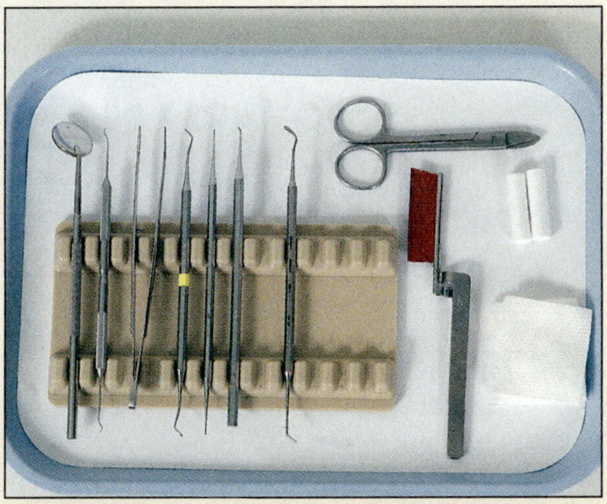

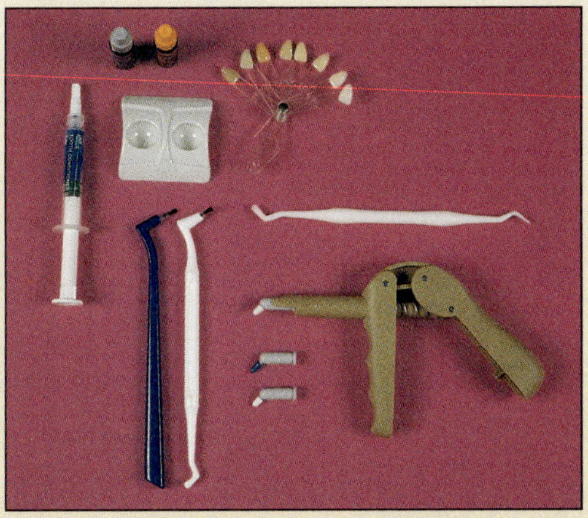

PROCEDURAL STEPS

Preparing the Tooth

1. Transfer the mouth mirror and explorer to the dentist.
   Purpose: The dentist examines the tooth to be prepared.
2. Assist in administration of the local anesthetic.
3. Assist in selection of the shade of the composite material.
4. Place and secure moisture-control techniques (cotton roll, dental dam).

Preparing the Cavity

1. Transfer the high-speed handpiece and hand cutting instruments so that the dentist can remove decayed tooth structure. Use the HVE to maintain a clear operating field.
2. Rinse and dry the tooth throughout the procedure. If indicated, place a cavity liner.

Etching, Bonding, and Composite Placement

1. After the preparation is etched, rinse and dry according to the manufacturer's instructions.
2. Assist in placing the matrix strip. If indicated, a wedge can also be placed.
3. Assist in the application of the primer and bonding resin, which are light-cured in accordance with the manufacturer's instructions.

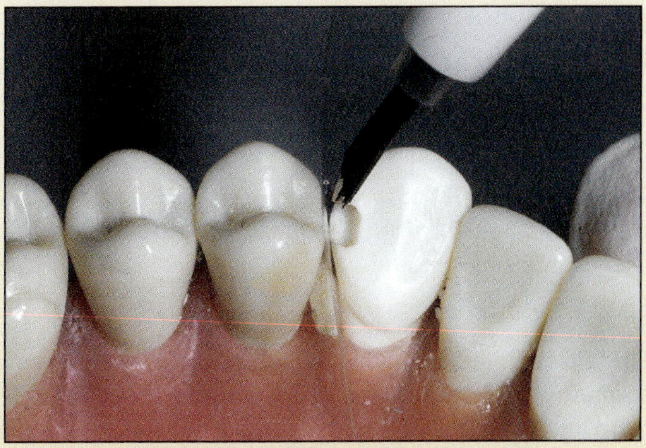

4. Dispense the composite material on a paper pad, or insert capsule into composite syringe, and transfer it along with the composite instrument to be placed into the preparation.

continued

Procedure 48-3 Assisting in a Class III or IV Restoration—cont'd

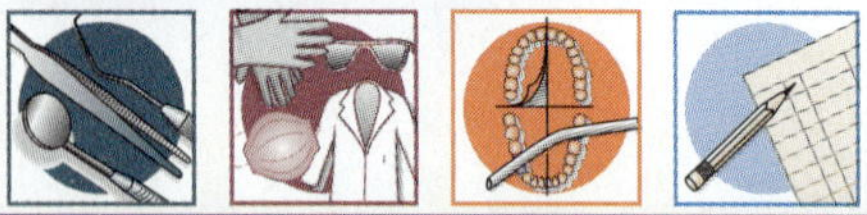

PROCEDURAL STEPS, cont'd

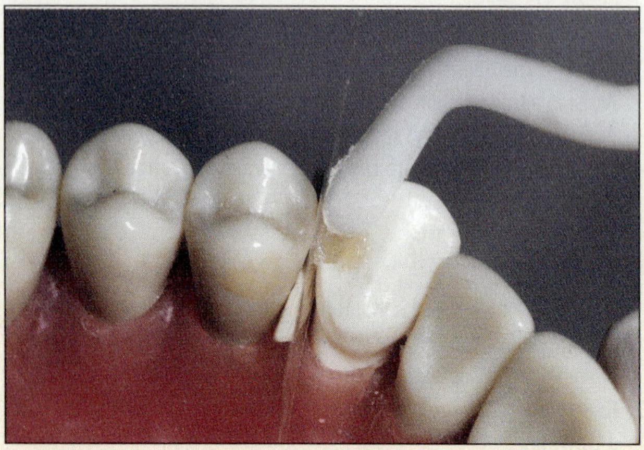

5. Assist as the matrix is pulled and held tightly around the tooth while the composite material is light-cured from the lingual and facial surfaces.

Finishing the Restoration

1. Remove the matrix strip and wedge.
2. Assist with transfers as the dentist uses finishing burs or diamonds in the high-speed handpiece to contour the restoration.
3. If indicated, transfer finishing strips for smoothing the interproximal surface.
4. Remove the moisture-control technique, and use articulating paper to check the occlusion. Adjustments are made as necessary.
5. Assist while the dentist uses polishing discs, points, and cups in the low-speed handpiece to polish the restoration.

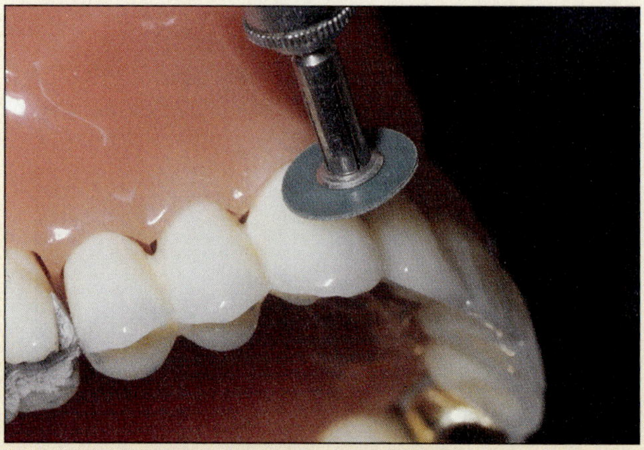

Date	Tooth	Surface	Charting Notes
7/20/05	8	MI	1 carpule Xylocaine w/o epi, cotton roll isolation, etching/bonding/Silux shade YL, Pt tolerated procedure fine. T. Clark, CDA/L. Stewart, DDS

Class V Restorations

The Class V restoration is classified as a *smooth surface restoration.* These decayed lesions occur in the gingival third of the facial or lingual surfaces of any tooth (Fig. 48-9). In the older population, class V lesions also tend to occur on the root of the tooth, near the cemento-enamel junction.

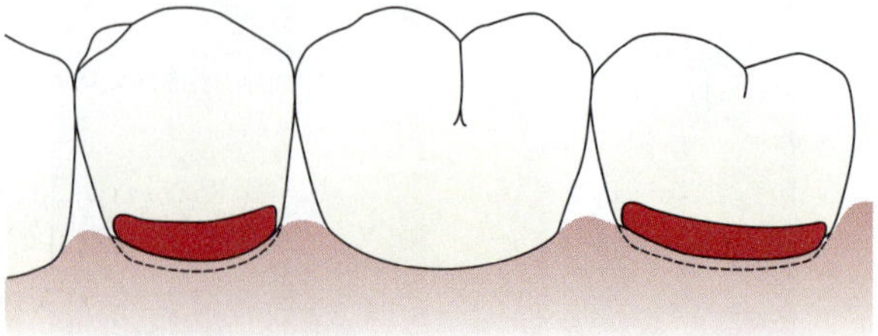

Fig. 48-9 Class V restoration. (From Baum L et al: *Textbook of operative dentistry,* ed 3, Philadelphia, 1995, Saunders.)

Tooth Preparation

As with the class I restorations, the class V lesion is prepared by having a smooth outline with no angles. The location of a class V lesion determines the type of material selected. The dentist would prefer to use a composite resin material for esthetic purposes, but the moisture-control factor in this area may prohibit its placement.

Special Considerations

One of the most important considerations for the dentist when restoring this area of the tooth is the proximity of the gingiva to the lesion. It is of utmost importance to be able to retract the gingiva away from the lesion during the preparation and restoration stages and keep the area as clean and dry as possible.

The application of the dental dam provides this added gingival retraction, but a cervical clamp should be used to move the dam subgingivally. If a dental dam is not placed, the dentist may select the placement of gingival retraction cord for better visibility and the reduction of moisture and hemorrhage from the area (see Procedure 48-4).

Procedure 48-4 Assisting in a Class V Restoration

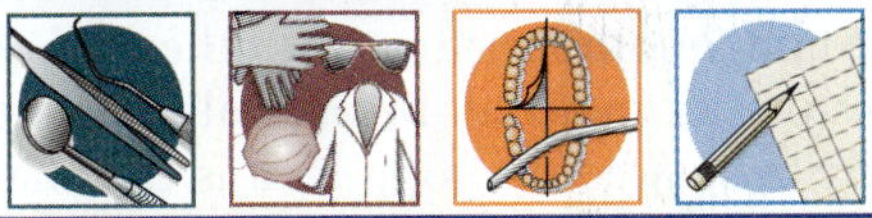

Equipment and Supplies

- Restorative tray (basic setup, hand cutting instruments, composite placement instrument, amalgam carrier, condensers, burnishers, carvers, articulating paper holder)
- Local anesthetic setup
- Dental dam setup (cervical clamp)
- Retraction cord and packer
- HVE tip
- Saliva ejector
- High-speed and low-speed handpieces
- Burs, assorted (dentist's choice)
- Cotton pellets, cotton rolls, 2-by-2–inch gauze
- Dental liners, base, sealers, bonding agents
- Permanent restorative material (composite or amalgam)
- Dental floss

PROCEDURAL STEPS

Preparing the Tooth

1. Transfer the mouth mirror and explorer to the dentist.
   Purpose: The dentist examines the tooth to be prepared.
2. Assist in administration of the topical and local anesthetic agent.
3. Place and secure cotton rolls or dental dam.

Preparing the Cavity

1. Transfer the mirror and the assembled high-speed handpiece with a cutting bur to the dentist.
2. During cavity preparation, use the HVE and air-water syringe, adjust the light, and retract the patient's cheek as necessary to maintain a clear field for the dentist.
   Purpose: With efficient placement and use of the HVE and the air-water syringe, the dentist will maintain a clear operating field, with comfort to the patient.
3. Transfer the explorer, excavators, and hand cutting instruments as needed throughout the cavity preparation.

Placing Dental Materials

1. Rinse and dry the preparation for evaluation. If a base, liner, or sealer is required, mix and transfer these materials in proper sequence.
2. After the tooth is etched and primed, prepare and transfer the bonding material to the dentist before the insertion of the permanent material.
3. If using amalgam, activate the capsule, place it in the amalgamator, close the cover, and mix according to the recommended time.
4. If using composite, place a small amount of universal color material on a paper pad, and cover it from the light.

Placing Permanent Material

1. With amalgam, fill the smaller end of the amalgam carrier and transfer the carrier to the dentist for placement, having the condenser in the transfer position ready for use.
2. Assist the dentist as the process of placing and condensing the amalgam is repeated until the preparation is slightly overfilled.
3. When the preparation is slightly overfilled, exchange the condenser for the burnisher so that the dentist can burnish the surface and margins of the restoration.
   Purpose: To strengthen the finished restoration by burnishing the excess mercury to the surface.
4. If using composite, carry the material to the transfer zone with the composite placement instrument. The dentist adds the material to the preparation in increments, following each placement with the curing light.
   Note: The depth of the restoration will determine how often the curing light is used.

Final Carving or Finishing

1. For amalgam, transfer the carvers until the carving is complete.
2. For composite, transfer the high-speed handpiece with finishing burs.
3. Keep the tip of the HVE close to the restoration during the carving and finishing process.
   Purpose: To remove all particles as soon as possible.
   Note: This step is especially important when a dental dam is not used.

Date	Tooth	Surface	Charting Notes
7/20/05	11	F	1 carpule Xylocaine w/o epi, dental dam isolation, etching/bonding/ Silux, shade Y, Pt tolerated procedure fine. T. Clark, CDA/L. Stewart, DDS

Recall

5. Where would you find a class I restoration in the mouth?
6. How many surfaces can be involved in a class II restoration?
7. Would a class II restoration be located in anterior or posterior teeth?
8. What restorative material would you set up for a class IV procedure?
9. What kind of moisture control is recommended for class III and IV restorations?
10. What population has a higher incidence of class V lesions?

COMPLEX RESTORATIONS

At times the loss of tooth structure will become greater than the remaining natural tooth structure. In these cases the dentist must decide whether to (1) move ahead and restore the tooth with a direct restorative material or (2) change the treatment plan and place an indirect restorative material. If the dentist and patient agree to move ahead with a direct restoration, there are additional techniques used to help in retaining the restoration.

Retention Pins

If decay has extended beyond a normal size or shape, it may be necessary for the dentist to use a stronger system for retaining and supporting the restoration other than retentive grooves or bonding materials. **Retention (retentive) pins** can provide this additional means. For example, a pin may be required when tooth decay has extended into the distolingual cusp, undermining the enamel and dentin. In general when using retention pins, one pin is placed for each missing cusp (Fig. 48-10).

Pins are available in several diameters (widths) and styles. The retention pin has deep threads that grip the dentin when screwed into tooth structure. The other end of the pin grips the restorative material. Because all pins are very small and easily misplaced or dropped, it is essential that the dental dam be in place during the process of preparing and placing the pins.

INTERMEDIATE RESTORATIONS

An intermediate restoration is a temporary restoration that can be placed for any tooth or surface for short-term placement (see Chapter 43). The use of this type of restoration is a preliminary step toward providing a patient with a permanent restoration. The dentist would recommend the placement of an intermediate restoration for three primary factors: (1) to determine the health of a tooth, (2) while waiting to receive a permanent restoration, or (3) for financial reasons.

Because this is for a short-term rather than a permanent restoration, many states have approved this procedure to be an *expanded function* of the certified dental assistant (see Procedure 48-5).

Procedure 48-5 Placing and Carving an Intermediate Restoration (Expanded Function)

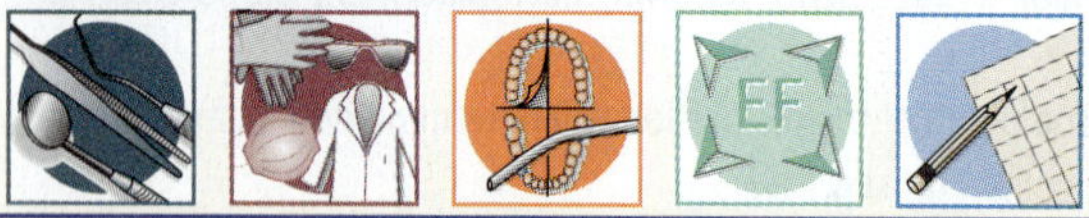

Equipment and Supplies

- Basic setup
- Tofflemire matrix retainer (for class II)
- Matrix band system (for classes II, III, and IV)
- Wedge (for classes II, III, and IV)
- Intermediate restoration material (IRM) setup (material, treated pad, spatula)
- Plastic instrument
- Condenser
- Discoid/cleoid carvers
- Hollenback carver
- Cotton pellet
- Articulating paper

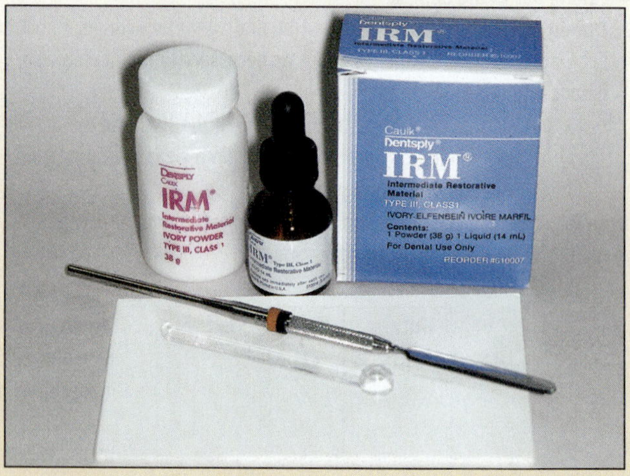

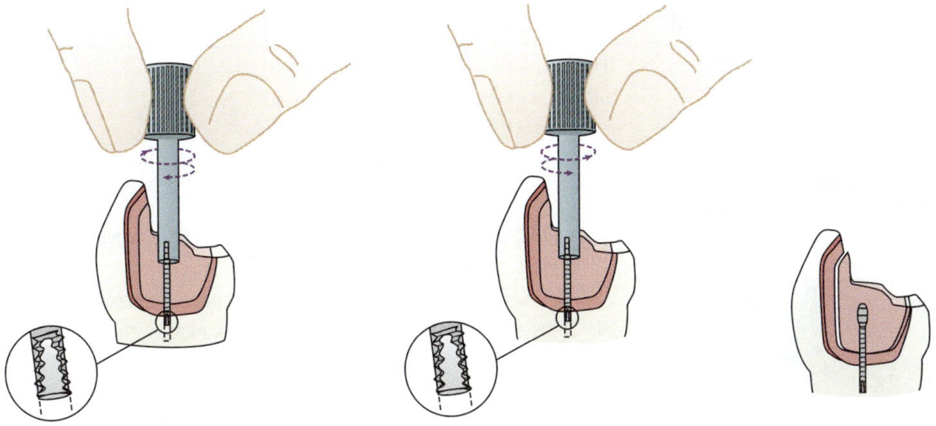

Fig. 48-10 Retention (retentive) pins placed in tooth structure for retaining and supporting a restoration.

Procedure 48-5 Placing and Carving an Intermediate Restoration (Expanded Function)—cont'd

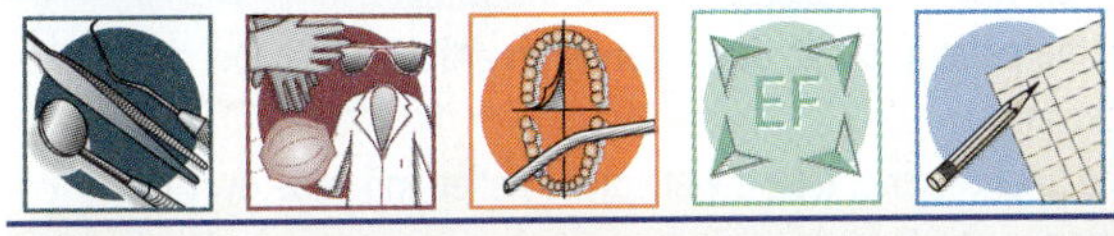

PROCEDURAL STEPS

1. Clean, dry, and isolate the site with either cotton rolls or dental dam.
2. Examine the tooth and preparation, being sure to keep a mental note of the outline of the preparation.
   Purpose: When you begin carving, you need to know how far to carve back to tooth structure.
3. If the preparation includes a proximal wall, you will need to place the appropriate matrix and wedge for the preparation. (See Chapter 49 for matrix selection and application.)
4. Mix the IRM to the appropriate consistency.
5. Using your plastic instrument, take increments of the materials to the preparation. If there is an interproximal box, begin filling this area first.
   Purpose: This area is more difficult to see, and material must be packed against the tooth for proper contour.

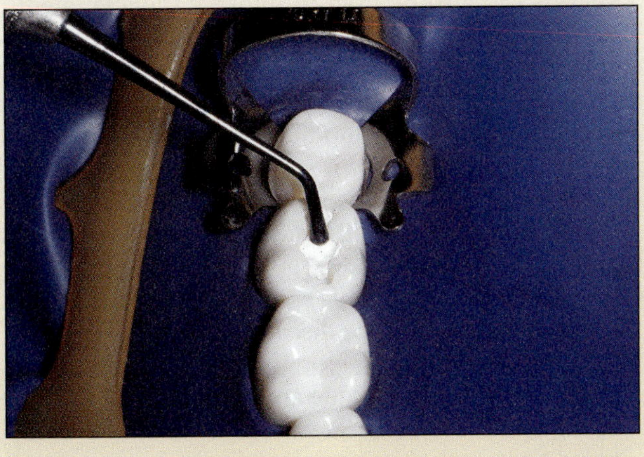

6. After each increment, condense the material using the small end of the condenser first.
7. Continue filling the preparation until it becomes overfilled.
   Purpose: You want enough material to be able to carve back to the tooth structure.

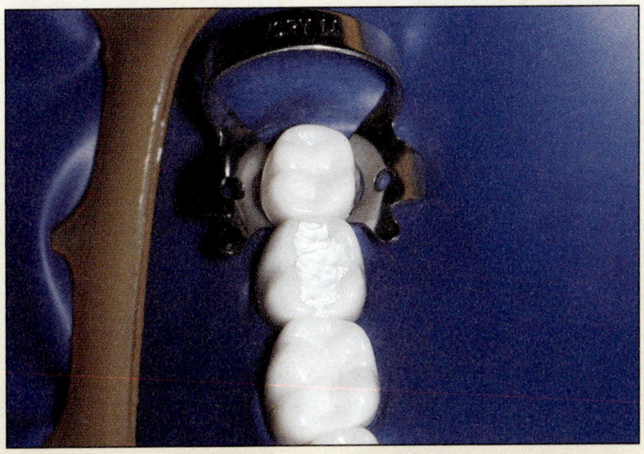

Carving Stage

1. While the material is still in putty form, use an explorer to run around the matrix band to remove any excess from the marginal ridge and proximal box.
2. Remove any excess material from the occlusal surface using the discoid/cleoid carver.

continued

Procedure 48-5 Placing and Carving an Intermediate Restoration (Expanded Function)—cont'd

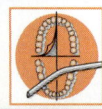

PROCEDURAL STEPS, cont'd

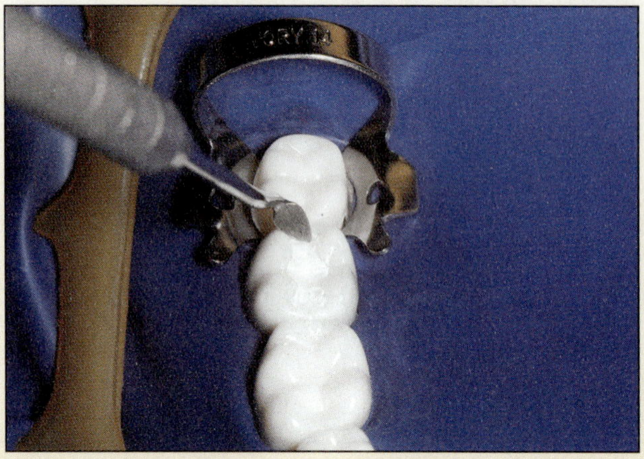

3. If a matrix system was used, remove it at this time, leaving the wedge in place.
   Purpose: To keep the interproximal space open for easier carving.
4. Complete the final carving of the occlusal surface with the discoid/cleoid carver, being sure to carve back to the tooth's normal anatomy.
   Note: Look at the same tooth on the opposite side of the arch for anatomic landmarks.
5. Using the Hollenback carver, remove any excess from the interproximal area, being sure not to create an overhang or indentation in the material.
6. Once all carving is completed, remove the wedge.
7. Instruct the patient to bite down gently on articulating paper to check the occlusion.
8. After the final carving, take a wet cotton pellet and wipe over the restoration.
9. Inform the patient that this restoration is "short-term," and instruct him or her not to chew sticky foods on that side.

Date	Tooth	Surface	Charting Notes
7/20/05	3	OL	Filling came out while chewing gum, cotton roll isolation, IRM placed. Instructed pt to reschedule for permanent rest. T. Clark, CDA/L. Stewart, DDS

Recall

11. What are three reasons for placing an intermediate restoration?
12. Is the placement of an intermediate restoration an expanded function of the dental assistant?

VENEERS

A **veneer** is a thin layer of tooth-colored material that is applied to the facial surface of a prepared tooth. A veneer may be placed on one or more anterior teeth to improve their appearance. Veneers are used to improve the appearance of teeth that are slightly abraded, eroded, discolored with intrinsic stains, or darkened after endodontic treatment (Fig. 48-11).

Veneers can also be used to improve the alignment of teeth or to close a **diastema** (Fig. 48-12). Use of a *direct* technique using composite resin creates a veneer that is bonded directly to the tooth surface. A porcelain veneer prepared in the dental laboratory and then cemented to the tooth surface is known as the *indirect technique.* (See Chapter 50 for the indirect technique and Procedure 48-6.)

Regardless of the type of veneer that is applied, the patient is advised of the following:

- Veneers have a limited life span and must be reapplied when wear, chipping, or discoloration occurs.
- Good oral hygiene is important to keep the surfaces and margins free of plaque and food debris.
- Biting on hard substances such as ice and hard candy could fracture the veneer.

A
B

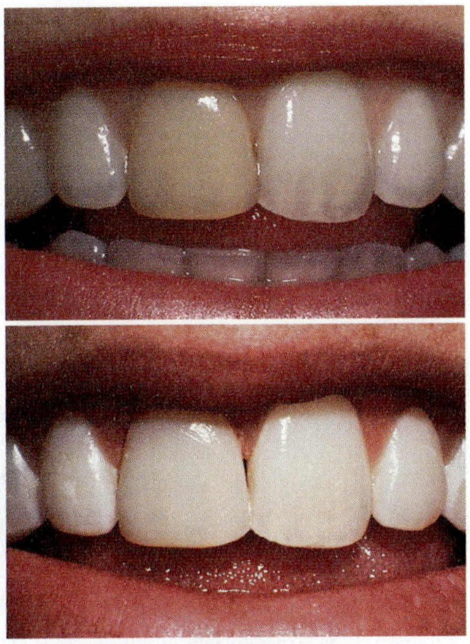

Fig. 48-11 **Veneers placed on teeth 8 and 9 to reduce discoloration and cover stain. A, Before placement. B, After placement.** (From Roberson T, et al: *Sturdevant's art and science of operative dentistry,* ed 4, St Louis, 2002, Mosby.)

A
B

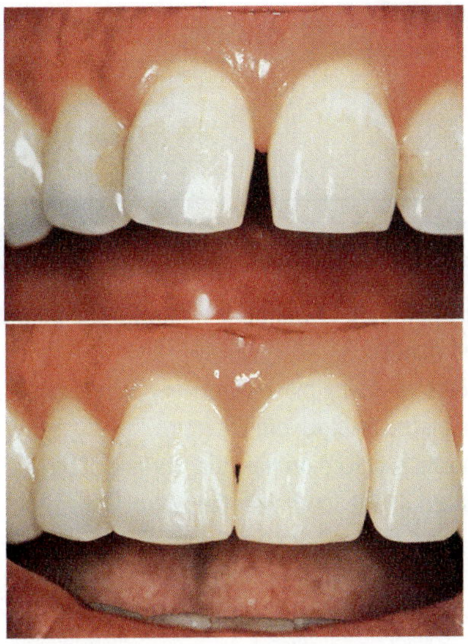

Fig. 48-12 **Veneers placed to close diastema.** (From Roberson T, et al: *Sturdevant's art and science of operative dentistry,* ed 4, St Louis, 2002, Mosby.)

Procedure 48-6 Assisting in the Placement of a Veneer

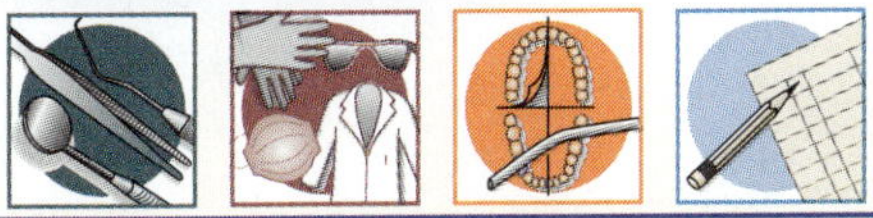

Equipment and Supplies

- Restorative tray (basic setup, hand cutting instruments, composite placement instrument, articulating paper holder)
- Composite shade guide
- Local anesthetic setup (if needed)
- Dental dam setup
- HVE tip
- Saliva ejector
- High-speed and low-speed handpieces
- Burs, assorted (dentist's choice)
- Mylar matrix setup
- Dental liners, base, sealers, bonding agents
- Composite material
- Curing light with protective shield
- Finishing burs and diamonds
- Dental floss
- Articulating paper
- Cotton pellets, cotton rolls, 2- × 2-inch gauze
- Dental floss
- Abrasive strips
- Articulating paper
- Polishing kit (disc and mandrel)
- Polishing paste

PROCEDURAL STEPS

1. A local anesthetic agent may not be required for this procedure, so proceed with moisture-control placement.
   Purpose: Because only a small amount of tooth structure is removed, it should not be uncomfortable for the patient.
2. The shade is selected; application of the dental dam is optional.
3. The tooth is measured to determine the appropriate crown form size. If necessary, the form is trimmed to fit the gingival contour.

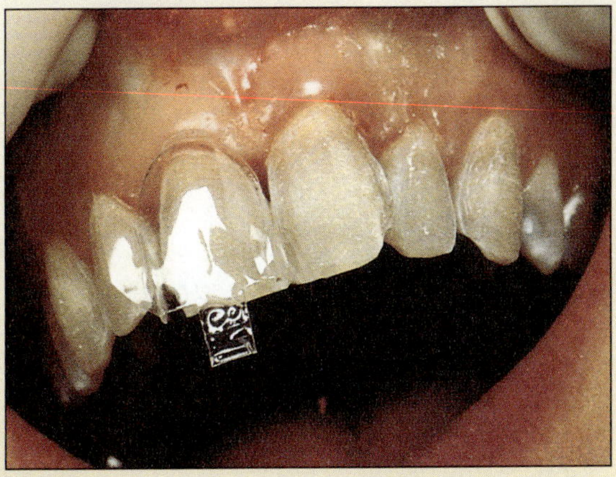

continued

Procedure 48-6 Assisting in the Placement of a Veneer—cont'd

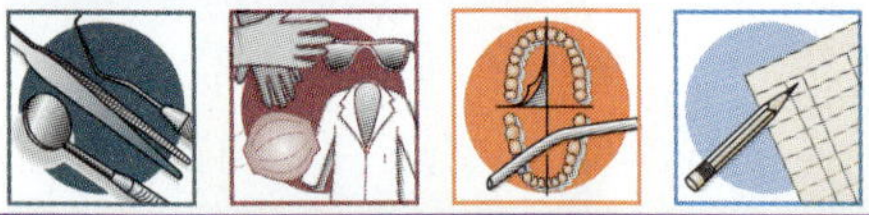

PROCEDURAL STEPS, cont'd

4. The required amount of enamel is removed, and then the tooth is etched and bonded.
5. If the veneers are being placed to cover dark stains, an opaque material may be placed to block out the stains.
6. The composite is placed on the inner surface of the crown form. The form is placed on the tooth with the matrix strips between the teeth. With one hand, the form is slowly pushed into place. With the other hand, the interproximal strips are pinched together at the lingual side of the tooth.

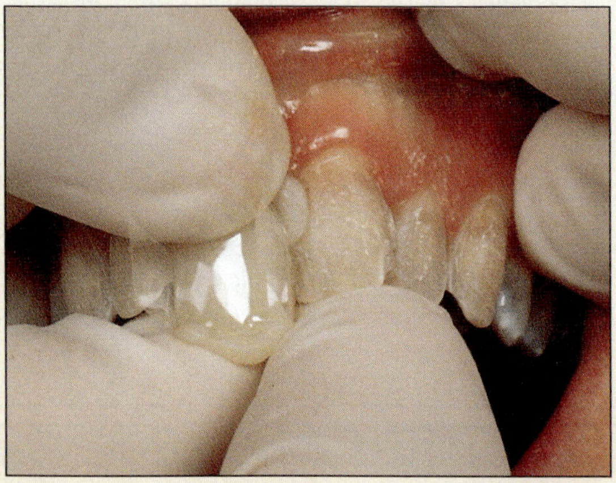

7. An explorer is used to trim away excess composite material that has extruded beyond the crown form.
8. With the crown form properly positioned, the material is light-cured for the time recommended by the manufacturer. When curing is complete, remove and discard the form.

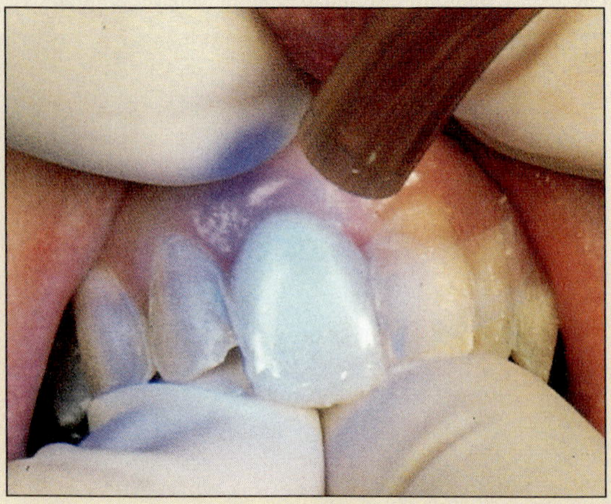

9. The dentist uses sandpaper discs to adjust the tooth to the proper length. Finishing burs are used to trim and smooth the veneer.

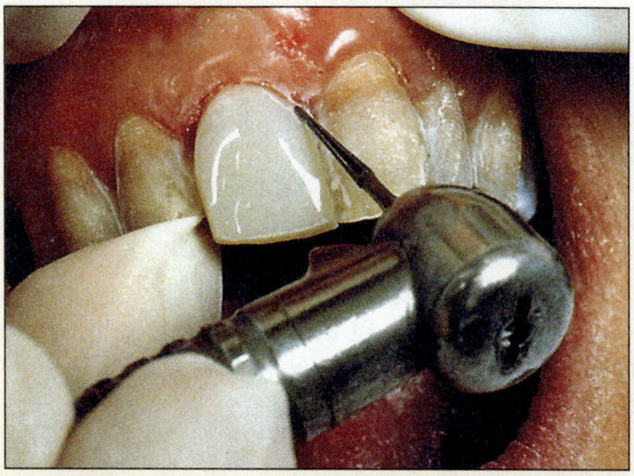

10. Assist as needed if these steps are repeated for each tooth that is to receive a veneer.

Date	Tooth	Surface	Charting Notes
7/20/05	8, 9	F	Veneer—dental dam isolation, etching/bonding/Silux shade YL, Pt tolerated procedure fine. T. Clark, CDA/L. Stewart, DDS

Recall

13. What tooth surface most often receives a veneer?
14. What is the difference between a direct and an indirect veneer?

TOOTH WHITENING

Tooth whitening, commonly known as *vital bleaching,* is a noninvasive method of lightening the color of dark or discolored teeth. Tooth whitening has become a routine procedure that includes both in-office options and professionally supervised at-home options. The three primary indications for having a tooth-whitening procedure are (1) extrinsic stains from foods, cigarette smoking, coffee, or tea (Fig. 48-13); (2) aged teeth, and (3) intrinsic stains, such as mild tetracycline stains and mild fluorosis (Fig. 48-14).

Tooth whitening is a type of treatment often requested by the patient. The patient must be aware that the results are not guaranteed and are not permanent. Most whitening systems last for 3 to 5 years. Chapter 43 describes the composition of whitening products and the basic facts of tooth whitening.

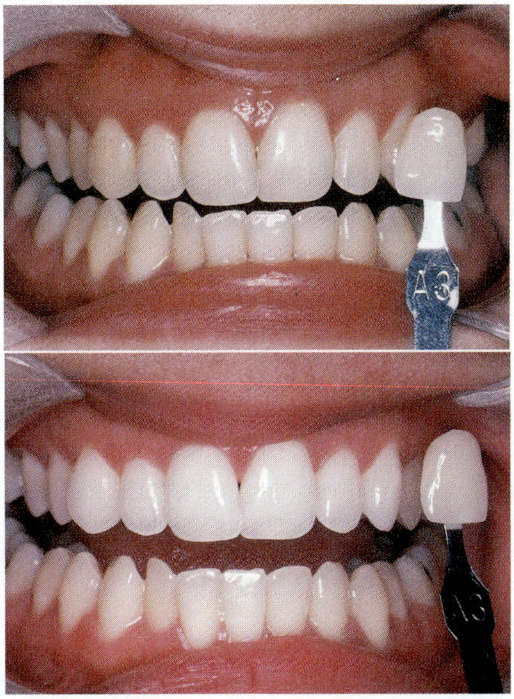

Fig. 48-13 **Before and after photos of tooth whitening used for extrinsic stains.**

Treatment Options

In-Office Treatment

Professionally applied tooth whitening can be accomplished by the dentist in as little as one hour. The patient will see results with the teeth becoming five shades lighter. This appointment includes the dental team following specific criteria in the application:

- Complete isolation of teeth involved (includes use of the dental dam, or a light-reflective resin barrier)
- Whitening agent at a higher concentration applied to facial surfaces of teeth.
- Light or laser source used to enhance the application.

At-Home Treatment

The decision to use a whitening product at home under the care of a dentist is another option for a patient wanting this procedure. The patient will see results within a couple of weeks, and can observe up to six shades lighter from this process. This includes the patient following specific criteria of application:

- Having a custom-fitted tray made in the dental office to hold the peroxide-based gel (see Fig. 43-25 in Chapter 43).
- Having a supply of peroxide-based gel for application for the suggested period of time.
- Usage regimens vary. Some products are used twice a day for two weeks, and others are intended for overnight use for one to two weeks.

Over-the-Counter Options

A variety of over-the-counter tooth-whitening products are available today. Most of the products that are manufactured

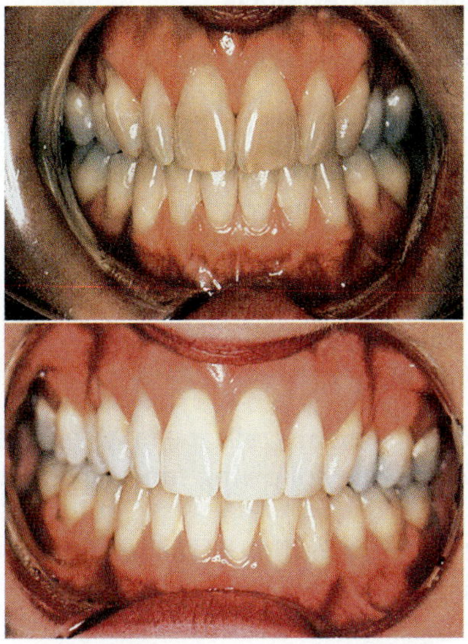

Fig. 48-14 **Before and after photos of tooth whitening used for intrinsic stains.** (From Roberson T, et al: *Sturdevant's art and science of operative dentistry,* ed 4, St Louis, 2002, Mosby.)

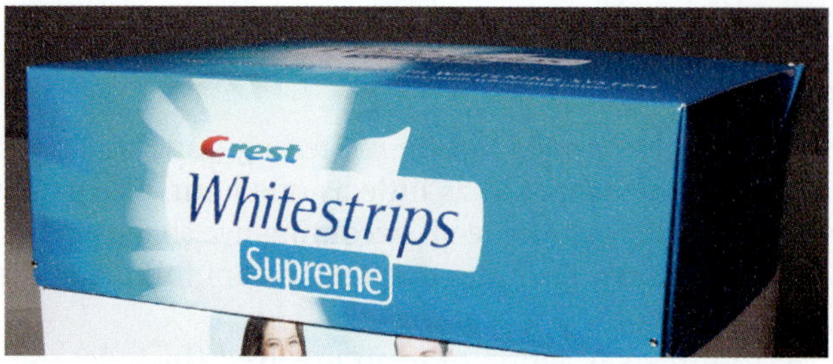

Fig. 48-15 An over-the-counter whitening product.

by the larger oral health companies are safe, reliable, and effective. However, these products will not achieve the dramatic changes that are available from the dentist-supervised products (Fig. 48-15). The three commonly used types of over-the-counter tooth-whitening systems available are:

- Brush-on whitening
- Strips to stick on the teeth
- Trays with bleaching gels

Whitening strips

The newest tooth-whitening product on the market is the tooth-whitening strip. These thin, flexible strips are coated with an adhesive hydrogen peroxide whitening gel. The patient peels off the backing like a bandage, and then presses the strip to the facial anterior teeth, being sure the upper edge of the strip is at the gingival margin. The remaining portion of the strip is folded onto the lingual surface. The patient is instructed to wear the strip for 30 minutes twice a day for 3 days.

Abuse of Whitening Products

With at-home and over-the-counter whitening products, the patient can have a higher potential for abuse. A patient will abuse a whitening product either by not following directions or by overuse to achieve whiter teeth. Most side effects are temporary, but on rare occasions, irreversible tooth damage can occur.

Assistant's Role and Patient Instructions in Tooth Whitening

The role of the dental assistant in the tooth-whitening process involves the following functions and procedural steps:

1. Assist in the recording of the medical and dental history.
2. Make the shade selection.
3. Take intraoral photographs before and after whitening procedure.
4. Take and pour up the preliminary impression for the custom tray.
5. Fabricate and trim the tray.
6. Provide postoperative instruction on the use of the material.
7. Assist in weekly or biweekly clinical visits.

Patient instructions for the gel tooth-whitening procedure include the following:

- Brush and floss before tray placement.
- Place gel in tray in an equal limited amount; less material is better than more.
- Seat tray.
- Do not eat or drink when wearing the tray.
- Wear the tray for the recommended time.
- Discontinue using the tray if side effects occur.
- Discuss side effects or other problems with the dentist.

Side Effects of Tooth Whitening

Thermal Hypersensitivity

The patient may experience sensitivity to hot and cold after removal of tray and material. Recommend that the patient use "sensitive teeth" toothpaste when completing this process.

Tissue Irritation

Gingival tissue may be exposed to excess gel because of improper fitting of the tray, allowing the material to ooze onto the gingiva. Advise the patient not to overfill the tray with material, and remind patient to remove any excess when seating the tray.

Recall

15. What are the three primary indications for tooth whitening?
16. What is used to hold whitening gel to the teeth?
17. What is the main ingredient of whitening strip products?
18. What side effects may a patient experience during tooth whitening?

Patient Education

The treatment and procedures discussed in this chapter involve the process of restoring teeth to their normal function as well as for esthetic purposes. Looking fit and healthy with an attractive smile is important in today's society regardless of age. Educating your patients in the way their smile can be improved is a service that helps them feel better about themselves.

Eye to the Future

The future of restorative dentistry seems unlimited with the new materials being designed today. As with tooth-whitening strips, many more dental products will be available over-the-counter for in-home use by the consumer. The dentist will then focus on the more complex procedures that will require dental expertise from the dental assistant, as well as the use of dental equipment.

Legal and Ethical Implications

One important reason a patient is a part of your dental practice is because of the type of dental work that is performed. It is the dental team's responsibility and obligation to update their knowledge of procedures and materials.

If it is legal in your state to perform expanded functions such as placement of liners and bonding agents, matrices, and intermediate restorations, ensure that you are trained in the new materials and techniques being used for restorative procedures. Remember that you are putting your patient, yourself, and your dentist at liability by performing these procedures.

Critical Thinking

1. The schedule indicates that you will assist in a class II procedure. What additional items do you need to set out for a class II procedure compared with other classifications?
2. Ms. Campbell will be coming in today to have a composite restoration replaced on tooth #10. Why would a patient have a restoration replaced?
3. A new patient indicates on his dental history form that he is unhappy with the appearance and color of his teeth. After the initial examination and further discussion about his habits, you find out that he drinks a lot of coffee. What procedures could be recommended to the patient to lighten the stains and color of his teeth?
4. You are assisting in a complex restoration on tooth #30 (MODF). During the final carving of the amalgam, a portion of the amalgam breaks off the distofacial cusp. What could the dentist have placed to create a better retention between the amalgam and tooth for such a large restoration?
5. Dr. Stewart is in the next operatory finishing a surgery that is taking longer than expected. She asks you to finish etching, place primer, and begin adding increments of composite to the small class I pit. What are you legally permitted to do in this procedure?

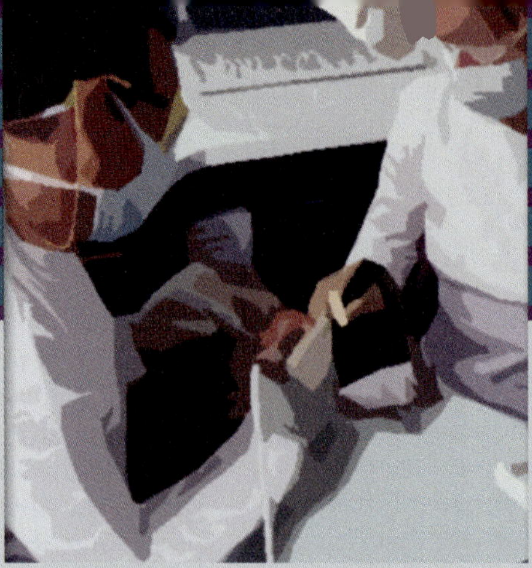

49 Matrix Systems for Restorative Dentistry

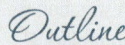

Outline

Posterior Matrix Systems
- Universal Retainer
- Matrix Band

Procedure 49-1: Assembling a Matrix Band and Universal Retainer
- Wedges

Procedure 49-2: Placing and Removing a Matrix Band and Wedge for a Class II Restoration (Expanded Function)

Anterior Matrix Systems

Procedure 49-3: Placing a Plastic Matrix for a Class III or Class IV Restoration (Expanded Function)

Alternative Matrix Systems
- Automatrix System
- Sectional Matrices
- Matrix Systems for Primary Teeth

Patient Education

Legal and Ethical Implications

Eye to the Future

Critical Thinking

KEY TERMS

Automatrix (*aw*-toe-**may**-triks) Matrix system designed to establish a temporary wall for tooth restoration without using a retainer.

Celluloid strip (**sel**-yuh-*loyd*) Clear plastic strip used in providing a temporary wall for the restoration of an anterior tooth.

Cupping Condition created by a concave tooth surface that has not been contoured properly.

Matrix (**may**-triks) Band that provides a temporary wall for a tooth structure to restore the proximal contours and contact to their normal shape and function.

Mylar (**my**-*lar*) Brand name for a clear plastic strip used to provide a temporary wall for restoration of an anterior tooth.

Overhang Excess restorative material extending beyond the cavity margin.

Palodent (**pa**-luh-dent) Small, oval-shaped matrix made of stainless steel used interproximally during tooth restoration.

Universal retainer Dental device used to hold a matrix band in place during a class II restoration.

Wedge Wooden or plastic triangular device placed in the embrasure to provide the contour needed during a class II restoration.

LEARNING OUTCOMES

On completion of this chapter, the student will be able to achieve the following objectives:

- Pronounce, define, and spell the Key Terms.
- Describe the use of a matrix system in class II, III, and IV restorations.
- Describe the type of matrices used for posterior restorations.
- Describe the type of matrices used for anterior restorations.
- Discuss the purpose and use of a wedge.
- Discuss alternative methods of matrix systems used in restorative dentistry.

PERFORMANCE OUTCOMES

On completion of this chapter, the student will be able to achieve competency standards in the following skills:

- Assemble a universal retainer and matrix band.
- Place and remove a matrix band and wedge for a class II restoration.
- Place and remove a matrix and wedge for a class III restoration.

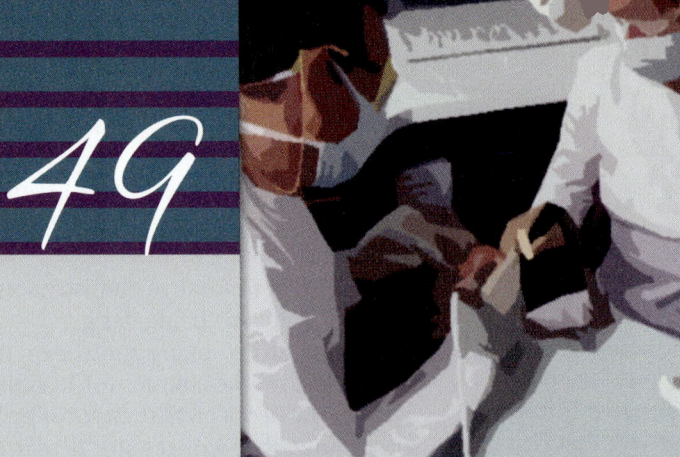

When a tooth has been prepared for a class II, III, or IV restoration, the tooth will have at least one interproximal wall removed. A matrix system creates a temporary wall for the amalgam, composite resin, or intermediate restorative material to be placed against (Fig. 49-1). The plural term for matrix is *matrices.* Additional functions of the matrix system are as follows:

- To restore the proximal anatomic contours and contact areas back into the tooth
- To create a smooth external surface for the restorative material

The placement and removal of the matrix system may be a legal expanded function in the state in which you are practicing. Pay special attention to the type of preparation, type of matrix system to prepare, and technique of placement and removal.

POSTERIOR MATRIX SYSTEMS

The most common matrix system used today for the class II restoration is the Tofflemire retainer and matrix band. To avoid unnecessary delay in a procedure, the assistant will have the retainer and band assembled at the beginning of the procedure.

Universal Retainer

The **universal retainer,** also referred to as the *Tofflemire retainer,* is a device that holds the matrix band snugly in position. This type of retainer is positioned most often from the *buccal* surface of the tooth being restored. If the dentist needs to restore a tooth that has an interproximal wall that extends onto the buccal surface, a contra-angle retainer has been designed with a slight bend in the body to accommodate positioning from the lingual surface.

Matrix Band

The **matrix** band is made of thin flexible stainless steel. The designs most commonly used are the *universal* and *extension* band (Fig. 49-2). The universal band is selected for a class II preparation where the proximal "box" is prepared to a minimum depth and width. The extension band is selected for a class II preparation with gingival extensions and where the height of the band cannot exceed the height of the tooth.

When you bring the ends of the curved band together, the band will form a circle. One side of the *circumference* (perimeter or outside edge) is smaller than the other. The circumference guides you in placing the band as follows:

- The *larger circumference* of the band is the *occlusal edge* and is always placed on the tooth toward the occlusal part of the tooth.
- The *smaller circumference* of the band is the *gingival edge* and is always placed toward the gingiva.

Contouring

In preparation for use, the center of the matrix band must be *contoured* (shaped) in the proximal contact area so that it will make proper contact with the adjacent tooth. To contour the band, place the band on a paper pad. Using a *burnisher* or end of the handle, rub against the inner surface of the band until the ends begin to curl (Fig. 49-3 and Procedure 49-1).

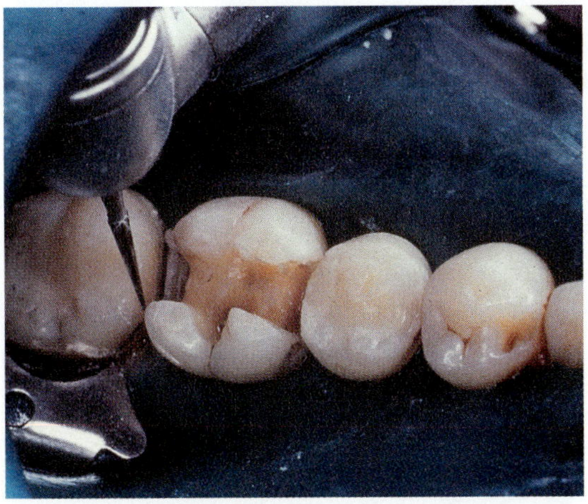

Fig. 49-1 Tooth preparation with mesial and distal proximal walls missing. (Courtesy Garrison Dental Solutions.)

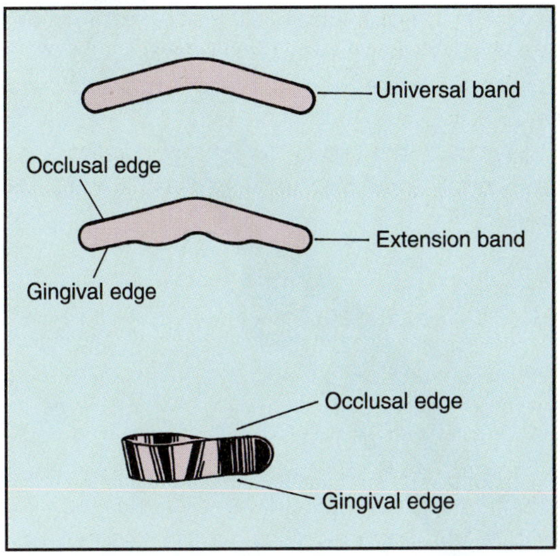

Fig. 49-2 Most commonly used posterior matrix bands.

Procedure 49-1 Assembling a Matrix Band and Universal Retainer

Equipment and Supplies

- Basic setup
- Universal retainer
- Matrix band
- Ball burnisher
- Paper pad

PROCEDURAL STEPS

1. Rinse and dry the preparation.
2. Examine the outline of the cavity preparation using a mirror and explorer.
3. Determine the size of matrix band to be used for the procedure.
   Purpose: The band is selected according to size of the tooth and depth of the cavity preparation.
4. Place the middle of the band on the paper pad, and burnish this area with a burnisher.
   Purpose: This creates a thin, slightly contoured area where the contact will be located.
5. Hold the retainer with diagonal slot facing you, and turn the *outer knob* counterclockwise until the end of the spindle is visible and away from the diagonal slot in the vise.

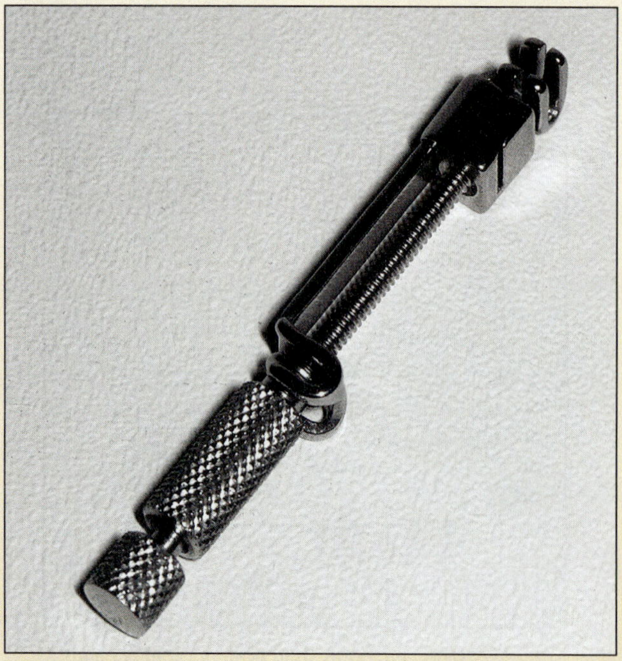

6. Turn the *inner knob* until the vise moves next to the guide slots.
   Purpose: The retainer is ready to receive the matrix band.
7. Bring together the ends of the band to identify the occlusal and gingival aspects of the matrix band. The occlusal edge has the larger circumference. The gingival edge has the smaller circumference.
8. With the diagonal slot of the retainer facing toward you, slide the joined ends of the band, *occlusal edge first,* into the diagonal slot on the vice.
9. Guide the band in the correct guide slots.
   Purpose: The band loop's position in the guide slots depends on whether the tooth being restored is maxillary, mandibular, right, or left.

Components of Universal Retainer

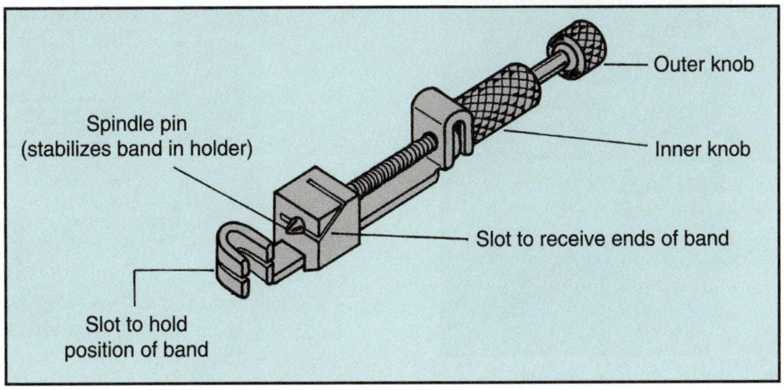

Outer knob: Used to tighten or loosen the spindle within the diagonal slot; this holds the matrix band securely in the retainer. To tighten the spindle, turn the outer knob away from you. To loosen the spindle, turn the outer knob toward you.

Be careful not to turn it too far, or the diagonal slot vise will fall off the spindle. If this happens, insert the end of the spindle into the diagonal slot vise and turn the outer knob away from you.

Inner knob: Used to increase or decrease the size of the matrix band loop. The size of the loop formed by the band depends on the tooth to be restored. When placing the band over the tooth, the size of the loop circumference should be larger than the tooth, and then tightened after placement.

Spindle: Internal screwlike pin that fits into the diagonal slot to hold the ends of the matrix band. When assembling the retainer, the spindle point must be clear of the slot while the band is slid into the slot, and then tightened.

Diagonal slot: Slot within the boxlike structure used to position the ends of the matrix band into the vise; the retainer is always positioned in the mouth with this slot facing *toward the gingiva.*

Outer guide slots: Also known as guide channels; they are located at the end of the retainer and serve as channels to guide the loop of the matrix band. The channel selected is determined by the quadrant being treated.

Recall

1. What classification(s) of cavity preparation uses a posterior matrix system?
2. What is the plural of matrix?
3. What is used to hold a posterior matrix band in position?
4. When placing a matrix band, where is the smaller circumference of the band placed?
5. What instrument is commonly used to contour the matrix band?

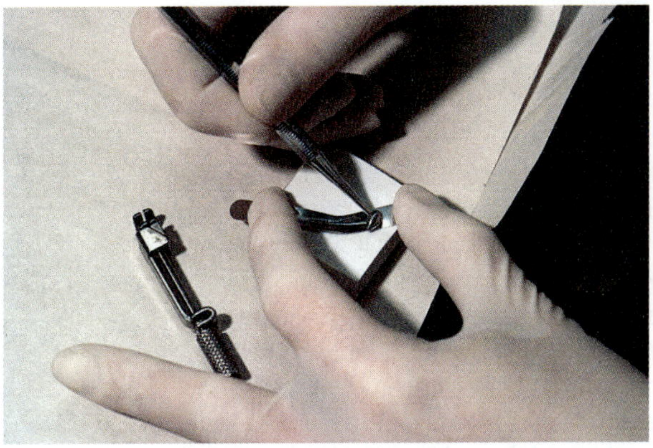

Fig. 49-3 Contouring the band assists in the restoration process.

Wedges

A class II restoration requires a matrix band to act as an artificial wall for that tooth, but the band alone does not provide the anatomic contour that is required interproximally. A **wedge** is inserted into the lingual embrasure to position the matrix band firmly against the gingival margin of the preparation (Fig. 49-4). This added pressure pushes the matrix against the proximal surface of the tooth so the contour of the finished restoration matches that of the natural tooth structure it replaces.

Wedges are made in various sizes, forms (triangular or round), and materials (wood and plastic). The most commonly used type of wedge is the triangular or round wooden wedge (Fig. 49-5). When selecting a wedge, specific considerations are:

- The wedge is wide enough to apply pressure to both the apical and gingival wall of the preparation.

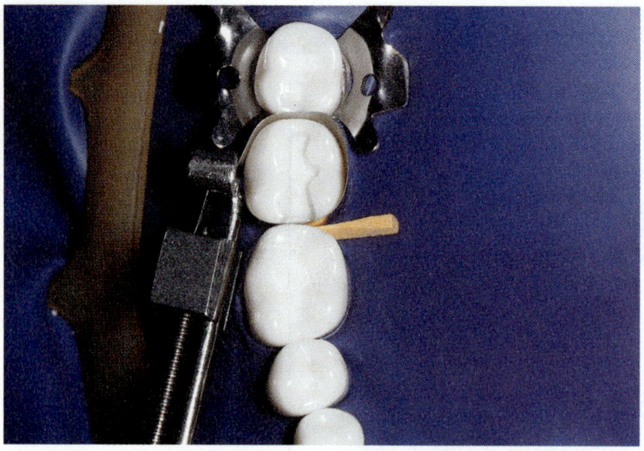

Fig. 49-4 Wedge correctly positioned interproximally.

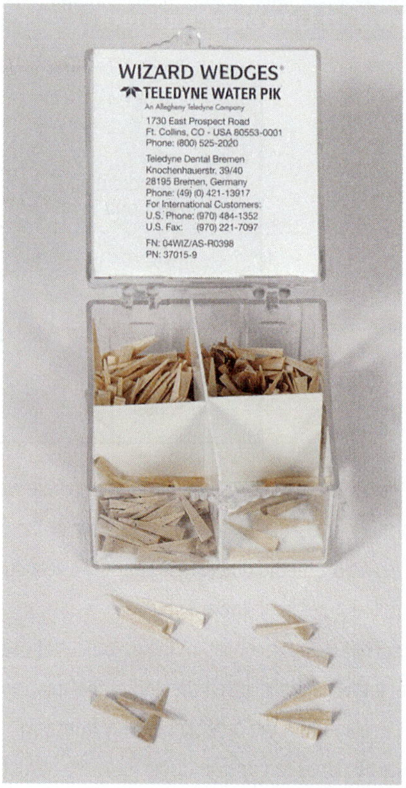

Fig. 49-5 Assortment of precontoured wedges.

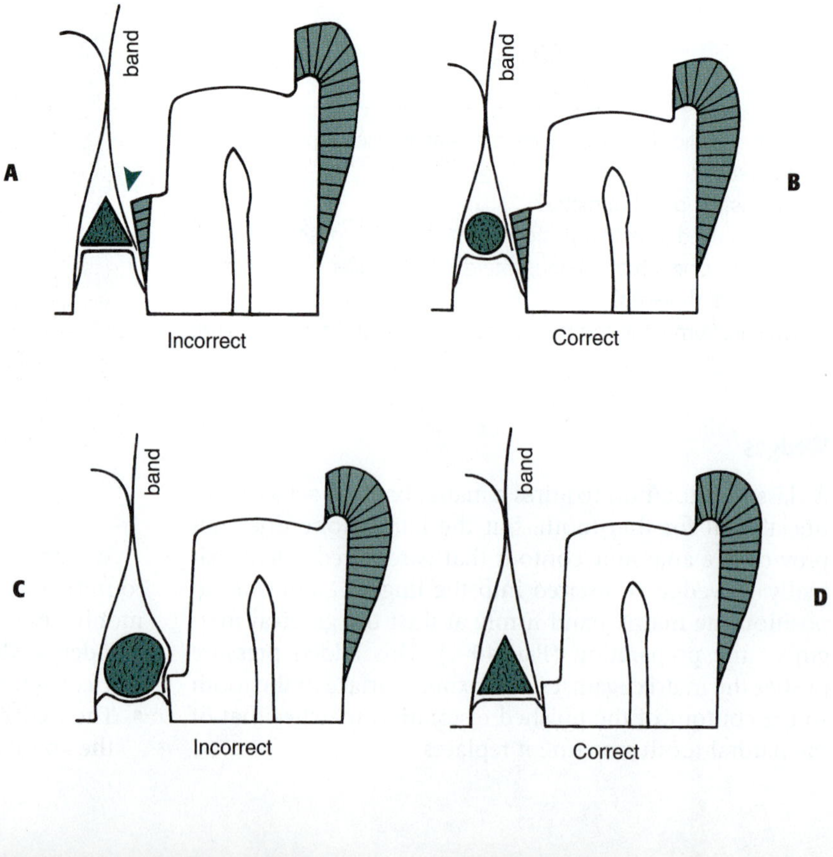

Fig. 49-6 The type of wedge placed is determined by the depth of the preparation. **A,** In a conservative preparation, a triangular wedge will not support the band against the margin. **B,** For a conservative preparation, a round toothpick wedge works best because it forms with the gingival margin. **C,** A deep preparation does not work with a round wedge. The contour of the wedge will buckle the matrix band. **D,** A triangular wedge works best with a deeper class II preparation. (From Roberson T, et al: *Sturdevant's art and science of operative dentistry,* ed 4, St Louis, 2002, Mosby.)

- The wedge presses the band against the tooth and causes a slight separation of the teeth.
- The wedge is slightly wider than the distance between the cervical portions of the adjacent teeth.

When positioning the wedge, cotton pliers or #110 (Howe) pliers are typically used to insert the wedge firmly into the embrasure. For posterior restorations, the wedge is positioned from the lingual side (see Procedure 49-2). Improper wedge and band placement can result in an **overhang** or in **cupping.** Neither condition is an acceptable replacement of tooth structure (Fig. 49-6).

Recall

6. What additional item is used in the matrix system to reestablish a proper contact with an adjacent tooth?
7. What can result from improper wedge placement?

Criteria for Placing the Posterior Matrix Retainer and Band

The diagonal slotted surface of the retainer is always positioned toward the gingiva.

The retainer is positioned from the buccal surface of the tooth.

The handle of the retainer extends out from the oral cavity at the corner of the lips.

The seated band extends approximately 1 mm below the gingival margin of the preparation.

The seated band extends no more than 1½ to 2 mm above the occlusal surface of the tooth.

Procedure 49-2 Placing and Removing a Matrix Band and Wedge for a Class II Restoration (Expanded Function)

Equipment and Supplies

- Basic setup
- Prepared matrix band and retainer
- Wedge for each proximal space involved
- #110 pliers

PROCEDURAL STEPS

Preparing the Band Size

1. If necessary, use the handle end of the mouth mirror to open the loop of the band.
   Purpose: The band can become flattened or bent during placement in the retainer, and will not slide easily onto the tooth preparation.

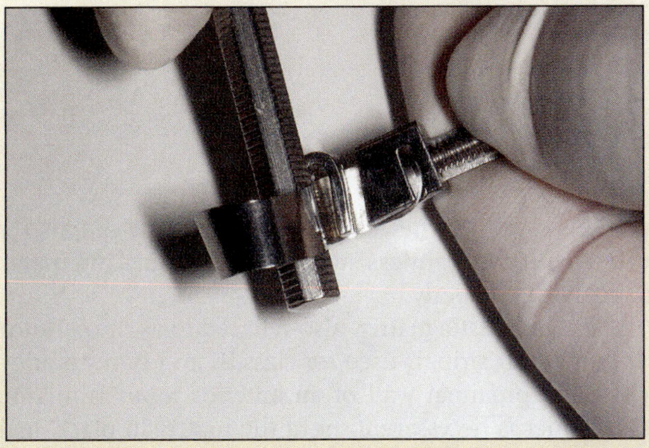

2. If necessary, adjust the size (diameter) of the loop by turning the *inner knob.*

Placing Matrix Band and Universal Retainer

1. Position and seat the band's loop over the occlusal surface, with the retainer parallel to the buccal surface of the tooth. Ensure that the band remains beyond the occlusal edge by approximately 1.0 to 1.5 mm.

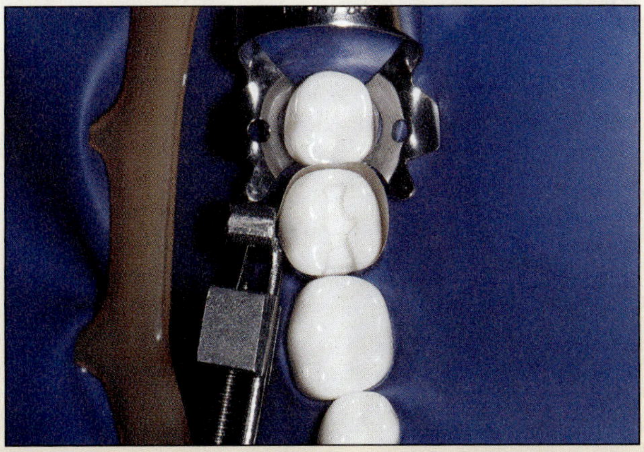

2. Hold the band securely in place by finger pressure over its occlusal surface. Turn the inner knob clockwise slowly to tighten the band around the tooth.
3. Use the explorer to examine the adaptation of the band.
   Purpose: Gingival tissue or dental dam material can become trapped between the band and the proximal box of the cavity preparation.

continued

Procedure 49-2 Placing and Removing a Matrix Band and Wedge for a Class II Restoration (Expanded Function)—cont'd

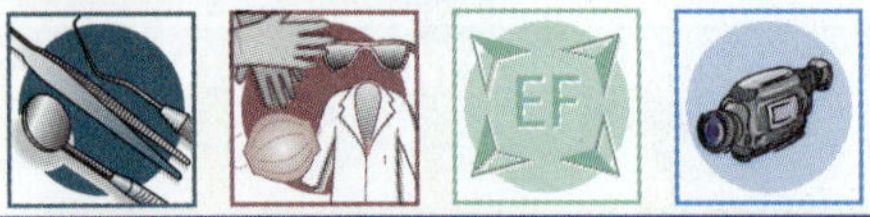

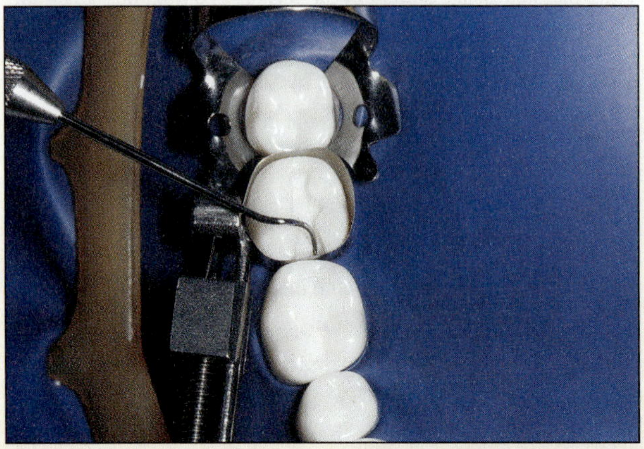

PROCEDURAL STEPS, cont'd

4. Use a burnisher to contour the band at the contact area, creating a slightly concave area.

Placing the Wedge

1. Select the proper wedge size and shape.
   Purpose: The size of the embrasure will determine the size and shape of the wedge for complete closure of the band and cavity preparation.
2. Place the wedge in the pliers so that the flat, wider side of the wedge is toward the gingiva.

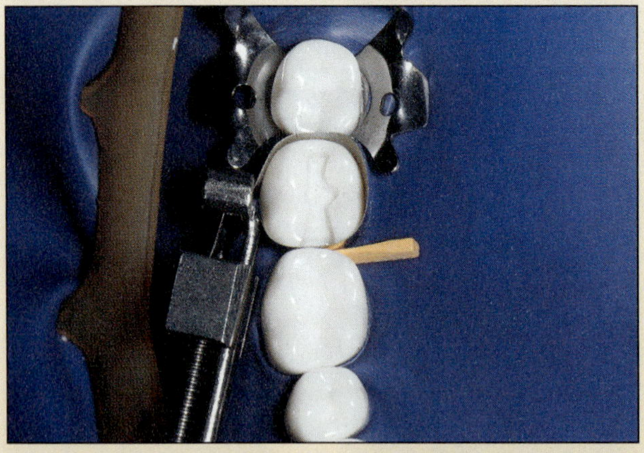

3. Insert the wedge into the lingual embrasure next to the preparation and the band.
   Note: If both proximal surfaces (mesial and distal) are being restored, a wedge is inserted for each open contact.
4. Check the proximal contact to ensure that the seal at the gingival margin of the preparation is closed.

Removing Universal Retainer, Matrix Band, and Wedge

1. After the dentist completes the initial carving, loosen the retainer from the band by placing a finger over the occlusal surface and slowly turning the *outer knob* of the retainer.
2. Carefully slide the retainer toward the occlusal surface, leaving the band around the tooth.
3. Gently lift the matrix band in an occlusal direction, using a seesaw motion.
   Purpose: To avoid fracturing the newly placed material.
4. Discard the matrix band into the "sharps" container.
5. Using #110 pliers, grasp the base of the wedge to remove it from the lingual embrasure.
   Purpose: The wedge remains in place to help prevent fracture of the restoration when the matrix band is removed.
6. The restoration is now ready for the final carving steps.
   Note: Some operators will prefer to take the wedge (or wedges) out before the matrix band is removed.

ANTERIOR MATRIX SYSTEMS

A clear plastic **matrix** is used with anterior composite resin or glass ionomer materials (Fig. 49-7). A different matrix system is used for anterior teeth because of the type of dental materials used. Composite resins have inorganic filler particles that can be scratched or marked by stainless steel. The newer bonding materials can also interfere with the stainless steel bands, causing the materials to set improperly.

The clear plastic matrix, also referred to as the **celluloid strip** or **Mylar** strip, is used for class III and IV restorations where the proximal wall of an anterior tooth is missing. No retainer is necessary to hold the matrix in place, making this system an easier application. The plastic matrix

Procedure 49-3 Placing a Plastic Matrix for a Class III or IV Restoration (Expanded Function)

Equipment and Supplies

- Basic setup
- Clear matrix strip
- Wedges
- #110 pliers

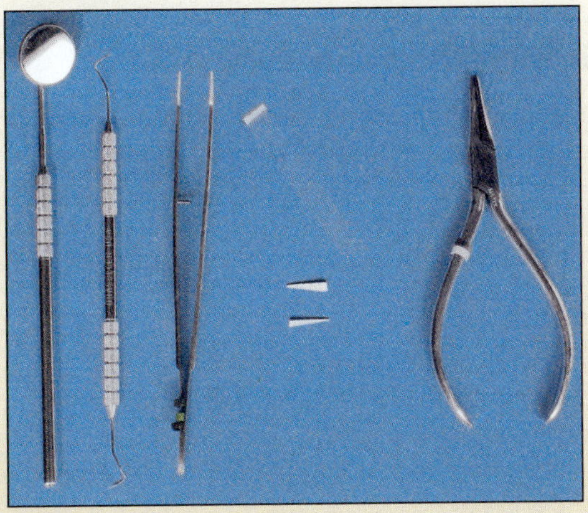

PROCEDURAL STEPS

1. Examine the contour of the tooth and preparation site, paying special attention to the outline of the preparation.
2. Contour the matrix strip.
3. Slide the matrix interproximally, ensuring that the gingival edge of the matrix extends beyond the preparation.

   Purpose: If the matrix does not completely cover the preparation, the cavity preparation could be filled incorrectly.

   Note: If placing a matrix during the etching process, make sure a new matrix is used for the placement of the composite resin material.
4. Using your thumb and forefinger, pull the band over the prepared tooth on the facial and lingual surfaces.
5. Using pliers, position the wedge into the gingival embrasure.

   Note: The wedge can be positioned from either the facial or the lingual side for anterior restorations.
6. After the preparation is filled and light-cured, the matrix is then removed.

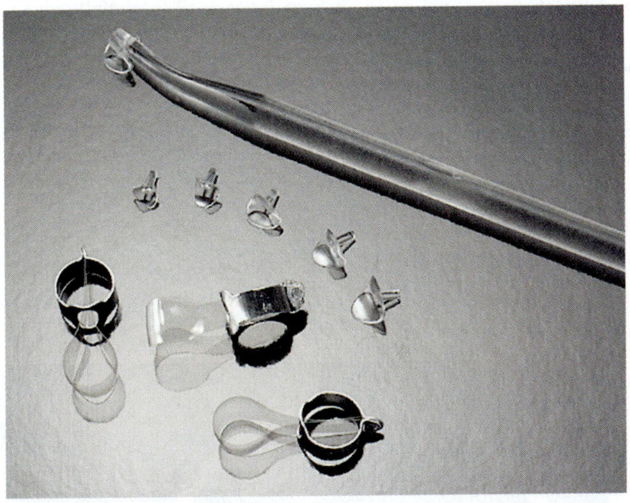

Fig. 49-7 A clear matrix system. (Courtesy Premier Dental Products.)

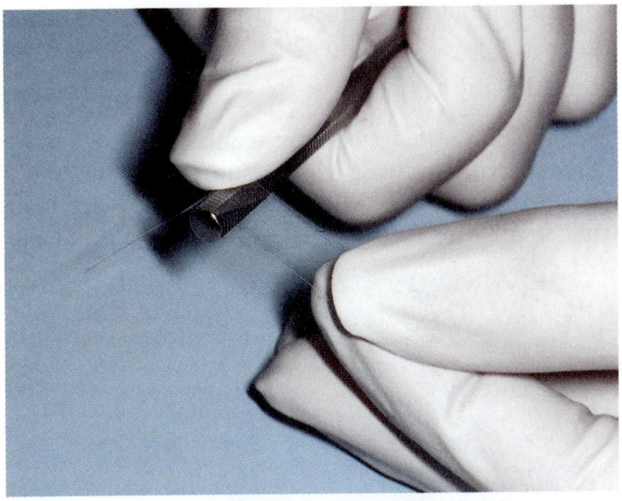

Fig. 49-8 Contouring a plastic matrix band.

and wedge serve the following three purposes during the restoration process:

1. The matrix is placed between the teeth before the etching and priming of the tooth *to protect adjacent teeth* from these materials.
2. After placement of the composite material, the matrix is pulled tightly around the tooth *to help in reconstructing* its natural contour.
3. The clear plastic allows the curing light to penetrate the material and *to complete the curing process.*

Because anterior teeth have a slight curvature of their interproximal surface, contouring the matrix before placement helps to keep it in place. To contour a plastic matrix strip, pull the matrix lengthwise over the rounded end of the cotton pliers (Fig. 49-8).

Once the matrix is securely placed and the material is adapted to the preparation, a wedge can be inserted from the facial or lingual surfaces to hold the matrix in place. When the restorative material has reached its final set, the matrix is removed for the finishing and polishing stages (see Procedure 49-3).

Recall

8. Why can't a stainless steel matrix band be used with composites?
9. What is another term for a clear plastic matrix?

ALTERNATIVE MATRIX SYSTEMS

Automatrix System

An alternative to the use of a Tofflemire retainer and band is the **automatrix** system (Fig. 49-9). This system has an advantage over the universal retainer in that no retainer is used to hold the band in place. The bands, which are already formed into a circle, are available in assorted sizes in both metal and plastic. Each band has a coil-like auto lock loop. The tightening wrench is inserted into the coil and turned clockwise to tighten the band. No additional retainer is necessary, and wedges are placed as indicated.

When the procedure is finished, the tightening wrench is inserted into the coil and turned counterclockwise to loosen the band. The removing pliers are used to cut the band. The band is removed and discarded with the sharps. The wedges are then removed. The tightening wrench and removing pliers are sterilized or disinfected in accordance with the manufacturer's instructions.

Sectional Matrices

Posterior composite restorations require a different type of matrix system than used with the universal band and retainer. With a wedge, a thin polished **Palodent**-type matrix band (small, oval-shaped stainless steel matrix), and a tension ring, this system is able to produce tight anatomic contact for composite resin materials (Fig. 49-10).

The most important goal for the dentist to consider when placing class II composites is to restore the contact back to its normal function with the adjacent tooth. The thin contoured *matrix band* is positioned first interproximally, and then the *wedge* is firmly placed to close the cervical margin. The prongs of the *tension ring* are placed between the band and the wedge, therefore creating a solid closure of the cavity preparation.

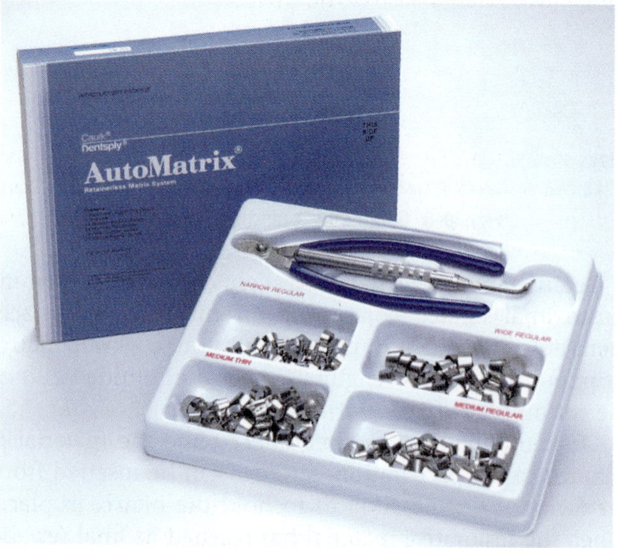

Fig. 49-9 Automatrix system. (Courtesy Dentsply Caulk.)

Matrix Systems for Primary Teeth

The universal retainer and matrix band do not fit primary molars properly because of the shape and size of these teeth. The T-band and the spot-welded band are two types of band systems designed to provide the correct width and depth needed for proper restoration of primary molars.

T-Band

The T-band is a copper band in the shape of a *T* (Fig. 49-11). When formed, the top portion of the *T* allows the straight portion to adjust and fit the circumference of the primary molar. Preparing the T-band matrix involves the following steps:

- Bend the wings of the T-band to form a *U*-shaped trough.
- Slip the free end of the band loosely through the *U* formation.
- Close the wings, and pull the free end to make a small loop of the band.
- Holding the free end toward the facial surface, place the band loop on the tooth to be prepared.

Spot-Welded Band

The spot-welded band is form-fitted around the tooth, using #110 pliers (Fig. 49-12). The band is then removed and

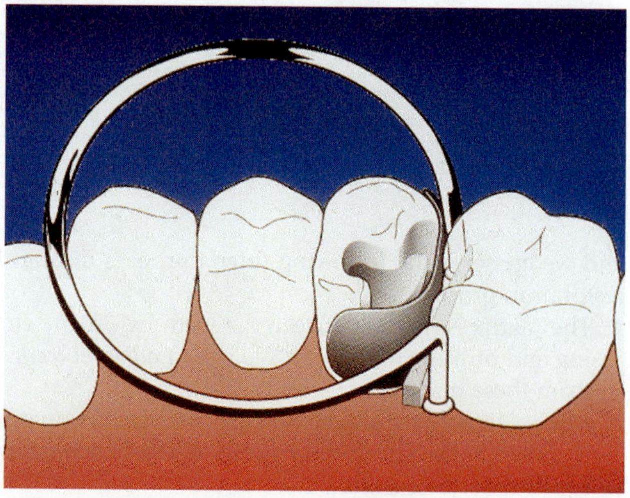

Fig. 49-10 Sectional matrix system. (Courtesy Garrison Dental Solutions.)

placed in the smaller form of a welder that fuses the metal to make a custom band.

Preparing a spot-welded matrix band involves the following steps:

- Measure ¾ to 1 inch of stainless steel matrix material.
- Fit the matrix material around the prepared tooth.
- Adapt the band with #110 pliers, ensuring that the ends of the matrix material are at the facial surface for visibility and control.
- Holding the ends tightly, remove the band in an occlusal direction.
- Place the band on the plate of the spot welder.
- Spot-weld the matrix at three positions.

Recall

10. What matrix system is an alternative to the universal retainer?

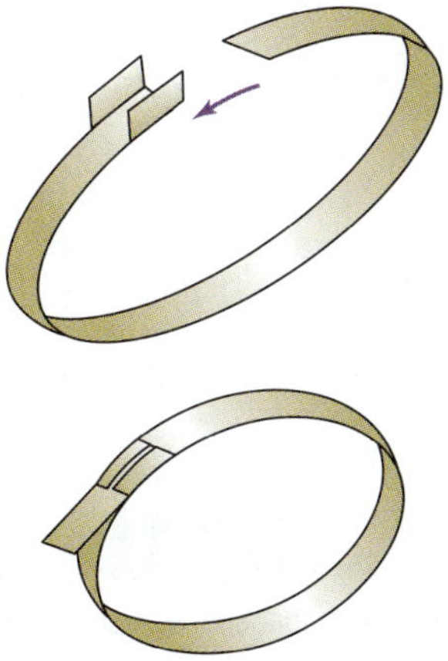

Fig. 49-11 Copper T-band used for primary molars.

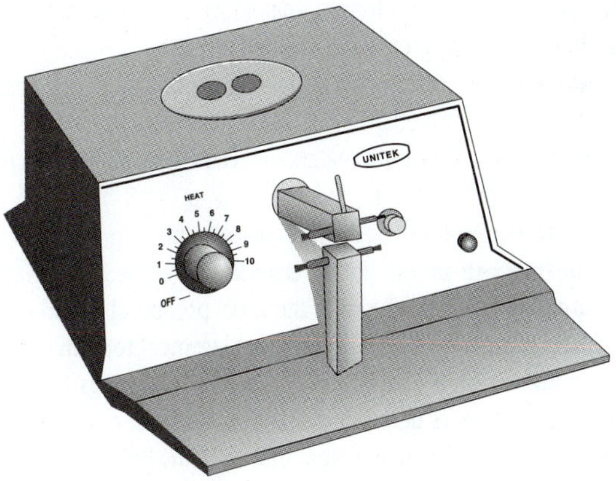

Fig. 49-12 Spot-welder used for primary molars. (Courtesy Unitek, Monrovia, California.)

Patient Education

Many instruments and supplies are used throughout a dental procedure in the restoration of a tooth. The patient may never have seen the matrix system. When assisting in a procedure that introduces a piece of dental equipment, such as the universal retainer or automatrix system, be sure to educate the patient in how it is used. This type of ongoing discussion will promote confidence in your patients, which will enhance their dental visit.

Legal and Ethical Implications

The placement of a matrix may be a legal expanded function in the state where you practice. If so, it is essential that you have training in the proper placement of matrix bands and the insertion of a wedge.

Do not let your dentist take for granted that you have placed a band or wedge correctly. Every time you complete this procedure, request that the dentist critique your work and offer advice about the application. This exchange improves communication in the office and makes you a more valuable member of the dental team.

Eye to the Future

The newer composite resin materials being placed for posterior restorations are requiring a different type of matrix system. The matrix is thinner, which provides a more accurate contact with the adjacent tooth or teeth. Always consult with a sales representative regarding what accessories are required for the type of restorative materials being selected and placed.

Critical Thinking

1. You are assisting in the restoration of a mesial-occlusal-distal (MOD) amalgam on tooth #13. How many wedges will you set out for this procedure? Where is a wedge positioned in the tooth preparation for proper contour? From what surface do you position the wedge?
2. You are to prepare the universal retainer and matrix band for tooth #29. When assembling the band into the retainer with the diagonal slot facing you, do you place the band in the guide slot in a right, straight, or left direction?
3. Before you assemble the matrix band and retainer or place the Mylar strip interproximally, what needs to be done to the band to enhance its contouring abilities?
4. The dentist has overfilled tooth #13, completed the initial carving, and is ready to complete the final carving of the occlusal and interproximal surfaces. Describe the sequence involved in the removal of the matrix band, retainer, and wedge.

50

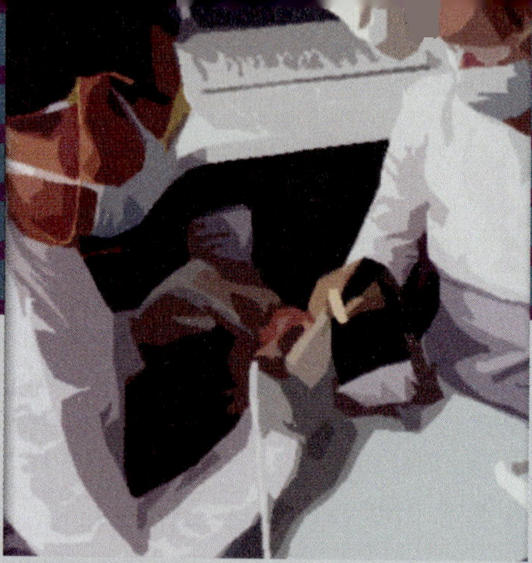

Fixed Prosthodontics

Outline

KEY TERMS

Abutment (ah-**but**-ment) Tooth, root, or implant used for the retention of a fixed or removable prosthesis.

Articulator (ahr-**tik**-u-lay-*ter*) Dental laboratory device that simulates the movements of the mandible and temporomandibular joint.

Bevel (**beh**-vul) Enamel margin of a tooth preparation.

Cast post Metal post placed into the root canal of an endodontically treated tooth to improve the retention of a cast restoration.

Chamfer (**cham**[p]-fur) Tapered finish line of the margin at the cervical area of a tooth preparation.

Core Portion of a post that extends above the tooth structure.

Die An accurate replica of the prepared portion of a tooth used in the laboratory during the fabrication of a cast restoration.

Fixed bridge Dental prosthesis with artificial teeth fixed in place and supported by attachment to natural teeth.

Full crown Cast restoration that covers the entire anatomic crown of the tooth.

Gingival retraction (**jin**-juh-vul ree-**trak**-shun) Means of displacing gingival tissue away from the tooth.

Hypertrophied (high-*per*-**tro**-feed) Pertaining to overgrown oral tissues.

Infuser (in-**fyu**-zer) Syringe that applies hemostatic solution on the gingival retraction cord.

Inlay (**in**-lay) Cast restoration designed for class II cavity.

Investment material Special gypsum product able to withstand extreme heat.

Master cast Cast created from a final impression used to construct baseplate, bite rims, wax setups, and finished prosthesis.

Onlay (**on**-lay) Cast restoration designed for occlusal crown and proximal surfaces of posterior teeth.

Opaquer (oh-**pay**-kur) Resin material placed under a porcelain restoration to mask tooth discoloration.

Pontic (**pon**-tik) Artificial tooth that replaces a missing natural tooth.

Porcelain-fused-to-metal (PFM) crown Indirect restoration in which a thin porcelain material is fused to the facial portion of a gold crown.

Prosthesis (pros-**thee**-sus) Fabricated replacement for a missing tooth.

Resin-bonded bridge Fixed dental prosthesis with wings that are bonded to the lingual surfaces of adjacent teeth; also known as *Maryland bridge.*

Shade guide Accessory dental item that contains different shades of teeth and is used to match the color of a patient's teeth for the laboratory technician.

KEY TERMS, cont'd

Shoulder Margins of a tooth preparation for a cast restoration.

Three-quarter crown Cast restoration that covers the anatomic crown of a tooth except for the facial or buccal portion.

Unit Each component of the fixed bridge.

Veneer (vuh-**nir**) Thin layer of composite resin or porcelain bonded or cemented to a prepared facial surface.

LEARNING OUTCOMES

On completion of this chapter, the student will be able to achieve the following objectives:

- Pronounce, define, and spell the Key Terms.
- List indications and contraindications for a fixed prosthesis.
- Identify the steps for a diagnostic workup.
- Identify the role of the laboratory technician.
- Describe the differences among full crowns, inlays, onlays, and veneer crowns.
- Identify the components of a fixed bridge.
- Describe the uses of porcelain for fixed prosthodontics.
- Describe the preparation and placement of a cast crown.
- Discuss the uses of core buildups, pins, and posts in crown retention.
- Describe the use of retraction cord before taking a final impression.
- Describe the function of provisional coverage for a crown or fixed bridge.
- Identify home care instructions for a permanent fixed prosthesis.

PERFORMANCE OUTCOMES

On completion of this chapter, the student will be able to achieve competency standards in the following skills:

- Demonstrate the placement and removal of gingival retraction cord.
- Assist in the preparation procedure of an indirect restoration.
- Assist in the cementation procedure of an indirect restoration.

Fixed prosthodontics, also referred to as *"crown and bridge"* is the specialized area of dentistry involved in replacing missing teeth with a gold or porcelain fixed **prosthesis** (adjective, *prosthetic*), which is cemented in place and cannot be removed by the patient. The *prosthodontist* is a doctor of dental surgery (DDS) with completion of an additional three years of clinical practice and research in the field of prosthodontics.

This chapter covers the preparation, making, and placement of indirect restorations that include inlays, onlays, veneers, single crowns, and bridges.

PLAN OF CARE

A patient's dental condition must be thoroughly evaluated before prosthodontic treatment is initiated. It is necessary to obtain detailed medical and dental histories, a thorough intraoral examination, diagnostic models, and a current series of full-mouth radiographs. The dentist can then determine a restorative treatment plan suited to the needs of the patient.

Recall

1. What are the more common terms used for fixed prostheses?
2. If a patient has poor dental hygiene habits, is fixed prosthodontics indicated?

Indications and Contraindications for Fixed Dental Prosthodontics

Indications

One or two adjacent teeth are missing in the same arch.

Supportive tissues are healthy.

Suitable abutment teeth are present.

Patient is in good health and wants to have the prosthesis placed.

Patient has the skills and motivation to maintain good oral hygiene.

Contraindications

Necessary supportive tissues are diseased or missing.

Suitable abutment teeth are not present.

Patient is in poor health or is not motivated to have the prosthesis placed.

Patient has poor oral hygiene habits.

Patient cannot afford the treatment.

INDIRECT RESTORATIONS

Indirect restorations, also known as *cast restorations,* are created in a commercial dental laboratory by a dental laboratory technician. A casting is permanent and cannot be reshaped; therefore the tooth structure that will hold the crown or bridge must be prepared to allow the casting to seat into place needing only minor adjustments by the dentist. The finished casting is delivered to the dental office ready to be bonded or cemented in place.

Inlays and Onlays

Inlays and onlays are cast restorations designed to fit snugly *within* a preparation of a tooth. An **inlay,** like a class II restoration, covers a portion of the occlusal and proximal surface (Fig. 50-1). An **onlay** covers the proximal surfaces and most or all of the occlusal surface (Fig. 50-2).

Gold is the strongest material available for these cast restorations, but gold does not match the color of the tooth. When esthetics is the primary concern, inlays and onlays are fabricated from porcelain, ceramic, or composite resin that can be made to exactly match the tooth color (Fig. 50-3).

Veneers

A **veneer** is a thin shell of tooth-colored material. There are two types of veneer restorations. The *direct veneer,* which was discussed in Chapter 48, also known as a *bonded veneer,* is created directly in the patient's mouth. An *indirect veneer* is fabricated in the dental laboratory on the basis of an impression taken of the prepared tooth.

Porcelain Veneers

Porcelain veneers are placed to improve the appearance of anterior teeth. Placement of veneers improves the appearance of a patient with intrinsic stains and anomalies such as *enamel hyperplasia* (Fig. 50-4).

An important factor in the creation and placement of an indirect veneer is matching the tooth color. Because of its translucence, the color of the finished veneer is also affected by the shade of the underlying tooth structure and by the color of the luting agent. The dentist must take these factors into account when selecting the shade for veneers.

The dentist uses specialized burs and discs to cut the preparation as conservatively as possible. After the preparation has been completed, gingival retraction is placed and a final impression is taken. Because only a thin layer of enamel is removed during the preparation on the facial surface, provisional coverage is not required.

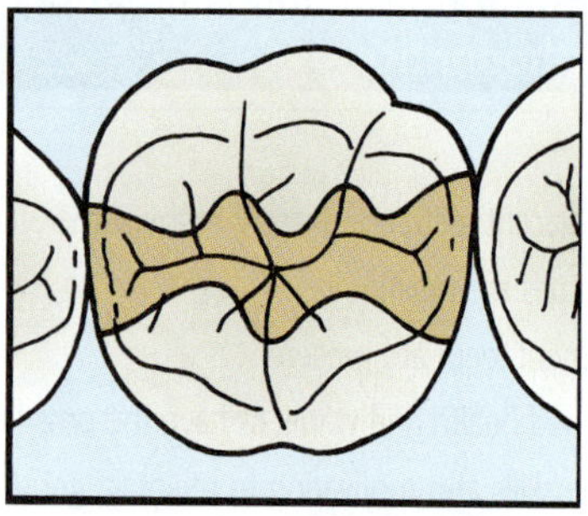

Fig. 50-1 Inlay cast restoration.

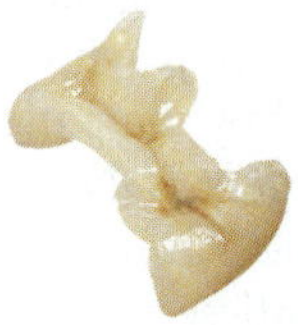

Fig. 50-3 Onlay fabricated from porcelain to match tooth color.

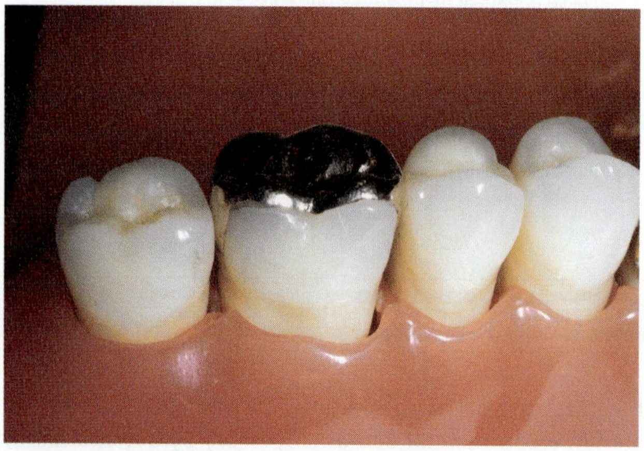

Fig. 50-2 Onlay cast restoration.

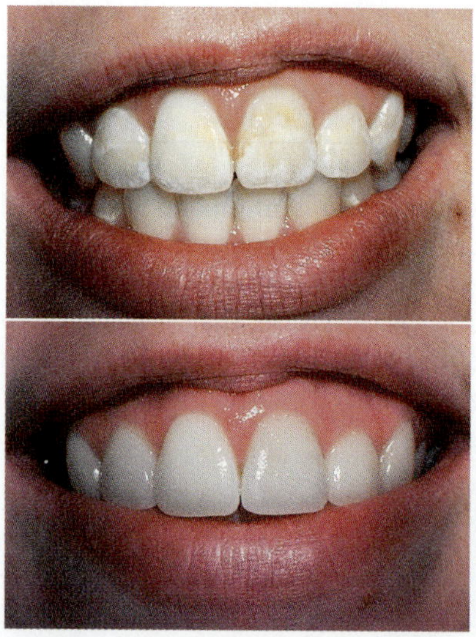

A

B

Fig. 50-4 **A** and **B,** Porcelain veneers placed to cover hypocalcification defects. (From Roberson T, et al: *Sturdevant's art and science of operative dentistry,* ed 4, St Louis, 2002, Mosby.)

At the cementation visit, the dentist tries the veneers for fit and color match. Before cementation, an **opaquer** may be placed on the tooth surface to block out underlying color and structural defects. The cement is also selected in a shade to enhance the color match. After etching and bonding, the veneers are then cemented in place. Any excess cement is removed, and final adjustments are made.

Crowns

A **full crown** completely covers the anatomic crown of an individual tooth (Fig. 50-5). The decision to place a full crown is made when a tooth is extremely decayed or fractured and cannot be reconstructed with a more conservative restoration. If a tooth is severely broken down, additional retention may be required with the use of retention pins or a post and core (see later in chapter for discussion).

The **three-quarter crown** differs from the full crown in that it does not cover the entire anatomic crown. Instead, the tooth is prepared so that the facial or buccal surface of the tooth is unchanged. When the crown is placed, the natural enamel on the facial surface is visible, and the crown covers the prepared portion.

A **porcelain-fused-to-metal (PFM) crown** is a full metal crown with outer surfaces covered with a thin layer of porcelain. This type of casting has the strength of a metal crown and the esthetic appeal of matching the natural tooth color (Fig. 50-6).

A *porcelain jacket crown* is constructed as a *very* thin metal shell covered by layers of porcelain built up to resemble the shading and translucence of the enamel of a natural tooth. These restorations are used on anterior teeth and are esthetically pleasing but lack the strength of a PFM crown.

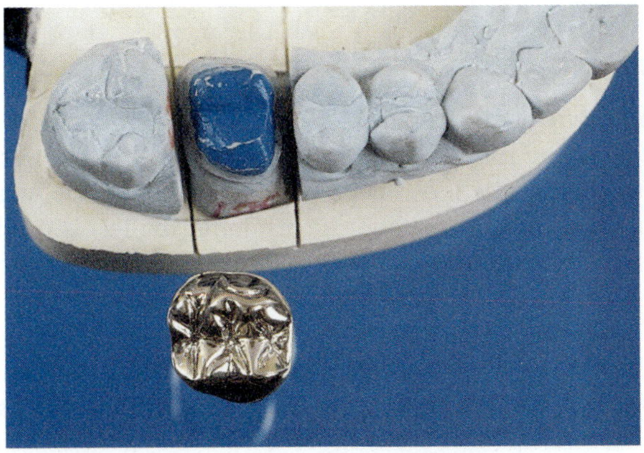

Fig. 50-5 Posterior gold crown.

Fixed Bridges

A **fixed bridge** is a type of prosthesis that is recommended when a tooth or teeth are missing within the same arch (Fig. 50-7). A fixed bridge consists of a series of units joined together for greater strength (Fig. 50-8). The bridge is cemented in place and cannot be removed by the patient. With proper oral hygiene habits, a fixed bridge will provide many years of excellent service.

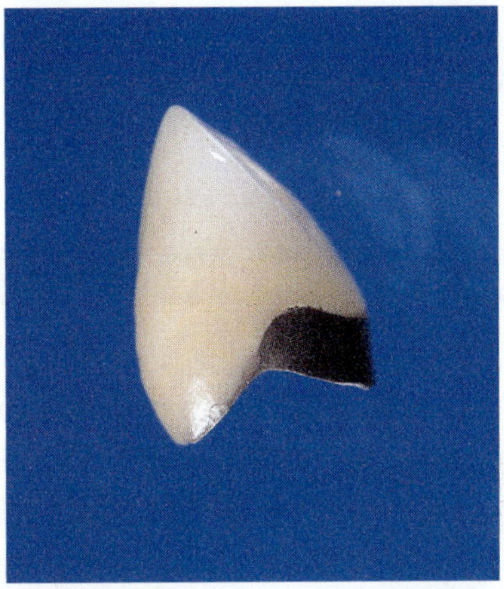

Fig. 50-6 Anterior porcelain-fused-to-metal (PFM) crown.

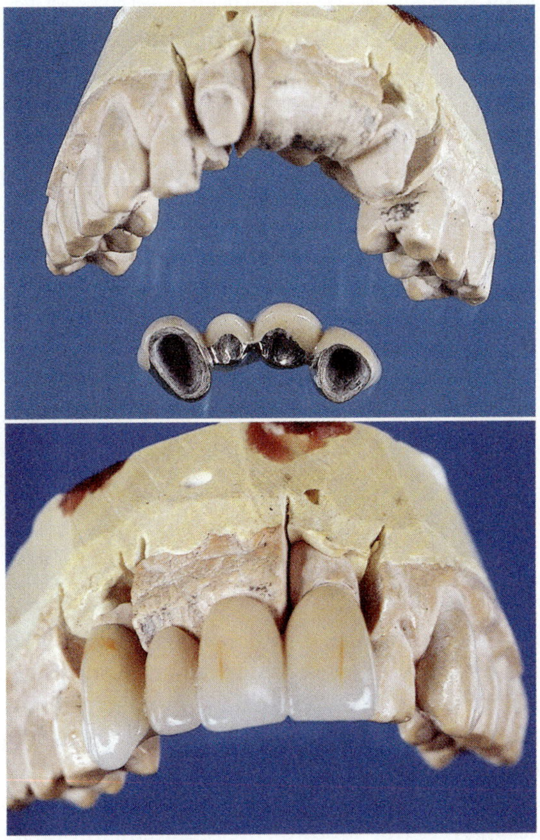

Fig. 50-7 Four-unit PFM anterior fixed bridge. The top photo shows the porcelain fused to the internal metal components. The lower photo shows the bridge seated on the working cast.

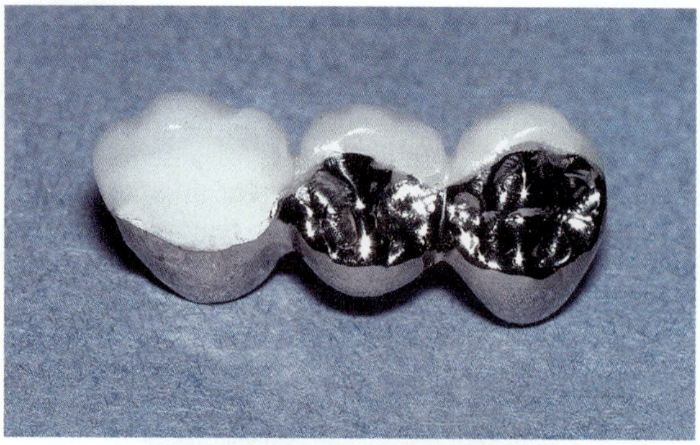

Fig. 50-8 Three-unit PFM bridge.

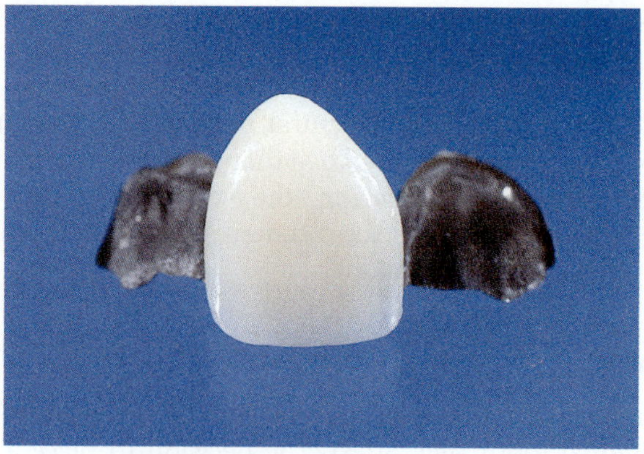

Fig. 50-9 Resin-bonded bridge.

Components of a Fixed Bridge

Unit

A bridge is described by the number of **units** (teeth) involved. For example, a bridge that replaces one missing tooth with its adjacent teeth holding the bridge in place would be a *three-unit bridge* because it consists of three parts (two abutments and a pontic).

Pontic

A **pontic** is the artificial tooth, or part of the dental appliance that replaces the missing natural tooth. When a bridge replaces more than one tooth, there is a pontic for each tooth being replaced.

Abutment

An **abutment,** also known as a *retainer,* is the natural tooth that serves as the support for the replacement tooth or teeth in a fixed bridge. There is *at least* one abutment at each end of the bridge. When a longer bridge is constructed to replace several teeth, two abutment teeth may be present at either end. The abutment tooth is commonly restored with an onlay or a cast crown. Because the completed bridge is placed in the mouth as a single piece, the abutment teeth must be in alignment to allow the bridge to slide into place without adding excessive width or length.

Resin-Bonded Bridge

A **resin-bonded bridge,** also known as a *Maryland bridge,* consists of a pontic having winglike extensions from the mesial and distal sides (Fig. 50-9). Bonding these extensions to the lingual surfaces of the adjacent teeth supports the pontic.

In selected situations, such as the replacement of a single missing anterior tooth or the replacement of congenitally missing lateral incisors, a bonded bridge is an attractive alternative to a traditional bridge. The dentist will decide if the patient is a candidate for this type of bridge.

The lingual surfaces of the adjacent teeth require limited preparation to accommodate the bridge supports. Some bonded bridges have very thin metal mesh extensions. Others have cast or PFM extensions that require more extensive tooth preparation so the natural contours of the abutment tooth are maintained when the completed bridge is bonded in place.

Recall

3. What type of indirect restoration is placed to improve the appearance of the facial surface of teeth?
4. What is the difference between an onlay and a three-quarter crown?

OVERVIEW OF A CROWN PROCEDURE

The placement of a cast restoration usually requires a minimum of two visits. The first appointment entails shade selection, preparation, impressions, and placement of provisional coverage. The second appointment involves cementation and finishing.

Shade Selection

If a crown or bridge is made of porcelain, matching the shade of the natural teeth is important and usually completed before the tooth is prepared. A **shade guide,** which contains samples of all of the available shades, is used to match the natural tooth color (Fig. 50-10). Most dentists prefer to take the shade selection while waiting for the local anesthetic agent to take effect.

The color sample is moistened and held close to the tooth to be restored. Because teeth are normally wet, this moisture helps achieve a more accurate match. To determine the shade, the match is checked in good light. Many

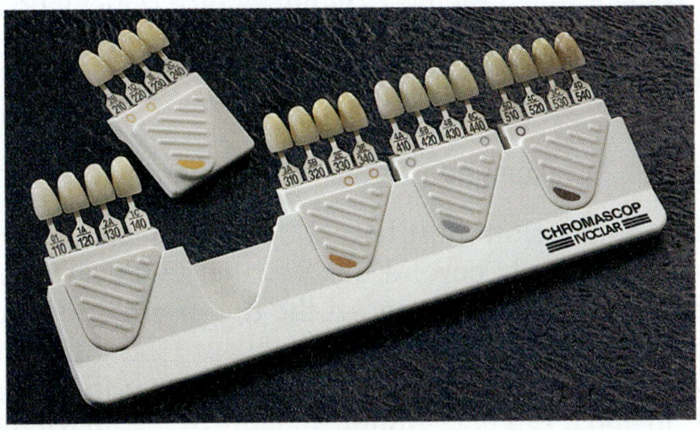

Fig. 50-10 **Shade guide, used to match the exact color of teeth.** (Courtesy Ivoclar Vivadent, Amherst, New York.)

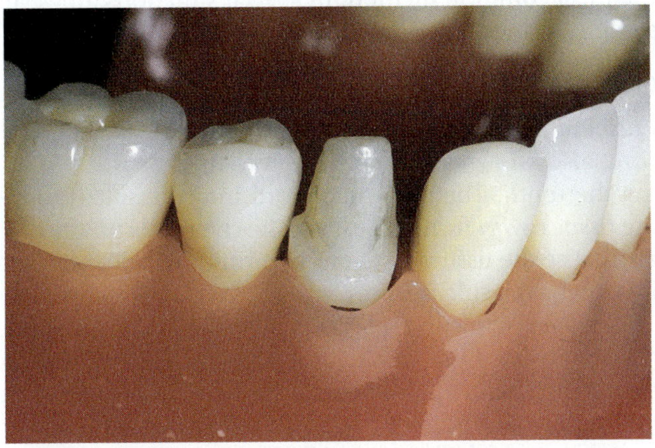

Fig. 50-11 **Prepared tooth structure showing height and contour.**

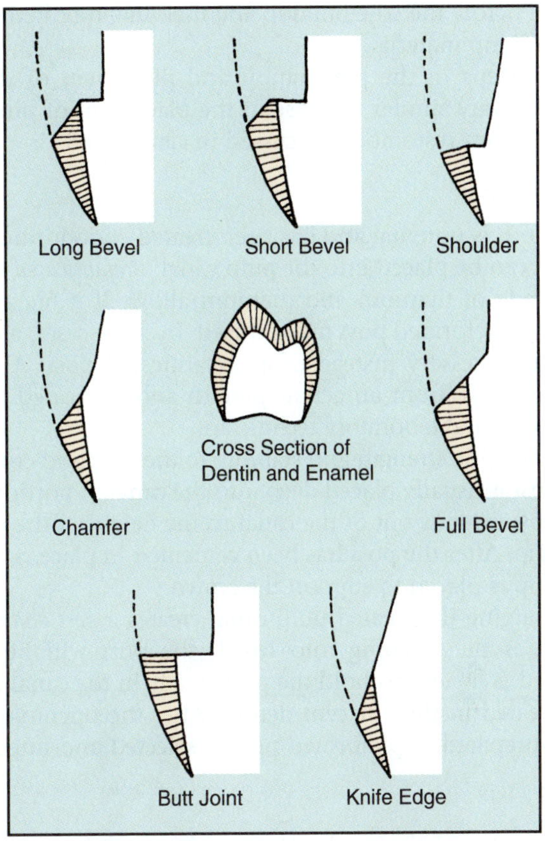

Fig. 50-12 **Prepared tooth structures showing different designs of the margin.** (From Baum RW, et al: *Textbook of operative dentistry,* ed 3, Philadelphia, 1995, Saunders.)

dentists prefer to use natural sunlight from a northern direction. The shade selected is identified by number from the shade guide and noted on the patient record and laboratory prescription.

The shade guide is a semicritical item that cannot withstand the heat of sterilization. After use, it is disinfected using a high-level EPA-registered disinfectant.

Preparation

During preparation, the dentist reduces the height and contour of the tooth with rotary instruments for a casting to have the necessary strength without increasing the overall size of the restored tooth (Fig. 50-11). The prepared tooth must also be designed so the cast restoration can slide into place and be able to withstand the forces of occlusion.

The gingival margins of the preparation are designed to provide a smooth, strong junction of the edges *(margins)* of the casting with the surface of the tooth. These margins are known by several terms, including the **bevel, chamfer,** and **shoulder** (Fig. 50-12).

Retention Aids for Crowns

When the coronal portion of a tooth is extensively decayed, fractured, or has been treated endodontically, it may be necessary to provide additional support for the crown to sit on.

Core Buildup

If the tooth is vital, a **core** buildup is used. This supports the cast crown and provides a larger area of surface retention for cementation of the crown. If an amalgam restoration is already in place, the restoration can be shaped and prepared (just like natural tooth structure) as the core (Fig. 50-13). If a restoration is not in place, a self-curing or light-cured composite material or reinforced glass ionomer cement is used for the buildup.

Retention Pins

Pin retention may be necessary to add strength to the core buildup for the crown. The type of crown and the location of the pulp determine the exact location of the pinholes and placement of the pins. When pins are used, they are placed before the core buildup and then incorporated into the buildup material.

The steps in the preparation and placement of these pins are very similar to those in the placement of pins in an amalgam restoration discussed in Chapter 48.

Post and Core

If a tooth is nonvital and has been treated endodontically, a post can be placed into the pulp canal. *Prefabricated posts* are made of titanium and titanium alloys. If it fits accurately, a preformed post may be used. In some cases, a **cast post** is necessary instead of a prefabricated post. A cast post is made from an acrylic pattern and fabricated by a trained dental laboratory technician.

To provide strength and stability to the post and crown, the post is usually placed deep into the canal. A portion of the post extends out of the canal to the height of the core buildup. After the post has been cemented in place, a core buildup is placed to support the crown.

Enlarging the treated pulp canal creates a *post channel*, which is the opening into which the post will be cemented. *Keyway slots* hold the post steady in the canal and are created in the adjacent dentin. After the opening has been prepared, a preformed post is selected and fitted. A *Lentulo spiral*, an endodontic instrument, is used to place the cement down the post channel. Once cementation of the post is complete, the dentist may proceed with the core buildup and tooth preparation.

Core Buildup Process

1. The core material is prepared.
2. The material is placed in an anatomic crown form and placed on the tooth.
3. After the initial set of the material, the crown form is slit and peeled away. The initial set time will vary depending on the material.
4. After the final set, approximately 10 minutes, the material is reduced to provide the foundation of the crown preparation.

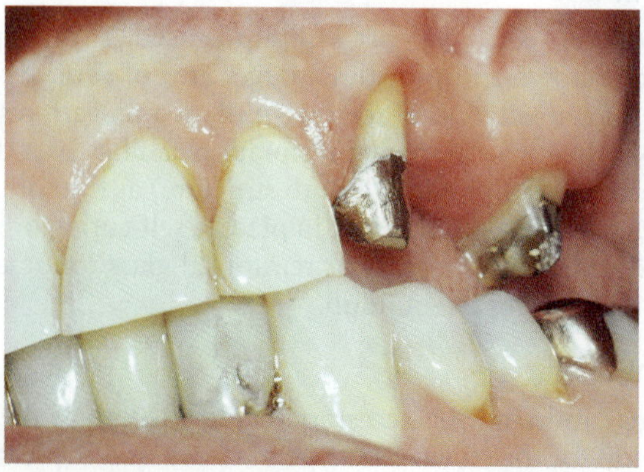

Fig. 50-13 An existing amalgam restoration is prepared for the core buildup designed to support the crown.

Gingival Retraction and Tissue Management

A final impression must have a detailed preparation that extends gingivally beyond the prepared tooth. Obtaining this detail is possible through the use of **gingival retraction.** Gingival retraction temporarily displaces the gingival tissue and widens the gingival sulcus so that the impression material can flow around all parts of the preparation.

Gingival retraction takes place *after* the preparation is complete and *just before* the final impression is taken. Chemical retraction through the use of retraction cord is the most common method. In special situations, however, surgical or mechanical retraction may be required.

Gingival Retraction Cord

Chemical retraction involves placing gingival retraction cord, also known as *packing cord,* into the sulcus surrounding the tooth. The packing of cord into the sulcus forces the tissues away from the tooth. The chemicals on the cord also cause the tissues to *contract* (shrink), which temporarily widens the sulcus.

Gingival retraction cords are available as untwisted *(plain)*, twisted, or braided. *Untwisted* cords must be twisted just before placement. *Twisted* and *braided* cords do not require additional twisting. Cords are available in various degrees of thickness, and the dentist will decide which thickness is needed (Fig. 50-14).

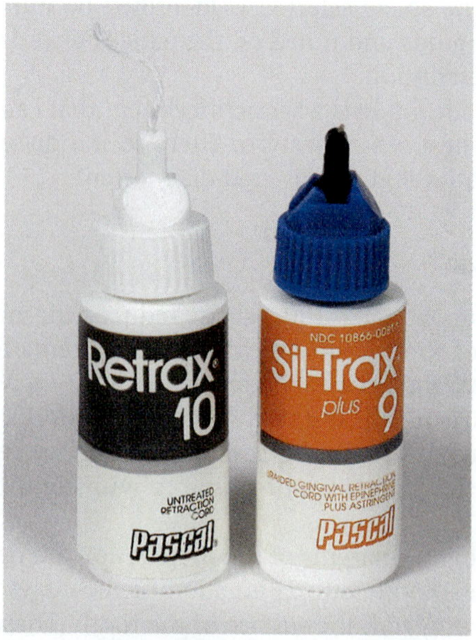

Fig. 50-14 Different types of gingival retraction cords.

Nonimpregnated retraction cord does not contain chemicals and retracts the tissues only by force. *Impregnated* retraction cord contains an astringent-vasoconstrictor agent that controls bleeding and causes the desired provisional shrinkage of the tissues.

Cords impregnated with a vasoconstrictor are contraindicated for patients with cardiovascular disease. For this reason, the patient's updated medical history is reviewed *before* the impregnated forms of retraction are used. If the use of epinephrine is contraindicated, a cord impregnated with aluminum chloride may be used instead. *Aluminum chloride* is a mineral astringent that does not produce undesirable cardiovascular effects.

A *hemostatic* solution also may be used to control bleeding in the area. The solution can be dispensed into a *dappen dish* and applied by lightly dabbing the area where bleeding is occurring with a cotton pellet moistened with the solution. Alternately, the solution can be dispensed with an **infuser** syringe with tips. Any solution that is dispensed but not used must be discarded.

Retraction Cord Packing

Retraction cord is placed with the use of a blunt cord-packing instrument. This instrument has a straight handle with a broad, rounded *(blunt)* working end used to place the retraction cord gently in the sulcus. Some operators use a plastic instrument with a blunted tip for this purpose. Regardless of the instrument used, the goal is to place the retraction cord *without* damaging the gingival tissues (see Procedure 50-1).

Procedure 50-1 Placing and Removing Gingival Retraction Cord

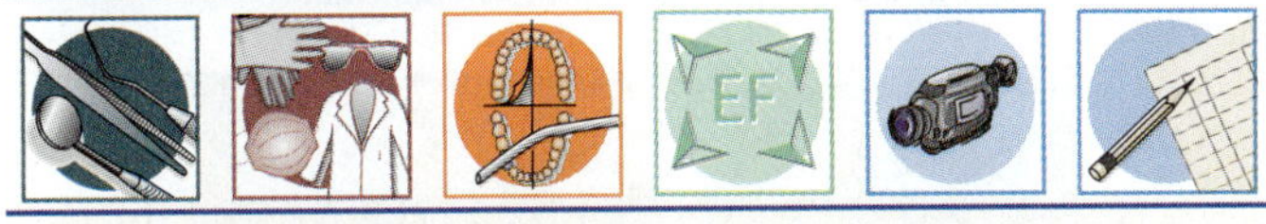

Equipment and Supplies

- Basic setup
- Cotton rolls
- Cord-packing instrument
- Gingival retraction cord
- Dappen dish
- Scissors

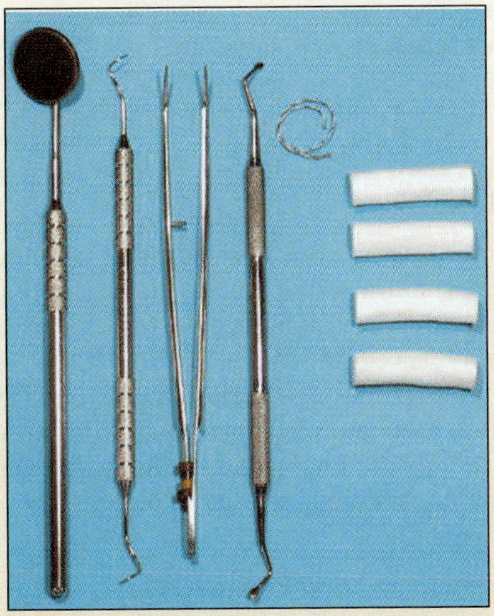

PROCEDURAL STEPS

Preparation

1. Rinse and gently dry the prepared tooth; isolate the quadrant with cotton rolls.
   Purpose: Dry tissue makes it easier to see the details of the gingival tissue and place the retraction cord.
2. Cut a piece of retraction cord 1 to 1½ inches in length, depending on the size and type of tooth under preparation.
   Note: The length is determined by the circumference of the prepared tooth and the placement technique to be used.
3. Use cotton pliers to form a loose loop of the cord.
   Purpose: This makes the cord easy to slip over the tooth, but the loop is not tied or knotted.

Placement

1. Make a loop in the retraction cord, slip it over the tooth, and position the loop in the sulcus around the prepared tooth.

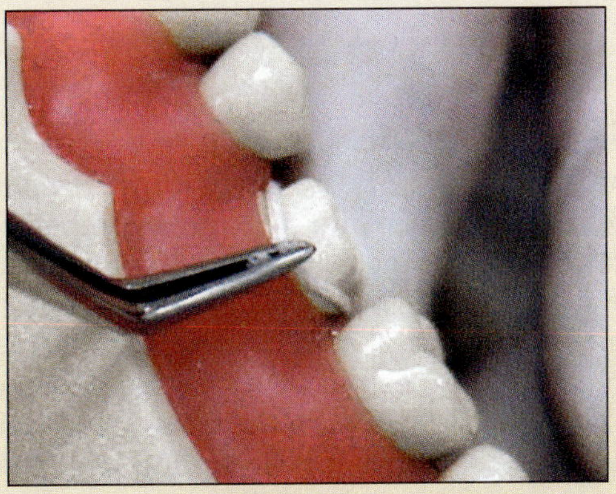

continued

Procedure 50-1 Placing and Removing Gingival Retraction Cord–cont'd

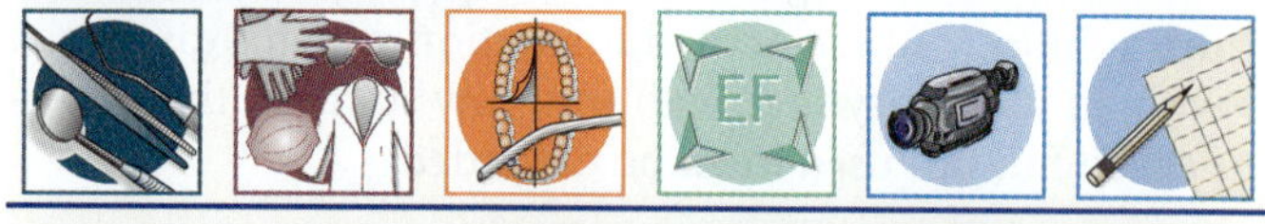

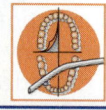

PROCEDURAL STEPS, cont'd

2. Using the cord-packing instrument and working in a *clockwise* direction, pack the cord gently into the sulcus surrounding the prepared tooth so that the ends are on the facial aspect.
   Purpose: The ends in this position are easier to reach for removal of the cord.

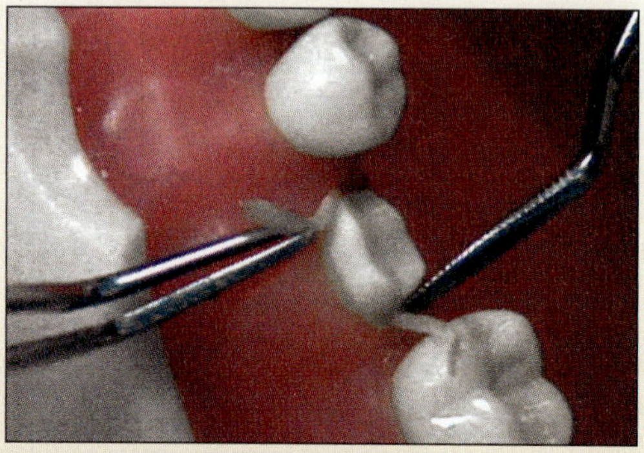

3. Pack the cord into the sulcus by gently rocking the instrument slightly backward as the instrument is moved forward to the next loose section of retraction cord. Repeat this action until the length of cord is packed in place.
4. Overlap the cord where it meets the first end of the cord. The ends may be tucked into the sulcus on the facial aspect.
   Note: An alternative is to leave a short length of the cord sticking out of the sulcus. This makes it easier to grasp and quickly remove the cord.
5. *Optional:* When a wider and deeper sulcus is required, two retraction cords may be placed with one on top of the other. *Before* the impression material is taken, remove the top cord. *After* the impression is completed, remove the second retraction cord.
6. The cord should be left in place for a maximum of five to seven minutes. Instruct the patient to remain still in order to keep the area dry.
   Purpose: The time allows the cord to push the tissue away from the tooth and stay in this position.
   Note: The exact time depends on the type of chemical retraction used.

Removal

1. Grasp the end of the retraction cord with cotton pliers, and remove it in a *counterclockwise* direction (the reverse of the method used in packing).
2. Remove the retraction cord just before the impression material is placed.
   Note: Usually the operator removes the cord while the assistant prepares the syringe-type impression material.

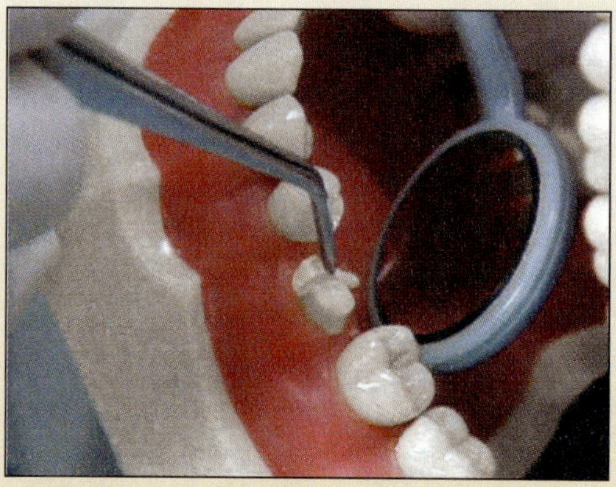

3. Gently dry the area, and apply fresh cotton rolls.
   Note: The impression is taken immediately.

The retraction cord is removed just before the impression material is placed. Often the operator removes the cord while the assistant prepares the syringe-type impression material.

Surgical Retraction

Surgical retraction may be necessary if **hypertrophied** tissue interferes with preparing and placing the restoration. This excess tissue may be removed electrosurgically or with a surgical knife. *Electrosurgery,* the most common method, is performed with a special electric tip that quickly cuts away the excess tissue and controls the bleeding. When using a surgical knife, the operator cuts the excess gingiva and frees it from the area. Bleeding may be profuse, and pressure or hemostatic material must be applied.

Mechanical Retraction

If other retraction methods are not suitable, the dentist may use mechanical retraction to force the tissue away from the tooth. A provisional crown, one that extends into the sulcus, is placed and worn by the patient for several days. It is removed just before the impression is taken.

The use of mechanical retraction requires an extra patient visit to take the final impressions. At the end of that visit, normal provisional coverage is placed.

Final Impression and Bite Registration

The final impression, also referred to as the *master impression,* for an indirect restoration must be accurate and detailed. If the impression is defective, the casting also will be defective. *Elastomeric materials* are generally used

Procedure 50-2 Assisting in a Crown and Bridge Restoration

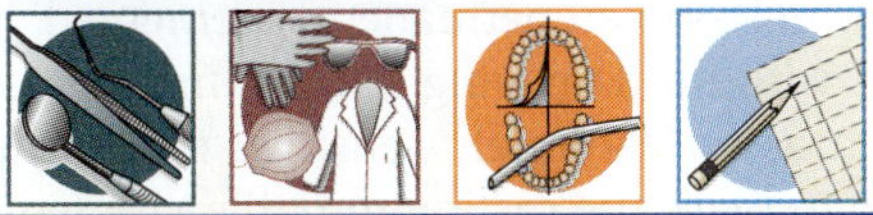

Equipment and Supplies

- Local anesthetic agent setup
- Alginate impression setup
- Shade guide (for tooth-colored restoration)
- Large spoon excavator
- Additional hand instruments (dentist's choice)
- Burs, diamond stones, and discs (dentist's choice)
- Gingival retraction setup
- Cotton rolls and gauze sponges
- High-volume oral evacuator (HVE) tip

At this visit, setups are also required for the following:

- Elastomeric impressions, which may include a custom tray
- Occlusal (bite) registration
- Provisional coverage fabrication, adjustment, and cementation supplies

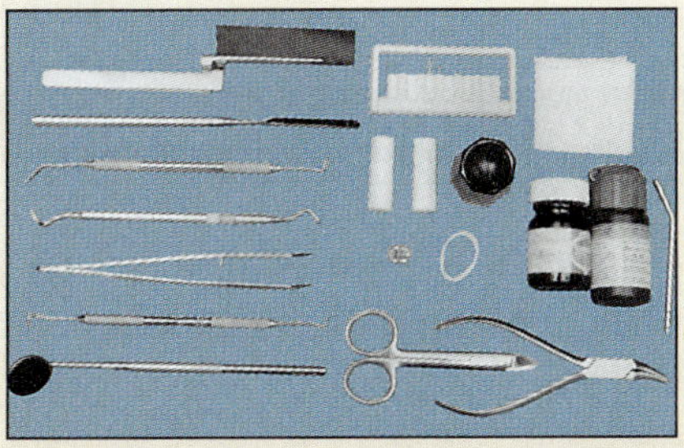

PROCEDURAL STEPS

Preliminary Steps

1. Assist in the administration of the local anesthetic agent.
2. If an alginate impression is needed to fabricate the provisional coverage, the impression is obtained at this time. In addition, an alginate impression is taken of the opposing arch (see Chapter 46).
3. If a silicone two-step impression method is used, the first impression is obtained at this time.
4. If this procedure involves a tooth-colored restoration, the shade is selected at this time.

Tooth Preparation

1. Throughout the preparation, maintain a clear operating field by using the HVE to retract the lips and tongue and to remove water and debris.
2. The dentist uses diamond stones in the high-speed handpiece to remove all decay or fractured portions of the tooth.
   Purpose: Diamond stones are used during crown preparation because they can rapidly remove tooth structure.
3. Assist in bur changes as necessary while the dentist reduces tooth bulk and completes the preparation using different-shaped burs.
4. When the preparation is complete, gingival retraction cord is placed.
5. Assist in readying the final impression material.
6. Before transferring the light-bodied material, transfer cotton pliers for the dentist to remove the gingival retraction cord.
   Note: The dentist may want to rinse and dry the sulcus before applying the light-bodied material.
7. While the dentist is applying the light-bodied material, ready the tray with heavy-bodied material.
8. Have the air-water syringe available for the dentist to "blow" air around the preparation.
   Purpose: This procedure thins out the material, allowing it to flow better in the sulcus and around the margins.
9. Retrieve the light-bodied material syringe from the dentist, and transfer the tray, ensuring that the dentist can grasp the handle and insert the tray properly.
10. After the recommended time for the material to set, the dentist will remove the tray.
11. The occlusal registration is obtained.
12. Provisional coverage is fabricated and temporarily cemented to protect the prepared teeth (see Chapter 51).
13. The patient is scheduled for a cementation appointment and then dismissed.
    Note: Ensure that the laboratory has sufficient time to fabricate the crown before scheduling the patient for another appointment.
14. After the dentist writes the laboratory prescription, prepare the case and send it to the laboratory.

Date	Tooth	Surface	Charting Notes
8/15/05	4	PFM	Crown prep, 2 carpules Xylocaine w/epi, final impression, temporary made and cemented with temp bond, Shade C2 for porcelain. Pt tolerated procedure well. Reschedule in 2 weeks for cementation. T. Clark, CDA/L. Stewart, DDS

to create these extremely accurate impressions. The dentist chooses the impression material to be used. It will also be necessary at this time to obtain a bite registration and an opposing-arch registration. Chapter 46 describes the mixing and application of final impressions and bite registrations.

Provisional Coverage

Provisional coverage is a protective temporary tooth covering that is placed after a tooth has been prepared and the final impression obtained. Chapter 51 illustrates the types of provisional coverage available, and the role of the expanded functions assistant in the fabrication.

The four specific rationales of provisional coverage are:

1. To reduce sensitivity and discomfort of the prepared tooth.
2. To maintain the function and esthetics of the tooth.
3. To protect the margins of the preparation.
4. To prevent shifting of adjacent or opposing teeth.

Generally, a provisional crown or bridge should maintain or restore function and keep the patient comfortable during the period from tooth preparation to final cementation, usually several days or a few weeks. Occasionally, patients are required to wear provisional coverage for a longer period to accommodate a more complex treatment plan (see Procedure 50-2).

Recall

5. How many appointments are required for a crown?
6. What part of the tooth is covered by a full crown?
7. What does the dentist use to reduce the height and contour of a tooth for a casting?
8. If a tooth is nonvital, what is fabricated and placed into the pulp for better retention of a crown?
9. What is used during a crown and bridge preparation to displace gingival tissue?
10. What type of agent is applied to retraction cord to control bleeding?
11. What other terms are used for overgrown tissue?
12. What types of impression are taken during crown preparation?

Delivery Appointment

Before a permanent restoration can be placed, the provisional coverage must be removed. A large spoon excavator, scaler, or Backhaus towel forceps may be used for this purpose. The provisional coverage should be placed aside in case it is needed again should a problem arise with the casting. The tooth preparation is examined, carefully cleaned, and dried.

When the casting has been fitted and is acceptable, the dentist cements it to the tooth with permanent cement. Great care must be taken during this step because once a cast restoration has been permanently cemented, it is almost impossible to remove it without damaging the casting, tooth, or both. In contrast, if the casting is not cemented properly, the margins may leak, decay may be recurrent, or the crown could slip off the preparation.

The cement selected for *luting* is the dentist's choice. Proper mixing of this cement in accordance with manufacturer's instructions, and placement of cement only on the interior surface of the crown are critical steps for the dental assistant. (See Chapter 45 and Procedure 50-3.)

Provisional Placement of a Permanent Casting

Once a cast restoration has been permanently cemented, it cannot be removed without damaging the casting. In special situations, such as an extremely sensitive tooth, the dentist may choose to place the casting initially with temporary cement, such as that used for provisional coverage. This provisional placement makes it possible to remove the casting without damage if a problem occurs with the tooth. If there are no problems, within a few weeks the crown is cemented into place with permanent cement.

Recall

13. What will the patient have on the prepared tooth while the laboratory is making a crown or bridge?
14. Who in the dental office is allowed to cement a crown or bridge permanently?

OVERVIEW OF A BRIDGE PROCEDURE

The preparation for a fixed bridge can be completed in two or three appointments: preparation, "try-in," and cementation.

Preparation Appointment

The first visit for a bridge is similar to the first visit for a crown but involves the preparation of at least two or more teeth. Also, a longer appointment is required. Depending on the case, the abutment teeth are usually prepared for either a full crown or an onlay.

After the preparations are complete, the final impressions, occlusal registration, and opposing arch impression must be taken. A custom provisional or temporary bridge is then placed. This bridge is prepared using the same technique as for coverage of an individual tooth.

Try-in Appointment

Before the second appointment, the assistant ensures that the case has been returned from the laboratory. At this stage the case consists of the castings for the abutment teeth without their tooth-colored covering. A local anesthetic agent is administered if necessary, and the provisional coverage is carefully removed, cleaned, and placed aside for reuse.

The castings are tried on the abutment teeth and checked carefully to determine their accurate fit. If the castings do not fit properly, final impressions are retaken and the try-in steps are repeated at the next appointment.

If they fit, the castings are left in place, and a polysiloxane impression is taken. When the impression is removed, the castings come off in the impression. This impression and castings are disinfected and returned to the dental laboratory for finishing. The provisional coverage is replaced, and the patient is scheduled for the final appointment.

In the laboratory, the technician uses this impression to assemble the bridge exactly as it will fit in the mouth. The units are soldered together, and the tooth-colored porcelain covering is added.

Cementation Appointment

Before the patient's appointment, the assistant ensures that the laboratory has returned the finished bridge. A local anesthetic agent is administered, if necessary. The provisional coverage is removed, and the completed bridge is tried on the prepared teeth. Adjustments are made as necessary, and the bridge is cemented in place (Fig. 50-15).

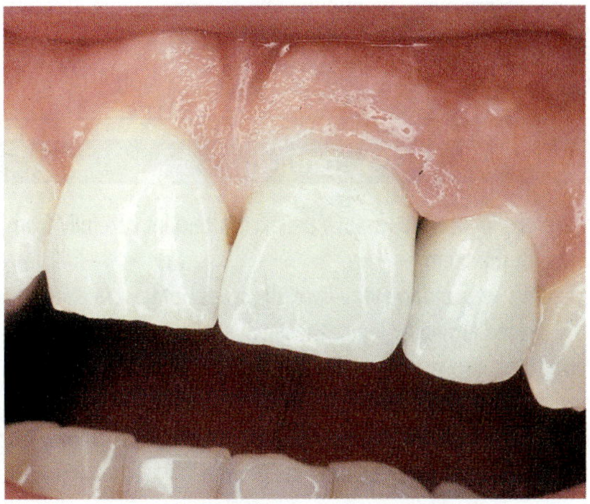

Fig. 50-15 Bridge cemented in place.

Procedure 50-3 Assisting in Delivery and Cementation of a Cast Restoration

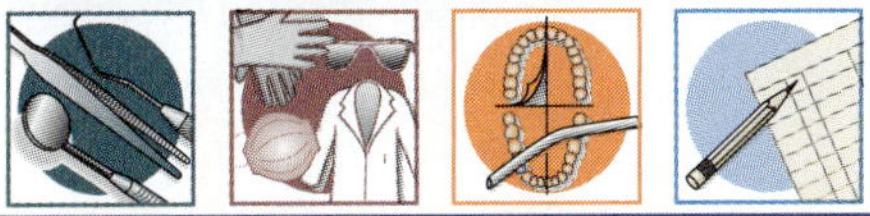

Equipment and Supplies

- Local anesthetic agent setup (if needed)
- Cast restoration
- Backhaus towel forceps (to remove provisional coverage)
- Large spoon excavator
- Cavity varnish/sealer and applicator (*optional*)
- Bonding supplies (dentist's choice)
- Cementation supplies (dentist's choice)
- Cotton rolls
- Saliva ejector (*optional*)
- Bite-stick
- Articulating paper and holder
- Polishing points and stones (dentist's choice)
- Scaler (to remove excess cement)
- Dental floss

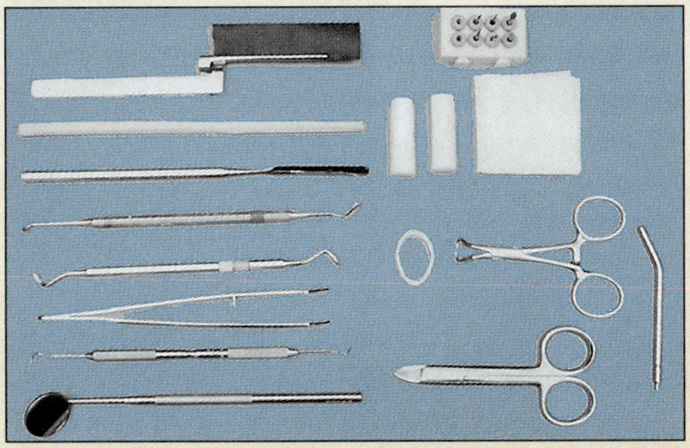

PROCEDURAL STEPS

1. Transfer cast restoration to the dentist to try on for fit. Transfer mirror and explorer.
2. When the dentist signals, mix the prepared cement.
3. Quickly apply the mixed cement in the internal surface of the casting, and transfer the prepared crown to the dentist.
4. The dentist places the crown on the prepared tooth, presses it into place, and then asks the patient to bite down on a wooden bite-stick or Burlew wheel to seat the restoration completely.

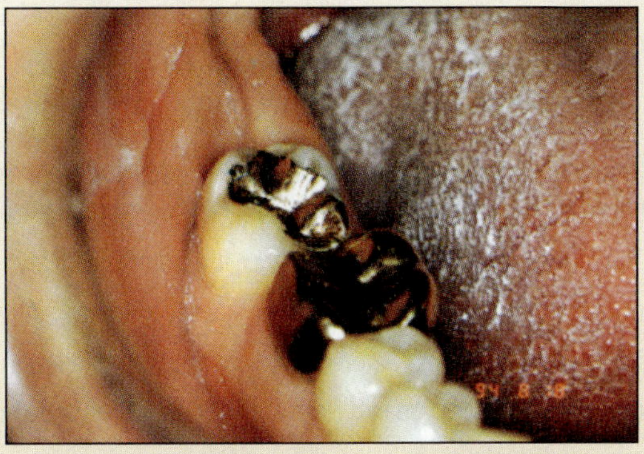

5. Instruct the patient to continue this biting pressure until the cement reaches the initial set, approximately 8 to 10 minutes.
6. *Optional:* Once the casting is firmly seated, a saliva ejector may be placed in the floor of the patient's mouth.
7. After the cement has set, remove the cotton rolls.

continued

Procedure 50-3 Assisting in the Delivery and Cementation of a Cast Restoration—cont'd

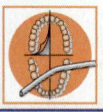

PROCEDURAL STEPS, cont'd

8. An explorer is used to remove the excess cement carefully from the crowns of the teeth.
   Note: This step is done very carefully so as not to scratch the newly placed crown or injure the gingiva.
9. A firm fulcrum is necessary for the hand that is holding the instrument.
   Purpose: The fulcrum prevents the instrument from slipping and consequently injuring the gingiva.
10. The tip of the instrument is placed at the gingival edge of the cement, and overlapping vertical strokes are used to remove the bulk of the cement.
11. Slight lateral pressure is applied (toward the tooth surface) to remove the remaining cement.
12. Dental floss with tied knots is passed between the teeth to remove excess cement from the interproximal areas.
   Purpose: The knots provide added bulk in removing the cement.
13. After the excess cement has been removed, the dentist may polish by using polishing points in the low-speed handpiece.

Date	Tooth	Surface	Charting Notes
9/03/05	4	—	Crown delivered, cemented with glass ionomer. Patient pleased with crown's fitting and appearance. T. Clark, CDA/L. Stewart, DDS

PATIENT INSTRUCTIONS

- Good home care is essential to the maintenance of a fixed prosthesis.
- The fixed prosthesis and supporting tissues must be brushed carefully each day.
- The other teeth are flossed as usual.
- A bridge threader is used to thread dental floss under the pontic and down into the sulcus at both abutments of the bridge.

Recall

15. How many appointments are required for a fixed bridge?
16. What accessory is used to help in flossing a bridge?
17. How is each unit of a bridge held together?

Laboratory Steps in Creating Indirect Restoration

1. The laboratory receives a prescription, final impression, and bite registration for the construction of an indirect restoration.
2. The final impression is poured to create the master casts. In the **master casts,** the prepared teeth are poured as **dies.** A **die** is an exact replica of the prepared portion of the tooth. The die is constructed so it can be taken in and out of the master cast.
3. The occlusal registration is used to position the casts properly on an **articulator** to simulate the patient's normal occlusion.
4. A wax pattern is created for the casting from the die of the prepared tooth.
5. The completed wax pattern is removed from the die, and a wax or plastic *sprue* is attached. In the casting process, the sprue forms a channel that allows the molten metal to flow into the mold.
6. The completed pattern and sprue are placed in a casting ring and *invested (encased)* in investment material. (*Investment material* is a special gypsum product that is able to withstand extreme heat.)
7. The casting ring is placed in a "burnout" oven. During the burnout process, the wax of the pattern and sprue is lost (burned away), and a negative pattern of the casting remains in the investment material.

Laboratory Steps in Creating Indirect Restoration—cont'd

8. The metal alloy is heated until it melts, and then centrifugal force is used to cause the molten metal to flow through the sprue opening and into the pattern. This creates the casting.
9. The cooled casting ring is placed in water to aid in removing the investment material, and the casting remains.
10. The *sprue button* (created when molten metal fills the sprue opening) is removed, and the casting is polished and completed.
11. To achieve a truly natural look on restorations, the dentist may instruct the laboratory technician to add characterization to the finished surface. These fine lines and small areas of slight discoloration resemble the stains or cracks that are present on the natural tooth.

ROLE OF THE DENTAL LABORATORY TECHNICIAN

A cast restoration is very precise, and must fit the prepared tooth exactly. A dental laboratory technician carefully fabricates a casting that meets the specific requirements stated on the laboratory prescription.

Laboratory Prescription

The laboratory technician can fabricate a casting only on the basis of a written prescription from the dentist (Fig. 50-16). The prescription should be detailed and precise in its description of the restoration or restorations to be fabricated. A copy of the prescription, also known as a *work order* or *requisition,* is included with the case, and a copy is retained with the practice records.

A laboratory prescription contains the following information:

- Dentist's name, license number, address, phone number, and signature
- Identification of the patient (name or case number)
- Type of prosthesis requested
- Type of alloy or other materials to be used
- Exact shade of restoration
- Anatomic characterization, if required
- Date on which the case is expected back at the dental practice

Laboratory Working Days

The laboratory requires a specific number of working days to complete the cast. These needs must be taken into consideration when the patient's return appointment is scheduled. Before the patient's next appointment, the assistant must determine whether the case has been completed and returned to the practice. If the case has not been returned or completed, it may be necessary to reschedule the patient's appointment.

MACHINE RESTORATIONS

Ceramic restoration systems are the newest technology available in many dental practices today. These systems combine the expertise of the dental laboratory technician and the proficiency of a computer. The two machining approaches for dental restorations are copy milling and CAD/CAM (computer aided design/computer assisted manufacturing) milling.

Copy milling works from a replica of the form to be fabricated. The dentist traces a pattern with a finger stylus, and the milling tool cuts the porcelain or ceramic into the shape. CAD/CAM uses digital information about the tooth preparation. The computer draws a three-dimensional design showing all margins and how the crown will look. Then the computer sends instructions to the milling tool to cut the restoration from a block of porcelain or ceramic (Fig. 50-17).

Recall

18. How does a dentist convey to a laboratory technician what type of crown to make?

19. What is the term for an exact replica of a tooth prepared by a laboratory technician?

20. What material does a laboratory technician use to create the pattern for a casting?

TRUE IMAGE BUSINESS FORMS 313377

PRECISION CERAMICS DENTAL LABORATORY

9591 Central Avenue • Montclair, CA 91763
(909) 625-8787 • (800) 223-6322
FAX: (909) 621-3125

TM FROM: DATE ______________

DR. ______________________ PHONE (____) ______________

ADDRESS ______________________ ACCT. NO. ______________

CITY ______________ STATE __________ ZIP __________

PATIENT'S NAME ______________________ AGE ____ SEX M F ____

TYPE OF CASE

☐ DICOR ☐ DICOR PLUS
☐ RENAISSANCE
☐ PORCELAIN ON METAL
☐ LAMINATE VENEER
☐ FULL CAST METAL
☐ MARYLAND BRIDGE
☐ ONLAY / INLAY
☐ PORCELAIN JACKET
☐ ACRYLIC JACKETS
☐ ACRYLIC ON METAL

TYPE OF METAL

☐ PREMIUM GOLD
☐ ECONOMY GOLD
Hard ☐ CLASS 4
☐ SEMI-PRECIOUS
☐ TITANIUM

GINGIVAL BANDS

☐ LINGUAL ONLY
☐ LINGUAL & FACIAL

CONTACTS

☐ NONE ☐ MEDIUM
☐ HEAVY

RIDGE RELIEF

☐ SLIGHT ☐ NONE
☐ MEDIUM ☐ SOCKET

☐ METAL TRY-IN ☐ BISQUE BAKE TRY-IN ☐ FINISH

	IN	OUT
DOCTOR'S MODELS (OPP)		
WORKING MODEL		
DIES		
IMPRESSIONS		
BITE		
ARTICULATOR		
SHADE GUIDE		
CROWN		
PARTIAL		
STUDY MODEL		
OTHER		
CHECK		

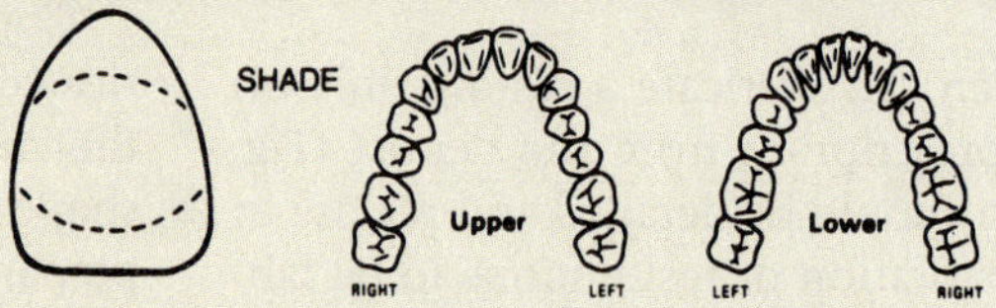

☐ OCCLUSAL STAIN Due In Your Office______________

PLEASE SEND: ☐ **BOXES** ☐ **Rx FORMS** ☐ **MAILING LABELS**
PLEASE CALL: ☐ ☐ **PARTIAL & DENTURE FORMS** ☐ **PRICE LIST**
CHECK NO:________ **VISA** ☐ **MC** ☐

*Signature*______________________ Lic. #______________

TERMS: Customer agrees to company policy as stated on reverse.

LAB COPY

Fig. 50-16 Laboratory prescription. (Courtesy Precision Ceramics, Montclair, California.)

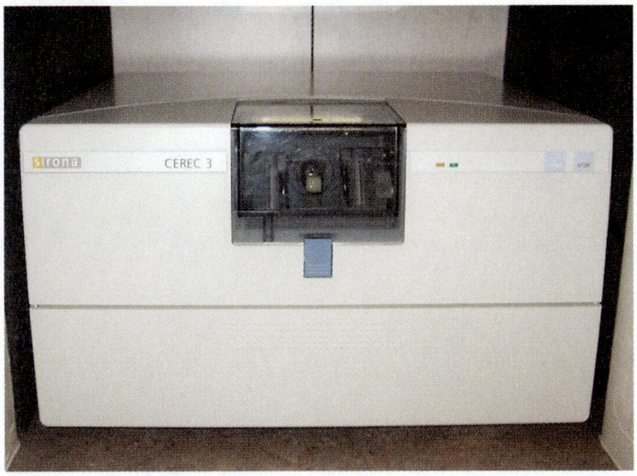

Fig. 50-17 CAD/CAM machine used to make ceramic dental restorations.

Patient Education

Your patients probably do not realize the amount of precise work that goes into the preparation, design, and fabrication of a crown or bridge. Delivery of a cast restoration to a patient truly involves a team, including the dentist, dental assistant, business manager, and dental laboratory technician.

Fixed prosthodontics is a tremendous investment for your patients. Acknowledge and educate your patients as they make positive decisions to take care of their oral health.

Legal and Ethical Implications

Because so many professionals are involved in the making of a cast restoration, communication is crucial in providing the best care to your patient. As an expanded-functions dental assistant, your involvement is important. You may be asked to take the preliminary impressions, place gingival retraction cord, fabricate and temporarily cement the provisional coverage, as well as assist in the series of appointments.

Remember always to review the patient record before treatment. Communicate with the dentist and dental laboratory technician, and practice only functions that are legal in your state.

Eye to the Future

The dental laboratory technician will be taking on a more important role in the future of dentistry. Until now, dentists received extensive training on the preparation of laboratory cases. Dental school curricula are changing and eliminating labwork. It will become common for certain dental specialties to hire a dental laboratory technician for patient casework.

Critical Thinking

1. Mrs. Cooper is coming in today for the preparation of a four-unit bridge to replace teeth #12 and #13. How many abutments and how many pontics will be present?
2. When placing the gingival retraction cord on tooth #20, from which surface of the tooth will the ends of the cord originate? From there, in which direction will you continue to pack the string?
3. The dentist has seated the finished crown and made all final adjustments. After mixing and loading the crown with cement, the dentist seats it, then notices that the crown is not seating completely. What do you think happened?
4. Your patient is diagnosed as having tetracycline stains. What type of procedure could the dentist recommend to this patient to cover and mask this anomaly?
5. A close friend of your family comes to you for advice about whether to spend "a lot of money" for a bridge or just have the teeth extracted and "get dentures." What would be your response?

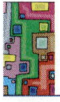

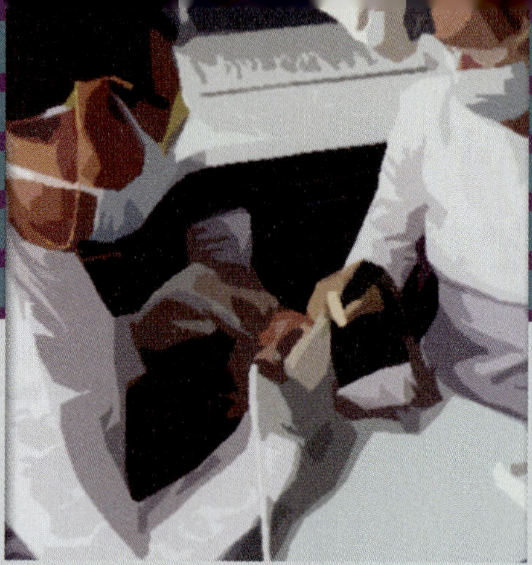

51 Provisional Coverage

Outline

KEY TERMS

Aluminum crown Thin crown used for provisional coverage on posterior teeth.

Custom provisional Pertaining to coverage designed from a preliminary impression or thermoplastic tray resembling the tooth being prepared.

Polycarbonate crown (*pah*-lee-**kahr**-bah-nate) Provisional crown made from a hard plastic tooth-colored material used for anterior teeth.

Polymer crown Provisional coverage designed in a shell-like form.

Preformed Pertaining to provisional coverage that is already shaped in the necessary appearance.

Provisional Pertaining to temporary coverage made for crown or bridge preparations and worn during cast preparation.

LEARNING OUTCOMES

On completion of this chapter, the student will be able to achieve the following objectives:

- Pronounce, define, and spell the Key Terms.
- Discuss the indications for provisional coverage for a crown or fixed-bridge preparation.
- Describe the types of provisional coverage.
- Discuss the dental assistant's role in making a provisional crown or bridge.
- Identify home care instructions for provisional coverage.

PERFORMANCE OUTCOMES

On completion of this chapter, the student will be able to achieve competency standards in the following skills:

- Fabricate a custom acrylic provisional crown.
- Fabricate a custom acrylic provisional bridge.
- Fabricate a direct provisional crown from a preformed polymer crown.
- Prepare and temporarily cement a polycarbonate crown.

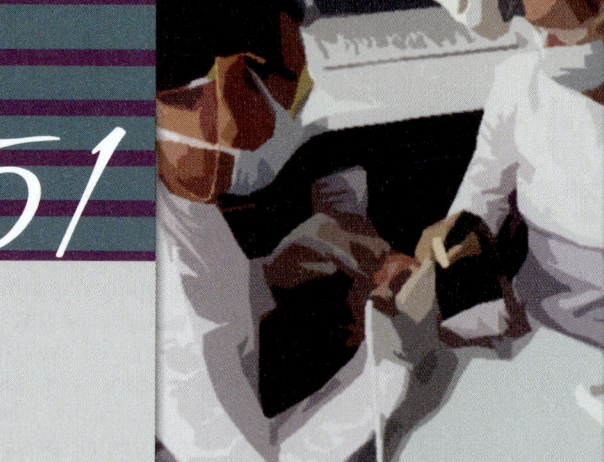

Provisional coverage is a *temporary* protective crown or bridge that is cemented to a prepared tooth for a single crown or to abutment teeth for a bridge. The patient wears provisional coverage while the dental laboratory technician prepares the fixed prosthesis.

A **provisional** crown or bridge restores and maintains function to that area of the mouth, as well as keeps the patient comfortable during the period from tooth preparation to final cementation. In most cases, this period can range from two weeks to one month. Occasionally, patients are required to wear a provisional prosthesis for a longer period to accommodate a more complex treatment plan. This type of treatment typically involves implants or periodontal therapy. Indications for provisional coverage are:

- To reduce sensitivity and discomfort of the prepared tooth and surrounding tissues.
- To maintain function and esthetics of the tooth.
- To protect the margins of the preparation.
- To prevent shifting of the adjacent or opposing teeth.

TYPES OF PROVISIONAL COVERAGE

Several types of provisional coverage are available. The dentist determines the type of coverage used on the basis of the patient's needs. The construction and temporary cementation of provisional coverage may be an *expanded function* in the state in which you practice. These procedures may be delegated to you as major roles in your clinical position.

Custom provisional represents the most common type of provisional coverage used for crown and bridge preparations (Fig. 51-1). Custom preparations can be the most time-consuming dental prostheses to make, but they provide the best-fitting and most natural-looking restorations. This custom technique can be used for either posterior or anterior crowns or bridges.

Preformed polymer crowns represent the type of provisional coverage used for posterior preparations (Fig. 51-2). These shell-like crowns are available for single crowns as well as for bridgework. The prostheses are supplied with a hybrid composite resin that bonds with the preformed crown.

Aluminum crowns are thin crowns made from a medium-hard aluminum for good durability. They are used for posterior teeth where strength is essential and a match with the tooth color is not a primary concern (Fig. 51-3).

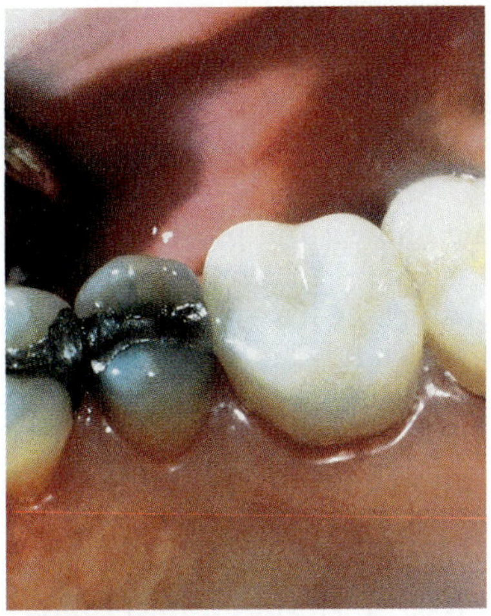

Fig. 51-1 Custom provisional coverage.

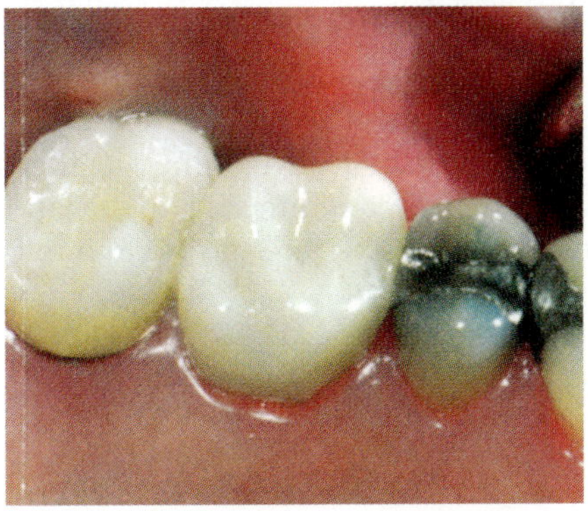

Fig. 51-2 Preformed polymer crown.

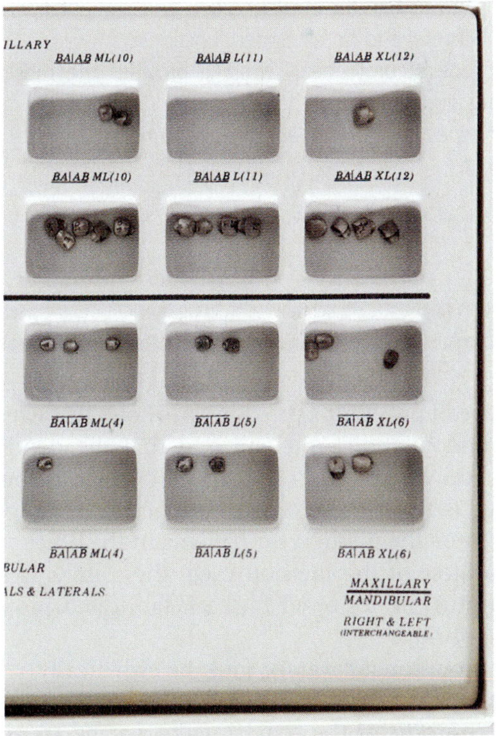

Fig. 51-3 Aluminum crown.

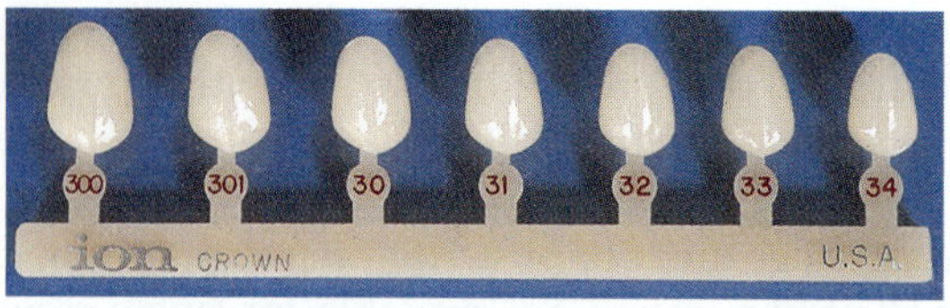

Fig. 51-4 Preformed polycarbonate crowns.

Preformed polycarbonate crowns are used where appearance is important. They are customized in varying sizes for anterior teeth (Fig 51-4).

Laboratory-fabricated coverage is used less frequently. When several teeth have been prepared, or when a long-span bridge is being created, a laboratory can complete the provisional prosthesis. A cast of the teeth before they are prepared is sent to the laboratory well in advance of the preparation appointment. When the laboratory approach is used, it is important to determine whether the provisional coverage has been returned from the laboratory and is ready for use.

Recall

1. What is the term for a temporary covering for a crown or bridge?
2. How long does a patient normally wear provisional coverage?
3. Why is it possible for the fabrication and cementation of provisional coverage to be expanded functions?
4. What type of provisional coverage provides the most natural-looking appearance?
5. What types of provisional coverage can be used for anterior teeth?

CRITERIA FOR PROVISIONAL FABRICATION

Each type of provisional prosthesis follows its own unique fabrication method. You will find that the dentist with whom you work will prefer a specific type of provisional coverage that works best for the practice. This approach will become the method for patients in the office.

Regardless of the method used, the following specific criteria must be followed for each fabricated provisional crown or bridge:

- The provisional coverage must be esthetically acceptable.
- The contours of the provisional coverage are similar to those of the natural tooth, with adequate interproximal contacts and appropriate alignment within the arch.
- The cervical margin of the provisional coverage is smooth and fits snugly, with no more than 0.5 mm of space between the crown margin and the finish line of the preparation.
- The provisional coverage does not extend below the margin of the preparation.
- The occlusal surface of the provisional coverage is aligned with the occlusal plane of the adjacent teeth.
- *Alternative:* To avoid trauma to the prepared tooth, the crown may be intentionally taken out of occlusion by making the occlusal surface slightly lower than the adjacent teeth.
- When temporarily cemented, the provisional coverage remains stable, stays in place, and is comfortable for the patient.
- The provisional coverage can be readily removed without damage to the tooth or adjacent tissues.

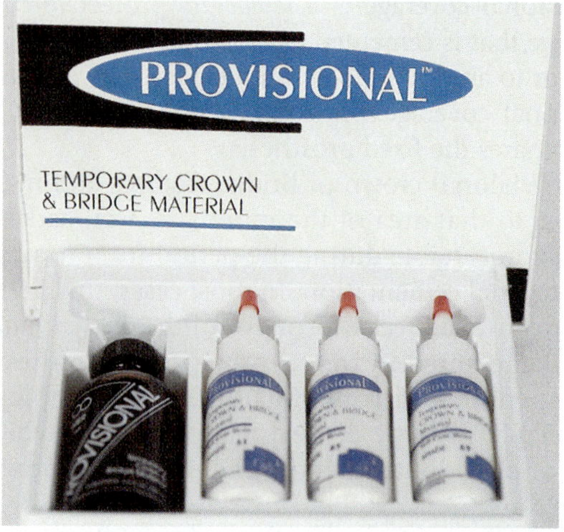

Fig. 51-5 Acrylic resin in powder/liquid form.

CUSTOM PROVISIONAL COVERAGE

In the making of a custom provisional crown or bridge, acrylic resin is placed in a preliminary alginate impression (see Chapter 46) or a vacuum-formed tray (see Chapter 47), which is taken and prepared for use prior to preparing the teeth for the final impression (see Procedures 51-1 and 51-2).

The most common material used for provisional coverage is *self-curing acrylic* (methylmethacrylate). This material is supplied as cartridges or as a liquid *(monomer)* and powder *(polymer)* (Fig. 51-5). The polymer comes in a variety of shades to match the color of the adjacent teeth.

Procedure 51-1 Fabricating and Cementing a Custom Acrylic Provisional Crown (Expanded Function)

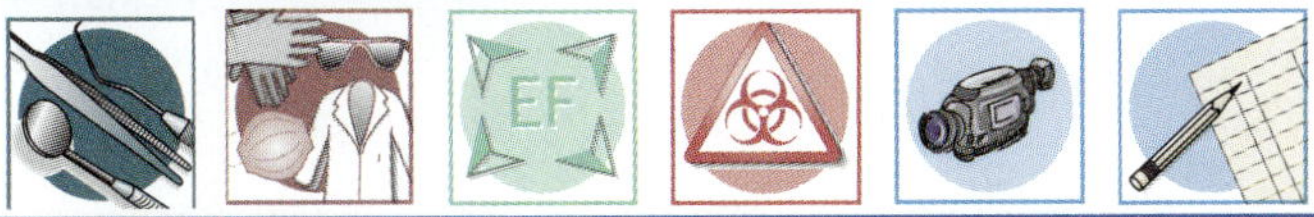

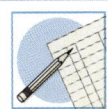

Equipment and Supplies

- Basic setup
- Spoon excavator
- Alginate impression (obtained *before* preparation of the teeth)
- Separating medium
- Cotton rolls
- Self-curing acrylic resin (liquid and powder)
- Spatula (small, cement type)
- Mixing container/dappen dish
- Scissors
- Surgical knife (optional)
- Burnisher ("beaver tail" or ball)
- Straight handpiece and mandrel
- Finishing diamond, discs, or burs
- Polishing discs or burs
- Articulating paper
- Pumice paste
- Lathe and sterile, white rag wheel
- Provisional cementation setup

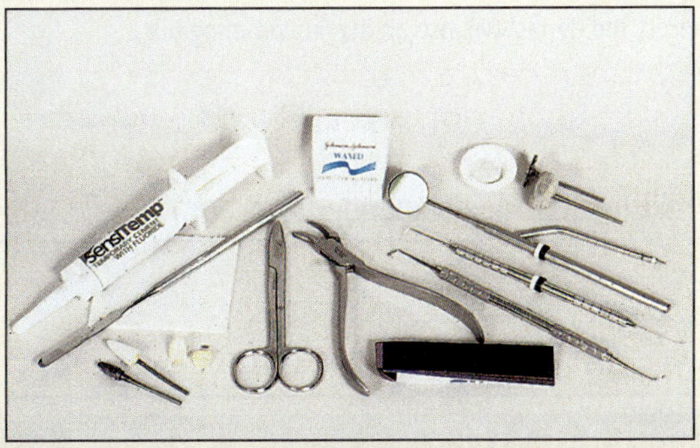

PROCEDURAL STEPS

1. Obtain an alginate impression of the arch *before* the teeth are prepared.
   Purpose: You want the provisional coverage to be a replica of the tooth before the dentist prepares it.
2. Check the impression to be sure it is free of debris and tears in the area selected for the construction of the provisional crown or bridge covering.
3. Disinfect the impression and keep moist until needed.
   Purpose: If allowed to dry, the impression will be distorted, and the provisional coverage will not fit.
4. Isolate the prepared tooth with cotton rolls to maintain moisture control.
5. Lightly apply petroleum jelly or a liquid medium to the prepared tooth to facilitate separating the acrylic dough from the preparations.
6. Place liquid monomer in the mixing container; 10 drops of liquid per unit is recommended. Quickly dispense the selected shade of self-curing powder (polymer) into the monomer until the powder is saturated.
   Important: Cover the monomer container immediately; this material is very volatile.
7. Use a small spatula to blend the powder and liquid to a homogeneous mix.
8. Set the mixed material aside for one to two minutes until the resin reaches a doughy, less glossy stage.
   Important: Do not let the resin cure beyond this point.
9. Unwrap the alginate impression, and gently dry the area of the teeth to receive provisional coverage.
10. Remove the resin from the mixing container with a small spatula, and immediately place it *within* the area of the prepared teeth.
    Optional: Express the acrylic resin from a cartridge directly into the impression.

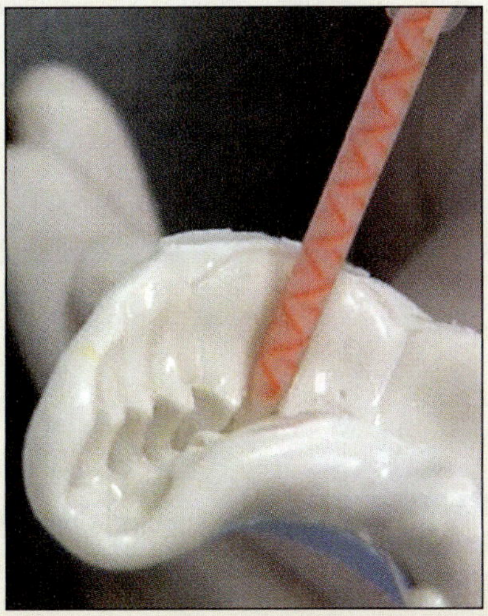

11. Place the acrylic-loaded impression back into the patient's mouth on the prepared tooth or teeth.
12. Allow the material to reach an initial set, approximately three minutes, and remove the tray from the patient's mouth.
13. Carefully remove the provisional coverage from the alginate impression, and place it onto the patient's teeth.
    Purpose: To avoid excess shrinkage during the final curing stage.

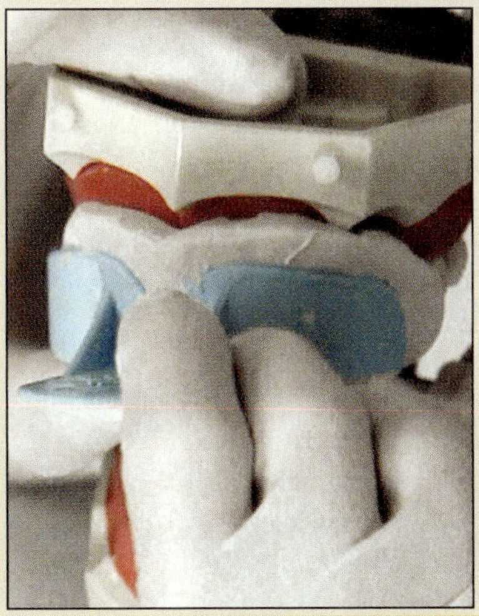

continued

Procedure 51-1 Fabricating and Cementing a Custom Acrylic Provisional Crown (Expanded Function)—cont'd

PROCEDURAL STEPS, cont'd

14. Mark the marginal border and contact points of the provisional coverage with a pencil to provide better visualization of the markings.

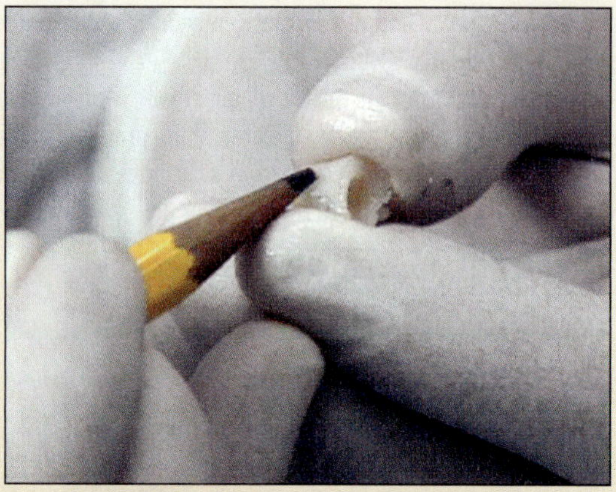

15. Trim the acrylic resin to within 1 mm of the gingival shoulder of the prepared tooth with an acrylic bur or stone.
    Note: Any trimming completed by the expanded-functions dental assistant (EFDA) must be completed outside the mouth with the low-speed handpiece and acrylic burs.
16. Check the occlusion, accuracy, and completeness of the provisional coverage, and adjust as necessary. Remove the provisional coverage from the prepared tooth, and complete the trimming with an acrylic bur.
17. Remove the provisional coverage and take it to the laboratory, where it is polished with a sterile white rag wheel and pumice on the laboratory lathe.
    Caution: Safety goggles *must* be worn throughout the trimming and polishing procedure. In addition, be aware that the rag wheel could remove a large bulk of acrylic or could overheat and cause distortion of the provisional coverage.
18. Temporarily cement the provisional coverage with provisional cement, such as zinc oxide–eugenol (Temp Bond) or intermediate restorative material.
19. Check the occlusion with articulating paper. If any reduction is required, the dentist will use an acrylic-trimming bur.

Procedure 51-2 Fabricating and Cementing a Custom Acrylic Provisional Bridge (Expanded Function)

Equipment and Supplies

- Basic setup
- Spoon excavator
- Alginate impression (obtained *before* preparation of the teeth)
- Separating medium
- Cotton rolls
- Self-curing acrylic resin (liquid and powder)
- Spatula (small, cement type)
- Mixing container/dappen dish
- Scissors
- Surgical knife (optional)
- Burnisher ("beaver tail" or ball)
- Straight handpiece and mandrel
- Finishing diamond, discs, or burs
- Polishing discs or burs
- Articulating paper
- Pumice paste
- Lathe and sterile, white rag wheel
- Provisional cementation setup

PROCEDURAL STEPS

1. Obtain an alginate impression of the arch *before* the teeth are prepared.
   Purpose: You want the provisional coverage to be a replica of the teeth before the dentist prepares it.

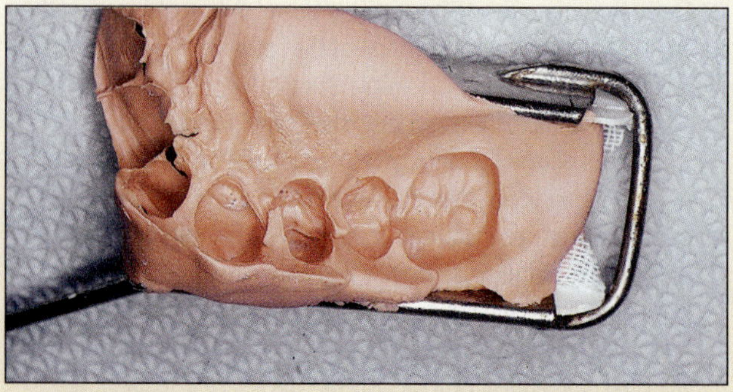

2. Check the impression to be sure it is free of debris and tears in the area selected for the construction of the provisional coverage.

Procedure 51-2 Fabricating and Cementing a Custom Acrylic Provisional Bridge (Expanded Function)—cont'd

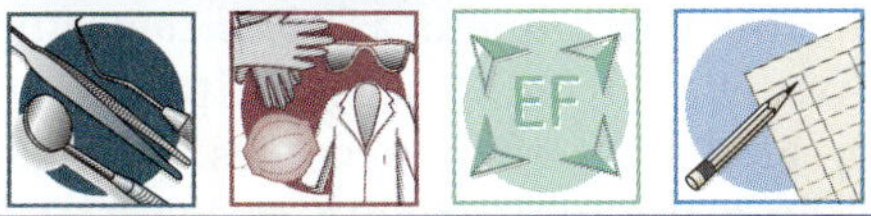

3. Disinfect the impression and keep moist until needed.
   Purpose: If allowed to dry, the impression will be distorted, and the provisional coverage will not fit.
4. Isolate the prepared teeth to maintain moisture control.

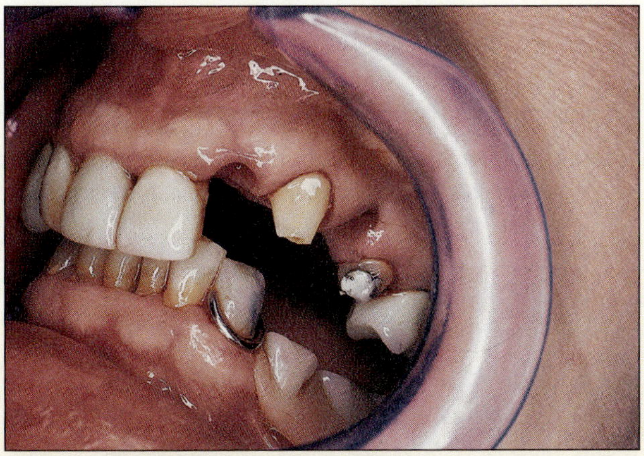

5. Lightly apply petroleum jelly or a liquid medium to the prepared tooth to facilitate separating the acrylic dough from the preparations.
6. Place liquid monomer in the mixing container; 10 drops of liquid per unit is recommended. Quickly dispense the selected shade of self-curing powder (polymer) into the monomer until the powder is saturated.
   Important: Cover the monomer container immediately; this material is very volatile.
7. Use a small spatula to blend the powder and liquid to a homogeneous mix, or prepare cartridge.
8. Set the mixed material aside for one to two minutes until the resin reaches a doughy, less glossy stage.
   Important: Do not let the resin cure beyond this point.
9. Unwrap the alginate impression, and gently dry the area of the teeth to receive provisional coverage.
10. Remove the resin from the mixing container with a small spatula, and immediately place it *within* the area of the prepared teeth. *Optional:* Express the acrylic resin from a cartridge directly into the impression.
11. Place the acrylic-loaded impression back into the patient's mouth on the prepared tooth or teeth.
12. Allow the material to reach an initial set, approximately 3 minutes, and remove the tray from the patient's mouth.
13. Carefully remove the provisional coverage from the alginate impression, and replace it onto the patient's teeth.
   Purpose: To avoid excess shrinkage during the final curing stage.
14. Mark the marginal border and contact points of the provisional coverage with a pencil to provide better visualization of the markings.
15. Trim the acrylic resin to within 1 mm of the gingival shoulder of the prepared tooth with an acrylic bur or stone.
   Note: Any trimming completed by the EFDA must be completed outside the mouth with the use of the low-speed handpiece and acrylic burs.
16. Check the occlusion, accuracy, and completeness of the provisional coverage, and adjust as necessary. Remove the provisional coverage from the prepared tooth and complete the trimming with an acrylic bur.
17. Remove the provisional coverage and take it to the laboratory, where it is polished with a sterile white rag wheel and pumice on the laboratory lathe.
   Caution: Safety goggles *must* be worn throughout the trimming and polishing procedure. In addition, be aware that the rag wheel could remove a large bulk of acrylic or could overheat and cause distortion of the provisional coverage.
18. Temporarily cement provisional coverage with provisional cement, such as zinc oxide–eugenol (Temp Bond) or intermediate restorative material.

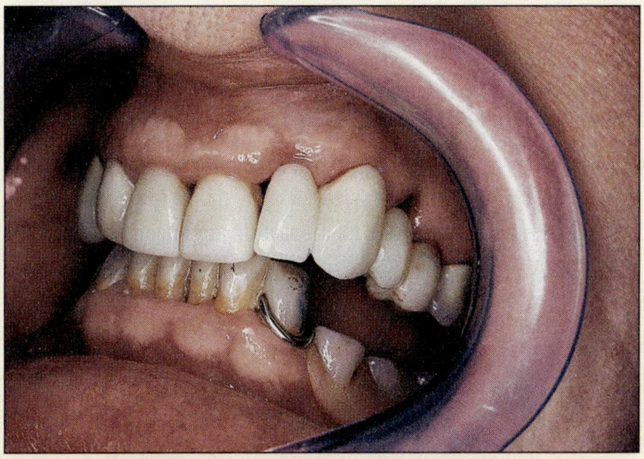

19. Check the occlusion with articulating paper. If any reduction is required, the dentist will use an acrylic-trimming bur.

PREFORMED POLYMER CROWNS

The preformed technique uses already-fabricated provisional shell-like crowns designed specifically for teeth. These shells are made from a polymer material and are designed with anatomic features of natural teeth. Having this shell reduces procedural steps by not requiring the preliminary impression or fabrication of a thermoplastic tray (Procedure 51-3).

The resin used in this technique is a *hybrid composite* resin-monomer mixture that has a setting time of 90 seconds. The resin and shell then becomes a single bonded unit, providing the patient with strength and optimal margins for the time required by provisional coverage.

Procedure 51-3 Fabricating and Cementing a Preformed Provisional Crown (Expanded Function)

Equipment and Supplies

- Basic setup
- Shell or bridge unit
- Composite resin mixture
- Dappen dish
- Laboratory spatula
- Low-speed handpiece
- Articulating paper and holder
- Acrylic burs
- Rubber wheels
- Temporary cement setup

PROCEDURAL STEPS

1. With the dentist, examine the prepared tooth for size and shape, and select the crown unit from the kit.
2. Mix the resin as directed and fill the shell, being sure not to trap any air bubbles in the material.

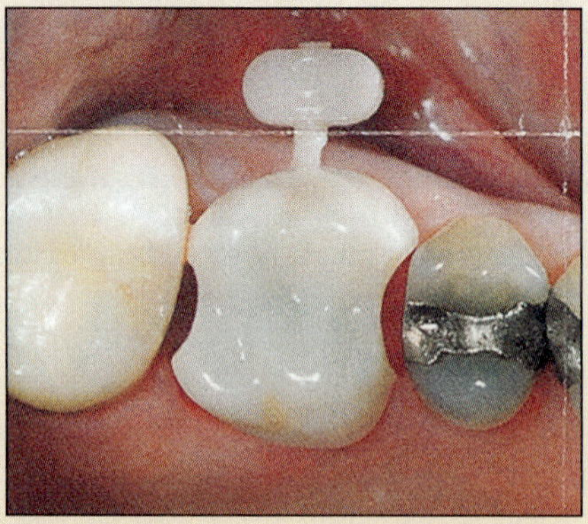

3. Seat the shell over the tooth or teeth, and ask the patient to bite down.

   Note: You will notice excess resin flowing from the shell into the margins and contacts.

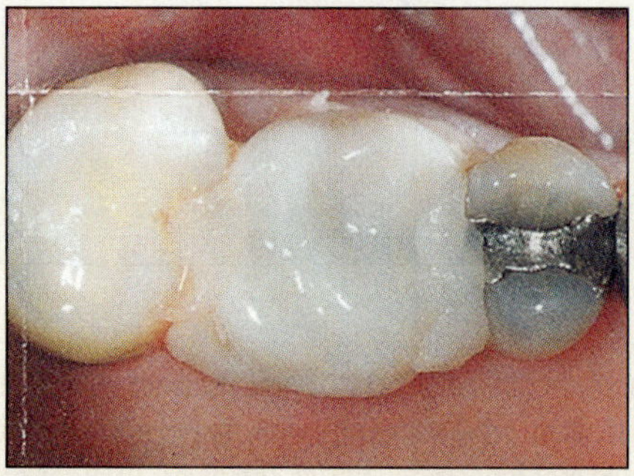

4. Use your fingers to apply pressure to the buccal and lingual areas of the crown.
5. Remove excess resin from the margins after 20 to 30 seconds.
6. Lift crown off and on tooth until the resin is hard. The time for this material is approximately 90 seconds.

   Purpose: To prevent the crown from locking onto the tooth.
7. Mark the patient's occlusion with articulating paper and with a pencil around the margins and contact points, and then adjust using acrylic burs, discs, and rubber wheels.

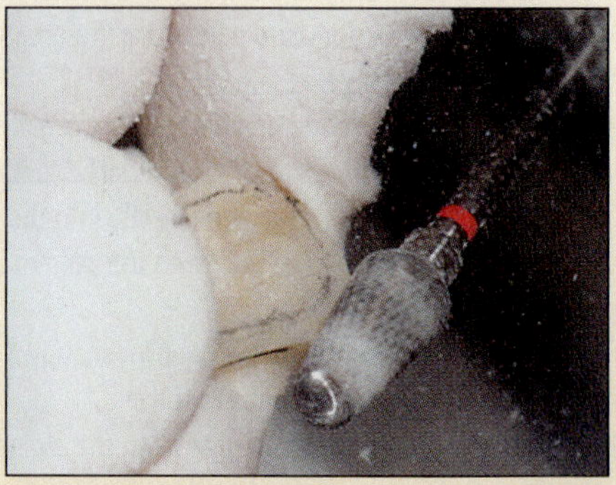

8. Finish the crown or bridge.
9. Cement with temporary cement.

PREFORMED POLYCARBONATE CROWNS

Tooth-colored preformed polycarbonate crowns are used on anterior teeth where appearance is important. These crowns are available in a variety of sizes, shapes, and shades and have an *identification tab* on the occlusal surface or incisal edge to indicate location of placement. This tab is removed once the crown has been selected. These crowns have the stability and appearance to remain on the tooth preparation as the temporary, or can also be used as a mold for acrylic resin as a custom temporary. If a preformed crown is tried in the mouth and *not* selected for use, it must be sterilized before reuse (see Procedure 51-4).

Procedure 51-4 Fitting and Cementing a Preformed Polycarbonate Crown (Expanded Function)

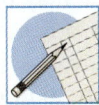

Equipment and Supplies

- Basic setup
- Selection of preformed polycarbonate crowns
- Crown scissors
- Acrylic-trimming stone or acrylic bur
- Burlew wheel
- Brush and pumice paste
- Articulating paper
- Provisional cementation setup

PROCEDURAL STEPS

Preparation

1. Select a crown of the appropriate shape and size, and check it for width, length, and adaptation at the margins.

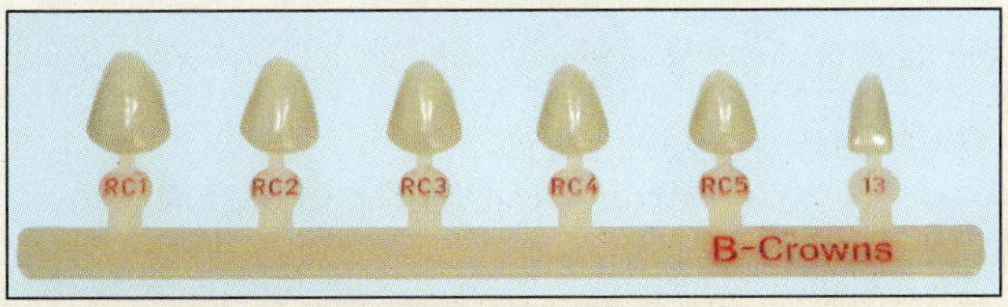

(From Duggal MS et al: *Restorative techniques in paediatric dentistry,* Philadelphia, 1995, Saunders.)

2. If necessary, use crown scissors to reduce the height (length) of the crown by trimming the cervical margin.
3. Smooth rough edges with an acrylic-trimming stone or acrylic bur, and polish with a Burlew wheel or a brush with pumice.

Cementation

4. Use provisional cement to hold the crown in place. Intermediate restorative material powder mixed with a small amount of petroleum jelly may be used.
   Purpose: The petroleum jelly facilitates removal of the crown.
5. Seat the crown on the prepared tooth.
6. Carefully remove excess cement with an explorer or a scaler.
7. Check the occlusion. If indicated, use a stone in the low-speed handpiece lightly to adjust the occlusion.

ALUMINUM CROWNS

A prepared posterior tooth can be protected by the placement of an aluminum crown. Such crowns are available in a range of sizes in aluminum or anodized gold. The crown surface may be *anatomic* (with simulated anatomic details) or *nonanatomic* (with no anatomic details). This technique has diminished in frequency, but can be used when cost and time are a factor.

Another type of temporary crown is the stainless steel crown. This crown can be used for long-term adult cases, but is commonly used for primary molars. To learn more about the fitting and cementing of stainless steel crowns, refer to Chapter 57.

Recall

6. What is required before tooth preparation in the making of custom provisional coverage?
7. What type of dental material is commonly used to fabricate custom provisional coverage?
8. After mixing the acrylic resin, where is it placed before seating it on the prepared tooth?
9. Why would an aluminum crown be selected for use?
10. Does a polycarbonate crown remain on a prepared tooth, or is it just a mold for the provisional coverage?

HOME CARE INSTRUCTIONS

For the patient with provisional coverage waiting for the delivery of a crown or bridge, the following instructions must be provided to the patient before he or she leaves the office:

- Bite and chew carefully on the provisional coverage, and avoid sticky foods.
- When flossing, do not "pop" the floss in and out of the contact. Once the floss is placed below the contact, pull the floss through the contact, to either the lingual or the facial side.
- If the provisional coverage is loose or lost, contact the office immediately to have it replaced.

Patient Education

Your patient has been informed that he or she will be wearing a "temporary" crown or bridge for the next couple of weeks. However, your patient most likely does not realize the importance of this coverage. If provisional coverage is not appropriately constructed to protect the margins, or if the prosthesis comes off and the dental office is not notified, the patient's crown or bridge preparation can be adversely affected. The crown or bridge may not fit properly, or the dentist may need to make adjustments in the preparation or restart the procedure.

Be sure to inform and educate your patient about the importance of the provisional coverage and appropriate home care.

LEGAL AND ETHICAL IMPLICATIONS

The EFDA can have a major role in the fabrication and temporary cementation of a provisional crown or bridge. It is the dentist's and your responsibility to remain current with the new provisional materials and techniques available. Remember that this procedure may be an *expanded function* and only legal for you to practice if your state permits. Check and keep current with your state's rulings and regulations.

Eye to the Future

As mentioned in Chapter 50, the dental laboratory technician will become increasingly involved in the dental practice setting. Many dental offices will have a complete laboratory setup with a dental laboratory technician on staff. By having the technician on hand, and with the availability of new indirect materials, there will be no need for provisional coverage. The dentist will be able to prepare the tooth structure while the technician is preparing the crown or bridge.

Critical Thinking

1. A patient comes in for a crown preparation for tooth #29. Because of the location of the crown, what type of provisional coverage would be recommended?
2. The dentist has anesthetized a patient and starts preparation for a crown on tooth #29. During the course of preparation, you realize that you did not obtain a preliminary impression. What would you do in regard to the making of a provisional crown?
3. After removing the provisional crown from a prepared tooth, you notice that the margins are too short. What is your plan of action in adjusting the crown so that it fits properly?
4. The dentist asks you to make provisional crowns for teeth #8 and #9. Your choice of coverage is the polycarbonate crown. Because you are preparing the maxillary centrals, what are your concerns regarding these provisional crowns?
5. What are the two most common temporary cements used for provisional coverage?

52

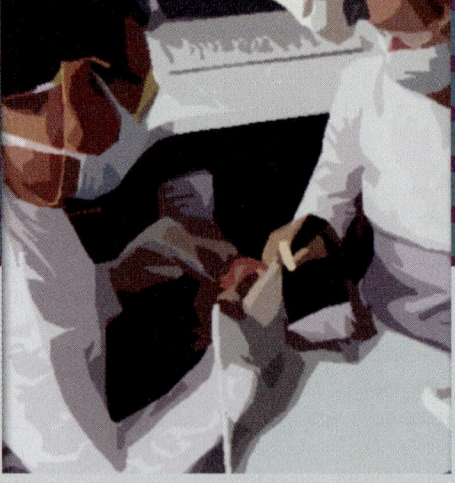

Removable Prosthodontics

Outline

KEY TERMS

Alveoplasty (al-**vee**-ah-o *plas*-tee) Surgical reduction and reshaping of the alveolar ridge.

Articulator (ahr-**tik**-u-*lay*-ter) Dental laboratory device that simulates the movements of the mandible and the temporomandibular joint.

Baseplate Rigid, preformed shape used during the fitting of a full denture to represent the base of the denture.

Border molding Process of using fingers to contour a closer adaptation of the margins of an impression while still in the mouth.

Centric relation (cen-tric) Having the jaws in a position that produces a centrally related occlusion.

Connector Piece of metal that joins the various parts of a partial denture; also called *bar.*

Coping (**ko**-ping, **kop**-ing) Thin metal covering or cap placed over a prepared tooth.

Edentulous (e-**den**-chuh-lus) Without teeth.

Festooning (fes-**too**-ning) Procedure to trim or shape a denture to simulate normal tissue appearance.

Flange (**flanj**) Parts of a full or partial denture that extend from the teeth to the border of the denture.

Framework Metal skeleton of a removable partial denture.

Full denture (**den**-chur) Prosthesis that replaces all of the teeth in one arch.

Immediate denture Temporary denture placed after the extraction of anterior teeth.

Lateral excursion (ek-**skur**-zhun) Sliding position of the mandible to the left or right of the centric position.

Mastication (*mas*-tah-**kay**-shun) Chewing.

Occlusal rim (ah-**klu**-sul) Rim built on the baseplate to register vertical dimension and occlusal relationship of the mandibular and maxillary arches.

Overdenture Full denture supported by two or more remaining natural teeth.

Partial denture Removable prosthesis replacing teeth within the same arch.

Post dam Seal in back of a full or partial denture that holds it in place; also called *posterior palatal seal.*

KEY TERMS, cont'd

Pressure points Specific areas in the mouth where a removable prosthesis may rub or apply more pressure.

Protrusion (pro-**tru**-zhun) Position of the mandible placed forward as related to the maxilla.

Rebasing (*re*-**bay**-sing) Procedure to replace the entire denture base material on an existing prosthesis.

Relining (*re*-**lie**-ning) Procedure to resurface the tissue side of a partial or full denture so that it fits more accurately.

Resorption (*re*-**sorp**-shun) The body's processes of eliminating existing bone or hard tissue structure.

Rest Metal projection on or near the retainer of a partial denture.

Retainer (ri-**tay**-ner) Device used to hold attachments and abutments of a removable prosthesis in place.

Retrusion (*re*-**tru** zhun) Position of the mandible posterior from the centric position as related to the maxilla.

Template (**tem**-plut) Clear plastic tray that represents the alveolus as it should appear after teeth have been extracted.

Tori (**tor**-*i*) Abnormal growths of bone in a specific area.

Tuberosity (*too*-buh-**rah**-seh-tee) Rounded area on the outer surface of the maxillary bones in the area of the posterior teeth.

LEARNING OUTCOMES

On completion of this chapter, the student will be able to achieve the following objectives:

- Pronounce, define, and spell the Key Terms.
- Differentiate between a partial and a full denture.
- Identify indications and contraindications for removable partial and full dentures.
- List the components of a partial denture.
- List the components of a full denture.
- Describe the steps in the construction of a removable partial denture.
- Describe the steps in the construction of a full denture.
- Discuss the construction of an overdenture and an immediate denture.
- Identify home care instructions for removable partial and full dentures.
- Identify the process of relining or repairing a partial or full denture.

PERFORMANCE OUTCOMES

On completion of this chapter, the student will be able to achieve competency standards in the following skills:

- Assist in the delivery of a partial denture.
- Assist in the try-in of the wax setup for a full denture.
- Assist in the delivery of a full denture.

Removable prosthodontics is the dental specialty in which missing teeth are replaced with a prosthesis that the patient can put in and take out of the mouth freely. There are two major types of removable prosthetics:

- *Removable* **partial denture,** commonly referred to as a *partial,* which replaces one or more teeth in the same arch (Fig. 52-1).
- *Removable full denture* commonly referred to as a *denture,* which replaces all the teeth in one arch (Fig. 52-2).

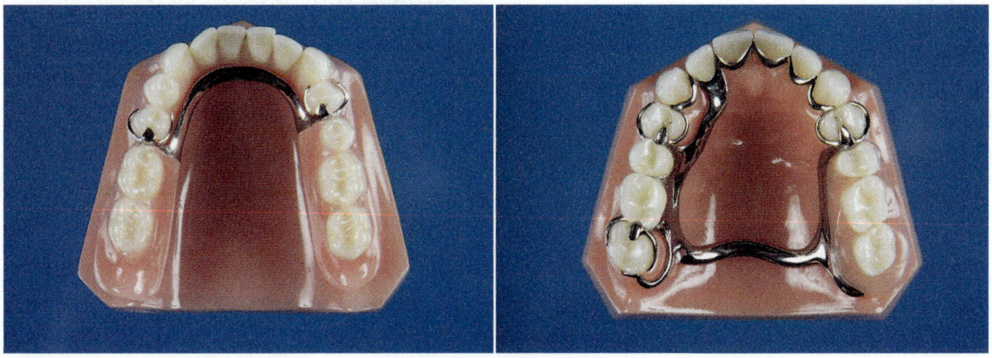

Fig. 52-1 Partial denture.

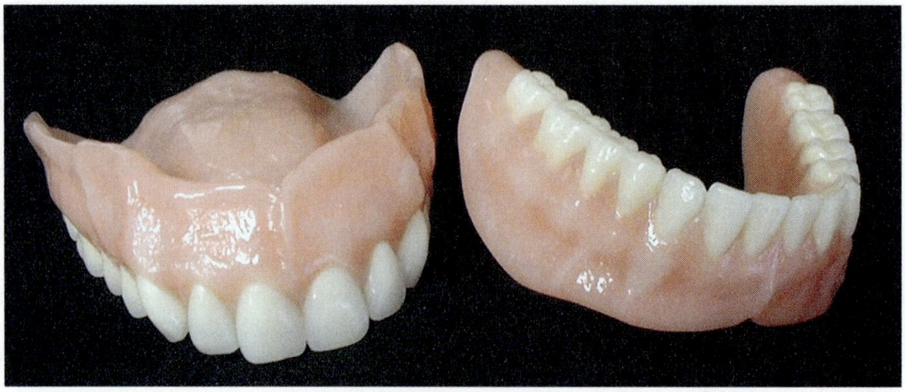

Fig. 52-2 Full denture. (Courtesy Ivoclar Williams, Amherst, New York.)

FACTORS INFLUENCING THE CHOICE OF A REMOVABLE PROSTHESIS

The dentist must advise patients who are considering a removable prosthesis that a prosthesis will never function as well as the natural dentition being replaced, regardless of how well it is constructed and fits. The dentist considers the following extraoral and intraoral factors before recommending a treatment plan for a patient.

Extraoral Factors

Although extraoral factors are usually beyond the control of the dentist, they cannot be ignored. These factors include the patient's physical and mental health, motivation, age, occupation, and dietary habits, as well as social and economic factors.

Physical Health

Certain physical conditions, such as diabetes, affect the ability of the tissues to tolerate the pressure of a removable prosthesis. Also, the patient who is in extremely poor health may be unable to cooperate during the fabrication of a new prosthesis or unable to adapt to wearing it.

Mental Health

Individuals with poor mental health may be irritated by and overly concerned about the denture in their mouth. Patients with severe mental disability or mental deterioration may not be able to keep the appliance in place or maintain adequate oral hygiene.

Patient Motivation

Occasionally, a patient's major reason for having teeth extracted and replaced with a prosthesis is *esthetic,* that is, only to improve appearance. The dentist explores all other acceptable alternative treatment options before giving serious consideration to the request.

Age

The design of a prosthesis for a young person must allow for growth and must accommodate new teeth as they erupt. If the patient is very active or plays contact sports, the strength of the appliance should also be an important factor.

A different challenge is found in the attitude of an older patient who associates the loss of teeth with age and has an unrealistic desire to retain teeth that are structurally unsound.

Dietary Habits

Healthy tissue is an important aspect of removable prosthodontic success. Patients with poor nutritional habits may have poor tissue response to the prosthesis, which could affect the overall tolerance and comfort of the prosthesis.

Social and Economic Factors

The patient's attitude toward the importance of replacing lost teeth and ability to pay for the treatment are major socioeconomic factors.

Occupation

Patients whose daily activities involve "meeting the public" are concerned about the possible change in their appearance during or after the transition to partial or full dentures. Appointments for surgery and the delivery of the prosthesis should be scheduled without seriously disrupting the patient's social and occupational activities.

Intraoral Factors

The condition of the tissues in the patient's mouth is a key factor in determining whether a removable partial or a complete denture can be recommended.

Musculature

Facial muscles contribute to the retention and functional control of the prosthesis. Strong muscle attachments with good muscle tone are important. Conversely, a large or very active tongue may cause difficulty in retention and wearing of the prosthesis. A patient with severe nervous, eccentric facial habits may have difficulty retaining and adjusting to a prosthesis. Extreme facial contortions will displace the denture by breaking the suction holding the denture in place, particularly the maxillary denture.

Salivary Flow

The presence of a new object such as a prosthesis in the oral cavity may stimulate an excessive flow of saliva. This response usually diminishes and is controlled as the patient becomes accustomed to wearing the prosthesis. However, the prosthesis may make saliva control more difficult in patients with partial paralysis of the facial muscles.

In contrast, a patient with a problem that severely inhibits the flow of saliva may find a prosthesis uncomfortable and difficult to wear. Physical conditions, medications, and radiation treatment may cause lack of adequate salivary flow.

Residual Alveolar Ridge

Successful wearing of a removable prosthesis depends mainly on the alveolar ridge for support. If high and evenly contoured, the alveolar ridge provides good support and even distribution for the stress of **mastication.** If the alveolar ridge has *resorbed,* it cannot provide adequate support. **Resorption** results in sore spots where the prosthesis rests on the mucosa. It also can cause the prosthesis to be loose, which affects proper mastication of food.

In some cases before placement of a prosthesis, it is necessary to recontour the alveolar ridge surgically to minimize such problems, using a procedure called **alveoplasty** (see Chapter 56). It is a normal ongoing process for the alveolar ridge to continue to decrease in size and change in shape after the teeth are lost. A well-fitted prosthesis minimizes these changes; a poorly fitting prosthesis accelerates the process. Because of these changes, it is important that the patient return periodically for an oral examination and reevaluation of the fit of the prosthesis.

Oral Mucosa

If the attached mucosa covering the residual ridge is altered by the patient's physical condition, the prosthesis may cause friction and irritation and be difficult for the patient to wear. Likewise, a poorly fitting prosthesis may cause irritation and sore spots, known as **pressure points,** on the oral mucosa. This patient should be seen promptly so the dentist can relieve these sore spots.

Oral Habits

Because oral habits such as clenching or grinding can cause extreme stress on the ridges and remaining teeth, this must be taken into account when planning a removable prosthodontic treatment. Mouth breathing may also affect the patient's ability to hold the appliance in place.

Tori

Tori are abnormal growths of bone in a specific area. If either mandibular or maxillary tori are present, they will affect the patient's ability to wear a prosthesis in that arch. Depending on the type of prosthesis required, it may be necessary to have the tori surgically removed before fabrication of the appliance is begun.

Recall

1. What type of removable prosthesis replaces one or more teeth?
2. How does a person's occupation affect the choice of a removable prosthesis?
3. How does the addition of a prosthesis affect the flow of saliva?
4. Why is it important that the alveolar ridge be evenly contoured for a removable prosthesis?
5. What oral habits can affect the choice of a removable prosthesis?

REMOVABLE PARTIAL DENTURE

A removable partial denture receives its support and retention from the underlying tissues and remaining teeth that serve as abutments. This type of prosthesis is designed to distribute the forces of mastication between these abutments and the supporting tissues.

Indications and Contraindications

The major indications for a removable partial denture are:

- To replace several teeth in the same quadrant or in both quadrants of the same arch.
- To serve as a temporary replacement for missing teeth in a child (as necessary, a new appliance is constructed to compensate for the child's growth).
- To avoid the reduction of tooth structure on primary or permanent dentition of children and adolescents.
- To replace missing teeth for a patient who cannot tolerate longer appointments and the extensive preparation required for the placement of a fixed bridge or implants.
- To provide the advantages of being removable, allowing the patient to maintain good oral hygiene easily.
- To serve through special design as a splint to support periodontally involved teeth.

Contraindications to a removable partial denture include the following:

- A lack of suitable teeth in the arch to support, stabilize, and retain the removable prosthesis
- Rampant caries or severe periodontal conditions that threaten the remaining teeth in the arch
- A lack of patient acceptance for esthetic reasons
- Chronic poor oral hygiene

Components of a Partial Denture

The basic components of a removable partial denture are the framework, connectors, denture base, retainers, rests, and artificial teeth (Fig. 52-3).

Framework

The **framework** is the cast metal skeleton that provides support for the remaining components of the prosthesis. The dental laboratory technician constructs this mesh-like portion of the partial denture to cover this framework with acrylic resin to mirror the appearance of gingiva.

Connectors

The **connectors,** or *bars,* join various parts of the partial denture together. The *major connector* is the piece of rigid metal that joins the right-and-left-quadrant framework of the partial denture. This connector also helps to form support for the remaining teeth so the stress is evenly distributed. A maxillary partial denture has a *palatal connector,* and a mandibular partial denture has a *lingual connector.*

A *stress-breaker* is a metal device built into a partial denture design that relieves the abutment teeth from excessive occlusal loads and stresses during mastication. A stress-breaker is advised for abutment teeth that have limited support in the alveolar ridge.

The *minor connector* links the major connector to the base and other areas, such as rests and clasps.

Retainer

A **retainer,** also known as a *clasp,* is the portion of the framework that directly supports and provides stability to the partial denture by partially encircling an abutment tooth.

The *I-bar retainer,* or *I-bar clasp,* approaches the tooth in a straight line from the apical direction and extends upward against the tooth (Fig. 52-4*A*). A *circumferential re-*

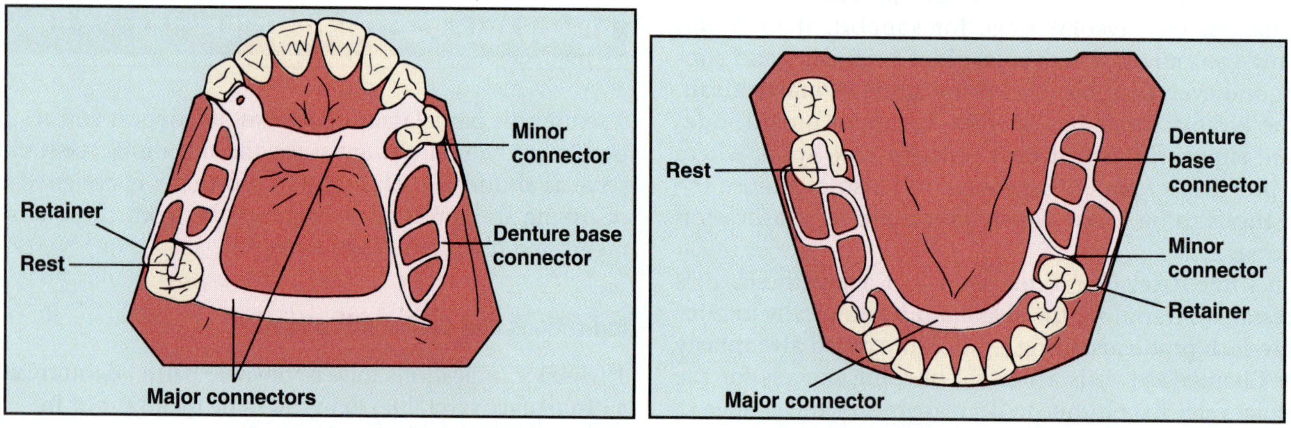

Fig. 52-3 Components of a partial denture. (Modified from Kratochvil FJ: *Partial removable prosthodontics,* Philadelphia, 1988, Saunders.)

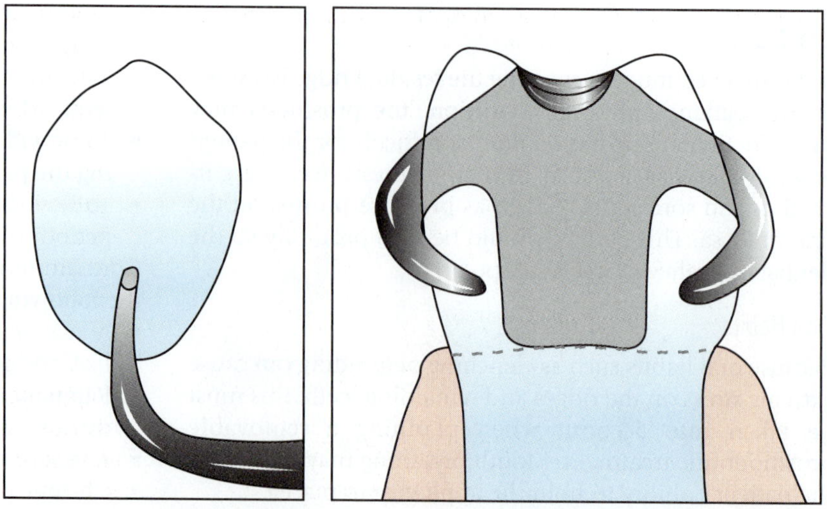

A

B

Fig. 52-4 Different types of clasps **A,** I-bar clasp. **B,** C-clasp.

tainer, or *C-clasp*, originates at the occlusal surface of the tooth and extends downward so that it partially encircles the tooth (Fig. 52-4*B*).

Rest

A **rest** is a metal projection designed to control the seating of a prosthesis as it is positioned in the mouth. Rests prevent the partial denture from moving in a gingival direction, which would add abnormal stress and wear on the abutment tooth. The rest also aids in distributing the retention load of the partial denture to several teeth, not just a single tooth. It also prevents passage of food between the abutment tooth and the retainer.

Rests are designed to lie in a prepared recess on the occlusal or lingual surface of a tooth. The recess is usually prepared in a cast restoration such as an onlay or crown. This cast restoration protects the tooth structure against wear caused by the movement of the rest. Although the rest fits into the casting, it is not attached to it. Two common types of rests are as follows:

- The *occlusal rest* is on the occlusal surface of the tooth. This placement minimizes trauma to the tooth by transmitting stress along the long axis of the tooth.
- The *lingual rest* is on the cingulum of the lingual surface of the tooth, where there is good support but no visibility.

Artificial Teeth

Artificial teeth can be constructed from either acrylic or porcelain (Fig. 52-5). *Acrylic teeth* are usually selected more often because they do not produce a clicking sound during chewing; however, acrylic teeth tend to wear faster and are more susceptible to staining. *Porcelain teeth* are more susceptible to fracture and tend to cause abrasion of the opposing natural teeth. Placement of acrylic teeth with natural or porcelain teeth in the opposing arch often is a satisfactory compromise.

Appointment Sequencing for a Partial Denture

The patient considering a partial denture must understand the sequencing of and commitment to the process of delivering a partial denture. A patient can expect five to six dental appointments before the prosthesis is delivered.

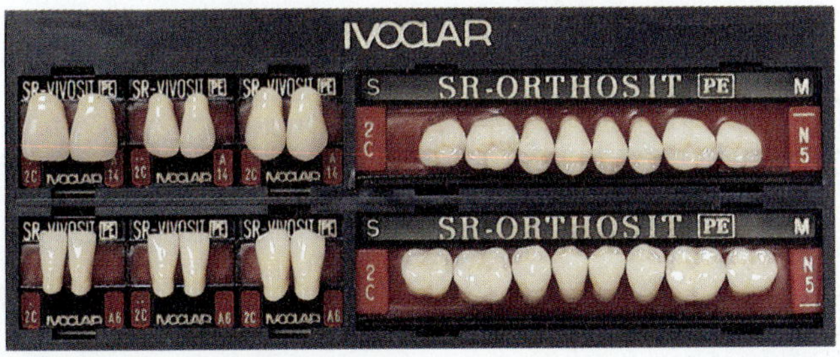

Fig. 52-5 Artificial teeth. (Courtesy Ivoclar Vivadent, Amherst, New York.)

Appointment One: Records

This appointment involves the preliminary steps listed in gathering the diagnostic tools that the dental team and laboratory technician will need to proceed.

- Updated health and dental *history*
- *Prophylaxis* completed by the dental hygienist
- *Preliminary impressions.* Casts are taken, poured up in stone, and sent to the dental laboratory for the making of custom trays.
- *Radiographs. Periapical* radiographs are prescribed for the evaluation of decay, periodontal problems, and other pathology that cannot be seen visually. A *panoramic* (Panorex) radiograph may be prescribed to evaluate the alveolar ridge and any additional structures.
- *Photographs.* It is always important to have intraoral and extraoral photographs for the case presentation and presentation of final results.

Appointment Two: Preparation

This appointment is the preparation appointment.

- *Preparation of the teeth.* The type of rest selected determines the preparation of the abutment teeth. This preparation may involve one of the following:
- Slight modification of the tooth
- Modification of an amalgam restoration, if present
- Placement of a cast metal restoration with a recessed area to receive the rest or precision attachment
- *Taking the final impression.* Because this must be an exact impression, an *elastomeric* material is used. A custom tray may be selected for taking the final impression to give the laboratory technician a better form of the surrounding structures.
- *Taking the bite and occlusal registration.* Jaw registration must be recorded to determine the relationship between the maxillary and mandibular arches.
- *Selecting the shade* and *mold of the teeth.* When choosing the tooth shade and mold, the dentist considers the patient's age and body size, length of the lip, and space to be occupied by the artificial tooth or teeth. The goal is to match as closely as possible the color, size, and shape of the patient's natural teeth. When the selection has been made, the mold and shade of the artificial teeth are written on the patient's chart.
- *Preparing the laboratory prescription.* Before the case is sent to the laboratory, the dentist prepares a written prescription that includes all details concerning the construction of the prosthesis (Fig. 52-6). The dentist must sign this prescription, and a copy is retained in the practice records.

Appointment Three: Try-in

An appointment is scheduled for the initial try-in of the prosthesis in the patient's mouth. At this point the appliance consists of the cast framework and the artificial teeth set in wax.

The dentist evaluates the fit, comfort, and function of the appliance. The shade, mold, and arrangement of the teeth are reviewed to ensure that the appearance is acceptable to the patient. If necessary, the dentist may alter the alignment of the teeth in the wax.

When the appliance is acceptable, another bite registration may be required to reflect any changes made during the try-in. Any changes in the partial denture design are noted on the laboratory prescription. The *wax-up* is disinfected and forwarded to the dental technician along with the prescription.

Appointment Four: Delivery

A 20- to 30-minute appointment is usually adequate for delivery of the partial denture. The day before the appointment, verify that the case has been returned from the laboratory (see Procedure 52-1).

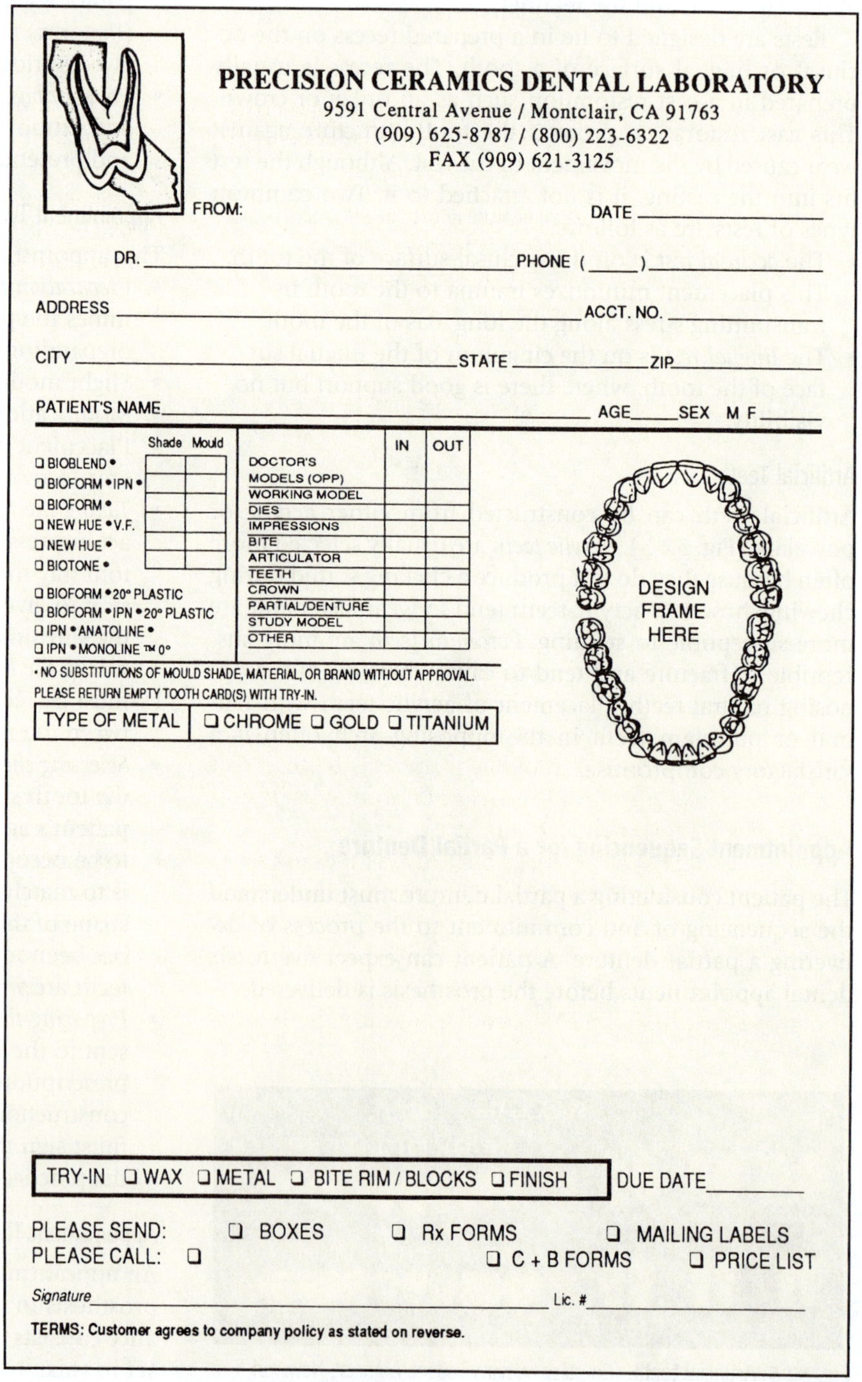

PRECISION CERAMICS DENTAL LABORATORY
9591 Central Avenue / Montclair, CA 91763
(909) 625-8787 / (800) 223-6322
FAX (909) 621-3125

FROM: DATE ______
DR. ______ PHONE (____) ______
ADDRESS ______ ACCT. NO. ______
CITY ______ STATE ______ ZIP ______
PATIENT'S NAME ______ AGE ____ SEX M F ____

	Shade	Mould
❑ BIOBLEND •		
❑ BIOFORM • IPN •		
❑ BIOFORM •		
❑ NEW HUE • V.F.		
❑ NEW HUE •		
❑ BIOTONE •		

❑ BIOFORM • 20° PLASTIC
❑ BIOFORM • IPN • 20° PLASTIC
❑ IPN • ANATOLINE •
❑ IPN • MONOLINE ™ 0°

	IN	OUT
DOCTOR'S MODELS (OPP)		
WORKING MODEL		
DIES		
IMPRESSIONS		
BITE		
ARTICULATOR		
TEETH		
CROWN		
PARTIAL/DENTURE		
STUDY MODEL		
OTHER		

DESIGN FRAME HERE

• NO SUBSTITUTIONS OF MOULD SHADE, MATERIAL, OR BRAND WITHOUT APPROVAL.
PLEASE RETURN EMPTY TOOTH CARD(S) WITH TRY-IN.

TYPE OF METAL ❑ CHROME ❑ GOLD ❑ TITANIUM

TRY-IN ❑ WAX ❑ METAL ❑ BITE RIM / BLOCKS ❑ FINISH DUE DATE ______

PLEASE SEND: ❑ BOXES ❑ Rx FORMS ❑ MAILING LABELS
PLEASE CALL: ❑ ❑ C + B FORMS ❑ PRICE LIST

Signature ______ Lic. # ______

TERMS: Customer agrees to company policy as stated on reverse.

Fig. 52-6 **Laboratory prescription.** (Courtesy Precision Ceramics, Montclair, California.)

Procedure 52-1 Assisting in the Delivery of a Partial Denture

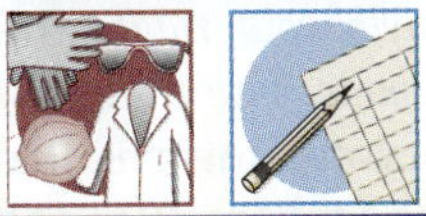

Equipment and Supplies

- Basic setup
- Articulating paper and holder
- Pressure indicator paste
- Low-speed and high-speed handpieces
- Acrylic burs
- Finishing burs
- Three-prong pliers

PROCEDURAL STEPS

1. Seat the patient.
2. The dentist places the new partial denture in the patient's mouth, and the patient is instructed to close his or her teeth together.
   Important: Before placing the prosthesis in the patient's mouth, it must be disinfected and rinsed with water.
3. To check the *occlusion,* assist in placing articulating paper on the occlusal surface of the mandibular teeth, and ask the patient to simulate chewing motions. If the occlusion is too high, the dentist reduces the artificial teeth with a small, round carbide bur.
4. To detect *pressure points* (high spots) that could cause discomfort to the patient, apply pressure-indicator paste on the tissue surface of the prosthesis. The prosthesis is placed in the patient's mouth. As necessary, these high spots on the prosthesis are adjusted.
5. The retainers are checked for tension on the natural abutment teeth. The dentist uses pliers very carefully to adjust the tension on the retainers.
6. After the adjustments, the partial denture is polished on the laboratory lathe, using the appropriate pastes and sterile buffing wheels.
7. Scrub the partial denture with soap, water, and a brush; disinfect and rinse; and return it to the treatment room for delivery to the patient.
8. Instruct the patient on the placement, removal, and care of the partial denture.

Date	Tooth	Surface	Charting Notes
8/20/05	—		Deliver maxillary partial, minor adjustments made. Pt pleased with appearance. Reschedule pt in 3 days for postdelivery check. T. Clark, CDA/L. Stewart, DDS

Appointment Five: Postdelivery Check

The patient is given an appointment to return within a few days after the delivery of the partial denture. A 10- to 20-minute appointment is usually adequate for this postdelivery visit. The dentist removes the partial denture and checks the mucosa for pressure areas and sore spots. If necessary, minor adjustments are made.

When the dentist and patient are satisfied that the prosthesis is functioning correctly, the patient is given a recall appointment for several months later. It is important that the patient return regularly for these recall visits so that the dentist can evaluate the fit, changes in the mucosa, function of the prosthesis, and effectiveness of the patient's oral hygiene.

As time passes, changes in the alveolar ridge and surrounding tissues may make it necessary to *reline* the partial denture (see later in the chapter for discussion).

Home Care Instructions

Patients with removable partials must be instructed to maintain good oral hygiene; the importance of this cannot be overemphasized. Patients should be given home care instructions verbally in the office as well as written instructions for the home to reinforce education after the patient leaves the office.

- Store the prosthesis in water or a moist, airtight container when not wearing it.
- After eating, remove the partial denture from the mouth, and brush or rinse the retainers, rests, and complete partial prosthesis.
- Carefully brush and floss the abutment teeth and the remaining natural teeth to keep them free of food debris and plaque.
- Do not adjust the partial denture. The patient should contact the dentist if he or she has any difficulties.

Recall

6. What is the term for the metal skeleton on a partial denture?
7. What is the term for the retainer on a partial denture?
8. What component on a partial denture controls the way it is seated in the mouth?
9. What impression material is typically used when taking a final impression for a partial denture?
10. What are the artificial teeth set in during the try-in appointment?

FULL (COMPLETE) DENTURE

Full dentures are designed to restore function and esthetics of the natural dentition when all of the natural teeth are missing. A complete denture receives all its support and retention from the underlying tissues, alveolar ridges, hard and soft palates, and surrounding oral mucosa.

Indications and Contraindications

The major indications for a full denture are:
- The patient is totally **edentulous.**
- The remaining teeth cannot be saved.
- The remaining teeth cannot support a removable partial denture, and no acceptable alternatives are available.
- The patient refuses alternative treatment recommendations.

Contraindications for a full denture include the following:
- Another acceptable alternative is available.
- Physical or mental illness affects the patient's ability to cooperate during fabrication of the denture and to accept or wear the denture.
- The patient is hypersensitive to denture materials (a hypoallergenic denture material may be indicated).
- The patient is not interested in replacing missing teeth.

Components of a Full Denture

The basic components of a denture include the base, flange, post dam, and artificial teeth (Fig. 52-7).

Base

The base is designed to fit over the residual alveolar ridge and surrounding gingival area. The base is commonly made from denture *acrylic.* To provide additional strength, however, it may be reinforced with a metal mesh embedded in the acrylic.

Flange

The **flange** is the part of the base that extends over the attached mucosa from the cervical margin of the teeth to the border of the denture. The flange of the mandibular denture base extends over the residual ridge and attached mucosa, down to the *oblique ridge* and *mylohyoid ridge,* and over the *genial tubercles* and *retromolar pads.* The flange of the maxillary denture base extends beyond the residual ridge and over the attached mucosa to the tuberosities and the junction of the hard and soft palates.

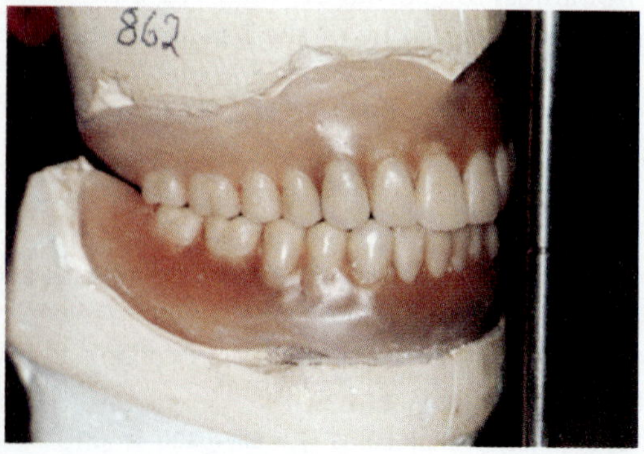

Fig. 52-7 Components of a full denture: base, flange, post dam, artificial teeth.

Post Dam

Retention of a maxillary denture depends on the suction seal known as the **post dam,** or the *posterior palatal seal.* The base of a maxillary denture covers the entire hard palate, and the seal is formed at the junction of the tissues and the posterior border of the denture. The post dam extends across the entire posterior portion of the denture from one buccal space across the back of the palate behind the maxillary **tuberosity** (rounded area on the outer surface of maxillary bones) to the opposite buccal space.

Retention for a mandibular denture depends on the support of the remaining alveolar ridge and the suction that can be achieved between the prosthesis and the tissues covering the ridge. Achieving good retention of a mandibular denture can be difficult. It lacks the broad suction area found in a maxillary denture, and the constant action of the tongue may dislodge it. For these reasons, retained teeth or implants are desirable to help hold the appliance in place.

Artificial Teeth

Denture teeth are fabricated from acrylic or porcelain and are designed to be retained in the acrylic base of the denture. Third molars are not included on dentures because space is needed in the posterior region to allow the patient to close, chew, swallow, and speak normally. A full denture has 14 teeth per arch, in which each arch constitutes a single unit, whereas a natural tooth functions as an individual unit.

Appointment Sequencing for a Full Denture

The patient considering a complete denture must understand the sequencing and commitment to the process of delivering a denture. It is common for a patient to have six dental appointments for the delivery of a denture.

Appointment One: Records

This appointment involves the preliminary steps in gathering the diagnostic tools the dental team and dental laboratory technician will require to proceed with the removable prosthodontic procedure:
- Updated health and dental *history.*
- *Preliminary impressions.* Taking alginate impressions of an edentulous arch differs from other alginate impressions in two ways: the height of the teeth is missing, and more extensive tissue details are needed. An *edentulous tray* is used to take this impression. This tray is

not as deep as other trays used for alginate impressions. In addition, attaching soft beading wax or similar material to the edges modifies the borders of the tray.

- The tray modification allows **border molding,** also known as *muscle trimming,* to achieve closer adaptation of the edges of the impression of the tissues in the mucobuccal fold. Border molding is performed after the impression tray is in place. The dentist uses his or her fingers to gently massage the facial area over these borders. This action shapes the tray's wax-covered edges so that they more closely approximate the tissues.
- *Radiographs.* A *panoramic* radiograph may be prescribed for the dentist to evaluate the underlying bone structure and observe any abnormal pathology that may not be visible.
- *Photographs.* It is always important to have intraoral and extraoral photographs for the case presentation and final results.

Appointment Two: Final Impression

The dental laboratory technician requires a final impression to create the base of a denture. Before taking the impression, a custom tray is fabricated. Because of the shape of the edentulous arch, custom trays are usually required for the final impression. Custom trays are constructed on the diagnostic casts and are prepared before the patient's appointment for the final impression (see Chapter 47). The edges of the custom tray for an edentulous arch are modified with beading wax to allow border molding. The edges of the tray should extend to 2 mm *short* of the mucobuccal fold.

Because accuracy is essential, an *elastomeric* impression material forms the final impression that will be used for the creation of the baseplates and occlusal rims (Fig. 52-8).

The **baseplate,** which is constructed on the master casts, is made of a semirigid material such as shellac and self-curing or heat-cured resins. If necessary for added stability, acrylic baseplates may be reinforced with wires or mesh metal sheets embedded in the material at processing.

The **occlusal rims** are built of wax on the alveolar crest of the baseplate and are sufficiently high and wide to occupy the space of the missing dentition.

Appointment Three: Try-in of Baseplate and Occlusal Rim

The baseplate–occlusal rim assembly is returned to the dental office on an **articulator,** a dental laboratory device that simulates movements of the mandible and temporomandibular joint. Before it is tried in the patient's mouth, the baseplate–occlusal rim is removed from the articulator, disinfected, and rinsed. On the occlusal rims, the dentist records the following:

- *Vertical dimension:* space occupied by the height of the teeth in normal occlusion
- *Occlusal relationship:* centric, protrusive, retrusive, and lateral excursions
- *Smile line:* line representing the area of teeth that is visible when the patient is smiling
- *Canine eminence:* vertical line indicating the location of the canines

Artificial teeth

At this appointment the mold, shade, and material of the artificial teeth to be placed in the denture are selected (Fig. 52-9). These factors are determined in the same way as for the teeth of a partial denture.

When placing the teeth in the denture, the laboratory technician is able to modify the arrangement as requested to produce a more natural appearance for the patient, for example, lightly overlapping the mesial incisal margin of the maxillary lateral incisor over the distal margin of the central incisor. In addition, the technician may set (position) the teeth to expose less or more of the cervical area of the teeth to emulate the natural setting of the teeth according to the patient's age. Less cervical area is shown in a younger patient; more area is visible in an older patient to simulate gingival recession.

Essentials of a Final Impression for Dentures

The impression material should be free of bubbles and distributed evenly over the tray and its margins so that the landmarks of the dental arches are accurately reproduced.

The maxillary impression should include the *hamular notches,* post dam, tuberosities, and *frenum attachments.*

The mandibular impression should include the retromolar pads, oblique ridge, outline of the mylohyoid ridge, genial tubercles, and the lingual, labial, and buccal frenula.

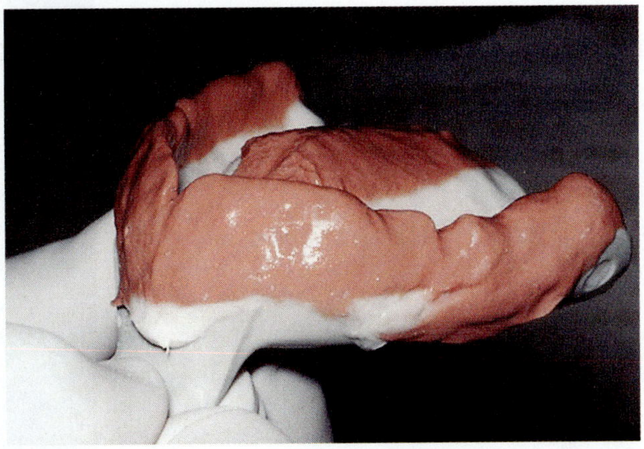

Fig. 52-8 Final impression for a full denture. (Courtesy Ivoclar Vivadent, Amherst, NY.)

Occlusal registration

During the construction of a complete denture, the laboratory technician must have an accurate and extensive record of the patient's occlusion. The technician uses this information to articulate the casts so that the completed prosthesis will replicate these normal motions.

The measurements most frequently used are the patient's bite registered in the following positions:

- **Centric relation** with the jaws closed, relaxed, and comfortably positioned
- **Protrusion** with the mandible placed as far forward as possible from the centric position
- **Retrusion** with the mandible placed as far posterior as possible from the centric position
- **Lateral excursion,** which is sliding the mandible to the left or right of the centric position

These exaggerated motions simulate the actual movements of the mandible as it functions in the acts of mastication, biting, yawning, and speaking. Various measuring devices are used to obtain these measurements.

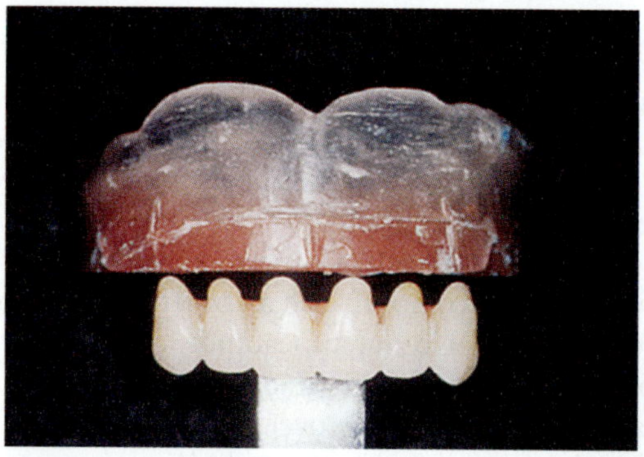

Fig. 52-9 Recording made from the baseplate–occlusal rim assembly: vertical dimensions, occlusal relationship, smile line, canine eminence.

Functionally generated path technique

The functionally generated path technique uses the patient's ability to create his or her own occlusal relationship by tracing in wax the movements of the mandible on the maxilla. Establishment of a functionally generated path involves the following steps:

1. Place the baseplates and occlusal rims for the new prosthesis in the patient's mouth.
2. Prepare a double thickness of specially formulated baseplate wax in a horseshoe shape, and lay it over the occlusal surface of the mandibular teeth.
3. Instruct the patient to close firmly into the wax and simulate the act of chewing as accurately as possible.
4. Remove the wax bite in approximately 20 to 30 seconds.
5. In the treatment room, rinse and disinfect the wax bite and place in a precaution bag.
6. In the laboratory, pour the wax bite with stone immediately after the patient's dismissal.

Appointment Four: Try-in

The wax setup consists of the baseplate with the artificial teeth set in wax that resembles gingival tissue. The shaping of the wax to simulate normal tissue contours, grooves, and eminences is known as **festooning.** The teeth are articulated according to the bite registration of the patient's occlusion, as established on the articulator through a functional-arch tracing.

The complete denture try-in, which has been fabricated in wax by the laboratory technician on an articulator, is returned to the dental office before the patient's appointment. The wax setup is removed from the articulator and disinfected before it is tried in the patient's mouth (Fig. 52-10 and see Procedure 52-2).

Patients may require more than one wax try-in appointment to achieve the esthetics they are seeking. It is

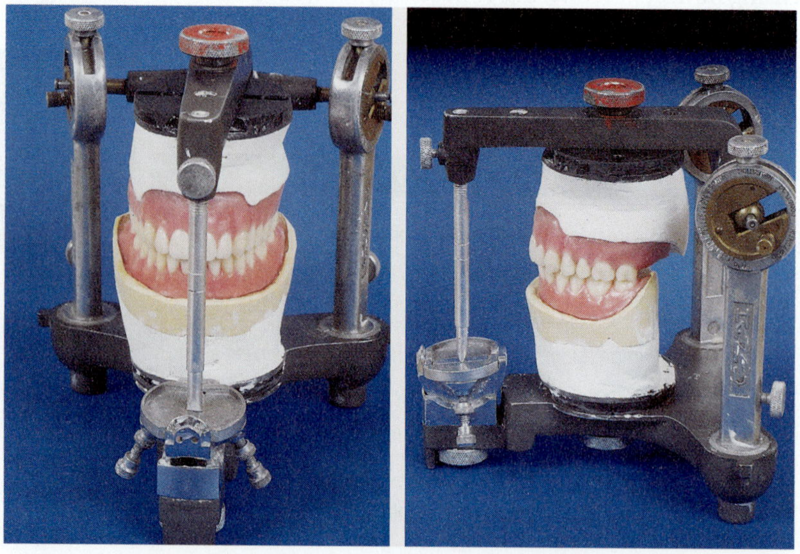

Fig. 52-10 Wax setup within the articulated cast.

Procedure 52-2 Assisting in a Wax Denture Try-in

Equipment and Supplies

- Denture wax setup
- Basic setup
- Articulating paper and holder
- Wax spatula
- Heat source
- Low-speed handpiece with acrylic burs, discs, and stones

PROCEDURAL STEPS

1. Assist in evaluating the wax setup of the denture for fit, comfort, and stability.
2. Verify the patient's acceptance of the appearance of the denture, including the shade, mold, and alignment of the teeth.
3. Check the retention of the denture setup as the patient verbalizes the *f, v, s,* and *th* sounds; swallows; and yawns.
4. Check the occlusion of the denture with the teeth of the opposing arch.
5. The dentist prepares the laboratory prescription for the completion of the denture. Disinfect the case, return it to the articulator, pack it, and return the case to the laboratory.

Date	Tooth	Surface	Charting Notes
8/20/05	—		Wax try-in of maxillary denture, base contoured and adjusted. Pt unhappy with canines. Noted on lab script for change in mold of #s 6 and 11. Centric occlusion evaluated and adjusted. Pt rescheduled for delivery in 1 week. T. Clark, CDA/L. Stewart, DDS

important for the dentist, laboratory technician, and patient to work together to achieve the patient's acceptance and satisfaction.

Appointment Five: Delivery

The completed dentures are delivered to the dental office in a sealed, moist container. The dentures must be disinfected before they are placed in the patient's mouth (see Procedure 52-3).

Appointment Six: Postdelivery

The patient is given an appointment to return in two to three days after the delivery of the full denture. A 10- to 20-minute appointment is usually adequate for this postdelivery visit.

The dentist removes the denture and checks the mucosa for pressure areas and sore spots. If necessary, minor adjustments are made to the denture. Patients usually need more than one adjustment appointment after the delivery of a complete denture. When the patient and dentist are satisfied that the prosthesis is functioning properly, the patient is given a recall appointment for several months later.

Home Care Instructions

As with partial dentures, the patient should be given home care instructions in writing to reinforce the verbal instructions:

- With the denture removed, thoroughly rinse the oral tissues at least once daily.
- On removal, thoroughly clean all surfaces of the denture; a special denture brush may be used. Avoid harsh abrasives such as toothpaste (Fig. 52-11).
- During cleaning, carefully hold the denture over a sink half-filled with cool water.
- Do not soak the denture in hot water or a strong solution such as undiluted bleach, because these liquids will damage the denture.
- When not in the mouth, store dentures in a moist, airtight container to prevent drying and warping. If the prosthesis is not stored in a safe container, it may be accidentally knocked to the floor, stepped on, or broken.
- Do not wear the denture at night.

Recall

11. What is the suction seal created between the denture and the mouth?
12. How many teeth are in a full set of dentures?
13. What technique does the dentist use to modify the borders of an impression?
14. What is a smile line?
15. What are the four jaw positions that the dentist measures when articulating a denture?

Procedure 52-3 Assisting in the Delivery of a Full Denture

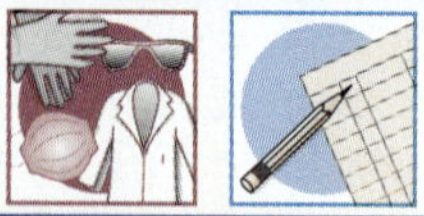

Equipment and Supplies

- Basic setup
- Dentures
- Hand mirror
- Articulating paper and holder
- High-speed and low-speed handpieces
- Finishing burs
- Acrylic burs

PROCEDURAL STEPS

1. Seat the patient.
2. The new denture is inserted into the patient's mouth, and the shade and mold of the artificial teeth are checked for natural appearance.
3. Ask the patient to perform the facial expressions and the actions of swallowing, chewing, and speaking, using *s* and *th* sounds.

   Note: These sounds also are appropriate for exercises to help the patient learn to speak normally with the new denture.
4. The occlusion is checked by using articulating paper.

   Purpose: Cusps that are too high in contact will be marked with the color of the articulating paper.
5. If the cusps are too high, the denture is removed from the mouth and adjusted with a stone mounted on a straight handpiece.
6. The denture is replaced in the mouth, and the procedure is repeated until the cusps appear to be in occlusion with the opposing arch.

   Note: If the denture must be taken into the laboratory for adjustment, it must be disinfected again before it is returned to the patient.
7. When the patient is pleased with the appearance, function, and comfort of the denture, another appointment is made for the postdelivery checkup.
8. Before dismissal, the patient is informed that learning to wear a new denture will take several days or weeks.

Date	Tooth	Surface	Charting Notes
8/28/05			Delivery of maxillary full denture. Pt pleased with change of canines. Teeth and shading good. Pt pleased with fit and appearance. Reschedule in 3 days for postdelivery check. T. Clark, CDA/L. Stewart, DDS

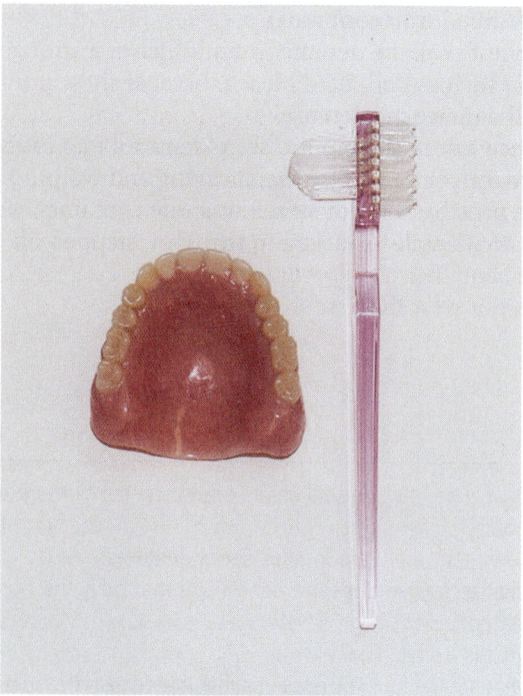

Fig. 52-11 Denture and denture brush.

IMMEDIATE DENTURES

Most often, an **immediate denture** is a prosthesis placed immediately after extraction of the patient's remaining anterior teeth. During the healing process, this type of denture serves as a compress and bandage to protect the surgical area. Although an immediate denture may be placed in either arch, placement of a *maxillary* immediate denture is more common because it restores function and spares the patient the embarrassment of being without teeth in that arch.

Before agreeing to receive an immediate denture, the patient must be aware that normal healing and resorption cause changes in the alveolar ridge. Because of these changes, the denture placed immediately after surgery must be replaced or relined in three to six months.

Construction

When a patient has the posterior teeth extracted and healing is complete, but before the extraction of the anterior teeth, the try-in of the wax setup includes only the posterior teeth. These teeth are aligned in the occlusal rims and checked for their ability to occlude with the opposing teeth. The denture, complete with the anterior teeth, is constructed, sterilized, and ready for placement at surgery.

Surgical Template

In addition to the denture, the laboratory prepares a surgical template. The surgical **template** resembles a clear plastic impression tray of the anterior area as this area should appear *after* the teeth have been extracted. The denture and template must be sterilized before surgery. After the anterior teeth have been extracted, the oral surgeon uses the surgical template as a guide in properly contouring the remaining alveolar ridge.

Placement

When the resulting alveolar ridge is satisfactory, the tissues are sutured in place. The sterilized denture is rinsed with saline solution and positioned in the mouth. The patient is given postsurgical instructions and home care instructions.

The patient returns in 24 hours for a postoperative checkup. During this time the denture should be worn continuously except when it is removed for cleaning. Daily visits continue until initial healing has started and the sutures are removed, usually 48 to 72 hours after surgery. During each visit the dentist irrigates the area with a mild antiseptic solution and checks the soft tissue for pressure points.

After the sutures have been removed and the dentist and patient are satisfied with the prosthesis, the patient is scheduled for another appointment within a few months.

Recall

16. When is an immediate denture used?
17. What is the normal length of time an immediate denture is worn?

OVERDENTURES

Patient satisfaction with a mandibular denture is increased when there are remaining teeth or *implants* to improve retention and stability (see Chapter 53). An **overdenture** is a full denture supported by the bony ridge and oral mucosa plus two or more remaining natural teeth or implants. Most often, these remaining teeth are canines.

Preparation and placement of the denture for use with implants and for an overdenture are similar. To permit the denture to fit snugly over the teeth without excessive bulk, the natural teeth are prepared by removing much of their bulk. The remaining tooth structure is protected with a **coping.** In the *long coping technique,* only a minimal amount of tooth structure is removed, and the length of tooth remains almost the same. In the *short coping technique,* which is used only on endodontically treated teeth, the tooth structure is greatly reduced and shortened.

The posts from an implant protrude through the gingiva much like teeth, and a casting is created to fit over the posts. In preparation for a mandibular denture, a *bar* to provide stability connects these castings; this forms the "male" portion of the appliance. The denture is prepared with a recessed *sleeve* in the anterior of the prosthesis, which serves as the receptor attachment; this is the "female" portion of the appliance. The denture is snapped over the bar and stabilized in alignment with the opposing arch.

The in-office steps in the fabrication of this special denture are similar to those for a normal denture.

DENTURE RELINING

Patients will assume that after completion of their denture they are free from future dental visits. In reality, a patient should be scheduled once a year to evaluate the fit and to examine the oral tissues for subclinical irritations and dysplasias. The clinical indications for relining or rebasing are as follows:

- Dentures are loose or ill-fitting.
- There is a loss in vertical dimension (angular cheilosis is an indication of this).
- Inflammatory hyperplasia is present.
- Traumatic ulcers appear after a long period of comfortable wear.

Relining is accomplished by placing a new layer of denture resin over the tissue surface of the appliance. **Rebasing** is a similar procedure that replaces the entire denture base material on an existing prosthesis without changing the occlusal relationship of the teeth. The difference is that a reline *resurfaces* the prosthesis, and a rebase *replaces* the denture base.

Tissue Conditioners

The process of relining a denture must be accurate to ensure a proper fit. The patient's supporting tissue must be healthy before impressions are taken. One method used to rehabilitate unhealthy supporting tissues is to place a tissue-conditioning material for a short period, usually three or four days.

This material is a soft *elastomer* composed of a powder and a liquid. The mixed material is placed in the prosthesis and adapts to the supporting tissues and ridge, resulting in a conditioning effect on unhealthy tissues.

Impression

At the preliminary appointment, when it is agreed that relining is necessary, the patient is informed that the denture will be unavailable for at least 8 to 24 hours while it is being processed in the laboratory. The impression is taken with the present (loose) denture used as the impression tray. The dentist flows a mix of zinc oxide–eugenol impression paste or an elastomeric impression material into the tissue side of the denture.

The denture is placed on the alveolar ridge, and the patient is instructed to close in normal occlusion and to hold the denture in place until the impression paste reaches a final set. The denture is removed from the mouth and disinfected. The denture and written prescription are sent to the laboratory technician for relining.

Delivery

When the relined denture is returned from the laboratory, it is disinfected before being returned to the patient's mouth. The relined denture rarely needs adjustment because the only alteration on the original prosthesis is the addition of material within the tissue side of the denture.

If necessary, minor trimming may be accomplished with an acrylic bur in a straight handpiece. Minor polishing may be done on the laboratory lathe with a sterile rag wheel with pumice paste; however, the tissue-bearing surfaces are *never* polished because this would alter the fit of the appliance.

The patient is dismissed and advised to return for a checkup of the tissue and the adaptation of the prosthesis within a period specified by the dentist.

Recall

18. How is an overdenture supported in the mouth?

19. What is the term for placing a new layer of resin over the tissue surface of a prosthesis?

DENTURE REPAIRS

A broken acrylic denture can be repaired. Simple repairs are sometimes handled in the dental office laboratory by using cold-cured acrylics. For more complicated repairs, particularly those involving the replacement of teeth or the complex fracture of the denture, dentures are usually sent to the dental laboratory technician.

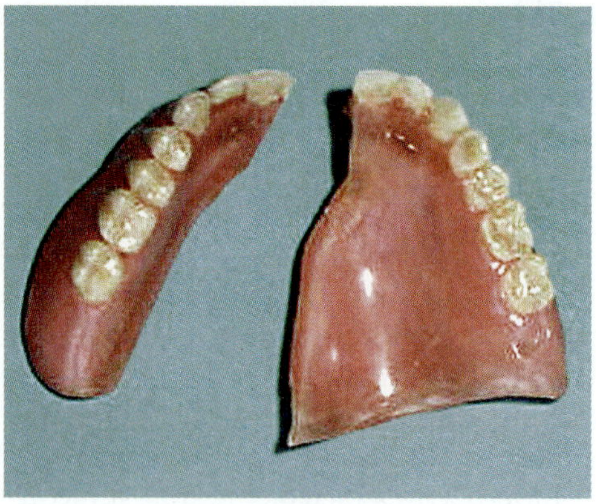

Fig. 52-12 Broken denture.

The patient with a broken denture tooth usually leaves the denture at the dental office (Fig. 52-12). In most cases, it is not necessary for the patient to be seen by the dentist at this time. If there has been more extensive damage to the denture, however, it may be necessary for the dentist to see the patient to obtain a new impression. When the repaired denture is returned, the patient is scheduled for a few minutes with the dentist to make certain the repair is satisfactory and the denture fits properly.

Recall

20. Who can repair a denture?

DENTURE DUPLICATION

Having a functional denture is important to the patient, and because dentures can break or require time for relining, the patient should have a duplicate denture. Although an extra expense, many patients find that a duplicate is an excellent investment because they will not be without their denture if the original is damaged. To prevent warpage while not in use, the spare denture should be stored in a moist, airtight container.

Patient Education

Removable prosthodontics is an area of dentistry that can actually change a patient's self-perception. Some patients have never really "liked" their teeth or have experienced a negative dental history regarding the care of their teeth. For these patients, a removable prosthesis may make a "new person" out of them. By educating patients on the importance of taking care of their prosthesis and following a structured recall schedule, you will make them ever grateful for your assistance in the provision of their dental needs.

Eye to the Future

With new advances in dental implants, patients requiring a prosthetic appliance will be able to have a prosthetic implant completed. Not only will this type of appliance be easier to maintain and be more natural looking for the patient, but the cost will be greatly reduced, making it an option in their treatment planning stages. Increasingly, general dentists will receive training in implantology, thus making it more readily available for a larger population.

Legal and Ethical Implications

On the other hand, wearing a removable prosthesis could be one of the most aggravating and worst experiences of a patient's life. If patients expect a removable prosthesis to feel and function just like their natural teeth did, they will not be satisfied. You will find that patients who experience this negative reaction do not want to wear the prosthesis because it fits poorly or the appearance is unappealing. If you have a patient who reacts in this manner, as part of the dental team you have not provided the knowledge and service that this patient expected.

Critical Thinking

1. Mr. Smith is scheduled for a lower partial denture. The partial will replace his molars on both sides. How many teeth will make up the partial denture? What teeth will become the abutment teeth for this prosthesis?
2. In reviewing the appointment stages for a partial and full denture, what additional step is included for the making of a full denture that is not in the making of a partial?
3. Describe the different structures of the oral cavity that the dental laboratory technician requires from a final impression for a removable prosthodontic appliance and compared to a fixed-prosthesis case.
4. Discuss the importance of an immediate denture.
5. Why would a patient with a full set of dentures be placed on a recall system? What would be completed during this procedure?

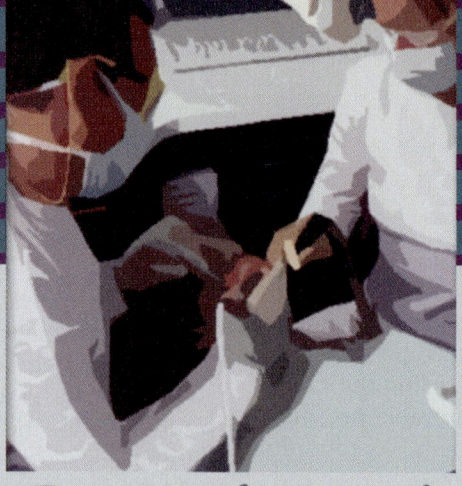

53 Dental Implants

Outline

Indications for Implants
Contraindications to Implants
The Dental Implant Patient
- Psychological Evaluation
- Dental Examination
- Medical History and Evaluation
- Specialized Radiographs
- Diagnostic Casts and Surgical Stents

Preparation for Implants
- Informed Consent
- Surgical Preparation

Types of Dental Implants
- Endosteal Implant
- *Procedure 53-1: Assisting in an Endosteal Implant Surgery*
- Subperiosteal Implant
- Transosteal Implant

Maintenance of Dental Implants
- Home Care
- Routine Office Visits

Patient Education
Legal and Ethical Implications
Eye to the Future
Critical Thinking

KEY TERMS

Circumoral (*ser*-kum-**ore**-ul) Surrounding the mouth.

Endosteal (en-*das*-tee-ul) Implant surgically embedded into the bone.

Implant Artificial teeth attached to anchors that have been surgically embedded into the bone or surrounding structures.

Osseointegration (*ahs*-ee-oh-*in*-te-**gray**-shun) Attachment of healthy bone to a dental implant.

Peri-implant tissue Gingival sulcus surrounding the implant.

Stent Clear acrylic template that is placed over the alveolar ridge to assist in locating the proper placement for dental implants.

Subperiosteal (*sub*-per-ee-**os**-tee-ul) Type of implant with a metal frame placed under the periosteum, but on top of the bone.

Titanium (tie-**tay**-nee-um) Type of metal used for implants because of its compatibility with bone and oral tissues.

Transosteal (*tranz*-**os**-tee-ul) Implant inserted through the inferior border of the mandible.

LEARNING OUTCOMES

On completion of this chapter, the student will be able to achieve the following objectives:

- Pronounce, define, and spell the Key Terms.
- Discuss the indications and contraindications for dental implants.
- Describe the selection of patients to receive dental implants.
- Identify the types of dental implants.
- Describe the surgical procedures for implantation.
- Give home care procedures and follow-up visits required after receiving dental implants.

PERFORMANCE OUTCOMES

On completion of this chapter, the student will be able to achieve competency standards in the following skill:

- Assist in implant surgery.

When natural teeth are lost, it is very difficult to duplicate their function and appearance. Dental **implants** are a natural-looking replacement for missing teeth that incorporates principles from both fixed and removable prosthodontics with the use of bone-anchored implants. Artificial teeth are attached to metal implants that are permanently placed in the jaw. The implants hold the artificial teeth in place as firmly as the root system holds natural teeth.

Dental implants are used to attach artificial teeth to anchors (similar to posts) that have been surgically embedded into the bone (Fig. 53-1). The implantation process involves several steps and may take from three to nine months to complete. Depending on the type of implant, the steps may vary. Most dental implant operations are performed in the dental office, but some may be performed in a hospital, depending on the patient's general health and the type of implant.

The placement of dental implants involves both surgery and placement of the prosthesis. Several specialists may perform the procedure, including the oral and maxillofacial surgeon, periodontist, prosthodontist, and *implantologist* (general dentist with specialized training). The experienced dental laboratory technician is also increasingly involved in this field of dentistry.

The type of specialist performing the procedure is less important than the *ability, experience,* and *education* of the clinician involved. The clinician must have in-depth knowledge of both surgical and prosthodontic aspects of implants. A coordinated effort among specialists and general practitioners is necessary to obtain optimal results when implants are being considered.

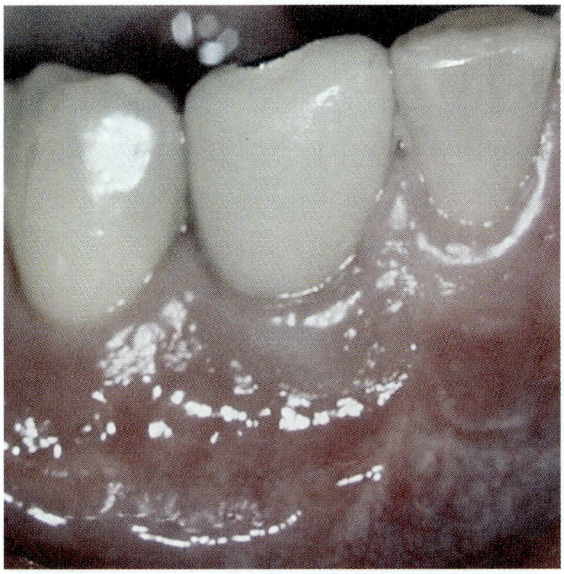

Fig. 53-1 Dental implant. (From Rose LF, Mealey BL, Genco RJ, et al.: *Periodontics: medicine, surgery, and implants.* St Louis, 2004, Mosby.)

INDICATIONS FOR IMPLANTS

Dental implants are often indicated as the treatment of choice. For example, lower full dentures have a very low rate of patient satisfaction, and implant dentistry has a very good chance of solving the problems associated with a mandibular denture. On the other hand, the placement of a three-unit fixed bridge has a very high success rate, so these patients are less likely to consider implants.

When properly placed, dental implants have a success rate of more than 90 percent. Effective home care and regular dental visits are essential to long-term success of dental implants, and this must be conveyed to the patient. Dental implants can last as long as 20 years and may last a lifetime.

The major indications for dental implants are:

- To replace one or more teeth as single units with crowns.
- To provide support for a partial denture.
- To increase the support, stability, and patient satisfaction for a full lower denture.
- To enhance the patient's comfort level when chewing.
- To increase the patient's confidence in smiling and speaking.
- To improve the patient's overall psychological health.
- To improve the esthetic appearance of the patient's teeth.

CONTRAINDICATIONS TO IMPLANTS

As with any dental procedure, dental implants involve some risk. Because each patient is unique, implant success cannot be guaranteed. The patient must be properly screened, and some patients are not good candidates for implants. The following contraindications should be considered when implant options are discussed:

- The financial investment is greater than that for a conventional bridge or denture.
- Treatment can take nine months or longer to complete.
- As with any surgical procedure, there is a risk of infection and other complications.
- Occasionally, an implant may loosen and require replacement.
- Emotionally, the implant procedure may be challenging for some patients.
- *Bruxism* is a significant component of failed implants.
- Patients with certain medical complications are not good candidates for dental implants.

Medical conditions that may contraindicate implants include diseases of the cardiovascular, respiratory, and gastrointestinal systems; seriously compromised immune system; and other chronic conditions that impede healing.

Recall

1. Which dental specialists have training in dental implants?
2. What is the success rate for dental implants?
3. How long can dental implants last?
4. Is the financial investment for an implant greater or less than for a fixed prosthesis?
5. How long can an implant procedure take to complete?

THE DENTAL IMPLANT PATIENT

Dental implants are not for everyone. The ideal candidate has good general health and adequate alveolar bone and is willing to commit to conscientious oral hygiene and regular dental visits. A comprehensive evaluation is essential to determine if the patient will benefit from dental implants.

Psychological Evaluation

The psychological evaluation takes place at the initial visit. The dentist assesses the patient's attitude, ability to cooperate during complex procedures, and overall outlook on dental treatment. The dentist also determines that the patient has realistic expectations about dental implants and the end results.

Dental Examination

During the examination, the dentist evaluates the condition of the teeth and soft tissues, areas of attached and unattached tissue, and the height and width of the edentulous alveolar bone ridge. This information is necessary to determine the best location to place the implants.

Medical History and Evaluation

The purpose of the medical history and evaluation is to assess any existing medical conditions that could worsen as a result of the stress of implant surgery. Any diseases that could interfere with normal healing must be carefully evaluated. Specific conditions that can interfere with implants are diabetes, suppressed immune system, and chemotherapy treatment for cancer.

Specialized Radiographs

Extraoral radiographs needed to evaluate the height, width, and quality of bone include *panoramic, cephalometric,* and *tomographic* views (see Chapter 42). These radiographs are useful in locating the exact position of anatomic structures such as the inferior alveolar nerve, mental foramen, maxillary sinus, nasal floor, and any abnormalities.

Diagnostic Casts and Surgical Stents

Diagnostic casts help the dentist in planning the implant procedure. In addition, the cast is used to make a surgical stent.

A surgical **stent** covers the area of surgery and is made from clear acrylic. Also known as a *template,* the stent acts as a guide during surgery to place the implants in their proper position (Fig. 53-2). The stent *must* be sterilized before use.

Recall

6. What are the three types of extraoral radiographs used by the dentist in evaluating the dental implant patient?
7. Why would a dentist use a surgical stent during implant surgery?

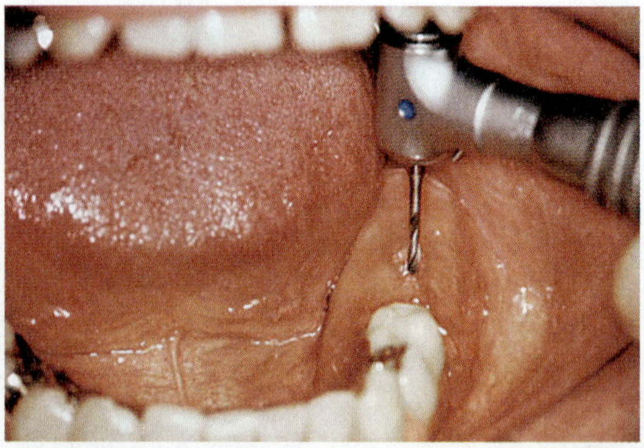

Fig. 53-2 Custom stent used to aid the dentist in placing an implant. (From Babbush CA: *Dental implants: Principles and practice,* Philadelphia, 1991, Saunders.)

Preliminary Patient Evaluation for Implants

- Psychological evaluation
- Dental evaluation
- Medical evaluation
- Radiographs
- Preliminary impressions

PREPARATION FOR IMPLANTS

Informed Consent

Written informed patient consent is required before treatment begins. The consent form should advise and educate the patient about (1) background information on implants, (2) complications of implant surgery, (3) prognosis, (4) time frame, (5) home care, and (6) follow-up appointments.

Surgical Preparation

Implant surgery must be completed under strict surgical sterile conditions with sterile instrumentation. The patient's mouth is rinsed with 0.1 percent chlorhexidine. The head is draped, and a sterile surgical drape is applied to the **circumoral** area, leaving only the mouth exposed.

It is recommended that the implant team consist of at least three persons: the clinician, the surgical dental assistant, and the nonsterile circulating assistant. The clinician and surgical dental assistant should be gowned and masked and should wear talcum powder-free *sterile* gloves.

The implants come in double-aseptic packaging. They must remain in this packaging until the actual placement. Just before placement, the inner vial is opened, and the implant is allowed to slide (untouched) onto a sterile surface.

Several treatment options are available to partially and completely edentulous patients. During treatment planning the restorative dentist and patient discuss the patient's needs, desires, and financial commitment. After these issues and existing problems are evaluated, the prosthesis that satisfies these goals is fabricated. The prosthesis may be fixed or removable depending on the existing oral conditions.

Depending on the type of implant to be placed, the surgical technique may vary slightly.

TYPES OF DENTAL IMPLANTS

Endosteal Implant

Endosteal implants, also known as *osseointegrated implants,* are surgically placed into the bone (Fig. 53-3). These implants have three components:

1. The *titanium implant* is surgically embedded into the bone during the stage I surgery.
2. The *titanium abutment screw* is screwed into the implant after osseointegration of the implant and during stage II surgery.
3. The *abutment post* or *cylinder* attaches to the artificial tooth or denture.

The implants and abutment screws are frequently made from the metal **titanium** because of its compatibility with bone and oral tissues. The titanium implants can be coated with *hydroxyapatite,* a ceramic substance that rapidly osseointegrates the implant to the bone.

Osseointegration is the process by which the living jawbone naturally grows around the implanted dental supports (*osseo* means bone). It refers to a bond that is developed between living bone and the surface of an implant fixture. Osseointegrated implants are used to support, stabilize, and retain removable dentures, fixed bridges, and, in some cases, single-tooth implants.

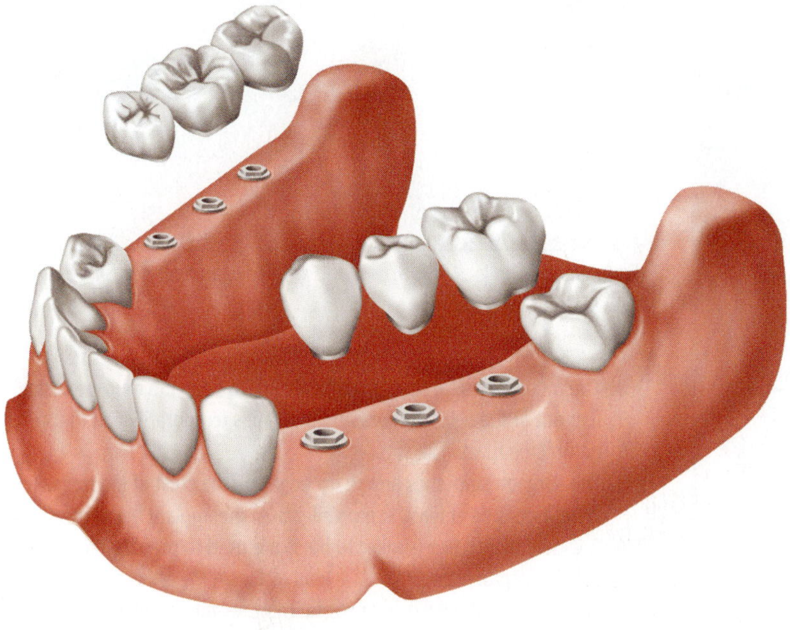

Fig. 53-3 Partially edentulous implant supported restorations. (From Rose LF, Mealey BL, Genco RJ, et al.: *Periodontics: medicine, surgery, and implants.* St Louis, 2004, Mosby.)

Two surgical procedures are required to place endosteal implants. At the *first surgery,* the implant fixtures are placed within receptor sites in the jawbone at predetermined locations. The mucosa is sutured over the fixtures. After a one- to two-week healing period, the existing prosthesis (when applicable) may be removed and relined to adapt to the healed ridge.

A period of three to six months, the *osseointegration period,* is required to permit the fixture to osseointegrate or bond to the bone. Care must be taken during this healing period to avoid trauma to the mucosa overlying the implant sites.

At the *second surgery,* the endosteal implant fixture is exposed, and the abutment screw is connected to the anchor. This portion protrudes through the mucosa and connects the fixture to the prosthesis.

After both surgeries are complete and tissues have healed, the patient begins the *restorative phase,* during which the final crown, bridge, partial denture, or full denture is fabricated. The entire implant process can require three to nine months to reach completion. Procedure 53-1 describes the surgical components of a *two-stage* standard osseointegrated implant system for a single tooth.

Procedure 53-1 Assisting in an Endosteal Implant Surgery

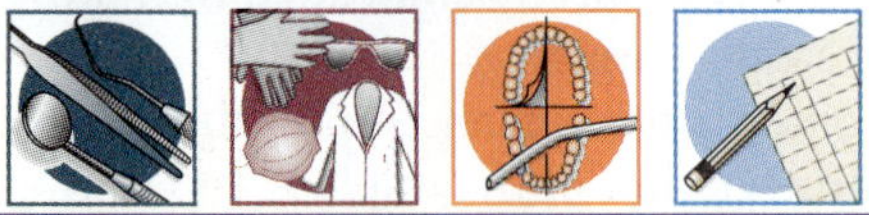

Equipment and Supplies

- Basic setup
- Local anesthetic
- Sterile surgical gloves
- Sterile surgical drilling unit
- Surgical irrigation tip
- Scalpel
- Periosteal elevator
- Implant instrument kit
- Implant kit
- Sterile saline solution
- Low-speed handpiece with contra-angle attachment
- Inserting mallet
- Suture setup
- Electrosurgical unit and tips (or tissue punch)
- 3 percent hydrogen peroxide with syringe
- Sterile cotton pellets
- Sterile 2- × 2-inch gauze sponges

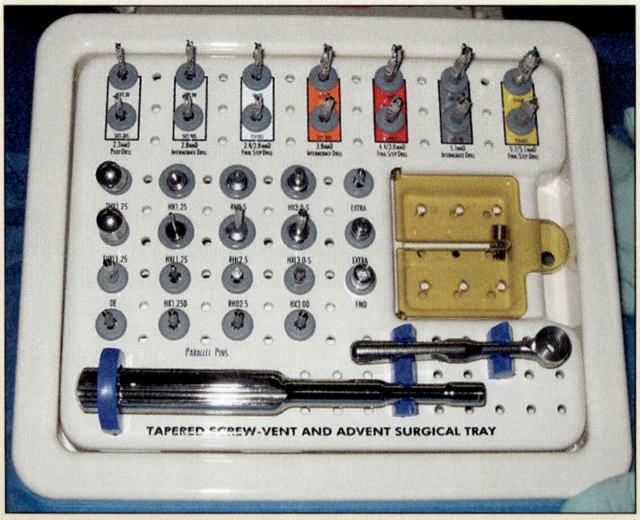

(From Weiss CM, Weiss A: *Principles and practice of implant dentistry,* St Louis, 2001, Mosby.)

PROCEDURAL STEPS

Stage I Surgery: Implant Placement

1. The surgical stent (template) is placed in position in the patient's mouth.
2. After achieving adequate anesthesia, the surgeon uses a "pilot drill" (similar to a pesso bur) to drill through the stent and into the soft tissue on the ridge. This creates a target point on the bone for the implant site.

   Note: All drilling of the bone is accomplished with generous amounts of sterile saline irrigation.
3. The surgeon removes the surgical stent and makes the incision at the implant site.

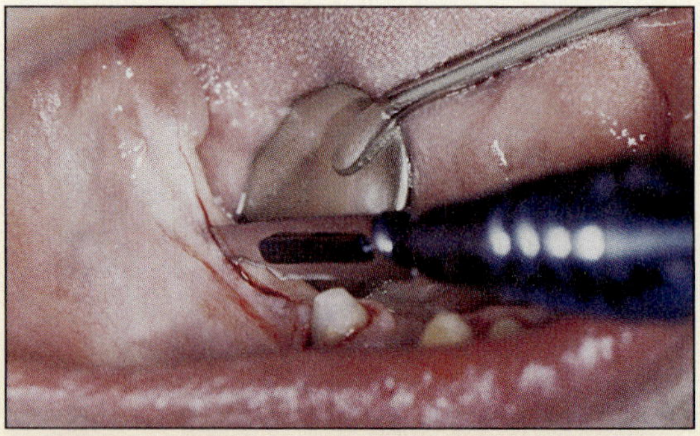

(From Weiss CM, Weiss A: *Principles and practice of implant dentistry,* St Louis, 2001, Mosby.)

4. The mucoperiosteal tissues are reflected. To keep the mucoperiosteal flap out of the field of operation, the flap is temporarily tied to the natural teeth with silk sutures.
5. The surgeon smoothes any sharp edges on the crest of the ridge. The crest should be at least 2 mm wider than the implant being used.
6. A variety of drill tips (similar to burs) are used to prepare the osseous receptor site.
7. The implant cylinder (with a plastic cap over the top of it) is partially inserted into the osseous receptor site.

Procedure 53-1 Assisting in an Endosteal Implant Surgery—cont'd

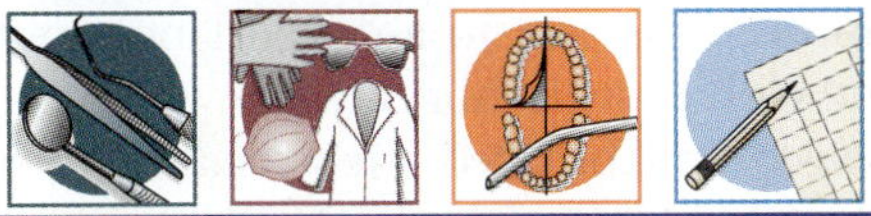

8. The plastic cap is removed, and the implant is tapped into its final position with the inserting mallet.
9. The sterile sealing screw (also called a *healing collar*) is placed into the implant cylinder with the contra-angle screwdriver. The final tightening of the sealing screw is accomplished with the handheld screwdriver.
10. The retraction suture is removed, and the mucoperiosteal flaps are repositioned and sutured in place. The implant receptor now is covered by the tissue and is not visible in the mouth.

Osseointegration Period

A period of three to six months is required to permit the fixture or fixtures to osseointegrate or bond to the bone. During this period, the existing denture or provisional coverage can be adapted to the healed alveolar ridge for temporary use, a procedure usually performed by the *restorative dentist*. The goal of the restorative dentist is to provide patients with beautiful teeth and a beautiful smile so they can continue their normal activities without delay.

Stage II Surgery: Implant Exposure

1. After local anesthesia is administered, the surgical stent (template) is repositioned.
2. A sharp instrument such as a periodontal probe is lowered through the opening in the stent to make bleeding points.

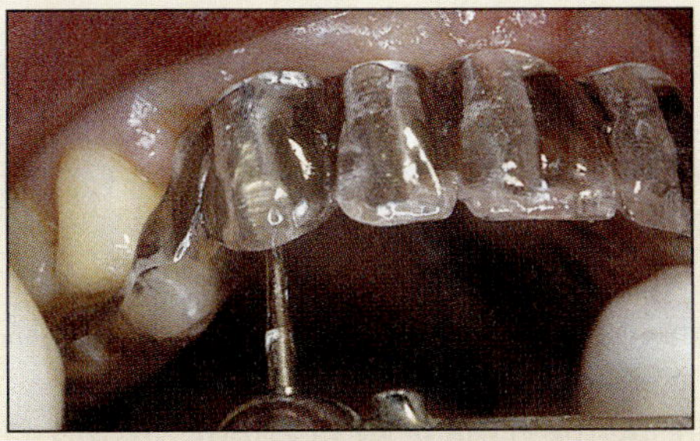

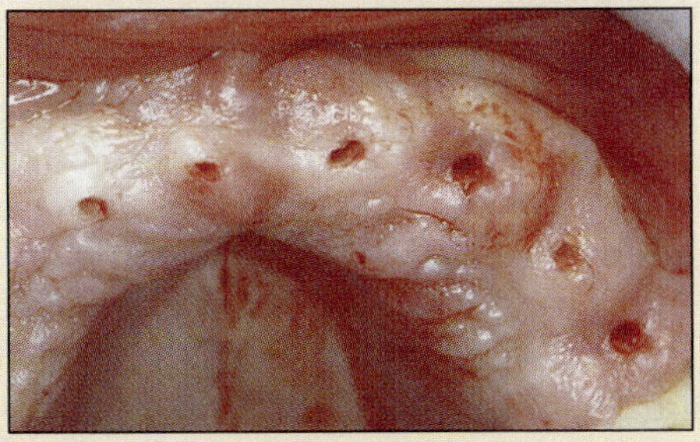

3. The stent is removed, and the mark on the soft tissue shows the position of the previously placed implant.
4. An electrosurgical loop is used to remove the soft tissue over the implant site by peeling it back one layer at a time until the titanium sealing screw is located. A special tissue punch also can be used to remove the tissue from over the implant.

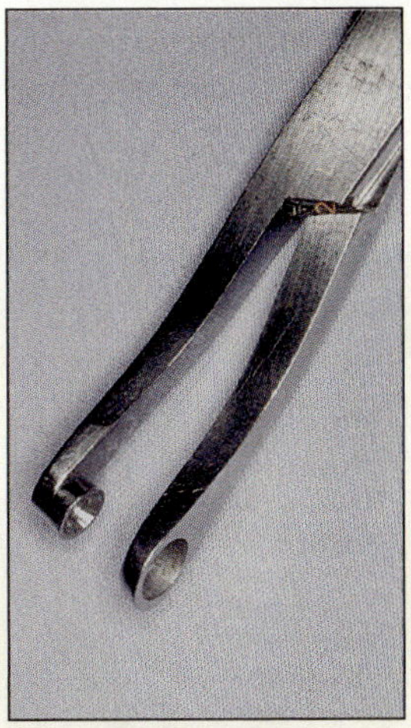

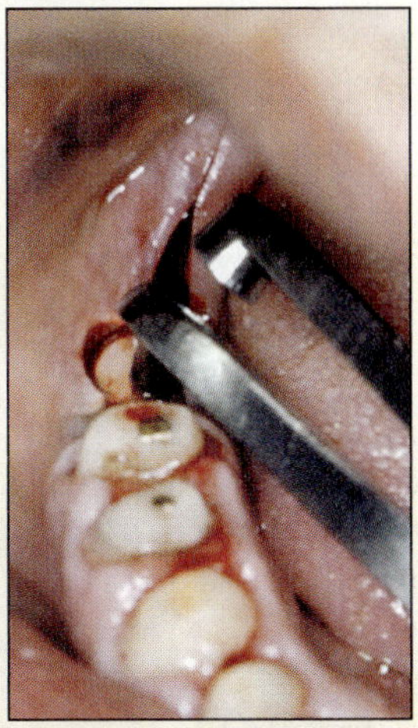

5. The implant is uncovered, and the sealing screw is removed.
6. The inside of the implant cylinder is cleaned with sterile cotton soaked in hydrogen peroxide.
7. A healing collar is screwed into the implant. This attachment will now extend above the mucosa.

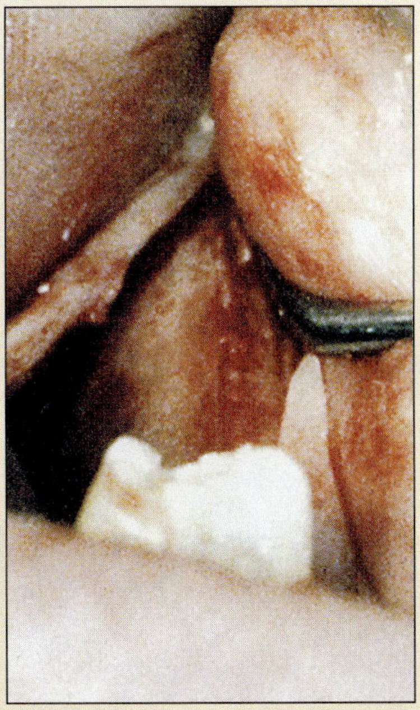

8. The soft tissues are allowed to heal for 10 to 14 days before the fabrication of a permanent crown.

Subperiosteal Implant

A **subperiosteal** implant is a metal frame that is placed under the periosteum and *on top* of the bone. Unlike an endosteal implant, the subperiosteal implant is *not* placed into the bone (Fig. 53-4).

Subperiosteal implants are indicated for patients who do not have sufficient alveolar ridge remaining to support the endosteal-type implant. This type of implant is used most frequently to support a mandibular complete denture (Fig. 53-5).

Two surgical procedures are required. During the *first surgery,* the alveolar ridge is exposed and impressions are taken of the alveolar ridge. After the impressions are taken, the tissue is repositioned over the ridge and sutured back into place. The impression is sent to a dental laboratory, where a metal frame with posts is fabricated.

After the frame has been fabricated, the *second surgery* is performed. The alveolar ridge again is surgically exposed, and the metal frame is placed over the ridge. When the frame is in place, the tissues are repositioned and sutured into place.

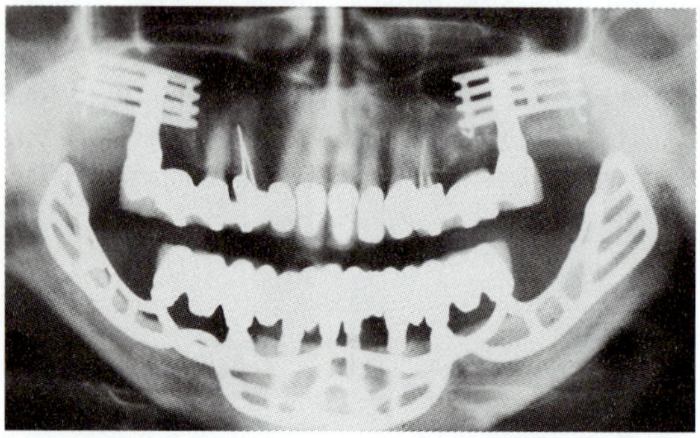

Fig. 53-4 Panoramic radiograph of a subperiosteal implant. (From Weiss CM, Weiss A: *Principles and practice of implant dentistry,* St Louis, 2001, Mosby.)

A

B

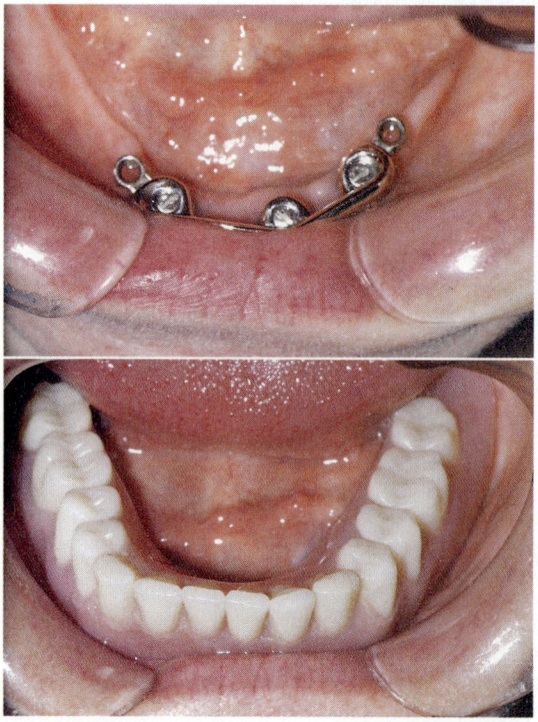

Fig. 53-5 Subperiosteal implant. **A,** Healed implant attachments. **B,** Denture in place.

Transosteal Implant

The **transosteal** implant is inserted through the inferior border of the mandible and into the edentulous area. The most common type is the *transmandibular staple implant,* or fixed mandibular implant. These implants are primarily used on patients with severely resorbed ridges and only when no other options exist.

Recall

8. What material is commonly used to make an implant?

9. What does *osseo* mean?

10. What component of the endosteal implant attaches to the artificial tooth or teeth?

11. When would a subperiosteal implant be recommended to a patient?

MAINTENANCE OF DENTAL IMPLANTS

Long-term maintenance for dental implant patients is an integral part of treatment. This maintenance includes home care by the patient and periodic maintenance visits to the dental office.

The health of the **peri-implant tissue** is a critical factor in the success of dental implants. It is similar to the gingival sulcus surrounding a natural tooth. Peri-implant tissue responds to bacterial plaque with inflammation and bleeding similar to gingival tissues around a normal tooth.

Many implant patients have lost their natural teeth because of chronic periodontal disease, caused in part by poor oral hygiene. The task of educating and motivating these patients to practice proper home care is difficult but critical to the long-term success of the implants.

Dental *plaque* and *calculus* form on implants just as on natural teeth. Because the surface of implants is very smooth, plaque is less adherent and more easily removed than it is from natural teeth. Calculus is relatively easy to remove from the implants because it cannot become embed-

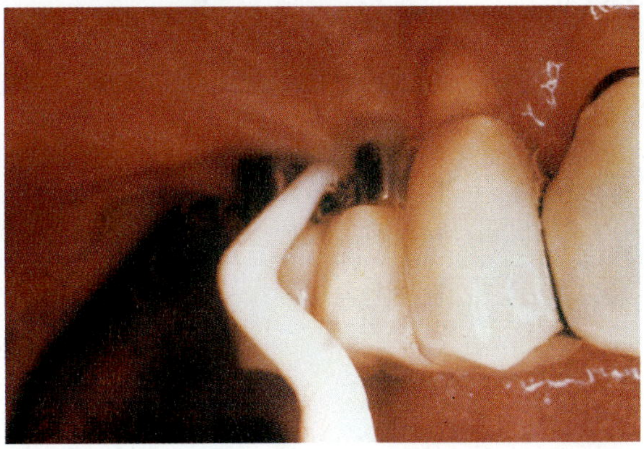

Fig. 53-6 Instruments used to remove calculus from a dental implant.

ded in the titanium surface. However, it is critical to remove plaque and calculus from the implant in such a way that the implant surfaces are not scratched (Fig. 53-6).

Home Care

As with all home care, the goal is to remove all plaque and debris at least once daily. Patients are instructed in the use of home care aids, and their progress is monitored regularly. As discussed in Chapter 15, the following devices are essential in plaque removal for implant patients:

- Toothbrushes, manual or electric
- Single-tufted toothbrushes
- Partial denture clasp brushes
- Interproximal brushes
- Floss (thick, thin, or fuzzy)
- Dental implant floss, with a stiff, curved end

Routine Office Visits

Recall visits are essential to the long-term success of implants. It is extremely important that patients understand the need to maintain optimum plaque control through meticulous home care and frequent professional recalls. Patients should be scheduled at regular intervals for examination, radiographs, prophylaxis, removal of fixed components, replacement of components, relines, and remakes as recommended.

Recall

12. Why are plaque and calculus easier to remove from an implant than from a natural tooth?

13. What cleaning accessories are used to clean implants?

Patient Education

In American culture, people are often judged by their facial expressions. A smile can be a sign of competence, inner reflections, thoughts, and emotions. A large population of people is not aware of dental implant procedures. By providing this information to all of your patients through brochures, educational videos, and patient discussion, you are furthering their knowledge of dental care.

Legal and Ethical Implications

With dental implants being such a large investment of money and time for a patient, it is important that the dental team present the complete plan of all stages of treatment. More and more dental insurance companies are handling dental implant procedures, but only for specific reasons. Dentists have a responsibility to their patients and should not deviate from the reasons for providing this procedure. This may cause undue harm to the patient through negligence in providing proper care.

Eye to the Future

Modern advances in implant technology have made immediate implant placement possible. Once a tooth is extracted, the bone underneath the space quickly starts to shrink back. If the implant is placed immediately at extraction and before any bone resorption has occurred, there is still a maximum amount of bone available for support. Because the implant is placed at the same time the tooth is extracted, there is no need for further surgical procedures and the implant can be placed while the patient is still anesthetized.

Critical Thinking

1. Describe your role as a clinical assistant in the procedure of implant surgery.
2. Discuss the reasoning behind using titanium metal for implants over other metals.
3. Your patient is considering implants. While updating the patient's medical and dental history, you find that the patient is taking fluoxetine (Prozac). For what condition is Prozac prescribed, and why would this information be important for the dentist to know before beginning the implant process?
4. Why is infection control so important in the preparation and procedure stages of implants?
5. Of all types of specialists involved in providing implants, what does each specialist bring to this area of dentistry?

54

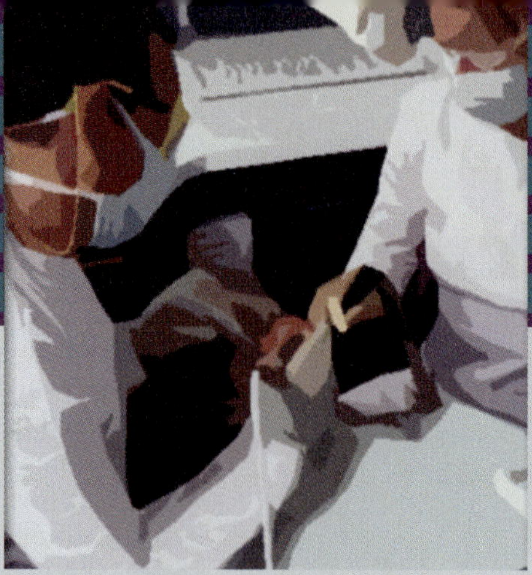

Endodontics

Outline

Causes of Pulpal Damage
Symptoms of Pulpal Damage
Endodontic Diagnosis
- Percussion and Palpation
- Thermal Sensitivity
- Electric Pulp Testing
- Radiographs

Procedure 54-1: Assisting in Electric Pulp Vitality Test
Diagnostic Conclusions
Endodontic Procedures
- Pulp Capping
- Pulpotomy
- Pulpectomy

Instruments and Accessories
- Hand Instruments
- Instruments for Pulp Preparation
- Ancillary Instruments

Medicaments and Dental Materials in Endodontics
- Irrigation Solutions
- Root Canal Filling Materials
- Root Canal Sealers

Overview of Root Canal Therapy
- Anesthesia and Pain Control
- Isolation and Disinfection of the Operating Field
- Access Preparation
- Debridement and Shaping the Canal
- Obturation

Procedure 54-2: Assisting in Root Canal Therapy
Surgical Endodontics
- Apicoectomy and Apical Curettage
- Retrograde Restoration
- Root Amputation and Hemisection

Patient Education
Legal and Ethical Implications
Eye to the Future
Critical Thinking

KEY TERMS

Abscess (**ab**-*ses*) Localized area of pus originating from an infection.

Acute (ah-**kyut**) Referring to a condition with a rapid onset.

Apical curettage (**a**-pi-kul *kyur*-uh-**tahzh**) Surgical removal of infectious material surrounding the apex of a root.

Apicoectomy (**a**-pi-ko-*ek*-teh-me) Surgical removal of the apical portion of a tooth through an opening made in the overlying bone and gingival tissues.

Chronic (**krah**-nik) Pertaining to disease symptoms that persist over a long time, as in periodontal disease.

Control tooth Healthy tooth used as a standard to compare questionable teeth of similar size and structure during pulp vitality testing.

Debridement (di-**breed**-munt) To remove or clean out the pulpal canal.

Endodontist A dentist who specializes in the prevention, diagnosis, and treatment of diseases of the dental pulp and the periradicular tissues.

Gutta-percha (guh-tah–per-chah) Plastic type of filling material used in endodontics.

Hemisection (**he**-mah-sek-shun) Surgical separation of a multirooted tooth through the furcation area.

Indirect pulp cap Placement of a medicament over a partially exposed pulp.

Irreversible pulpitis (puhl-**pi**-tis) Infectious condition in which clinical diagnostic findings show that the pulp is incapable of healing, indicating root canal therapy or extraction as the only treatment option.

Nonvital Not living, as in oral tissue and tooth structure.

Obturation (*ahb*-tyah-**ray**-shun) Process of filling a root canal.

Palpation (pal-*pay*-shun) Examination technique of the soft tissues with the examiner's hand or fingertips.

Percussion (per-**kuh**-shun) Examination technique that involves tapping on the incisal or occlusal surface of a tooth to determine vitality.

Perforation (per-fah-**ray**-shun) Making a hole, as in breaking through and extending beyond the apex of the root.

Periodontal abscess An inflammatory reaction to bacteria trapped in the periodontal sulcus.

KEY TERMS

Periradicular (per-ee-ruh-**di**-kyuh-ler) Referring to the area of nerves, blood vessels, and tissues that surround the root of a tooth.

Periradicular abscess An inflammatory reaction to pulpal infection.

Periradicular cyst A cyst that develops at or near the root of a necrotic tooth.

Pulp cap Application of dental material to a cavity preparation with an exposed or nearly exposed dental pulp.

Pulpectomy (puhl-**pek**-tah-me) Complete removal of the vital pulp from a tooth.

Pulpitis (puhl-**pi**-tis) Inflammation of the dental pulp.

Pulpotomy (puhl-**pah**-tah-me) Removal of the coronal portion of the vital pulp from a tooth.

Retrograde restoration (**re**-trah-*grade res*-tah-**ray**-shun) Small restoration placed at the apex of a root.

Reversible pulpitis Form of pulpal inflammation in which the pulp may be salvageable.

Root amputation (*am*-pyuh-**tay**-shun) Removal of one or more roots without removing the crown of the tooth.

Root canal therapy Process of removing the dental pulp and filling the canal with material.

LEARNING OUTCOMES

On completion of this chapter, the student will be able to achieve the following objectives:

- Pronounce, define, and spell the Key Terms.
- Describe the diagnostic testing performed for endodontic diagnosis.
- List the conclusions of the subjective and objective tests in the endodontic diagnosis.
- Describe diagnostic conclusions for endodontic therapy.
- List the types of endodontic procedures.
- Discuss the medicaments and dental materials used in endodontics.
- Provide an overview of root canal therapy.
- Describe surgical endodontics and how it affects treatment.

PERFORMANCE OUTCOMES

On completion of this chapter, the student will be able to achieve competency standards in the following skills:

- Assist in electric pulp vitality test.
- Assist in root canal therapy.

Endodontics is the specialty of dentistry that manages the prevention, diagnosis, and treatment of the dental pulp and the **periradicular** tissues that surround the root of the tooth. *Endodontic treatment,* often referred to as **root canal therapy,** provides an effective means of saving a tooth that might otherwise have to be extracted.

The general dentist is skilled and qualified to perform endodontic treatment; however, dentists will refer patients in need of this treatment to an **endodontist,** a dentist who specializes in this area. An endodontist is a general dentist who has continued training for a minimum of three years in the clinical skill and research of pulp therapy.

CAUSES OF PULPAL DAMAGE

The two sources of pulpal nerve damage occur from either physical irritation or trauma. *Physical irritation* is most often caused by extensive decay that has moved into the pulp carrying bacteria. When bacteria reach the nerves and blood vessels, infection will result in an **abscess,** which is a localized area of pus (Fig. 54-1).

Trauma, such as a blow to a tooth or the jaw, can cause damage to the surrounding tissues. Over time this damage will affect the nerve tissue and blood vessels of the pulp (Fig. 54-2).

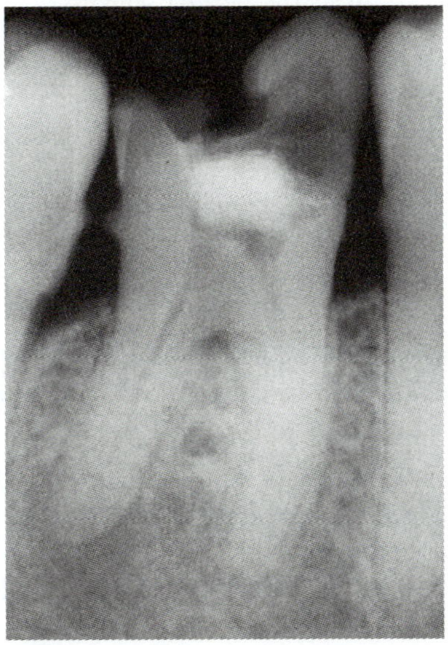

Fig. 54-1 Radiograph showing extensive decay into the pulp. (From Johnson W: *Color atlas of endodontics,* Philadelphia, 2002, Saunders.)

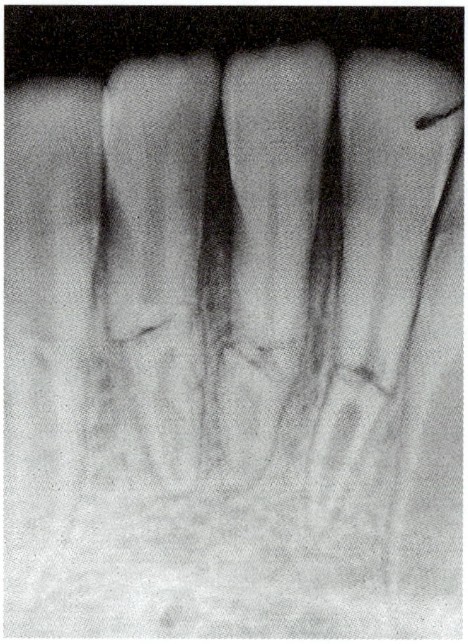

Fig. 54-2 **Radiograph of a necrotic tooth resulting from trauma.** (From Johnson W: *Color atlas of endodontics,* Philadelphia, 2002, Saunders.)

SYMPTOMS OF PULPAL DAMAGE

A patient experiencing sensitivity, discomfort, and pain may be experiencing symptoms of *pulpal nerve damage.* Even though patients experience symptoms differently, the most common signs and symptoms of pulpal damage are:

- Pain when occluding
- Pain during mastication
- Sensitivity to hot or cold beverages
- Noticeable facial swelling

Recall

1. What are periradicular tissues?
2. What specialist performs root canal therapy?
3. What will result if bacteria reach the nerves and blood vessels of a tooth?

ENDODONTIC DIAGNOSIS

The diagnosis of a tooth that requires endodontic treatment is based on an examination that has both subjective and objective components.

The *subjective examination* includes an evaluation of symptoms or problems *described by the patient,* which include:

- Chief complaint
- Character and duration of pain
- Painful stimuli
- Sensitivity to biting and pressure

The *objective examination* is conducted by the endodontist, who evaluates the status of the tooth and surrounding tissues in regard to the following:

- Extent of decay
- Periodontal conditions surrounding the tooth in question
- Presence of an extensive restoration
- Tooth mobility
- Swelling or discoloration
- Pulp exposure

Several techniques are used to test pulp vitality in determining whether endodontic therapy is required or the pulp is vital and able to repair itself. When testing a questionable tooth, a **control tooth** is selected for comparison. A healthy tooth, usually of the same type, in the opposite quadrant is selected as a control tooth. For example, if the maxillary right first premolar is the *suspect tooth,* the control tooth would be the maxillary left first premolar. The use of a control tooth shows that the stimulus is capable of achieving a response.

Percussion and Palpation

Percussion and palpation tests are used to determine whether the inflammatory process has extended into the periapical tissues. A positive response to these tests indicates that there is inflammation in the periodontal ligament and that endodontic treatment is most likely required.

The dentist performs the **percussion** *test* by tapping on the incisal or occlusal surface of the tooth in question with the end of the mouth mirror handle, which is held parallel to the long axis of the tooth (Fig 54-3).

The dentist performs the **palpation** *test* by applying firm pressure to the mucosa above the apex of the root (Fig. 54-4). The dentist will note any sensitivity and swelling.

Thermal Sensitivity

Tests with temperature extremes are another method of determining the status of the pulp. A thermal stimulus is *never* placed on a metallic restoration or the gingival tissue. The application of extreme temperatures will result in an abnormal response and possible damage to the tissues.

In the *cold test,* the dentist uses ice, dry ice, or carbon dioxide to determine the response of a tooth to cold. First, the control tooth and the suspect tooth are isolated and dried. Next, the source of cold is applied first to the cervical area of the control tooth, then to the cervical area of the suspect tooth (Fig. 54-5).

A necrotic pulp will *not* respond to cold. Irreversible pulpitis is suspected when the cold relieves the pain; however, cold in teeth with irreversible pulpitis also can initiate severe, lingering pain.

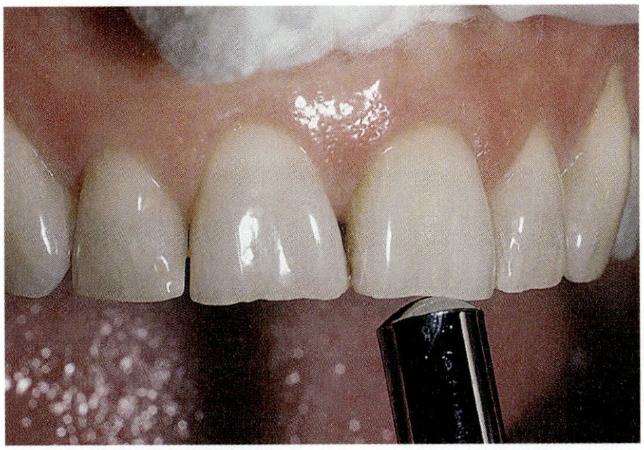

Fig. 54-3 Percussion test. (From Johnson W: *Color atlas of endodontics,* Philadelphia, 2002, Saunders.)

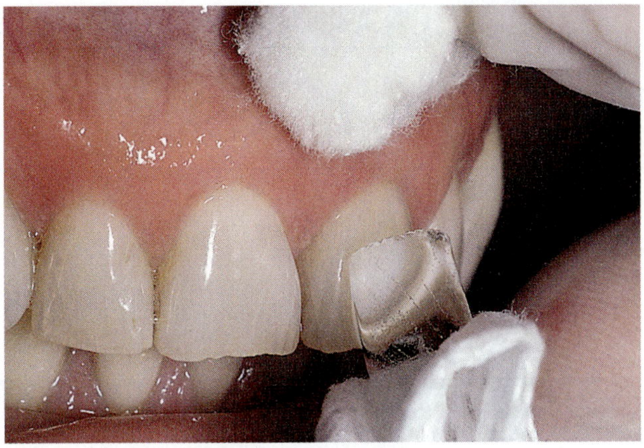

Fig. 54-5 Ice used for testing thermal sensitivity. (From Johnson W: *Color atlas of endodontics,* Philadelphia, 2002, Saunders.)

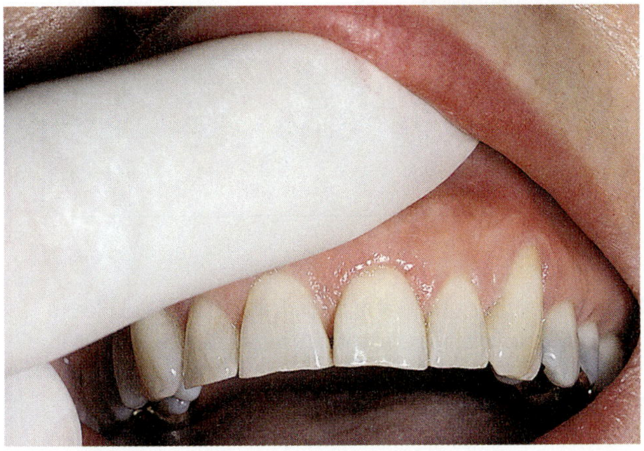

Fig. 54-4 Palpation test. (From Johnson W: *Color atlas of endodontics,* Philadelphia, 2002, Saunders.)

The *heat test* is generally the least useful of the vitality tests because a painful response to the heat could indicate *either* reversible pulpitis or irreversible pulpitis. A necrotic pulp will not respond to heat. A small (pea-sized) piece of **gutta-percha** is heated in a flame and applied to the facial surface of the tooth. Another method is to heat the end of an instrument and place it on the tooth. Petroleum jelly should be applied to the tooth surface before testing to prevent the material from sticking to the tooth surface.

Electric Pulp Testing

Electric pulp testing is used in endodontic diagnosis to determine whether a pulp is vital or **nonvital.** Like other testing devices, the pulp tester can produce a *false-positive* or *false-negative* response (test result that shows a positive or negative response incorrectly). Therefore the test results must be supported by other diagnostic findings (see Procedure 54-1).

Electric pulp testers deliver a small electrical stimulus to the pulp. Factors that influence the reliability of the pulp tester include:

- Teeth with extensive restorations can vary in response.
- Teeth with more than one canal can have one vital canal and other nonvital canals.
- A failing pulp can produce a variety of responses.
- Control teeth may not respond as anticipated.
- Moisture on the tooth during testing may produce an inaccurate reading.
- The batteries in the tester may weaken over time.

Radiographs

Radiographs are a necessity for diagnostic testing as well as for root canal therapy. Good-quality radiographs are required for optimal information (Fig. 54-6). (See Chapters 40 and 42.) The following films are required for the diagnosis and completion of endodontic treatment:

- *Initial radiograph.* A periapical radiograph is taken during the diagnostic stages before treatment.
- *Working length film.* A periapical radiograph is taken once the pulp is opened. This film is used to determine the length of the canal. It is easier to detect canal length with the file remaining in the tooth.
- *Final instrumentation film.* A periapical radiograph is taken with the final size files in all canals receiving treatment.
- *Root canal completion film.* A final periapical radiograph is taken of the completed root filling after the tooth has been temporized and the dental dam removed.
- *Recall films.* Radiographs are taken at posttreatment evaluations.

Procedure 54-1 Assisting in Electric Pulp Vitality Test

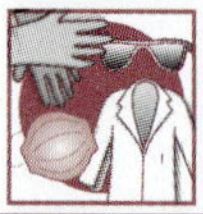

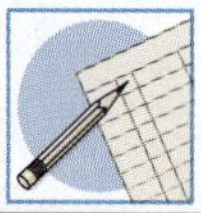

Equipment and Supplies

- Electric pulp tester
- Toothpaste
- Electric pulp testing kit

PROCEDURAL STEPS

1. Describe the procedure to the patient, and explain that the patient may feel a tingling or a warm sensation.
2. Identify the teeth to be tested (suspect tooth and control tooth), then isolate these teeth and thoroughly dry.

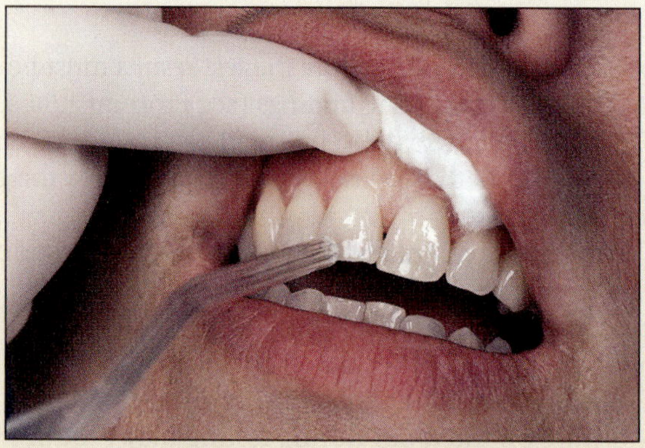

3. Set the dial (current level) at zero.
4. Place a thin layer of toothpaste on the tip of the pulp tester electrode.
   Purpose: To provide adequate contact to conduct a current from the pulp tester to the tooth.
5. Test the control tooth first.
6. Place the tip of the electrode on the facial surface of the tooth at the *cervical third.*

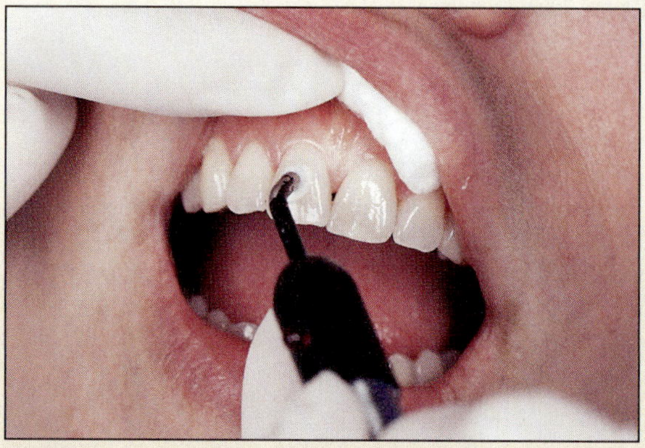

7. Gradually increase the level of the current until the patient feels a sensation. Document on the patient's record the level at which the response occurred.
8. Repeat the procedure on the suspect tooth.

Date	Tooth	Surface	Charting Notes
8/12/05	8	—	Pt complained of pain. Tooth #13 used as control tooth. Vitality tester showed tooth still responding to sensation. Periapical radiograph showed decay extending into pulp. T. Clark, CDA/L. Stuart, DDS

Requirements of Endodontic Films

1. Show 4 to 5 mm beyond the apex of the tooth and the surrounding bone or pathologic condition.
2. Present an accurate image of the tooth without elongation or foreshortening.
3. Exhibit good contrast so all pertinent structures are readily identifiable.

Recall

4. Is pain a subjective or objective component of a diagnosis?
5. Tooth #21 is being tested for possible endodontic treatment. What tooth would be used as a control tooth?
6. When the dentist taps on a tooth, what diagnostic test is being performed?
7. How many radiographs may be taken through the course of root canal therapy?

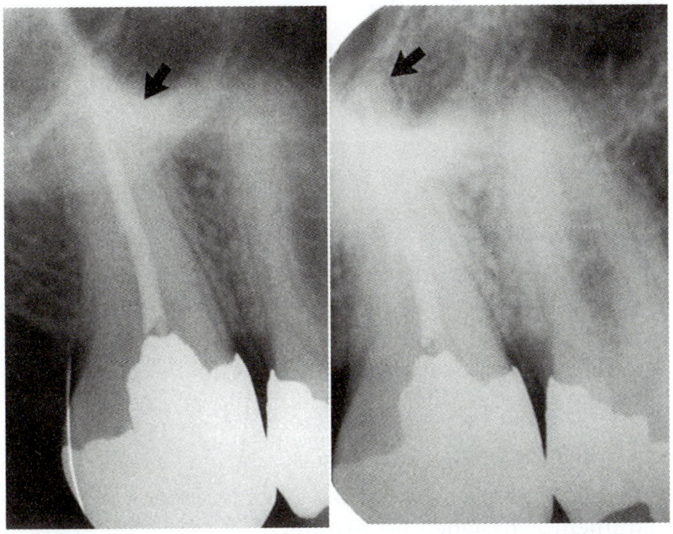

Fig. 54-6 Good-quality radiographs are necessary for endodontic evaluation. *Left,* Showing good contrast around the apex; *right,* showing poor contrast around the apex.

DIAGNOSTIC CONCLUSIONS

Once the subjective and objective tests are complete, a diagnosis is presented to the patient.

Normal pulp indicates no subjective symptoms or objective signs. The tooth responds normally to sensory stimuli, and a healthy layer of dentin surrounds the pulp.

Pulpitis indicates that pulpal tissues have become inflamed. Pulpitis can be clinically described as follows:

- **Reversible pulpitis** is when the pulp is irritated and the patient is experiencing pain to thermal stimuli. With reversible pulpitis, eliminating the irritant and placing a sedative material may save the pulp.
- **Irreversible pulpitis** displays symptoms of lingering pain. Clinical diagnostic findings show that the pulp is incapable of healing, indicating root canal therapy or extraction as the only treatment option.

Periradicular abscess is an inflammatory reaction to pulpal infection. **Chronic** periradicular abscess is characterized by the presence of a draining sinus tract. The lesion is asymptomatic with little or no discomfort, and an intermittent discharge of pus may be noticed. **Acute** periradicular abscess is an inflammatory response with pain, tenderness of the tooth to pressure, pus formation, and swelling of the tissue resulting from necrosis.

Periodontal abscess is an inflammatory reaction frequently caused by bacteria entrapped in the periodontal sulcus. Most often a patient will experience rapid onset, pain, tenderness of the tooth to pressure, pus formation, and swelling.

Periradicular cyst develops at or near the root of a necrotic tooth. These types of cysts develop as an inflammatory response to pulpal infection and necrosis of the pulp.

Pulp fibrosis is the decrease of living cells within the pulp, causing fibrous tissue to take over the pulpal canal. Fibrosis is seen in older patients as well as in patients with traumatic injury to a tooth.

Necrosis, also referred to as **necrotic** or **nonvital,** is used to describe a tooth that does not respond to sensory stimulus. These terms are inaccurate, because even though the tooth may be considered "dead," the tooth continues to be attached to the alveolus by way of the cementum and periodontal ligaments, which are still living.

Recall

8. What diagnosis is given when pulpal tissues are inflamed?
9. What is another term for necrotic or necrosis?

ENDODONTIC PROCEDURES

The choice of endodontic treatment depends on the diagnosis. The first line of treatment is *pulpal therapy,* which is an attempt to stimulate pulpal regeneration and save the pulp. When pulpal therapy is not effective, the endodontist will move to more extreme measures, including root canal therapy or surgery.

Pulp Capping

In an attempt to save the pulp, a covering of calcium hydroxide is placed over an exposed or nearly exposed pulp to encourage the formation of irritated dentin at the site of injury.

Indirect pulp cap is indicated when a thin partition of dentin is still intact. The pulp has not yet been exposed, but the pulp may become exposed when removing decay near the pulp. The goals are (1) to promote pulpal healing by removing most of the decay and (2) to stimulate the production of reparative dentin through placement of calcium hydroxide.

Direct pulp cap is indicated when the pulp has been slightly exposed. With a direct pulp cap the tooth is still vital. However, it may become infected and require additional treatment or become necrotic and require root canal therapy. When a direct pulp cap is performed, it is necessary to inform the patient that problems may develop later and that periodic monitoring is necessary.

Pulpotomy

A **pulpotomy** involves the removal of the coronal portion of an exposed vital pulp. This procedure is done to preserve the vitality of the remaining portion of the pulp within the root of the tooth. Pulpotomy is often indicated for vital primary teeth, teeth with deep carious lesions, and emergency situations (see Chapter 57).

Pulpectomy

A **pulpectomy**, also referred to as *root canal therapy*, involves the complete removal of the dental pulp (see later in the chapter for complete discussion).

Recall

10. What dental material is used for pulp capping?
11. How much of the pulp is removed in a pulpotomy?

INSTRUMENTS AND ACCESSORIES

Endodontic instruments and accessories are designed to be flexible and to fit into the pulpal canal.

Hand Instruments

Explorer

The endodontic explorer is a double-ended instrument that is long and straight. The working ends are at an angle to the handle (Fig. 54-7). The unique design of the endodontic explorer helps to locate canal openings.

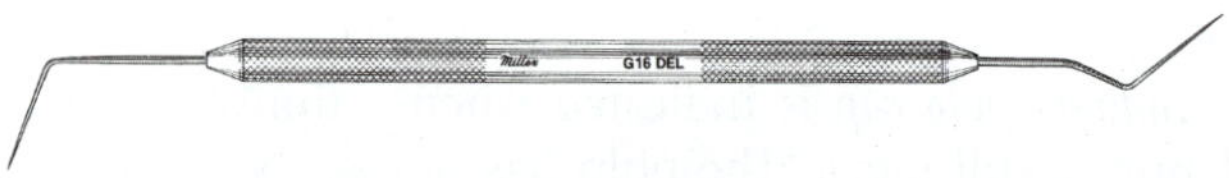

Fig. 54-7 **Endodontic explorer.** (Courtesy Miltex Inc., York, PA.)

Endodontic Spoon Excavator

The double-ended endodontic spoon excavator is similar to other spoon excavators. However, the endodontic spoon has a very long shank allowing it to reach deep into the tooth and canal to remove coronal pulp tissue, decay, and temporary cements (Fig. 54-8).

Spreaders and Pluggers

These instruments are used **in the obturation** of the canal. They condense and adapt the gutta-percha points into the canals. Pluggers and spreaders look similar but differ at the tip (Fig. 54-9). The *pluggers* have a flat tip like a condenser, and the *spreaders* have a pointed tip like an explorer.

Glick Number 1

The paddle-shaped end of the Glick Number 1 dental instrument is designed for placement of temporary restorations, and the rod-shaped plugger at the opposite end is ideal for removal of excess gutta-percha. The plugger end is graduated at 5-mm increments and can be heated for placement or removal of gutta-percha.

Instruments for Pulp Preparation

There are three classifications of endodontic instruments for pulp preparation.

Hand-Operated and Finger-Operated Files

Broaches

A broach is a thin, flexible, tapered metal hand instrument. Broaches have tiny fishhook-like projections along the shaft that are used to remove vital, inflamed hemorrhagic

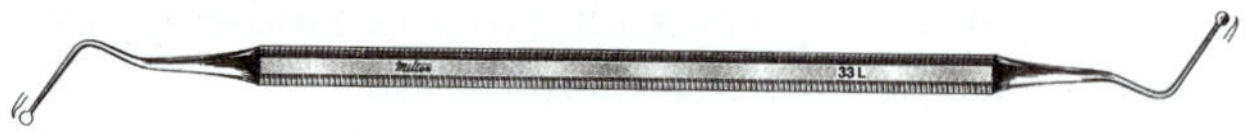

Fig. 54-8 **Endodontic spoon excavator.** (Courtesy Miltex Inc., York, PA.)

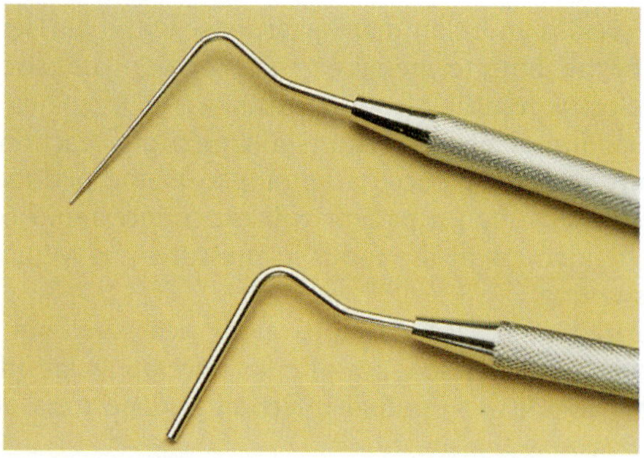

Fig. 54-9 **Spreader and plugger used to obturate the canal.**

pulp tissue from the canal (Fig. 54-10*A*). Although broaches are used less frequently, they are still used to remove objects such as cotton pellets and paper points. Broaches should be discarded after a single use because of their fragile makeup.

K-type file

The *K-type file* has a twisted design and is used in the initial debridement (cleaning) of the canal and in the later stages of shaping and contouring the canal. The *conventional* K-type file has a "stiff" feel that is very effective for straight canals. For narrow canals and curved canals, some dentists prefer the *flexible K-type file* (Fig. 54-10*B*).

Hedstrom file

The *Hedstrom file* provides greater cutting efficiency because of its design (Fig. 54-10*C*). The Hedstrom file can be used for final enlargement of the canal after a Gates-Glidden bur or Pesso reamer has been used (see later discussion). The H-type file has its spiral edges arranged so that cutting occurs only on the pulling stroke, making the dentinal walls smooth and easier to fill.

Both K-type and Hedstrom files are available in stainless steel or nickel-titanium (Ni-Ti) alloy. Although more expensive than stainless steel files, the Ni-Ti files have the advantages of (1) *extreme flexibility,* which enables them to better follow the contour of the canal; (2) *good strength,* which is an important safety factor to keep the instrument from breaking while in the canal; and (3) a *longer working life.*

Sizes and color codes

To provide uniformity among manufacturers, the American Dental Association (ADA) has standardized the numbering and color-coding system for intracanal instruments.

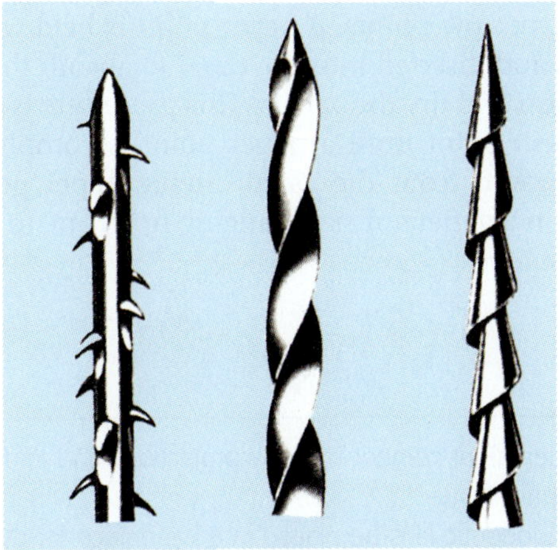

A B C

Fig. 54-10 Hand-operated and Finger-operated files. **A,** Dental broach. **B,** K-type file. **C,** Hedstrom file.

Files are supplied in different diameters ranging from size 08 (the smallest) to size 140 (the largest). Box 54-1 shows how colors are used to code handles of the instruments according to diameter.

Instruments Attached to the Low-Speed Handpiece

Gates-Glidden burs, also known as *Gates-Glidden drills,* have a football-shaped working end with a very long shank (Fig. 54-11). They are used in a handpiece, with a latch-type attachment, and are operated in a clockwise direction. These burs are designed to have the cutting edge on the sides, not on the end.

Pesso reamers, which work in the same manner as the Gates-Glidden burs, are shaped slightly to have their blades long and parallel with the noncutting ends. These files are used primarily when the tooth requires a post preparation for placement of the final restoration.

Box 54-1 Color Coding and Sizing of Hand-Operated Files

Handle color	Diameter
Gray	08
Purple	10
White	15–49–90
Yellow	20–50–100
Red	25–55–110
Blue	30–60–120
Green	35–70–130
Black	40–80–140

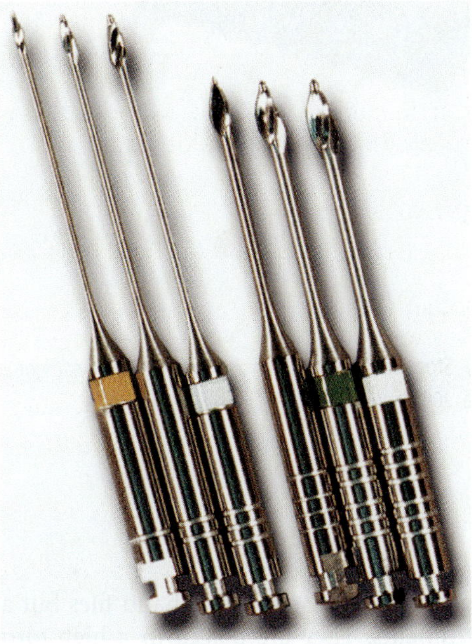

Fig. 54-11 Gates-Glidden burs. (From Johnson W: *Color atlas of endodontics,* Philadelphia, 2002, Saunders.)

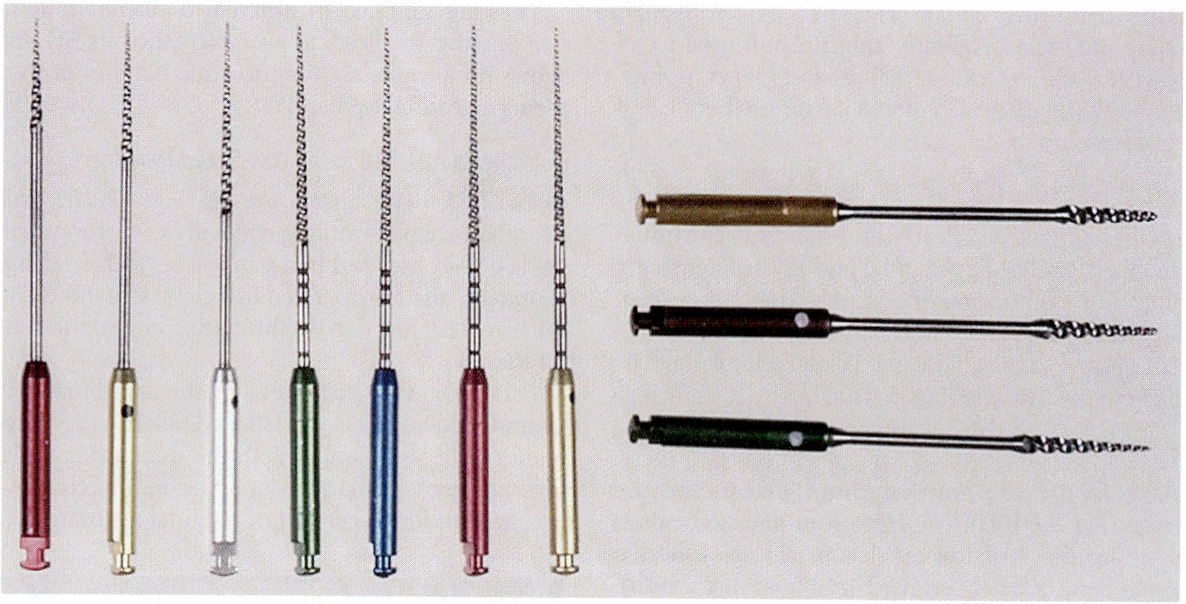

Fig. 54-12 **Rotary instruments used during endodontic therapy. Profile series.** (From Johnson W: *Color atlas of endodontics,* Philadelphia, 2002, Saunders.)

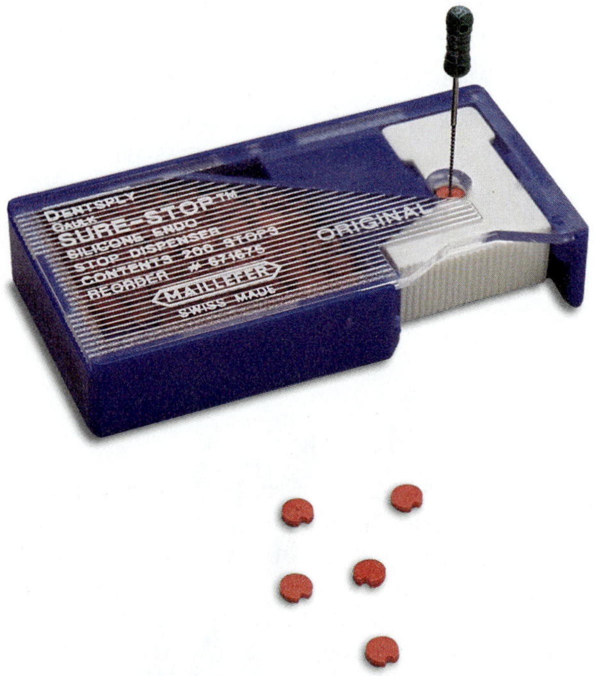

Fig. 54-13 **Stop dispenser.** (From Johnson W: *Color atlas of endodontics,* Philadelphia, 2002, Saunders.)

Rotary Files

Rotary instruments are similar to hand files but are latch-type instruments. They are placed in a high-torque, low-rpm handpiece designed for nickel titanium rotary instruments. These groups of instruments are becoming more popular in use because of their makeup, ease in use, and efficiency. Common types of these instruments are Profile and LightSpeed (Fig. 54-12).

Ancillary Instruments

Rubber Stops

A *stop* is a small, round piece of rubber, silicone, or plastic that is slid onto the intracanal instrument to prevent **perforation** of the apex of the tooth during instrumentation (Fig. 54-13). The lengths of the files are carefully measured on a radiograph, and the stop is placed precisely at the predetermined working length of the canal.

Paper Points

Paper points are sterile absorbent pieces of paper rolled into long, narrow points. A paper point is held with locking pliers and inserted into the canal to absorb the irrigating solution and dry the canals. This procedure is repeated with a fresh point until a paper point is completely dry when removed from the canal. Sterile paper points are available in a variety of sizes ranging from fine to coarse.

Recall

12. What dental instrument has tiny projections and is used to remove pulp tissue?
13. Can endodontic files be placed in a handpiece for use?
14. What type of file is best suited for canal enlargement?
15. Why is a rubber stop used on a file?
16. What does obturate mean?

MEDICAMENTS AND DENTAL MATERIALS IN ENDODONTICS

Medicaments and dental materials used in endodontics include irrigation solutions, root canal filling materials, and root canal sealers (Fig. 54-14).

Irrigation Solutions

In endodontics, irrigating the canal facilitates the removal of materials from the canal and provides tissue dissolution, bleaching, deodorizing, and hemorrhage control. The following solutions are used to provide this process.

Sodium hypochlorite, commonly known as household bleach, is diluted with equal parts of sterile water for use as an irrigation solution. A 5-ml to 6-ml disposable plastic syringe with a special 27-gauge needle is used for irrigation. This solution is an antimicrobial agent and has a solvent action on necrotic pulp tissue and organic debris. It must be used with caution because a bleach solution causes skin irritation, and drips or splashes can ruin the patient's clothing.

Hydrogen peroxide is a clear, colorless liquid with disinfectant and bleaching properties for endodontics.

Parachlorophenol (PCP) is a colorless, crystalline toxic phenol compound used as an antimicrobial agent for disinfection of the pulp canal.

Root Canal Filling Materials

Gutta-percha points are made from a rubber material taken from the *Palaquium gutta* tree. Gutta-percha is an organic substance that is solid at room temperature and becomes soft and pliable when heated. Gutta-percha points are used to obturate the pulpal canal after treatment has been completed. This *radiopaque* material is supplied in various sizes and used with a sealer.

Root Canal Sealers

A *root canal sealer* is a cement-type material that seals out the unfilled voids during the obturation process. Several cements can be used as a sealer for root canal therapy, including calcium hydroxide, zinc oxide–eugenol, and glass ionomer (see Chapter 45). These materials must have very little shrinkage. They also must be easy to place, radiopaque for detection on a radiograph, nonstaining to the teeth, bacteriostatic, gentle on the periapical tissues that surround them, and able to resist moisture.

Formocresol is a mixture of formaldehyde and cresol in a water-glycerin base. This type of solution is used as a sealer for pulpotomy of deciduous teeth and as an intracanal medicament for permanent teeth during root canal therapy.

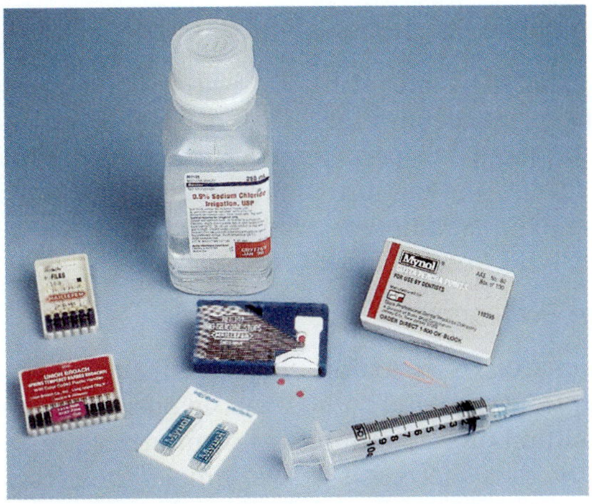

Fig. 54-14 Materials needed for preparing and obturating the pulpal canal. *Top,* Sterile irrigating solution; *Bottom,* sterile paper points and syringe used with irrigating solution; *Left,* files; *Right,* gutta-percha.

Recall

17. Which irrigation solution is most often used during root canal therapy?

OVERVIEW OF ROOT CANAL THERAPY

The procedure of root canal therapy involves specific steps of treatment (see Procedure 54-2).

Anesthesia and Pain Control

The anesthesia techniques of choice for endodontic treatment are *infiltration* for maxillary teeth and *nerve blocks* for mandibular teeth (see Chapter 37). A local anesthetic agent is administered any time there is vitality remaining in the tooth to be treated. If the tooth is nonvital, the endodontist may advise the patient that a local anesthetic agent is not necessary.

After the pulp has been removed, a local anesthetic agent may or may not be administered during subsequent visits, depending on the patient's preference. Inflamed and infected tissues are difficult to anesthetize. Because endodontic treatment procedures generally involve inflamed pulp, periapical tissues, or both, obtaining an adequate level of anesthesia can be a problem. It may be necessary to inject additional local anesthetic solution directly into the pulp. In addition, *sedatives* (oral or inhalation) may be used for patients who are extremely apprehensive.

Isolation and Disinfection of the Operating Field

The standard of care established by the ADA for endodontic treatment requires the use of a *dental dam.* Once the dam is placed, it is necessary to disinfect the tooth, dental dam clamp, and the surrounding dental dam material using an iodine solution or a sodium hypochlorite solution.

Access Preparation

During access preparation, the dentist uses a high-speed handpiece and round bur to create an opening in the coronal portion of the tooth for the instrumentation to reach the root canals. Access is gained through the occlusal surfaces of posterior teeth and the lingual surfaces of anterior teeth.

Estimated Working Length

The dentist must know the length of the completed canal preparation and root canal filling. Problems that result from inaccurate measurement of length include (1) perforation of the apex, (2) overinstrumentation or underinstrumentation of the canal length, (3) overfilling or underfilling of the canal, and (4) postoperative pain (Fig. 54-15).

Because exact apex locations vary, and because these variations are not always visible on radiographs, the working length is estimated and is termed the *estimated working length.* The estimated working length is determined by selecting a reference point on the tooth, usually the highest point on the incisal or occlusal surface. On a periapical radiograph, a millimeter endodontic ruler is used to measure the distance from the reference point to the apex of the tooth. It is extremely important that the tooth length as represented on the radiograph be accurate and not distorted.

Debridement and Shaping the Canal

The purposes of **debridement** and shaping the canal are (1) to remove bacteria, necrotic tissue, and organic debris from the root canal and (2) to smooth and shape the canal so that the filling material can be completely adapted to the walls of the canal.

Obturation

After the canal has been filed to the desired size and shape, it is debrided and dried. The canal now is ready to be filled by the endodontist. If the tooth has more than one canal, each canal is filled individually, with each requiring a properly fitted and sealed gutta-percha point.

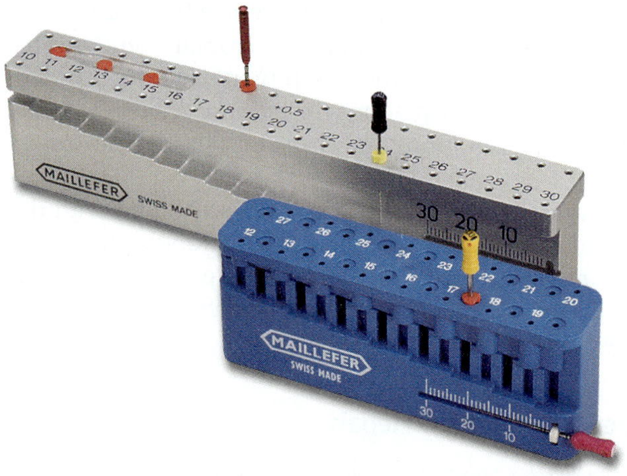

Fig. 54-15 Two types of stop setting and measuring devices. (From Johnson W: *Color atlas of endodontics,* Philadelphia, 2002, Saunders.)

Procedure 54-2 Assisting in Root Canal Therapy

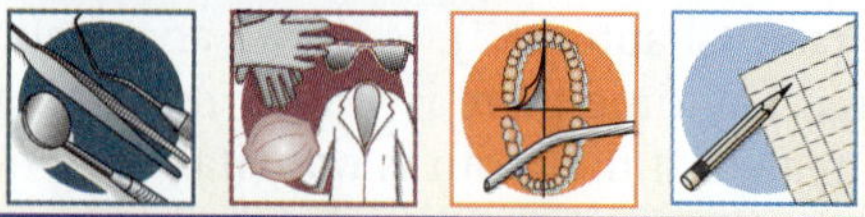

Equipment and Supplies

- Basic setup
- Local anesthetic agent setup (*optional*)
- Dental dam setup
- High-speed handpiece with burs (dentist's choice)
- Low-speed handpiece with latch attachment
- 5-ml to 6-ml syringe with 27-gauge needle
- Broaches and Hedstrom/K-type files (assorted sizes and lengths)
- Rubber instrument stops
- Paper points
- Gutta-percha points
- Endodontic sealer supplies
- Endodontic spoon excavator
- Endodontic explorer
- Glick Number 1
- Lentulo spiral
- Millimeter ruler
- Locking cotton pliers
- Sodium hypochlorite solution
- Hemostat
- High-volume oral evacuator (HVE) tip

Procedure 54-2 Assisting in Root Canal Therapy—cont'd

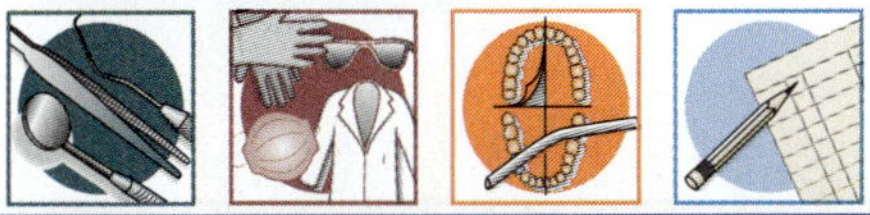

PROCEDURAL STEPS

Preparing the Field of Operation

1. Assist in administration of the local anesthetic agent (if applicable).
2. Assist with preparation and placement of the dental dam (expose only the tooth being treated).
3. Swab the antiseptic solution over the exposed tooth, the clamp, and the surrounding dental dam.

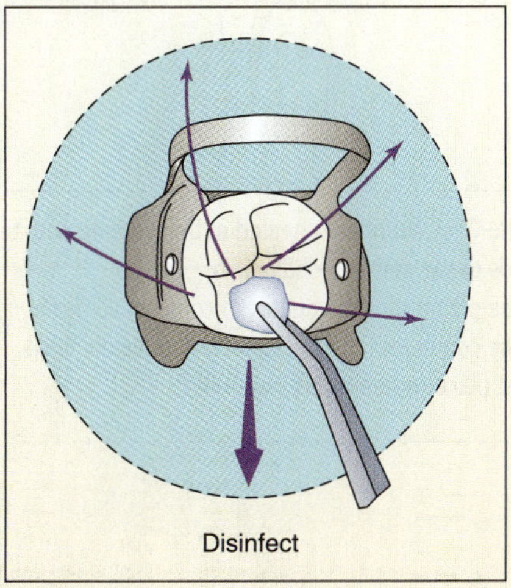

Removing the Pulp

1. The dentist enters the coronal portion of the tooth with a carbide bur, removing decay and infected tooth structure.

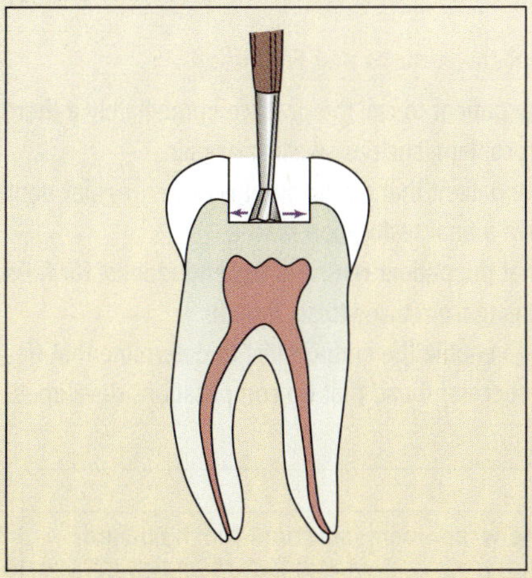

2. Once the canals are located with the endodontic explorer, the pulp tissue is removed with intracanal instruments.

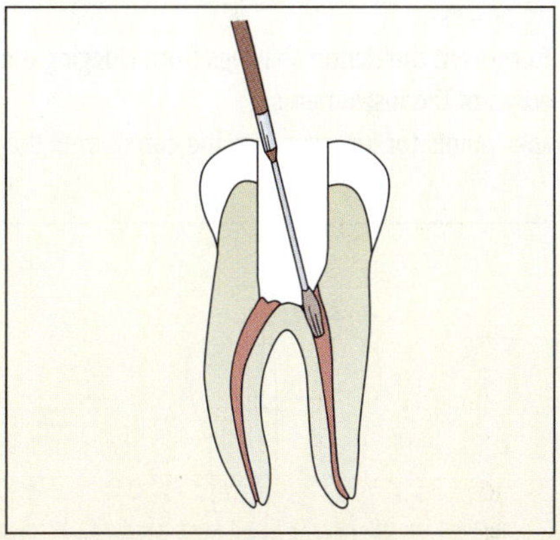

3. The canals are irrigated gently with the sodium hypochlorite solution. Excess solution is removed with the HVE tip.
4. The dentist uses a small endodontic file to rub the irrigation solution against the walls of the canal and pulp chamber.
   Purpose: The solution acts as a disinfectant to destroy bacteria in the canal and to wash away debris. This step is called *biochemical cleaning.*

Cleaning and Shaping the Canal

1. The dentist inserts files into the canal and moves them up and down with short strokes.
   Purpose: During this motion, the cutting edges of the files will remove dentin and debris from the walls of the canal.

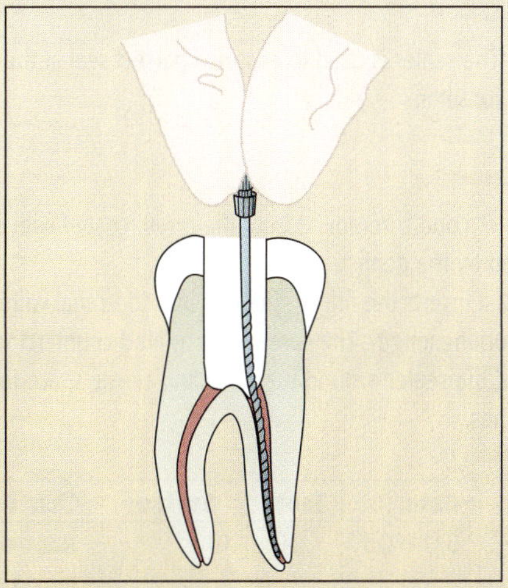

2. Transfer larger files to dentist to clean and shape the canals.
   Purpose: The increase in size is to enlarge the diameter of the canal.
3. The rubber stop must be placed on the file at the desired working length for each canal.

continued

Procedure 54-2 Assisting in Root Canal Therapy—cont'd

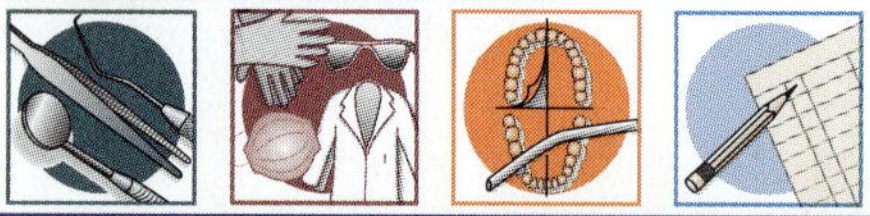

PROCEDURAL STEPS, cont'd

4. Irrigate the canals thoroughly at frequent intervals during this shaping and cleaning process.
   Purpose: To prevent the dentin shavings from clogging the cutting edges of the instruments.
5. Transfer paper points for insertion into the canals until the points come out dry.

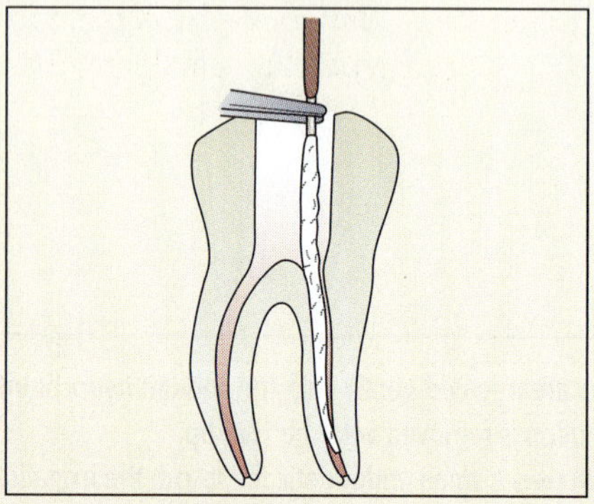

Preparing to Fill the Canal

1. Select the appropriate-sized gutta-percha point, and cut it to the predetermined length. This is called the *trial point.*
2. Take a periapical radiograph of the tooth with the trial point in the canal. This is the *working-length radiograph.*
3. If the radiograph does not show the tip of the trial point within 1 mm of the apex of the root, the point is repositioned and another radiograph taken.
4. At the signal from the dentist, prepare a thin mix of sealer on a sterile glass slab.
   Purpose: The sealer is used to ensure a perfect seal at the apical foramen.

Filling the Canal

1. The master cone is removed from the canal, coated with sealer, and reinserted by the dentist.
2. The dentist inserts the finger spreader into the canal within 1 mm of the working length. The spreader is rotated counterclockwise to spread the sealer around the canal and create space for the other cones.
3. Continue transferring gutta-percha points to fill the canal.

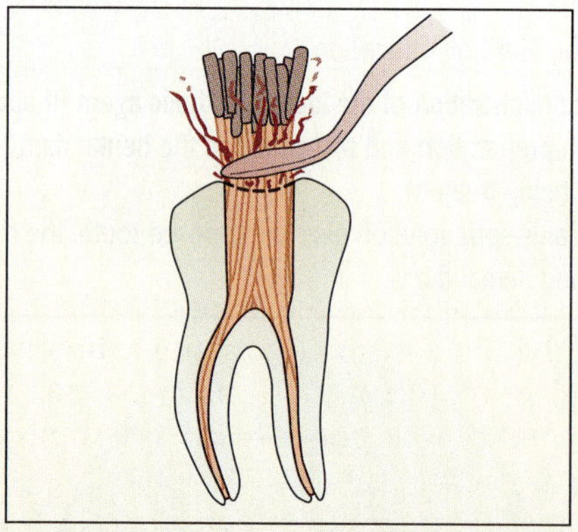

4. Transfer the Glick Number 1, heated at the working end, to remove the excess ends of the gutta-percha points.
5. Transfer the plugger for the dentist to compact vertically.
6. This routine continues until the canal is completely filled.
7. The dentist places a temporary restoration.

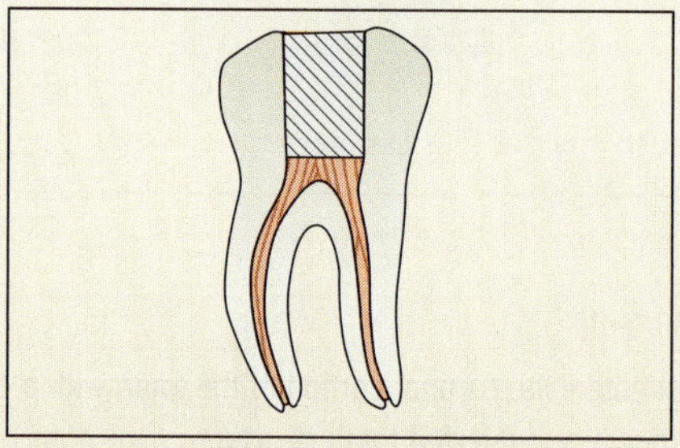

8. Expose a posttreatment radiograph.
9. The dentist checks the occlusion and adjusts as needed.

Posttreatment Instructions and Follow-up

1. Instruct the patient to call the practice immediately if there are indications of a problem, such as swelling or pain.
2. Remind the patient that a return to his or her regular dentist is necessary to have a final restoration placed.
3. Request that the patient return to the endodontist for follow-up at intervals ranging from three to six months.
   Purpose: To enable the endodontist to determine that treatment was successful and that no complications developed.

Date	Tooth	Surface	Charting Notes
8/14/05	30		Root canal therapy, 2 carp. Xylocaine w/epi, dam isolation, tooth opened, maximum file used #70, working length 24 mm, formocresol pellet, gutta-percha fill, closed with cavit, initial, working/post treatment radiographs. Pt tolerated procedure well. Return for postop check in 1 week. T. Clark, CDA/L. Stuart, DDS

Recall

18. What material is used for obturation of a canal?

19. What type of moisture control is recommended for root canal therapy?

20. What surface of an anterior tooth does the dentist enter when performing root canal therapy?

SURGICAL ENDODONTICS

Root canal therapy is successful approximately 90 to 95 percent of the time. In some situations, however, surgical endodontic techniques must be used to save a tooth from extraction. Indications for surgical intervention include the following:

- *Endodontic failure.* Failure of nonsurgical endodontics may be caused by persistent infection, severely curved roots, perforation of the canal, fractured roots, extensive root resorption, pulp stones, or accessory canals that cannot be treated.
- *Exploratory surgery.* Surgery may be necessary to determine why healing has not occurred after root canal therapy. Canal medications that extend beyond the apex and into the periapical tissues may be the cause.
- *Biopsy.* A tissue sample for a biopsy may be required (see Chapter 56).

Apicoectomy and Apical Curettage

Apicoectomy involves surgically removing the apical portion of the root with the use of a tapered fissure bur in a high-speed handpiece (Fig. 54-16). The dentist then can examine the apex for signs of (1) inadequate sealing of the canal, (2) accessory (additional) canals, and (3) fractures of the root.

Once the endodontist has entered the apical area of a tooth, **apical curettage** may be required to remove the pathologic soft tissue around the root apex. *Curettage* means the removal of diseased tissue through scraping with a curette.

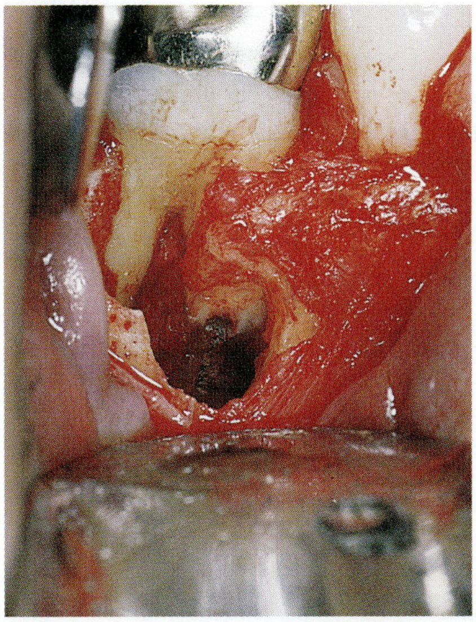

Fig. 54-16 The apex of this mesiofacial root has been surgically removed. (From Johnson W: *Color atlas of endodontics,* Philadelphia, 2002, Saunders.)

Retrograde Restoration

Retrograde restoration, also referred to as *root end filling,* is completed when the apical seal is not adequate. A small preparation is made at the apex and is sealed with filling materials such as gutta-percha, amalgam, or composite (Fig. 54-17).

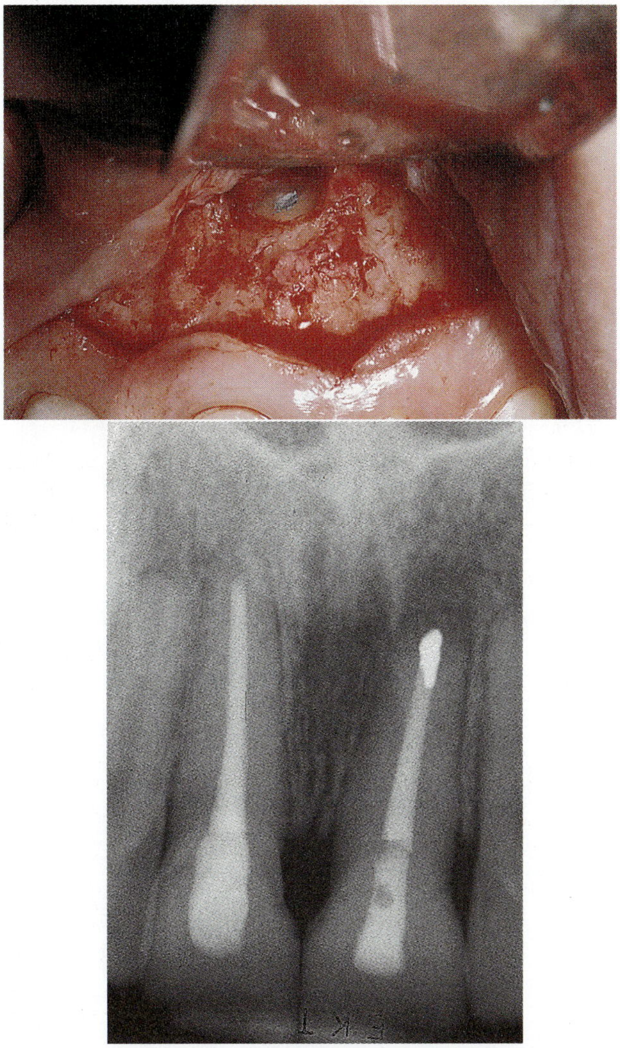

Fig. 54-17 Root end filling is completed on a central incisor. (From Johnson W: *Color atlas of endodontics.* Philadelphia, 2002, Saunders.)

Root Amputation and Hemisection

Root amputation is a surgical procedure used to remove one or more roots of a multirooted tooth without removing the crown (Fig. 54-18*A* and *B*). The amputation occurs at the point at which the root joins the crown. Root amputation is most often performed on maxillary molars.

Hemisection is a procedure in which the root and the crown are cut lengthwise and removed (Fig. 54-18*C*). Hemisections are most often performed on mandibular molars.

Recall

21. What is the success rate of root canal therapy?

22. What surgical procedure involves the removal of the apex of a root?

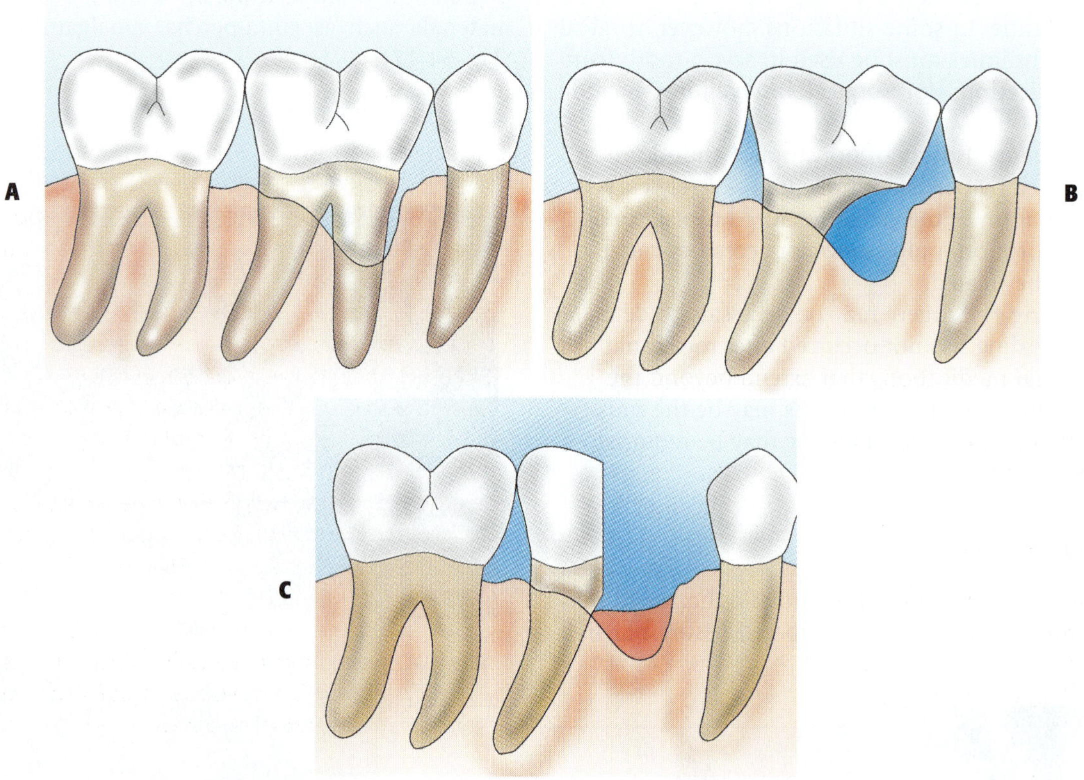

Fig. 54-18 A, Periodontal loss involving the mesial root. **B,** Root amputation. **C,** Hemisection. (From Johnson W: *Color atlas of endodontics,* Philadelphia, 2002, Saunders.)

Patient Education

Endodontics is an area of dentistry in which you are almost always working with a patient who is in pain. Many people are apprehensive about endodontic treatment, and good patient education helps to relieve this uneasiness. The patient must be provided with sufficient information to give informed consent for endodontic treatment.

Always provide positive communication when discussing pulp therapy with a patient. *Do not say the following:*

- "All root canals are successful."
- "There is no pain in having a root canal."
- "Once the root canal is completed, the tooth will last forever."
- "There may be extreme pain and swelling from root canal treatment."

Legal and Ethical Implications

For root canal therapy to be completed properly, it is imperative to remember that *accuracy* is the number-one criterion when exposing diagnostic and working radiographs, as well as in the measurement and placement of rubber stops on endodontic files.

Endodontics is deemed the "emergency room" of dentistry, and your patient may not always understand all that is being conveyed. Make sure you review the diagnostic findings with the patient, and review the patient consent form. If the patient seems to be hesitant, stop and review again.

Eye to the Future

New technology such as the apex finder, vitality scanner, and ultrasonic handpiece is providing endodontists the ability to diagnose and treat patients more efficiently and accurately. Because the dental laser is becoming a standard instrument in the field of dentistry, the next ideal area for its application will be endodontics. The dental laser will be introduced in endodontics as a quick, pain-free method to remove diseased pulpal tissue.

Critical Thinking

1. You have a new patient who requires root canal therapy. When discussing the procedure, she immediately says she will not allow radiographs to be taken because "they are harmful and of no use." How would you explain the necessity of x-rays to her, knowing the importance of radiographs during root canal therapy?
2. In root canal therapy, it is discussed that anesthesia may or may not be used in a procedure. Discuss why a dentist would *not* anesthetize the tooth and area before root canal therapy.
3. Why is it so important to use a dental dam in root canal therapy? Why is it imperative to keep saliva and other moisture away from a pulp exposure?
4. You are assisting the dentist in an endodontic diagnosis. The dentist is placing ice on the suspected tooth. The patient says that "the pain goes away" when the ice is on the tooth. What diagnostic conclusion would the dentist most likely reach?
5. You are assisting the endodontist in the therapy of a mandibular second molar. The patient record indicates that all roots will require treatment. How many roots are in a mandibular second molar? How would these roots appear on a periapical radiograph?

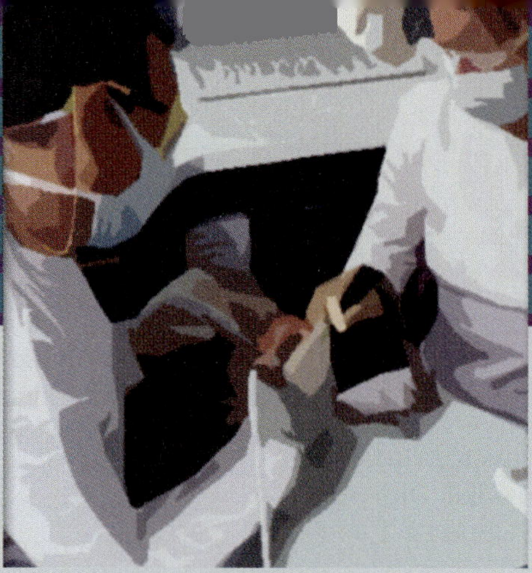

55 Periodontics

Outline

KEY TERMS

Bleeding index Method of scoring the amount of bleeding present.

Chisel scaler Instrument used to remove *supragingival* calculus in the contact area of anterior teeth. The blade is curved slightly to adapt to tooth surfaces.

Cosmetic dentistry Therapy limited to improving patients' appearance.

Curette (ku-**ret**) Surgical instrument used to remove tissue from the tooth socket; also *curet.*

File A metal tool of varying size and form with numerous ridges or teeth on its cutting surfaces.

Gingivectomy (*jin*-jah-**vek**-tah-me) Surgical removal of diseased gingival tissues.

Gingivoplasty (**jin**-jah-vah-*plas*-tee) Surgical reshaping and contouring of gingival tissues.

Gracey curette An area-specific curette with one cutting edge; it is designed to adapt to specific tooth surfaces (mesial or distal).

Hoe scaler Type of scaler used to remove heavy supragingival calculus; it is most effective on buccal and lingual surfaces of posterior teeth.

Kirkland knife Double-ended knife with kidney-shaped blades commonly used in periodontal surgery.

Laser (**lay**-zur) Highly concentrated beam of light; acronym for *light amplification by stimulated emission of radiation.*

Mobility To have movement.

Occlusal trauma Abnormal occlusal relationships of the teeth, causing injury to the periodontium.

Orban knife Knife with a spearlike shape and cutting edges on both sides of the blade; it is used to remove tissue from interdental areas.

Osseous surgery (**ah**-see-us) Surgical specialty in which bone defects are removed.

Ostectomy (ahs-**tek**-tah-me) Surgery involving the removal of bone.

Osteoplasty (**ahs**-tee-oh-*plas*-tee) Surgery in which bone is added, contoured, and reshaped.

Periodontal charting (*per*-ee-oh-**dahn**-tul) Commonly accepted notations that are made to the patient's chart to indicate the condition, position, and restorative history of individual teeth.

KEY TERMS, cont'd

Periodontal dressing (Perio Pak) Surgical dressing applied to a surgical site for protection; similar to a bandage.

Periodontal explorer Fine thin instrument that is easily adapted around root surfaces.

Periodontal flap surgery (flap surgery) Incisional surgery performed when excisional surgery is not indicated. Tissues are not removed, but are pushed away from the underlying tooth roots and alveolar bone, similar to the flap of an envelope.

Periodontal pocket Deepening of the gingival sulcus beyond normal, resulting from periodontal disease.

Periodontal probe Probe used to locate and measure the depth of periodontal pockets tapered to fit into the gingival sulcus with a blunt or rounded tip.

Periodontics (*per*-ee-oh-**dahn**-tiks) Dental specialty involved with the diagnosis and treatment of diseases of the supporting tissues.

Periodontist (*per*-ee-oh-**dahn**-tist) Dentist with advanced education in the specialty of periodontics.

Root planing Procedure that smoothes the surface of a root by removing abnormal toxic cementum or dentin that is rough, contaminated, or permeated with calculus.

Scaling Removal of calcareous deposits from the teeth using suitable instruments.

Sickle scaler Hook-shaped instrument available in various sizes and shapes used for removal of tenacious supragingival calculus deposits.

Ultrasonic scaler Device used for rapid calculus removal that operates on high-frequency sound waves.

Universal curette Hand instrument used to treat subgingival surfaces; it has a blade with an unbroken cutting edge that curves around the toe and a flat face set at a 90-degree angle to the lower shank.

LEARNING OUTCOMES

On completion of this chapter, the student will be able to achieve the following objectives:

- Pronounce, define, and spell the Key Terms.
- Describe the role of the dental assistant in a periodontal practice.
- Explain the procedures necessary for a comprehensive periodontal examination.
- Identify and describe the instruments used in periodontal therapy.
- Identify the indications for placement of periodontal surgical dressings, and describe the technique for proper placement.
- Describe the role of radiographs in periodontal treatment.
- Describe the indications and contraindications for the use of the ultrasonic scaler.
- Describe the types of nonsurgical periodontal therapy.
- Describe the goals of nonsurgical periodontal therapy.
- Describe the types of surgical periodontal therapy.

PERFORMANCE OUTCOMES

On completion of this chapter, the student will be able to meet competency standards in the following skills:

- Assist with a dental prophylaxis procedure.
- Demonstrate periodontal charting.
- Assist with gingivectomy and gingivoplasty.
- Prepare and place noneugenol periodontal dressings (expanded function).
- Remove a periodontal surgical dressing (expanded function).

Periodontics is the dental specialty involved with the diagnosis and treatment of diseases of the supporting tissues.The dental assistant in a periodontal specialty office must have a thorough understanding of periodontal diseases and the types of periodontal instruments and procedures. In a periodontal practice, the dental assistant assists with periodontal charting and periodontal surgeries and provides home care instructions to the patient. Depending on the particular state's dental practice act, the dental assistant may also place and remove periodontal dressings, remove sutures, perform coronal polishes, take impressions for study models, and administer topical fluoride applications.

This chapter will focus on the *treatment* of periodontal diseases, and will include a discussion of the instruments and procedures commonly performed in a periodontal specialty office. It is recommended that you refer to Chapter 14 to review the types of periodontal disease, the risk factors, and the systemic factors that influence the progression of periodontal disease.

THE PERIODONTAL PRACTICE

Patients are usually referred to a periodontist's office by a general dentist or dental hygienist for treatment of a periodontal condition that requires the skill and knowledge of a specialist. After periodontal treatment, the patient will return to the general dentist for routine dental care.

Frequently a periodontal patient will alternate periodontal maintenance (cleaning and follow-up) appointments between the periodontist's office and the general dentist's office. The staff in both offices must coordinate periodontal maintenance therapy between the two practices to provide the most comprehensive care for the patient.

THE PERIODONTAL EXAMINATION

In addition to a thorough dental examination (see Chapter 28), specialized periodontal examinations are necessary to diagnose periodontal disease and to determine the proper treatment. A periodontal examination includes the patient's medical and dental history, radiographic evaluation, examination of the teeth, examination of the oral tissues and supporting structures, and periodontal charting.

Periodontal charting includes pocket readings, furcations, tooth mobility, exudate (pus), and gingival recession. The clinical findings of the periodontal examination are recorded on the periodontal chart (Fig. 55-1). Software programs are also available that provide computerized printouts of the periodontal charting (Fig. 55-2).

Medical and Dental History

The **periodontist** reviews the medical history to detect any systemic conditions that may influence periodontal treatment. Systemic diseases, such as acquired immunodeficiency syndrome (AIDS), human immunodeficiency virus (HIV) infection, or diabetes, can lower resistance of the tissue to infection. Lowered resistance makes periodontal disease more severe and more difficult to treat.

The dental history is used to gather information about conditions that could indicate periodontal disease. For

Early Signs of Periodontal Disease

- Changes in the gingiva (color, size, shape, texture)
- Gingival inflammation
- Gingival bleeding
- Evidence of exudates
- Development of periodontal pockets

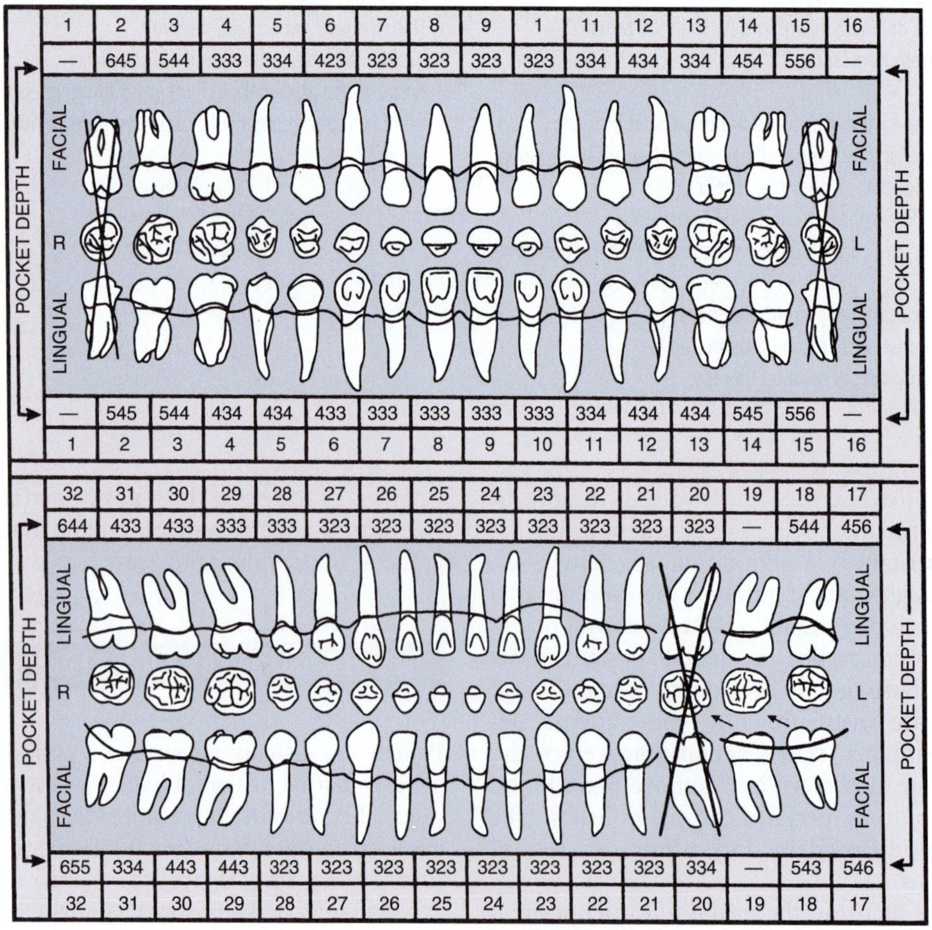

Fig. 55-1 Periodontal charting for a 40-year-old patient. (Courtesy Colwell, a division of Patterson Supply, Inc., Champaign, Illinois.)

example, patients with periodontal disease often complain of bleeding gums, loose teeth, or a bad taste. They may describe a dull pain after eating or a burning sensation in the gingival tissue.

Dental Examination

The dental examination focuses on the teeth for indications of periodontal disease or factors that could contribute to periodontal disease (Box 55-1).

Mobility

Teeth normally have a slight amount of **mobility** (tooth movement) due to the cushioning effect of the periodontal membranes. However, excessive mobility can be an important sign of periodontal disease (Fig. 55-3).

Oral Tissues and Supporting Structures

The periodontal examination includes an assessment of the amounts of plaque and calculus, changes in the gingival health and bleeding, assessment of the level of bone, and the detection of periodontal pockets (Box 55-2).

Box 55-1 Dental Conditions that Contribute to Periodontal Disease

Condition	Description
Pathologic migration	Shift in the position of the teeth caused by loss of periodontal support.
Clenching or grinding *(bruxism)*	Bruxism places excessive biting forces on the teeth and may accelerate bone loss.
Defective restorations or bridgework	Dental prostheses may retain plaque and increase the risk of periodontal disease.
Mobility	All teeth have some mobility (see Fig. 55-3). Mobility is recorded with the following scale: *0,* normal; *1,* slight mobility; *2,* moderate mobility; *3,* extreme mobility.
Occlusal interferences	Certain tooth areas can prevent the teeth from occluding properly. These interferences do not directly cause periodontal disease but can contribute to mobility, migration, and temporomandibular joint pain.

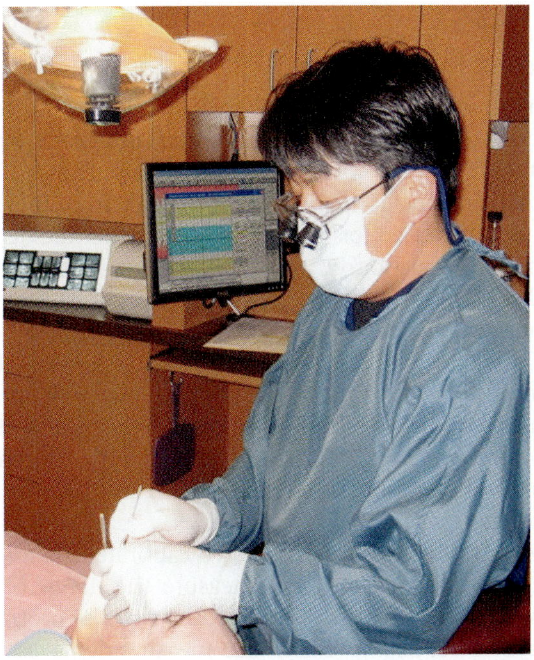

Fig. 55-2 A periodontal chart on a computer screen. This periodontist can easily refer to the chart as he treats the patient.

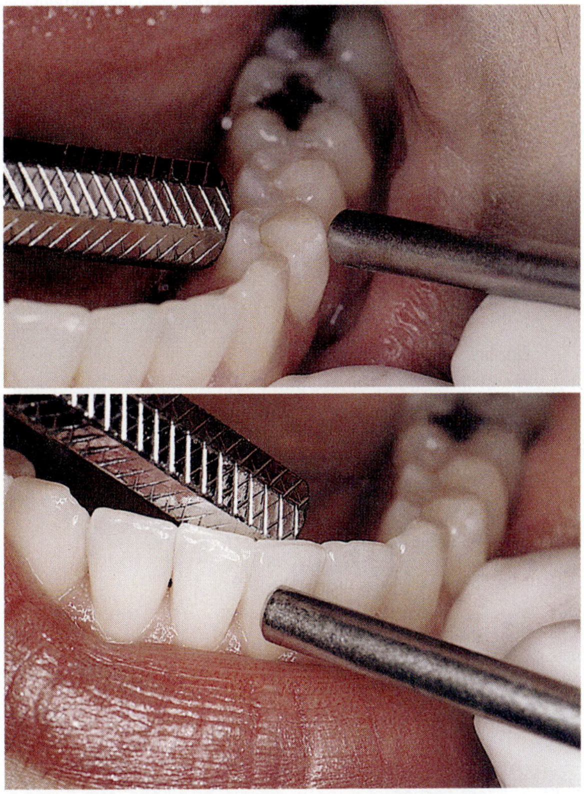

Fig. 55-3 Mobility is detected with the blunt ends of two instruments. (From Daniel SJ, Harfst SA: *Mosby's dental hygiene: concepts, cases, and competencies, 2004 update,* St Louis, 2004, Mosby.)

Box 55-2 Periodontal Examination of Gingiva and Supporting Tissues

Assessment	Description
Plaque	Plaque is the primary cause of gingival inflammation and most other forms of periodontal disease.
Calculus	Calculus is hard mineralized plaque. Calculus may be *supragingival* (above the gingivae) or *subgingival* (below the gingivae). Calculus adheres to the surfaces of natural teeth, crowns, bridges, and dentures. It is a contributing factor in periodontal disease because it is always covered with plaque.
Gingival recession	As disease progresses, the gingiva may recede, leaving portions of the roots of the teeth exposed below the cementoenamel junction. Gingival recession levels can be visualized on the chart by drawing a dotted or colored line to indicate the gingival margin (see Fig. 55-1).
Bleeding index	Severity of gingival inflammation is measured by the amount of bleeding observed during probing. There are several different indices to measure bleeding. Each system is based on the principle that healthy gingivae do not bleed.
Measurement of periodontal pockets	A periodontal pocket occurs when the disease causes the normal gingival sulcus to become deeper than normal. (A normal sulcus is 3 mm or less.)
Assessment of bone level	Radiographs and probing measurements are used to assess the patient's bone level. These may also be visualized on the chart by drawing a colored line to indicate the bone level (see Fig. 55-1).
Radiographs	• Detect interproximal bone loss. • Show the changes in the bone as periodontitis progresses. • Locate furcation involvements. • Measure the crown-to-root ratio (the length of the clinical crown compared with the length of the root of the tooth). • Show signs of traumatic occlusion.

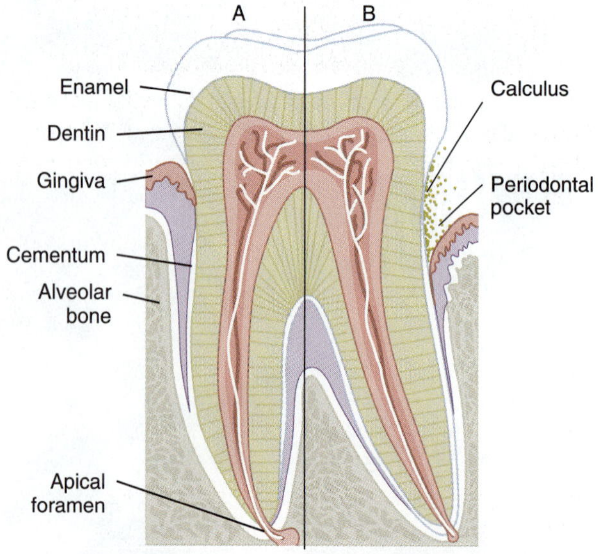

Fig. 55-4 Cross-section of a tooth, gingiva, and bone. The *A* side shows normal sulcus depth. The *B* side shows a periodontal pocket.

Periodontal Probing

A **periodontal pocket** occurs when the disease causes the gingival sulcus to become deeper than normal. A normal sulcus is 3 mm or less (Fig. 55-4). The purpose of periodontal probing is to measure how much epithelial attachment has been lost to disease. The greater the depth of the periodontal pocket, the greater the loss of epithelial attachment and bone, and therefore the more severe the periodontal disease.

When periodontal pockets are present, it is very difficult and may be impossible for the patient to keep the pockets clean and free from bacteria and debris. The bacteria in the periodontal pockets will multiply, and if left untreated, the disease will progress until the tooth is ultimately lost to periodontal disease.

Periodontal probes, which are calibrated in millimeters, are used to locate and measure the depth of periodontal pockets (Fig. 55-5). On some types of probes, the tip is color-coded to make the measurements easier to read. The periodontal probe is tapered to fit into the gingival sulcus and has a blunt or rounded tip. Six measurements are taken and recorded for each tooth (Fig. 55-6).

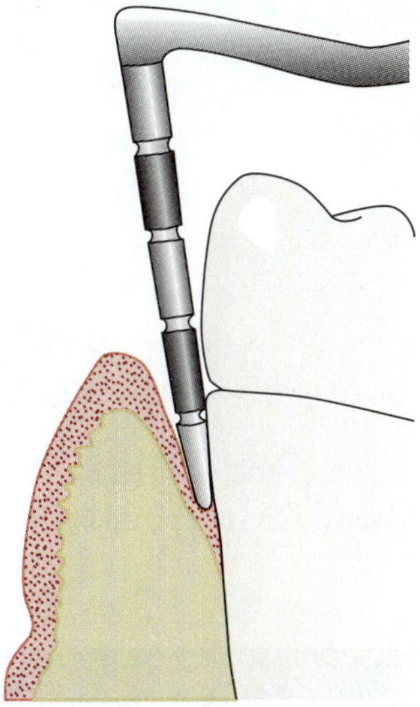

Fig. 55-5 **Diagram showing probing of the periodontal pocket depth. The millimeter measurement indicates the distance from the gingival margin to the base of the pocket.** (From Perry D, Beemsterboer P, Taggart E: *Periodontology for the dental hygienist,* Philadelphia, 2001, Saunders.)

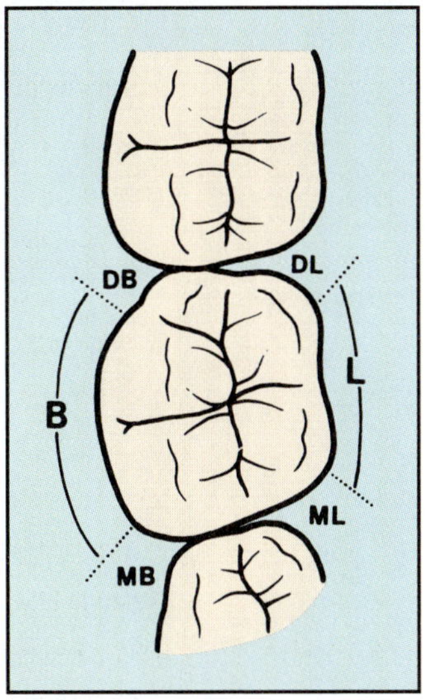

Fig. 55-6 **Six probing depths are taken for each tooth.** ***DB,*** **Distobuccal;** ***B,*** **buccal;** ***MB,*** **mesiobuccal;** ***DL,*** **distolingual;** ***L,*** **lingual;** ***ML,*** **mesiolingual.** (From Perry DA, Beemsterboer P, Carranza FA: *Techniques and theory of periodontal instrumentation,* Philadelphia, 1990, Saunders.)

Periodontal probes are available in many designs, and selection depends on the operator's personal preference.

Bleeding Index

The severity of gingival inflammation can be measured by the **bleeding index,** or the amount of bleeding observed during probing. Several different systems of recording bleeding scores are used. Each system is based on the principle that healthy gingiva does not bleed.

Occlusal Adjustment

The patient's bite is evaluated for areas of unequal pressure. If there is excessive biting pressure in a specific area, **occlusal trauma** can result. Occlusal adjustment, or *occlusal equilibration,* is a procedure that adjusts the patient's bite so that occlusal forces are equally distributed over all the teeth. Articulating paper, occlusal wax, stones, and burs are used to adjust the occlusion. Several appointments may be necessary to adjust the occlusion properly.

Occlusal trauma does *not cause* periodontal pocket formation, but it can cause tooth mobility, destruction of bone, migration of teeth, and temporomandibular joint pain.

Radiographic Analysis

Radiographs are a valuable aid for evaluating periodontal disease. The accuracy of the radiographs is critical in the diagnosis of periodontal disease because distortion of the image can result in incorrect diagnosis (Fig. 55-7).

The *bite-wing radiograph* is particularly valuable because it can accurately depict the bone height along the root surface. Vertical bite-wing radiographs are excellent for determining the extent of crestal bone loss (Fig. 55-8).

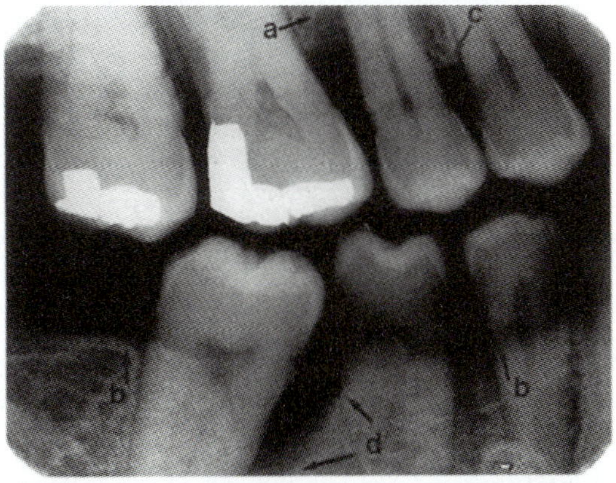

Fig. 55-7 **Bone loss in periodontal disease: A, Vertical bone defect. B, Crestal ridge at near-normal height. C, Alveolar crest. D, Severe vertical defect.** (From Miles DA, et al: *Radiographic imaging for dental auxiliaries,* ed 3, Philadelphia, 1999, Saunders.)

Recall

1. How do patients most often seek periodontal care?
2. What information is included in the periodontal charting?
3. Should teeth have any mobility?
4. What is the depth of a normal sulcus?
5. What units of measurement are used on the periodontal probe?
6. What type of radiograph is especially useful in periodontics?

A

B

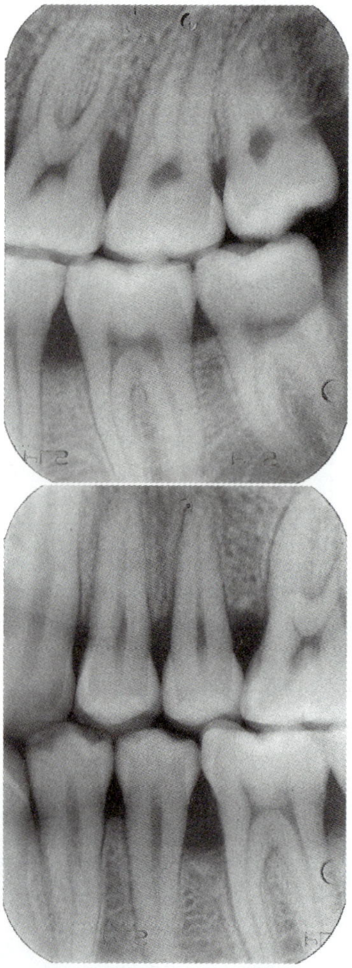

Fig. 55-8 **A,** Molar vertical bite-wing. **B,** Premolar vertical bite-wing.

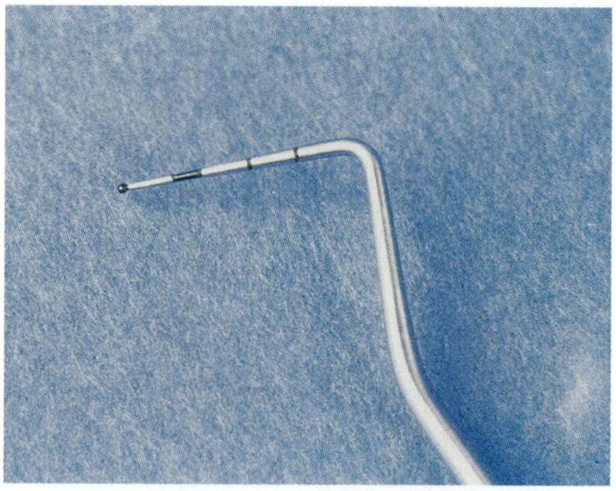

Fig. 55-9 Working end of a periodontal probe.

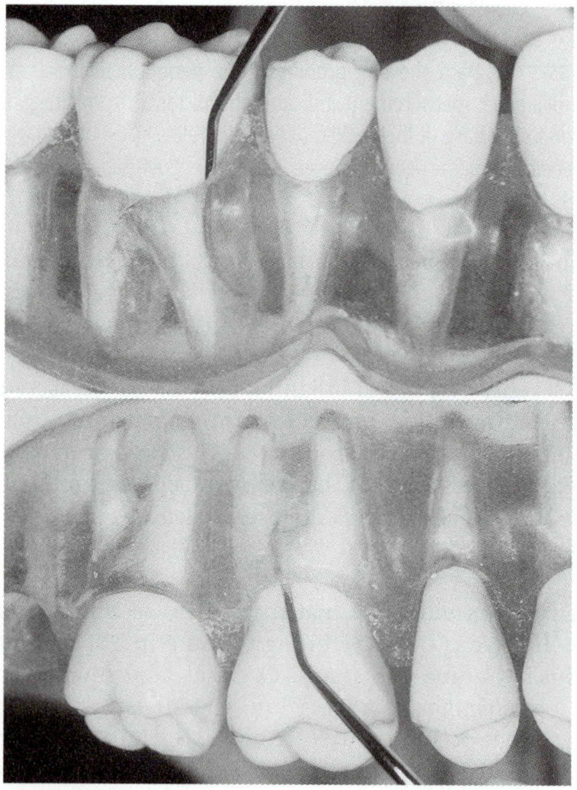

A

B

Fig. 55-10 Various styles of periodontal explorers. **A,** EXC 11/12 AF explorer allows access to pockets deeper than 5 mm for evaluating root surfaces. **B,** Elongated design is useful for exploring the furcation area. (Courtesy Hu-Friedy Manufacturing, Chicago, Illinois.)

PERIODONTAL INSTRUMENTS

Periodontal therapy requires the use of specialized instruments to remove calculus, smooth root surfaces, measure periodontal pockets, and perform periodontal surgery. These instruments must be sharp to perform periodontal procedures such as *scaling, root planing,* and *periodontal surgery.* In general, the dentist or registered dental hygienist who uses these instruments takes responsibility for maintaining their sharpness. The use of periodontal probes is discussed earlier in this chapter (Fig. 55-9).

Explorers

Periodontal explorers are used in periodontics to locate deposits of calculus that may be either *supragingival* or *subgingival.* Explorers also provide tactile information to the operator about the roughness or smoothness of the root surfaces.

Many styles of explorers are used in periodontal treatment. Periodontal explorers are longer and more curved than explorers used for caries detection. (See Chapter 34 for other types of explorers.)

The working ends of periodontal explorers are thin, fine, and easily adapted around root surfaces. They also are long enough to be capable of reaching to the base of deep pockets and furcations (Fig. 55-10). A *furcation* is the point at which the roots of a multirooted tooth diverge.

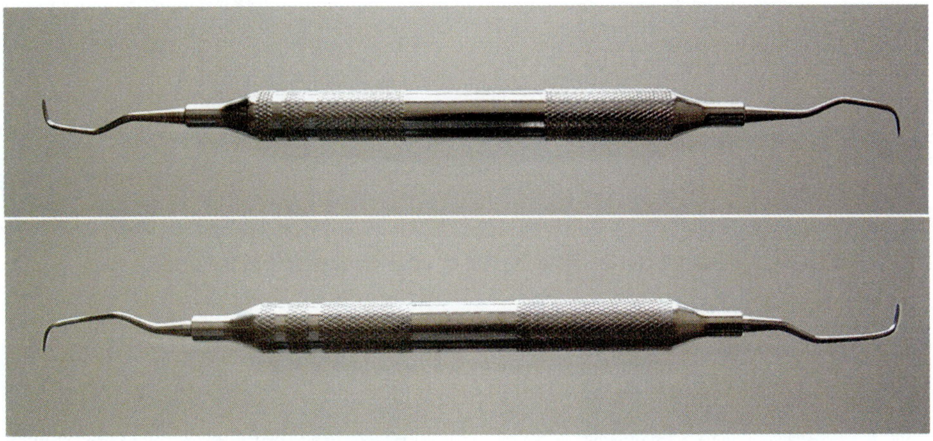

Fig. 55-11 **A,** Anterior curette. **B,** Posterior curette.

Scalers and Files

Sickle scalers are used primarily to remove large deposits of *supragingival* calculus. A sickle scaler with a long, straight shank is used to remove calculus from the anterior areas of the oral cavity. A *contra-angle* sickle scaler, which is angled at the shank, is designed to remove calculus from the posterior teeth.

Chisel scalers are used to remove *supragingival* calculus in the contact area of anterior teeth. The blade on the chisel scaler is curved slightly to adapt to the tooth surfaces.

Hoe scalers are used to remove *heavy supragingival* calculus. Hoes are most effective when used on buccal and lingual surfaces of posterior teeth.

Files are used to crush or fracture *extremely heavy* calculus. The fractured calculus then is removed from the tooth surface with curettes.

NOTE: *The chisel, hoe, and files are less frequently used in periodontal procedures.*

Curettes

Curettes are used to remove *subgingival* calculus, smooth rough root surfaces *(root planing)*, and remove the diseased soft tissue lining of the periodontal pocket *(soft tissue curettage)* (Fig 55-11). Unlike a scaler, which has a pointed end, curettes have a rounded end (Fig. 55-12). There are two basic designs of curettes.

Universal curettes are designed so that one instrument is able to adapt to all tooth surfaces. These curettes have *two cutting edges,* one on each side of the blade. Universal curettes resemble the spoon excavators used in restorative dentistry (Fig. 55-13).

Gracey curettes, which have only *one cutting edge,* are *area-specific;* they are designed to adapt to specific tooth surfaces (mesial or distal). Treatment of the entire dentition requires the use of several Gracey curettes (Fig. 55-14).

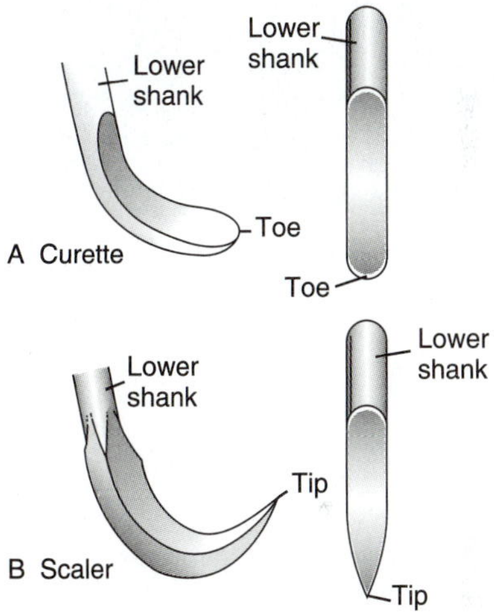

Fig. 55-12 Comparison of the end of a scaler (pointed) and the end of a curette (rounded).

Surgical Knives

Kirkland knives are one of the most common types of surgical knives used in periodontal surgery. These instruments are usually double-ended with kidney-shaped blades. **Orban knives** are used to remove tissue from *interdental* areas. These knives have a spearlike shape and cutting edges on both sides of the blade (Fig. 55-15).

Pocket Markers

Pocket markers are similar in appearance to cotton pliers; however, one tip is smooth and straight, and the other tip is sharp and bent at a right angle. The smooth tip of the pocket marker is inserted at the base of the pocket. When pressure is applied to the instrument, the sharp tip makes small perforations in the gingiva. These perforations make *bleeding points* that are used to mark the area for an incision on the gingiva (Fig. 55-16).

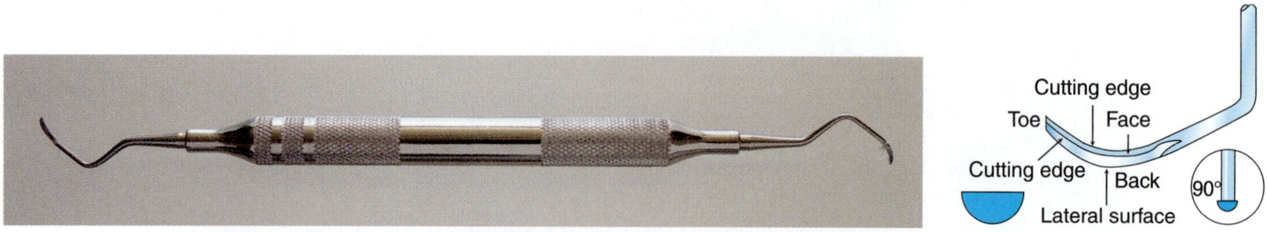

Fig. 55-13 Universal curette. Note the cutting edge on each side of the blade.

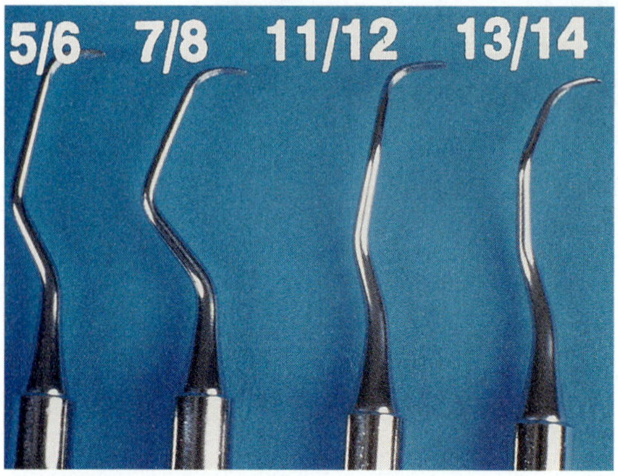

Fig. 55-14 Assorted Gracey curettes. (Courtesy Hu-Friedy Manufacturing, Chicago, Illinois.)

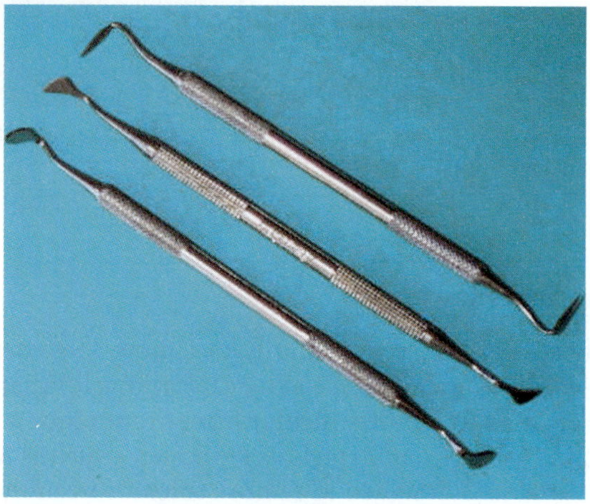

Fig. 55-15 Kirkland and Orban interdental knives.

Recall

7. What instruments are used to remove calculus from supragingival surfaces?
8. What instruments are used to remove calculus from subgingival surfaces?
9. What is the purpose of explorers in periodontal treatment?
10. What is the difference between a Universal curette and a Gracey curette?
11. What is the purpose of a periodontal pocket marker?

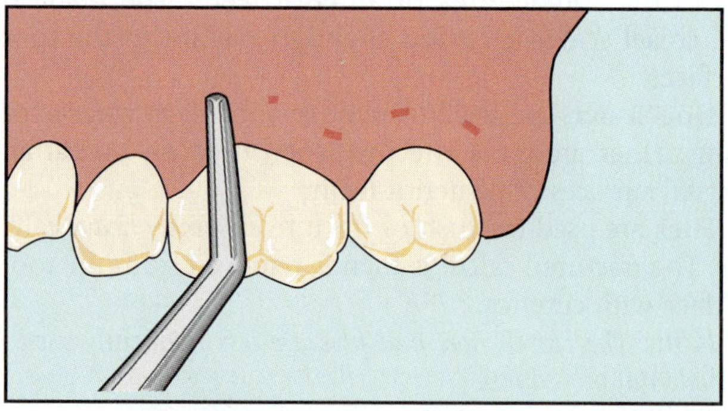

Fig. 55-16 Periodontal pocket marker makes pinpoint perforations that indicate the line for a surgical incision.

Ultrasonic Scaler

The **ultrasonic scaler** provides rapid calculus removal and reduces hand fatigue for the operator. Newer styles and slimmer instrument tips have been designed to allow better access to subgingival pockets. The use of these devices is rapidly increasing in periodontics (Fig. 55-17).

The ultrasonic scaler works by converting very-high-frequency sound waves into mechanical energy in the form of extremely rapid vibrations (20,000 to 40,000 cycles per second) at the tip of the instrument. A spray of water at the tip prevents the buildup of heat and continuously flushes debris and bacteria from the base of the pocket (Fig. 55-18).

Because of this spray of water at the tip, however, a large amount of potentially contaminated aerosol spray is released into the dental office environment. The operator of an ultrasonic scaler should have the dental assistant use the high-volume evacuator (HVE) to minimize aerosol contamination.

Indications and Contraindications

Indications for use of an ultrasonic scaler include the following:

1. Removal of supragingival calculus and difficult stains
2. Removal of subgingival calculus, attached plaque, and endotoxins from the root surface
3. Cleaning of furcation areas
4. Removal of deposits before periodontal surgery

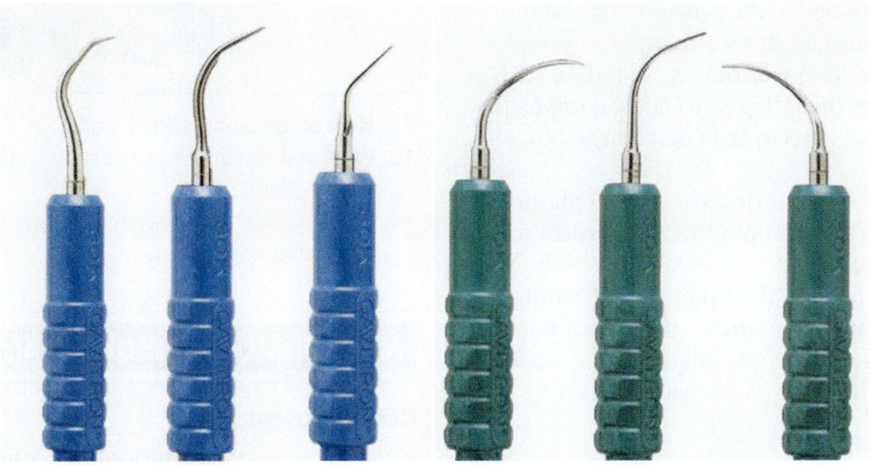

Fig. 55-17 **A series of ultrasonic tips designed to reach every area of the mouth.** (Courtesy Dentsply, York, PA.)

Hand Scaling versus Ultrasonic Scaling

Advantages of hand scaling

Increased tactile sensitivity

Greater control

Area-specific designs to enhance access

Advantages of ultrasonic scaling

Improved healing time from lavage effect

Operating field kept clean by water delivery

Repetitive motions minimized with proper use

Less tissue distention

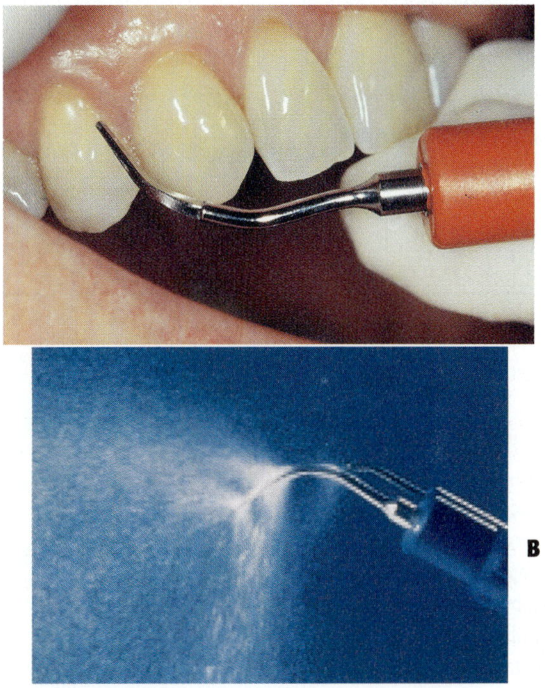

Fig. 55-18 **A, Positioning of the ultrasonic scaler. B, Ultrasonic scaler with water source turned on.** (Courtesy Hu-Friedy Manufacturing, Chicago, Illinois.)

5. Removal of orthodontic cements, or *debonding*
6. Removal of overhanging margins of restorations

Contraindications to use of the ultrasonic scalers include the following *general health considerations:*

1. *Communicable disease.* Patients with a known communicable disease, such as tuberculosis, can transmit contaminated aerosols. It is important to use an HVE to remove these aerosols.
2. *Patient susceptible to infection.* Medically compromised patients are more susceptible to infection, such as patients receiving chemotherapy or with HIV infection, uncontrolled diabetes, debilitation, or organ transplants.
3. *Respiratory problems.* Materials can be aspirated into the lungs of patients with chronic pulmonary disease, including asthma or other breathing problems, emphysema, and cystic fibrosis.
4. *Swallowing difficulty.* Patients with muscular dystrophy, multiple sclerosis, paralysis, or amyotrophic lateral sclerosis may have swallowing problems or may have a severe gag reflex. The water flow and spray can be very uncomfortable for some patients.
5. *Cardiac pacemaker.* Consultation with the patient's cardiologist is necessary because theoretically an ultrasonic scaler can disrupt a pacemaker, although no actual cases have been reported. The newer models of ultrasonic scalers have protective coatings to prevent this.

Oral conditions *may also be contraindications to the ultrasonic scalers, as follows:*

1. *Demineralized areas.* The vibrations of the ultrasonic scaler may remove the areas of remineralization that begin to cover the demineralization.

2. *Exposed dentinal surfaces.* Tooth structure may be removed and may cause tooth sensitivity.
3. *Restorative materials.* Some restorative materials, such as esthetic restorations including porcelains, composite resins, and laminate veneers, may be damaged by ultrasonic scalers.
4. *Titanium implant abutments.* Unless a special plastic sheath is used to cover the tip, ultrasonic scalers will damage titanium surfaces.
5. *Narrow periodontal pockets.* The tip of the ultrasonic scaler will not fit into very narrow subgingival pockets without interfering with proper angulation of the tip and limiting visibility.

Precautions for Children

Young tissues are very sensitive to ultrasonic vibrations. The vibrations and heat may damage the pulp tissue of primary and newly erupted permanent teeth, which have large pulp chambers. Therefore the use of ultrasonic scalers is contraindicated on primary and newly erupted permanent teeth.

Recall

12. How do ultrasonic scalers work?
13. What oral conditions would contraindicate the use of an ultrasonic scaler?
14. Should an ultrasonic scaler be used on a patient with a communicable disease?

NONSURGICAL PERIODONTAL TREATMENT

Dental Prophylaxis

A dental prophylaxis procedure, commonly referred to as *prophy* or *cleaning,* is the complete removal of calculus, soft deposits, plaque, and stain from all supragingival and unattached subgingival tooth surfaces. The dentist and dental hygienist are the *only* dental health team members licensed to perform a prophylaxis (see Procedure 55-1).

A prophylaxis is indicated for patients with healthy gingiva as a preventive measure and is most often performed

Procedure 55-1 Assisting with a Dental Prophylaxis

Goal

To assist competently with a dental prophylaxis procedure.

Equipment and Supplies

- High-volume evacuator (HVE) tip or saliva ejector
- Basic instrument setup
- Scalers, universal curette
- "Prophy" angle
- Rubber polishing cup and brushes
- Polishing agent
- Dental floss/tape
- Preprocedural mouthrinse

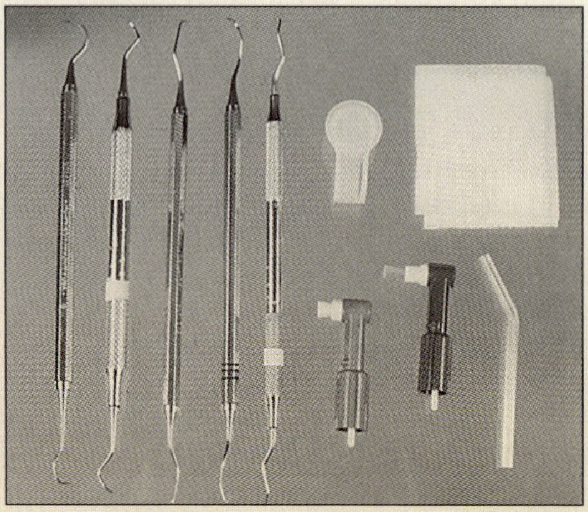

PROCEDURAL STEPS

1. Assist with transfers as the operator uses an explorer to locate interproximal and subgingival calculus.
   Note: The operator must have good access and visibility during this procedure.
2. Use the HVE as necessary and retract the lips, tongue, and cheeks to improve visibility and access as the operator uses scalers and curettes to remove all calculus and plaque.
3. The operator checks for and removes any remaining calculus.
4. The operator polishes the teeth using polishing paste, a rubber cup, and bristle brushes.
5. The operator removes any remaining interproximal debris with dental floss or tape.
6. Provide oral hygiene instructions appropriate to the individual needs of the patient.

during recall appointments. A dental prophylaxis also is the primary treatment for gingivitis.

Scaling and Root Planing

Scaling and root planing are done as part of a periodontal debridement. The goal of debridement is to remove the deposits on the tooth and to reduce the bioburden within the pocket. This procedure will help return the tissues to a healthy state.

A local anesthetic is usually administered before performing these procedures (Fig. 55-19).

Scaling is done to remove *supragingival* calculus from the tooth surface with periodontal scalers. Curettes are used to remove *supragingival* and *subgingival* calculus. Areas on the root surface may remain rough after calculus removal because the cementum has become necrotic (dead) or because the scaling has produced grooves and scratches in the cementum.

Root planing follows scaling procedures to remove any remaining particles of calculus and necrotic cementum embedded in the root surface. After root planing, the surfaces are smoother and free from endotoxins. Smooth root surfaces are easier for the patient to keep clean.

Gingival Curettage

In addition to scaling and root planing, which involve treating the surfaces of the tooth, some patients also require gingival curettage. *Curettage* involves scraping or cleaning the gingival lining of the pocket with a sharp curette to remove necrotic tissue from the pocket wall. Gingival curettage is also referred to as *subgingival curettage.*

Antimicrobial and Antibiotic Agents

The periodontist may prescribe antimicrobial agents and antibiotics for use with periodontal treatment.

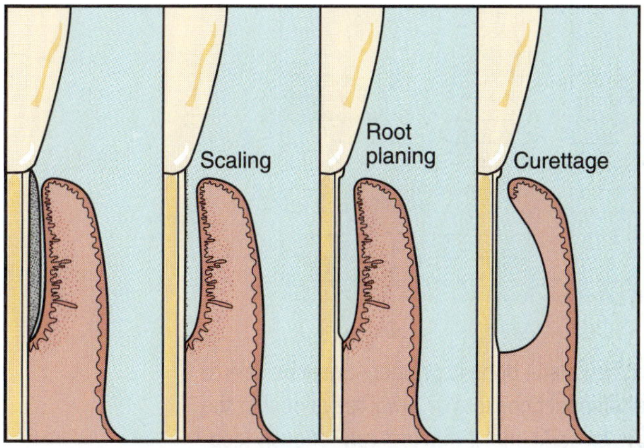

Fig. 55-19 Scaling, root planing, and curettage. (From Perry DA, Beemsterboer P, Carranza FA: *Techniques and theory of periodontal instrumentation,* ed 2, Philadelphia, 1990, Saunders.)

Tetracycline is a particularly useful antibiotic for the treatment of early-onset periodontitis as well as rapidly destructive periodontitis. An important side effect of tetracycline is that it interferes with the effectiveness of birth-control pills (oral contraceptives).

Penicillin is less effective against periodontal disease infections because many periodontal pathogens are resistant to it.

Fluoride mouthrinses have been shown to reduce bleeding by delaying bacterial growth in the periodontal pockets.

Chlorhexidine rinse twice daily is the most effective antimicrobial therapy available to reduce plaque and gingivitis. Chlorhexidine can cause temporary brown staining of the teeth, tongue, and resin restorations. This stain can be removed by polishing.

Locally Delivered Antibiotics

New methods can now apply antibiotics directly into the periodontal pockets. In one technique, a fiber that contains tetracycline is packed into periodontal pockets that have not responded to other methods. This procedure is similar to placing a retraction cord before an impression. These fibers must be removed and are most effective in pockets greater than 7 mm.

Other methods include using a syringe to insert *dissolvable materials* such as a gel (that contains an antibiotic similar to tetracycline) into the pocket. As the gel heats to body temperature, it becomes a semisolid. The material releases the antibiotic as it dissolves and does not have to be removed. In another technique a dissolvable chip that releases chlorhexidine is inserted into deep pockets.

The advantages of these methods are easy insertion and no need for removal. This local delivery of medications is particularly useful for patients with isolated areas of recurrent periodontitis and in the treatment of medically compromised patients who cannot tolerate systemic medications (Fig. 55-20).

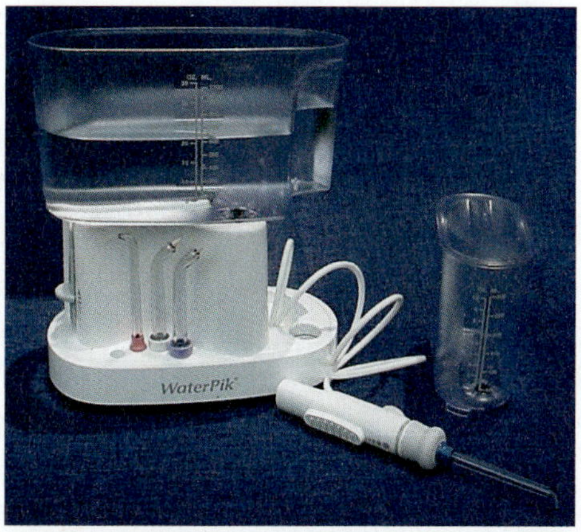

Fig. 55-20 Irrigator. Unit is shown with supragingival and marginal irrigation tips and two reservoirs. The larger reservoir is on top of the unit and is designed for chemotherapeutic agents (e.g., chlorhexidine) and is tinted to reduce light degradation. (Courtesy Waterpik Technologies, Fort Collins, Colorado.)

Recall

15. What are the more common terms for dental prophylaxis?
16. Who can legally perform a dental prophylaxis procedure?
17. What are three nonsurgical periodontal treatments?
18. How is tetracycline used in periodontal treatment?

SURGICAL PERIODONTAL TREATMENT

When nonsurgical treatment is ineffective in stopping the disease process, periodontal surgery is indicated to control the progress of periodontal destruction and loss of attachment.

Advantages and Disadvantages

The primary advantage of periodontal surgery is to *gain access* to the root surface by removing or lifting the gingival tissues. When the root surfaces are exposed, they can be more easily and thoroughly scaled and root-planed. Surgery also improves access for the patient to clean difficult areas.

Many new surgical techniques are being used to improve patients' dental and oral esthetics by altering the position of the gingival margin. These new techniques are used extensively in **cosmetic dentistry** procedures.

Disadvantages and contraindications to periodontal surgery include the patient's health status or age as well as limitations of the procedures. From the patient's point of view, the disadvantages of surgery usually include time, cost, esthetics, and discomfort. The dental assistant usually has developed a good rapport with the patient and is in a unique position to discuss these concerns.

Remaining Bone

The amount of bone remaining around a tooth is an important consideration in the decision to perform periodontal surgery. When there are large amounts of bone around a tooth, the dentist may take a "wait-and-see" approach to postpone or avoid periodontal surgery. When this approach is taken, it is important for the patient to maintain excellent home care techniques and seek routine dental care. If the amount of bone is already reduced, delaying the surgery may drastically reduce the chance to save the tooth (Fig. 55-21).

Excisional Surgery

Excisional periodontal surgery is a type of surgery that *removes* the excess tissue. It is the most rapid method for reduction of periodontal pockets. Gingivectomy and gingivoplasty are common types of excisional surgeries.

Gingivectomy

Gingivectomy is the surgical removal of diseased gingival tissues. This procedure is performed when it is necessary to reduce the depth of the periodontal pocket and to remove fibrous gingival tissue. The procedure involves making bleeding points with pocket markers and removing the gingival tissues with periodontal knives and scissors. Recently, dental laser equipment has become popular for gingivectomy (see later discussion). After healing, the pockets are reduced and it is easier for the patient to clean the area.

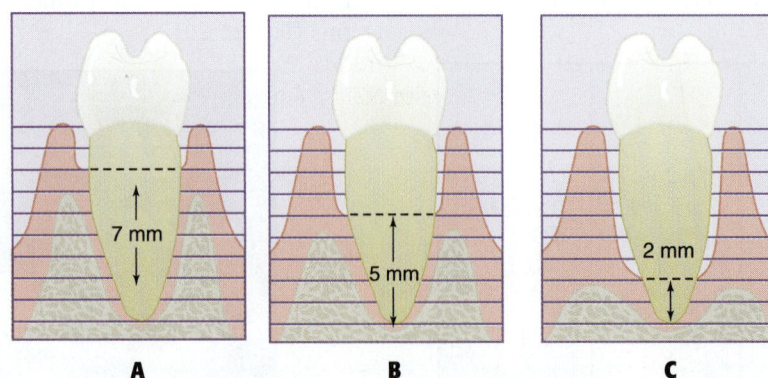

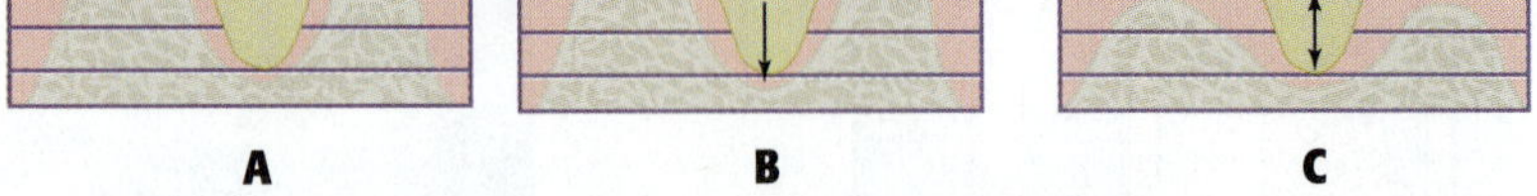

Fig. 55-21 Prognosis based on amount of bone loss. **A,** When some bone is present, it may be safe to postpone surgery and take a wait-and-see approach. An additional bone loss of 2 mm may not alter the prognosis of the tooth. **B,** When half the bone has been lost, an additional 2-mm loss can seriously jeopardize the tooth; therefore surgery is highly recommended. **C,** With advanced bone loss, surgery may be performed in an effort to save the tooth, but the prognosis is poor. (From Perry D, Beemsterboer P, Taggart E: *Periodontology for the dental hygienist,* Philadelphia, 2001, Saunders.)

Gingivoplasty

Gingivoplasty involves the surgical reshaping and contouring of the gingival tissues. The presence of *deep periodontal pockets* with fibrous tissue is the main indication for both gingivectomy and gingivoplasty. Often *both procedures* are performed simultaneously (see Procedure 55-2).

During gingivoplasty the gingivae are recontoured using periodontal knives, rotary diamond burs, curettes, and surgical scissors. Gingival margins are thinned and given a scalloped edge.

Incisional Surgery

Incisional surgery, also known as **periodontal flap surgery** or simply **flap surgery,** is performed when excisional surgery is not indicated (Fig. 55-22). In flap surgery the tissues *are not removed,* but are pushed away from the underlying tooth roots and alveolar bone, similar to the flap of an envelope.

When the flap is elevated (lifted up), the dentist may perform one or more of the following procedures:

- Thorough scaling and root planing of exposed root surfaces
- Moving the flap laterally (to the side) to cover the root surfaces of an adjacent tooth that does not have adequate tissue coverage (laterally sliding flap)
- Recontouring (reshaping) the underlying bone

After the procedure is completed, the flap is closed and sutured into place (Fig. 55-23). A periodontal dressing usually is placed after flap surgery.

Osseous Surgery

Osseous (bone) **surgery** is performed to *remove* defects and *restore* normal contours in the bone. The two primary bone surgeries are *osteoplasty* and *ostectomy.* Each requires surgically exposing the bone and recontouring it with a rotary diamond bur or a bone chisel.

Osteoplasty

In **osteoplasty,** or *additive bone surgery,* bone is contoured and reshaped. In addition, bone may be added either through *bone grafting* (taking bone from one area and placing it in another) or *placement of artificial bone-substitute materials.* This procedure is useful for patients with bone defects caused by periodontal disease.

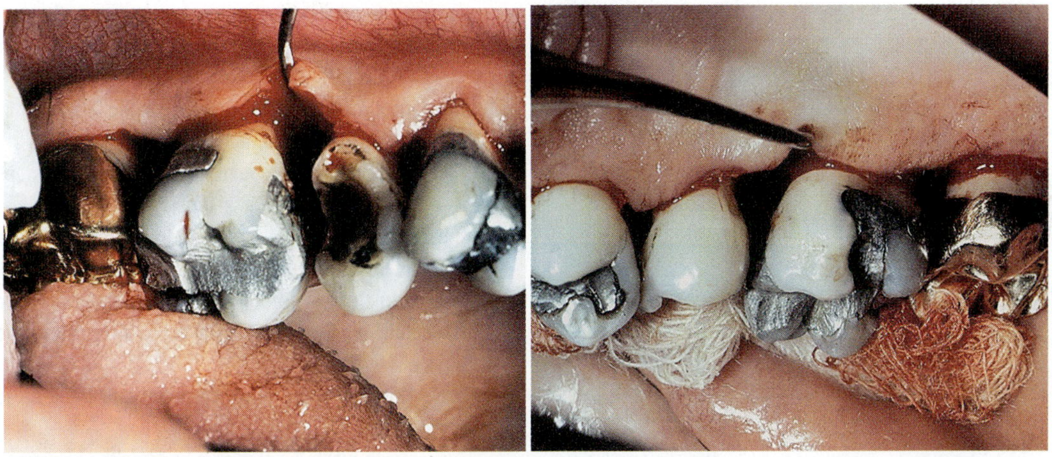

Fig. 55-22 Modified Widman flap surgery.

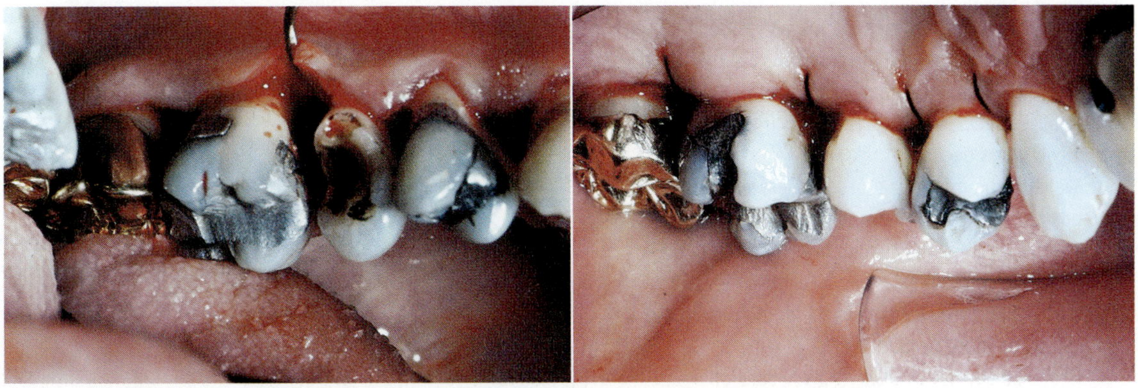

Fig. 55-23 Periodontal flap procedure. (Courtesy James F. Coggan, DDS.)

Procedure 55-2 Assisting with Gingivectomy and Gingivoplasty

Goal

To assist the dentist competently in performing gingivectomy and gingivoplasty periodontal procedures.

Equipment and Supplies

- HVE tip and surgical aspirating tip
- Local anesthetic setup
- Scalpel and blades
- Surgical periodontal knives
- Surgical tissue retraction forceps
- Periodontal pocket marker
- Tissue tweezers
- Scalers and curettes
- Diamond burs and sterile stones
- Suture needle and sutures
- Hemostat and surgical scissors
- Periodontal surgical dressing materials
- Sterile gauze sponges
- Sterile irrigation solution (water or saline)

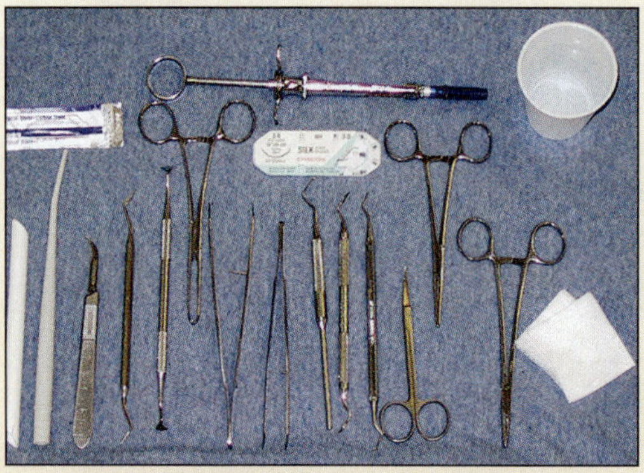

PROCEDURAL STEPS

Role of the Dental Assistant

1. Set out the patient's health history, radiographs, and periodontal chart.
   Purpose: The dentist needs to review the case before surgery.
2. Assist in the administration of local anesthetic.
3. Anticipate the dentist's needs, and be prepared to transfer and retrieve surgical instruments when needed.
   Purpose: To save time and make the procedure less stressful.
4. Have gauze ready to remove tissue from the instruments as necessary.
   Purpose: Periodontal surgery can generate heavy bleeding.
5. Provide oral evacuation and retraction.
   Purpose: Good access and visibility are critical for the dentist, and the patient will be more comfortable.
6. Irrigate with sterile saline.
   Purpose: To keep the surgical site clean and free of debris.
7. If sutures are used, prepare the suture needle and suture material and position them in a hemostat or needle holder. Transfer them to the dentist when requested.
   Purpose: To simplify the procedure for the dentist, and to aid in patient comfort.
8. Place, or assist with placement of, the periodontal dressing.
   Purpose: The dressing acts as a bandage to protect the surgical site.
   Note: Check your state's dental practice act before placing a periodontal dressing without assistance.
9. Wipe any blood or debris from the patient's face. Provide postoperative instructions to the patient.
   Purpose: To ensure that the patient clearly understands the postoperative instructions as necessary for personal well-being, and to address legal considerations.

Role of the Dentist

1. The dentist administers the local anesthetic.
   Purpose: In addition to pain control, local anesthetic aids visibility by constricting blood vessels so there is less blood at the surgical site.
2. The dentist marks the pockets on both the facial and the lingual gingivae by using the periodontal pocket marker.
   Purpose: The bleeding points indicate the pocket depth and thus the point for the initial incision.
3. The dentist uses a scalpel or periodontal knife to incise the gingiva at a 45-degree angle following along the bleeding points. The incision is beveled to create a normally contoured, free gingival margin.
4. The dentist removes the gingival tissue along the incision line using surgical knives.
5. The dentist tapers the gingival margins and creates a scalloped marginal outline.
   Purpose: To create an attractive and healthy appearance.
6. The dentist shapes the interdental papillae using interdental knives.
   Purpose: To contour the interdental grooves.
7. The dentist performs scaling and root planing of the root surfaces.
   Purpose: To remove any residual calculus that was inaccessible before surgery.
8. The dentist places sutures if needed.
9. The dentist irrigates the surgical site and then covers it with a periodontal dressing.
   Purpose: To protect the surgical site.
   Note: In some states, placement and removal of the periodontal dressing are delegated to the dental assistant (expanded function).

Ostectomy

In **ostectomy,** or *subtractive bone surgery,* bone is removed. This procedure is necessary when the patient has large *exostoses* (bony growths). For example, an ostectomy is performed if a patient needs a full denture and the bony growth would interfere with the comfort and fit of the denture.

Postsurgical Patient Instructions

After periodontal surgery, the periodontist will most likely prescribe an analgesic (pain medication) and possibly an antibiotic. Many periodontists recommend the use of an antibacterial rinse twice daily to help with plaque control. A chlorhexidine mouthwash may also be used during the first week to freshen the mouth and inhibit plaque formation during the early stages of healing.

Postoperative instructions should be given to the patient to ease discomfort and promote healing.

Patient Instructions After Periodontal Surgery

Activity: Limit your activities to those requiring minimal exertion for the next few days.

Rinsing: Do not rinse your mouth for 24 hours.

Bleeding: Some slight bleeding may occur during the first 4 or 5 hours after the operation. This bleeding is not unusual. If bleeding continues, apply firm pressure for 20 minutes with a piece of gauze. Repeat as necessary. Do not remove the gauze during this period. Do not rinse with water to stop the bleeding. If bleeding persists, call the office.

Discomfort: Some discomfort is to be expected when the anesthesia wears off. If you have been given a prescription, fill it and take the medication as directed. If discomfort persists, call the office.

Eating: Limit yourself to a soft diet immediately after surgery. Avoid chewing in the area of surgery. Do not drink very hot beverages the first day. You may return to your regular diet as soon as you feel comfortable. Highly seasoned or spicy foods may irritate the area of surgery.

Dressing: A dressing material may have been placed around your teeth. It will become hard within about 2 hours and should not be disturbed. Although the dressing may remain in place until your next appointment, small parts may chip off. If a large portion of the dressing comes off, call the office for instructions.

Swelling: Swelling is expected after some procedures. You may use an ice pack on the outside of your face, 15 minutes on and 15 minutes off, for the next 4 hours. If you have excessive swelling in your neck or under your chin, call the office.

Smoking: Do not smoke. Smoking may interfere with the healing process and produce poor results.

Home care: If a surgical dressing is present, brush the top of the dressing lightly with a soft toothbrush. If no dressing is present, gently use a soft toothbrush to clean the area of surgery for the first few days. You may rinse gently with a medicated mouthwash if it was prescribed or warm salt water starting the day after surgery.

IF YOU HAVE ANY QUESTIONS OR CONCERNS, CALL THE OFFICE.

Telephone number:

Recall

19. What is the primary goal of periodontal surgery?
20. From a patient's point of view, what are the primary disadvantages of periodontal surgery?
21. What is a gingivectomy?
22. What is the purpose of osseous surgery?

Periodontal Surgical Dressings

A **periodontal dressing (Perio Pak)** serves as a bandage over the surgical site. Periodontal dressings, also known as *periopacks,* are used for the following purposes:

1. To hold the flaps in place
2. To protect the newly forming tissues
3. To minimize postoperative pain, infection, and hemorrhage
4. To protect the surgical site from trauma during eating and drinking
5. To support mobile teeth during the healing process

There are a variety of materials on the market for periodontal dressings. The dressings most often used are those made with zinc oxide–eugenol (ZOE) and those made without eugenol.

Zinc Oxide–Eugenol Dressing

The ZOE dressing is supplied as a powder and a liquid that are mixed before use. The material can be mixed beforehand, wrapped in wax paper, and frozen for future use (Fig. 55-24).

ZOE has a slow set, which allows for a longer working time. It sets to a firm and heavy consistency and provides good support and protection for tissues and flaps. Some patients are allergic to the eugenol and will experience redness and burning pain in the area of the dressing.

Noneugenol Dressing

The noneugenol dressing is the most widely used type of periodontal dressing. This material is supplied in two tubes, one for the base material and the other for the accelerator.

Noneugenol material is easy to mix and place and has a smooth surface for patient comfort. This material has a rapid setting time if exposed to warm temperatures, and it *cannot be mixed* and *stored in advance* (Fig. 55-25). (See Procedures 55-3 and 55-4.)

Recall

23. What is the function of a periodontal surgical dressing?

24. What are the most common materials used for periodontal dressings?

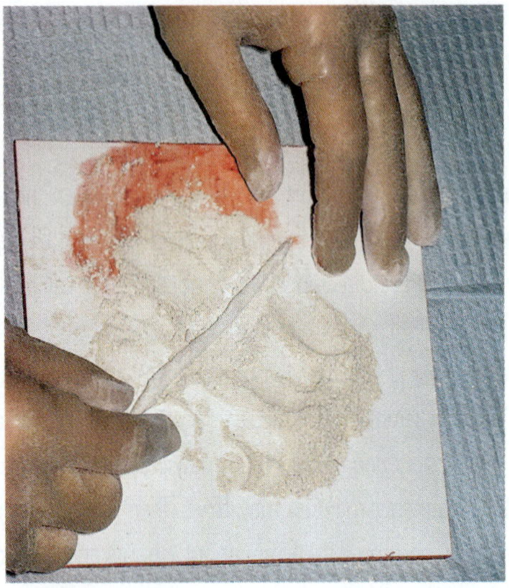

Fig. 55-24 Zinc oxide powder and liquid eugenol are mixed in advance.

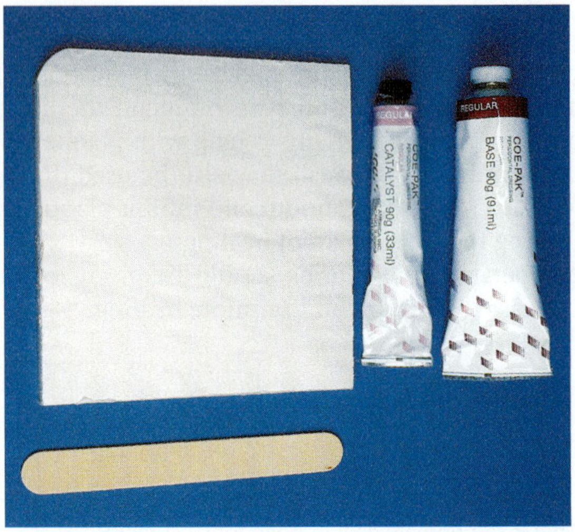

Fig. 55-25 Paste for noneugenol dressing is ready to be mixed.

Procedure 55-3 Preparing and Placing Noneugenol Periodontal Dressing

Goal

To prepare and assist the dentist in placing a noneugenol periodontal dressing.

Equipment and Supplies

- Paper mixing pad (supplied by manufacturer)
- Wooden tongue depressor
- Noneugenol dressing (base and accelerator)
- Paper cup filled with room-temperature water
- Saline solution
- Plastic-type filling instrument

PROCEDURAL STEPS

Mixing the Material

1. Extrude equal lengths of the two pastes on the paper pad.
2. Mix the pastes with a wooden tongue depressor until a uniform color has been obtained (two to three minutes).
3. When the paste loses its tackiness, place it in the paper cup filled with room-temperature water.
4. Lubricate gloved fingers with saline solution.
   Purpose: To prevent the material from sticking to the gloves.
5. Roll the paste into strips approximately the length of the surgical site.

Placing the Dressing

1. Press small triangle-shaped pieces of dressing into the interproximal spaces.

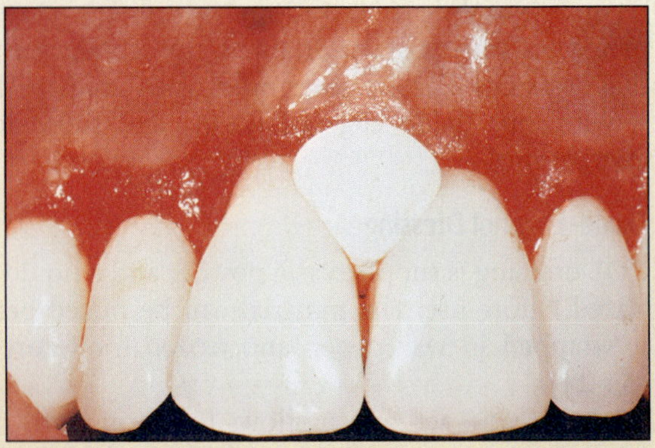

Procedure 55-3 Preparing and Placing Noneugenol Periodontal Dressing—cont'd

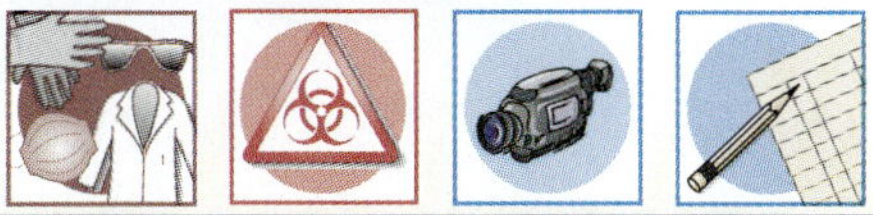

2. Adapt one end of the strip around the distal surface of the last tooth in the surgical site.
3. Bring the remainder of the strip forward along the facial surface, and gently press the strip along the incised gingival margin.
4. Gently press the strip into the interproximal areas.

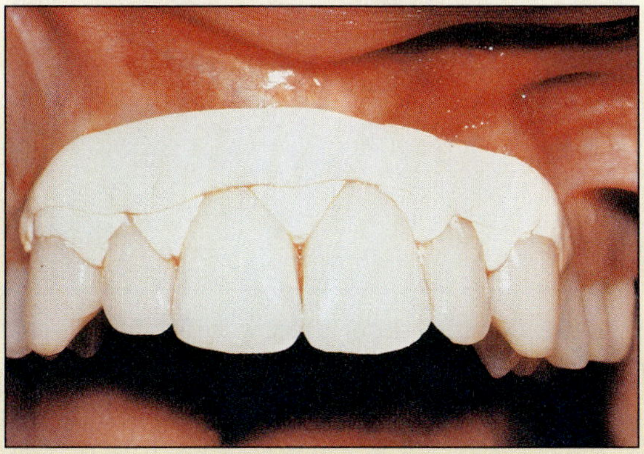

5. Apply the second strip in the same manner from the lingual side.
6. Join the facial and lingual strips at the distal surface of the last tooth at both ends of the surgical site.
7. Apply gentle pressure on the facial and lingual surfaces.
8. Check the dressing for overextension and interference with occlusion.
   Purpose: Excess packing irritates the mucobuccal fold and floor of the mouth.
9. Remove any excess dressing, and adjust the new margins to remove any roughness.
   Purpose: If the pack is not adapted properly, it can break off.

Procedure 55-4 Removing a Periodontal Dressing

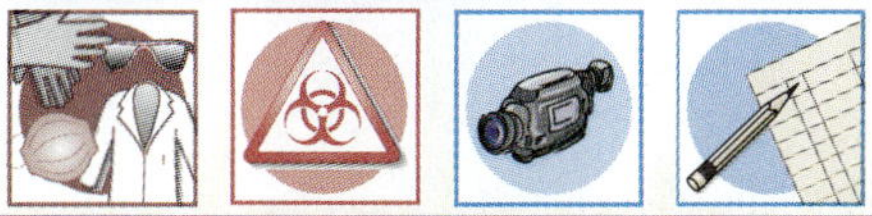

Goal

To remove a periodontal dressing.

Equipment and Supplies

- Spoon excavator
- Suture scissors (for sutures if present)
- Dental floss
- Warm saline solution
- Irrigating solution
- High-volume evacuator (HVE) tip or saliva ejector

PROCEDURAL STEPS

1. Gently insert the spoon excavator under the margin.
2. Use lateral pressure to pry the dressing gently away from the tissue.
   Purpose: The area may still be sensitive, and the newly healed tissue is delicate and easily injured.

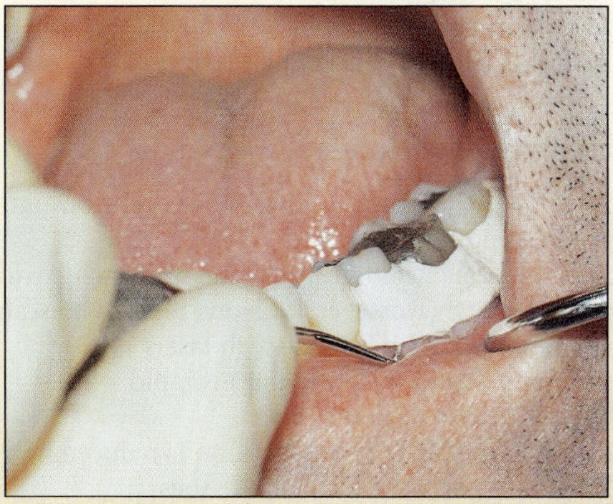

continued

Procedure 55-4 Removing a Periodontal Dressing—cont'd

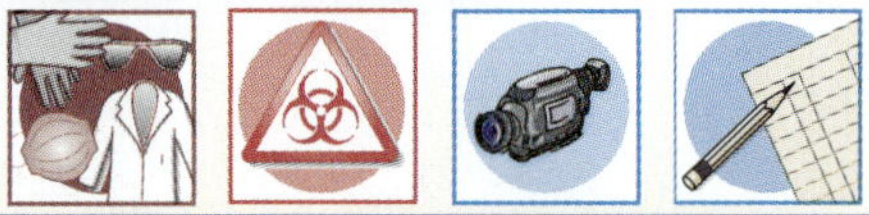

3. If sutures are embedded in the dressing material, cut the suture material free. Remove the sutures gently from the tissue.
   Purpose: Accidentally pulling the sutures could be painful for the patient and might open the wound.
4. Gently use dental floss to remove all fragments of dressing material from the interproximal surfaces.
   Purpose: Remaining fragments could cause discomfort for the patient and result in tissue irritation.
5. Irrigate the entire area gently with warm saline solution to remove superficial debris.

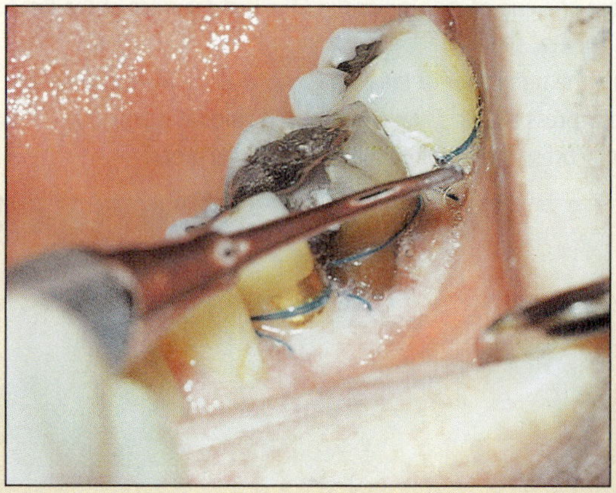

6. Use the HVE tip or saliva ejector to remove the fluid from the patient's mouth.

LASERS IN PERIODONTICS

The term **laser** is an acronym for *light amplification by stimulated emission of radiation.* A laser beam is a highly concentrated beam of light. The power of this beam can be adjusted to enable it to cut, vaporize, or cauterize tissue (Fig. 55-26).

The use of lasers is a promising new technology for dentistry. Research is continuing that may lead to more widespread uses of lasers in clinical dentistry. The periodontal applications of lasers on soft tissue include the following:

- Removal of tumors and lesions
- Vaporization of excess tissues, as in gingivoplasty, gingivectomy, and *frenectomy*
- Removal of or reduction in hyperplastic tissues
- Control of bleeding in vascular lesions

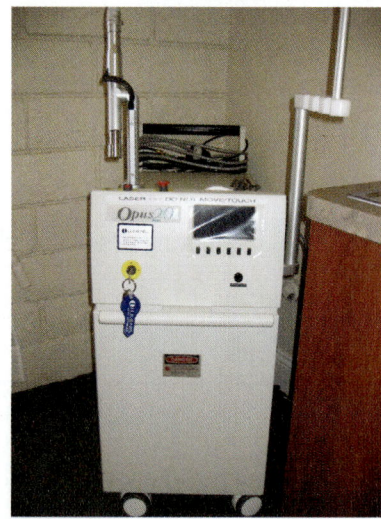

Fig. 55-26 The Opus 20 is a laser that is used in periodontal surgery. (Courtesy Dr. Peter Pang, Sonoma, CA.)

Advantages of Laser Surgery

Lasers offer the following advantages over conventional surgical techniques:

1. Laser incisions heal faster than incisions made with electrosurgery. (However, incisions made with scalpels heal faster than those made with lasers.)
2. *Hemostasis* (control of bleeding) is rapid.
3. Surgical field is relatively dry.
4. Risk of bloodborne contamination is reduced.
5. Less trauma occurs to adjacent tissues.
6. Postsurgical swelling, scarring, and pain are reduced.
7. Some procedures can be performed more quickly.
8. Patients who are afraid of "surgery" may accept laser therapy.

Laser Safety

Precautions must be taken to protect both the patient and the dental staff during laser procedures. Any person who operates a laser or assists during a laser operation must be thoroughly trained in the use of this powerful instrument (Fig. 55-27).

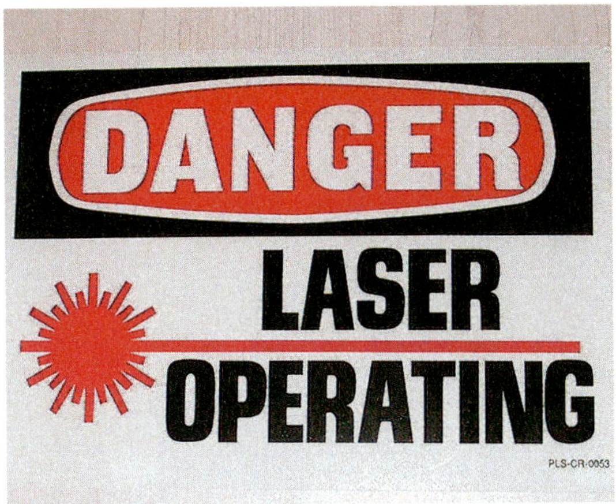

Fig. 55-27 To prevent injury to the eyes of persons who are not wearing special light filter glasses, warning signs must be placed in areas where lasers are used.

Guidelines for laser safety include the following protective devices and measures:

- *Shielded eyeglasses.* The dental staff and patient must wear special shielded eyeglasses to protect the eyes.
- *Matte-finished instruments.* Reflective surfaces such as instruments, mirrors, and even polished restorations can reflect laser energy. Matte-finished (nonshiny) instruments are recommended to avoid this reflection.
- *Protection of nontarget tissues.* Nontarget oral tissue (tissues not being treated with the laser) should be shielded with wet gauze packs.
- *High-volume evacuation.* HVE should be used to draw off the *plume* (cloud) created when tissue vaporizes. This plume could be infectious.

Recall

25. Are there any training requirements for persons working with lasers?

Patient Education

The dental assistant can play an important role in a periodontal office. Patients must be educated about the cause of their disease and how to incorporate new oral hygiene techniques that will help them achieve periodontal health (see Chapters 14 and 15).

Periodontal patients usually require more complex home care procedures than simple toothbrushing and flossing. These patients often have areas of attachment loss caused by the disease process or as a result of periodontal surgery. It can be very challenging for the patient to clean furcations, periodontal pockets, and areas of root exposure.

Patient Education—cont'd

Patients with periodontal disease usually have had poor oral hygiene most of their lives that has contributed to their disease process. The dental assistant can help motivate the periodontal patient to begin and continue a lifelong process of improved daily oral hygiene. Thorough home care may require an additional 15 to 30 minutes a day. It is not easy for patients to change lifetime habits, and the dental assistant must be patient, understanding, and encouraging to each patient.

Legal and Ethical Implications

Two of the most common types of malpractice suits result from the failure to *diagnose* periodontal disease and the failure to *refer* patients to a periodontist when it is necessary.

The accurate diagnosis of periodontal disease requires a comprehensive clinical examination. This examination should include extraoral, intraoral, oral mucosal, oral hygiene, and comprehensive periodontal and dentition assessments. Each of these assessments must be *documented.* It is unacceptable to assess the patient's oral health without documenting that information in the patient's record. Documentation serves many purposes, including a historical record, patient education tool, and guide to treatment planning. It may also serve as an important part of a legal defense.

Eye to the Future

New evidence suggests that periodontal disease is a *risk factor* in the development and management of serious systemic disease. In particular, periodontal infections have been implicated in cardiovascular diseases, conditions affecting preterm low-birthweight infants, and bacterial pneumonia. In addition, it appears to be more difficult to control non–insulin-dependent diabetes in patients with severe periodontitis.

Studies conducted by the National Institutes of Health suggest that in people over 40 years of age, there is a relationship between periodontal conditions and history of heart attacks. The inflammatory response in periodontal disease may influence buildup in the arterial walls. Research regarding the relationship between heart disease and periodontal disease will continue. It is obvious, however, that a healthy mouth is necessary for a healthy body.

Critical Thinking

1. Mrs. Camp has been a patient in your general dental office for more than 20 years. She has a history of missing her regular appointments for dental cleanings, and her home care is not ideal. At her most recent visit, the dentist told Mrs. Camp that she is developing periodontal pockets of 4 to 6 mm and should be referred to a periodontist. Mrs. Camp does not want to seek periodontal care and promised that she will faithfully brush and floss her teeth. What do you think the dentist will say to her? Why?
2. Why do you think the dental hygienist in your office may ask you to assist with suction when she uses the ultrasonic scaler?
3. What would you say to a very nervous patient who has just been referred to a periodontist for a gingivectomy?

56

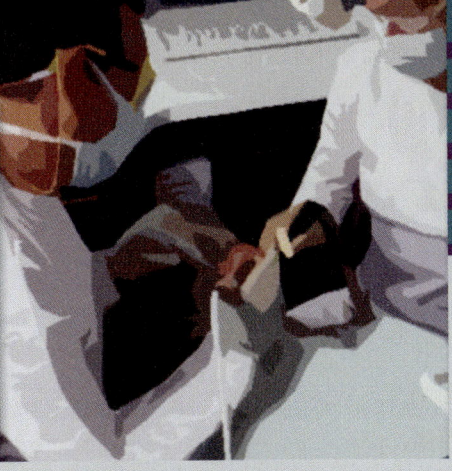

Oral and Maxillofacial Surgery

Outline

Indications for Oral and Maxillofacial Surgery
The Oral Surgeon
The Surgical Assistant
The Surgical Setting
- Private Practice
- Operating Room

Specialized Instruments and Accessories
- Elevators
- Forceps
- Surgical Curette
- Rongeur
- Bone File
- Scalpel
- Hemostat
- Needle Holder
- Surgical and Suture Scissors
- Retractors
- Mouth Props
- Chisel and Mallet
- Surgical Burs

Surgical Asepsis
- Sterile Field
- Surgical Scrub

Procedure 56-1: Preparing a Sterile Field for Instruments and Supplies
Procedure 56-2: Performing a Surgical Scrub
- Proper Gloving

Procedure 56-3: Performing Sterile Gloving
Surgical Preparation
Surgical Procedures
- Forceps Extraction

Procedure 56-4: Assisting in Forceps Extraction
- Multiple Extractions and Alveoplasty
- Removal of Impacted Teeth

Procedure 56-5: Assisting in Multiple Extraction and Alveoplasty
Procedure 56-6: Assisting in Removal of an Impacted Tooth
- Biopsy

Sutures
- Suture Placement

Procedure 56-7: Assisting in Suture Placement
- Suture Removal

Procedure 56-8: Performing Suture Removal (Expanded Function)
Postoperative Care
- Control of Bleeding
- Control of Swelling

Postsurgical Complications
- Alveolitis

Procedure 56-9: Assisting in the Treatment of Alveolitis
Patient Education
Legal and Ethical Implications
Eye to the Future
Critical Thinking

KEY TERMS

Alveolitis (*al*-vee-ah-**li**-tis) Inflammation and infection associated with the disturbance of a blood clot following an extraction of an impacted tooth.

Alveoplasty (al-**vee**-o-*plas*-tee) Surgical reduction and reshaping of the alveolar ridge.

Bone file Surgical instrument used to smooth rough edges of bone structure.

Chisel Surgical instrument used for cutting or severing a tooth and bone structure.

continued

KEY TERMS, cont'd

Curette (ku-**ret**) Surgical instrument used to remove tissue from the tooth socket; also *curet.*

Donning Act of placing on an item, such as gloves; dressing.

Elevator Surgical instrument used to reflect and retract the periodontal ligament and periosteum.

Excisional biopsy (ik-**sizh**-nul, ek-**sizh**-ah-nul **bi**-*ahp*-see) Surgical procedure in which tissue is cut from a suspect oral lesion for analysis.

Exfoliative biopsy (eks-**fo**-lee-*a*-tiv) Diagnostic procedure in which cells are scraped from a suspect oral lesion for analysis.

Forceps (**for**-seps) Surgical instrument used to grasp and hold onto teeth for their removal.

Hard tissue impaction (im-**pak**-shun) Oral condition in which a tooth is partly to fully covered by bone and gingival tissue.

Hemostat (**he**-mah-*stat*) Surgical instrument used to hold or grasp items.

Impacted tooth Tooth that has not erupted.

Incisional biopsy (in-**sizh**-ah-nul, in-**si**-zhah-nul) Section of suspect oral lesion that is removed for evaluation.

Luxate (**luk**-sate) To dislocate, as a tooth from its socket.

Mallet Hammerlike instrument used with a chisel to section teeth or bone.

Needle holder Surgical instrument used to hold the suture needle.

Oral and maxillofacial surgeon (OMFS) (mak-***si***-*loh*-**fay**-shul) Dentist who has specialized in surgeries of the head and neck region.

Oral and maxillofacial surgery Dental specialty concerned with the treatment of the head and neck.

Outpatient Patient seen and treated by a physician, then sent home for recovery.

Retractor (ri-**trak**-tur) Surgical instrument used to hold back soft tissue.

Rongeur (raw-**shur**) Surgical instrument used to cut and trim the alveolar bone.

Root tip picks Surgical instrument used for the removal of root tips or fragments in the surgical site.

Scalpel (**skal**-pul, skal-**pel**) Surgical knife.

Soft tissue impaction Oral condition in which a tooth is partially to fully covered by gingival tissue.

LEARNING OUTCOMES

On completion of this chapter, the student will be able to achieve the following objectives:

- Pronounce, define, and spell the Key Terms.
- Describe the specialty of oral and maxillofacial surgery.
- Discuss the role of an oral surgery assistant.
- Discuss the importance of the chain of asepsis during a surgical procedure.
- Identify specialized instruments used for basic surgical procedures.
- Describe surgical procedures typically performed in a general practice.
- Describe postoperative care given to a patient after a surgical procedure.
- Discuss possible complications from surgery.

PERFORMANCE OUTCOMES

On completion of this chapter, the student will be able to achieve competency standards in the following skills:

- Prepare a sterile field.
- Perform a surgical scrub.
- Perform sterile gloving.
- Assist in a simple extraction.
- Assist in a multiple extraction procedure with alveoplasty.
- Assist in removal of an impacted tooth.
- Assist in suture placement.
- Perform suture removal.
- Assist in the treatment of alveolitis (dry socket).

The specialty of **oral and maxillofacial surgery** is involved in the diagnosis and surgical treatment of diseases, injuries, and defects. These surgeries are performed on the basis of functional challenges and esthetic aspects of the hard and soft tissues of the head and neck.

INDICATIONS FOR ORAL AND MAXILLOFACIAL SURGERY

- Extraction of decayed teeth that cannot be restored
- Surgical removal of impacted teeth
- Extraction of nonvital teeth
- Preprosthesis surgery to smooth and contour the alveolar ridge
- Removal of teeth for orthodontic treatment
- Removal of root fragments
- Removal of cysts and tumors
- Biopsy
- Treatment of fractures of the mandible or maxilla
- Surgery to alter the size or shape of the facial bones
- Surgery of the temporomandibular joint
- Reconstructive surgery
- Cleft lip and cleft palate repairs
- Salivary gland surgery
- Surgical implant procedures

THE ORAL SURGEON

An **oral and maxillofacial surgeon (OMFS),** also referred to as an *oral surgeon,* is a dentist who has received four to six additional years of postgraduate training in a hospital-based residency. The oral surgeon completes a core surgical-medical year before completion, with an emphasis on surgical techniques, anesthesiology, and oral medicine. The surgeon must pass a national standardized examination by the American Board of Oral and Maxillofacial Surgery in order to practice. Most current surgeons have obtained their medical license as well.

The general dentist receives basic training in simple oral surgery procedures and can perform these in the private practice setting. For specific areas of the mouth and more complicated procedures, however, many dentists will refer the patient to a specialist.

THE SURGICAL ASSISTANT

The surgical assistant is one of the most important members of the surgical team. Because most surgical procedures are more invasive and in-depth, the surgical assistant must have advanced knowledge and skill in (1) patient assessment and monitoring, (2) specialized instruments, (3) surgical asepsis, (4) surgical procedures, and (5) pain-control techniques.

After completion of a general dental assisting program, dental assistants can further their education and training in either a specialized program for surgical dental assistants, or by acquiring additional on-the-job training. Dental assistants that assist the oral surgeon in the operating room often first become certified in advanced cardiac life support.

THE SURGICAL SETTING

The surgical team will complete procedures in two specific settings: the private dental office and the hospital operating room.

Private Practice

An oral surgeon's private-practice medico-dental-surgical office consists of treatment areas similar to those in a general practice. In addition to the treatment areas, the office has a *surgical suite* that resembles the operating room, but on a much smaller scale. Specific items used only for surgical procedures, such as monitoring equipment, pain-control units, and mobile trays, replace items of the general dentist.

The patient who receives surgical care from an OMFS in an office setting is receiving *minor surgery* and is seen as an **outpatient.** The patient arrives a short time before surgery, receives surgical treatment, recovers, and then is escorted home to complete the recovery.

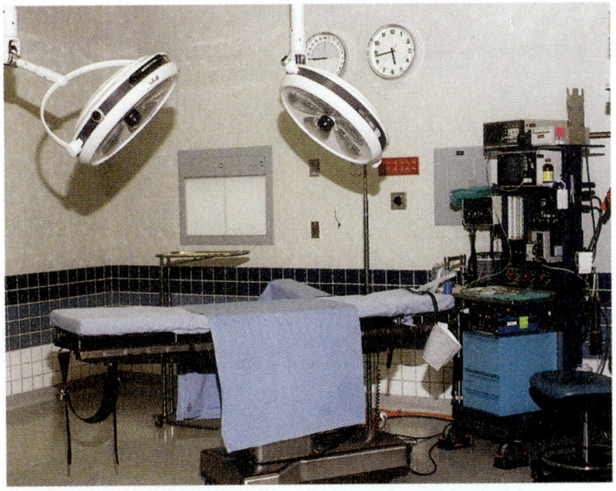

Fig. 56-1 The operating room. (Courtesy Fresno Surgery Center, Fresno, California.)

Operating Room

The operating room of a hospital is quite different from the private practice (Fig. 56-1). The surgeon first submits an application for privileges to practice at that institution. The hospital grants privileges to physicians and dentists based on their training, competence, and experience.

The environment is spacious enough to accommodate the (1) operating table; (2) anesthesiology equipment; (3) mobile surgical trays, holding instruments, and supplies; (4) overhead lighting; (5) monitoring equipment; and (6) standing room for the surgeon, surgical assistant, roving assistant, and anesthesiologist.

Recall

1. Can a general dentist perform extractions?
2. How can surgical assistants further their profession?
3. In which two settings can a patient receive oral surgery?
4. Are outpatient oral and maxillofacial surgical procedures considered major or minor surgeries?

SPECIALIZED INSTRUMENTS AND ACCESSORIES

It is critical for the surgical assistant to have a working knowledge and understanding of surgical instruments. Such knowledge prepares them for the sterilization and preparation of a surgical setup, but when a surgeon requests an instrument, they also will be ready to assist.

Surgical instruments are designed to separate the tooth from the socket, retract surrounding tissue, loosen and

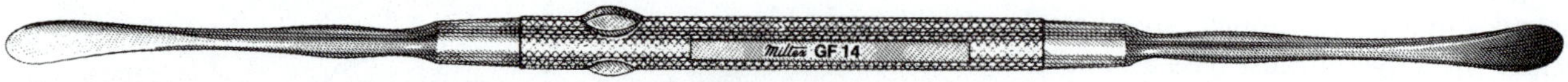

Fig. 56-2 Periosteal elevators. (Courtesy Miltex, Inc., York, PA.)

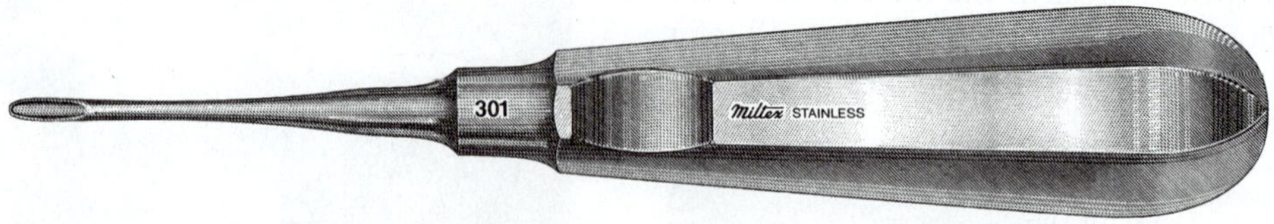

Fig. 56-3 Straight elevator. (Courtesy Miltex, Inc., York, PA.)

elevate the tooth within the socket, or extract the tooth from the socket. The instruments discussed in this chapter are the oral surgical instruments most commonly used. All surgical instruments are classified as *critical instruments* and must be sterilized after each use.

Elevators

Periosteal **elevators** are available in many designs, but they all provide the same basic function (Fig. 56-2). They are used to reflect *(separate)* and retract the *periosteum* from the surface of the bone. Before the surgical forceps is placed around the tooth, the dentist uses a periosteal elevator to detach the gingival tissues from around the cervix *(neck)* of the tooth.

Straight elevators are used to apply leverage against the tooth to loosen it from the periodontal ligament and ease the extraction (Fig. 56-3). Additional uses include the removal of residual root fragments and removal of teeth that have been sectioned with a surgical handpiece and bur.

Root tip picks are instruments for the removal of root tips or fragments that may break away from the tooth during the extraction procedure (Fig. 56-4).

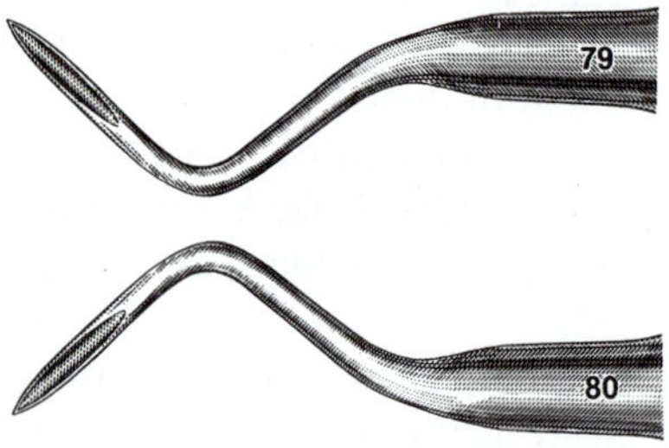

Fig. 56-4 Root tip picks. (Courtesy Miltex, Inc., York, PA.)

Forceps

Extraction **forceps** are available in many different shapes and designs able to accommodate the oral surgeon's needs in grasping teeth with different crown shapes, root configurations, and location in the mouth. The goal is to remove the tooth in one piece with the crown and root intact.

The beaks of the forceps are shaped to grasp the crown of the tooth firmly at or below the cervical line. The inner surface of the beaks may be either *plain* (smooth finished) or *serrated* (rough finished) to provide additional grasping power when a tooth is extracted. The handles can be either *horizontal* (side by side) or *vertical.*

Forceps are used to remove teeth from the alveolus after they have been slightly loosened in the sockets by the application of elevators. The handles, which are held firmly in a palm grasp, provide the dentist with the leverage necessary to **luxate** and remove the tooth.

Universal forceps are designed to allow the surgeon to use the same instrument for either the left or right side of the same arch, as well as for a specific tooth. Fig. 56-5 shows commonly used forceps for specific areas of the mouth.

Surgical Curette

The surgical **curette** resembles a large spoon excavator. It is a double-ended, scoop-shaped instrument with sharp edges that is used with a scraping motion. Curettes are used after extractions to scrape the interior of the socket to remove diseased tissue or abscesses. Curettes come in varying sizes, and the shanks are straight or angled to reach different areas of the mouth (Fig. 56-6).

Rongeur

The **rongeur** is similar in its size to forceps, and the design resembles that of fingernail clippers. The rongeur has a spring between the handles and blades with sharp cutting edges. The blades of the rongeur may be end cutting or side cutting, depending on the design (Fig. 56-7).

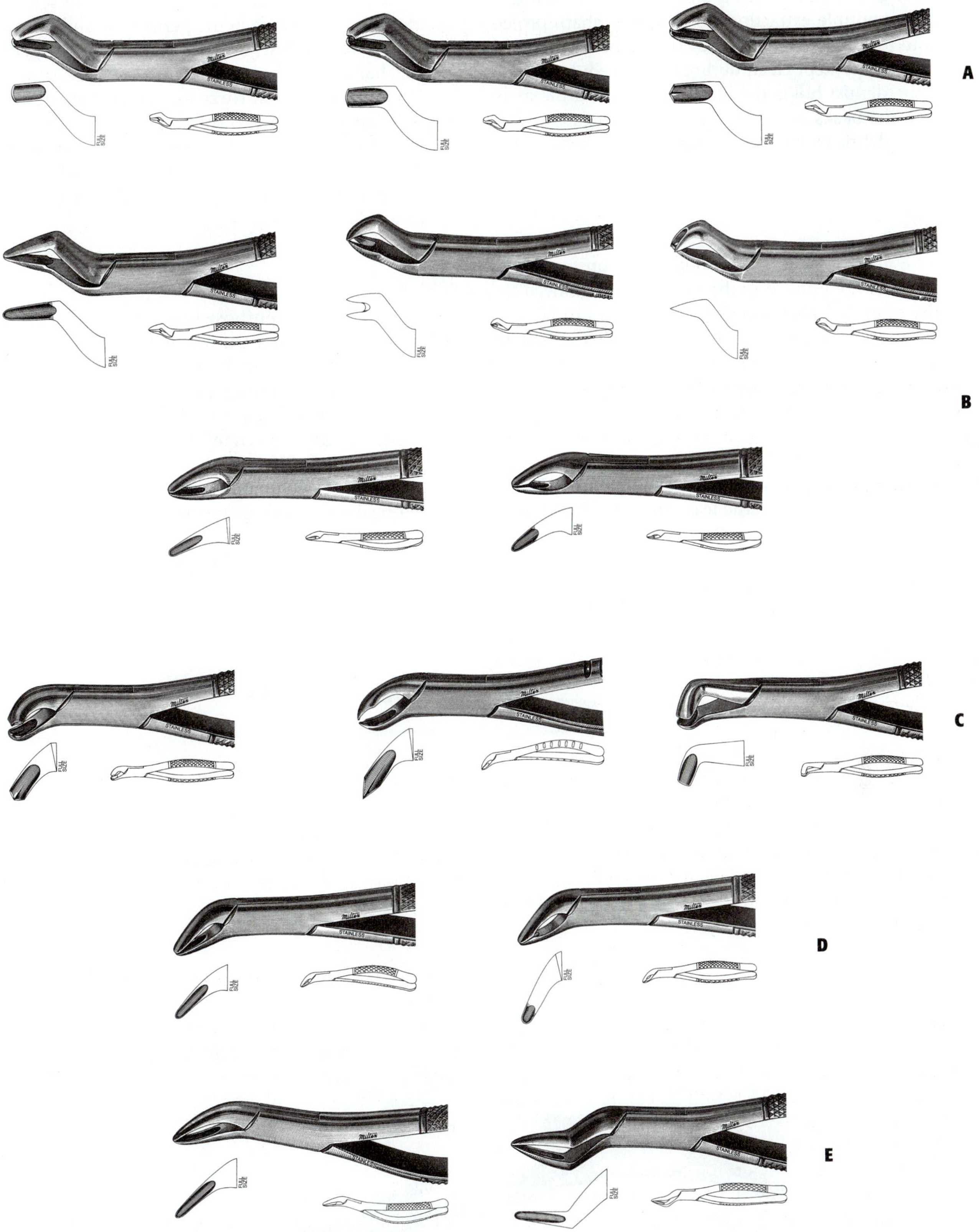

Fig. 56-5 Types of extraction forceps. **A,** Maxillary molar extraction forceps. **B,** Maxillary anterior extraction forceps. **C,** Mandibular molar extraction forceps. **D,** Mandibular anterior extraction forceps. **E,** Root tip extraction forceps. (Courtesy Miltex, Inc., York, PA.)

The rongeur is used to trim alveolar bone. It is widely used after multiple extractions to eliminate sharp projections and to shape the edentulous ridge. The beaks of the rongeur must be kept clean during the procedure. As necessary, the dentist holds the instrument toward the assistant with the beaks open. The assistant then carefully removes the debris by wiping the beaks with a sterile gauze sponge.

Bone File

The **bone file** is used with a push-pull motion to smooth the surface of the bone after the rongeur has removed the majority of undesirable bone. Bone files also can be used to smooth rough margins of the alveolus after an extraction. The working ends of bone files are very rough and are available in a variety of shapes and sizes (Fig. 56-8).

Scalpel

The **scalpel** is a surgical knife used to make a precise incision into soft tissue with the least amount of trauma to the tissue. The size and shape of the blade selected depend on the procedure being performed and on the dentist's preference (Fig. 56-9). Disposable scalpels have plastic handles with metal blades and are supplied in sterile sealed packages. These instruments are designed to be used once and then discarded into the "sharps" container. Care must be taken to avoid injury while the blades are attached and removed. The use of a mechanical scalpel blade remover helps avoid injury during the removal of scalpel blades.

Hemostat

Hemostats are multipurpose instruments that are used to grasp and hold things. During oral surgery a hemostat is used to grasp soft tissue, bone, and tooth fragments that have been removed during the procedure. A **hemostat** has grooves in its beak that are used for grasping and holding. The handles have a mechanical lock to hold an object or tissue securely in the beaks (Fig. 56-10). These instruments are available in a variety of sizes, with straight and curved beaks and with different handle lengths.

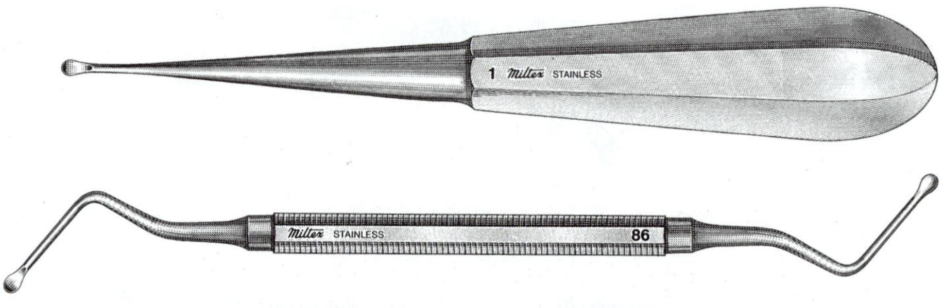

Fig. 56-6 Surgical curettes. (Courtesy Miltex, Inc., York, PA.)

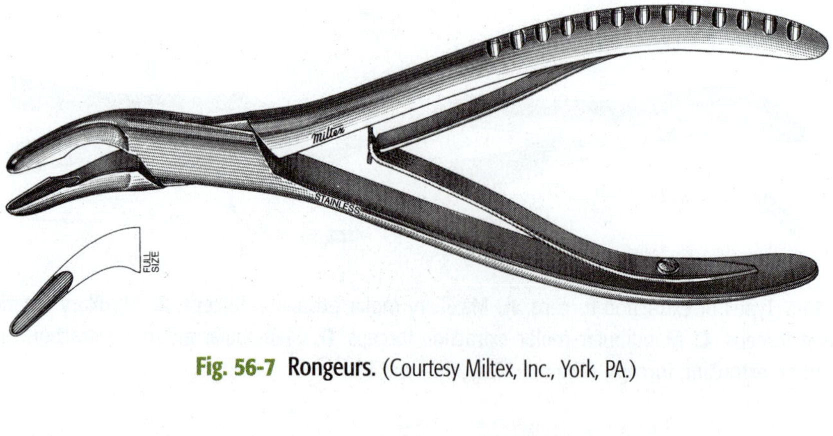

Fig. 56-7 Rongeurs. (Courtesy Miltex, Inc., York, PA.)

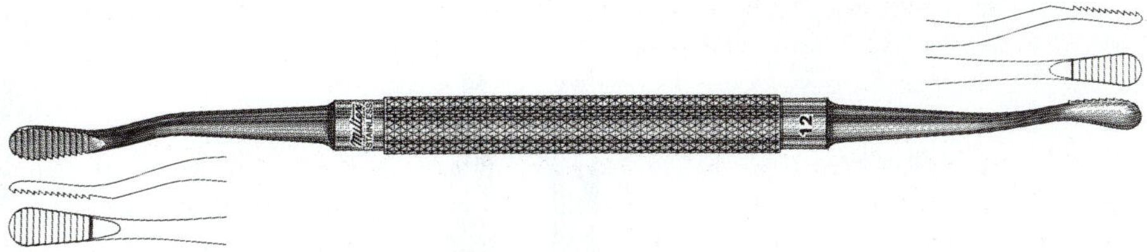

Fig. 56-8 **Bone files.** (Courtesy Miltex, Inc., York, PA.)

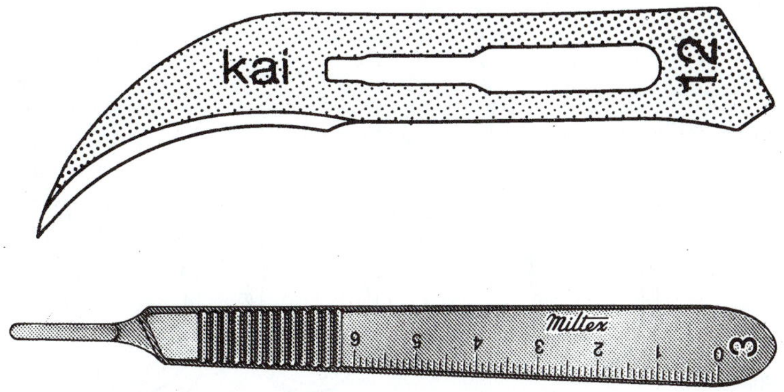

Fig. 56-9 **Scalpel handles and blades.** (Courtesy Miltex, Inc., York, PA.)

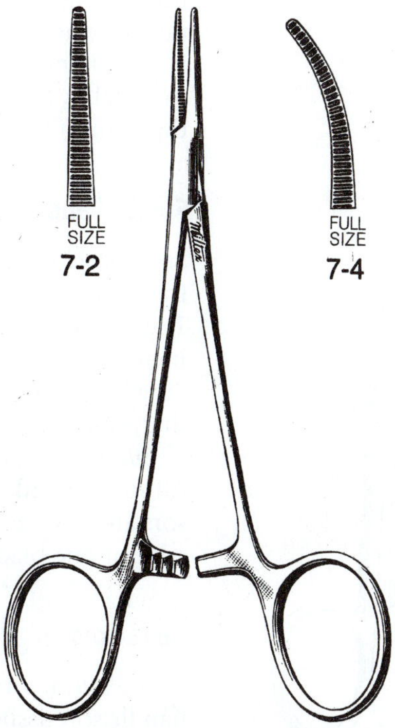

Fig. 56-10 **Hemostats.** (Courtesy Miltex, Inc., York, PA.)

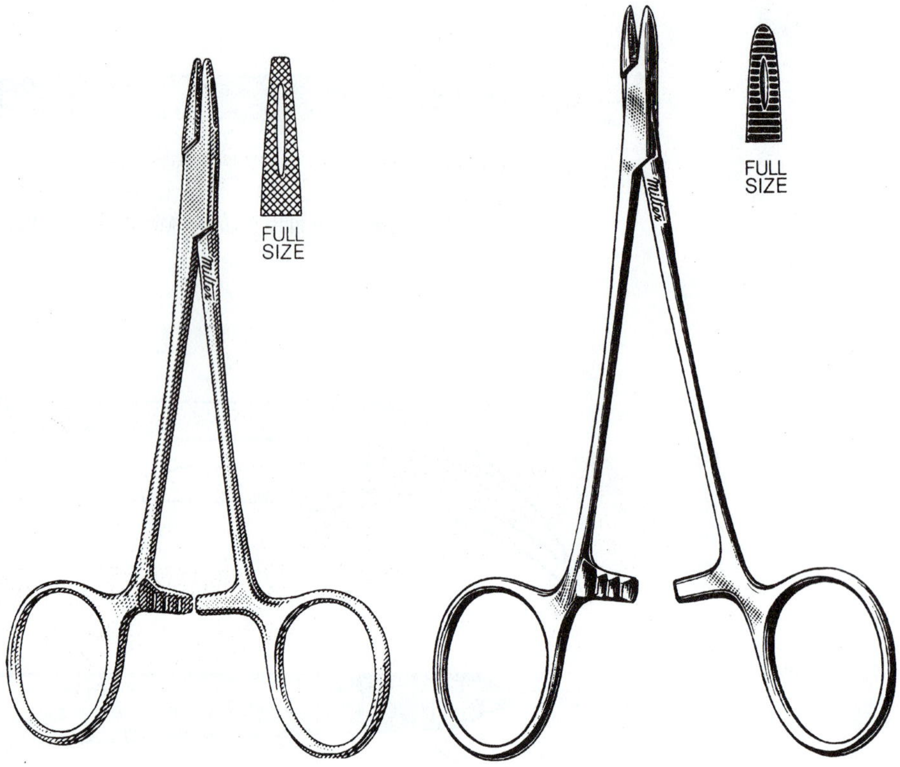

Fig. 56-11 **Needle holders.** (Courtesy Miltex, Inc., York, PA.)

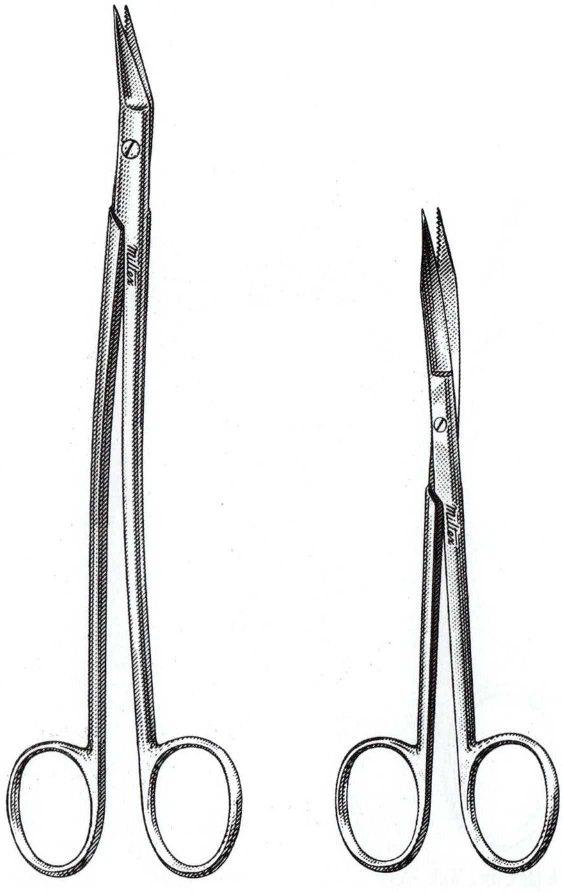

Fig. 56-12 **Surgical scissors.** (Courtesy Miltex, Inc., York, PA.)

Needle Holder

The **needle holder** looks and operates similar to a hemostat. The beaks are straight with cross-pattern serrations on the surface allowing the surgeon to grasp a suture needle firmly (Fig. 56-11). The handles are held in place by a ratchet action that holds an object until the dentist releases it. This handle design allows the dentist to tie the suture material by using the needle holder without snagging it in the joint of the instrument.

Surgical and Suture Scissors

Surgical scissors are available with straight or curved blades that have smooth or serrated cutting edges (Fig. 56-12). The handles range in length from approximately $3^1/_2$ to $6^1/_4$ inches. These delicate scissors are used to trim soft tissue. Surgical scissors should never be used for nonsurgical tasks that would dull the cutting surfaces.

Suture scissors are designed to cut only suture material. Although similar in design to surgical scissors, suture scissors are sturdier and may have a small notch on the cutting edge of one blade.

Retractors

Tissue **retractors** are used during surgical procedures to handle soft tissue as carefully as possible to prevent trauma that may delay healing. These instruments resemble cotton pliers that have notched tips (Fig. 56-13).

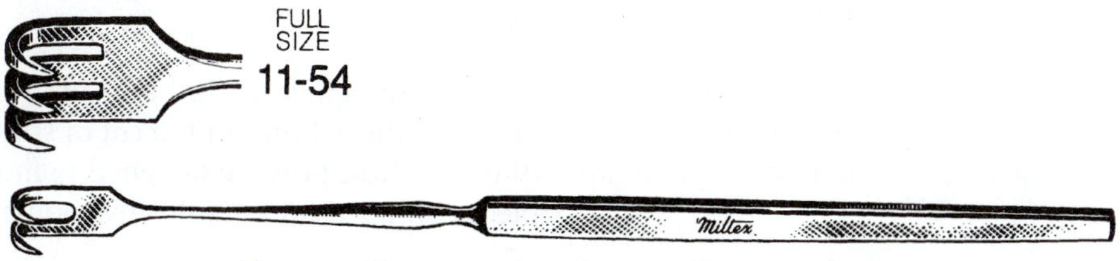

Fig. 56-13 **Tissue retractors.** (Courtesy Miltex, Inc., York, PA.)

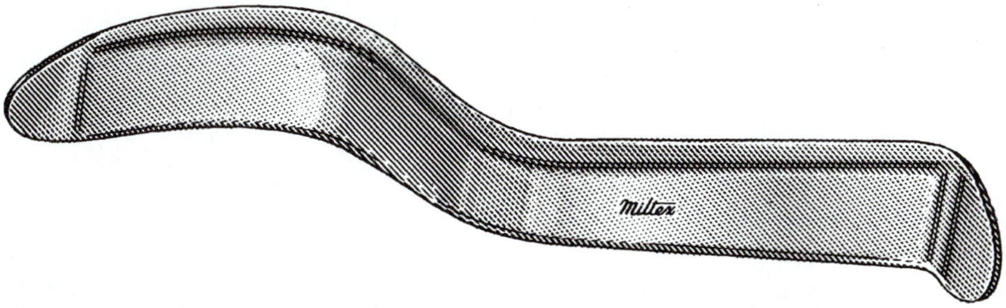

Fig. 56-14 **Cheek and tongue retractor.** (Courtesy Miltex, Inc., York, PA.)

Cheek and tongue retractors are designed to hold and retract the cheeks and tongue during surgical procedures. They are large, curved, angled instruments made of metal or plastic. If plastic retractors are used during surgery, they must be able to withstand heat sterilization (Fig. 56-14).

Mouth Props

During a surgical procedure a rubber mouth prop, also known as a *bite-block,* allows the patient to rest and relax the jaw muscles (Fig. 56-15). The mouth prop is placed on the opposite side of the mouth from that being treated. A patient receiving nitrous oxide/oxygen, intravenous sedation, or general anesthesia should have a mouth prop to prevent involuntary closure of the patient's mouth.

Chisel and Mallet

When there is a need to remove or reshape bone, a surgical chisel and mallet can be used (Fig. 56-16). Surgical **chisels** are available in either a single-bevel or bibevel

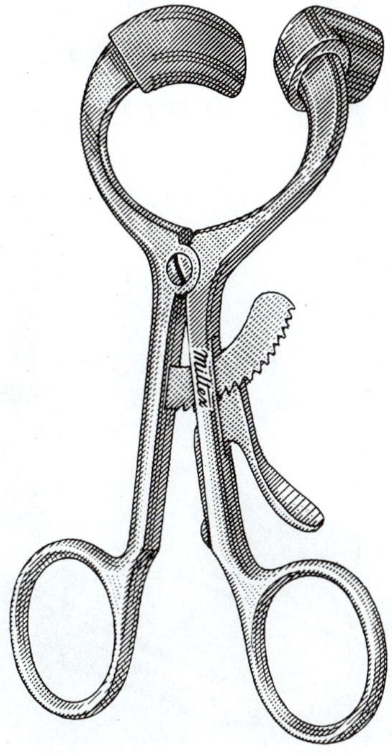

Fig. 56-15 **Mouth props.** (Courtesy Miltex, Inc., York, PA.)

design. The single-bevel type (bevel on one side of the edge) is used for removing bone. The bibevel type (bevel on both sides of the edge) is used for splitting teeth. Some chisels are designed for use with a hand **mallet.** Another type is driven by a surgical handpiece operated by an electrical system.

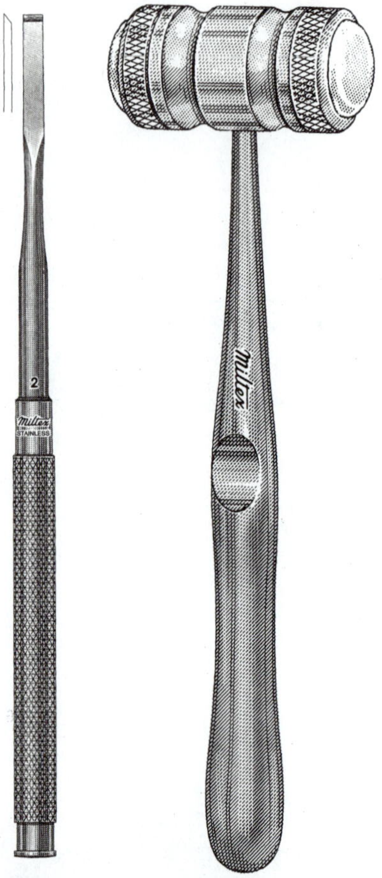

Fig. 56-16 Chisel and mallet. (Courtesy Miltex Instruments, Bethpage, New York.)

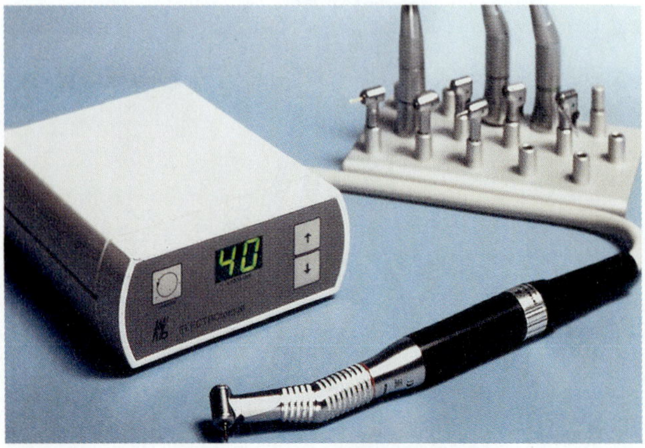

Fig. 56-17 Surgical handpiece.

Surgical Burs

Specially designed surgical burs with extra-long shanks are used to remove bone and to cut or split the crowns or roots of teeth. These burs are designed to fit into a surgical handpiece equipped for a sterile environment (Fig. 56-17).

Recall

5. What does the periosteal elevator reflect and retract?
6. What number is given to the universal forceps?
7. What surgical instrument resembles a spoon excavator?
8. What surgical instrument is used to trim and shape bone?
9. What is the difference between a hemostat and a needle holder?
10. When using the chisel, what additional surgical instrument must be used?

SURGICAL ASEPSIS

You have become skilled with infection-control practices in the general dentistry environment, but when a surgical procedure is performed, the surgical team must take these preventive measures a step further.

Establishing and maintaining the *chain of asepsis* for a procedure requires that the instruments, surgical drapes, and gloved hands of the surgical team must be sterile. Contact with nonsterile objects or surfaces breaks the chain of asepsis and contaminates the surgical area. Once established, the chain of asepsis must not be broken. Because surgical procedures invade open tissue, the surgical team *must* follow a sterile technique. The purpose of this method of asepsis is to minimize the number of organisms that can enter an open wound.

Sterile Field

A sterile field is prepared to hold surgical instruments and accessories that will be used during a surgery. Sterile setups are prepared just before assistants prepare themselves and begin a procedure. If a surgical setup has been opened for more than an hour because of delays or changes, the setup is considered unsterile at that point and should not be used (see Procedure 56-1).

Surgical Scrub

A surgical scrub is used to lessen the chance of infection. Even though sterile gloves will be used for a surgical procedure, the number of organisms must be decreased on a person's hands in case of a tear or break in the gloves (see Procedure 56-2).

Procedure 56-1 Preparing a Sterile Field for Instruments and Supplies

PROCEDURAL STEPS

1. Wash and dry hands.
2. Position the mobile cart behind the patient chair, and place a sterile pack on the tray.
3. Turn the outside wrapping so that the first section of the packaging will be opened away from you.

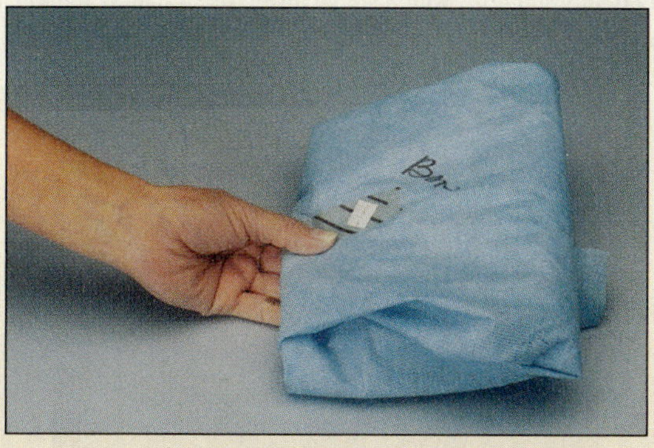

(From Young AP, Kennedy DB: *Kinn's the medical assistant: an applied learning approach,* ed 9, Philadelphia, 2003, Saunders.)

4. Allow the paper to open completely so that the sterile field is facing up.
5. Holding the outside flaps of the internal wrapping, allow the sterile contents to fall onto the tray.

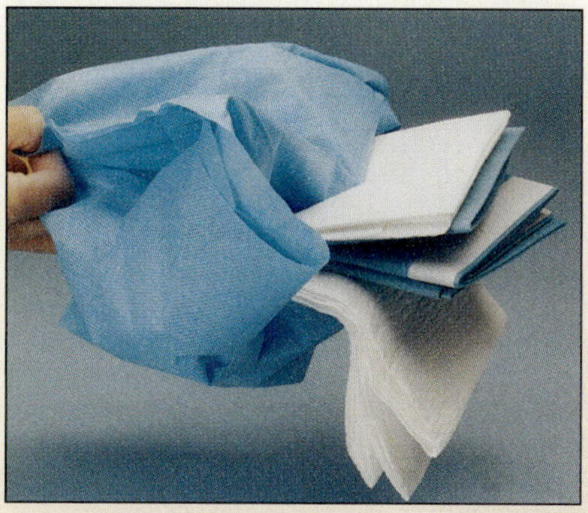

(From Young AP, Kennedy DB: *Kinn's the medical assistant: an applied learning approach,* ed 9, Philadelphia, 2003, Saunders.)

6. You can now begin adding items to the sterile field, such as additional surgical instruments and suture material.

Procedure 56-2 Performing a Surgical Scrub

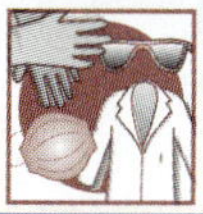

Equipment and Supplies

- Orange stick
- Antimicrobial soap (such as chlorhexidine gluconate)
- Sterile surgical scrub brush
- Sterile disposable towels

PROCEDURAL STEPS

1. Have your hair covered and don protective eyewear and mask before performing a surgical scrub.
   Purpose: Once your hands are scrubbed, they should not touch anything.
2. Remove all jewelry.
3. With water running, use the orange stick to clean under your nails. Discard the stick and rinse your hands without touching the faucet or inside of the sink.

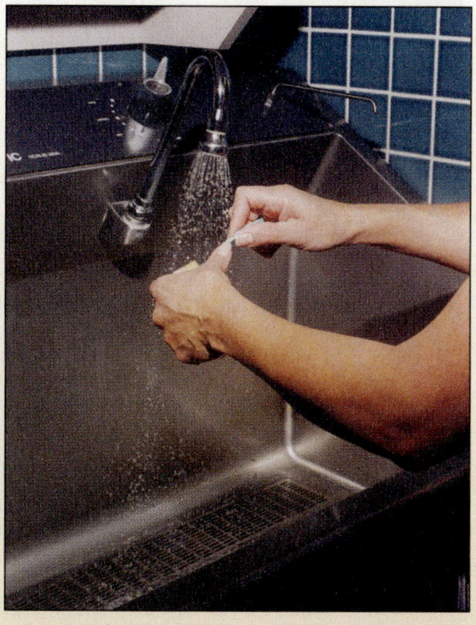

(From Young AP, Kennedy DB: *Kinn's the medical assistant: an applied learning approach,* ed 9, Philadelphia, 2003, Saunders.)

continued

Procedure 56-2 Performing a Surgical Scrub—cont'd

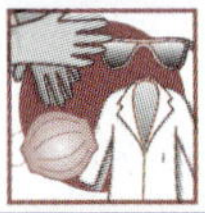

PROCEDURAL STEPS, cont'd

4. Wet hands and forearms up to the elbows with warm water, then dispense about 5 ml of antimicrobial soap into cupped hands.

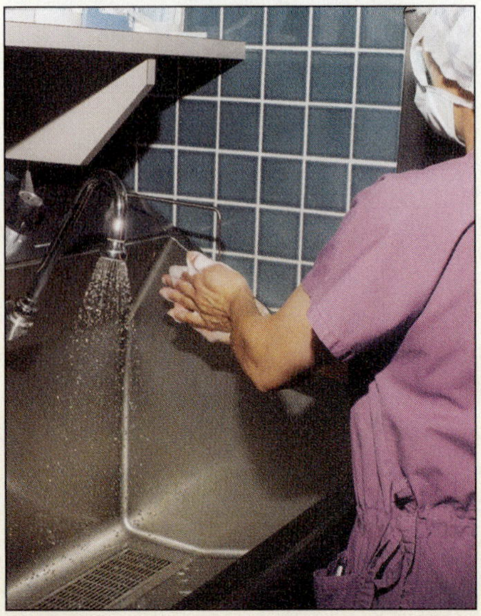

(From Young AP, Kennedy DB: *Kinn's the medical assistant: an applied learning approach,* ed 9, Philadelphia, 2003, Saunders.)

5. Use the surgical scrub brush to scrub hands and forearms for seven minutes.

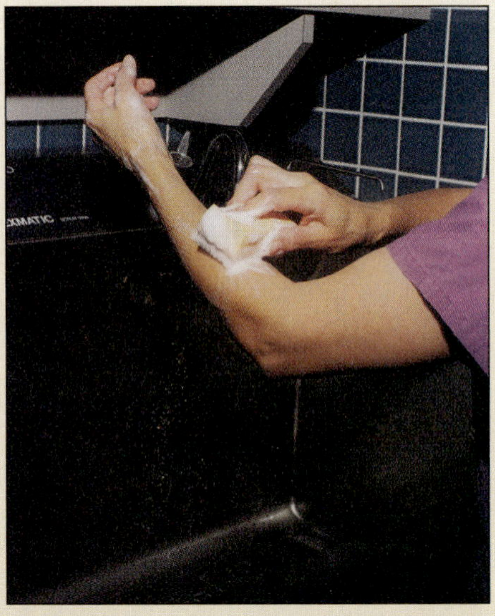

(From Young AP, Kennedy DB: *Kinn's the medical assistant: an applied learning approach,* ed 9, Philadelphia, 2003, Saunders.)

6. Rinse thoroughly with warm water. Keep your hands up and above waist level.
   Purpose: This allows the water to run toward the elbows, keeping hands clean.
7. Dispense another 5 ml of antimicrobial soap, and repeat the scrub.
8. Wash for an additional seven minutes without using a brush. Rinse so the contaminated water runs down the arms and off the elbows.
9. Dry hands and arms with a sterile towel. Use a patting motion, and continue up the forearms.

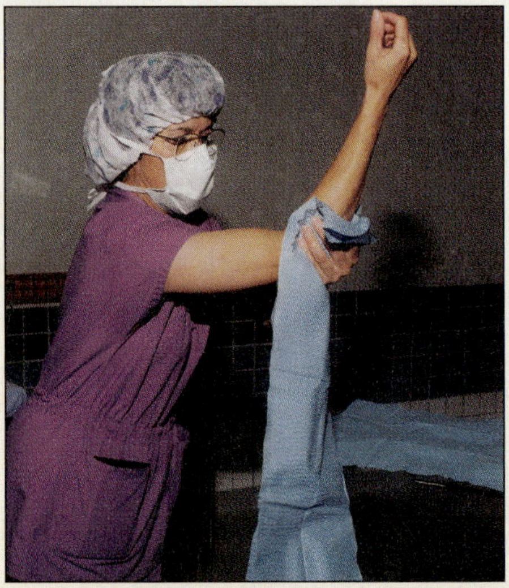

(From Young AP, Kennedy DB: *Kinn's the medical assistant: an applied learning approach,* ed 9, Philadelphia, 2003, Saunders.)

10. Keep your hands above your waist before donning your sterile gown.

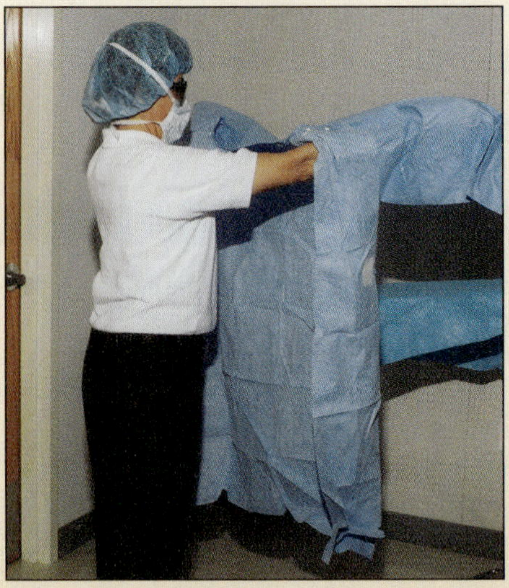

(From Young AP, Kennedy DB: *Kinn's the medical assistant: an applied learning approach,* ed 9, Philadelphia, 2003, Saunders.)

Proper Gloving

Sterile gloves are prepackaged gloves that come in different sizes. When you are assisting in an invasive procedure, you must wear sterile gloves. The process of **donning** sterile gloves is important in the noncontamination process (see Procedure 56-3).

Recall

11. What equipment is used when performing a surgical scrub?
12. What does the term donning mean?

Procedure 56-3 Performing Sterile Gloving

PROCEDURAL STEPS

1. The glove package should already be opened before the surgical scrub. Be sure to touch *only* the inside of the package at this point.
   Purpose: The open glove pack is a sterile field.
2. Glove your *dominant* hand first.
   Purpose: Applying the second glove is more difficult, and you have more dexterity with your dominant hand.
3. Pull the glove over the hand, touching only the folded cuff.
   Purpose: Remember that you want to touch only the *inside* of the glove.

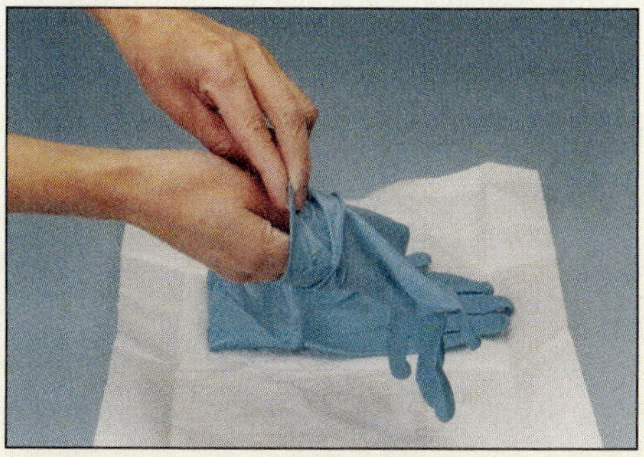

(From Young AP, Kennedy DB: *Kinn's the medical assistant: an applied learning approach,* ed 9, Philadelphia, 2003, Saunders.)

4. With your dominant hand gloved, slide your forefingers under the cuff of the other glove.
   Purpose: You can only touch the sterile portion of the glove with your dominant hand.

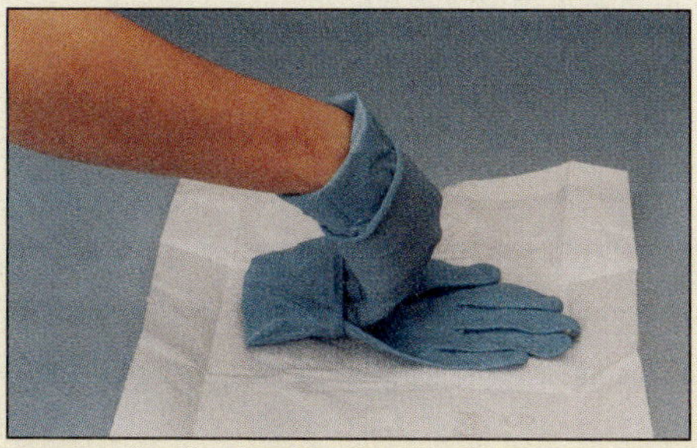

(From Young AP, Kennedy DB: *Kinn's the medical assistant: an applied learning approach,* ed 9, Philadelphia, 2003, Saunders.)

5. Pull the glove up over your other hand.

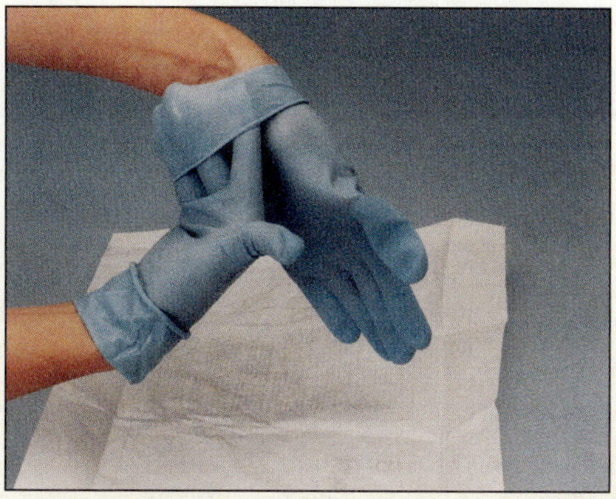

(From Young AP, Kennedy DB: *Kinn's the medical assistant: an applied learning approach,* ed 9, Philadelphia, 2003, Saunders.)

6. Unroll the cuff from your gloves.

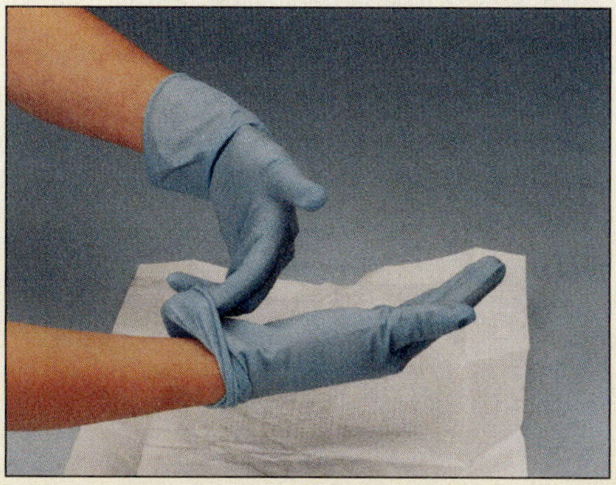

(From Young AP, Kennedy DB: *Kinn's the medical assistant: an applied learning approach,* ed 9, Philadelphia, 2003, Saunders.)

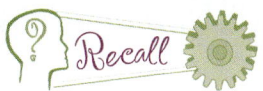

SURGICAL PREPARATION

Whether surgical procedures are performed in a private practice or the operating room, an understanding of aseptic protocol, knowledge of needed supplies, and familiarity with the instruments used for a procedure are critical to the surgical assistant's role. The surgical team will follow a routine each time a patient is seen, and this routine should not be altered.

When preparing for a surgery, specific criteria must be met for smooth, efficient performance of procedural steps. Every surgical procedure requires preparation and advance planning by the dental team.

SURGICAL PROCEDURES

Forceps Extraction

Forceps extractions are often described as "routine" or "simple" extractions. These terms are misleading because all extractions are *surgical* procedures. The use of these terms implies that the extraction can be completed without extensive instrumentation. A forceps extraction is performed on a tooth that is fully erupted and has a solid, intact crown that can be grasped firmly with the forceps. Most "routine" forceps extractions do not require placement of sutures (see Procedure 56-4).

Surgical Assistant's Role in Oral Surgery

Advanced preparation

Check that patient record and radiographs are in order.

Have necessary consent forms signed and available for review.

Verify that any information requested from the patient's physician has been received.

If a prosthesis will be delivered to the patient, determine whether the dental laboratory has returned it.

Verify that the appropriate surgical setups have been prepared and sterilized.

Contact the patient and provide preoperative instructions for taking any premedication and for eating or drinking after midnight.

Treatment room preparation

Prepare the treatment room by placing protective barriers on anything that may be touched during the procedure.

Keep surgical instruments in their sterile wraps until ready for use. If a surgical tray has been set out, open it and place a sterile towel over the instruments.

Have the appropriate pain-control medications ready for administration (local anesthesia, nitrous oxide/oxygen inhalation, intravenous sedation).

Have the necessary postoperative instructions ready to provide to the patient.

Patient preparation

Update patient's medical history and all laboratory reports.

Check that the patient has taken prescribed premedication. If not, the surgeon should be alerted immediately.

Place radiographs on view box.

Take vital signs to determine a baseline.

Patient preparation, cont'd

Seat and drape the patient. (To protect the patient's clothing, a large drape is often used in addition to a patient towel.)

Adjust the chair into a comfortable reclining position. If general anesthesia is to be administered, place the patient in a supine position.

During the surgery

Maintain the chain of asepsis.

Transfer and receive instruments.

Aspirate and retract as needed.

Maintain a clear operating field with adequate light.

Monitor patient's vital signs.

Steady the patient's head and mandible if necessary during the use of a mallet and chisel.

Observe the patient's condition, and anticipate the surgeon's needs.

After surgery

Stay with the patient until he or she has recovered sufficiently to leave the office.

Give verbal and written postoperative instructions to the patient and the responsible person accompanying the patient.

Confirm postoperative visit as directed by the dentist.

Update the patient's treatment records, including a copy of any new prescription given to the patient.

Return the patient's records to the business assistant.

Break down and disinfect the treatment area.

Transport all contaminated items to the sterilization center.

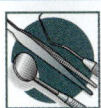

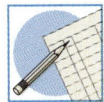

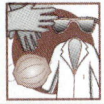

Procedure 56-4 Assisting in Forceps Extraction

Equipment and Supplies

- Local anesthetic agent setup
- Basic setup
- Periosteal elevator
- Elevator (dentist's choice)
- Forceps (dentist's choice)
- Surgical curette
- Sterile gauze sponge
- Surgical aspirator tip

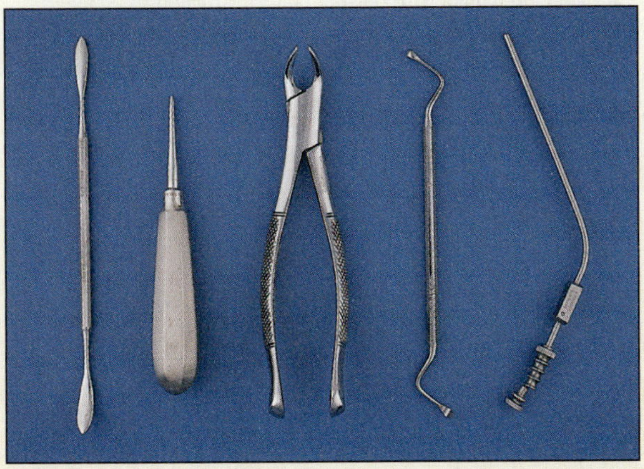

PROCEDURAL STEPS

1. The local anesthetic agent is administered.
2. Transfer explorer for the dentist to probe the area to determine the level of anesthesia.
3. Transfer the periosteal elevator for the dentist to loosen the gingival tissue gently and to compress the alveolar bone surrounding the neck of the tooth.
4. Transfer an elevator (most often a straight) as requested by the dentist to loosen the tooth.
5. The dentist places the beaks of the forceps on the tooth and firmly grasps the tooth around and below the cementoenamel junction.

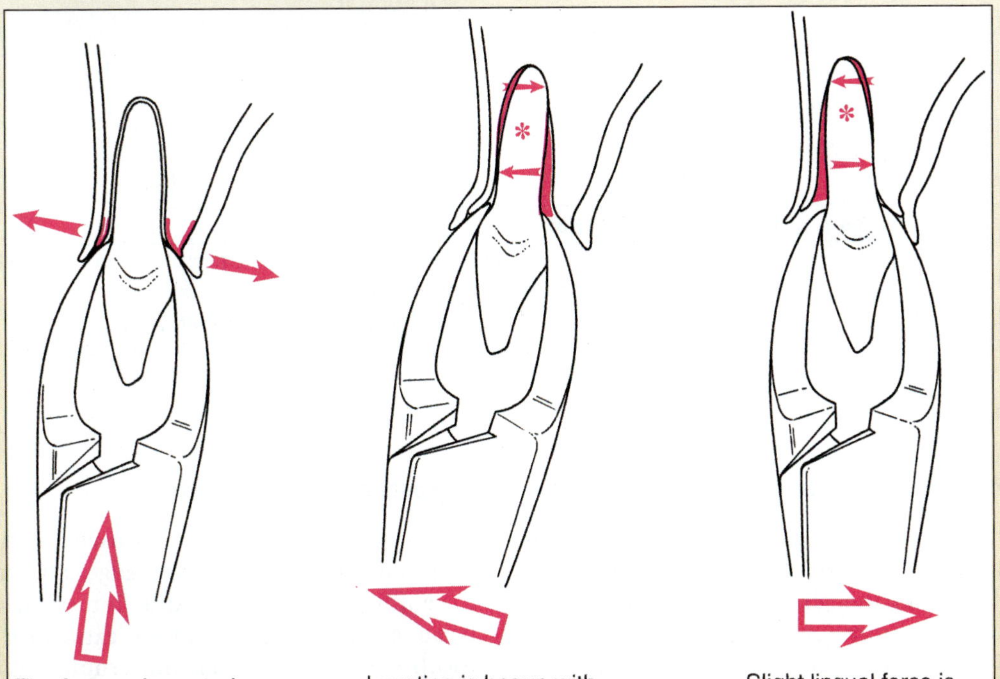
The forceps is seated as far apically as possible.
Luxation is begun with labial force.
Slight lingual force is used.

(From Peterson LJ, et al.: *Contemporary oral and maxillofacial surgery,* ed 4, St Louis, 2003, Mosby.)

continued

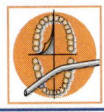

Procedure 56-4 Assisting in Forceps Extraction—cont'd

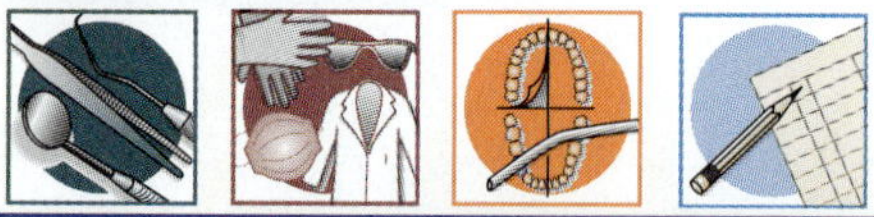

PROCEDURAL STEPS, cont'd

6. The tooth is luxated in the socket to compress the bone and enlarge the socket. When this is complete, the tooth can be freely lifted from the socket.

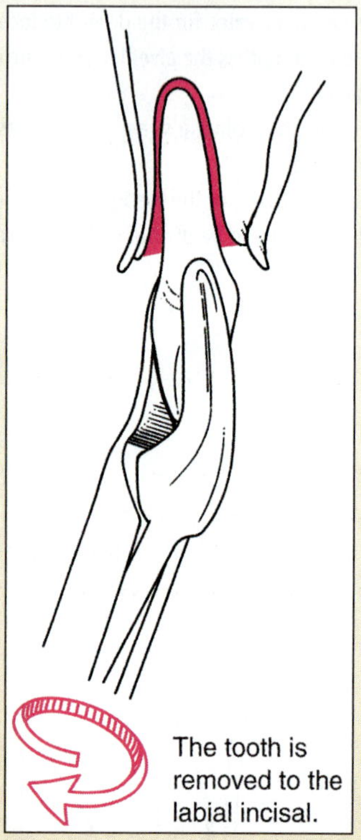

The tooth is
removed to the
labial incisal.

(From Peterson LJ, et al.: *Contemporary oral and maxillofacial surgery*, ed 4, St Louis, 2003, Mosby.)

7. The dentist examines the tooth to ensure the root is intact.
8. When the tooth is removed, use the aspirating tip to debride the surgical site.
9. Fold several sterile gauze sponges into a tight pad to form a pressure pack. Retract the cheek, and place the folded gauze over the extraction site.
10. Instruct the patient to bite firmly on the pack for at least 30 minutes.
    Purpose: This pressure aids in control of bleeding and in blood clotting.
11. Slowly move the dental chair to an upright position.
12. Provide the patient with postoperative instructions.

Date	Tooth	Surface	Charting Notes
8/26/05	4	—	Extraction, 2 carpules Xylocaine 1/50,000. Pt tolerated procedure well, Postop instructions given. Pt instructed to return in 1 week. T. Clark, CDA/L. Stewart, DDS

Multiple Extractions and Alveoplasty

A multiple extraction procedure is most commonly indicated when a patient will be receiving a partial denture, full denture, or implants. Even though the teeth are fully erupted and the procedure is a routine forceps extraction procedure, the end result of the patient's alveolar ridge changes the completion of the procedure. When several teeth have been extracted, the alveolar crest is still intact, and the surgeon must perform an **alveoplasty** to contour and smooth the affected area (see Procedure 56-5).

Removal of Impacted Teeth

The term *complex extraction* is used when conditions require additional skill, knowledge, and instrumentation to remove a tooth. The extraction of an impacted tooth is an example of a complex extraction. An **impacted tooth** is a tooth that has not erupted. A **soft tissue impaction** indicates that the tooth is under the gingival tissue. A **hard tissue impaction** indicates that the tooth is partially or totally covered by tissue and bone (see Procedure 56-6).

Procedure 56-5 Assisting in Multiple Extraction and Alveoplasty

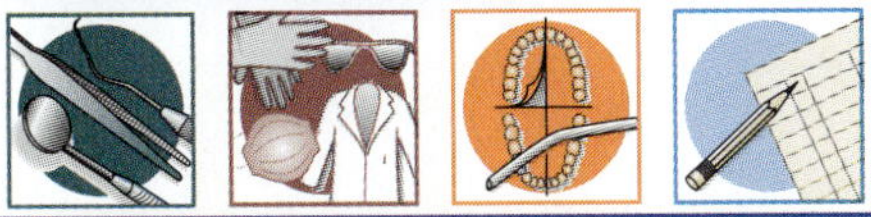

Equipment and Supplies

- Forceps extraction setup
- Additional elevators and forceps (dentist's choice)
- Rongeur
- Curettes
- Bone file
- Scalpel
- Suture material and needle
- Needle holder or hemostat
- Suture scissors
- Sterile saline solution

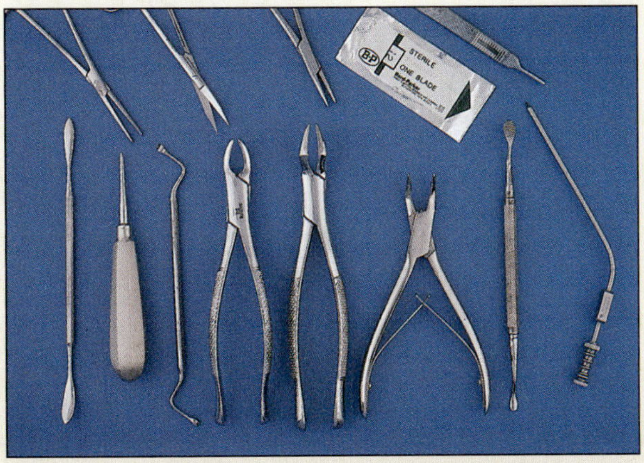

PROCEDURAL STEPS

1. Follow steps 1 through 9 in **Assisting in Forceps Extraction** (see Procedure 56-4) until all teeth have been extracted.
2. After the teeth have been extracted, the dentist uses the rongeur to trim the alveolus. After each cut with the rongeur, have a sterile gauze available to remove debris carefully from the cutting ends.

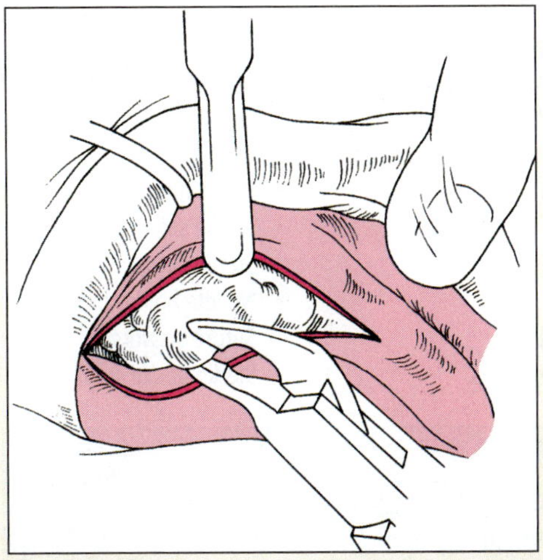

(From Peterson LJ, et al.: *Contemporary oral and maxillofacial surgery,* ed 4, St Louis, 2003, Mosby.)

3. After the rongeur, transfer the bone file for the dentist to finish smoothing rough margins. After each stroke with the file, use a clean sterile gauze square to remove debris from the grooves.
4. Irrigate and aspirate the surgical site with sterile saline solution to remove bone fragments.
5. The dentist repositions the mucosa over the ridge and sutures it into place.

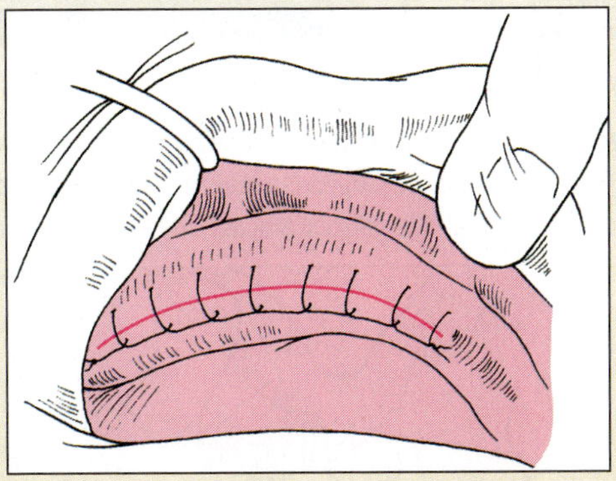

(From Peterson LJ, et al.: *Contemporary oral and maxillofacial surgery,* ed 4, St Louis, 2003, Mosby.)

6. Place pressure packs made of sterile gauze sponges as needed. Provide the patient with postoperative instructions, both verbal and written, and complete the patient's dismissal.

Date	Tooth	Surface	Charting Notes
8/26/05	4-13	—	Vitals: P 90, BP 140/90. Multiple extractions, 3 carpules Xylocaine 1:20,000, alveoplasty, 8 nylon sutures placed. Pt tolerated procedure well. Postop instructions given. Pt to return in 1 wk for suture removal and check. T. Clark, CDA/ L. Stewart, DDS

Procedure 56-6 Assisting in Removal of an Impacted Tooth

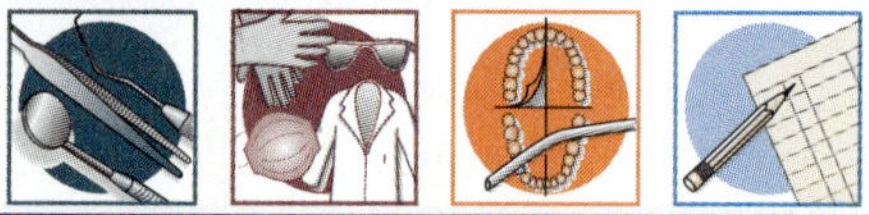

Equipment and Supplies

- Forceps extraction setup
- Scalpel, #15 blade and handle
- Additional elevators and forceps (surgeon's choice)
- Rongeur
- Bone file
- Curettes
- Root tip picks
- Surgical scissors
- Conventional high-speed handpiece with surgical bur or mallet and chisel
- Irrigating syringe
- Sterile saline solution
- Sterile suture material and needle
- Needle holder or hemostat
- Suture scissors
- Sterile gauze sponges

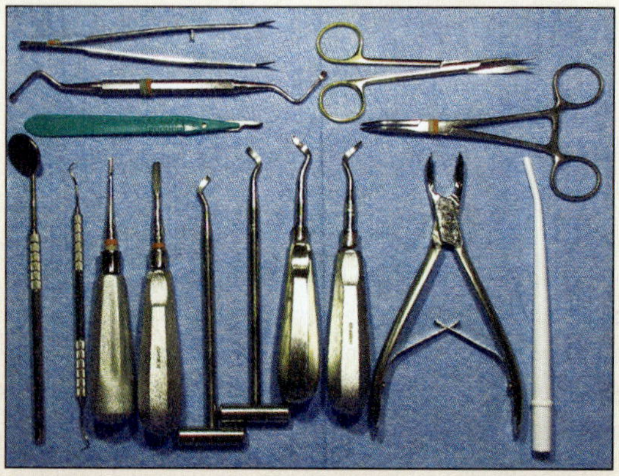

PROCEDURAL STEPS

Surgical Preparation

1. The surgeon determines that adequate anesthesia has been achieved.
2. Transfer the scalpel for the surgeon to make the initial incision along the ridge through both the gingival mucosa and the periosteum.

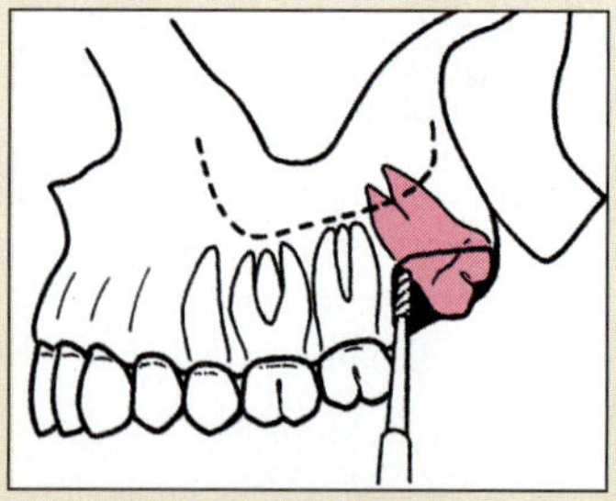

(From Peterson LJ, et al.: *Contemporary oral and maxillofacial surgery,* ed 4, St Louis, 2003, Mosby.)

3. The periosteal elevator is used to retract the tissues away from the bone.
4. Once the incision is made, continuously evacuate blood, debris, and saliva from the surgical site.
5. A surgical mallet and chisel or a surgical handpiece with surgical burs will be used to remove the bony covering from the impacted tooth.

Removing the Impacted Tooth

1. When the surgeon has uncovered the impacted tooth, it can be luxated and lifted from the alveolus with an elevator or extraction forceps.

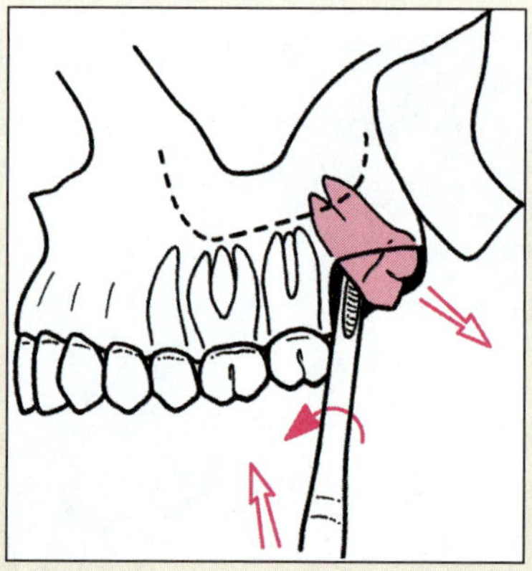

(From Peterson LJ, et al.: *Contemporary oral and maxillofacial surgery,* ed 4, St Louis, 2003, Mosby.)

2. In some cases the tooth is lodged between bone and another tooth. This may necessitate sectioning the crown of the impacted tooth with the mallet and chisel or a surgical bur.
3. After the tooth has been removed, the surgical site is curetted, irrigated, and evacuated to remove all debris and infectious material.
4. After a thorough debridement, the surgeon returns the mucoperiosteal flap to its normal position over the wound and sutures it into place.
5. Return the patient slowly to an upright position.
6. Provide the patient with postoperative instructions.

Date	Tooth	Surface	Charting Notes
8/26/05	17, 32	—	Vitals: P 80, BP 130/82. Extraction, N_2O sedation, 4 carpules Xylocaine 1:20,000; incision using #12 blade, teeth removed in sections; 2 gut sutures placed per site. Pt tolerated procedure well. Pt to return in 1 wk. Postop instructions given. T. Clark, CDA/L. Stewart, DDS

Biopsy

A *biopsy* is a process in which tissue is removed and examined to distinguish malignancies *(cancerous)* from other nonmalignant *(noncancerous)* lesions in the oral cavity. The three most common biopsy procedures used in dentistry are incisional biopsy, excisional biopsy, and exfoliative biopsy.

Incisional Biopsy

When a lesion is located in an area that would be cosmetically or functionally impaired by surgery, an **incisional biopsy** often is indicated. An incisional biopsy is also indicated when the lesion is larger than 1 cm in all dimensions. The surgeon cuts a wedge of tissue from the lesion, along with some normal tissue to be used for comparison. Complete surgical removal of the lesion is not performed until a final diagnosis of the type of lesion is made.

Excisional Biopsy

An **excisional biopsy** involves the removal of the entire lesion plus some adjacent normal tissue. This procedure is ideal for small lesions when complete removal would not create esthetic or functional problems. For example, a small, nonhealing sore on the labial mucosa may be completely removed during the biopsy.

Exfoliative Biopsy

An **exfoliative biopsy** is a nonsurgical technique that is becoming more accepted by dental practitioners. A sterile flat-ended brush is used to gather the surface cells from a suspect oral lesion (Fig. 56-18). The cutting edges of the brush are placed against the lesion and rotated several times. The cells are spread onto a glass slide for microscopic examination or computer-assisted analysis. Exfoliative biopsy is minimally invasive, requires no anesthesia, and definitively distinguishes benign from precancerous and cancerous lesions.

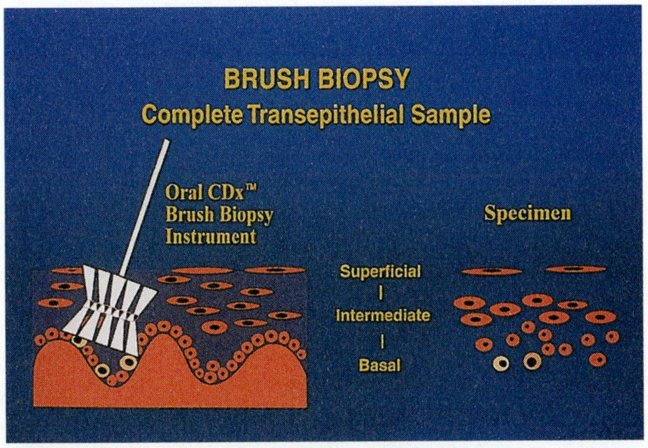

Fig. 56-18 Brush used to gather surface cells. (From Darby ML, Walsh MM: *Dental hygiene theory and practice*, ed 2, Philadelphia, 2003, Saunders.)

Biopsy Results

The pathology report indicates whether the lesion is malignant or benign. Nonmalignant tumors and cysts are removed if their size and location interfere with appearance and normal function. If they do not interfere and do not pose a threat to the patient, removal may be postponed. However, the situation must be reviewed regularly to determine whether the tumor has changed in size or shape.

Informing the patient of a malignant tumor requires kindness, empathy, and special tact from the dentist. In general, this is not done by phone; ideally, the dentist informs the patient in person with a close family member present. A malignant tumor dictates immediate treatment by a qualified specialist.

Recall

13. What procedure is completed after the removal of multiple teeth in the same quadrant or arch?

14. Which type of impaction occurs when a tooth is directly under the gingival tissue?

15. Which type of biopsy is done when a surface lesion is scraped to attain cells?

SUTURES

The term *suture* refers to the act of stitching. As a rule, if a scalpel has been used, sutures will be placed to control bleeding and promote healing. Therefore, when a scalpel is on the setup tray, suture equipment will be added.

Suture Placement

Suture needles usually are supplied already threaded and in a sterile pack (Fig. 56-19). Suture material is available in both absorbable and nonabsorbable varieties.

Absorbable suture materials dissolve and become absorbed by the body's enzymes during the healing process. The most common types of absorbable suture materials are (1) *plain catgut,* which provides the fastest healing for mucous membrane and subcutaneous tissues; (2) *chromic catgut,* which provides a much slower healing, allowing the internal tissues to heal first; and (3) *polyglactin 910* (Vicryl), which is a synthetic absorbable material.

Nonabsorbable suture materials include (1) *silk,* for its strength and easy application; (2) *polyester fiber,* which is one of the strongest sutures; and (3) *nylon,* for its strength and elasticity. Nonabsorbable sutures are usually removed five to seven days after surgery (see Procedure 56-7).

Procedure 56-7 Assisting in Suture Placement

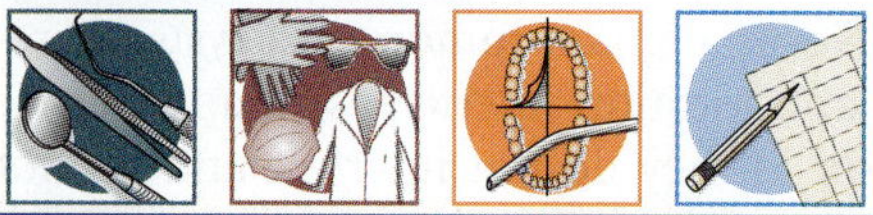

Equipment and Supplies

- Suture material
- Hemostats
- Needle holder
- Suture scissors
- Sterile gauze sponges

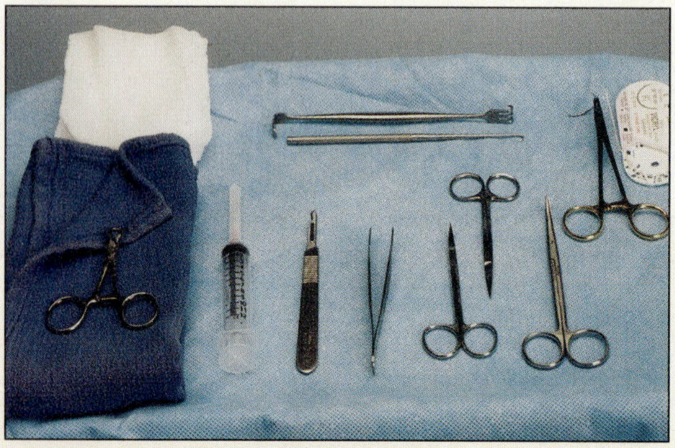

(From Young AP and Kennedy DB: *Kinn's the medical assistant: an applied learning approach,* ed 9, St Louis, 2003, Saunders.)

PROCEDURAL STEPS

1. Remove the suture material from its sterile package.
2. Using the needle holder, clamp the suture needle at the upper third.

Purpose: If you clamp too close to the thread, you may cause the suture to detach from the needle; if you clamp too close to the needle end, you may damage the needle point.

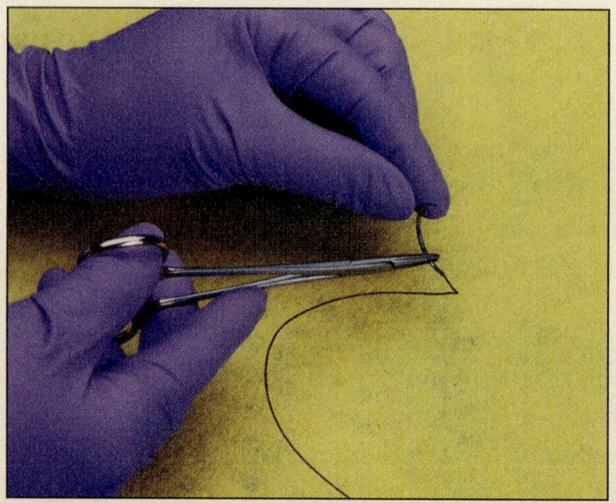

(From Young AP and Kennedy DB: *Kinn's the medical assistant: an applied learning approach,* ed 9, St Louis, 2003, Saunders.)

3. Transfer the needle holder to the surgeon with you grasping the hinge, allowing the surgeon to grasp the handle of the instrument.

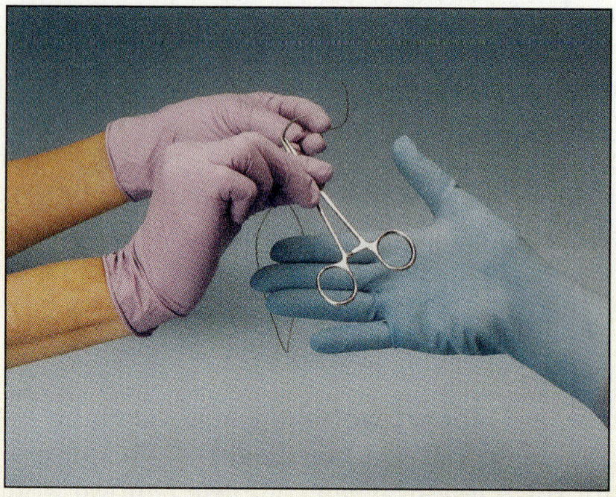

(From Young AP and Kennedy DB: *Kinn's the medical assistant: an applied learning approach,* ed 9, St Louis, 2003, Saunders.)

4. Retract the tongue or cheek to provide a clear line of vision for the surgeon as the sutures are placed.
5. After the tying of each suture, if directed by the surgeon, use the suture scissors to cut the sutures, leaving approximately 2 to 3 mm of suture material beyond the knot.
6. Retrieve the suturing supplies from the surgeon, and replace them on the surgical tray.
7. Record the number and types of sutures placed in the patient's record.

Suture Removal

If nonabsorbable sutures were placed, the patient will be scheduled to return to have the sutures removed in approximately five to seven days. Suture removal may be an *expanded function* in the state in which you practice. If so, there are specific steps in the suture removal process (see Procedure 56-8).

Recall

16. To what does the term suture refer?
17. What are the three types of nonabsorbable suture material?
18. What is the approximate time frame for removing nonabsorbable sutures?

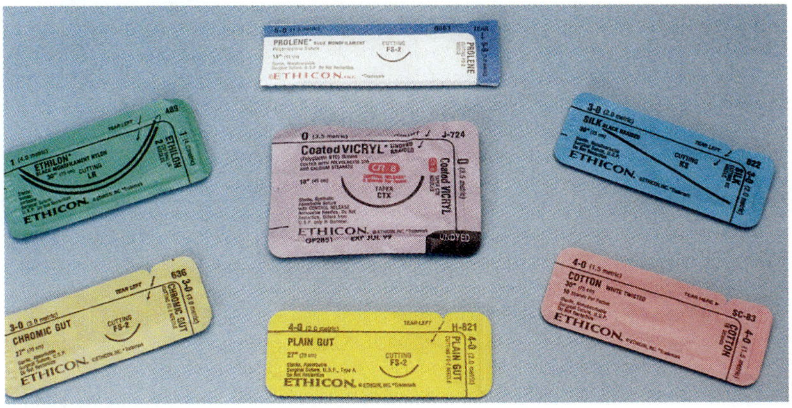

Fig. 56-19 **Types of suture material labeled according to size, type, length, and type of needle.** (From Young AP, Kennedy DB: *Kinn's the medical assistant: an applied learning approach,* ed 9, Philadelphia, 2003, Saunders.)

Procedure 56-8 Performing Suture Removal (Expanded Function)

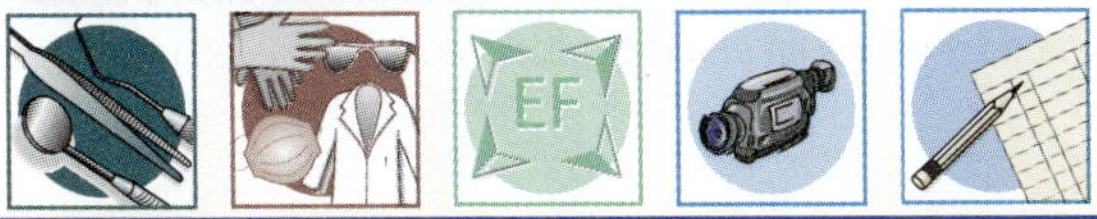

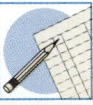

Equipment and Supplies

- Basic setup
- Suture scissors
- Sterile cotton gauze
- Cotton tip applicator

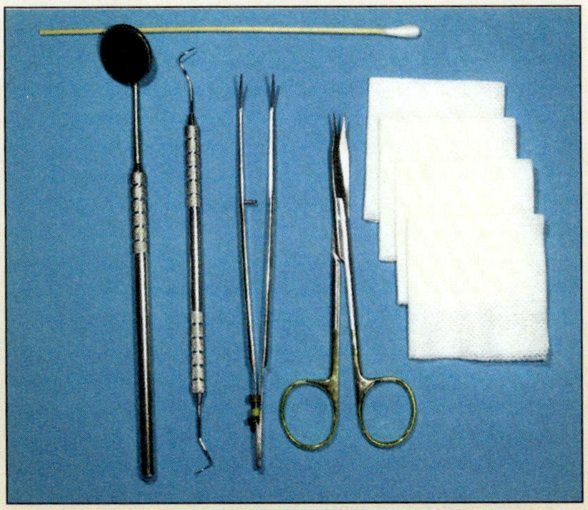

PROCEDURAL STEPS

1. Surgeon examines the surgical site to evaluate healing. If healing is satisfactory, the sutures may be removed.
2. Swab the site with an antiseptic agent to remove any debris.

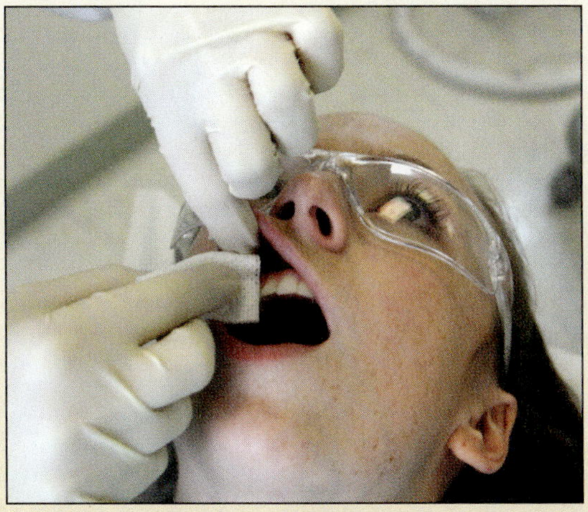

continued

Procedure 56-8 Performing Suture Removal (Expanded Function)—cont'd

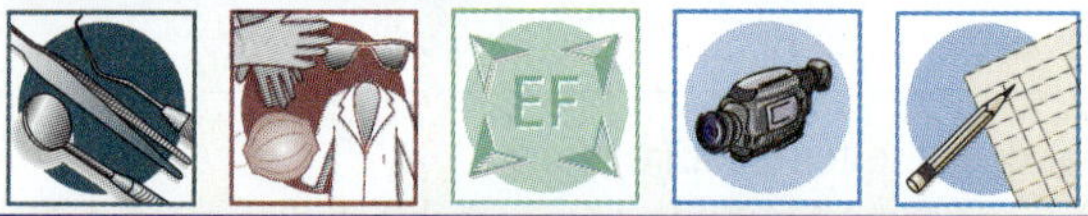

PROCEDURAL STEPS, cont'd

3. Use cotton pliers to hold the suture gently away from the tissue to expose the attachment of the knot.
4. Slip one blade of the suture scissors gently under the suture. Cut near the tissue.

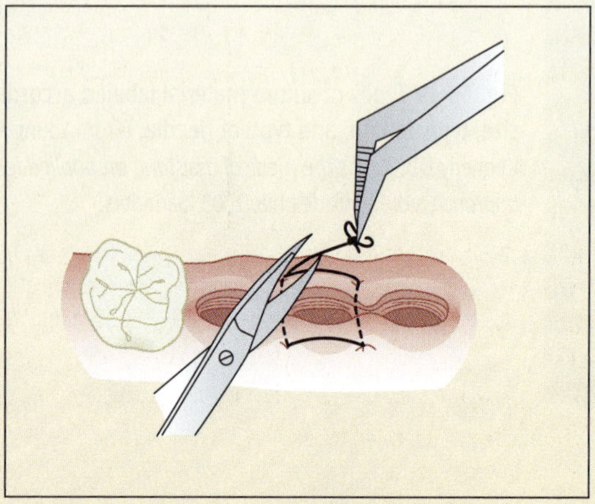

5. Use the cotton pliers to grasp the knot, and gently tug it so that the suture slides through the tissue.
   Note: Never *pull* ("yank") the knot through the tissue.

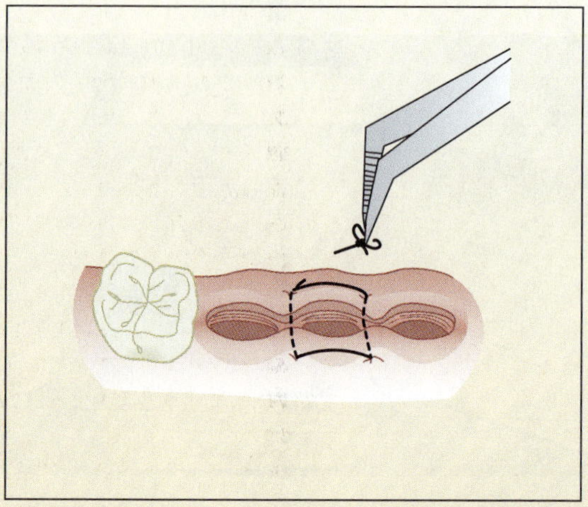

6. If there is bleeding, irrigate the surgical site with an antiseptic solution or warm saline solution. Apply a compress briefly to the surgical site to promote clotting.
7. Count the sutures that have been removed, and compare this number with the number indicated on the patient's record.

Date	Tooth	Surface	Charting Notes
9/3/05	—	—	Suture removal, 4 nylon sutures removed. Pt. healing well, with no complications. T. Clark, CDA/L. Stewart, DDS

POSTOPERATIVE CARE

When a surgery is completed, the patient will be escorted to the recovery area to rest and to allow sedation to wear off. Postoperative care and instructions are provided for the *total* recovery period, not only during immediate care before the patient leaves the office. In addition to the directions from the dentist, the assistant routinely provides the postoperative instructions to the patient and the individual accompanying him or her. Instructions for home care should be provided in writing and verbally.

Control of Bleeding

Immediately after an extraction, sterile 2- × 2-inch gauze is folded and placed over the socket to control bleeding and to promote clot formation and healing. The pack must stay in place to control bleeding, and the patient is given the following instructions:

- Keep the pack in place for at least another 30 minutes. If the pack is removed too soon, it could disturb clot formation and may increase bleeding.
- If bleeding continues and does not stop, call the dental office.
- Do not disturb the clot with your tongue or by rinsing your mouth vigorously.
- Restrict strenuous work or physical activity for that day.

Control of Swelling

After extensive surgery, expected swelling can be controlled with cold packs. The patient is given the following instructions regarding the control of swelling:

- If recommended by the dentist, take ibuprofen before and after surgery to help prevent and control swelling as well as to relieve pain.
- During the first 24 hours, place a cold pack in a cycle of 20 minutes on and 20 off.
- After the first 24 hours, apply external heat to the area of the face to increase circulation in the tissues and to promote healing.
- After the first 24 hours, begin gently rinsing the oral cavity with warm saline solution (1 tsp. salt to 8 oz. warm water) every two hours to promote healing.

Recall

19. How long should a pressure pack remain on a surgical site to control bleeding?
20. What analgesic may be prescribed for swelling?
21. Would you instruct a patient to use a hot compress or cold compress for swelling?

POSTSURGICAL COMPLICATIONS

Alveolitis

Once a tooth has been extracted, healing begins immediately, with blood filling the socket and forming a clot. The clot is important because it protects the wound and is later replaced by granulation tissue and ultimately bone.

Failure of the healing process can result in **alveolitis,** also known as a *dry socket.* This extremely painful condition usually occurs two to four days after removal of the tooth. Causes include (1) inadequate blood supply to the socket, (2) trauma (injury) to the socket, (3) infection within the socket, and (4) dislodgment of the clot from the socket.

Procedure 56-9 Assisting in the Treatment of Alveolitis

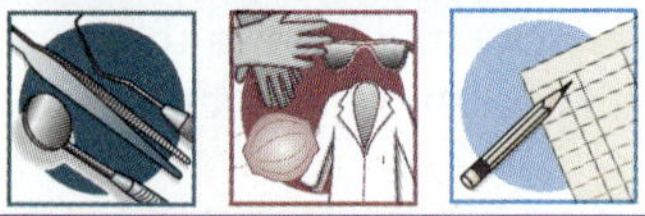

Equipment and Supplies

- Basic setup
- Scissors
- Irrigation syringe
- Warm saline solution
- Iodoform gauze
- Medicated dressing
- High-volume oral evacuator (HVE) tip

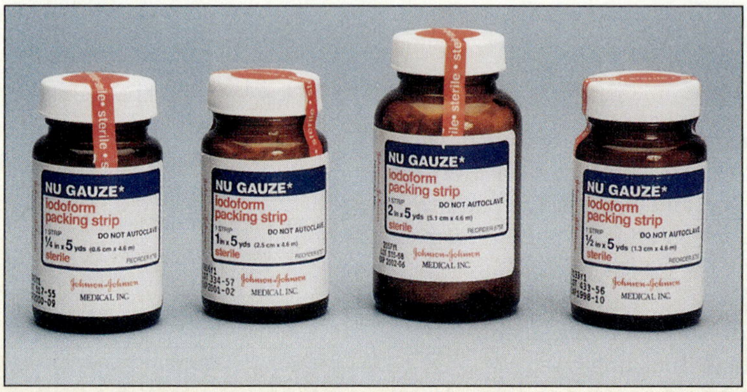

(Courtesy Johnson & Johnson Medical, Inc., Arlington, Texas.)

PROCEDURAL STEPS

1. The socket is gently irrigated with warm saline solution.
   Purpose: To remove accumulated debris from the alveolus.
2. A narrow strip of iodoform gauze is cut to a length to fill the socket.
   Purpose: Iodoform gauze contains a topical antiseptic that prevents infections.
3. The gauze is dipped in the medication and gently packed into the socket.
   Purpose: The medication soothes the nerve endings in the exposed bone. Packing the gauze in the socket prevents food from becoming lodged in the wound.
4. The dentist may prescribe analgesics to relieve the pain, antibiotics to treat the infection, or both.
5. The patient is instructed to return every one to two days to repeat this procedure and to evaluate healing.

Date	Tooth	Surface	Charting Notes
9/4/05	—	—	Pt having discomfort from surgery. Diagnosed with alveolitis. Surgical site irrigated with warm saline solution, iodoform gauze packed into socket, prescription for Tylenol with codeine. Have pt return tomorrow for evaluation and change of dressing. T. Clark, CDA/L. Stewart, DDS

Patient Education

When preparing for surgery, patients have many fears and apprehensions. Some have heard "stories" from friends or family who had the same surgery with a negative outcome. As the surgical assistant, one of your many important roles is to talk with the patient, answer any questions, and help eliminate any fears. Be sure that you are confident and explicit when providing preoperative and postoperative instructions to a patient.

Eye to the Future

The oral and maxillofacial surgeon will become the medicodental expert in head and neck diseases and treatment. No longer will a patient seek care from a medical surgeon regarding head and neck diseases.

Because of advances in surgical dentistry, surgical assistants will need to expand their knowledge and skill to maintain their level of competence. Because more time will be spent in the operating room than in the office setting, it is advantageous for the surgical assistant to acquire additional credentialing.

Legal and Ethical Implications

When a surgical procedure moves from the hospital operating room to the treatment room of a private practice, legal awareness and responsibilities become more consequential for the oral surgeon and the surgical team. Before beginning any surgery, confirm the following with the patient:

- The surgeon has explained the procedure and answered all questions.
- The patient has signed all consent forms, with a witness along with the surgeon's signature and date.
- Another person is present to escort the patient home.
- All postsurgical instructions have been given verbally and in writing.

Critical Thinking

1. You are in the middle of a surgical procedure, and an instrument has dropped on the floor. There is no duplicate available on the tray. What do you do?
2. A patient is scheduled to have multiple extractions and an alveoplasty. What may be the patient's concerns about the procedure? How can you alleviate these concerns?
3. You are assisting in a forceps extraction. List what you would place on the tray setup for this procedure.
4. Which personality traits are required for a surgical assistant? Do you think you have the necessary traits to make a good surgical assistant?
5. Contrast the operating room in a hospital with the treatment area of a private practice.

57

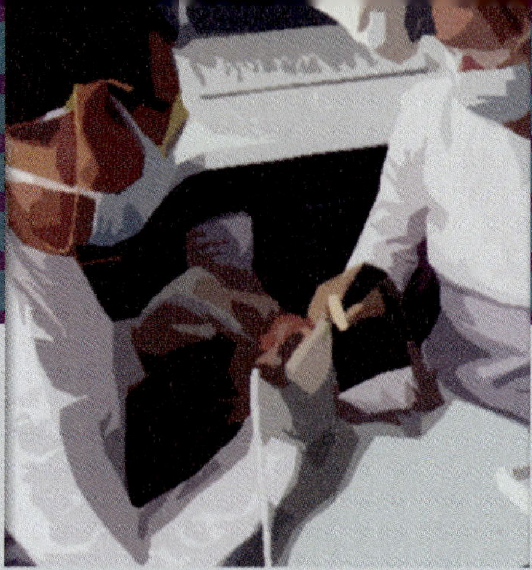

Pediatric Dentistry

Outline

The Pediatric Dentist
The Pediatric Dental Assistant
The Pediatric Dental Office
The Pediatric Patient
- Stages of Childhood
- Behavior Management

Patients with Special Needs
- Mental Retardation
- Down Syndrome
- Cerebral Palsy

Diagnosis and Treatment Planning
- Medical and Dental History
- Initial Clinical Exam

Preventive Dentistry for Children
- Oral Hygiene
- Fluorides
- Diet
- Sealants
- Orofacial Development
- Sports Safety

Pediatric Procedures
- Restorative Procedures
- Endodontic Procedures
- Prosthodontic Procedures

Procedure 57-1: Assisting in Pulpotomy of a Primary Tooth
Procedure 57-2: Assisting in Placement of a Stainless Steel Crown
Dental Trauma
- Fractured Anterior Teeth
- Traumatic Intrusion
- Extrusion and Lateral Luxation Injuries
- Avulsed Teeth

Child Abuse
Patient Education
Legal and Ethical Implications
Eye to the Future
Critical Thinking

KEY TERMS

Analogy (ah-**na**-leh-jee) Comparison of similarities between things that are otherwise unlike.

Athetosis (*ath*-ah-**toe**-sis) Type of involuntary movement of the body, face, and extremities.

Autonomy (aw-**tah**-neh-me) Childhood process of becoming independent.

Avulsed (ah-**vulst**) Torn away or dislodged by force.

Cerebral palsy (suh-**ree**-bruhl **pawl**-zee) Neural disorder of motor function caused by brain damage.

Chronologic age (*krah*-nah-**lah**-jik) Actual age (in months, years) of pediatric patients.

Contour (**kahn**-toor) To shape or conform an object.

Crossbite Condition that occurs when a tooth is not properly aligned with its opposing tooth.

Down syndrome Chromosomal defect resulting in abnormal physical characteristics and mental impairment; also called *trisomy 21.*

Emotional age Measure of the level of emotional maturity of pediatric patients.

Extrusion (ek-**stru**-zhun) Displacement of a tooth *from* its socket as a result of injury.

Festooning (fes-**too**-ning) Procedure to trim or shape a denture to simulate normal tissue appearance.

Frankl scale (**frang**-kul) Scale designed to evaluate patient behavior.

Intrusion (in-**tru**-zhun) Displacement of a tooth *into* its socket resulting from injury.

Luxation (*luk*-**say**-shun) Dislocation.

Mental age Measure of the level of intellectual capacity and development of pediatric patients.

Mental retardation Disorder in which an individual's intelligence is underdeveloped.

Neural (**nur**-ahl) Referring to the brain, nervous system, and nerve pathways.

Open bay Concept of open design used in pediatric dental practices.

Papoose board (pa-**poos**) Type of restraining device to hold a pediatric patient's hands, arms, and legs still.

KEY TERMS, cont'd

Pediatric dentistry (pee-dee-**a**-trik) Dental specialty concerned with neonatal through adolescent patients, as well as patients with special needs in these age groups.

Postnatal (post-**nay**-tuhl) After birth.

Prenatal Before birth.

Pulpotomy (puhl-**pah**-tah-me) Removal of the coronal portion of the vital pulp from a tooth.

Spasticity (spa-**sti**-seh-tee) Exaggerated movement by the arms and legs.

T-band Type of matrix band used for primary teeth.

LEARNING OUTCOMES

On completion of this chapter, the student will be able to achieve the following objectives:

- Pronounce, define, and spell the Key Terms.
- Describe the appearance and setting of a pediatric dental office.
- Give the stages of childhood from birth through adolescence.
- Discuss the specific behavior techniques that work as positive reinforcement when treating children.
- Describe why children and adults with special needs are treated in a pediatric practice.
- Describe what is involved in the diagnosis and treatment planning of a pediatric patient.
- Discuss the importance of preventive dentistry in pediatrics.
- Give the types of procedures for the pediatric patient compared with the treatment of patients with permanent teeth.

PERFORMANCE OUTCOMES

On completion of this chapter, the student will be able to achieve competency standards in the following skills:

- Assist in a pulpotomy of a primary tooth.
- Assist in the placement of a stainless steel crown.

Pediatric dentistry is the specialized area of dentistry limited to the care of children from birth through adolescence, with additional focus on providing oral health care to patients with special needs. The emphasis of the pediatric dental practice is prevention, early detection, diagnosis, and treatment of the child and adolescent. Although many of the procedures completed for children are similar to those for adult patients, pediatric patients require special adaptations and techniques in the methods used (Fig. 57-1).

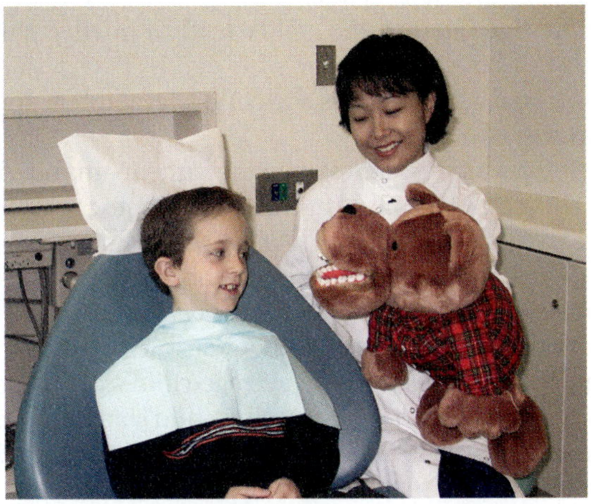

Fig. 57-1 Patient at a pediatric dental office.

THE PEDIATRIC DENTIST

Pediatric dentists continue their education for 3 additional years after dental school in an accredited pediatric program based in a dental school setting. The most important aspect of pediatric dentistry is understanding and respecting young people.

THE PEDIATRIC DENTAL ASSISTANT

The dental assistant in a pediatric setting must have compassion, patience, and enjoyment when working with children and adolescents. Pediatric dentistry provides a clinical practice ("hands on") environment with a more active role in *preventive* dental care. Many pediatric dental offices hire the certified dental assistant to provide the preventive procedures that are legal to perform. If coronal polishing, application of sealants, and taking of preliminary impressions are legal functions within the particular state, these *expanded functions* would also become responsibilities of the credentialed dental assistant.

THE PEDIATRIC DENTAL OFFICE

The successful pediatric dental office displays cheerfulness and a pleasant environment with a nonthreatening decor. Many offices have a "theme" in the overall decor, such as a rain forest, outer space, or even a popular movie character (Fig. 57-2).

When entering a pediatric dental practice, you will notice that the treatment areas are not confining or structured. Many practices are designed with the **open bay** concept, in which several dental chairs are arranged in one large area. The advantage of this design is that it provides reassurance by allowing pediatric patients to see other children receiving care. This can be psychologically effective, because children often are hesitant to express fear or to misbehave in the presence of other children.

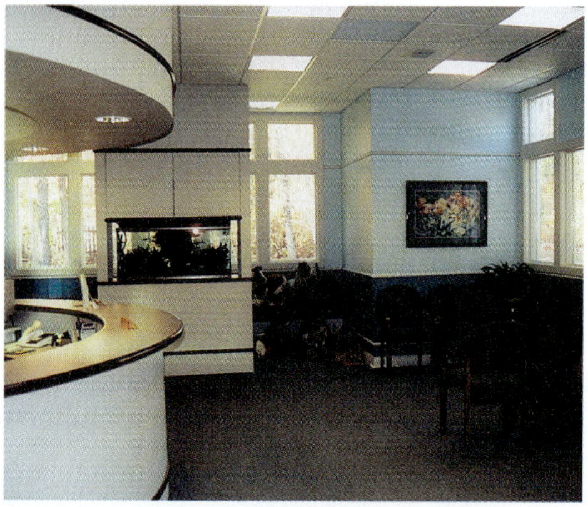

Fig. 57-2 Example of pleasing, patient-friendly reception area of a pediatric dental office.

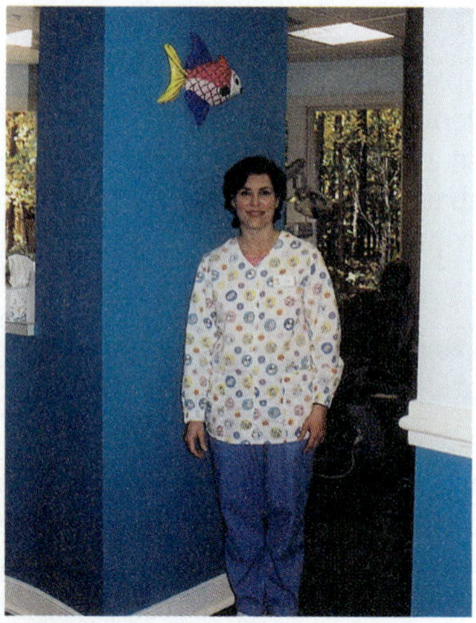

Fig. 57-3 Clinical assistants should dress professionally but in a nonthreatening manner for the pediatric dental patient.

If an isolated area is required for patient care, most practices use a "quiet room." This room is separate from the open area and is used for children whose behavior may upset other children.

A variety of reading materials should be available, such as magazines and educational brochures, for both the pediatric patient and the parent. Some offices will install computer and video equipment with programs intended for patient education and entertainment.

Many pediatric offices are less "medical looking" in regard to how the dental personnel dress. It is common for "scrubs" to be worn in bright coordinating colors or even with a design (Fig. 57-3). Nametags worn by the staff may even resemble a tooth with the assistant's name inscribed.

Recall

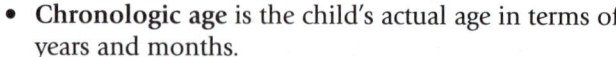

1. Would you expect to see a 17-year-old patient in a pediatric office?
2. What is unique about the treatment areas of a pediatric practice?
3. What types of patients are seen in a pediatric practice?

THE PEDIATRIC PATIENT

Children constitute an important and special group of the dental population. As with adults, children have individual likes and dislikes, as well as fears and complex personalities. The pediatric patient must be treated with the same respect for dignity and individuality as provided to an adult. The child must be understood in terms of his or her chronologic, mental, and emotional ages, as follows:

- **Chronologic age** is the child's actual age in terms of years and months.
- **Mental age** refers to the child's level of intellectual capacity and development.
- **Emotional age** describes the child's level of emotional maturity.

These ages are not necessarily the same in an individual child. For instance, a child at the chronologic age of 6 may have a mental age of 8 (i.e., *mentally,* the child is comprehending information at the level of the average 8-year-old) and an emotional age of 4 (i.e., *emotionally,* he or she is reacting at the level of the average 4-year-old).

A guideline (*norm*) for the average child's development can be used as a crude index to the child's anticipated behavior level at a certain age. A child who differs widely from these norms may have a physical or emotional challenge. However, many children under the stress of a dental appointment may temporarily regress to a more immature level of behavior.

Stages of Childhood

Birth Through Age 2 Years

During this period, children learn to sit, stand, walk, and run. Vocally, they progress from babbling to using simple sentences. Socially, they learn to identify familiar faces and alternate through periods of being friendly or being fearful of strangers. From the age of 1 to 2 years, children have basic fears such as separation from the parent and the related fear of strangers.

These "toddlers" are too young to be expected to cooperate in a dental treatment. It is easier for the parent to be with the child during the initial examination. If further treatment is required, the child most likely will be premedicated.

Ages 3 Through 5 Years

A child of this age has two primary and somewhat conflicting needs. First, the child needs to be allowed to develop **autonomy** and initiative. Second, this child requires control and structure in the environment. Children are able to follow simple instructions, and they welcome having an active role in the treatment experience. The child's role is to help by following directions and "sitting still," "keeping your hands by your side," and "opening your mouth wide."

By allowing the child to have choices, the dental team shows regard for the child's need for autonomy and initiative.

Ages 6 Through 11 Years

This is the period of *socialization,* which involves learning to "get along" with people, learning the rules and regulations of society, and learning to accept them. Through their experiences with others, these children have learned to overcome fears of objects and situations that were once quite frightening to them. They have learned that situations are less threatening than they had imagined and that they need not be afraid.

Examples of Including a Young Child in a Procedure

Ask the child, "Which tooth would you like to start with?"

Have the child point to the tooth that was "smiling for the camera" (radiograph).

Allow the child to choose the flavor of fluoride.

Ask the child to hold the saliva ejector during the procedure.

Behavior Management

The initial examination is important for both the child and the dental team. Remember that this often is the first dental experience for the child. The rapport developed during the initial examination can establish an attitude toward dental health that will last for a child's lifetime.

Many dentists follow a *behavior scale* early in the treatment of a pediatric patient. The child's behavior can then be evaluated and followed with the child's experience in the practice. Dr. Spencer Frankl developed one of the most widely used systems, the **Frankl scale,** to measure a pediatric patient's behavior (Box 57-1).

Guidelines for Child Behavior

The development of trust between the parent/child and the dentist is the basis for a productive, effective means of dental health care. Dental procedures can be accomplished for patients of all ages if the dental team practices the following procedural guidelines in behavior confidence:

- *Be honest with the child.* Make sure what is said to the child is true from the child's point of view.
- *Consider the child's point of view.* Words that unnecessarily evoke fear in the child should be avoided. Also, the child must understand the words that are used. For example, it is better to use a word such as "pinch" rather than "mosquito bite," especially if the child does not clearly understand that a "mosquito bite" hurts.
- *Always "tell, show, and do." Tell* the child what is to be done, *show* the child what is to be done, and then proceed to *do* exactly what the child has been led to expect. The dental team should not assume that a procedure or instrument is so harmless that it will not

Box 57-1: Frankl Scale for Pediatric Dental Patient Behavior

Rating	Definition	Patient behavior
1	Definitely negative	Refusal of treatment; crying forcefully; fearful; other evidence of extreme negativism
2	Negative	Reluctance to accept treatment; uncooperative; some evidence of negative attitude but not pronounced, that is, no sudden withdrawal
3	Positive	Acceptance of treatment; cautious at times; willingness to comply, at times with reservation, but follows directions
4	Definitely positive	Good rapport with dentist; interested in dental procedures; laughing and enjoying the situation

Courtesy Dr. Spencer Frankl.

concern a child. The team should include this "tell, show, and do" process in any new procedure.

- *Give positive reinforcement.* Reinforce and reward appropriate behaviors; avoid rewarding undesirable behavior.

The Challenging Patient

In some situations, a child will remain uncooperative despite the fact that the dental team has used every possible approach to provide a positive dental experience. Treating an anxious, fearful, uncooperative child can be challenging for the dentist, assistant, parents, and especially for the child.

In certain cases, some form of restraint may be required for the patient's protection. *Restraints* are physical or pharmacologic means used to restrict a patient's movement or activity. If the dentist knows restraint will be needed, premedication can be prescribed to calm and ease the patient before treatment. The use of nitrous oxide/oxygen is a method of mild sedation that can help calm a patient for treatment (see Chapter 37).

Physical restraint can be as simple as the dentist or assistant holding a child's hands during treatment. By holding the child's hands, you can prevent a possible injury to the child, dentist, and yourself if, for instance, the child were to quickly reach for the syringe during an injection or for the dentist's arm that is using the handpiece.

Further steps in restraining a child can be taken by using a **papoose board.** This device gently "hugs" the child during a procedure. The papoose board has Velcro straps that fasten over the child and restrain the movement of the child's hands, arms, and legs (Fig. 57-4). This device is excellent for the younger child who has been sedated and thus has less control of his or her movement.

When the dentist takes steps in using pharmacologic or physical restraints with a child, the parents must be made aware and provide consent. An immediate and documented explanation should be given to the parents as to why such actions must be provided. The child should also be informed appropriately.

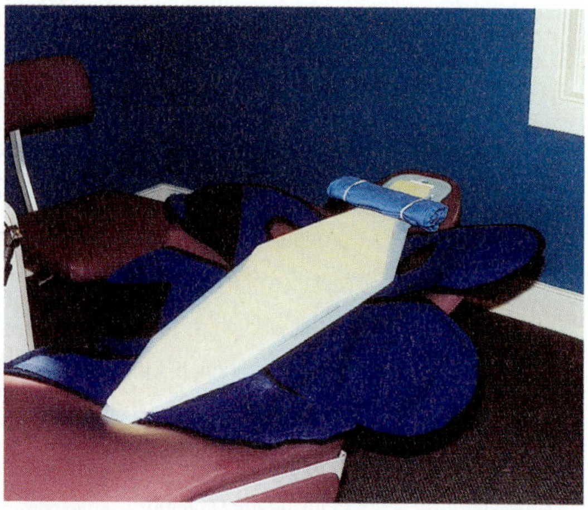

Fig. 57-4 Papoose board is a form of restraint used to prevent pediatric patients from hurting themselves.

Recall

4. Is it possible for a child to be 10 years old but to act like an 8-year-old? If so, what are you describing about this patient?
5. At what developmental stage do children first want control and structure of their environment?
6. How would Dr. Frankl describe a "positive" child?
7. When would a papoose board be used?

PATIENTS WITH SPECIAL NEEDS

Certain physical and mental disorders can slow or challenge a child's psychologic and social growth. When a child has been diagnosed with mental retardation, Down syndrome, or cerebral palsy, parents and families become responsible for maintaining more of their daily physical and oral health needs.

The environment of a pediatric dental office better suits a patient who has been diagnosed with special needs. The severity of each individual patient's disorder dictates whether treatment is provided in the pediatric dental office or the hospital setting. An evaluation of a patient's medical and social history will help determine necessary modifications to the treatment plan.

Mental Retardation

Mental retardation is a particular state of functioning that begins in childhood and is characterized by limitation in both intelligence and adaptive skills. For descriptive purposes, *mentally challenged* persons are classified into four groups that reflect their degree of intellectual impairment: mild, moderate, severe, and profound.

Mild mental retardation describes individuals with intelligence quotients (IQs) ranging from 50 up to 70. These individuals typically develop social and communication skills during the preschool years, have minimal impairment in sensorimotor areas, and often are indistinguishable from normal children until a later age. These patients are capable of receiving dental care in the usual manner. Because comprehension is slow, a patient may require extra patience, understanding, and reassurance. With help from the dental team, a person with mild mental retardation can become a good dental patient.

Moderate mental retardation describes individuals with IQs ranging from 35 up to 55. These individuals will talk or learn to communicate during the preschool years. They may profit from vocational training and, with moderate supervision, can take care of themselves; however, they are unlikely to progress beyond the second-grade level in academic subjects. They adapt well to life in the community, but they need supervision and guidance when under stress and usually live in supervised group homes. A patient with moderate mental retardation will probably require special care in receiving dental treatment, including premedication, restraints, or care while under general anesthesia.

Severe mental retardation describes individuals with IQs ranging from 20 up to 40. During the preschool period, they display poor motor development and acquire little or no communicative speech. In their adult years, they may be able to perform simple tasks under close supervision. Specialized dental treatment involving general anesthesia is frequently necessary for patients with severe mental retardation.

Profound mental retardation describes individuals with IQs below 20 to 25. During the early years, these children display minimal capacity for sensorimotor functioning. A highly structured environment with constant aid and supervision is necessary throughout life. These individuals require specialized dental care, which is usually provided in an institutional setting.

Down Syndrome

Patients with **Down syndrome,** also known as *trisomy 21,* have a chromosomal defect that commonly results in certain abnormal physical characteristics and mental impairment. The mental impairment may range from mild to moderate retardation. Not all the physical characteristics of Down syndrome are found in all patients with Down syndrome. Typically, however, the back of the head is flattened, the eyes are slanted and almond shaped, and the bridge of the nose is slightly depressed. Muscle strength and muscle tone are usually reduced, and one third of these children will be diagnosed with heart problems.

Frequently, patients with Down syndrome have abnormalities in dental development. Eruption of teeth may be delayed, with the primary incisors not erupting until after 1 year of age. Teeth may be small and peg-shaped, often with malocclusion. Periodontal problems are common because of malaligned teeth, mouth breathing, or poor dental care at home. The forward position of the mandible and the underdeveloped nasal and maxillary bones do not provide sufficient space for the tongue. The resulting open-mouth, forward-tongue position gives the appearance of an enlarged tongue.

Dental treatment for patients with Down syndrome depends on the person's psychologic development and physical problems. The patient should be approached in terms of *mental* age and abilities, not chronologic age.

Cerebral Palsy

Cerebral palsy is a broad term used to describe a group of nonprogressive **neural** disorders caused by **prenatal** or **postnatal** brain damage before the central nervous system has reached maturity. The resultant brain damage *manifests* (presents) as a malfunction of motor centers and is characterized by paralysis, muscle weakness, lack of coordination, and other disorders of motor function.

In addition to their motor disabilities, many individuals with cerebral palsy have other symptoms of brain damage, such as seizure disorders, mental retardation, and sensory and learning disorders. These conditions may be complicated further by behavioral and emotional disorders.

Cerebral palsy is most often classified according to the type of *motor disturbance.* The two most common types are spasticity and athetosis. **Spasticity** is characterized by a state of increased muscle tension manifested by an exaggerated stretch reflex. **Athetosis** is marked by uncontrollable, involuntary, purposeless, and poorly coordinated movements of the body, face, and extremities; grimacing, drooling, and speech defects are present.

Premedication is frequently used to help control and relax the patient with cerebral palsy. Along with patience, understanding, and flexibility by the dental team, premedication makes routine dental care possible. For some patients, however, general anesthesia may be necessary.

Oral hygiene in most cerebral palsy patients is poor, partly because of the nature of their disease and the resulting physical limitations. The patient and the caregiver should receive a thorough orientation to a home care program, with modifications as necessary to meet the patient's special needs. Frequently, an electric toothbrush can be used effectively. Special adaptations of toothbrush handles and other aids to hygiene also may be helpful.

Recall

8. What types of skills are limited in a mentally challenged child?
9. What is another term for Down syndrome?
10. Is it possible for a 2-year-old child to have cerebral palsy?

DIAGNOSIS AND TREATMENT PLANNING

The first dental appointment for a child should take place at about 2 years of age. This appointment is scheduled to collect information, introduce the child to the dentist, and help the child feel comfortable in the office surroundings. It also gives the dental team an opportunity to educate the parents in prevention and knowledge of pediatric care. Once dental care has begun, the patient returns every 6 months for recall appointments.

The child's parent or legal guardian must give consent before any dental care is provided for a child under the age of 18 years. Introduce yourself to both the child and the parent, and welcome them to the office. While interacting with the parent and the child, establish a friendly but professional rapport to aid in the development of confidence in the dental team.

Medical and Dental History

The medical and dental history should include information about the child's general medical and dental health background, which is reviewed with the parent and child.

Initial Clinical Exam

Depending on the child's age, the dentist completes a radiographic examination, an extraoral examination, an intraoral soft tissue examination, and a clinical examination, which includes charting of the teeth.

Radiographic Exam

In general, children require radiographs more often than adults. Because their mouths grow and change rapidly, children are more susceptible to tooth decay. The American Academy of Pediatric Dentistry (AAPD) recommends radiographic examinations every 6 months for children with a high risk for tooth decay (less frequently in children at low risk).

A radiographic examination is necessary to make a complete diagnosis. Young children often have difficulty cooperating with the radiographic procedure, which may need to be postponed until the child is better able to withstand the size of the film in the mouth and refrain from any movement. When radiographs are possible, the following steps are helpful in introducing the child to the procedure:

- Use words such as "camera" and "taking a picture" as an **analogy** to explain the equipment and process.
- Use the "tell, show, do" concept. By positioning the film and x-ray unit, you can determine whether the child will sit for the exposure without actually exposing the child to unnecessary radiation.
- Match the size of the film to the level of comfort for the child. In some cases, bending the anterior corners helps for bite-wing placement.
- Expose the easiest films first. Usually, occlusal projections are the most comfortable for the child.

Extraoral Exam

The extraoral examination is used to evaluate the patient's profile to determine skeletal characteristics. Any facial deviation or asymmetry of the eyes, ears, or nose may be symptoms of an undiagnosed syndrome, and the child should be referred to an appropriate professional for a complete evaluation.

Intraoral Soft Tissue Exam

It is important for the dentist or hygienist to evaluate the child's gingiva and periodontium through the use of a gingival score and/or periodontal plaque score (see Chapter 55).

Examination and Charting of Teeth

The initial clinical examination requires the use of a mouth mirror and explorer. Very young children may be hesitant in allowing the dentist or hygienist to place an instrument and instead may allow "only fingers" in their mouth.

The primary or mixed dentition is examined with the occlusion to determine spacing and crowding of teeth. Chapter 28 describes the type of charting system used with the primary dentition.

Specific Information Noted in the Pediatric Medical and Dental History

Medical history

Past hospitalizations and procedures while under general anesthesia
Date of last visit to the physician and current treatment
Medications taken in the past
Daily medications
Unfavorable reaction to any medicine
Allergies, including any prescribed or over-the-counter medications taken
Weight at birth and any problems at birth
Parental report on level of learning

Dental history

Primary concern about the child's dental health
Satisfaction with appearance of teeth
Bleeding gums with brushing
Finger, thumb, or pacifier habits
Fluoride and toothbrush habits
Inherited family dental characteristics

Recall

11. When should a child first see a dentist?
12. If a patient is at high risk for decay, how often should radiographs be taken?

PREVENTIVE DENTISTRY FOR CHILDREN

Prevention is one of the most encompassing areas for a pediatric dental practice. It not only involves the complete dental team in educating the patient and parents but also reaches to the community and local school systems. The role of the pediatric dentist is to communicate preventive dental health in such areas as oral hygiene, fluoride use, diet, and preventive procedures.

Oral Hygiene

Oral hygiene instructions are geared to improving a child's brushing and flossing techniques. This teaching eventually will lead to cleaner teeth and healthier gums, thus preventing decay. By teaching children the habit of brushing effectively twice a day with fluoride toothpaste and flossing once a day, children will maintain proper oral habits throughout their lives (see Chapter 15).

The AAPD recommends a dental checkup at least twice a year for most children (Fig. 57-5). Some children need more frequent dental visits because of increased risk for tooth decay, unusual growth patterns, or poor oral hygiene.

Fluorides

Fluoride is safe and necessary, but only at appropriate levels. Children between 6 months and 16 years of age should have the intake of fluoride daily. Ensure proper fluoride intake through drinking water, fluoride products, or fluoride supplements (see Chapter 15).

Fluoride Varnish

Some patients are more susceptible to decay, and fluoride rinses are not as beneficial. Fluoride varnish has been used in Europe and Canada for many years for caries prevention and is now being adopted in the United States. The varnish is a gel-like substance designed to release fluoride on enamel and root structure (Fig. 57-6).

Diet

A healthy diet is one that is balanced and naturally supplies all the nutrients a child needs to grow. Chapter 16 describes the types of foods that children should eat for normal growth and identifies foods that may increase caries activity.

Sealants

Sealants protect the grooved and pitted surfaces of teeth, especially the chewing surfaces of back teeth, where most cavities in children are found. Made of clear or shaded plastic, sealants are applied to the teeth to help keep them cavity-free (see Chapter 59).

Orofacial Development

It is never too early to start evaluating a child's oral and facial (*orofacial*) development. The pediatric dentist is the first to identify malocclusion, crowded or crooked teeth, and habits that can affect the dentition. The pediatric dentist can actively intervene or refer the patient to an orthodontist to guide the teeth as they emerge in the mouth. Early preventive and interceptive orthodontic treatment can avoid more extensive treatment later.

Preventive orthodontics allows the dentist to prevent or eliminate irregularities and malpositions in the developing dentofacial region. Preventive orthodontics includes the following:

- Control of decay to prevent the premature loss of primary teeth, which may result in loss of space for the eruption of permanent teeth.
- Use of a *space maintainer* to save space for the eruption of permanent teeth (Fig. 57-7). Space maintainers are most often cemented in place and retained until the permanent tooth erupts.
- Use of appliances cemented in place to correct oral habits such as thumb sucking that may be damaging to the permanent dentition (Fig. 57-8).
- Early detection of genetic and congenital anomalies that may influence dental development.
- Supervision of the natural *exfoliation* (shedding) of the primary teeth. If retained for too long, primary teeth may cause the permanent teeth to erupt out of alignment or to be impacted.

Interceptive orthodontics allows the dentist to intercede or correct problems as they develop. For example, a **crossbite** occurs when one or both sides of the maxillary teeth are positioned lingual to the mandibular teeth. Interceptive orthodontics includes the following:

- Extraction of primary teeth that may be contributing to malalignment of the permanent dentition.
- Correction of a crossbite through the use of a removable or fixed appliance (Fig. 57-9).
- Correction of a jaw size discrepancy through the use of a removable or fixed appliance (Fig. 57-10).
- Extraction of primary or permanent teeth to correct overcrowding.

Sports Safety

The fields of sports medicine and dentistry have documented the benefits of wearing protective face equipment during recreational sports that might injure the mouth area. Mouth protectors are an important piece of protective face gear. Many states have regulations that require all athletes in school contact sports to wear protective mouth

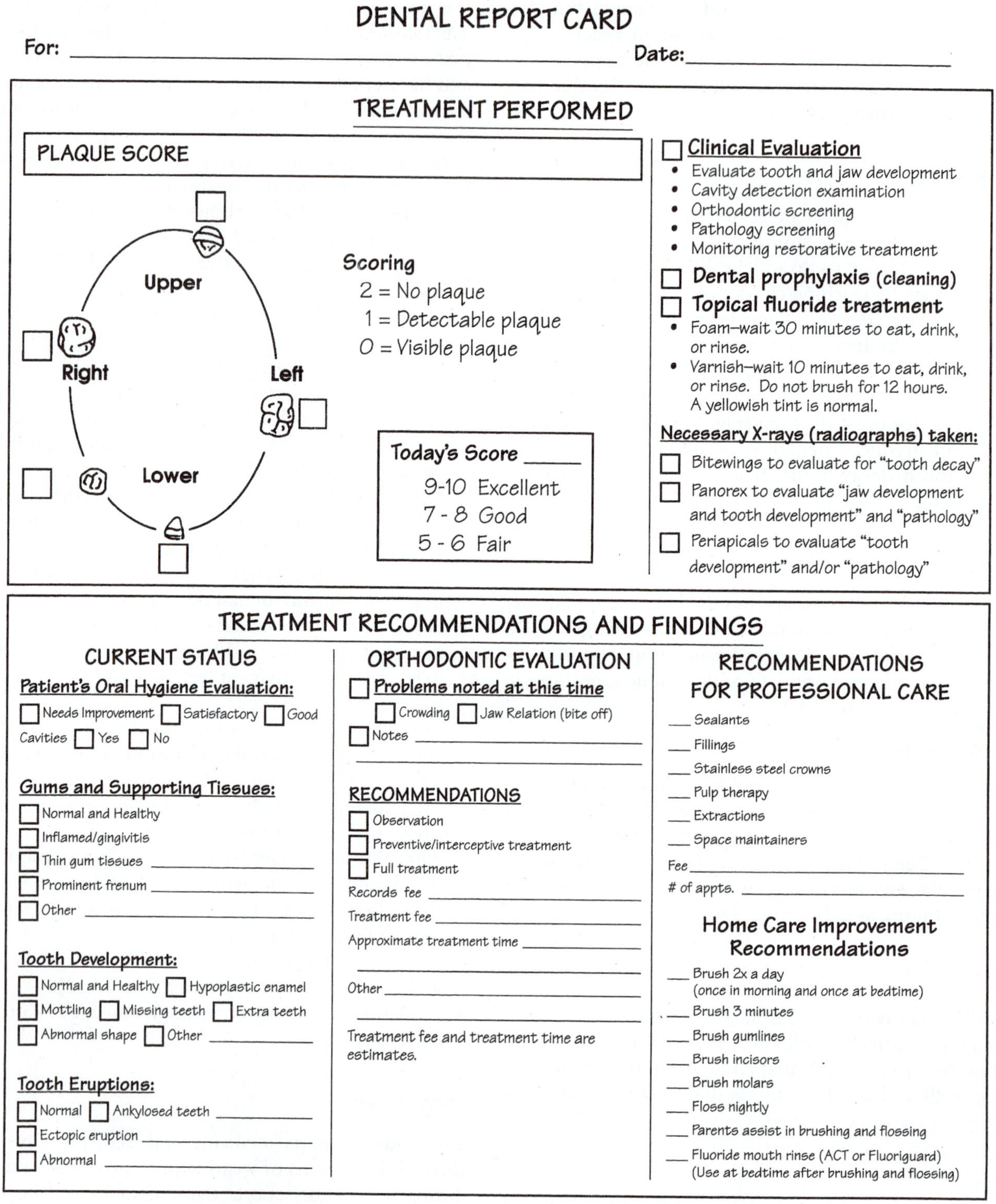

DENTAL REPORT CARD

For: ______________________ Date: ______________

TREATMENT PERFORMED

PLAQUE SCORE

Scoring
2 = No plaque
1 = Detectable plaque
0 = Visible plaque

Today's Score ____
9-10 Excellent
7 - 8 Good
5 - 6 Fair

☐ Clinical Evaluation
- Evaluate tooth and jaw development
- Cavity detection examination
- Orthodontic screening
- Pathology screening
- Monitoring restorative treatment

☐ Dental prophylaxis (cleaning)

☐ Topical fluoride treatment
- Foam–wait 30 minutes to eat, drink, or rinse.
- Varnish–wait 10 minutes to eat, drink, or rinse. Do not brush for 12 hours. A yellowish tint is normal.

Necessary X-rays (radiographs) taken:
☐ Bitewings to evaluate for "tooth decay"
☐ Panorex to evaluate "jaw development and tooth development" and "pathology"
☐ Periapicals to evaluate "tooth development" and/or "pathology"

TREATMENT RECOMMENDATIONS AND FINDINGS

CURRENT STATUS

Patient's Oral Hygiene Evaluation:
☐ Needs Improvement ☐ Satisfactory ☐ Good
Cavities ☐ Yes ☐ No

Gums and Supporting Tissues:
☐ Normal and Healthy
☐ Inflamed/gingivitis
☐ Thin gum tissues ____________
☐ Prominent frenum ____________
☐ Other ____________

Tooth Development:
☐ Normal and Healthy ☐ Hypoplastic enamel
☐ Mottling ☐ Missing teeth ☐ Extra teeth
☐ Abnormal shape ☐ Other ____________

Tooth Eruptions:
☐ Normal ☐ Ankylosed teeth ____________
☐ Ectopic eruption ____________
☐ Abnormal ____________

ORTHODONTIC EVALUATION

☐ Problems noted at this time
☐ Crowding ☐ Jaw Relation (bite off)
☐ Notes ____________
____

RECOMMENDATIONS
☐ Observation
☐ Preventive/interceptive treatment
☐ Full treatment
Records fee ____________
Treatment fee ____________
Approximate treatment time ____________
____
Other ____________
____
Treatment fee and treatment time are estimates.

RECOMMENDATIONS FOR PROFESSIONAL CARE

___ Sealants
___ Fillings
___ Stainless steel crowns
___ Pulp therapy
___ Extractions
___ Space maintainers
Fee ____________
# of appts. ____________

Home Care Improvement Recommendations

___ Brush 2x a day (once in morning and once at bedtime)
___ Brush 3 minutes
___ Brush gumlines
___ Brush incisors
___ Brush molars
___ Floss nightly
___ Parents assist in brushing and flossing
___ Fluoride mouth rinse (ACT or Fluoriguard) (Use at bedtime after brushing and flossing)

Fig. 57-5 Example of dental report card used for recall appointments. (Courtesy Dr. John Christensen.)

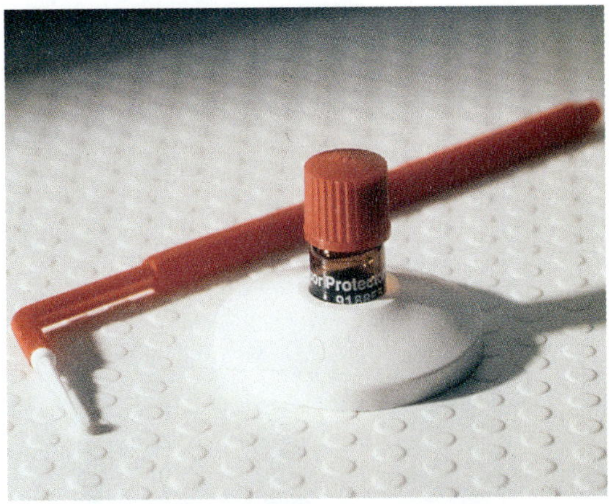

Fig. 57-6 **Fluoride varnish (Vivadent) is a new fluoride system that is being introduced in the United States.** (Courtesy Ivoclar Vivadent.)

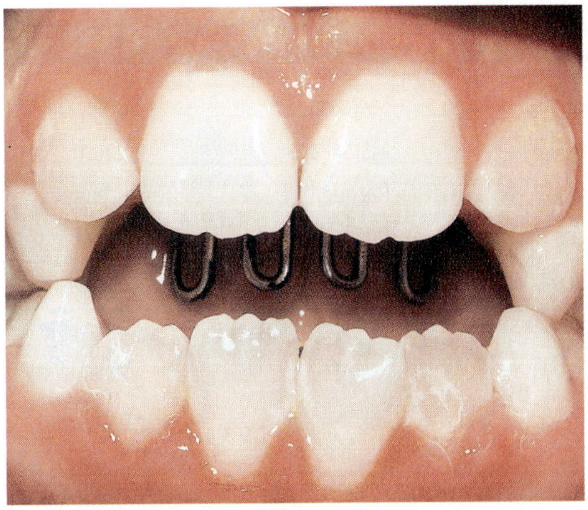

Fig. 57-8 **Example of fixed appliance to discourage thumb sucking.** (Courtesy Dr. Frank Hodges.)

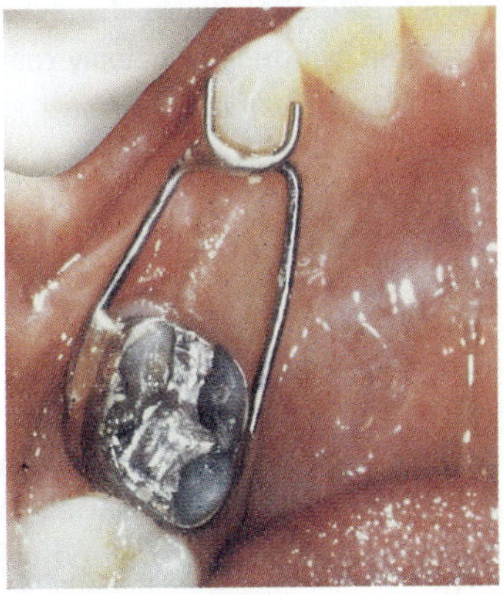

Fig. 57-7 **Space maintainer used to "reserve" the space until the permanent tooth erupts.**

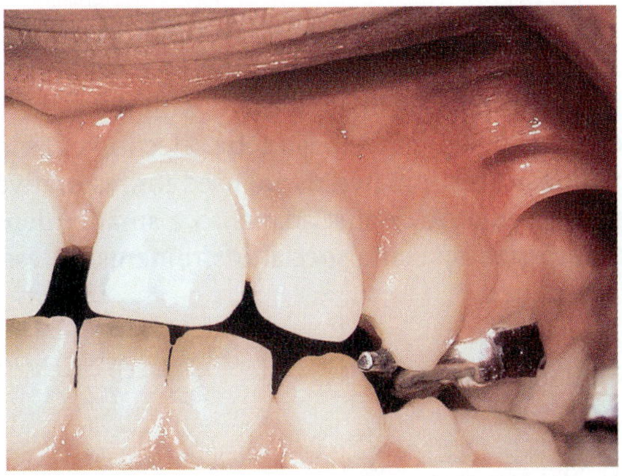

Fig. 57-9 **Example of fixed appliance to correct crossbite.** (Courtesy Dr. Frank Hodges.)

guards to help prevent traumatic injuries to the teeth. Professional athletes in sports that expose them to potential oral injury are required to wear mouth guards.

Three types of mouth guards are used: commercial mouth guards, mouth-formed protectors, and custom-fitted vacuum-formed guards. Custom mouth guards can be easily fabricated in the dental office.

Recall

13. How is fluoride varnish used?
14. What procedure is recommended for children to protect the pits and fissures of posterior teeth?
15. Is an appliance that is placed to stop a patient from sucking the thumb considered interceptive or preventive orthodontics?
16. If you are a competitive swimmer, should you wear a mouth guard?

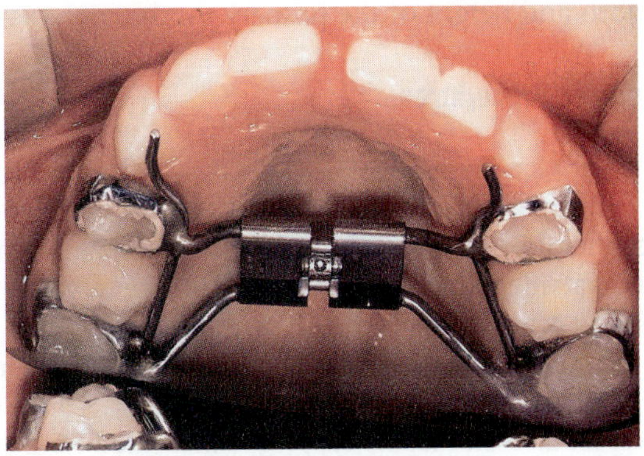

Fig. 57-10 **Palatal expansion appliance used to widen the maxillary arch.** (Courtesy Dr. Frank Hodges.)

Sports Requiring Mouth Protection

Acrobatics	Lacrosse	Soccer
Basketball	Martial arts	Squash
Boxing	Racquetball	Surfing
Discus	Rugby	Throwing sports
Football	Shotputting	Volleyball
Gymnastics	Skateboarding	Water polo
Handball	Skiing	Weightlifting
Hockey	Skydiving	Wrestling

PEDIATRIC PROCEDURES

The basic principles of operative or restorative treatment of primary teeth are generally the same as those for permanent teeth. Primary teeth are charted with the same classifications as permanent teeth, and the selection of amalgam and composite resin materials are used for restorative purposes. The pediatric dentist adapts to a smaller dentition and mouth size by using special instruments, accessories, and techniques.

Restorative Procedures

Instrument Size

Dental instruments, handpieces, and rotary instruments are scaled down in size for use with the pediatric patient. The smaller sizes allow the dentist easier access to areas within the mouth and also do not require the child to open the mouth as wide.

Matrix System

Two types of matrices are used when restoring primary teeth: the **T-band** and the spot-welded band (see Chapter 49). Both of these custom bands are designed to better fit the width and height of the primary tooth.

Endodontic Procedures

Pulp Therapy

Pulp therapy is an attempt to stimulate and preserve pulpal regeneration in primary teeth. The two most common factors that affect the pulpal health of young teeth are deep caries and traumatic injuries. Deep caries is much more likely to affect the posterior teeth, and trauma is much more likely to affect the anterior teeth.

Indirect and direct *pulp capping* is indicated for a young permanent tooth to promote pulpal healing and stimulate the production of reparative dentin (see Chapter 54).

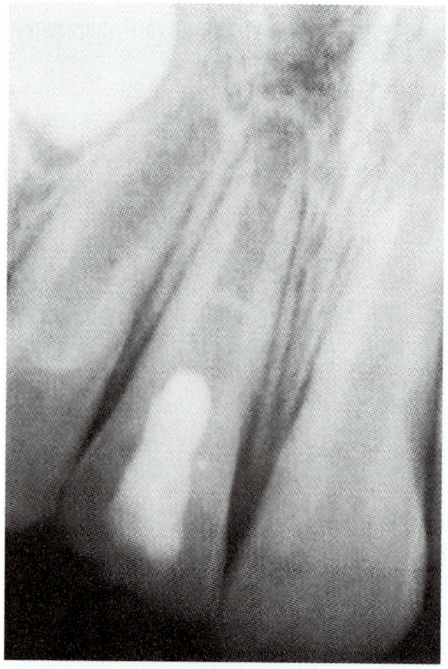

Fig. 57-11 A deep calcium hydroxide pulpotomy completed on central incisor. (From Cohen S, Burns R: *Pathways of the pulp,* ed 8, St Louis, 2002, Mosby.)

Pulpotomy

Pulpotomy is the complete removal of the coronal portion of the dental pulp. The goal of this procedure is to remove the portion of the pulp that is inflamed but to maintain the healthy vital pulp tissue in the canals of the primary tooth. A pulpotomy can be accomplished using two different types of medicaments.

The *formocresol pulpotomy* is the procedure most often used for primary teeth. This medicament is a 50:50 formulation of 19 percent formaldehyde and 35 percent cresol in an aqueous glycerin solution (see Procedure 57-1).

The *calcium hydroxide pulpotomy* is used primarily for young permanent teeth with open apices (Fig. 57-11). A common indication on the fractured tooth is significant exposure of the pulp. This type of treatment allows continued apical development so that endodontic treatment can be performed later.

Prosthodontic Procedures

Stainless Steel Crown

Because of the importance of maintaining primary teeth throughout adolescent years, the dentist requires a crown system to cover severely decayed and endodontically treated teeth without the cost and time investment of a fixed prosthesis. A stainless steel crown is the restoration of choice for the following reasons:

- Stainless steel crowns can be prepared and placed at a single appointment, which is especially important in young children, patients with behavioral problems, and patients with special needs.

Procedure 57-1 Assisting in Pulpotomy of a Primary Tooth

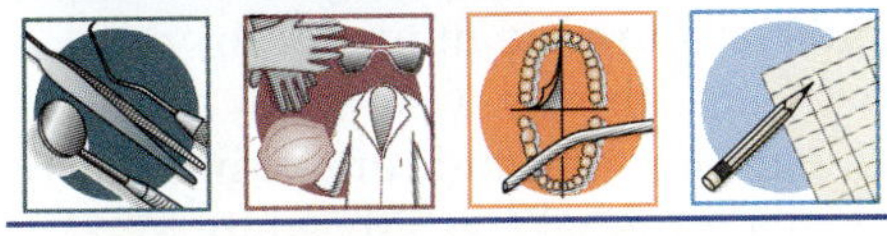

Equipment and Supplies

- Local anesthetic agent setup
- Basic setup
- Dental dam setup
- Low-speed handpiece
- Round burs
- Spoon excavators (various sizes)
- Sterile cotton pellets
- Formocresol
- Zinc oxide–eugenol (ZOE) base
- Final restorative material and instruments for placement

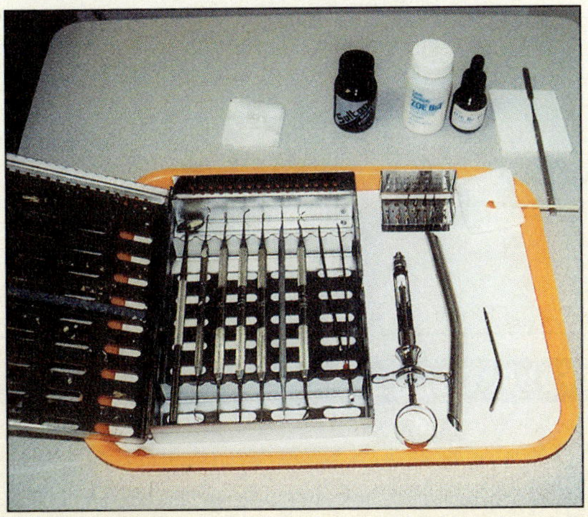

PROCEDURAL STEPS

1. The local anesthetic agent is administered.
2. The dental dam is placed.
3. The dentist will use a round bur in the low-speed handpiece to remove the dental caries and expose the pulp chamber.
4. Transfer a spoon excavator for the dentist to remove all pulp tissue inside the coronal chamber.
5. Transfer a sterile cotton pellet moistened with the formocresol for the dentist to place in the pulp chamber for approximately 5 minutes to control hemorrhaging.
6. Once bleeding is controlled, the pulp chamber is filled with ZOE paste, to which a drop of formocresol has been added.
7. The ZOE base and final restoration are placed.

Date	Tooth	Surface	Charting Notes
9/4/05	C	—	Pulpotomy, 1 carpule Xylocaine, 1:100,000 w/o epi. Dam isolation, tooth opened, formocresol placed. ZOE base, amalgam. Pt tolerated procedure well. T. Clark, CDA/L. Stewart, DDS

- The crowns are sufficiently durable to last until the primary teeth are replaced with the permanent teeth.
- The crowns are almost always well tolerated by the gingivae of young patients.
- Stainless steel crowns are much less expensive than cast restorations.

Types of Crowns

Stainless steel crowns are available in a variety of sizes for the various primary and permanent teeth (Fig. 57-12). The two types typically used in pediatric dentistry are the pretrimmed and the precontoured stainless steel crowns.

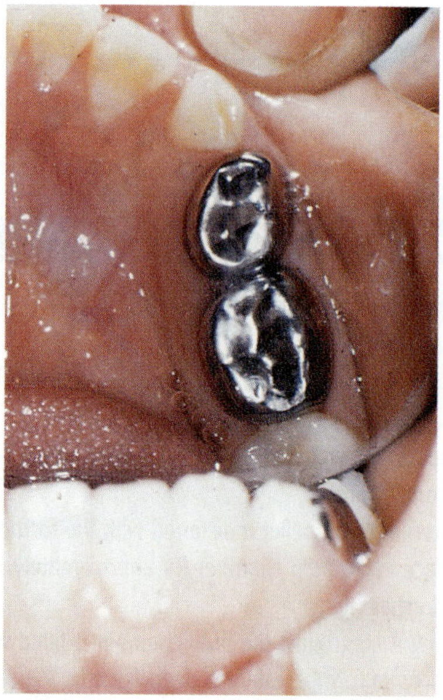

Fig. 57-12 Stainless steel crowns are trimmed and contoured to fit properly.

Pretrimmed crowns have straight sides but undergo **festooning** to follow a line parallel to the gingival crest. They must be trimmed and **contoured** to fit the tooth.

Precontoured crowns are already festooned and contoured. Some additional trimming and contouring may be necessary but are usually minimal (see Procedure 57-2).

Recall

17. What types of matrices are used on primary teeth?
18. What endodontic procedure is commonly performed on primary teeth?
19. Would a child be referred to a prosthodontist for the placement of a stainless steel crown?

Procedure 57-2 Assisting in Placement of a Stainless Steel Crown

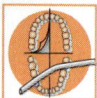

Equipment and Supplies

- Basic setup
- Local anesthetic agent setup
- Dental dam setup
- Low-speed and high-speed handpieces
- High-volume oral evacuator (HVE) tip
- Friction grip burs (dentist's choice of diamond or carbide)
- Spoon excavator
- Selection of stainless steel crowns
- Crown and bridge scissors
- Contouring and crimping pliers
- Mandrel
- Finishing and polishing discs
- Mounted green stones
- Cotton rolls
- Cementation setup
- Dental floss
- Articulating paper and holder

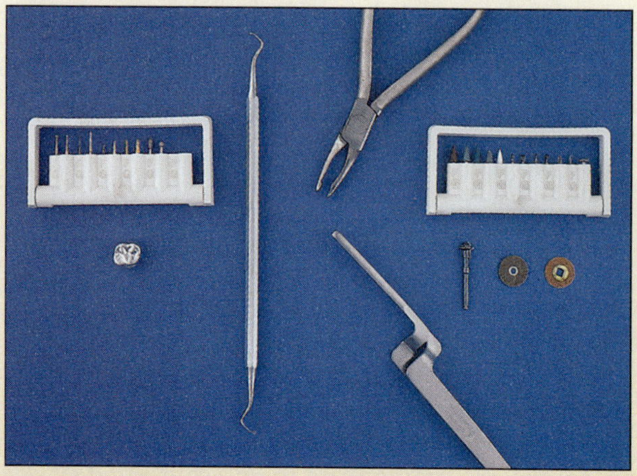

PROCEDURAL STEPS

Preparing the Tooth

1. After the local anesthetic agent has been administered and taken effect, the dental dam is applied.
2. The dentist will use the high-speed handpiece and a tapered diamond or carbide bur to prepare the tooth in a method similar to that for a cast crown (see Chapter 50).
3. The dentist reduces the entire circumference of the tooth, as well as the height of the tooth.
4. All dental caries are removed with hand instruments and burs.

Selecting and Sizing the Stainless Steel Crown

1. The crown is selected and tried on the prepared tooth for fit.
2. The stainless steel crown is properly sized when it fits snugly on the prepared tooth and has *both* mesial and distal contact.
3. Clean and sterilize any crowns that were tried in the mouth but not used; then return them to storage.

Procedure 57-2 Assisting in Placement of a Stainless Steel Crown—cont'd

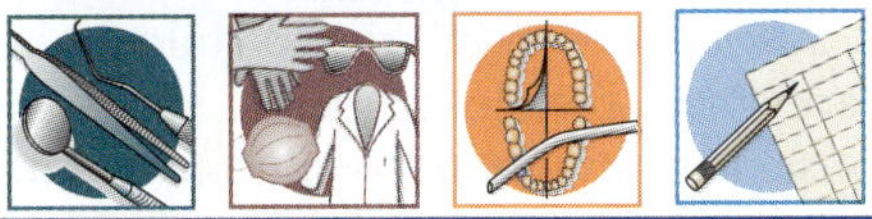

Trimming and Contouring the Crown

1. The dentist will use a crown and bridge scissors to reduce the height of the crown until it is approximately the same height as the adjacent teeth.

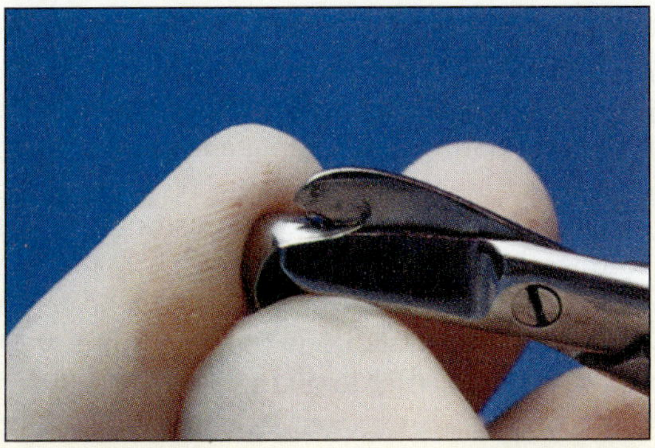

(From Duggal MS, et al: *Restorative techniques in paediatric dentistry,* Philadelphia, 1995, Saunders.)

2. The dentist may use a green stone to smooth the rough edges of the crown along the cervical margin.
3. The cervical margin of the crown may be polished with a rubber abrasive wheel.
4. The occlusion is checked and adjusted as needed.
5. The dentist uses the contouring pliers to crimp the cervical margins of the crown toward the tooth to obtain a tight fit and a proper cervical contour.

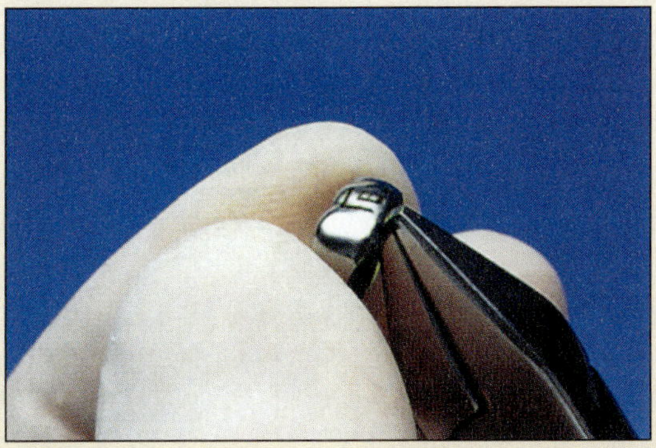

(From Duggal MS, et al: *Restorative techniques in paediatric dentistry,* Philadelphia, 1995, Saunders.)

Cementation

1. Rinse and dry the tooth thoroughly. Place cotton rolls to maintain dry conditions.
2. Mix the permanent cement (polycarboxylate is often selected).
3. Line the crown with the cement and transfer to the dentist for placement.

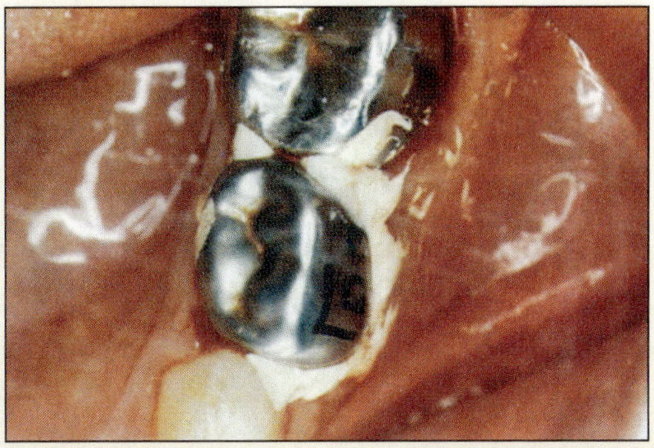

(From Duggal MS, et al: *Restorative techniques in paediatric dentistry,* Philadelphia, 1995, Saunders.)

4. Transfer an explorer to the dentist to remove the excess cement from around the tooth.
5. Use dental floss to remove any remaining cement from the interproximal areas.
6. Use the air-water syringe and HVE tip to rinse the patient's mouth before dismissal.

Date	Tooth	Surface	Charting Notes
9/5/05	B		Stainless steel crown, 1 carpule Xylocaine 1:100,000 w/o epi. Cotton roll isolation, cemented crown w/ Duralon. Pt tolerated procedure well. T. Clark, CDA/L. Stewart, DDS

DENTAL TRAUMA

An injury to the tooth of a young child can have serious and long-term consequences, including discoloration and possible loss. Many injuries to primary teeth occur at 1 to $2^1/_2$ years of age, the "toddler" stage. The teeth most frequently injured in the primary dentition are the maxillary central incisors (Fig. 57-13).

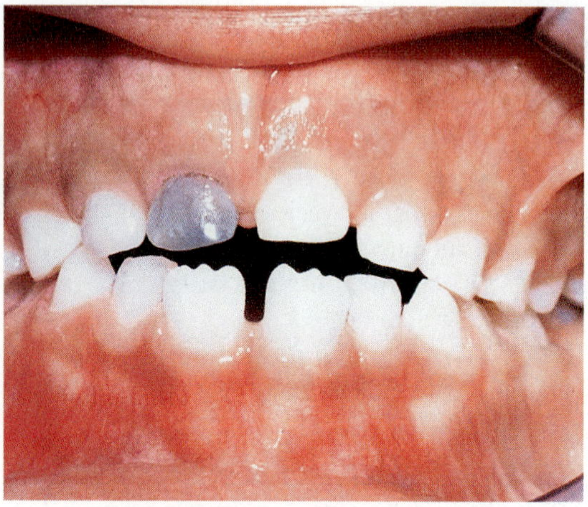

Fig. 57-13 **Traumatized maxillary incisor.** (Courtesy Dr. Frank Hodges.)

The concern with these injuries is that the permanent tooth developing directly under the injured tooth may also become damaged. Causes of dental injuries to children include automobile accidents, bicycle accidents, sports injuries, and child abuse. It is important to educate parents and school nurses on proper actions to take when a dental emergency occurs (Fig. 57-14).

Fractured Anterior Teeth

Fractures of the anterior teeth are common emergencies in a pediatric dental practice (Fig. 57-15). The dentist should see children with fractured teeth as soon as possible. Complete documentation of the accident, clinical examination, vitality testing, and radiographic examination are usually done at the emergency visit.

The dentist often prefers to delay restorative treatment for 3 to 6 weeks to avoid any further trauma to the pulp of an injured tooth. This time gives the delicate pulp an opportunity to recover without additional injury. During this recovery period the dentist (1) provides temporary relief by covering all exposed dentin with calcium hydroxide to prevent thermal sensitivity and (2) places an interim covering of resin material. Radiographs and vitality tests are taken at subsequent appointments to determine the status of the injured tooth. If the pulp is

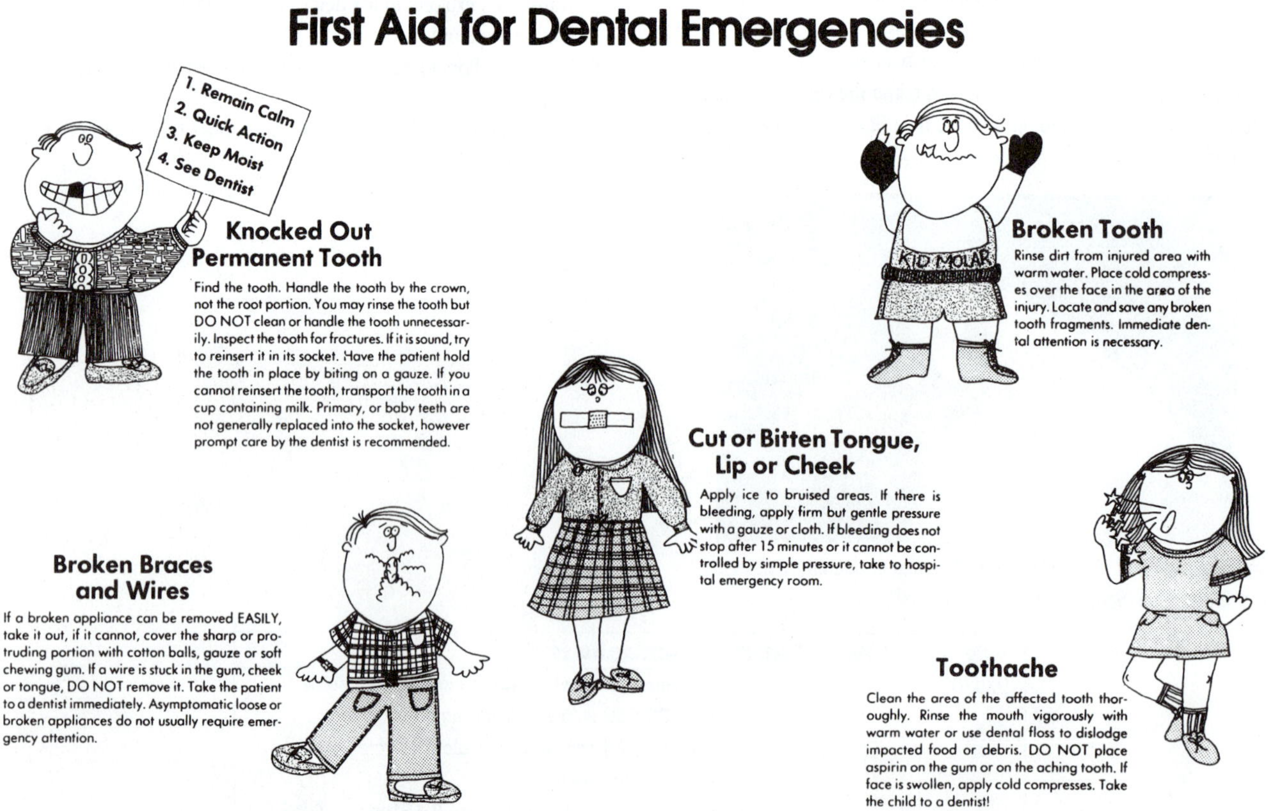
First Aid for Dental Emergencies
1. Remain Calm
2. Quick Action
3. Keep Moist
4. See Dentist
Knocked Out Permanent Tooth
Find the tooth. Handle the tooth by the crown, not the root portion. You may rinse the tooth but DO NOT clean or handle the tooth unnecessarily. Inspect the tooth for fractures. If it is sound, try to reinsert it in its socket. Have the patient hold the tooth in place by biting on a gauze. If you cannot reinsert the tooth, transport the tooth in a cup containing milk. Primary, or baby teeth are not generally replaced into the socket, however prompt care by the dentist is recommended.
Broken Tooth
Rinse dirt from injured area with warm water. Place cold compresses over the face in the area of the injury. Locate and save any broken tooth fragments. Immediate dental attention is necessary.
KID MOLAR
Cut or Bitten Tongue, Lip or Cheek
Apply ice to bruised areas. If there is bleeding, apply firm but gentle pressure with a gauze or cloth. If bleeding does not stop after 15 minutes or it cannot be controlled by simple pressure, take to hospital emergency room.
Broken Braces and Wires
If a broken appliance can be removed EASILY, take it out, if it cannot, cover the sharp or protruding portion with cotton balls, gauze or soft chewing gum. If a wire is stuck in the gum, cheek or tongue, DO NOT remove it. Take the patient to a dentist immediately. Asymptomatic loose or broken appliances do not usually require emergency attention.
Toothache
Clean the area of the affected tooth thoroughly. Rinse the mouth vigorously with warm water or use dental floss to dislodge impacted food or debris. DO NOT place aspirin on the gum or on the aching tooth. If face is swollen, apply cold compresses. Take the child to a dentist!

Fig. 57-14 **Flyer on actions to take in a dental emergency distributed to school personnel.** (Courtesy Dr. John Christensen.)

still vital, more definitive restorative procedures can be performed.

Traumatic Intrusion

Traumatic **intrusion** results from an injury during which the tooth is forcibly driven into the alveolus so that only a portion of the crown is visible. Traumatic intrusion can occur to primary and permanent dentition. Teeth that are intruded should be allowed to re-erupt naturally; these teeth often require endodontic treatment later. Damage to the developing permanent tooth can occur when a primary tooth is intruded. The extent of damage to the permanent tooth cannot be determined until it erupts.

Extrusion and Lateral Luxation Injuries

Extrusion and lateral **luxation** injuries occur when the teeth are displaced from their position. Severe damage to the periodontal ligaments usually occurs with these injuries. The dentist repositions the displaced teeth as soon as possible. A temporary splint of resin material or ligature wire is used to stabilize the repositioned permanent teeth.

Endodontic treatment often is required later for these teeth. Primary teeth tend to undergo root resorption more quickly after injuries of this type, and they tend to become mobile. These teeth should be observed for signs of infection and removed if indicated.

Avulsed Teeth

Permanent teeth that have been **avulsed** can be replanted with varying degrees of success (Fig. 57-16). Primary teeth are not usually replanted. The more quickly a tooth can be replanted, the greater the chance for success. Therefore, when an injury of this type occurs, the adult present should be instructed to do the following:

- Recover the tooth immediately.
- Wrap the tooth in moistened gauze.
- Go immediately to the dentist's office.

Replanting an Avulsed Tooth

The success rate for replantation of permanent teeth is highest when the tooth is replanted within 30 minutes of the accident. The procedure for replantation is as follows:

- The local anesthetic agent is administered.
- Radiographs are taken. Often, both periapical and occlusal radiographs are indicated to reveal any fragments of tooth or bone.
- Clotted blood is removed from the alveolus (socket) with a surgical curette.
- The avulsed tooth is washed in saline solution and inserted into the alveolus.
- The tooth is splinted in place with wire, acrylic, or orthodontic splints.
- Postoperative radiographs are taken.
- Endodontic treatment is performed 6 to 8 weeks after replantation.

Recall

20. Which teeth are most frequently injured in the mouth?
21. What happens when a tooth is avulsed?
22. How would a dentist stabilize a tooth after an injury?

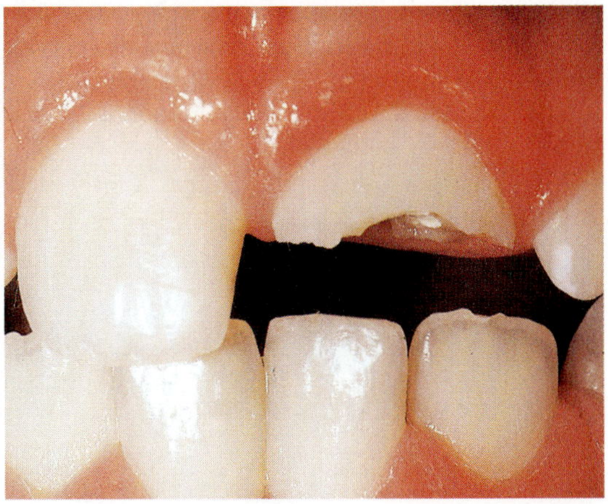

Fig. 57-15 Fracture of an anterior tooth. (Courtesy Dr. Frank Hodges.)

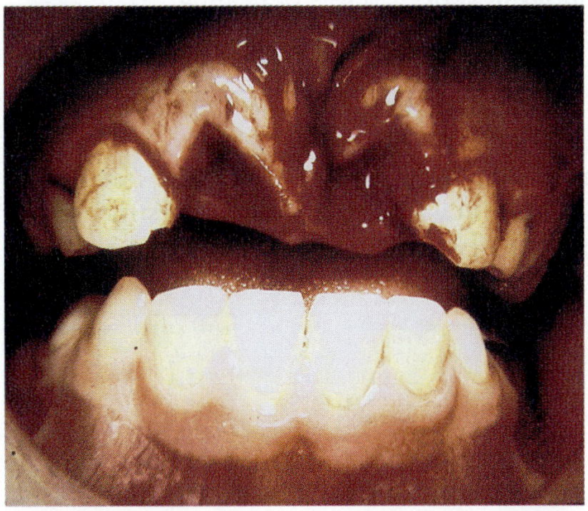

Fig. 57-16 Avulsion of maxillary central incisors. (Courtesy Dr. Frank Hodges.)

What to Include When Reporting Child Abuse

1. Name, address, gender, age, height, and weight of the child
2. Name and address of the adult who has custody of the child
3. Description of the current physical and emotional abuse or neglect of the child
4. Evidence of previous injuries or negligence
5. Information that may assist in establishing the cause of the injuries
6. Sketches or photographs documenting the nature and location of the injuries

CHILD ABUSE

By law, in all 50 states, healthcare professionals (physicians, dentists, nurses, and social workers) are required to report any case in which they suspect that a child is being neglected or abused. The state or county child protective services agency is the government body to contact.

The name of the person making the report will not be revealed. Although dental assistants and clerical staff are not legally required to report abuse, each member of the dental team has a moral responsibility to report known or suspected abuse cases to the dentist. Reporting of suspected child abuse may be done by telephone, in person, or in writing. Specific information is required to file a report.

For various reasons—because of embarrassment, fear of losing custody of the child, or the wish to avoid a fine or imprisonment—abusive parents tend to make up stories about how the child "fell" or sustained some other injury to the head. Child abuse must be suspected as the cause when a child presents with unexplained signs such as the following:

- Injuries in various stages of healing
- Repeated injuries
- Chipped or injured teeth
- Scars inside the lips or on the tongue
- Tears of labial frena
- Battering or other injuries around the head and neck
- Facial bruising, swelling of the facial structures, or blackened eye(s)
- Fractured nose
- Bite marks
- Injuries not consistent with the explanation presented by the parent

Injuries in various stages of healing indicate that the trauma has occurred over time rather than being a single incident.

Recall

23. Are you legally required to report child abuse?
24. Could a fractured or broken nose be a result of child abuse?
25. Who in the dental office should report child abuse?

Patient Education

Children are spongelike in that they absorb and remember everything you say and do. Always be mindful of their presence when they are in the dental chair. Allow children to feel comfortable about asking questions. When you answer their questions, think about their age, how they grasp concepts, and how can you make them more interested in taking better care of their oral health.

Legal and Ethical Implications

Because the clinical assistant takes on such an important role in prevention with the pediatric patient, it is easy to acquire responsibilities that may not be legal for an assistant to practice in your state. Review your state laws and discuss with your dentist what role you want to take in the practice. Come up with a plan for how you can be legally involved to your maximum potential.

Eye to the Future

For many years the rate of tooth decay has declined, primarily because of water fluoridation and products with fluoride. However, pediatric and general dentists are now seeing a comeback in problems of rampant decay in teenagers. The problem is candy, sodas, fruit juices, and sports drinks. Preteens and teenagers are taking in large amounts of sugar-containing products, and therefore interproximal and cervical decay rates are rising. Caries has become such an epidemic that the American Dental Society and the American Academy of Pediatric Dentistry are emphasizing that dental professionals must educate their patients about diet.

Critical Thinking

1. You are assisting with a new patient named Katie today. After reviewing the patient registration form, you see that she is 3 years old. When you go out to call Katie, she runs to her mother and clings to her arm. What can you do to encourage her to come with you for her appointment?
2. You are applying sealants to the primary molars of a 6-year-old boy. Your choice of moisture control is cotton rolls. When you place the cotton roll on the lower lingual side, the boy pushes it up with his tongue. How can you maintain a dry area and still complete the procedure?
3. An emergency patient has just arrived. The patient, 1-year-old Lori, has fallen and hit her front tooth. You have been asked to take a periapical radiograph of the area. How will you take a periapical view of this very young girl?
4. Your next oral hygiene patient is Luke, a 10-year-old boy with Down syndrome. Describe how you will prepare for this special needs patient and identify what techniques you can use to make Luke feel more comfortable and have a positive experience.
5. Explain why a different type of matrix system is used with primary teeth. Which additional supplies would you require to set up this system?

58

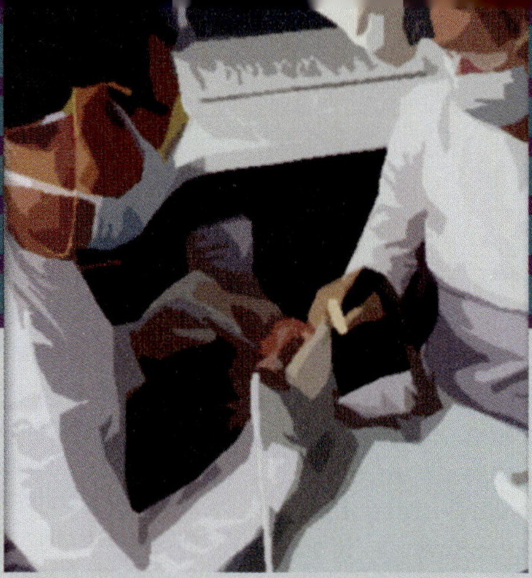

Coronal Polishing

Outline

Selective Polishing
Dental Stains
- Types of Stains
- Methods of Removing Plaque and Stains

Handpieces and Attachments for Coronal Polishing
- Polishing Cups
- Bristle Brushes

Abrasives
Polishing Esthetic Restorations
Prophylaxis Angle and Handpiece
- Grasping the Handpiece
- Handpiece Operation
- The Fulcrum and Finger Rest

Coronal Polishing Steps
- Polishing Stroke
- Positioning the Patient and Operator

Procedure 58-1: Rubber Cup Coronal Polishing (Expanded Function)
Sequence of Polishing
Flossing After Polishing
Evaluation of Polishing
Patient Education
Legal and Ethical Implications
Eye to the Future
Critical Thinking

KEY TERMS

Calculus (**kal**-kyou-lus) Calcium and phosphate salts in saliva that become mineralized and adhere to tooth surfaces.

Clinical crown That portion of the tooth that is visible in the oral cavity.

Coronal polishing (cuh-**rone**-uhl) A technique used to remove plaque and stains from the coronal surfaces of the teeth.

Endogenous stains (en-**doj**-en-us) Stains developed from within the structure of the tooth.

Exogenous stains (ex-**oj**-en-us) Stains developed from external sources.

Extrinsic stains (ex-**trin**-zik) Stains that occur on the *external* surfaces of the teeth and that may be removed by polishing.

Fulcrum (**ful**-krum) Finger rest used when holding an instrument or handpiece for a specific time.

Intrinsic stains (in-**trin**-zik) Stains that occur within the tooth structure and that cannot be removed by polishing.

Oral prophylaxis (*pro*-fuh-**lax**-is) The complete removal of calculus, debris, stain, and plaque from the teeth.

Rubber cup polishing A technique used to remove plaque and stains from the coronal surfaces of the teeth.

LEARNING OUTCOMES

On completion of this chapter, the student will be able to achieve the following objectives:

- Pronounce, define, and spell the Key Terms.
- Explain the difference between a prophylaxis and coronal polishing.
- Explain the indications for and contraindications to a coronal polish.
- Name and describe the types of extrinsic stains.
- Name and describe the two categories of intrinsic stains.
- Describe types of abrasives used for polishing the teeth.
- Describe the types of abrasives used for porcelain esthetic restorations.
- Name materials to avoid when polishing esthetic restorations.
- Describe the technique for polishing esthetic restorations.
- Demonstrate safety precautions during coronal polish.
- In states where it is legal, demonstrate coronal polishing technique.

PERFORMANCE OUTCOMES

On completion of this chapter, the student will be able to achieve the competency standards in the following skills:

- Demonstrate the handpiece grasp and positioning for the prophy angle.
- Demonstrate the fulcrum or finger rest used in each quadrant during a coronal polish procedure.
- Demonstrate the proper seating positions for the operator and the assistant during a coronal polish procedure.
- Be able to determine that the teeth are free from stains and plaque.
- Complete coronal polishing without causing tissue trauma.

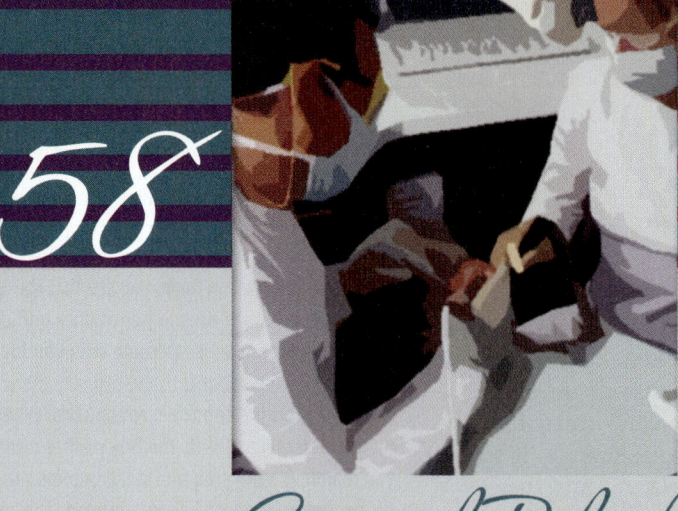

Coronal polishing is a technique used to remove plaque and stains from the coronal surfaces of the teeth. (Refer to Chapter 15 for a discussion of dental plaque.) Polishing the crowns of teeth is considered to be a mainly cosmetic procedure. However, there are instances in which coronal polishing has therapeutic value also. Patients like the feeling of smooth, polished teeth. Coronal polishing is done with the use of a dental handpiece with a prophy angle (Fig. 58-1), a rubber cup, and an abrasive agent. There are specific indications and contraindications for doing a coronal polish (Box 58-1).

Coronal polishing is strictly limited to the clinical crowns of the teeth. (The **clinical crown** is that portion of the tooth that is visible in the oral cavity.) In some states, coronal polishing is delegated to registered or expanded-function dental assistants (EFDAs) who have had special training in this procedure.

It is very important to understand the difference between a prophylaxis and a coronal polishing. A coronal polish is **NOT** a substitute for an oral prophylaxis. An **oral prophylaxis,** commonly known as a *prophy* or a *cleaning,* is the complete removal of calculus, debris, stain, and plaque from the teeth. (**Calculus** is a hard-mineralized deposit attached to the teeth.) In almost every state, the dentist and the registered dental hygienist are the only members of the dental team licensed to perform an oral prophylaxis.

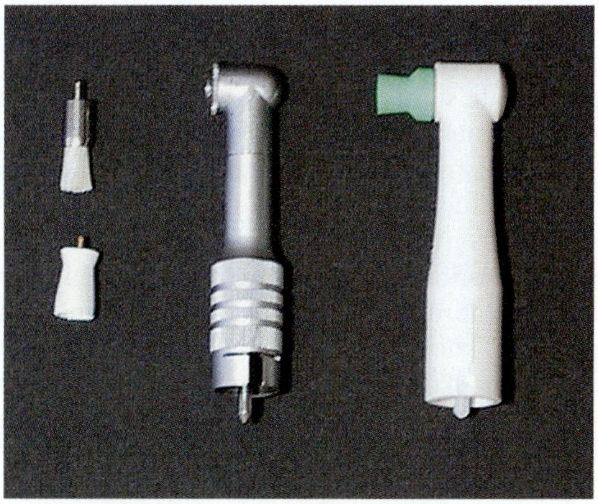

Fig. 58-1 Various types of handpieces.

SELECTIVE POLISHING

Selective polishing is a procedure in which *only* those teeth or surfaces with stain are polished. Studies have shown that the abrasive agent used during coronal polishing actually removes a small amount of the fluoride-rich outer enamel layer. The purpose of selective polishing is to avoid removing even small amounts of the surface enamel unnecessarily. Therefore, when the stain is very light and not of esthetic concern to the patient, selective *polishing* should be considered. The basic principle of selective polishing is not to polish teeth unless it is necessary. For some individuals, stain removal may cause dentinal hypersensitivity during and after the appointment. The needs of the patient always must be reviewed before stain removal. If you encounter a patient who does not have visible stain but is accustomed to polishing and chooses to have it done, you should use a very fine abrasive such as commercial toothpaste.

Historically, teeth were polished to remove all soft deposits and stains before the application of fluoride, because it was believed that there would be greater uptake of the fluoride into the enamel. As scientific knowledge has evolved, it has been shown that polishing *does not* improve the uptake of professionally applied fluoride. Therefore polishing is no longer necessary prior to fluoride application.

In addition to cosmetic value, coronal polishing can have a therapeutic value. *Therapeutic polishing* refers to polishing of the root surfaces that have been exposed during periodontal surgery. (Refer to Chapter 55 for a review of periodontal surgery.) The polishing will reduce

Box 58-1 Indications and Contraindications to Coronal Polishing

Indications	Contraindications
Before placement of dental sealants	When no stain is present
Before placement of the dental dam	Patients who are at high risk for dental caries, such as nursing bottle caries, root caries, or areas of thin demineralized enamel (because small amounts of enamel are removed during the polishing procedure)
Before cementation of orthodontic bands	Sensitive teeth (because abrasive agents can increase the areas of sensitivity)
Before application of acid etching solution on enamel (if indicated by the manufacturer's instructions)	Newly erupted teeth (because the mineralization of the surfaces may be incomplete)
Before cementation of crowns and bridges	

Box 58-2 Possible Damaging Effects of Coronal Polishing

Tooth surfaces	Gingival tissues	Restorations
Newly erupted teeth are incompletely mineralized, and excessive polishing with an abrasive could remove a small amount of surface enamel.	Potential to damage the gingival tissue if the cup is run at a high speed and applied too long.	Abrasive pastes can leave scratches or rough surfaces on gold, composite restorations, acrylic veneers, and porcelain-filled surfaces.
Avoid polishing exposed cementum in areas of recession because cementum is softer than enamel and is more easily removed.	Potential with fast rotation to force particles of the polishing agent into the sulcus and create a source of irritation.	
Avoid polishing areas of demineralization due to possibility of loss of surface enamel.		

From Robinson D, Bird D: *Essentials of dental assisting,* ed 3, Philadelphia, 2001, Saunders.

Benefits of Coronal Polishing

Polishing prepares the teeth for placement of dental sealants.
Smooth tooth surfaces are easier for the patient to keep clean.
Formation of new deposits is slowed.
Patients appreciate the smooth feeling and clean appearance.
Polishing prepares the teeth for placement of orthodontic brackets and/or bands.

the endotoxins and the bacteria on the cementum. Whether polishing for cosmetic or therapeutic purposes, it is important to understand the polishing process and the effects on the tooth surface (Box 58-2).

DENTAL STAINS

Stains are primarily an esthetic problem. Some types of stains can be removed, whereas others cannot. It is important for the dental assistant to be able to correctly identify stains to help provide the patient with accurate information about the cause of the stains and possible options to remove them. For stains that cannot be removed, there are other treatment options for patients. These include professional and at-home bleaching procedures, enamel microabrasion, or cosmetic restorative procedures such as laminate veneers or composite restorations.

Types of Stains

Dental stains are categorized as either endogenous or exogenous in nature.

- **Endogenous stains** originate within the tooth from developmental and systemic disturbances. Types of endogenous stains include those caused by an excessive amount of fluoride during the formation of the tooth. Another example of an endogenous stain would be from medications taken by the mother or child during tooth development. Tetracycline is an example of a medication known to cause developmental staining. Endogenous stains may be seen in both deciduous and permanent dentitions and cannot be removed by polishing (Figs. 58-2 through 58-6).
- **Exogenous stains** are those that originate outside the tooth and are caused by environmental agents. They can be subdivided even further as extrinsic or intrinsic stains, depending on whether or not the stain can be removed.
  - **Extrinsic stains** are those stains that are on the exterior of the tooth and *can* be removed. Examples include staining from food, drink, and tobacco. In these cases, the source of the stain is external and the stain may be removed (Table 58-1).
  - **Intrinsic stains** are those that are caused by an environmental source but *cannot* be removed because the stain has become incorporated into the structure of the tooth. Examples include tobacco stains from smoking, chewing, or dipping and stains from dental amalgam that have become incorporated into the tooth structure. The dental assistant must be able to recognize these conditions because these stains cannot be removed by polishing or scaling (Table 58-2).

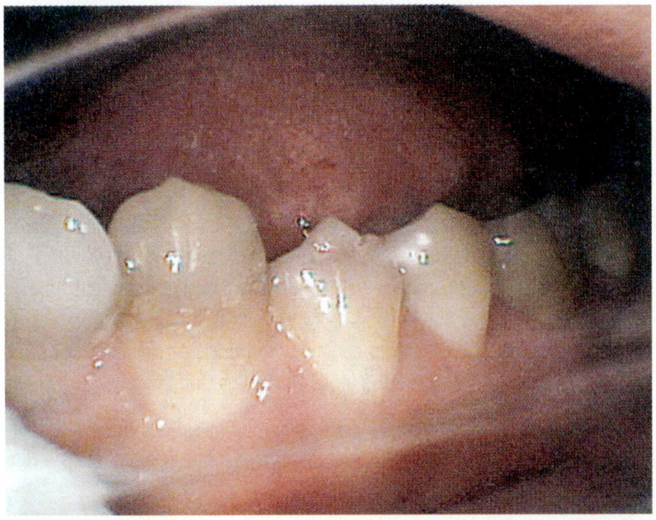

Fig. 58-2 Endogenous developmental stain: tetracycline. Notice how the stained area corresponds to the period of tooth development and the time the drug was taken. (Courtesy Santa Rosa Junior College, Santa Rosa, Calif.)

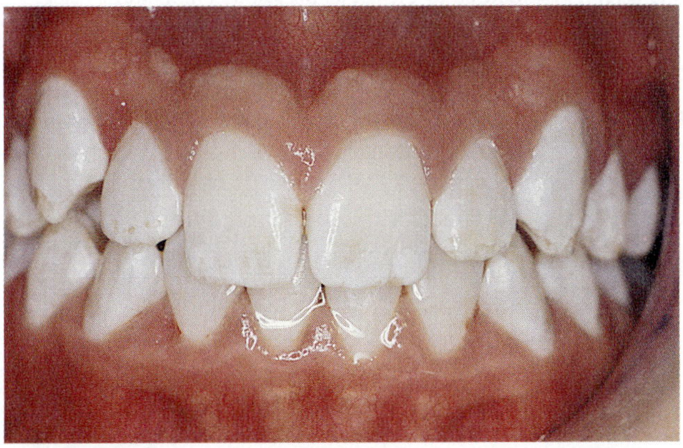

Fig. 58-3 Endogenous developmental stain: enamel hypoplasia. (From Daniel SJ, Harfst SA: *Mosby's dental hygiene: concepts, cases, and competencies–2004 update,* St Louis, 2004, Mosby. Courtesy Dr. George Taybos, Jackson, Miss.)

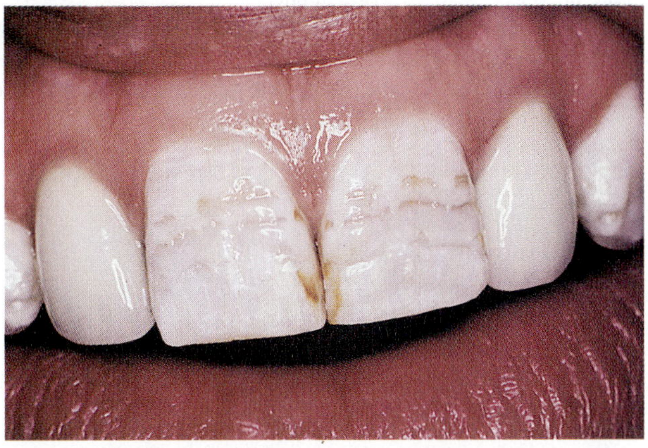

Fig. 58-4 Endogenous developmental stain: dental fluorosis. (From Daniel SJ, Harfst SA: *Mosby's dental hygiene: concepts, cases, and competencies–2004 update,* St Louis, 2004, Mosby. Courtesy Dr. George Taybos, Jackson, Miss.)

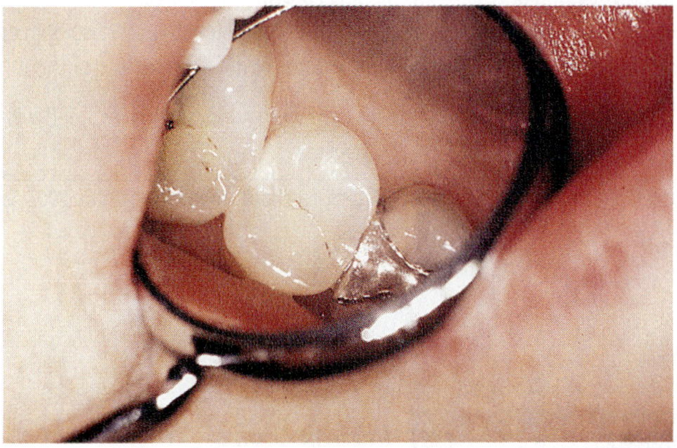

Fig. 58-5 Endogenous developmental stain: secondary caries. (From Daniel SJ, Harfst SA: *Mosby's dental hygiene: concepts, cases, and competencies–2004 update,* St Louis, 2004, Mosby. Courtesy Dr. George Taybos, Jackson, Miss.)

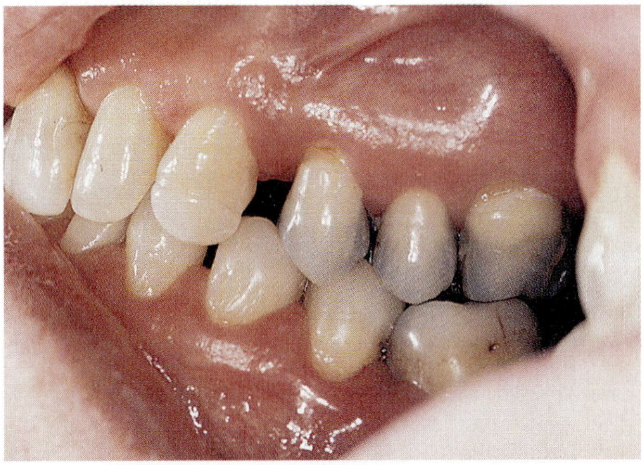

Fig. 58-6 Endogenous stain: amalgam restoration. (From Daniel SJ, Harfst SA: *Mosby's dental hygiene: concepts, cases, and competencies–2004 update,* St Louis, 2004, Mosby. Courtesy Dr. George Taybos, Jackson, Miss.)

Tooth Stains

Stains of the teeth occur in three basic ways:

1. The stain adheres directly to the surface of the tooth.
2. The stain is embedded in calculus and plaque deposits.
3. The stain is incorporated within the tooth structure.

Recall

1. What is a coronal polish?
2. What is the difference between a coronal polish and an oral prophylaxis?
3. What is the purpose of selective polishing?
4. What is an extrinsic stain?
5. What is an intrinsic stain?

Table 58-1 ***Extrinsic Stains***

Type of Stain	Appearance	Cause
Black stain	Thin black line on the teeth near the gingival margin. More common in girls. Frequently found in clean mouths. Difficult to remove.	Caused by natural tendencies.
Tobacco stain	A very tenacious dark brown or black stain.	Caused by the products of coal tar in the tobacco and from the penetration of tobacco juices into pits and fissures, enamel, and dentin of the teeth. Use of any tobacco-containing products causes tobacco stains on the teeth and restorations.
Brown or yellow stain	Most commonly found on the buccal surfaces of the maxillary molars and the lingual surfaces of the lower anterior incisors.	Cause by poor oral hygiene or using a toothpaste with inadequate cleansing action.
Green stain	Appears as a green or green-yellow stain usually occurring on the facial surfaces of the maxillary anterior teeth. Most common stain in children.	Caused by poor oral hygiene when bacteria or fungi are retained in the bacterial plaque.
Dental plaque agents	Reddish brown stain appears on the interproximal and cervical areas of the teeth. It can also appear on restorations, in plaque, and on the surface of the tongue.	Caused by the use of prescription mouthrinses that contain chlorhexidine. (Chlorhexidine is a disinfectant with broad antibacterial action.)
Food and drink	Light brownish stain. Stain is lessened with good oral hygiene.	Caused by tea, coffee, colas, soy sauce, berries, and other foodstuff.

From Robinson D, Bird D: Essentials of dental assisting, *ed 3, Philadelphia, 2001, Saunders.*

Table 58-2 ***Intrinsic Stains***

Type of Stain	Appearance	Cause
Pulpless teeth	Not all pulpless teeth discolor. A wide range of colors exists: light yellow, gray, reddish brown, dark brown, or black; sometimes an orange or greenish color is seen.	Blood and pulpal tissues break down as a result of bleeding in the pulp chamber or death of the pulp tissue. Pigments from the blood and tissue penetrate the dentin and show through the enamel.
Tetracycline antibiotics	Light green to dark yellow or a gray brown. Discoloration depends on the dosage, length of time the drug was used, and the type of tetracycline.	Can occur in the child when the mother is given tetracycline during the third trimester of pregnancy or when given in infancy and early childhood.
Dental fluorosis	Also termed "mottled enamel," it results from ingestion of excessive fluoride during the mineralization period of tooth development.	Varying degrees of discoloration ranging from a few white spots to extensive white areas or distinct brown stains.
Imperfect tooth development	Teeth are yellowish brown or gray brown. Teeth appear translucent or opalescent and vary in color.	May result from genetic abnormality or environmental influences during development.
Silver amalgam	Appears as a gray or black discoloration around a restoration.	Metallic ions from the amalgam penetrate into the dentin and enamel.
Other systemic causes	Appears as a yellowish or greenish discoloration in the teeth.	Conditions of prolonged jaundice early in life and erythroblastosis fetalis (Rh incompatibility).

From Robinson D, Bird D: Essentials of dental assisting, *ed 3, Philadelphia, 2001, Saunders.*

Methods of Removing Plaque and Stains

Two methods of stain removal are **air-powder polishing** and the **rubber cup polishing** technique.

With any type of stain and plaque removal procedure, you must be careful not to remove surface enamel of the tooth and to avoid trauma to the gingiva.

Remember, you must check the regulations in your state regarding whether coronal polishing is delegated to qualified dental assistants and, if so, which technique is permitted.

Air-Powder Polishing

The air-powder polishing technique uses a specially designed handpiece with a nozzle that delivers a high-pressure stream of warm water and sodium bicarbonate.

Under the high pressure, the powder and water remove stains rapidly and efficiently. The flow rate is adjusted to control the rate of abrasion.

Rubber Cup Polishing

The most common technique for removing stains and plaque and polishing the teeth is the use of an abrasive polishing agent in a *rubber polishing cup* that is rotated slowly and carefully by a prophy angle attached to the slow-speed handpiece. This is the form of coronal polishing described in detail in this chapter.

HANDPIECES AND ATTACHMENTS FOR CORONAL POLISHING

Polishing Cups

Soft, webbed polishing cups are used to clean and polish the smooth surfaces of the teeth. The polishing cup attaches to the reusable prophy angle by either a snap-on or screw-on attachment.

Polishing cups are made from either natural or synthetic rubber. The natural rubber polishing cups are more resilient and do not stain the teeth. The synthetic polishing cups are stiffer than the natural polishing cups. Synthetic polishing cups should be used for patients with latex allergies.

Bristle Brushes

Bristle brushes are made from either natural or synthetic materials and may be used to remove stains from deep pits and fissures of the enamel surfaces. Bristle brushes can cause cuts on the gingivae and must be used with special care. Brushes are *not* recommended for use on exposed cementum or dentin because these surfaces are soft and easily grooved.

Bristle Brush Polishing Stroke

1. If necessary, soak stiff brushes in hot water to soften them.
2. Apply a mild abrasive polishing agent to the brush and, using a light-wiping stroke, spread the polishing agent over the occlusal surfaces to be polished.
3. Use the free hand and fingers to both retract and protect the cheek and tongue from the revolving brush.
4. Establish a firm finger rest and bring the brush almost into contact with the tooth surface before activating the brush.
5. Using the slowest speed, apply the revolving brush lightly to the occlusal surfaces. Take care to avoid contacting the gingiva.
6. Use a short-stroke brushing motion, moving from the inclined planes to the cusps of the tooth.
7. Move frequently from tooth to tooth to avoid generating frictional heat.
8. Replenish the supply of polishing agent frequently to minimize frictional heat.

ABRASIVES

Dental abrasives (polishing materials) are used to remove stains and polish natural teeth, prosthetic appliances, restorations, and castings.

Abrasives are available in various grits. (*Grit* refers to the degree of coarseness of an agent.) Abrasives are available in extra coarse, coarse, medium, fine, and extra fine. The coarser the agent, the more abrasive the surface.

Even a fine-grit agent removes small amounts of the enamel surface. Therefore the goal is to always use the abrasive agent that will produce the *least* amount of abrasion to the tooth surface.

Abrasives are available as commercial premixed pastes or as powders mixed with water or mouthwash to form slurry used on the polishing cup. The powder abrasives should be as wet as possible (i.e., the texture should be similar to moist cake mix) to minimize frictional heat. If the mixture is too wet, spatter will occur, and it will be difficult to keep the material in the cup. The commercial type of premixed pastes is available in ready-to-use packages (Box 58-3).

Factors Influencing the Rate of Abrasion

The amount of abrasive agent used (the more agent used, the greater the degree of abrasion)

The amount of pressure applied to the polishing cup (the lighter the pressure, the less abrasion)

The rotation speed of the polishing cup (the slower the rotation of the cup, the less abrasion)

Box 58-3 Commonly Used Abrasives

Agent	Action
Silex	Fairly abrasive and is used for cleaning more heavily stained tooth surfaces.
Super-fine silex	Used for removal of light stains on tooth enamel.
Fine pumice	Mildly abrasive and is used for more persistent stains, such as tobacco stains.
Zirconium silicate	Used for cleaning and polishing tooth surfaces (this material is highly effective and does not abrade tooth enamel).
Chalk	Also known as *whiting;* chalk is precipitated calcium carbonate (it is frequently incorporated into toothpaste and polishing pastes to whiten the teeth).
Commercial premixed preparations	Contain an abrasive, water, a humectant (to keep the preparation moist), a binder (to prevent separation of the ingredients), flavoring agents, and color. Some commercial preparations are available in small plastic containers or individual packets that contribute to the cleanliness and sterility of the procedure.
Fluoride prophylaxis pastes	Replace some of the fluoride that is lost from the surface layer during the polishing process. These pastes are not a substitute for topical application of fluoride. Use of fluoride paste is contraindicated before acid etching of the enamel when followed with bonding of sealants or other bonded materials.

From Robinson D, Bird D: *Essentials of dental assisting,* ed 3, Philadelphia, 2001, Saunders.

POLISHING ESTHETIC RESTORATIONS

Esthetic dentistry has become an important part of today's dental practice, and this trend will continue to grow. Many patients have crown and bridge restorations, and many are choosing to have cosmetic resin, composite, bonding, and veneers placed to enhance their smile (Fig. 58-7).

Improper oral care can quickly damage many of these types of restorations. Dental assistants who perform rubber cup coronal polishing must understand the maintenance requirements associated with esthetic dentistry.

Coarse polishing paste, use of acidulated phosphate fluorides, and even hard toothbrushing with abrasive toothpaste can be destructive to the surfaces of restorative mate-

A

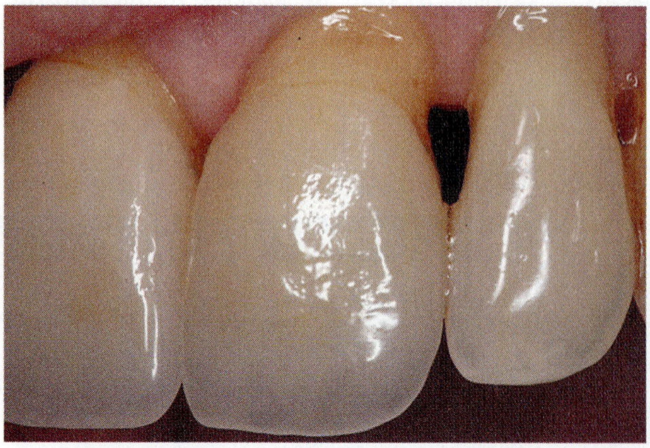

B

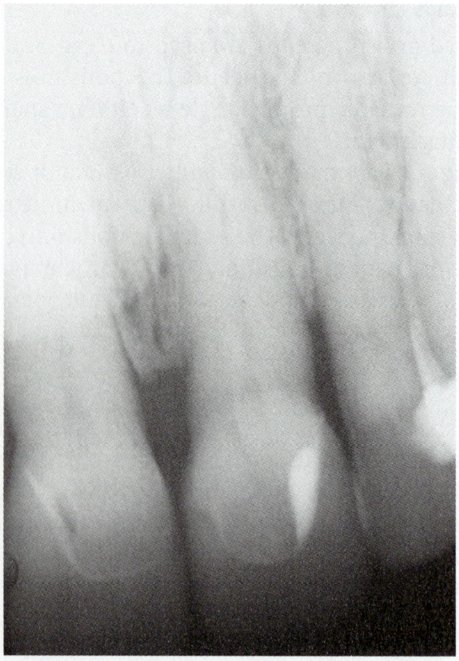

Fig. 58-7 A, It can be difficult to detect esthetic restorations. Two of these teeth have crowns. **B,** Note the opaque white line of cement on teeth #8 and #9, showing that these teeth have porcelain crowns. (Courtesy Dr. Peter Pang, Sonoma, Calif.)

rials. A diamond paste, aluminum oxide paste, or low-abrasive toothpaste should be used for these restorations. The polishing agent should be applied directly to the restoration and then polished thoroughly using a rubber cup for 30 seconds. Diamond-polishing paste is suggested when only porcelain is being polished. Aluminum oxide paste is recommended for use on filled hybrid composites and resin restorations.

Esthetic and porcelain restorations should be polished first. Then the remaining teeth may be polished using the appropriate methods for any stain present. This is to reduce the possibility of having a coarse abrasive remain in the rubber cup when polishing the esthetic restorations.

PROPHYLAXIS ANGLE AND HANDPIECE

The prophylaxis angle, commonly called a *prophy angle,* attaches to the low-speed handpiece (see Chapter 35).

The two basic types of prophy angles are the *reusable* and *disposable.* The reusable type of prophy angle must be properly cleaned and sterilized after each use. (Handpiece maintenance is discussed in Chapter 35.) The disposable angle is simply discarded after a single use. The disposable angle is manufactured with either a polishing cup or a brush already attached.

When attaching the polishing cup or brush to the reusable type prophy angle, ensure that the polishing cup or brush is securely fastened. If a polishing cup or brush falls off during the procedure, the patient could swallow or aspirate it.

Grasping the Handpiece

The handpiece and prophylaxis angle are held in a pen grasp with the handle resting in the U-shaped area of the hand between the thumb and index finger (Fig. 58-8).

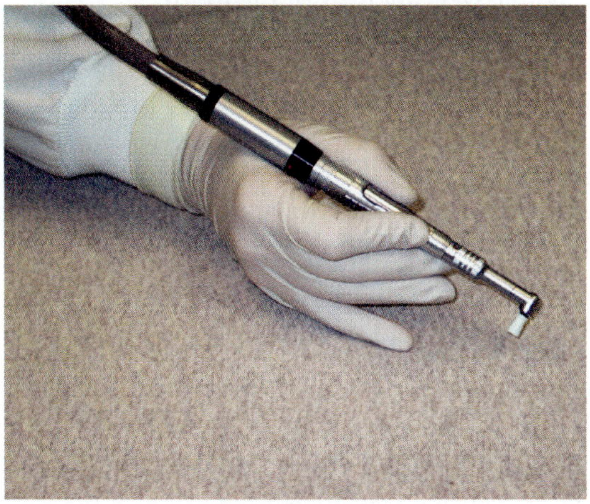

Fig. 58-8 Close-up of hand with handpiece and proper grasp.

A proper grasp is important; if the grasp is not secure and comfortable, the weight and balance of the handpiece can cause a loss of control and result in hand and wrist fatigue.

Handpiece Operation

1. A low-speed handpiece that operates at a maximum of 20,000 revolutions per minute (rpm) is recommended. The low speed minimizes frictional heat and gingival trauma from the polishing cup.
2. The rheostat (foot pedal) is used to control the speed (rpm) of the handpiece.
3. The toe of the foot is used to activate the rheostat. The sole of the foot remains flat on the floor. This is similar to operating a gas pedal on a car.
4. Apply a steady pressure with the toe on the rheostat to produce a slow, even speed. Release the rheostat immediately when the handpiece is removed from the tooth for more than a moment. This will prevent prophy paste and saliva from splattering.
5. Use intermittent pressure on the tooth to allow the heat that is generated to dissipate between strokes. Constant pressure of the rubber cup or brush on the tooth builds up frictional heat that may cause discomfort and possible pulpal damage.
6. The speed of the cup is important both in minimizing frictional heat and in effective polishing. Operating the cup at high speeds is harmful and ineffective.

The Fulcrum and Finger Rest

The terms **fulcrum** and *finger rest* are used interchangeably to describe the placement of the third, or ring, finger of the hand, which holds the instrument or handpiece.

The fulcrum provides stability for the operator and must be placed in such a way as to allow for movement of the wrist and forearm.

Polishing Tips

Use approximately one cupful of polishing agent for one or two teeth. An empty cup generates more heat.

Use moderate intermittent pressure to permit heat dissipation. Heavy pressure creates more heat and more abrasion to the tooth.

Use the lowest possible handpiece speed that will move the cup or brush against the tooth without stalling. A whine or whistle in the handpiece indicates excessive speed.

Usually 20 pounds per square inch (psi) of air pressure is sufficient for stain removal.

Polish each tooth approximately 3 to 5 seconds. The more time spent polishing a tooth, the more the abrasive effect.

The fulcrum is repositioned throughout the procedure as necessary and usually is maintained as close as possible to the working area. The fulcrum may be either intraoral or extraoral, depending on a variety of circumstances:

- The presence or absence of teeth
- The area of the mouth being treated
- The patient's ability to widen the mouth when open

When possible, an intraoral fulcrum is preferable. Improper positioning of the hand and fingers greatly increases operator fatigue and can cause painful inflammation of the ligaments and nerves of the wrist over time.

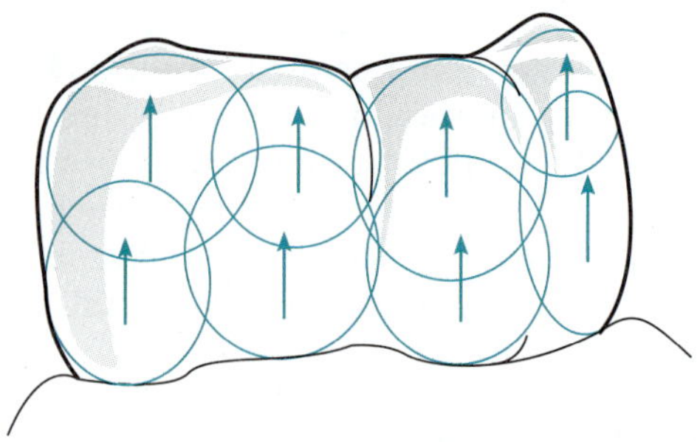

Fig. 58-9 Use overlapping strokes to ensure complete coverage of the tooth.

Recall

6. Which is the most common technique for stain removal?
7. Which type of grasp is used to hold the handpiece?
8. What is the purpose of a fulcrum?
9. What precaution should be taken when polishing esthetic type restorations?

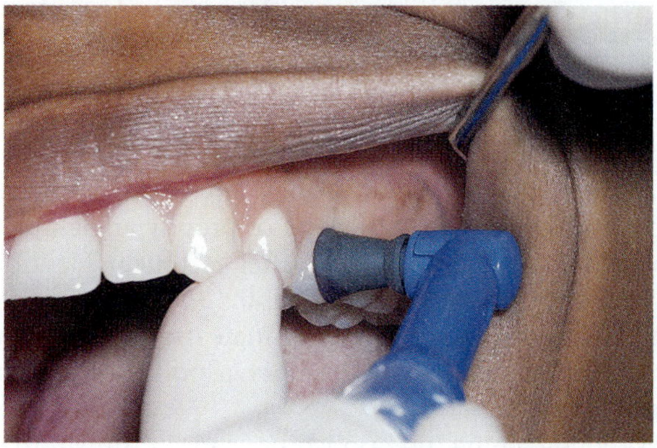

Fig. 58-10 Stroke from the gingival third with just enough pressure to cause the cup to flare.

CORONAL POLISHING STEPS

Polishing Stroke

1. Begin with the distal surface of the most posterior tooth in the quadrant and work forward toward the anterior.
2. The stroke should be from the gingival third toward the incisal third of the tooth (Fig. 58-9).
3. Fill the polishing cup with the polishing agent and spread it over several teeth in the areas to be polished.
4. Establish a finger rest and place the cup almost in contact with the tooth.
5. Using the slowest speed, apply intermittent strokes with the revolving cup lightly to the tooth surface for approximately 1 to 2 seconds between strokes. *Purpose:* Higher speeds produce frictional heat that can damage the tooth and burn the gingiva. Intermittent strokes allow the heat to dissipate.
6. Use intermittent pressure that is sufficient to cause the edges of the polishing cup to flare slightly. Each tooth should be completed in approximately 3 to 5 seconds (Fig. 58-10).
7. Move the cup to another area on the tooth, using a patting, wiping motion and an overlapping stroke. *Purpose:* This motion avoids creating heat that could harm the tooth.
8. Reapply polishing agent frequently as needed.
9. Turn the handpiece to adapt the polishing cup to fit every area of the tooth. *Purpose:* Doing so ensures that the cup covers all areas of the tooth.
10. If you are using two polishing agents with different degrees of coarseness, always use a separate polishing cup for each. Use the most abrasive agent first; then finish with the finest (least abrasive). Always rinse between polishing agents. *Purpose:* The finer abrasive will remove tiny scratches left by the more coarse abrasive.

Positioning the Patient and Operator

Proper positioning of both the operator and patient during coronal polishing procedures is necessary for maximum comfort and efficiency (see Procedure 58-1).

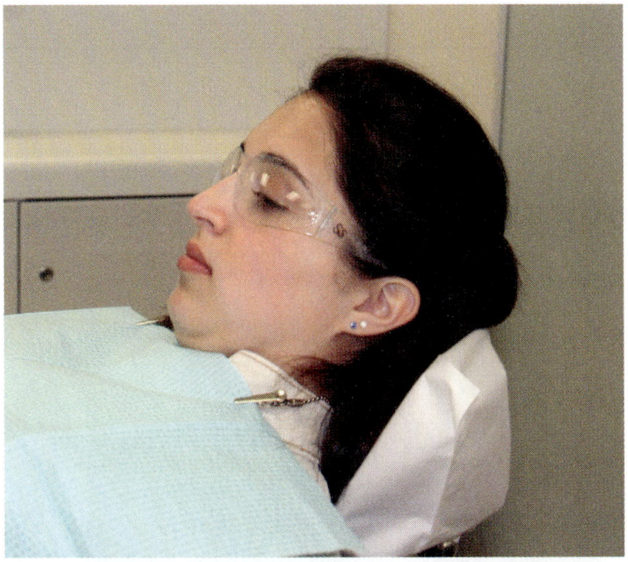

Fig. 58-11 For the mandibular arch, the patient's head is positioned so that the lower jaw is parallel to the floor when the mouth is open.

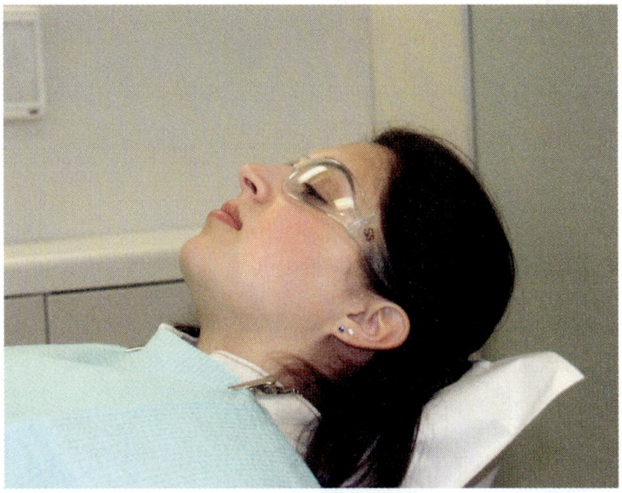

Fig. 58-12 For access to the maxillary arch, position the patient's head with the chin up.

Positioning the Patient

- The dental chair is adjusted so that the patient is approximately parallel to the floor with the back of the chair raised slightly.
- The movable headrest is adjusted for patient comfort and operator visibility.
- For access to the *mandibular arch,* position the patient's head chin down. When the mouth is open, the lower jaw is parallel to the floor (Fig. 58-11).
- For access to the *maxillary arch,* position the patient's head with the chin up (Fig. 58-12).

Positioning the Operator

The operator positions described in this chapter refer to the face of a clock. (This concept is discussed in Chapter 33.)

- The operator should be seated comfortably at the patient's side and must be able to move around the patient to gain access to all areas of the oral cavity.
- The seated operator's feet should be flat on the floor with the thighs parallel to the floor.
- The operator's arms should be at waist level and even with the patient's mouth.
- When performing a coronal polish procedure, the right-handed operator generally begins by being seated at the eight o'clock or nine o'clock position (Fig. 58-13).
- When performing a coronal polish procedure, the left-handed operator generally begins by being seated at the three o'clock or four o'clock position.

Tip: For maximum support and safety, keep the fulcrum as close to the area you are polishing as possible, preferably on the same dental arch.

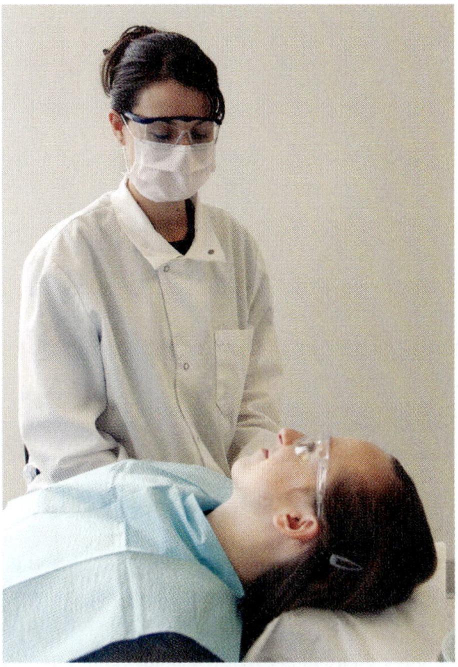

Fig. 58-13 The right-handed operator is seated at the nine o'clock position.

Procedure 58-1 Rubber Cup Coronal Polishing

Equipment and Supplies

- Prophy angle, sterile or disposable
- Polishing cup accessory, snap-on or screw-on
- Bristle brush, snap-on or screw-on
- Prophy paste or other abrasive in slurry
- HVE tip or saliva ejector
- Disclosing agent (tablets, gel, or solution)
- Cotton-tipped applicator (if disclosing solution is used)
- Dental tape
- Dental floss
- Bridge threader
- Air-water syringe and sterile tip

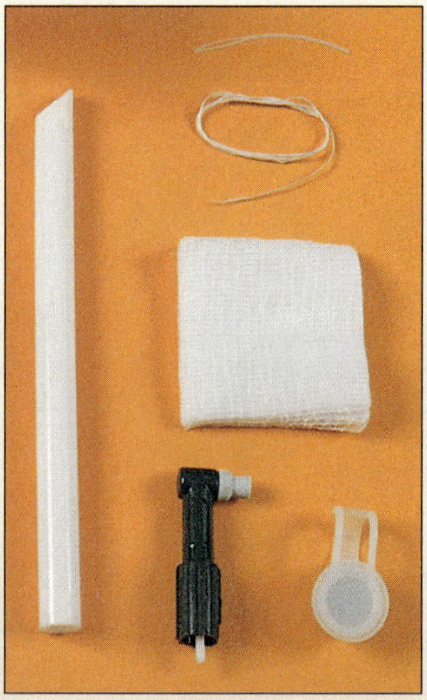

PROCEDURAL STEPS

1. Check the patient's medical history for any contraindications to the coronal polish procedure.
2. Seat and drape the patient with a waterproof napkin. Ask the patient to remove any dental prosthetic appliance that he or she may be wearing. Provide the patient with protective eyewear.
3. Explain the procedure to the patient and answer any questions.
4. Inspect oral cavity for lesions, missing teeth, tori, etc.
5. Apply a disclosing agent to identify areas of plaque.

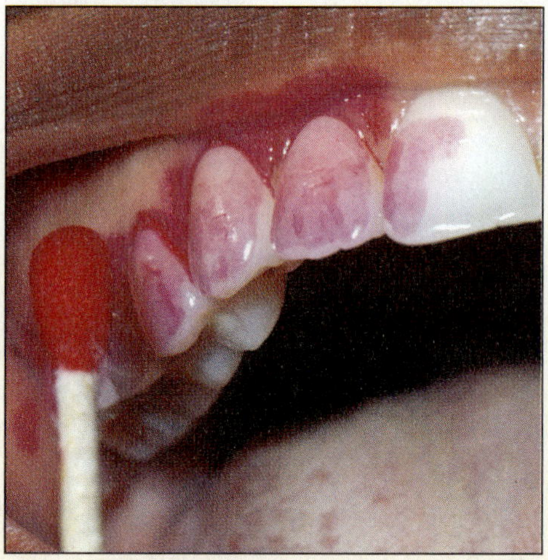

Maxillary Right Posterior Quadrant, Buccal Aspect (Eleven O'clock or Twelve O'clock Position May Also Be Used)

1. Sit in the eight o'clock to nine o'clock position.
2. Ask the patient to tilt the head up and turn slightly away from you.
3. Hold the dental mirror in your left hand. Use it to retract the cheek or for indirect vision of the more posterior teeth.

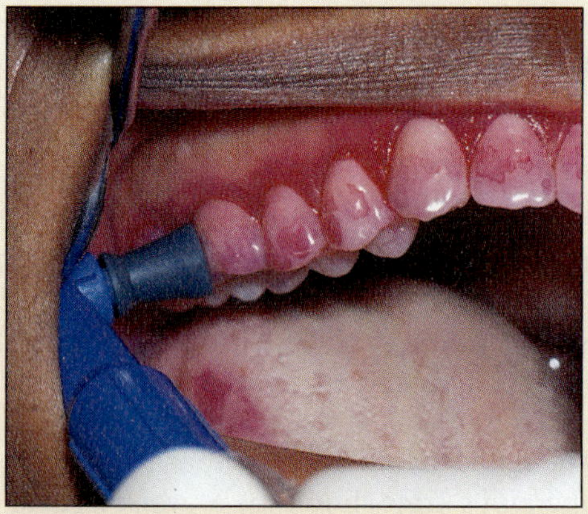

4. Establish a fulcrum on the maxillary right incisors.

Maxillary Right Posterior Quadrant, Lingual Aspect (Eleven O'clock or Twelve O'clock Position May Also Be Used)

1. Remain seated in the eight o'clock to nine o'clock position.
2. Ask the patient to turn the head up and toward you.
3. Hold the dental mirror in your left hand. Direct vision in this position and the mirror provides a view of the distal surfaces.
4. Establish a fulcrum on the lower incisors and reach up to polish the lingual surfaces.

Procedure 58-1 Rubber Cup Coronal Polishing—cont'd

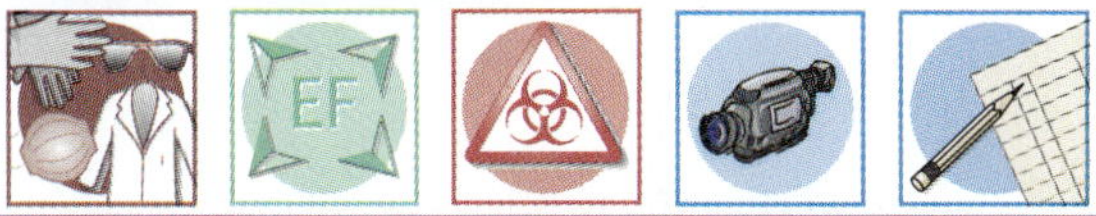

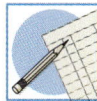

Maxillary Anterior Teeth, Facial Aspect

1. Remain in the eight o'clock to nine o'clock position.
2. Position the patient's head tipped up slightly and facing straight ahead. Make necessary adjustments by turning the patient's head either slightly toward or away from you.
3. Use direct vision in this area.
4. Establish a fulcrum on the incisal edge of the teeth adjacent to the ones being polished.

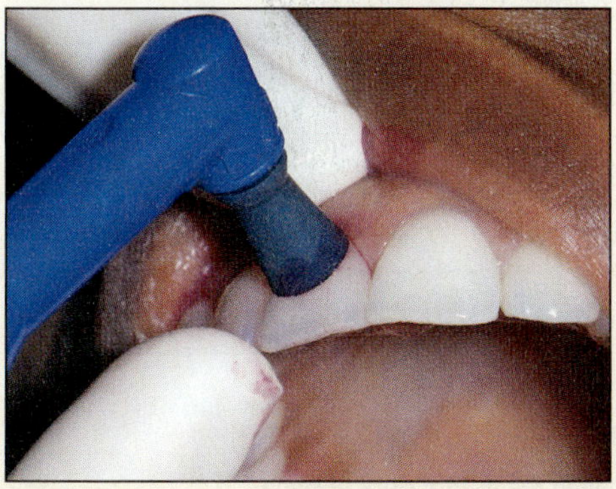

Maxillary Anterior Teeth, Lingual Aspect

1. Remain in the eight o'clock to nine o'clock position or move to the eleven o'clock to twelve o'clock position.
2. Position the patient's head so that it is tipped slightly upward.
3. Use the mouth mirror for indirect vision and to reflect light on the area.

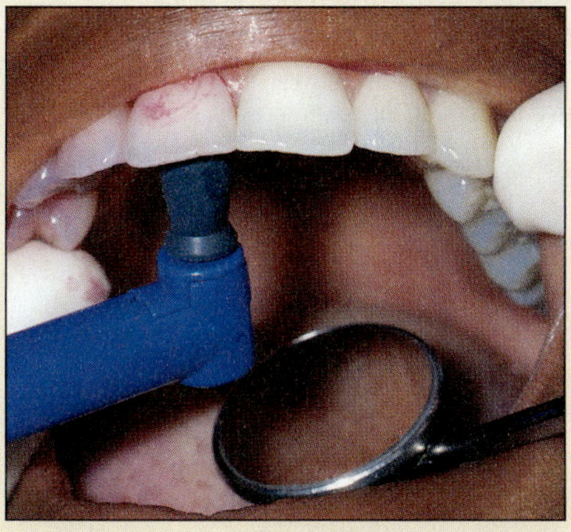

4. Establish a fulcrum on the incisal edge of the teeth adjacent to the ones being polished.

Maxillary Left Posterior Quadrant, Buccal Aspect

1. Sit in the nine o'clock position.
2. Position the patient's head tipped upward and turned slightly toward you to improve visibility.
3. Use the mirror to retract the cheek and for indirect vision.
4. Rest your fulcrum finger on the buccal occlusal surface of the teeth toward the front of the sextant.
   Alternative: Rest your fulcrum finger on the lower premolars and reach up to the maxillary posterior teeth.

Maxillary Left Posterior Quadrant, Lingual Aspect

1. Remain in the eight o'clock to nine o'clock position.
2. Ask the patient to turn the head away from you.
3. Use direct vision in this position. Hold the mirror in your left hand for a combination of retraction and reflecting light.
4. Establish a fulcrum on the buccal surfaces of the maxillary left posterior teeth or on the occlusal surfaces of the mandibular left teeth.

Mandibular Left Posterior Quadrant, Buccal Aspect (Eleven O'clock or Twelve O'clock Position May Also Be Used)

1. Sit in the eight o'clock to nine o'clock position.
2. Ask the patient to turn the head slightly toward you.
3. Use the mirror to retract the cheek and for indirect vision of distal and buccal surfaces.
4. Establish a fulcrum on the incisal surfaces of the mandibular left anterior teeth and reach back to the posterior teeth.

Mandibular Left Posterior Quadrant, Lingual Aspect

1. Remain in the nine o'clock position.
2. Ask the patient to turn the head slightly away from you.
3. For direct vision, use the mirror to retract the tongue and reflect more light to the working area.
4. Establish a fulcrum on the mandibular anterior teeth and reach back to the posterior teeth.

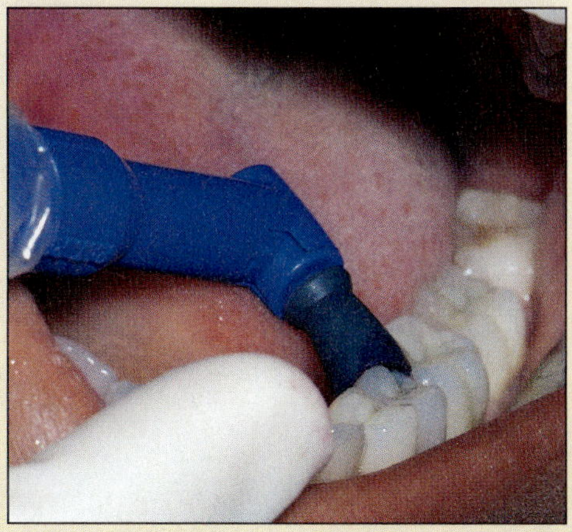

continued

Procedure 58-1 Rubber Cup Coronal Polishing—cont'd

Mandibular Anterior Teeth, Facial Aspect

1. Sit in either the eight o'clock to nine o'clock position or in the eleven o'clock to twelve o'clock position.
2. As necessary, instruct the patient to make adjustments in the head position by turning either toward or away from you or by tilting the head up or down.
3. Use your left index finger to retract the lower lip. Both direct and indirect vision can be used in this area.
4. Establish a fulcrum on the incisal edges of the teeth adjacent to the ones being polished.

Mandibular Anterior Teeth, Lingual Aspect

1. Sit in either the eight o'clock to nine o'clock position or in the eleven o'clock to twelve o'clock position.
2. As necessary, instruct the patient to make adjustments in the head position by turning either toward or away from you or by tilting the head up or down.
3. Use the mirror for indirect vision, to retract the tongue, and to reflect light onto the teeth. Direct vision is often used in this area when the operator is seated in the twelve o'clock position, but indirect vision can also be helpful.
4. Establish a fulcrum on the mandibular cuspid incisal area.

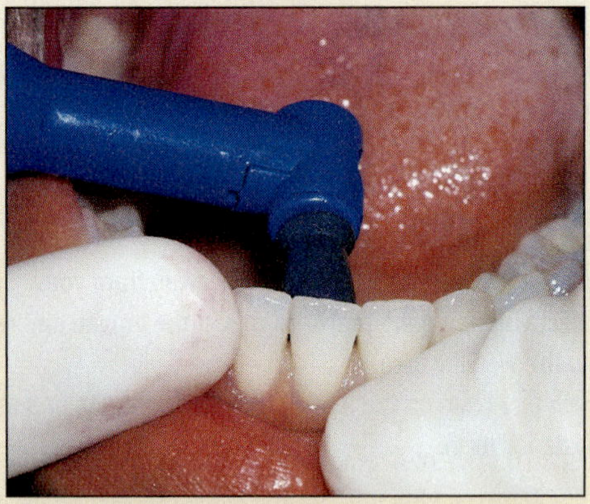

Mandibular Right Quadrant, Buccal Aspect

1. Sit in the eight o'clock position.
2. Ask the patient to turn the head slightly away from you.
3. Use the mirror to retract tissue and reflect light. The mirror may also be used to view the distal surfaces in this area.
4. Establish a fulcrum on the lower incisors.

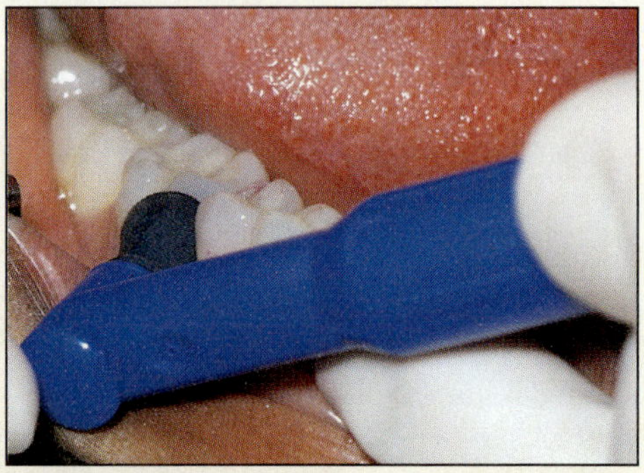

Mandibular Right Quadrant, Lingual Aspect

1. Remain in the eight o'clock position.
2. Ask the patient to turn the head slightly toward you.
3. Retract the tongue with the mirror.
4. Establish a fulcrum on the lower incisors.

Mandibular Right Quadrant, Lingual Aspect (Eleven O'clock or Twelve O'clock Position May Also Be Used)

1. Sit in the eight o'clock to nine o'clock position.
2. Ask the patient to turn the head slightly toward you.
3. Retract the tongue with the mirror.
4. Establish a fulcrum on the lower incisors.

SEQUENCE OF POLISHING

If full-mouth coronal polishing is indicated, it must be done in a predetermined sequence to be certain that no area is missed. The best sequence is based on the operator's preference and the individual needs of the patient.

One very effective sequence is described in Procedure 58-1. The positions and fulcrums described are for a right-handed operator. The concepts of direct and indirect vision are discussed in Chapter 33.

The patient's mouth is rinsed with water from the air-water syringe as necessary to maintain patient comfort throughout the procedure. The high-volume evacuation (HVE) tip is used to removes excess water and debris.

Recall

10. In which direction should the polishing stroke move?
11. What damage can result from using the prophy cup at a high speed?
12. How should the patient's head be positioned for accessing the maxillary mandibular arch?

FLOSSING AFTER POLISHING

Dental floss or tape can be used after coronal polishing to polish the interproximal tooth surfaces and to remove any abrasive agent or debris that may be lodged in the contact area.

To polish these areas, abrasive is placed on the contact area between the teeth, and the floss or tape is worked through the contact area with a back-and-forth motion. Because operators' and patients' preferences for floss and tape vary, many types are available. When used properly, floss and tape (or both) are equally effective.

After the interproximal surfaces are polished, a fresh piece of dental floss or tape is used to remove any remaining abrasive particles between the teeth.

If necessary, a floss threader can be used to pass the floss under any fixed bridgework to gain access to the abutment teeth. Flossing techniques are further discussed in Chapter 15.

EVALUATION OF POLISHING

When you have completed polishing and flossing, evaluate the effectiveness of your technique by reapplying the disclosing agent and checking for the following criteria:

- After drying the tooth surfaces with air, no disclosing agent remains on any of the tooth surfaces.
- The teeth are glossy and reflect light from the mirror uniformly.
- There is no evidence of trauma to the gingival margins or any other soft tissues in the mouth.

Patient Education

Most patients are self-conscious about stains on their teeth and appreciate any tips you can give them about how they can keep their teeth as white as possible.

You can explain to the patient that the causes of extrinsic stains are often controllable sources, such as coffee, tea, and tobacco. Patients may then want to eliminate the causes of the stains or have you show them how to improve their oral hygiene procedures. It is important that patients understand the cause of stains on their teeth. When stains are intrinsic, the dentist may want you to mention possible cosmetic dental care options to satisfy the desire for attractive and stain-free teeth.

Legal and Ethical Implications

Laws regarding dental assistants performing coronal polishing vary widely among states. In some states, the dental assistant may have to be certified or registered to perform this function. It is your responsibility to understand and comply with the regulations of your state.

It is also important to remember that a coronal polish is not the same as a prophylaxis. Dental assistants are not allowed to perform a prophylaxis. A dentist or a dental hygienist must do this procedure.

Eye to the Future

Every day, patients see and hear advertisements in the media for products that will clean, polish, whiten, and remove stains from their teeth. Some of the products are effective; many are not. This trend of consumer interest will continue to grow, and patients will look to the dental professionals who provide their care to help them make wise choices. The role of the dental healthcare professional is to help patients realize that good oral health means more than just white teeth.

Critical Thinking

1. Prior to performing a coronal polish on Michelle, a 16-year-old girl, the certified dental assistant (CDA) notices in the health history that Michelle was given the drug tetracycline as a very young child. Michelle states that she took the drug repeatedly during several months. What, if any, conditions might the CDA expect to see on Michelle's teeth?
2. The dentist asks the CDA to perform a coronal polish on a patient who will have some orthodontic brackets placed. The CDA notices some light calculus formation on the facial surfaces of the anterior teeth. What should the CDA do?
3. You are getting ready to perform a coronal polish procedure by beginning on the facial surfaces of the maxillary right quadrant. How would you position yourself and your patient?

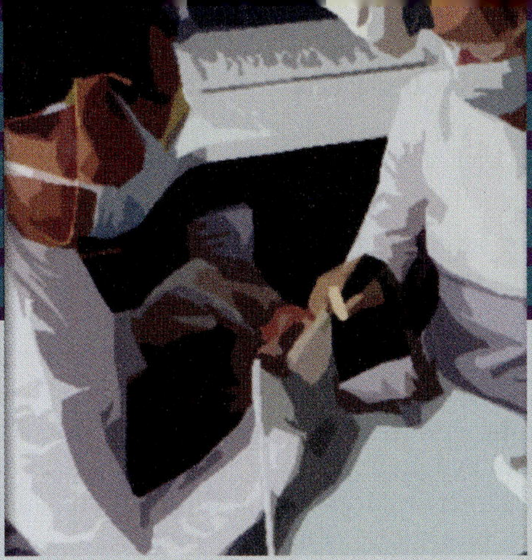

59 Dental Sealants

Outline

KEY TERMS

Acrylate (ak-**ri**-late) A salt or ester of acrylic acid.
Dental sealant Coating that covers the occlusal pits and fissures of teeth.
Filled resin (**re**-zin) Sealant material that contains filler particles.
Light-cured Type of material that is polymerized by a curing light.
Microleakage (**my**-cro-*leak*-age) Microscopic leakage at the interface of the tooth structure and the sealant or restoration.
Polymerization (puh-*lim*-er-i--**za**-shun) Process of changing a simple chemical into another substance containing the same elements.
Sealant retention The sealant firmly adhering to the tooth surface.
Self-cured Type of material that is polymerized by chemical reactions.
Unfilled resin (**re**-zin) Sealant material that does not contain filler particles

LEARNING OUTCOMES

On completion of this chapter, the student will be able to achieve the following objectives:

- Pronounce, define, and spell the Key Terms.
- Describe the purpose of dental sealants.
- Describe the clinical indications for dental sealants.
- Describe the contraindications to dental sealants.
- Discuss the rationale for filled and unfilled sealant materials.
- Describe the two types of polymerization.
- Explain the most important factor in sealant retention.

PERFORMANCE OUTCOMES

On completion of this chapter, the student will be able to achieve competency standards in the following skills:

- Demonstrate the steps in the application of dental sealants.
- Describe and demonstrate the safety steps necessary for the patient and operator during sealant placement.

The National Institutes of Health reports that pit and fissure caries account for at least 88 percent of the total caries experienced by school children in the United States.

Dental sealants are highly effective in preventing dental caries in the pit and fissure areas of the teeth. Although fluorides have the ability to increase the enamel's resistance to decay, the pits and fissures do not benefit from the effect of fluoride as much as smooth enamel surfaces do. Studies have shown 100 percent caries protection when dental sealants are properly placed and retained on the tooth surface.

Dental sealants are made of a resin material and are applied to the pits and fissures of teeth to prevent dental caries. A dental sealant is successful *only* if it firmly adheres to the enamel surface and protects the pits and fissures from the oral environment. Pits and fissures are the fossa and grooves that failed to fuse during development (see Chapter 8).

The narrow width and uneven depth of pits and fissures make them ideal places for the accumulation of acid-producing bacteria (Fig. 59-1). Saliva, which helps to remove food particles from other areas of the mouth, cannot clean deep pits and fissures in molars. The pits and grooves on the teeth are so small that even a single toothbrush bristle is too large to enter and clean pits and fissures (Fig. 59-2). The sealant acts as a physical barrier that prevents oral bacteria and dietary carbohydrates from creating the acid conditions that cause demineralization and ultimately dental caries. Placement of a dental sealant is a noninvasive technique that preserves the tooth structure and also prevents dental decay (Fig. 59-3).

In many states, application of dental sealants is a duty that may be delegated to the educationally qualified dental assistant (see Procedure 59-1).

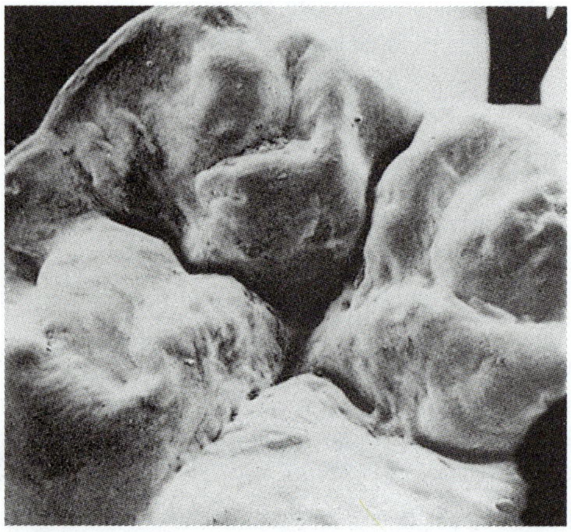

Fig. 59-1 Scanning electron micrograph (SEM) of occlusal pits and fissures. (From Daniel SJ, Harfst SA: *Mosby's dental hygiene: concepts, cases, and competencies–2004 update,* St Louis, 2004, Mosby.)

Recall

1. What is the purpose of dental sealants?
2. Why are pits and fissures susceptible to caries?

DENTAL CARIES AND SEALANTS

On occasion, teeth with very small initial carious lesions may be inadvertently sealed, or some bacteria will remain beneath the sealant. It was once believed that if this were to occur, decay would develop under the sealant. However, numerous studies have shown that this does not occur. Bacteria cannot survive beneath a *properly placed sealant* because the ingested carbohydrates they need to survive cannot reach them. Studies have shown that the number of bacteria in small, existing carious lesions that had been sealed actually *decreased* dramatically with time. The most important factor is that the sealant be properly placed.

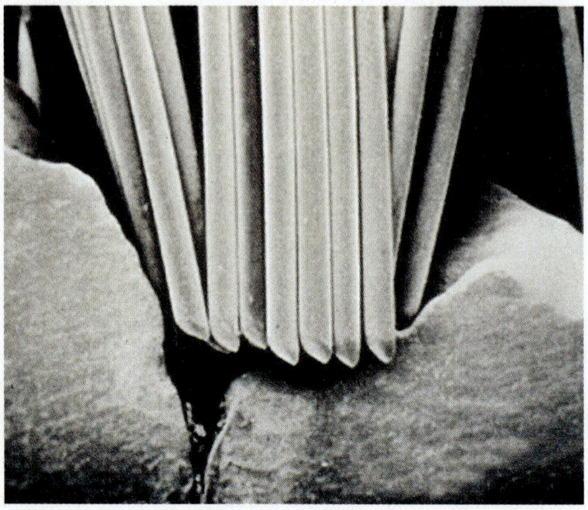

Fig. 59-2 Micrograph showing toothbrush bristle in a groove.

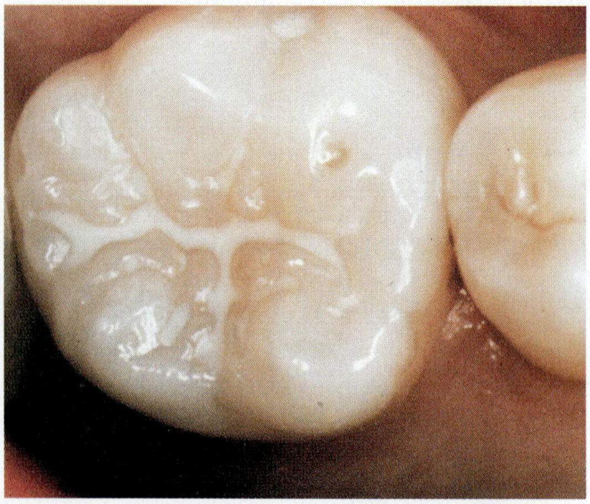

Fig. 59-3 Molar with a properly placed sealant.

However, surfaces on teeth that have large, overt dental caries should *not* be sealed. Scientific research on the use of pit and fissure sealants has proven that sealants are an effective way to prevent the development of dental caries.

INDICATIONS FOR SEALANTS

Sealants are used primarily on children, but in certain circumstances, adults can also benefit from their use. The dental professional must exercise proper patient selection and application techniques. Pit and fissure sealants are especially useful through the caries-active period (i.e., ages 6 to 15 years) and may delay the need for an occlusal restoration unless a proximal lesion develops.

Sealants are indicated for teeth with deep pits and fissures, preferably in recently erupted teeth (i.e., less than 4 years). Sealants should be used as part of a preventive program that includes the use of fluorides, dietary considerations, plaque control, and regular dental examinations (see Chapter 15).

CONTRAINDICATIONS TO SEALANTS

The contraindications to sealant placement include the following:

- Lack of deep pits and fissures
- Obvious dental decay
- Any proximal surface decay
- Insufficiently erupted teeth
- Primary teeth expected to be lost soon
- Poor patient cooperation in the dental chair

The cooperation of the patient during sealant placement is very important because proper placement requires a well-isolated, dry field. Patients and their parents should be advised that dental sealants are not a substitute for other caries control measures. Dental sealants are an *additional* part of the patient's overall preventive care.

TYPES OF SEALANT MATERIALS

A wide variety of sealant materials are available. The dental assistant should have a thorough understanding of the types and characteristics of the various sealant products (Fig. 59-4).

Method of Polymerization

One major difference among the materials is the method of **polymerization** (setting or curing). Some brands are self-cured, whereas others are light-cured. Both types are comparable in bond strengths and rates of retention.

Self-cured materials are supplied as a two-part system (base and catalyst). When these pastes are mixed together, they quickly polymerize *(harden)*. This usually occurs within 1 minute, and the material must be in place before the initial setting occurs.

Light-cured sealants do not require mixing. They cure when exposed to ultraviolet light. Currently, a one-step delivery system is available in which the material is provided in a light-protected preloaded syringe and is ready for direct application to the tooth. After the material is applied to the tooth, the curing light activates the setting of the material.

Color

Sealants may be clear, tinted, or opaque (white). Tinted or opaque sealants are more popular because they are easier to see during application and when checking for sealant retention on subsequent office visits. Some brands have a tint that is visible during the application but then turns clear after polymerization.

Fillers

Sealant materials are available as **filled** or **unfilled resins.** The purpose of filler material in the sealant is to reduce the occlusal wear. However, filled and unfilled sealants penetrate the fissures equally well. There is no difference in **microleakage** (leakage between the tooth surface and the sealant material), and they have similar rates of retention.

Some dentists believe that a filled sealant is better because of a lower wear rate on occlusal surfaces. Other dentists believe that the occlusal wear is insignificant because sealants flow deep into the pits and fissures to form a barrier.

An important clinical consideration between the two types is that the unfilled sealant material *does not* require

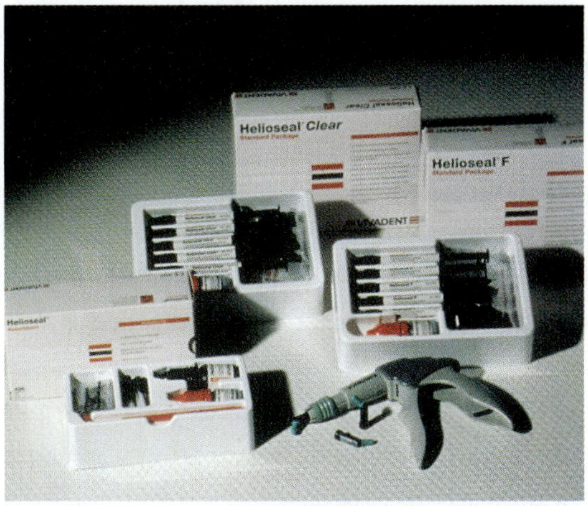

Fig. 59-4 **Helioseal Clear sealant material.** (Courtesy Ivoclar Vivadent, Amherst, NY.)

occlusal adjustment after placement because the natural wear is sufficient to establish occlusion, whereas a filled resin sealant *does* require checking the occlusion and possible adjustment with a stone or bur.

Recall

3. Should sealants be the only preventive measure used?
4. What are the two types of polymerization?
5. Why is clear sealant material less desirable?
6. Is there a difference in retention rates between filled and unfilled sealants?

Fluoride Release

Some brands of sealant materials contain fluoride that is released after polymerization. The theory is that the fluoride released from the sealant may create a fluoride-rich layer at the base of the sealed groove, helping remineralize incipient enamel caries. This fluoride-rich layer is also thought to make the pit or fissure more resistant to decay if the sealant is lost. Clinical studies are still underway comparing the effectiveness of these two types of sealants.

Some manufacturers recommend that fluoride-containing polishing paste not be applied to the enamel surface immediately before a sealant procedure. Other manufacturers do not consider fluoride polishing pastes to be contraindicated. Always follow the sealant manufacturer's instructions for each product you use.

STORAGE AND USE

Because products and recommendations differ among manufacturers, it is very important that you read the instructions specific to the brand being used. The following are some general tips on sealant materials:

- Replace caps on syringes and bottles immediately after use.
- Do not expose materials to air or light.
- Do not store materials in proximity to eugenol-containing products.
- Most etchant and sealant materials are designed to be used at room temperature. Check the manufacturer's recommendations.
- The shelf life of most sealant products at room temperature ranges from 18 to 36 months.
- Some brands of sealants must be stored in a refrigerator.

Manufacturer's Instructions

Always read and carefully follow the manufacturer's instructions when applying dental sealants. The application technique and etching times may vary among manufacturers. For example, some manufacturers recommend against using a polishing paste that contains fluoride. Other manufacturers do not consider fluoride polishing pastes to be contraindicated.

PRECAUTIONS FOR DENTAL PERSONNEL AND PATIENTS

Etchant Precautions

Etching agents contain phosphoric acid. Patients and dental personnel should always wear protective eyewear when using etchants. Avoid contact with oral soft tissue, eyes, and skin. In case of accidental contact, flush immediately with large amounts of water. If eye contact is involved, immediately rinse with plenty of water and seek medical attention.

Sealant Precautions

Sealant material contains **acrylate** resins. *Do not* use sealants on patients with known acrylate allergies. To reduce the risk for an allergic response, minimize the exposure to these materials. In particular, avoid exposure to uncured resin. Use of protective gloves and a *no-touch technique* is recommended. If skin contact occurs, wash skin with soap and water. Acrylates may penetrate gloves. If the sealant contacts the gloves, remove and discard the glove, wash hands immediately with soap and water, and then put on new gloves. If accidental eye contact or prolonged contact with oral soft tissue should occur, flush with large amounts of water. If irritation persists, contact a physician.

Protective glasses should be used by operators when using either the ultraviolet or visible light-cured resins. Protective eyewear should also be provided for the patient during sealant procedures.

FACTORS IN SEALANT RETENTION

The effectiveness of dental sealants depends on how well and how long the sealant remains on the tooth. This is referred to as **sealant retention.** Dental caries will not occur if the sealant remains in place and completely covers the pits and fissures.

Moisture contamination is the *primary cause* of failure of sealant retention. Inadequate etching is also a factor in loss of sealant retention. Dental sealants should be examined at each recall visit to be certain that the sealant material is not partially or totally lost. When dental sealants are *properly placed,* it is not uncommon for them to last from 5 to 10 years.

Recall

7. What is the reason for putting fluoride in dental sealant material?
8. What is the range of shelf-life of sealant materials?
9. What are two patient safety precautions to keep in mind when using sealants?
10. What determines the effectiveness of dental sealants?

Procedure 59-1 Application of Dental Sealants

Goal

The student will apply a light-cured dental sealant according to the manufacturer's instructions and within the scope of the state dental practice act.

Equipment and Supplies

- Protective eyewear
- Basic setup
- Cotton rolls or rubber dam setup
- Etching agent (liquid or gel)
- Sealant material
- Applicator syringe or device
- Prophy brush
- Pumice and water
- High-volume oral evacuator (HVE)
- Curing light and appropriate shield
- Low-speed dental handpiece with contra-angle attachment
- Articulating paper and holder
- Round white stone (latch type)
- Dental floss
- Materials for occlusal adjustments (when using a filled resin product)

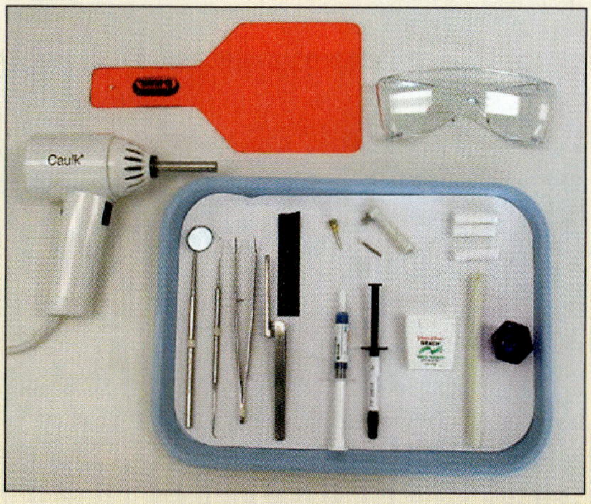

PROCEDURAL STEPS

1. Select teeth. The teeth must have deep pits and fissures and be sufficiently erupted so that a dry field can be maintained.
   Purpose: The teeth must be sufficiently erupted for sealant placement.
2. Check air-water syringe. Blow a jet of air from the syringe onto a mirror or glove. If small droplets are visible, the syringe must be adjusted so that *only* air is expressed.
   Purpose: Any moisture contamination during certain steps of this procedure can cause the retention of the sealant to fail.
3. Clean the enamel. Thoroughly clean the teeth with pumice and water to remove plaque and debris from the occlusal surface. Rinse thoroughly with water.
   Note: Do not use any cleaning agents that contain oils. Check the manufacturer's instructions to see whether a fluoride-containing prophy paste is contraindicated for cleaning the enamel.
   If you use an air polish device that uses sodium bicarbonate for cleaning, the etching step should be repeated for a second time, or 3 percent hydrogen peroxide should be applied to the surface for 10 seconds to neutralize the sodium bicarbonate and then thoroughly rinsed with water prior to applying the etch.

continued

Procedure 59-1 Application of Dental Sealants–cont'd

PROCEDURAL STEPS, cont'd

4. Isolate and dry the teeth. The rubber dam provides the best isolation; however, cotton rolls are acceptable. Use a saliva ejector or high-volume evacuation.
   Purpose: Excess saliva is uncomfortable for the patient and may contaminate the tooth to be sealed.

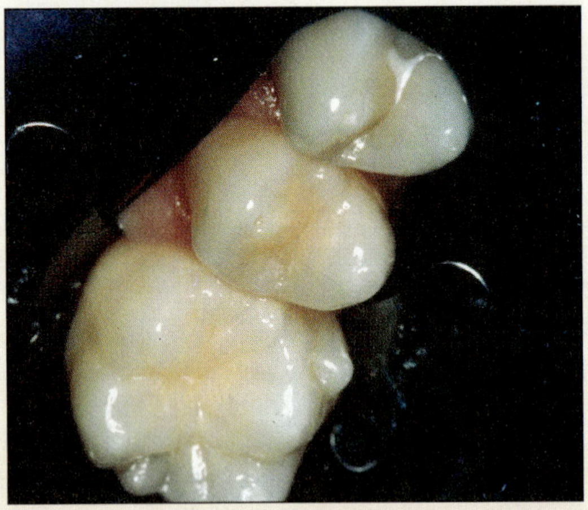

5. Etch enamel. Use the syringe tip, or device, to apply a generous amount of etchant to all enamel surfaces to be sealed, extending slightly beyond the anticipated margin of the sealant. Etch for a minimum of 15 seconds but no longer than 60 seconds.
   Purpose: The sealant will not adhere to surfaces not thoroughly etched.

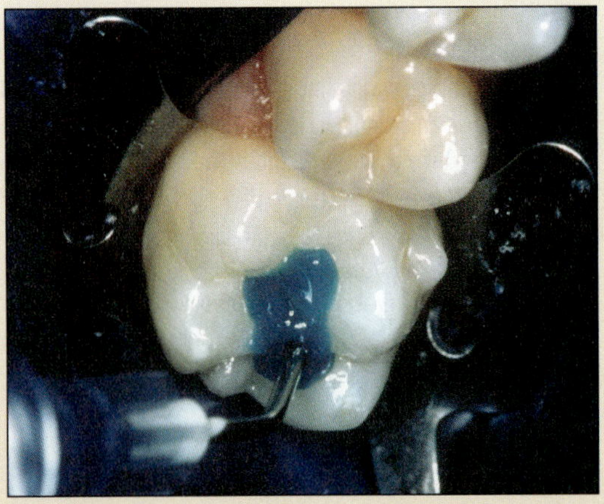

6. Rinse etched enamel. Thoroughly rinse teeth with the air-water syringe to remove etchant. Remove the rinse water with suction. Do not allow the patient to swallow or rinse.
   Note: If saliva contacts the etched surfaces, re-etch for 5 seconds and rinse again.
   Purpose: Saliva will contaminate the etched surface, and the sealant will not properly adhere to the enamel.

7. Dry etched enamel. Thoroughly dry the etched surfaces using the air-water syringe. The air from the syringe should be dry and free from oil and water. The dry etched surfaces should appear as a matte frosty white. If not, repeat steps 5 and 6. *Do not allow the etched surface to be contaminated.*
   Purpose: Moisture contamination of etched surfaces is the main cause of failure of pit and fissure sealants.

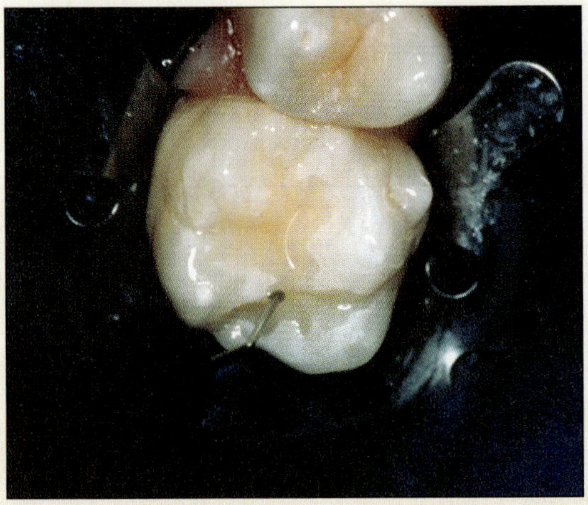

8. Apply sealant. Using the syringe tip or a brush, slowly introduce sealant into the pits and fissures. Do not let sealant flow beyond the etched surfaces. Stirring the sealant with the syringe tip or brush during or after the placement will help eliminate any possible bubbles and increase the flow into the pits and fissures. An explorer may also be used. Remember to check the manufacturer's recommendations for the most effective technique for sealant placement.
9. Cure the sealant. Hold the tip of the light as close as possible to the sealant without actually touching the sealant. A 20-second exposure is needed for each surface.

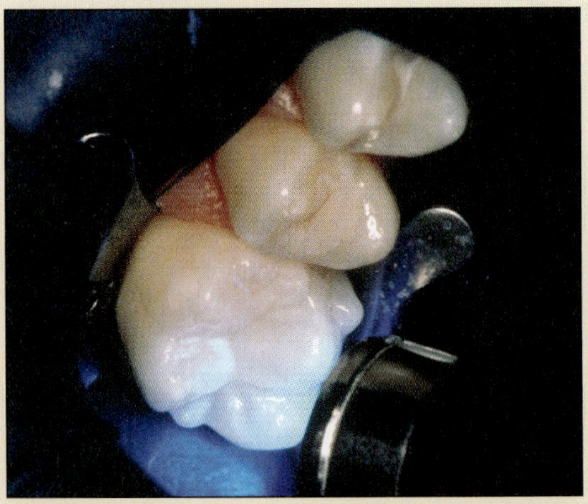

Procedure 59-1 Application of Dental Sealants—cont'd

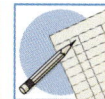

10. Evaluate the sealant. Carefully inspect the sealant for complete coverage and voids. If the surface has not been contaminated, additional sealant material may be placed. If contamination has occurred, re-etch and dry prior to placing more sealant material. Check the interproximal areas using dental floss to make certain there is no sealant material in the contact area.

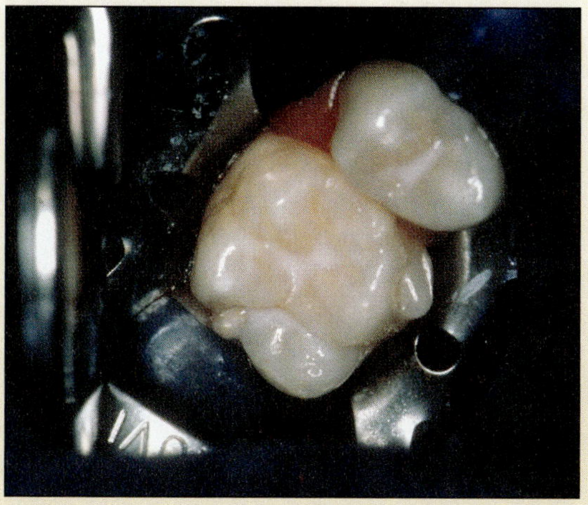

11. **Completion.** Wipe the sealant with a cotton applicator to remove the thin, sticky film on the surface. Check occlusion using the articulating paper and adjust if required.
12. Document the procedure in the patient's chart

Date	Charting Notes	Signature
5/10/05	Application of sealants to #3, 14, 19, 30.	PJL

Legal and Ethical Implications

Application of dental sealants is considered to be an expanded function for dental assistants in many states. In other states, however, dental assistants are allowed only to assist with the placement of dental sealants. It is your professional responsibility to check the regulations in your state and to practice accordingly.

Whether or not you are legally allowed to actually *place* sealants, you can certainly educate your patients about the importance of sealants, explain the process, and answer their questions.

Eye to the Future

Dental sealants also protect the margins of dental restorations. Microleakage can occur around the margins of composite restorations because the material shrinks slightly during the visible-light curing process. These tiny gaps can lead to recurrent decay and marginal staining. Clinical researchers have shown that sealing the margins of amalgam and composite restorations with unfilled resins will (1) reduce microleakage, (2) arrest the progression of caries, (3) preserve existing restorations, and (4) preserve tooth structure.

This type of treatment may increase the longevity of the restoration, especially if the sealant is reapplied at 1-year intervals.

Critical Thinking

1. Carol Tyler is a single mom with limited financial means. Her young son, Phillip, has deep grooves and pits on his newly erupted first molars, and the dentist has recommended dental sealants. After the dentist leaves the room, Carol explains that she is on a very tight budget and asks you why it is necessary to add sealants when the teeth have just erupted and there is no decay. What will you tell her?
2. Emily Schmidt is a very lively 6-year-old child who does not sit still in the dental chair. About 6 months ago, when two dental sealants were placed, Emily was very uncooperative and difficult to manage. Now, on her 6-month recall, the dentist notes that one of the two sealants is gone. What do you think might have happened to make the sealant fail in such a short period?
3. Lorraine Yee and her friend Margaret Printz are talking about their children's first dental visit to Dr. McNeal's office. Both children are 5 years old, and both of them saw Dr. McNeal. Lorraine was advised to have dental sealants placed on her child's teeth; however, Dr. McNeal did not tell Margaret that her child needed sealants. Why would Dr. McNeal recommend sealants for one child, but not for another?

60

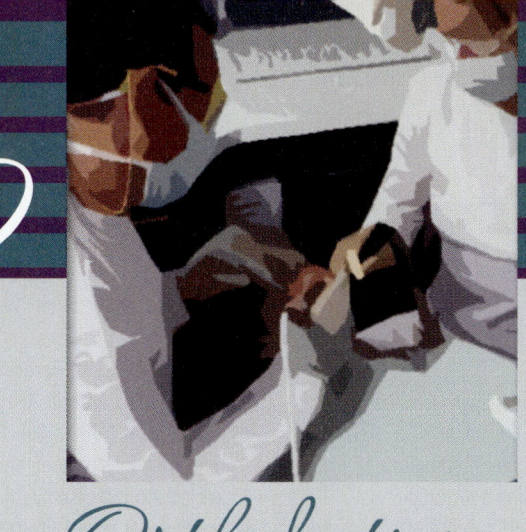

Orthodontics

Outline

KEY TERMS

Arch wire A contoured metal wire that provides force when guiding teeth in movement for orthodontics.

Auxiliary (aug-**zil**-er-ee) Type of attachments located on brackets and bands that hold arch wires and elastics.

Band Stainless steel ring attached to molars to hold the arch wire and auxiliaries for orthodontics.

Braces Another term for fixed orthodontic appliances.

Bracket A small device bonded to teeth to hold the arch wire to the teeth.

Cephalometric radiograph (*sef*-uh-lo-**me**-trik) An extraoral radiograph of the bones and tissues of the head.

Crossbite Condition that occurs when a tooth is not properly aligned with its opposing tooth.

KEY TERMS, cont'd

Crowding Condition that occurs when teeth are not aligned properly within the arch.

Dentofacial Describes structures including the teeth, jaws, and surrounding facial bones.

Distoclusion A class II malocclusion in which the mesiobuccal cusp of the maxillary first molar occludes (by more than the width of a premolar) mesial to the mesiobuccal groove of the mandibular first molar.

Fetal molding Pressure applied to the jaw, causing a distortion.

Headgear An external orthodontic appliance used to control growth and tooth movement.

Ligature tie (**lig**-a-chure) Light wire used to hold the arch wire in its bracket.

Malocclusion (**mal**-o-clu-zhun) Occlusion that is deviated from a class I normal occlusion.

Mesioclusion (**mez**-i-o-clu-zhun) Term used for class III malocclusion.

Occlusion (oh-*klu*-zhun) The natural contact of the maxillary and mandibular teeth in all positions.

Open bite A lack of vertical overlap of the maxillary incisors, creating an opening of the anterior teeth.

Orthodontics (orth-o-**don**-tics) Specialty within dentistry that focuses on preventing, intercepting, and correcting skeletal and dental problems.

Overbite An increased vertical overlap of the maxillary incisors.

Overjet An excessive protrusion of the maxillary incisors.

Positioner An appliance used to retain teeth in their desired position.

Retainer An appliance used for maintaining the positions of the teeth and jaws after orthodontic treatment.

Separator A device made from wire or elastic and used to separate molars before the fitting and placement of orthodontic bands.

LEARNING OUTCOMES

On completion of this chapter, the student will be able to achieve the following objectives:

- Pronounce, define, and spell the Key Terms.
- Describe the environment of an orthodontic practice.
- Describe the types of malocclusion.
- Discuss corrective orthodontics and describe what type of treatment is involved.
- List the types of diagnostic records used to assess orthodontic problems.
- Describe the components of the fixed appliance.
- Describe the use and function of headgear.
- Describe ways to convey the importance of good dietary and oral hygiene habits in the treatment of orthodontics.

PERFORMANCE OUTCOMES

On completion of this chapter, the student will be able to achieve competency standards in the following skills:

- Place and remove brass wire separators.
- Place and remove steel separating springs.
- Place and remove elastomeric ring separators.
- Assist in the fitting and cementation of orthodontic bands.
- Assist in the direct bonding of orthodontic brackets.
- Place an archwire.
- Place and remove ligature ties.
- Place and remove elastomeric ties.

Orthodontics is the specialty of dentistry concerned with the supervision, guidance, and correction of the growing and mature **dentofacial** structures. This area of dentistry encompasses all ages of the population. As insurance companies increase benefits for continued orthodontic care, more people will choose orthodontic treatment throughout their lifetime.

THE ORTHODONTIST

The orthodontist works very closely with the pediatric and general dentist in providing an opportunity to change a person's "smile." As a specialist, the orthodontist continues education after dental school. Most accredited orthodontic programs are 3 years in length. The emphasis of study for the orthodontist is orofacial growth and development, new techniques, and research. After receiving a certificate or master's degree, the orthodontist either sets up private practice or remains in academia.

THE ORTHODONTIC ASSISTANT

If you are looking for an area of dentistry with more autonomy, orthodontics is the specialty of choice. The orthodontic assistant is able to participate in many "hands-on" skills. Depending on the expanded functions legally permitted in the state in which you practice, the assistant is able to participate in various procedures involving diagnostic records, preliminary appointments, and adjustment visits.

If advancing further in the profession of orthodontics is your goal, you can (1) continue in specialized training within a program or (2) sit for the Dental Assisting National Boards in Orthodontic Assisting. After passing this exam, your professional title would be certified orthodontic assistant (COA).

THE ORTHODONTIC OFFICE

An orthodontic office is designed to accommodate many patients at a time. Because very little equipment is required in orthodontic procedures, the orthodontic office follows the "open bay" concept as with pediatric dentistry. The patient care area of the office is sectioned off to serve three functions: (1) to obtain records and create a more private setting, (2) to take radiographs, and (3) to provide patient care for all stages of treatment. In larger practices, it is common to see up to 30 patients a day. Longer appointments, such as those to obtain records, are scheduled in the mornings; shorter appointments, such as adjustments and emergencies, are kept for the afternoon.

One area of the practice that is *more* expansive in the orthodontic setting is the dental lab. Most orthodontic practices pour and trim diagnostic models and fabricate fixed and removable appliances.

UNDERSTANDING OCCLUSION

To comprehend the importance of **occlusion,** it is necessary to understand differences among individuals in the size and shape of the jaws, occlusions, and the reasons that some teeth become crowded. In most cases, malocclusion and dentofacial deformities result from moderate distortions of normal development. The orthodontic problems of most people come from an interaction of developmental, genetic, environmental, and functional influences.

Developmental Causes

Disturbances of dental development can accompany major congenital defects; however, they occur more frequently as isolated findings. The most commonly encountered developmental disturbances include the following:

- Congenitally missing teeth
- Malformed teeth
- Supernumerary teeth
- Interference with eruption (e.g., an impaction in which eruption is blocked or the tooth is forced to erupt into an abnormal position)
- *Ectopic* eruption

Genetic Causes

Genetic causes are responsible for malocclusion when there are discrepancies in the size of the jaw and/or the size of the teeth. This happens more commonly when the child inherits a small jaw from one parent and larger teeth from the other parent. If you have a missing tooth, it is likely that one of your parents or grandparents has the same missing tooth.

Environmental Causes

Birth Injuries

Injuries can occur at birth in two major categories: fetal molding and trauma during birth.

Fetal molding occurs when an arm or leg of the fetus is pressed against another part of the body, such as when an arm is abnormally pressed against the mandible. This pressure can lead to distortion of rapidly growing areas.

Trauma during birth, such as an injury to the jaw, may occur during the actual birth, particularly from the use of forceps in delivery.

Injury Throughout Life

Trauma to the teeth can also occur throughout life. Dental trauma can lead to the development of malocclusion in three ways:

1. Damage to permanent tooth buds when an injury to primary teeth has occurred
2. Movement of a tooth or teeth as a result of the premature loss of a primary tooth
3. Direct injury to permanent teeth

Habits

Habits that contribute to malalignment must be corrected if orthodontic treatment is to be successful. As a general rule, sucking habits that involve the thumb, tongue, lip, or finger during the primary dentition years are considered normal. These habits have few, if any, long-term effects beyond the mixed dentition; however, if they persist beyond this stage, it may be necessary to seek guidance in eliminating the habit. Box 60-1 describes habits that affect the dentition.

Recall

1. What age groups seek orthodontic care?
2. What could be a genetic cause for malocclusion?

Box 60-1 Habits Affecting the Dentition

Tongue thrusting	*Anterior tongue thrust*–The tongue rests on the lingual surfaces of the maxillary teeth. The pressure causes the teeth to move forward. *Lateral tongue thrust*–The pressure of the tongue causes the bite to close down, preventing the permanent teeth from erupting. *Fan tongue thrust*–The tongue thrusts out at the occlusal surfaces.
Tongue thrust swallowing	The tongue presses forward against the anterior teeth with each swallow, placing a forward pressure against the teeth.
Thumb and finger sucking	Beyond the age of 5, the facial structure will be affected, particularly the maxillary arch, the palate, and the anterior teeth.
Bruxism	The involuntary grinding or clenching of the teeth in movements other than chewing. This occurs most frequently during sleep. The grinding of teeth causes unnatural wear of the enamel and pressure on the periodontium.
Mouth breathing	May be a result of the narrowing of the maxilla, which can cause a pinched facial appearance. Mouth breathing prolonged over a number of years can cause a change in the dentofacial structure of the child.

OCCLUSION

As described in Chapter 12, the maxillary and mandibular teeth, when closed correctly, are referred to as being *occluded* or having *normal occlusion* or *class I occlusion* (Fig. 60-1, *A* and *B*). Orthodontists are concerned with teeth that do not occlude properly because of the size of the jaws, crowding, or displacement of teeth. **Malocclusion** refers to this abnormal or malpositioned relationship of the maxillary teeth to the mandibular teeth when occluded.

Malocclusion

According to Angle's classification, any deviation from class I occlusion is considered to be malocclusion.

Class II Malocclusion

In class II malocclusion, also known as **distoclusion,** the body of the mandible is in an abnormal distal relationship to the maxilla. This frequently gives the appearance of the maxillary anterior teeth protruding over the mandibular anterior teeth. A common lay term for this condition is

A

B

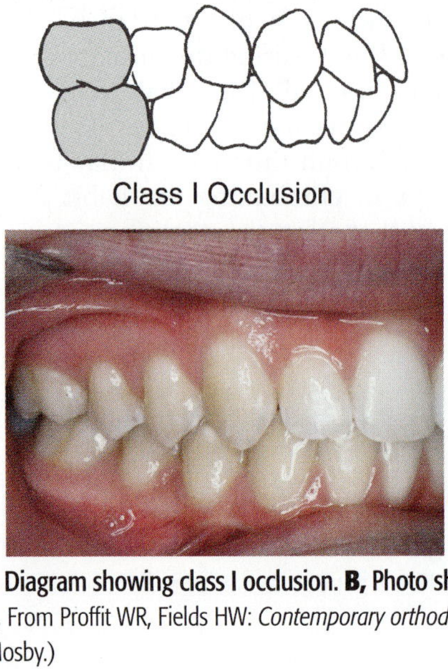

Fig. 60-1 A, Diagram showing class I occlusion. **B,** Photo showing class I occlusion. (A, From Proffit WR, Fields HW: *Contemporary orthodontics,* ed 3, St Louis, 2000, Mosby.)

A

B

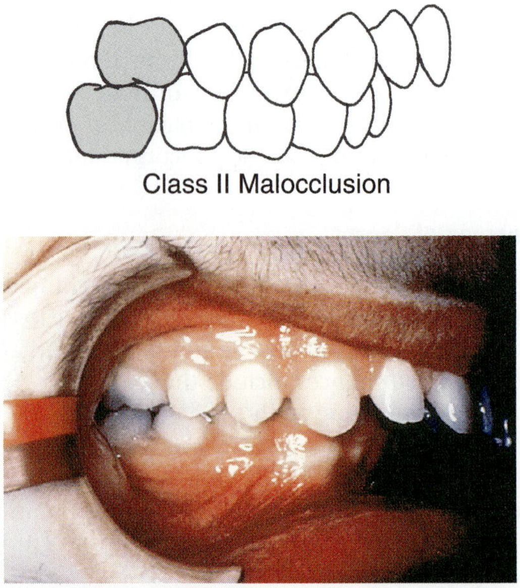

Fig. 60-2 A, Diagram showing class II malocclusion. **B,** Photo showing class II malocclusion. (A, From Proffit WR, Fields HW: *Contemporary orthodontics,* ed 3, St Louis, 2000, Mosby.)

buckteeth. The mesiobuccal cusp of the maxillary first molar occludes in the interdental space between the mandibular second premolar and the mesial cusp of the mandibular first molar (Fig. 60-2, *A* and *B*).

Class III Malocclusion

In class III malocclusion, also known as **mesioclusion,** the body of the mandible is in an abnormal mesial relationship to the maxilla. This frequently gives the appearance of the mandibular anterior teeth protruding in front of the maxillary anterior teeth, also referred to as an *underbite.* The mesiobuccal cusp of the maxillary first molar occludes in the interdental space between the distal cusp of the mandibular first permanent molar and the mesial cusp of the mandibular second permanent molar (Fig. 60-3, *A* and *B*).

Malaligned Teeth

In addition to evaluating a patient's occlusion, the orthodontist examines specific alignment of the teeth and arches. The most common malalignment problems are as follows:

- **Crowding** is the most common contributor to malocclusion. One or many teeth can be involved in misplacement (Fig. 60-4).
- **Overjet** is an excessive protrusion of the maxillary incisors, causing space or distance between the facial surface of the mandibular incisors with the lingual surface of the maxillary incisors (Fig. 60-5).
- **Overbite** is an increased vertical overlap of the maxillary incisors. In an extreme overbite, the mandibular incisors may not be visible (Fig. 60-6).
- **Open bite** is a lack of vertical overlap of the maxillary incisors, creating an opening of the anterior teeth when the posterior teeth are closed (Fig. 60-7).
- **Crossbite** indicates that a tooth is not properly aligned with its opposing tooth. An example of this is when a person closes the teeth; the maxillary arch should be

A

B

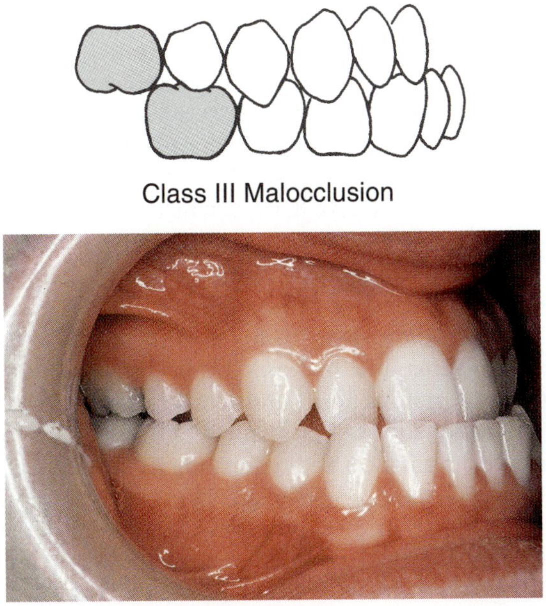

Fig. 60-3 A, Diagram showing class III malocclusion. **B,** Photo showing class III malocclusion. (A, From Proffit WR, Fields HW: *Contemporary orthodontics,* ed 3, St Louis, 2000, Mosby.)

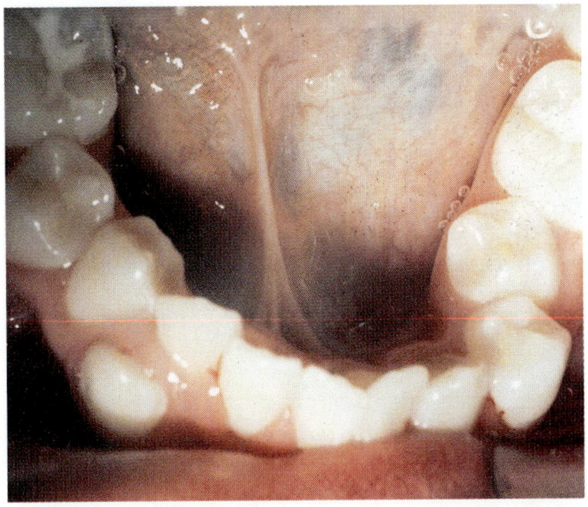

Fig. 60-4 Crowding of teeth in the mandibular arch.

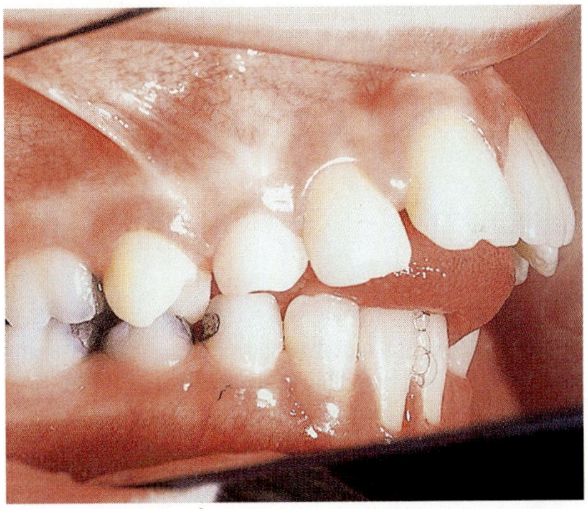

Fig. 60-5 Excessive protrusion of the maxillary incisors creates an overjet.

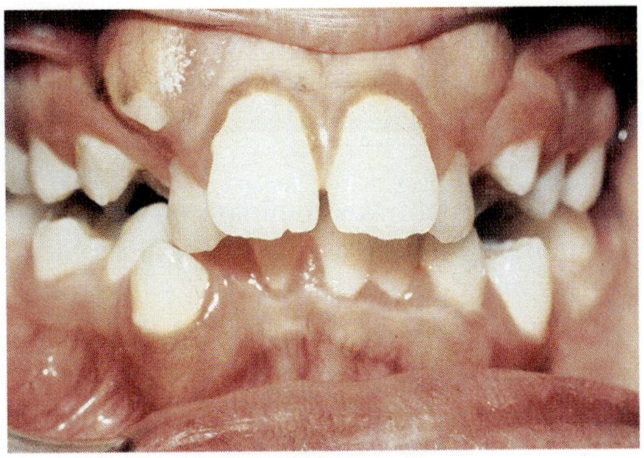

Fig. 60-6 Overbite.

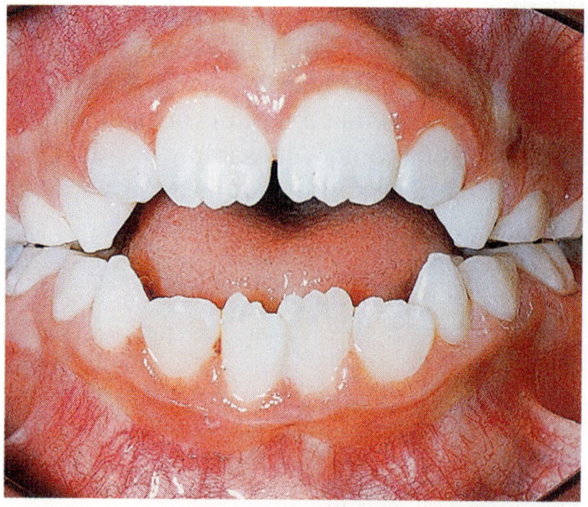

Fig. 60-7 An open bite is created when patient's anterior teeth make an opening.

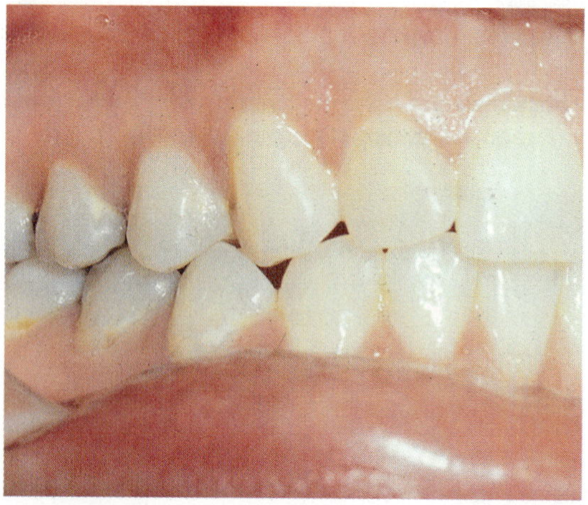

Fig. 60-8 An example of a crossbite showing an improper alignment of the maxillary canine and mandibular premolar.

slightly wider and longer so that it properly occludes the mandibular arch. If a maxillary tooth is inward or touching end to end with another tooth, then a crossbite exists (Fig. 60-8).

BENEFITS OF ORTHODONTIC TREATMENT

Orthodontic treatment can eliminate or reduce adversity for the patient in three areas: psychosocial problems, oral malfunction, and dental disease.

Psychosocial Influences

Severe malocclusion and dental facial deformities can be a social handicap. The impact of these types of problems may have a strong influence on patients' self-esteem and their positive feelings about themselves.

Oral Function

Malocclusion can compromise all aspects of oral function:

- Chewing can be difficult if teeth do not occlude properly.
- Jaw discrepancies can force changes in the manner of swallowing.
- Malocclusion can make it more difficult for certain speech sounds to be made.
- Temporomandibular joint pain can arise from minor imperfections in occlusion that trigger clenching and grinding activities.

Dental Disease

Malocclusion can contribute to both dental decay and periodontal disease. When the teeth and tissues do not receive the benefits of normal occlusion and natural cleansing, proper plaque removal becomes difficult.

Recall

3. What term is used for abnormal occlusion?
4. What tooth determines a person's occlusion?
5. If a tooth is not properly aligned with its opposing tooth, it is said to be in ___________.
6. If a person occludes and you cannot see the mandibular anteriors, what is that patient's diagnosis?

MANAGEMENT OF ORTHODONTIC PROBLEMS

Pediatric and general practitioners are trained in the recognition and treatment of preventive and interceptive orthodontic cases (see also Chapter 57). More extensive cases, however, are referred to the orthodontist for diagnosis and treatment.

Corrective Orthodontics

The scope of corrective orthodontics includes conditions that require the movement of teeth and the correction of malrelationships and malformations. These adjustments between and among teeth and facial bones are made by the application of fixed appliances with force and sometimes with stimulation and redirection of functional forces within the dentofacial structure. The responsibilities of personnel in the orthodontic practice include the treatment of all forms of malocclusion of the teeth and surrounding structures.

Corrective orthodontics includes:

- Fixed appliances (e.g., cemented or bonded in place; cannot be removed by the patient)

- Removable appliances for the correction or maintenance of orthodontic treatment
- Orthognathic surgery when the orthodontic problem is too severe to be corrected by other means

ORTHODONTIC RECORDS AND TREATMENT PLANNING

The first step in determining a treatment plan is for the orthodontist to learn as much about the orthodontic condition as possible. The patient's first orthodontic appointment is devoted to obtaining records. These records are needed for the orthodontist to make a diagnosis and devise a treatment plan.

Medical and Dental History

Careful medical and dental histories are necessary to provide a comprehensive understanding of the physical condition and to evaluate specific orthodontically related concerns.

Physical Growth Evaluation

Because orthodontic treatment in children is closely related to growth stages, it is necessary to evaluate the child's physical growth status. Questions are asked about how rapidly the child has grown recently and about signs of sexual maturation.

Social and Behavioral Evaluation

Motivation for seeking treatment is very important. What does the patient expect as a result of treatment? How cooperative or uncooperative is the patient likely to be? A major motivation for orthodontic treatment of children is the parent's desire for treatment; however, it is essential that the child be willing and cooperative. The typical child accepts orthodontic treatment in a positive way.

Adults tend to seek orthodontic treatment for themselves for other reasons, including the need to improve personal appearance or function of the teeth. It is important to explore the reasons why an adult patient seeks treatment.

Clinical Examination

The purpose of the orthodontic clinical examination is to document, measure, and evaluate the facial aspects, the occlusal relationship, and the functional characteristics of the jaws. At the initial (records) visit, the orthodontist decides which diagnostic evaluations are required for the patient.

Evaluation of Facial Esthetics

A reasonable goal for orthodontic treatment is to recognize and improve facial symmetry by correcting disproportion.

In *frontal evaluation,* the face is examined for:

- Bilateral symmetry
- Size proportions of midline to lateral structures
- Vertical proportionality

In the *profile evaluation,* the profile relationship is analyzed for the following reasons:

- To determine whether the jaws are proportionately positioned
- To evaluate lip protrusion (excessive lip protrusion is most often caused by protrusion of the incisors)
- To evaluate the vertical facial proportions and the mandibular plane angle

Evaluation of Oral Health

A thorough hard and soft tissue examination, as well as an oral hygiene assessment and prophylaxis, must be completed before any orthodontic treatment begins. Any charting of periodontal pockets must be noted. If necessary, the patient is referred for the treatment of these problems before orthodontic treatment is started.

Evaluation of Jaw and Occlusal Function

The orthodontist examines the patient's occlusion and palpates the temporomandibular joint (TMJ) to evaluate its function. Lateral or anterior shifts of the mandible on closure are of special interest for orthodontic purposes.

Diagnostic Records

Before the clinical evaluation can be completed, diagnostic records are required in the form of photographs, radiographs, and diagnostic models. When possible, it is best to have these available at the time of the intraoral examination. Diagnostic records document features such as tooth angulation, dental crowding, and the presence of unerupted teeth.

Photographs

Photographs capture the color, shape, texture, and characteristics of intraoral and extraoral structures. Photography also is useful as an aid in patient identification, treatment planning, case presentation, case documentation, and patient education.

Two standard extraoral photographs are taken (Fig. 60-9):

- The frontal view, with the lips in a relaxed position
- A profile view of the patient's right side, with the lips in a relaxed position

Three standard intraoral photographs are required (Fig. 60-10, *A* to *C*):

- The full direct view, which includes all teeth in occlusion
- The maxillary occlusal view, which includes the palate and all maxillary occlusal surfaces

- The right buccal view, which includes the distal of the canine to the distal of the last molar view

When intraoral photographs are taken, it is important that the cheeks and lips are retracted sufficiently to show all these structures.

Radiographs

The type of radiograph that is most commonly exposed for an orthodontic patient is the **cephalometric radiograph.** This extraoral radiograph makes it possible to evaluate the anatomic bases for malocclusion, skull, bones, and soft

A

B

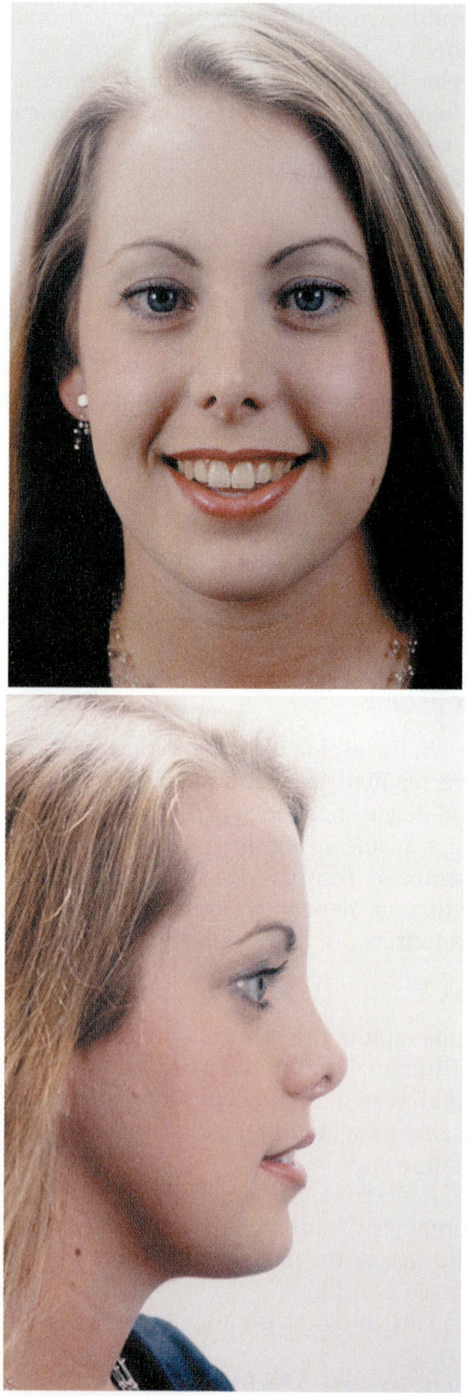

Fig. 60-9 A and B, Standard extraoral photographs. (From Proffit WR, White RP, Sarver DM: *Contemporary treatment of dentofacial deformity,* St Louis, 2003, Mosby.)

A

B

C

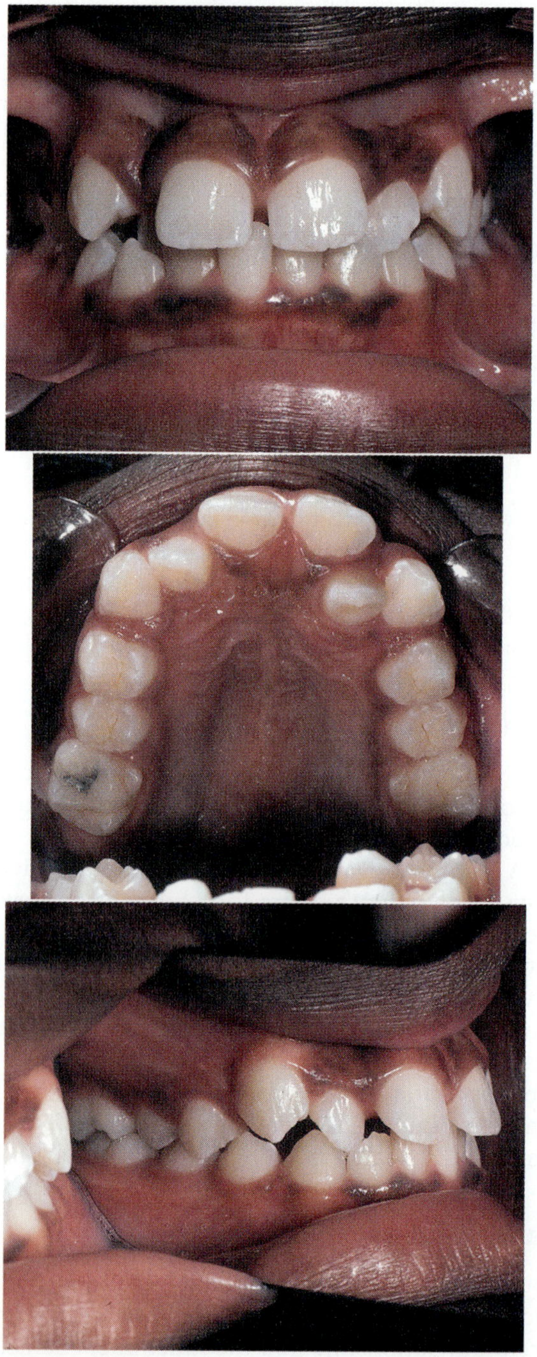

Fig. 60-10 Intraoral photographs showing a patient's front view in occlusion **(A)**, maxillary occlusal view **(B)**, and right buccal view **(C)**.

tissue (Fig. 60-11, *A*). Serial cephalometric radiographs taken at intervals before, during, and after treatment can be superimposed to study changes in jaw and tooth positions. (See Chapter 42 for techniques in exposing the cephalometric radiograph.)

Cephalometric analysis

Cephalometric analysis is not completed on the radiograph but instead as either a tracing or a computerized drawing that emphasizes the relationship of selected points. Cephalometric landmarks are represented as a series of points, making it possible for the orthodontist to compute mathematical descriptions and measurement of the status of the skull (Fig. 60-11, *B*). From these measurements the orthodontist can analyze growth patterns, which will determine the type of treatment for the patient.

A

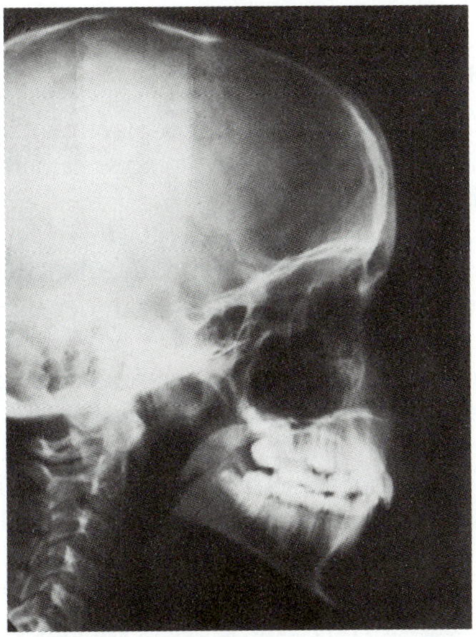

B

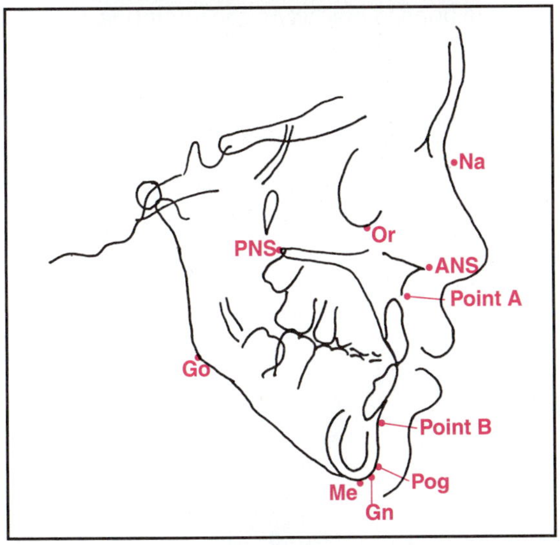

Fig. 60-11 **A,** Cephalometric radiograph. **B,** Cephalometric analysis.

Diagnostic Models

Diagnostic models are used for the diagnosis and case presentation of the orthodontic patient. The diagnostic model for orthodontics is most commonly made from plaster and is constructed in a more precise and finished manner (Fig. 60-12). Chapter 47 gives detailed instruction in the taking of preliminary impressions and the fabrication of diagnostic models.

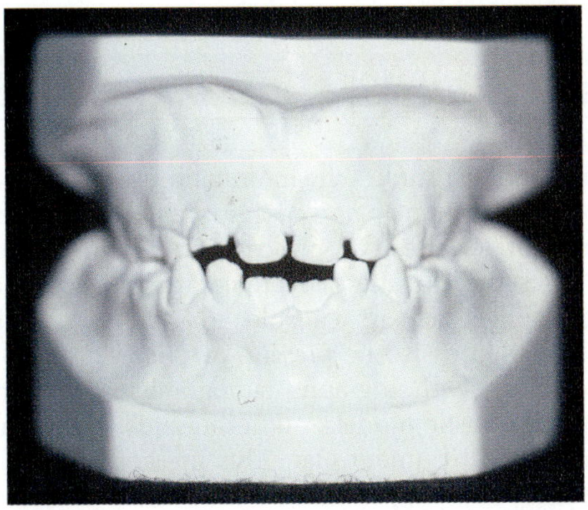

Fig. 60-12 Diagnostic model.

Cephalometric Landmarks and Points

Anterior nasal spine (ANS): the median bony process of the maxilla at the lower margin of the anterior nasal opening

Gonion (Go): the center of the inferior contour of the mandibular angle

Gnathion (Gn): the center of the inferior contour of the chin

Menton (Me): the most inferior point on the mandibular symphysis (the bottom of the chin)

Nasion (Na): the anterior point of the intersection between the nasal and frontal bones

Orbitale (Or): the lowest point on the inferior margin of the orbit

Pogonion (Pog): the most anterior point on the contour of the chin

Point A: the innermost point on the contour of the premaxilla between the anterior nasal spine and the incisor

Point B: the innermost point on the contour of the mandible between the incisor and the bony chin

Posterior nasal spine (PNS): the tip of the posterior spine of the palatine bone, at the junction of the hard and soft palate

Recall

7. What two positions does the orthodontist evaluate for facial symmetry?
8. What type of radiograph is most commonly taken in orthodontics?
9. How many photographs are taken during the records appointment?
10. What gypsum material is most commonly used for fabricating diagnostic models in an orthodontic office?

CASE PRESENTATION

The orthodontist studies the information gathered and develops a treatment plan and cost estimate for the patient in preparation for the case presentation. Approximately 1 hour is reserved for the case presentation visit. If the patient is younger than 18 years old, an adult responsible for the child should also be present. At this visit, the orthodontist uses the photographs, radiographs, cephalometric tracing, diagnostic models, and other aids to present the diagnosis and treatment plan. This presentation includes the approximate length of treatment and a clear statement of the responsibility of the patient in helping to ensure successful completion.

Once treatment has been accepted, the adult or legal guardian signs a consent form. This consent form clearly states the information presented during the case presentation.

Financial Arrangements

In addition to the case presentation and consent form, a formal contract for payment of the treatment fee is presented and discussed with the individual responsible for the finances. The most frequently used payment plan involves divided payments. Once the patient and responsible persons agree that treatment should proceed, the person legally responsible for the account signs the contract.

Some dental insurance plans cover the cost of orthodontic treatment. When insurance coverage exists, it is usually the responsibility of the subscriber, not the orthodontic practice, to submit periodic progress claims for reimbursement.

SPECIALIZED INSTRUMENTS AND ACCESSORIES

Orthodontics requires the use of highly specialized instruments. The following are the most commonly used types of instruments and pliers:

Intraoral Instruments

The *orthodontic scaler* aids in bracket placement, removal of elastomeric rings, and removal of excess cement or bonding material (Fig. 60-13, *A*).

The *ligature director* guides the elastic or wire ligature tie around the bracket. Additionally, the operator can tuck the twisted and cut ligature tie under the arch wire (Fig. 60-13, *B*).

The **band** plugger has a round serrated end to help seat a molar band for a fixed appliance (Fig. 60-13, *C*).

The *bite stick* consists of a molded plastic handle with a triangular stainless-steel serrated working area. This is used to aid in seating a molar band for a fixed appliance (Fig. 60-13, *D*).

Bracket placement tweezers are long-tipped, reverse-action tweezers with fine serrated beaks. They are used to carry and place the bonded bracket on the tooth (Fig. 60-13, *E*).

A

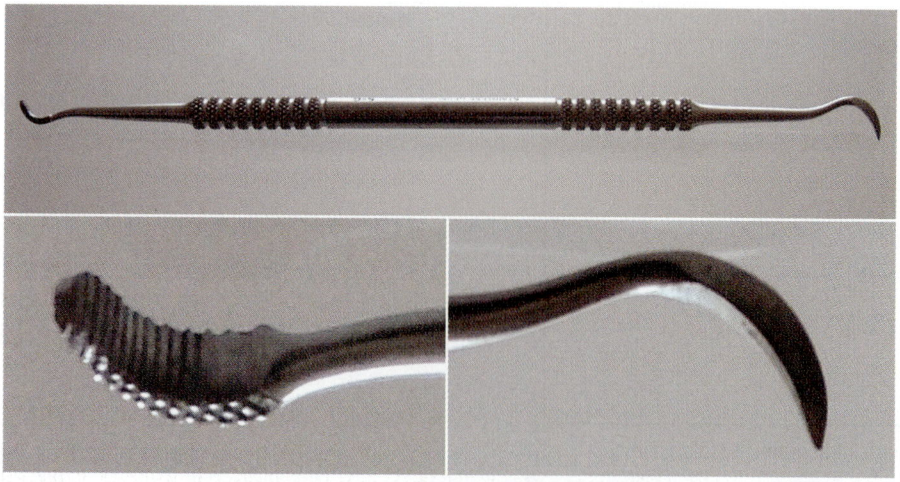

Fig. 60-13 Intraoral instruments. **A,** Orthodontic scaler.

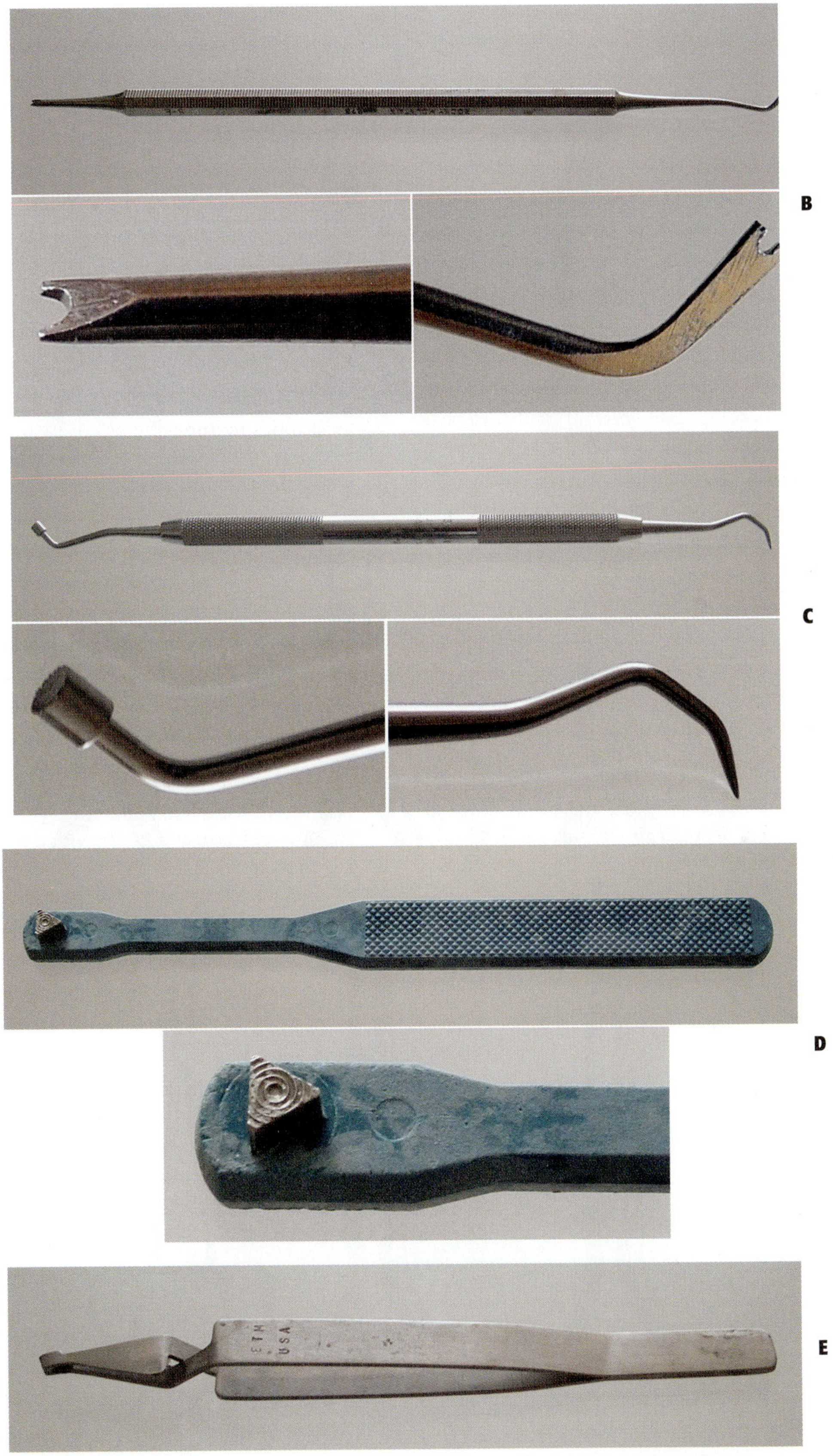

Fig. 60-13, cont'd Intraoral instruments. **B,** Ligature director. **C,** Band plugger. **D,** Bite stick. **E,** Bracket placement tweezers. (From Boyd LR: *Dental instruments: a pocket guide*, ed. 2, Saunders, St. Louis, 2005.)

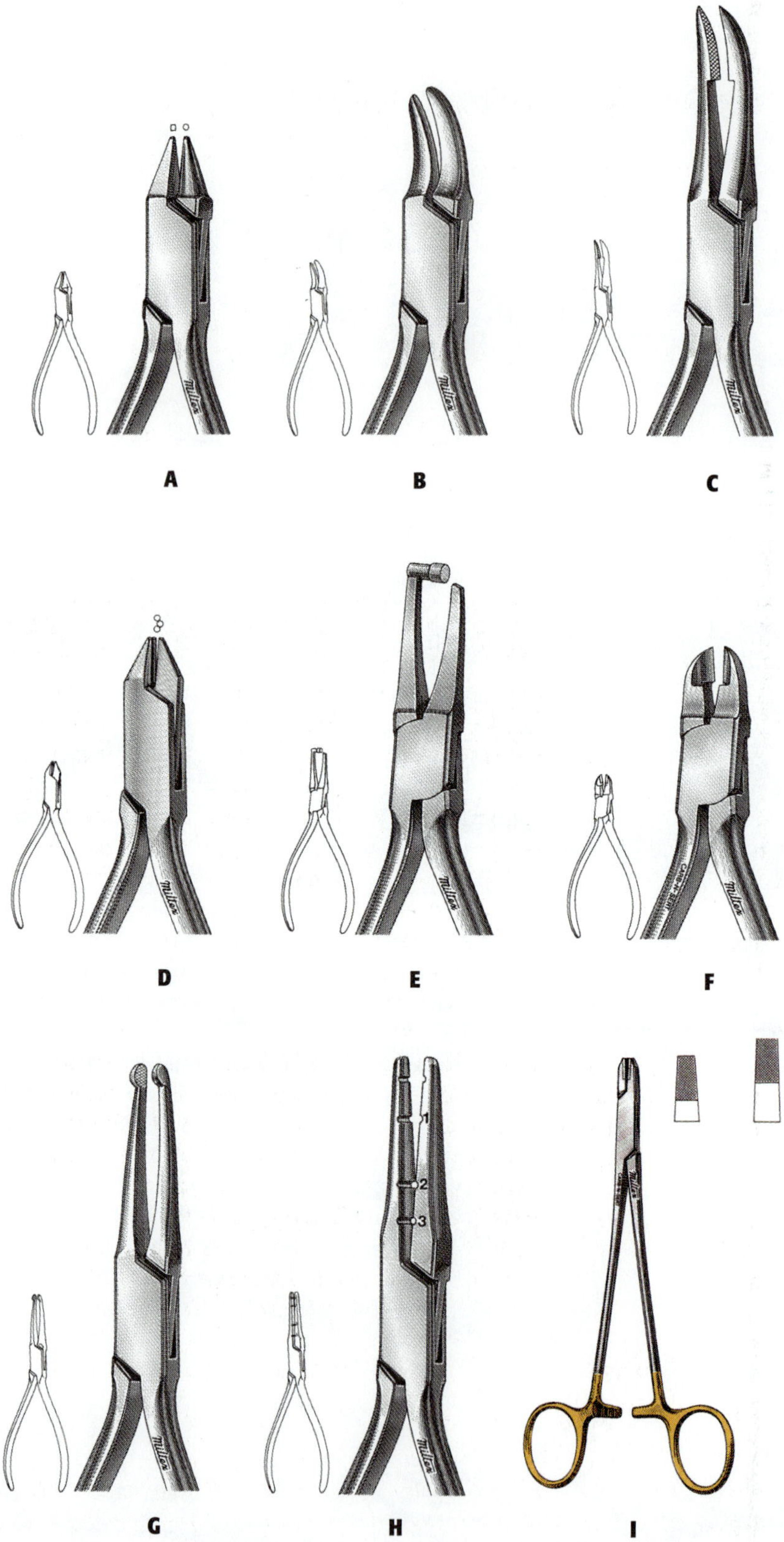

Fig. 60-14 Pliers. **A,** Bird-beak pliers. **B,** Contouring pliers. **C,** Weingart utility pliers. **D,** Three-prong pliers. **E,** Posterior band remover. **F,** Ligature pin-and-ligature cutter. **G,** Howe (110) pliers. **H,** Wire bending pliers. **I,** Ligature-tying pliers. (Courtesy Miltex, Inc., York, PA.)

Pliers

Bird-beak pliers are useful in forming and bending wires for either fixed or removable appliances (Fig. 60-14, *A*).
Contouring pliers aid in fitting bands for fixed or removable appliances (Fig. 60-14, *B*).
Weingart utility pliers have finely serrated narrow beaks, allowing accessibility to all areas. They are used in placing arch wires (Fig. 60-14, *C*).
Three-prong pliers are used primarily in closing and adjusting of clasps (Fig. 60-14, *D*).
Posterior band remover pliers remove bands without placing stress on the tooth or providing discomfort to the patient (Fig. 60-14, *E*).
Pin-and-ligature cutter cuts the ligature wire once it has been ligated around the bracket (Fig. 60-14, *F*).
Howe (110) pliers have a flat, rounded serrated tip that allows placement and removal or creation of adjustment bends in the arch wire (Fig. 60-14, *G*).
Wire bending pliers are used for holding and bending and adjusting arch wires to create movement (Fig. 60-14, *H*).
Ligature-tying pliers have finely serrated narrow beaks to allow ease in ligature tying (Fig. 60-14, *I*).

Recall

11. What instruments are used to seat a molar band?
12. Is the orthodontic scaler used for removing calculus from around the fixed appliance?
13. What is another name for 110 pliers?

ORTHODONTIC TREATMENT

Orthodontic treatment is the use of fixed or removable appliances or a combination of both types. This type of treatment is performed to mechanically move the teeth or jaw.

Fixed Appliances

Fixed appliances, also referred to as **braces,** are a combination of bands, brackets, arch wires, and auxiliaries that can move a tooth in six directions: mesially, distally, lingually, facially, apically, and occlusally (Fig. 60-15).

Auxiliaries are attachments to the brackets and bands, such as tubes and hooks, which make it possible to attach arch wires and elastics to the tooth and give strength in movement of the tooth.

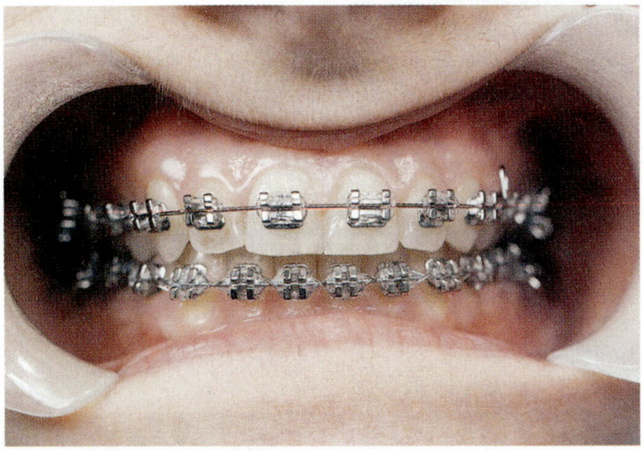

Fig. 60-15 Full braces.

Sequence of Appointments for the Orthodontic Patient

1. Placement of separators
2. Cementation of molar bands
3. Bonding of brackets
4. Insertion of arch wire and tying in with ligature ties or elastomeric ties
5. Adjustment checks
6. Removal of appliance
7. Retention of teeth

The **arch wire** is attached to the brackets and bands and serves as a pattern for the dental arch. Bending the arch wire creates force and pressure, thus causing the tooth or teeth to move in the desired direction.

Separators

Tight interproximal contacts can make it impossible to properly seat a band; therefore the teeth must be separated before fitting bands. A **separator** is used for this purpose. Although separators are available in many varieties, the principle is the same in each case: a device is placed to force or wedge the teeth apart long enough for initial tooth movement to occur. The separator slightly separates the teeth *before* the appointment during which bands are to be fitted. It is important to instruct the patient to call the office promptly if a separator falls out and to schedule an appointment to have it placed again.

The three main methods of separation used for posterior teeth are brass wire separators, steel separating springs, and elastomeric separators (see Procedures 60-1, 60-2, and 60-3).

Procedure 60-1 Placing and Removing Brass Wire Separators

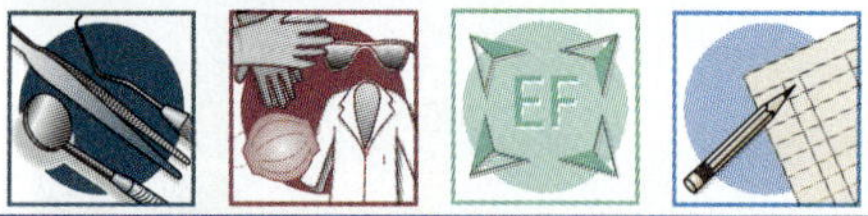

Equipment and Supplies

- Soft brass wire
- Hemostat
- Ligature wire cutter
- Orthodontic scaler

PROCEDURAL STEPS

Placing Brass Wire Separators

1. Bend a 20-mm soft brass wire into an open hook shape.

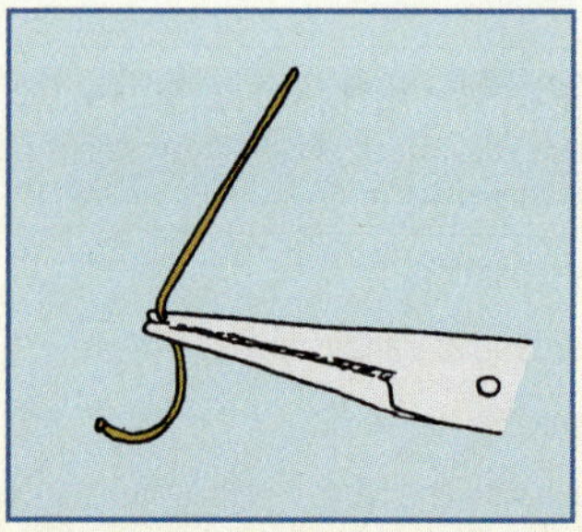

2. Use a hemostat to pass the wire beneath the contact from the lingual side.

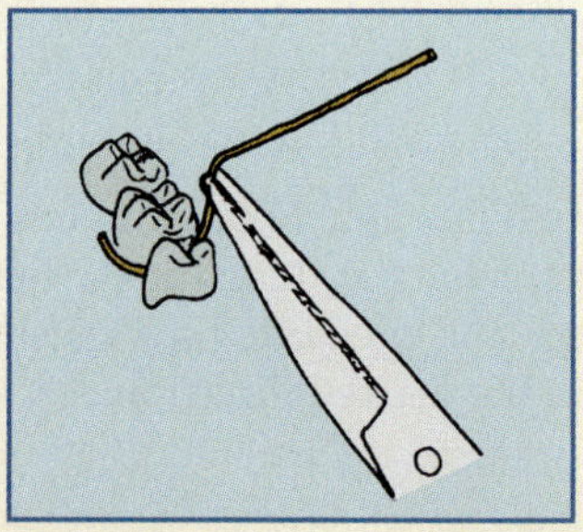

3. Bring the wire back over the contact and twist it slightly.

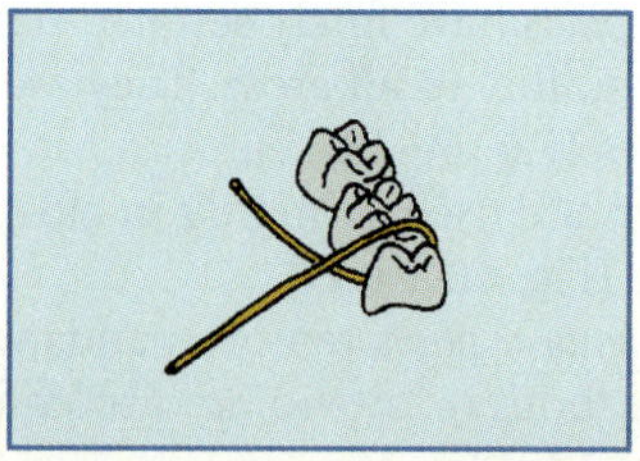

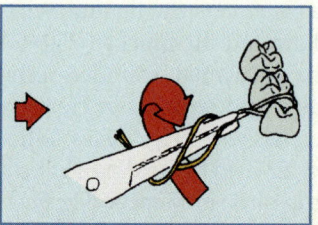

4. Use a ligature wire cutter to cut the twisted pigtail to 3 mm in length. Tuck the pigtail into the gingival crevice between the teeth.

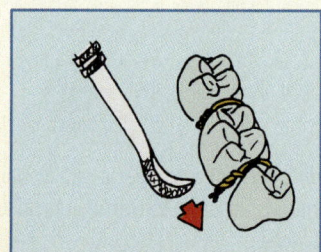

5. This type of separator is normally left in place for 5 to 7 days.

Removing Brass Wire Separators

1. Use a ligature wire cutter to carefully cut the twisted pigtail.

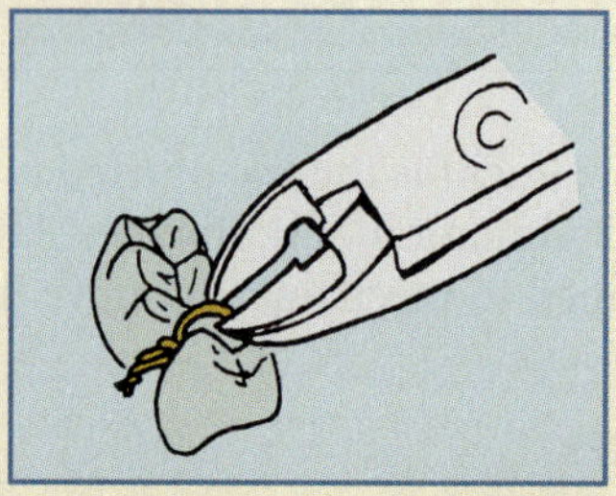

2. Use a hemostat to carefully remove the wire from under the contact from the facial side.

Procedure 60-2 Placing and Removing Steel Separating Springs

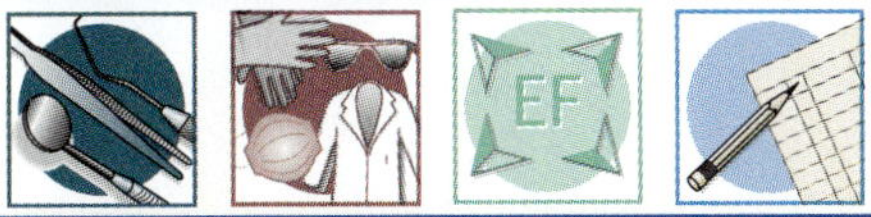

Equipment and Supplies

- Separating springs
- Bird-beak pliers
- Orthodontic scaler

PROCEDURAL STEPS

Placing Steel Separating Springs

1. Grasp the spring with bird-beak pliers at the base of its shorter leg.

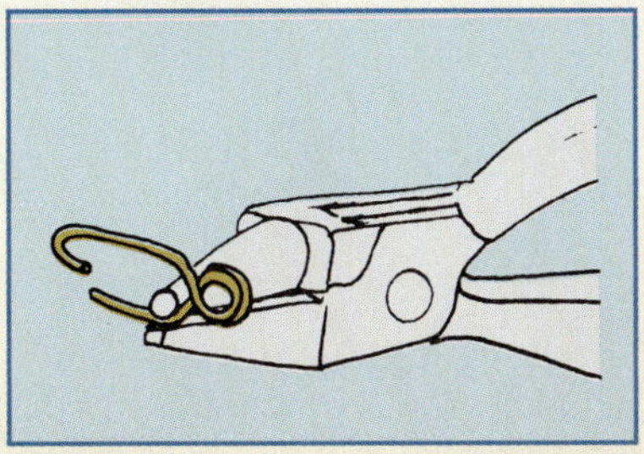

2. Place the bent-over end of the longer leg in the lingual embrasure. Pull the spring open so that the shorter leg can slip beneath the contact from lingual to facial.
3. Slip the spring into place with the helix to the facial side.
4. This type of separator is normally left in place for 3 to 5 days.

Removing Steel Separating Springs

1. During this procedure, keep the fingers of the other hand over the separator to prevent it from coming off the tooth unexpectedly.

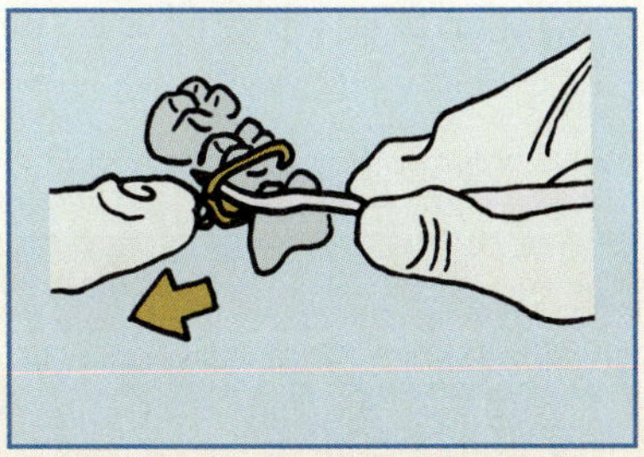

2. Use an orthodontic scaler to engage the helix of the separator. Lift upward until there is space between the upper arm and the occlusal aspect of the marginal ridge.

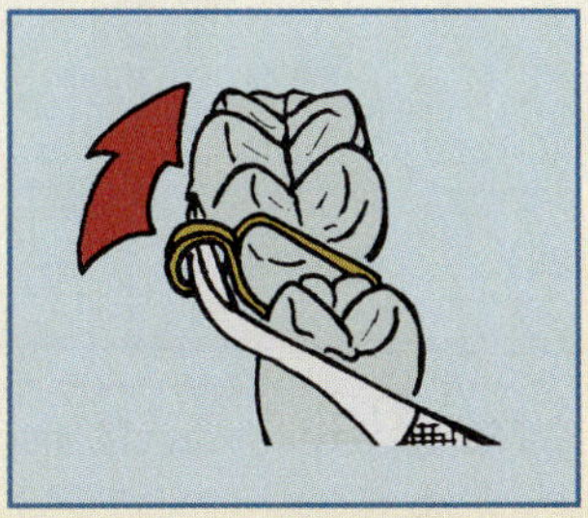

3. Support the separator on the helix with the index finger. Disengage the upper arm from the lingual embrasure and pull the separator toward the facial surface.

Procedure 60-3 Placing and Removing Elastomeric Ring Separators

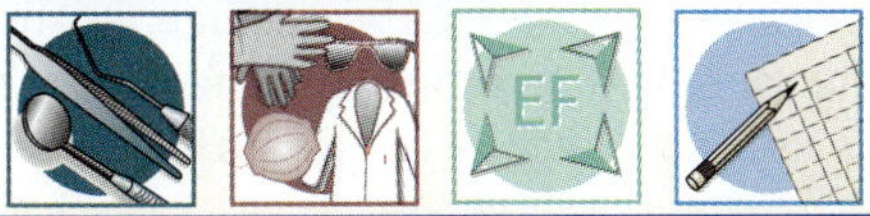

Equipment and Supplies

- Elastomeric separators
- Separating pliers
- Floss
- Orthodontic scaler

PROCEDURAL STEPS

Placing Elastomeric Ring Separators

1. Place the separator over the beaks of separating pliers.
2. Stretch the ring; then use a see-saw motion to gently force it through the contact.

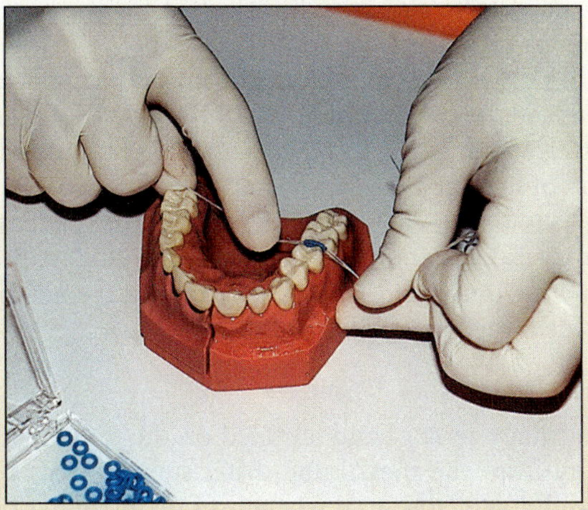

continued

Procedure 60-3 Placing and Removing Elastomeric Ring Separators—cont'd

PROCEDURAL STEPS, cont'd

3. An alternative method is to use two loops of dental floss to stretch the ring and guide it into place.
4. This type of separator can be left in place for up to 2 weeks.

Removing Elastomeric Ring Separators

1. Slide an orthodontic scaler into the doughnut-shaped separator.
2. Use slight pressure to remove the ring from under the contact.

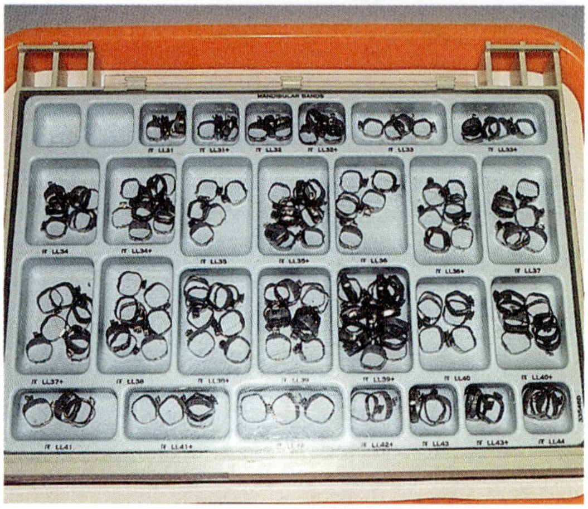

Fig. 60-16 Varying sizes of bands.

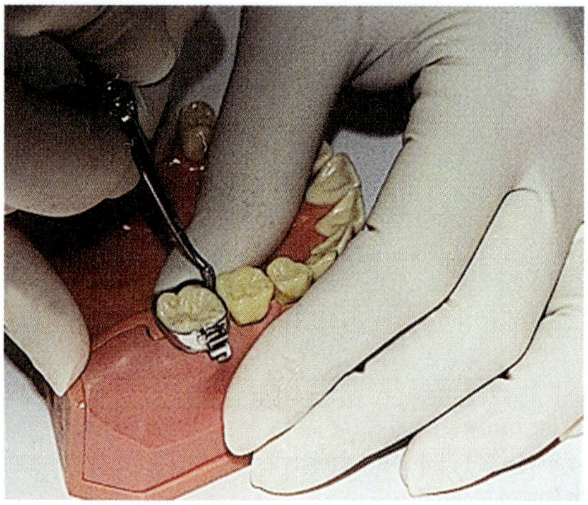

Fig. 60-17 The band pusher is used to seat the band interproximally.

Orthodontic Bands

Bands are preformed stainless steel rings that are fitted around the teeth and cemented in place. Most commonly, bands are placed on the first and second molars. The bands are divided into maxillary and mandibular, and right and left, to compensate for individual tooth differences. The occlusal edge of the band is slightly rolled or contoured, whereas the gingival edge is straight and smooth. Buttons, tubes, and cleats also may be attached for the arch wire and power products.

Bands to be fitted are selected from the manufacturer's tray with sterile cotton pliers (Fig. 60-16). At the chairside, bands can be selected through visual inspection and estimation of the size of the tooth and then fitted, or an alternative is to select, adapt, and fit bands on the patient's diagnostic cast. This method eliminates the lengthy process at chairside, and minor alterations can be accomplished at chairside as necessary.

Fitting Molar Bands

The maxillary molar band is seated on the tooth by finger pressure from the mesial and distal surfaces. This brings the band down close to the height of the marginal ridges. The band pusher is used on the mesiobuccal and distolingual edges to seat the band into place (Fig. 60-17). Mandibular molar bands are designed to be seated initially with finger pressure on the proximal surfaces. Then a band seater is placed along the buccal margins, and the patient's heavy biting force is used to drive the band into place.

Cementation of Orthodontic Bands

Cementation of orthodontic bands is similar to cementation of a cast restoration; the difference is that the cementation is exclusively to enamel. Cement that is selected must have the strength to aid in retention with enamel and have properties, including a time-released fluoride that aids in preventing decay under the band.

The cement to be used is determined by the orthodontist. The type selected must be mixed in accordance with the manufacturer's directions (see Procedure 60-4).

Bonded Brackets

The bonded **bracket** is the most common type of attachment for fixed appliances (Fig. 60-18). Most commonly,

Procedure 60-4 Assisting in the Fitting and Cementation of Orthodontic Bands

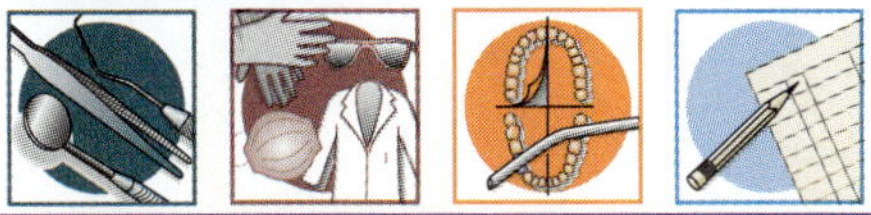

Equipment and Supplies

- Basic setup
- Preselected orthodontic bands
- Chilled glass slab
- Spatula (stainless steel)
- Gauze sponges
- Band pusher
- Band seater
- Scaler
- Band remover
- Contouring pliers
- Isopropyl alcohol
- Masking tape
- Chapstick or utility wax
- Selected cement

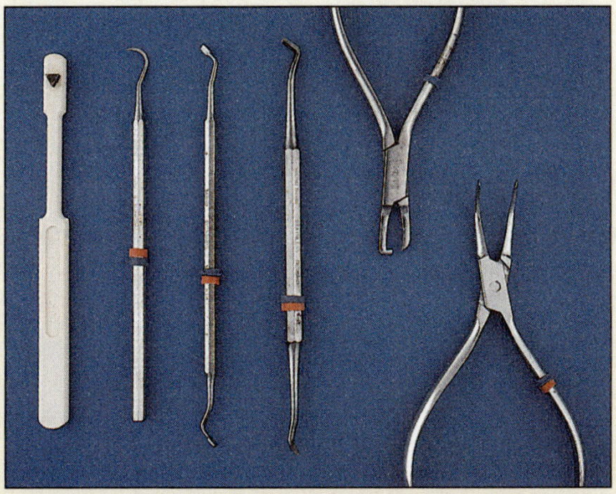

PROCEDURAL STEPS

Preparation

1. Place each preselected orthodontic band on a small square of masking tape with the occlusal surface on the tape and the gingival margin of the band upright.
   Purpose: This keeps the bands in order and prevents the cement from flowing out the other side.
2. Wipe any buccal tubes or attachments with Chapstick or utility wax.
   Purpose: This prevents cement from getting into or around these areas.

Mixing and Placing the Cement

1. The teeth are isolated and dried.
2. At a signal from the orthodontist, dispense the cement according to the manufacturer's directions; then quickly mix the cement until it is homogeneous.
3. Hold the band by the margin of the masking tape. The gingival surface is upright, and the cement spatula is placed on the margin of the band.
4. Wipe the spatula over the margin, allowing the cement to flow into the circumference of the band.

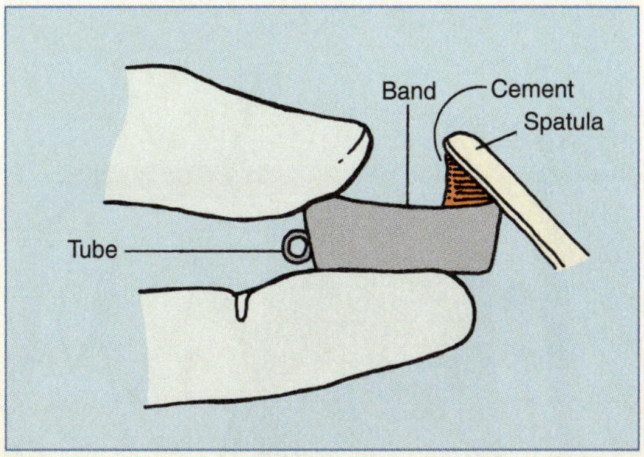

5. Transfer the cement-filled band to the orthodontist, who inverts the band over the tooth.
6. Transfer the band seater. The orthodontist places it on the buccal margin of the band.
7. The patient is instructed to bite gently on the band. This action forces the band down onto approximately the middle third of the tooth crown.
8. Excess cement is forced out from under the gingival and occlusal margins of the bands and is allowed to harden.
9. This process is repeated until all of the bands have been seated.

Removing Excess Cement

1. After the cement has reached its final stage of setting, a scaler or explorer is used to remove the excess cement on the enamel surfaces.
2. The patient's mouth is rinsed, flossed, and checked to ensure that all of the excess cement has been removed.

Date	Tooth	Surface	Charting Notes
9/6/05			Upper and lower bands cemented w/ glass ionomer on first molars, UR-22, UL-24, LL-21, LR-22. Schedule for bonding. T. Clark, CDA / L. Stewart, DDS

Procedure 60-5 Assisting in the Direct Bonding of Orthodontic Brackets

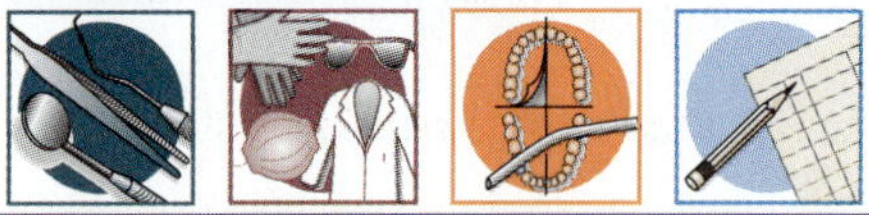

Equipment and Supplies

- Brackets (type specified by the orthodontist)
- Cotton rolls or lip retractors
- Prophy cup
- Pumice
- Bonding setup
- Bracket placement tweezers
- Orthodontic scaler

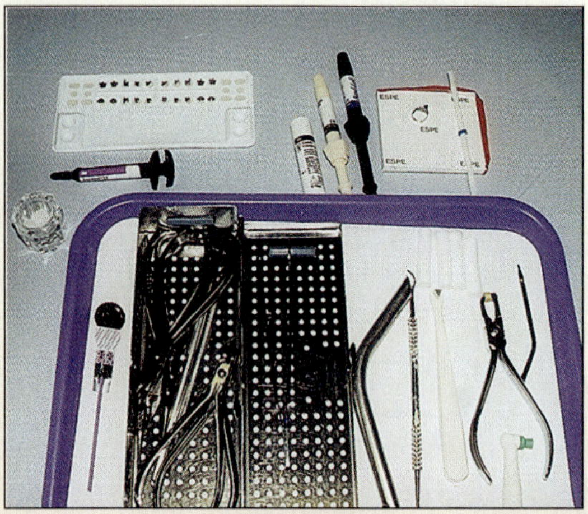

PROCEDURAL STEPS

Preparing the Teeth

1. The tooth surface must be cleaned with prophy cup and pumice slurry and then rinsed and dried.
2. Use either cotton rolls or retractors to isolate the teeth.
3. An etchant gel is placed on the facial area of the tooth that is to receive bonding. This remains on the tooth for the manufacturer's specified time and then is rinsed and dried thoroughly.

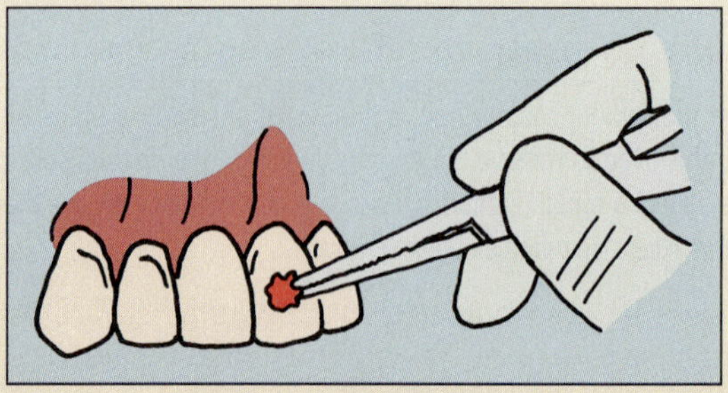

Bonding the Brackets

1. The orthodontist applies a liquid sealant, usually the monomer of the bonding agent, to the prepared tooth surface.
2. Mix a small quantity of bonding material and place it on the back of the bracket. Bracket placement tweezers are used to transfer the bracket to the orthodontist.

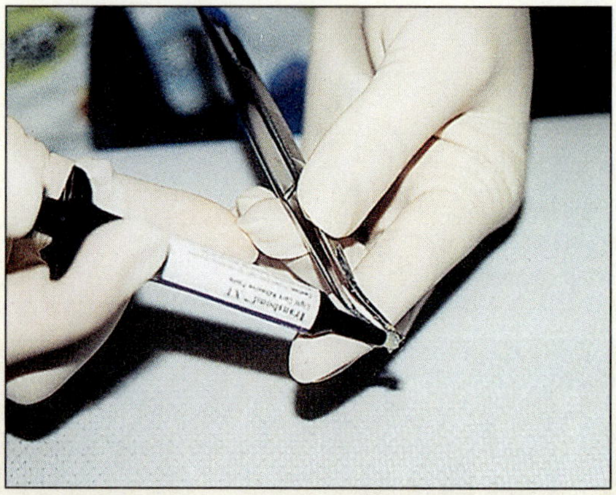

3. Transfer the orthodontic scaler. The orthodontist will place the bracket and move it into final position with a scaler.
4. The orthodontist uses the scaler to immediately remove the excess bonding material before light-curing the material.

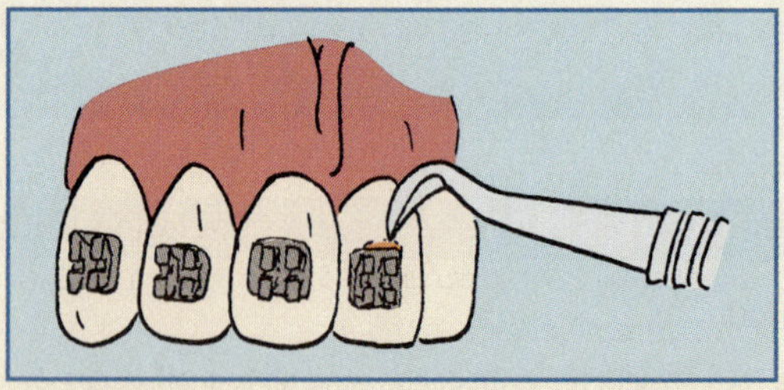

Date	Tooth	Surface	Charting Notes
9/7/05			Edgewise brackets bonded on Max. 5-1/1-5 and Mand. 4-1/1-4. Light arch wire placed. T. Clark, CDA / L. Stewart, DDS

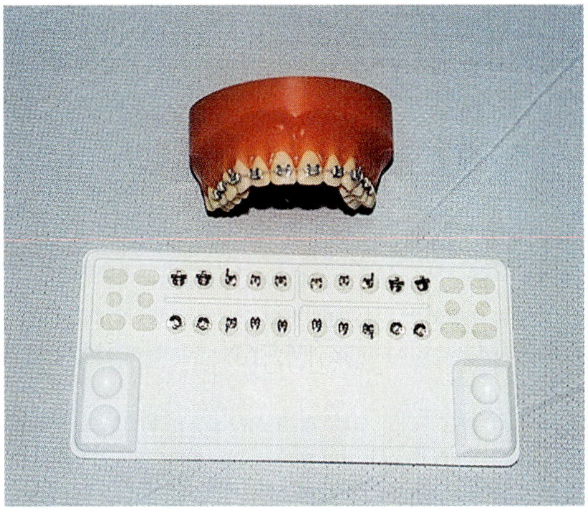

Fig. 60-18 Bonded bracket.

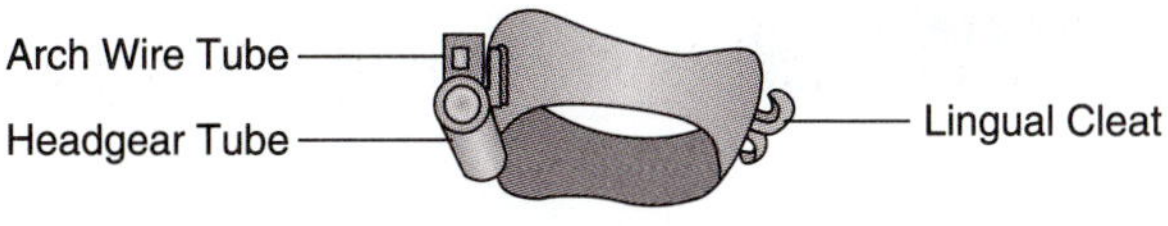

Fig. 60-19 Auxiliary attachment on a molar band.

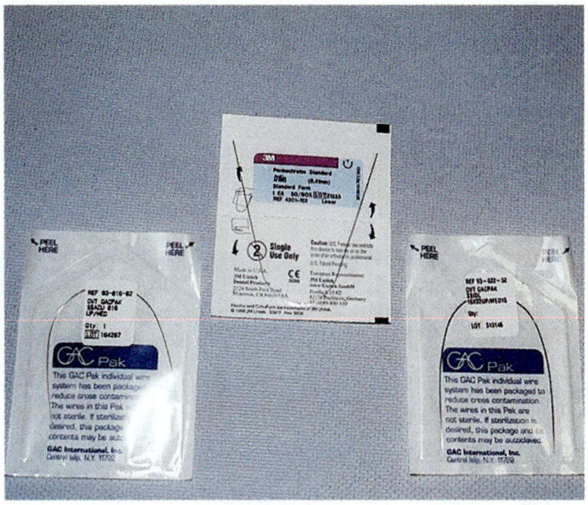

Fig. 60-20 An assortment of arch wires.

brackets are bonded onto the anterior teeth and premolars. The bracket is attached to a stainless steel backing pad that is bonded to the enamel of the tooth. The bonded bracket is designed with four tie wings so that the arch wire is placed horizontally through the wings of the bracket and then *ligated* in place. This stabilization of the arch wire initiates tooth movement by allowing the forces from the arch wire to be transmitted to the tooth (see Procedure 60-5).

Auxiliary Attachments

Auxiliary attachments are an integral part of the contemporary edgewise appliance. They can be attached to molar bands or single brackets (Fig. 60-19).

Headgear tubes are round tubes placed routinely on maxillary first molar bands. They are used for the insertion of the inner bow of a facebow appliance.

Edgewise tubes are rectangular tubes placed gingival to the plane of the main arch wire. These tubes should be present on the facial surfaces of the upper and lower first molars to receive the arch wire.

Labial hooks are located on the facial surfaces of the first and second molar bands for both arches. These hooks hold the interarch elastics.

Lingual arch attachment is a button or bracket located on the lingual portion of the bands to stabilize the arch and to reinforce anchorage and tooth movement.

Arch Wire

The arch wire is an essential component of fixed orthodontics. The arch wire is the pattern from which the dental arch will take its shape. When the arch wire is placed into the slots of each bracket and then held into position by a ligature or elastomeric tie, a force is created that guides the teeth in movement (see Procedure 60-6).

Several shapes and materials are used in the design of arch wires. Each type has properties that are unique to a particular application (Fig. 60-20).

Types of Arch Wires

Nickel titanium is very useful for movement because of its flexibility. This type of arch wire is used during the initial stages of tooth movement for malaligned and/or crowded teeth.

Stainless steel wire, which is stiffer and stronger than other types of wire, is used to apply more force and give better stability to control the teeth. It can withstand greater forces and is called the *working arch wire.*

Beta titanium (TMA) provides a combination of strength, flexibility, and memory. The orthodontist may choose this type of arch wire when many bands need to be placed.

Optiflex is a newer type of arch wire made from a composite material with a top coating of optical glass fibers, making it esthetically pleasing. This type of wire is used for light force in the initial stages of alignment.

Shapes of Arch Wires

Round wires are normally used in the initial and intermediate stages of treatment. Their main functions are to correct crowded and crooked teeth and to level the arch. They also can be used in opening a bite and sliding teeth along to close spaces.

Square or *rectangular* wires are used during the final stages of treatment to position the crown and root in the correct maxillary and mandibular relationship. These wires also give the tooth more stability and apply more force.

Procedure 60-6 Placing Arch Wires

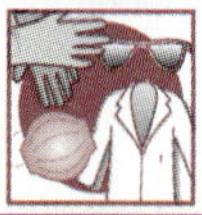

Equipment and Supplies

- Preformed arch wires
- Patient's diagnostic casts (or previously used arch wire)
- Weingart pliers
- Bird-beak pliers
- Torquing pliers
- Distal end cutter

PROCEDURAL STEPS

Measuring the Arch Wire

1. Preformed wires are measured before they are placed in the mouth. The wire should be long enough to extend past the end of the buccal tube on the molar band but not so long that it injures the patient's tissues.
2. Measure the wire by trying it on the patient's diagnostic model or by holding it against the arch wire that is being replaced.
3. If the orthodontist needs to place any bends in the wire, additional wire must be allowed for the length.

Positioning the Arch Wire

1. Locate the mark at the center of the arch wire.
   Purpose: This indicates the midline or center of the arch form.
2. Position the wire in the mouth with the mark between the central incisors.
3. Place the arch wire in the main arch wire slot of the buccal tube.
4. Use Weingart pliers to slide the wire in on either side of the arch and to position the wire in the bracket slots.
5. Check the distal ends to determine whether they are securely positioned or either too long or too short.

Ligating the Arch Wire

Once the arch wire has been positioned, it must be ligated to be held in place. The methods used are either ligature ties or elastomeric ties. Ligature ties are thin wires that are twisted around the bracket to hold the arch wire in place.

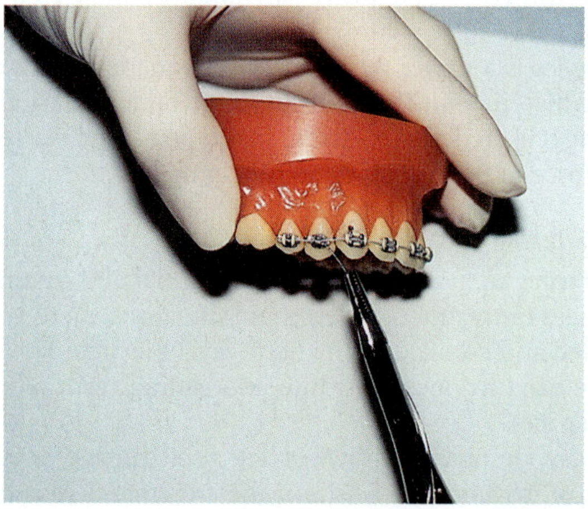

Fig. 60-21 A ligature tie can be placed around one bracket or placed in a figure-8 pattern to create a chain around several brackets.

Elastomeric ties are made of plastic or a rubber-like material stretched around the bracket to hold the arch wire in place (see Procedures 60-7 and 60-8).

Ligature ties are 0.01-gauge stainless steel wires used to "tie" arch wires in two unique ways. The dentist can either indicate each bracket to be tied with a ligature tie or designate a quadrant or group of teeth to be tied with one ligature tie, creating a figure-8 to form a chain (Fig. 60-21). With either application, the operator begins from the most posterior tooth and works toward the midline. This makes for a much easier application process and more uniformity in technique.

Kobyashi hooks are ligature ties that have been spot-welded at the tip to form a hook for the attachment of elastics. These hooks are ligated on a bracket as necessary to attach elastics (Fig. 60-22).

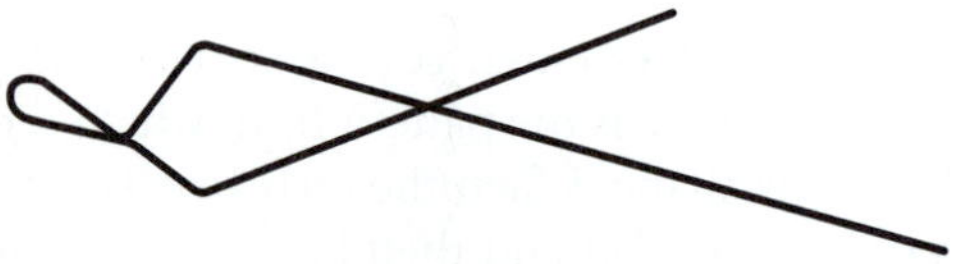

Fig. 60-22 The Kobyashi hook has a welded hook at the end of a ligature tie that is used to hold auxiliaries.

Procedure 60-7 Placing and Removing Ligature Ties

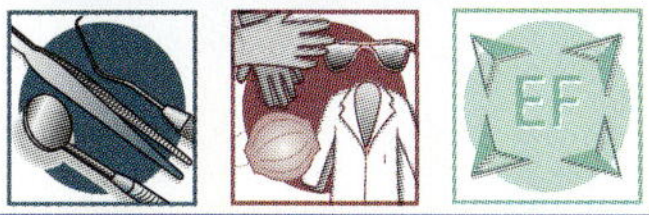

Equipment and Supplies

- Ligature ties
- Ligature director
- Hemostat
- Ligature cutter

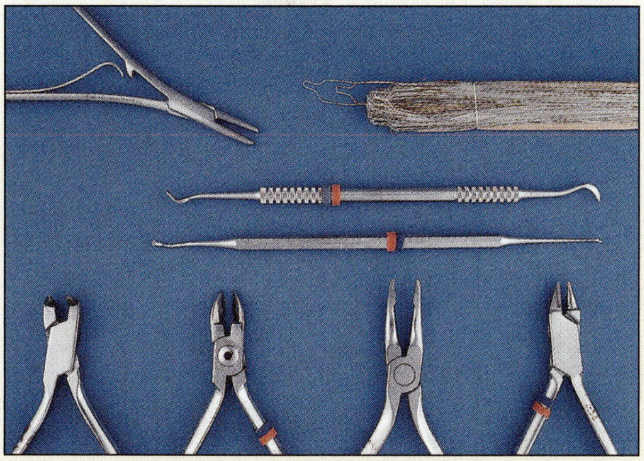

Placing Wire Ligatures

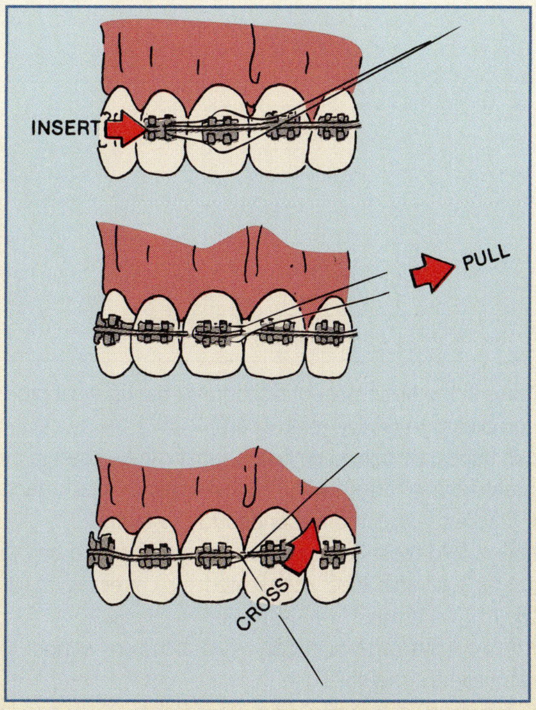

1. Holding the ligature between the thumb and index finger, slide the wire between these fingers so that only the section that wraps around the bracket is exposed. Make sure to work toward the midline.
2. Slide the ligature around the bracket, using the ligature director to push the wire against the tie wing.
3. Twist together the ends of the ligature. Place the hemostat about 3 to 5 mm from the bracket and twist the wire snugly against the bracket.
4. After all teeth have been ligated, use a ligature cutter to remove the excess wire, leaving a 4- to 5-mm pigtail.
5. Use the ligature director to tuck the pigtails under the arch wire toward the gingiva at the interproximal space.
6. Repeat this procedure until all ligatures have been cut and tucked away.
7. Run a finger along the arch to make sure there are no protruding wires that could injure the patient.

Removing Ligature Ties

1. Using the ligature cutter, place the beaks of the pliers at the end of the twisted wire and snip it off, making sure to hold on to the cut portion.
2. Carefully remove the portion of the wire.
3. Do not twist or pull as you cut and remove the ligatures.

Procedure 60-8 Placing and Removing Elastomeric Ties

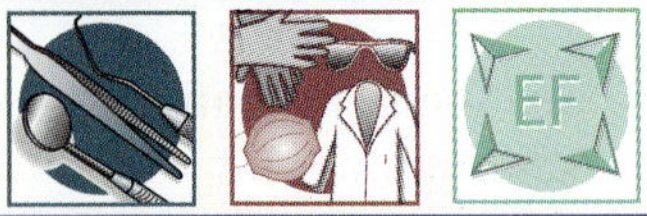

Equipment and Supplies

- Elastomeric tie for each bracket
- Hemostat
- Orthodontic scaler

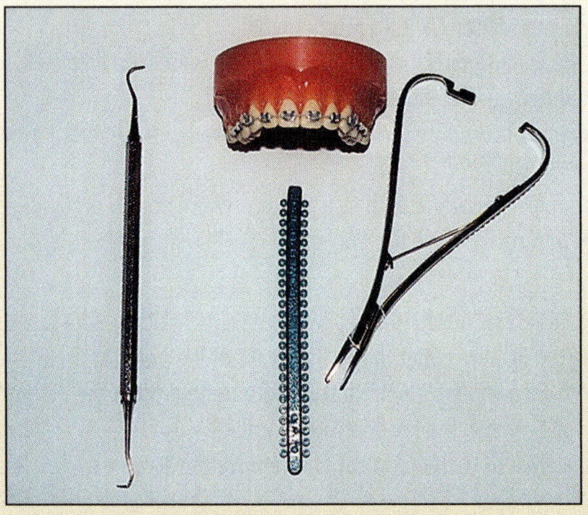

Placing Elastomeric Ties

1. Use a hemostat to place the pliers' beak on a tie; lock the pliers.
2. Do not place the beaks too closely to the center of the "O," or else it will be impossible to stretch the tie around the bracket.
3. Place the tie on the occlusal portion of one tie wing; then slide the tie under the edge of the bracket.
4. To get the tie started, support it with your finger.
5. Pull the tie up and over the tie wing and then over and down the other tie wing.
6. Release the pliers.

Removing Elastomeric Ties

1. Use an orthodontic scaler held in a pen grasp.
2. Place the scaler tip between the bracket tie wings and pull the tie at the occlusal position with a rolling motion.
3. Remove the tie in a gingival direction.

Power Products

Power products are accessory items made of elastic materials that help in tooth movement.

Elastic chain ties are continuous "Os" that form a chain. They are used to close space between teeth or to correct rotated teeth.

Elastics, commonly referred to as *rubber bands,* are placed from one tooth to another in the same arch or from one tooth to another tooth in the opposing arch. Elastics help in closing space between teeth and correcting occlusal relationships. The placement is determined by the orthodontist to create a specific direction of movement.

Elastic thread is a type of tubing used to close space or aid in the eruption of impacted teeth.

Comfort tubing aids in patient comfort by covering an arch wire that may be causing discomfort.

Recall

14. To ease in the placement of orthodontic bands, what procedure is completed to wedge teeth apart?
15. When bands are being cemented, what can be used to prevent cement from getting into the buccal tubes or attachments?
16. Are brackets cemented or bonded to the tooth?
17. Where would most auxiliary attachments be found on braces?
18. What type of arch wire is indicated for correcting malaligned teeth?
19. What two ways can you measure an arch wire without placing it in a patient's mouth?
20. Besides using ligature ties, what other technique is used to hold an arch wire in place?

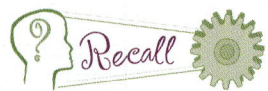

HEADGEAR

Another aspect of the treatment phase in fixed appliances is the **headgear.** This is an orthopedic device used to control growth and tooth movement. Headgear is composed of two parts: the facebow and the traction device.

Facebow

The facebow is used to stabilize or move the maxillary first molar distally and create more room in the arch. The intraoral part of the facebow fits into the buccal tubes of the maxillary first molars. The outer part of the bow attaches to the traction device.

Traction Devices

Traction devices apply the extraoral force used to achieve the desired treatment results. Fig. 60-23 describes the four types of traction.

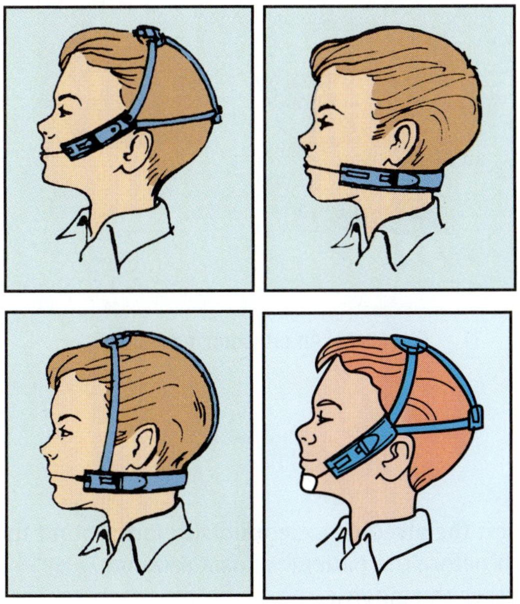

Fig. 60-23 **A,** High-pull headgear. The high-pull traction device is a cap-like device that fits around the top of the patient's head and hooks perpendicular to the occlusal plane. It can be used in controlling the growth of the maxilla or retraction of anterior teeth. **B,** Cervical traction. The cervical traction device fits around the patient's neck. The exerted force is parallel to the occlusal plane of the patient's teeth. This type of traction is used when the maxillary first molars are stabilized or moved distally. **C,** Combination headgear. A combination traction device combines the features of the high-pull and cervical traction devices. It exerts a force along the occlusal plane and upward. **D,** Chin cap. The chin cap traction device is a combination of a high-pull strap and a chin cup that fits on the mandible. This helps control the growth of the mandible in patients with class III malocclusion.

ADJUSTMENT VISITS

Throughout active orthodontic treatment, the patient must return regularly for adjustment. At these appointments, the orthodontist reviews the patient's progress and makes adjustments as necessary.

Checking the Appliance

At each adjustment appointment, it is the responsibility of the chairside assistant to check the patient's appliance to determine whether any of the following exist:

- Broken or missing arch wires
- Loose brackets and bands
- Loose, broken, or missing ligatures
- Loose, broken, or missing elastics

ORAL HYGIENE AND DIETARY INSTRUCTIONS

Orthodontic appliances offer areas for food and plaque to be trapped and hidden, and they make brushing more difficult. Good oral hygiene during orthodontic treatment is imperative. If the patient does not take care of his or her mouth properly, the results can be disastrous, including rampant decay, hypocalcification, and periodontal disease.

A concern with patients in orthodontic treatment is poor eating habits. The patient should be urged to use good sense in selecting foods and to avoid eating anything that can loosen a band, pop off a bracket, or bend an arch wire. Table 60-1 provides simple dietary guidelines to follow during orthodontic treatment.

Toothbrushing Instructions

Floss your teeth using a floss threader for easy application.

Brush your teeth at least once every day.

After brushing, rinse and swish water around your mouth to remove any debris.

Inspect your teeth and braces carefully to make sure they are spotless.

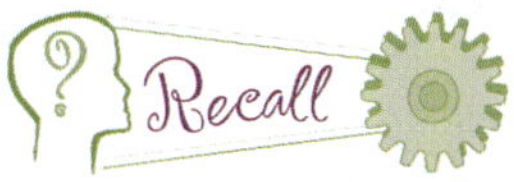

21. What additional appliance might the orthodontist use to control growth and tooth movement?
22. How can hard foods possibly harm braces?
23. How can a patient make flossing easier with braces?

Table 60-1 Dietary Habits and Orthodontics

Types of Foods to Avoid	Reasons	Examples
Sugar-containing foods	Weakens cement beneath bands, causing bands to loosen. Attacks tooth enamel, causing cavities.	Candy, cookies, cakes, pies, ice cream, soda, sugar-coated cereals, candy apples.
Sticky foods	Loosens bands, pulls out ligature ties, may bend arch wires.	Caramel, caramel corn, taffy, licorice, Gummy Bears, Starbursts, Sugar Daddies, chewy fruit snacks.
Hard foods	Loosens bands and bends and occasionally breaks arch wires.	Ice, hard breads, hard-shell tacos, jawbreakers, peanut brittle, chips, frozen candy bars.
Husk foods	May lodge between bands and beneath arch wires, causing irritation to gum tissues.	Peanuts, popcorn, corn on the cob, meat on the bone.
Chewing gum	Loosens bands, pulls out the wires, and bends arch wires.	Large pieces of gum.

COMPLETED TREATMENT

Once the patient has completed the treatment phase of orthodontics, the bands and bonded attachments are removed.

- Band removal is accomplished by breaking the seal of cement and lifting the bands off the tooth with the band remover.
- Bonded brackets are removed by creating a fracture within the resin bonding material. This is completed carefully so as not to damage the enamel surface.
- Any cement or resin material can be removed with a scaling instrument or an ultrasonic scaler.

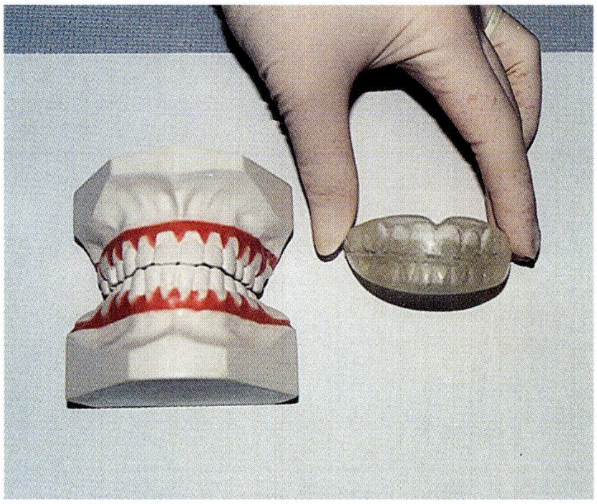

Fig. 60-24 An orthodontic positioner.

Retention

A patient may think that the treatment is complete when the fixed appliances are removed, but at that point an important stage in orthodontic treatment still lies ahead. Orthodontic control of tooth position and occlusal relationships must be withdrawn gradually, not abruptly, if excellent long-term results are to be achieved. Retention is necessary for the following reasons:

- To allow gingival and periodontal tissues the required time for reorganization
- To support the teeth that are in an unstable position so that the pressure of the cheeks and tongue does not cause a relapse
- To control changes caused by growth

Orthodontic Positioner

The **positioner** is a custom appliance made of rubber or pliable acrylic that fits over the patient's dentition after orthodontic treatment (Fig. 60-24). The positioner is designed to accomplish the following:

- Retain the teeth in their desired position
- Permit the alveolus to rebuild support around the teeth before the patient wears a **retainer**
- Massage the gingiva

Hawley Retainer

The Hawley retainer is the most commonly used removable retainer. This is worn to passively retain the teeth in their new position after the removal of the fixed appliances. The retainer also allows for some tooth movement to close band spaces and provides control of the incisors (Fig. 60-25). A Hawley retainer is constructed of clear, self-polymerizing acrylic that is designed to hold wire clasps on molar teeth. On a maxillary retainer, the acrylic portion is placed over the palate. On a mandibular retainer, the acrylic portion is placed on the anterior floor of the mouth.

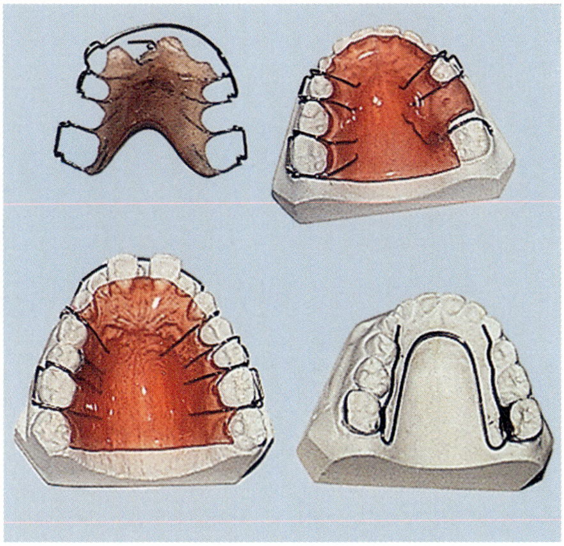

Fig. 60-25 Examples of Hawley retainers.

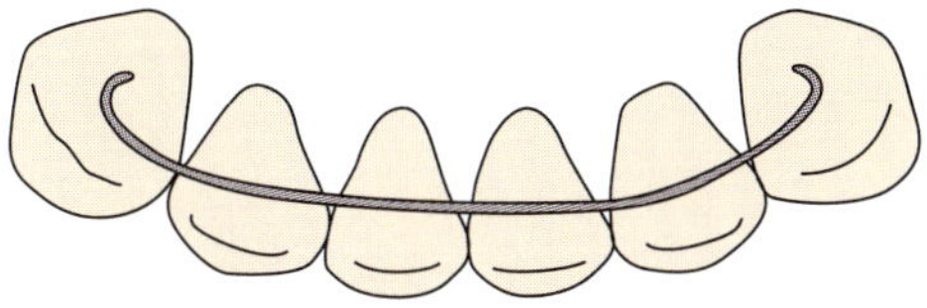

Fig. 60-26 The lingual retainer is bonded in place.

The anterior facial wire of the retainer should rest lightly on the facial surfaces at the midline of the anterior maxillary teeth and the lingual surface of the anterior mandibular teeth. The wire should fit lightly between the contact areas of the canines and first premolars.

Lingual Retainer

A fixed lingual canine-to-canine retainer is designed to be bonded to the lingual surfaces (Fig. 60-26). This provides lower incisor position during late growth. The fabrication is light steel wiring bent so that it rests against the flat portion of the lingual surface of the incisors with a long loop over the cingulum of the canines.

Recall

24. When a patient's braces come off, does that mean treatment is over?

25. Give an example of a retention appliance.

TREATMENT OPTIONS

Recent technology has devised a new way to straighten teeth without fixed appliances. This type of system does not work in all cases of malocclusion. A series of clear "aligners" (similar in design and fit to the thermoplastic vacuum-formed tray) is designed by computer. The customized aligners are then fabricated and worn at 2-week intervals. The patient's teeth gradually move from the pressure that the aligner creates until the desired result is achieved.

Patient Education

Most individuals that have had "braces" believe that their orthodontist was the "greatest." Patients seek orthodontic treatment because they want to, not because they are in pain. Because of this attitude, in most cases you will find patients to be willing participants in their treatment. The problem occurs when a patient is receiving orthodontic treatment because it is *someone else's* decision, such as a parent. When this takes place, your patient will probably not be as compliant in oral hygiene care and diet and the dental team will have to take on a more enforcing role through the process of treatment.

Legal and Ethical Implications

Patients receiving orthodontic care may be seen in the office every month for several years. Because of such an extensive relationship with your patients, they will become very comfortable with you and your role in their treatment. Being an orthodontic assistant allows you to become more involved in the care and treatment of your patients. Regardless, *always* make sure that the functions you carry out on patients are ones that are legal for you to perform in the state in which you are practicing.

Eye to the Future

One of the newest developments in orthodontics is the use of magnets. These magnets, which measure 3 to 4 mm, are attached to upper and lower molars. Then opposing magnetic forces are used to help move teeth. In some cases, the magnets may even replace orthodontic headgear. Research shows that with the use of magnet therapy, treatment time is shorter than with conventional braces, especially when bringing embedded teeth through a bony barrier.

Critical Thinking

1. As a certified orthodontic assistant, what expanded functions could you potentially be responsible for during the records appointment?
2. A patient is scheduled to have separators placed. The patient record notes that bands are to be placed on the permanent first and second molars. How many separators will be placed, and where?
3. When you sit down to examine a patient at an adjustment appointment, you notice that the patient's buccal mucosa is inflamed and irritated. What could be the cause of this? How could this be corrected?
4. Amy is 12 years old and will soon be getting braces. She is very concerned about her appearance once she gets them. How can you help her through this adjustment period? How can braces become more personalized?
5. Sheila is 35 years old and has always been unhappy with her teeth because of crowding. Because of financial reasons, she was unable to get braces as a child, but now she has orthodontic coverage through her job. Since Sheila is an adult patient, what issue(s) would not be a concern in her case (as opposed to a child patient)?

Part 11

Dental Administration and Communication Skills

The business aspect of a dental practice must be managed and operated proficiently. A career as a dental business assistant can provide the opportunity to practice your business skills while working in the dental field.

The chapters in this section will provide an overview of communicating with colleagues and patients, learning the communication systems used in the dental setting, managing the financial aspects of a practice, and marketing your personal skills for lifelong learning.

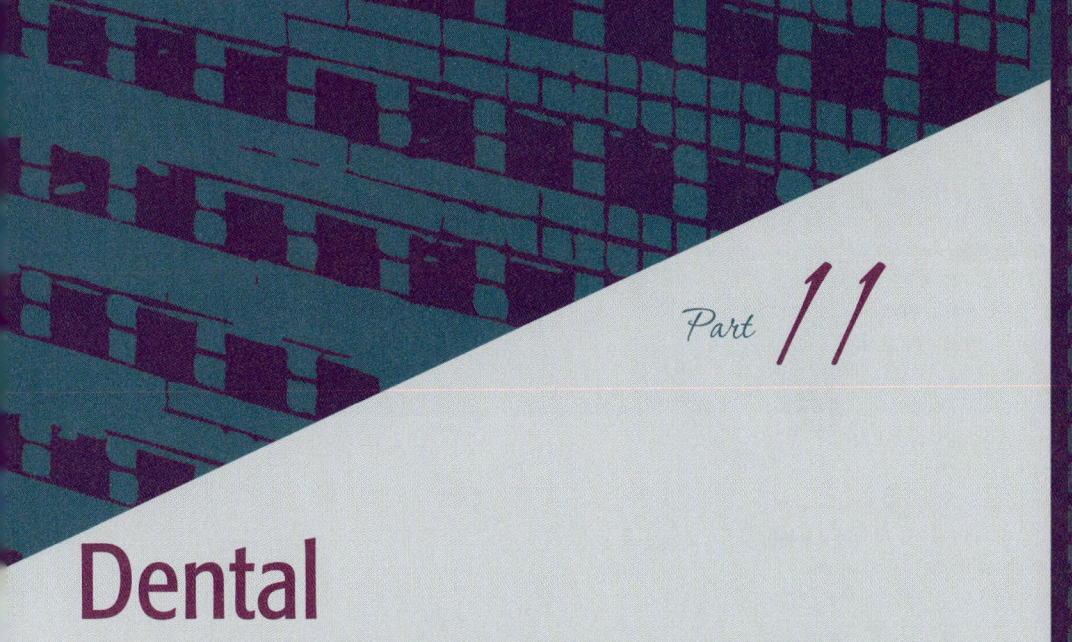

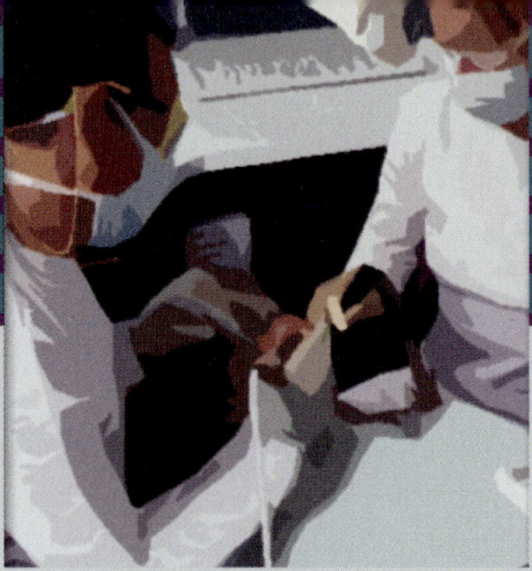

61 Communication in the Dental Office

Outline

KEY TERMS

Copier A business machine that can make duplicates (copies) from an original.

Fax machine A business machine that is attached to a phone line and transmits hard-copy written messages (handwritten or typed); "fax" is short for "facsimile."

HIPAA The Health Insurance Portability and Accountability Act of 1996, which specifies federal regulations ensuring privacy of a patient's healthcare information.

Letterhead The part of a letter (or printed stationery) that contains the name and address of the person sending the letter.

Marketing A way of advertising or recruiting people to a business.

Nonverbal communication Type of communication in which body language is used as a form of expression.

Salutation (sal-u-**ta**-shun) The part of a letter that contains the introductory greeting.

Verbal communication Type of communication in which words are used as a form of expression.

Word processing software A computer program designed to create most types of business documents.

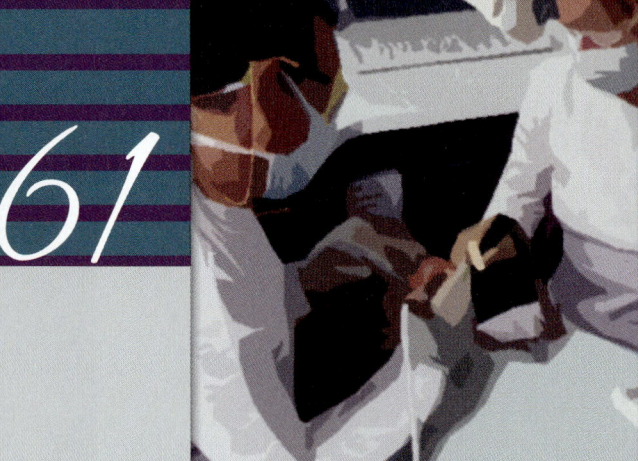

LEARNING OUTCOMES

On completion of this chapter, the student will be able to achieve the following objectives:

- Pronounce, define, and spell the Key Terms.
- Describe the type of relationship the patient and dental team should have.
- Discuss oral communications and identify the differences between verbal and nonverbal communications.
- Describe good phone courtesy.
- Describe and compare the handling of different types of phone calls.
- Describe external and internal marketing.
- Discuss stress in the dental practice.
- Discuss the team concept for bettering communication.

PERFORMANCE OUTCOMES

On completion of this chapter, the student will be able to meet competency in the following skills:

- Use correct phone techniques when talking with a patient.
- Compose a business letter that includes the appropriate parts of a letter.

Good communication, in all forms, is the backbone of a well-run organization. With effective interpersonal skills, the dental staff is able to enhance the quality of relationships, establish connections, solve problems, and create possibilities. Interpersonal communication teaches you how to communicate and interpret what others say and do; this trait is important to everyday social and business relationships.

The following chapter presents the importance of oral and written communication, focusing on the details of effective use of communication skills in a dental practice.

COMMUNICATION PATHWAYS

Effective communication may be one of the most important aspects of a dental assistant's job. We spend a majority of our working day communicating with others.

Communication is the sending of a message by one individual and the receiving of the same message by another individual. Every message we send has two parts, which must coincide in time:

- The *statement proper,* or the "This is what I have told you" portion, consists of the words being used.
- The *explanation,* or the part of the message that conveys "Now, this is how I expect you to understand it." This part of the message is sent nonverbally.

We communicate with words, facial expressions, appearance, gestures, mannerisms, listening, voice inflection, attitudes, and actions. The two parts of the message identified above are grouped into the two general categories of verbal and nonverbal communication.

Verbal Communication

Verbal communication is made up of the words we use. Most verbal communication is perceived by the ear.

Words Are Important

Words are verbal symbols used to represent an object or a meaning. Unfortunately, these verbal symbols are not usually checked against the things they represent; the result is often confusion, distortion of meaning, or misunderstanding.

It is also important to remember that words mean different things to different people—and they can mean different things at different times. Good verbal communication depends on the foundation of a common language, in which the sender and receiver are using words they both understand to have the same meaning.

When speaking to a dental patient, take care to select words that the individual understands rather than confuse the person with the technical language and specialized jargon of dentistry. Be careful to select words that will not frighten, intimidate, or upset the patient. Box 61-1 lists effective words for patient interaction.

Voice Quality

Voice quality accounts for more than one third of the impact of the total message and reveals much about the individual.

Box 61-1 Effective Words

Instead of this ...	Try this ...
Pain	Discomfort
Shot	Anesthetic
Pull	Remove
Drill	Prepare tooth
Filling	Restoration
False teeth	Denture
Operatory	Treatment area
Waiting room	Reception area

Table 61-1 ***Nonverbal Communication***

Message	Low-Level Behavior	High-Level Behavior
Empathy	Frown resulting from lack of understanding	Positive head nods; facial expressions that reflect the content of the conversation
Respect	Mumbling; patronizing tone of voice	Devoting full attention
Warmth	Apathy; fidgeting; signs indicating a desire to leave	Smiling; physical contact
Genuineness	Avoidance of eye contact	Congruence between verbal and nonverbal behavior
Self-disclosure	Bragging gestures; pointing to oneself	Gestures that minimize references to oneself
Confrontation	Pointing a finger or shaking a fist; speaking in a loud tone of voice	Speaking in a natural tone of voice

From Kinn ME, Woods M: The medical assistant, *ed 8, Philadelphia, 1999, Saunders.*

You should cultivate a pleasant voice (tone) quality and speak slowly, distinctly, and loud enough to be heard easily without being harsh or too loud.

In the event of a true emergency in the dental office, it is particularly important that you be extremely careful to keep your voice calm, because it is not *what* is said, but *how* it is said that may alarm the patient or the person accompanying the patient.

Asking Questions

Questions are used to gather information. Often, the way you phrase a question determines the kind of answer you get. By being aware of this, you can be more effective both in information gathering and in helping patients to feel more at ease.

Closed-ended questions are ones that can be answered with "Yes" or "No." These questions are best used to confirm information, to limit a conversation, or to close a conversation. Closed-ended questions often begin with the words *is, do, has, have, can,* or *will.* For example, "Is next Monday at 9 a.m. convenient for you, Mr. Thomas?" is a closed-ended question that can simply be answered "Yes" or "No."

Open-ended questions are ones that require more than "Yes" or "No" for an answer. These questions are best used to obtain information, maintain control of the conversation, or build rapport. Open-ended questions usually begin with words such as *what, when, how, who, where,* or *which.* For example, "Mrs. Jackson, what time of day is best to schedule your next appointment?" is an open-ended question.

Nonverbal Communication

Nonverbal communication is perceived at an almost subconscious level through all the senses. Nonverbal communication is conveyed by our body language. Body language consists of the messages that we send, the way we carry ourselves, and how we move about.

Posture, movements, and attitudes transmit major messages. For example, the person who is depressed often moves slowly with a restrained gait that reflects his or her mental attitude. The happy, healthy individual with a bright outlook on life tends to demonstrate this attitude with a free-moving walk that mirrors a sense of well-being. Hands grasping chair arms and restless shifting of body position are reliable indicators of inner tension and uneasiness in a patient. Rapid, shallow breathing also is a sign of tension and stress, and you can help the patient relax by encouraging him or her to breathe slowly and deeply in a more normal pattern. Table 61-1 describes specific behaviors observed in nonverbal communication.

Facial expressions indicate a wide variety of emotional states at which words can only hint. The eyes are particularly expressive of emotion and the patient's mental state of well-being.

Although many patients become capable of hiding their true emotions, the assistant should be aware of the signs of tension, stress, pain, boredom, lack of interest, or anxiety. At chairside, be careful not to convey a feeling of alarm on your face as a reaction to operative or surgical procedures, because this response could unnecessarily alarm the patient.

Listening Skills

It has been estimated that 90 percent of all spoken words are never heard; indeed listening is one of the greatest arts of communication and one of the most difficult to master. Good listening requires that you concentrate entirely on the patient.

Recall

1. What type of communication describes our body language?
2. What percentage of spoken words do we never hear?
3. Can anxiety be communicated through facial expression?
4. Give a more effective word for "pulling" a tooth.

Being a Good Listener

Do not let your mind wander. Put aside personal concerns while the patient is talking.

Do not concentrate on formulating a reply. Instead, concentrate on what the patient is actually saying. This shows the patient that you care.

Look as well as listen. In this way, pick up both the verbal and nonverbal information the patient is transmitting.

Do not stereotype. A person's appearance, cultural background, race, or religion should not influence your response to what they are saying.

Be careful of selective hearing. Sometimes we hear only parts of what someone is saying.

Do not get impatient. When you are in a hurry or trying to obtain a specific answer, it is easier to become annoyed with a patient, especially if the patient is a child or older adult.

COMMUNICATING WITH PATIENTS

A solid foundation of excellence in dental care and communication skills is necessary to achieve the goals of a dental practice and to fulfill the needs of the patients at all levels. Effective communication is important in achieving patient satisfaction. Patients who have good relationships with their dentist and the staff are likely to stay with the practice, accept the treatment presented to them, pay for the treatment on time, and refer other patients to the practice (Fig. 61-1).

Patient Needs

Patients build a relationship with their dentist and their staff through confidence and trust. Patients base their perceptions about a practice on the following factors:

- How they are treated on the phone
- How they are greeted
- How they are made to feel in the office
- How efficiently the staff manages business aspects, such as billing and insurance

Establishing a positive professional-patient relationship is part of understanding the needs of the patient. As a dental professional, it is necessary to recognize that patients are different and have different needs.

Psychologic Needs

Psychologic reactions are more obvious when a patient appears tense, suspicious, apprehensive, and resistant to suggested treatment. All individuals have emotional needs,

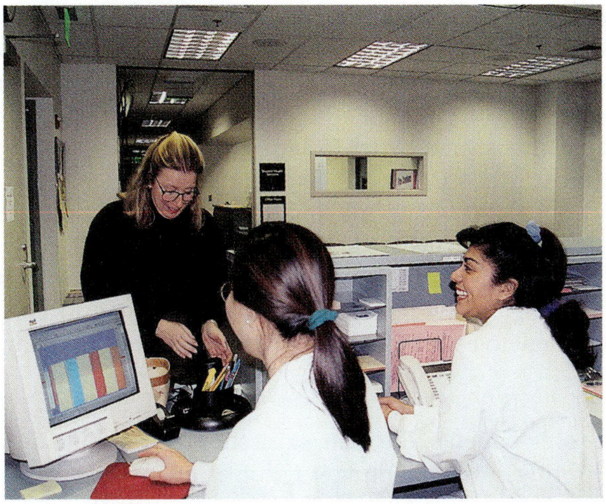

Fig. 61-1 Communication is the most important tool in a practice.

and these needs must be considered even when a patient seems confident, comfortable, and agreeable. One factor of major importance is the patient's current life situation; this includes the many stresses, tensions, conflicts, and anxieties that may be present in any part of the patient's life.

Other important factors that influence the patient's reactions to the current situation are his or her *previous dental experiences* and the patient's *attitudes and beliefs* about the importance of his or her teeth. These attitudes and beliefs are strongly influenced by the patient's socioeconomic and cultural background, as well as by the attitudes of peers or relatives. For example, if a patient grew up in a family in which going to the dentist was a dreaded experience, he or she may have difficulty overcoming this attitude.

Anxiety and fear of pain

The fear of pain is a frequently stated cause of anxiety concerning dental treatment. For many patients, however, it is the *expectation* of pain, not *actual* pain, that causes the greatest distress. Unfortunately, the more fearful and anxious the patient becomes, the more sensitive he or she may be to pain.

Subjective fears, also known as *acquired fears,* are based on feelings, attitudes, and concerns that have developed at the suggestions of peers, siblings, parents, or other individuals. These fears are based on anecdotal evidence (hearing stories or seeing dental care depicted in movies or television shows). Subjective fears, imaginative as they are, can cause irreparable damage to a patient's composure and conduct during a routine dental visit. Small children, especially, have an intense fear of the unknown. Whether the patient is a child or an adult, he or she should be informed in a general and positive way about the dental procedure, the use of equipment, and the sequence of events that can be expected.

Objective fears, also known as *learned fears,* are those related to the patient's experiences and his or her own memories of those experiences. If the experience was traumatic, the patient dreads subsequent treatment. If the experience was a positive one, the patient will not be fearful. The best way to address objective fear is to be honest when communicating to the patient. Never lie to a patient. For example, it is always better to say, "This will pinch for just a moment," than to say, "This won't hurt at all."

Despite their concerns and feelings of uneasiness, the majority of patients are able to seek and receive treatment. The dental team can help these patients by seeking to understand patient behavior and actively working to enable the patient to cope with the experience in a positive manner.

Dental-phobic patients

For some patients, the mere suggestion of a routine dental visit brings overwhelming sensations of panic and terror. These patients are termed *dental-phobic*. Patients with the most severe cases of dental phobia avoid routine treatment completely and seek urgent or emergency treatment only with the most aggravated of dental symptoms.

Patient's responses

The patient's responses to dental treatment and to the dental team are not limited to what is being said and done at the moment; rather, responses are influenced by the patient's total personality and his or her background experiences. When working with patients, it is particularly important to remember the following:

- The patient's response to the situation results primarily from causes that are not part of the present situation.
- These causes probably are not fully understood by the patient and probably will remain largely unknown to the dental team.
- The patient's anxieties concerning treatment may result in hostile, irrational, and inappropriate behavior.
- This hostility is an expression of the patient's anxieties and is not caused by, or directed at, dental personnel.

Physical and Mental Needs

The maintenance of high standards of care includes sensitivity to the patient's physical and mental needs. The patient registration form and medical-dental history form should include questions concerning the patient's dental and medical health. With this information, it is easier to determine whether a patient requires extra attention because of specific physical needs. Patients with physical or mental impairments have complicated and special needs that must be considered before and during dental treatment.

Financial Needs

Often, a major obstacle to patient acceptance is the cost of the treatment. Patients may believe that the fees are too high, that they are unable to afford the treatment, or that they do not need the treatment. Employment, payment, and insurance information are all relevant to patient care. Many people do not equate dental care with basic human needs such as shelter and food. Getting patients to understand the benefits and advantages of appropriate treatment is a part of good communication skills.

Meeting Patient Needs

The following sections describe ways to help the dental team meets patients' needs.

Positive Atmosphere

The physical appearance of the office speaks very clearly to patients. To ensure that patients feel welcome, create an environment and decor that reflect a warm, hospitable atmosphere. Worn or shabby floor covering should be replaced or cleaned when necessary. Plants and fresh floral arrangements reflect a healthy and inviting practice atmosphere. Plants, magazines, and other reception area amenities must be well maintained to keep this area as comfortable and pleasant as a living room in a private home.

Sincerity

Every action and word that takes place in the dental office is a reflection of the dental practice's level of sincerity. Patients are especially sensitive to tone of voice and remarks that could be misinterpreted (for example, a humorous remark could be mistaken as serious). Every member of the dental team must make a conscious effort to think before speaking or acting.

Showing Respect

Patients prefer to be treated as "friends of the practice." Every effort should be made to help patients feel welcome and important. It is advisable to address adults as "Mr.," "Mrs.," "Miss," or "Ms." at the initial greeting. If, after that time, the patient expresses a desire to be called by a first name or a nickname, then do so. (Make a note of this on the patient's chart for future reference.)

Respecting the Patient's Time

Patients expect the value of their time to be respected and not wasted in unnecessary waiting. Scheduling of appointments and staying on time are thus two essential components of helping patients feel welcome. By keeping a patient "waiting," the dental office is sending the message that the patient's time is not important.

Resolving Complaints and Misunderstandings

It has been estimated that 95 percent of patients who are unhappy or dissatisfied never say so; they simply leave the practice. Thus it makes good sense to listen carefully to those few patients who do attempt to express dissatisfaction. One of the best ways to calm an irate patient is to listen silently, use good eye contact, and occasionally nod the head. Do not interrupt. Let the patient finish. Often, this helps the patient calm down slowly. It then is appropriate to say to the patient, for example, "If I hear correctly what you are saying, Mr. Harris, you feel upset about the charge that appeared on last month's statement. Is that right?" This will give the patient a sense of control over the situation.

Make sure that all misunderstandings and concerns are resolved quickly, professionally, and pleasantly. If the patient insists on speaking with the dentist, tell the patient that the dentist will contact the patient by a specific time (later that same day, ideally); then take steps to ensure that this indeed takes place. (Dentists should only be interrupted to take calls that meet specific predetermined criteria. See further discussion below.)

Remaining Approachable

Many patients are afraid of approaching professionals or about asking questions that they fear may seem "dumb." One of the best communication techniques the dental office can practice is to display a sense of approachability at all times. Patients' questions should be encouraged. The dental team should respond to the patient with a sense of genuine care and concern. If the dentist has a "call-in" or "call-back" time each day for handling phone calls, this time should be used to reach patients. Most patients want to feel reassured that the dental team cares about them.

Respecting Patient Confidentiality

In a time of increasing litigation, it is more important than ever to keep conversations and patient records confidential. If patients believe that their concerns are not taken seriously or if they detect or sense a lack of confidentiality, the practice-patient relationship may experience irreparable damage (see Chapters 4 and 5).

Recall

5. How can a patient be psychologically influenced by others' attitudes?
6. Are objective fears acquired or learned?
7. What are some of the best ways to calm an irate patient?

CULTURAL DIVERSITY

Another aspect of effective communication is our respect for a highly diverse society. Social diversity is an important factor to consider as a professional. Differences in race, gender, cultural heritage, age, physical abilities, and spiritual beliefs are variations that must be appreciated and understood when working with patients and other staff members.

Verbal and nonverbal language varies among cultures. When working with such a diverse population as exists in the United States, it is advantageous to have someone in the practice that is bilingual. Encourage all members of the team to learn various culture traditions and to always show respect to these traditions when providing patient care.

If there is no one in the office that speaks another language, have a multiple-language dictionary on hand.

Basic Dental Terms in Spanish

English	Spanish
mouth	la boca
tooth	el diente
pain	el dolor
open	abierto/a
bite	la mordedura
decay	la descomposición
filling	la empastadura
x-ray	la radiografía

PHONE SKILLS

The phone is your most important tool in public relations. Most patients make their first contact with the dental office by phone. Based on this first contact, the patient forms an opinion of the practice. This opinion reflects on the dentist and dental team and even on the quality of care provided—although no actual care has yet been provided.

The business assistant is responsible for answering the phone and for ensuring that this and all patient contacts are positive experiences (Fig. 61-2).

Courtesy

Phone calls should be governed by the same rules of courtesy that apply to face-to-face meetings. This courtesy should begin with a prompt and pleasant response to the ring of the phone and should continue until the receiver is gently replaced at the end of the call. When answering the phone, your voice should convey the equivalent of a warm smile and the perceived message should be, "I'm glad you called!" You never want to send the message that the call is an unwanted interruption or that you are tired, angry, preoccupied, or in a hurry. Remember the following:

- Smile; it shows in your voice.
- Never chew gum, eat, drink, or have a pen or pencil in your mouth while talking on the phone.
- Speak directly into the receiver (mouthpiece), keeping your mouth 1 to 2 inches away.
- Speak clearly and slowly; guard against slurring your words.

- Get the name of the person who is calling, and talk to him or her, not to the phone.
- Use the caller's name in the conversation and give him or her your complete attention.
- When completing a call, always allow the person originating the call to hang up first.

Incoming Calls

The phone should be answered promptly, preferably after the first ring. Use the wording preferred by the dentist at your practice.

- Greet the patient pleasantly.
- Identify the practice and yourself. (Properly identifying yourself at the beginning of the conversation will prompt the caller to identify himself or herself as well.)
- Ask how you may help the caller.

Placing a Caller on Hold

Before placing a caller on hold, ask for his or her permission: "May I put you on hold for just a moment, Mr. Johnson?" Then wait for the caller's response before pressing the "hold" or "mute" button.

Always be courteous and do not expect the caller to remain on hold for more than a few moments. If necessary, ask whether you can return the call and give a specific time when you will do so.

On-Hold Message Systems

On-hold message systems consist of recorded messages or music used by the practice to make "on-hold" time educational and more pleasant for callers than a waiting signal. These messages may explain a variety of treatments and services available at the practice. The messages or musical interludes are broken occasionally by recordings by professional announcers who apologize for any delay and thank the caller for waiting.

Callers Wanting to Speak to the Dentist

The dentist should not be interrupted at chairside to come to the phone. Phone interruptions (1) reduce productivity and cause treatment delays, (2) are inconsiderate to the seated patient, and (3) make it difficult for the dental team to maintain infection-control protocols.

The most common exceptions for a dentist to come to the phone are to talk to another dentist, the dental laboratory technician, or an immediate family member. It is the business assistant's responsibility to know the dentist's policy on this and to handle all other calls tactfully.

Select your words and phrases with care. If a caller requests to speak with the dentist does not meet the dentist's specified criteria for interruption, be polite. A statement such as "Dr. Garcia is with a patient. How may I help you?" is appropriate.

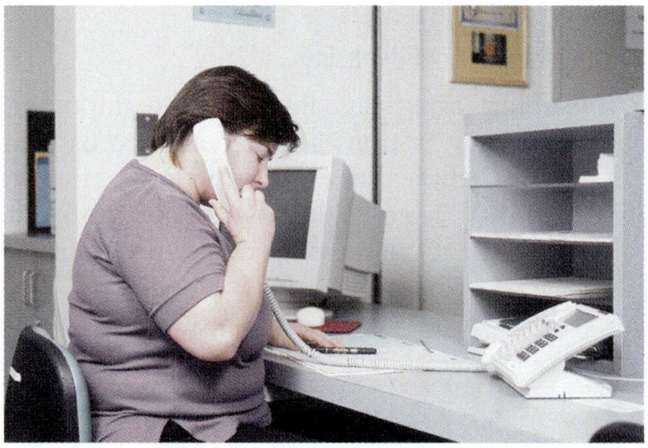

Fig. 61-2 The business assistant answers the phone.

Procedure 61-1 Answering the Phone

Equipment and Supplies

- Phone
- Message pad
- Pen or pencil
- Appointment book

PROCEDURAL STEPS

1. Answer the phone on the first ring.
   Purpose: This shows the patient that your office is prompt and ready to please.
2. Speak directly into the receiver with your mouth approximately 1 inch from the mouthpiece.
3. Identify the office and yourself.
   Purpose: This lets the caller know whether they have reached the correct number.
4. Acknowledge the caller by name.
   Purpose: This shows interest in the call and initiates the first relationship.
5. Follow through on the caller's request by answering specific questions about new patient information, appointments, or financial information.
6. Take a message if appropriate.
7. Complete the call in a professional manner and replace the receiver after you hear that the caller has done so.

Taking Messages

Make a written notation of all incoming calls, particularly those that require further action. Many practices use a printed form or a phone log to organize this information (Fig. 61-3). Many of these types of form systems create a duplicate copy of the message as you write, so that the original message can be torn off and delivered. At the beginning of the conversation, note the caller's name and then ask the appropriate questions. Be sure to record the information completely and accurately. After you take a message, deliver it promptly and accurately.

If you promise to follow through on a call, be sure to do just that! Do not promise that the dentist will call back at a certain time unless you are positive that this is possible and that the dentist will be willing to follow through. When the dentist is expected to return a call to a patient, have the appropriate patient records ready for the dentist when you deliver the message (see Procedure 61-1).

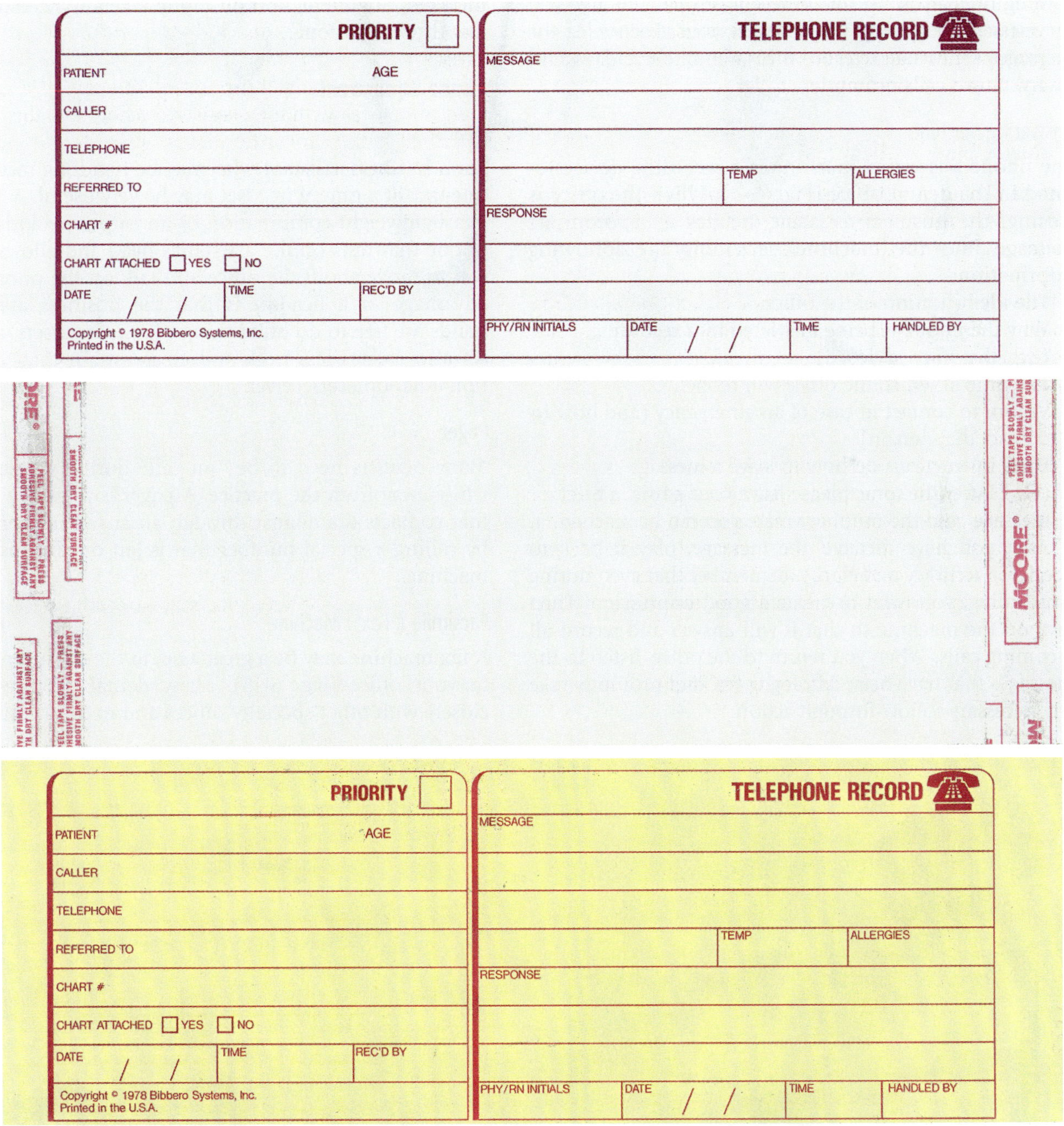
PRIORITY

PATIENT AGE

CALLER

TELEPHONE

REFERRED TO

CHART #

CHART ATTACHED ☐ YES ☐ NO

DATE / / TIME REC'D BY

Copyright © 1978 Bibbero Systems, Inc.
Printed in the U.S.A.

TELEPHONE RECORD

MESSAGE

TEMP ALLERGIES

RESPONSE

PHY/RN INITIALS DATE / / TIME HANDLED BY

PRIORITY

PATIENT AGE

CALLER

TELEPHONE

REFERRED TO

CHART #

CHART ATTACHED ☐ YES ☐ NO

DATE / / TIME REC'D BY

Copyright © 1978 Bibbero Systems, Inc.
Printed in the U.S.A.

TELEPHONE RECORD

MESSAGE

TEMP ALLERGIES

RESPONSE

PHY/RN INITIALS DATE / / TIME HANDLED BY

Fig. 61-3 An example of a printed form for taking messages. (Courtesy Bibbero Systems, Inc., Petaluma, Calif.)

Phone Message Systems

Answering Service

When the dental office is closed, some form of phone coverage must be provided. If an answering service is used, learn how to use the services properly. In general, it is necessary to call the service and notify them when the office is closing. Relay the following information to the service:

- When the office will reopen
- Whom to contact in case of an emergency (and how to contact that person)

When the office reopens, call the service immediately to notify them that you are back and will be taking the incoming calls again. At this time, the service will give you the messages they have taken during your absence. As the messages are dictated, record them accurately and, as necessary, return calls promptly.

Answering Machine

The phone answering machine is a recording device located in the dental office (Fig. 61-4). When the office is closing, the business assistant dictates an appropriate message into the machine, providing the following information:

- The identification of the office
- Why the phone is being answered by a recording (e.g., the office is closed)
- The time at which the office will reopen
- Whom to contact in case of an emergency (and how to contact that person)
- Basic instructions on how to leave a message (e.g., "After the tone, please leave your name, a brief message, and the number where you can be reached.")

After you have dictated the message, play it back to check for accuracy and clarity. Remember that even during a recording, you want to create a good impression. Then turn on the machine so that it will answer and record all incoming calls. When you return to the office, listen to the messages that have been left, log them, and promptly take any necessary follow-through action.

Voice Mail

Many dental practices prefer to use a voice mail service to allow the caller to select a variety of options. These services are usually contracted through the company who provides the practice's local phone service. As a rule, calls may be forwarded directly to various parties to answer questions, or the caller may leave a message for the dentist or one of the assistants. Voice mail services allow you to leave a recorded greeting similar to that used with an answering machine; however, there is no physical machine kept in the dental office. Instead, the messages are retrieved by calling an access number and entering a security code number. As with the other message systems, listen to the messages, log them, and promptly take any necessary follow-through action.

Phone Equipment

Headsets

For a business assistant who may be handling more than one task at a time, a headset may be very useful. A headset is a lightweight combination of an earphone and microphone that rests on the assistant's head and allows a person to move about the office and talk on the phone. The advantage of a headset is that the business assistant's hands are free to do other things. For many users, a headset also creates less neck and elbow strain than a traditional handpiece/receiver.

Pager

Many dentists need to be "on call" during weekends or while away from the practice. A pager is a mobile system that contacts the dentist through an answering service or by calling a special number that is left on the answering machine.

Facsimile ("Fax") Machine

A **fax machine** may be a great asset to the communication in your office (Fig. 61-5). Many dental practices work closely with other specialty offices and need to convey pa-

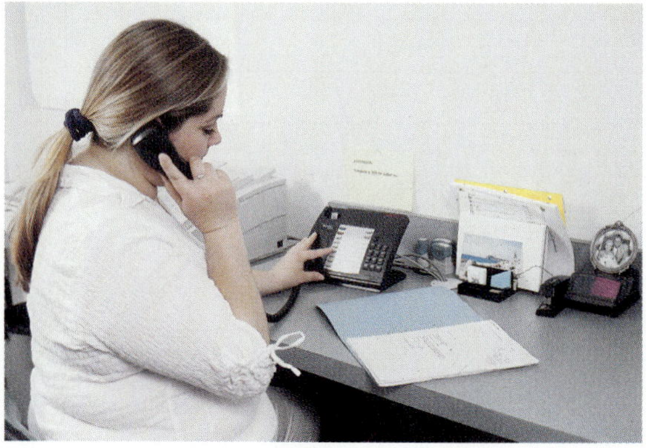

Fig. 61-4 An answering machine.

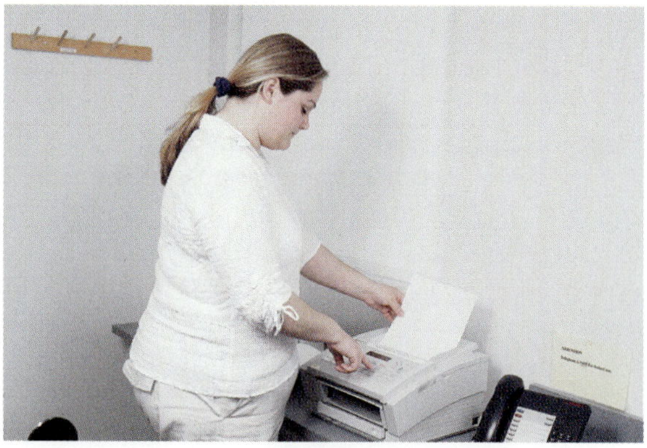

Fig. 61-5 A facsimile (fax) machine.

tient information to dentists or with other healthcare professionals. Sending this information by fax can save time and labor. The fax unit is hooked into the phone system and is used to electronically send and receive hard-copy messages (handwritten or typed).

Uses of the fax machine in the dental office can include placing orders with suppliers, relaying and receiving patient information, and sending information to insurance companies. When sending a fax, remember that it should be neat and professional in appearance (just like other forms of written communication).

Recall

8. What is the most important piece of equipment used for public relations?
9. On which ring should you answer the phone?
10. When the dental office is closed, how are messages obtained?
11. What piece of equipment allows you to transmit hard-copy written messages?

WRITTEN COMMUNICATIONS

Many types of written communications originate from the dental practice. It is important to realize that, other than speaking with someone on the phone, written communication is the most important public relations tool of a practice. Thus the practice's image or the perception it creates is based to a great degree on the type and quality of the printed communications it generates.

Equipment

If one of your responsibilities in the dental office is to correspond through written communication, you will be required to learn how to use the necessary business equipment within the office (Fig. 61-6).

The *computer* is the system most offices use today for written communication (Fig. 61-7). This useful and most versatile piece of equipment allows the business assistant to handle all written communication procedures, as well as any marketing, scheduling, insurance, ordering, and billing procedures. Today, many dental software companies are available to come in and set up a customized program for the dental office. Learning basic keyboarding is useful for writing effectively with the computer.

A **copier** allows you to make duplicates (copies) of documents that need to be sent to a patient, another dentist, dental laboratory, or supply company. Maintenance of copy machines can be time-consuming and costly. Make sure the office invests in a copier that will withstand the amount of work for that practice.

Business Letters

Sending high-quality letters is essential to convey a professional image. Every letter or correspondence must be produced on high-quality, professionally designed stationery. These letters must be concise, accurate, neat, and proofread for spelling and grammatical errors. Misspelled words and poor grammar convey the image of an office that does not care about quality. Patients and referring dentists may see this as unprofessional and even as a reflection on the quality of dental care provided.

Parts of a Letter

The structure of a letter and its layout on the page are standardized into four parts: heading, opening, body, and closing (Fig. 61-8).

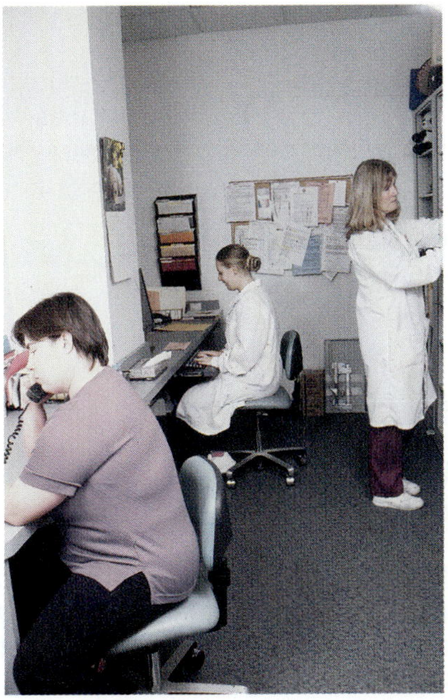

Fig. 61-6 Business equipment is set up within the office management area.

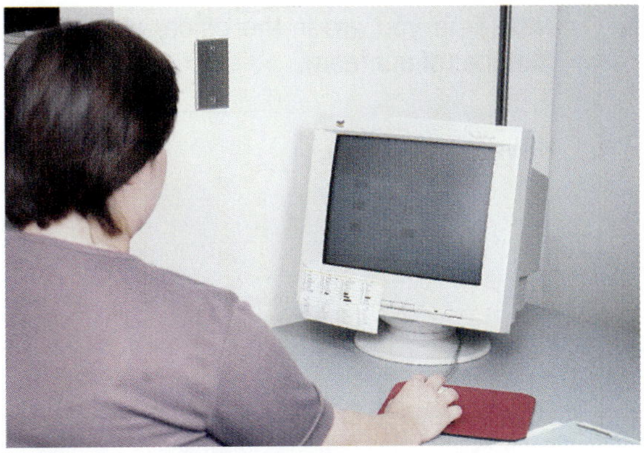

Fig. 61-7 A desktop computer system used in the office.

1. *Heading:* The heading of a letter consists of the **letterhead,** which is most commonly preprinted or embossed on the stationery. The letterhead usually appears at the top of the page and may include the dentist's name and title, address, and phone number. If the dentist is in practice with other associates, these names may also be included.

2. *Opening:* The opening of a letter consists of the inside address, date, and salutation. The inside address is the person or organization to whom the letter is being written. This should include the person's name and appropriate title, street address, city, state, and zip code.

   The date of the letter is inserted directly above or to the right of the inside address. The date includes the

Children's Pediatric Dental Associates
693 Professional Drive
Chapel Hill, North Carolina 27514

June 2, 2005

Ms. Nancy Campbell
945 Branch Road
Chapel Hill, NC 27516

Dear Nancy:

We are pleased to announce our exciting news! Children's Pediatric Dental Associates will be taking on a new associate.

Dr. Kim Chi will be seeing patients beginning in August. She comes to us from Norfolk, Virginia, where she graduated from the University of Virginia with a Bachelor's of Science in Chemistry, and then attended and completed her DDS and Pediatric residency from the University of North Carolina in 2003.

Because of this timely addition of Dr. Chi, the office will now be able to offer extended hours to accommodate your busy schedules with work, school and after-school activities. When you call for your next appointment, inquire about the extended times and scheduling with Dr. Chi.

Next time you are in the office, please take a minute to meet Dr. Chi and get to know the newest member of our team.

Have a good day,

Sincerely,

Jim R. Stewart, D.D.S.

Fig. 61-8 A business letter.

month, day, and year. Abbreviation of any part of the date is not recommended.

The **salutation** is the introductory greeting. The type of salutation used depends on the level of formality appropriate for each individual letter.

3. *Body:* The body of the letter deals with the subject of the correspondence. Its length depends on the type of correspondence. It is often best to provide an introductory paragraph, give specific details about the subject in the second paragraph, and then provide a conclusion in the third paragraph.
4. *Closing:* The final section of the letter is the closing. The closing consists of just a few polite words, essentially saying goodbye to the reader. It is common to see words such as *sincerely, cordially,* or *best regards* in the closing. Below the closing is the typewritten name of the person sending the letter. Make sure to leave several spaces below the closing for a handwritten signature; this makes the letter personal and legal.

Types of Business Letters

Many practices send letters to their patients for a variety of reasons:

- Welcome to the practice
- Congratulations
- Acknowledgment of a referral
- Completion of an extensive case
- Continuing care (recall)
- Missed appointment
- Proposed treatment
- Collection of payment (see Chapter 63)

To save time when composing letters, many practices keep sample letters on file under specific headings. Other commercially prepared sample letters (often called "templates") are available in books ("hard copy" format) or in electronic format (disks, CDs, or downloadable files) for use with a **word processing software** program. The word processing program enables users to quickly create form letters and personalize them automatically by merging appropriate information from patient data files.

Letters to Colleagues

Dentists frequently communicate with other professionals in writing. It is the job of the alert dental assistant to ensure that these communications take place in an expedient and a professional manner. Letters to the dentist's colleagues may include examination findings or referral to specialists. It is important to double-check for spelling accuracy and consistency when sending written communications to other professional practices.

Letters to Insurance Carriers

When completing written correspondence to insurance carriers, make sure that the following is included:

- Patient identification information: Patient's name, address, contract number or identification number. (NOTE: Be careful not to include a patient's social security number when submitting information.)
- Case information: Nature and extent of the case, any unusual circumstances or conditions, and an estimate of the fees to be incurred
- Radiographs: Only included if required

Recall

12. What part of a letter includes the salutation?
13. In addition to the patient, to whom else might you send a business letter?

Procedure 61-2 Composing a Business Letter

Equipment and Supplies

- Computer
- Letterhead paper
- Pen

PROCEDURAL STEPS

1. Prepare a draft of the letter by hand; then have a peer review it and make comments.
   Purpose: This provides practice in writing skills and also helps develop your verbal and nonverbal skills with another person.
2. Check the draft for correct information, grammar, spelling, and punctuation.
3. Using your word processor, set your margins, font, spacing, and order of the letter (if this is a function of your particular software).
4. Create the final letter from the corrected draft.
5. Type your name and sign by hand (or, if you are writing the letter for someone else, type the sender's name at the closing and have that person sign by hand).

MARKETING YOUR DENTAL PRACTICE

The term **marketing** usually brings to mind large advertising campaigns; however, that is not how this term applies to dentistry. In dentistry, marketing encompasses all activities involved in attracting and retaining satisfied patients in the practice. Communication skills are an essential part of the marketing of a dental practice.

Initiation and development of a marketing plan are the responsibilities of the dentist; however, for a marketing plan to be successful, all members of the dental team must be actively and enthusiastically involved in planning, implementing, and monitoring that plan.

Although this is a team effort, one person (usually the office manager or business assistant) may be given the responsibility for ensuring the overall smooth functioning of the marketing program.

Goals of Practice Marketing

A primary goal of any marketing plan is to create a positive image of the practice as a place where patients receive quality treatment in a caring atmosphere. The positive and cooperative attitudes of all staff members are vital to successfully creating this image; however, the business assistant is a key person because he or she usually has the all-important first contact with the patient.

A secondary goal is to enroll new patients at the practice. An important part of achieving this goal is to determine the perceived needs of potential patients and to seek out ways to meet these needs.

Logistics of Marketing

The majority of practices with successful marketing programs attribute this success to good organization, attention to detail, determination of a budget, and tracking of the results.

The Plan

For a marketing plan to succeed, written goals and dates must be established. Attention to detail is essential.

Marketing Budget

The average amount of investment budgeted by dentists for a practice marketing plan ranges between 3 and 5 percent of the previous year's gross revenues.

Tracking Responses

Tracking determines the success of the marketing plan. Specific tracking gives a response to each marketing activity. This may be accomplished by counting the number of new patient referrals that result from a marketing promotion; for example, "Thirty new patients entered the practice after [a specific] marketing event" is a measurable response of success.

Types of Practice Marketing

External marketing activities are those that take place outside of the office and are directed to people who are not patients. These activities include health fairs and presentations to school children or senior citizen groups. These external marketing activities may require staff members' participation in the community. If so, they are expected to cooperate in an enthusiastic and a fully professional manner. The dental team is an extension of the practice at all times, especially when representing the practice in public.

Internal marketing strategies are those activities and promotions targeted to current patients of the practice. These also may require staff participation. Such activities may include, but are not limited to, the following:

- Publishing a practice newsletter
- Developing promotional materials for insertion into monthly statements
- Sending flowers or other appropriate "thank you" gifts to those who refer new patients to the practice
- Sending birthday or other special occasion cards to patients
- Sponsoring giveaways, office open houses, and other promotional events

Practice Newsletter

The newsletter represents a valuable communication tool for the practice. Patients enjoy reading about new techniques available and learning about the "human" side of the practice. The purposes of a practice newsletter include the following:

- Keeping patients aware of technologic and treatment advances
- Keeping in touch with the dentist and members of the dental team
- Listing patients' names as referral sources or contest winners. (NOTE: Names are used *only* with the patient's permission.)
- Announcing other changes that have taken place in the practice

Most practices that publish a newsletter for their patients do so on a quarterly basis. A number of professional newsletter preparation organizations are available to produce a newsletter that incorporates the dentist's masthead and practice information.

Patient Education Materials

Printed pamphlets, brochures, and statement "stuffers" are other printed communication tools that have been used successfully by many dental practices. When these materials are dispensed, it is essential to include the dentist's name, address, and phone number on each printed piece. Another effective marketing mechanism is to write the patient's name on the educational material because this increases the likelihood the patient will actually review the material and refer to it later.

Recall

14. Which members of the dental office should be involved in the marketing of the practice?
15. How much should a practice invest in marketing?
16. Give an example of an external marketing activity.

COMMUNICATING WITH COLLEAGUES

Most Americans spend more time with their coworkers than with their own families. Working in a positive, challenging, and stress-free environment is what everyone wants from their place of employment. How you communicate and get along with your coworkers will be evident to your patients and their perception of the practice (Fig. 61-9). A patient can tell right away what kind of harmony exists in a dental setting.

Being a Team Member

Be flexible and receptive to altering the way duties are performed.

Be self-confident and use self-initiative when it is time to get things done. Do not wait to be told what to do.

Show appreciation to coworkers; do not take advantage of them.

Think before speaking.

Do not let your emotions get overly involved.

Remember that the first impression is not always the right one.

Share the ups and downs of the day.

Remember that your way is not always the right way.

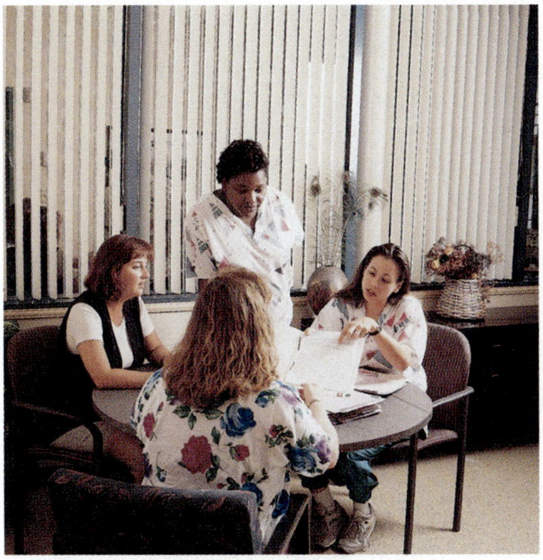

Fig. 61-9 Team meeting.

The one key to a successful work environment is teamwork. Teamwork exists when everyone feels needed and respected and is given an opportunity to fulfill his or her role with the others in a specific setting.

Stress in the Dental Office

An important aspect of good communication is how you handle stress in your personal life and at work. The dental atmosphere can be a very stressful environment and can affect the way you deal with your patients and coworkers.

Causes

Stress is common in the workplace. Many dental team members feel stressed at times and need to find an outlet for their emotions. Causes of stress in the dental office include, but are not limited to, the following:

- Lack of sufficient staff
- Appointment overbooking
- Multiple tasks required simultaneously
- Lack of good communication
- Perceived lack of job advancement

Methods of Stress Reduction

You can reduce stress by a lifestyle that includes engaging in regular exercise, taking time for yourself, leaving the office behind at the end of the day, eating properly, and setting realistic expectations. Learning to control stress will enable you to make intelligent decisions regarding patient management, patient care, and patient relationships.

If differences among colleagues within the office setting are creating stress, learn how to work through those differences by engaging in team-building dialogue. Almost every dental team problem can be dealt with by following these five basic steps: (1) voice the problem, (2) list possible solutions, (3) eliminate the solutions you know won't work, (4) select a solution to try, and (5) evaluate. After the first four steps have been put into action, bring the dental team back together to evaluate (step 5). If the solution worked, there is no longer a problem. If it did not work, choose another solution and plan to reevaluate.

Learning to control stress will enable you to make intelligent decisions regarding patient management, patient care, and patient relationships.

Recall

17. What is the key to a successful work environment?
18. Describe stressors in a dental office.

Patient Education

The dental team is the front door to a practice. Everything you say and do represents the dentist and the practice. The entire staff should work as a team to create an atmosphere of patient confidence and trust. Offer information about appointment schedules, billing, insurance services, phone hours, office hours, and emergency coverage. Information about fees and office policies should be readily available to patients. The more information you can offer to your patients, the more they will feel confident in the dental practice's care.

Legal and Ethical Implications

Remember that all communication with patients is confidential, whether by phone, through written letters, or in the documentation in a patient's record. The Health Insurance Portability and Accountability Act **(HIPAA)** of 1996 has increased our awareness of privacy when speaking with a patient. Be sure that you are discreet in discussing specific treatment or financial information. Every means of communication should project a professional image.

Eye to the Future

Technology allows us to communicate with people very easily. For example, a dental practice can maintain its own website that introduces the staff, philosophies of practice, and the specialty or focus of the practice. Through the use of the Internet, most information in the future will be conveyed via email. As patients update their patient registration forms, they will be required to include their email address. The business assistant can then email appointment reminders, recall notification, insurance information, and billing questions.

Critical Thinking

1. Go through your personal "junk mail"; select examples that show a powerful marketing technique to get your attention.
2. Write down a specific dialogue that you might use when answering the phone in a dental office.
3. Think back to your last visit to the dentist or doctor and discuss how the business of the office was handled. Describe how the reception area was maintained and how the staff members treated one another.
4. List some possible reasons why a patient might feel apprehensive about visiting the dentist.
5. Have you ever observed a situation in which someone was being discriminated against by another person? If so, describe the situation, your feelings, and ways this could have been prevented.

62

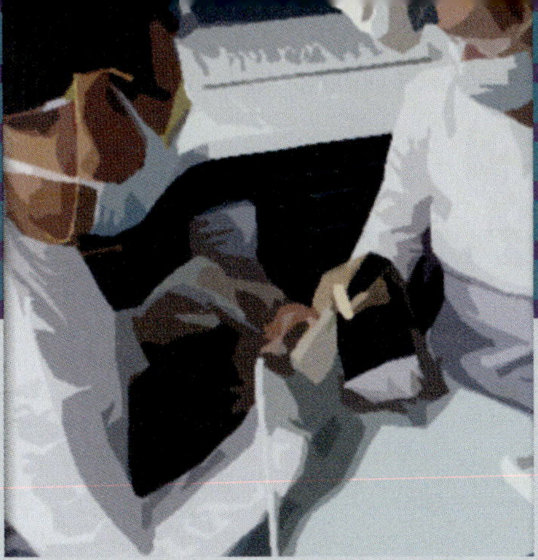

Business Operating Systems

Outline

Operating Procedure Manual
- HIPAA Compliance
- Personnel Manual

Computer Applications in the Dental Office

Record-Keeping
- Types of Records and Files

Guidelines to Efficient Filing
- Basic Filing Systems
- Active and Inactive Files
- Purge Tabs
- Record Protection and Confidentiality

Appointment Scheduling
- Computerized or Manual Scheduling
- The Appointment Book
- Guidelines for Scheduling
- Outlining the Appointment Book
- Making Appointment Book and Appointment Card Entries
- Special Considerations for Scheduling
- Confirmation of Appointments
- Patient Circumstances
- Daily Treatment Area Schedule

Preventive Recall Programs
- Types of Recall Systems

Inventory Management
- Inventory Systems
- Guidelines for Ordering Dental Supplies
- Dental Supply Budget

Equipment Repairs
- Equipment Records

Legal and Ethical Implications

Eye to the Future

Critical Thinking

KEY TERMS

Active files Files of patients who have been seen within the past 2 to 3 years.

Buffer time Time reserved on the schedule for emergency patients.

Call list List of patients who can come in for an appointment on short notice.

Chronologic file Filing system that divides materials into months (and possibly days of the month).

Cross-reference file A file is which each item is listed in alphabetic order by name and includes its document number.

Daily schedule Printed schedule that is copied and placed throughout the office for viewing by staff only.

Downtime Waiting period between patient procedures.

File guides An insert placed between files, displaying the letters or numbers of the patient records that follow it.

Filing The act of classifying and arranging records to be easily retrieved when needed.

HIPAA The Health Insurance Portability and Accountability Act of 1996, which specifies federal regulations ensuring privacy regarding a patient's healthcare information.

Inactive files Files of patients who have not been seen in the past 3 years.

Lead time A time estimate to allow for delays in ordering or shipping of materials.

Ledger A financial statement that maintains all account transactions.

Outguide Device used for a filing system; similar to a bookmark.

Patient of record Individual who has been examined and diagnosed by the dentist and has had treatment planned.

Purchase order A form that authorizes the purchase of products from a supplier.

continued

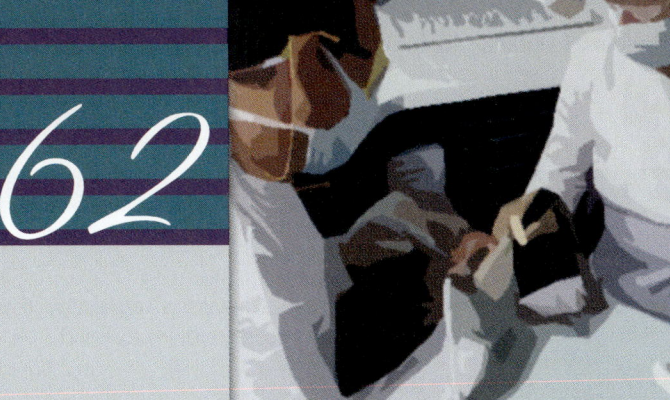

KEY TERMS, cont'd

Rate of use The quantity of a product that is used within a given time.

Requisition (reh-kwi-**zi**-shun) A formal request for supplies.

Reorder tags A notation system that is used when the supply of a certain item is getting low and the item needs to be reordered.

Shelf life How long a product may be stored prior to use.

Units of time Time increments used in planning appointments.

Want list A list of supplies to be ordered and questions to be asked of the representative.

Warranty A written statement explaining the manufacturer's responsibility for replacing and/or repairing a product.

LEARNING OUTCOMES

On completion of this chapter, the student will be able to achieve the following objectives:

- Pronounce, define, and spell the Key Terms.
- Discuss the role of the office manager/business assistant in the dental office.
- Identify types of practice records and files.
- Identify how to use these filing systems: alphabetic, numeric, cross-reference, chronologic, and subject.
- Describe the process of scheduling appointments for maximum productivity.
- Identify three types of preventive recall systems and state the benefits of each.
- Describe the function of computerized practice management systems and manual bookkeeping systems.
- Discuss the management of inventory systems.

The business office is the core of the business side of a dental practice. Effective management is necessary to achieve organizational goals, team-oriented employee satisfaction, and financial success. This chapter introduces business operating systems that are vital to the day-to-day operations of a dental practice. Efficient and effective business systems can increase productivity, decrease stress, and increase patient confidence.

Depending on the size of the practice, the business portion of the office may consist of one business assistant or several individuals who handle different aspects of the business. In a large practice, responsibilities may be divided among the receptionist, bookkeeper, appointment clerk, file clerk, insurance clerk, and secretary. In a smaller practice, one individual may handle all of these responsibilities; that person is usually titled the administrative or business assistant.

Role of the Business Assistant

Many important responsibilities and roles are filled by the business assistant. These duties may include, but are not limited to, the following:

- Greeting patients and answering the telephone
- Scheduling patients
- Managing patient records
- Managing accounts receivable and accounts payable
- Managing the recall and inventory control systems
- Overseeing and monitoring practice marketing activities
- Managing payroll
- Presenting fees and making financial arrangements

OPERATING PROCEDURE MANUAL

It is essential for a smooth-running dental practice to have an office procedure manual on hand. This manual includes policies and procedures that the dentist wants the staff to follow within the practice. The manual should outline individual job descriptions for the business and clinical assistants. Information included in this office manual may include, but is not limited to, the following:

- Objective or purpose of the manual
- Office communications
- Staff policies
- Employment policies
- Office records
- OSHA and infection-control policy
- Clinical procedures
- Professional organizations

HIPAA Compliance

The introduction of the Health Insurance Portability and Accountability Act of 1996 (commonly known as **HIPAA**) was adopted to enhance and protect the rights of patients. Knowing the state and federal law requirements eases the implementation of this act into the dental practice.

The American Dental Association (ADA) has been an integral part in the implementation of HIPAA. With the ADA's involvement, dental practices have the flexibility to create their own privacy procedures tailored to fit the size and needs on an individual basis.

The dentist must follow a specific format when putting HIPAA policies into practice. The dental staff must be informed of specific security and confidentiality issues. HIPAA-related training of existing dental staff must be reinforced continuously. New staff need to be trained as soon as possible.

Personnel Manual

Personnel issues may be included in the employment section of the office procedure manual or in a separate personnel manual. Personnel topics include the job description for each employee, pay periods, working hours, and information concerning employee benefits such as paid holidays, vacation, and sick leave. Also included might be policies on provisional employment, maternity leave, disciplinary measures, sexual harassment, and termination.

Some practices use a commercially prepared manual, whereas others customize their own personnel manual. Whichever type is preferred, it is helpful to use a ring binder, which allows pages to be added or deleted as office policy is updated or information becomes obsolete. To prevent miscommunication among staff, make sure that each new employee reviews the office manual during the first weeks of employment and that all employees continue to review any new information that is added. Any areas that are not clear should be addressed during that time.

COMPUTER APPLICATIONS IN THE DENTAL OFFICE

The use of computers in the dental practice continues to replace many of the manual tasks that were completed by the business assistant for so many years. The computer, which can receive, store, process, and send information, can handle nearly all the business aspects of the practice. Here are some specific applications that the computer can handle:

- Appointment scheduling
- Health information records
- Word processing
- Networking
- Bookkeeping entries
- Database management
- Billing and collection
- Patient ledger
- Processing insurance claims

HIPAA ***HIPAA Privacy Compliance List***

Specific areas that must be included in the procedure manual:

- Know the law. Become familiar with HIPAA regulations. Know the requirements of your state privacy laws.
- Adopt or develop the required forms to put into action the privacy policies and procedures.
- Train the dental staff on the privacy policies and procedures and designate a privacy officer and a contact person to receive complaints. Make sure to document the training.
- Notify patients of the new policies by posting and distributing a Notice of Privacy Practice, and obtain written permission by the patient's Acknowledgment of Receipt of Notice of Privacy Practice.
- Make sure policies and procedures are fully implemented and up to date. If changes need to be made, make sure the modifications are documented.

NOTE: Information modified from the ADA HIPAA Privacy Kit.

Recall

1. Is overseeing financial activities the responsibility of the clinical assistant or the business assistant?
2. What is the best way for a new employee to learn about office protocol?
3. What continues to replace the "handwritten" operating procedures in the handling of business?

RECORD-KEEPING

The maintenance of adequate records is one of the business assistant's most important responsibilities. Because so much information is maintained in files, the office must decide what type of records and filing system best suits the needs of the practice. The maintenance of accurate and complete records is a sign of quality care.

Types of Records and Files

Patient Dental Records

The patient record includes the patient registration, medical and dental history form, examination findings, diagnosis and treatment plans, a record of all treatment provided, correspondence, consent forms, and radiographs (see Chapter 26 for more information).

Patient Financial Records

Financial information regarding a patient's account is maintained separately as part of the practice business records. This information should never be filed with patient clinical records.

A patient statement, or **ledger,** contains all of the financial information for each patient or family (Fig. 62-1). The ledger statement is also available on a dental management software program for the office computer. Within the program, the patient account screen allows the business assistant to enter or review all aspects of financial charges, payments, and insurance transactions (Fig. 62-2).

In both the ledger card system and the software program, the standard design includes columns for the date, patient's name, description of service, charges, payments, and balance. An additional column can provide for an insurance summary.

Practice Business Records

Accurate financial and business records enable the dentist to operate the practice in a well-organized and business-like manner. These records are usually stored through the use of a subject file system; that is, they are filed under categories such as "laboratory expenses" and "business office supplies." Business records include, but are not limited to, the following:

- Accounts receivable records
- Practice expenses awaiting payment
- Expense records (receipts and paid bills)
- Payroll records
- Business correspondence
- Canceled checks and bank statements
- Records of income and expenses
- Financial statements, tax records, and possibly corporate records
- Computer printouts of practice reports

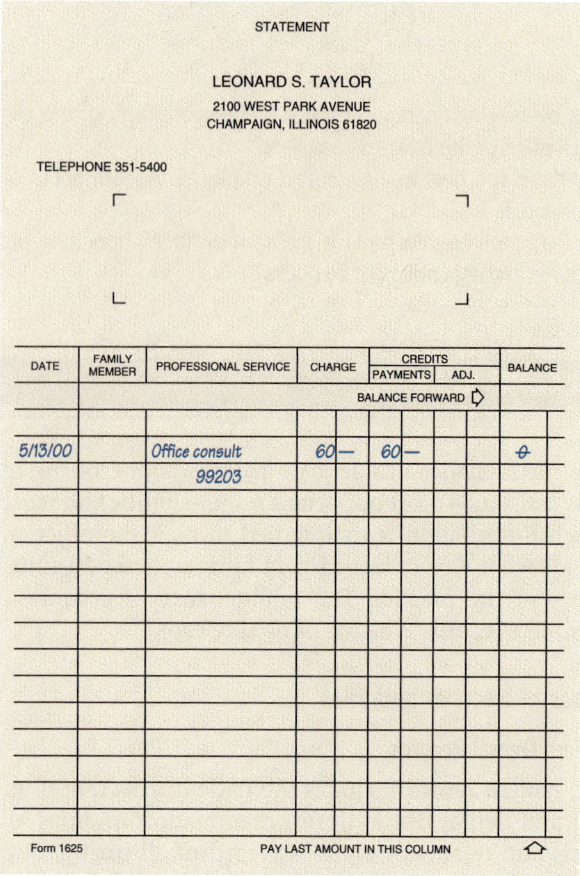

Fig. 62-1 **Patient ledger.** (Courtesy Colwell, a division of Patterson Companies, Inc., 1-800-637-1140.)

Recall

4. What is another term used for a patient statement?

GUIDELINES TO EFFICIENT FILING

Filing is the act of classifying and arranging records so that they are preserved safely and can be quickly retrieved when needed. The specific guidelines in filing are as follows:

- *Keep the filing system simple.* The simpler the system, the easier it is to work with. For most practices, alphabetic filing with color-coding is the simplest and most efficient system (Fig. 62-3).
- *Label folders clearly.* Each file folder should have a neatly typed label showing the patient's full name. This saves time in having to go through the chart to make certain that you have the right one. Use an adequate number of **file guides.** There should be approximately 1 file guide for every 5 to 10 folders, depending on the size of the folders.

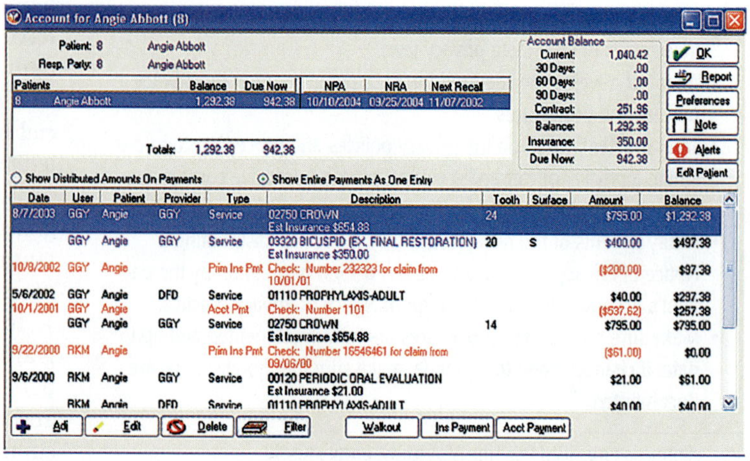

Fig. 62-2 **Computerized patient account summary.** (Courtesy Eaglesoft, a division of Patterson Dental, Inc.)

- *Leave adequate working space within each file.* If too little space is allowed for each file, papers become tightly wedged, which slows the process of filing, makes records more difficult to find, and may damage filed materials. Leave at least 4 inches of working space on each shelf or in each drawer.
- *Label shelves or drawers.* All files should be clearly, neatly, and accurately labeled as to the contents or other appropriate designation (Fig. 62-4).
- *Use outguides.* An **outguide** is like a bookmark for the filing system. When a folder is removed from the file, place an outguide to mark its place. This makes it faster to return records to the file and easy to spot where records are missing (Fig. 62-5).
- *Presort.* Presorting folders into approximate order before starting to file will speed the filing process.

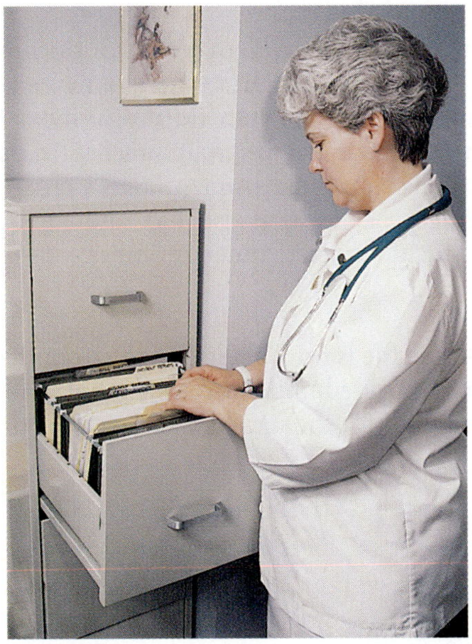

Fig. 62-4 **Label drawers.** (From Chester GA: *Modern medical assisting,* Philadelphia, 1998, Saunders.)

Basic Filing Systems

The basic methods of filing used in dental offices are alphabetic by last name, numeric, color-coding, and chronologic.

Alphabetic

The alphabetic filing system is by far the easiest and most commonly used system for filing patient records and ledger cards. In alphabetic filing, all items are filed in straight alphabetic (A-B-C) order in accordance with the basic rules of indexing. Standard rules must be followed for this system. Table 62-1 provides the rules for alphabetic filing.

Color-Coding

Color-coding is used to make filing and retrieving patient records easier and faster (Fig. 62-6). With color-coding, the tabs combine colors and letters, which are used to indicate the first two letters of the patient's last name. In addition to speeding up filing and finding records, color-coding makes it easier to spot a misfiled record. Color-coding may be used with numeric filing; in this case, the color tabs are labeled with the last two digits of the chart number.

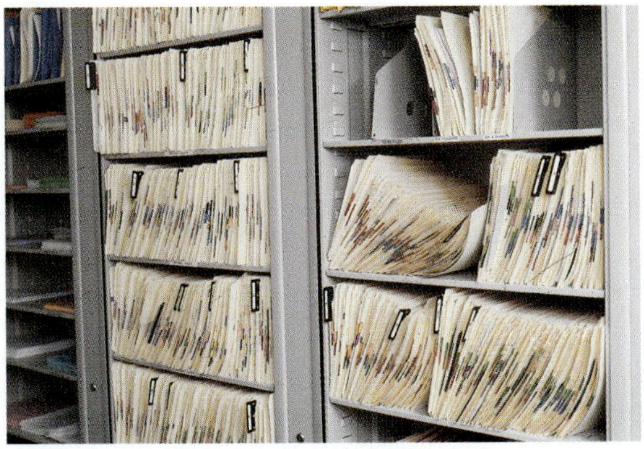

Fig. 62-3 **Keep filing systems simple.**

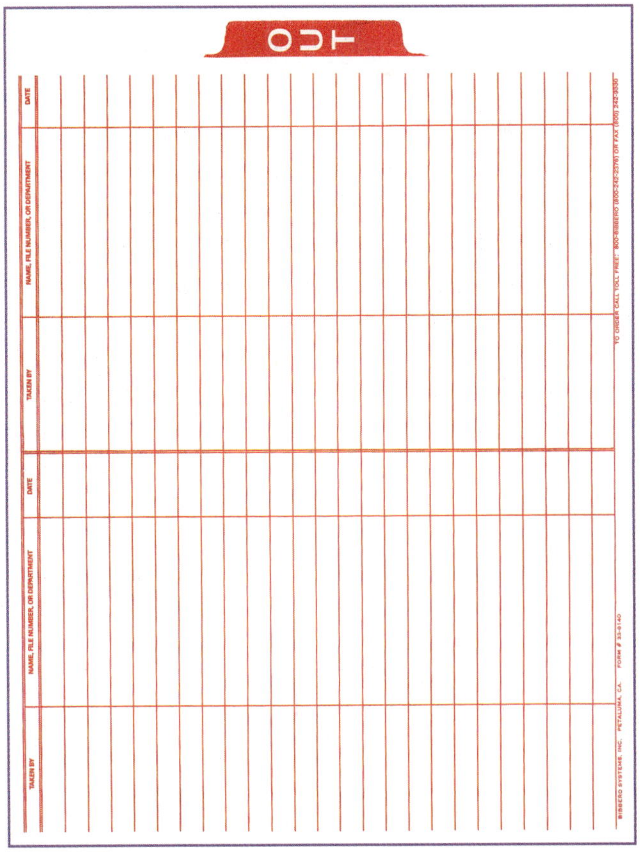

Fig. 62-5 **Use an outguide.** (Courtesy Bibbero Systems, Inc, Petaluma, Calif.)

Numeric

In numeric filing, each patient record or document is assigned a number. In straight numeric filing, all items are filed in strict 1-2-3 order. Numeric filing is most often used for patient records in a large group practice. In this system, to locate items, you must also maintain a **cross-reference file,** in which each item is listed in alphabetic order by name and includes its document number.

Chronologic

A **chronologic file** is usually divided into months and may be further subdivided into days of the month. This kind of file may be used for the recall system or as a "tickler" system for miscellaneous tasks, such as routine maintenance, which must be performed at specific times during the year. Other special files may be maintained for purposes such as cross-reference files, inventory control files, and short-notice appointment lists.

Electronic

You will most likely use at least one type of electronic filing or storage system. Electronic files are stored on the computer's hard drive (at least temporarily); they should additionally be stored on either floppy disks, zip disks, or CDs. To keep track of these files, label each unit with a subject name or number.

Table 62-1 ***Indexing* Rules for Alphabetic† Filing***

Indexing Rules	Unit 1‡ (Caption)§	Unit 2	Unit 3	Unit 4
Names	Brown *(surname)*	John *(first name)*	William *(middle name)*	Senior *(term denoting seniority)*
Married woman	Brown *(surname)*	Mary *(her first name)*	Harris *(her middle name or maiden name)*	Mrs. John W. *(for information only, not an indexing unit)*
Nothing comes before something	Brown			
	Brown	J.		
	Brown	John		
	Brown	John	W.	
	Brown	John	William	
	Brown	John	William	Senior
The prefix is part of surname, not a separate unit *(maintain strict alphabetical order!)*	Macdonald	Peter		
	McDonald	Paul		
Abbreviated prefix *(index as if spelled out)*	St. Andrew *(Saint Andrew)*	Francis	Lee	
Hyphenated names *(treat as one unit)*	Vaughan-Eames	Henry	David	
Titles are not indexing units	Douglass	James	Richard	Ph.D. *(for information only, not for indexing)*

**__Indexing__ is the process of selecting a caption under which a paper will be filed. It is also the process of determining the order in which the units of that name are to be considered.*

†__Alphabetizing__ is the arrangement of captions and indexing units in strict alphabetical order: A-B-C.

‡A __unit__ is a single important element in a name or subject. Material to be indexed is handled in units. A name can be arranged out of normal order for indexing; however, once it is assigned a unit number, the units are then handled in their normal numerical order.

§The __caption__ is the name or phrase under which a paper is filed. This constitutes the first indexing unit.

Active and Inactive Files

Patient records are *permanent records* of the dental practice, which means they should never be discarded or destroyed without the dentist's specific instruction. To reduce the number of charts to be sorted through daily, many practices subdivide patient records into active and inactive files.

Active files are files of patients who have been seen recently (usually within the past 2 to 3 years). These are maintained in the areas of easiest accessibility.

Inactive files are records of patients that have not been seen in the last 3 years. These files are maintained in a less convenient area but can be accessed if needed.

Purge Tabs

Color-coded purge tabs, also known as *aging tabs,* make it easier to sort records into active and inactive categories. For example, at a patient's first visit in 2004, a red 2004 tag is placed on the folder. At the first visit in 2005, a green 2005 tag is placed over the previous one. When it is time to sort out the charts for all patients not seen since 2004, it is easy to go through the file and quickly identify those folders still labeled with only a red 2004 tag.

Record Protection and Confidentiality

The destruction of records through loss, fire, or other catastrophe could seriously handicap a dental practice. For this reason, it is vital that all records be protected at all times. Patient records and all other practice information are confidential and should be treated with appropriate care.

HIPAA Safeguards

Safeguards need to be in place to ensure the confidentiality and protection of electronic files. Specific protocol of HIPAA compliance states that the dental office must have physical and technical safeguards to ensure the safety and confidentiality of the patient's personal information. Passwords should be put into practice and changed often. It is important to maintain up-to-date antivirus protection software on your computer system. Firewalls should be constructed if you are working from a network. Also, the business area must not have computer screens in plain sight of patients. Even if you are certain that your computer screen is out of public sight, never leave patient files open on your screen unless you are currently using them. Once you have finished using a file, close it.

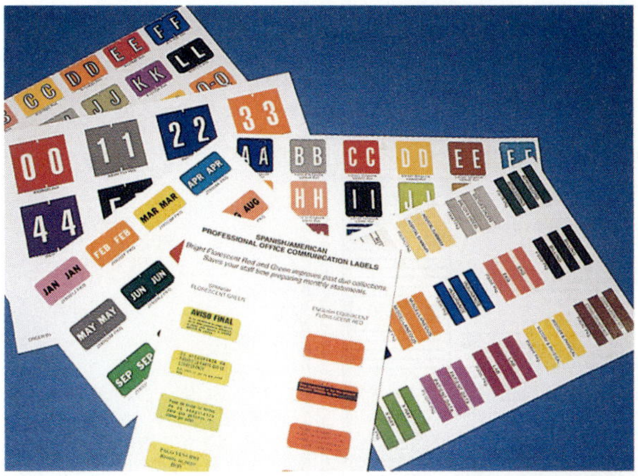

Fig. 62-6 A variety of coding systems are used for filing patient records. (From Chester GA: *Modern medical assisting,* Philadelphia, 1998, Saunders.)

Protecting Electronic Files

If the practice system is computerized, it is advisable to back up all files at the end of each business day. To *back up* means to make a copy of the computer files. The backup file is then available in case there is a problem with the system. Many practices keep two sets of backup files: one set in the office and a second set in a safe place outside of the office. Thus, in the event of fire or other catastrophe, a remaining set of files is available.

Protecting Paper Files

Never leave paper records outside their appropriate file space. As you finish using a record, return it to its proper place. When leaving for the day, make certain that all records are protected in file cabinets and that the cabinets are properly closed. Precautions also should be taken to prevent cross-contamination when files are moved from the treatment area and returned to the business area.

Recall

5. How much free space should be left on each shelf of a filing cabinet?
6. What is used to mark a space from which a record has been taken?
7. What is the easiest filing system to use?
8. If a patient has not been seen within the last 3 years, would that patient be considered active or inactive?

APPOINTMENT SCHEDULING

Effective appointment scheduling is vital to the smooth functioning and success of the entire dental practice.

Scheduling is most effective when one person is responsible for all appointment planning and all entries in the appointment book. This responsibility is usually given to the business assistant, but in a larger practice, more than one person must be involved. In this case, a system should be established to determine who schedules each appointment in case of a communication breakdown regarding scheduling policies.

Computerized or Manual Scheduling

Appointment control may be managed with a computerized scheduling system or manually with a traditional appointment book. Regardless of the system used, the basic understanding and guidelines are the same: the appointment book format must be selected, the days must be outlined, and the patients must be scheduled effectively to make the best possible use of time (Fig. 62-7).

Efficient Appointment Scheduling

- *Patients are seen on time.* Making patients wait is discourteous and shows a lack of respect for their time.
- *The patient load is well balanced.* This provides an even pace, and the day is completed without undue tension or hurry.
- *The dentist and staff are able to make good use of their time.* This enables them to maximize their productivity while providing quality care for patients.
- *The stress level is decreased when production goals are reached and patients are happy with good customer service.*

The Appointment Book

If a manual appointment book is used, it must be selected to ensure sufficient space for all necessary entries and to facilitate the efficient scheduling of patients for the dental practice. The most efficient format is the so-called week-at-a-glance design. This allows the business assistant to view all days of the week at once. Ideally, the book should have ring binders or be spiral-bound to allow it to lie flat when fully open. Additional options include the following:

- With or without printed dates
- Number of columns, depending on the needs of the practice
- Units of time (10-, 15-, or 30-minute intervals)

If an electronic appointment system is selected, you have the advantage of selecting a software program that will make the business assistant's job of scheduling, canceling, rescheduling, and shifting appointments much easier. Furthermore, you can set production goals by controlling when and where specific procedures are performed. Additional options include the following:

- *Autoscheduler,* which allows for a quick search of appointment openings.
- *Patient record,* which allows you to view the demographics and patient information.
- *Daily appointment screen,* which allows you to color-code columns as they relate to patient care.

Guidelines for Scheduling

Units of Time

The basic time increments used in planning appointments are described as **units of time.** A unit of time may be 10, 15, or 30 minutes, depending on the dentist's preference.

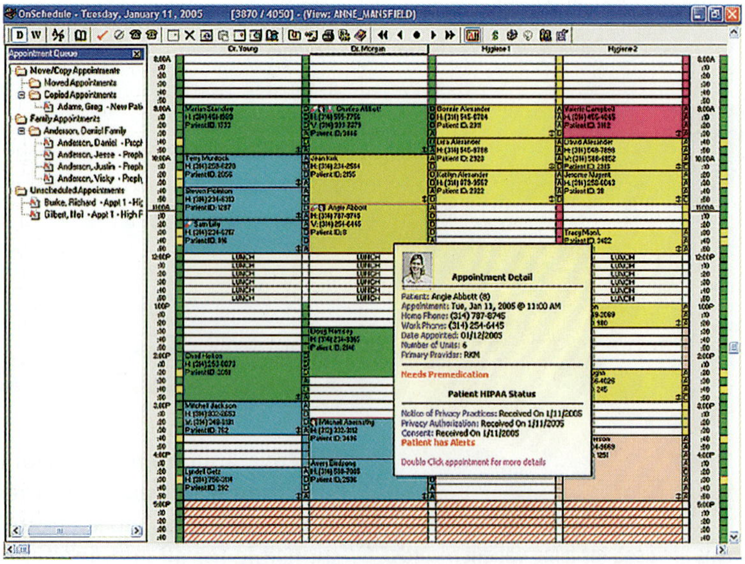

Fig. 62-7 Computerized schedules. (Courtesy Eaglesoft, a division of Patterson Companies, Inc.)

With 10-minute increments, there are six units per hour. With 15-minute increments, there are four units per hour. And with 30-minute increments, there are two units per hour. Most dental practices use 15-minute units because they provide maximum flexibility in scheduling, which allows for more productivity.

The key to efficient patient scheduling is to schedule patients according to the time necessary for their complete procedure rather than by trying to fit all procedures into a standard 30-minute or 1-hour formula. If a 15-minute time unit is used in the practice and a patient must be scheduled for a procedure that will take about 40 minutes to complete, the dentist should then request that this patient be given a "three-unit" appointment.

Columns Per Day

Appointment scheduling for each day will be assigned to a separate column designated specifically for each operator, with each column representing an operatory. An "operator" may be the dentist, a hygienist, or an assistant with expanded-function responsibilities. For example, in a typical solo practice, one column per day is scheduled for the dentist, and one is scheduled for the dental hygienist. If an expanded-functions assistant is also employed in the practice, a separate column may be designated for that person.

To make most efficient use of their time, many dentists prefer to use several treatment areas simultaneously. This preference is reflected in the appointment book by having one column represent each operatory. In larger practices with many providers, it is necessary to use a computerized system or multiple appointment books.

Outlining the Appointment Book

The business assistant should go through the appointment book several months in advance and outline basic information (Fig. 62-8). The four basic elements to be outlined are as follows:

- Office hours
- Buffer time
- Meetings
- Holidays

Computer scheduling allows the business assistant to block out operatories and times for specific procedures; this helps the practice to customize the schedule to meet specific production goals. Manual entries should be made

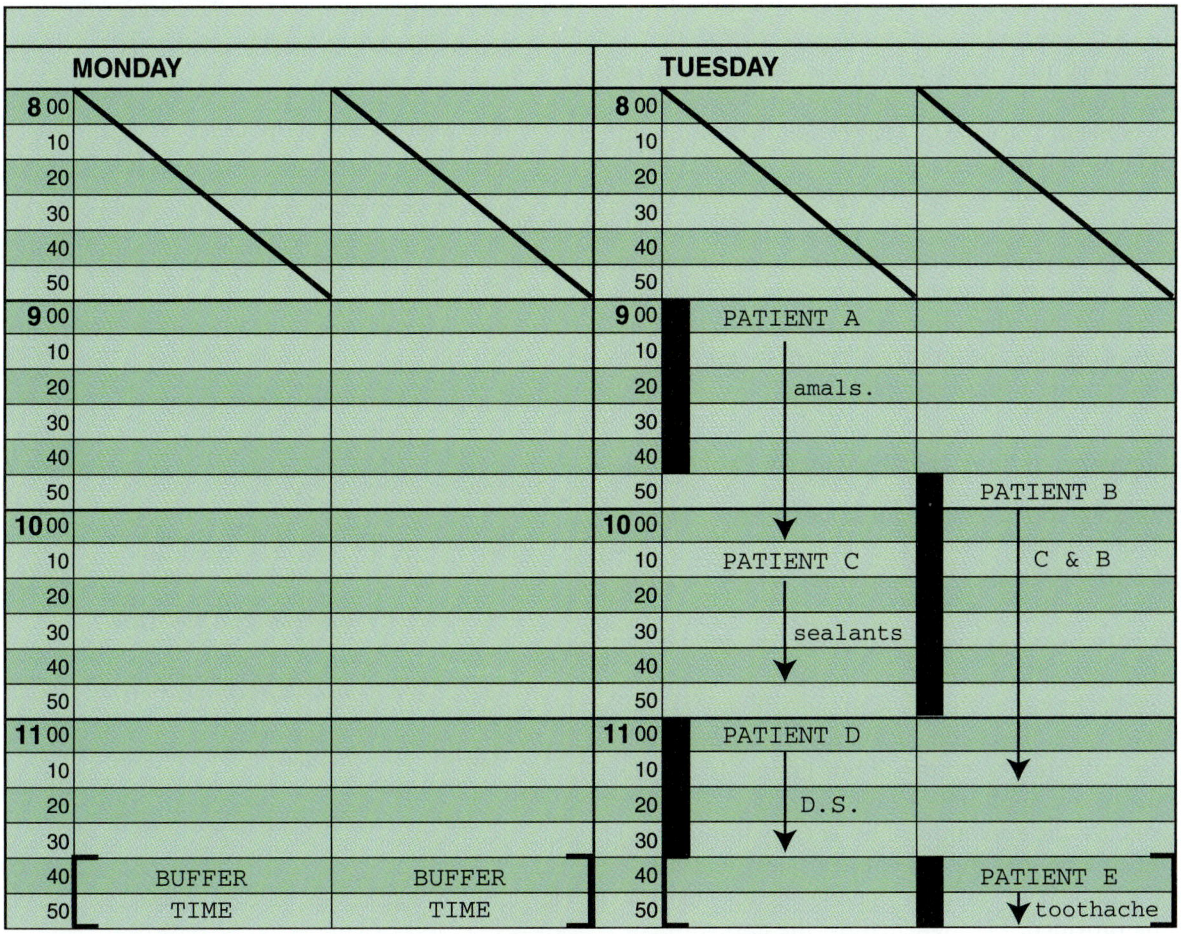

Fig. 62-8 A typical daily format for scheduling.

in pencil that is sufficiently dark to be seen but easily erasable in case of change.

Office Hours

Office hours are the hours that a practice is open for business. They do not include the hours when the practice is opening or closing, the lunch hour, and routine days off. A diagonal line is drawn through these time periods on the schedule to indicate that they are not available for scheduling patients.

Buffer Time

Buffer time is the time reserved each day for scheduling emergency patients. In many practices, there is a buffer period of one or two units scheduled in the late morning or in the afternoon. These times are bracketed or highlighted in the appointment book. Buffer time not needed for emergencies may be used at the last minute for short appointments, such as denture adjustments or suture removal. This time should *not* be filled more than 24 hours in advance.

An experienced business assistant may not need specific buffer times actually marked in the appointment book. The assistant can determine the best time to schedule a patient just by looking at the existing appointment sequence.

Meetings

Regular meetings that occur during the working day or those that require the dentist to leave the office early should be marked. The time for staff meetings also should be blocked out well in advance.

Holidays

Major holidays on which the office is closed also should be crossed out. Other holidays and school vacations, when school is closed but the office is open, should also be noted. These times may be more convenient for scheduling school children and working people.

Making Appointment Book and Appointment Card Entries

All appointment book entries must be *accurate, legible, complete,* and *in pencil.*

- Entries must be clearly written so that they are easy to read.
- Entries must be made in pencil that is sufficiently dark to read yet erasable if necessary.
- Entries must be complete and accurate so that it is clear exactly who is scheduled and for what treatment.

The entries should be complete but limited to the information directly applicable to the scheduled appointment. Generally, the appointment book entry includes (1) the patient's name, (2) the patient's business and home telephone numbers, (3) an abbreviated code for the treatment to be provided, (4) the length of the appointment, and (5) special notations such as whether the patient is new or requires premedication.

The proper sequence of recording entries is as follows:

1. Make the complete entry in the appointment book.
2. Write the appointment card for the patient.
3. Double-check to ensure the information is the same in both places.

When the appointment book entry is complete, the patient is given an appointment card that states the day, date, and time of the appointment (Fig. 62-9). As the business assistant hands this to the patient, he or she orally confirms that the patient understands the information.

Special Considerations for Scheduling

Higher-stress procedures, such as extensive crown and bridge preparation, implants, or surgery, require careful scheduling. These types of procedures are often scheduled in the morning when the dentist and staff members are at their highest energy levels. Scheduling also must be engineered so as to allow efficient use of "idle" time for greater productivity. For example, during a restorative

Daily Scheduling Rules

- Do not schedule too many difficult procedures close together. This can place additional stress and strain on the dentist and staff.
- Allow time for treatment area cleanup. Remember that the treatment area must be prepared, broken down, and disinfected before a patient can be seated. How long does this take in your practice?
- Educate your patients about treatment times; reinforce this teaching regularly.
- Protect the appointment book from the eyes of others; this is private information.

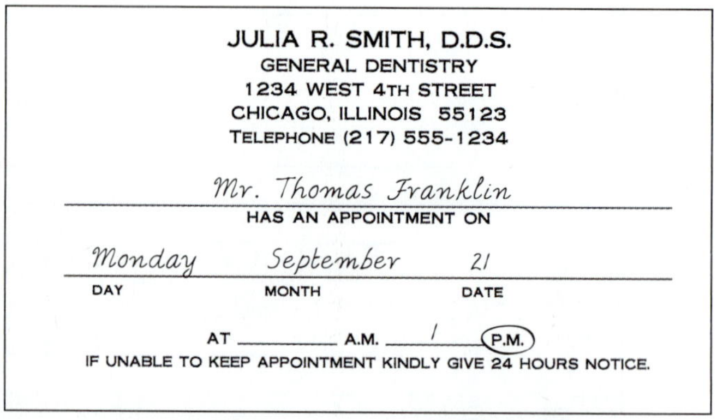

JULIA R. SMITH, D.D.S.
GENERAL DENTISTRY
1234 WEST 4TH STREET
CHICAGO, ILLINOIS 55123
TELEPHONE (217) 555-1234

Mr. Thomas Franklin
HAS AN APPOINTMENT ON

Monday September 21
DAY MONTH DATE

AT ______ A.M. 1 P.M.
IF UNABLE TO KEEP APPOINTMENT KINDLY GIVE 24 HOURS NOTICE.

Fig. 62-9 An appointment card is completed. (Courtesy Colwell, a division of Patterson Companies, Inc., 1-800-637-1140.)

procedure, the dentist will inject the patient with a local anesthetic agent and then wait 3 to 5 minutes for the anesthetic agent to take effect. This waiting period is referred to as **downtime.** During the downtime, if the dentist's time is well scheduled, he or she can check a hygiene patient, make a prosthetic adjustment, see an emergency patient, return a telephone call, or meet with a sales representative.

New Patients

New patients should be scheduled as soon as possible after they call for an appointment, even if it is not an emergency. Some practices accomplish this by reserving a "new patient time" each day. New patients should be asked to come to the dental office at least 15 minutes before the beginning of their appointment time so that they can complete the necessary patient registration forms. Some practices also send an introductory packet of information to new patients before the first appointment. This packet may contain information such as:

- A letter welcoming the patient to the practice
- Practice information such as the dentist's educational and licensure credentials
- Office policies such as payment plans and management of insurance claims
- A map or printed directions to the office (including information about parking facilities if applicable)
- Patient registration forms (so that the patient can fill them out before the appointment)

Scheduling for the Dental Hygienist

Effective appointment scheduling for the dental hygienist is important. The business assistant must pay close attention to the time needed for these appointments. It is recommended that the hygienist and business assistant work out a list of average times required for certain types of hygiene visits. Examples for scheduling hygiene patients are as follows:

- New adult patient
- New child patient
- Adult prophylaxis
- Child prophylaxis
- Fluoride treatment
- Pit and fissure sealants

The scheduling list should cover all the types of procedures commonly performed by the hygienist and should include the time required for the dentist to check the hygiene patient. On the basis of this information, the business assistant can schedule hygiene patients for the correct amount of time so that the hygienist is neither rushed nor wasting time waiting for the next patient.

Recall Patients

Recall patients are customarily scheduled with the hygienist for a prophylaxis, review of home care, and routine radiographs. However, it is also necessary to allow time in this appointment for the dentist to see the patient. A recall patient must always be asked whether there have been any changes in his or her health history, address, or insurance coverage and whether the patient is taking any new or different medications.

Children

Young children are usually at their best in the morning, so most dentists prefer to schedule them early in the day. Whenever possible, older school children are scheduled after school or at times when school is closed. Having a copy of the school calendar is helpful in planning such appointments. Sometimes it is necessary to have a child dismissed from school for dental treatment. To minimize the disruption of the school day, it is best to schedule the child either at the beginning of the day (before he or she goes to school) or near the end of the school day.

Emergency Patients

Emergency patients must be seen as quickly as possible. Buffer time is reserved in the appointment book for this purpose. Regardless of buffer time, a patient with an acute emergency must be seen immediately. An emergency can obviously delay the treatment of the regularly scheduled patients. If this happens, the situation should be explained to the scheduled patients, and their cooperation should be requested. If necessary, the scheduled patients should be offered the option of rescheduling.

The patient in pain who has been seen before in the practice should be scheduled as soon as possible. This caller is known as a **patient of record,** and failure to accommodate him or her could leave the dentist open to charges of abandonment. Emergency callers who are not patients of record may become regular patients. For this reason, many practices make every effort to accommodate them as well. However, if the dentist is out of town or unavailable, another dentist should be on call to take care of emergencies.

When you receive a telephone call from a patient in pain, gather as much information as possible that will help the dentist diagnose the patient's problem. For example:

- Where is the pain?
- How long has it continued?
- Is there fever or swelling?
- Is the pain constant or "on and off"?
- Is the pain in response to heat? Cold? Sweets? Chewing? Pressure?
- Has there been recent treatment or injury in the area of the pain?

A patient with a true emergency will generally come at the first available time. If a patient tries to negotiate a time that is more convenient, it may not be a true emergency. The business assistant must use good judgment to determine whether the patient is a true emergency case.

Scheduling an Appointment Series

Certain procedures, such as the fabrication of a prosthetic device or the restoration of multiple teeth, may require a series of appointments. It is more efficient to plan the entire series at the beginning of treatment. To do this, the business assistant must answer the following:

- How many appointments will be required?
- How long (the number of units) will each appointment take?
- How many laboratory working days must be allowed between appointments?

When scheduling a series of appointments, try to give the patient the same day of the week and same time of day for each appointment. This makes it easier for the patient to remember the appointments. With the exception of prosthodontics, it is not generally recommended to schedule more than two appointments in advance. Otherwise, the dentist's schedule becomes overbooked and appointment time is not available for new patients and emergencies. In addition, there is a greater chance of a patient missing an appointment if it is scheduled too far in advance.

Scheduling for an Expanded-Functions Dental Assistant

When scheduling for an expanded-functions dental assistant, entries in the appointment book are made "by the chair." To do this, a separate appointment book column is designated for each operatory. Appointments must also be planned so that only one patient is scheduled per chair and per expanded-functions assistant. Before scheduling an appointment, the business assistant must answer the following:

- What treatment is planned?
- How much time must be reserved for the entire appointment?
- Which units of the visit will be spent with the dentist? Which units will be solo time for the expanded-functions assistant before the dentist enters or after the dentist leaves the treatment room? For example, a patient having teeth prepared for the placement of a bridge must first have an alginate impression taken to create a diagnostic cast that can be used in fabricating provisional coverage. The first 10 minutes of the appointment may be scheduled with the assistant who can legally perform this function.

Confirmation of Appointments

One of the greatest obstacles to good appointment control is failure by the patient to keep the appointment. Sometimes these missed appointments are unavoidable; however, confirming all appointments by telephone the day before the appointment catches many cancellations far enough in advance to allow the time to be used effectively. Noting the patient's telephone number next to his or her name in the appointment book facilitates the task of placing these confirmation calls. Confirming your patients' appointments by email is another alternative.

Patient Circumstances

Late Patients

An office that consistently runs late is disrespectful of its patients' time. In turn, the dentist will soon find that patients begin to come in late for their appointments rather than having to wait. If the dentist is able to see patients on time, the same courtesy should be expected of the patients. Patients who are chronically late should be tactfully reminded that their tardiness is depriving them, as well as others, of treatment.

Canceled Appointments

If a patient has not appeared within 10 minutes of the appointed time, the patient should be contacted immediately in the hope that he or she will still be able to be seen for the remainder of the scheduled time. If not, the patient is usually offered another appointment, and every effort is made to schedule another patient into the remainder of the reserved time.

When a patient fails to keep an appointment, the information should be recorded on the patient record as "BA" (broken appointment) with the date. This is important clinical data because in case of a malpractice suit, repeatedly breaking appointments can be considered contributory negligence on the part of the patient.

Short-Notice Appointments

Although scheduling patients on short notice is not as efficient as careful prior planning, it is to the office's advantage to maintain a list of patients who are available to take an appointment on short notice. Information on such available patients may be placed on file cards or kept as a **call list.** This listing should include the patient's name, work and home telephone numbers, notes of the treatment to be provided, and the times when the patient is available.

The list should be kept up to date at all times, and the patient's name should be removed when he or she no longer needs an appointment. A patient who comes in on short notice should be thanked for changing his or her plans for the convenience of the dental office.

Daily Treatment Area Schedule

Appointment book information for the next day is transferred to the **daily schedule** form (Fig. 62-10). A sufficient number of copies are produced so that one can be posted in each treatment area, the laboratory, and the dentist's private office. On this form, the patient's name and an abbreviated code for treatment should be provided next to the appointment time. However, remember the HIPAA privacy rules, and do not indicate specific types of appointments for other patients to see. This list is updated throughout the day as changes in the schedule are made. A check mark is placed to the left of the patient's name when the appointment has been confirmed. A circle around the time indicates that the appointment has not been confirmed.

Prior Appointment Preparations

At the end of the day, the business assistant must make certain preparations for patients who are scheduled for the next day.

Daily Meeting

Many practices make a point of starting each workday with a team meeting. This is usually a brief meeting of 5 to 10 minutes during which the dentist and staff review the daily schedule and any specific treatment procedures or patient concerns.

Recall

9. What are the most common time lengths used for scheduling units of time in a dental practice?
10. What four elements should be outlined in an appointment book?
11. If a patient does not keep an appointment, where should this be recorded?

PREVENTIVE RECALL PROGRAMS

Regularly scheduled preventive care is important for a patient's dental health. The recall system, which is also referred to as the *continuing care program,* is designed to help patients return in a timely manner for treatment. It is the responsibility of the business assistant to ensure that patients are placed on recall and that those who are due to return are notified promptly.

The patient should be placed on recall when current dental treatment is completed or on instruction from the dentist. Box 62-1 can be used to calculate when a patient is due to return. The most common period of recall is 6 months; however, patients requiring more periodic visits may be placed on a 3- or 4-month recall. All steps necessary to place the patient on recall should be completed before the patient's treatment is filed for insurance. Doing this helps to ensure that the patient's information is indeed placed into the recall system.

Tues. 3/21	Dr. Edwards	Vivian (hyg)
8 00	Louise Brook	
15		Carrie James
30	f.imp	
45		
9 00	Dorothy Starr	Al Parker
15		
30	Comp, 8 & 9	
45	Francisco Lopez	Maria Gonzales
10 00	Cr. Prep 30	
15		
30		Jody Tan
45	Maria Gonzales	
11 00		
15	Amal. 14 & 18	Sarah Martin
30	*	
45	*	
12 00		
15		
30		
45		
1 00	Lloyd Barber	Mark Kemp
15	Try-in	
30	Jim Becker	
45	Ext	Sue Le
2 00	(tp 1:45 pre-med)	
15		
30	Mary Thomas	Anita Vasquez
45	Amal 3 & 4	
3 00	Comp 7	
15		Larry Smith
30		
45		
4 00		Rob Hills
15		
30		
45		
5 00		
15		
30	6:30 ADAA meeting	
45	Canyon View Civic Center	
6 00	Dr. Wagner, Patient	
15	Management	
30		
45		

Fig. 62-10 A daily schedule. (Courtesy Colwell, a division of Patterson Companies, Inc., 1-800-637-1140.)

Box 62-1 Calculating 6-Month Recall Time

Jan. (1)	Feb. (2)	March (3)	April (4)	May (5)	June (6)
July (7)	Aug. (8)	Sept. (9)	Oct. (10)	Nov. (11)	Dec. (12)

From the first half of the year, add 6 to the number of the month.
From the second half of the year, subtract 6 from the number of the month.

Types of Recall Systems

Continuing Appointment System

This method is also known as the *advance* or *preappointment recall* appointment system. At the time of the last visit in the current series, the patient is given a specific appointment time and date for the recall visit. This is noted in the appointment book, and the patient is given an appointment card. These appointments are coded in the appointment book so that the patient can be sent a reminder 2 weeks before the appointment. These appointments should also be confirmed by telephone.

Written Recall Notification

Many practices send a recall card or postcard to remind the patient to return for continuing care. With a computerized recall system, the cards for each month are quickly prepared by the system (Fig. 62-11). With a manual system, at the time of the last visit in the current series, the patient may be asked to self-address a recall card. This card is then filed behind the month of recall. At the beginning of each month, the business assistant removes the cards from the file for that month and mails them to the patients.

Recall by Telephone

Another option is to maintain a list of the names and telephone numbers of all patients due to be recalled each month. As time permits, the business assistant calls each patient and tries to schedule the recall appointment. A note is made next to the patient's name regarding the results of the call, and the patient's name is crossed out when he or she has been contacted. Although recall by telephone is time-consuming, it is usually more effective than repeatedly sending written reminders.

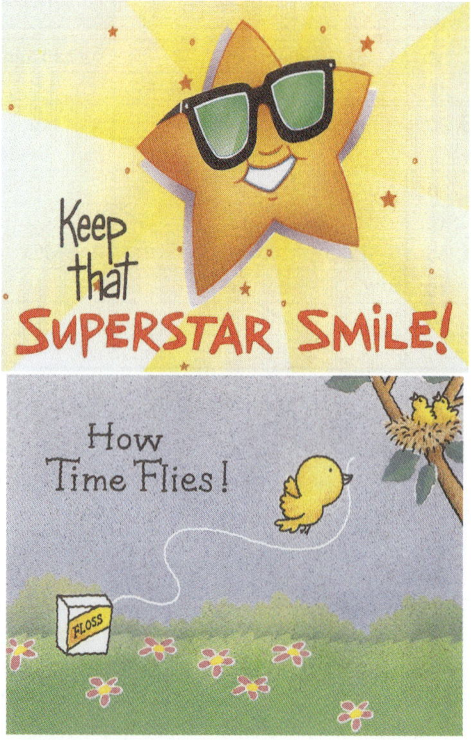

Fig. 62-11 Recall postcards are mailed. (Courtesy Colwell, a division of Patterson Companies, Inc., 1-800-637-1140.)

Recall

12. What is the most common time period for recall?
13. If a patient was last seen in March, when would be their recall time?

INVENTORY MANAGEMENT

Running out of supplies can create embarrassing situations and unnecessary crises in the dental office. Therefore an adequate quantity of all necessary dental supplies available at all times is essential for the smooth functioning of the practice (Fig. 62-12).

Inventory Systems

An inventory system should be simple, readily workable, and kept up to date at all times; it is advisable that one person be responsible for maintaining the inventory control and ordering supplies. However, the cooperation of the entire staff is necessary if the system is to work. Frequently,

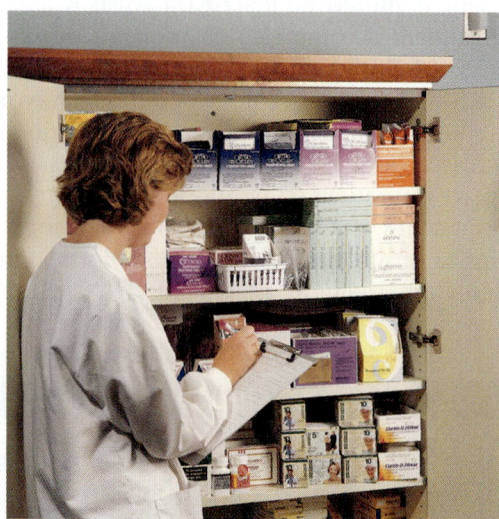

Fig. 62-12 Supplies available for the practice. (From Kinn ME, Woods M: *The medical assistant,* ed 8, Philadelphia, 1999, Saunders.)

the coordinating assistant or clinical assistant is assigned to handle the inventory of clinical area supplies, and the business assistant is assigned to manage the inventory of business office supplies.

Of major concern in organizing the inventory system are the expendable and disposable items that are used up in a relatively short time and must be reordered regularly; these include restorative and impression materials, disposable needles, local anesthetic solutions, radiographic film, laboratory supplies, paper products, and business office supplies. A simple system should be developed with the following information for ordering a product:

- Full brand name of the product
- All applicable descriptive information, such as name of the manufacturer, size, gauge, color, grit, length, shank type, fast or regular set, or container size
- Reorder point for that product
- Purchase source, including the name, telephone number, and if necessary, the address of the supplier of that product (it also is helpful to note the name of the contact person who usually handles the order)
- Any necessary catalog numbers for that product
- Quantity purchase rates and reorder quantity

Reorder Point

The reorder point for any given item is the minimum amount that represents an adequate reserve for that product. Thus, a reorder point, or minimum quantity, should be established for each expendable item used in the practice. This point, which ensures an adequate supply while the new order is being processed, is based on two factors:

1. The **rate of use** of the product on a daily, weekly, or monthly basis.
2. The **lead time** necessary to order and receive a new supply of that product; this time estimate should include a generous allowance for delays in ordering or shipping or the possibility of backordering

Marking the reorder point

The reorder point for each item should be clearly marked on the supply of that item. This task can be accomplished with **reorder tags.** These tags, also known as *red flag reorder tags* or *tie tags,* are usually bright red. The reorder tag is attached to the minimum quantity of the item with a rubber band or tape or by being placed into a stack of a flat product (such as a supply of ledger cards). This tag may be marked with the name of the product only, or it may contain full reordering information. When the reorder point is reached, this tag is removed and immediately processed for reordering.

Automatic shipments

Many suppliers offer dentists the advantage of bulk quantity pricing with automatic shipments of a portion of the total order. This ensures the practice a constant supply of the amount of a product necessary to meet the practice's need. It also eliminates bulk storage problems and spreads the billing over a sequence of monthly or quarterly payments.

Bar code reorder system

An automated supply reorder system uses bar code technology for commonly used dental supply items. The assistant uses a bar code wand to "read" the product and reorder information, which then is transmitted electronically to the supplier.

Quantity Purchase Rate

The quantity purchase rate is a saving that can be effective by purchasing a product in larger quantities. The price break is the point at which the greater savings become effective. Although it is often wise for the office manager to take advantage of the best price per unit on supplies, it also is necessary to take into consideration the available storage space in the office and the rate at which the product is used.

Reorder Quantity

Reorder quantity is the maximum quantity of a product to be ordered at one time. This should be reviewed periodically and increased or decreased, depending on changes in these determining factors. The reorder quantity is determined by the following:

- Rate of use
- **Shelf life** and any storage problems for that product
- Availability of storage space: a consideration with bulky items that take up a lot of space (e.g., patient bibs)
- Availability of proper storage conditions: a concern with items that are particularly sensitive to heat and light (e.g., radiograph film)
- Best quantity purchase rate
- Investment involved (e.g., the purchase of a large quantity of a supply may tie up too much of the practice's cash flow to make it a "good buy")

Guidelines for Ordering Dental Supplies

Supplies may be ordered (1) through a dental supply sales representative, (2) from a catalog by telephone, fax, mail order, or bar code scanning, and (3) online (by Internet). When you are ordering and managing dental supplies in the office, it is important to keep all items in one central storage place. This eliminates the need to look through several places in the office to locate a needed product. It also makes treatment room restocking and tray setups more efficient. Many offices make use of alphabetically labeled and arranged plastic storage bins to keep supplies neat and organized. The dentist should specify his or her preference as to the purchase source, quantity, and brand information.

Journals and catalogs should be reviewed for ideas that can be adapted to the needs of the practice. The assistant should check regularly with the sales representative and make a point to review the exhibits at dental meetings for new products and ideas.

Backorders

When an item is not available for delivery with the rest of an order, it is placed on *backorder* and will be delivered as soon as it becomes available. A backorder notice is usually sent to the dentist to advise him or her of this situation. If sufficient lead time has been allowed, a backorder does not create a major problem. However, if the item is in critically short supply, it may be necessary to purchase it elsewhere. In this case, to avoid duplication, the backorder must be canceled.

Order Exchange, Return, or Replacement

Sometimes it is necessary to exchange, return, or replace a product ordered. This may occur as a result of a variety of factors, including the following:

- The wrong item was ordered.
- The right item was ordered, but the wrong item was shipped.
- The size, color, or quantity was wrong.
- The product was broken or damaged in shipment.

When it is necessary to correct the supply order, the office manager must contact the supplier regarding the order and the reason for the exchange, replacement, or request for a credit on account. Until the supplier has made good on the request, a record should be maintained to trace and, if necessary, follow up on the transaction.

Requisitions and Purchase Orders

In a large group practice, institution, or clinic with a central supply source, dental supplies are obtained by **requisition.** The requisition form usually is completed in duplicate. One copy is submitted to procure the supplies, and the person requesting the supplies retains the other copy. In institutions with central purchasing, a requisition may be submitted to the purchasing agent, who in turn issues a **purchase order**. These forms are numbered, and when an order is placed, the supplier may refer to the purchase order number.

Dental Supply Budget

Institutions and well-organized practices operate on a budget. The budget request for dental supplies is based on how much money was spent in the previous year and an estimate of the increased rate of use, plus consideration for inflation.

When Ordering Supplies

- *Be prepared.* Have a *want list* ready and check with the dentist before the sales representative is due to call.
- *Be specific.* Know what you need and how much is needed. Be sure to supply all the necessary information, including the correct catalog or item number, descriptive information, and the quantity desired.
- *Be alert.* Be on the lookout for "specials" and authentic savings (a special on something that is not needed or not used is no bargain). The assistant should plan ahead to take advantage of seasonal savings and convention specials.
- *Be informed.* Just as the dentist will want to keep abreast of new product information, the assistant should be alert for new products and ideas that can make business office responsibilities easier to manage.

Consumables and Disposables

Consumable supplies are those that are literally "used up" as part of their function, such as restorative and impression materials. Disposables are items that are used once and then discarded, such as a disposable local anesthetic agents, needle, a saliva ejector, and cotton rolls.

Expendables

Expendable items are materials of relatively low cost that are used up in a short time. Minor dental instruments, such as mouth mirrors and burs, are examples of expendable items. For budget purposes, expendable items may be classified as those items that cost less than a certain amount, such as $50, and are ordered regularly. In some institutions, consumable, disposable, and expendable items are classified together under the single heading of "Expendables."

Nonexpendables

Nonexpendable items are smaller pieces of equipment or instruments that will eventually be replaced as the items wear out or are broken, such as a calculator or a curing light.

Major Equipment

This category includes larger pieces of equipment that are costly to purchase and will depreciate over a 5- to 10-year period. In the treatment area, this includes items such as dental chairs, radiograph units, and the air compressor. In the business office, this might include the computer and printer.

Recall

14. What two factors must be determined when a product needs to be reordered?
15. How is an item marked for reorder?
16. Identify three ways that supplies can be ordered.
17. If an item you ordered is not currently available from a supply company, the item is placed on _____.
18. Is a handpiece considered an expendable item? Why or why not?

EQUIPMENT REPAIRS

The breakdown of dental equipment can result in major expense, loss of income, and inconvenience for the dental staff and the patients. The best way to control this situation is through a sound preventive maintenance program.

Equipment Records

When a new piece of equipment is purchased, the following information regarding that equipment should be entered on a service record:

- Date of purchase
- Name of supplier
- Expiration date of manufacturer's warranty
- Model and serial numbers

A **warranty** is a written statement explaining the manufacturer's responsibility for replacement and/or repair of a piece of equipment over a limited time. A warranty card, which registers this warranty with the manufacturer, is usually enclosed with the instruction manual. This should be completed and mailed promptly. Instructions for the use, care, and cleaning of the equipment should be filed systematically so that they are available for ready reference. The people responsible for the preventive maintenance of a piece of equipment should read the instructions and care manual thoroughly and add this item to the preventive maintenance schedule.

Service Contracts

Some dental equipment is protected by a service contract. Under the terms of this contract, emergency repairs and possibly some routine maintenance are provided on a fixed-fee basis. An example would be a service contract for a computer system that guarantees emergency service within a specified period.

Service Call

The expense of service calls is high because the cost is based on mileage, time, expertise of the technician, and the materials and parts involved. Naturally, service calls should be avoided if possible. If a piece of equipment does not work, check the following points *before* calling for repair service:

- Is the equipment properly plugged in and turned on?
- Is there a *reset* button that must be pushed?
- Did you check the equipment for a blown fuse?
- Did someone check the fuse box or circuit breaker to ensure that the electrical circuit is functioning properly?

If you must still call for service after checking these points, be prepared to give complete information so that the service technician may make best use of his or her time and to help avoid the need for a second trip. The necessary information includes the following:

- The brand name of the piece of equipment
- The model number and approximate age or year of installation
- A brief description of the problem

Legal and Ethical Implications

When discussing dental information or financial information about a patient, it is important to understand the ownership of the documents. Patient records and financial statements belong to the dentist; the information that is placed in these documents belongs to the patient. Always make certain that every paper placed in a file has the date, name of the patient, and name of the person who entered the information.

Eye to the Future

More and more, the business aspects of dentistry and the smooth day-to-day operation of a dental practice are accomplished by computer. In the future, these functions will become completely computerized. Because of these challenges, the role of the business assistant will require new levels of skill and knowledge. It has always been advantageous for the business assistant to first be a dental assistant or dental hygienist. Having this background allows the business assistant to be knowledgeable when answering questions about patients' dental needs. However, in the future, the business assistant will also be required to have a background in technology to operate new equipment.

Critical Thinking

1. Describe how color-coding can speed up the filing and retrieval of patient records.
2. When preparing the daily schedule for the treatment areas, what two items will you include in addition to the patient's name?
3. Describe three common reasons why patients fail to keep appointments, and discuss how the business assistant should deal with each of these situations.
4. Discuss the importance of buffer time. Where in the daily schedule is this time best suited?
5. Discuss why the number of patients seen in a dental practice may determine the type of filing method used.

63

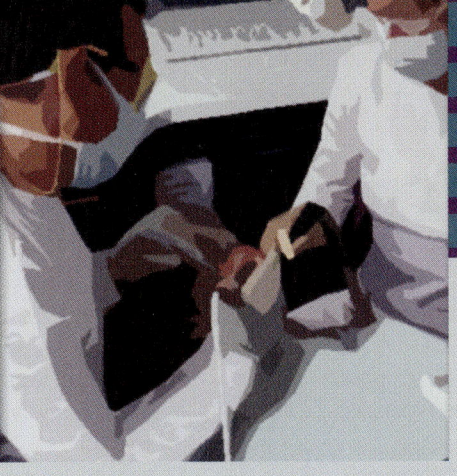

Financial Management in the Dental Office

Outline

KEY TERMS

Accounting A system designed to maintain financial records of a business.

Accounts payable Expenses and disbursements paid out from a business.

Audit trail Method of tracking the accuracy and completeness of bookkeeping records.

Bonding Form of insurance that reimburses an employer for a loss resulting from theft by an employee.

Bookkeeping The process of managing financial accounts of a business.

Carrier The insurance company that pays the claims and collects premiums.

Change fund Fixed amount of cash.

Check A draft or an order drawn on a bank account for payment in a specific amount of money.

Check register Record of all checks issued on and deposits made to a specific account.

Coordination of benefits (COB) Coordinating insurance coverage between two insurance carriers.

Current Dental Terminology (CDT) Publication that lists the procedure codes assigned to dental services for the process of dental insurance.

continued

KEY TERMS, cont'd

Customary fee A fee that is within the range of the usual fee charged for the service.

Deposit slip An itemized memorandum of the funds to be deposited into the bank.

Disbursements Payments on any outstanding accounts payable.

Expenses The overhead costs of a business to keep operating.

Fixed overhead Business expenses that are ongoing.

Gross income The total of all professional income received.

Invoice An itemized list of goods specifying the prices and terms of sale.

Ledger A financial statement that maintains all account transactions.

Net income Gross income minus expenses.

Packing slip An itemized listing of shipped goods.

Payee The person (or business) named on the check as the recipient of the amount shown.

Pegboard system A manual bookkeeping system.

Petty cash A limited amount of cash that is kept on hand for small daily expenses.

Posted Describes the documentation of money transactions within a business.

Provider The dentist that provides the treatment to the patient.

Reasonable fee A fee that is considered justified for an extensive or complex treatment.

Responsible party Person who has agreed to pay for services or for an account.

Statement A summary of all charges, payments, credits, and debits for the month.

Transaction Any charge, payment, or adjustment made to a financial account.

Usual fee A fee that the dentist charges for a specific service.

Variable overhead Business expenses that change depending on the type of services needed.

Walk-out statement A written indication of any balance due on an account, given to a patient as he or she leaves the practice at the end of an appointment.

LEARNING OUTCOMES

On completion of this chapter, the student will be able to achieve the following objectives:

- Pronounce, define, and spell the Key Terms.
- Describe the function of computerized practice management systems and manual bookkeeping systems.
- Demonstrate making financial arrangements with a patient.
- Describe the importance and management of collections in the dental office.
- Describe check writing.
- Explain the purpose of business summaries.
- Identify common payroll withholding taxes and discuss the financial responsibility of the employer.
- Discuss the purpose of dental insurance.
- Identify insurance fraud.
- Identify the parties involved with dental insurance.
- Identify the types of prepaid dental programs.
- Define managed care.
- Discuss and define basic dental terminology.
- Explain dual coverage.
- Identify dental procedures and coding.
- Detail claim forms processing.
- Describe the procedure and purpose of claim forms follow-up.

The business records of a dental practice are the foundation to managing finances of a dental office. The business assistant has the responsibility of maintaining complete, accurate, and up-to-date financial records for the following:

- Billing and collection procedures
- Financial planning
- Declaring money earned to federal and state agencies

ACCOUNTING

Accounting is the means or process of recording, classifying, and summarizing financial transactions. **Bookkeeping** is the recording of the accounting process. The business assistant conducts bookkeeping procedures daily to maintain dental practice accounts. The two types of bookkeeping systems used in a dental practice are the accounts receivable and the accounts payable systems.

PREVENTIVE ACCOUNT MANAGEMENT

Preventive account management begins with clearly defined financial policies established by the dentist. Once these guidelines have been determined, it is the responsibility of the business assistant to follow through with them. Basic practice financial policies should cover gathering financial information, presenting the fee, making financial arrangements with the patients, and collecting overdue accounts.

Gathering Financial Information

When the patient calls for an appointment, ask whether he or she has dental insurance. If so, request that the identification card and benefits booklet be brought to the first visit. These should be reviewed to determine eligibility and available benefits. At the patient's first visit, ask him or her to complete a registration form. This form gathers all the basic financial information needed to manage the account history and complete the patient identification portion of an insurance claim form (Fig. 63-1).

This information includes the following:

- The name, address, telephone number(s), and place of employment of the person responsible for the account
- Information concerning the patient's coverage under a dental insurance plan
- Identification information for all individuals included in the account

Credit Reports

In some practices, a credit report of the responsible party may be requested. If it is the dentist's policy, the responsible party should be informed before the credit report is requested. Consumer credit reporting agencies, commonly referred to as *credit bureaus* or *agencies,* provide a financial profile of the patient. The report covers the record of his or her paying habits and accounts placed for collection, plus other pertinent information such as lawsuits, judgments, and bankruptcies.

Fee Presentation

Before a case presentation, an estimate must be developed of the basis of the treatment plan to be presented. According to planned treatment information provided by the dentist, this responsibility is usually assigned to the business assistant. This estimate is prepared in duplicate: one copy is given to the patient, and the other is retained with the office records.

The fee charged represents a fair return to the dentist for professional treatment provided. After the dentist has completed the case presentation to the patient, the business assistant may be asked to handle the discussion of the fees involved. At this time, the business assistant presents the necessary fee information and makes financial arrangements with the patient to the satisfaction of both the dentist and the patient.

Making Financial Arrangements

Financial arrangements must be made with each patient for whom professional services are performed. These arrangements should be made before treatment is initiated, except in such instances as emergency treatment. Realistic financial arrangements should be made with the person responsible for the account in an unhurried manner. These arrangements are confidential and should be made in a private setting where others cannot overhear the discussion.

When making financial arrangements, it is necessary to take into consideration the dentist's stated payment plans

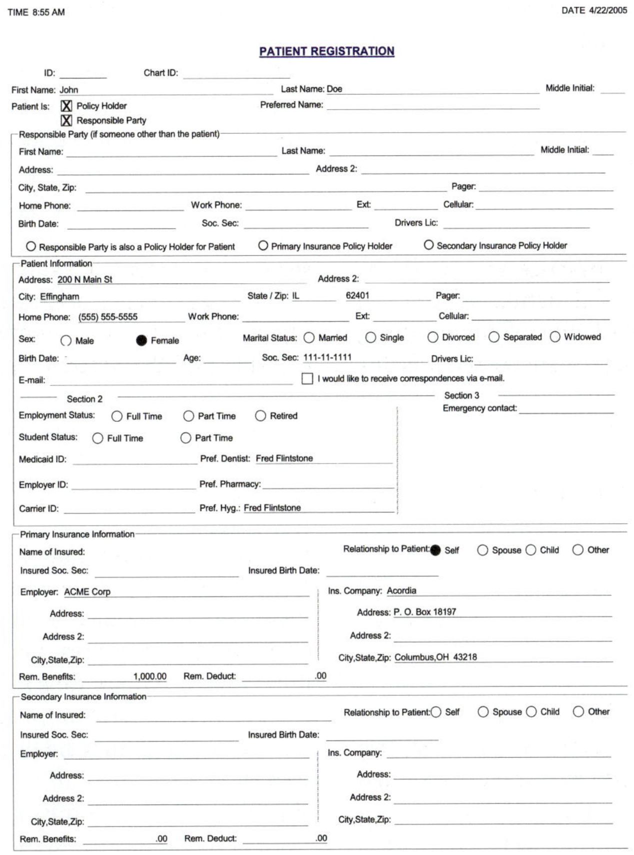
TIME 8:55 AM
DATE 4/22/2005
PATIENT REGISTRATION
ID: Chart ID:
First Name: John Last Name: Doe Middle Initial:
Patient Is: [X] Policy Holder Preferred Name:
[X] Responsible Party
Responsible Party (if someone other than the patient)
First Name: Last Name: Middle Initial:
Address: Address 2:
City, State, Zip: Pager:
Home Phone: Work Phone: Ext: Cellular:
Birth Date: Soc. Sec: Drivers Lic:
○ Responsible Party is also a Policy Holder for Patient ○ Primary Insurance Policy Holder ○ Secondary Insurance Policy Holder
Patient Information
Address: 200 N Main St Address 2:
City: Effingham State / Zip: IL 62401 Pager:
Home Phone: (555) 555-5555 Work Phone: Ext: Cellular:
Sex: ○ Male ● Female Marital Status: ○ Married ○ Single ○ Divorced ○ Separated ○ Widowed
Birth Date: Age: Soc. Sec: 111-11-1111 Drivers Lic:
E-mail: ☐ I would like to receive correspondences via e-mail.
Section 2
Employment Status: ○ Full Time ○ Part Time ○ Retired
Student Status: ○ Full Time ○ Part Time
Medicaid ID: Pref. Dentist: Fred Flintstone
Employer ID: Pref. Pharmacy:
Carrier ID: Pref. Hyg.: Fred Flintstone
Section 3
Emergency contact:
Primary Insurance Information
Name of Insured: Relationship to Patient: ● Self ○ Spouse ○ Child ○ Other
Insured Soc. Sec: Insured Birth Date:
Employer: ACME Corp Ins. Company: Acordia
Address: Address: P. O. Box 18197
Address 2: Address 2:
City,State,Zip: City,State,Zip: Columbus,OH 43218
Rem. Benefits: 1,000.00 Rem. Deduct: .00
Secondary Insurance Information
Name of Insured: Relationship to Patient: ○ Self ○ Spouse ○ Child ○ Other
Insured Soc. Sec: Insured Birth Date:
Employer: Ins. Company:
Address: Address:
Address 2: Address 2:
City,State,Zip: City,State,Zip:
Rem. Benefits: .00 Rem. Deduct: .00

Fig. 63-1 Computerized registration form. (Courtesy Colwell, a division of Patterson Companies, Inc.)

and the sound business principles used in the management of the practice. However, it is also necessary to consider the patient's ability to pay. The resulting arrangements should be equitable to both parties. The patient must realize that once these arrangements have been made, he or she is responsible for following through as agreed. All financial agreements should be recorded on the account **ledger.**

The dentist may request that the patient sign a contract for the agreed-on amount. If a contract is signed, a copy is given to the patient, and the original is retained with the office records.

Recall

1. What two types of bookkeeping systems are used in dental practices?
2. What form in the patient record is used to gather financial information from a patient?
3. Where should the business assistant discuss financial arrangements with a patient?

ACCOUNTS RECEIVABLE

The accounts receivable system manages all money owed to the practice. Accounts receivable management, which is frequently referred to as *bookkeeping,* involves maintaining financial records regarding all **transactions** related to collecting fees for professional services provided to the patient. This information must be arranged systematically so that it is accurate at all times and provides data needed to effectively manage these financial matters. Accounts receivable activities are not difficult; however, in carrying out these activities, the business assistant assumes the responsibility of handling other people's money. In this way, he or she is responsible for making every effort to keep this money safe, to record it accurately, and to respect the confidence in which all of this information must be held.

The dentist may obtain **bonding** insurance on staff members who handle practice funds, such as receiving and banking patient payments or writing checks. Although this insurance will cover a loss, the employee can be prosecuted under the law for any such theft.

Types of Accounts Receivable Systems

The most frequently used type of accounts receivable bookkeeping system in dental practices is a computerized system or a manual **pegboard system.** Increasingly, offices are switching to computer practice management systems because they are capable of integrating technologies with bookkeeping capabilities.

Pegboard Accounts Receivable Management

Pegboard accounting, also known as a *one-write system,* is a manual bookkeeping system in which all records are completed with a single entry. By positioning the daily journal page, ledger card, and a carbonized receipt, all financial records for each patient visit are completed by writing the information just one time (Fig. 63-2). Entries for additional records, such as the daily totals and monthly summaries, must be completed manually. The totals must then be calculated and verified for accuracy.

Computerized Accounts Receivable Management

With a computerized accounts receivable system, data entered into the system are used to maintain account histories and practice records (Fig. 63-3). It is essential that the information be entered into the system accurately because it is used to generate account totals and daily and monthly summaries. These and other management reports are automatically calculated and produced by the system. It also is important that the data stored in the hard drive of the computer be protected by being backed up (copied for safekeeping) at least once daily. An additional set of backup files (disks or CDs) should be stored in a safe place outside of the office. These backup records are vital in the event of theft, fire, or other disaster that makes it necessary to reconstruct information that has been lost from the system.

Accounts Receivable Management Basics

Whether you are using a manual or computerized system, the same information requirements and organizational format are necessary. Learning to use either system begins with understanding the basics of accounts receivable bookkeeping. The accounting process begins when the patient leaves the treatment area.

Charge Slips

Charge slips are used to transmit financial information between the treatment area and the business office. This form usually shows the current account balance; if there is an overdue or very large balance, the dentist or office manager may choose to discuss this with the patient. The charge slip has space for the dentist or assistant to note the treatment provided at each patient visit (Fig. 63-4). The completed charge slip is returned to the business office, and the information is **posted** to the accounts receivable system. With a computerized system, the alternative is to enter the data directly from a terminal in the treatment area.

Charge slips are numbered as part of the **audit trail.** A charge slip should be generated for each patient. At the end of the day, a number must account for each charge slip. This way, the dentist knows that all patient visits have been entered into the system.

DAILY LOG OF CHARGES AND RECEIPTS

DATE 1/31/99 SHEET NUMBER ________

	DATE	FAMILY MEMBER	PROFESSIONAL SERVICES	CHARGE (A)	CREDITS PYMTS. (B1)	CREDITS ADJ. (B2)	NEW BALANCE (C)	PREVIOUS BALANCE (D)	NAME
1	1/31	Rose	ins. pmt./adj.		98 00	12 00	80 00	190 00	Rose Budd
2	1/31	Frank	NSF	80 00	—	—	80 00	⊖	Frank Williams
3	1/31	Jodi	payment	—	62 00	—	<22 00>	40 00	Jodi Coulson
4	1/31	Dawn	Restorative	230 00	⊖	—	240 00	10 00	Dawn Johnson
5	1/31	Maria	prophy/c.pmt.	62 00	62 00	—	⊖	⊖	Marie Gonzales
6	1/31	Angela	FMX		62 00	—	80 00	62 00	Angela Brown
7	1/31	Mark	Composite	246 00	—	24 00	221 40	⊖	Mark Vail
8	1/31	Lois	ins. pmt.	—	630 00	20 00	171 00	821 00	Lois Tract
9									
10									
11									
12									
13									
14									
15									
16									
17									
18									
19									
20									
21									
22									
23									
24									
25									
26									
27									
28									
29									
30									
31									
32									

TOTALS	Col. "A"	Col. "B-1"	Col. "B-2"	Col. "C"	Col. "D"
THIS PAGE	698 00	914 00	56 60	850 40	1123 00
PREVIOUS PAGE	3240 00	2163 00	<21 10>	5419 10	4321 00
MONTH-TO-DATE	3938 00	3077 00	35 50	6269 50	5444 00

PROOF OF POSTING	
COL. D TOTAL	$ 1123.00
PLUS COL. A TOTAL	$ 698.00
SUB TOTAL	$ 1821.00
LESS COLS. B-1 & B-2	$ 970.60
MUST EQUAL COL. C	$ 850.40

ACCOUNTS RECEIVABLE CONTROL	
PREVIOUS DAY'S TOTAL	$ 1098.10
PLUS COL. A	$ 698.00
SUB TOTAL	$ 1796.10
LESS COLS. B-1 & B-2	$ 970.60
TOTAL ACCTS. REC.	$ 825.50

ACCOUNTS RECEIVABLE PROOF	
ACCTS. REC. 1ST OF MONTH	$ Ø
PLUS COL. A.-MO. TO DATE	$ 3938.00
SUB TOTAL	$ 3938.00
LESS B-1 & B-2 MO. TO DATE	$ 3112.50
TOTAL ACCTS. REC.	$ 825.50

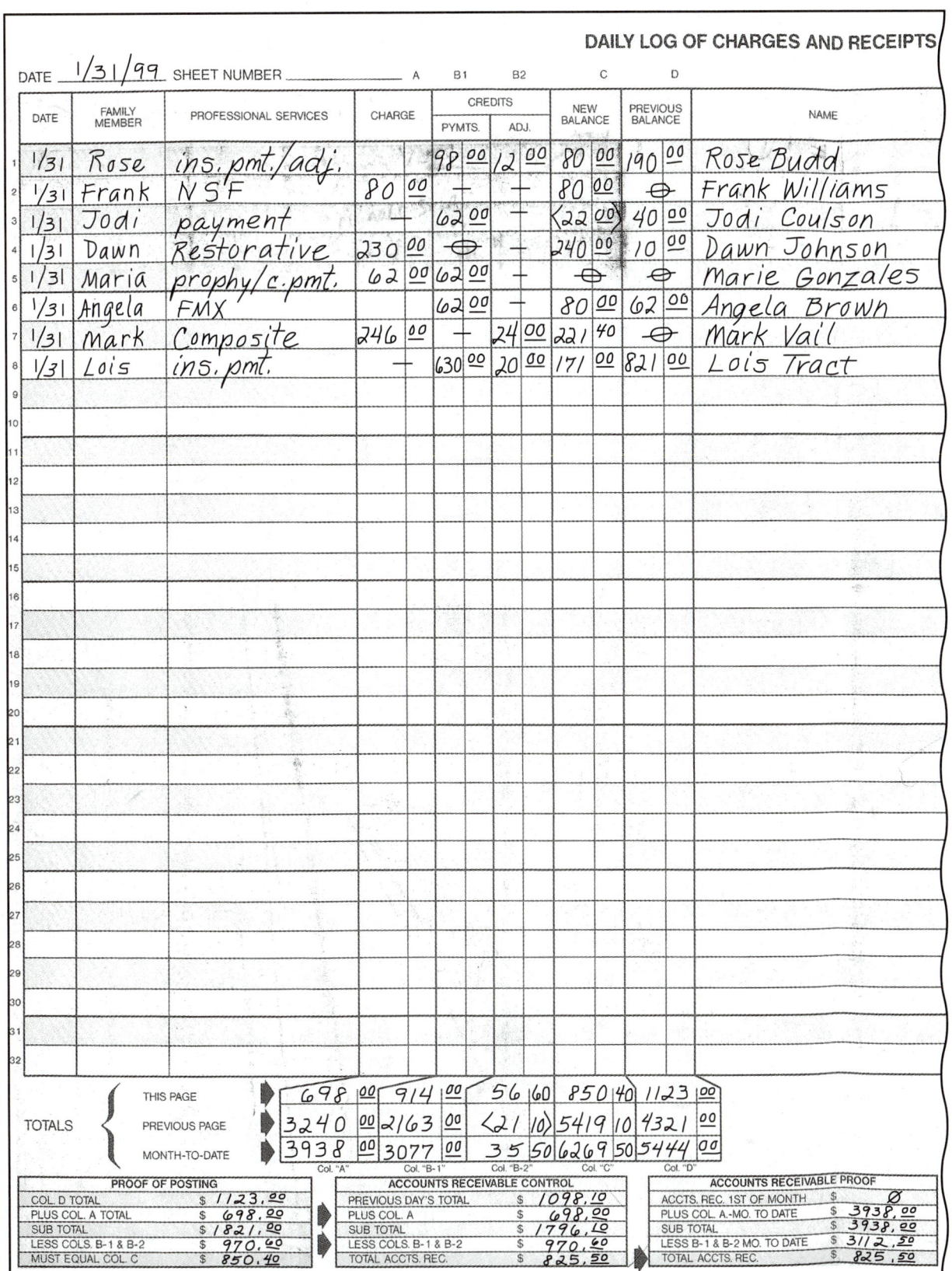

Fig. 63-2 Manual pegboard system. (From Gaylor LH: *The administrative dental assistant,* Philadelphia, 2000, Saunders.)

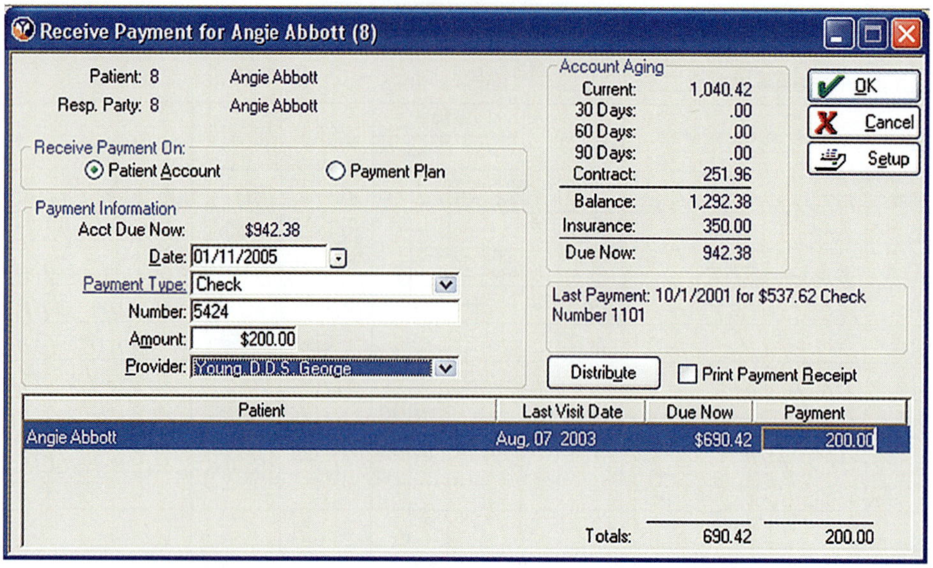

Fig. 63-3 Computerized accounts receivable management system. (Courtesy Eaglesoft, a division of Patterson Companies, Inc.)

Daily Journal Page

The daily journal page is the practice record of all transactions for the patients seen each day; this includes the name of each patient seen and any charges, payments, and adjustments to that account. Throughout the day, all transactions are posted to the bookkeeping system. In addition to maintaining the patient account record, this posting generates the daily journal page entry. A computerized system automatically totals this form and uses the information to generate the other practice reports.

Receipts and Walk-Out Statements

The charge slip is usually printed in duplicate. One copy is used to enter charges and payments into the bookkeeping system. It then is saved as part of the practice records. The other copy is completed and serves as a receipt, a **walk-out statement,** or both for the departing patient. A **walk-out statement** is similar to a receipt except that it shows the current account balance. It is given to the patients who do not make payment in full. A walk-out statement is provided with a postage-paid reply envelope, and the patient is requested to mail the outstanding payment as soon as possible. The use of walk-out statements improves cash flow because it speeds payments. It also reduces the number of statements that must be prepared and mailed at the end of the month.

Recording Payments

All payments must be entered promptly into the bookkeeping system so that they are recorded in the account history and on the daily journal page. Payments received by mail are entered in the same manner as those made in person. As a safeguard, checks should be stamped immediately with a *restrictive endorsement,* which prevents anyone from cashing a check if it is stolen.

Patient Account Records

Patient account records are organized based on information regarding the responsible party. The **responsible party,** also known as the *guarantor,* is the person who has agreed to be responsible for payment of the account. This is not always the patient. The patient account record is used to track all account transactions. A current account balance is maintained at all times, and this information is used to generate statements, insurance claims, and other collection efforts. In a manual system, the patient account records are maintained on account ledger cards. In a computerized system, they are organized as account histories or ledgers.

Payment

There are several ways in which patients' accounts can be handled; these include payment at the time of treatment, payment by monthly statements, and divided payments. Dental insurance may be considered another method of payment, although it must be emphasized that the patient is responsible for the balance not covered by the insurer. To help alleviate concern for the patient, a pretreatment estimate form can be submitted to the insurance carrier. This would provide information on what the insurance company covers and any additional patient payment or copayments.

Payment at the Time of Treatment

Under this payment policy, patients are asked to make payment in full for treatment provided at each visit. This

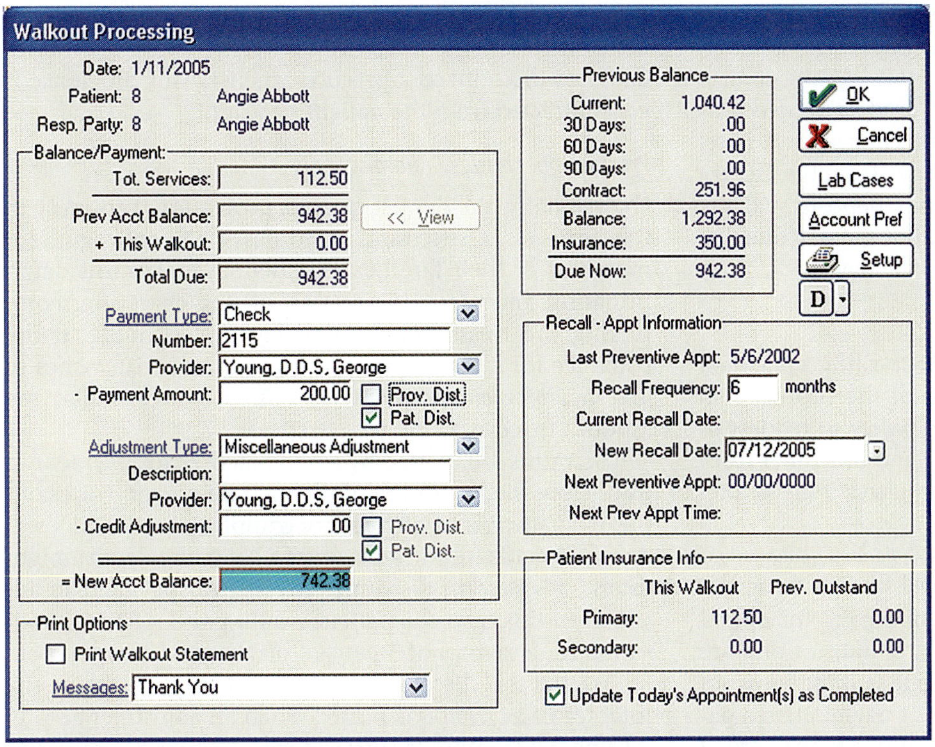

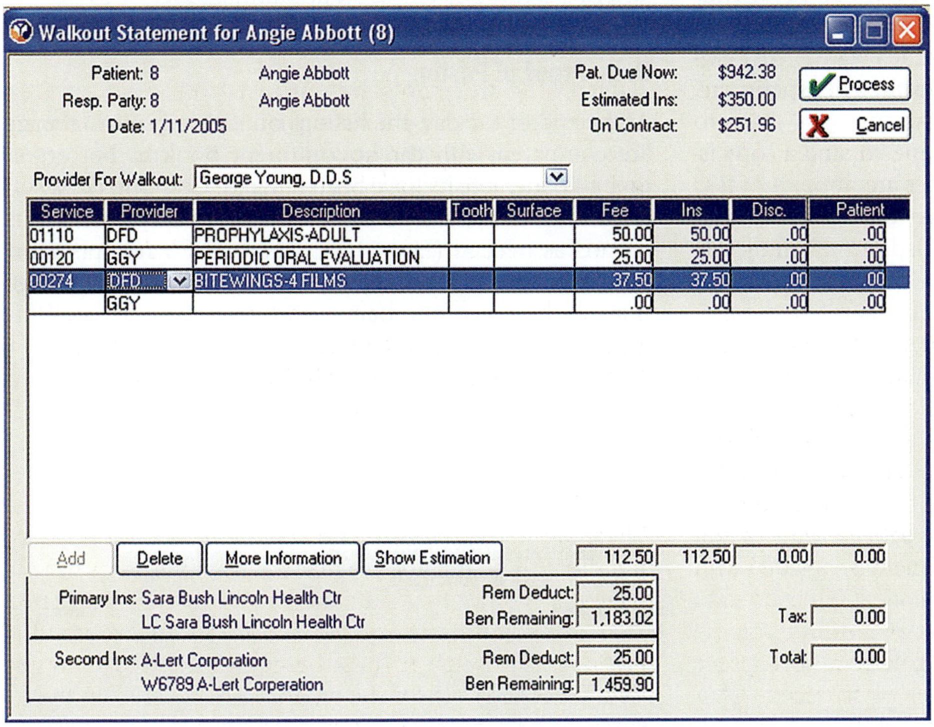

Fig. 63-4 **A charge slip is given to the patient to take to the front desk. A printout of this provides a walk-out statement for the patient.** (Courtesy Eaglesoft, a division of Patterson Companies, Inc.)

system helps control practice costs by improving cash flow and reducing the cost of sending statements or other collection methods. Patients must be notified of this payment plan before the first visit. In many practices, this is done during the initial telephone conversation. Under this plan, cash, checks, and credit cards are usually all accepted for payment.

Cash

Although few patients pay for dental treatment in cash, it is necessary to be alert to the needs of cash-paying patients. When accepting payment in cash for services, it is essential to ensure that the correct change is available and that it is counted out to the patient. The patient paying cash must be given a written (or computer-generated) receipt.

A **change fund** is a fixed amount of cash (usually $50 or less) that is maintained in small bills to have money available when a patient pays cash. Each morning, the change fund is placed in the cash drawer and used as needed during the day. At the end of the day, the change fund is removed and placed in safekeeping. Money from the change fund does *not* become part of the daily deposit, and the amount in the change fund at the end of the day must be the same as it was at the beginning of the day.

Check

Many patients pay for dental services by writing a personal check to the dentist or to the name of the professional practice. In some practices, it is office policy to request to see the payer's driver's license number and one other form of identification. The patient paying by check is given a receipt on request.

Credit cards

The patient may choose the option of paying for dental services with a credit card. Credit card transactions are listed as payments, but the posting code is different from that for cash or a check. Before accepting payment on a patient's credit card, it is necessary to verify that the card is valid and that the credit limit has not been exceeded. This can be done electronically or verbally with the participating bank card company. When a dentist agrees to be a bankcard merchant, the participating bank will explain the procedure of verification and submittal.

The credit card charge form is completed, and a copy is given to the patient. Credit card charges are not part of the regular bank deposit. Instead, they are managed in accordance with the instructions from the institution issuing the credit card. The bank charges a percentage rate as a service fee for handling these transactions. This is referred to as *discounting* because at the end of the month, the service charge is deducted, or discounted, from these funds. An adjustment entry is made in the checkbook to accommodate this discount as a practice expense. This difference is *not* subtracted from the patient's account.

Professional courtesy and discounts

Occasionally, the dentist extends professional courtesy in the form of a discount to professional colleagues or members of their families. The dentist makes this determination and places a notation on the chart after completing the treatment for the day. For example, if the usual fee for a procedure is $50 and the dentist wishes to give a *professional courtesy* of $10, this means that the amount owed is $40.

Discounts are offered by some practices for payment in full before the beginning of planned treatment. For example, if a patient is having a set of complete upper and lower dentures made for the amount of $1250, the dentist might extend a 5 percent discount ($62.50) for payment in advance. In this case, the patient would pay $1187.50 in advance, for a savings of 5 percent off the total charge.

To enter this discount into the bookkeeping system, the total fee of $1250.00 is posted. Then an adjustment representing the discount is entered for $62.50. This adjustment acts as a credit and leaves an account balance of $1187.50.

Daily Proof of Posting

At the end of the day, the listings on the daily journal page are compared with the appointment book to be certain that all patient visits have been entered. Computerized systems total all figures automatically and can print various reports as needed (Fig. 63-5). The total for receipts must match the amount in the cash drawer minus the change fund. If these two numbers do not match, or "balance," it is necessary to go back and find the mistake.

TIME 9:26 AM — George Young, D.D.S. — DATE 1/11/2005

DEPOSIT REPORT WITH ITEMIZED CASH

Bank Account: 123456

	Date	Payment		Amount
Cash Deposits				
Deanna Bond	1/11/2005	Cash		$50.00
			Total Cash:	$50.00
Check Deposits				
Angie Abbott	1/11/2005	Number 5424		$200.00
Charles Abbott	1/11/2005	Number 3422		$350.00
Julie Bennett	1/11/2005	Number 1245		$13.60
Harvey Abraham	1/11/2005	Number 3628		$85.00
			Total Check:	$648.60
			TOTAL DEPOSIT:	$698.60

Fig. 63-5 A daily proof of posting allows the business assistant to compare the total for receipts.

Bank Deposits

All receipts should be deposited every day. When the amount of receipts exactly matches the amount of the deposits, the account has met the auditor's critical test to verify bookkeeping accuracy. A **deposit slip** is an itemized memorandum of the currency and checks taken to the bank to be credited to the practice's account (Fig. 63-6). This slip is generated from the computer after all checks have been posted. After the deposit has been made, the date and amount of the deposit should be entered in the practice check register as follows:

- The deposit slip must be imprinted with the practice name, address, and account number.
- The information on the deposit slip must be legible.
- All cash (bills and coins) is listed together under "Currency."
- Checks are listed separately, usually by the last name and first initial of the person writing the check. Computer systems do this automatically when posted.
- In many practices, the deposit slip is completed in duplicate so that a copy can be retained with the practice records.

Monthly Statement

The monthly statement represents a request for payment of the balance due on the account receivable. Under this plan, the patient is expected to pay the balance in full on receipt of the statement. With a manual system, this statement frequently is a photocopy of the ledger card showing the information about charges for treatment provided, payments, and account adjustments. A computer-generated statement shows these data, plus an age analysis of the account balance. Financial arrangements also can be printed on a computer-generated statement. Some practices add a finance charge (usually 1 percent) to accounts that are not paid within 30 days of receipt of the first statement.

When such a charge is made or there are more than four payment installments, the patient must be notified of this policy in advance with a *Truth in Lending* form.

Cycle Billing

Statements should be routinely mailed at the same time each month. If the task is too large to be handled at one time, the practice may use cycle billing. In cycle billing, the alphabet is divided into parts, and statements for patients with last names in each part of the alphabet are mailed at specified times during the month.

Divided Payment Plans

Divided payment plans are arrangements by which the patient pays a fixed amount on a regular basis. For example, orthodontic treatment is usually paid for on a divided payment plan. These arrangements are made at the time of the case presentation. After the patient has accepted the proposed treatment plan, the business assistant may be asked to work with the patient to develop a divided payment plan. When a divided payment plan is set up, the primary information to be determined is as follows:

- Total fee for services to be rendered
- Balance after deduction of the down payment; the resulting amount is to be financed
- Annual percentage rate of the finance charge (if there is one)
- Number of payments to be made
- Amount of each payment
- Date on which each payment is due

Once this information has been determined, the payment plan agreement is completed, and both the patient

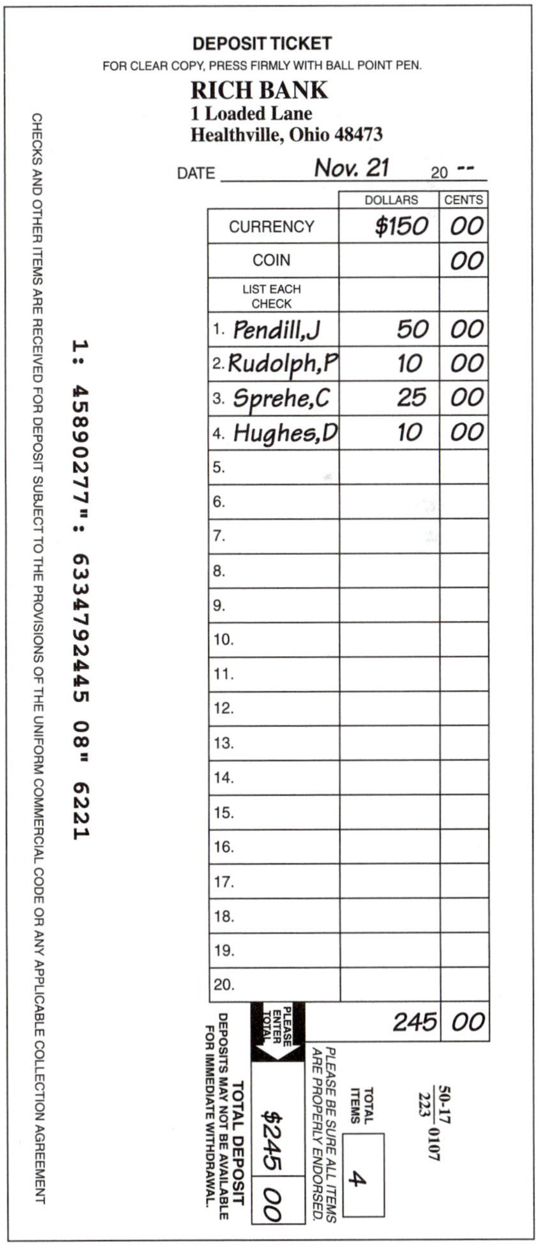
DEPOSIT TICKET
FOR CLEAR COPY, PRESS FIRMLY WITH BALL POINT PEN.
RICH BANK
1 Loaded Lane
Healthville, Ohio 48473
DATE Nov. 21 20 --

	DOLLARS	CENTS
CURRENCY	$150	00
COIN		00
LIST EACH CHECK		
1. Pendill,J	50	00
2. Rudolph,P	10	00
3. Sprehe,C	25	00
4. Hughes,D	10	00
5.		
6.		
7.		
8.		
9.		
10.		
11.		
12.		
13.		
14.		
15.		
16.		
17.		
18.		
19.		
20.		
	245	00

50-17 / 223 0107
TOTAL ITEMS 4
PLEASE BE SURE ALL ITEMS ARE PROPERLY ENDORSED.
PLEASE ENTER TOTAL
$245 00
TOTAL DEPOSIT
DEPOSITS MAY NOT BE AVAILABLE FOR IMMEDIATE WITHDRAWAL.
1: 45890277": 6334792445 08" 6221
CHECKS AND OTHER ITEMS ARE RECEIVED FOR DEPOSIT SUBJECT TO THE PROVISIONS OF THE UNIFORM COMMERCIAL CODE OR ANY APPLICABLE COLLECTION AGREEMENT

Fig. 63-6 Deposit slip.

and the dentist sign it. A copy is given to the patient, and the original is kept in the dental office.

Recall

4. Is money that is owed to the practice considered part of accounts payable?
5. If a dental office does not have a computerized accounts receivable system, what type of system would be used?
6. What form is used to transmit a patient's fee from the treatment area to the business office?
7. What methods of payment can a patient use to pay on an account?
8. How often should bank deposits be made?

COLLECTIONS

It is essential that amounts owed to the practice be collected in a timely and organized manner.

Accounts Receivable Report

The accounts receivable report is a valuable management report that shows the total balance due on each account plus an analysis of the "age of the account." This shows how much of the balance is current (recent charges not yet billed), 30 days old, 31 to 60 days old, 61 to 90 days, and older. This information is helpful in tracking and taking action on overdue accounts.

A computer can automatically generate this report with a breakdown of the account age (Fig. 63-7). Although creation of the report is not automatic with a pegboard system, it is possible to generate one manually.

Management of Collection Efforts

All collection efforts must be handled tactfully and in keeping with the dentist's wishes and policies, because the dentist is ultimately responsible for the actions of his or her employees. The dentist does not want to lose a patient's good will because of poor collection tactics. Under

Collection Follow-Through

Below is a collection follow-through timetable that is used in many practices:

30 days: The regular statement, sent at the end of the month, within 30 days, or on completion of treatment with financial arrangements printed on the statement.

60 days: A second statement, with a kindly printed collection message or a telephone call.

75 days: Another telephone call and an amiable collection letter.

90 days: A third statement with a stronger note or a collection letter; often, this letter states that unless payment is made within 10 days, the account will be turned over to a collection agency for action.

105 days: Another telephone call; in this call, the message should be "Unless the account is paid by the specified date, it will be necessary to turn the account over to a collection agency for action."

120 days: If no payment has been made and promises have not been kept, the account is turned over to a collection agency for action.

TIME 9:35 AM | George Young, D.D.S. | DATE 1/11/2005

ACCOUNTS RECEIVABLE BY RESPONSIBLE PARTY

Responsible Party		Current	30 Days	60 Days	90 Days	Contract	Total A/R	- Est. Ins.	= Due Now
8	Abbott, Angie	$840.42	$0.00	$0.00	$0.00	$251.96	$1,092.38	$350.00	$742.38
3446	Abbott, Charles	$1,972.52	$0.00	$0.00	$0.00	$0.00	$1,972.52	$585.70	$1,386.82
3431	Abbott, James	$2,169.13	$0.00	$0.00	$29.00	$0.00	$2,198.13	$844.00	$1,354.13
3434	Abernathy, Bryan	$198.00	$0.00	$0.00	$19.12	$0.00	$217.12	$0.00	$217.12
3021	Abrams, Debra	$0.00	$0.00	$0.00	$85.00	$0.00	$85.00	$0.00	$85.00
3675	Adams, Fester	$0.00	$0.00	$0.00	$109.50	$0.00	$109.50	$0.00	$109.50
9	Adams, Greg	$0.00	$0.00	$0.00	$53.60	$0.00	$53.60	$0.00	$53.60
2889	Ahuja, Kishore	$0.00	$0.00	$0.00	$68.60	$0.00	$68.60	$0.00	$68.60
1453	Albin, Conrad	$0.00	$0.00	$0.00	$443.00	$0.00	$443.00	$0.00	$443.00
1120	Alexander, Cathy	$0.00	$0.00	$0.00	$80.00	$0.00	$80.00	$0.00	$80.00
15	Allen, Avery	$0.00	$0.00	$0.00	$150.00	$0.00	$150.00	$0.00	$150.00
2539	Allen, Daniel	$100.80	$0.00	$0.00	$0.00	$0.00	$100.80	($0.00)	$100.80
2393	Allen, Rita	$0.00	$0.00	$0.00	$15.00	$0.00	$15.00	$0.00	$15.00
20	Allsop, Margie	$0.00	$0.00	$0.00	$59.00	$0.00	$59.00	$0.00	$59.00
23	Ambuehl, Jackie	$0.00	$0.00	$0.00	$78.60	$0.00	$78.60	$0.00	$78.60
25	Ambuehl, Nikki	$0.00	$0.00	$0.00	$80.12	$0.00	$80.12	$0.00	$80.12
26	Ames, Greg	$190.04	$0.00	$0.00	$0.00	$0.00	$190.04	$0.00	$190.04
30	Amsbary, Roxanne	$0.00	$0.00	$0.00	$12.60	$0.00	$12.60	$0.00	$12.60
31	Anderson, Daniel	$0.00	$0.00	$0.00	$14.50	$0.00	$14.50	$0.00	$14.50
3488	Ankney, Andrew	$0.00	$0.00	$0.00	$63.00	$0.00	$63.00	$0.00	$63.00
39	Ard, Tina	$0.00	$0.00	$0.00	$56.80	$0.00	$56.80	$0.00	$56.80

Fig. 63-7 Accounts receivable report. (Courtesy Eaglesoft, a division of Patterson Dental, Inc.)

the federal *Fair Debt Collection Practice Act,* it is illegal for anyone to do the following:

- Telephone the debtor at inconvenient hours (e.g., between 5:00 and 8:00 P.M. is considered an acceptable time)
- Threaten violence or use obscene language
- Use false pretenses to get information
- Contact the debtor's employer, except to verify employment or residence

Collection Letters

All collection letters should be phrased in firm, positive, businesslike terms that make every effort to persuade the patient to pay the debt, to help him or her pay it, and to allow the patient to avoid embarrassment while doing so (Box 63-1).

Collection Telephone Calls

Telephone calls are more effective than letters because they are a direct contact with the debtor and therefore are not as easily ignored. When placing a collection call, be certain to speak only to the person responsible for the account. Never leave a message that could be misunderstood, could reveal confidential information, or could be considered damaging!

Once the proper person has been reached, the business assistant should identify himself or herself and wait. The person being called knows what is wanted, and it is best to let that person make the first statement. The debtor may react with anger or hostility. It is important to remember that these are part of a defense mechanism and not a personal attack. Regardless of what the debtor says or does, do not become argumentative or defensive. Try to be understand-

Box 63-1 Suggestions for Composing Collection Letters

1. Your account has always been paid promptly in the past, so this must be an oversight. Please accept this note as a friendly reminder of your account due in the amount of $__________.
2. Since your care in this office in March, we have had no word from you in regard to how you are feeling or your account due. If it is impossible for you to pay the full amount of $__________ at this time, please call this office before June 15 so that satisfactory arrangements can be worked out.
3. Medical bills are payable at the time of service unless special credit arrangements are made. Please send your check in full or call this office before June 30.
4. If you have some question about your statement, we will be happy to answer it for you. If not, may we have a payment before the end of this month?
5. Unless some definite arrangement is made to reduce your balance of $__________, we can no longer carry your account on our books. Delinquent accounts are turned over to our collection agency on the 25th of the month.
6. **When a payment plan has been established, it can be reinforced by recognizing the first remittance with a letter of acknowledgment:**
   Thank you for the recent payment of $__________ on your account. We are glad to cooperate with you in this arrangement for clearing your account. We will look for your next check at about the same time next month, and your final payment the following month.
7. **When a payment schedule has been arranged by a telephone call, it can be confirmed by letter.**
   As agreed upon in our telephone conversation today, we will expect you to mail a payment of $50 on February 10; $50 on March 10; and the balance on April 10. If some emergency should prevent your making one of these payments on time, please notify us immediately by telephone.

DO'S AND DON'TS

DO:

1. Individualize letters to suit the situation.
2. Design your early letters as mere reminders of debt.
3. Always imply that the patient has good intentions to pay, until lack of response over a period of time proves otherwise.
4. Send letters with a firmer tone only after you have sent one or two friendly reminders.

DON'T

1. Use the same collection letter for a patient with good paying habits as for one who is known to neglect financial obligations.
2. Place an overdue notice of any kind on a postcard or on the outside of an envelope. This is an **invasion of privacy.**

From Young AP, Kennedy DB: *Kinn's The medical assistant: an applied learning approach,* ed 9, St. Louis, 2003, Saunders.

ing but firm and never permit yourself to be insulting, no matter what the provocation. Note any agreement made over the telephone on the patient's account ledger. Promises should be followed up carefully, and if they are not kept, the account should be taken to the next step in the collection process.

Final Collection Options

The final decision concerning turning accounts over for collection must be made by the dentist, and an account is never turned over without the dentist's specific approval.

Collection Agency

A collection agency makes additional efforts to collect the balance on an overdue account. The agency's charge is a percentage of the amount collected, and this is deducted before the balance is remitted to the dental office. Some attorneys also attempt to collect overdue accounts in exchange for a percentage of the amount collected.

Small Claims Court

Another option is to take the debtor to small claims court. Sometimes, arrangements are made so that the business assistant, not the dentist, appears for the hearing. One drawback to the option of seeking a small claims court judgment is that even if the court rules that the debtor must pay, it is still up to the practice to collect the amount of the judgment.

Recall

9. After how much time should an office begin collection efforts?

10. Give four ways that a business can follow through on the collection of fees.

ACCOUNTS PAYABLE MANAGEMENT

Accounts payable systems manage all of the money that is owed by the practice. Expenses and disbursements determine the cost of doing business in the dental practice. **Expenses** are called *overhead,* which is the actual cost of doing business. As these expenses are incurred, they become *accounts payable.* **Disbursements** are the payments of these accounts payable. It is the responsibility of the office manager or business assistant to ensure accuracy in all accounts payable transactions within the practice.

Dental Office Overhead

Dental office overhead consists of all expenses incurred in running of the dental practice; these expenses are categorized as *fixed overhead* and *variable overhead.* Fee schedules must reflect both of these overhead factors, plus a fair return to the dentist.

Fixed Overhead

Fixed overhead includes business expenses that continue at all times; these are costs (such as the rent or mortgage, utilities, insurance, and salaries) that are incurred regardless of whether the dentist is in the office and whether professional services are actually being provided.

NOTE: Not all salaries are part of fixed overhead. Salaries that are not fixed are those of professionals who work as independent contractors, on a commission basis, or as part-time workers who are employed on an hourly rate "as needed."

Variable Overhead

Variable overhead expenses are those that change depending on the type of services procured or obtained—for example, dental and stationery supplies, independent contractor fees, laboratory fees, and equipment repair fees.

Gross Versus Net Income

The return the dentist receives for professional services rendered is calculated as **gross income** (the total of *all* professional income received). Gross income minus the payment of all practice-related expenses yields the dentist's **net income** from the practice. Unless the dentist earns an adequate net income, he or she will not be able to afford to maintain a practice.

A *certified public accountant* often is employed on a retainer basis. It is his or her responsibility to handle the major financial records, such as annual profit and loss statements, tax returns, and other government reports. These reports are based on financial information supplied by the dental practice. This information must be accurate, up to date, complete, and presented in a usable format. The business assistant or office manager is usually responsible for the management of the day-to-day expenses and disbursements. He or she also helps the accountant by having the required information and records in good order and ready on time.

Disbursements

The effective management of a dental practice requires organized handling and prompt payment of all bills for practice-related expenses. The payment of major expenses should be made by check, with records kept up to date and balanced at all times. Minor expenses are handled through the use of petty cash. All expenses should be documented as completely as possible with bills and receipts or canceled checks.

Packing Slips, Invoices, and Statements

A **packing slip** is an itemized listing of the goods shipped; it is enclosed with the delivery. It does not contain price information, and an invoice or a statement is sent separately. When materials are received, they should be carefully checked against the packing slip to ensure that everything has been received as ordered and is in safe condition. Discrepancies or damage should be reported immediately to the supplier.

An **invoice** may be included with the shipment, or it may be mailed separately. Once an invoice has been verified, it should be paid promptly unless other arrangements have been made.

A **statement** is a summary of all invoices (charges), payments, credits, and debits for the month.

Organizing Expenditure Records

Statements and invoices that have not yet been paid are placed in the *accounts payable folder.* As part of the organization of expenditure records, expenses are classified into categories; these usually include groups such as professional supplies, laboratory fees, salaries, rent and maintenance, utilities, and business office supplies. The category headings, which are determined by the dentist, are used on file folders to store the expense records in an organized manner. At the end of the year, this expense documentation is removed and filed, in the same categories, with other business records for that year.

The same categories are used to organize disbursements in the check register and for budget purposes. If the practice has a computer system that handles disbursements, this information is entered by category and used when disbursements are made and records for the financial management of the practice are maintained.

Payment of Accounts

In the dental office, the accounts payable are routinely paid once or twice a month. Before writing checks to pay these accounts, the business assistant removes all invoices and statements from the accounts payable folder. The statements and invoices are verified by checking the numbers and amounts of the invoices received from each supplier during that period against the monthly statement. It also is necessary to verify that all payments, credits, and returns have been properly entered. To facilitate the handling and storage of records, the invoices are stapled to the statement covering them.

The dentist should review and approve all bills before payment is made. Once these accounts have been approved for payment, the business assistant writes the necessary checks. As each statement is paid, the number of the check and the date that payment was made are noted on the statement. Customarily, the business assistant writes the checks but does not sign them; the prepared checks are given to the dentist for his or her signature. The office manager who has been given limited power of attorney by the dentist and has proper authorization on file with the bank may sign checks.

Cash on Delivery

Sometimes goods are shipped cash on delivery (C.O.D), which means that at the time of delivery, the person receiving the goods must pay the cost of the merchandise plus a C.O.D. handling fee. Some delivery services handling C.O.D. merchandise will accept a check for the exact amount; others insist on cash. If a check is acceptable, it should be made out to the supplier and not to the delivery service.

The business assistant should never accept a C.O.D. package unless it is something that has been ordered and is expected. When paying for a C.O.D. delivery, the business assistant should receive a signed receipt of payment.

Petty Cash

Petty cash is a limited supply of funds kept on hand to meet frequent small expenses for which immediate cash is needed (e.g., postage due). The amount in the fund should be large enough to last about 1 month but not sufficiently large to invite theft. In most offices, this amount is no more than $50. If more than this is needed within 1 month, it is likely that the concept of petty cash is misunderstood or being misused.

A petty cash voucher must be submitted for all payments made from the fund. Each voucher must include the date, the amount spent, to whom it was paid, for what it was spent, and who spent it. A receipt should be attached to each voucher (Fig. 63-8).

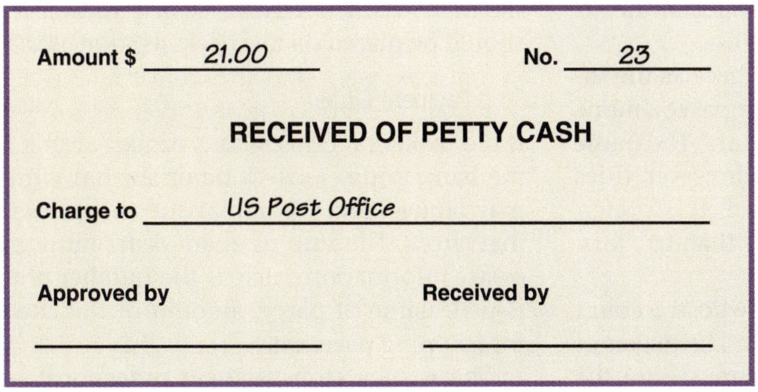
Amount $ 21.00 No. 23

RECEIVED OF PETTY CASH

Charge to US Post Office

Approved by ______ Received by ______

Fig. 63-8 Petty cash voucher.

Replenishing petty cash funds

Petty cash should be balanced and replenished on a regular basis, usually at the beginning of the month. Because there is a voucher for each petty cash payment, the sum of all the vouchers plus the cash on hand should always equal the total amount of the petty cash fund. When these have been balanced, a check is written to refill the fund. If the fund is balanced, the check (which will return the fund to its original amount) should be for a sum equal to that of the vouchers for that month. The vouchers and attached receipts are stapled together, and the date and total are noted. These are filed under the "Business Office" expense category.

Recall

11. Give an example of fixed overhead.
12. After a dental practice pays all practice-related expenses, what type of income is rendered?
13. What type of itemized listing of goods may be included in a shipment of supplies?
14. What does C.O.D. mean?

WRITING CHECKS

Some practices have computerized check-writing capabilities. The advantages of computerized check writing are savings in time, the reduced possibility of error, and the ease of storage and retrieval of specific information. Other practices use a manual pegboard check-writing system or a business checkbook.

Check Terminology

A **check** is a draft, or an order, drawn on a specific bank account for payment of a certain sum of money to the payee or to the bearer. Payment is on demand; that is, when the check is presented to the bank, that amount of money must be paid provided there are sufficient funds in the account to cover the amount of the check.

The **payee** is the person named on the check as the intended recipient of the amount shown. The payee's name is written after the words "Pay to the order of." The name of the payee should be written out in full; however, titles such as Mr., Mrs., and Ms. are best omitted. It is preferable to make a check out to "Mary Jones" than to "Mrs. John Jones."

The *maker* of the check is the one from whose account the amount of the check will be withdrawn. The maker of the check, or his or her authorized agent, must sign the check on the signature line. The **check register** is a record of all checks issued and deposits made to the account. The check register entry should be made *before* the check is written. It should include the following:

- Date (a check should be dated for the day it is written and never be predated or postdated)
- Number of the check
- Name of the payee
- Amount and purpose of the check

Whether a manual or a computerized system is used to process check writing, the utmost care should be taken in stating the amount of the check in both figures and words and in making certain that the amount stated agrees in the following three places (Fig. 63-9):

1. On the check register
2. In numbers on the right side of the check next to the dollar sign
3. Written out in words on the line before the word dollars; the number of cents is usually written as a fraction so that there can be no mistake about the placement of the decimal point.

Checks that are written carelessly or with conflicting numbers can be "raised" or otherwise altered. A *raised check* is one on which extra numbers have been added, for example changing the check's value from $100.00 to $1000.00. Having the amount specified accurately in both words and numbers is one way of safeguarding against this.

Check Endorsement

Before the payee can receive cash for the check, he or she must endorse *(sign)* it. Endorsement is made on the back left side of the check and must match the name shown on the face of the check. A check signed in this manner has a *blanket endorsement,* and anyone holding that check may cash it (including someone who may have stolen it).

With a *restrictive endorsement,* which may read "For deposit only to the account of [*the name of the payee*]," the check can be deposited only to the account of the named individual. This type of endorsement makes the check nonnegotiable; that is, it can be deposited only to that account, and if it is stolen, it cannot be cashed.

A rubber stamp with the appropriate restrictive phrase and the payee's name may be used in place of the payee's signature. As a safeguard, such a restrictive endorsement should be placed on all checks as soon as they are received.

Stop Payment Order

If the maker of a check, for various reasons, does not want the bank to pay a check he or she has written, the maker may request that the bank issue a stop payment order for that check. The stop payment order must give all the necessary information, such as the number of the check, date issued, name of payee, amount of the check, and reason for stopping payment.

The written stop payment order must reach the bank bookkeeper before the check is presented for payment.

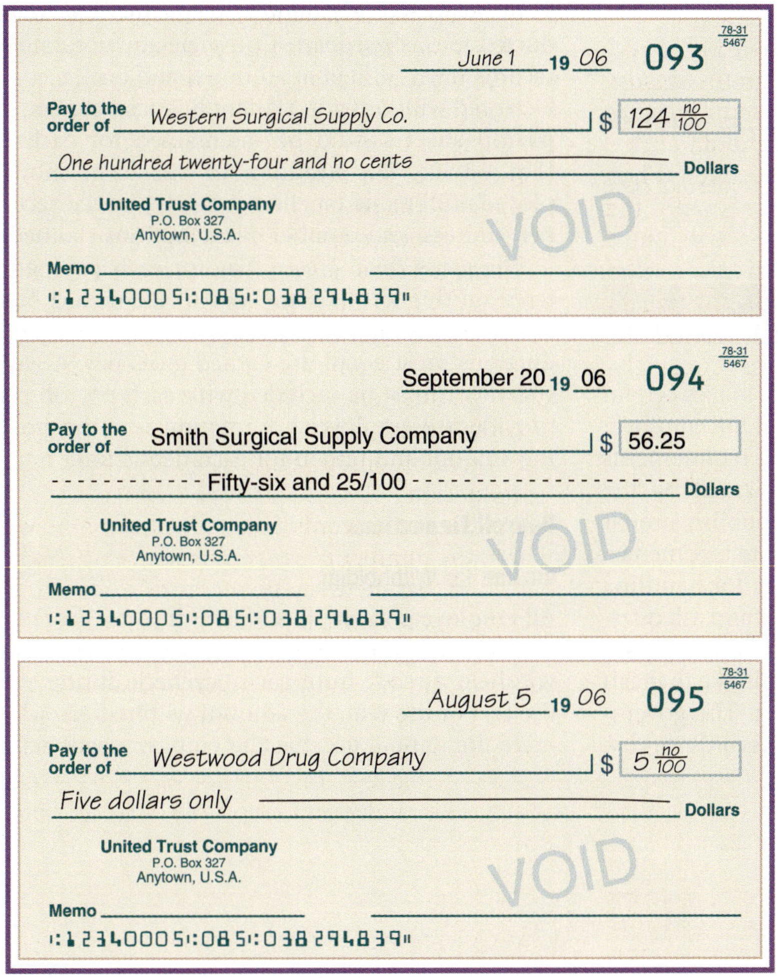

Fig. 63-9 Correct way to write a check.

These orders are usually in force for 90 days, and the bank charges for this service.

Nonsufficient Funds

A check written for more than the amount in the maker's account will usually be refused when presented for payment. The check will then be returned to the payee marked *N.S.F. (nonsufficient funds)*. This means there is not enough money in the account to cover the check, and the payee cannot collect any of the amounts due. A check that has been returned for this reason is known as a *returned item;* however, it is commonly referred to as having "bounced" *(come back)*. The bank makes a charge against the account of the person (or company) who wrote the N.S.F. check; however, there usually is no charge to the person who received the check.

When a check from a patient is returned, the amount of that check must be "charged back" against the patient's account. Do this by making an entry in the ledger, noting the date on which the check was returned. Then make an adjustment, which acts as a charge and increases the account balance by the amount of the returned check. It also is necessary to make a check register entry; here, the amount of the returned check is subtracted from the checking account balance.

Often a telephone call to the maker will resolve the problem, and the check may be redeposited. A check that must be redeposited should be listed on a separate deposit slip and clearly marked so that it is not credited twice to income. When the check is redeposited, this should be noted on the account history, and the amount of the check should again be subtracted from the balance.

If a returned check cannot be redeposited, there is an outstanding balance on the account that requires immediate attention.

Business Summaries

All checks must be accounted for in a specific expense category. With a computerized system, posting to the appropriate category is part of the check-writing process. With pegboard check writing, expenses are posted into categories at the time the check is written. Totals from monthly summaries are carried forward to an annual summary. Through the keeping of these records, the dentist and the accountant can at any time quickly tell what the practice expenses have been to date. This is important information for management, budgeting, and tax purposes.

Recall

15. Where in the checkbook do you record the checks written and deposits made on an account?

16. What term is used to indicate that an account does not have enough money in it to cover a check?

PAYROLL

Federal regulations require that an employer makes certain deductions from an employee's pay and that the employer also pays certain payroll taxes. These federal requirements are explained in the *Circular E* booklet issued by the Internal Revenue Service (IRS). Most states publish similar booklets explaining the requirements for state income tax.

The business assistant who is responsible for handling payroll should study these booklets carefully and ask questions about any point that is not clear. It is better to ask questions first than to make an expensive mistake that can be corrected only with great difficulty later. The government requires that each employer keep records of the hours worked, the amount paid, and the amounts deducted for tax purposes. Complete and accurate employee records must be kept at all times, and back records should be stored with other important financial papers. A separate payroll sheet should be maintained for each employee (Fig. 63-10). The headings of this form show the employee's full name (spelled correctly), social security number, address, and number of exemptions claimed.

The gross *(total pretax)* pay for each pay period is entered on this form, as are each of the deductions and the net *(gross pay minus all deductions)* pay. Net pay plus deductions must equal the earned gross pay. A withholding statement must be included with each payroll check. This provides the employee information as to the gross pay and the amount and reason for each deduction.

Payroll Deductions

Income Tax Withholding

All employees must file a federal income tax return before April 15 of each year. A portion of the estimated tax is withheld directly from each paycheck during the year. By the end of the year, the amount withheld should approximate the annual tax that the employee will actually owe.

NAME Patricia Andrews, CDA	Social Sec. Number 123-45-6789		
STREET 305 Oak Drive	Phone Number 933-0111	No. of Exempt 1	
CITY Centerville, NJ 08511	Date Started 7/1/9X Date Left	M	F X

Record of Pay Rate Changes	
DATE	RATE
7/1/9X	9.00
1/1/9X	10.00

DATE	HOURS reg	HOURS over	GROSS AMOUNT	DEDUCTIONS Social Sec.	Fed. Inc. Tax	State Inc. Tax				NET AMOUNT
1/8/9X	40		400.00	33.20	40.00	8.50				318.30
1/15/9X	40		400.00	33.20	40.00	8.50				318.30
1/22/9X	40		400.00	33.20	40.00	8.50				318.30
1/29/9X	40		400.00	33.20	40.00	8.50				318.30
JANUARY TOTALS			1600.00	132.80	160.00	34.00				1273.20

GROSS EARNINGS

NET EARNINGS

EMPLOYER MAKES MATCHING CONTRIBUTION

Fig. 63-10 Payroll report. (Courtesy Eaglesoft, a division of Patterson Companies, Inc.)

Amounts withheld are determined from a schedule in Circular E. These amounts are based on earnings and the number of exemptions claimed. It is the responsibility of the employer to withhold this tax and to remit it to an authorized bank or directly to the IRS.

Each employee must complete an *employee's withholding exemption certificate (W-4 form)* at the following times: (1) on the beginning of employment, (2) within 10 days of any change of status (such as marriage), and (3) before December 1 for the following year. This form authorizes the employer to deduct the tax and indicates the number of exemptions that the employee is claiming. These completed forms must be kept with other payroll records.

Federal Insurance Contributions Act

Under the *Federal Insurance Contributions Act (FICA)*, commonly known as *social security*, the employer is required to deduct a certain percentage of the employee's gross pay. This is a fixed amount regardless of the number of exemptions. The employer is also required to match the contribution. Thus for each FICA dollar withheld from the employee's wages, the employer also contributes a dollar. Both contributions are forwarded quarterly to the federal government to be credited to the employee's account.

For FICA earnings to be properly credited, it is important to keep the Social Security Administration informed of any change of name. The employee will receive a *Statement of Earnings* from the Social Security Administration annually. This is a written record of the amount "credited" to the employee's account. Should there be an error here, it must be reported and corrected through the Social Security Administration.

Other Deductions

Additional federal, state, and local taxes may be withheld from the employee's pay. The person in charge of payroll computations is responsible for having current information about the regulations governing these deductions. Personal deductions, such as the employee's contribution to health or life insurance coverage, an automatic personal savings plan, or pretax retirement contributions, may be taken directly from the employee's earnings.

The employer must pay additional payroll taxes such as *workers' compensation, federal unemployment taxes (FUTA), and state unemployment insurance (SUI)*. These amounts are not deducted from the employee's earnings, except in states in which a portion of the SUI tax is paid by the employee.

Government Remittance

All government reports must be completed accurately and neatly (preferably typewritten or computer generated) and filed *on time*. Stiff penalties are issued for late reports. All employers are required to file an "Employer's Quarterly Federal Tax Return." This is a report of all taxable wages paid during the quarter. Withheld taxes and FICA contributions must be deposited regularly; the frequency of these deposits depends on the total amount owed.

Within 30 days of the end of the calendar year or on termination of employment, the employee must be furnished with a statement of total earnings and taxes withheld for that year (W-2 form). Many computer systems have the capabilities to process payroll and taxes; this allows computer-generated reports and business summaries that fit the individual practice.

DENTAL INSURANCE

Dental insurance is a plan that assists the patient or family with the cost of dental care. A person can obtain dental insurance two ways: (1) from an employer or spouse's employer as a benefit through a group plan or (2) as an individual plan. The individual plan is most commonly a much higher premium than a group plan. A group policy usually provides better benefits and is more affordable for the employer and employee.

Dental insurance is designed to make dental care more accessible by reducing the cost to the patient. Although it reduces the cost of care, insurance is not intended to cover all of the expenses. Under most plans, the patient remains responsible for any portion of the fee not covered by the insurance. In most practices, reimbursement from dental insurance plans is a major source of practice income; therefore it is important that claims be prepared accurately and completely and filed promptly so that all fees are collected from the appropriate party in a timely manner.

Parties Involved in Dental Insurance

A working knowledge of the parties involved in dental insurance is necessary to comprehend basic insurance concepts. In most instances, the following are the parties involved: The person receiving the treatment can be the *subscriber* who carries the dental plan or a *dependent* of the subscriber, such a spouse or child. The *group* is the union or employment organization that has negotiated the dental insurance as part of its benefits package. The **carrier** is the party (usually an insurance company) that pays the claims and collects the premiums. The **provider** is the dentist who renders treatment to the patient.

Types of Prepaid Dental Programs

Many types of dental insurance coverage are available today. The three most commonly used methods of calculating fee-for-service benefits are (1) usual, customary, and reasonable (UCR) fees, (2) schedule of benefits, and (3) fixed fee schedule.

Usual, Customary, and Reasonable Fees

The term **usual fee** refers to a fee that the dentist charges private patients for a given service. These fees are determined by the individual dentist and are the fees that are routinely charged in the practice. The dentist files a confidential list of these fees with the carrier. The carrier uses this information, called *prefiled fees,* to determine the customary fee for the area.

A **customary fee** is one that is within the range of the usual fees charged for the same service by dentists with similar training and experience within the same geographic area (such a city or county). Using the information from the prefiled fees, the carrier determines what is customary on the basis of a percentile of the fees charged by dentists within that area.

A **reasonable fee** is one that is considered justified by special circumstances necessitating extensive or complex treatment. These are the unusual cases for which the dentist would charge more than the usual fee, even to a private patient, because of the extent of treatment involved. For instance, a particularly difficult extraction might justify an unusual fee. In these instances, the dentist is able to charge whatever is *reasonable* for the situation; however, the carrier may request written documentation to explain why the unusual fee was necessary.

In a UCR system, the payment can still be low, and the patient usually is responsible for the difference between the insurance payment and the dentist's fee. The **limitations** of the policy also influence the amount that the dentist receives from the carrier and how much the patient must pay.

Schedule of Benefits

This also is known as a *table of allowances* or a *schedule of allowances.* A schedule of benefits is a list of fixed specified amounts that the carrier will pay toward the cost of *covered services.* A schedule of benefits is not related in any way to the dentist's actual fee schedule. Under most schedule of benefit plans, the patient is responsible for the difference between what the carrier will pay and what the dentist actually charges.

Fixed Fee Schedule

A fixed fee schedule is an established fee for any treatment received by the patient. Under government programs, such as Medicaid, the dentist must accept the amount paid by the carrier as payment in full and may not bill the patient for the difference.

Alternative Payment Plans

Capitation programs

This means that the dentist has contracted to provide all or most of the dental services covered under the program to subscribers in return for payment on a per capita basis. Under this plan, payment to the dentist is *not* based on services rendered. Instead, the dentist receives a fixed rate per covered member regardless of the services provided.

Capitation plans are widely used in *health maintenance organizations (HMOs) or dental maintenance organizations (DMOs);* in these organizations, dentists who are employed by the HMO or DMO may provide dental care. An alternative form of capitation is to have services provided by a dentist who has a contract with the HMO or DMO. In both situations, the subscriber's choice of dentist is limited to those who are under contract with the HMO or DMO.

Direct reimbursement plans

A direct reimbursement plan is a self-funded program in which the individual is reimbursed by his or her employer on the basis of a percentage of dollars spent for dental care provided. This type of plan allows beneficiaries to seek treatment from the dentist of their choice. Under a direct reimbursement plan, no insurance carrier is involved. Instead, the employee pays the dentist, and the employer reimburses a portion of this expense. The amount of reimbursement depends on the benefit design established by the employer.

Individual practice associations

An individual practice association (IPA) is an organization formed by groups of dentists or, in some cases, dental societies for the primary purpose of collectively entering into contracts to provide dental services to the enrolled populations. Frequently, services are provided on a capitation basis. These dentists may practice in their own offices. In addition to treating patients enrolled in the IPA, they may provide care to patients who are not covered by the contract. Treatment of the patients who are not covered is provided in the traditional fee-for-service basis.

Preferred provider organizations

A preferred provider organization (PPO) is a formal agreement between a purchaser of a dental benefits program and a defined group of dentists for the delivery of dental services to a specific patient population, in which discounted fees are used for cost savings. This is a variation of a fee-for-service practice. A dentist may join a PPO in the hope of attracting more new patients or in an effort to retain his or her current patients who are covered by the PPO plan. These patients are seen in the dentist's office. The dentist may also continue to see other fee-for-service patients who are not part of the PPO contract. The fee-for-service patients are still charged the dentist's usual fees.

Managed Care

Managed care is a method of providing low- to medium-cost healthcare coverage to everyone. The idea is to provide excellent care more efficiently and less expensively than what is otherwise offered. Under these plans, the type, level, and frequency of treatment can be limited and disease prevention is encouraged. The plans also try to control the level of reimbursement for services. Capitation plans, DMOs, HMOs, IPAs, and closed panels are considered managed care plans.

Escalating medical and dental premiums continue to affect the healthcare system, and managed care will continue to be a source of discussion and negotiation. It is extremely important for the dental healthcare worker to stay up to date on dental healthcare plan policies and procedures. Box 63-2 provides an alphabetical list of the terms most commonly used for dental insurance.

Determining Eligibility

Dental plans do not pay for care rendered to patients who are not eligible to receive benefits. When a subscriber starts a new job, there usually is a 30- to 60-day waiting period before coverage comes effective. If a subscriber changes jobs, is laid off, or retires, his or her coverage is customarily terminated within 30 days of the change. However, the subscriber has the option to continue coverage under the Consolidated Omnibus Budget Reconciliation Act (COBRA) of 1985. This entitles the subscriber to continue the same coverage, but he or she is responsible for paying the premiums. If there is any question concerning eligibility, the carrier should be contacted *before* routine dental care is started.

The rules for eligibility under other government programs, such as Medicaid and the Civilian Health and Medical Program of the Uniformed Services (CHAMPUS), vary greatly. Medicare does **not** include dental coverage.

When working with clients enrolled in government programs, you must be familiar with the specific form of iden-

Box 63-2 Basic Dental Insurance Terminology

Term	Description
Assignment of benefits	The patient authorizes payment of the dental benefits directly to the provider. The patient, or subscriber if the patient is a minor, signs the insurance form or has a signature on file starting with the first visit.
Carrier	An insurance company that agrees to pay benefits claimed under a dental plan. A single carrier may offer several different dental plans.
Coinsurance/copayment	A provision of a dental benefits program by which the beneficiary shares in the cost of covered services, generally on a percentage basis. This percentage is expressed in terms of how much the carrier will pay. For example, the expression "80% coinsurance" means that the carrier will pay 80% of the cost on the basis of the carrier's method of payment (UCR or schedule of benefits). The patient pays the remaining 20% plus any balance not covered by the carrier. The percentages vary from one plan to another. Under some plans, the carrier pays 100% for preventive services (such as recall prophylaxis and examination), 80% for routine or basic services (such as restorations), and 50% for major services (such as crown and bridge). When patients are enrolled in managed care programs, they are typically responsible for a small copayment such as $5 or $10, and the insurance company pays the balance based on a fixed fee.
Deductible	Specified amount that the insured must pay toward the cost of dental treatment *before* the benefits of the plan go into effect. The amount and type of deductible depend on the contract. There may be an individual deductible; this means that each family member must meet this amount before he or she becomes eligible for benefits. Alternatively, there may be a family deductible. Under this plan, the first family member or members meeting the dollar value will satisfy the deductible for the entire family.
Dependent	Child or spouse of the subscriber. Coverage for a child usually ceases when the child reaches a certain age as indicated in the contract. (This age varies but is usually 18 or 19 unless the child is still a full-time student.)
Eligibility	The process of determining whether the patient is eligible for benefits. This should be done before treatment is started.
Exclusions	Services not covered by a dental policy. Some policies exclude certain services, such as cosmetic dentistry and orthodontics. In this context, *cosmetic dentistry* is defined as services provided that are aimed at improving appearance but are not deemed by the carrier to be necessary for the patient's dental health. This does not mean that the dentist may not provide these services. It simply means that the carrier will not pay for this treatment. The patient may still receive the treatment but is responsible for the entire fee.

continued

Box 63-2 Basic Dental Insurance Terminology—cont'd

Maximum	The maximum dollar amount a benefits plan will pay toward the cost of dental care over a specific period of time (usually one calendar year), such as $1000 annually per patient. The carrier will not pay for any treatment beyond that amount—even if the treatment is a covered service. The carrier may also establish a lifetime maximum for certain procedures. For example, the plan may include a lifetime maximum of $2000 for orthodontic treatment. This means that the carrier will not pay more than this amount in orthodontic benefits for this patient regardless of how long the treatment takes.
Predetermination of benefits	Also known as a *pretreatment estimate,* it is an administrative procedure that may require the dentist to submit a treatment plan to the insurance company before treatment begins. The carrier returns the treatment plan indicating the patient's eligibility, covered services, and benefit amounts that are payable. Most commonly, this step is required if the planned treatment exceeds a certain dollar limit. The request for predetermination should be submitted to the carrier immediately after the patient's first visit. The response from the carrier should be received before the case presentation visit. In this way, both the dentist and the patient know the amount of benefits available to help with the cost of the recommended treatment. If the carrier requests radiographs with the treatment plan for predetermination, a dual film packet should be used when the films are taken. The extra set of radiographs is sent to the carrier. If these are not available, the original radiographs are duplicated, and the duplicates are submitted to the carrier. Under no circumstances are the original radiographs submitted because they can be lost.
Provider	The dentist who renders treatment to the patient.
Subscriber	Also known as the *insured,* this is the person who represents the family unit in relation to the dental plan. (This usually is the employee who is earning these benefits.)

tification to request to determine eligibility. This usually is an identification card or a proof-of-eligibility sticker. Because the individual's eligibility may change from month to month, it is essential that this identification be verified at each visit.

Determining Benefits

The employer who purchases the coverage as a benefit for the employees negotiates the limitations and benefits of these plans. The carrier is responsible for covering *only* the level of treatment that is included in that plan. Information explaining the coverage under a specific plan is found in the *benefits booklet* supplied to the subscriber. The patient is asked to bring this booklet to the first dental visit so that coverage can be reviewed and discussed before the start of treatment.

The two major factors that determine how much the carrier will pay and how much the patient must pay are the *method of payment* and the *limitations* within the plan.

Limitations

In addition to different methods of payment, other factors influence the amount of benefits that the beneficiary is entitled to receive under the plan and how much he or she must pay as a share of these costs.

Least-expensive alternative treatment

The least-expensive alternative treatment (LEAT), also known as an *alternative benefit policy,* is a limitation in a dental plan that allows benefits only for the least-expensive treatment. For example, the patient needs a replacement for a missing tooth. The treatment alternatives are a fixed bridge costing $3000 or a removable partial denture for $1200. Under LEAT, the carrier will pay benefits only for the partial denture. The patient may choose to have the bridge, but the carrier will pay only $1200 (as if the patient had a partial denture made), and the patient is responsible for the difference in the fee.

Dual coverage

If a patient has dental insurance coverage under more than one plan, this is known as *dual coverage.* In this case, it is necessary to take steps to be certain that the appropriate benefits are paid.

Determining primary and secondary carriers. With situations involving dual coverage, it is necessary to determine which carrier is *primary* (and should pay first) and which carrier is *secondary* (and should pay at least a portion of the balance). Specific questions on a claim form ask for this information. When the *patient* is the insured, his or her carrier is always primary and the spouse's carrier is secondary. When there is spousal coverage for patients with insurance of their own, their insurance must be billed first. After payment from the primary insurance company is received, a claim is sent to the other insurance company if any balance is still due.

Birthday rule. The birthday rule was established to explain which insurance carrier is the primary carrier when both parents have insurance to cover the child. The rule stipulates that when a child is covered under both parents' plans, the plan of the parent whose birthday (month and day, not year) falls earlier in the calendar year is billed first. This rule applies to parents who are *not* divorced. Other factors are considered when parents are divorced or separated and when step-parents are involved. It is important to work with the parents to determine the sequencing of insurance form filing by clearly defining the office billing policies to the parent accompanying the child.

Coordination of benefits. Under *coordination of benefits (COB)*, the patient will receive payment from both carriers, but the total received may **not** be more than 100 percent of the actual dental expenses. For example, the fee is $250. Benefits from the primary carrier are $175 for this service. No matter what benefits the secondary carrier usually pays for this service, under coordination of benefits, the second carrier will pay no more than the difference between the fee and the amount paid by the primary carrier. This comes to $75, after which the patient has been reimbursed for 100 percent of the fee.

Nonduplication of Benefits

Under plans that call for nonduplication of benefits, which is also known as *benefit-less-benefit*, a provision relieves the carrier from responsibility for paying for services that are covered under another program. Under these plans, reimbursement is limited to the higher level allowed by the two plans rather than a total of 100 percent of the charges. For example, the fee is $250. The primary carrier allows $175 for this service. The secondary carrier allows $190 for this service. In this situation, the primary carrier pays $175. The secondary carrier pays only $15, which is the total amount of the allowed benefit minus the amount that has already been paid. If the primary carrier allowed the higher of the two benefits, the secondary carrier would not pay anything. The result is that the patient is reimbursed for the higher of the two allowed amounts but not for 100 percent of the fee.

Many patients are not aware of the nonduplication of benefits clause, which can cause confusion regarding their benefits. It is important to explain this clause to patients after their predetermination results return.

Dental Procedure Codes

The *Code on Dental Procedures and Nomenclature* was developed by the American Dental Association (ADA) to speed and simplify the reporting of dental procedures. These codes are published in **Current Dental Terminology (CDT)**, which is published and periodically updated by the ADA. These codes are *very* specific. The CDT should be reviewed carefully before specific dental treatment is coded. Each procedure has a designated code number. The codes are divided into categories of service and are listed in Box 63-3.

Box 63-3 Dental Procedure Codes

Diagnostic D0100-D0999
Preventive D1000-D1999
Restorative D2000-D2999
Endodontics D3000-D3999
Periodontics D4000-D4999
Prosthodontics, removable D5000-D5899
Maxillofacial prosthetics D5900-D5999
Implant services D6000-D6199
Prosthodontics, fixed D6200-D6999
Oral surgery D7000-D7999
Orthodontics D8000-D8999
Adjunctive general services D9000-D9999

In many practices, encounter forms (also known as *charge slips* or *routing slips*) are preprinted with the codes used in the practice. One of these forms is clipped to the outside of the patient's file folder before the dentist sees the patient. After the visit, the dentist simply checks the boxes for services and charges and makes any notations. This reduces the possibility of coding errors by the clinical assistant or front office personnel.

Claim Forms

Claim Form Preparation

Claims for dental treatment are filed in one of two ways: by submission on a claim form that is mailed to the carrier (paper claim) or by electronic transmission, in which information is submitted electronically to the carrier (electronic claim). Both types of transmission require the same three primary areas of information: patient and subscriber identification, dentist identification, and details concerning the treatment provided.

Paper Claim

If completed manually, a dental insurance claim form is used either to submit a predetermination of benefits for planned treatment or to request payment of claims for services that have been rendered. The ADA provides a standardized claim form that is accepted by most carriers (Fig. 63-11).

The completed claim form is generated in duplicate; one copy is submitted to the carrier, and the other copy is retained with the practice records. The claim form includes

ADA Dental Claim Form

HEADER INFORMATION

1. Type of Transaction (Check all applicable boxes)

☐ Statement of Actual Sevices ☐ Request for Predetermination/Preauthorization

☐ EPSDT/Title XIX

2. Predetermination/Preauthorization Number

PRIMARY PAYER INFORMATION

3. Name, Address, City, State, Zip Code

OTHER COVERAGE

4. Other Dental or Medical Coverage? ☐ No (Skip 5-11) ☐ Yes (Complete 5-11)

5. Other Insured's Name (Last, First, Middle Initial, Suffix)

6. Date of Birth (MM/DD/CCYY) | 7. Gender ☐M ☐F | 8. Subscriber Identifier (SSN or ID#)

9. Plan/Group Number | 10. Patient's Relationship to Other Insured (Check applicable box) ☐ Self ☐ Spouse ☐ Dependent ☐ Other

11. Other Carrier Name, Address, City, State, Zip Code

PRIMARY INSURED INFORMATION

12. Name (Last, First, Middle Initial, Suffix), Address, City, State, Zip Code

13. Date of Birth (MM/DD/CCYY) | 14. Gender ☐M ☐F | 15. Subscriber Identifier (SSN or ID#)

16. Plan/Group Number | 17. Employer Name

PATIENT INFORMATION

18. Relationship to Primary Insured (Check applicable box) ☐ Self ☐ Spouse ☐ Dependent Child ☐ Other | 19. Student Status ☐FTS ☐PTS

20. Name (Last, First, Middle Initial, Suffix), Address, City, State, Zip Code

21. Date of Birth (MM/DD/CCYY) | 22. Gender ☐M ☐F | 23. Patient ID/Account # (Assigned by Dentist)

RECORD OF SERVICES PROVIDED

	24. Procedure Date (MM/DD/CCYY)	25. Area of Oral Cavity	26. Tooth System	27. Tooth Number(s) or Letter(s)	28. Tooth Surface	29. Procedure Code	30. Description	31. Fee
1								
2								
3								
4								
5								
6								
7								
8								
9								
10								

MISSING TEETH INFORMATION

34. (Place an 'X' on each missing tooth)

	Permanent																Primary									
	1	2	3	4	5	6	7	8	9	10	11	12	13	14	15	16	A	B	C	D	E	F	G	H	I	J
	32	31	30	29	28	27	26	25	24	23	22	21	20	19	18	17	T	S	R	Q	P	O	N	M	L	K

32. Other Fee(s)

33. Total Fee

35. Remarks

AUTHORIZATIONS

36. I have been informed of the treatment plan and associated fees. I agree to be responsible for all charges for dental services and materials not paid by my dental benefit plan, unless prohibited by law, or the treating dentist or dental practice has a contractual agreement with my plan prohibiting all or a portion of such charges. To the extent permitted by law, I consent to your use and disclosure of my protected health information to carry out payment activities in connection with this claim.

X

Patient/Guardian signature Date

37. I hereby authorize and direct payment of the dental benefits otherwise payable to me, directly to the below named dentist or dental entity.

X

Subscriber signature Date

ANCILLARY CLAIM/TREATMENT INFORMATION

38. Place of Treatment (Check applicable box) ☐ Provider's Office ☐ Hospital ☐ ECF ☐ Other

39. Number of Enclosures (00 to 99) Radiograph(s) ☐ Oral Image(s) ☐ Model(s) ☐

40. Is Treatment for Orthodontics? ☐ No (Skip 41-42) ☐ Yes (Complete 41-42) | 41. Date Appliance Placed (MM/DD/CCYY)

42. Months of Treatment Remaining | 43. Replacement Prosthesis? ☐ No ☐ Yes (Complete 44) | 44. Date Prior Placement (MM/DD/CCYY)

45. Treatment Resulting from (Check applicable box) ☐ Occupational illness/injury ☐ Auto accident ☐ Other accident

46. Date of Accident (MM/DD/CCYY) | 47. Auto Accident State

BILLING DENTIST OR DENTAL ENTITY (Leave blank if dentist or dental entity is not submitting claim on behalf of the patient or insured/subscriber)

48. Name, Address, City, State, Zip Code

49. Provider ID | 50. License Number | 51. SSN or TIN

52. Phone Number ( )

TREATING DENTIST AND TREATMENT LOCATION INFORMATION

53. I hereby certify that the procedures as indicated by date are in progress (for procedures that require multiple visits) or have been completed and that the fees submitted are the actual fees I have charged and intend to collect for those procedures.

X

Signed (Treating Dentist) Date

54. Provider ID | 55. Liscense Number

56. Address, City, State, Zip Code

57. Phone Number ( ) | 58. Treating Provider Specialty

J515 (Same as ADA Dental Claim Form – J516, J517, J518, J519)

To Reorder, call 1-800-947-4746 or go online at www.adacatalog.org

Fig. 63-11 ADA standard claim form.

two boxes for patient signatures. These are for the release of information and the assignment of benefits.

Release of information regarding the patient's treatment is confidential and may be done only with the patient's written consent. The patient's signature in the "release of information" box gives the dentist permission to reveal to the insurance carrier information regarding the patient's dental treatment.

Assignment of benefits is a procedure by which the subscriber authorizes the carrier to make payment of allowable benefits directly to the dentist. If there is no assignment of benefits, the check goes directly to the patient. To assign the benefits, the subscriber signs the appropriate box on the insurance claim form. If there is no assignment of benefits, financial arrangements are made for the total amount of the fee, just as if the patient did not have dental insurance.

Signature on file

The patient registration form has signature boxes similar to those on the claim form; specific signature authorization forms can also be used. The patient should sign these when completing the form. These signatures are kept on file, and when the claim form is prepared, "Signature on File" can be used. When claims are submitted electronically, there is no place for a patient signature. The "Signature on File" option covers the need to have the patient's permission for the release of this information.

Electronic Claim

With electronic claims processing, data already stored in the practice's computer are used to generate and submit claims from the practice's computer to the carrier's computer (Fig. 63-12). This has the advantages of speeding claim submission and payment and reducing paperwork and the possibility of errors. As part of claims preparation on the computer, the system checks each claim for missing information before electronic submission. When the claims have been verified as complete, they are transmitted by modem. This transmission may be directly to the carrier's computer; however, because a practice deals with many carriers, the claims are usually transmitted through a clearinghouse that is set up through the individual practice software. Your software vendor will assist you with this information.

Dental practices that see a large number of patients transmit their claims on a daily basis. Dentists who see a small number of patients per day may decide to transmit their claims once a week. Although there is no paper claim generated, the practice must have a record of each claim that was submitted. Transmission problems can arise periodically when submitting electronic claims. Therefore this record is essential in the event that a claim is lost or disputed and must be submitted again. It also is important in tracking claims for payment. A daily or weekly status report of claims is sent electronically from the clearinghouse to check against your record.

HIPAA and Electronic Transactions

Under the Health Insurance Portability and Accountability Act of 1996 (or **HIPAA**), the Department of Health and Human Services (HHS) implemented transaction standards to protect the integrity and promote the standardization of electronic claims submissions. The goal of the program is to allow one standardized format for each specific transaction, with a standard set of procedure codes. By doing this, electronic data transmissions are more efficient, which results in a cost savings for healthcare providers. For dentistry, the CDT codes are used to simplify transaction processing.

Dental offices that are not filing electronically are not affected by this particular section of the law but must still comply with the privacy rule and with the other aspects of administrative simplification that address security standards. Medicaid accepts only electronic claims, so any office that accepts Medicaid will need to submit all insurance claims electronically.

HIPAA *Electronic Transfers*

Under HIPAA, electronic claim submissions must be standardized. For dentistry, the CDT codes are used to standardize submission processing.

Claim Form Processing

At the end of the patient's visit, all charges are entered into the patient's account history or ledger (with or without insurance). A claim for payment then is submitted to the insurance company. If this is the patient's first visit, it also may be necessary to file a predetermination for planned additional treatment. If so, the predetermination is submitted on a separate claim. Make definite financial arrangements with the patient for payment of his or her portion of the fee.

Tracking Claims in Process

Insurance claims are another form of accounts receivable—that is, money that has been earned and must now be collected. It is important that these claims be handled in a businesslike manner. Most computerized programs generate the reports needed to track these claims; these include reports of the following:

- Claims that have been submitted for predetermination but have not yet been returned
- Claims that have been submitted for payment but have not yet been paid
- Charges for claims that have been generated but have not yet been submitted
- Claims that have been returned for any reason and have not yet been resubmitted

These reports should be printed and reviewed on a regular basis. It is important that you follow up promptly on

ADA Dental Claim Form

HEADER INFORMATION

1. Type of Transaction (Check all applicable boxes)
[X] Statement of Actual Services [ ] Request for Predetermination/Preauthorization
[ ] EPSDT/Title XIX

2. Predetermination/Preauthorization Number

PRIMARY PAYER INFORMATION

3. Name, Address, City, State, Zip Code
Ralph Henderson
287 Oak Drive
Centerville, IL 61822

OTHER COVERAGE

4. Other Dental or Medical Coverage? [X] No (Skip 5-11) [ ] Yes (Complete 5-11)

5. Other Insured's Name (Last, First, Middle Initial, Suffix)

6. Date of Birth (MM/DD/CCYY): 04/25/1960
7. Gender: [X] M [ ] F
8. Subscriber Identifier (SSN or ID#): 543-20-9765

9. Plan/Group Number: FBOC
10. Patient's Relationship to Other Insured (Check applicable box): [X] Self [ ] Spouse [ ] Dependent [ ] Other

11. Other Carrier Name, Address, City, State, Zip Code

PRIMARY INSURED INFORMATION

12. Name (Last, First, Middle Initial, Suffix), Address, City, State, Zip Code
Ralph Henderson
287 Oak Drive
Centerville, IL 61822

13. Date of Birth (MM/DD/CCYY): 04/25/1960
14. Gender: [X] M [ ] F
15. Subscriber Identifier (SSN or ID#): 543-20-9765

16. Plan/Group Number: FBOC
17. Employer Name: First Bank of Centerville

PATIENT INFORMATION

18. Relationship to Primary Insured (Check applicable box): [X] Self [ ] Spouse [ ] Dependent Child [ ] Other
19. Student Status: [ ] FTS [ ] PTS

20. Name (Last, First, Middle Initial, Suffix), Address, City, State, Zip Code
Ralph Henderson
287 Oak Drive
Centerville, IL 61822

21. Date of Birth (MM/DD/CCYY): 04/25/1960
22. Gender: [X] M [ ] F
23. Patient ID/Account # (Assigned by Dentist): 543-20-9765

RECORD OF SERVICES PROVIDED

	24. Procedure Date (MM/DD/CCYY)	25. Area of Oral Cavity	26. Tooth System	27. Tooth Number(s) or Letter(s)	28. Tooth Surface	29. Procedure Code	30. Description	31. Fee
1	01/10/20xx					D0150	Comprehensive oral evaluation	70 00
2	01/10/20xx					D0210	Intraoral FMS - Complete Series	80 00
3	01/10/20xx					D1330	Oral Hygiene Instructions	35 00
4	01/10/20xx					D1110	Prophylaxis - adult	80 00
5	01/10/20xx					D0470	Diagnostic Casts	75 00
6								
7								
8								
9								
10								

MISSING TEETH INFORMATION

34. (Place an 'X' on each missing tooth)

	Permanent																Primary									
	1	2	3	4	5	6	7	8	9	10	11	12	13	14	15	16	A	B	C	D	E	F	G	H	I	J
	32	31	30	29	28	27	26	25	24	23	22	21	20	19	18	17	T	S	R	Q	P	O	N	M	L	K

32. Other Fee(s)
33. Total Fee: 340 00

35. Remarks

AUTHORIZATIONS

36. I have been informed of the treatment plan and associated fees. I agree to be responsible for all charges for dental services and materials not paid by my dental benefit plan, unless prohibited by law, or the treating dentist or dental practice has a contractual agreement with my plan prohibiting all or a portion of such charges. To the extent permitted by law, I consent to your use and disclosure of my protected health information to carry out payment activities in connection with this claim.

X Signature on File — 2/1/XX
Patient/Guardian signature — Date

37. I hereby authorize and direct payment of the dental benefits otherwise payable to me, directly to the below named dentist or dental entity.

X Signature on File — 2/1/XX
Subscriber signature — Date

ANCILLARY CLAIM/TREATMENT INFORMATION

38. Place of Treatment (Check applicable box): [ ] Provider's Office [ ] Hospital [ ] ECF [ ] Other
39. Number of Enclosures (00 to 99): Radiograph(s) Oral Image(s) Model(s)

40. Is Treatment for Orthodontics? [ ] No (Skip 41-42) [ ] Yes (Complete 41-42)
41. Date Appliance Placed (MM/DD/CCYY)

42. Months of Treatment Remaining
43. Replacement Prosthesis? [ ] No [ ] Yes (Complete 44)
44. Date Prior Placement (MM/DD/CCYY)

45. Treatment Resulting from (Check applicable box): [ ] Occupational illness/injury [ ] Auto accident [ ] Other accident

46. Date of Accident (MM/DD/CCYY)
47. Auto Accident State

BILLING DENTIST OR DENTAL ENTITY (Leave blank if dentist or dental entity is not submitting claim on behalf of the patient or insured/subscriber)

48. Name, Address, City, State, Zip Code
Leonard S Taylor
2100 W. Park Avenue
Champaign, IL 61820

49. Provider ID
50. License Number: IL-3456
51. SSN or TIN: 203-55-9278

52. Phone Number (217) 351-5400

TREATING DENTIST AND TREATMENT LOCATION INFORMATION

53. I hereby certify that the procedures as indicated by date are in progress (for procedures that require multiple visits) or have been completed and that the fees submitted are the actual fees I have charged and intend to collect for those procedures.

X
Signed (Treating Dentist) — Date

54. Provider ID
55. License Number

56. Address, City, State, Zip Code

57. Phone Number ( )
58. Treating Provider Specialty

Fig. 63-12 Computerized claim form submitted for payment.

any claims process that has not been completed in a reasonable period of time.

Payments from Insurance Carriers

Checks received from insurance carriers should be accompanied by an explanation of benefits explaining which benefits have been paid and which have been denied. The explanation of benefits breaks down how payment was determined and contains the following information:

- Patient's name and policy number
- Provider of services
- Dates of services
- Procedures
- Amount billed by the provider
- Amount allowed by the insurance carrier
- Amount disallowed or not eligible for payment
- The deductible deducted
- Copayment or coinsurance amount due from the patient
- Total amount paid by the insurance carrier
- Comments explaining why payment was denied, asking for more information, or specifying coordination of benefits

This report should be reviewed carefully to determine whether further action is necessary. Each check is entered into the bookkeeping system by patient account with a notation showing the source of the payment. If, after this payment, the patient owes a balance, he or she should be notified that the insurance carrier has paid its portion and that the patient is now responsible for the unpaid balance.

Occasionally, it is necessary to make adjustments in the bookkeeping system to write off *(deduct)* amounts that cannot be collected. The balance of the patient's account is reduced by the amount of the adjustment.

Handling Overpayments

If the patient has paid his or her account and a check also arrives from the insurance carrier, this procedure must be followed to handle the resulting overpayment:

- Credit the check from the carrier to the patient's account, and deposit it as any other payment on account. Crediting the check to the patient's account will create a credit; insurance carriers report to the IRS how much they paid to each dentist, and it is important that the practice records show the receipt of these funds.
- Write a check from the practice to the patient to refund the amount of the overpayment. This check is from the accounts payable system and shows up as a practice expense.
- Make an entry on the account ledger showing that the check was sent. This will eliminate the credit balance on the account.
- Because the funds received and the refund check are equal, the total amount of taxable income for the practice is not increased.

Insurance Fraud

The business assistant is responsible for accurate and honest claims submission. It is important for the assistant to understand the consequences of submitting fraudulent claims even if it is the dentist's idea. An assistant cannot escape liability by pleading ignorance; therefore it is necessary to understand what constitutes fraud. To commit fraud is to lie or deceive someone for unlawful gain. Some examples of dental insurance fraud are as follows:

- Billing for services not provided
- Changing fees on a claim form to obtain a higher payment
- Disregarding a copayment or deductible, accepting only the insurance payment, and writing off the difference

Recall

17. What are the three most commonly used methods of calculating fee-for-service benefits?
18. ____________ is a specified amount of money that an insured person must pay before the insurance goes into effect.
19. A child or spouse of an insurance subscriber is considered to be a ____________.
20. Is it possible to be covered under two insurance policies?
21. How is insurance submitted?
22. What category of service would include radiographs?
23. What category of service would include amalgam restorations?
24. What category of service would include a full denture?
25. What category of service would include root planing and curettage?

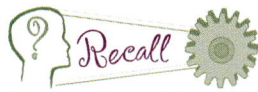

Patient Education

The office manager or business assistant has the important task of discussing financial obligations with a patient. The discussion of money can be one of the most time-consuming and stressful parts of your job. Because discussing finances involves the personal realm of a patient, it is important to remember that patients must be respected for who they are, not for what they have. Try to present as much information as possible prior to treatment—for example, asking about insurance coverage, explaining what the patient is responsible for, and discussing how payments can be handled.

Eye to the Future

In the area of financial matters, you will never see an automatic self-checkout in the medical and dental setting as you have probably seen in some grocery and department stores. Dental and medical services are personal and require a more respectful and individual way of handling finances. Even so, with the increasing use of debit cards, the traditional paper check will one day be a thing of the past, and deductions will be made directly from one of the patient's personal accounts.

Legal and Ethical Implications

The responsibility placed on the business assistant in keeping the financial records current and up to date shows a great trust in that person. It is in turn important to keep accurate and completed daily procedures for all accounts receivable and accounts payable systems. Keep an open communication network with the dentist and accountant regarding all transactions of the day-to-day business of a dental practice.

Critical Thinking

1. A patient is checking out and wishes to pay today's fees ($76.00), as well as an outstanding account ($320.00). The patient writes a check for $400.00. How do you record this payment?
2. It takes an enormous amount of fortitude and courage to collect money from a patient. Examine your thoughts and feelings regarding collections and describe your style of asking for payment on an account.
3. Discuss your thoughts on searching a patient's credit background. When do you think it would not be necessary and when would it be necessary in a dental practice?
4. As the business assistant for the office, one of your job responsibilities is to prepare the staff payroll. Do you think that this should be a job of the business assistant? Why or why not? If so, how important is it for you to maintain confidentiality of each staff member's salary?
5. A woman who is not a patient of the practice came in today for an emergency. When checking out, she hands you her dental insurance card. Your dental office does not accept this type of insurance, and she does not have any other means of payment. How could this have been prevented, and what do you do now?

64

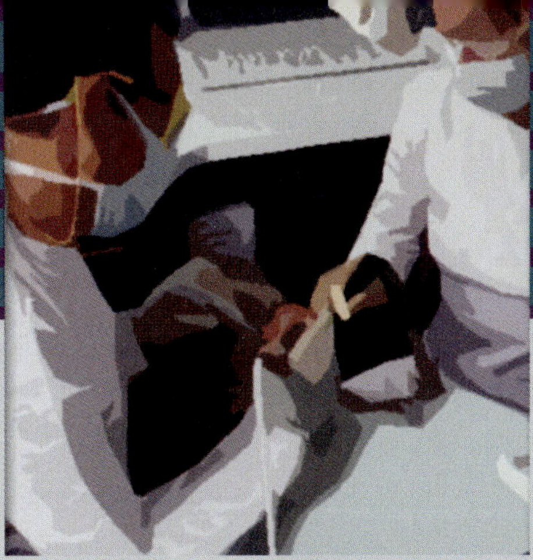

Marketing Your Skills

Outline

LEARNING OUTCOMES

On completion of this chapter, the student will be able to achieve the following objectives:

- Determine career goals and develop a personal philosophy.
- Identify potential career opportunities.
- Describe the preparation and demeanor needed for a job interview.
- Prepare a follow-up letter.
- Discuss factors to consider in salary negotiations.
- Discuss the elements of an employment agreement.
- Describe the steps for achieving career objectives.
- Describe the steps for job termination.

PERFORMANCE OUTCOMES

On completion of this chapter, the student will be able to achieve competency in the following skills:

- Prepare a letter of application.
- Prepare a professional resume.

As you complete your education, you will begin to identify and assess the kind of employment you will be seeking. Your knowledge, skills, and attitude will enable you to select a career in which your needs and capabilities are met and a setting in which you will be recognized as a valuable employee.

YOUR PROFESSIONAL CAREER

You have many resources to offer to a potential employer. It is important to analyze your qualifications and career direction. From this, you can determine what type of employment you are looking for and what type of environment is compatible with your needs.

Goals and Philosophy

Ultimately, you are responsible for your personal and professional development. This means that you need to ask yourself what you want to accomplish in your work and your personal life. You can establish concrete professional goals that focus on your talents and accomplishments. Your personal philosophy should reflect your commitments, values, and concerns as they relate to future employment.

Career Opportunities

Given your education and the many opportunities available within dental assisting, you have a wide range of employment choices from which to choose. This range of choices will open doors to new and exciting career choices.

Private Practice

Traditionally, independent private practitioners have delivered dental care in the United States. These practitioners provide a wide range of professional services for their patients. A private practice can take the form of a solo practice or a nonsolo practice; a nonsolo practice can involve additional dentists as associates, a partnership, or a group practice. The American Dental Association definition states that a nonsolo dentist works "in a practice with at least one other dentist. Some of these dentists may be employed by the owner dentist in the practice."

A nonsolo practice may be composed of almost any number and variety of general practitioners and specialists working in a shared facility. The benefits of being employed in a larger group include:

- Opportunities to develop more specialized skills
- Professional stimulation and sociability of working with many other auxiliaries
- Greater opportunity for advancement
- Potential for a more extensive program of employee benefits than can be offered by a solo practitioner

Insurance

Dental insurance companies are continually looking for skillful dental assistants to contribute to their organizations. Depending on your skills and interests, you could consider a challenging career in business and administrative procedures that incorporates your knowledge of dentistry, the processing of claims, and customer service.

Sales

There are many dental manufacturing companies that will seek out individuals with a background in dentistry. If you are outgoing, find it easy to approach new people, have experience in dental assisting, and like to travel, you may find sales to be a rewarding career.

Research

Hospitals hire dental assistants to work in their dental clinics or within research laboratories. These positions generally require you to be responsible for researching, report writing, and calculating and analyzing a wide range of data.

Management Consulting

Experienced dental assistants with managerial and clinical backgrounds bring their expertise to dental practices through consulting firms. Many assistants either join an existing consulting firm or provide the resources and support to start their own. Their purpose is to develop customized practice management concepts for individual dental practices that are interested in increasing employee satisfaction, achieving economic success, and improving communication and management skills.

Teaching

Employment as an instructor in a dental assisting program is a challenging and rewarding career option for the ambitious dental assistant. Each school and state has requirements for teacher certification. These vary and may include prescribed college courses in educational methodology, at

Factors to Remember When Seeking Employment

You want to feel physically, psychologically, and socially comfortable in your work environment.

You want to select an employer whom you respect and whose philosophy of practice parallels your beliefs.

You want to find the type of employment situation that will be the most stimulating, interesting, and rewarding for you—one that will provide professional and personal growth.

You want to be able to work well with other members of the dental health team to achieve mutual respect and shared values.

least a bachelor's degree, and certification or registration as a dental assistant.

An assistant who would enjoy teaching should continue taking college courses in related sciences and education on a part-time basis while simultaneously gaining valuable work experience in the dental office.

Dental Schools

Educationally qualified and experienced dental assistants are employed by dental schools to work in clinical settings to provide dental students with experience in four-handed dentistry. Employment in a dental school provides the assistant with the stimulation of working in an educational setting with faculty, students, and patients.

Hospitals

Dental care often is provided in hospitals for those special situations in which general anesthesia and the other resources of a hospital are required. Some hospitals hire qualified assistants to participate in these special situations.

Public Health and Government Programs

Public health and other government-supported dental facilities function at the federal, state, and local levels. Dental public health programs promote dental health through organized community efforts. Dental assistants may be employed in programs in which dental services are provided at no cost or minimal cost to patients who are eligible to receive care. Public health practices almost always involve a team effort with other professionals such as physicians, nurses, social workers, and nutritionists.

These settings generally also collect data and report statistics on specific public health issues and services such as fluoridation, incidence of acquired immunodeficiency syndrome (AIDS), and care for older adults or specific population groups, including Native Americans and migrant workers.

Recall

1. List the nine basic employment choices from which a dental assistant may choose.

LOCATING EMPLOYMENT OPPORTUNITIES

Once you have determined potential areas of employment, it is important to be knowledgeable about employment sources. This will assist you in finding the position and employer you seek.

Newspaper Advertisements

Newspaper advertisements are an excellent employment source. Frequently, dentists place classified advertisements describing the position available and the requirements. The employer will include a telephone number if he or she wishes to speak to you directly or ask that you send your letter of application and resume to a box address. This is known as a *blind box* advertisement; it gives the employer an opportunity to screen prospective employees before scheduling an interview.

Campus Placement

If you are attending a formal dental assisting program, the school usually offers a placement service or has a list of employment opportunities with practicing dentists in the area. Dentists frequently contact dental assisting schools for new employees.

Employment Agencies

Employment agencies are found in almost all regions, and most states offer employment services and employment opportunity information free of charge. Private employment agencies charge a fee if they help you find a position, but over the past decade, employment agencies have changed their fee policy from applicant-paid to employer-paid. The agencies are paid on a contingency-fee basis, and the placement fees are calculated based on a percentage of the projected monthly or annual starting salary of the applicant.

Temporary Agencies

Temporary employment can be an ideal route to finding permanent employment. It is not always possible to be certain on the basis of a resume and one interview whether the dental practice and the prospective employee are a good match for each other. By working temporarily in a variety of settings, you have a chance to evaluate firsthand the responsibilities and challenges involved in a given position.

Many assistants prefer temporary work because it is usually short-term or part-time and ideal for employees with the responsibility of young children. However, most temporary services offer a temporary-to-permanent conversion if desired.

Dental Supply Companies

The sales representatives who call on dental offices in the area frequently know when a dentist is looking for a qualified assistant. When you are seeking employment, inform the salesperson about the type of employment you prefer.

Professional Organizations

Local dental society and dental assistant organizations frequently serve as informal employment information centers. Many local dental societies publish monthly news bulletins in which it may be possible to place a classified advertisement or be placed on a hiring list. Professional journals also have a classified section of possible job opportunities.

Recall

2. Where might a dentist advertise for a job position?

SEEKING EMPLOYMENT

As you embark on your job search, you need to represent and sell your qualifications to warrant an employment interview. Given below are the specific stages that will assist you in your job search.

Telephone Contact

Your first contact with a prospective employer will probably be by telephone. When you call, identify yourself and explain your reasons for calling. The first impression over the telephone is very important because if you do not make a good impression here, you may not get a second chance to prove yourself in an interview. You may be asked to submit a completed application or a resume before the interview.

Letter of Application

A well-written cover letter, or letter of application, serves to introduce you to your prospective employer and markets your skills and qualifications at the same time. It also serves to create interest on the part of the reader to look at your resume. A variety of approaches and styles are available, but the following are some general guidelines (Fig. 64-1):

- Your letter should be brief, professional, and neat. One page is sufficient.
- The letter should be printed on white or ivory bond paper.
- Address your letter to a specific person.
- If responding to an advertisement, identify the advertisement and its source, such as the newspaper in which it appeared.
- Identify the position for which you are applying.
- Request an interview.
- Give appropriate contact numbers where you can be reached.
- Thank the recipient for his or her consideration.

A letter of application can be completed in three paragraphs. The first paragraph serves to introduce yourself, states how you found out about the position, and your interest in applying for the position. The second paragraph tells why you feel you deserve the position. The third paragraph invites the dentist to contact you. Let the employer know that you are available for an interview *at his or her convenience.* Make sure the phone number you give is a number where you can be reached personally.

Resume

The resume is a very important marketing tool that is designed to interest prospective employers (Fig. 64-2). It should present a summary of your skills and qualifications in a positive and professional manner. The primary purpose of the resume is to convince a potential employer that you are a qualified candidate for employment and that it would be well worth his or her time to interview you in person. There are different resume styles to consider, but the style you choose should fit the type of job you want, your qualifications, and the actual job opening. The appearance of the resume is extremely important because it may represent the first physical contact with a prospective employer; therefore a well-organized, concise, neat resume is vital. Include the following information:

Heading

This consists of three items: your full name (with credentials if appropriate), complete address, and appropriate telephone number or numbers; this information is most often centered at the top of the page.

Professional Objective

This is a clear statement of the type of job you are seeking; however, it should not be so narrowly stated that it limits your job opportunities.

Professional Experience

List your work experiences in order, beginning with the most recent. For each job, provide the dates (month and years only) of your employment, your position or title, the employer's name and location, and your responsibilities and accomplishments.

Education

List your most recent educational level obtained. You may list all degree programs you have completed, but if you have a college degree, do not list your high school graduation. If you took special courses or received honors that may be of interest to your potential employer, you may want to make note of them here.

Alicia Moore, CDA
121 Pleasant Drive
Any City, US 27740
(000) 555-1212
almoore@internet.com

Date, 20XX

Dr. Name
123 Cherry Lane
Any City, US 27740

Re: Clinical Assistant Position

Dear Dr. Name:

I am applying for the Clinical Assistant position advertised in the Any City newspaper.

I am a Certified Dental Assistant and a graduate of the Area Accredited School of Dental Assisting. My enclosed resume provides additional information about my experience and background in the dental field.

I would appreciate the opportunity to schedule an interview with you and your staff at your earliest convenience. I can also be reached on my cell phone at (000) 965-1255.

Thank you in advance for your consideration, and I look forward to hearing from you.

Sincerely,

Alicia Moore, CDA

Fig. 64-1 Letter of application.

Certifications

List your licensure, cardiopulmonary resuscitation (CPR) certification, and any other appropriate certification information. Emphasize career-related affiliations. It is not recommended that personal data be included on your resume.

Under federal Equal Employment Opportunity regulations, employers may not ask questions regarding race, color, religion, gender, national origin, marital status, and child care arrangements unless they relate to bona fide occupational qualifications. However, you may be required to submit verification of citizenship or appropriate alien status.

It is not recommended that "References on Request" be included on the resume, but you may have a list of references available if the prospective employer requests them.

Electronic Resume

Many companies process incoming resumes by using electronic scanners and computers. Knowing how to post your resume on the Internet will be beneficial as an increasing number of dental offices go online to look for potential employment candidates. For more details, see Procedure 64-1.

Alicia Moore, CDA
121 Pleasant Drive
Any City, US 27740
(000) 555-1212
almoore@internet.com

PROFESSIONAL OBJECTIVE:

Clinical Assistant with a pediatric or general dental practice.

PROFESSIONAL EXPERIENCE:

6/20XX to Present	**Clinical Assistant**, Dr. Janice Davison, New City, US Part-time employment (List your responsibilities and accomplishments here)
6/20XX to 9/20XX	**Coordinating Assistant**, Dr. Harold Randolph, Top City, US (List your responsibilities and accomplishments here)
1/20XX to 5/20XX	**Student Intern**, Dr. Janice Davison, New City, US (List your responsibilities and accomplishments here)

EDUCATION:

9/20XX to 6/20XX	Area Accredited School of Dental Assisting, Any City, US Graduated on Dean's List.
20XX to 20XX	Any City High School, Graduate City, US

CERTIFICATIONS:

Date, 20XX	Currently Certified Dental Assistant
Date, 20XX	Applied for Registered Dental Assistant
Date, 20XX	Treasurer of local Dental Assistants' Society, Any City, US

Fig. 64-2 An example of a professional resume.

Completing a Job Application Form

Before your interview, you may be asked to complete an application form. This will serve as the initial basis of your conversation with the interviewer. In completing this form, be sure that you *follow directions exactly* and that the information you give is accurate, neat, and complete.

The Interview

The employment interview is an all-important exchange of information and impressions. This is when you gather information to help you determine whether you would be happy working for this dentist, with his or her staff, and in this practice. At the same time, the dentist is trying to determine whether you are the right employee for this position. If you have not already sent a resume, take a cover letter and resume along when you go to the interview, and leave it with the interviewer.

Appearance

Your appearance is very important. In selecting your clothing, you want your appearance to reflect the fact that you are a neat, well-organized, and competent professional. Do not wear your dental assisting uniform to an interview. It is best to wear conservative business attire. Keep jewelry and make-up to a minimum.

Procedure 64-1 Preparing a Professional Resume

Goal

To prepare a resume to be used for seeking employment.

PROCEDURAL STEPS

1. Keep the resume to one page (see Fig. 64-2).
2. Use a standard $8\frac{1}{2}$- × 11-inch white or ivory rag paper.
3. Use common typefaces.
4. Use 1-inch margins on all sides.
5. Use a 12-point font size.
6. Ensure that the resume is neat and error-free.
7. Make the resume concise and easy to read.

Presenting Yourself Professionally

You should plan to arrive 10 to 15 minutes before the scheduled time of the interview. If the interview is scheduled in a geographic area with which you are unfamiliar, it is advisable to take a "dry run" to find the office before the interview. In addition, make sure you arrive alone; you may think you need moral support, but you will appear unprofessional.

Interviewing Professionally

The first 10 minutes of your interview are the most critical because during this time, both you and the interviewer will have formed first impressions. You may be nervous, but try to relax and be natural. You can create a positive and professional impression by smiling, maintaining direct eye contact, offering a firm yet gentle handshake, and using words such as, "Hi, I'm [first name, last name]; it's a pleasure to meet you" (Fig. 64-3).

During the interview, many questions will be asked and answered on both sides. Try to answer all questions courteously, completely, and honestly. Be prepared for a variety of questions, and feel free to ask questions yourself if it seems to be an appropriate time. Remember that your attitude and motivation during the interview are important determining factors. You want to convey a positive attitude without overselling yourself.

Concluding the Interview

Let the prospective employer (or office manager) conclude the interview. If you believe the interview has concluded, you could say, "Do you have any other questions you would like to ask at this time?" Usually, the interviewer stands up to signal the conclusion of the interview. Make sure to extend your hand for a final handshake, and again use direct eye contact as you say, "I look forward to hearing from you." Within the first week after the interview, you will have developed some intuition of how the interview went, as well as whether the office is one in which you would like to pursue employment.

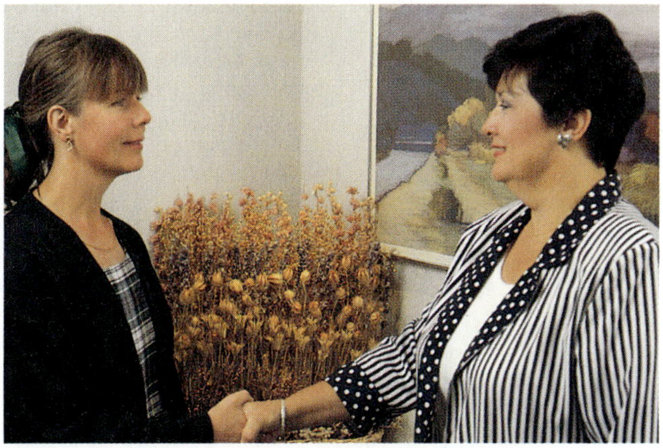

Fig. 64-3 Your first impression is very important.

Follow-Up Letter

A thank-you letter is an excellent way to follow up with an employer after an interview. It serves to remind the employer of your interview, to accentuate your qualifications, to reaffirm your interest in the position, and to help you stand out in the interviewer's mind. The letter should be sent within 48 hours, be addressed to the person with whom you interviewed, and reaffirm your interest in the position in the practice. Make sure the letter is thoughtful and sincere (Fig. 64-4).

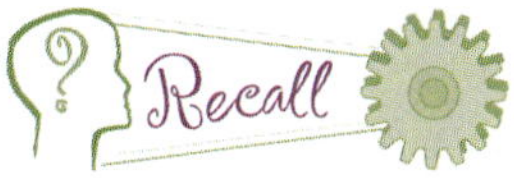

3. What is the most common means of communication for your first contact with a future employer?
4. What does a cover letter do?
5. Should a resume list your gender, race, religion, and marital status?
6. How many pages should a resume be?
7. When is the most critical part of the interview?

Alicia Moore, CDA
121 Pleasant Drive
Any City, US 27740
(000) 555-1212
almoore@internet.com

Date, 20XX

Dr. Name and Staff
123 Cherry Lane
Any City, US 27740

Dear Dr. Name and Staff:

Thank you for taking time out of your busy schedule to interview me last Tuesday, October 25th. I enjoyed our conversation and am very enthusiastic about the possibility of working with you and your staff.

I know that my clinical and communication skills would be an asset to your practice. Please do not hesitate to call me should you have any other questions.

Again, thank you for your consideration. I look forward to hearing from you in hopes that you have reached a decision favorable to both of us.

Sincerely,

Alicia Moore

Alicia Moore, CDA

Fig. 64-4 An example of a follow-up letter.

SALARY NEGOTIATIONS

Although salary and benefits are not the only factors to be considered when you are accepting a job, they are very important issues that need to be clarified. The interviewer may ask, "What do you expect in terms of salary?" If you have a definite and realistic idea, by all means state it. Keep in mind that education, experience, and skills are important factors that should be considered in a fair and equitable salary and benefits package.

As you negotiate your compensation package with the dentist, you should realize the importance of the total dollar value when benefits are added to salary, the amount of hours you will be working, and working conditions. This is an excellent opportunity to ask about the frequency of reviews, salary increases, and the opportunity to advance with the practice. Specific benefits to inquire about are:

- Health insurance
- Dental care for self and family
- Retirement plan
- Uniform allowance
- Dues toward professional organizations
- Travel expenses for professional meetings
- Bonuses

EMPLOYMENT AGREEMENT

Before you accept a position, there are several topics that you need to explore with the dentist or office manager. Reaching a clear understanding of these topics when you are offered the position is important because it can prevent later misunderstandings.

This process is best managed through the completion of an employment agreement. An **employment agreement** is prepared in duplicate and is signed by both employer and employee (Fig. 64-5). One copy is retained in the personnel file, and the other is given to the employee for his or her records. The agreement should cover the following topics:

Job Description Your job description states specifically what your employment duties and responsibilities will be.

Work Schedule This is a list of the hours and days you will routinely be expected to work. If this schedule varies, it is important to know how far in advance these changes will be announced.

EMPLOYMENT AGREEMENT

(Complete form in duplicate: one copy for the employer; one copy for the employee.)

EMPLOYEE'S NAME Debbie Quigley, CDA

Date 11/08/XX Full time/Part Time fulltime

JOB TITLE Chairside assistant to Dr. Hernandez

See attached list for details of duties and responsibilities:

PRACTICE WORK SCHEDULE

(Your hours will be scheduled within these times.)

Usual days per week: S ___ M ✓ T ✓ W 1/2 Th ✓ F ✓ S 1/2

Usual working hours: 8:30 to 5:30; lunch 1 hr; breaks ___.

Work schedules are posted: two weeks in advance. Assigned hours may vary

SALARY AND BENEFITS

Pay days: every other friday Starting rate: $XX. per hour

Basis for increases: review at 6 months, then annually

Vacation days: 5; Sick days: 5; Personal time: 2.

Additional benefits: group insurance is available retirement plan after 3 years

TERMINATION

For each new employee, the first 6 weeks are a provisional period of employment. During this time, the new employee may leave or be dismissed without notice.

After this period, the employee is expected to give 2 weeks notice.

If dismissed, the employee will receive 2 weeks notice or the equivalent in severance pay.

In the event of fraud, theft, illegal drug use, or unprofessional conduct, the employee may be dismissed without notice or severance pay.

Debbie Quigley, CDA — Employee's signature

J. Hernandez, DDS — Employer's signature

Fig. 64-5 An example of an employment agreement.

Compensation This section covers agreements regarding salary and benefits plus provisions for performance reviews and salary increases. It may also cover items such as payment of required registration fees, association dues, and continuing education costs.

Professional Attire Required personal protective equipment must be provided and maintained by the employer. If there are other uniform requirements, you need to know who is responsible for supplying and maintaining them.

Termination Most employers routinely consider the first several weeks to 90 days as provisional employment, during which either party may terminate the relationship without notice. At the end of this period, the new employee should receive a performance review.

Summary Dismissal Summary dismissal is termination without notice or severance pay. The causes for summary dismissal include stealing, the use of illegal drugs, or any other form of unprofessional behavior.

Giving Notice The agreement should clarify how much notice you are expected to give should you decide to terminate your employment. The agreement should also cover what happens if the dentist decides to terminate your employment. One common agreement is that you will receive 2 weeks' notice or severance pay.

Recall

8. What time frame is usually considered provisional employment?
9. What is the term for termination without notice or severance pay?

AMERICANS WITH DISABILITIES ACT

The 1992 American with Disabilities Act (ADA) is commonly believed to pertain only to disabled people seeking access to public accommodations and health care, but the act also applies to job applicants and current employees.

Title I of the act specifically makes it illegal for an employer to discriminate against prospective job applicants on the basis of disability. An employer is required to make an accommodation to the known disability of a qualified applicant or employee if it would not impose an "undue hardship" on the operation of the employer's business. Undue hardship is defined as an action requiring significant difficulty or expense when considering factors such as an employer's size, financial resources, and the nature and structure of the operation. An employer is not required to lower quality or production standards to make an accommodation, nor is an employer obligated to provide personal use items such as glasses or hearing aids.

Title I also makes it illegal for the employer to discriminate against employees of the practice who may become disabled. If a dental staff member becomes disabled while in the employment of the dentist, the law requires that the employer make reasonable accommodations (i.e., take action within reason) to continue employment of that person at the same rate of pay. The dentist may not discharge an employee on the basis of disability without the employee's consent.

This law applies to companies that employ at least 15 people and thus may not apply to the practice for which you work. However, legal and economic realities are pushing small businesses into realizing the value of skilled workers with disabilities.

JOB TERMINATION

If it becomes necessary to terminate employment, it should be done in keeping with the terms of the employment agreement. The most common time frame is 2 weeks' notice. If you are leaving under friendly conditions, give adequate notice and, if asked, help select and train your replacement. It also is appropriate to request a letter of recommendation that may be helpful in finding other employment. If you are leaving under other circumstances, it is best to leave quickly and quietly.

If your employer terminates your employment, your departure should be handled in accordance with the terms of your employment agreement. Severance pay, which is the equivalent of salary for the notice period, is paid if you are asked to leave immediately on being notified of your dismissal. This is usually paid with the final paycheck. Your benefits termination also should be outlined in the employment agreement.

ACHIEVING CAREER OBJECTIVES

Achieving and maintaining career objectives and employment represent a two-sided situation. Team members have responsibilities as employees, and the dentist (or other group) has responsibilities as the employer. Before accepting employment, try to determine, through observation and by talking to other employees, whether the dentist does indeed carry out the responsibilities of a good employer. If it is apparent that the dentist does not, perhaps you should consider employment elsewhere.

Positive Attitude

A positive attitude is important in all aspects of our lives, including work. No single factor is more important in determining your professional success and achieving your career objectives than your own attitude. As a team player, a positive attitude goes a long way. It can reduce stress with the dental team and enhance your communication skills with the patients.

Professional Responsibilities

The dental assistant has many responsibilities as an employee of a dental practice. The following is a list of the responsibilities of a truly professional employee:

- To comply with the local, state, and federal laws and regulations governing the practice of dentistry in which the practice is located.
- To acquire and maintain all required professional credentials, such as in CPR and appropriate state registration.
- To maintain high personal and professional ethical standards that result in pleasant, respectful, and professional interactions with *all* patients and staff members.
- To be honest, cooperative, and responsible.
- To be punctual and on duty at all assigned times. (If an absence is unavoidable, the employee should make advance arrangements to ensure that his or her position is covered.)
- To carefully follow the instructions given and work to the best of his or her ability.
- To realize that supervision, feedback, and criticism are occasionally necessary and to be able to respond to these in a constructive manner.
- To give proper due notice to the employer should it become necessary to seek other employment.

The dentist also has responsibilities as the employer of the practice. The following are some of the duties of a true professional employer:

- The employer must comply with the local, state, and federal laws and regulations governing the practice of dentistry and the hiring of employees.
- The employer must treat all employees with professional and personal dignity and respect in an atmosphere that will motivate and encourage employees to do their best.
- The employer must establish and maintain fair employment policies and practices to provide safe and pleasant working conditions for all.
- The employer or office manager should conduct a performance review for each employee at least once a year. This review, which is conducted in private, is a discussion of the employee's job skills, attitudes, contributions to the practice, and areas of strength and weakness. A written copy of this report is given to the employee, and another copy is maintained in the personnel file.

Physical Well-Being

Physical well-being is reflected in all aspects of your life. Maintaining a healthy lifestyle is an important part of successful employment. As a dental professional, you need to focus on areas of your life that will lead to a lifelong commitment to sound physical and mental health. In day-to-day terms, the attainment and maintenance of health include exercising regularly, making wise food choices, getting sufficient sleep, maintaining friendships, and indulging in a diversity of interests.

Your professional image is very important. You should always look professional by having healthy skin, a neat and clean hair style that does not fall in your face or in that of the patient, and appropriate clothing. Clinical personnel should follow Occupational Safety and Health Administration (OSHA) regulations, and business personnel should dress in professional businesslike clothes. As a healthcare professional, you should be a reflection of the quality of care provided in your practice.

Recall

10. What is the most important factor in determining your professional success?

Patient Education

As a professional healthcare provider, it will be up to you to educate your patients about your profession. Your patients are unaware of your educational background, your qualifications, and your role in a dental practice. Begin by displaying your credentials, describing your role in their care when they first come to the practice, and introducing new techniques as you use them. The more patients are aware of their surroundings, the more they feel confident in the care that is provided for them.

Legal and Ethical Implications

As an employee, plan to observe all office protocols such as presenting yourself professionally, working the scheduled hours, practicing business or clinical functions, and representing the dentist and his or her practice. If the state in which you will practice has regulations and guidelines, know those boundaries so that you perform only what is legal for you to practice.

Eye to the Future

Developments in technology, procedures, new materials, and research will continue to challenge the practice of dentistry. The role of the dental assistant will become more complex and efficient. Research has shown that the productivity and income of dentists can be greatly improved with the use of qualified assistants and hygienists. This should encourage states to permit a wider range of expanded functions and challenging job opportunities for assistants.

Critical Thinking

1. Review the Wednesday or Sunday classified section of your local newspaper. Select the dental assisting job opportunities that interest you. Discuss why those ads appeal to you.
2. List the strengths and weaknesses of your extern sites. Based on these, try to develop criteria for your ideal working environment.
3. Your instructor has told you that a local dentist has a clinical position available. What is your plan of action in pursuing this position?
4. You have been on the job now for 2 weeks, and you are just not happy with your position. What should you do?
5. At the end of the day, your dentist calls you into his or her office and asks you to have a seat. The dentist indicates that you are not working out as well as hoped and that your last day will be this Friday. You are completely shocked by this comment and are not sure why this has happened. How do you handle this situation?

References

Abrahams PH, Marks SC Jr, and Hutchins RT: *McMinn's color atlas of human anatomy,* ed 5, St Louis, 2003, Mosby.

American Association of Dental Schools: Function, aging, oral health for professionals, 1989.

Bath-Balogh MJ, Fehrenbach MB: *Illustrated embryology, histology, and anatomy,* ed 2, St Louis, 2005, Saunders.

Bernie M: Get the facts on tooth whitening, ADHA Factsheet.

Berthold M: Anesthesia color codes: new system helps recognition, increases safety. *Journal of the American Dental Association,* June 2003.

Best Practice for Sealants, *Dimensions of Dental Hygiene,* July 2004.

Black T: Incorporating a professional whitening program in your practice. *California Dental Hygienists Association Journal,* volume 16, no 2.

Budenz A: Local anesthetics and medically complex patients, *Journal of the California Dental Association,* August 2000.

CDA: Waste management guide for dental offices, California Dental Association, March 2004.

Centers for Disease Control and Prevention: *MMWR Morbidity, and Mortality Weekly Report,* 19 December 2003.

Daniel SJ and Harfst SA: *Mosby's dental hygiene: concepts, cases, and competencies-2004 update,* St Louis, 2004, Mosby.

Darby M, Walsh M: *Dental hygiene: theory and practice,* ed 2, Philadelphia, 2003, Saunders.

Featherstone JBD: The caries balance: contributing factors and early detection, *Journal of the California Dental Association,* February 2003.

Fehrenbach MJ, Herring SW: *Illustrated anatomy of the head and neck,* ed 2, Philadelphia, 2001, Saunders.

Finkbeiner B: Four handed dentistry revisited, *Journal of Contemporary Dental Practice,* November 2000.

Haring J, Jansen Howerton L: *Dental radiography: principles and techniques,* ed 3, Philadelphia, 2005, Saunders.

Ibsen O, Phelan J: *Oral pathology for the dental hygienist,* ed 4, St Louis, 2004, Saunders.

Johnson W: *Color atlas of endodontics,* St Louis, 2002, Saunders.

Lynch H, Milgrom P: Xylitol and dental caries: an overview for clinicians, *Journal of the California Dental Association,* March 2003.

Malamed SF: *Handbook of local anesthesia,* ed 5, St Louis, 2004, Mosby.

Miller C, Palenik C: *Infection control and management of hazardous materials for the dental team,* ed 3, St Louis, 2004, Mosby.

Mosby: *Spanish terminology for the dental team,* St Louis, 2003, Mosby.

National Institutes of Health Consensus Statement: Diagnosis and management of dental caries throughout life, 2001.

National Institutes of Health: The Seventh Report of the Joint National Committee on Prevention, Detection, Evaluation, and Treatment of High Blood Pressure: Hypertension Guidelines (brochure), 2003.

Organization for Safety and Asepsis Procedures (OSAP): OSAP from policy to practice: OSAP's Guide to the Guidelines, March 2003.

Ring ME: *Dentistry: an illustrated history,* St Louis, 1985, Abradale Press, Mosby.

Roberson T, et al: *Sturdevant's art and science of operative dentistry,* St Louis, 2002, Mosby.

Samaranayake LP: *Essential microbiology for dentistry,* ed 2, St Louis, 2001, Churchill Livingstone.

Spolarich A: Adverse drug effects, *Access,* December 1995.

Spolarich A: Drugs used to manage medical emergencies, *Access,* March 2000.

Spolarich A: Managing emergencies, *Access,* September 2002.

Sultanov D: Full denture relining using Tokuso rebase, *Dental Products Report,* April 2001.

Glossary

Abandonment Withdrawing a patient from treatment without giving reasonable notice or providing a competent replacement. (5)
Abdominal cavity Contains the stomach, liver, gallbladder, spleen, and most of the intestines. (6)
Abdominopelvic Part of the ventral cavity containing the abdominal and pelvic cavities. (6)
Abducens nerve (ab-**doo**-sens) Sixth cranial nerve, which serves eye muscle. (9)
Abscess (**ab**-*ses*) A localized accumulation of pus in a cavity formed by tissue disintegration. (17) (54)
Absorption The passage of a substance into the interior of another by solution or penetration. (30)
Abutment (ah-**but**-ment) A tooth, root, or implant used for support and retention of a fixed or removable prosthesis. (50)
Accounting A system designed to maintain financial records of a business. (63)
Accounts payable A dollar amount owed to creditors for items or services purchased from them. (63)
Acquired immunity Immunity that is developed during a person's lifetime. (19)
Acrylate (ak-**ri**-late) A salt or ester of acrylic acid. (59)
Active files Patients that have been seen within the past 2 to 3 years. (62)
Acute (ah-**kyut**) Pertaining to a traumatic, pathologic, or physiologic phenomenon or process having a short and relatively severe course. (31, 54)
Acute exposure High levels of exposure over a short period. (23)
Acute infection An infection of short duration that is often severe. (19)
Adhere To stick or glue two items together. (43)
Administrative law Category of law that involves regulations established by government agencies. (5)
Aerobes (**air**-ohbz) A variety of bacteria that require oxygen in order to grow. Compare with anaerobes and facultative. (18)
Agar (**a**-gar) Gelatin type material derived from seaweed. (46)
Ala (**ah**-la) Winglike tip of the outer side of each nostril; plural *alae.* (10)
ALARA concept Acronym for As Low As Reasonably Achievable; pertains to radiation exposure encountered when taking x-rays. This idea requires that every possible precaution is taken to limit radiation levels when exposing the patient or technician to radiation. (38)
Alert To bring attention to by making someone aware. (26)
Alginate (**al**-jeh-nate) A salt of alginic acid (for example, sodium alginate), which, when mixed with water in accurate proportions, forms an irreversible hydrocolloid gel used for making impressions. (46)
Allergen (**a**-ler-jen) A substance capable of producing an allergic response. Comon allergens are pollens, dust, drugs, and foods. (31)
Allergy (**a**-ler-jee, **al**-er-jee) A hypersensitive reaction of the body to an allergen; an antigen-antibody reaction is manifested in several forms – anaphylaxis, asthma, hay fever, urticaria, angioedema, dermatitis, and stomatitis. (31)
Alloy A solution composed of two metals dissolved in each other when in the liquid state. (43)
Aluminum crown Thin aluminum crown used for provisional coverage on posterior teeth. (51)
Alveoplasty (al-**vee**-o-*plas*-tee) The surgical shaping and smoothing of the margins of the tooth socket after extraction of the tooth, generally in preparation for the placement of a prosthesis. (52, 56)
Alzheimer's disease (**als**-hi-merz) A presenile dementia characterized by confusion, memory failure, disorientation, restlessness, agnosia, hallucinosis, speech disturbances, and the inability to carry out purposeful movement. The disease usually begins in later middle life with slight defects in memory and behavior that become progressively more severe. (29)
Amalgam (ah-**mal**-gum) An alloy, one of the constituents of which is mercury. (43)
Ameloblasts (a-**mel**-o-*blasts*) Epithelial cells associated with the tooth bud which, during tooth formation, secretes the tooth enamel. (8)
American Dental Assistants Association (ADAA) An organization representing the professional interests of dental assistants. (2)
American Dental Association (ADA) A nonprofit professional association whose membership is made up of dentists in the United States. Its purpose is to assist its members in providing the highest professional and ethical care to the citizens of the United States and to serve as an advocate for the advancement of the profession. (22)
Amino acids (ah-**me**-no) Compounds in proteins used by the body to build and repair tissue. (16)
Anaerobes (**a**-nuh-robz) Microorganisms that can exist and grow only in the partial or complete absence of molecular oxygen. (18)
Analgesia (*a*-nul-**jee**-zee-ah, *a*-nul-**jee**-zhuh) Insensibility to pain without loss of consciousness; a state in which painful stimuli are not perceived or interpreted as pain; usually induced by a drug, although trauma or a disease process may produce a general or regional analgesia. (37)
Analogy (ah-**na**-leh-jee) Comparison of similarities between things that are otherwise unlike. (57)
Anaphylaxis (*a*-nah-fah **lak**-sis) A violent allergic reaction characterized by sudden collapse, shock, or respiratory and circulatory failure after injection of an allergen. (19, 31)
Anatomic (*a*-neh-**tah**-mik) Pertaining to the anatomy of a structure. (47)
Anatomic crown That portion of dentin covered by enamel. (8)
Anatomical (anatomic) position (*an*-eh-**tom**-i-kul, *an*-eh-**tom**-ik) The human body is standing erect and facing forward, with the arms at the sides and the palms facing up. (6)
Anatomy (ah-**nat**-eh-mee) The science of the form, structure, and parts of animal organisms. (6)
Anemia (ah-**nee**-me-ah) A term indicating that the concentration of hemoglobin or the number of red blood cells is below the accepted normal value with respect to age and sex. In true anemia the total concentration of hemoglobin, or the total number or erythrocytes, is below normal regardless of concentration values. Symptoms, which may not be evident, include weakness, pallor, anorexia, and those related to the cause of anemia. (29)
Anesthesia (*a*-nuhs-**the**-zee-ah, *a*-nuhs-**the**-zhuh) Temporary loss of feeling or sensation. (37)
Anesthetic A drug that produces the temporary loss of feeling or sensation. (37)
Angina (an-**ji**-nah) Chest pain caused by inadequate oxygen to the heart. (31)
Angle of the mandible The lower posterior of the ramus. (10)
Angulation Alignment of central ray of x-ray beam in horizontal and vertical planes. (41)
Anode (**a**-node) The positive electrode in the x-ray tube. (38)
Anorexia nervosa (*a*-neh-**rek**-see-ah ner-**voh**-sah) Eating disorder caused by an altered self-image. (16)
Antecubital space (*an*-teh-**ku**-bi-tul) Small groove or fold in the inner arm, at or in front of *(anti)* the elbow *(cubitus).* (27)
Anterior Toward the front surface. (6, 11)
Anterior faucial pillar Anterior arch of the soft palate. (10)
Anterior jugular vein Vein that begins below the chin, descends near the midline, and drains into the external jugular vein. (9)
Anterior naris (**na**-ris) The nostril; plural *nares.* (10)
Antibodies Immunoglobulins produced by lymphoid tissue in response to a foreign substance. (31)
Antigen (**an**-ti-jen) A substance introduced into the body to stimulate the production of an antibody. (31)
Antiretraction device A mechanism that prevents entry of fluids and microorganisms into waterlines as a result of negative water pressure; also called "suck back." (24)
Antiseptic Substances for killing microorganisms on the skin. (20)
Apex Tapered end of each root tip. (8)

Apical curettage (**a-**pi-kul *kyur*-uh-**tahzh**) Surgical removal of infectious material surrounding the apex of a root. (54)

Apical foramen A natural opening in root. (8)

Apicoectomy (**a-**pi-ko-*ek*-teh-me) Surgical removal of the apical portion of the tooth through a surgical opening made in the overlying bone and gingival tissues. (54)

Appendicular (*ap*-pen-**dik-**u-ler) Referring to the body region that consists of the arms and legs. (6)

Appendicular skeleton (*ap*-pen-**dik-**u-ler) Portion of the skeleton that consists of the upper extremities and shoulder girdle plus the lower extremities and pelvic girdle. (7)

Arch wire A contoured metal wire that provides force when guiding teeth in movement for orthodontics. (60)

Arrhythmia (a-**rith-**me-a) Irregularity in the force or rhythm of the heartbeat. (27)

Arteries Large blood vessels that carry blood away from the heart. (7)

Arthritis (ar-**thri-**tis) Inflammation of a joint or many joints resulting in pain and swelling. (29)

Articular space (ar-**ti-**cue-lar) Space between the capsular ligament and between the surfaces of the glenoid fossa and the condyle. (9)

Articulations (*ahr*-tik-u-**lay-**shuns) Another term for joints. (7)

Articulator (ar-**ti-**kyuh-*lay*-tur) Dental laboratory device that simulates mandibular and temporomandibular joint movement when models of the dental arches are attached to it. (47, 50, 52)

Artifact An image on a radiograph that is not a structure but is caused by the technique. (40)

Artificially acquired immunity Immunity that results from a vaccination. (19)

Aspirate (**as-**puh-*rate*) To draw back or to draw within. (36, 37)

Aspiration (*as*-pah-**ray-**shun) The act of inhaling, or ingesting, as of a foreign object. (31)

Assessment Process of making an official evaluation of someone or a situation. (26)

Asthma (**az-**mah) Respiratory disease often associated with allergies and characterized by sudden recurring attacks of labored breathing, chest constriction, and coughing. (29, 31)

Athetosis (*ath*-ah-**toe-**sis) Type of involuntary movement of the body, face, and extremities. (57)

Atom The basic unit of matter. (38)

Atrophy (**a-**trah-fee) A wasting away or deterioration. (29)

Audit trail Method of tracking the accuracy and completeness of bookkeeping records. (63)

Autoclave (**aw-**toe-klave) Instrument for sterilization by means of moist heat under pressure. (21)

Auto-cured Hardened or set by a chemical reaction of two materials. (43)

Automatic processor Device that automates all film processing steps. (39)

Automatrix (*aw*-toe-**may-**triks) Matrix system designed to establish a temporary wall for tooth restoration without using a retainer. (49)

Autonomy (aw-**tah-**neh-me) Childhood process of becoming independent. (57)

Auxiliary (aug-**zil-**er-ee) Attachments located on brackets and bands that hold arch wires and elastics. (60)

Avulsed (ah-**vulst**) Torn away or dislodged by force. (57)

Axial (**ak-**see-al) Referring to the body region that comprises the head, neck, and trunk. (6)

Axial skeleton Portion of the skeleton that consists of the skull, spinal column, ribs, and sternum. (7)

Axial wall Internal surface of a cavity preparation positioned in the same vertical direction as the pulp within the tooth. (48)

Bacteremia (bak-tah-**ree-**me-ah) Presence of bacteria in the blood. (29)

Band Stainless steel ring attached to molars to hold the arch wire and auxiliaries for orthodontics. (60)

Base Foundation or the basic ingredient of a material. (46)

Baseplate Rigid, pre-formed shape used during the fitting of a full denture to represent the base of the denture. (52)

Beam alignment device Assists in the positioning of the PID. (39)

Bevel (**beh-**vul) Enamel margin of a tooth preparation. (50)

Beveled (**be-**vuld, **bev-**uld) Characterized by an angle of a surface that meets another angle. (34, 36)

Bicanineate Form of mandibular second premolar: two-cusp type. (12)

Bioburden Blood, saliva, and other body fluids. (20)

Biofilm (**buy-**oh-film) Slime-producing bacterial communities that may also harbor fungi, algae, and protozoa a. (24)

Biologic indicators Vials or strips, also known as *spore tests,* that contain harmless bacterial spores; used to determine if sterilization has occurred. (21)

Biologic monitor Verifies sterilization by confirming that all spore-forming microorganisms have been destroyed. (21)

Biopsy (**bi-**ahp-see) Removal of tissue from living patients for diagnostic examination. (17)

Bisecting (bisection of the angle) **technique** Intraoral technique of exposing periapical films. (41)

Bite-wing Radiographic view that shows the crowns of both arches on one film. (39)

Bite-wing film Type of film used in the interproximal examination. (41)

Blade Flat edge of instrument sharp enough to cut. (34)

Bleeding index Method of scoring the amount of bleeding present. (55)

Blood pressure Pressure exerted by the blood against the walls of the blood vessels. (27)

Board of dentistry State agency that adopts rules and regulations and implements the specific state's dental practice act. (5)

Bonding Form of insurance that reimburses an employer for a loss resulting from theft by an employee. (63)

Bone file Surgical instrument used to smooth rough edges of bone structure. (56)

Bone marrow Gelatinous material that produces either white blood cells, red blood cells, or platelets. (7)

Bookkeeping The process of managing financial accounts of a business. (63)

Border molding Process of using fingers to contour a closer adaptation of the margins of an impression while still in the mouth. (46,52)

Bow Rounded part of clamp that extends through the dental dam. (36)

Braces Another term for fixed orthodontic appliances. (60)

Brachial (**bray-**kee-ahl) Relating to the arm *(brachium),* as in *brachial artery.* (27)

Bracket A small device bonded to teeth to hold the arch wire to the teeth. (60)

Broad-spectrum activity Capable of killing a wide range of microbes. (20)

Bronchitis (brahn-**ki-**tis) Inflammation of the mucous membrane of the bronchial tubes. (29)

Buccal (**buke-**ul, **buh-**kul) Referring to structures closest to the inner cheek. (9)

Buccal surface Facial surface closest to the inner cheek. (11)

Buccal vestibule Area between cheeks and the teeth or alveolar ridge. (10)

Buffer time Time reserved on the schedule for emergency patients. (62)

Bulimia (boo-**lee-**me-ah) Eating disorder characterized by binge eating and self-induced vomiting. (16)

Calcium tungstate Common type of phosphor. (39)

Calculus (**kal-**kyou-lus) Calcium and phosphate salts in saliva that become mineralized and adhere to tooth surfaces. (14, 58)

Call list List made up of patients that can come in for an appointment on short notice. (62)

Cancellous bone (kan-**sil-**us) More lightweight bone found in the interior of bones. (7)

Candidiasis (kan-duh **die**-ah-sus) Superficial infection caused by a yeast like fungus. (17)
Canine eminence (e-meh-nen[t]s) External vertical bony ridge on the labial surface of the canines. (12)
Cannula (**kan**-yuh-lah) Flexible tube inserted into a body opening. (29)
Canthus (**kan**-thus) Fold of tissue at the corner of the eyelids. (10)
Capillaries A system of microscopic vessels that connect arterial and venous system. (7)
Carcinoma (kar-sih-**no**-muh) Malignant tumor in epithelial tissue. (17)
Cardiopulmonary resuscitation (CPR) (*kar*-dee-oh-**pul**-mah-nare-ee ri-*seh*-sah-**tay**-shun) A planned action for restoring consciousness or life. (31)
Caries (**kar**-ez) Tooth decay. (13)
Cariogenic Producing or promoting tooth decay. (16)
Carotid (ka-**rot**-id) Relating to either of the two major arteries on each side of the neck that carry blood to the head. (27)
Carpal tunnel syndrome (CTS) Pain associated with continued flexion and extension of the wrist. (25)
Carrier The insurance company that pays the claims and collects premiums. (63)
Cartilage Tough connective, nonvascular, elastic tissue. (7)
Cassette Holder for extraoral films during exposure. (39)
Cast post Metal post placed into the root canal of an endodontically treated tooth to improve the retention of a cast restoration. (50)
Catalyst (**ka**-tul-ust) Substance that modifies or increases the rate of a chemical reaction. (46)
Cathode (**ka**-thode) The negative electrode in the x-ray tube. (38)
Cavitation (ka-veh-**tay**-shun) Formation of a cavity or hole. (13)
Cavity Pitted area in a tooth caused by decay. (48)
Cavity preparation Process of decay removal and tooth design in the preparation for restoring a tooth. (48)
Cavity wall Internal surface of a cavity preparation. (48)
CDT Procedure codes that are assigned to dental services for the process of dental insurance. (63)
Cellulitis (sel-yuh-**lie**-tus) Inflammation of cellular or connective tissue. (17)
Celluloid strip (**sel**-yuh-*loyd*) Clear plastic strip used in providing a temporary wall for the restoration of an anterior tooth. (49)
Cementoblasts (se-**men**-to-blasts) Cells that form cementum. (8)
Cementoclasts (se-**men**-to-*klasts*) Cells that resorb cementum. (8)
Cementum Specialized, calcified connective tissue that covers the anatomic root of a tooth. (8)
Cental ray X-rays at center of beam. (38)
Centers for Disease Control and Prevention (CDC) Federal agency that is nonregulatory and issues recommendations on health and safety. (22)
Central groove Most prominent developmental groove on posterior teeth. (12)
Central nervous system (CNS) The brain and spinal cord. (7)
Central ray Central portion of the primary beam of radiation. (41)
Centric (**cen**-trik) Having an object centered, such as maxillary teeth centered over mandibular teeth in correct relation. (46)
Centric occlusion Maximum contact between the occluding surfaces of the maxillary and mandibular teeth. (11)
Centric relation (cen-tric) Having the jaws in a position that produce a centrally related occlusion. (52)
Cephalometric (**seph**-uh-loh-meh-trik) An extraoral radiograph of the bones and tissues of the head. (60)
Cephalometric film Shows the bony and soft tissue areas of the facial profile. (39)
Cephalostat Special devices that allow the operator to easily position both film and patient. (42)
Ceramic Hard, brittle, heat and corrosive resistant material such as clay. (43)
Cerebral palsy (suh-**ree**-buhl **pawl**-zee) Neural disorder of motor function caused by brain damage. (57)
Certified dental assistant (CDA) The nationally recognized credential of the dental assistant who has passed the DANB certification examination and keeps up current practice through continuing education. (2)
Certified dental technician Technician who has passed the proper written exam. (3)
Chamfer (**cham**-fur) Tapered finish line of the margin at the cervical area of a tooth preparation. (50)
Chancre A painless ulcerating sore. (18)
Change fund Fixed amount of cash. (63)
Charge-coupled device (CCD) Image receptor found in the intraoral sensor. (42)
Check A draft or an order on a bank for payment in a specific amount of money. (63)
Check register Record of all checks issued and deposits made on a specific account. (63)
Chemical inventory Comprehensive list of every product used in the office that contains chemicals. (23)
Chemical vapor sterilizer (**ster** uh-lie-zur) Instrument for sterilization by means of hot formaldehyde vapors under pressure. (21)
Chisel Surgical instrument used for cutting or severing a tooth and bone structure. (56)
Chisel scaler Instrument used to remove *supragingival* calculus in the contact area of anterior teeth. The blade on the chisel scaler is curved slightly to adapt to the tooth surfaces. (55)
Chlorine dioxide Effective, rapid-acting environmental surface disinfectant or chemical sterilant. (20)
Chronic Persisting over a long period of time. (26, 54)
Chronic exposure Repeated exposures, generally to lower levels, over a long time. (23)
Chronic infection An infection of long duration. (19)
Chronologic Arranged according to time of occurrence; earliest to most recent. (26)
Chronologic age (*krah*-nah-**lah**-jik) Actual age (months, years) of pediatric patients. (57)
Chronological file Filing system that divides materials into months and possible days of the month. (62)
Cingulum (sin[g]-gu-lum) Raised, rounded area on the cervical third of the lingual surface. (12)
Circumoral (*ser*-kum-**ore**-ul) Surrounding the mouth. (53)
Circumvallate lingual papillae (sur-kum-**va**-late,-let **lin**-gwul pah-**pi**-lay) Large tissue projections on the tongue. (9)
Civil law Category of law that deals with the relations of individuals, corporations, or other organizations. (5)
Clean area Place where sterilized instruments, fresh disposable supplies, and prepared trays are stored. (21)
Clinical contact surface Surfaces touched by contaminated hands, instruments, spatter during dental treatment. (20)
Clinical crown That portion of the tooth that is visible in the oral cavity. (8, 58)
Code of ethics Voluntary standards of behavior established by a profession. (4)
Colloid (**kol**-loid, **kah**-loid) A suspension of particles in a dispersion medium such as water. Its two phases are sol and gel. (46)
Colony-forming units (CFUs) Number of separable cells on the surface of a semisolid agar medium that create a visible colony. (24)
Commission on Dental Accreditation of the American Dental Association Commission that accredits dental, dental assisting, dental hygiene, and dental laboratory educational programs. (1)
Commissure (**kom**-i-sure, **ka**-mih-shur) Angle at the corner of the mouth where the upper and lower lips join. (10)

Communicable disease Condition caused by an infection that can be spread from person to person or from contact with body fluids. (19)
Compact bone Outer layer of the bones, where needed for strength. (7)
Concave Curved inward. (11)
Conception Union of the male sperm and the ovum of the female. (8)
Condensation (*kahn*-duhn-**say**-shun) Process by which liquid is removed from vapor. (32)
Congenital disorder (kun-**je**-nah-tul) A disorder that is present at birth. (17)
Connective tissue The major support material of the body. (6)
Connector Piece of metal that joins the various parts of a partial denture; also called *bar.* (52)
Console (**kahn**-sole) Freestanding cabinet that holds contents or control device, as for laser handpiece. (35)
Consultation room (*kahn(t)*-suhl-**tay**-shun) Meeting room or specified area where diagnostic and treatment information is discussed with the patient. (32)
Contact area Area of tooth that touches adjacent tooth in the same arch. (41)
Contaminated area Place where contaminated items are brought for precleaning. (21)
Contaminated waste Items such as gloves and patient napkins that may contain the potentially infectious body fluids of patients. (19, 23)
Contour (**kahn**-tur) To shape or conform an object. (57)
Contract law Category of law that involves an agreement for services in exchange for a payment (*contract*). (5)
Contrast The differences in degrees of blackness on a radiograph. (38)
Control tooth Healthy tooth used as a standard to compare questionable teeth of similar size and structure during pulp vitality testing. (54)
Convenience form Cavity preparation step that allows the dentist easier access when restoring a tooth. (48)
Convex Curved outward. (11)
Convulsion (kun-**vul**-shun) An involuntary muscular contraction. (31)
Coordination of benefits (COB) Coordinating insurance coverage between two insurance carriers. (63)
Copier A business machine that can make copies from an original. (61)
Coping (**ko**-ping, **kop**-ing) Thin metal covering or cap placed over a prepared tooth. (52)
Core Portion of the post that extends above the tooth structure. (50)
Coronal polish (cuh-**rone**-uhl) A technique used to remove plaque and stains from the coronal surfaces of the teeth. (58)
Coronavirus (core-o-na virus) Type of virus that causes respiratory infections. (18)
Coronal pulp Part that lies within crown portion of tooth. (8)
Coronal suture The line of articulation between the frontal bone and the parietal bones. (9)
Cortical plate The dense outer covering of the spongy bone that makes up the central part of the alveolar process. (8)
Cosmetic dentistry Therapy limited to improving patients' appearance. (55)
Coupling agent Agent that strengthens resin by bonding filler to the resin matrix. (43)
Cranial cavity (**kray**-nee-ul) Space that houses the brain. (6)
Cranium (**kray**-nee-um) Eight bones that cover and protect the brain. (9)
Crestal bone Coronal portion of alveolar bone found between the teeth. (41)
Creutzfeldt-Jacob disease (**kroits**-fuhlt–**yah**-kop) Rare chronic brain disease with onset in middle to late life (40 to 60 years). (18)
Criminal law Category of law that involves violations against the state or government. (5)
Critical instrument Item used to penetrate soft tissue or bone. (21)
Crossbite A tooth is not properly aligned with its opposing tooth. (57, 60)
Cross-reference file A file is listed in alphabetical order by name and gives its document number. (62)
Crowding Teeth that are not aligned properly within the arch. (60)
Crystallization (*kris*-tah-lah-**zay**-shun) Chemical process in which crystals form a structure. (47)
Cumulative trauma disorders (CTDs) (**kyu**-myeh-luh-tiv) Painful conditions resulting from ongoing stresses to muscles, tendons, nerves, and joints. (25)
Cupping Condition created by a concave tooth surface that has not been contoured properly. (49)
Cured Preserved, or finished by a chemical or physical process. (43)
Curette (ku-**ret**) Surgical instrument used to remove tissue from the tooth socket; also *curet.* (55, 56)
Curve of Spee The curvature formed by the maxillary and mandibular arches in occlusion. (11)
Curve of Wilson The cross-arch curvature of the occlusal plane. (11)
Cusp Major elevation on the masticatory surface of canines and posterior teeth. (12)
Custom provisional Coverage designed from a preliminary impression or thermoplastic tray resembling the tooth being prepared. (51)
Customary A fee that is within the range of the usual fee charged for the service. (63)
Cyst (**sist**) Closed cell or pouch with a definite wall. (17)
Cytoplasm (**si**-toe-*plaz*-em) Gel-like fluid inside the cell. (6)
Daily schedule Printed schedule that is copied and placed throughout the office for easy viewing. (62)
Debridement (di-**breed**-munt) To remove or clean out the pulpal canal. (54)
Deciduous teeth (di-**si**-jeh-wus) First dentition of 20 teeth, often called "baby" or *primary* teeth. (11)
Delegate To authorize or entrust another person to perform a specific skill or procedure. (33)
Dementia (di-**men[t]**-shah) A mental disorder with loss of memory, concentration, and judgment. (29)
Demineralization (de-mi-neh-ra-leh-**zay**-shun) Loss of minerals from the tooth. (13)
Demographics Personal information about patients, such as address, and work; also, statistical characteristics of populations. (26)
Density The overall darkness or blackness of a radiograph. (38)
Dental assistant Oral healthcare professional trained to provide supportive procedures to the dentist and patients. (3)
Dental Assisting National Board (DANB) National agency responsible for administering the certification examination and issuing the credential of Certified Dental Assistant (CDA). (2)
Dental auxiliary (ox-**zil**-yah-ree) Dental assistants, dental hygienists, and dental laboratory technicians. (5)
Dental equipment technician Specialist who installs and maintains dental equipment. (3)
Dental hygienist (hy-**jen**-ist) Licensed oral healthcare professional who provides preventive, therapeutic, and educational services. (3)
Dental laboratory technician Professional who performs dental laboratory services such as fabricating crowns, bridges, and dentures, as specified by the dentist's written prescription. (3)
Dental lamina A thickened band of oral epithelium following the curve of each developing arch. (8)
Dental operatory (**op**-er-ah-*tor*-ee) Dental treatment room and control center of the clinical area. (32)
Dental papilla Small nipple shaped elevation. (8)
Dental public health Specialty that promotes oral health through organized community efforts. (3)
Dental radiography (*ray*-dee-**ah**-greh-fee) Process of making radiographs of the teeth and adjacent structures by exposure to radiographs. (38)
Dental sac Connective tissue that envelops the developing tooth. (8)

Dental sealant Coating that covers the occlusal pits and fissures of teeth. (15, 59)
Dental spa A new trend in dentistry where once inside the dental office, patients are treated to a variety of amenities including massages and herbal masks, in a spa-like atmosphere. (3)
Dental supply person Representative of dental supply company providing dental supplies, product information, services and repairs. (3)
Dental treatise (**tree-**tiz) Formal article or book based on dental evidence and facts. (1)
Dental unit waterline (DUWL) Small- bore tubing usually made of plastic, used to deliver dental treatment water through a dental unit. (24)
Dentinal fiber Fibers found in dentinal tubules. (8)
Dentinal tubules Microscopic canals found in dentin. (8)
Dentist Oral healthcare provider licensed to practice dentistry. (3)
Dentition (den-**ti-**shun) Natural teeth in the dental arch. (11)
Dentofacial Structures that include the teeth, jaws, and surrounding facial bones. (60)
Deposition The process of the body adding new bone. (8)
Depth In respiration, amount of air in a breath. (27)
Deposit slip An itemized memorandum of the money to be deposited into the bank. (63)
Desiccate (**de-**si-kate) To remove all moisture from an item, or to dry out. (44)
Detail person Representative of a specific company providing information concerning that specific company's product. (3)
Detection Act or process of discovering tooth imperfections or decay. (28)
Developmental disability Impairment of mental or physical functioning that occurs before age 22 and lasts indefinitely. (41)
Diabetes mellitus (die-ah-**bee-**tez **me-**leh-tus, meh-**lie-**tus) Metabolic disorder characterized by high blood glucose and insufficient insulin. (29)
Diagnosis To identify or determine the nature and cause of a disease or injury through the evaluation of a patient's history and examination. (26)
Diagnostic quality Referring to radiographs with the proper images and necessary density, contrast, definition, and detail for diagnostic purposes. (41)
Diastema (*di*-uh-**stee-**muh) A space between two teeth. (12, 48)
Diastolic (*di*-a-**stahl-**ik, *di*-eh-**stah-**lik) Normal rhythmic relaxation and dilatation of the heart chambers. (27)
Die An accurate replica of the prepared portion of a tooth used in the laboratory during the fabrication of a cast restoration. (47, 50)
Differentiation Term for the specialization function of cells. (6)
Diffuse (di-**fyuz**) To spread from an area of high concentration to one of low concentration. (37)
Digital radiography Filmless imaging system that uses a sensor to capture images, break them into electronic pieces, and store the images in a computer. (42)
Digitize (**di-**jeh-*tize*) To convert an image into a digital form that in turn can be processed by a computer. (42)
Dihydrate (di-**hi-**drate) Relating to gypsum products and indicating two parts of water to one part of calcium sulfate. (47)
Dimensionally stable (dah-**mench-**nah-lee) Resistant to change in width, height, and length. (47)
Direct contact Touching or contact with the patient's blood or saliva. (19)
Direct supervision Level of supervision in which the dentist is physically present when the dental auxiliary performs delegated functions. (5, 33)
Disbursements To pay out on an account. (63)
Disclosing agent Coloring agent that makes plaque visible when applied to teeth. (15)
Disclosure Process of informing the patient about x-ray procedures. (40)
Disinfectant Chemical used to reduce or lower the number of microorganisms on living objects. (20)
Dissipate (**di-**sah-pate) To cause something to scatter, or become dispersed, and gradually disappear. (45)
Distal Farther away from the trunk of the body; opposite of *proximal.* (6)
Distal surface Surface of tooth distant from midline. (11)
Distoclusion (dist-o-**clu-**shun) Term used for Class II malocclusion. (60)
Distribution Action by which a drug is released throughout the body. (30)
Donning Act of placing on an item, such as gloves; dressing. (56)
Dorsal cavity Cavity located in back of body. (6)
Dosage Amount of drug to be administered in a specific time, often according to body weight. (30)
Dose 1. A specified quantity of a drug or medicine. (30); 2. The amount of energy absorbed by tissues. (38)
Down syndrome Chromosomal defect resulting in abnormal physical characteristics and mental impairment; also *trisomy 21.* (57)
Downtime Waiting period between patient procedures. (62)
Droplet infection An infection that occurs through mucosal surfaces of the eyes, nose, or mouth. (19)
Drug A substance used in the diagnosis, treatment, or prevention of a disease. (30)
Dry heat sterilizer Instrument for sterilization by means of heated air. (21)
Dual-cured Prepared, preserved, or finished by a chemical or physical process. (43)
Due care Just, proper, and sufficient care, or the absence of negligence. (5)
Duplicating film Film designed for use in film duplicating machines. (39)
Duration (duh-**ray-**shun) Time from induction to complete reversal of anesthesia. (37)
Ecchymosis (e-ki-**mo-**sis) Technical term for *bruising.* (17)
Edentulous (*e*-**den-**chuh-lus) Without teeth. (52)
Elastomeric (*i*-*las*-tuh-**mer-**ik) Material having elastic properties from rubber. (46)
Electrocardiogram (e-*lek*-tro-**kahr-**de-o-*gram*) Instrument used in the detection and diagnosis of heart abnormalities. It generates a record of the electrical currents associated with heart muscle activity. (27)
Electron A negatively charged particle in the atom. (38)
Elevator Surgical instrument used to reflect and retract the periodontal ligament and periosteum. (56)
Embrasure (im-**bray-**zhur) Triangular space in a gingival direction between the proximal surfaces of two adjoining teeth in contact. (11)
Embryo Organism in the earliest stages of development. (8)
Embryology (*em*-bre-**ahl-**eh-jee) The study of prenatal development. (8)
Embryonic period (*em*-bre-**on-**ik) Stage of human development that extends from the beginning of the second week to the end of the eighth week. (8)
Emotional age Measure of the level of emotional maturity of pediatric patients. (57)
Emphysema (em[p]-feh-**zee-**mah) Abnormal increase in the size of the air spaces in the lungs, resulting in labored breathing and an increased susceptibility to infection. (29)
Employment An activity or service performed, usually for payment. (64)
Emulsion (ei-**mul-**shun) A layer on the x-ray film that contains the radiograph–sensitive crystals. (39)
Enamel organ Part of a developing tooth destined to produce enamel. (8)
Endocarditis (*en*-doe-kahr-**die-**tus) Inflammation of the endocardium. (29)
Endodontics (*en*-do-**don-**tiks) Dental specialty that diagnoses and treats diseases of the pulp. (3)
Endogenous stains (en-**doj**–en-us) Stains developed from within the structure of the tooth. (58)
Endospore A resistant, dormant structure, formed inside of some bacteria that can withstand adverse conditions. (18,21)
Endosteal (en-**das-**tee-ul) Implant surgically embedded into the bone. (53)
Energy The ability to do work. (38)
Environmental Protection Agency (EPA) Federal regulatory agency. (22, 23)

Environmental surface Surfaces within a healthcare facility that are not directly involved in patient care, but may be contaminated during the course of treatment (e.g., countertops, floors, walls, instrument control panels, etc.). (20)

Epidemiological studies (ep-i-de-mi-o-log-i-cal) The study of the patterns and causes of diseases. (19)

Epilepsy (**eh-**pah-*lep*-see) Neurologic disorder with sudden recurring seizures of motor, sensory, or psychic malfunction. (29, 31)

Epithelial tissue (*ep*-i-**thee-**lee-ul) Type of tissue that forms the covering of all body surfaces. (6)

Ergonomics (er-guh-nah-miks) Adaptation of the human body to the work environment. (25)

Erosion Wearing away of tissue. (17)

Erythema (*er*-ah-**thee-**mah) Skin redness, often caused by inflammation or infection. (31)

Esthetic (aesthetic) (es-**the-**tik) Artistically pleasing and beautiful appearance. (43)

Esthetic dentistry (es-**theh-**tik) Type of dentistry that improves the appearance of teeth by camouflaging defects and whitening teeth. (48)

Etchant (**eh-**chunt) Chemical agent used in etching. (44)

Etching (**ech-**ing) Process of cutting into a surface by the use of an acid product. (44)

Ethical drug A drug that requires a prescription. (30)

Ethics Moral standards of conduct; rules or principles that govern proper conduct. (4)

Eugenol (**yu-**jeh-nol) Colorless liquid made from clove oil used for its soothing qualities. (44)

Event-related packaging Instruments in packages should remain sterile indefinitely unless an event causes them to become contaminated (e.g., torn or wet packaging). (21)

Excisional biopsy (ik-**sizh-**nul, ek-**sizh-**ah-nul **bi-***ahp*-see) Surgical procedure in which tissue is cut from a suspect oral lesion. (56)

Excretion (ik-**skree-**shun) Action by which a drug leaves the body. (30)

Exfoliation (eks-*fo*-le-**a-**shun) Normal process of shedding the primary teeth. (8)

Exfoliative biopsy (eks-**fo-**lee-*a*-tiv) Diagnostic procedure in which cells are scraped from a suspect oral lesion for analysis. (56)

Exogenous stains (ex-**oj-**en-us) Stains developed from external sources. (58)

Exothermic (*ek*-so-**thur-**mik) Characterized by the release heat from a chemical reaction. (45)

Expanded functions Specific intraoral functions delegated to an auxiliary that require advanced skill and training. (5, 33)

Expenses The overhead of a business to keep operating. (63)

Exposed Referring to selected teeth visible through the dam; *isolated.* (36)

Exposure controls Adjust the milliamperage and kilovoltage settings. (42)

Expressed contract A contract that is established through verbal or written words. (5)

External auditory meatus Bony passage of the outer ear. (9)

Extraoral Outside the oral cavity. (28)

Extraoral film Film designed for use in cassettes. (39)

Extraoral radiographs Taken when large areas of the skull or jaw must be examined. (42)

Extrinsic stain (ex-**trin-**zik) Stains that occur on the *external* surfaces of the teeth and may be removed by polishing. (58)

Extrude (ik-**strude**) To push or force out. (46)

Extrusion (ik-**stru-**zhun) Displacement of a tooth *from* its socket as a result of injury. (57)

Facebow Portion of articulator used to measure the upper teeth compared to the temporomandibular joint. (47)

Facial surface Surface of teeth closest to the face. (11)

Facultative anaerobes Organisms that can grow with or without oxygen. (18)

Fats Lipids. (16)

Fax machine A business machine attached to the phone line that transmit written or typed materials. (61)

Felony Major Crime such as fraud or drug abuse. Conviction can result in imprisonment of 1 year or more. (5)

Fermentable carbohydrates (fur-**men-**teh-bull) Simple carbohydrates, such as sucrose, fructose, lactose, and glucose. (13)

Festooning (fes-**too-**ning) Procedure to trim or shape a denture to simulate normal tissue appearance. (52, 57)

Fetal molding Pressure applied to the jaw, causing a distortion. (60)

Fetal period Stage starting at the ninth week and lasting until birth. (8)

Fibroblasts Type of cell in connective tissue responsible for the formation of the intercellular substance of pulp. (8)

File A metal tool of varying size and form with numerous ridges or teeth on its cutting surfaces. (55)

File guides An insert between files, giving the letters or numbers of the patient records that follow it. (62)

Filing The act of classifying and arranging records to be easily retrieved when needed. (62)

Filled resin (**re** zin) Sealant material that contains filler particles. (59)

Filler Inorganic material that adds strength and other characteristics to composite resins. (43)

Film holder Device used to position and hold dental x-ray films. (39)

Film speed The sensitivity of the emulsion on the film to radiation. (39)

Fixed bridge Dental prosthesis with artificial teeth fixed in place and supported by attachment to natural teeth. (50)

Fixed overhead Business expenses that are ongoing. (63)

Flange (**flanj**) Parts of a full or partial denture that extend from the teeth to the border of the denture. (52)

Flutes Blades on the working end of a finishing rotary instrument, which resembles pleats. (35)

Focal trough (**trof**) Imaginary three-dimensional horseshoe-shaped zone used to focus panoramic radiographs. (42)

Food and Drug Administration (FDA) Federal regulatory agency. (22)

Force To cause a physical change through energy and strength. (43)

Forceps (**for-**seps) Surgical instrument used to grasp and hold onto teeth for their removal. (56)

Fordyce's spots (**For-**dies-ez) Normal variations that may appear on the buccal mucosa. (10)

Forensic (fo-**ren-**zik) To establish the identity of an individual based on scientific methods. (26)

Forensic dentistry (fo-**ren-**zik) Area of dentistry that establishes the identity of an individual based on dental evidence such at dental records, impressions, bite marks, etc. (1)

Fossa (fos-ah, faw-seh) Wide, shallow depression on the lingual surface of anterior teeth. (12)

Four-handed dentistry Process of the operator and assistant working together to perform clinical procedures in an ergonomically structured environment. (33)

Framework Metal skeleton of a removable partial denture. (52)

Frankfort plane Imaginary plane that passes through the top of the ear canal and the bottom of the eye socket. (42)

Frankyl scale (**frang-**kul) Scale designed to evaluate patient behavior. (57)

Frontal plane Vertical plane that divides the body into anterior (front) and posterior (back) portions. (6)

Fulcrum (**ful-**krum) Finger rest used when holding an instrument or handpiece for a specified time. (33, 58)

Full crown Cast restoration that covers the entire anatomic crown of the tooth. (50)

Full denture (**den-**chur) Prosthesis that replaces all of the teeth in one arch. (52)

Functional occlusion The contact of the teeth during biting and chewing movements. (11)
Furcation (fur-kay-shun) Area between two or more root branches. (12, 28)
Gait A particular way of walking, or *ambulating.* (31)
Galvanic (gal-**va**-nik) An electrical current that takes place when two different or dissimilar metal come together. (43)
Gauge Standard dimension or measurement of the thickness of an injection needle. (37)
General supervision Level of supervision in which the dental auxiliary performs delegated functions according to the instructions of the dentist, who is not necessarily physically present. (5)
Generic drug (jeh-**ner**-ik) Drug that is sold without a brand name or trademark. (30)
Genetic effects (juh-**neh**-tik) Effects of radiation that are passed on to future generations through genetic cells. (38)
Gestation (jes-**ta**-tion) The period from fertilization to birth. (8)
Gingiva (**jin**-jeh-vah) Masticatory mucosa that covers the alveolar processes of the jaws and surrounds the necks of the teeth; plural *gingivae.* (10)
Gingival retraction (**jin**-juh-vul ri-**trak**-shun) The means of displacing gingival tissue away from the tooth. (50)
Gingivectomy (*jin*-jah-*vek*-tah-me) Surgical removal of diseased gingival tissues. (55)
Gingivitis (*jin*-jih-**vi**-tis) Inflammation of the gingival tissue. (14)
Gingivoplasty (**jin**-jah-vah-*plas*-tee) Surgical reshaping and contouring of gingival tissues. (55)
Glabella (glah-**bel**-ah) Smooth surface of the frontal bone; also, the anatomic part directly above the root of the nose. (10)
Glenoid fossa In the temporal bone in which condyles of the mandible articulate with the skull. (9)
Glossitis (glaw-**sigh**-tus) General term used to describe inflammation of the tongue. (17)
Glutaraldehyde (glut-er-al-da-hide) EPA registered high level disinfectant. (20)
Gold A soft, yellow, corrosive-resistant metal used in the making of indirect restorations. (43)
Gracey curette Curette with one cutting edge, "area specific"; they are designed to adapt to specific tooth surfaces (mesial or distal). (55)
Granuloma (gran-yuh-**lo**-muh) A granular tumor or growth. (17)
Grasp The correct way an instrument or handpiece is held. (33)
Greater palatine nerve (**pa**-lah-tine) Nerve that serves the posterior hard palate and posterior lingual gingiva. (9)
Grid Device used to reduce the amount of scatter radiation that reaches an extraoral film. (42)
Gross income The total of all professional income received. (63)
Gurney (**gur**-nee) Mobile table to transport patients. (56)
Gutta-percha (guh-tah–per-chah) Plastic type of filling material used in endodontics. (54)
Gypsum (**jip**-sum) Mineral used in the formation of plaster of paris and stone. (47)
Handle Part of a dental instrument that the operator grasps. (34)
Hard tissue impaction (im-**pak**-shun) Oral condition in which a tooth is partly to fully covered by *bone* and gingival tissue. (56)
Hazard Communication Standard OSHA standard regarding employees' "right to know" about chemicals in the workplace. (23)
Hazardous waste Waste posing a risk to humans or the environment. (19, 23)
Headgear An external orthodontic appliance used to control growth and tooth movement. (60)
Hematoma (he-muh-**toe**-muh) Swelling or mass of blood collected in one area or organ. (17)
Hemihydrate (*he*-mi-**hi**-drate) Removal of one-half part water to one part of calcium sulfate, forming the powder product of gypsum. (47)
Hemisection (**he**-mah-sek-shun) Surgical separation of a multirooted tooth through the furcation area. (54)
Hemophilia (*heh*-meh-**fi**-lee-ah, *heh*-mo-**fil**-ee-ah) Blood coagulation disorder in which the blood fails to clot normally. (29)
Hemostat (**he**-mah-*stat*) Surgical instrument used to hold or grasp items. (56)
Heterotrophic bacteria **(het-er-o-top-ik)** Bacteria that use organic carbon as a source of nutrients. Priotozoa, fungi, and most bacteria fall into this category. (24)
High-level disinfectant Hospital disinfectant with tuberculocidal activity. (20)
HIPAA The Health Insurance Portability and Accountability Act of 1996 specifies federal regulations ensuring privacy regarding a patient's healthcare information. (2, 4, 26, 61, 62, 63)
Histology (his-**tahl**-eh-jee) The study of the structure and function of body tissues on a microscopic level. (8)
Hoe scaler Type of scaler used to remove heavy supragingival calculus, most effective when used on buccal and lingual surfaces of the posterior teeth. (55)
Homogenous (ho-**mah**-jah-nus), **homogeneous** (*ho*-mah-jah-**ne**-us) Having a uniform quality and consistency throughout. (47)
Horizontal plane Plane that divides the body into superior (upper) and inferior (lower) portions. (6)
Hospital disinfectant Has the ability to kill *Staphylococcus aureus, Salomonella choleraesuis,* and *Pseudomonas aeruginosa.* (20)
Housekeeping surface Surfaces not contaminated during dental treatment (e.g., floors, walls). (20)
Hybrid (**hi**-brud) Material that produces a similar outcome to its natural counterpart. (44)
Hydro- Prefix meaning "water." (46)
Hydroxyapatite Mineral compound which is the principal inorganic component of bone and teeth. (8)
Hyoid arch The second branchial arch. (8)
Hyperglycemia (*hi*-per-gly-**see**-me-ah) Abnormally high blood glucose level. (31)
Hyperplasia (*hi*-per-**play**-zh[ee-]ah) Abnormal increase in the number of cells in an organ or a tissue. (29)
Hypersensitivity State of being excessively sensitive to a substance, often with allergic reactions. (31)
Hyperthyroidism (*hi*-per-**thi**-roid-iz-em, *hi*-per-**thi**-roi-di-zem) Condition resulting from excessive activity of the thyroid gland. (29)
Hypertrophied (*hi*-per-**tro**-feed) Referring to overgrown oral tissues. (50)
Hyperventilation Abnormally fast or deep breathing. (31)
Hypoglycemia (*hi*-poe-gly-**see**-me ah) Abnormally low blood glucose level. (31)
Hypotension (*hi*-poe-**ten**-shun) Abnormally low blood pressure. (31)
Hypothyroidism (*hi*-poe-**thi**-roid-iz-em, *hi*-poe-**thi**-roi-di-zem) Condition resulting from severe thyroid hormone insufficiency. (29)
Imbibition (*im*-bah-**bi**-shun) Absorption of water, causing an object to swell. (46)
Imbrication lines (im-breh-kay-shun) Slight ridges that run mesiodistally in the cervical third of teeth. (12)
Immediate denture Temporary denture placed after the extraction of anterior teeth. (52)
Immersion disinfectants Disinfectants to be used for immersion (soaking) of heat-sensitive instruments. (20)
Immunity (i-**mu**-neh-tee) Ability of the body to resist disease. (19)
Impacted tooth Tooth that has not erupted. (56)
Implant Artificial teeth attached to anchors that have been surgically embedded into the bone or surrounding structures. (53)
Implied consent Consent in which the patient's action indicates consent for treatment. (5)

Implied contract A contract that is established by actions, not words. (5)

Inactive files Files of patients that have not been seen in the past three years. (62)

Incipient caries (in-**si-**pee-eunt) Tooth decay that is beginning to form or become apparent. (13)

Incisal edge Ridge on permanent incisors that appears flattened on labial, lingual, or incisal view after tooth eruption. (12)

Incisal surface Chewing surface of anterior teeth. (11)

Incisive papilla Pear shaped pad of tissue that covers the incisive foramen. (10)

Incisional biopsy (in-**sizh-**ah-nul, in-**si-**zhah-nul) Section of suspect oral lesion that is removed for evaluation. (56)

Inclined cuspal planes Sloping areas between the cusp ridges. (12)

Indirect contact Touching or contact with a contaminated surface or instrument. (19)

Indirect pulp cap Placement of a medicament over a partially exposed pulp. (54)

Indirect supervision To oversee an assistant's work by being in the immediate area. (33)

Indirect vision Viewing an object through the use of a mirror. (33)

Induction (in-**duhk-**shun) Time from injection to effective anesthesia. (37)

Infectious disease A disease that is communicable. (19)

Infectious waste Waste capable of transmitting an infectious disease. (19, 23)

Inflammation Protective response of the tissues to irritation or injury. (17)

Informed consent Permission granted by a patient after being informed about the details of a procedure. (5, 40)

Infraction Minor offense that usually results in only a fine. (5)

Infraorbital (*in*-frah-**or-**bi-tul) Region of the head below the orbital region. (9)

Infuser (in-**fyu-**zer) Syringe that applies hemostatic solution on the gingival retraction cord. (50)

Inherited immunity Immunity that is present at birth. (19)

Inlay (**in-**lay) Cast restoration designed for class II cavity. (50)

Innervation (*i*-ner-**vay-**shun) Supply or distribution of nerves to a specific body part. (37)

Inscription On a prescription, the name and quantity of a drug. (30)

Insulating Preventing the passage of heat or electricity. (44)

Integumentary system (in-teg-yu-**men-**ta-re) The skin system. (7)

Intensifying screen Device used to convert x-ray energy into visible light, which in turn exposes screen film. (39)

Intermediate-level disinfectant A liquid disinfectant with the EPA registration as a hospital disinfectant with tuberculocidal activity. It is used for disinfecting operatory surfaces. (20)

Interproximal Between two adjacent surfaces. (41)

Interproximal space (in-ter-**prawk-**sah-mul) The area between adjacent tooth surfaces. (11)

Intersecting To cut across or through. (41)

Intraoral Within the oral cavity. (28)

Intraoral film Film designed for placement in the patient's mouth. (39)

Intrinsic stain (in-**trin-**zik) Stains that occur within the tooth structure and may be removed by polishing. (58)

Intrusion (in-**tru-**zhun) Displacement of a tooth *into* its socket resulting from injury. (57)

Invert (in-**vert**) To reverse the position, order, or condition. To turn inside out or upside down. (36)

Investment material Special gypsum product able to withstand extreme heat. (50)

Invoice An itemized list of goods specifying the prices and terms of sale. (63)

Involuntary muscles Muscles that function automatically, without conscious control. (7)

Iodophor (i-oh-duh-for) EPA-registered, intermediate-level hospital disinfectant. (20)

Ion (**i-**on) An electrically charged particle. (38)

Ionization (*i*-eh-nuh-**zay-**shun) Process by which electrons are removed from atoms, causing the harmful effects of radiation in humans. (38)

Ionizing radiation (**i-**ah-*nize*-ing) Radiation that produces ionization, resulting in harmful effects. (38)

Irregular Not straight, uniform or symmetrical. (43)

Irreversible pulpitis (puhl-**pi-**tis) Infectious condition in which the pulp is incapable of healing requiring a root canal. (54)

Isolated Referring to selected teeth visible through the dam; *exposed.* (36)

Isthmus of fauces The opening between the two arches of the soft palate. (10)

Jaws Part of clamp shaped into four prongs that help stabilize the clamp on the tooth. (36)

Joints Structural areas where two or more bones come together. (7)

Kilovoltage peak (kVp) (**ki-**luh-*vole*-tij) Highest voltage of radiograph tube used during an radiograph exposure. (38)

Kirkland knife Double ended knife with kidney-shaped blades commonly used in periodontal surgery. (55)

Korotkoff sounds (**korot-**kof) Specific sounds heard when taking a blood pressure. (27)

Label side Colored side of the film that faces the tongue. (39)

Labia The gateway to the oral cavity commonly known as "lips". (10)

Labial commissure The angle at the corner of the mouth where the upper and lower lips join. (10)

Labial frenum (**lay-**bee-ul **fre-**num) Band of tissued that passes from the facial oral mucosa at the midline of the arch to the midline of the inner surface of the lip; also called *frenulum;* plural *frenula.* (10)

Labial surface Facial surface closest to the lips. (11)

Lacrimal bones (**lak-**ri-mul) Paired facial bones that help form the medial wall of the orbit. (9)

Lactobacilli (*lak*-toe-bah-**sil-**eye) Bacteria that produce lactic acid from carbohydrates. (13)

Laser (**lay-**zur) Highly concentrated beam of light. (55)

Latent Dormant. (18)

Latent image (**lay-**tunt) The invisible image on the x-ray film after exposure but before processing. (39)

Latent infection (**lay-**tunt) Persistent infection with recurrent symptoms that "come and go." (19)

Latent period (**lay-**tunt) Time between exposure to ionizing radiation and appearance of symptoms. (38)

Lateral excursion (ik-**skur-**zhun) Sliding position of the mandible to the left or right of the centric position. (52)

Lateral pterygoid plate The point of origin for the internal and external pterygoid muscles. (9)

Lathe (**layth**) Machine used for cutting or polishing dental appliances. (47)

Laws Minimum standards of behavior established by statues for a population or profession. (4)

Lead apron Device used to protect the reproductive and blood forming tissues from scatter radiation. (38)

Lead time A time estimate to allow for delays in ordering or shipping of back-ordered materials. (62)

Ledger A financial statement that maintains all account transactions. (62, 63)

Legionella (lee-jeh-**nel-**a) Genus of bacteria responsible for the disease *legionellosis.* (24)

Lesion (**lee-**zhun) An area of pathology. (17)

Letterhead A part of a letter that contains the name and address of the person sending the letter. (61)

Leukemia (lu-**kee-**me-ah) A progressive disease in which the bone marrow produces an increased number of immature or abnormal white cells. (17, 29)

Leukoplakia (lew-ko-**play-**kee-ah) Formation of white spots or patches on the oral mucosa. (17)

Liable Accountable or legally responsible. (40)

Licensure License to practice in a specific state. (5)
Lichen planus (**li**-kun, **li**-chun) Benign, chronic disease affecting the skin and oral mucosa. (17)
Ligature tie (**lig**-a-chure) Light wire used to hold the arch wire in its bracket. (60)
Light cured Type of material that is polymerized by a curing light. (59)
Line angle Junction of two walls in a cavity preparation. (11, 48)
Linea alba Normal variation noted on the buccal mucosa. (10)
Lingual surface Surface of teeth closest to the tongue. (11)
Litigation (li-teh-**gay**-shun) Act of initiating legal proceedings, as in a lawsuit. (26)
Long axis of the tooth Imaginary line dividing the tooth longitudinally into two equal halves. (41)
Low-level disinfectant Agent that destroys certain viruses and fungi; used for general housecleaning (e.g., walls, floors). (20)
Lumen (lu-**mun**) The hollow center of the injection needle. (37)
Luting agent (**lut**-ing) Cement-type substance used to seal a surface. (45)
Luxate (**luk**-sate) To dislocate, as a tooth from its socket. (56)
Luxation (*luk*-**say**-shun) Dislocation. (57)
Lymphadenopathy (lim-**fad**-**nop**-athy) Disease or swelling of the lymph nodes. (9, 17)
Lymphoma (lim-**fo**-ma) Malignant disorder of the lymphoid tissue. (17)
Malaligned (*mal*-eh-**lined**) Displaced out of line, especially teeth displaced from normal relation to line of the dental arch; *maloccluded.* (36)
Malleability (*may*-lee-ah-**bi**-leh-tee) The ability of a material to withstand permanent deformation under compressive stress without permanent damage. (43)
Mallet Hammerlike instrument used with a chisel to section teeth or bone. (56)
Malocclusion (**mal**-o-clu-shun) Occlusion that is deviated from a Class I normal occlusion. (11, 60)
Malpractice Professional negligence. (5)
Mamelon (mam-ah-lon) Rounded enamel extension on the incisal ridge of incisors. (12)
Mandated reporters Designated professionals who are required by law to report known or suspected child abuse. (5)
Mandibular arch (man-**di**-bu-ler) The lower jaw. (8, 11)
Mandrel (**man**-druhl) Metal shaft on which a sandpaper disk or other abrasive materials are mounted on. (35)
Marginal ridge Rounded, raised border on the mesial and distal portions of the lingual surface of anterior teeth and the occlusal table of posterior teeth. (12)
Marketing A way of advertising or recruiting people to a business. (61)
Masseter (ma-**se**-tur) Most obvious and strongest muscle of mastication. (9)
Master cast Cast created from a final impression used to construct baseplate, bite rims, wax setups, and finished prosthesis. (50)
Master switch, Indicator light, Selector buttons, Exposure button Components of control panel. (38)
Mastication (*mas*-tah-**kay**-shun) Chewing. (52)
Masticatory mucosa (**mas**-ti-kah-*tor*-e) Oral mucosa that covers the hard palate, dorsum of the tongue, and gingiva. (8)
Masticatory surface (**mas**-ti-kah-tor-ee) The chewing surface of the teeth. (11)
Mastoid process Projection on the temporal bone located behind the ear. (9)
Material safety data sheet (MSDS) Form that provides health and safety information regarding materials that contain chemicals. (23)
Matrix (**may**-triks) Foundation binding a substance together; continuous phases (organic polymer) in which particles of filler are dispersed in composite resin. (43)
Matrix band (**may**-triks) Band that provides a temporary wall for a tooth structure to restore the proximal contours and contact to normal shape and function. (49)
Matter Anything that occupies space and has form or shape. (38)
Maxillary arch (**max**-sah-lair-ee) The upper jaw. (11)
Maximum horizontal reach The reach created when the upper arm is fully extended. (25)
Maximum vertical reach The reach created by the vertical sweep of the forearm while keeping the elbow at midtorso level. (25)
Medial Toward or nearer to the midline of the body. (6)
Medial pterygoid plate Plate that ends in hook shaped hamulus. (9)
Meiosis (mi-**oh**-sis) Reproductive cell production that ensures the correct number of chromosomes. (8)
Mental age Measure of the level of intellectual capacity and development of pediatric patients. (57)
Mental protuberance Part of the mandible that forms the chin. (10)
Mental retardation Disorder in which an individual's intelligence is underdeveloped. (57)
Mesial surface Surface of tooth toward the midline. (11)
Mesioclusion (**mez**-i-o-clu-shun) Term used for Class III malocclusion. (60)
Metabolism (me-**tab**-eh-*liz*-um) Physical and chemical processes that occur within a living cell or organism that are necessary for the maintenance of life. (27, 30)
Metastasize (muh-**tas**-tah-size) Spreading of disease from one part of the body to another. (17)
Microbiology The study of microorganisms. (18)
Microfiltration Use of membrane filters to trap microorganisms suspended in water. (24)
Microleakage (**my**-cro-**leak**-age) Microscopic leakage at the interface of the tooth structure and the sealant or restoration. (43, 59)
Micromechanical (*my*-kro-mi-**ka**-ni-kul) Means for a material and structure to lock onto one another through minute cuttings. (44)
Midsagittal plane Imaginary line that divides the patient's face into right and left sides. (6, 42)
Milliampere (mA) (*mi*-lah-**am**-pir) One one-thousandth (1/1000) of a ampere, a unit of measurement used to describe the intensity of an electric current. (38)
Misdemeanor Offense that might result in imprisonment of 6 months to 1 year. (5)
Mobility To have movement. (28, 55)
Model Replica of the maxillary and mandibular arches made from an impression. (47)
Molars Teeth located in the posterior aspect of the upper and lower jaws. (12)
Monomer (**ma**-nah-mur) A molecule that, when combined with other molecules, forms a polymer. (47)
Morphologically (mor-fah-**lahj**-i-kul-lee), morphologic (mor-fah-**lah**-jik), morphology (mor-**fol**-eh-jee, mor-**fah**-leh-jee) Branch of biology that deals with the form and structure. (28)
Morphology (mor-fah-leh-jee) Study of the form and shape, as of the teeth. (12)
Mucobuccal fold Base of vestibule where the buccal mucosa meets the alveolar mucosa. (10)
Mucogingival (*mu*-ko-**jin**-ji-vul) Below the gingival tissue that surrounds a tooth. (28)
Mucogingival junction Distinct line of color change in the tissue where the alveolar membrane meets with attached gingivae. (10)
Multi-parameter indicators Strips placed into packages that change colors when exposed to a combination of heat, temperature, and time. Also known as process integrators. (21)
Muscle insertion Location where the muscle ends; the portion away from the body's midline. (7)
Muscle origin Location where the muscle begins; the portion toward the body's midline. (7)
Muscle tissue Tissue with the ability to lengthen or shorten to provide movement to body parts. (6)

Musculoskeletal disorders (MSDs) (mus-kyu-loh-skeh- leh-tul) Painful conditions affecting both the muscles and bones, such as neck or back pain and carpal tunnel syndrome. (25)

Mutans streptococci (*strep*-toe-**kok**-si) Type of bacteria primarily responsible for caries. (13)

Mylar (**mi**-*lar*) Brand name for clear plastic strip used in providing a temporary wall for restoration of an anterior tooth. (49)

Myocardial infarction (*mi*-oh-**kahr**-dee-ul in-**fark**-shun) Also referred to as a *heart attack,* where there is damage to the muscular tissue of the heart, commonly caused by obstructed circulation. (29, 31)

Nasion (**nay**-ze-on) Midpoint between the eyes just below the eyebrows. (10)

Nasolabial sulcus The groove extending upward between each labial commissure and nasal ala. (10)

National Institute for Occupational Safety and Health (NIOSH) Federal agency that is nonregulatory. (22)

National Institute of Dental and Craniofacial Research (NIDCR) (22)

National Institutes of Health (NIH) (22)

Naturally acquired immunity Immunity that occurs when a person has contracted and is recovering from a disease. (19)

Needle holder Surgical instrument used to hold the suture needle. (56)

Nerve tissue Responsible for coordinating and controlling body activities. (6)

Net income Income minus the expenses that are taken out. (63)

Neural (**nur**-ahl) Referring to the brain, nervous system, and nerve pathways. (57)

Neutral position The position when the body is properly aligned and the distribution of weight throughout the spine is equal. (25)

Nib Blunt point or tip. (34)

NIDCR Federal agency whose mission is to improve oral, dental, and craniofacial health through research, research training, and the dissemination of health information.

NIH One of the world's foremost research centers.

NIOSH Federal agency that is nonregulatory and provides national and worldwide leadership to prevent work-related illnesses and injuries.

Noncritical instrument Item that comes into contact with intact skin only. (21)

Nonpathogenic (*non*-pa-thuh-**jeh**-nik) Referring to microorganisms that do *not* produce disease. (18)

Nonsuccedaneous (non-suk-se-day-ne-us) Referring to a tooth that does not replace a primary tooth. (12)

Nonverbal communication Type of communication in which body language is used as a form of expression. (61)

Nonvital Not living, as in oral tissue and tooth structure. (54)

Normal horizontal reach The reach created by the sweep of the forearm with the upper arm held at the side. (25)

Nucleus (**noo**-klee-us) "Control center" of the cell. (6)

Neurons Direct nerve impulses. (7)

Nutrients (**new**-tree-unts) Organic and inorganic chemicals in food that supply energy. (16)

Obliterating (uh-**bli**-tur-ate-ing) Removing something completely. (44)

Obturation (*ahb*-tyah-**ray**-shun) Process of filling a root canal. (54)

Occipital (ok-**sip**-i-tul) Region of the head overlying the occipital bone and covered by the scalp. (9)

Occlusal radiographic View that shows large areas of the maxilla or mandible. (39)

Occlusal registration (ah-**klu**-sul, a-**klu**-zul) Reproduction of a patient's bite using wax or elastomeric material. (46)

Occlusal rim (ah-**klu**-sul) Rims built on the baseplate to register vertical dimension and occlusal relationship of the mandibular and maxillary arches. (52)

Occlusal surface Chewing surface of posterior teeth. (11)

Occlusal technique Used to examine large areas of the upper or lower jaw. (41)

Occlusal trauma Abnormal occlusal relationships of the teeth, causing injury to the periodontium. (55)

Occlusion (oh-**klu**-zhun) The natural contact of the maxillary and mandibular teeth in all positions. (11, 60)

Occupational exposure Any reasonably anticipated skin, eye, or mucous membrane contact or percutaneous injury with blood or any other potentially infectious materials. (19)

Occupational Safety and Health Administration (OSHA) Federal regulatory agency. (22)

Odontoblasts (o-**don**-to-blasts) Cells that form dentin. (8)

Odontogenesis (o-*don*-to-**jen**-eh-sis) Formation of new teeth. (8)

Onlay (**on**-lay) Cast restoration designed for occlusal crown and proximal surfaces of posterior teeth. (50)

Opaquer (oh-**pay**-kur) Resin material placed under a porcelain restoration to mask tooth discoloration. (50)

Open bay Concept of open design used in pediatric dental practices. (57)

Open bite A lack of vertical overlap of the maxillary incisors, creating an opening of the anterior teeth. (60)

Operating zones Concept using the clock when positioning the dental team, equipment and supplies. (33)

Operative dentistry Common term used when describing restorative and esthetic dentistry. (48)

Oral and maxillofacial radiology (*ray*-de-**ol**-o-gee) Dental specialty that deals with the diagnosis of disease through various form of imaging, including x-ray films (radiographs). (3)

Oral and maxillofacial surgeon (OMFS) (mak-***si***-*loh*-**fay**-shul) Dentist who has specialized in surgeries of the head and neck region. (56)

Oral and maxillofacial surgery (mak-***sil*-o-fay**-shul) Dental surgical specialty that diagnoses and treats conditions of the mouth, face, upper jaw (maxilla), and associated areas. (3, 56)

Oral candidiasis (kan-dah-**die**-uh-sis) Yeast infection of the oral mucosa. (18)

Oral cavity proper The space on the tongue side within the upper and lower dental arches. (10)

Oral pathology (pa-**thol**-o-gee) Dental specialty that diagnoses and treats diseases of the oral structures. (3)

Oral prophylaxis (pro-**fuh**-lax-is) The complete removal of calculus, debris, stain, and plaque from the teeth. (58)

Orban knife Knife with a spearlike shape and cutting edges on both sides of the blade used to remove tissue from the *interdental* areas. (55)

Organelle (*or*-guh-**nel**) Specialized part of a cell that performs a specific function. (6)

Organic (or-**ga**-nik) Food products that have been grown without the use of chemical pesticides, herbicides, or fertilizers. (16)

Organization for Safety and Asepsis Procedures (OSAP) The premier infection control education organization in dentistry. (22)

Orthodontics (orth-o-**don**-tics) Specialty of dentistry designed to prevent, intercept, and correct skeletal and dental problems. (3, 60)

OSHA Bloodborne Pathogens Standard Guidelines designed to protect employees against occupational exposure to bloodborne pathogens. (19)

Osseointegration (*ahs*-ee-oh-*in*-te-**gray**-shun) Attachment of healthy bone to a dental implant. (53)

Osseous surgery (**ah**-see-us) Surgical specialty to remove defects in bone. (55)

Ostectomy (ahs-**tek**-tah-me) Surgery involving the removal of bone. (55)

Osteoblasts (**os**-te-o-*blasts*) Cells that form bone. (7, 8)

Osteoclasts (**os**-te-o-*klasts*) Cells that resorb bone. (8)

Osteoplasty (**ahs**-tee-oh-*plas*-tee) Surgery in which bone is added, contoured, and reshaped. (55)

Outguide Similar to a bookmark for a filing system. (62)

Outline form Design and initial depth of sound tooth structure used by the dentist when restoring a tooth. (48)
Outpatient Patient seen and treated by a physician, then sent home for recovery. (56)
Overbite An increased vertical overlap of the maxillary incisors. (60)
Overhang Excess restorative material extending beyond the cavity margin. (49)
Overjet An excessive protrusion of the maxillary incisors. (60)
Oximetry (ok-**sim-**uh-tree) Measurement of oxygen concentration in the blood. (37)
Packing slip An itemized listing of shipped goods. (63)
Palatal surface Lingual surface of maxillary teeth. (11)
Palladium (puh-**lay-**dee-um) Soft, steel-white, tarnish-resistant metal that occurs naturally with platinum. (43)
Palodent (**pa-**luh-dent) Small, oval-shaped matrix made of stainless steel used interproximally during tooth restoration. (49)
Palpate (**pal-**pate) To examine or explore by touching. (27)
Palpation (pal-**pay-**shun) To touch or feel for abnormalities within soft tissue. (28, 54)
Panoramic film Provides a wide view of the upper and lower jaws. (39)
Papoose board (pa-**poos**) Type of restraining device to hold a pediatric patient's hands, arms, and legs still. (57)
Parallel Moving or lying in the same plane, always separated by the same distance. (41)
Paralleling technique Intraoral technique of exposing periapical films. (41)
Parietal (pah-**rye-**ih-tul) Pertaining to the walls of a body cavity. (6)
Parotid duct (pah-**rot-**id) Duct associated with the parotid salivary gland, which opens into the oral cavity at the parotid papilla. (9)
Parotid papilla A small elevation of tissue located on the inner surface of the cheek. (10)
Partial denture Removable prosthesis replacing teeth within the same arch. (52)
Patent medicine Drug that can be obtained without a prescription; also called *over-the-counter drug.* (30)
Pathogen (**pah-**thuh-jehn), Disease-producing microorganisms. (18, 19)
Pathology (pa-**tha-**lah-jee) The study of disease. (17)
Patient of record Individual who has been examined and diagnosed by the dentist and has had treatment planned. (5, 62)
Payee The person named on the check as the recipient of the amount shown. (63)
Pediatric dentistry (pee-dee-**a-**trik) Dental specialty concerned with neonatal through adolescent patients as well as patients with special needs in these age groups. (3, 57)
Pegboard system A manual bookkeeping system. (63)
Pegged laterals Incisors with a pointed or tapered shape. (12)
Pellicle (**pe-**leh-kul) Thin film coating of salivary materials deposited on tooth surfaces. (13)
Pelvic cavity Contains portions of the large and small intestines, the rectum, urinary bladder, and reproductive organs. (6)
Penumbra (puh-**num-**bruh) The blurred or indistinct area that surrounds an image. (38)
Percussion (per-**kuh-**shun) Examination technique that involves tapping on the incisal or occlusal surface of a tooth to determine vitality. (54)
Percutaneous (per-que-tan-eous) Through the skin, such as a needle stick, cut, or human bite. (18, 19)
Perforation (per-fah-**ray-**shun) Making a hole, as in breaking through and extending beyond the apex of the root. (54)
Periapical radiographic (*per*-e-**a-**pi-kul) View that shows the crown, root tip, and surrounding structures. (39)
Pericardium (*per*-i-**kahr-**dee-um) Double-walled sac that encloses the heart. (7)
Peri-implant tissue Gingival sulcus surrounding the implant. (53)
Periodontal (*per*-e-oh-**don-**tul) Referring to the periodontium. (14)
Periodontal charting (*per*-ee-oh-**dahn-**tul) Commonly accepted notations that are made to the patient's chart to indicate the condition, position, and restorative history of individual teeth. (55)
Periodontal disease (*per*-e-o-**don-**tul) Infections and other conditions of the structures that support the teeth (gums and bone). (1)
Periodontal dressing (Perio Pak) Surgical dressing applied to the surgical site for protection, similar to a bandage. (55)
Periodontal explorer Thin, fine instrument that is easily adapted around root surfaces. (55)
Periodontal flap surgery (flap surgery) Incisional surgery performed when excisional surgery is not indicated. In flap surgery the tissues *are not removed,* but are pushed away from the underlying tooth roots and alveolar bone, similar to the flap of an envelope. (55)
Periodontal pocket Deepening of the gingival sulcus beyond normal, resulting from periodontal disease. (55)
Periodontal probe Probe used to locate and measure the depth of periodontal pockets tapered to fit into the gingival sulcus with a blunt or rounded tip. (55)
Periodontics (*per*-ee-oh-**dahn-**tiks) Dental specialty involved in with the diagnosis and treatment of diseases of the supporting tissues. (55)
Periodontist (*per*-ee-oh-**dahn-**tist) Dentist with advanced education in the specialty of periodontics. (55)
Periodontitis (*per*-e-oh-*don*-**ti-**tis) Inflammatory disease of the supporting tissues of the teeth. (14)
Periodontium (*per*-e-oh-**don-**she-um) Structures that surround, support, and are attached to the teeth. (8, 14)
Perioscopy (per-e-os-co-py) Procedure using a dental endoscope subgingivally. (14)
Periosteum (*per*-e-**ahs-**tee-um) Specialized connective tissue covering all bones of the body. (7)
Peripheral nervous system (PNS) Cranial nerves and spinal nerves. (7)
Periradicular (pear-ee-ruh-**di-**kyuh-ler) Referring to the area of nerves, blood vessels, and tissue that surround the root of a tooth. (54)
Peristalsis (*per*-i-**stahl-**sis) Rhythmic action that moves food through the digestive tract. (7)
Permeate (**per-**me-ate) To spread or flow throughout. (37)
Permucosal (per-mu-**ko-**sul) Contact with mucous membranes, such as the eyes or mouth. (19)
Perpendicular Intersecting at or forming a right angle. (41)
Personal protective equipment (PPE) Items such as protective clothing, masks, gloves, and eyewear to protect employees. (19)
Pestle (**pe-**sul, **pes-**tul) An object that moves vertically pounding or pulverizing a material. (43)
Petechiae (pe-teak-ea) Small, pinpoint red spot on the skin or mucous membrane. (17)
Petty cash A small amount of cash that is kept on hand for small daily expenses. (63)
Pharmacology A branch of medicine concerned with the uses, effects and action of drugs. (30)
Philtrum (**fil-**trum) Rectangular area from under the nose to the midline of the upper lip. (10)
Photon (**fo-**tahn) A minute (tiny) bundle of pure energy that has no weight or mass. (38)
Physical disability Problems with vision, hearing, or mobility. (41)
Physiology (*fiz*-ee-**ahl-**eh-jee) The study of the functions of the human body. (6)
Plane Flat or level surface. (34)
Planes Three imaginary lines used to divide the body into sections. (6)
Planktonic bacteria (plank-**tah-**nik) Bacteria that is freely floating in water. (24)
Plaque (**plak**) Soft deposit on teeth that consists of bacteria and bacterial byproducts. (13,14)

Platinum (**plat-**num) Silver-white noble metal that does not corrode in air. (43)
Point Sharp or tapered end. (34)
Point angle Formed by the junction of three surfaces. (11)
Polycarbonate crown (*pah*-lee-**kahr-**bah-nate) Provisional crown made from a hard plastic tooth-colored material used for anterior teeth. (51)
Polymer (**pah-**leh-mur) Compound of many molecules. (47)
Polymerization (poli mer ih **za** shun) Process of changing a simple chemical into another substance containing the same elements. (59)
Polymerize (pah-**li-**meh-rize) To subject a material to the bonding process of two or more monomers. (44)
Pontic (**pon-**tik) Artificial tooth that replaces a missing natural tooth. (15, 50)
Porcelain (**por-**su-lun) Hard, white, translucent ceramic made by firing and then glazing it. (43)
Porcelain-fused-to-metal (PFM) **crown** Indirect restoration in which a thin porcelain material is fused to the facial portion of a gold crown. (50)
Porous (**pore-**us) An object with minute openings that allow the passage of gas or fluid. (37)
Positioner An appliance used to retain teeth in their desired position. (60)
Post dam Seal in back of a full or partial denture that holds it in place; also called *posterior palatal seal.* (52)
Posted A term used for documenting money transactions within a business. (63)
Posterior Toward the back. (11)
Posterior faucial pillar Posterior arch of the soft palate. (10)
Postnatal (post-**nay-**tuhl) After birth. (57)
Preceptorship (pri-**sep-**tor-ship) Study under the guidance of a dentist or other professional. (1)
Precleaning Removal of bioburden before disinfection. (20)
Pre-formed Referring to provisional coverage that is already shaped in the appearance needed. (51)
Preimplantation period Stage of development during the first week after fertilization. (8)
Prenatal Before birth. (57)
Prenatal development (pre-**nay-**tul) Stage of human development from the start of pregnancy until birth. (8)
Prescription A written order for a specific drug. (30)
Pressure points Specific areas in the mouth where a removable prosthesis may rub or apply more pressure. (52)
Preventive dentistry Program of patient education, use of fluorides, application of dental sealants, proper nutrition, and plaque control. (15)
Primary cementum Formed outward from the cementodentinal junction for the full length of the root. (8)
Primary beam The most penetrating beam produced at the target of the anode. (38)
Primary palate The shelf seperating the oral and nasal cavities. (8)
Primary radiation Same as primary beam. (38)
Prions (**pry-**ons) Infectious particles of proteins that lack nucleic acids. (18)
Prism A calcified column or rod. (8)
Probing Use of a slender, flexible instrument to explore and measure the periodontal pocket. (28)
Process indicator Tapes, strips, or tabs with heat-sensitive chemicals that change color when exposed to a certain temperature. (21)
Process integrator Strips placed into packages that change colors when exposed to a combination of heat, temperature, and time. (21)
Processing A series of steps that changes exposed film into a radiograph. The steps include developing, rinsing, fixing, washing, drying. (39)
Professional Person who meets the standards of a profession. (2)
Prophylaxis (pro-fah-**lak-**sus) Administration of drugs to prevent disease or protect a patient. (30)
Prosthesis (praus-**thee-**sus) Fabricated replacement for a missing tooth. (50)
Prosthodontics (*pros*-tho-**don-**tiks) Dental specialty that provides restoration and replacement of natural teeth. (3)
Protozoa (pro-tuh-**zo-**uh) Single-celled microscopic animals without a rigid cell wall. (18)
Protrusion (pro-**tru-**zhun) Position of the mandible placed forward as related to the maxilla. (52)
Provider The dentist that provides the treatment to the patient. (63)
Provirus Virus that is hidden during the latency period. (18)
Provisional Referring to temporary coverage made for crown or bridge preparations and worn during cast preparation. (45, 51)
Proximal Closer to the trunk of the body. (6)
Pterygoid process Process of the sphenoid bone, consisting of two plates. (9)
Pulp chamber The space occupied by the pulp. (8)
Pulpal wall (**puhl-**puhl) Surface of the cavity preparation perpendicular to the pulp of a tooth. (48)
Pulp cap Application of dental material to a cavity preparation with an exposed or nearly exposed dental pulp. (54)
Pulpectomy (puhl-**pek-**tah-me) Complete removal of a vital pulp from a tooth. (54)
Pulpitis (puhl-**pi-**tis) Inflammation of the dental pulp. (54)
Pulpotomy (puhl-**pah-**tah-me) Removal of the coronal portion of a vital pulp from a tooth. (54, 57)
Pulse Rhythmic throbbing of the arteries produced by the regular contractions of the heart. (27)
Purchase order A form that authorizes the purchase of supplies from the supplier. (62)
Quadrant One quarter of the dentition. (11)
Quality assurance A plan to ensure that the dental office will produce consistent, high quality images with a minimum of exposure to patients and personnel. (40)
Quality control tests Specific tests used to ensure quality in dental x-ray equipment, supplies, and film processing. (40)
Radial Relating to the radius (bone) or forearm *(antebrachium),* as in *radial artery.* (27)
Radiation Forms of waves of energy emission through space or a material. (38)
Radicular pulp The other portion of pulp known as root pulp. (8)
Radiograph (**ray-**dee-oh-*graf*) Image produced on photosensitive film by exposing the film to radiation and then processing it. (38, 39)
Radiology (*ray*-dee-**ah-**luh-jee) The science or study of radiation as used in medicine. (38)
Rampant caries (**ram-**puent) Decay that develops rapidly and is widespread throughout the mouth. (13)
Rate A quantity measured, as in breaths and heartbeats. (27)
Rate of use The quantity of a product that is used within a given time. (62)
Reasonable A fee that is considered reasonable for an extensive or complex treatment. (63)
Rebasing (*re*-**bay-**sing) Procedure to replace the entire denture base material on an existing prosthesis. (52)
Recession Process of withdrawl or wearing away from its normal location. (28)
Reciprocity (re-sa-**prah-**si-tee) System that allows individuals in one state to obtain a license in another state without retesting. (5)
Registration The act of completing forms with personal information. (26)
Regulated waste Infectious waste that requires special handling, neutralization, and disposal. (23)
Relining (*re*-**lie-**ning) Procedure to resurface the tissue side of a partial or full denture so that it fits more accurately. (52)
Remineralization Replacement of minerals in the tooth. (13)
Reorder tags A notation system that is placed when a certain item is close to being low and needs to be reordered. (62)
Requisition (reh-**kwi-zi-**shun) A formal request for supplies. (62)

Res gestae (Latin, "things done") Statements made by any person present at the time of an alleged negligent act that are admissible as evidence in a court of law. (5)

Res ipsa loquitur (Latin, "the thing speaks for itself") (5)

Residual activity Action that continues long after initial application, as with disinfectants. (20)

Resin-bonded bridge Fixed dental prosthesis with wings that are bonded to the lingual surfaces of adjacent teeth; also known as *Maryland bridge.* (50)

Resistance form (ri-**zis**-tun[t]s) Shape and placement of cavity walls in the preparation of tooth restoration. (48)

Resorption (*re*-**sorp**-shun) The body's processes of eliminating existing bone or hard tissue structure. (8, 52)

Respiration Act or process of inhaling and exhaling; breathing. (27)

Respondeat superior (Latin, "Let the master answer") Legal doctrine that holds the employer liable for the acts of the employee. (5)

Responsible party Person who has agreed to pay for an account. (63)

Rest Metal projection on or near the retainer of a partial denture. (52)

Restoration (*res*-tuh-**ray**-shun) The use of a dental material to restore a tooth or teeth to a functional permanent unit. (28, 48)

Restorative (ri[reh]-**stor**-eh-tiv) To restore or bring back to its natural appearance. (43)

Restorative dentistry (ri-**stor**-ah-tiv) Type of dentistry that restores teeth by removing decay and restoring defects. (48)

Retainer (ri-**tay**-ner) 1. Device used to hold attachments and abutments of a removable prosthesis in place. (52); 2. An appliance used for maintaining the positions of the teeth and jaws after orthodontic treatment. (60).

Retard (re-**tard**) To slow down a process. (45)

Retention (ri-ten[t]-shun) The result of adhesion, mechanical locking or both. (43, 44)

Retention form (ri-**ten**[t]-shun) The shaping of the cavity walls to aid in retaining the restoration. (48)

Retention (retentive) pin Basis of a stronger system used to retain and support a tooth restoration. (48)

Retractor (ri-**trak**-tur) Surgical instrument used to hold back soft tissue. (56)

Retrograde restoration (**re**-trah-*grade res*-tah-**ray**-shun) Small restoration placed at the apex of a root. (54)

Retrusion (*re*-**troo** zhun) Position of the mandible posterior from the centric position as related to the maxilla. (52)

Reuse life The time period that a disinfectant should remain effective during use and reuse. (20)

Reversible pulpitis Form of pulpal inflammation in which the pulp may be salvageable. (54)

Rheostat (**ree**-uh-*stat*) Foot-controlled device to operate dental handpieces. (32)

Rhythm A sequence or pattern, as the heartbeat or breathing. (27)

Right angle Angle of 90 degrees formed by two lines perpendicular to each other. (41)

Rongeur (**ron**-gore, raw-**shur**) Surgical instrument used to cut and trim the alveolar bone. (56)

Root Facial landmark commonly called the "bridge" of the nose. (10)

Root amputation (*am*-pyuh-**tay**-shun) Removal of one or more roots without removing the crown of the tooth. (54)

Root canal therapy Removal of the dental pulp and filling the canal with material. (54)

Root planing Procedure that smooths the surface of a root by removing abnormal toxic cementum or dentin that is rough, contaminated, or permeated with calculus. (55)

Rotary (**roh**-teh-ree) Part or device that rotates around an axis. (35)

Rubber cup polishing A technique used to remove plaque and stains from the coronal surfaces of the teeth. (58)

Sagittal suture Located at the midline of the skull where the two parietal bones are joined. (9)

Salutation (sal-u-**ta**-shun) A part of the letter that contains the introductory greeting. (61)

Sarcoma (sar-**ko**-ma) Malignant tumor in connective tissue such as muscle or bone. (17)

Scaling The removal of calculus deposits from the teeth using suitable instruments. (55)

Scalpel (**skal**-pul, skal-**pel**) Surgical knife. (56)

Scatter radiation A form of secondary radiation that occurs when an x-ray beam has been deflected from its path by interaction with matter. (38)

Sealant retention The sealant firmly adhering to the tooth surface. (59)

Secondary cementum Formed on the apical half of the root. (8)

Secondary palate The final palate formed during embryonic development. (8)

Secondary radiation X-radiation that is created when the primary beam interacts with matter. (38)

Sedative (**se**-dah-tiv) Having a soothing effect. (44)

Seizure A sudden attack, spasm, or convulsion, that occurs in specific disorders. (29)

Self-contained water reservoir Container attached to a dental unit that is used to hold and supply water or other solutions to handpieces and air-water syringes. (24)

Self-cured Type of material that is polymerized by chemical reactions. (59)

Semicritical instrument Item that comes in contact with oral tissues but does not penetrate soft tissue or bone. (21)

Sensor Small detector that is placed intraorally to capture a radiographic image. (42)

Separator A device made from wire or elastic used to separate molars prior to fitting and placement of orthodontic bands. (60)

Septum (**sep**-tuhm) 1. Dental dam material located between the holes of the punched dam. (36); 2. Tissue that divides the nasal cavity into two nasal fossae. (10)

Serrated (*sur*-**ray**-ted) Having notchlike projections extending from a flat surface. (34)

Sextant One sixth of the dentition. (11)

Shade guide Accessory dental item that contains different shades of teeth and is used to match the color of a patient's teeth for the laboratory technician. (50)

Shank Part of an instrument or bur that attaches to the working end. (34, 35)

Sharpey's fibers Tissues that anchor the periosteum to the bone. (7)

Sharpness How well the radiograph reproduces the fine details or outlines of an object. (38)

Sharps Pointed or cutting instruments, including needles, scalpel blades, orthodontic wires, and endodontic instruments. (19)

Shelf life How long a product may be stored prior to use. (20, 62)

Shoulder Margins of a tooth preparation for a cast restoration. (50)

Sickle scaler A hook shaped instrument available in various sizes and shapes used for the removal of tenacious supragingival deposits of calculus. (55)

Signature Instructions on a prescription of how to take a specific medicine. (30)

Silver amalgam paste (a-mal-gum) A mixture of mercury, silver, and tin. (1)

Single-parameter indicators Tapes, strips, or tabs with heat-sensitive chemicals that change color when exposed to a certain temperature. Also known as process indicators. (21)

Slurry (**slur**-ee) Mixture of gypsum and water used in the finishing of models. (47)

Smear layer Very thin layer of debris on newly prepared dentin. (44)

Sodium hypochlorite (hi-po-klor-ite) Surface disinfectant commonly known as *household bleach.* (20)

Soft tissue impaction Oral condition in which a tooth is partially to fully covered by gingival tissue. (56)

Solder joint (**sah-**der) Point or junction where two metal objects are fused, such as on a bridge. (50)

Somatic effects (so-**ma-**tik) Effects of radiation that cause illness and are responsible for poor health (such as cancer, leukemia, and cataracts) but are not passed on to offspring. (38)

Spasticity (spa-**sti-**seh-tee) Exaggerated movement by the arms and legs. (57)

Spatulate (**spa-**chu-late) To mix using a spatula-type instrument. (45)

Sphenoid sinuses Located in the sphenoid bone. (9)

Spherical (**sfer-**i-kul) Round in shape. (43)

Sphygmomanometer (*sfig*-mo-ma-**nom-**eh-tur) Instrument for measuring blood pressure in the arteries. (27)

Splash, spatter, and droplet surface Surface that does not contact members of the dental team or contaminated instruments or supplies. (20)

Sporicidal Capable of killing bacterial spores. (20)

Sprains Injuries caused by a sudden twist or wrenching of a joint with stretching or tearing of ligaments. (25)

Standard of care The level of knowledge, skill, and care comparable to that of other dentists treating similar patients under similar conditions. (5)

Standard precautions A standard of care designed to protect healthcare providers from pathogens that can be spread by blood or any other body fluid, excretion, or secretion. Expands upon the concept of Universal Precautions. (19)

Staphylococci Cocci that form irregular groups or clusters. (18)

State dental practice act Document of law that specifies the legal requirements to practice dentistry in the particular state. (5)

Statement A summary of all charges, payments, credits, and debits for the month. (63)

Statutory law Law enacted by legislation through United States Congress, state legislature, or local legislative bodies. (5)

Stent Clear acrylic template that is placed over the alveolar ridge to assist in locating the proper placement for dental implants. (53)

Stepwedge Device constructed of layered aluminum steps to demonstrate the film densities and contrasts. (40)

Sterilant (**ster** uh-lunt) Agent capable of killing all microorganisms. (20, 21)

Sterilization (ster-uh-luh-**zay-**shun) Process that kills all microorganisms. (21)

Sternocleidomastoid (*stir*-no-*kli*-doe-**mass-**toid) Major cervical muscle. (9)

Stethoscope Instrument used for listening to sounds produced within the body. (27)

Stomodeum The primitive mouth. (8)

Strain The distortion or change produced as a result of stress. (43)

Strains Injuries caused by extreme stretching of muscles or ligaments. (25)

Stratified squamous epithelium (**skwa-**mus) Layers of flat, formed epithelium. (8)

Stress The internal reaction or resistance to an externally applied force. (43)

Stroke A sudden loss of brain function caused by a blockage or rupture of a blood vessel to the brain; also called *cerebrovascular accident.* (29)

Stylus (**sti-**lus) Sharp, pointed tool used for cutting. (36)

Subgingival Referring to the area below the gingiva. (14)

Subperiosteal (*sub*-per-ee-**os-**tee-ul) Type of implant with a metal frame placed under the periosteum, but on top of the bone. (53)

Subscription Directions to the pharmacist for mixing the medication; now seldom done. (30)

Subsupine position (*sub*-**sue-**pine) Lying-down position where the patients head is lower than the feet (below the heart); used in emergency situations. (32)

Succedaneous teeth (*suk*-se-**day-**ne-us) Permanent teeth that replace primary teeth. (8, 11)

Sudoriferous (soo-door-IF-er-us) Sweat glands widely distributed over the body. (7)

Superficial On or near the surface. (6)

Superior Above another portion, or closer to the head. (6)

Superscription The patients name, address, date, and Rx symbol on a prescription. (30)

Supine position (**sue-**pine) Lying-down position with patient's head, chest, and knees at the same level. (32)

Supragingival (*soo*-preh-**jin-**jih-vul) Referring to the area above the gingiva. (14)

Surface barrier Fluid-resistant material used to cover surfaces likely to become contaminated. (20)

Symmetric (si **meh-**trik) Balanced or even on both sides. (28)

Symphysis menti (**sim-**fa-sis **men-**te) The separation of the mandible at the chin at birth. (9)

Syncope (**sing-**keh-pee) Loss of consciousness caused by insufficient blood to the brain. (31)

Syneresis (seh-**ner-**eh-sus) Loss of water, causing something to shrink. (46)

Synthetic phenol compound (sin-theh-tik fee-nol) EPA-registered intermediate-level hospital disinfectant with broad-spectrum disinfecting action. (20)

Systemic (sis-**tee-**mik) Referring to a drug that affects a specific system of the body. (30)

Systemic fluoride Fluoride that is ingested and then circulated throughout the body. (15)

Systemic toxicity (sis-**tee-**mik *tawk*-**sis-**i-tee) A substance or condition that is poisonous to a body system, or typically the entire body. (37).

Systolic (sis-**tahl-**ik, sis-**tah-**lik) Rhythmic contraction of the heart, especially of the ventricles. (27)

Tactile (**tak-**t[uh]l) Having a sense of touch or feeling. (34)

T-band Type of matrix band used for primary teeth. (57)

Temperature Degree of hotness or coldness of a body or an environment. (27)

Tempering (**tem-**p[uh-]ring) Bringing a material to a desired consistency. (46)

Template (**tem-**plut) Clear plastic tray that represents the alveolus as it should appear after teeth have been extracted. (52)

Temporomandibular joint (TMJ) (*tem*-pah-ro-man-**dib-**u-ler) Joint on each side of head that allows for movement of the mandible. (9, 42)

Termination The end of an employee/employer relationship which can be initiated by the employee or employer. (64)

Thenar eminence (**thee-**nar **e-**meh-nents) Fleshy mound on the palm at the base of the thumb. (25)

Thermal (**thur-**mul) Relating to heat. (44)

Thermometer Instrument for measuring temperature. (27)

Thoracic cavity Contains the heart, lungs, esophagus, and trachea. (6)

Three-quarter crown Cast restoration that covers the anatomic crown of a tooth except for the facial or buccal portion. (50)

Thyroid collar A flexible lead shield that is placed securely around the neck. (38)

Tidal volume Amount of air inhaled and exhaled with each breath. (37)

Titanium (ti-**tay-**nee-um) Type of metal used for implants. (53)

Titrate (**tie-**trate) The process of determining the concentration of a substance. (37)

Titration The exact amount of a drug or substance that would be used to achieve a desired level of sedation. (37)

Tomography (toe-**mah-**greh-fee} Radiographic technique that allows imaging of one layer or section of the body while blurring images from structures in other planes. (42)

Tooth buds Enlargements produced by the formation of dental lamina. (8)

Topical fluoride Fluoride that is applied directly to the tooth. (15)

Tori (**tor-***i*, **tor-***ee*) Abnormal growths of bone in a specific area. (52)

Torque (**tork**) Twisting or turning force. (35)

Tort law Involving an act that brings harm to a person or damages to property. (5)

Touch surfaces Surfaces directly touched and contaminated during procedures. (20)
Toxic waste Waste that can have a poisonous effect. (23)
Tragus (**tray-**gus) Cartilaginous projection anterior to the external opening of the ear. (10)
Transaction Change, payment, or adjustment made to a financial account. (63)
Transfer surface Surfaces not directly touched, but often contacted by contaminated instruments. (20)
Transosteal (*tranz-***os-**tee-ul) Implant inserted through the inferior border of the mandible. (53)
Trapezius (trah-**pee-**zee-us) Major cervical muscle. (9)
Tricanineate Form of mandibular second premolar: three-cusp type. (12)
Trifurcation Area in which three roots divide. (12)
Triglycerides Nuetral fats. (16)
Triturate (**trich-**ur-ate, **tri-**chuh-*rate*) The process of mechanically mixing a material, as in using an amalgamator to mix an alloy and mercury to create dental amalgam. (32)
Trituration (*tri*-chuh-**ray-**shun) To mix together, as in the process of mixing an alloy with mercury to form an amalgam. (43)
Tube side Solid-white side of the film that faces the x-ray tube. (39)
Tubehead, Extension arm, Control panel Three primary components of all machines. (38)
Tuberculocidal (too-bur-ku-lo-si-dul) Capable of inactivating tuberculosis. (20)
Tuberosity (*too*-buh-**rah-**seh-tee) Rounded area on the outer surface of the maxillary bones in the area of the posterior teeth. (52)
Tungsten target A focal spot in the anode. (38)
Tympanic (tim-**pan-**ik) Relating to or resembling a drum, as in the *tympanic membrane,* or eardrum. (27)
Tyndallization (*tin*-duhl-i-**zay-**shun) Intermittent, or fractional, sterilization. (18)
Ultrasonic (*uhl*-treh-**sah-**nik) Mechanical radiant energy of water and sound vibrations used to break down materials or tissue. (35)
Ultrasonic cleaner Instrument that loosens and removes debris by sound waves traveling through a liquid. (21)
Ultrasonic scaler Device used for rapid calculus removal that operates on high-frequency sound waves. (55)
Unfilled resin (**re** zin) Sealant material that does not contain filler particles. (59)
Unit Each component of the fixed bridge. (50)
Unit time Time increments used in planning appointments. (62)
Universal Referring to same clamp that can be placed on same type of tooth in the opposite quadrant. (36)
Universal curette Hand instrument used to treat subgingival surfaces that has a blade with an unbroken cutting edge that curves around the toe and a flat face that is set at a 90 degree angle to the lower shank. (55)
Universal precautions Guidelines based on treating all human blood and body fluids (including saliva) as potentially infectious. (19)
Universal retainer Dental device used to hold a matrix band in place during restoration of a class II cavity. (49)
Upright position (up-right) Vertical position of a seated patient with the back of dental chair upright at 90-degree angle. (32)
Use-life Duration that a germicidal solution is effective after prepared for use. (21)
Usual A fee that the dentist charges for a specific service. (63)
Uvula Pear shaped projection at the end of the soft palate. (10)
Vasoconstrictor (**vay-**zoh-kun-**strik-**tor) Type of drug that constricts (narrows) blood vessels; used to prolong anesthetic action. (37)
Veins Blood vessels that carry blood to the heart. (7)
Veneer (vuh-**nir**) Thin layer of composite resin or porcelain bonded or cemented to a prepared facial surface. (48, 50)
Ventral cavity Cavity located in front of body. (6)
Ventricular fibrillation (ven-**tri-**kyeh-ler *fi*-breh-**lay-**shun) Abnormal cardiac rhythm that prevents the heart from pumping blood. (31)
Verbal communication Type of communication in which words are used as a form of expression. (61)
Vermilion border (ver-**mil-**yun) Darker-colored border around the lips. (10)
Vestibule Space between the teeth and the inner mucosal lining of the lips and cheeks. (10)
Viewbox Necessary equipment for the interpretation of dental radiographs. (40)
Virucidal Capable of killing some viruses. (20)
Virulence (**vir-**eh-lents) Strength of an pathogen's ability to cause disease; also known as *pathogenicity.* (19)
Virulent (**veer-**uh-luhnt) Capable of causing serious disease. (18)
Viruses Ultramicroscopic infectious agents that contain either DNA or RNA. (18)
Visceral (**vis-**er-ul) Pertaining to internal organs or the covering of organs. (6)
Viscosity (vis-**kah-**suh-tee) Physical property of fluids for resistance to flow. (43, 46)
Volatile (**vah-**leh-tul) Evaporates easily and is very explosive. (47)
Volume Quantity or amount, as in force of a heartbeat. (27)
Walkout statement Similar to a receipt that gives an account balance. (63)
Want list A list of those supplies to be ordered and questions to be asked of the representative. (62)
Warranty A written statement outlining the manufacturer's responsibility for replacing and repair of the product. (62)
Wedge Wooden or plastic triangular device placed in the embrasure to provide the contour needed when restoring a class II lesion. (49)
Wetting Covering or soaking something with a liquid. (43)
Word processing software A computer program designed to create most types of business documents. (61)
Working end Part of a dental instrument that is used on the tooth or dental materials. (34)
Written consent Consent that involves a written explanation of the diagnostic findings, prescribed treatment, and reasonable expectations about treatment results. (5)
Xerostomia (zir-oh-**sto-**me-ah) Dryness of the mouth caused by reduction of saliva. (9, 13, 17, 29)
X-radiation High-energy ionizing electromagnetic radiation. (38)
Zygote Fertilized egg. (8)

Index

Page numbers followed by f indicate figures; t, tables; b, boxes and boxed material.

A

B

P

S

X

Y

Z